D0852212

Disorders of Voluntary Muscle

For Churchill Livingstone:

Publisher: Michael Parkinson
Project Editor: Dilys Jones
Copy Editor: Pat Croucher
    Indexer: June Morrison
Project Controller: Nancy Arnott
Sales Promotion Executive: Maria O'Connor

Disorders of Voluntary Muscle

Edited by

John Walton (Lord Walton of Detchant)
Kt TD MA MD DSc FRCP
Honorary Fellow and Former Warden,
Green College, Oxford, UK;
Former Professor of Neurology and Dean of Medicine,
University of Newcastle upon Tyne;
Honorary Consulting Neurologist, Oxford Hospitals

George Karpati MD FRCP(C)
Isaac Walton Killam Chair of Neurology,
Montreal Neurological Institute, McGill University,
Montreal, Canada

David Hilton-Jones MD MRCP
Consultant Neurologist, Department of Clinical Neurology,
Radcliffe Infirmary, Oxford, UK

SIXTH EDITION

CHURCHILL LIVINGSTONE
EDINBURGH LONDON MADRID MELBOURNE NEW YORK TOKYO 1994

CHURCHILL LIVINGSTONE
Medical Division of Longman Group Limited

Distributed in the United States of America by Churchill
Livingstone Inc., 650 Avenue of the Americas, New York,
N.Y. 10011, and by associated companies, branches and
representatives throughout the world.

© J & A Churchill Ltd 1964
© Longman Group Limited 1981, 1994

All rights reserved. No part of this publication may be
reproduced, stored in a retrieval system, or transmitted in any
form or by any means, electronic, mechanical, photocopying,
recording or otherwise, without either the prior permission of
the publishers (Churchill Livingstone, Robert Stevenson
House, 1–3 Baxter's Place, Leith Walk, Edinburgh EH1 3AF),
or a licence permitting restricted copying in the
United Kingdom issued by the Copyright Licensing Agency
Ltd, 90 Tottenham Court Road, London, W1P 9HE.

First edition 1964
Second edition 1969
Third edition 1974
Fourth edition 1981
Fifth edition 1988
Sixth edition 1994

ISBN 0-443-04624-7

British Library Cataloguing in Publication Data
A catalogue record for this book is available from the British
Library.

Library of Congress Cataloging in Publication Data
A catalog record for this book is available from the Library of
Congress.

The
publisher's
policy is to use
**paper manufactured
from sustainable forests**

Printed in Great Britain by The Bath Press, Avon

Contents

Contributors

Zohar Argov MD
Associate Professor, Department of Neurology, Hebrew University and Hadassah Medical School, Jerusalem, Israel

Robert L. Barchi MD PhD
David Mahoney Professor of Neurological Sciences and Professor of Neurology, University of Pennsylvania School of Medicine, Philadelphia, USA

David D. Barwick MB FRCP FRCPE
Consultant Clinical Neurophysiologist and Consultant Neurologist, Regional Neurosciences Centre, Newcastle General Hospital, Newcastle upon Tyne, UK

L. A. Bindoff Bsc MB BS MD
Lecturer in Neurology, Department of Clinical Neuroscience, The Medical School, University of Newcastle, Newcastle upon Tyne, UK

Katharine M. D. Bushby MB ChB MSc MRCP
MRC Clinician Scientist, Department of Human Genetics, University of Newcastle upon Tyne, UK

Malcolm J. Campbell MB FRCP
Consultant Neurologist, Frenchay Healthcare Trust, Bristol; Clinical Lecturer, University of Bristol, Bristol, UK

Stirling Carpenter MD
Neuropathologist, Montreal Neurological Hospital, Montreal, Quebec; Professor, Department of Neurology, Neurosurgery and Pathology, McGill University, Montreal, Canada

Barry J. Cooper BVSc PhD
Professor, Department of Pathology; Director, Neuromuscular Diseases Laboratory, College of Veterinary Medicine, Cornell University, New York, USA

Michael J. Cullen MA DPhil
Principal Research Associate, University of Newcastle upon Tyne School of Neurosciences, Muscular Dystrophy Research Laboratories, Newcastle General Hospital, Newcastle upon Tyne, UK

S. Currie MA MD B Chir FRCP
Consultant Neurologist, St James's University Hospital; Clinical Lecturer, University of Leeds, UK

Patrick Doherty BSc PhD
Senior Lecturer, Department of Experimental Pathology, United Medical and Dental Schools, Guy's Hospital, London, UK

Victor Dubowitz BSc MD PhD FRCP
Professor of Paediatrics, Royal Postgraduate Medical School, Hammersmith Hospital, London, UK

Richard H. T. Edwards PhD FRCP
Professor of Medicine and Head, Department of Medicine, University of Liverpool, Liverpool, UK

Alan E. H. Emery MD DSc PhD MDhc (Naples) FRCP HonFACMG FLS FRS(E)
Research Director, European Neuromuscular Centre, Baarn, The Netherlands

Peter R. W. Fawcett BSc MB BS FRCP
Consultant Clinical Neurophysiologist, Department of Clinical Neurophysiology, Regional Neurosciences Centre, Newcastle General Hospital; Clinical Lecturer in Neurology, University of Newcastle upon Tyne, UK

Charles S. B. Galasko MSc ChM FRCS (Eng) FRCS (Ed)
Professor of Orthopaedic Surgery, University of Manchester; Consultant Orthopaedic Surgeon, Hope Hospital and Royal Manchester Children's Hospital, Salford, Manchester, UK

David Gardner-Medwin MD FRCP
Paediatric Neurologist, Newcastle General Hospital, Newcastle upon Tyne, UK

John Gergely MD PhD
Director, Boston Biomedical Research Institute; Biochemist, Massachusetts General Hospital; Associate Professor of Biological Chemistry and Molecular Pharmacology, Harvard Medical School, Boston, USA

Robert C. Griggs MD
Professor of Neurology, Medicine, Pathology and Pediatrics and Chairman of Neurology, University of Rochester School of Medicine and Dentistry, Rochester, New York, USA

Peter S. Harper MA DM FRCP
Professor of Medical Genetics, University of Wales College of Medicine, Cardiff

John B. Harris PhD MRPharmS FIBiol
Professor of Experimental Neurology, University of Newcastle upon Tyne; Director of the Muscular Dystrophy Group Laboratories, Newcastle General Hospital, Newcastle upon Tyne, UK

David Hilton-Jones MD MRCP
Consultant Neurologist, Department of Clinical Neurology, Radcliffe Infirmary, Oxford, UK

P. Hudgson MB BS FRCP FRACP
Consultant Neurologist, Northern Region and Newcastle Health Authorities; Senior Lecturer in Neurology, University of Newcastle; Clinical Director, Muscular Dystrophy Research Laboratories, Newcastle General Hospital, Newcastle upon Tyne, UK

Sandra Jackson BSc
Research Associate, Department of Clinical Neuroscience, The Medical School, University of Newcastle, Newcastle upon Tyne, UK

Byron Arthur Kakulas AO MD (Hon Athens) MD(WA) FRACP FRCPath FRCPA
Professor of Neuropathology, Department of Pathology, University of Western Australia; Head, Department of Neuropathology, Royal Perth Hospital; Medical Director, Australian Neuromuscular Research Institute, Queen Elizabeth II Medical Centre, Nedlands, Western Australia, Australia

George Karpati MD FRCP(C)
Isaac Walton Killam Chair of Neurology, Montreal Neurological Institute, McGill University, Montreal; Professor of Pediatrics, McGill University, Montreal, Canada

D. N. Landon MB BS BSc
Professor of Neurology, Institute of Neurology, London, UK

Paul D. Lewis DSc MD FRCP FRCPath
Consultant Neuropathologist, Charing Cross Hospital; Emeritus Reader in Histopathology, Royal Postgraduate Medical School; Honorary Consultant Pathologist and Neurologist, Hammersmith Hospital, London, UK

Robert P. Lisak MD
Professor and Chairman of Neurology and Professor of Immunology and Microbiology, Wayne State University School of Medicine; Neurologist-in-Chief, Detroit Medical Center; Chief of Neurology, Harper Hospital, Detroit, USA

F. L. Mastaglia MD FRACP FRCP
Professor of Neurology, University of Western Australia; Consultant Neurologist, Queen Elizabeth II Medical Centre, Perth, Western Australia

Richard T. Moxley III MD
Professor of Neurology and Pediatrics, Director of Neuromuscular Disease Center, Department of Neurology, University of Rochester School of Medicine and Dentistry, Rochester, USA

Theodore L. Munsat MD
Professor of Neurology and Pharmacology, Tufts University; Director of Neuromuscular Research, New England Medical Center, Boston, USA

John Newsom-Davis MD FRCP FRS
Professor of Neurology, University of Oxford,
Department of Clinical Neurology, Radcliffe
Infirmary, Oxford, UK

Louise V. B. Nicholson MSc PhD
Action Research Lecturer in Experimental
Neurology, Muscular Dystrophy Group Research
Laboratories, Regional Neurosciences Centre,
Newcastle General Hospital, Newcastle upon
Tyne, UK

Christopher Pallis MA DM FRCP
Reader Emeritus in Neurology, Royal
Post-graduate Medical School, London, UK

Lewis P. Rowland MD
Henry and Lucy Moses Professor and Chair,
Department of Neurology, Columbia University
College of Physicians and Surgeons; Director,
Neurology Service, Neurological Institute,
Presbyterian Hospital, Columbia-Presbyterian
Medical Center, New York City, USA

Ian S. Schofield MB BMedSci FRCP
Consultant Clinical Neurophysiologist, Regional
Neurosciences Centre, Newcastle General
Hospital, Newcastle upon Tyne, UK

Caroline A. Sewry BSc PhD
Lecturer, Neuromuscular Unit, Royal
Postgraduate Medical School, Hammersmith
Hospital, London, UK

Clarke R. Slater PhD
William Leech Senior Lecturer in Clinical
Science and Head of Division of Neurobiology,
University of Newcastle upon Tyne, UK

P. K. Thomas CBE DSc MD FRCP FRCPath
Emeritus Professor of Neurological Science in the
University of London, Royal Free Hospital
School of Medicine and Institute of Neurology,
London, UK

D. M. Turnbull MB BS MD PhD FRCP
Professor of Neurology, Division of Clinical
Neuroscience, The Medical School, University of
Newcastle upon Tyne, UK

Frank S. Walsh BSc PhD
Sir William Dunn Professor of Experimental
Pathology, United Medical and Dental Schools,
Guy's Hospital, London, UK

John Walton (Lord Walton of Detchant), Kt, TD, MA,
MD, DSc, FRCP FRCP(Ed) FRCPath FRCPsych
Honorary Fellow and Former Warden, Green
College, Oxford; Former Professor of Neurology
and Dean of Medicine, University of Newcastle
upon Tyne; Honorary Consultant Neurologist,
Oxford Hospitals, UK

D. Wray BA MSc DPhil
Professor and Head of Department of
Pharmacology, Leeds University, Leeds, UK

Preface to the Sixth Edition

Since *Disorders of Voluntary Muscle* was first published in 1964, there have been remarkable developments in our understanding of neuromuscular function in health and disease and many of these have been highlighted in previous editions of this book, which I have had the privilege of editing in each of the last five editions. Having now retired from active clinical practice, and after consulting my colleagues at Churchill Livingstone, I decided that for this sixth edition the time had come when it would be appropriate to recruit two co-editors who would not only share the responsibility for the writing, revision and editing of chapters for this new edition, but who would also be willing to accept editorial responsibility for seeing the book through any subsequent editions which may be required. I was therefore delighted when Dr George Karpati of Montreal and Dr David Hilton-Jones of Oxford willingly agreed to accept this responsibility and I welcome them on board as co-editors of this edition and as editors of subsequent editions as this is the last in which I shall personally be involved.

While the structure of the book is much the same as in the last edition in that there are four sections dealing respectively with anatomy, physiology and biochemistry, pathology, clinical problems in neuromuscular disease, and electrodiagnosis, developments in knowledge have necessitated several major changes with new chapters being included and others being omitted. Thus in section one, new chapters on the cell biology of muscle (by Professor F. B. Walsh and Dr P. Doherty of London) and on the molecular biology of muscle (by Dr Louise Nicholson of Newcastle upon Tyne) are included, giving detailed and scholarly reviews of the remarkable advances in knowledge which have occurred since the last edition was published in 1988. In the second section on pathology, Dr Stirling Carpenter of Montreal has contributed a new chapter on the light microscopic morphological abnormalities in skeletal muscle disease. Chapter 12 on experimental disorders of muscle by Professor Byron Kakulas of Perth has been substantially expanded and now includes a major section on animal models of human neuromuscular disease, contributed by Dr. Barry Cooper of New York, who joins Professor Kakulas as co-author of this chapter. In the third large section on clinical problems in neuromuscular disease, I am delighted that Professor L. P. Rowland of New York has joined me as a co-author of Chapter 13 on clinical examination, differential diagnosis and classification. He has been a tower of strength and his work on updating the international classification of neuromuscular diseases, prepared on behalf of the Research Group on Neuromuscular Diseases of the World Federation of Neurology, has been in every way exemplary and invaluable. In checking that classification, Professor P. K. Thomas of London and Professor J. G. McLeod of Sydney, Australia, have also given substantial help; the classification has also been published in a supplement to the Journal of the Neurological Sciences and I am most grateful to the editor, Professor J. F. Toole, and the publishers, Elsevier, for permission to reproduce that classification as an appendix to Chapter 13. In Chapter 14 on the muscular dystrophies, my colleague Dr David Gardner-Medwin now becomes the senior author, and in Chapter 16 Professor Karpati joins Dr Simon Currie of Leeds in updating the contribution on the inflammatory myopathies. Since Dr Andrew Engel no longer wished to continue to write a comprehensive chapter reviewing all of the metabolic myopathies, we decided to divide that chapter from the previous edition into two and are grateful to Dr Richard Moxley of Rochester, New York, for contributing a new chapter on metabolic and endocrine myopathies; a second on the mitochondrial and lipid storage diseases of muscle has been contributed by Drs L.A. Bindoff, S. Jackson and Professor D. M. Turnbull of Newcastle upon Tyne. These new contributions, like those in the previous section by Drs Carpenter and Cooper, are in our view admirable and up-to-date reviews. We were also very grateful to learn that following Professor J. A. Simpson's retirement, Professor John Newsom-Davis of Oxford, widely acknowledged as a major international authority on myasthenia and related disorders, was willing to contribute the appropriate chapter on these conditions, and we also much appreciate the willingness of Dr R. C. Griggs of Rochester, New York, who agreed to collaborate with Professor Richard Edwards of Liverpool in updating Chapter 22 on the medical and psychological management of neuromuscular disease. Similarly, we welcome Professor T. L. Munsat of Boston as co-author, with Dr M. J. Campbell of Bristol, of Chapter 24 on the motor neurone diseases, and were very glad that Professor P. K. Thomas of London was willing to update Chapter 25 on peripheral nerve diseases in view of the fact that his co-author, Professor W. G. Bradley of Miami, felt unable to continue as a contributor to this edition. Yet another new author, Dr Kate Bushby of Newcastle upon Tyne, has joined Professor Alan Emery of Edinburgh in producing a superb update in Chapter 26 on genetic aspects of neuromuscular diseases, and Dr. David Hilton-Jones has taken over from Dr J. B. Foster of Newcastle Chapter 27 dealing with the clinical features of some miscellaneous neuromuscular disorders.

Finally, in section IV on electrodiagnosis, we felt that there was no need to continue to have a separate chapter on integration and analysis of the EMG and the study of the reflexes, as contributed in the last edition by the late Dr J. A. R. Lenman and Dr I. T. Ferguson. Relevant material from that chapter has now been integrated into the two chapters in this section written by Drs Barwick, Fawcett and Schofield of Newcastle. I also wish, on behalf of myself and my co-editors, to thank all of the other authors not mentioned above who have updated and in some cases largely rewritten their

contributions to this edition, which I hope will continue to be the single most comprehensive one-volume reference text on disorders of muscle. Readers will note that this edition no longer contains a chapter on the pathological anatomy of the neuromuscular junction, and I am grateful to Professor Coërs of Brussels and Dr Chou for agreeing that relevant material should now be included in Chapters 7 and 8 by Carpenter on the one hand and Sewry and Dubowitz on the other. Similarly, Drs K.-E. Aström, R. D. Adams, H. A. John and K. W. Jones and Dr R. J. T. Pennington, for whose contributions to previous editions I would like to express my sincere personal gratitude, are no longer among our authors as material which they previously contributed has been replaced at their request or integrated into other contributions. We also felt that there was no need in this new edition to have a separate chapter on neuromuscular disease in animals in view of Dr Cooper's contribution in Chapter 12 on animal models, and accordingly I would like to thank Drs Bradley and McKerrell and Professor Barnard for their admirable contributions to previous editions.

In the course of this revision, many illustrations have been replaced and new ones have been added, some from other publications but others original. Where appropriate, acknowledgments to original sources are given either in the captions to the illustrations or at the end of individual chapters. Inevitably, as in previous editions, there is in this one some duplication and overlap between different chapters in that many diseases are commented upon in several chapters but from different standpoints and with varying emphasis upon their clinical, pathological, biochemical and physiological characteristics. This, as in the past, is necessary in order that each individual chapter can stand as a comprehensive essay upon the topic to which it is devoted. I trust that this will continue to make the book invaluable as a work of reference.

Finally, may I express my gratitude to my co-editors for their invaluable help throughout, to the staff of Churchill Livingstone and to my secretary, Rosemary Allan, for their patient and willing co-operation and for all the help they have given during the preparation of this edition.

1994   J. W.

Preface to the First Edition

The last fifteen years have seen a world-wide awakening of interest in diseases of muscle and during this period several outstanding books upon this subject have been published. At first sight, therefore, a new text-book devoted to this group of disorders may seem to be superfluous. However, the excellent work on *Diseases of Muscle* by Adams, Denny-Brown and Pearson, now in its second edition, approaches the subject primarily from the pathological standpoint, while the three-volume work on *Structure and Function of Muscle,* edited by Geoffrey Bourne, consists of a series of comprehensive essays of encyclopaedic scope, invaluable for reference by the research worker but perhaps too weighty for the general reader. Furthermore, the volume on *Neuromuscular Disorders,* embodying the proceedings of the 1958 meeting of the Association for Research in Nervous and Mental Disease, is primarily a commentary upon research in this field, while the recent work *Muscular Dystrophy in Man and Animals* edited by Bourne and Golarz, surveys only the problem of muscular dystrophy.

In designing the present volume, therefore, it has been my aim and that of the other twenty-four contributors, each an acknowledged expert in the field, to give an up-to-date and comprehensive yet concise view of disorders of muscle from several standpoints. The book is aimed primarily at the clinician, whether he be a general physician, paediatrician or neurologist, a post-graduate student studying for a higher examination or any doctor wishing to expand his knowledge of this group of disorders. The first section of the book is devoted to a consideration of modern views of the structure and function of muscle, the second to the changes, both structural and biochemical, which may occur in disease, and the third contains a series of essays on the clinical and genetic aspects of muscle disease in man with a chapter describing the related disorders which occur in animals; the final section deals with electrical methods of investigation of muscular disease. Throughout, references are given not only to original sources of information but also to current research.

In the preparation of this volume I am indebted to the contributors; I am sure that many of them, like myself, are grateful for the help they have obtained from previous publications, pre-eminent among which are the four volumes to which I have referred above. More detailed acknowledgements of sources of material contained in this volume are given, where necessary, at the end of individual chapters. I wish personally to thank Mr J. Rivers, Mr A. S. Knightley and the staff of J. and A. Churchill Ltd for all the patience and understanding they have shown during the process of publication and, as always, I am deeply indebted to my secretary, Miss Rosemary Allan, for her unfailing willingness and efficiency.

Newcastle upon Tyne,
1964
J. W.

Anatomy, physiology and biochemistry

1. The anatomy and physiology of the motor unit

C. R. Slater   J. B. Harris

INTRODUCTION

Skeletal muscle fibres are innervated by motor neurones whose cell bodies lie within the central nervous system and whose axons extend peripherally to the muscles. A single motor neurone and the many muscle fibres uniquely innervated by it are known as a *motor unit*. Because a nerve impulse in a motor neurone normally elicits the contraction of all the muscle fibres it innervates, the motor unit is the elementary basis of neuromuscular function; under normal circumstances, all voluntary muscle contractions result from the activation of a number of complete motor units.

Each motor unit consists of a large number of cells whose anatomical and physiological properties are closely matched so that the unit as a whole is specialised to do a particular kind of work. This matching results largely from interactions between nerve and muscle which continue throughout life to promote both the formation and the maintenance of a well-integrated yet still adaptable neuromuscular system.

In this chapter, we shall first describe the basic features of the cells that make up motor units and their role in the generation of voluntary movements. We will then indicate some of the ways in which these cells interact throughout life so that in spite of major changes resulting from varied patterns of use, ageing, injury or disease, the motor unit remains functionally adequate.

ANATOMICAL ORGANISATION OF THE MOTOR UNIT

Nerve

The activity of the motor unit is coordinated by

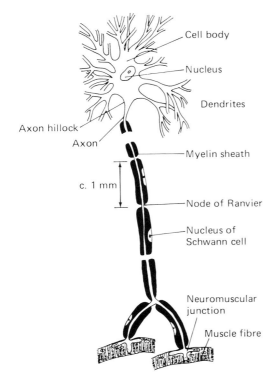

Fig. 1.1 A diagrammatic view of a spinal motor neurone. The cell body and its dendrites lie within the spinal cord. The single axon emerges from the enlarged axon hillock and lies mainly outside the cord. Schwann cells wrapped around the axon form the myelin sheath which is interrupted at the nodes of Ranvier. At the neuromuscular junction the axon loses its myelin and branches to form the presynaptic terminal.

the *motor neurone* (Fig. 1.1). The *cell body* of the motor neurone contains the nucleus and the intracellular organelles associated with protein synthesis; ribosomes and rough endoplasmic reticulum (the Nissl substance of neurohistology). Neural inputs to motor neurones are made at synapses located either on the cell body or on the many elongated *dendrites* which extend from it. When the summed effects of these inputs are sufficiently great, a nerve impulse is generated in the initial segment of the single *motor axon* and propagates away from the spinal cord to the muscle fibres.

The cytoplasm within the motor axon contains a prominent cytoskeleton. This is composed primarily of two types of proteinaceous fibres, *neurofilaments* and *microtubules* (Alberts et al 1989). Neurofilaments are a neurone-specific

form of 10 nm diameter 'intermediate filament'. Like the other keratin-related proteins of this class, they form extremely stable intracellular fibres which are thought to provide the mechanical rigidity necessary to maintain the elongated form of the axon. Microtubules are much more dynamic structures found in almost all cells. Each microtubule is a helical polymer, 25 nm in diameter, of the protein tubulin. The main role of microtubules in axons appears to be to provide a track along which membrane-bound vesicles move carrying material between the cell body and the periphery (see below).

Surrounding each axon is an insulating *myelin sheath* formed of many layers of plasma membrane of the *Schwann cells*, a type of glial cell. Each Schwann cell is typically about 1 mm long, so a motor axon innervating distal limb muscles may be associated with several hundred Schwann cells. A gap in the myelin sheath, the *node of Ranvier*, is present at the boundary between adjacent Schwann cells. Each individual axon, together with its associated Schwann cells, is surrounded by a connective tissue sheath. This consists of a mesh-like basal lamina together with associated fibrous components of the extracellular matrix including collagen and elastin.

The spinal motor neurones innervating an individual muscle lie in a more or less well-defined 'column', two to three segments long, within the anterior horn of the spinal cord (Romanes 1940, 1941, Sharrard 1955) (Fig. 1.2). The columns for more proximal muscles tend to lie medial to those supplying more distal muscles, although there is a good deal of overlap. The motor axons leave the spinal cord at discrete points where they gather together to form the ventral roots, each root containing axons destined for many muscles. Motor axons of the ventral roots join with sensory axons of the dorsal roots to form the *peripheral nerves*. A cross-section of a peripheral nerve (Fig. 1.3) reveals that the myelinated axons normally form two distinct size populations. The largest axons, some 8–20 μm in diameter in man, include the alpha motor axons that innervate the muscle fibres of the motor units, and the sensory afferents from the specialised intrafusal muscle fibres of the muscle spindles and the Golgi tendon organs (see below). The smallest

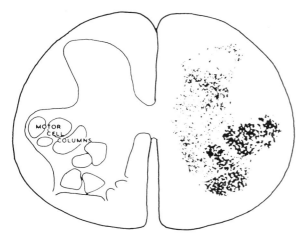

muscle come together and separate from the main trunk to form a well-defined muscle nerve. In most muscle nerves, about half of the myelinated axons are motor and half sensory (Boyd & Davey 1968). Until such a nerve reaches its target muscle, the axons rarely branch. Within the muscle, extensive branching at the nodes of Ranvier leads to the formation of numerous intra-muscular nerve bundles from which individual axons split off to innervate each muscle fibre.

Peripheral nerves are surrounded by a tough connective tissue sheath, the *epineurium*. Within the nerve, axons are grouped into fascicles, each surrounded by a further sheath, the *perineurium* (Fig. 1.3a). Each individual motor axon is in turn intimately surrounded by an *endoneurium*.

Fig. 1.2 Cell chart showing the grouping of the large motor neurones in the anterior horns of the spinal cord. The outlines of the column of motor neurones innervating individual muscles, determined from the study of polio patients, is shown on the left (from Sharrard, 1955, by courtesy of H.A. Sissons: *Disorders of Voluntary Muscle*, 3rd edn).

axons, 1–8 μm in diameter, include the gamma motor axons that innervate the intrafusal muscle fibres and small sensory axons.

In the periphery, the axons destined for a single

Muscle

Each motor neurone innervates a large number of *skeletal muscle* fibres (Fig. 1.4), all contained within the same muscle. In man most motor units contain 100–1000 muscle fibres but some may have as many as 10 000 (Cooper 1966). Individual muscle fibres are usually between 10 and 100 μm

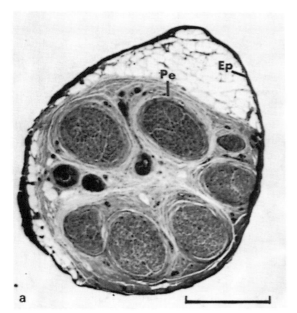

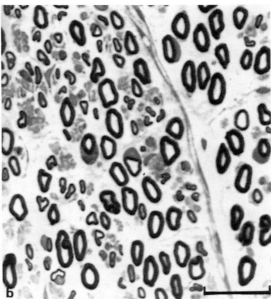

Fig. 1.3 The structure of peripheral nerve (human sural nerve). **a** Low-power view of transverse section showing fascicles, epineurium (Ep), and perineurium (Pe) (scale bar = 0.5 mm). **b** Higher-power view showing large and small diameter myelinated axons. Scale bar = 25 μm. **c** Frequency distribution of myelinated nerve fibre diameters (after Asbury & Johnson 1978).

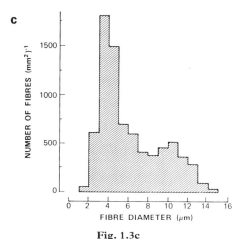

Fig. 1.3c

in diameter and between a few millimetres and several centimetres long.

Under the light microscope, muscle fibres exhibit transverse striations. These result from alternating arrays of two types of longitudinally oriented contractile filaments. The *thin filaments* are composed mainly of the protein *actin*, while the *thick filaments* are based on *myosin*. The repeating unit, from the *Z-line* at the centre of one group of thin filaments to that at the centre of the next group, is the *sarcomere*, and is usually 2.5–3.5 μm long. Sarcomeres are assembled longitudinally to form a myofibril. Muscle contraction results from an interaction between the thin filaments and molecular 'cross-bridges' protruding from the thick filaments. This interaction generates a force which causes the filaments to slide past each other, making the muscle fibre shorten or develop tension. The stability of the myofibrils is maintained by non-contractile, highly elastic proteins such as titin (sometimes known as connectin) and nebulin. Adjacent myofibrils are connected, predominantly at the level of the Z-line, by a number of cytoskeletal proteins including the

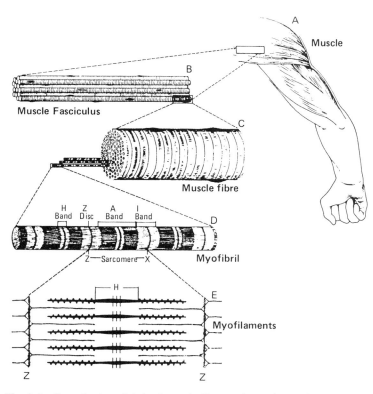

Fig. 1.4   Organisation of skeletal muscle. Progressing, at increasing magnifications, from the whole muscle (A), to a fascicle (B) and a single muscle fibre (C). At the subcellular level, the muscle fibre contains myofibrils (D) which are bundles of contractile filaments (E) (after Bloom & Fawcett 1968).

intermediate filament protein desmin. As a result, adjacent myofibrils are kept in register.

The cytoskeletal proteins also provide an organised structure for the attachment of myofibrils to the sarcolemma. A number of proteins are involved in this function including vinculin, spectrin, α-actin and, possibly, dystrophin. Spectrin, dystrophin and vinculin are also major components of the subsarcolemmal cytoskeleton, providing a physical scaffold for the muscle fibre. The details of the organisation and function of the cytoskeletal and non-contractile myofibrillar proteins have yet to be determined. In particular, carefully coordinated studies of both localisation and changes in orientation during contraction are required. There is little doubt of the importance of such studies in view of the growing awareness of the involvement of the non-contractile proteins in development, growth, regeneration and disease.

Muscle fibres arise during development by the fusion of numerous myogenic cells and therefore contain many nuclei within a common cytoplasm. There are usually about 100 nuclei per millimetre of muscle fibre length. Each muscle fibre is contained within a stocking-like layer of extracellular matrix, the *basal lamina*, strengthened with fibres of collagen.

Closely associated with each muscle fibre, lying within the basal lamina sheath, are numerous *satellite cells*. (These are myogenic cells which fail to fuse with the muscle fibre during its initial formation (see below). During muscle growth or regeneration, the satellite cells may become 'activated', replicating their DNA and dividing to provide a supply of new muscle-forming cells, some of which fuse with the muscle fibres.) The number of satellite cells associated with a given muscle fibre varies, but is usually between 1% and 10% of the number of myonuclei. The ends of each muscle fibre are connected to the tendons by an elaboration of the connective tissue sheath, joined to the fibre at the myo-tendinous junction.

Muscle fibres are grouped within the muscles into fascicles, each with its own vascular supply and connective tissue sheath (*perimysium*). Fascicles vary greatly in size, but in man typically contain about a thousand fibres. Each fascicle contains fibres belonging to a number of motor units, and these are extensively intermixed.

Indeed, in most normal muscles, it is rare for a muscle fibre to lie adjacent to another fibre from the same motor unit (Edström & Kugelberg 1968). Though widely dispersed, the fibres of an individual motor unit generally occupy only a part of the total muscle cross-section. The muscle as a whole is enclosed in a tough *epimysium*.

Several distinct classes, or 'types', of muscle fibre are present in most muscles, each of which is characterised by a functionally inter-related set of properties which suit it for a particular form of contraction (see below). An important principle of motor unit organisation is that all the fibres of any one motor unit have very similar properties. Thus, each motor unit can itself be considered as being of a particular type, to be used in a characteristic way, appropriate to its functional properties.

Neuromuscular junction

Nerve impulses are transmitted to an individual muscle fibre at a highly specialised site of contact, the *neuromuscular junction*, also referred to as the *motor end-plate* (Fig. 1.5). At these junctions, the nerve action potential causes the release of a chemical transmitter, acetylcholine, which acts on specialised proteins in the membrane of the muscle fibre to initiate an action potential in the muscle fibre. This, in turn, leads to the rapid activation of the contractile apparatus of the muscle cell (see Ch. 3 for details of the process of neuromuscular transmission).

In mammalian muscle fibres, a single neuromuscular junction about 25–50 μm long is normally present, approximately equidistant from the fibre ends. As a motor axon makes contact with the muscle, it forms a number of fine unmyelinated terminal branches. These branches are accommodated in depressions ('gutters') in a dome of specialised cytoplasm and capped by extensions of the terminal Schwann cells. With the electron microscope (see Ch. 4), it can be seen that the plasma membrane of the axon terminal remains separated from that of the postsynaptic membrane of the muscle fibre by a gap of about 50 nm and a single layer of specialised synaptic basal lamina. The postsynaptic membrane is thrown into numerous tight folds, about 1 μm deep, initially recognised with the light microscope

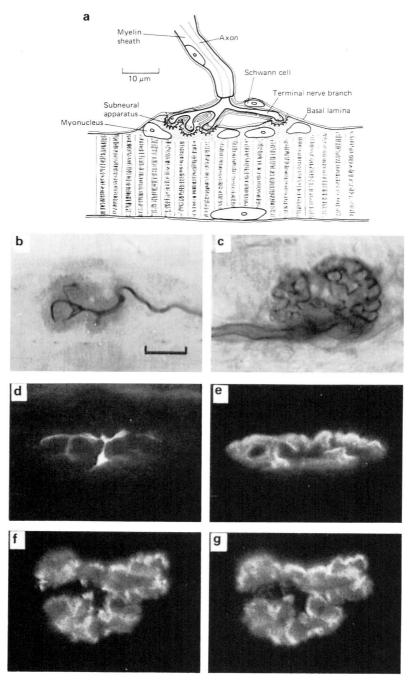

Fig. 1.5 The neuromuscular junction. **a** The principal cellular and subcellular components. **b** Silver stain shows the axon and its terminal branches (human). **c** The myelin is stained with Sudan black and the postsynaptic region with a histochemical reaction for AChE (rat). **d, e** Two views of a rat junction in which the nerve is stained with an antibody to neurofilament protein (**d**) and the AChR with a fluorescent conjugate of alpha-hungarotoxin (fl-BgTx) (**e**). **f, g** Two views of another rat junction in which the AChE is stained with a fluorescent antibody (**f**) and the AChR with fl-BgTx (**g**). **h, i** Views of a human junction in which the cluster of myonuclei have been stained with a fluorescent dye (**h**) and the AChR with fl-BgTx (**i**). The scale bar in b = 10 μm and applies to frames b–i.

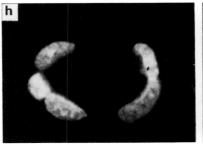 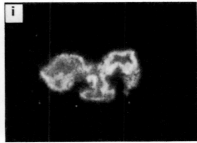

Fig. 1.5 h & i

and referred to as the 'subneural apparatus' (Couteaux 1960).

Recent studies of human neuromuscular junctions have made it clear that they are significantly smaller than those in lower vertebrates. At the same time, the intensity of postsynaptic folding is considerably greater (Slater et al 1992). The likely functional significance of these structural features of human junctions is discussed below.

Within the synaptic region, a number of functionally important molecules are present in high density at the muscle fibre surface, including acetylcholine receptors, voltage-dependent Na^+ channels and the enzyme acetylcholinesterase (see below for further details). In recent years, the use of methods which allow these components to be visualised has shown how closely their distribution is matched to the regions of contact with the motor axon terminal and to each other (Fig. 1.5).

Beneath the postsynaptic membrane is an accumulation of a number of components of the cytoskeleton, including ankyrin, spectrin, dystrophin and structurally similar proteins (Froehner 1986, Flucher & Daniels 1989, Bewick et al 1992). These subsynaptic components may help to maintain the high local concentration of a number of synaptic molecules such as the acetylcholine receptors (see below). A further factor in maintaining this molecular differentiation is the specialised pattern of genes expressed by the 5–10 myonuclei clustered at the junction. The best studied examples of this are the genes for the subunits of the acetylcholine receptor which are normally expressed at a much higher level in the junctional region than elsewhere (e.g. Simon et al 1992).

Sensory structures

In addition to the cells of the motor unit proper, each muscle contains sensory structures which convey information about muscle length and tension to the central nervous system (Nicholls et al 1992). The cell bodies of the sensory neurones associated with these structures are located in the dorsal root ganglia. From there they send one process centrally to make synaptic contact with as many as 300–400 spinal motor neurones, while their peripheral axon forms the sensory afferent.

Muscle spindles consist of a bundle of four to six specialised *intrafusal muscle fibres*. The endings of sensory axons make contact with these fibres and generate nerve impulses when the length of the muscle changes. Two types of sensory neurone innervate each spindle; large-diameter Group IA afferents form *primary endings* near the centre of each intrafusal fibre and smaller Group II afferent axons make less elaborate *secondary endings*. The two types of ending and the structures associated with them are generally specialised to allow them to respond either to the absolute length of the muscle or to changes in that length. The intrafusal fibres also receive motor innervation from small *gamma motor neurones*. While contraction of these fibres generates little tension, it serves to keep the spindle taut when the muscle contracts and thus allows the sensory ending to respond to stretch over a range of muscle lengths. The discharge from the spindle afferents is relayed directly to the ipsilateral spinal motor neurones innervating the muscle in which the spindle is found.

Golgi tendon organs are located at the ends of the

muscle fibres. Each tendon organ is formed from a common tendon to which a number of muscle fibres are attached. The sensory nerve ending wraps around this tendon and responds when tension is generated by contraction of any of the muscle fibres ending on it. The discharge from a Golgi tendon organ is also 'fed' to the ipsilateral alpha motor neurones where it is inhibitory.

FUNCTIONAL ORGANISATION OF THE MOTOR UNIT

Motor neurone

The dexterity typical of voluntary movements in mammals requires the precise control of the motor units in each muscle. The nerve impulses that trigger motor unit contraction arise as a result of the combined effects of as many as 10 000 excitatory and inhibitory synaptic inputs impinging on each motor neurone. These inputs originate from higher levels in the central nervous system, interneurones within the spinal cord, and sensory neurones innervating muscle, joints and skin (Kandel et al 1991, Nicholls et al 1992).

Motor neurones have a resting membrane potential of about −70 mV. Propagated action potentials are generated only when the membrane potential is reduced to a threshold level of about −60 mV (Aidley 1989). Since a typical excitatory synaptic input generates a postsynaptic depolarisation of less than 250 µV, action potentials are only generated in a motor neurone when a large number of different excitatory inputs discharge more or less synchronously (spatial summation) or a smaller number of inputs discharge at a high frequency so that the individual synaptic potentials sum (temporal summation). Inhibitory synaptic inputs also exhibit spatial and temporal summation, but their effect is primarily to decrease the electrical resistance of the cell membrane and to stabilise the membrane potential at a value near to the resting potential. In the spinal motor neurone, the inhibitory input causes an increase in K^+ and Cl^- conductances, normally leading to a small hyperpolarisation.

When the net effect of excitatory and inhibitory inputs is a depolarisation which exceeds the threshold, a regenerative, Na^+-dependent action

potential is generated at the *axon hillock*, the site of origin of the motor axon (see Fig. 1.1). This region is particularly sensitive to depolarisation because it has a very high local density of the voltage-sensitive Na^+ channels which are responsible for the regenerative nature of the action potential (Aidley 1989). This property is shared with action potential-generating regions in other cells such as the node of Ranvier of myelinated axons and the postsynaptic membrane of the neuromuscular junction.

In the face of strong excitatory input, most motor neurones generate repetitive action potentials. However, the resulting pattern of action potentials differs in motor neurones innervating muscle fibres of different types. These patterns of activity are largely determined by the differing tendencies of motor neurones to remain hyperpolarised for a time after each nerve impulse, and thus incapable of generating a further action potential. This property is in turn a consequence of the type and density of ion channels, particularly those permeable to K^+, in the motor neurone membrane (Hille 1992). These differences are discussed further below.

Motor axon

The motor axon and the Schwann cells associated with it act together as a functional unit, the physiological behaviour of the axon being determined as much by the presence of the myelin as by the basic properties of the axonal membrane. In unmyelinated axons, impulses propagate continuously; the ionic currents generated by activity in one region spread along the axon and excite the adjacent nerve membrane. The speed of nerve impulse propagation is determined by the rate at which such currents can depolarise the membrane to the threshold for action potential generation. This is limited both by the resistance to the flow of current through the axoplasm and the amount of current taken up in charging the large electrical capacitance of the plasma membrane. In larger diameter unmyelinated axons, because the longitudinal resistance to current flow is less, impulses are conducted faster than in smaller axons (Hursh 1939).

In a myelinated axon, the insulation afforded by

the myelin sheath restricts the flow of current across the membrane and greatly reduces the membrane's effective capacitance. As a result, most of the current entering the axon in an active region leaves the axon by crossing the naked membrane at the nodes of Ranvier. To take advantage of this situation, voltage-dependent Na^+ channels are normally concentrated in the nodal membrane but are largely absent in the internodal region (Waxman & Ritchie 1985). The net effect is that the nerve impulse 'jumps' rapidly from one node to the next ('saltatory' conduction) and the overall conduction velocity is much faster than for an unmyelinated axon of the same size.

The velocity of action potential propagation in myelinated axons is influenced by several structural factors. As in unmyelinated axons, the larger the diameter of the axon the greater the conduction velocity. In addition, increasing the thickness of the myelin sheath improves its insulating properties and this, too, speeds conduction. On biophysical grounds, Rushton (1951) pointed out that there should be an optimal ratio between the diameter of the axon and the external diameter of the myelin sheath, and that this ratio should be the same irrespective of the actual size of the nerve fibre. In practice, for large axons this is true, and the ratio is approximately 0.7 (Gasser & Grundfest 1939).

Conduction velocity is also influenced by the distance between successive nodes of Ranvier, since this determines the length of the 'jumps' taken by the nerve impulse. In general, internodal length is proportional to axon diameter (Fig. 1.6a), though the constant of proportionality is not the same in all nerves (Bradley 1974). Action potentials in larger diameter nerve fibres therefore move in longer jumps. However, since current spreads more rapidly in large axons, the time taken for each jump is roughly constant (about 15 μs for limb nerves). The combined effect of all these relationships is that there is a direct proportionality between action potential conduction velocity and nerve fibre diameter in myelinated nerves (Fig. 1.6b) as in unmyelinated ones, though for somewhat different reasons. For most myelinated axons, the constant of proportionality is 6 m/s/μm diameter (Hursh 1939).

It follows from what has been said above that

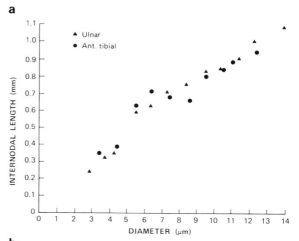

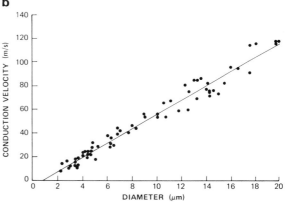

Fig. 1.6 Properties of myelinated axons. **a** Internodal length is directly related to nerve fibre diameter (data from Vizoso, 1950, for human ulnar and anterior tibial nerves). **b** Action potential conduction velocity is similarly related to fibre diameter (after Hursh 1939).

action potentials in large myelinated axons may travel at more than 100 m/s, while those in the smaller axons travel at about 6–60 m/s. Since the main peak of the action potential lasts about 1 ms, it may 'occupy' a distance of up to 100 mm (equivalent to about 100 internodes) in a large diameter axon. Thus, although the process of excitation moves discontinuously from node to node, the resulting potential change travels more smoothly.

Axonal transport of material. As in most cells, the synthesis of macromolecules in motor neurones occurs in the vicinity of the nucleus. An important feature of the motor neurone is that the synthesis of new proteins occurs only in the cell body. To enable proteins, as well as other new membrane components and mitochondria, to reach the axon and its terminals, specialised transport mechanisms are present within the axon (Grafstein & Forman 1980, Alberts et al 1989).

Two mechanisms of axonal transport have been discovered (Vallee & Bloom 1991). One operates at a rate of about 1 mm/day ('slow' transport) and represents the rate of synthesis and 'extrusion' of new components of the axonal cytoplasm. These include the main elements of the cytoskeleton and many soluble cytoplasmic proteins. The second mechanism is much faster (100–400 mm/day) and involves the movement of membrane-bound vesicles containing the transported substances along the axonal microtubules. This process now appears to be mediated by mechanoprotein cross-links between the vesicles and the microtubules which are probably analogous in their operation to the myosin cross-bridges in muscle. This 'fast' transport also operates in a retrograde direction, conveying to the cell body material which enters the axoplasm at the terminal.

Neuromuscular junction

At the neuromuscular junction, both the nerve and muscle cells are highly specialised to carry out the process of neuromuscular transmission, which is described in Chapter 5. Within the axon terminal, the neurotransmitter acetylcholine (ACh) is synthesised from choline and acetylCoA in a reaction catalysed by the enzyme cholineacetyl-transferase (ChAT; EC 2.3.1.6). Up to 90% of the total active ChAT in muscle is located within the nerve terminals. It is transported there from its site of synthesis in the cell body.

The resting concentration of choline in cholinergic neurones is much higher than typical concentrations for plasma or interstitial fluid and is maintained at such a high level partly because there is a continual turnover of phospholipids in cells and partly because cholinergic neurones possess a high affinity uptake system for the accumulation of free choline from the interstitial fluid. At times of accelerated ACh synthesis, as during high levels of synaptic activity, the uptake of choline is enhanced so that the choline released

by hydrolysis of ACh in the synaptic cleft (see below) can be reutilised. The details of ACh release are considered in the next chapter.

The postsynaptic surface of the muscle cell is also highly differentiated. Of most immediate significance to neuromuscular transmission is the presence of a high density of ACh receptors (AChR). On binding ACh, these complex membrane proteins form an ion channel which allows a net entry of positive ions into the muscle fibre, thus generating a local depolarisation, the *end-plate potential*. As at the motor axon hillock and the node of Ranvier, a high density of voltage-dependent Na^+ channels is present in the muscle fibre membrane at the neuromuscular junction (Angelides 1986) and allows the end-plate potential to generate a muscle fibre action potential.

Acetylcholine is released from the nerve terminal in packets of several thousand molecules. In normal circumstances, many such packets are released by a single nerve impulse and considerably more transmitter is released than is necessary to bring the muscle fibre to the action potential threshold. As a result of this high *safety factor*, the process of neuromuscular transmission is normally very reliable, even during repetitive activity when the amount of transmitter released may decline somewhat (Elmqvist & Quastel 1965).

Recent studies have shown that the number of packets of transmitter released in experimental conditions from human neuromuscular (20–25) junctions is considerably less than from those of lower vertebrates (50–200) (Slater et al 1992). It seems likely that this is due to the smaller extent of synaptic contact at human junctions mentioned above. While this might be expected to result in a reduced safety factor in human neuromuscular transmission, there is no clear evidence that this is the case. Rather, it seems likely that the particularly extensive postsynaptic folds in humans harbour a high density of voltage-dependent Na^+ channels and that these serve to amplify the relatively weak postsynaptic currents induced by the direct action of the transmitter (Slater et al 1992).

The activity of the ACh released by a nerve impulse is terminated by hydrolysis by the enzyme acetylcholinesterase (AChE; 3.1.1.7) and by diffusion out of the synaptic cleft. AChE is a highly polymorphic enzyme and numerous forms exist in skeletal muscle (Massoulié & Bon 1982). Most of the functionally significant AChE is located not in the muscle fibre itself, but in the synaptic basal lamina (McMahan et al 1978). Because the synaptic gap is very narrow, most of the ACh released from the nerve is able to reach and bind to AChRs before it can be hydrolysed by the intervening AChE. However, as individual ACh molecules dissociate from AChR, they are generally broken down before they are able to bind a second time. Drugs that block AChE activity allow individual ACh molecules to bind repeatedly and thus prolong the synaptic currents that flow as a result of ACh action.

Skeletal muscle

An action potential generated at the neuromuscular junction propagates towards the ends of the muscle fibre at a velocity of about 5 m/s. The wave of depolarisation is carried to the interior of the muscle fibre by tubular invaginations of the plasma membrane, the *transverse tubules* (or *T-tubules*). Depolarisation of the T-tubules causes the release of Ca^{2+} from the extensive sarcoplasmic reticulum (SR), a specialised form of endoplasmic reticulum, into the cytoplasm. When the concentration of free Ca^{2+} in the vicinity of the contractile filaments reaches about 10^{-6}M (it is normally about 10^{-8}M), interaction between myosin cross-bridges and the thin filaments can take place and contraction ensues. This sequence of events is known as *excitation-contraction (EC) coupling*.

At the heart of EC coupling are two membrane proteins; a 'voltage sensor' in the T-tubule membrane and a 'dihydropyridine receptor' in the SR membrane controlling Ca^{2+} permeability. Considerable progress has been made recently in characterising these protein complexes but the exact nature of their interaction remains unclear. The structural aspects of EC coupling are described in Chapter 4.

The cyclic making and breaking of actin-myosin cross-bridges which accounts for contraction is powered by the hydrolysis of ATP, in a reaction catalysed by ATPase activity associated with the myosin cross-bridges. The interaction between thick and thin filaments comes to an end and the muscle relaxes when the Ca^{2+} released into the cytoplasm is reaccumulated by the SR. (See Ch. 4 and Ch. 6 for further details of the ultrastructural and molecular basis of muscle contraction.)

Isometric contractions. Most experimental studies of muscle contraction are made with the ends of the muscle rigidly fixed so that shortening does not occur. In these *isometric* conditions the response to a single muscle fibre action potential is a *twitch*, an increase in tension which rises to a peak in less than 100 ms and decays slightly more slowly. If the muscle is stimulated repetitively at a frequency greater than about 5 Hz, successive twitches sum and a greater maximum tension is produced than in a single twitch. As the frequency of stimulation is increased to about 50–200 Hz, the individual responses 'fuse' to form a tetanus, a smooth and rapid increase in tension rising to a stable plateau (Fig. 1.7). At still higher frequencies there is no further increase in peak tension, although the rate of rise of tension may continue to increase (Harris & Wilson 1971).

The characteristics of the isometric response depend not only on the contractile events themselves, but also on the high degree of elasticity associated with the muscle. This elasticity, which is effectively in series with the contractile apparatus, is present both in the tendons and connective tissue sheaths, and within the sarco-

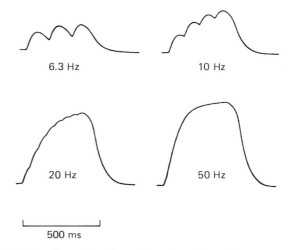

Fig. 1.7 Generation of tetanic tension at increasing frequencies of stimulation. Rat soleus muscle stimulated at 6.3, 10, 20 and 50 impulses/s (adapted from A. J. Buller: *Disorders of Voluntary Muscle*, 3rd edn. Fig. 2.1).

meres themselves. If it were possible to remove all of the elasticity from the muscle, a muscle action potential would result in the prompt generation of all the tension the contractile component could bear. Repetitive stimulation would merely prolong the period of tension and would have no effect on the amount of tension recorded. As it is, the series elasticity must be stretched before the full tension generated by the contractile component can be recorded.

Hill (1949) considered the amount of tension a muscle could bear at any moment (as opposed to the amount that could be recorded) as a measure of the intensity of the 'active state'. In a single twitch, the active state lasts for only a few ms (in a mammalian muscle it may not even be fully expressed after a single action potential). Because it takes a relatively long time to stretch the elastic component, the active state begins to decline as the tension is still rising. With repetitive stimulation, the active state is prolonged, the elastic component becomes more fully stretched, and more tension is recorded. At the appropriate frequency, the developed tension reaches the maximum the contractile component can generate. This maximal tetanic tension is often referred to as 'P_o' and in mammalian muscle is typically 5–10 times greater than the tension in a twitch.

The absolute amount of tension generated in a contraction is proportional to the number of interfilament cross-bridges that can be made. This depends in turn on two structural features of the muscle. The first is the cross-sectional area of the contractile material. In general, most of the bulk of the muscle fibre is occupied by the thick and thin filaments which are very regularly spaced. As a result, the total tension a muscle can generate is closely related to its total cross-sectional area.

The magnitude of the contraction is also dependent on the length of the muscle. This property may be studied by constructing a length–tension diagram as shown in Fig. 1.8. First the passive tension, which results solely from the elastic component, is measured in the unstimulated muscle at different muscle lengths. Next the total tension during a maximal tetanic contraction is measured at a variety of muscle lengths. This tension represents the sum of both elastic and contractile components. By subtracting the

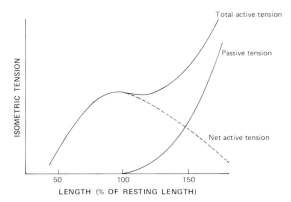

Fig. 1.8 Length–tension diagram for isometric contractions. Passive tension is measured in the unstimulated muscle. Total active tension is the tension generated during maximal tetanic stimulation at each length. Net active tension, the difference between the two other curves, is the tension generated by the contractile component itself.

passive tension from the total tension ('net active tension'), the tension generated by the contractile component itself is obtained. This curve shows that a muscle can only generate its maximal active tension over a narrow range of lengths. The optimal length, at which the muscle generates the greatest tension, is that at which the thin filaments just completely overlap the region of the thick filaments which bears the cross-bridges, and thus permits the maximum number of cross-bridge interactions to occur (Gordon et al 1966).

Isotonic contractions. If an active muscle is allowed to shorten against a constant load, the contraction is said to be isotonic. The rate of shortening is maximal when no load is being lifted but decreases as the load is increased (Aidley 1989). Pure isometric or isotonic contractions rarely occur in the body. Most contractions are hybrids involving both load-bearing and shortening. Moreover, many are 'eccentric', a term applied to the condition where a muscle is stretched while it is still developing tension. During normal daily activities, most eccentric contractions probably occur while walking downstairs or downhill. In these situations, the load-bearing muscles are stretched as the body is lowered. The muscle pain and stiffness that result from unusual activity of this kind (such as the overenthusiastic participation in step-aerobics by untrained individuals) is a manifestation of damage caused by eccentric contractions.

Eccentric contractions are highly demanding in terms of energy and they result in the particularly rapid onset of fatigue (Edwards et al 1981). They are poorly understood, and the features that allow elongation without causing major damage have not been well studied.

MOTOR UNIT SPECIALISATIONS AND PATTERNS OF USE

Muscle fibre diversity

Mammalian motor units contract at different speeds (Close 1972). In most muscles, two distinct classes, or 'types', of unit can be distinguished, 'slow-twitch' or type I, and 'fast-twitch', or type II (Fig. 1.9). The precise speed of contraction varies greatly from animal to animal. In a mouse, for example, a typical fast motor unit reaches its peak tension (T_c) after a single stimulus in about 6 ms, while in a cat T_c is typically 25 ms and in man about 35 ms. The T_c of slow units in these species is typically 20 ms, 75 ms and 90 ms respectively. In man, and possibly in several other species, the differentiation of motor units into fast-twitch and slow-twitch is rather arbitrary because in most muscles there is a continuum of motor unit twitch speeds rather than two distinct populations (Freund 1983). Muscles which have a marked predominance of one type of muscle fibre are themselves either fast or slow. Since slow muscles tend to be reddish in appearance, due to a large amount of myoglobin, the terms 'slow, red' and 'fast, white' have entered the scientific vocabulary.

Two factors are chiefly responsible for determining the speed of contraction of an individual muscle fibre. The first is the particular species of contractile proteins present (Pette & Vrbová 1985). Both actin and myosin, as well as most of the regulatory proteins associated with them, exist in several closely related 'isoforms' (see Ch. 3). Myosin has been most carefully studied in this respect; distinct isoforms exist in fast and slow muscle fibres, as well as in fetal and neonatal muscles. Because the ATPase activity of slow myosin is less than that of fast, appropriate histochemical methods for the demonstration of ATPase activity can distinguish fast from slow fibres. More recently, monoclonal antibodies specific for the different myosin isoforms have come to be used for the same purpose.

While the contractile proteins present determine the speed of contraction, the speed of relaxation, and hence the frequency of repetitive stimulation a muscle fibre can 'follow', is largely determined by the rate of calcium uptake into the SR. Fast fibres have more extensive SR than slow (Eisenberg & Kuda 1976) and are much richer in the Ca^{2+}–Mg^{2+} ATPase that is responsible for Ca^{2+} uptake (Pette & Vrbová 1985).

Fast and slow muscle fibres have also long been known to differ in their patterns of energy metabolism. Slow-twitch muscle fibres rely on oxidative mechanisms for the generation of energy while fast-twitch fibres rely on glycolysis, either on its own ('fast, glycolytic' or type IIB fibres) or in combination with oxidative mechanisms ('fast, oxidative-glycolytic' or type IIA fibres). In keeping with these patterns, slow-twitch fibres have more mitochondria and are more highly vascularised than fast-twitch fibres (Eisenberg & Kuda 1976).

Closely related to the pattern of energy metabolism is the ability of the muscle to sustain contraction. While muscle fibres with oxidative metabolism are able to produce substantial tension for

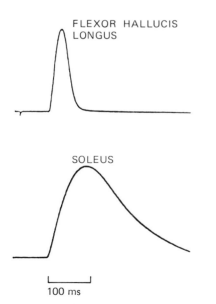

FLEXOR HALLUCIS LONGUS

SOLEUS

100 ms

Fig. 1.9 Isometric twitches in a fast (flexor hallucis longus) and a slow (soleus) muscle of the cat (from Buller & Lewis 1963).

some minutes ('fatigue-resistant'), those utilising glycolytic pathways fatigue rapidly in the face of sustained stimulation ('fatiguable'). Because metabolic and contractile properties are normally closely coupled in individual muscle fibres, histochemical procedures which demonstrate the activity of mitochondrial enzymes, such as succinate dehydrogenase, show higher activity in those fibres with low myosin-ATPase activity while procedures for enzymes of glycolysis, such as phosphorylase, show greater activity in high-ATPase fibres.

The general correlation between the speed of contraction of a muscle and the metabolic properties of its muscle fibres suggested to Henneman and his colleagues that individual motor units might be composed of fibres of a single metabolic type (Henneman & Olsen 1965, Wuerker et al 1965). This was subsequently elegantly confirmed by a number of studies (Edström & Kugelberg 1968, Burke et al 1973, Nemeth et al 1981). These all demonstrated that whether one considers molecules related to the speed of contraction or to energy metabolism, all the muscle fibres in a given motor unit are essentially identical. Thus the motor unit itself may be considered to be 'fast, fatiguable', 'slow, fatigue-resistant' or to be of an intermediate type.

Fatigue of muscles. It is a common experience that sick people complain of feeling 'tired', 'weak' or 'fatigued', but it is clear that these expressions do not always refer to muscle fatigue itself. In the normal healthy person, however, muscle 'fatigue' usually follows a period of extremely strenuous activity, or a period of continuous low-level activity. We may therefore define fatigue as the condition in which muscles fail to maintain tension, or fail to develop constant tension, in response to stimulation at a constant frequency. The stimulus may be imposed or generated voluntarily.

Muscle fatigue in healthy people does not result from a failure of neuromuscular transmission or from a failure of the action potential mechanism in nerve or muscle, because the relevant safety factors are too high. Rather, fatigue arises either from a failure of excitation–contraction coupling (Edwards et al 1977) or from a depletion of energy resources (Dawson et al 1978). These two alter-

natives are not mutually exclusive, but Fitch and McComas (1985) have presented compelling evidence that, at least during relatively high rates of stimulation (electrical stimulation of the nerve at 20 Hz or maximal voluntary contractions lasting 90 s), the dominant factor is the depletion of energy resources.

Vascular supply. The different patterns of energy metabolism of fast and slow motor units require that the microcirculation is appropriately organised. Ranvier (1874) is credited with being the first to observe that red muscles have a higher capillarity than white, a feature now documented by many others. As a result of the higher capillarity, blood flow through the predominantly slow soleus muscle of the cat during normal standing (approximately 50 ml/100 g/min) is much higher than through the gastrocnemius (approximately 14 ml/100 g/min) (Hilton et al 1970). In mixed muscles, blood flow at rest tends to be proportional to the number of slow fibres. As muscle activity increases, blood flow increases to become proportional to the number of fast muscle fibres, and particularly the fast oxidative-glycolytic fibres (Laughlin & Armstrong 1982). This increase in blood flow does not result simply from the selective dilatation of small blood vessels to fast fibres; blood supply to the viscera is decreased and cardiac output is also increased.

In some quadrupeds, there is a clear segregation of slow motor units into those muscles that are involved with posture, such as soleus, and fast motor units into those muscles concerned with rapid movements, such as extensor digitorum longus. In humans, the extent of such segregation is not so clear. None the less, there is great variation in the proportions of the various muscle fibre types in human muscles and it is reasonable to assume that this is of functional significance.

Motor neurone diversity

Motor neurones, as well as muscle fibres, show considerable diversity of form and function. One of the most important properties to show variation is the size of the cell body. The functional significance of cell size derives from its electrical consequences; the resistance of a cell is inversely related to its size. A given synaptic current therefore generates a larger voltage change in a small cell than in a large one. For a given intensity of excitatory synaptic input to the 'pool' of motor-neurones innervating a single muscle, small cells are more likely to reach threshold than large ones (Kernell 1966, Burke 1967). By the same token, a given inhibitory input has a more powerful effect on a small cell than on a large one. This effect of cell size on excitability influences the order in which motor units are recruited as the strength of muscle activation is increased (see below), as well as the order in which they 'drop out' as activation decreases (see summary by DeLuca 1985).

Low threshold motor neurones, presumed to be relatively small in size, also have relatively small diameter axons. Because action potential conduction velocity is inversely related to axon diameter (see above), action potentials generated in low threshold neurones are conducted more slowly than those in high threshold neurones. Furthermore, action potentials in 'slow' motor neurones, but not in 'fast', are followed by a characteristic 'after-hyperpolarisation' which prolongs the 'refractory period' during which another action potential cannot be generated (Eccles et al 1958, Aidley 1989). Thus, the motor neurones innervating 'fast' and 'slow' muscle fibres have distinctive functional properties and are themselves 'fast' and 'slow', though in a different sense to the muscle fibres they innervate.

The presynaptic terminals of fast and slow motor neurones differ in structural complexity. Those of fast neurones have more terminal branches and synaptic boutons than those of slow neurones (Korneliussen & Waerhaug 1973, Ogata & Yamasaki 1985). The functional significance of these structural differences is not yet known.

Matching of nerve and muscle properties

Not surprisingly, the functional properties of the motor neurone and muscle fibres comprising a given motor unit are carefully matched. Slowly contracting motor units are innervated by low-threshold motor neurones whose axons conduct relatively slowly. The long after-hyperpolarisation in these neurones helps to ensure that the frequency of firing is relatively low. In contrast, rapidly contracting units are innervated by

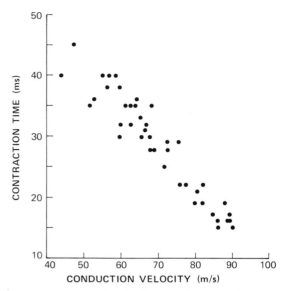

Fig. 1.10 Inverse relationship between the speed of contraction of a motor unit (the time to peak tension of an isometric twitch) and the conduction velocity of the motor axon in the first superficial lumbrical muscle of the cat (data from Appelberg & Emonet-Dénand 1967).

relatively high-threshold motor neurones with rapidly conducting action potentials which can occur in high-frequency bursts. As a result, when a large number of motor units is studied, there is a close correlation between motor axon conduction velocity and contraction speed (Fig. 1.10).

A second important aspect of nerve–muscle matching is that 'large' motor neurones innervate 'large' motor units. More strictly, the tension generated by motor units innervated by high-threshold, rapidly conducting motor neurones is generally greater than that generated by units innervated by low-threshold, slowly conducting neurones (see below).

Patterns of motor unit use

The strength of muscle contraction can be increased by the central nervous system in two ways; either by changing the number of active motor units ('recruitment') or by altering the frequency of firing so that successive twitches begin to sum and the tension generated by individual units increases ('frequency coding') (Freund 1983).

Recruitment order. In a given set of circumstances, the order in which motor units are
recruited is relatively constant and related to their
'size', as defined by the amount of tension they
generate. As a muscle is activated from rest, the
first units to be recruited are usually the weakest.
As increasing strength of contraction is called for,
larger and larger units are recruited. As a result of
this pattern of excitation, each newly recruited unit
adds a roughly constant proportion of the
background contractile strength (Fig. 1.11). The
orderly recruitment of motor units according to
their size ('size principle') has been considered
in detail by Henneman and his colleagues
(Henneman et al 1965) and has been shown to
apply in many, though not all (e.g. Sica &
McComas 1971, Wyman et al 1974), situations. In
any case, the precise order in which motor units are
recruited is not rigidly fixed. In muscles in which a
range of movements is possible, the particular order
of recruitment may depend on the movement
being made (Denier van der Gon et al 1982),
probably as a consequence of differing descending
inputs to the motor neurones for each different
class or direction of movement.

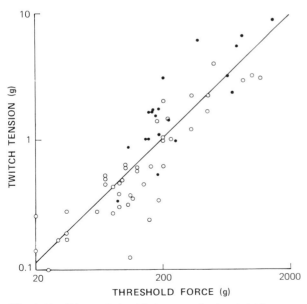

Fig. 1.11 Direct relationship between the threshold force at
which a particular motor unit is normally excited, and the
twitch tension of the motor unit, determined in the first dorsal
interosseous muscle of man (from Milner-Brown et al 1973).

Although the order in which motor units are
recruited is relatively fixed for a particular
movement, the absolute tension at which recruitment occurs depends very much on the speed with
which the movement is made. As the speed
increases the threshold for all units falls with the
result that large units are used transiently when it
is necessary to develop tension rapidly (Freund
1983).

Firing patterns. Many early studies (reviewed
by Freund 1983) pointed to differences in the
firing patterns of motor neurones. Eccles and his
colleagues showed that in cats, the motor neurones
innervating postural muscles such as the soleus
were active in quiet standing and inhibited when
the flexors were excited (Eccles et al 1958). Burke
and his colleagues showed that even in mixed
muscles, slow units were active during quiet
standing, and that during movement, when fast
units were activated, slow units were inhibited
(Burke et al 1970). This was an important observation since it indicated that the pattern of activity
of a motor unit is related to its functional type
regardless of the particular muscle it is in.

During activity, the firing patterns of fast and
slow motor units differ considerably. In general,
slow motor neurones discharge continuously at a
frequency of about 10–20 Hz. In contrast, fast
motor neurones usually discharge in short, high-
frequency (up to 100 Hz) bursts. Henning &
Lømo (1985) made a detailed study of the
relationship between firing patterns and motor
unit tension in fast and slow muscles of the rat.
They found that the slow motor units of the soleus
muscle fired more or less continuously at about
20 Hz, at which rate they generate 50–80% of their
maximal tetanic force. Similarly, fast motor units,
when active, fired at a mean frequency of about
80 Hz at which rate they, too, generate 50–80% of
their maximal force. In units of both types, small
changes in frequency of activation lead to substantial changes in tension. These results show that, to a
first approximation, the firing pattern of a motor
neurone is well matched to the contractile properties of the muscle fibres it innervates.

The view of motor neurones with fixed firing
patterns which are matched to the contractile
properties of the muscle fibres they innervate seems
to make good functional sense but is clearly an

oversimplification. Newer studies of motor neurone firing patterns are revealing abrupt transitions in firing rate, apparently determined by descending inputs, possibly mediated by 5-hydroxytryptamine (Kiehn 1991). These studies suggest that motor neurones may be able to exist in alternative states of excitability which can be selected by appropriate central commands. The true significance of such alternative states remains to be established.

The distinctions between slow and fast motor units, involving excitation threshold, pattern of activity, contractile speed and pattern of energy metabolism, suit them to distinctive physiological roles. Slow-twitch units are easily activated. Through their reliance on abundantly available energy stores of carbohydrate and fat, in combination with a good oxygen delivery system, they are able to maintain tension for prolonged periods. However, they lack the ability to contract rapidly. They are thus well suited for the moderate but continuous contractions required to maintain posture and in prolonged exertion. By contrast, fast-twitch units are specialised for explosive, short-term activity where considerable loads are to be borne and their energy source, glycogen, is rapidly available, but relatively quickly exhausted.

The central control of motor unit activity is beyond the scope of this chapter. Clearly, the activity of sensory receptors in the muscle, joints and skin, the interneurones and recurrent motor axon collaterals in the spinal cord, and descending pathways from higher centres all influence the pattern of motor unit activation (see, for example, Nicholls et al 1992).

MOTOR UNIT PLASTICITY

So far, we have considered the motor unit as if the properties of its cells, and the relationships between them, were fixed. In most biological systems, including the neuromuscular system, functional interrelationships are maintained by the interplay of numerous dynamic interactions. This gives the overall system the advantage of adaptability. There are two main ways in which the performance of the neuromuscular system adapts to changes in conditions. One is through alterations in the patterns of motor unit activation by the central nervous system and is beyond the scope of this chapter. The other is through changes in the properties of the units themselves. In the rest of this chapter, we will consider how the properties of motor units vary during development, the nature and limits of their adaptability in the mature individual, the response of the motor unit to injury, and finally, how the adaptive potential of the motor unit helps to reduce the functional impact of the loss of motor units during ageing.

Development of the motor unit

The formation of the neuromuscular system, though a continuous process, can be divided into two distinctive phases. In the first, the various cells that give rise to nerve and muscle interact to form a system that is immature, but none the less functional. In the second phase, this immature system undergoes numerous transformations that shape the fully mature motor units. The cell–cell interactions involved in the first phase precede the development of a functional system. By contrast, the events of the second phase depend critically on how the system is used.

Early events. Motor neurones are among the first nerve cells to be 'born' (Jacobson 1978). Like other newly formed neurones, they migrate away from the basal surface of the neural epithelium and lodge in the marginal zone of the ventrolateral quadrant of the developing spinal cord. Soon afterwards, the motor axon grows away from the neuraxis toward the muscles. In limb regions, the motor axons from several segments contribute to the formation of the plexuses. Within the plexus, the relative positions of the axons change so that those destined for anatomically related muscles come together. At the time this happens, the target muscles have not yet formed. This supports the view, derived from a variety of experiments (Lance-Jones & Landmesser 1980), that the factors governing the formation of the main divisions of the peripheral nerves are independent of the muscles themselves. Recent studies suggest that the development of the spatial patterns of muscle innervation are strongly influenced by the presence of characteristic molecules, such as nerve cell adhesion molecules (N-CAMs) and polysialic acid, in the surface of the immature nerve and muscle cells (Rutishauser & Landmesser 1991).

Skeletal muscles arise from the myotomal cells of the segmented embryonic somites (Alberts et al 1989). As development proceeds, some of these cells become fibroblasts. Others, though still dividing, become committed to making muscle. The commitment of these cells to myogenesis appears to be controlled by the expression of individual genes coding for members of the helix-loop-helix class of transcriptional regulators, including *MyoD* and *myogenin* (Weintraub et al 1991). Apparently as a result of environmental cues, cells from this myogenic line eventually stop dividing and become postmitotic myoblasts. The formation of muscle fibres begins with the alignment and subsequent fusion of myoblasts so that their nuclei come to occupy a common cytoplasm. It appears that in all cases, some myoblasts remain unfused and persist in association with the muscle fibre as satellite cells (see above). Neither the factors that ensure the persistence of such quiescent myogenic cells, nor the factors that cause them to become activated during muscle injury, are understood. The multinucleated cells thus formed are called myotubes.

Soon after myotubes form, the pattern of protein synthesis coded by their nuclei changes dramatically. Particularly notable is the appearance of the proteins that make up the contractile filaments, metabolic proteins such as creatine kinase, integral membrane proteins such as the acetylcholine receptor, and the various components of the basal lamina. Although the expression of the different genes for these various proteins is not inextricably linked, during normal development their products appear as a closely associated cohort that accounts for the coordinated appearance of muscle properties.

Motor axons are present in muscle-forming regions of the embryo before myotubes first appear. Myotubes become innervated very soon (less than 1 day) after they first appear (Bennett & Pettigrew 1974). Although this early innervation is very immature, activity in the nerve is almost immediately able to elicit muscle contraction and to exert an important influence on subsequent muscle development.

The first axon to innervate each muscle fibre does so at a discrete spot apparently chosen at random along the length of the still very short (<1 mm) muscle fibre. This axon is soon joined at the same spot by the terminals of several other axons, each of which becomes able to elicit muscle contraction. This early state of polyneuronal innervation stands in marked contrast to the adult condition in which each muscle fibre is innervated by a single axon (Bennett 1983, Purves & Lichtman 1985).

As muscle fibres are being innervated, approximately half of the motor neurones initially produced die (Oppenheim 1991). The extent of this cell death is greatly influenced by the amount of muscle available for innervation. Removing limb buds prior to innervation causes nearly all the motor neurones to die, while enlarging the bulk of muscle 'rescues' substantial numbers of neurones that would normally die. As there is very little indication that growing motor neurones ever innervate the 'wrong' muscle, motor neurone death seems designed to ensure the survival of appropriate numbers of neurones, rather than to eliminate qualitative errors of connectivity.

The nature of the events leading to motor neurone death is still poorly understood. The dependence on target muscles, particularly in immature animals, suggests that *trophic factors* produced by muscles are taken up by the neurones and are required for their survival. If such factors were present in limiting amounts, the number of neurones surviving might be matched to the size of the target. A clear precedent for such a mechanism is provided by the neurones of the autonomic and sensory systems which depend for their survival on adequate supplies of *nerve growth factor* (*NGF*) (Purves & Lichtman 1985). However, in spite of strenuous efforts, no 'motor neurone growth factor' has yet been unambiguously identified.

Maturation of the motor unit. Many properties of nerve and muscle cells change dramatically during the first few weeks after initial nerve–muscle contacts form. The dendrites of the motor neurones increase in extent and complexity and many synapses form on them, while other synapses are lost from the region of the axon hillock (Ronnevi & Conradi 1974). The motor axon increases in diameter and length, and myelin forms as individual Schwann cells wrap themselves around the axon (Geren 1954). This results in an increase in the speed of conduction of nerve impulses and in the frequency with which they can be generated and propagated.

Newly innervated muscle fibres grow rapidly in length and girth and begin to express the properties that mark them as belonging to a particular 'type'. Increase in length is accompanied by continued fusion of myogenic cells, derived, it is thought, from satellite cells (Ontell 1979). Muscle growth depends critically on the integrity and activity of the nerve supply. Denervation during muscle formation arrests growth (Harris 1981) and may lead to death of muscle fibres that have already formed (Jaros & Johnstone 1983).

The mature pattern of muscle fibre innervation arises during this period by the gradual elimination of supernumary nerve–muscle contacts (Fig. 1.12). This process, which lasts several weeks and is enhanced by activity, determines the sets of muscle fibres that make up the adult motor units (Jansen & Fladby 1990, Brown et al 1991). As the redundant innervation is lost, the terminal of the 'sole-surviving' axon at each neuromuscular junction expands and takes on its adult form (Slater 1982). Extensive folding of the muscle fibre surface occurs, as does an increase in the metabolic half-life of the acetylcholine receptors in the muscle membrane and an increase in the speed of operation of the ionic channels associated with them (Scheutze & Role 1987). These events fail to occur if the nerve is cut at an early stage in development, suggesting that maturation of the junction requires a continuing interaction between nerve and muscle cells.

Although the main period of developmental motor neurone death occurs when muscles are first being innervated, motor neurones of rodents remain dependent for their survival on contact with muscle fibres for a week or so after birth (Lowrie & Vrbová 1992). While most motor neurones in adult rats or mice survive for a long time without functional contact with muscle, most motor neurones in newborn animals will die in the same circumstances. Like the studies of motor neurone death earlier in development, these observations suggest that muscle fibres release 'trophic factors' which are required by immature motor neurones for their survival.

While it is likely that such trophic factors are

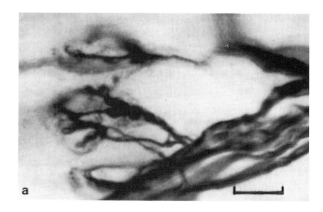

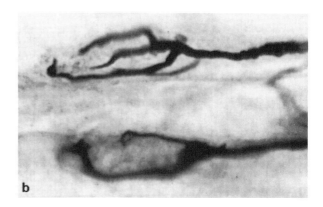

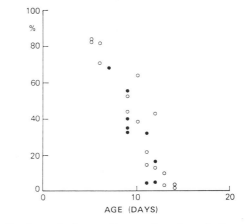

Fig. 1.12 Loss of polyaxonal innervation of muscle fibres during development (mouse). **a** Multiple axons innervate most muscle fibres 1 week after birth (silver stain). **b** A single, more robust axon innervates most muscle fibres by 2 weeks of age. **c** Time-course of the loss of polyaxonal innervation in the mouse soleus muscle, determined both by physiological and anatomical criteria (experimental details in Slater 1982) (scale bar = 10 μm).

normally produced by muscle fibres, recent experiments suggest that Schwann cells may be an alternative source. The ciliary neurotrophic factor (CNTF), present in mature Schwann cells, can prevent much of the motor neurone death induced by nerve section in immature animals (Thoenen 1991). The absence of this putative 'lesion factor' from immature peripheral nerves may account for the inability of mature motor neurones to survive isolation from their normal target.

The 'type-specific' properties of fully mature muscle fibres, such as the speed of contraction and the molecular factors that underlie it, develop during the first few weeks after birth in laboratory mammals (Buller et al 1960a, Close 1964). Several factors seem to govern the expression of these properties. One is the pattern of activity imposed by the nerve (see below). However, some recent studies indicate that muscle fibres may express type-specific properties at a very early stage in development.

Evidence from several sources, including studies of immature myogenic cells grown in culture and muscles that develop in situ in the absence of innervation, indicate that at least some muscle fibres can develop appropriate type-specific characteristics in the absence of innervation (Miller & Stockdale 1987, Sanes 1987). If this is generally true, it suggests that the matching of motor neurone and muscle fibre types that is such an important feature of the mature neuromuscular system arises during development by the preferential innervation of muscle fibres by motor neurones of an appropriate type (Thompson 1986, Jasen & Fladby 1990). It may well be that one of the main functions of the initial period of polyneuronal innervation is to promote this matching by allowing competition between motor neurones of varying degrees of functional matching with individual muscle fibres.

Neural control of muscle fibre properties

The influence of innervation on muscle properties persists into adulthood (Pette & Vrbová 1985). A dramatic demonstration of this is the atrophy of muscle which follows paralysis resulting from immobilisation or denervation (see below). While the alterations in motor unit properties which accompany specialised training are more modest, they too reflect the response of motor unit properties to changing use. Between these extremes lie modifications of motor unit properties which are associated with recovery from injury or disease.

Much of our current thinking about the nature of the effect of innervation on the properties of mature muscle stems from a series of animal experiments in which the nerve supply to predominantly fast and slow muscles was cut and then surgically redirected so that the 'fast' nerve reinnervated the 'slow' muscle and vice versa. Effective 'cross re-innervation' was accompanied by a change in the speed of contraction of each muscle so that it came to resemble that of the muscle of the opposite type (Fig. 1.13) (Buller et al 1960b). These changes in the speed of contraction are now known to reflect alterations of many muscle fibre properties including the myosin isoforms, metabolic enzyme profiles and the extent of vascularisation (Pette & Vrbová 1985).

In contrast to the changes in muscle that occur in these experiments, the motor neurones retain

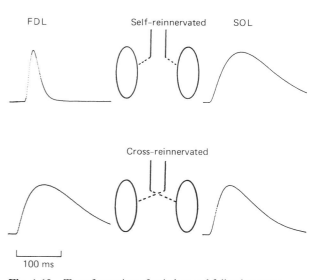

Fig. 1.13 Transformation of twitch speed following cross-reinnervation in the cat. **a** Twitches of the fast flexor hallucis longus (FDL) and the slow soleus (SOL) muscles, reinnervated by their own nerves. **b** Twitches of the same muscles after their nerve supplies had been experimentally crossed (adapted from Buller 1972)

their characteristic type-specific properties. Thus the after-hyperpolarisation and relatively slow conduction velocity of 'slow' motor neurones are preserved even when they innervate what had been a fast muscle (Kuno et al 1974). This suggests that while the type-specific properties of muscle fibres can be modified by the nerve, those of the motor neurones themselves are more stable and largely independent of the particular type of muscle fibre they innervate.

The nature of the neural influence on muscle. Two distinct views have emerged over the years to explain how motor nerves exert long-term control over the muscles they innervate. The first is that nerves exert a 'trophic' influence on muscle, most clearly seen in the maintenance of muscle bulk, which is mediated by chemical messengers released from the nerve which acts on the muscle. The second view is that muscles alter their properties in response to changes in the pattern and amount of their own activity, which is normally imposed on them by their innervation. Strong evidence for control of target tissues by one 'trophic' substance, nerve growth factor, has emerged from studies of those parts of the peripheral nervous system that derive from the neural crest (Purves & Lichtman 1985). While much work is currently underway to determine whether or not similar factors may account for nerve–muscle interactions, no clear picture has yet emerged.

In contrast, it is now well established that the amount and pattern of muscle activity, whether elicited by nerve impulses or by direct electrical stimulation of denervated muscles, has profound effects on many muscle fibre properties (Pette and Vrbová 1985). In general, if muscles are stimulated directly or through the nerve with a pattern of activity characteristic of slow motor units (e.g. continuous 10 Hz) their properties come to resemble those of slow units, whereas stimulation with short, high-frequency bursts, characteristic of fast units, induces the properties of fast units. Detailed analysis of this transformation has shown that while the pattern of activity influences many type-specific muscle properties, these do not all change at the same rate or equally completely. Changes in the proteins of energy metabolism and calcium sequestration can be detected within a week, when the earliest slowing of the contractile

response are seen, but changes in the contractile proteins, and myosin isoforms in particular, do not occur until some weeks later.

There are numerous isoforms of myosin and a minimum of four may be expressed in a single muscle. For example, at various stages of its development and growth, the rat soleus muscle expresses embryonic, neonatal, adult fast and adult slow isoforms, and individual muscle fibres can express multiple isoforms. In all, approximately 20 distinct myosin genes have been identified.

The regulation of this large multigene family is not well understood. There is no doubt that there are underlying patterns to the sequence of gene activation and expression and that there is a high degree of developmental regulation, but the precise factors involved (which include neural activity, endocrine status and age) have not been determined.

A second important example of the effect of activity on muscle fibre properties concerns the postsynaptic acetylcholine receptors. In normal muscle, these are normally restricted to the immediate postsynaptic membrane and the genes controlling their synthesis are expressed almost exclusively by the myonuclei in the vicinity of the neuromuscular junction (e.g. Simon et al 1992). It has been known for many years that following denervation, AChRs appear all over the muscle fibre surface (Scheutze & Role 1987 and see below). It is now clear that this results from the expression of AChR genes by many of the myonuclei along the length of the paralysed muscle fibres, and that this can be suppressed by artificial stimulation of such denervated muscles (Goldman et al 1988). Recent studies have shown that the effect of muscle activity on AChR gene expression involves an intracellular second messenger cascade. When denervated rat muscles, which express genes for AChR subunits at a high rate, are stimulated directly, a significant decrease in the rate of AChR subunit gene expression can be seen within less than 30 min. This is accompanied by an even more rapid activation of protein kinase C (Huang et al 1992). This suggests that activation of protein kinase C may lead to phosphorylation of a regulatory protein that, more or less directly, inhibits AChR subunit gene expression. Whether a similar mechanism is involved in controlling the type-specific properties of muscle fibres is not yet known.

Effects of training on motor unit properties

While mature muscle fibres are capable of nearly complete transformation from one fibre type to another in experimental situations, extremes of imposed activity have to be used that lie well beyond what is possible during normal voluntary movement. None the less, the intense training programmes undertaken by top-class athletes can induce significant modifications of motor unit properties.

Broadly speaking, training programmes are usually aimed at increasing either endurance or maximum power, but usually not both. For endurance training, activities such as long-distance running are pursued, in which the muscles work against relatively modest loads but undergo considerable changes in length. This predominantly isotonic exercise leads to an increase in the rate of oxygen utilisation and is accompanied by an increase in the content of mitochondria and the density of capillaries around the muscle fibres. In general, however, even very rigorous and prolonged endurance training leads to relatively little change in muscle fibre diameter or in the proportion of slow to fast fibres as determined by the intensity of myofibrillar ATPase activity (Ingjer 1979, Larsson & Ansverd 1985).

The fact that training has little effect on fibre-type composition raises the interesting question of the importance of genetic influence on muscle composition. It has been reported that the limb muscles of top-class long-distance runners have an unusually high proportion of type I muscle fibres. These fibres, even in the resting state, are high in oxidative capacity, well endowed with a dense capillary network and have a large number of mitochondria. It seems probable that genetic factors confer a muscle composition that is favourable to 'endurance' or 'strength' training and that training itself simply reinforces that predisposition.

To increase strength, it is necessary to increase the cross-sectional area of muscle. Weight training involves exertion against heavy loads with relatively little length change. This predominantly isometric activity increases muscle fibre diameter and hence, capacity for generating force. In experimental circumstances, increasing the load on a particular muscle, even if it is denervated, leads to what is known as 'compensatory hypertrophy' (Gutmann et al 1971). It appears to be a general principle that tension on muscles, however imposed, leads to hypertrophy.

Hormonal effects on muscle

Endocrinologists have often reported that a number of factors other than activity may influence muscle development. For example, certain highly specialised muscles like the *levator ani* in quadrupeds develop only in the presence of an adequate level of testosterone. In other circumstances, however, endocrine disturbances are either without effect on muscle, or they affect muscle growth, rather than muscle fibre production or differentiation (see Hudgson & Hall 1982).

In contrast, there is compelling evidence that the level of circulating thyroid hormones is a significant determinant of muscle differentiation. It has been known for many years that hypothyroidism in both man and animals results in a slowing of the muscle twitch (Wilson & Walton 1959, Gold et al 1970). It now appears that hypothyroidism results in the transformation of fast-twitch muscle fibres expressing fast forms of myosin and troponin into muscle fibres expressing slow forms of these proteins (Johnson et al 1980, Dhoot & Perry 1981). Moreover, Nwoye & Mommaerts (1981) reported that the subunit composition of lactate dehydrogenase was also susceptible to the effects of changes in thyroid status. Hyperthyroidism results in the transformation of slow into fast muscle fibres, but in the rat at least, the transformation is incomplete, and results primarily from a change in the capacity of the muscle fibres to utilize oxidative rather than glycolytic metabolic pathways.

While the effects of hypothyroidism are dependent on an intact nerve supply, and can be blocked by surgical denervation (Johnson et al 1980), it is not clear whether the thyroid hormones act directly on muscle fibres or indirectly, via the regulation of growth hormone levels and the somatomedins (Butler-Browne et al 1984, Whalen et al 1985).

RESPONSE OF THE MOTOR UNIT TO DAMAGE

The greatest test of the motor unit's ability to respond to changing circumstances comes when injury or disease cause damage to the nerve or muscle cells. The regenerative capacity of peripheral nerve and skeletal muscle is highly developed and allows many forms of damage to be adequately compensated. Although traumatic injury may lead to simultaneous damage of nerve and muscle, some injuries, and many diseases, have a more selective effect and it is useful to consider the response to damage of nerve and muscle separately.

Nerve section

When a peripheral nerve is severed, a characteristic sequence of events is initiated, both in the nerve and in the muscle, which promote effective reinnervation. An appreciation of these events forms the basis for interpretation of less complete nerve damage, such as occurs in the early stages of anterior horn cell disorders.

Nerve degeneration. When a peripheral axon is cut, its distal segment degenerates, a process known as Wallerian degeneration after the author who provided the first detailed account of it (Waller 1850). The first part of the axon to break down is the synaptic terminal; the more proximal portion of the isolated axon segment breaks down more slowly (Miledi & Slater 1970). Axonal degeneration is accompanied by activation and proliferation of Schwann cells within the basal lamina tube surrounding each nerve fibre and recruitment of macrophages which play an important part in removing axonal debris. While it is generally assumed that the degenerating axon must produce diffusable signals that influence the behaviour of Schwann cells and macrophages, the nature of these signals is not yet known.

The response to nerve injury is greatly slowed in the mutant mouse *Ola* (Lunn et al 1989). In these animals, very slow axonal degeneration is accompanied by a substantial failure of macrophage invasion. Since *Ola* macrophages behave normally when implanted into genetically normal hosts, it seems that the primary defect is in the axon itself (Perry et al 1990). A better understanding of the mode of action of the *Ola* gene product might point the way to reducing the time required for recovery from peripheral nerve injury.

Nerve regeneration. Within hours after damage, axonal sprouts begin to emerge from the proximal stump. If the basal lamina tubes remain intact, as when the nerve has been crushed, they provide a direct channel for axonal growth. If, however, the nerve is cut and the ends retract, the growing sprouts may wander aimlessly for weeks. The rate of axonal regeneration is usually close to that of the slow component of axonal transport, about 1 mm/day, presumably because it depends on the assembly of a new cytoskeletal framework. Axonal growth usually continues unabated until the axons reach an appropriate target, even if this takes months.

A number of changes, known collectively as *chromatolysis*, occur in the cell body of the motor neurone following axonal damage (Kandel et al 1991). These include a dispersal of the protein synthetic apparatus of the cell, and a peripheral movement of the nucleus. In addition, the after-hyperpolarisation of 'slow' motor neurones is reduced (Kuno et al 1974) and many of the synaptic inputs to the motor neurone are withdrawn. These changes are associated with an altered pattern of protein synthesis by the cell body, presumably related to the changing demands associated with growth (Kandel et al 1991). Many of these changes are reversed if the regenerating axon makes functional contact with a muscle.

Denervation effects on muscle. Within a few days of nerve section, a sequence of events is initiated in the muscle fibres which brings them to a state of great sensitivity to the effects of regenerating axons (Nicholls et al 1992). The resting membrane potential falls from about −75 mV to about −60 mV, approaching the threshold for action potential generation (this is one of the factors that accounts for the spontaneous fibrillation of denervated muscle fibres). As already mentioned, denervation also leads to the appearance of AChRs over most of the muscle fibre surface, resulting in a generalised 'denervation sensitivity' to acetylcholine which resembles that of embryonic muscle fibres (Diamond & Miledi 1962, Scheutze & Role 1987). Recent studies show that another component of the surface of embryonic muscle fibres, N-CAM, also appears after denervation of mature muscle (Sanes et al 1986). It seems likely that these components favour the formation of new synaptic contacts by regenerating axons.

On a longer time-scale, denervation leads to profound muscle fibre atrophy. This results from alterations in the normal balance of synthesis and breakdown of many muscle constituents, often increasing the rate of turnover of muscle components as well as tipping the balance in favour of net loss.

Reinnervation of muscle. Regenerating motor axons usually reinnervate denervated muscle fibres at the site of the original neuromuscular junction. This tendency may well be related to the presence of an accumulation of factors in the synaptic basal lamina that induce the growing axon tip to differentiate into a presynaptic terminal (Sanes et al 1978). Of particular interest is a largely synapse-specific form of laminin, S-laminin, which appears to stabilise the tips of growing axons at old synaptic sites (Hunter et al 1989, Sanes 1989).

Neuromuscular transmission is usually restored within a day or two after the arrival of the regenerating axon. At the earliest stages of reinnervation, spontaneous transmitter release is restored prior to the restoration of effective neuromuscular transmission. Thereafter, there follows a period when the combination of low resting membrane potential and high input resistance of the atrophied muscle fibres ensures that the safety factor for transmission is higher than normal, even though the quantal content of nerve-evoked transmitter release is low (see Ch. 5 for a discussion of the microphysiology of neuromuscular transmission). Thus even 'immature' regenerating synapses are robust and capable of functioning without the onset of transmission failure, over a period of several weeks, in parallel with maturation of the nerve terminal structure and the loss of any aberrant nerve sprouts that may have formed.

Reinnervation is very effective if it occurs soon after nerve damage, but it becomes less so as the time between damage and the arrival of the growing nerve at the muscle increases (Gutmann & Young 1944). In man, it may take many months after injuries far from the muscle before nerves reach their targets, by which time it may have become impossible for fully effective reinnervation to occur. Even when effective synaptic contacts are restored after damage, their functional significance depends on the accuracy of reinnervation. If the nerve has been cut through, the axons may enter basal lamina tubes destined for inappropriate muscles. Because there appears to be little ability of regenerating motor nerves in adults to distinguish between different muscles, reinnervation of an inappropriate muscle may ensue. There is apparently no mechanism for the correction of such an error of regeneration which may render the reinnervation worse than useless.

Restoration of muscle properties after reinnervation. Effective reinnervation of muscle is followed by reversal of the effects of denervation. The resting potential returns to normal, extrajunctional sensitivity to acetylcholine is lost, and with time, the muscle fibres regain their original dimensions. Because direct electrical stimulation of denervated muscles can prevent or reverse most of the changes associated with denervation (Lømo 1976), it seems that the loss of muscle activity plays a key role in the induction of denervation-induced changes. At the same time, a number of observations suggest that there may be significant consequences of denervation other than paralysis.

Partial denervation. Diseases of the motor neurone often result in the death of a fraction of the cells innervating a given muscle. The presence of denervated muscle fibres scattered throughout the muscle appears to promote the outgrowth of sprouts from the surviving axons, either at the nodes of Ranvier or from the axon terminal itself, and the reinnervation of the denervated muscle fibres with which they make contact (Brown et al 1991).

An important consequence of this response is that new muscle fibres are added to the surviving motor units. Often, the properties of such added fibres will not be appropriate to their new nerve supply. In time, however, the activity pattern of the new innervation will cause them to come to match the rest of the muscle fibres in the unit. The result of this process is that distinctive clusters of muscle fibres of similar type appear. This fibre type grouping is often a useful indication of a neurogenic disturbance.

Muscle injury

A number of events can cause muscle fibres to degenerate. Some of the most obvious are mechanical trauma and primary myopathic diseases such as the muscular dystrophies. It is often the case that destruction of the muscle fibres leaves a substantial number of satellite cells intact. So long as this number is large enough, muscle regeneration can occur and in favourable cases can largely restore the lost tissue. As with damage to peripheral nerves, survival of intact basal lamina sheaths does much to aid regeneration of muscle and its subsequent reinnervation.

Muscle necrosis. Any event that leads to either the physical breakdown of the plasma membrane or to a loss of function of ion-selective channels will result in the movement of inorganic ions along their respective concentration gradients. In the case of small lesions, the damage may involve only a part of the muscle fibre's length. It is generally accepted that a common step in the breakdown of the muscle fibre is the entry of Ca^{2+} into the cells and the activation of Ca^{2+}-dependent proteases and phospholipases. This may not be completely accurate. There is growing evidence that the activation of the lysosomal enzymes and of some other non-Ca^{2+}-dependent neutral proteases occurs very rapidly, implying that these enzymes are involved in the very earliest stages of proteolytic activity. Furthermore, it is also probable that most endogenous phospholipase activity in muscle cells is not Ca^{2+}-dependent.

The first proteins to be hydrolysed during a degenerative episode are the cytoskeletal proteins and the non-contractile proteins of the myofibrils. The contractile proteins, myosin and actin, are hydrolysed relatively late.

When the vascular supply to a damaged mammalian muscle remains substantially intact, muscle fibre breakdown is accompanied within a day or two by an invasion of phagocytic cells originating in the blood. These cells cross the intact basal lamina sheaths and ingest muscle fibre debris. Within a few days, the bulk of this debris has been disposed of and the phagocytic cells have departed. In other circumstances, especially when the vascular supply is damaged and access of phagocytic cells is impaired, the removal of debris may take much longer. In these cases regeneration is impaired, and muscles may even enter a second phase of degeneration when fibres that survived the initial insult may succumb to the ischaemia caused by the disruption of the circulation.

Muscle regeneration. Even before muscle fibre breakdown is complete, satellite cells within the basal lamina sheath begin to divide, producing the myogenic progeny that will form new muscle fibres. In favourable experimental circumstances in mammals the original population of muscle fibre nuclei can be replaced within a few days, the new cells promptly fusing to form myotubes within the basal lamina tube. If the nerve supply remains intact, these myotubes become innervated within a day or two. After 2–3 weeks, they have grown to the size of normal muscle fibres (Harris et al 1975).

The rapid and complete regeneration of damaged muscle cells depends on several factors. If an insufficient number of satellite cells survives damage, regeneration is not possible. If the basal lamina tubes are disrupted, as in experiments in which the muscle is 'minced' or in severe trauma, the cellular events leading to new muscle fibre formation are spatially disorganised, and regeneration is much less effective. If reinnervation is prevented or delayed, the regenerated muscle fibres fail to grow after their initial formation but may survive until effective nerve regeneration can occur. The restoration may not be complete, however, because a regenerating muscle that is ischaemic during the early stages of regeneration may become extremely fibrotic.

Regeneration of the neuromuscular junction

When muscle fibres regenerate within the original basal lamina sheath, the specialised features of the neuromuscular junction are rapidly reconstructed. Although the formation of mature postsynaptic specialisations takes several weeks during normal development, it can occur within a few days during muscle regeneration in adult mammals. This is true even if damage to the nerve results in the absence of the nerve terminal during the regeneration process (Jirmanová & Thesleff 1972, Slater & Allen 1985).

The basal lamina plays a key role in promoting

rapid and effective restoration of functional inner-vation. The involvement of synaptic basal lamina in the recognition and reinnervation of original synaptic sites by regenerating axons has already been mentioned. Surviving basal lamina also promotes the formation of synaptic folds and the accumulation of AChR at original synaptic sites on regenerating muscle fibres, even if the nerve supply and Schwann cells have been destroyed (Burden et al 1979, McMahan & Slater 1984). Newer studies show that in addition to its ability to organise the postsynaptic membrane, the synaptic basal lamina can also influence the expression of AChR genes in the underlying myonuclei (Brenner et al 1992, Jo & Burden 1992).

The molecular basis of the ability of the synaptic basal lamina to organise the postsynaptic region of the muscle fibre is becoming increasingly well understood. Of key importance is a protein called agrin, first identified as a component of the extracellular matrix, which is able to cause the aggregation of acetylcholine receptors in non-innervated muscle cells. Agrin is synthesised by motor neurones and then transported to the periphery where it is released from the presynaptic terminal and incorporated into the basal lamina, tagging it as 'synaptic' (McMahan & Wallace 1989). Whether agrin mediates the effect of synaptic basal lamina on the expression of synapse-specific genes is not yet known. Although originally sought as a factor that could explain the success of the reconstruction of the postsynaptic region after muscle damage, it now seems likely that it plays a crucial role in the events of synapto-genesis (McMahan 1990).

Changes in muscle innervation in old age

There is strong evidence that the number of motor units declines in old age (Campbell et al 1973, McComas et al 1973) (Fig. 1.14). This loss of motor units results from the death of motor neurones, for reasons that are not understood. In contrast to muscle, there is no mechanism for the replacement of neurones. The sporadic death of motor neurones leaves muscle fibres denervated and evokes sprouting of the surviving motor neurones similar to that already discussed in the context of partial denervation.

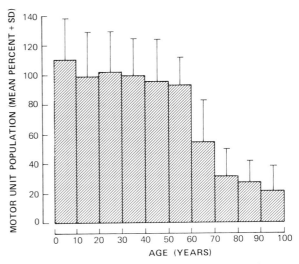

Fig. 1.14   Loss of motor units with age in humans. The estimated number of motor units in various muscles in humans at different ages, relative to that at 20–30 (from McComas et al 1973)

Initially, the surviving neurones take over the denervated fibres. The motor units increase in size and the transformation of the properties of the reinnervated fibres leads to increasing fibre type grouping. As the number of surviving motor neurones falls, they become unable to reinnervate all the denervated muscle fibres. As a result, both the delicacy of control and, eventually, overall strength, are lost. Ultimately, some muscles may become completely denervated.

CONCLUSION

We are able to use our muscles to create an almost infinite variety of movements, differing in speed, force and direction. Because motor commands from the central nervous system can only take the form of action potentials in the motor axons, this variety depends critically on the patterns of connections of those axons with the muscle fibres. While each motor neurone controls a set of muscle fibres with very similar properties, motor units vary from those specialised for relatively slow, maintained contractions of limited force to those specialised for fast but brief and powerful efforts. Because the speed of action potential propagation in the motor axon and the contractile properties of the muscle fibres in each motor unit are closely related to the excitability of the motor neurone, the set of motor units innervating a muscle has an inherent functional order which ensures that increasing demand is met with smoothly graded contractions over a wide range of speeds and forces.

The matching of properties between the motor neurone, its associated Schwann cells, and the muscle fibres it innervates arises during development as a result of a complex set of poorly understood cell–cell interactions.   One component of these interactions is the pattern of activity of the motor unit itself, which has an important influence on the development of the specific properties of the muscle fibres in the mature motor unit. The survival into adulthood of the sensitivity of muscle fibres to the way they are used endows the mature motor unit with the ability to adapt its properties to meet changing demands.

Following damage to the motor unit, many cellular activities which play an important role in development are reactivated. These allow the regeneration of damaged motor axons and muscle fibres, and reinnervation of muscle fibres denervated as a consequence of motor neurone death. While the extent of functional recovery after certain forms of damage can be impressive, there are very definite limits; motor neurones themselves cannot be replaced and there appears to be no peripheral mechanism to correct the reinnervation of inappropriate muscles by the wayward growth of regenerating axons.

The many interacting relationships between the cells within individual motor units and between the motor units of individual muscles provide an important background against which the details of any disorder of voluntary muscle may be viewed.

REFERENCES

Aidley D J 1989 The physiology of excitable cells, 3rd edn. Cambridge University Press, Cambridge

Alberts B, Bray D, Lewis J, Raff M, Roberts K, Watson J D 1989 Molecular biology of the cell, 2nd edn. Garland, New York

Angelides K J 1986 Fluorescently labelled Na^+ channels are localized and immobilized to synapses of innervated muscle fibres. Nature 321: 63

Appelberg B, Emonet-Dénand F 1967 Motor units of the first superficial lumbrical muscle of the cat. Journal of Neurophysiology 30: 154

Asbury A K, Johnson P C 1978 Pathology of peripheral nerve. W B Saunders, Philadelphia

Bennett M R 1983 Development of neuromuscular synapses. Physiological Reviews 63: 915

Bennett M R, Pettigrew A G 1974 The formation of synapses in striated muscle during development. Journal of Physiology (London) 241: 515

Bewick G S, Nicholson L V B, Young C, O'Donnell E, Slater C R 1992 Different distributions of dystrophin and related proteins at nerve–muscle junctions. NeuroReport 3: 857

Bloom W, Fawcett D W 1968 A textbook of histology, 9th edn. W B Saunders, Philadelphia

Boyd I A, Davey M R 1968 Composition of peripheral nerves. Livingstone, Edinburgh

Bradley W G 1974 Disorders of peripheral nerves. Blackwell Scientific Publications, Oxford

Brenner H R, Herczeg A, Slater C R 1992 Synapse-specific expression of acetylcholine receptor genes and their products at original synaptic sites in rat soleus muscle fibres regenerating in the absence of innervation. Development 116: 41

Brown M C, Hopkins W G, Keynes R J 1991 Essentials of neural development, 2nd edn. Cambridge University Press, Cambridge

Buller A J 1972 The neural control of some characteristics of skeletal muscle. In: Downman C B B (ed) Modern trends in physiology, 1. Butterworth, London, pp 72–85

Buller A J, Eccles J C, Eccles R M 1960a Differentiation of fast and slow muscles in the cat hind limb. Journal of Physiology (London) 15: 399

Buller A J, Eccles J C, Eccles R M 1960b Interaction between motoneurones and muscles in respect of their characteristic speeds of their responses. Journal of Physiology (London) 150: 417

Buller A J, Lewis D M 1963 Factors affecting the differentiation of mammalian fast and slow muscle fibres. In: Gutmann E, Hnik P (eds) The effect of use and disuse on neuromuscular functions. Publishing House of the Czechoslovak Academy of Sciences, Prague, pp 149–159

Burden S J, Sargent P B, McMahan U J 1979 Acetylcholine receptors in regenerating muscle accumulate at original synaptic sites in the absence of the nerve. Journal of Cell Biology 82: 412

Burke R E 1967 Motor unit types of the cat triceps surae muscle. Journal of Physiology (London) 193: 141

Burke R E, Jankowska E, tenBruggencate G 1970 A comparison of peripheral and rubrospinal input to slow and fast twitch motor units of triceps surae. Journal of Physiology (London) 207: 709

Burke R E, Levine D N, Tsairis P, Zujac F E 1973 Physiological types and histochemical profiles in motor units of the cat gastrocnemius. Journal of Physiology (London) 234: 723

Butler-Browne G S, Herlicoviez D, Whalen R G 1984 Effects of hypothyroidism on myosin isozyme transitions in developing rat muscle. FEBS Letters 166: 71

Campbell M J, McComas A J, Petito F 1973 Physiological changes in ageing muscles. Journal of Neurology, Neurosurgery and Psychiatry 36: 174

Close R 1964 Dynamic properties of fast and slow skeletal

muscles of the rat during development. Journal of Physiology (London) 173: 74

Close R 1972 Dynamic properties of mammalian skeletal muscles. Physiological Reviews 52: 129

Cooper S 1966 Muscle spindles and motor units. In: Andrew B L (ed) Control and innervation of skeletal muscle. University of St Andrews, St Andrews, pp 9–16

Couteaux R 1960 Motor end plate structure. In: Bourne G H (ed) Structure and function of muscle, vol I. Academic, New York, p 337

Dawson M J, Gadian D G, Wilkie D R 1978 Muscle fatigue investigated by phosphorus nuclear magnetic resonance. Nature (London) 247: 861

DeLuca C J 1985 Control properties of motor units. Journal of Experimental Biology 115: 125

Denier van der Gon J J, Gielen C C A M, ter Harr Romeny B M 1982 Changes in recruitment threshold of motor units in the human biceps muscle. Journal of Physiology (London) 328: 28P

Dhoot G K, Perry S V 1981 Effect of thyroidectomy on the distribution of the fast and slow forms of troponin I in rat soleus muscle. FEBS Letters 133: 225

Diamond J, Miledi R 1962 A study of foetal and new-born rat muscle fibres. Journal of Physiology (London) 162: 393

Eccles J C, Eccles R M, Lundberg A 1958 The action potentials of the alpha motoneurones supplying fast and slow muscles. Journal of Physiology (London) 142: 275

Edström L, Kugelberg E 1968 Histochemical composition, distribution of fibres and fatigability of single motor units. Journal of Neurology, Neurosurgery and Psychiatry 31: 424

Edwards R H T, Hill D K, Jones D A, Merton P A 1977 Fatigue of long duration in human skeletal muscle after exercise. Journal of Physiology (London) 272: 769

Edwards R H T, Mills K R, Newham D J 1981 Greater low frequency fatigue produced by eccentric than concentric muscle contractions. Journal of Physiology (London) 317: 17P

Eisenberg B R, Kuda A M 1976 Discrimination between fiber populations in mammalian skeletal muscle using ultrastructural parameters. Journal of Ultrastructural Research 54: 76

Elmqvist D, Quastel D M J 1965 A quantitative study of end-plate potentials in isolated human muscle. Journal of Physiology (London) 178: 505

Fitch S, McComas A 1985 Influence of human muscle length on fatigue. Journal of Physiology (London) 272: 769

Flucher B E, Daniels M P 1989 Distribution of Na^+ channels and ankyrin in neuromuscular junctions is complementary to that of acetylcholine receptors and the 43 kd protein. Neuron 3: 163

Freund H J 1983 Motor unit and muscle activity in voluntary motor control. Physiological Reviews 63: 387

Froehner S C 1986 The role of the postsynaptic cytoskeleton in AChR organization. Trends in Neurosciences 9: 37

Gasser H S, Grundfest H L 1939 Axon diameters in relation to the spike dimensions and the conduction velocity in mammalian A fibres. American Journal of Physiology 127: 393

Geren B 1954 The formation from the Schwann cell surface of myelin in the peripheral nerves of chick embryos. Experimental Cell Research 7: 558

Gold H K, Spann J F, Braunwald E 1970 The effect of alterations in the thyroid state on the intrinsic contractile properties of isolated rat skeletal muscle. Journal of Clinical Investigation 49: 849

Goldman D, Brenner H R, Heinemann S 1988 Acetylcholine receptor α-, β-, γ-, and δ-subunit mRNA-levels are regulated by muscle activity. Neuron 1: 329

Gordon A M, Huxley A F, Julian F J 1966 The variation in isometric tension with sarcomere length in vertebrate muscle fibres. Journal of Physiology (London) 184: 170

Grafstein B, Forman D S 1980 Intracellular transport in neurons. Physiological Reviews 60: 1167

Gutmann E, Young J Z 1944 Reinnervation of muscle after various periods of atrophy. Journal of Anatomy 78: 15

Gutmann E, Schiaffino S, Hanzliková V 1971 Mechanism of compensatory hypertrophy in the skeletal muscle of the rat. Experimental Neurology 31: 451

Harris A J 1981 Embryonic growth and innervation of rat skeletal muscles. I. Neural regulation of muscle fibre numbers. Philosophical Transactions of the Royal Society London (Biology) 293: 257

Harris J B, Wilson P 1971 Mechanical properties of dystrophic mouse muscle. Journal of Neurology, Neurosurgery, and Psychiatry 34: 512

Harris J B, Johnson M A, Karlsson E 1975 Pathological responses of rat skeletal muscle to a single subcutaneous injection of a toxin isolated from the venom of the Australian tiger snake, Notechis scutatus scutatus. Clinical and Experimental Pharmacology and Physiology 2: 383

Henneman E, Olsen C B 1965 Relations between structure and function in the design of skeletal muscles. Journal of Neurophysiology 28: 581

Henneman E, Somjen G, Carpenter D O 1965 Functional significance of cell size in spinal motoneurons. Journal of Neurophysiology 28: 560

Hennig R, Lømo T 1985 Firing patterns of motor units in normal rats. Nature (London) 314: 164

Hill A V 1949 The abrupt transition from rest to activity in muscle. Proceedings of the Royal Society London (Biology) 136: 399

Hille B 1992 Ionic channels in excitable membranes, 2nd edn. Sinauer Associates, Sunderland, MA

Hilton S M, Jeffries M G, Vrbová G 1970 Functional specialisation of the vascular bed of the soleus muscle. Journal of Physiology (London) 206: 543

Huang C-F, Tong J, Schmidt J 1992 Protein kinase C couples membrane excitation to acetylcholine receptor gene inactivation in chick skeletal muscle. Neuron 9: 671

Hudgson P, Hall R 1982 Endocrine myopathies. In: Walton J N, Mastaglia F L (eds) Skeletal muscle pathology. Churchill Livingstone, Edinburgh, pp 393–498

Hunter D D, Shah V, Merlie J B, Sanes J R 1989 A laminin-like adhesive protein concentrated in the synaptic cleft of the neuromuscular junction. Nature (London) 338: 229

Hursh J B 1939 Conduction velocity and diameter of nerve fibers. American Journal of Physiology 127: 131

Ingjer F 1979 Effects of endurance training on muscle fibre ATP-ase activity, capillary supply and mitochondrial content in man. Journal of Physiology (London) 294: 419

Jacobson M 1978 Developmental neurobiology. Plenum, New York

Jansen J K S, Fladby T 1990 The peripheral reorganization of the innervation of skeletal muscle in mammals. Progress in Neurobiology 34: 39

Jaros E, Johnstone D 1983 Effect of denervation upon muscle fibre number in normal and dystrophic (dy/dy) mice. Journal of Physiology (London) 343: 104P

Jirmanová I, Thesleff S 1972 Ultrastructural study of experimental degeneration and regeneration in the adult rat. Zeitung fur Zellforschung und Mikroskopische Anatomie 131: 77

Jo S A, Burden S J 1992 Synaptic basal lamina contains a signal for synapse-specific transcription. Development 115: 673

Johnson M A, Mastaglia F L, Montgomery A G, Pope B, Weeds A G 1980 Changes in myosin light chains in the rat soleus after thyroidectomy. FEBS Letters 110: 230

Kandel E R, Schwartz J H, Jessell T M 1991 Principles of neuroscience, 3nd edn. Elsevier Science Publishing, New York

Kernell D 1966 Input resistance, electrical excitability and size of ventral horn cells in cat spinal cord. Science, New York 152: 1637

Kiehn O 1991 Plateau potentials and active integration in the 'final common pathway' for motor behaviour. Trends in Neurosciences 14: 68

Korneliussen H, Waerhaug O 1973 Three morphological types of motor nerve terminals in the rat diaphragm, and their possible innervation of different muscle fibre types. Zeitschrift für Anatomie und Entwicklungsbiologie 140: 73

Kuno M, Miyata Y, Munos-Martinez E J 1974 Properties of fast and slow motoneurones following motor reinnervation. Journal of Physiology (London) 242: 273

Lance-Jones C, Landmesser L 1980 Motoneurone projection patterns in the chick hind limb following early partial reversals of the spinal cord. Journal of Physiology (London) 302: 581

Larsson L, Ansverd T 1985 Effects of long-term physical training and detraining on enzyme histochemical and functional skeletal muscle characteristics in man. Muscle and Nerve 8: 714

Laughlin M H, Armstrong R B 1982 Muscular blood flow distribution patterns as a function of running speed in rats. American Journal of Physiology 243: 296

Lømo T 1976 The role of activity in the control of membrane and contractile properties of skeletal muscle. In: Thesleff S (ed) Motor innervation of muscle. Academic, London pp 289–321

Lowrie M B, Vrbová G 1992 Dependence of postnatal motoneurones on their targets: review and hypothesis. Trends in Neurosciences 15: 80

Lunn E R, Perry V H, Brown M C, Rosen H, Gordon S 1989 Absence of Wallerian degeneration does not hinder regeneration in peripheral nerve. European Journal of Neuroscience 1: 27

McComas A J, Upton A R M, Sica R E P 1973 Motoneurone disease and ageing. Lancet ii: 1477

McMahan U J 1990 The agrin hypothesis. Cold Spring Harbor Symposia on Quantitative Biology 50: 407

McMahan U J, Sanes J R, Marshall L M 1978 Cholinesterase is associated with the basal lamina at the neuromuscular junction. Nature (London) 271: 172

McMahan U J, Slater C R 1984 Influence of basal lamina on the accumulation of acetylcholine receptors at synaptic sites in regenerating muscle. Journal of Cell Biology 98: 1453

McMahan U J, Wallace B 1989 The agrin hypothesis. Developmental Neuroscience 11: 227

Massoulié J, Bon S 1982 The molecular forms of cholinesterase and acetylcholinesterase in vertebrates. Annual Reviews of Neuroscience 5: 57

Miledi R, Slater C R 1970 On the degeneration of rat neuromuscular junctions after nerve section. Journal of Physiology 207: 507

Miller J B, Stockdale F E 1987 What muscle cells know that nerves don't tell them. Trends in Neurosciences 10: 325

Milner-Brown H S, Stein R B, Yemm R 1973 The orderly recruitment of human motor units during voluntary isometric contractions. Journal of Physiology (London) 230: 359

Nastuk M A, Fallon J R 1993 Agrin and the molecular choreography of synapse formation. Trends in Neurosciences 16: 72

Nemeth P M, Pette D, Vrbová G 1981 Comparison of enzyme activities among single muscle fibres within defined motor units. Journal of Physiology (London) 311: 489

Nicholls J G, Martin A R, Wallace B G 1992 From neuron to brain, 3nd edn. Sinauer Associates, Sunderland, MA

Nwoye L, Mommaerts W F H M 1981 The effects of thyroid status on some properties of rat fast-twitch muscle. Journal of Muscle Research and Cell Motility 2: 307

Ogata T, Yamasaki Y 1985 The three-dimensional structure of motor endplates in different fiber types of rat intercostal muscle. Cell and Tissue Research 241: 465

Ontell M 1979 The source of 'new' muscle fibers in neonatal muscle. In: Mauro A (ed) Muscle regeneration. Raven, New York, pp 137–146

Oppenheim R W 1991 Cell death during development of the nervous system. Annual Review of Neuroscience 14: 453

Perry V H, Brown M C, Lunn E R, Tree P, Gordon S 1990 Evidence that very slow Wallerian degeneration in C57BL/Ola mice is an intrinsic property of the peripheral nerve. European Journal of Neurosciences 2: 802

Pette D, Vrbová G 1985 Neural control of phenotypic expression in mammalian muscle fibres. Muscle and Nerve 8: 676

Purves D, Lichtman J W 1985 Principles of neural development. Sinauer Associates, Sunderland, MA

Ranvier L 1874 De quelques faits relatifs á l'histologie et á la physiologie des muscles striés. Archives Physiologie Normale et Pathologique 6: 1

Romanes G J 1940 Cell columns in the spinal cord of the human foetus of fourteen weeks. Journal of Anatomy (London) 75: 145

Romanes G J 1941 The development and significance of the cell columns in the ventral horn of the cervical and upper thoracic spinal cord of the rabbit. Journal of Anatomy (London) 76: 112

Ronnevi L-O, Conradi S 1974 Ultrastructural evidence for spontaneous elimination of synaptic terminals on spinal motorneurones in the kitten. Brain Research 80: 335

Rushton W A H 1951 A theory of the effects of fibre size in medullated nerve. Journal of Physiology (London) 115: 101

Rutishauser U, Landmesser L 1991 Polysialic acid on the surface of axons regulates patterns of normal and activity-dependent innervation. Trends in Neurosciences 14: 528

Sanes J R 1987 Cell lineage and the origin of muscle fibre types. Trends in Neurosciences 10: 219

Sanes J R 1989 Extracellular matrix molecules that influence neural development. Annual Review of Neuroscience 12: 491

Sanes J R, Marshall L M, McMahan U J 1978 Reinnervation of muscle fiber basal lamina after removal of myofibers. Journal of Cell Biology 78: 176

Sanes J R, Schachner M, Couvalt J 1986 Expression of several adhesive molecules (N-CAM, L1, J1, NILE, uvomorulin, laminin, fibronectin, and a heparan sulfate proteoglycan) in embryonic, adult and denervated adult skeletal muscle. Journal of Cell Biology 102: 420

Scheutze S M, Role L W 1987 Developmental regulation of

nicotinic acetylcholine receptors. Annual Review of Neuroscience 10: 403

Sharrard W J W 1955 The distribution of the permanent paralysis in the lower limb in poliomyelitis. Journal of Bone and Joint Surgery 38B: 540

Sica R E P, McComas A J 1971 Fast and slow twitch units in a human muscle. Journal of Neurology, Neurosurgery, and Psychiatry 34: 113

Simon A M, Hoppe P, Burden S J 1992 Spatial restriction of AChR gene expression to subsynaptic nuclei. Development 114: 545

Slater C R 1982 Post-natal maturation of nerve–muscle junctions in hindlimb muscle of the mouse. Developmental Biology 94: 11

Slater C R, Allen E G 1985 Acetylcholine receptor distribution on regenerating mammalian muscle fibres at sites of mature and developing nerve–muscle junctions. Journal de Physiologie (Paris) 80: 238

Slater C R, Lyons P R, Walls T J, Fawcett P R W, Young C 1992 Structure and function of neuromuscular junctions in man: a motor point biopsy study in two patient groups. Brain 115: 451

Thoenen H 1991 The changing scene of neurotrophic factors. Trends in Neurosciences 14: 165

Thompson W 1986 Changes in the innervation of mammalian skeletal muscle fibers during postnatal development. Trends in Neurosciences 9: 25

Vallee R B, Bloom G S 1991 Mechanisms of fast and slow axonal transport. Annual Review of Neuroscience 14: 59

Vizoso A D 1950 The relationship between internodal length and growth in human nerves. Journal of Anatomy (London) 82: 110

Waller A V 1850 Experiments on the section of the glossopharyngeal and hypoglossal nerves of the frog, and observations of the alterations produced thereby in the structure of their primitive fibres. Philosophical Transactions of the Royal Society 140: 423

Waxman S G, Ritchie J M 1985 Organization of ion channels in the myelinated nerve fiber. Science, New York 228: 1502

Weintraub H, Davis R, Tapscott S et al 1991 The MyoD gene family: nodal point during specification of the muscle cell lineage. Science 25: 761

Whalen R G, Toutant M, Butler-Browne G S, Watkins S C 1985 Hereditary pituitary dwarfism in mice affects skeletal and cardiac myosin isozyme transitions differentially. Journal of Cell Biology 101: 603

Wilson J, Walton J N 1959 Some muscular manifestations of hypothyroidism. Journal of Neurology, Neurosurgery and Psychiatry 22: 320

Wuerker R B, McPhedran A M, Henneman E 1965 Properties of motor units in a heterogeneous pale muscle (m. gastrocnemius) of the cat. Journal of Neurophysiology 28: 85

Wyman R J, Waldron I, Wachtel G M 1974 Lack of fixed order of recruitment in cat motoneuron pools. Experimental Brain Research 20: 101

2. Cell biology of muscle

F. S. Walsh   P. Doherty

INTRODUCTION

For many years neuromuscular diseases appeared to be intractable problems and thus it was felt that answers about pathogenesis would come about from analyses of diseased muscle or body fluids. While studies on the cell biology of muscle were carried out they were not thought to be directly related to the problem although interesting in their own right from a cellular and biochemical standpoint. Much effort was devoted to attempting to find molecular 'defects' in cell cultures of muscle cells from a diverse set of diseases that may be specific to these conditions. Two developments in recent years have completely changed our thinking about muscle cell biology. The first of these is the major advances in knowledge that have come about regarding the origins, developmental potential, plasticity, regulation of gene expression and fusion of myoblasts. The second is that through the use of reverse genetics the molecular pathology of one major neuromuscular disease, namely Duchenne muscular dystrophy, has been elucidated and the cause of the disease is now known to be due to mutations in the gene for the protein dystrophin. The coming together of these two sets of data has given impetus to the development of strategies such as myoblast transfer and gene transfer that utilise the results gleaned from basic science approaches to attempt to design rational therapies for Duchenne muscular dystrophy. In this chapter we review aspects of the cell biology of muscle that relate to the current interest in therapeutic approaches.

MYOBLASTS ORIGINATE FROM THE MESODERM

Multinucleate skeletal muscle fibres arise during early development by a highly specific process of cell fusion of precursor cells called myoblasts. Figure 2.1 shows in outline some of the events that probably occur at the cellular level. A multi-potential stem cell in the mesoderm gives rise to cells that subsequently become determined or committed to the myogenic lineage. These cells, now called myoblasts, undergo a programme of differentiation that ultimately leads to the forma-tion of myotubes. Further differentiation of these cells, particularly under the influence of nerve, leads to the appearance of mature myofibres. The somite is the main area of the embryo that gives rise to skeletal muscle of the body while the precordial plate gives origin to some of the head muscles. Detailed studies of somite formation have been carried out in the chick embryo (Lash & Ostrovsky 1986), but similar processes probably occur in mammals (Buckingham 1992). It is possible to observe somites in the mouse embryo from about day 8 following a process of segmenta-tion of the paraxial mesoderm. Figure 2.2 shows some of the morphological events associated with somite formation. The nascent somite contains an epithelial wall structure with core cells at the centre. This structure progresses rapidly to form the dermamyotome which differentiates to form the skin and skeletal muscle while the sclerotome

becomes the skeleton. The dermamyotome segre-gates into the dermatome and myotome following cell migration of precursor cells. The myotome results from the migration of cells from the dorso-medial edge of the dermamyotome. The limb premuscle masses arise from migration from the ventrolateral somite edge. Recent studies using in situ hybridisation have provided the molecular correlates of the formation of the myotomes (reviewed in Buckingham 1992). Some of the earliest markers of the somites and myotomes are cardiac actin and the myogenic regulatory factors (see later) myf-5 and myogenin (Sassoon et al 1989, Bober et al 1991, Hinterberger et al 1991, Ott et al 1991, Cusella-de Angelis et al 1992). Of these, myf-5 appears to be the earliest marker of the muscle lineage and as such it may play a role in commitment of cells to this lineage. This is because the Myf-5 transcript is found in the dor-somedial edge of the somite before the myotome is formed (Ott et al 1991).

DIVERSITY OF MYOBLASTS

Adult muscle fibres are extremely heterogeneous and can be placed in a number of 'fibre types'. These are characterised by both physiological and biochemical criteria, such as expression of unique patterns of enzymes or contractile protein isoforms. In general the nomenclature has reflected muscle function. Fast muscle fibres (Type II) are involved in rapid but brief movements, while slow (Type I)

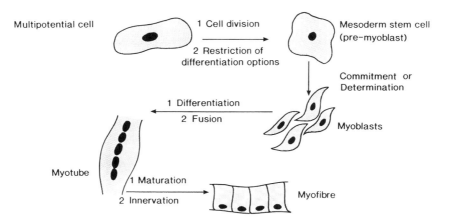

Fig. 2.1   Diagram showing some of the key regulatory events that occur at the cellular level during the development of skeletal muscle.

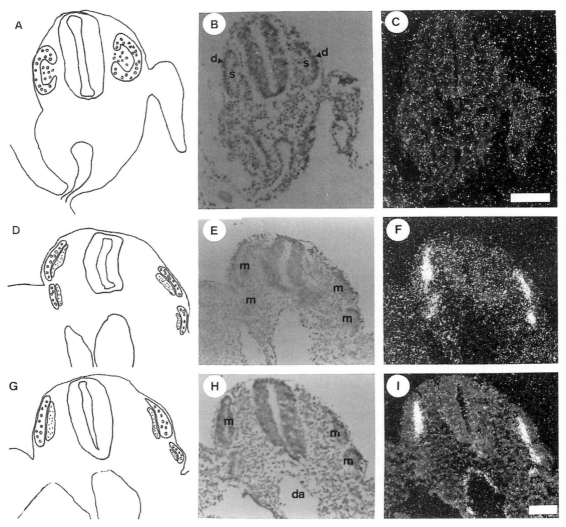

Fig. 2.2 Myotome formation in the mouse embryo can be monitored by the expression of specific gene transcripts. A–I Transverse sections of mouse embryos which have been hybridized with several cRNA probes. **A, D** and **G** represent schematic drawings of the brightfield micrographs in **B, E** and **H**, respectively. The diagrams show the locations of the somites in relation to the neural tube. Hybridization of probes to the sections is indicated in the darkfield micrographs in **C, F** and **I** by the presence of silver grains. A–C illustrate the early stages of somite development. The somites on either side of the neural tube have started to differentiate into sclerotomes (s) and dermamytomes (d). The myotome has not yet formed as the section was hybridized with a muscle cadherin probe (Moore & Walsh, 1993). Several myotomes (m) have formed and stain specifically with this probe (F). The myotomal specificity of the muscle cadherin probe is confirmed in G, H and I. Here a section adjacent to that in E was hybridized with the cardiac α-actin probe. The staining of the myotomes (m) is nearly identical in F and I. Cells lining the dorsal aorta (da) were also stained with the cardiac α-actin probe (scale bars = 100 μm).

fibres are involved in more prolonged movements. The more popular typing schemes have used the ATPase activity of myosin heavy chain (MHC) isoforms or specific antibodies to these isoforms of MHC. These studies have indicated that in partic-

ular the Type II fibres can be subdivided into a large number of subgroups.

The activity of motor neurones can clearly alter the contraction rate and fibre type of muscle fibres. A large body of physiological experiments have confirmed this observation using cross-innervation or chronic stimulation paradigms. The implication has therefore been that all myoblasts and myofibres are multipotential and that the nerve determines fibre type solely via its activity pattern. The alternative hypothesis, that there are a number of myoblast populations that are predetermined to form the different types of muscle fibres, has not until recently received a large amount of experimental support. A number of experiments could not easily be reconciled with the innervation model. The first was that there is a degree of fibre type development in animals that have had part of the neural tube removed (Butler et al 1982). Paralysis by curare was found to have a similar effect (McLennan 1983, Crow & Stockdale 1986a). It therefore seems that some of the early events of myofibre differentiation are nerve-independent while there is no doubt that later stages require a neural influence (Sanes 1987). In broad outline these two phases may correspond to the two phases of myogenesis that have been observed, namely primary and secondary myotube formation (reviewed in Miller 1991). The first burst of myotube formation in the embryo leads to the formation of primary myotubes at about E13–14 in the mouse embryo and E3–8 in the chick embryo. At slightly later stages (E16–17 in the mouse and E8–14 in the chicken) new fibres called secondary myotubes form in the same basal lamina sheath parallel to the primary fibres. These form all around the primary myotubes, are electrically coupled and in intimate contact with the primary myotubes. However, as development proceeds, the two types of fibre become indistinguishable and form their own basal lamina. A major question has therefore been whether the diversity of fibre types might reflect intrinsic diversity in myoblast populations. Recent studies by Stockdale & colleagues in the avian system have provided an answer to this question (Crow & Stockdale 1986b, Miller & Stockdale 1986, Stockdale et al 1988, Stockdale 1989). Using single cell myoblast cloning methods in conjunction with MHC fibre-specific antibodies, it has been possible to ask questions about the origin of fibre types in a system where all the myotubes result from the fusion of myoblasts of a single type. The results showed that for primary (innervation-independent) myotube formation about 70% of the myoblast clones fused to form fast MHC-containing myotubes, while about 30% expressed both fast and slow MHC characteristics. A small percentage in the order of 1–2% expressed slow MHC. These antigenic phenotypes were stable and heritable and led to the suggestion that there are three types of myoblast in embryonic chick muscle, namely fast, fast-slow and slow. These three populations are intrinsically different from one another in that they are committed to form myotubes of one type only. At later stages of development corresponding to innervation-dependent or secondary or fetal myogenesis a different picture emerges. These myotubes are morphologically distinct from the embryonic (primary) myotubes, being much larger with over 100 nuclei compared to under 10 nuclei for the embryonic myotubes. In addition, they require media conditioned by muscle cells to grow into colonies while embryonic myoblasts do not. These characteristics are similar to the 'late' myoblasts described by White & Hauschka (1971). In terms of fibre types fetal myoblasts produce fast myotubes only. However this phenotype can be modulated in culture and often fast MHC-expressing myotubes start to express slow MHC. The third stage of myogenesis occurs in the adult when a population of myoblasts called satellite cells can be activated to repair muscle damage. Satellite cells are in contact with muscle fibres and sit beneath the basal lamina (Mauro 1961). Culture of satellite cells at clonal density results in the formation of fast fibres and a second population with fast/slow characteristics. These studies on avian muscle (summarised in Fig. 2.3) have shown clearly that different types of myoblast exist but a number of key experiments and predictions still remain to be carried out. We do not know if the behaviour of myoblasts in cell culture truly reflects what goes on in vivo. It is possible that fetal myoblasts will not fuse with embryonic myoblasts while satellite cells might fuse with both types of myofibre. Alternatively it is possible, especially in the case of satellite cells, that they might adopt the phenotype of the pre-existing fibre due to the type of trans-acting transcription factors present in the fibre.

Studies on mammalian muscle are not as far

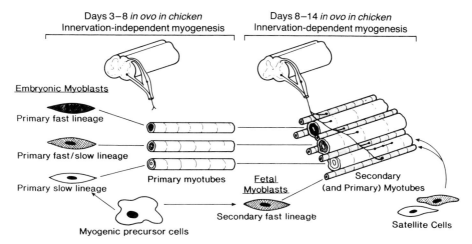

Days 3–8 *in ovo in chicken*
Innervation-independent myogenesis

Days 8–14 *in ovo in chicken*
Innervation-dependent myogenesis

Embryonic Myoblasts

Primary fast lineage

Primary fast/slow lineage

Primary slow lineage

Primary myotubes

Fetal Myoblasts

Secondary (and Primary) Myotubes

Secondary fast lineage

Satellite Cells

Myogenic precursor cells

Fig. 2.3 A model showing how myotubes expressing different fibre types develop. Although based on work in the chicken by Stockdale and colleagues, it is likely that similar events occur in mammals (adapted from Millar & Stockdale 1986).

advanced as those on the avian models, none the less various types of myoblast have been found. A number of different types of myoblast, each with their own culture requirements, have been identified (Cossu & Molinaro 1987, Vivarelli et al 1988) in the mouse. Human myoblasts also appear to be heterogeneous with respect to growth factor and media requirements (Haushka 1974, Webster et al 1988). It appears that in postnatal muscle development in the rat there is no lineage restriction to myoblast fusion. Hughes & Blau (1992) have shown that satellite cells marked via a retroviral vector can fuse with both fast and slow muscle fibres. Thus the MHC expressed by the satellite cell once it has fused into the myofibre is dictated by the fibre type of that fibre. This study pertains only to postnatal muscle development when the fibre types have been laid down. However, it still seems likely that the development of fibre types in the mammalian embryo is due to the presence of distinct lineages. No evidence has been found for selective fusion of embryonic myoblasts, so it possible that the fibre type is dictated by the phenotype of the first myoblasts to fuse. These questions should be resolved when the retroviral marking experiments are extended to embryonic muscle development.

An additional level of complexity in the muscle system is the positional identity of myoblasts. All muscles are not equal and there are clearly differ-

ences in shape, location, fibre types and density of innervation (Miller 1992). A recent study by Donoghue et al (1992) has emphasised the role of positional identity in myofibre development. Transgenic mice carrying a reporter construct consisting of the chloramphenicol acetyltransferase (CAT) gene linked to the myosin light chain (MLC)1 promoter with a MLC1/3 enhancer region show a rostrocaudal gradient of transgene expression (Donoghue et al 1988, 1991a, b, 1992). Analysis of the diaphragm shows the highest level of expression in the caudal region with low transgene expression in the rostral regions. Thus it seems likely that the transgene is sensing positional cues in the different muscles. However the MLC1 mRNA does not exhibit a similar gradient of expression, showing that this gene must be under the control of other regulatory elements. Clonal analysis of myoblasts from regions with different levels of transgene expression shows that this is indeed a heritable property. This depends on the position of the satellite cells rather than any other interactions the myoblasts may be involved in. These studies suggest a more complex scenario than previously shown and may suggest a greater degree of clonal diversity. However it still has to be shown that the myoblasts at different parts of the gradient are indeed functionally different and that this correlates to some important property such as selective innervation of intercostal muscles.

MYOGENIC REGULATORY GENES

The formation, differentiation and maturation of skeletal muscle is associated with the expression of a large number of cell type-specific gene families. Recently a family of proteins called myogenic regulatory factors that are regulators of commitment to the myogenic lineage has been identified (reviewed in Olson 1990, Funk et al 1991). These factors were shown to be capable of converting multipotential fibroblast cells to cells indistinguishable from skeletal muscle myoblasts and these could then go on to fuse. A large body of evidence inferred the existence of myogenic regulatory genes. One such strategy was heterokaryon analysis which is outlined in Figure 2.4 (Blau et al 1985). In these experiments a mouse muscle cell line called C2 was artificially fused either at the myoblast or the myotube stages of differentiation with human non-muscle cells such as fibroblasts using polyethylene glycol. As species-specific antibodies are available to a number of human muscle gene products, these can be used to assess whether the human cells can be reprogrammed (Blau et al 1985). The results have been dramatic and clear. The mouse muscle cell can reprogramme the fibroblast to express components of the myogenic lineage. These involve muscle

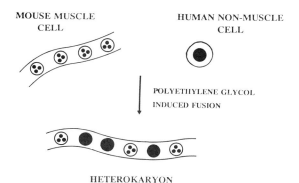

MOUSE MUSCLE CELL

HUMAN NON-MUSCLE CELL

POLYETHYLENE GLYCOL INDUCED FUSION

HETEROKARYON

Fig. 2.4 Heterokaryon analysis has been of great value in defining factors controlling muscle differentiation. The experimental model generally uses multinucleate myotubes of mouse muscle cells to fuse with human non-muscle cells. Activation of human genes by transacting factors in the muscle cells can generally be analysed by methods such as species-specific antibodies. The dye Hoechst 33258 binds to mouse nuclei in a speckled manner while human nuclei appear smoothly stained. This is used to determine the percentage of each type of nucleus in the heterokaryon following polyethylene glycol-induced fusion.

surface proteins such as NCAM, enzymes such as M-creatine kinase and various contractile protein genes (Blau et al 1985). Other studies showed that the cell-line C3H10T $\frac{1}{2}$ could be converted to the myogenic lineage by treatment with 5-azacytidine (Konieczny & Emerson 1984) at a frequency suggesting that a single regulatory gene might be involved. Since then four regulatory genes have been identified which on their own can convert non-muscle cells to the myogenic lineage. These are Myo D, myogenin, myf-5 and myf-6 (MRF-4) (reviewed in Olson 1990, Funk et al 1991, Buckingham 1992). These proteins all locate to the nucleus and have the property of being able to bind to the regulatory region of a number of muscle-specific genes and to activate their expression even in a non-muscle background. The studies on the ability of MyoD to activate a programme of muscle gene activation in non-muscle cells led to the idea that it was the master regulator of muscle gene expression (Weintraub et al 1991). However, support for this idea has not been forthcoming. For instance the identification of the three other structurally related but separate myogenic regulatory genes, all of which can activate the same programme of myogenesis as MyoD, showed that MyoD was not unique. Additionally the transformation of some cells to the myogenic lineage by MyoD is not complete. This is most dramatically seen in non-mesodermal kidney cell lines (Schafer et al 1990) where it is not possible to activate completely the muscle programme by MyoD, yet when these cells are fused with fibroblasts they can activate the muscle programme. Thus positive activators other than MyoD are required for full conversion to the myogenic lineage.

The basic structure of the myogenic regulatory factors is similar and is outlined in Figure 2.5. All four factors share two structural motifs called the helix-loop-helix (HLH) domain and a highly basic region (Weintraub et al 1991). Both regions are required for MyoD-mediated myogenesis following dimerising with other HLH proteins and with themselves. For instance activation of the M-creatine kinase gene is more efficient in the presence of other products of the E2A gene called E12 and E47. A negative regulator of these interactions has been identified in the form of the Id

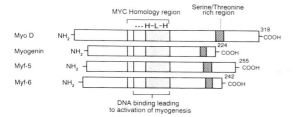

Fig. 2.5 Comparison of the protein structure of the four main myogenic regulatory factors. Although each protein has a different size ranging from 224 to 318 amino acids, they share a number of structural motifs. These include a region of homology to the MYC protein. This region is divided into other regions, two of which show specific motifs such as a basic region and a helix-loop-helix (H-L-H) homology region. The region in MyoD that will activate myogenesis following DNA binding is shown at the bottom of the diagram. Further towards the COOH terminus there is a serine-threonine rich region (adapted from Olson 1990).

protein which binds to E12 and inhibits its interaction with MyoD. In its role as a transcriptional activator MyoD binds to the consensus sequence — CANNTG — which was originally defined in the immunoglobulin gene as an enhancer region. The activation of the muscle genes by myogenic regulatory factors has best been studied in systems where the regulatory region of the gene of interest has been analysed via a reporter gene following addition of the pure myogenic factor. The consensus sequences for the factors other than MyoD have not been described yet in detail. It seems likely that each myogenic regulatory protein has the capacity to regulate a unique subset of muscle proteins. Developmentally there are clearly distinct patterns of expression for the myogenic factors (reviewed in Buckingham 1992), and this is shown schematically in Table 2.1. The earliest detectable transcript is myf 5 which can be found

in the somites at E8. MyoD, in contrast, does not appear until about E10.0. Myf 6 is transiently expressed from E9 to E11. Additionally these factors show different patterns of expression in the somites and limb buds. The ratio of the myogenic factors is also different in adult versus embryonic muscle for myf-6 and MyoD. Thus it is likely that the level of these factors and other positive and negative regulatory factors will give the specific temporal pattern of activation of the different genes that define the myogenic phenotype. A number of questions, however, still remain unanswered with respect to the temporal pattern of expression of muscle genes. For instance, although all four of the above factors are expressed at E10.5, it is not until much later, around E13, that well-studied genes such as M-creatine kinase are expressed at the mRNA level. Thus in vivo the regulation of genes is much more complex than indicated by studies on isolated promoter regions. There are also genes such as NCAM which are expressed in skeletal muscle (see later) and are developmentally regulated but do not have binding sites for MyoD. In contrast, the acetylcholine receptor whose profile of expression overlaps that of NCAM has a well-defined MyoD binding site. It also seems likely that the different myogenic regulatory factors can cross-activate each other. The known myogenic regulatory factors are, however, specific to skeletal muscle and are not expressed by cardiac muscle. Thus the regulatory factors that control cardiac muscle gene expression remain to be determined and in this context attempts to isolate MyoD homologues have failed to date.

A large number of cell structure studies have shown that muscle differentiation is controlled by

Table 2.1 Expression of the myogenic regulatory factors in vivo. Techniques such as in situ hybridisation (see Fig. 2.2) have been extremely valuable in analysing the comparative expression patterns of the myogenic regulatory factors (reviewed in Buckingham 1992). A + indicates that its expression is below detectable levels. There appear to be interesting differences in expression patterns between the myotomes and limb buds with respect to myogenin and MyoD

	Embryonic expression in somites and myotubes							Postnatal expression	Expression in limb buds		
	E8	E8.5	E9	E10.5	E11	E12	E15		E10.5	E11	E12
MyoD	−	−	−	+	+	+	+	−	−	+	+
Myogenin	−	+	+	+	+	+	+	−	−	+	+
Myf5	+	+	+	+	+	+	+	−	+	+	−
Myf6	−	−	+	+	+	−	+	+			

the nature and level of mitogens or growth factors in the culture media. These factors act in the opposite manner to MyoD, but over-expression of MyoD appears to be able to suppress mitogen action (reviewed in Olson 1990). It is possible that MyoD could suppress the activation of the immediate early genes such as c-*fos* which may be the initial targets of growth factor action. MyoD can also be phosphorylated, so this may also be a mechanism for growth factors to inhibit or alter MyoD function. The identification of members of the myogenic regulatory gene family has been an enormous stimulus to research in the area of control of muscle gene expression. However there are likely to be more parts of the regulatory network to be identified and many questions about the origin of muscle cells and the role of neural factors remain unanswered.

MYOBLAST FUSION

Multinucleate myotubes arise by fusion of the cell membranes of myoblasts (reviewed in Wakelam 1988). This is a very rare event in nature and occurs in only a few systems such as fertilization. While myoblasts are mitotic cells, myotubes are postmitotic. The transition from myoblast to myotube is associated with the activation of a large number of muscle-specific genes with the eventual synthesis and formation of the myofibrillar apparatus. The fusion process is complex and multistage and has been subjected to extensive analysis. However a complete molecular picture is not yet available.

Figure 2.6 shows some of the main features of myoblast fusion as observed in tissue culture at the light microscope level. When plated, myoblasts

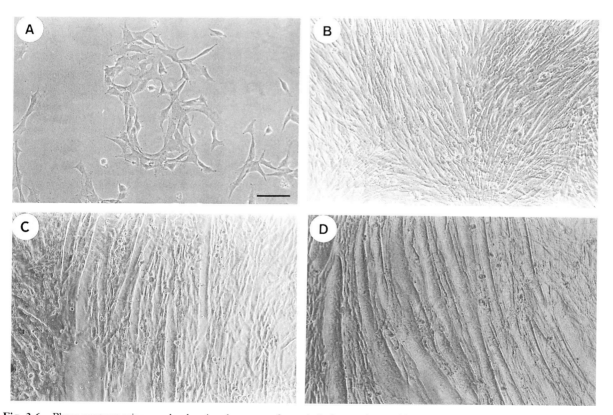

Fig. 2.6   Phase contrast micrographs showing the stages of muscle fusion as observed in tissue culture. When plated (**A**) myoblasts attach to the culture dish which is usually coated with collagen and start to divide. After a number of cell divisions the membranes come in contact with others and the cells start to align (**B**). This is followed by fusion of the myoblasts to form multinucleate myotubes (**C**). These then mature further (**D**) and often exhibit spontaneous contractions.

from some species will adhere strongly to the extra-cellular matrix and rapidly assume a bipolar morphology. Following this the myoblasts align and subsequently fuse at their ends. In the well-studied chick system it is possible to observe fusion after only 30–40 hours and this is complete by 60 hours. However human myoblasts do not have such rapid kinetics of fusion or align in the same manner. One clear requirement for fusion is the presence of extracellular Ca^{2+}. Removal of Ca^{2+} from the medium allows myoblasts to align but blocks their fusion. This characteristic has been used to obtain synchronised populations of myoblasts which fuse rapidly when Ca^{2+} is restored.

The process of fusion has been studied from a morphological standpoint. Areas of cytoplasmic continuity have been identified in cultures while fusing and exhibit weak electrical coupling probably via gap junction-like complexes. However these are clearly the initial stages of the process as they can occur under conditions where overt fusion is blocked, thus emphasising the multicomponent nature of the process. One study (Kalderon & Gilula 1979) has suggested that fusion occurs in protein- and particle-free areas of the cell membrane. Proteins would be cleared in an active process in order to mediate fusion of lipid bilayers. However this type of structure has not been found in all studies on fusion (Funagalli et al 1981). Myoblast fusion appears to have major restrictions in terms of the types of cells that will participate in the process. The prime require-ment is for a cell to be of the muscle lineage. However even within this definition there are differences, because secondary myoblasts do not appear to be able to fuse with primary myofibres. In the muscle system the second major cell type is the fibroblast and these cells never fuse with myoblasts. An exception to this rule are fibroblasts from mice with muscular dysgenesis (Chaudhari et al 1990) which appear to be able to fuse with myoblasts at low frequency. However the true nature of these fibroblasts and their mechanism of fusion is not clear. There does not seem to be any species restriction to myoblast fusion as human myoblasts can fuse with cells from other species including the mouse.

As the fusion of myoblasts is such a dramatic morphological event, and one that can be readily measured, a large number of inhibitor studies have been carried out. A number of agents that alter the differentiation state of myoblasts such as the growth factors FGF and TGFβ block fusion. Agents that alter cell-surface proteins such as the glycosylation inhibitor tunicamycin or the enzyme phosphatidylinositol-specific phospholi-pase C (PIPLC) also modulate fusion, as do agents that alter the sites of membrane contact or the attachment of cytoskeletal proteins (reviewed in Knudsen 1990). Agents that fall into the latter class include cytochalasin B and trifluoroperazine. While all these inhibitor studies have provided insights into the complex nature of fusion, they have not as yet provided a molecular description, although various models have been presented (Wakelam 1988). As the process occurs specifically between two cell membranes it is likely that the specific interactions occurring at the cell surface such as recognition and adhesion are of crucial importance, at least in the very first steps of the process.

MOLECULAR BASIS OF MYOBLAST CELL–CELL INTERACTIONS

Two distinct adhesive systems can be observed on the surface of myoblasts. One of these shows a dependence on Ca^{2+} while the second does not. The Ca^{2+}-dependent system appears to involve a strengthening of adhesion in that initial aggregates of myoblasts can be dispersed by removal of Ca^{2+}, while after a few hours they become resistant. Two studies (Gibralter & Turner 1985, Pizzey et al 1988) have identified a Ca^{2+}-independent compo-nent of adhesion in addition to the Ca^{2+}-depen-dent system. Experimentally one or other of the adhesion systems can be destroyed by trypsin treatment in the absence or presence of Ca^{2+}.

These adhesion-based studies can now be reinterpreted in the light of the fact that a number of the components in the myoblast membrane that mediate these interactions have now been identified. In addition, a number of proteins involved in myoblast–extracellular matrix interac-tions have now been characterised. Table 2.2 provides a list of the better characterised adhesion molecule systems that have been analysed in skeletal muscle.

Table 2.2   A list of some of the main characteristics and patterns of expression of some of the adhesion molecules that have been identified in skeletal muscle. While the data in vitro are easier to compile, the data in vivo are more difficult because of the results of the different techniques (generally immunocytochemistry and in situ hybridisation analyses) used

CAM	Molecular weight (kDa)	Expression pattern	
		In vitro	*In vivo*
NCAM	140 (transmembrane)	Myoblasts	Myotome to E14
NCAM	180 (transmembrane)	ND	Myotome to E13
NCAM	125 (GPI anchored)	Myotubes	Myofibres up to PN8 (by protein analysis)
N-cadherin	124 (transmembrane)	Myoblasts Myotubes	Myotome to E14
M-cadherin	124 (transmembrane)	Myoblasts Myotubes	Myotome to E16
T-cadherin	90 (GPI anchored)	Myoblasts Myotubes	ND
β_1-integrin	130 (transmembrane)	Myoblasts Myotubes	ND
VLA-4 α4 integrin chain	150 and 180	Myoblasts	Primary myotubes
V-CAM-1	95	Myoblasts Myotubes	Secondary myoblasts Satellite cells

The neural cell adhesion molecule

One of the best characterised Ca^{2+}-independent CAMs in muscle is the neural cell adhesion molecule (NCAM) (reviewed in Walsh & Doherty 1991). Although originally identified in neural tissue, a number of studies have reported on the expression of NCAM in skeletal muscle. NCAM is a member of the immunoglobulin (Ig) super-family of recognition molecules and operates via a homophilic (self) binding mechanism. This means that the receptor for NCAM is NCAM itself. Sequence analysis predicts a domain structure. In the extracellular region there are five Ig-like domains of the C2 type starting at the amino terminus. Downstream of these are two fibronectin Type III repeat regions proximal to a membrane-association region. NCAM can be attached to the cell membrane by two mecha-nisms, either a transmembrane spanning region or by a glycosylphosphatidylinositol (GPI) anchor. This is determined by differential alter-native splicing and in muscle this is developmen-tally regulated. The transmembrane form is of 140 kDa and predominates on myoblasts. The GPI-anchored forms are 125 kDa in muscle and these predominate on myotubes and developing myofibres (Moore et al 1987). The switch from myoblast to myotube is associated with an upreg-ulation of expression of the NCAM gene, being about four to five times more NCAM on myotubes than myoblasts. Although in vivo NCAM is present on both primary and secondary myofibres, as development proceeds there is a progressive loss of the protein from mature myofibres. In the rat this occurs postnatally around day 10. After that time the main site of expression of NCAM is at the neuromuscular junction (Moore & Walsh 1986) (see later). There is one additional difference between the NCAM on myotubes as compared to myoblasts; alternative splicing leads to insertion in the extra-cellular region of a small set of four exons which when used together inserts 37 amino acids between the fibronectin Type III repeats. The sequence is used uniquely by muscle and has been named the MSD1 region, although the first exon is shared between brain and muscle. Insertion of the MSD1 region has two conse-quences. The first is to introduce a bend or kink in the protein which may assist homophilic inter-actions, and secondly it endows NCAM with a site of O-linked carbohydrate attachment with the preponderance of serine and threonine residues providing the site of carbohydrate attachment. The function of this region is not clear at present but it may be a spacer region or be involved in CIS interactions between NCAM in the membrane (Peck & Walsh 1993).

To date, NCAM has been shown to have two

clear functions in skeletal muscle. The first of these is the process of myoblast fusion (Knudsen 1990, Knudsen et al 1990, Dickson et al 1991) and the second is in nerve–muscle interactions (see below). Antibody perturbation strategies have implicated NCAM as one of the molecules that is involved in fusion, although the process is clearly multicomponent. Less direct evidence is the observation that PIPLC will inhibit fusion significantly under conditions where GPI-linked NCAM is removed (Knudsen et al 1989). However, the best evidence for a role in cell fusion comes from gene transfer studies. Initial studies showed expression of NCAM cDNAs encoding a human GPI-linked muscle isoform to promote fusion following transfection into the C2-myoblast cell line (Dickson et al 1990). More recent results have shown that other NCAM isoforms can also stimulate fusion and that the 140 kDa transmembrane isoform is more active than the GPI anchored form (Peck & Walsh 1993). The increased activity of the transmembrane isoform may be due to some effects on cell signalling and/or direct interaction with the cytoskeleton.

Another interesting isoform of NCAM that has been detected transiently in muscle is the 180 kDa transmembrane form. This form has a large cytoplasmic domain and was thought to be expressed only by neurones. Some studies have suggested that it may have a restricted distribution in the plasma membrane as a consequence of linkage to the cytoskeleton. An in situ hybridisation study has shown that in myotomes from their formation to about day 13 in the mouse embryo there is specific expression of this isoform (Lyons et al 1992). This may alter the migratory properties of myoblasts at this time.

Expression of Ca^{2+}-dependent CAMs in muscle: the cadherins

The second main adhesive system in muscle is Ca^{2+}-dependent. Recent studies have identified the molecular components responsible for this system. These are a class of proteins known as the cadherins (Takeichi 1991). Originally it was thought that there was only one cadherin in skeletal muscle called N-cadherin (Knudsen 1990). This is the main cadherin found in the brain, although it can be found in skeletal muscle and cardiac muscle also. In terms of structure cadherins (with one exception) are transmembrane proteins of about 124 kDa. The extracellular domain has a number of sites that probably bind Ca^{2+}. One of the sites required for homophilic interactions has been identified about 100 amino acids from the amino terminus and contains the amino acids -His-Ala-Val in most cases (Takeichi 1991). The intracellular domain of the transmembrane cadherins interacts with the actin cytoskeleton via linker proteins called the catenins. A deletion mutagenesis strategy has shown that these interactions are essential for the adhesive functions of cadherins to be operational. Two additional cadherins have been found to be expressed in skeletal muscle: M (muscle) cadherin (Donalies et al 1991, Moore & Walsh 1993) and T (truncated) cadherin (Ranscht & Bronner-Fraser 1991). M-cadherin is unique in that it is expressed exclusively in skeletal muscle with no transcript being found in cardiac muscle or brain (Moore & Walsh 1993). While N-cadherin is expressed in postnatal tissues such as brain, M-cadherin is lost from the embryo as assessed by in situ hybridisation analysis at about E18 in the mouse, having been present on myotubes from about embryonic day 10. Its structure is similar in outline to that of N-cadherin but it does not contain the His-Ala-Val sequence. Whether M-cadherin can cross-bind with N-cadherin is not known. The third cadherin to be found in muscle is T-cadherin. This cadherin is unusual in that it is attached to the cell membrane via a GPI anchor. No other cadherin has been found to date to have this type of membrane association. Although T-cadherin has been found to participate in homophilic interactions it also does not express the His-Ala-Val homophilic binding site.

The relative roles of the three cadherins in muscle have not been elucidated. Most studies have concentrated on N-cadherin where blocking antibodies and synthetic peptides modelled around the sequence His-Ala-Val sequence will partially block myoblast fusion, again emphasising the multicomponent nature of the process (Knudsen 1990).

Extracellular matrix receptors

The development of skeletal muscle is intimately dependent on the interaction of skeletal muscle myofibres with components of the extracellular matrix (ECM). The endomysium of skeletal muscle contains two quite distinct layers. These are the outer reticular lamina that contains fibronectin and collagens I–III and the basal lamina that contains laminin, collagen type IV, entactin and heparin sulphate proteoglycans. Although many studies have reported on the in vivo expression of the ECM proteins, most can also be studied in tissue culture systems where ECM components are assembled on the surface of myoblasts and myotubes (Anderson and Fambrough 1983, Kuhl et al 1986). Interest in the ECM has increased in recent years with the observation that dystrophin is a component of the sub-sarcolemmal cytoskeleton and may be involved in maintaining the structural integrity of the myofibre through interactions with membrane glycoproteins and ECM components (Dickson et al 1992). This has been studied in detail by Campbell and colleagues who have identified a class of membrane glycoproteins that co-purify with dystrophin. These integral membrane proteins are of 50 kDa, 43 kDa, 35 kDa and 25 kDa with two other peripheral proteins of 59 kDa and 156 kDa present also (Ervasti & Campbell 1991). The 150 kDa glycoprotein is believed to be a high affinity laminin-binding protein with features of a cell surface proteoglycan (Ibraghimov-Beskrovnaya et al 1992). There therefore appears to be a transmembrane linkage system that connects dystrophin on the inner face of the sarcolemma with laminin in the basal lamina. Loss of dystrophin presumably leads to a cascade of events that leads finally to muscle fibre destruction.

The integrins are a large family of heterodimers that have been shown to be one class of receptor for ECM proteins (Reichardt & Tomaselli 1991, Hynes 1992). The integrins are composed of one α-chain and a second β-chain. These are non-covalently associated with each other and both chains are transmembrane proteins. A large number of α-chains (at least 14) and β-chains (at least eight) can associate together to give a high degree of structural diversity. In skeletal muscle the β-chain is of the β_1 class and a number of studies have analysed its role in cell attachment and fusion. One antibody that reacts with chick β_1-integrin has been most valuable. The hybridoma-secreting CSAT antibody has been placed in chick embryos and has been shown to cause muscle abnormalities due to defective migration (Jaffredo et al 1988). The cell stratum attachment antibody (CSAT) will also cause detachment of myoblasts from culture dishes (Horwitz et al 1985) and will also block myoblast fusion (Menko & Boettiger 1987) by not allowing myoblasts to leave the cell cycle. The nature of the α-subunits in muscle has been less clear until recently. Although myoblasts synthesise and accumulate fibronectin on their surface, no evidence has been found for the classic $\alpha5\beta_1$-fibronectin receptor in human muscle cultures (G. Dickson, personal communication). Recently an $\alpha7$-integrin chain has been found in rat muscle. This corresponds to the antigen originally identified by a monoclonal antibody called H36 (Song et al 1992). The $\alpha7$-integrin chain is present on myoblasts in tissue culture but is upregulated in myotubes. Its expression pattern in vivo overlaps with that of laminin and this may suggest that $\alpha7$ might also be part of the complex that links dystrophin with laminin. Although likely, this idea has not been formally proven at present.

Interactions between integrins and members of the immunoglobulin superfamily have been found to occur in the immune system (Springer 1990). One such interaction has been proposed between the immunoglobulin superfamily member VCAM-1 and VLA-4 (corresponding to the integrin $\alpha4\beta_1$) in rat muscle. $\alpha4$ has not yet been found on human muscle so it is not clear if its expression in mouse muscle is a species-specific event. Rosen et al (1992) have proposed a model where the integrin VLA-4 ($\alpha4$) and VCAM-1 may partly control the alignment of secondary myoblasts on primary myotubes and the fusion potential of secondary myoblasts. Indirect immunofluorescense staining showed VLA4 ($\alpha4$) to be present on myotubes in vivo with weak expression on primary myoblasts and secondary myotubes. VCAM, in contrast, is present on secondary myoblasts and myotubes. Adult satellite cells express VCAM-1 but not VLA4 ($\alpha4$). Based on this data it is possible to speculate that this adhesion-based system may impart some specificity to the interaction of primary myotubes and secondary myoblasts. Antibodies to VCAM-1 and VLA4 (α4) will partially block myoblast fusion. As the block is of the same degree as antiNCAM, Rosen et al (1992) suggest that this adhesive system may be as important as NCAM.

MYOBLAST TRANSFER THERAPY

The last decade has witnessed a dramatic increase in our knowledge about the cell biology of the myoblast. This has proceeded to the stage, as already discussed, of having a large amount of information about the origins, developmental potential and fusion characteristics of myoblasts both from animal systems and also normal and pathological human material. An additional feature of myoblasts is that they can fuse with and integrate into muscle fibres when injected into suitable animal hosts. The incidence of this event increases dramatically in muscle which is undergoing regeneration, as in a number of muscle disease states. This is an inherent property of skeletal muscle and one in which the muscle satellite cell normally participates. The experiments suggest that direct injection of normal healthy myoblasts into skeletal muscle leads to the formation of mosaic fibres that may be able to overcome the deleterious effects of loss of important gene products. The idea has gained particular popularity in the case of Duchenne muscular dystrophy (DMD) (Partridge et al 1989, Partridge 1991). Here loss of dystrophin is the first step in a cascade in muscle that ultimately results in loss of the myofibre. A constant cycle of degeneration and regeneration is then set up with activation of satellite cells followed by integration of these cells into damaged fibres and also the generation of new fibres. The basic question is whether it is technically feasible to devise systems of cell replacement in diseases such as DMD using human myoblasts as the donor cells (reviewed in Griggs & Karpati 1990). The term myoblast transfer therapy arises from the observations that it is possible to inject populations of myoblasts into muscle and obtain integration. If the efficiency was such that it could lead to clinical improvement then it could be regarded as a therapy. The starting point for any procedure involving human myoblasts is a muscle biopsy (Dubowitz 1985). For experimental purposes it is unlikely that a needle biopsy could provide the necessary number of cells for transfer. The exact number of cells required is difficult to predict and would depend on the range of procedures being contemplated. Most exploratory studies to date have used in the region of 10^8 myoblasts (Gussoni et al 1992). This is easily possible using a muscle biopsy from a patient or an unaffected family member, followed by extensive subculturing. From a 0.3 g biopsy our own group have routinely produced 5×10^4 to 3×10^5 mononucleate cells using standard procedures of tissue dissociation (Yasin et al 1977, Hurko et al 1986). In contrast dissociation of human fetal muscle obtained from abortion material can yield much larger numbers of cells ($>2 \times 10^6$). It is not clear, however, whether the adult satellite cell cultures and fetal cultures have the same developmental potential or whether there might be lineage-specific restrictions to growth and differentiation. Another major question is how many cell divisions one can expect from cells of different sources. In general human cells will divide from 30 to 60 times before senescing. However, for any procedure it is clearly more beneficial to be starting with myoblasts of the lowest cell division numbers as these will have the greatest proliferative potential.

Growth and purification of myoblasts

For myoblast transfer therapy to have any chance of success it is essential to be able to grow large populations of myoblasts and either before or after culture to be able to purify the myoblasts away from contaminating non-myogenic cells. Muscle is a particularly difficult tissue from which to cultivate large numbers of cells. As mentioned above, there is the problem of cells with different numbers of cell divisions before they senesce so it is not possible to obtain a synchronised culture.

Additionally there is the question of whether all myoblasts are equal in their developmental capacities. There is also the problem that at any time myoblasts will leave the cell cycle and commit to fusion if their growth requirements are not ideal for proliferation compared to differentiation. Most standard procedures for the culture of human muscle cells use serum and chick embryo extract in conjunction with a basal culture medium such as F10 or DMEM. The substrates used have generally been collagen or gelatin (Yasin et al 1977, Blau & Webster 1981), and with these basic procedures it has generally been possible to obtain cultures that can be cloned down to the single level and which additionally showed good fusion characteristics (Yasin et al 1977, Blau & Webster 1981, Walsh & Ritter 1981, Yasin et al 1982, Blau et al 1983, Hurko et al 1987). A new cell culture medium for the growth of human myoblasts has recently been formulated (Ham et al 1988, Ham & St Clair 1989, Ham et al 1990). This medium, called MCDB120, supports good clonal growth of human myoblasts and is serum-free. The medium is supplemented with a number of defined components including epidermal growth factor which stimulates cell division rather than differentiation. With this medium it has been possible to carry out direct single cell cloning experiments from biopsies, but more importantly it allows mass cultures of myoblasts to be produced. Replacement of the MCDB120 medium with serum-containing media or low insulin-containing media results in the rapid fusion of myoblasts (Ham et al 1990).

The next major problem to be approached is the purification of myoblasts from contaminating cells. The percentage of contaminating cells in biopsies varies enormously. Estimates range from 40% to 90% of non-fusing cells which are presumably fibroblasts. A number of procedures are available for the purification of myoblasts, as it is generally believed that the purer the sample the greater the chances of functional improvement in myoblast transfer therapy. Single cell cloning procedures can be used to obtain myoblast clones, but this is tedious and many cells are lost when test samples are set up for fusion assays in order to prove the myogenic nature of specific clones. The nature of the procedure means that no more than 10^6–10^7 cells per clone can easily be obtained and by this time many rounds of cell division have been used up. Pooling of clones is possible but is time-consuming.

A more efficient procedure is to use antibody markers to isolate cell populations. In principle this can operate by either negative or positive selection methods. The only major requirement is to have a cell type-specific surface marker. Most successful has been positive selection of myoblasts by surface markers such as the NCAM protein in conjunction with a fluorescence-activated cell sorter (FACS) or cell panning. NCAM is present on myoblasts and myotubes but not on fibroblasts, so it is a useful candidate antigen (Walsh 1990, Walsh & Doherty 1991). The results to date (Hurko et al 1987, Webster et al 1988) show that it is possible to purify relatively large numbers of myoblasts by FACS analysis. The resulting cell population is >99% pure and is capable of achieving a number of cell divisions before the cells senesce. The fusion competence of the pure population is also high. Problems associated with the technique are the high losses, sometimes in the order of 50%, and the concern that not all myoblasts are being selected. NCAM levels rise by about three-fold on myoblasts as they become committed to differentiating (Moore et al 1987). This may mean that some cells are not selected by the procedure as they may be below threshold levels. Alternative markers have not been tried yet but the protein M-cadherin (Donalies et al 1991) looks particularly promising owing to its muscle specific expression pattern (Moore & Walsh 1993).

A second procedure that has been used to purify myoblasts for mouse muscle is cell panning (Jones et al 1990). Here a tissue culture dish is coated with a specific antibody and the cell suspension is allowed to come into contact with it. After gentle washing the unbound cells are removed, leaving the tightly bound cells behind. These can be removed by a gentle shear force. A recent study on mouse muscle (Jones et al 1990) used an antibody to NCAM and neonatal mouse muscle. Good separation was made between the two cell populations and myogenic cells preferentially attached to the antibody. It is not yet clear whether the procedure could be scaled up sufficiently or whether some myoblasts do not attach sufficiently well to the dish and are lost.

The problem of lack of sufficient myoblasts with good proliferative capacity and developmental potential has not yet been solved and all the present results should be viewed as pilot studies. It may be possible to increase the number of myoblasts available for therapy by genetic means. As discussed earlier it is possible to transform fibroblasts to fusion-competent myoblasts via transfection with MyoD or myogenin cDNA constructs.

This could even be extended to skin biopsies if the conversion was efficient and complete. A number of pilot studies have proceeded to the extent that boys with DMD have been injected with purified myoblasts. All studies have used first degree relatives to minimise the problems of immune rejection. Gussoni et al (1992) showed that it was possible using the polymerase chain reaction to detect expression of dystrophin mRNA in muscle injected with 10^8 purified myoblasts. One month after transplantation was the time chosen for the biopsy and there was evidence of dystrophin mRNA at 6 months also. While this result is encouraging there are still questions about the efficiency of the procedure. PCR is a very sensitive procedure, yet it required 40 cycles to obtain specific bands on agarose gels. Hopefully these studies will be complemented by more detailed immunocytochemical studies. A second more extensive study (Karpati et al 1993) has not yielded positive results yet. This study used a similar procedure of FACS purification of myoblasts, although the differentiation capacity of the purified myoblasts was not high. In contrast a third study has yielded positive results (Lan et al 1991), although there have been questions raised about its validity (Thompson 1992a). In a progressive disease, such as DMD, there is always the question of the ethics of double-blind trials. However placebo effects are possible if this is not done, as in the study by Lan et al (1991). In the future more effort should be put into standardising the type and nature of the myoblasts to be injected and the clinical assessments to be used. The results of these three pilot studies and more recent follow-up studies have been reviewed with concern by a group of scientists working in the field (Thompson 1992b). A plea for a halt to this type of study has been made until more controlled animal experiments are carried out. The lack of efficacy of the procedure to date is worrying and it is likely that it will have to be rethought from first principles.

DYSTROPHIN GENE TRANSFER

A variant strategy to myoblast transfer is to use gene transfer approaches (reviewed in Dickson & Dunckley 1993). There are a number of possible options for gene therapy approaches. One would be to introduce into DMD myoblasts, which are deficient in their ability to synthesise dystrophin when they fuse, a copy of a functional dystrophin gene, generally in the form of a cDNA. The myoblasts would be obtained from the DMD patient and following gene transfer reintroduced by injection back into the major muscle masses. The recent cloning of full-length and truncated dystrophin cDNAs and their subsequent expression in a variety of cellular backgrounds (Dickson et al 1991, Lee et al 1991, Dickson et al 1992) shows that this strategy is feasible to contemplate in the future if enough myoblasts could be obtained from boys with DMD and the procedure could be carried out with high efficiency and safety. Two dystrophin constructs have generally been used in cell culture studies to date. These are either full-length constructs which are of the order of 12 kb and which can direct the synthesis of the full 427 kDa protein (Dickson et al 1991). An alternative is to use a mutant gene which may be fully or at least partially functional. The one chosen so far corresponds to a Becker muscular dystrophy patient (England et al 1990). This is a patient with a deletion in the central rod domain of dystrophin and although over 40% of the mature protein sequence is missing in the patient he has shown a relatively mild disease. This latter gene construct is generally known as the dystrophin 'mini-gene' (England et al 1990). There are a number of alternatives to transfection of DMD myoblasts with various dystrophin constructs. The first of these is the direct injection of plasmid DNA into muscle fibres. Wolff et al (1990, 1991) have reported the remarkable finding that injection of plasmid DNA into muscle can lead to the uptake and stable expression of the construct. Although the number of fibres that are transformed is small, of the order of 1–2%, this none the less is a possible vehicle for introduction of genes into muscle. Ascadi et al (1991) have now reported that dystrophin can be re-expressed in the sarcolemma of *mdx* myofibres following injection of DNA constructs under the control of the rous sarcoma virus promoter. An alternative to the direct injection strategy is to use viral-mediated gene transfer. Two vehicles look most promising. The first of these is to use adenovirus; a recent pilot study in cystic fibrosis has highlighted the possibilities with this system (Rosenfeld et al 1991, 1992), and recent studies on *mdx* muscle also look promising (Ragst et al 1982, Vincent et al 1993). Studies on muscle have also been carried out using retroviral vectors (Dunckley et al 1991). The problem with these viral-based systems is that the packaging capacity of the virus is low and below the size of the full dystrophin mRNA. However the Becker 'mini-gene' has been cloned into a murine leukaemia virus-based system. *Mdx* myoblasts have now been infected with this construct and dystrophin can now be found at the sarcolemma of myotubes. Interestingly direct injection of high titre virus into *mdx* myofibres in vivo results in the conversion of a significant number of myofibres greater to or certainly the equal of the direct injection methods (Dunckley et al 1992, 1993). Although retroviruses require active cell division for integration it is likely that the environment found in *mdx* or DMD muscle with a large amount of regeneration would fulfil these requirements.

Although these studies with different vectors have shown that it is possible to obtain expression of dystrophin in *mdx* myofibres, they have not, with one exception (Vincent et al 1993), addressed the issue of whether there is any change in the ongoing pathology. Two studies have now reported that germ line expression of dystrophin using transgenic animals reverses some aspects of the pathology in *mdx* mice (Wells et al 1992, Cox et al 1993). The dystrophin 'mini-gene' was introduced into *mdx* mice and low levels of expression of the truncated protein found at the sarcolemma. A marked reduction in myofibre necrosis and consequent regeneration was observed, suggesting that the 'mini-gene' was at least partially functional at the early time points analysed. By contrast, high-level expression of dystrophin, via the strong M-creative kinase promoter, reversed many of the pathological changes in *mdx* mice.

Rapid progress is likely to be made in the area of dystrophin gene transfer in the *mdx* mouse. This should give an indication as to which constructs, promoter and delivery systems work best. This should be followed by studies in one of the larger animal models of DMD like the *xmd* dog (Cooper et al 1988). Only if the requirements for safety and efficiency can be met should studies on DMD boys be contemplated.

ESTABLISHING PATTERNS OF MUSCLE INNERVATION

Innervating neurones and target cells clearly cooperate to form and maintain the mature neuromuscular system (for anatomy and physiology see Ch. 1). In this section we will consider the molecular basis whereby muscle cells can influence both the survival of motor neurones and also their ability to grow into the developing limb. Most information concerning both events has been obtained from studies on the chick (e.g. see Oppenheim 1989, Dahm & Landmesser 1988). However, where available, data from other species, including humans, suggests that the same molecular mechanisms are highly conserved. Nerve fibre ingrowth and ramification into limb muscle occurs over a very similar developmental period as that of naturally occurring motor neurone cell death (stages 27–36 or embryonic day 5–10). During this period nerve and muscle become functionally coupled, spontaneous miniature end-plate potentials can be observed and electrical stimulation of the nerve results in muscle contraction (e.g. see Landmesser et al 1988). However at this stage (stages 32–33) contraction is likely to depend on diffusion of acetylcholine from neurones to clusters of receptors on myotubes and not on the function of classical synapses, as very few are present at this time.

Very little is known about the precise molecular basis of classical synapse formation and it will not be considered here. However, the initial clustering of acetylcholine receptors on myotubes is likely to involve the release of molecules from nerve terminals (Phillips et al 1991, Ferns et al 1992).

The temporal sequence of events leading to the innervation of the chick hindlimb

A detailed picture of the temporal course of motor neurone ingrowth and ramification within the iliofibularis muscle in the chick thigh has been built up from the work of Lynn Landmesser's group (e.g. see Lance-Jones & Landmesser 1980, 1981a,b, Dahm & Landmesser 1988, Landmesser et al 1988, 1990, Tang et al 1992). Very briefly, motor neurones from the medial and lateral columns exit the spinal cord at stages 17–22 and grow to the crural or sciatic plexus. Subgrouping of motor neurones that will eventually go on to innervate specific muscle groups are 'sorted out' within the plexus regions and thereby emerge into either the dorsal or ventral nerve trunks. They subsequently (stages 24–26) leave the main trunk and innervate their appropriate muscle target. Motor neurone development, axonal growth and segregation within the plexus occurs normally in the absence of target muscle (Tosney & Landmesser, 1984). Individual neurones grow into and ramify within respective muscles in a highly stereospecific and reproducible manner and this is illustrated for the iliofibularis muscle in Figure 2.7. In the adult, individual motor neurones normally innervate large groups of muscle fibres

(the motor unit); the fibres themselves normally receive a single synaptic input. In addition to growth and ramification of the nerve with the muscle (Figure 2.7), there are two other major events that are clearly influenced by the muscle. First, over half of the motor neurones projecting to the muscle die over the short development period widely termed that of 'naturally occurring cell death' (~stages 28–36 in the chick). Secondly, multiple innervation of fast muscles is lost, leaving singly innervated muscle fibres. The latter process is activity-dependent and apparently takes place in the absence of any further cell death. The physiological significance of motor neurone cell death is not clear, however; obvious explanations could include the elimination of inappropriately projecting neurones and/or the matching of fast and slow motor neurones to the appropriate fast/slow muscle fibres. The importance of muscle in these events is evident from the observation that experimental manipulation of the muscle mass can influence the number of motor neurones that die during this period (see below)

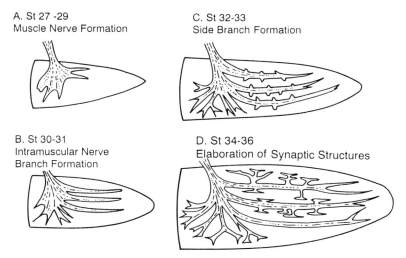

A. St 27 -29
Muscle Nerve Formation

C. St 32-33
Side Branch Formation

B. St 30-31
Intramuscular Nerve
Branch Formation

D. St 34-36
Elaboration of Synaptic Structures

Fig. 2.7   A schematic illustration of the stages in the innervation of the iliofibularis muscle of the chick hindlimb adapted from Landmesser et al (1988). At the stage illustrated in **A** the nerve has grown into the muscle and the muscle will contract upon nerve stimulation even though classical synapses have not yet formed. At **B** some of the axons start to form transversely running fascicles. At **C** collateral branching from these fascicles results in the outgrowth of side-branches of axons that intimately contact the muscle surface. This process is particularly susceptible to inhibition of NCAM function by blocking antibodies or by removal of PSA from neuronal NCAM. At **D** individual axonal branches have been elaborated from the small side-branches and single axons can be found in contact with the muscle surface. The period of motor neurone cell-death is coming to an end and the muscle is ready to generate secondary myotubes.

and the fact that retraction of polyneural innervation is inhibited by paralysis of the target muscle.

Evidence for a muscle-derived trophic factor

Hamburger has written a brief overview providing
a historical perspective for the development of the
theory that the target can influence the survival of
the neurones that project to it (1988). The origin
lies in the work of Shorey and Lillie that demonstrated that destruction of the developing limb
bud of the chick resulted in hypoplasia of the
motor column and the spinal ganglia. The subsequent work of Hamburger and his associates
confirmed and extended these observations by
showing that supernumary limbs could induce
hyperplasia and that cell numbers in the spinal
cord and ganglia are independently regulated by
the size of their muscle and skin targets respectively
(Hamburger 1934, Hollyday and Hamburger
1976). It is now well established that substantial
cell death is a natural phenomenon that most, if not
all, neuronal populations are subject to and that
this can be regulated to a considerable extent by
the target tissue (reviewed in Oppenheim 1989).

A molecular postulate to explain the above
observations followed from the identification and
extensive studies on a polypeptide growth factor
called nerve growth factor or NGF (reviewed in
Thoenen 1991). This factor is present in limiting
amounts in the targets of sympathetic and some
sensory neurones, primarily at the time when the
axons of the neurones invade their respective
targets (e.g. see Heumann et al 1984, Davies et al
1987). It is widely accepted that up to half of the
neurones that project to the target will be
successful in the competition for the 'limiting'
amounts of NGF and thereby obtain sufficient
'trophic' support to survive the critical period of
naturally occurring cell death. Crucial experimental support for this postulate includes the
demonstration that appropriate neurones bear
high affinity receptors for NGF and that NGF can
support their survival in vitro. Perhaps more critically exogenous NGF administered to the developing embryo can specifically rescue the above
neurones from death, and a reduction in the availability of endogenous NGF (by administering
blocking antibodies) essentially prevents any of the

respective neurones from surviving this period. The
fact that NGF supports only a small number of
neuronal cell types led to the hypothesis that a
family of perhaps related molecules would exist
with individual members governing the survival of
unique populations of neurones. The purification
and cloning of brain-derived neurotrophic factor
(BDNF) led to experiments which broadly
substantiated the general 'neurotrophic hypothesis'. For example, BDNF can support the
survival both in vitro and in vivo of neurones that
are not responsive to NGF and its presence in low
amounts at the appropriate times in development
suggests that it also is a target-derived trophic
factor (reviewed in Barde 1989). Structural
similarities between NGF and BDNF allowed
for the development of genetic strategies to identify other family members. To date two new
molecules have been cloned (termed neurotrophins 3 and 4). Perhaps not surprisingly these
factors can interact with a family of structurally
related receptors that in some instances can bind
and transduce information from more than one
neurotrophin (reviewed in Bothwell 1991). The
more strict aspects of the general neurotrophic
factor hypothesis do not apparently hold up in that
individual neurones can be rescued by more than
one neurotrophin (at least in vitro) and some
neurotrophins are expressed in relatively large
amounts in a wide variety of tissues.

One thing that is clear is that there remains only
scant evidence that the neurotrophic theory can
account for muscle-dependent survival of motor
neurones. Purified motor neurones cannot be
rescued in vitro by NGF, BDNF or any of the
neurotrophins tested to date. Also there is no
evidence that any of the identified neurotrophins
shows a pattern of expression in the developing
muscle consistent with them subserving the role of
a target-derived neurotrophic factor. Muscle
extracts undoubtedly contain factors that can
support motor neurone survival both in vitro
(reviewed in Henderson 1988) and in vivo (see
below). However treatments of muscle that are
associated with substantial reductions in the
degree of motor neurone cell death (e.g. paralysis
of muscle) are not associated with corresponding
increases in the content of survival activity
as measured in both in vitro (Tanaka 1987) and in

vivo assays (Houenou et al 1989). This suggests that motor neurone survival may be controlled by processes other than amount of trophic factor in the muscle, such as limited access to any such trophic factor (for review see Oppenheim 1989).

Although many groups have failed to purify a neurotrophic factor from skeletal muscle (reviewed in Henderson 1988), there is perhaps one notable exception. A 22 kDa polypeptide termed ChAT development factor (CDF) has been purified (but not cloned) from rat skeletal muscle by conventional chromatography (McManaman et al 1990). This factor can promote survival and increases ChAT activity in cultures of purified motor neurons. Perhaps more importantly this factor can rescue motor neurones from death following injection into the developing embryo.

Sympathetic neurones can exhibit either an adrenergic or cholinergic phenotype and this can be determined by molecules present in the target (e.g. see Patterson & Chun 1977). A cholinergic differentiation factor (unfortunately also known by the acronym CDF) originally purified by Weber (1981) has recently been cloned and found to be identical to an independently studied factor called leukaemia inhibitory factor (LIF) (Martinou et al 1992). This factor may be secreted by muscle cells in culture and the recombinant molecule again has very pronounced effects on motor neurone survival and ChAT activity in vitro. The factor has not yet been tested in in vivo bioassays.

A third factor that may be produced within developing muscle and may contribute to the regulation of both myoblast proliferation and motor neurone survival is the fibroblast growth factor (FGF) (reviewed in Gospodarowicz 1988). This factor is remarkable in that it essentially contains none of the hallmarks of a hypothetical target-derived factor. For example it is very widely expressed and lacks a conventional signal sequence for secretion from cells. However recombinant FGF (both basic and acidic) can support the survival of a large number of neuronal cell types in culture, including highly purified populations of motor neurones (Unsicker et al 1987). This final observation has not as yet been confirmed by others working in this field.

A final factor which like FGF is highly abundant and relatively widely distributed is the ciliary neurontrophic factor (CNTF) originally purified from sciatic nerve (Manthorpe et al 1986). Again the trophic activity of this factor is relatively broad as regards responsive neurones; however this molecule can also prevent both the in vivo and in vitro death of avian motor neurones (Oppenheim et al 1991). Unfortunately, this factor does not show a pattern of expression consistent with it being a muscle-derived trophic agent.

In summary, although the evidence remains consistent with a muscle-derived trophic factor determining the extent of motor neurone cell death, it seems likely that access to the factor rather than the amount of factor may control the process. For example, the nature of the branching pattern of motor neurones may allow some but not all neurones to obtain the factor via intimate contact with the muscle. However, it is worth noting that at least in the chick hindlimb, conventional synapses and the production of secondary myotubes occur after the period of motor neurone cell death. A more extreme view would be for the survival to be governed by a generally available non-muscle factor (like CNTF), with a specific interaction between nerve and muscle regulating the competence or ability of the neurone to respond to such a factor. In any case, the acceptance of any agent as the elusive target-derived motor neurone survival factor will require a demonstration that a reduced availability of the factor mimics the motor column hypoplasia first demonstrated by limb removal by Shorey in 1908 (see Hamburger 1988).

MOLECULES ON THE MUSCLE MEMBRANE THAT AFFECT AXONAL GROWTH

As discussed above, during the period of cell death the motor neurones are actively growing and branching within the developing muscle. At stage 36 branching of fascicles is at an end and single axons diverge to contact the myotubes. Whereas the ability of muscle to promote the survival of motor neurones is likely to depend on the retrograde transport of soluble factors, the ability of axons to bundle and branch is likely to be controlled by contact-dependent interactions mediated by cell-recognition molecules present on the surface of neuronal growth cones and myotubes. In this section we will discuss the molecular basis of contact-dependent axonal growth.

General classes of molecules mediating contact-dependent axonal growth

In order to identify the molecules that promote contact-dependent axonal growth over muscle, Bixby & colleagues cultured chick ciliary ganglion motor neurones over monolayers of primary muscle cells (Bixby et al 1987). Neurite outgrowth was assessed in cultures treated with antibodies that block the function of neuronal integrin receptors which recognise components of the extracellular matrix (e.g. laminins, collagens and fibronectin) and antibodies that block the function of NCAM and N-cadherin on both muscle and the nerve. When added individually each of the antibodies had little effect on neurite outgrowth. However, when added in combination, all three were required for a maximal inhibition of neurite outgrowth, suggesting that multiple receptors can act in concert to promote neurite outgrowth. An identical experimental paradigm was used by other groups to determine the nature of receptors used by other neurones that extend axons on monolayers of Schwann cells, muscle cells, astrocytes or fibroblasts.

The results of these studies (reviewed in Doherty and Walsh 1989) clearly established four important points. First, blocking the function of integrins, NCAM, N-cadherin and the L1 adhesion molecule can substantially inhibit neurite outgrowth over the most efficacious of all the substrata (Schwann cells). By contrast, inhibition of integrins, NCAM and N-cadherin was sufficient to block neurite outgrowth over muscle cells and astrocytes, whereas inhibition of integrins was sufficient to inhibit neurite outgrowth over fibroblasts. A second important point was that if differing populations of neurones are grown on the same cellular monolayer, the inhibitory profile of the blocking of antibodies is not always the same. For example E8 chick ciliary neurones did not respond to NCAM on astrocytes, whereas E11 chick retinal neurones did. Thus individual populations of neurones can respond in their own unique manner to an identical set of recognition

molecules present on one cell type. Thirdly, neurones can respond to a single CAM present on one cell type but not another. For example, whereas ciliary neurones respond to NCAM on muscle they fail to respond to NCAM on astrocytes. Finally the ability of neurones to respond to a fixed set of recognition cues can change as a function of developmental age of the neurone. For example, integrin antibodies can perturb neurite outgrowth from E8 but not E14 chick ciliary ganglion neurones. Thus even though a small number of receptors are involved in general growth a remarkable degree of variability in responsiveness can be observed and this is likely to depend on a number of factors, including the level of an individual CAM on both the neurone and the substratum.

Regulation of neurite outgrowth via changes in expression of NCAM on myotubes

As discussed above, muscle cells express differing isoforms of NCAM at various stages of development and these isoforms can differentially contribute to myoblast fusion. N-cadherin and integrins also contribute to myoblast fusion (see above). Thus the same set of cues can influence not only muscle–muscle cell interactions but also muscle–nerve interactions.

Although blocking antibodies can be used to identify cell recognition molecules involved in neurite outgrowth, more direct assays are required to address questions concerning the relationship between the level of CAM expression and response, the effects of post-translational modifications on function, the relative efficacy of different isoforms on function and finally the postrecognition events that underlie signal transduction and neurite outgrowth.

To address the above questions, we have used the molecular genetic approach described above for the study of molecules that promote myoblast fusion. NIH-3T3 fibroblasts have been transfected with plasmid vectors containing cDNAs encoding several individual isoforms of human NCAM and the single isoform of chick N-cadherin (reviewed in Doherty & Walsh 1991). Clones of 3T3 cells that stably express NCAM and/or N-cadherin are then selected and characterised to determine the relative level of expression of

NCAM and/or N-cadherin. The ability of a variety of neuronal cell types to extend neurites over confluent monolayers of parental 3T3 cells and 3T3 cells expressing known levels of the various isoforms of NCAM can then be determined. The data obtained to date has shown that the two main isoforms of NCAM found in developing skeletal muscle (the 140 kDa transmembrane isoform and the 125 kDa GPI-anchored isoform that contains the MSD1 region) both show similar efficacy in promoting neurite outgrowth from chick or rat neurones. Neurite outgrowth could be blocked by species-specific antibodies that bound exclusively to NCAM in the monolayer or to NCAM in the neurones. Thus a homophilic binding mechanism can account for NCAM-dependent neurite outgrowth. Neurones grow equally well on cells expressing NCAM isoforms that did not contain the MSD1 region, but did not respond to NCAM that was directly secreted from 3T3 cells into the culture media. From these results we can conclude that alternative splicing of NCAM during skeletal muscle development has more important functional consequences for muscle–muscle interactions than muscle–nerve interactions. These data also suggest that muscle is more likely to modulate NCAM-dependent neurite outgrowth by changing the level of expression of NCAM. In this context, when neurones are grown over a panel of 3T3 cells expressing differing amounts of transfected NCAM, there is a highly cooperative relationship between the level of NCAM expressed and neurite outgrowth. A discrete threshold value of NCAM expression was required before neurite outgrowth was stimulated, and above this value relatively small changes in NCAM expression were found to have substantial effects on neurite outgrowth. As discussed above there are quite dramatic changes in NCAM expression during the development of skeletal muscle, with the temporal pattern of expression suggesting that a rapid increase in NCAM on myotubes may indeed trigger the growth of motor axons over the muscle. For example in a detailed study of the differing stages of innervation of the iliofibularis muscle in the chick (see Fig. 2.7), the level of NCAM on myotubes increases between stages 30 and 34 and this correlates with the sprouting of axons from the main branches to form small side-branches from which individual axons diverge to grow over and form neuromuscular junctions on individual myotubes (Tosney et al 1986, Dahm & Landmesser 1988). Direct evidence that NCAM on muscle might trigger this response comes from the observation that injection of anti-NCAM antibodies into the developing limb can reduce the length of side-branches by up to 60% (Landmesser et al 1988). As discussed above, NCAM expression is down-regulated and becomes restricted to the neuromuscular junction region following synapse formation. Most of the NCAM in adult muscle and at the synapse is of the 140 kDa form and this may function to stabilise the structure (Kobayashi et al 1992).

Not all isoforms of NCAM promote neurite outgrowth following transfection and expression in 3T3 fibroblasts. For example the 180 kDa isoform of NCAM which is expressed primarily by post-mitotic neurones but can also be seen (by in situ hybridisation) in early migrating myoblasts (see above) is relatively poor at stimulating neurite outgrowth (Doherty et al 1992a). This isoform has an identical extracellular structure to the 140 kDa isoform and differs only by use of a single exon (number 18) which encodes an ~250 amino acid block that is expressed within the cytoplasmic domain. As the main difference between the 180 kDa isoform and the others is reduced lateral mobility due, perhaps, to specific interaction with cytoskeletal components (Pollerberg et al 1987), this observation suggests that lateral diffusion of a CAM in the substratum can affect its ability to promote neurite outgrowth, and cautions against using purified CAMs as immobilised substrate-associated molecules for studying their function. As discussed above there are two sites where alternative splicing changes the extracellular structure of membrane-bound NCAM. Insertion of the MSD block of 37 amino acids (by use of four small exons) between the FNIII repeats did not affect transfected NCAM's ability to stimulate neurite outgrowth. In contrast, use of the VASE or π exon in Ig domain 4 substantially inhibits NCAM's ability to promote neurite outgrowth (Doherty et al, 1992b). The percentage of transcripts containing the VASE exon increases from ~3% to 50% during development of the central nervous system over a time-course that suggests VASE-containing isoforms may regulate synaptic plasticity in a negative manner (Small and Akeson 1990, Walsh et al 1992). VASE is not expressed in skeletal muscle or most other regions of the periphery. Thus whereas the ability of muscle to regulate NCAM-dependent neurite outgrowth primarily involves changing the level of NCAM expression, pathway and targets in the central nervous system have the added ability to do so by expressing alternatively spliced variants of NCAM.

NCAM on the motor neurone

Neurones express transmembrane isoforms of NCAM of 140 and 180 kDa. Antibodies that bind to and block the function of NCAM on neurones inhibit neurite outgrowth that is stimulated by NCAM in the substratum, but not neurite outgrowth stimulated by other CAMs (Doherty & Walsh 1991). NCAM in neurones is subjected to dynamic changes in its patterns of post-translational processing. In particular at some stages in development NCAM contains one or more chains of $\alpha2$–8 linked polysialic acid (PSA), each up to 200 residues long. PSA expression on NCAM is generally high in many parts of the nervous system during periods of axonal growth, with subsequent down-regulation after appropriate connections have been made (e.g. see Chuong and Edelman 1984, Schlosshauser et al 1984). PSA expression on NCAM remains high in several regions in the central nervous system where neurogenesis and associated axonal growth continue into adulthood. Removal of PSA from embryonic NCAM substantially increases NCAM-dependent adhesion and also adhesion mediated by other molecules (Acheson et al 1991). NCAM expression on chick motor neurones has also been studied in considerable detail by Landmesser's lab (e.g. see Tang et al 1992). NCAM, but not PSA, is present on motor neurones when they initially send axons towards the nerve plexus at the base of the limb (stages 20–21). Just prior to entering the plexus where specific populations of motor neurones sort their axons into bundles for projection to their appropriate targets, PSA expression is dramatically increased (stages 23–34). At this stage there are differences in the relative level of PSA on differing groups of axons, but no changes in the level of NCAM polypeptide. The level of NCAM and PSA on the motor neurones then remains relatively stable during growth and branching into the muscle. Shortly after the major period of growth within the muscle (stages 27–36), PSA expression is downregulated independently of NCAM polypeptide expression. Over subsequent developmental stages NCAM polypeptide expression on motor neurones is also down-regulated; however expression of non-sialyated NCAM remains at the neuromuscular junction (see above).

From the above detailed descriptions of NCAM expression on myotubes and motor neurones it is clear that changes in NCAM on muscle rather than nerve most likely trigger side-branching from axon fascicles. However the dynamic regulation of PSA on neuronal NCAM during development in general, and in the muscle in particular, raises questions as to the functional significance of this particular post-translational modification.

We have observed that the ability of three independent populations of neurones (chick retinal ganglion cells, rat cerebellar and hippocampal neurones) to respond to fixed levels of NCAM expressed in a cellular monolayer is lost over relatively short developmental periods. At the stage when these neurones are most responsive to NCAM they all express PSA. Removal of PSA (by use of a specific enzyme called endoneuraminidase N) dramatically inhibits their ability to respond to NCAM in the monolayer, but not their ability to respond to extracellular matrix molecules (via integrin receptors) nor their ability to respond to transfected N-cadherin or L1 expressed in the same cellular monolayers (for review see Walsh & Doherty 1992). Thus PSA on neurones is required for NCAM-dependent neurite outgrowth and this post-translational modification can act as a highly specific modulator of NCAM function.

Studies have also been conducted on the effects of the specific removal of PSA for neuronal NCAM during the innervation of limb muscles in the chick (Landmesser et al 1988, 1990, Tang et al 1992). These studies are difficult to interpret at the molecular level as alterations in NCAM function can affect nerve fasciculation per se as well as nerve–muscle interactions. The former event is likely to be capable of indirectly affecting the latter. However several important observations have been made. First, removal of PSA during axonal segregation in the plexus (but not following this) resulted in motor neurones making projection errors. Therefore NCAM (via differences in PSA levels on sub-groups of motor neurones) can contribute to pathway selection. Secondly, removal of PSA at the stages of development when side-branch formation was taking place (see Figure 2.7) had an almost identical effect to that of antibodies that block NCAM function in that it substantially inhibited this process. Endo-N had no effects on branching patterns in muscles where NCAM function had already been functionally inactivated with specific antibodies. This suggests that removal of PSA specifically affects NCAM-mediated functions (Landmesser et al 1988). Thus, although the in vivo situation is complex, these data also suggest that PSA is required for, and can specifically promote, NCAM-dependent neurite outgrowth, during development of the neuromuscular junction.

The role of integrins and N-cadherin in nerve–muscle interactions

Muscle cells synthesise a complex basal lamina that contains many extracellular matrix components such as collagens and laminins that are known to be capable of promoting axonal growth from purified motor neurons in vitro (see Reichardt & Tomaselli 1991). There may also be components of the extracellular matrix that are inhibitory for axonal growth, and one of these called S-laminin is found localised at synapses. Neurones recognise and respond to extracellular matrix molecules by increased neurite outgrowth via integrin receptors. These molecules are heterodimers composed of covalently associated α and β subunits. A recent extensive review documents the presence of several α and β subunits expressed in various combinations by neurones together with their ligand specificity (Reichardt & Tomaselli 1991). As discussed above, the ability of a variety of neurones to disperse axons over a wide range of cell types can be partially inhibited by blocking the function of β_1-class integrins. However the precise nature of individual integrin receptors on motor neurones and the exact contribution that various compo-

nents of the muscle extracellular matrix make to neurite outgrowth, both in vitro and in vivo, remain to be determined.

Muscle cells also express a variety of cadherins (N-cadherin, M-cadherin and T-cadherin — see above); however, to date only the function of N-cadherin has been investigated in bioassays in vitro of muscle fusion and neurite outgrowth. Blocking the function of N-cadherin reduces neurite outgrowth from a number of neuronal types cultured on muscle (see above). Also chick N-cadherin expressed via gene transfer in both L-cells and 3T3 fibroblasts can promote neurite outgrowth from a variety of neurones (Matsunaga et al 1988, Doherty et al 1991). However in contrast to NCAM-transfected cells, clones expressing relatively low levels of N-cadherin had positive effects on neurite outgrowth. The magnitude of the neurite outgrowth response increased in a linear manner as a function of the relative level of N-cadherin expression in the transfected fibroblasts, and this is fundamentally different from the threshold effect and highly cooperative nature of the NCAM dose–response curve. Thus, neuronal responsiveness to NCAM may be more dramatically regulated than responsiveness to N-cadherin and this may explain the more widespread role that N-cadherin has in supporting neurite outgrowth from virtually all tested neurones, irrespective of developmental age, grown on a variety of cellular monolayers (reviewed in Doherty & Walsh 1989, 1991).

NCAM and N-cadherin are co-expressed on muscle cells with immuno-electron microscopy showing that both CAMs frequently co-localise in clusters on the myoblast plasma membrane (Soler & Knudsen 1991). In order to test for functional co-operativity between these molecules in promoting neurite outgrowth, we generated a panel of cells expressing both human NCAM and chick N-cadherin. The data clearly showed that 'sub-threshold' levels of NCAM which do not normally stimulate neurite outgrowth on their own, do so in cells when functional levels of N-cadherin are also present (Doherty et al 1991). Therefore, in addition to changes in the level of NCAM expression, changes in NCAM isoforms, and changes in post-translational processing of NCAM, a fourth parameter can modulate NCAM-dependent neurite outgrowth, that is expression of an accessory CAM that in this instance was N-cadherin.

Again the exact role that the extracellular matrix and the cadherins play during normal development will require more studies. However there is considerable ingrowth of axons into muscle prior to the expression of NCAM on myotubes and antibodies that block NCAM function do not perturb this (Landmesser et al 1988). In addition, antibodies to NCAM only partially inhibit side-branch formation (see above). Thus, other molecules, and the cadherins and extracellular matrix are attractive candidates, and clearly function in concert with NCAM to regulate the innervation of skeletal muscles.

Contact-dependent axonal growth is controlled by calcium influx into neurones

The designation of NCAM and other CAMs as adhesion molecules is derived from observations made in non-physiological assay systems. Although adhesion per se is likely to be important in maintaining contacts between cells (such as those that maintain axon bundling in fascicles and those found at the synapse), a large body of recent evidence has shown that there is no correlation between adhesive strength and axonal growth stimulated by extracellular matrix molecules (Gundersen 1987), axonal growth stimulated by various NCAM forms (Doherty et al 1990, Doherty & Walsh 1992) and also in a comparison between integrin and CAM (N-cadherin and L1)-dependent axonal growth (Payne et al 1992). For example, whereas all of the NCAM isoforms can support NCAM-dependent adhesion, the use of exon 18 or the VASE exon specifically prevents NCAM-dependent neurite outgrowth. In addition, whereas removal of PSA from NCAM increases its ability to mediate adhesion (Hoffman & Edelman 1983, Acheson et al 1991), it can dramatically and specifically reduce NCAM-dependent neurite outgrowth (Doherty et al 1990).

A considerable amount of evidence now suggests that contact-dependent axonal growth stimulated by a variety of CAMs (NCAM, N-cadherin and L1), but not by extracellular matrix components, depends on the activation of a CAM-specific second messenger pathway in neurones rather than on adhesion per se. The key effector in this pathway is calcium and CAMs appear to operate by simulating the opening of both N- and L-type calcium channels in neurones. Evidence for this includes the observation that NCAM-, N-cadherin- and L1-stimulated axonal growth can be inhibited by reducing extracellular calcium to 0.25 mM, by blocking N- and L-type calcium channels, or by pretreating neurones with a chelator of intracellular calcium. None of the above inhibit the ability of the same neurones to extend neurites in response to integrins, NGF or agents that increase intracellular cAMP (reviewed in Doherty & Walsh 1992).

A key experiment suggests that contact-dependent activation of the above second messenger pathway is solely responsible for CAM-dependent neurite outgrowth. Direct activation of calcium influx through N- and L-type channels following K^+-depolarisation fully mimics, in a non-additive way, CAM-dependent neurite outgrowth. It follows that adhesion per se does not contribute to the response (Saffell et al 1992; Williams et al 1992).

The details of the mechanism whereby the homophilic binding of NCAM on, for example, muscle to NCAM on a motor neurone growth cone, results in the opening of neuronal calcium channels remains to be determined. Pretreatment of neurones with pertussis toxin results in a complete inhibition of contact-dependent axonal growth stimulated by CAMs but not that stimulated by extracellular matrix molecules, NGF or K^+ depolarisation. Similarly, inhibitors of tyrosine kinases such as the erbstatim analogue can specifically inhibit CAM-dependent neurite outgrowth (Williams et al 1994). This implicates both a heterotrimeric G-protein and tyrosine kinase in the pathway and recent studies suggest that an important tyrosine kinase in the pathway is the FGF-receptor. It is involved in transmitting signals via CIS-interactions with NCAM (Doherty & Walsh 1994). It is also clear that some isoforms of NCAM have been adapted to promote plasticity via activation of the above pathway, whereas others may serve to maintain stable connections between cells through direct adhesive interactions.

In summary, although it is clear that muscle can influence nerve function via release of soluble molecules and via intimate cell contact, a considerable amount of work is required to establish how the intricacies of the interplay between nerve and muscle result in the formation and maintenance of neuromuscular connections.

ACKNOWLEDGEMENTS

We acknowledge the assistance of Dr Robert Moore for producing Figure 2.2 and Dave Peck for producing Figure 2.6.

REFERENCES

Acheson A, Sunshine J L, Rutishauser U 1991. NCAM polysialic acid can regulate both cell–cell and cell–substrate interactions. Journal of Cell Biology 114: 143

Anderson M J, Fambrough D M 1983 Aggregates of acetylcholine receptors are associated with plaques of basal lamina heparan sulphate proteoglycan on the surface of skeletal muscle fibres. Journal of Cell Biology 97: 1396

Arakawa Y, Sendtner M, Thoenen H 1990 Survival effect of ciliary neurotrophic factor (CNTF) on chick embryonic motoneurons in culture; comparisons with other neurotrophic factors and cytokines. Journal of Neuroscience 10: 3501

Ascadi G, Dickson G, Love D R et al 1991 Human dystrophin expression in *mdx* mice after intramuscular injection of DNA constructs. Nature 352: 815

Barde Y A 1989 Trophic factors and neuronal survival. Neuron 2: 1525

Bixby J L, Pratt R S, Lilien J, Reichardt L F 1987 Neurite outgrowth on muscle cell surfaces involves extracellular matrix receptors as well as Ca^{2+}-dependent and independent cell adhesion molecules. Proceedings of the National Academy of Sciences of the USA 84: 2555

Blau H M, Pavlath G K, Hardeman E C et al 1985 Plasticity of the differentiated state. Science 230: 758

Blau H M, Pavlath G K, Rich K, Webster S G 1990 Localization of muscle gene products in nuclear domains: does this constitute a problem for myoblast transfer therapy. In: Griggs R C, Karpati G (eds) Myoblast transfer therapy. Plenum, New York, pp 167–172

Blau H M, Webster C 1981 Isolation and characterisation of human muscle cells. Proceedings of the National Academy of Sciences 78: 5623

Blau H M, Webster C, Chiu C-P, Guttman S, Chandler F 1983 Differentiation properties of pure populations of human dystrophic muscle cells. Experimental Cell Research 144: 495

Bober E, Lyons G E, Braun T, Cossu G, Buckingham M, Arnold H-H 1991 The muscle regulatory gene Myf-6 has a biphasic pattern of expression during early mouse development. Journal of Cell Biology 113: 1255

Bothwell M 1991 Keeping track of neurotrophin receptors. Cell 65: 915

Buckingham M 1992 Making muscles in mammals. Trends in Genetics 8: 144

Butler J, Cosmos E, Brierly J 1982 Differentiation of muscle fiber types in aneurogenic brachial muscles of the chick embryo. Journal of Experimental Zoology 224: 65

Chaudhari N, Delay R, Beam K G 1990 Fibroblasts fuse with myotubes developing in culture. In: Griggs R C, Karpati G (eds) Myoblast transfer therapy. Plenum, New York, pp 131–137

Chuong C-M, Edelman G M 1984 Alterations in neural cell adhesion molecules during development of different regions of the nervous system. Journal of Neuroscience 4: 2354

Cooper B J, Winand N J, Stedman H et al 1988 The homologue of the Duchenne locus is defective in X-linked muscular dystrophy of dogs. Nature 334: 154

Cossu G, Molinaro M 1987 Cell heterogeneity in the myogenic lineage. Current Topics in Developmental Biology 23: 185

Covault, Sanes J R. Neural cell adhesion molecule (NCAM) accumulates in denervated and paralysed skeletal muscles. Proceedings of the National Academy of Sciences USA 82: 4544

Cox G A, Cole N M, Matsumurak et al 1993 Overexpression of dystrophin in transgenic *mdx* mice eliminates dystrophic symptoms without toxicity. Nature 364: 725

Crow M T, Stockdale F E 1986a The developmental program of fast myosin heavy chain expression in avian skeletal muscle. Developmental Biology 118: 333

Crow M T, Stockdale F E 1986b Myosin expression and specialization of the earliest muscle fibers of the developing avian limb. Developmental Biology 113: 238

Cusella-de Angelis M G, Lyons G, Sonnino C et al 1992 MyoD, myogenin independent differentiation of primordial myoblasts in mouse somites. Journal of Cell Biology 116: 1243

Dahm L M, Landmesser L 1988 The regulation of intramuscular nerve branching during normal development and following activity blockade. Developmental Biology 130: 621

Davies A M, Bandtlow C, Heumann R, Korsching S, Rohrer H, Thoenen H 1987 Timing and site nerve growth factor synthesis in developing skin in relation to innervation and expression of receptor. Nature 326: 353

Dickson G, Peck D, Moore S E, Barton C H, Walsh F S 1990 Enhanced myogenesis in NCAM transfected mouse myoblasts. Nature 344: 348

Dickson G, Azad A, Morris G E, Simon H, Noursadeghi M, Walsh F S 1992 Co-localization and molecular association of dystrophin with laminin at the surface of mouse and human myotubes. Journal of Cell Science 103: 1223

Dickson G, Love D R, Davies K E, Wells K E, Piper T A, Walsh F S 1991 Human dystrophin gene transfer: production and expression of a functional recombinant DNA-based gene. Human Genetics 88: 53

Dickson G, Dunckley M 1993 Human dystrophin gene transfer. In: Partridge T (ed) Genetic correction of dystrophin deficiency in molecular and cell biology of skeletal muscle. Chapman and Hall, London p 283–302

Doherty P, Walsh F S 1989 Neurite guidance molecules. Current Opinion in Cell Biology 1: 1102

Doherty P, Walsh F S 1991 The contrasting roles of NCAM and N-cadherin as neurite outgrowth promoting molecules. Journal of Cell Science 15: 13

Doherty P, Walsh F S 1992 CAMs, second messengers and

axonal growth. Current Opinion in Neurobiology 2: 595

Doherty P, Walsh F S 1994 Signal transduction events underlying neurite outgrowth stimulated by cell adhesion molecules. Current Opinion in Neurobiology 4: 49

Doherty P, Cohen J, Walsh F S 1990 Neurite outgrowth in response to transfected NCAM changes during development and is modulated by polysialic acid. Neuron 5: 209

Doherty P, Moolenaar C E C K, Ashton S V, Michalides R J A M, Walsh F S 1992a Use of the VASE exon down-regulates the neurite growth promoting acitivity of NCAM 140. Nature 356: 791

Doherty P, Rimon G, Mann D A, Walsh F S 1992b Alternative splicing of the cytoplasmic domain of neural cell adhesion molecule alters its ability to act as a substrate for neurite outgrowth. Journal of Neurochemistry 58: 2338

Doherty P, Rowett L H, Moore S E, Mann D A, Walsh F S 1991 Neurite outgrowth in response to transfected NCAM and N-cadherin reveals fundamental differences in neuronal responsiveness to CAMs. Neuron 5: 209

Donalies M, Cramer M, Ringwald M, Starzinski-Powitz A 1991 Expression of M-cadherin, a member of the cadherin multigene family, correlates with differentiation of skeletal muscle cells. Proceedings of the National Academy of Sciences USA 88: 8024

Donoghue M, Ernst H, Wentworth B, Nadal-Ginard B, Rosenthal N 1988 A muscle specific enhancer is located at the 3' end of the myosin light-chain 1/3 gene locus. Genes Development 2: 1779

Donoghue M J, Merlie J P, Rosenthal N, Sanes J R 1991a A rostrocaudal gradient of transgene expression in adult skeletal muscle. Proceedings of the National Academy of Sciences USA 88: 5847

Donoghue M J, Alvarex J D, Merlie J P, Sanes J R 1991b Chloramphenicol acetyltransferase (CAT) transgene detected with a novel histochemical stain for CAT. Journal of Cell Biology 115: 423

Donoghue M J, Morris-Valero R, Johnson Y R, Merlie J P, Sanes J R 1992 Mammalian muscle cells bear a cell-autonomous, heritable memory of their rostrocaudal position. Cell 69: 67

Dubowitz V 1985 Muscle biopsy. A practical approach. Balliére Tindall, London

Dunckley M G, Love D R, Davies K E, Walsh F S, Morris G E, Dickson G 1992 Retroviral-mediated transfer of a dystrophin minigene into mdx myoblasts in vitro. FEBS Letters 296: 128

Dunckley M G, Wells D J, Morris G E, Walsh F S, Dickson G 1993 Direct retroviral-mediated transfer of a dystrophin minigene into regenerating mdx mouse muscle in vivo. Human Molecular Genetics 2: 717

England S B, Nicholson L V B, Johnson M A et al 1990 Very mild muscular dystrophy associated with deletion of 46% of dystrophin. Nature 343: 180

Ervasti J M, Campbell K P 1991 Membrane organization of the dystrophin–glycoprotein complex. Cell 66: 1121

Ferns M, Hoch W, Campanelli J T, Rupp F, Hall Z W, Scheller R H 1992 RNA splicing regulates agrin-mediated acetylcholine receptor clustering activity on cultured myotubes. Neuron 8: 1079

Funagalli G, Brigonzi A, Tachikawa T, Clements F 1981 Rat myoblast fusion: morphological study of membrane apposition, fusion and fission during controlled myogenesis in vitro. Journal of Ultrastructure Res. 75: 112

Funk W D, Ouelette M, Wright W E 1991 Molecular biology of myogenic regulatory factors. Molecular Biology and Medicine 8: 185

Gibralter D, Turner D C 1985 Dual adhesion systems of chick myoblasts. Developmental Biology 112: 292–307

Gospodarowicz D 1988 Molecular and developmental biology aspects of fibroblast growth factor. In: Kudlow J E, Maclinnan D H, Bernstein A, Gotlied A I (eds) Biology of growth factors, vol 234. New York: Plenum, pp 23–39

Griggs R C, Karpati G 1990 Myoblast transfer therapy. Plenum. New York

Gundersen R W 1987 Response of sensory neurites and growth cones to patterned substrata of laminin and fibronectin in vitro. Developmental Biology 121: 423

Gussoni E, Pavlath G K, Lanctot A M et al 1992 Normal dystrophin transcripts detected in Duchenne muscular dystrophy patients after myoblast transplantation. Nature 356: 435

Ham R G, St Clair J A 1989 Differentiation and partial maturation of human skeletal muscle cells in serum-free culture. In Vitro Cellular and Developmental Biology 25: 44A

Ham R G, St Clair J A, Meyer S D 1990 Improved media for rapid clonal growth of normal human skeletal muscle satellite cells. In: Griggs R C, Karpati G (eds) Myoblast transfer therapy. Plenum, New York, pp 193–199

Ham R G, St Clair J A, Webster C, Blau H M 1988 Improved media for normal human muscle satellite cells: serum-free clonal growth and enhanced growth with low serum. In Vitro Cellular and Developmental Biology 24: 833

Hamburger V 1934 The effects of wing bud extirpation on the development of the central nervous system in the chick embryo. Journal of Experimental Zoology 68: 449–494

Hamburger V 1988 Ontogeny of neuroembryology. Journal of Neuroscience 8: 3535

Hauschka S D 1974 Clonal analysis of vertebrate myogenesis. IV Developmental changes in the muscle colony-forming cells of the human fetal limb. Developmental Biology 37: 345

Henderson C E 1988 The role of muscle in the development and differentiation of spinal motoneurons: in vitro studies. In: Selective neuronal death. Ciba Foundation Symposium 126: 65

Heumann R, Korsching S, Scott J, Thoenen H 1984 Relationship between levels of nerve growth factor (NGF) and its messenger RNA in sympathetic ganglia and peripheral target tissues. EMBO Journal 3: 3183

Hinterberger T J, Sassoon D A, Rhodes S J, Konieczny S F 1991 Expression of the muscle regulatory factor MRF4 during somite and skeletal myofiber development. Developmental Biology 147: 144

Hoffman S, Edelman G M 1983 Kinetics of neuronal binding by E and A forms of neural cell adhesion molecule. Proceedings of the National Academy of Sciences USA 80: 5762

Hollyday M, Hamburger V 1976 Reduction of the naturally occurring motor neuron loss by enlargement of the periphery. Journal of Comparative Neurology 170: 311

Horwitz A, Duggan K, Greggs R, Decker C, Buck C 1985 The cell substrate attachment (CSAT) antigen has properties of a receptor for laminin and fibronectin. Journal of Cell Biology 101: 2134

Houenou L, Prevette D, Oppenheim R 1989 Motoneuron

survival in vivo following treatment with extracts from active and inactive muscle. Soc Neurosci Abstr 15: 436

Hughes S M, Blau H M 1992 Muscle fiber pattern is independent of cell lineage in postnatal rodent development. Cell 68: 659

Hurko O, McKee L, Zuurveld J G E M 1986 Transfection of human skeletal muscle cells with SV40 large T antigen gene coupled to a metallothionein promoter. Annals of Neurology 20: 573

Hurko O, McKee L, Zuurveld J, Swick H M 1987 Comparison of Duchenne and normal myoblasts from a heterozygote. Neurology 37: 675

Hynes R 1992 Integrins: versatility, modulation and signalling in cell adhesion. Cell 69: 11

Ibraghimov-Beskrovnaya O J M, Ervasti C-J, Leveille C A, Slaughter S W, Sernett, Campbell K P 1992 Primary structure of dystrophin-associated glycoproteins linking dystrophin to the extracellular matrix. Nature 355: 696

Jaffredo T, Horwitz A F, Buck C A, Rong P M, Dieterlen-Lievre F 1988 Myoblast migration specifically inhibited in the chick embryo by grafted CSAT hybridoma cells secreting an anti-integrin antibody. Development 103: 431

Jones G E, Murphy S J, Watt D J 1990 Segregation of the myogenic cell lineage in mouse muscle development. Journal of Cell Science 97: 659

Kalderon N, Gilula N B 1979 Membrane events involved in myoblast fusion. Journal of Cell Biology 81: 411

Karpati et al 1993 Myoblast transfer in Duchenne muscular dystrophy. Annals of Neurology 34: 8

Knudsen K A 1990 Cell adhesion molecules in myogenesis. Current Opinion in Cell Biology 2: 902

Knudsen K A, McElwee S, Myers L 1990 A role for the neural cell adhesion molecule, NCAM, in myoblast interaction during myogenesis. Developmental Biology 138: 159

Knudsen K A, Smith L, McElwee S 1989 Involvement of cell surface phosphatidylinositol-anchored glycoproteins in cell–cell adhesion of chick embryo myoblasts. Journal of Cell Biology 109: 1779

Kobayashi H, Robbins N, Rutishauser U 1992 Neural cell adhesion molecule in aged mouse muscle. Neuroscience 48: 237

Konieczny S F, Emerson C P Jr 1984 5-Azacytidine induction of stable mesodermal stem cell lineages from 10T cells: evidence for regulatory genes controlling determination. Cell 38: 791

Kuhl U M, Ocalan R, Timpl, Von Der Mark K 1986 Role of laminin and fibronectin in selecting myogenic versus fibrogenic cells from skeletal muscle cells in vitro. Developmental Biology 117: 628

Lan P K, Goodwin T G, Fang Q et al 1991 Myoblast transfer therapy for Duchenne Muscular Dystrophy. Acta Paediatrica Japan 33: 206

Lance-Jones C, Landmesser L 1980 Motoneuron projection patterns in the chick hindlimb following early partial spinal cord reversals. Journal of Physiology 302: 581

Lance-Jones C, Landmesser L 1981a Pathway selection by embryonic chick motoneurons in an experimentally altered environment. Proceedings of the Royal Society of London. Series B: Biological Sciences 214: 19

Lance-Jones C, Landmesser L 1981b Pathway selection by chick lumbosacral motoneurons during normal development. Proceedings of the National Academy of Sciences USA 214: 1

Landmesser L, Dahm L, Schultz K, Rutishauser U 1988 Distinct roles for adhesion molecules during innervation of embryonic chick muscle. Developmental Biology 130: 645

Landmesser L, Dahm L, Tang J C, Rutishauser U 1990 Polysialic acid as a regulator of intramuscular nerve branching during embryonic development. Neuron 4: 655

Lash J W, Ostrovsky D 1986 On the formation of somites In: Browder L W (ed) Developmental biology. A comprehensive treatise. Vol 2. The cellular basis of morphogenesis. Plenum, New York p 547

Lee C C, Pearlman J A, Chamberlain J S, Caskey C T 1991 Expression of recombinant dystrophin and its localisation to the cell membrane. Nature 349: 334

Lyons G E, Moore R, Yahara O, Buckingham M E, Walsh F S 1992 Expression of NCAM isoforms during skeletal myogenesis in the mouse embryo. Developmental Dynamics 194: 94

Manthorpe M, Skaper S D, Williams L R, Varon S 1986 Purification of adult rat sciatic nerve ciliary neurontrophic factor. Brain Research 367: 282

Martinou J-C, Martinou I, Kato A C 1992 Cholinergic differentiation factor (CDF/LIF) promotes survival of isolated rat embryonic motoneurons in vitro. Neuron 8: 737

Matsunaga M, Hatta K, Nagafuchi A, Takeichi M 1988 Guidance of optic nerve fibres by N-cadherin adhesion molecules. Nature 334: 62

Mauro A 1961 Satellite cells of skeletal muscle fibres. Journal of Biophysical and Biochemical Cytology 9: 493

McLennan I S 1983 Differentiation of muscle fiber types in the chicken hindlimb. Developmental Biology 97: 222

McManaman J L, Oppenheim R W, Prevette D, Marchetti D 1990 Rescue of motoneurons from cell death by a purified skeletal muscle polypeptide: effects of the ChAT development factor, CDF. Neuron 4: 891

Menko A S, Boettiger D 1987 Occupation of the extracellular matrix receptor, integrin, is a control point for myogenic differentiation. Cell 51: 51

Miller J B 1991 Myoblasts, Myosins, MyoDs, and the diversification of muscle fibers. Neuromuscular Disorders 1: 7

Miller J B 1992 Myoblast diversity in skeletal myogenesis: how much and to what end. Cell 69: 1

Miller J B, Stockdale F E 1986 Developmental origins of skeletal muscle fibers: clonal analysis of myogenic cell lineages based on fast and slow myosin heavy chain expression. Proceedings of the National Academy of Sciences USA 83: 3860

Miller J B, Stockdale F E 1987 What muscle cells know that nerves don't tell them. Trends in Neuroscience 10: 325

Moore S E, Thompson J, Kirkness V, Dickson J G, Walsh F S 1987 Skeletal muscle neuronal cell adhesion molecule (NCAM). Changes in protein and mRNA species during myogenesis of muscle cell lines. Journal of Cell Biology 105: 1377

Moore S E, Walsh F S 1986 Nerve dependent regulation of neural cell adhesion molecule expression in skeletal muscle. Neuroscience 18: 499

Moore R, Walsh F S 1993 The cell adhesion molecule M-cadherin is specifically expressed in developing and regenerating, but not denervated muscle. Development 117: 1409

Olson E N 1990 MyoD family: a paradigm for development? Genes and Development 4: 1454

Oppenheim R W 1989 The neurotrophic theory and naturally occurring motoneuron death. Trends in Neuroscience 12: 252

Oppenheim R W, Prevette D, Qin-Wei Y, Collins F, MacDonald J 1991 Control of embryonic motoneuron survival in vivo by ciliary neurotrophic factor. Science 251: 1616

Ott M-O, Bober E, Lyons G, Arnold H, Buckingham M 1991 Early expression of the myogenic regulatory gene Myf-s in precursor cells of skeletal muscle in the mouse embryo. Development 111: 1097

Partridge T A 1991 Myoblast transfer: a possible therapy for inherited myopathies. Muscle and Nerve 14: 197

Partridge T A, Morgan J E, Coulton G R, Hoffman E P, Kunkel L M 1989 Conversion of *mdx* myofibres from dystrophin negative to positive by injection of normal myoblasts. Nature 337: 176

Patterson P H, Chun L L Y 1977 The induction of acetylcholine synthesis in primary cultures of dissociated rat sympathetic neurons. Effects of conditioned medium. Developmental Biology 56: 263

Payne H R, Burden S M, Lemmon V 1992 Modulation of growth cone morphology by substrate-bound adhesion molecules. Cell Motility and the Cytoskeleton 21: 65

Peck D, Walsh F S 1993 Differential effects of over-expressed neural cell adhesion molecule isoforms on myoblast fusion. Journal of Cell Biology 123: 1587

Phillips W P, Kopta C, Blount P, Gardner P D, Steinbach J H, Merlie J P 1991 Ach receptor-rich membrane domains organized in fibroblasts by recombinant 43-kilodalton protein. Science 251: 568

Pizzey J A, Jones G E, Walsh F S 1988 Requirements for the Ca^{2+} independent component in the initial intercellular adhesion of C2 myoblasts. Journal of Cell Biology 107: 2307

Pollerberg G E, Burridge K, Krebs K E, Goodman S R, Schachner M 1987 The 180-kD component of the neural cell adhesion molecule NCAM is involved in cell–cell contacts and cytoskeleton–membrane interactions. Cell and Tissue Research 250: 227

Ragot T, Vincent N, Chafey P et al 1992 Efficient adenovirus mediated transfer of a human minidystrophin gene to skeletal muscle of *mdx* mice. Nature 361: 647

Ranscht B, Bronner-Fraser M 1991 T-cadherin expression alternates with migrating neural crest in the trunk of the avian embryo. Development 111: 15

Reichardt L F, Tomaselli K J 1991 Extracellular matrix molecules and their receptors: functions in neural development. Annual Review of Neuroscience 14: 531

Rosen G D, Sanes J R, Lachance R, Cunningham J M, Roman J, Dean D C 1992 Roles for the Integrin VLA-4 and its counter receptor VCAM-1 in myogenesis. Cell 69: 1107

Rosenfeld M A, Siegfried W, Yoshimura K et al 1991 Adenovirus-mediated transfer of a recombinant alpha-1 antitrypsin gene to the lung epithelium in vivo. Science 252: 431

Rosenfeld M A, Yoshimura K, Trapnell B C et al 1992 In vivo transfer of the human cystic fibrosis transmembrane conductance regulator gene to the airway epithelium. Cell 68: 143

Saffell J, Walsh F S, Doherty P 1992 Direct activation of second messenger pathways mimic cell adhesion molecule-dependent neurite outgrowth. Journal of Cell Biology 118: 663

Sanes J R 1987 Cell lineage and the origin of muscle fibres. Trends in Neurosciences 10: 219

Sassoon D, Lyons G, Wright W E et al 1989 Expression of two myogenic regulatory factors, myogenin and MyoD1 during mouse embryogenesis. Nature 341: 303

Schafer B W, Blakely B T, Blau H M 1990 Cell history dictates response to myogenic regulators. Nature 344: 454

Schlosshauer B, Schwartz U, Rutishauser U 1984 Topological distribution of different forms of neural cell adhesion molecule in the developing chick visual system. Nature 310: 141

Small S J, Akeson R 1990 Expression of the unique NCAM VASE exon is independently regulated in distinct tissues during development. Journal of Cell Biology 111: 2089

Soler A P, Knudsen K A 1991 Colocalization of NCAM and N-cadherin in avian skeletal myoblasts. Developmental Biology 148: 389

Song K-S, Wang W, Foster R H, Bielser D A, Kaufman S J 1992 H36-α7 is a novel integrin alpha chain that is developmentally regulated during skeletal myogenesis. Journal of Cell Biology 117: 643

Springer T A 1990 Adhesion receptors of the immune system. Nature 346: 425

Stockdale F E 1989 Skeletal muscle fiber specification during development and the myogenic cell lineage. In: The assembly of the nervous system. Plenum, New York, pp 37–50

Stockdale F E, Miller J B, Feldman J L, Hager J 1988 Myogenic cell lineages. Commitment and modulation during differentiation of avian muscle. In: Stockdale F E, Kedes L (eds) Cellular and molecular biology of muscle development, vol 29. Alan R Liss, New York, pp 213–223

Takeichi M 1991 Cadherin cell adhesion receptors as a morphogenic regulator. Science 251: 1451

Tanaka H 1987 Chronic application of curare does not increase the level of motoneurone survival-promoting activity in limb muscle extracts during naturally occurring motoneurone cell death period. Developmental Biology 124: 347

Tang J, Landmesser L, Rutishauser U 1992 Polysialic acid influences specific pathfinding by avian motoneurons. Neuron 8: 1031

Thoenen H 1991 The changing scene of neurotrophic factors. TINS 14: 165

Thompson L 1992a Cell-transplant results under fire. Science 257: 472

Thompson L 1992b Researchers call for time out on cell-transplant research. Science 257: 738

Tosney K W, Landmesser L 1984 Pattern and specificity of axonal outgrowth following varying degrees of chick limb bud ablation. Journal of Neuroscience 4: 2518

Tosney K W, Watanabe M, Landmesser L, Rutishauser U 1986 The distribution of NCAM in the chick hindlimb during axon outgrowth and synaptogenosis. Journal of Developmental Biology 114: 1464

Unsicker K, Reichert-Preibesch H, Schmidt R, Pettman B, Labroudette G, Sensenbrenner M 1987 Astrological and fibroblast growth factors have neurotrophic functions for cultured peripheral and central nervous system neurons. Proceedings of the National Academy of Sciences USA 84: 5459

Vincent N, Ragot T, Gilgen Krantz H et al 1993 Long term correction of mouse dystrophic degeneration by adenovirus mediated transfer of a minidystrophin gene. Nature Genetics 5: 130

Vivarelli E, Brown W E, Whalen R G, Cossu G 1988 The expression of slow myosin during mammalian somitogenesis and limb bud differentiation. Journal of Cell Biology 107: 2191

Wakelam M J O 1988 Myoblast fusion – a mechanistic analysis. Current Topics in Membranes and Transport 32: 87

Walsh F S 1990 N-CAM is a target cell surface antigen for the purification of muscle cells for myoblast transfer therapy. In: Griggs R C, Karpati G (eds) Myoblast transfer therapy. Plenum, New York, pp 41–46

Walsh F S, Doherty P 1991 Structure and function of the gene for neural cell adhesion molecule. Seminars in the Neurosciences 3: 271

Walsh F S, Doherty P 1992 Second messenger underlying cell contact dependent axonal growth stimulated by transfer NCAM, N-cadherin or L1. Cold Spring Harbor Symposium on Quantitative Biology 57: 431

Walsh F S, Furness J, Moore S E, Ashton S, Doherty P 1992 Use of the NCAM VASE exons by neurons is associated with a specific down regulation of NCAM dependent neurite outgrowth in the developing cerebellum and hippocampus. Journal of Neurochemistry 59: 1959

Walsh F S, Ritter M A 1981 Surface antigen differentiation during human myogenesis culture. Nature 289: 60

Weber M 1981 A diffusible factor responsible for the determination of cholinergic functions in cultured sympathetic neurons. Journal of Biological Chemistry 246: 3447

Webster C, Pavlath G K, Parks D R, Walsh F S, Blau H M 1988a Isolation of human myoblasts with the fluorescence-activated cell sorter. Experimental Cell Research 174: 252

Webster S, Travis M, Webster C, Rich K, Silberstein L, Blau H M 1988b Spatial and temporal regulation of myosin heavy chain isoform expression during human skeletal muscle development. Journal of Cell Biochemistry 12C: 345

Weintraub H, Davis R, Tapscott S 1991 The myo-D gene family: nodal point during specification of the muscle cell lineage. Science 251: 761

Wells D J, Wells K E, Walsh F S et al 1992 Human dystrophin expression corrects the myopathic phenotype in transgenic mdx mice. Human Molecular Genetics 1: 35–40

White N K, Hauschka S D 1971 Muscle development in vitro. A new conditioned medium effect on colony differentiation. Experimental Cell Research 67: 479

Williams E J, Doherty P, Turner G, Reid R A, Hemperly J J, Walsh F S 1992 Calcium influx into neurons can solely account for cell-contact dependent neurite outgrowth stimulated by transfected L1. Journal of Cell Biology 119: 883

Williams E J, Walsh F S, Doherty P 1994 Tyrosine kinase inhibitors can differentially inhibit integrin-dependent and CAM stimulated neurite outgrowth. Journal of Cell Biology 124: 1029

Wolff J A, Malone R W, Williams P et al 1990 Direct gene transfer into mouse muscle in vivo. Science 247: 1465

Wolff J A, Williams P, Acsadi G, Jiao S, Jani A, Chong W 1991 Conditions affecting direct gene transfer into rodent muscle in vivo. Biotechniques 11: 474

Yasin R G, Van Beers G, Nurse K, Landon D N, Thompson E J 1977 A quantitative technique for growing human adult skeletal muscle in culture starting from mononucleated cells. Journal of the Neurological Sciences 32: 347

3. Molecular biology of muscle — the generation of protein diversity

Louise V. B. Nicholson

INTRODUCTION

When myoblasts fuse to become myotubes and, eventually, mature muscle fibres, the organisation and control of gene and protein expression changes. While myoblasts are single cells with individual nuclei which are capable of division, mature muscle fibres are multinucleated cells which have turned from division to differentiation. The degree of coordination that is required for effective gene expression becomes very obvious when one considers that a 1 cm segment from a single muscle fibre may contain over 1 000 myonuclei (Landing et al 1974). Terminally differentiated fibres have particular characteristics: they are very large (a single fibre from a human sartorius muscle may be over 30 cm long with a volume of cytoplasm which totals several microlitres), very long-lived (repairing themselves rather than reproducing), and very complex with a well-defined organisation of overlapping thick and thin filaments which give skeletal muscle its characteristically striated appearance. The fibres interact with nerves at neuromuscular junctions, and these regions require localized concentrations of particular proteins. Superimposed upon this is the need to respond to changing requirements and altered patterns of activity, for example, during development, or during intensive training for a sporting activity. The aim of this chapter is to describe how skeletal muscle generates diverse forms of proteins to cope with these changing requirements, and to review the categories of factors which may control or influence the choice of protein expressed.

Unlike the prokaryotic genes of bacteria, the eukaryotic genes of higher animals have exons or expressed sequences which are interspersed with non-coding introns. Skeletal muscle contains the largest gene identified to date (dystrophin, ~2 500 000 base pairs), the longest intron (~180 000 bp) and the largest number of exons (~79) which are also found in dystrophin (Koenig et al 1987, den Dunnen et al 1989). A gene with the largest number of exon permutations identified so far — 32 different combinations for exons 4–8 — is present in one of the troponin T genes (Breitbart et al 1987). Vertebrate striated muscle also has the longest known single-chain protein (titin, with a molecular mass of ~3000 kDa). Single titin molecules are long enough to stretch from the Z-disc to the M-line, a length of over 1 μm in resting muscle, and may form the template for the assembly of other proteins into the thick filament (Fulton & Isaacs 1991).

Individual nuclei may control the production of proteins present in their immediate vicinity, and the restricted distribution of some proteins, particularly at neuromuscular junctions, has led to the concept of 'nuclear domains' where protein synthesis is compartmentalized and controlled by individual nuclei within the syncytium (Pavlath et al 1989, Ralston & Hall 1992, Simon et al 1992).

The flow diagram in Figure 3.1 indicates the hierarchical stages in the production of a protein with the opportunities that can arise to generate diversity or alter expression. Genes which are encoded by mitochondrial DNA are not considered in this chapter. Each of the factors or mechanisms which can alter the diversity of protein expression is considered in turn in the following sections.

CHROMOSOMES AND DNA CONFORMATION

The DNA in metaphase chromosomes, such as those seen in pictures of a karyotype, is highly condensed relative to the extended linear length. Such highly coiled and condensed DNA, whether present in chromosomes or in the heterochromatin of interphase nuclei, is almost never transcriptionally active. The ratio of extended to compressed length is known as the 'packing ratio' and whereas the DNA in chromosomes and heterochromatin has a packing ratio in the range

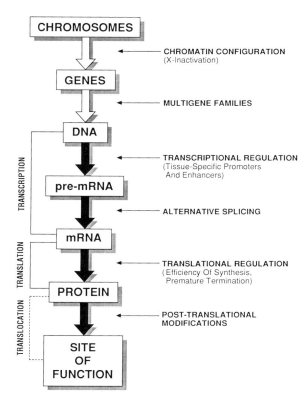

Fig. 3.1 Flow diagram of the stages involved in the production of a protein and the opportunities that arise to generate diversity or alter expression. Filled arrows indicate the formal stages of protein synthesis. Transcription and translation always occur, translocation may be required to transport a newly synthesised protein to its site of function.

of 1 000–10 000, the DNA from which mRNAs are transcribed in interphase nuclei has a packing ratio of only 1–10 (Hall 1992). A classic example of the regulatory power of chromatin configuration is in X-chromosome inactivation (Lyon 1962), in which one of the two chromosomes in cells that are genetically female is rendered constitutively heterochromatic (appearing in the nucleus as 'Barr bodies') so that almost none of the genes on such inactivated X-chromosomes are transcribed.

One practical aspect of X-inactivation involves women who are carriers of X-linked diseases. In any cell, the active X-chromosome may be either the normal or abnormal one. If, by chance, there is a non-random distribution and a high proportion of active abnormal-X, the carriers themselves may show some disease symptoms. Thus women

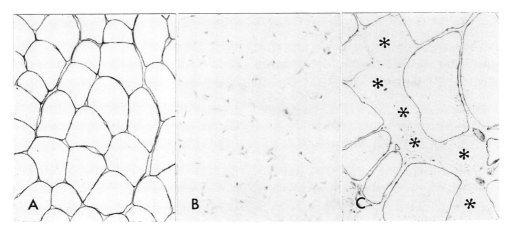

Fig. 3.2 Immunolabelling of dystrophin in transverse sections of skeletal muscle. **A** Control showing uniform labelling at the periphery of all fibres. **B** Patient with Duchenne muscular dystrophy (DMD) who has a mutation of the Xp21 locus and dystrophin-negative muscle fibres. **C** Manifesting carrier of DMD with a mixture of dystrophin-positive and -negative fibres. Fibres which do not express dystrophin (indicated with asterisks) have the normal X-chromosome inactive so that protein expression is controlled by the defective X-chromosome bearing the DMD mutation. Indirect peroxidase labelling, magnification × 140 (photographs by courtesy of Dr Margaret Johnson and Mr Martin Barron).

who carry mutations of the dystrophin gene may manifest the clinical signs of muscular dystrophy (Bonilla et al 1988, Arahata et al 1989). This may be particularly striking in pairs of female identical twin carriers, where one may manifest severe clinical symptoms while the other does not. Each severely affected twin appears to have skewed or non-random X-inactivation patterns so that a high proportion of their muscle fibres have the mutant X active (Burn et al 1986, Richards et al 1990, Lupski et al 1991). The possible effects of X-inactivation on dystrophin expression in female carriers are demonstrated in Figure 3.2, which shows the uniform dystrophin labelling at the periphery of muscle fibres in a control male subject (A), the absence of dystrophin in the muscle of a Duchenne muscular dystrophy (DMD) patient (B), and a mixture of the two types of labelling in a manifesting carrier (C) who has the normal X active in the dystrophin-positive fibres and the mutated X active in the dystrophin-negative fibres.

MULTI-GENE FAMILIES

In evolutionary terms, current multigene families arose from gene duplications which were found to be advantageous (or at least not disadvantageous),

and were therefore selected in subsequent generations. In some instances the genes remained clustered, but if the duplication event was followed by crossing over and recombination between non-homologous chromosomes, the genes are translocated to a different chromosome. Pseudogenes are evolutionary 'blind alleys' which may be derived from a duplication event which then mutated into a gene which was missing some or all of the signals required for successful transcription, splicing or translation (Lewin 1990).

Skeletal muscle shares some common features with other excitable tissues (cardiac and smooth muscle, tissues of the nervous system) and many of the proteins in adult skeletal muscle have homologous counterparts (chains, subunits, isoforms) in these other tissues. One obvious way to generate protein diversity is to have different genes encoding related products and skeletal muscle has many examples of multigene families.

Genes on different chromosomes

Myosin is a hexameric ATPase composed of two heavy chains (MHC), two non-phosphorylated alkali light chains and two phosphorylatable regulatory light chains (MLC). Each of the three myosin subunits is encoded by multigene families which are specifically expressed according to tissue, developmental stage or physiological requirement (Buckingham et al 1986). In humans, genes for skeletal muscle MHCs have been assigned to chromosomes 17 and 7 (Karsch-Mizrachi et al 1989, 1990), those for cardiac MHCs to chromosome 14 (Matsuoka et al 1989, Qin et al 1990, Matsuoka et al 1990), and non-muscle isoforms to chromosomes 22 and 17 (Simons et al 1991, Toothaker et al 1991). Among the myosin light chains, fast skeletal MLC1/3 is assigned to chromosome 2 (Cohen-Haguenauer et al 1988), cardiac MLCs have been mapped to chromosomes 3, 12 and 17 (Cohen-Haguenauer et al 1989b, Seharaseyon et al 1990, Macera et al 1992), with a cardiac-like isoform assigned to chromosome 8 (Balazs et al 1985). A novel MLC isoform which is found in adult retina, cerebellum, basal ganglia and fetal skeletal muscle has recently been mapped to chromosome 4 (Collins et al 1992).

Other examples of human multigene families with protein isoforms in muscle include actin (Miwa et al 1991), tropomyosin (Lees-Miller & Helfman 1991), the troponins (see Emerson et al 1986), the acetylcholine receptor (AChR) subunits (Cohen-Haguenauer et al 1989a, Beeson et al 1990), creatine kinase (Kaye et al 1987, Nigro et al 1987), sodium channels (Agnew & Trimmer 1989), calcium channels (Biel et al 1991), potassium channels (Ghanshani et al 1992), spectrin (Winkelmann et al 1990, Liebhaber et al 1992), and several members of the family of cell adhesion molecules including the cadherins (Donalies et al 1991) and the integrins (Hynes 1992).

Gene clusters

Some members of gene families are organised together on the same chromosome, rather than being on different chromosomes. In humans, several adult, perinatal and embryonic isoforms of skeletal muscle myosin heavy chain (MYH1, MYH2, MYH3, MYH4 and MYH8) are clustered on the short arm of chromosome 17, while both the α and β cardiac MHC isoforms (MYH6 and MYH7) are assigned to the long arm of chromosome 14 (HGM 11 1991). Although the skeletal MHC genes are physically linked to

each other and are sequentially expressed during development, they do not appear to be activated in a coordinate manner and transcription of each gene is independently regulated, as in the corresponding rodent gene cluster (Cox et al 1991). The genes coding for the α, γ, δ subunits of the skeletal muscle AChR have all been localized to the region of 2q24-qter (Cohen-Haguenauer et al 1989a, Beeson et al 1990) and the genes for a group of myogenic determination factors (myf) are also clustered, on chromosome 12 (Braun et al 1990).

Genes within genes

Where does an isoform end and a new protein begin? Isoforms are derived from a common gene and generally represent subtle variations on a theme with an overall structure/function which is not vastly different from the basic molecule. Alternatively, proteins which are products of different genes but which share a family resemblance in terms of structure or function are said to be homologues. Thus α-actinin, spectrin and dystrophin are homologous members of the family of rod-like actin-binding proteins. Several examples now exist, however, of proteins which are encoded by parts of the same gene but which have such vastly different size, structure (and therefore presumably function) and tissue distribution, that it is tempting to regard them as different proteins. In general these 'genes within genes' result from rather extreme forms of alternative splicing and are initiated by their own promoters.

Dystrophin, the protein product of the gene which is defective in Duchenne/Becker muscular dystrophy (Hoffman et al 1987), has a 'standard' molecule of about 427 kDa which is primarily expressed in skeletal and cardiac muscle, and to a lesser extent in smooth muscle and brain. This molecule has a globular amino domain, a central rod-like domain of triple helical repeats, a region which is relatively cysteine-rich and a globular carboxy terminal domain (Koenig et al 1988). This gene product is synthesized from a 14 kb transcript using one of three 5' promoters (Chelly et al 1990, Górecki et al 1992). Recently, however, alternative transcripts of 6.5 kb (Bar et al 1990)

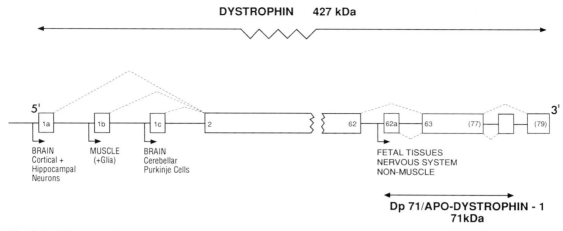

Fig. 3.3 Diagrammatic representation of the alternative promoters and two major products of the dystrophin gene. The numbers indicate exons, which are not drawn to scale. The numerous variations produced by cassette-type alternative splicing which have been reported for the large dystrophin transcript are not shown. The organization of the exons at the 3' end of the gene has not been confirmed, and the inferred exon numbers are shown in parentheses.

and/or 4.5–4.8 kb (Blake et al 1992, Hugnot et al 1992) have been identified which originate from a promoter in the intron between exons 62 and 63 of the full-size molecule (Fig. 3.3). This transcript (or transcripts) appears to encode a protein with a molecular mass of only ~71 kDa. The short transcript has a unique first exon and then shares the remaining cysteine-rich and C-terminal exons of full-length dystrophin (with an alternative terminus), but is without the exons forming the actin-binding amino domain or central rod domain (Lederfein et al 1992, Hugnot et al 1992). The short distal transcript (Dp71: Lederfein et al 1992, apo-dystrophin-1: Blake et al 1992) was not detected in adult skeletal muscle but was more abundant than the full-length 14 kb transcript in brain, tissue containing smooth muscle (stomach, lung, skin and testis) and many fetal tissues (Hugnot et al 1992, Rapaport et al 1992b). In addition, the distal transcript and a protein of about 70–80 kDa were identified in tissues where the full-length protein is not generally synthesized: liver, kidney and spleen, plus hepatoma, lymphoblastoid and Schwannoma cell lines (Bar et al 1990, Blake et al 1992, Rapaport et al 1992b). The function of full-length dystrophin in muscle is thought to be related to the fact that it forms a link between actin on the inside of fibres (e.g. Levine et al 1992) and laminin in the extracellular matrix on the outside of the sarcolemma,

via a complex of six proteins, four of which are glycoproteins (Ervasti & Campbell 1991, Ibraghimov-Beskrovnaya et al 1992). The central rod domain may act as a 'spacer' between adjacent glycoprotein complexes. Since the protein product of the small distal transcript lacks both the actin-binding domain and the rod-like spacer domain, and is found in different tissues from 'standard' dystrophin, it is likely to have a different function. At present that function is unknown, but its abundance in brain has led to the suggestion that it may be implicated in the intellectual impairment which has long been recognised as a feature of Duchenne dystrophy (reviewed by Emery in 1988).

Around the same time that the dystrophin 'gene within a gene' was being investigated, other examples of the independent expression of the carboxy terminal domains of proteins were described. Calspermin, a small acidic protein identified in rat testis, represents the independent expression of the carboxy terminus of a Ca^{2+}/calmodulin-dependent protein kinase which is found in cerebellar granule cells (Means et al 1991, Ohmstede et al 1991). Similarly, the carboxy terminal domain of smooth muscle myosin light chain kinase (MLCK) was found to be expressed as one or more separate proteins named 'telokin' (Ito et al 1989) or kinase-related protein, KRP (Collinge et al 1992).

CONTROL OF TRANSCRIPTION

Eukaryotic genes are of three types, each transcribed by a different RNA polymerase. Class l genes are tandemly linked ribosomal RNA genes which are clustered in the nucleolus. Class II genes produce messenger RNA (mRNA) and are characterised by a promoter region at the 5' end and the presence of introns. Enhancers are commonly found at the 5' end, although they may be internal or lie downstream of the gene (Fig. 3.4). Transcription factor binding sites are also found at the 5′ end of the gene. Class III genes, which include those producing transfer RNA (tRNA), are physically small and characterized by internal promoters (reviewed by Lewin 1990, Beebee & Burke 1992).

Transcription of Class II genes starts with the core promoter, which is located just upstream of the transcript start site or 'cap site', so named because the 5' ends of eukaryotic mRNAs are modified or capped by the addition of a methylated G residue (Fig. 3.4). Elements in the promoter are recognised, and bound in turn, by the initiation proteins TFIID, TFIIA, TFIIB, the class-specific RNA polymerase pol II, TFIIE and TFIIF. Once assembled, this very large complex (with a total molecular mass of over 900 kDa) is poised to unwind locally the DNA template and initiate transcription. Initiation requires the hydrolysis of an ATP molecule and the formation of a 'rapid start complex'. Elongation of the primary transcript commences with the phosphorylation of pol II and is accompanied by the binding of another protein, TFIS. The rate of transcription depends upon the binding of yet more regulatory factors. A sequence which codes for the polyadenylation signal (AAUAAA) is found just before the end of the transcript. The end of the pre-mRNA is clipped and a stabilising poly(A) tail is added to the mature mRNA about 20–30 bp after this signal (Fig. 3.4).

cis-acting elements

Although the same genes are present in all cells, ultilization of specific cis-acting DNA sequences and trans-acting factors allows gene transcription to be regulated in a tissue- or developmental stage-specific manner. cis-acting modulators exert an effect on their own gene (e.g. promoters and enhancers), whereas trans-acting factors or proteins are not an integral part of the gene themselves. Among the best characterised of the general cis elements are the TATA box (frequently required for the correct initiation at the transcription start site), and the CAAT and/or GC boxes (which play a role in controlling the frequency of initiation) (Beebee & Burke 1992). Specific patterns of DNA methylation around promoter regions may also play a role in controlling tissue- or developmental-

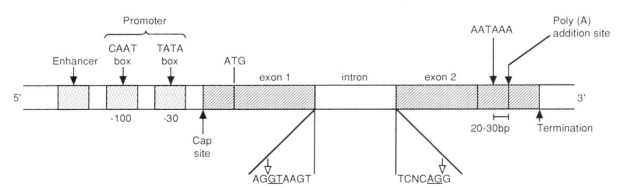

Fig. 3.4 Organisation of a Class II gene. A typical gene is characterised by a promoter region at the 5' end and the presence of introns. In some cases the CAAT and TATA consensus sequences are absent. Transcription factor binding sites are found at the 5' end of the gene, as are many enhancer elements. The exon/intron splice sites are indicated with open arrows. The left junction (splice donor) and right junction (splice acceptor) consensus sequences are shown with the most invariant dinucleotides underlined. See text for other details (modified from an illustration in Beebee & Burke 1992, by permission of Oxford University Press).

specific promotion of gene expression (Lloyd et al 1987, Lamson & Stockdale 1989, Edwards 1990).

A number of muscle-associated regulatory elements have been described and the best characterized of these is the CArG box, originally identified in the promoters of cardiac and skeletal muscle α-actin (Miwa et al 1987, Muscat & Kedes 1987), but found subsequently, by deletion and mutational analysis, to be required for the muscle-specific activation of genes for myosin light chain (Arnold et al 1988, Kurabayashi et al 1990), troponin T (Mar et al 1988), troponin C (Parmacek & Leiden 1989), creatine kinase (Sternberg et al 1988) and dystrophin (Klamut et al 1990, Gilgenkrantz et al 1992). Multiple CArG boxes may be present which interact with each other and with the initiating TATA sequence (Miwa & Kedes 1987). Such cis-acting elements may also be found after the first exon (Ng et al 1989, Nikovits et al 1990), and at the 3' end of the gene (Donoghue et al 1988) as well as in the conventional position upstream of the cap site.

Another potentially 'muscle-specific' promoter element is the MCAT (muscle-CAT) consensus CATTCCT and disruption of only one or two of these sequence elements can abolish the ability to direct muscle-specific transcription (Mar & Ordahl 1988). The promoters or enhancers of many muscle genes also contain a consensus sequence referred to as an E-box (CANNTG), which forms the binding site for many of the basic-helix-loop-helix (bHLH) regulatory factors described in the next section. Multiple E-boxes or their homologues are found in the 5' regions of genes for myosin heavy chain (Vosberg et al 1992), troponin I (Lin et al 1991), muscle creatine kinase (Yi et al 1991) and the acetylcholine receptor subunits (Gilmour et al 1991, Prody & Merlie 1991). The gene for the immature AChR γ-subunit contains two adjacent CANNTG sequence motifs that appear to be essential for muscle-specific transcriptional activity. The gene for the mature ε-subunit carries only a single CANNTG motif which is not required for the positive expression in muscle cells, but is necessary for repressing transcription in non-muscle cells (Numberger et al 1991). Promoter elements may also play a role in restricting transcription to synaptic nuclei (Klarsfeld et al 1991).

Many tissue-specific promoters are associated with alternative 5' exons. Figure 3.3 (see earlier section) illustrates the promoters that have been identified to date for dystrophin. The most 5' promoter (e.g. associated with the exon labelled 1a in Fig. 3.3) is active in brain and transcripts have been localised to cortical and hippocampal neurones (Chelly et al 1990, Górecki et al 1992). Interestingly, the loss of this promoter does not seem to be associated with intellectual impairment (Boyce et al 1991, den Dunnen et al 1991, Rapaport et al 1992c). The first promoter appears to be quite restricted in its activity compared with the next promoter (associated with exon 1b), which is active in skeletal, cardiac and smooth muscle and, to a lesser extent, in some neurones and cultured glial cells. This promoter is 'leaky' and low levels of transcription ('illegitimate' or 'ectopic'), may occur in fibroblasts and lymphocytes (Chelly et al 1990). The muscle promoter contains a TATA box, a GC-rich motif, and several conserved motifs which have been found in muscle-specific genes (Klamut et al 1990, Gilgenkrantz el al 1992). In contrast, the brain promoter does not contain any of these elements, and may use a less defined 'initiator' element instead (Makover et al 1991). The third 5' promoter (plus its associated exon labelled 1c) is reported to be specific for cerebellar Purkinje neurones (Górecki et al 1992). As discussed in the previous section the fourth, distal, promoter (with its exon labelled 62a) appears to direct transcription in fetal tissues, a number of nervous tissues, and non-muscle tissues or cell lines.

trans-acting factors

trans-factors which may bind to promoter or enhancer elements include the bHLH superfamily of regulatory transcription factors which all have a DNA-binding basic sequence adjacent to a helix-loop-helix domain which is required for the formation of dimers. The MyoD (myogenic determination) family is a group of muscle-associated bHLH transcription factors which include MyoD1, myogenin, myf-5 and MRF4 (myf-6 or herculin) (see reviews by Olson 1990, Buckingham 1992). These proteins associate into homodimers, or sometimes more effectively into heterodimers with other members of the MyoD family or with members of the more ubiquitous E-protein class of bHLH factors which includes the E12 and E47 proteins, ITF2 and HEB (Hu et al 1992). Conversely, when another bHLH protein, Id (inhibitor of differentiation), binds to E12, dimerization with MyoD family members is prevented and transcription is inhibited (Benezra et al 1990). Proliferin, a protein with homology to prolactin and growth hormone, has also been identified as a selective inhibitor of bHLH *trans*-activators in the actin multigene family (Muscat et al 1991).

The genes for many muscle proteins are not equally sensitive to the various members of the MyoD family (Yutzey et al 1990). Thus, muscle-specific processing of tropomyosin transcripts can continue in the absence of myogenin, unlike the expression of muscle actin and skeletal myosin heavy chain (Saitoh et al 1990). Transcription of some acetylcholine receptor subunit genes requires MyoD muscle-specific activation (Piette et al 1990, Gilmour et al 1991, Prody & Merlie 1991), while expression of genes for cardiac myosin heavy chain (Thompson et al 1991), cardiac/slow myosin light chain (Lee et al 1992) and dystrophin (Gilgenkrantz et al 1992) can be activated through MyoD-independent pathways.

Other factors which have the potential to regulate transcription in skeletal muscle include the muscle actin promoter factors or MAPFs (Walsh 1989, Ernst et al 1991), myocyte nuclear factors (MEF-1 and -2) which are protein homologues of MyoD1 (Buskin & Hauschka 1989, Gossett et al 1989), TA-rich recognition protein TARP (Horlick et al 1990), and DNA-binding proteins from skeletal muscle extracts identified as muscle factor 3 (Santoro et al 1991) and distal regulatory factors DRF-1, 2 and 3 (Muscat et al 1992), plus a new factor detected in rat cardiac and skeletal muscle, which has been rather humorously named Myomy (Gupta et al 1992).

RNA SPLICING

Constitutive splicing

Precise excision of intron sequences from the primary pre-mRNA transcript and concomitant ligation of the exons is accomplished in the nucleus through a sequence of splicing processes. In a simple gene, each exon present is incorporated into one mature mRNA transcript through the invariant joining of consecutive pairs of donor and acceptor splice sites, thereby producing a single gene product from each transcriptional unit (reviewed in Beebee & Burke 1992, Arnstein & Cox 1992).

The mechanisms of pre-mRNA splicing are the subject of much current interest and examples of erroneous splicing may be informative in this context. Thus, in dystrophin Kobe, the deletion of 52 bp near the 5' splice donor site within exon 19 of the dystrophin gene leads to the skipping of exon 19 during mRNA splicing, to disruption of the open reading frame and to premature termination of translation (Matsuo et al 1990, 1991). Although this deletion does not affect the splice site directly, it abolishes the formation of an intra-exonic hairpin structure which the wild-type dystrophin mRNA precursor is able to produce in its secondary structure. The hairpin structures were also found in a further 22 separate exons indicating that they may be essential components for constitutive splicing of dystrophin mRNA (Matsuo et al 1992). Other dystrophin gene defects which lead directly to defective RNA splicing and exon skipping include a single base change in the 3' splice site of intron 6, resulting in the skipping of exon 7 in dystrophin-deficient Golden Retriever dogs (Sharp et al 1992).

A variant of osteogenesis imperfecta is caused by a point mutation which alters a constitutive splice site in one of the pro-α chains of type 1 collagen. This results in the skipping of exon 28 and, although the open reading frame is maintained, the loss of the exon prohibits subunit assembly and results in a lethal phenotype (Tromp & Prockop 1988).

Alternative splicing

In many genes expressed in muscle, constitutive RNA splicing is enriched by varieties of alternative splicing which generate multiple forms of protein from a single gene (see reviews by McKeown 1990, Nadal-Ginard et al 1991). Figure 3.5 illus-

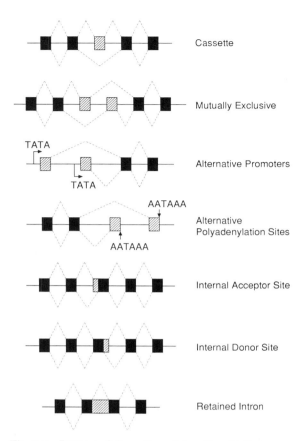

Cassette

Mutually Exclusive

Alternative Promoters

Alternative Polyadenylation Sites

Internal Acceptor Site

Internal Donor Site

Retained Intron

Fig. 3.5 Patterns of alternative splicing. Constitutive exons (black), alternative sequences (striped), and introns (solid lines) are spliced according to different pathways (dotted lines). Alternative promoters (TATA) and polyadenylation signals (AATAAA) are indicated (reproduced, with permission, from the Annual Review of Biochemistry Vol. 56, © 1987 by Annual Reviews Inc. (Breitbart et al 1987)).

trates the various mechanisms which result in the production of alternative transcripts.

Combinatorial cassette exons. While exons which are included in all transcripts are constitutive, individual whole exons which may or may not be included are said to be combinatorial cassettes (Breitbart et al 1987). Troponin T, which is a component of the Ca²⁺ sensitive complex that regulates the interactions of tropomyosin with the actin filaments in striated muscle, contains several such exons. The fast skeletal troponin T gene in the rat contains a group of five exons which may be assembled together in 32 different combinations (Fig. 3.6)

(Breitbart et al 1987). Although several different transcripts may be detected at the same time in the same fibre, the default splicing pattern is the exclusion of exons 4–8 and their inclusion is controlled by the state of differentiation and physiological demand (Breitbart & Nadal-Ginard 1989). The extreme heterogeneity caused by the alternative splicing of exons 4–8 may be important in modulating interactions of TnT within the troponin/tropomyosin complex (Breitbart & Nadal-Ginard 1989). The extent of alternative splicing among the human troponin genes has not yet been fully elucidated, but it has been demonstrated in the genes for slow skeletal TnT (Gahlmann et al 1987) and slow and fast skeletal TnC (Schreier et al 1990).

The neural cell adhesion molecule (NCAM) is expressed in neurones, glia and skeletal muscle, after transient expression in a number of early embryonic structures. In skeletal muscle NCAM is implicated in several aspects of myogenesis including innervation and synaptogenesis (see Ch. 2). The human gene for NCAM is extensively spliced and processed in a tissue-specific manner, and a block of 4 exons (the smallest exon coding for a single amino acid) is spliced in between exons 12 and 13 of the brain transcript, to form a 'muscle-specific domain' in the extracellular domain of the molecule (Dickson et al 1987). Vinculin is another protein associated with cell–cell interactions and a larger form of the protein, meta-vinculin, is found only in smooth and skeletal muscle. Like NCAM, this 'muscle-specificity' is generated by the splicing of an additional exon into the basic transcript (Koteliansky et al 1992).

A number of alternatively spliced transcripts have been identified in the dystrophin gene. In addition to alternative proximal and distal promoters with inital exons, a number of splice variants have been detected in the C-terminal domain (Feener et al 1989, Geng et al 1991, Bies et al 1992) and in the central rod domain (Geng et al 1991). The variation seems to be most extensive in non-muscle tissues, particularly in the brain (Bies et al 1992), and possibly in the retina (Ray et al 1992) and other synaptic sites including Purkinje conduction fibres in the heart (Bies et al 1992).

Cassette exons have also been found for the

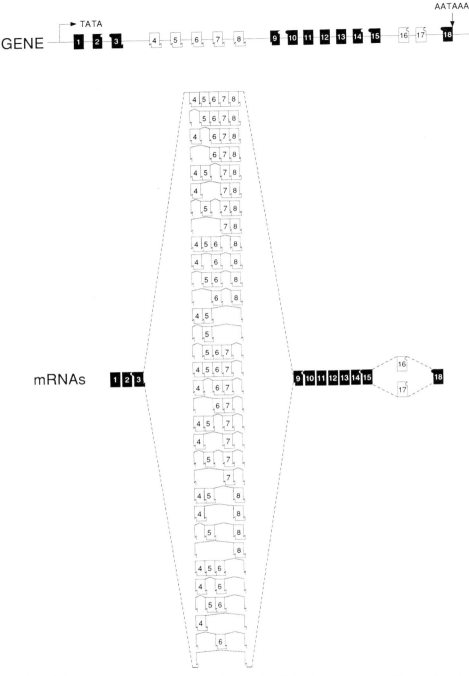

Fig. 3.6   Alternative splicing patterns among the 18 exons of the rat fast skeletal muscle troponin T gene. Constitutive exons are indicated by black boxes and alternative sequences are indicated by open boxes. The shape of each box represents the codon position of the exon boundary — sawtooth edges indicate boundaries which lie between the first and second nucleotide of the codon, concave/convex shapes are boundaries between the second and third nucleotide, and straight edges indicate exon boundaries lying between intact codons. Each mRNA comprises the constitutive sequences, one of the 32 combinations of exons 4–8, and either exon 16 or 17. The total number of possible mRNA species is therefore 64 (reproduced, with permission, from the Annual Review of Biochemistry, Vol. 56 © 1987 by Annual Reviews Inc. (Breitbart et al 1987)).

muscle isoforms of human tropomyosin (MacLeod & Gooding 1988), L-type calcium channels (Biel et al 1991), insulin receptors (Moller et al 1989) and agrin. Agrin is a component of the synaptic basal lamina and alternative use of cassette exons in a region near the C-terminus generates four isoforms which are implicated in the mediation of acetylcholine receptor clustering. Two isoforms are active in cluster formation by themselves but the other two require some form of interaction with proteoglycans in the basal lamina before they are active (Ferns et al 1992).

Mutually exclusive exons. Exons which are never spliced together in the same transcript are mutually exclusive. Exons 16 and 17 of the rat troponin T gene are organised like this (see Fig. 3.6). Tropomyosin (TM), in skeletal muscle, contains α and β subunits which are assembled into homo- and heterodimers in variable proportions depending on the fibre type (Schachat et al 1985). Analogous pairs of mutually exclusive exons in the rat α- and β-TM genes encode different internal domains that specify, in part, the skeletal and smooth or non-muscle TM isoforms (Helfman et al 1986). The human α-TM gene has two mutually exclusive versions of exon 5, one of which is expressed specifically in skeletal muscle (Graham et al 1992). Other genes with mutually exclusive exons include myosin light chain 1/3 (Periasamy et al 1984), pyruvate kinase (Noguchi et al 1986) and phosphorylase kinase (Harmann et al 1991).

Several different mechanisms have been proposed to account for alternative splice site selection in these genes. These include the relative strengths of 5' and 3' splice sites, intron size, the pyrimidine content of 3' splice site, the location, number and sequence of branch points, intron sequences between a 3' splice site and upstream branch point, exon sequences and sequence-specific RNA-binding proteins (reviewed in McKeown 1990).

Alternative promoters and/or polyadenylation sites. Alternative 5' and 3' end sequences arise through the differential utilization of promoters or cleavage sites, each associated with their own exons. This can generate variability in the amino acid sequences of the amino- and carboxy-

terminal domains which, in turn, may regulate interactions with other proteins, in a tissue-specific manner. In dystrophin, for example, three tissue-related promoters and exons have been identified at the 5' end of the gene plus a fourth distal promoter plus exon (see Fig. 3.3). In addition, alternative 3' exons generate other tissue and developmentally regulated isoforms (e.g. Feener at al 1989, Geng et al 1991).

Alternative promoter selection dictates the splicing pattern of the gene for myosin light chain 1_F and 3_F (Periasamy et al 1984) and produces a muscle-specific isoform of aldolase (Maire et al 1987) and phosphofructokinase (Yamasaki et al 1991), while examples of alternative 3' exons and polyadenylation sites are found in tropomyosin (Helfman et al 1986) and myosin heavy chain (Saez et al 1990). Human erythrocyte and skeletal muscle β-spectrin are transcribed from the same gene, but in skeletal muscle the C-terminal exon of the erythrocyte form (which is involved in phosphorylation-dependent αβ subunit interactions) is spliced out and replaced with four longer exons (Winkelmann et al 1990). The presence of such a different C-terminal domain in skeletal muscle β-spectrin may indicate an association with a different membrane protein complex from that found in erythrocytes.

Alternative acceptor and donor splice sites. Many of the examples already cited include the utilization of alternative splice sites. The alternative production of calcitonin in thyroid C cells and calcitonin gene-related peptide neurones of the central and peripheral nervous system is primarily regulated by *cis*-active elements near the calcitonin-specific 3'-splice junction (Emeson et al 1989). Similarly, the transcripts for erythroid and non-erythroid β-spectrin differ in C-terminal splice site selection (Winkelmann et al 1990), and some of the sodium channel isoforms in brain, cardiac and skeletal muscle utilize alternative donor splice sites (Schaller et al 1992), as do isoforms of the acetylcholine receptor β-subunit (Goldman & Tamai 1989).

Retained introns. This is not a very common occurrence in mammals, but examples may be found in the genes for fibronectin (Schwarzbauer et al 1987), acetylcholinesterase in haematopoietic cells (Li et al 1991) and platelet-derived growth factor (Collins et al 1987, Tong et al 1987).

TRANSLATION

Proteins are synthesised from the amino- to the carboxy-terminus on ribosomes which move along the mRNA. In eukaryotes, mRNA translation starts with Met-tRNA binding to the 40S subunit of a ribosome together with initiation factors and guanosine 5'-diphosphate (GDP). This initiation complex then binds the mRNA at the cap structure, and scans along until the initiation codon AUG is reached (see Fig. 3.4 in earlier section). The 60S ribosomal subunit then binds and elongation of the polypeptide chain ensues. To become a substrate for protein synthesis, free amino acids are activated by coupling with the adenylic moiety of ATP and covalent linkage to transfer RNA via aminoacyl-tRNA synthetase. The resulting aminoacyl-tRNA is used by the ribosome as a substrate and the energy of the chemical bond between the amino acid residue and tRNA is used for forming a peptide bond (reviewed in Spirin 1986, Arnstein & Cox 1992).

The efficiency of translation may depend on several factors including sequences in the 5' untranslated region immediately preceding the initiation codon (Frances et al 1992), transcript secondary structures formed in the vicinity of the initiation codon (Murtagh et al 1991), and motifs in the 3' untranslated region (Baumann et al 1990). Translational efficiency is a useful regulatory process. Thus, although there are two genes for adult haemoglobin α-chain and only one for the β-chain, reduced efficiency of transcription and, particularly, of translation, ensures that there is not a significant overproduction of α-chains for assembly with β-chains in the final $\alpha_2\beta_2$ complex (Arnstein & Cox 1992, Liebhaber et al 1992).

Open reading frame and premature termination

The instruction to synthesize any particular amino acid (and to terminate synthesis) is defined by adjacent triplets of RNA nucleotides or codons. The open reading frame is the name given to the alignment, usually starting with the AUG initiation codon, which will divide the mRNA nucleotide sequence into triplets which are potentially translatable (reviewed in Lewin 1990).

In some genes a truncated isoform of the full-length protein is produced by the introduction of a premature stop codon. Thus a novel secreted form of NCAM is produced in skeletal muscle and brain by the inclusion of a discrete exon which induces a premature in-frame stop codon. The truncated polypeptide lacks either of the C-terminal hydrophobic domains necessary for interaction with the plasma membrane (Gower et al 1988). Similarly, vascular smooth muscle expresses a truncated isoform of the Na^+,K^+-ATPase α-1 subunit, which may play a role in active ion transport (Medford et al 1991).

Premature termination of translation and the production of a truncated polypeptide may, however, produce disastrous results. In patients with Duchenne muscular dystrophy unintentional stop codons may be generated in the dystrophin gene by deletions or duplications which shift the open reading frame by one or two nucleotides. This appears to produce a polypeptide which, if synthesized at all, is very rapidly degraded, resulting in a state of severe dystrophin deficiency in most patients (Monaco et al 1988, Hoffman & Kunkel 1989).

Co- and post-translational processing

During or following synthesis, polypeptide chains may be modified in various ways to produce mature forms of protein. Such processing may involve proteolytic cleavage, covalent alterations to the carbon chains of certain amino acids like proline, lysine or glutamic acid, or chemical substitution of amino acid residues by sugars or acyl, carboxyl, alkyl, methyl, phosphate or sulphate groups (reviewed in Harding 1985, Arnstein & Cox 1992). In some cases more than one class of processing takes place.

Proteolytic cleavage. Cleavage by proteolytic enzymes is a common processing event among the precursors of many hormones and enzymes (e.g. insulin, adrenocorticotropin/β-lipotropin) or neuroendocrine peptides (e.g. substance P, enkephalin) (see Hall 1992). In skeletal muscle a recent example is dystroglycan, which is processed into two of the dystrophin-associated glycoproteins (DAGs) which form part of the complex at the muscle membrane (Ervasti & Campbell 1991). A 97 kDa precursor polypeptide is synthesized which is then split into two polypeptides of about 56 kDa and 41 kDa (Fig. 3.7). The 56 kDa polypeptide undergoes extensive *O*-glycosylation, forming a mature 156 kDa protein which is an extracellular, laminin-binding component of the DAG complex. A putative N-terminal signal peptide, which may be used to ensure translocation, may also be cleaved. The 41 kDa polypeptide undergoes some *N*-glycosylation, to form a mature 43 kDa protein with a single trans-membrane domain and a cytoplasmic tail (Ibraghimov-Beskrovnaya et al 1992).

Modification of side-chains. Various covalent modifications to amino acid residues occur in muscle proteins. Disulphide bonds, between or within chains, are important for the tertiary and quaternary structure of some proteins. The anchorage of acetylcholinesterase to the extracellular matrix is achieved via disulphide bridges (Silman & Futerman 1987). The hydroxylation of certain proline and lysine residues occurs in the biosynthesis of collagen for the extracellular matrix of muscle (Pihlajaniemi et al 1991). Similarly, some proteins involved in calcium-dependent interactions have been found to contain glutamate residues (Glu) that have been modified by post-translational carboxylation to γ-carboxyglutamate (Gla), which is able to chelate calcium (Arnstein & Cox 1992).

Chemical substitution of residues. Mono- or oligo-saccharide chains may be attached via the amino group of asparagine (*N*-glycosylation), or through the hydroxyl group of serine, threonine or hydroxylysine residues (*O*-glycosylation). As mentioned above, most of the proteins in the dystrophin-associated complex are glycosylated, one so extensively that its apparent molecular mass increases nearly three-fold. The extent of glycosylation may vary between muscle and non-muscle tissues (Ibraghimov-Beskrovnaya et al 1992). The muscle-specific domain of the cell adhesion molecule, NCAM, has *O*-linked oligosaccharides (Walsh et al 1989), which may have functional significance in terms of an extended structure which would lift the NCAM molecule above the glycocalyx of muscle cells to a position where it could more effectively mediate specific interactions (Walsh & Doherty, 1991).

Many skeletal muscle proteins contain phosphate groups linked to the hydroxyl groups of serine, threonine or tyrosine residues. Protein phosphorylation is the most common post-translational modification, and reversible phosphorylation modifies the action of many enzymes, mediators and regulatory factors involved in movement, cell growth and metabolic regulation (Arnstein & Cox 1992). In skeletal muscle there are many phosphorylatable proteins like the regulatory myosin light chains, phospho-fructokinase, acetylcholine receptor subunits, ion channels, titin, nebulin, desmin, vimentin and

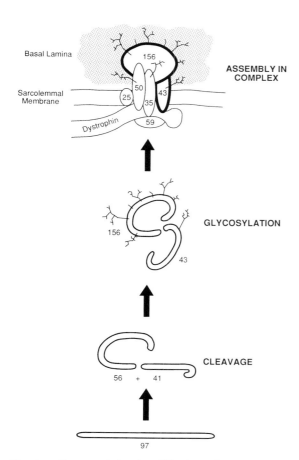

Fig. 3.7 Post-translational modifications of the dystroglycan polypeptide (97 kDa) to produce two mature proteins of 156 kDa and 43 kDa

dystroglycan (O'Conner et al 1981, Somerville & Wang 1988, Chen & Lo 1991, Hill et al 1991, Gao et al 1992, Ibraghimov-Beskrovnaya et al 1992). The pattern of phosphoprotein expression is different in fast- and slow-twitch muscles and this appears to be controlled by neuronal activity rather than by trophic factors (Nicholson et al 1990). Altered patterns of calcium channel phosphorylation may contribute to the phenotype in *dy/dy* murine muscular dystrophy (Senni et al 1990). In myotonic dystrophy (see Ch. 15) the causal mutation is in a protein kinase gene and thus defective protein phosphorylation may underlie the disease. In contrast to phosphorylation, methylation is not a frequent modification; nevertheless, both skeletal muscle myosin and actin in muscle undergo this process (Huszar 1975).

Acylation of a variety of specific proteins by fatty acids is a common post-translational modification. The binding of lipid to vinculin is implicated in the reversible association of the protein with plasma membranes (Burn & Burger 1987), and the co-translational myristoylation of the acetylcholine receptor-associated 43 K protein affects the affinity with which the protein is anchored in the plasma membrane (Musil et al 1988).

A number of membrane-associated proteins are attached to the cell surface via glycosyl-phosphatidylinositol (GPI) anchors (Low 1989). Thus the hydrophobic anchorage of acetylcholinesterase in the lipid bilayer of muscle plasma membranes is achieved by the covalent attachment of single phosphatidylinositol residues (Silman & Futerman 1987). Similarly, most of the NCAM in skeletal muscle is a GPI-anchored isoform, while the larger isoforms of NCAM in neurones have trans-membrane domains (Walsh & Doherty 1991).

Targeting and translocation

There are two main routes for proteins to arrive at their site of function, involving the synthesis of polypeptides either by ribosomes bound to the endoplasmic reticulum (ER) or by free cytosolic ribosomes. In the first pathway, protein synthesis is accompanied by insertion of the nascent protein into the ER membrane followed by translocation into the lumen. After any processing that is required, the protein is then transported through the Golgi network to various destinations depending on the particular protein. The second major route involves synthesis on non-membrane-bound ribosomes, and many water-soluble globular proteins destined for housekeeping use in the cytoplasm use this pathway (Austin & Westwood 1991)

In the environment that a protein encounters inside the cell, there are many possibilities for incorrect interactions with other macromolecules and 'chaperones' keep the nascent polypeptide, literally, on the straight and narrow. Chaperones are additional proteins that help assembly and folding, but which are not part of the final structure. They form stable complexes with precursor proteins, preventing them from folding prematurely and maintaining an open conformation for translocation across membranes (reviewed in Gatenby 1992).

The transcription and translation of proteins which are composed of several subunits that are encoded by different genes is coordinated. The five subunits of mature acetylcholine receptors, $\alpha_2\beta\delta\varepsilon$, ($\alpha_2\beta\gamma\delta$ in immature form) are translocated to the inside of the endoplasmic reticulum. Here they are assembled into α-ε (or α-γ) and α-δ heterodimers which associate with the β subunit and with each other to gain the correct stoichiometry (Blount et al 1990, Yu & Hall 1991). The fully assembled functional unit then enters the Golgi apparatus and is transported to the muscle membrane (Smith et al 1987).

INFLUENCE OF EXTERNAL FACTORS ON PROTEIN EXPRESSION

Development and regeneration

The effects of myogenic regulatory factors (MyoD, myogenin, myf-5, MRF4) on gene expression during development are discussed in Chapter 2. During myogenesis, muscle contractile protein gene expression is induced and the products are used to assemble the contractile apparatus characteristic of striated muscle. The different muscle proteins are accumulated in a fixed stoichiometric ratio according to their organisation in the contractile apparatus. It appears, however, that the maintenance of stoichiometry between the contractile proteins is largely regulated by the accumulation of mRNA from each of the gene families (Long & Ordahl 1988, Wade et al 1990). As muscle differentiates and matures, the expression of genes for embryonic-type proteins is repressed, possibly by the inhibition of translation by other RNA species (Vanderburg & Nathanson 1988).

Studies on mRNA from 21 contractile proteins have shown that each protein has its own determinants for accumulation, and that the acquisition of particular skeletal muscle fibre phenotypes occurs late in development (Sutherland et al 1991). Many specialised gene products appear late in development: the transcript for the small C-terminal form of dystrophin is expressed in the pluripotent stem cells which give rise to the entire embryo, long before the full-length transcripts are expressed in their own differentiated cells (Rapaport et al 1992a).

Embryonic and fetal isoforms of skeletal muscle proteins may be re-expressed during regeneration, as the fibres repair themselves after injury. For example, injury may cause a decrease in the trans-membrane ionic potential which results in the loss of glutamine and reduced gene transcription (Fong et al 1991). The effects of myogenic regulatory factors on satellite cells is also under investigation (Eftimie et al 1991, Russell et al 1992). Studies with mRNA in site hybridization show that increases in mRNA concentrations are found near nuclei in damaged regions and at the subcellular sites being repaired in the middle of skeletal muscle fibres (Russell et al 1992).

Innervation

Myofibres can differentiate in the total absence of nerves, but the maintenance of the differentiated state and continuing growth and maturation require innervation. Recent studies suggest, however, that innervation or denervation can trigger a rather complex set of gene regulatory mechanisms. As embryonic myotubes become innervated by motor neurones, the changes in gene expression are selective, thus innervation down-regulates a subset of muscle synaptic proteins (including acetylcholine receptor subunits, voltage-gated sodium channels and adhesion molecules) but does not affect the expression of other enzymes or structural proteins (e.g. creatine kinase, myosin light chain, α-actin) (see Frail et al 1989, Eftimie et al 1991). This selective effect may be mediated via the family of myogenic factors. The mRNA for myogenin, MyoD and MRF4 are regulated by nerve-induced muscle activity, and these factors may directly influence transcription of certain synaptic protein genes, including those for AChR subunits (Eftimie et al 1991, Witzemann & Sakmann 1991, Asher et al 1992).

Innervation appears to activate two pathways of transcriptional regulation for AChR subunits. One pathway is triggered by signals associated with fibre depolarisation, and these signals act to repress subunit gene expression in extrajunctional nuclei (Goldman et al 1988, Witzemann et al 1990, Martinou & Merlie 1991, Simon et al 1992). Transcription in synaptic nuclei is maintained and ε subunit expression replaces that of the immature γ subunit (Mishina et al 1986, Martinou et al 1991, Numberger et al 1991). Denervation reverses the repression so that AChR subunits are expressed again in non-synaptic regions (Goldman et al 1988, Goldman & Staple 1989, Witzemann et al 1991). A second pathway is triggered by an unknown signal that is synapse-specific and persists after denervation (Brenner et al 1990, Simon et al 1992). There is evidence to suggest that the factors which induce synapse-specific AChR gene expression are stably bound to synaptic basal lamina (Brenner et al 1992).

Load bearing and activity

Skeletal muscle can adapt to changing requirements. In an animal or human undergoing a programme of physical training which consists of at least 30 min of running a day, the skeletal muscles used in running exhibit an adaptive increase in mitochondrial density without an increase in muscle mass (Holloszy & Booth 1976). If, however, the training is a resistance exercise like weight lifting, the recruited muscles undergo an increase in mass with unchanged or reduced mitochondrial density (Schantz & Kallman 1989, Tesch et al 1989). Such observations imply that there is a differential expression of muscle genes in response to alterations in the inherent type of contractile activity. The lack of adaptation in muscles not recruited during running or weight training supports the idea that differential gene expression is a consequence of the specific pattern of contractile activity (Booth & Kirby 1991).

It appears that multiple, complex controls of gene regulation underlie the adaptive changes in protein quantity associated with alterations of the inherent amount of contractile activity in adult skeletal muscle. Investigations of increased contractile activity by running and resistance exercise, as well as recovery from the reduced contractile activity of limb immobilisation, suggest that the control of the alterations of gene expression are initially at the level of translation. Likewise, experimental models which do not closely mimic human physical training (e.g. electrical stimulation and chronic overload) produce early alterations in the translational control of gene expression. More prolonged changes in contractile activity (disuse or prolonged physical training), induce altered gene expression via changes in controls at the level of transcription as well as translation (Howard et al 1989, Booth & Kirby 1991, 1992, Goldspink et al 1992).

Hormones

It is now well established that the terminal differentiation of muscle cells in vitro is subject to control by hormones and growth factors present in serum supplements to the incubation medium (Florini & Magri 1989). Phenotypic expression of many muscle genes is known to be influenced by thyroid hormone (Izumo et al 1986, Mahdavi et al 1987), which may also induce precocious muscle maturation and the expression of adult myosin heavy chains in human fetal skeletal muscle (Butler-Browne et al 1990). The addition and subsequent withdrawal of insulin to cultured muscle cells may also produce profound changes. Addition induces massive increases in myosin, creatine kinase, tropomyosin and muscle actin (see Emerson et al 1986). Furthermore, the increase in transcription rate is accompanied by an even greater increase in

stability of the induced mRNA (Pontecorvi et al 1988). Hormone withdrawal causes rapid degradation of induced mRNA, which is selective in that there is, for example, an almost total loss of mRNA for creatine kinase while myosin mRNA is not affected (Pontecorvi et al 1988).

Other hormones which modify muscle gene expression include insulin-like growth factors, transforming growth factor-β, somatotropin and fibroblast growth factor (Muntz, 1990). Calcitonin gene-related peptide (CGRP) increases transcription of the acetylcholine receptor α-subunit gene, but has no effect on the other subunit genes. This effect is thought to be mediated by a CGRP-induced rise in intracellular cAMP (Moss et al 1991). Glucocorticoid administration increases transcription of the rat phosphofructokinase gene by acting as a *trans*-factor on an enhancer element (Lange et al 1989, 1992), as does thyroid hormone on the human skeletal α-actin gene (Collie & Muscat 1992).

CONCLUSION

In this chapter examples have been shown of the ways gene and protein expression can be modified to generate diversity. In the past, research has tended to focus on the study of genes *or* proteins, but recent advances in the techniques of molecular biology have made it possible to integrate these approaches. For example, techniques which permit the simultaneous demonstration of mRNA and protein expression (by a combination of in situ hybridization and immunocytochemistry) are likely to find increased use in the next few years (e.g. Morley & Hodes 1987, Bursztajn et al 1990, Taneja et al 1992). Analysis of the *cis*-acting elements and *trans*-acting factors which direct tissue-specific transcription is another rapidly developing area. Techniques are also being developed whereby gene expression in mouse embryonic stem cells may be manipulated so that a target gene is 'knocked out' (Waldman 1992). By disabling a specific gene it would be feasible to generate a murine model of a genetic disease and by studying the effects of the absence or malproduction of a protein, the function of the native protein might be deduced. Alternatively, if an animal model with a defective gene already exists, it may be possible to correct the defect by introducing a functional gene via an assortment of routes. Thus gene therapy experiments have been undertaken in animal models of cystic fibrosis (Hyde et al 1993), Parkinson's disease (Jiao et al 1993) and Duchenne muscular dystrophy (Ascadi et al 1992, Wells et al 1992, Ragot et al 1993). In summary, skeletal muscle has much to offer those interested in gene and protein expression, and there are many exciting areas of research currently under development which are likely to provide us with a much greater understanding of the complex nature of muscle gene and protein expression in the future.

REFERENCES

Acsadi G, Dickson G, Love D R et al 1992 Human dystrophin expression in mdx mice after intramuscular injection of DNA constructs. Nature 352: 815

Agnew W S, Trimmer J S 1989 Molecular diversity of voltage-sensitive Na channels. Annual Review of Physiology 51: 401

Arahata K, Ishihara T, Kamakura K et al 1989 Mosaic expression of dystrophin in symptomatic carriers of Duchenne's muscular dystrophy. New England Journal of Medicine 320: 138

Arnold H H, Tannich E, Paterson B M 1988 The promoter of the chicken cardiac myosin light chain 2 gene shows cell-specific expression in transfected primary cultures of chicken muscle. Nucleic Acids Research 16: 2411

Arnstein H R V, Cox R A 1992 Protein biosynthesis — in focus. IRL/Oxford University Press, Oxford

Asher O, Fuchs S, Zuk D, Rapaport D, Buonano A 1992 Changes in the expression of mRNAs for myogenic factors and other muscle-specific proteins in experimental autoimmune myasthenia gravis. FEBS Letters 299: 15

Austin B M, Westwood O M R 1991 Protein targeting and secretion — in focus. IRL/Oxford University Press, Oxford

Balazs I, Nicholas L, Siddiqui M A Q, Greschik K H 1985 Chromosome mapping and characterization of human cDNA sequences homologous to cardiac myosin light chain gene. Cytogenetics and Cell Genetics 40: 574

Bar S, Barnea E, Levy Z, Neuman S, Yaffe D, Nudel U 1990 A novel product of the Duchenne muscular dystrophy gene which greatly differs from the known isoforms in its structure and tissue distribution. Biochemistry Journal 272: 557

Baumann M, Baumann H, Fey G H 1990 Molecular cloning, characterization and functional expression of the rat liver interleukin 6 receptor. Journal of Biological Chemistry 265: 19853

Beebee T, Burke J 1992 Gene structure and transcription — in focus, 2nd edn. IRL/Oxford University Press, Oxford

Beeson D, Jeremiah S, West L F, Povey S, Newsom Davis J 1990 Assignment of the human nicotinic acetylcholine receptor genes: the α and δ subunit genes to chromosome 2 and the β subunit gene to chromosome 17. Annals of Human Genetics 54: 199

Benezra R, Davis R L, Lockshon D, Turner D L, Weintraub H 1990 The protein Id: a negative regulator of helix-loop-helix DNA binding proteins. Cell 61: 49

Biel M, Hullin R, Freundner S et al 1991 Tissue-specific expression of high-voltage-activated dihydropyridine-sensitive L-type calcium channels. European Journal of Biochemistry 200: 81

Bies R D, Phelps S F, Cortez M D, Roberts R, Caskey C T, Chamberlain J S 1992 Human and murine dystrophin mRNA transcripts are differentially expressed during skeletal muscle, heart, and brain development. Nucleic Acids Research 20: 1725

Blake D J, Love D R, Tinsley J et al 1992 Characterisation of a 4.8 kb transcript from the Duchenne muscular dystrophy locus expressed in Schwannoma cells. Human Molecular Genetics 1: 103

Blount P, Smith M M, Merlie J P 1990 Assembly intermediates of the mouse muscle nicotinic acetylcholine receptor in stably transfected fibroblasts. Journal of Cell Biology 111: 2601

Bonilla E, Schmidt B, Samitt C E et al 1988 Normal and dystrophin-deficient fibres in carriers of the gene for Duchenne muscular dystrophy. American Journal of Pathology 133: 440

Booth F W, Kirby C R 1991 Control of gene expression in adult skeletal muscle by changes in the inherent level of contractile activity. Biochemical Society Transactions 19: 374

Booth F W, Kirby C R 1992 Changes in skeletal muscle gene expression consequent to altered weight bearing. American Journal of Physiology 262: R329

Boyce F M, Beggs A H, Feener C A, Kunkel L M 1991 Dystrophin is transcribed in brain from a distant upstream promoter. Proceedings of the National Academy of Science USA 88: 1276

Braun T, Bober E, Winter B, Rosenthal N, Arnold H H 1990 Myf-6, a new member of the human gene family of myogenic determination factors: evidence for a gene cluster on chromosome 12. EMBO J 9: 821

Breitbart R E, Andreadis A, Nadal-Ginard B 1987 Alternative splicing: a ubiquitous mechanism for the generation of multiple protein isoforms from single genes. Annual Review of Biochemistry 56: 467

Breitbart R E, Nadal-Ginard B 1989 Tissue specific alternative splicing in the troponin T multigene family. In: Renkawitz R (ed) Tissue specific gene expression. VCH Verlagsgessellschaft, Weinheim, p 199

Brenner H R, Witzemann V, Sakmann B 1990 Imprinting of acetylcholine receptor mRNA accumulation in mammalian neuromuscular synapses. Nature 344: 544

Brenner H R, Herczeg A, Slater C R 1992 Synapse-specific expression of acetylcholine receptor genes and their products at original synaptic sites in rat soleus muscle fibres regenerating in the absence of innervation. Development 116: 41

Buckingham M E, Alonso S, Barton P et al 1986 Actin and myosin multigene families: their expression during the formation and maturation of striated muscle. American Journal of Medical Genetics 25: 623

Buckingham M E 1992 Making muscle in mammals. Trends in Genetics 8: 144

Burn J, Povey S, Boyd Y et al 1986 Duchenne muscular dystrophy in one of monozygotic twin girls. Journal of Medical Genetics 23: 494

Burn P, Burger M M 1987 The cytoskeletal protein vinculin contains transformation-sensitive, covalently bound lipid. Science 235: 476

Bursztajn S, Berman S A, Gilbert W 1990 Simultaneous visualization of neuronal protein and receptor mRNA. Biotechniques 9: 440

Buskin J N, Hauschka S D 1989 Identification of a myocyte nuclear factor that binds to the muscle-specific enhancer of the mouse muscle creatine kinase gene. Molecular and Cellular Biology 9: 2627

Butler-Browne G S, Barbet J P, Thornell L E 1990 Myosin heavy and light chain expression during human skeletal muscle development and precocious muscle maturation induced by thyroid hormone. Anatomy and Embryology 181: 513

Chelly J, Hamard G, Koulakoff A, Kaplan J-C, Kahn A, Berwald-Netter Y 1990 Dystrophin gene transcribed from different promoters in neuronal and glial cells. Nature 344: 64

Chen X Y, Lo T C Y 1991 Involvement of a cell surface protein and an ecto-protein kinase in myogenesis. Biochemistry Journal 279: 475

Cohen-Haguenauer O, Barton P J, Nguyen V C et al 1988 Assignment of the human fast skeletal muscle myosin alkali light chains gene (MLC1F/MLC3F) to 2q 32.1–2qter. Human Genetics 78: 65

Cohen-Haguenauer O, Barton P J, Buonanno A et al 1989a Localization of the acetylcholine receptor γ subunit gene to human chromosome 2q32----qter. Cytogenetics and Cell Genetics 52: 124

Cohen-Haguenauer O, Barton P J, Van Cong N et al 1989b Chromosomal assignment of two myosin alkali light-chain genes encoding the ventricular/slow skeletal muscle isoform and the atrial/fetal muscle isoform (MYL3, MYL4). Human Genetics 81: 278

Collie E S, Muscat G E 1992 The human skeletal α-actin promoter is regulated by thyroid hormone: identification of a thyroid hormone response element. Cell Growth and Differentiation 3: 31

Collinge M, Matrisian P E, Zimmer W E et al 1992 Structure and expression of a calcium-binding protein gene contained within a calmodulin-regulated protein kinase gene. Molecular and Cellular Biology 12: 2359

Collins C, Schappert K, Hayden M R 1992 The genomic organisation of a novel regulatory myosin light chain gene (MYL5) that maps to chromosome 4p 16.3 and shows different patterns of expression between primates. Human Molecular Genetics 1: 727

Collins T, Bonthron D T, Orkin S H 1987 Alternative RNA splicing affects function of encoded platelet-derived growth factor A chain. Nature 328: 621

Cox R D, Weydert A, Barlow D, Buckingham M E 1991 Three linked myosin heavy chain genes clustered within 370 kb of each other show independent transcriptional and post-transcriptional regulation during differentiation of a mouse muscle cell line. Developmental Biology 143: 36

den Dunnen J T, Grootscholten P M, Bakker E et al 1989 Topography of the Duchenne muscular dystrophy (DMD) gene: FIGE and cDNA analysis of 194 cases reveals 115 deletions and 13 duplications. American Journal of Human Genetics 45: 835

den Dunnen J T, Casula L, Kakover A et al 1991 Mapping of dystrophin brain promoter: a deletion of this region is compatible with normal intellect. Neuromuscular Disorders 1: 327

Dickson G, Gower H J, Barton C H et al 1987 Human muscle neural cell adhesion molecule (N-CAM): identification of a muscle-specific sequence in the extracellular domain. Cell 50: 1119

Donalies M, Cramer M, Ringwald M, Starzinski-Powitz A 1991 Expression of M-cadherin, a member of the cadherin multigene family, correlates with differentiation of skeletal muscle cells. Proceedings of the National Academy of Sciences USA 88: 8024

Donoghue M, Ernst H, Wentworth B, Nadal-Ginard B, Rosenthal N 1988 A muscle-specific enhancer is located at the 3' end of the myosin light-chain 1/3 gene locus. Genes and Development 2: 1779

Edwards Y H 1990 CpG islands in genes showing tissue-specific expression. Philosophical Transactions of the Royal Society of London 326: 207

Eftimie R, Brenner H R, Buonanno A 1991 Myogenin and MyoD join a family of skeletal muscle genes regulated by electrical activity. Proceedings of the National Academy of Sciences USA 88: 1349

Emerson C, Fischman D, Nadal-Ginard B, Siddiqui M A Q (eds) 1986 Molecular Biology of Muscle Development — UCLA Symposia on Molecular and Cellular Biology 29. Alan R Liss, New York

Emery A E H 1988 Duchenne muscular dystrophy, revised edn. Oxford University Press, Oxford

Emeson R B, Hedjran F, Yeakley J M, Guise J W, Rosenfeld M G 1989 Alternative production of calcitonin and CGRP mRNA is regulated at the calcitonin-specific splice acceptor. Nature 341: 76

Ernst H, Walsh K, Harrison C A, Rosenthal N 1991 The myosin light chain enhancer and the skeletal actin promoter share a binding site for factors involved in muscle-specific gene expression. Molecular and Cellular Biology 11: 3735

Ervasti J M, Campbell K P 1991 Membrane organization of the dystrophin–glycoprotein complex. Cell 66: 1121

Feener C A, Koenig M, Kunkel L M 1989 Alternative splicing of human dystrophin mRNA generates isoforms at the carboxy terminus. Nature 338: 509

Ferns M, Hoch W, Campanelli J T, Rupp F, Hall Z W, Scheller R H 1992 RNA splicing regulates agrin-mediated acetylcholine receptor clustering activity on cultured myotubes. Neuron 8: 1079

Florini J R, Magri K A 1989 Effects of growth factors on myogenic differentiation. American Journal of Physiology 256: C701

Fong Y M, Minei J P, Marano M A et al 1991 Skeletal muscle amino acid and myofibrillar protein mRNA response to thermal injury and infection. American Journal of Physiology 261: R536

Frail D E, Musil L S, Buonanno A, Merlie J P 1989 Expression of RAPsyn (43 K protein) and nicotinic acetylcholine receptor genes is not coordinately regulated in mouse muscle. Neuron 2: 1077

Frances V, Morle F, Godet J 1992 Identification of two critical base pairings in 5' untranslated regions affecting translation efficiency of synthetic uncapped globin mRNAs. Biochimica et Biophysica Acta 1130: 29

Fulton A B, Isaacs W B 1991 Titin, a huge, elastic sarcomeric protein with a probable role in morphogenesis. BioEssays 13: 157

Gahlmann R, Troutt A B, Wade R P, Gunning P, Kedes L 1987 Alternative splicing generates variants in important functional domains of human slow skeletal troponin T. Journal of Biological Chemistry 262: 16122

Gao Z H, Moomaw C R, Hsu J, Slaughter C A, Stull J T 1992 Autophosphorylation of skeletal muscle myosin light chain kinase. Biochemistry 31: 6126

Gatenby A A 1992 Protein folding and chaperonins. Plant Molecular Biology 19: 677

Geng Y, Sicinski P, Gorecki D, Barnard P J 1991 Developmental and tissue-specific regulation of mouse dystrophin: the embryonic isoform in muscular dystrophy. Neuromuscular Disorders 1: 125

Ghanshani S, Pak M, McPherson J D et al 1992 Genomic organization, nucleotide sequence, and cellular distribution of a Shaw-related potassium channel gene, Kv3.3, and mapping of Kv3.3 and Kv3.4 to human chromosomes 19 and 1. Genomics 12: 190

Gilgenkrantz H, Hugnot J -P, Lambert M, Chafey P, Kaplan J -C, Kahn A 1992 Positive and negative regulatory DNA elements including a CCArGG box are involved in the cell type-specific expression of the human muscle dystrophin gene. Journal of Biological Chemistry 267: 10823

Gilmour B P, Fanger G R, Newton C, Evans S M, Gardner P D 1991 Multiple binding sites for myogenic regulatory factors are required for expression of the acetylcholine receptor γ-subunit gene. Journal of Biological Chemistry 266: 19871

Goldman D, Brenner H R, Heinemann S 1988 Acetylcholine receptor α-, β-, γ- and ∂-subunit mRNA levels are regulated by muscle activity. Neuron 1: 329

Goldman D, Staple J 1989 Spatial and temporal expression of acetylcholine receptor mRNAs in innervated and denervated rat soleus muscle. Neuron 3: 219

Goldman D, Tamai K 1989 Coordinate regulation of RNAs encoding two isoforms of the rat muscle nicotinic acetylcholine receptor β-subunit. Nucleic Acids Research 17: 3049

Goldspink G, Scott A, Loughna P T, Wells D J, Jaenicke T, Gerlach G F 1992 Gene expression in skeletal muscle in response to stretch and force generation. American Journal of Physiology 262: R356

Górecki D C, Monaco A P, Derry J M, Walker A P, Barnard E A, Barnard P J 1992 Expression of four alternative dystrophin transcripts in brain regions regulated by different promoters. Human Molecular Genetics 1: 505

Gossett L A, Kelvin D J, Sternberg E A, Olson E N 1989 A new myocyte-specific enhancer-binding factor that recognizes a conserved element associated with multiple muscle-specific genes. Molecular and Cellular Biology 9: 5022

Gower H J, Barton C H, Elsom V L et al 1988 Alternative splicing generates a secreted form of N-CAM in muscle and brain. Cell 55: 955

Graham I R, Hamshere M, Eperon I C 1992 Alternative splicing of a human α-tropomyosin muscle-specific exon: identification of determining sequences. Molecular and Cellular Biology 12: 3872

Gupta M, Smeekens S P, Gupta M P, Zak R 1992 Isolation and characterization of a rat ventricular cDNA expressed specifically in cardiac and skeletal muscles. Biochemical and Biophysical Research Communications 183: 176

Hall Z W (with 11 contributors) 1992 An introduction to molecular neurobiology. Sinauer Associates, Sunderland, MA

Harding J J 1985 Nonenzymatic covalent posttranslational modification of proteins in vivo. Archives of Protein Chemistry 37: 247

Harmann B, Zander N F, Kilimann M W 1991 Isoform diversity of phosphorylase kinase α and β subunits generated by alternative RNA splicing. Journal of Biological Chemistry 266: 15631

Helfman D M, Cheley S, Kuismanen E, Finn L A, Yamawaki-Kataoka Y 1986 Nonmuscle and muscle tropomyosin isoforms are expressed from a single gene by alternative RNA splicing and polyadenylation. Molecular and Cellular Biology 6: 3582

HGM 11 1991 Eleventh International Workshop On Human Gene Mapping. Cytogenetics and Cell Genetics 58: 8

Hill J A, Nghiem H O, Changeux J P 1991 Serine-specific phosphorylation of nicotinic receptor associated 43 K protein. Biochemistry 30: 5579

Hoffman E P, Brown R H, Kunkel L M 1987 Dystrophin: the protein product of the Duchenne muscular dystrophy locus. Cell 51: 919

Hoffman E P, Kunkel L M 1989 Dystrophin abnormalities in Duchenne/Becker muscular dystrophy. Neuron 2: 1019

Holloszy J O, Booth F W 1976 Biochemical adaptations to endurance exercise in muscle. Annual Review of Physiology 38: 273

Horlick R A, Hobson G M, Patterson J H, Mitchell M T, Benfield P A 1990 Brain and muscle creatine kinase genes contain common TA-rich recognition protein-binding regulatory elements. Molecular and Cellular Biology 10: 4826

Howard G, Steffen J M, Geoghegan T E 1989 Transcriptional regulation of decreased protein synthesis during skeletal muscle unloading. Journal of Applied Physiology 66: 1093

Hu J S, Olson E N, Kingston R E 1992 HEB, a helix-loop-helix protein related to E2A and ITF2 that can modulate the DNA-binding ability of myogenic regulatory factors. Molecular and Cellular Biology 12: 1031

Hugnot J P, Gilgenkrantz H, Vincent N et al 1992 Novel products of the dystrophin gene: a distal transcript initiated from a unique alternative first exon encoding a 75 kDa protein widely distributed in non-muscle tissues. Proceedings of the National Academy of Science USA 89: 7506

Huszar G 1975 Tissue-specific biosynthesis of -N-monomethyllysine and -N-trimethyllysine in skeletal and cardiac muscle myosin: a model for the cell-free study of post-translational amino acid modifications in proteins. Journal of Molecular Biology 94: 311

Hyde S C, Gill D R, Higgins C F et al 1993 Correction of the ion transport defect in cystic fibrosis transgenic mice by gene therapy. Nature 362: 250

Hynes R O 1992 Integrins: versatility, modulation, and signaling in cell adhesion. Cell 69: 11

Ibraghimov-Beskrovnaya O, Ervasti J M, Leveille C J, Slaughter C A, Sernett S W, Campbell K P 1992 Primary structure of dystrophin-associated glycoproteins linking dystrophin to the extracellular matrix. Nature 355: 696

Ito M, Dabrowska R, Guerriero V, Hartshorne D J 1989 Identification in turkey gizzard of an acidic protein related to the C-terminal portion of smooth muscle myosin light chain kinase. Journal of Biological Chemistry 264: 13971

Izumo S, Nadal-Ginard B, Mahdavi V J 1986 All members of the MHC multigene family respond to thyroid hormone in a highly tissue-specific manner. Science 231: 597

Jiao S, Gurevich V, Wolff J A 1993 Long-term correction of rat model of Parkinson's disease by gene therapy. Nature 362: 450

Karsch-Mizrachi I, Travis M, Blau H, Leinwand L A 1989 Expression and DNA sequence analysis of a human embryonic skeletal muscle myosin heavy chain gene. Nucleic Acids Research 17: 6167

Karsch-Mizrachi I, Feghali R, Shows T B, Leinwand L A 1990 Generation of a full-length human perinatal myosin heavy-chain-encoding cDNA. Gene 89: 289

Kaye F J, McBride O W, Battey J F, Gazdar A F, Sausville E A 1987 Human creatine kinase-B complementary DNA. Nucleotide sequence, gene expression in lung cancer, and chromosomal assignment to two distinct loci. Journal of Clinical Investigation 79: 1412

Klamut H J, Gangopadhyay S B, Worton R G, Ray P N 1990 Molecular and functional analysis of the muscle-specific promoter region of the Duchenne muscular dystrophy gene. Molecular and Cellular Biology 10: 193

Klarsfeld A, Bessereau J -L, Salmon A -M, Triller A, Babinet C, Changeux J -P 1991 An acetylcholine receptor α-subunit promoter conferring preferential synaptic expression in muscle of transgenic mice. EMBO Journal 10: 625

Koenig M, Hoffman E P, Bertelson C J, Monaco A P, Feener C A, Kunkel L M 1987 Complete cloning of the Duchenne muscular dystrophy (DMD) cDNA and preliminary genomic organization of the DMD gene in normal and affected individuals. Cell 50: 509

Koenig M, Monaco A P, Kunkel L M 1988 The complete sequence of dystrophin predicts a rod-shaped cytoskeletal protein. Cell 53: 219

Koteliansky V E, Ogryzko E P, Zhidkova N I et al 1992 An additional exon in the human vinculin gene specifically encodes meta-vinculin-specific difference peptide: cross-species comparison reveals variable and conserved motifs in the meta-vinculin insert. European Journal of Biochemistry 204: 767

Kurabayashi M, Komuro I, Shibasaki Y, Tsuchimochi H, Takaku F, Yazaki Y 1990 Functional identification of the transcriptional regulatory elements within the promoter region of the human ventricular myosin alkali light chain gene. Journal of Biological Chemistry 265: 19271

Lamson G, Stockdale F E 1989 Developmental and muscle-specific changes in methylation of the myosin light chain LC1f and LC3f promoters during avian myogenesis. Developmental Biology 132: 62

Landing B H, Dixon L G, Wells T R 1974 Studies on isolated human skeletal muscle fibres: including a proposed pattern of nuclear distribution and a concept of nuclear territories. Human Pathology 5: 441

Lange A J, Kummel L, el Maghrabi M R et al 1989 Sequence of the 5'-flanking region of the rat 6-phosphofructo-2-kinase/fructose 2,6-bisphosphatase gene: regulation by glucocorticoids. Biochemical and Biophysical Research Communications 162: 753

Lange A J, Espinet C, Hall R et al 1992 Regulation of gene expression of rat skeletal muscle/liver 6-phosphofructo-2-kinase/fructose-2,6-bisphosphatase. Isolation and characterization of a glucocorticoid response element in the first intron of the gene. Journal of Biological Chemistry 267: 15673

Lederfein D, Levy Z, Augier N et al 1992 A 71 kd protein is a major product of the Duchenne muscular dystrophy gene in brain and other non-muscle tissues. Proceedings of the National Academy of Science USA 89: 5346

Lee K J, Ross R S, Rockman H A et al 1992 Myosin light chain-2 luciferase transgenic mice reveal distinct regulatory programs for cardiac and skeletal muscle-specific expression of a single contractile protein gene. Journal of Biological Chemistry 267: 15875

Lees-Miller J P, Helfman D M 1991 The molecular basis for tropomyosin isoform diversity. BioEssays 13: 429

Levine B A, Moir A J G, Patchell V B, Perry S V 1992 Binding sites involved in the interaction of actin with the N-terminal region of dystrophin. FEBS Letters 298: 44

Lewin B 1990 Genes IV. Oxford University/Cell Press, New York/Cambridge, MA

Li Y, Camp S, Rachinsky T L, Getman D, Taylor P 1991 Gene structure of mammalian acetylcholinesterase. Alternative exons dictate tissue-specific expression. Journal of Biological Chemistry 266: 23083

Liebhaber S A, Cash F, Eshleman S S 1992 Translation inhibition by an mRNA coding region secondary structure is determined by its proximity to the AUG initiation codon. Journal of Molecular Biology 226: 609

Lin H, Yutzey K E, Konieczny S F 1991 Muscle-specific expression of the troponin I gene requires interactions between helix-loop-helix muscle regulatory factors and ubiquitous transcription factors. Molecular and Cellular Biology 11: 267

Lloyd J, Brownson C, Tweedie S, Charlton J, Edwards Y H 1987 Human muscle carbonic anhydrase: gene structure and DNA methylation patterns in fetal and adult tissues. Genes and Development 1: 594

Long C S, Ordahl C P 1988 Transcriptional repression of an embryo-specific muscle gene. Developmental Biology 127: 228

Low M G 1989 Glycosyl-phosphatidylinositol: a versatile anchor for cell surface proteins. FASEB Journal 3: 1600

Lupski J R, Garcia C A, Zoghbi H Y, Hoffman E P, Fenwick R G 1991 Discordance of muscular dystrophy in monozygotic female twins: evidence supporting asymmetric splitting of the inner cell mass in a manifesting carrier of Duchenne dystrophy. American Journal of Medical Genetics 40: 354

Lyon M F 1962 Sex chromatin and gene action in the mammalian X-chromosome. American Journal of Human Genetics 14: 135

Macera M J, Szabo P, Wadgaonkar R, Siddiqui M A, Verma R S 1992 Localization of the gene coding for ventricular myosin regulatory light chain (MYL2) to human chromosome 12q23-q24.3. Genomics 13: 829

MacLeod A R, Gooding C 1988 Human hTM α gene: expression in muscle and nonmuscle tissue. Molecular and Cellular Biology 8: 433

Mahdavi V, Izumo S, Nadal-Ginard B 1987 Developmental and hormonal regulation of sarcomeric myosin heavy chain gene family. Circulation Research 60: 804

Maire P, Gautron S, Hakim V, Gregori C, Mennecier F, Kahn A 1987 Characterization of three optional promoters in the 5' region of the human aldolase A gene. Journal of Molecular Biology 197: 425

Makover A, Zuk D, Breakstone J, Yaffe D, Nudel U 1991 Brain-type and muscle-type promotors of the dystrophin gene differ greatly in structure. Neuromuscular Disorders 1: 39

Mar J H, Antin P B, Cooper T A, Ordahl C P 1988 Analysis of the upstream regions governing expression of the chicken cardiac troponin T gene in embryonic cardiac and skeletal muscle cells. Journal of Cell Biology 107: 573

Mar J H, Ordahl C P 1988 A conserved CATTCCT motif is required for skeletal muscle-specific activity of the cardiac troponin T gene promoter. Proceedings of the National Academy of Science USA 85: 6404

Martinou J-C, Falls D L, Fischbach G D, Merlie J P 1991 Acetylcholine receptor-inducing activity stimulates expression of the epsilon-subunit gene of the muscle acetylcholine receptor. Proceedings of the National Academy of Sciences USA 88: 7669

Martinou J -C, Merlie J P 1991 Nerve-dependent modulation of acetylcholine receptor-subunit gene expression. Journal of Neuroscience 11: 1291

Matsuo M, Masumura T, Nakajima T et al 1990 A very small frame-shifting deletion within exon 19 of the Duchenne muscular dystrophy gene. Biochemical and Biophysical Research Communications 170: 963

Matsuo M, Masumura T, Nishio H, Nakajima T, Kitoh Y 1991 Exon skipping during splicing of dystrophin mRNA precursor due to an intraexon deletion in the dystrophin gene of Duchenne muscular dystrophy Kobe. Journal of Clinical Investigation 87: 2127

Matsuo M, Nishio H, Kitoh Y, Francke U, Nakamura H 1992 Partial deletion of a dystrophin gene leads to exon skipping and to loss of an intra-exon hairpin structure from the predicted mRNA precursor. Biochemical and Biophysical Research Communications 182: 495

Matsuoka R, Yoshida M C, Kanda N, Kimura M, Ozasa H, Takao A 1989 Human cardiac myosin heavy chain gene mapped within chromosome region 14q11.2–q13. American Journal of Medical Genetics 32: 279

Matsuoka R, Yoshida M C, Takao A 1990 Molecular cloning and chromosomal localization of a gene coding for human cardiac myosin heavy-chain. Japanese Circulation Journal 54: 1206

McKeown M 1990 Regulation of alternative splicing. Genetic Engineering 12: 139

Means A R, Cruzalegui F, LeMagueresse B, Needleman D S, Slaughter G R, Ono T 1991 A novel Ca^{2+}/calmodulin-dependent protein kinase and a male germ cell-specific calmodulin-binding protein are derived from the same gene. Molecular and Cellular Biology 11: 3960

Medford R M, Hyman R, Ahmad M et al 1991 Vascular smooth muscle expresses a truncated Na^+,K^+-ATPase α-1 subunit isoform. Journal of Biological Chemistry 266: 18308

Mishina M, Takai T, Imoto K et al 1986 Molecular distinction between fetal and adult forms of muscle acetylcholine receptor. Nature 321: 406

Miwa T, Boxer L M, Kedes L 1987 CArG boxes in the human cardiac α-actin gene are core binding sites for positive trans-acting regulatory factors. Proceedings of the National Academy of Science USA 84: 6702

Miwa T, Manabe Y, Kurokawa K et al 1991 Structure, chromosome location, and expression of the human smooth muscle (enteric type) γ-actin gene: evolution of six human actin genes. Molecular and Cellular Biology 11: 3296

Miwa T, Kedes L 1987 Duplicated CArG box domains have positive and mutually dependent regulatory roles in expression of the human α-cardiac actin gene. Molecular and Cellular Biology 7: 2803

Moller D E, Yokota A, Caro J F, Flier J S 1989 Tissue-specific expression of two alternatively spliced insulin receptor mRNA's in man. Molecular Endocrinology 3: 1263

Monaco A P, Bertelson C J, Liechti-Gallati S, Moser H, Kunkel L M 1988 An explanation for the phenotypic differences between patients bearing partial deletions of the DMD locus. Genomics 2: 90

Morley D J, Hodes M E 1987 In situ localization of amylase mRNA and protein. An investigation of amylase gene activity in normal human parotid gland. Journal of Histochemistry and Cytochemistry 35: 9

Moss S J, Harkness P C, Mason I J, Barnard E A, Mudge A W 1991 Evidence that CGRP and cAMP increase transcription of AChR α-subunit gene, but not of other subunit genes. Journal of Molecular Neuroscience 3: 101

Muntz L 1990 Cellular and biochemical aspects of muscle differentiation. Comparative Biochemistry and Physiology 97B: 215

Murtagh J J Jr, Eddy R, Shows T B, Moss J, Vaughan M 1991 Different forms of Go α mRNA arise by alternative splicing of transcripts from a single gene on human chromosome 16. Molecular and Cellular Biology 11: 1146

Muscat G E, Perry S, Prentice H, Kedes L 1992 The human skeletal α-actin gene is regulated by a muscle-specific enhancer that binds three nuclear factors. Gene Expression 2: 111

Muscat G E O, Gobius K, Emery J 1991 Proliferin, a prolactin/growth hormone-like peptide represses myogenic-specific transcription by the suppression of an essential serum-response factor-like DNA-binding activity. Molecular Endocrinology 5: 802

Muscat G E O, Kedes L 1987 Multiple 5'-flanking regions of the human α-skeletal actin gene synergistically modulate muscle-specific expression. Molecular and Cellular Biology 7: 4089

Musil L S, Carr C, Cohen J B, Merlie J P 1988 Acetylcholine receptor-associated 43 K protein contains covalently bound myristate. Journal of Cell Biology 107: 1113

Nadal-Ginard B, Smith C W, Patton J G, Breitbart R E 1991 Alternative splicing is an efficient mechanism for the generation of protein diversity: contractile protein genes as a model system. Advances in Enzyme Regulation 31: 261

Ng S Y, Gunning P, Liu S H, Leavitt J, Kedes L 1989 Regulation of the human β-actin promoter by upstream and intron domains. Nucleic Acids Research 17: 601

Nicholson G A, Hawkins S, McLeod J G 1990 Effect of neural activity on skeletal muscle phosphoproteins. Muscle and Nerve 13: 675

Nigro J M, Schweinfest C W, Rajkovic A et al 1987 cDNA cloning and mapping of the human creatine kinase M gene to 19q13. American Journal of Human Genetics 40: 115

Nikovits W Jr, Mar J H, Ordahl C P 1990 Muscle-specific activity of the skeletal troponin I promoter requires interaction between upstream regulatory sequences and elements contained within the first transcribed exon. Molecular and Cellular Biology 10: 3468

Noguchi T, Inoue H, Tunaka T 1986 The M1 and M2 type isoforms of rat pyruvate kinase are produced from the same gene by alternative RNA splicing. Journal of Biological Chemistry 261: 13807

Numberger M, Durr I, Kues W, Koenen M, Witzemann V 1991 Different mechanisms regulate muscle-specific AChR γ- and epsilon-subunit gene expression. EMBO Journal 10: 2957

O'Conner C M, Gard D L, Asal D J, Lazarides E 1981 Phosphorylation of the intermediate filament proteins desmin and vimentin in muscle cells. Cold Spring Harbor Conferences on Cell Proliferation 8: 1157

Ohmstede C -A, Bland M M, Merrill B M, Sahyoun N 1991 Relationship of genes encoding Ca^{2+}/calmodulin-dependent protein kinase Gr and calspermin: a gene within a gene. Proceedings of the National Academy of Science USA 88: 5784

Olson E N 1990 MyoD family: a paradigm for development? Genes and Development 4: 1454

Parmacek M S, Leiden J M 1989 Structure and expression of the murine slow/cardiac troponin C gene. Journal of Biological Chemistry 264: 13217

Pavlath G K, Rich K, Webster S G, Blau H M 1989 Localization of muscle gene products in nuclear domains. Nature 337: 570

Periasamy M, Strehler E E, Garfinkel L I, Gubits R M, Ruiz-Opazo N, Nadal-Ginard B 1984 Fast skeletal muscle myosin light chains 1 and 3 are produced from a single gene by a combined process of differential RNA transcription and splicing. Journal of Biological Chemistry 259: 13595

Piette J, Bessereau J L, Huchet M, Changeux J P 1990 Two adjacent MyoD1-binding sites regulate expression of the acetylcholine receptor α-subunit gene. Nature 345: 353

Pihlajaniemi T, Myllyla R, Kivirikko K I 1991 Prolyl 4-hydroxylase and its role in collagen synthesis. Journal of Hepatology 13 Suppl 3: S2

Pontecorvi A, Tata J R, Phyillaier M, Robbins J 1988 Selective degradation of mRNA: the role of short-lived proteins in differential destabilization of insulin-induced creatine phosphokinase and myosin heavy chain mRNAs during rat skeletal muscle L_6 cell differentiation. EMBO Journal 7: 1489

Prody C A, Merlie J P 1991 A developmental and tissue-specific enhancer in the mouse skeletal muscle acetylcholine receptor α-subunit gene regulated by myogenic factors. Journal of Biological Chemistry 266: 22588

Qin H, Kemp J, Yip M Y et al 1990 Localization of human cardiac β-myosin heavy chain gene (MYH7) to chromosome 14q12 by in situ hybridization. Cytogenetics and Cell Genetics 54: 74

Ragot T, Vincent N, Chafey P et al 1993 Efficient adenovirus-mediated transfer of a human minidystrophin gene in skeletal muscle of mdx mice. Nature 361: 647

Ralston E, Hall Z W 1992 Restricted distribution of mRNA produced from a single nucleus in hybrid myotubes. Journal of Cell Biology 119: 1063

Rapaport D, Fuchs O, Nudel U, Yaffe D 1992a Expression of the Duchenne muscular dystrophy gene products in embryonic stem cells and their differentiated derivatives. Journal of Biological Chemistry 267: 21289

Rapaport D, Lederfein D, den Dunnen J T et al 1992b Characterization and cell type distribution of a novel, major transcript of the Duchenne muscular dystrophy gene. Differentiation 49: 187

Rapaport D, Passos-Bueno M R, Takata R I et al 1992c A deletion including the brain promoter of the Duchenne muscular dystrophy gene is not associated with mental retardation. Neuromuscular Disorders 2: 117

Ray P N, Bulman D E, D'Souza V N et al 1992 Dystrophin expression in the human retina is required for normal function. American Journal of Human Genetics 51: A7

Richards C S, Watkins S C, Hoffman E P et al 1990 Skewed X inactivation in a female MZ twin results in Duchenne muscular dystrophy. American Journal of Human Genetics 46: 672

Russell B, Dix D J, Haller D L, Jacobs-El J 1992 Repair of injured skeletal muscle: a molecular approach. Medical Science of Sports and Exercise 24: 189

Saez C G, Myers J C, Shows T B, Leinwand L A 1990 Human nonmuscle myosin heavy chain mRNA: generation of diversity through alternative polyadenylylation. Proceedings of the National Academy of Sciences USA 87: 1164

Saitoh O, Olson E N, Periasamy M 1990 Muscle-specific RNA processing continues in the absence of myogenin expression. Journal of Biological Chemistry 265: 19381

Santoro I M, Yi T M, Walsh K 1991 Identification of single-stranded-DNA-binding proteins that interact with muscle gene elements. Molecular and Cellular Biology 11: 1944

Schachat F, Bronson D, McDonald O 1985 Heterogeneity of contractile proteins. Journal of Biological Chemistry 260: 1108

Schaller K L, Krzemien D M, McKenna N M, Caldwell J H 1992 Alternatively spliced sodium channel transcripts in brain and muscle. Journal of Neuroscience 12: 1370

Schantz P G, Kallman M J 1989 NADH shuttle enzymes and cytochrome b_5 reductase in human skeletal muscle: effect of strength training. Journal of Applied Physiology 67: 123

Schreier T, Kedes L, Gahlmann R 1990 Cloning, structural analysis, and expression of the human slow twitch skeletal muscle/cardiac troponin C gene. Journal of Biological Chemistry 265: 21247

Schwarzbauer J E, Patel R S, Fonda D, Hynes R O 1987 Multiple sites of alternative splicing of the rat fibronectin gene transcript. EMBO Journal 6: 2573

Seharaseyon J, Bober E, Hsieh C L et al 1990 Human embryonic/atrial myosin alkali light chain gene: characterization, sequence, and chromosomal location. Genomics 7: 289

Senni M I, De Angelis L, Nervi C et al 1990 Altered protein phosphorylation in murine muscular dystrophy. Journal of the Neurological Sciences 96: 303

Sharp N J H, Kornegay J N, van Camp S D et al 1992 An error in dystrophin mRNA processing in Golden Retriever muscular dystrophy, an animal homologue of Duchenne muscular dystrophy. Genomics 13: 115

Silman I, Futerman A H 1987 Posttranslational modification as a means of anchoring acetylcholinesterase to the cell surface. Biopolymers 26: S241

Simon A M, Hoppe P, Burden S J 1992 Spatial restriction of AChR gene expression to subsynaptic nuclei. Development 114: 545

Simons M, Wang M, McBride O W et al 1991 Human nonmuscle myosin heavy chains are encoded by two genes located on different chromosomes. Circulation Research 69: 530

Smith M M, Lindstrom J, Merlie J P 1987 Formation of the α-bungarotoxin binding site and assembly of the nicotinic acetylcholine receptor subunits occur in the endoplasmic reticulum. Journal of Biological Chemistry 262: 4367

Somerville L L, Wang K 1988 Sarcomeric matrix of striated muscle: in vivo phosphorylation of titin and nebulin in mouse diaphragm muscle. Archives of Biochemistry and Biophysics 262: 118

Spirin A A 1986 Ribosome structure and protein biosynthesis. Benjamin/Cummings, Menlo Park, California

Sternberg E A, Spizz G, Perry W M, Visard D, Well T, Olson E N 1988 Identification of upstream and intragenic regulatory elements that confer cell-type-restricted and differentiation-specific expression on the muscle creatine kinase gene. Molecular and Cellular Biology 8: 2896

Sutherland C J, Elsom V L, Gordon M L, Dunwoodie S L, Hardeman E C 1991 Coordination of skeletal muscle gene expression occurs late in mammalian development. Developmental Biology 146: 167

Taneja K L, Lifshitz L M, Fay F S, Singer R H 1992 Poly(A)RNA codistribution with microfilaments: evaluation by in situ hybridization and quantitative digital image microscopy. Journal of Cell Biology 119: 1245

Tesch P A, Thorsson A, Essen-Gustavsson B 1989 Enzyme activites of FT and ST muscle fibres in heavy-resistance trained athletes. Journal of Applied Physiology 67: 83

Thompson W R, Nadal-Ginard B, Mahdavi V 1991 A MyoD1-independent muscle-specific enhancer controls the expression of the β-myosin heavy chain gene in skeletal and cardiac muscle cells. Journal of Biological Chemistry 266: 22678

Tong B D, Auer D E, Jaye M et al 1987 cDNA clones reveal differences between human glial and endothelial cell platelet-derived growth factor A-chains. Nature 328: 619

Toothaker L E, Gonzalez D A, Tung N et al 1991 Cellular myosin heavy chain in human leukocytes: isolation of 5' cDNA clones, characterization of the protein, chromosomal localization, and upregulation during myeloid differentiation. Blood 78: 1826

Tromp G, Prockop D J 1988 Single base mutation in the proα2(I) collagen gene that causes efficient splicing of RNA from exon 27 to exon 29 and synthesis of a shortened but in-frame proα2(I) chain. Proceedings of the National Academy of Science USA 85: 5254

Vanderburg C R, Nathanson M A 1988 Posttranslational control of embryonic rat skeletal muscle protein synthesis: control at the level of translation by endogenous RNA. Journal of Cell Biology 107: 1085

Vosberg H P, Horstmann Herold U, Wettstein A 1992 The regulation of the human β myosin heavy-chain gene. Basic Research in Cardiology 87 Suppl 1: 161

Wade R, Sutherland C, Gahlmann R, Kedes L, Hardeman E, Gunning P 1990 Regulation of contractile protein gene family mRNA pool sizes during myogenesis. Developmental Biology 142: 270

Waldman A S 1992 Targeted homologous recombination in mammalian cells. Critical Reviews in Oncology and Haematology 12: 49

Walsh F S, Parekh R B, Moore S E et al 1989 Tissue-specific O-linked gycosylation of the neural cell adhesion molecule (NCAM). Development 105: 803

Walsh F S, Doherty P 1991 Structure and function of the gene for neural cell adhesion molecule. Seminars in the Neurosciences 3: 271

Walsh K 1989 Cross-binding of factors to functionally different promoter elements in c-fos and skeletal actin genes. Molecular and Cellular Biology 9: 2191

Wells D J, Wells K E, Walsh F S et al 1992 Human dystrophin expression corrects the myopathic phenotype in transgenic mdx mice. Human Molecular Genetics 1: 35

Winkelmann J C, Costa F F, Linzie B L, Forget B G 1990 β-spectrin in human skeletal muscle: tissue-specific differential processing of 3'β spectrin pre-mRNA generates a β spectrin isoform with a unique carboxyl terminus. Journal of Biological Chemistry 265: 20449

Witzemann V, Stein E, Barg B et al 1990 Primary structure and functional expression of the α-, β-, γ-, ∂- and ε-subunits of the acetylcholine receptor from rat muscle. European Journal of Biochemistry 194: 437

Witzemann V, Brenner H R, Sakmann B 1991 Neural factors regulate AChR subunit mRNAs at rat neuromuscular synapses. Journal of Cell Biology 114: 125

Witzemann V, Sakmann B 1991 Differential regulation of MyoD and myogenin mRNA levels by nerve-induced muscle activity. FEBS Letters 282: 259

Yamasaki T, Nakajima H, Kono N et al 1991 Structure of the entire human muscle phosphofructokinase-encoding gene: a two-promoter system. Gene 104: 277

Yi T M, Walsh K, Schimmel P 1991 Rabbit muscle creatine kinase: genomic cloning, sequencing, and analysis of upstream sequences important for expression in myocytes. Nucleic Acids Research 19: 3027

Yu X M, Hall Z W 1991 Extracellular domains mediating epsilon subunit interactions of muscle acetylcholine receptor. Nature 352: 64

Yutzey K E, Rhodes S J, Konieczny S F 1990 Differential trans activation associated with the muscle regulatory factors MyoD1, myogenin, and MRF 4. Molecular and Cellular Biology 10: 3934

4. The normal ultrastructure of skeletal muscle

M. J. Cullen   D. N. Landon

INTRODUCTION

This chapter describes the ultrastructure of skeletal muscle, concentrating in particular on the muscle fibres and their modifications from one type of motor unit to another. The structure of muscle is exactly tuned to its function, and slight differences in activity from muscle to muscle and from fibre to fibre are associated with subtle differences in their fine structure. When electron micrographs are examined it is important to remember that they have been obtained from a functioning dynamic tissue and represent more than the flat two-dimensional image that they are usually taken to portray.

The basic ultrastructure of the skeletal muscle fibre was largely established during the 1950s and 1960s. In the last decade there has been a resurgence of interest in filling in the details of its fine structure, using new techniques such as immuno-labelling to identify the location of many of the minor proteins. Much of this new information is only now being fitted into the general body of information about the motor unit and in this chapter coverage is limited to those features that are accepted to be a normal part of the structure of nerve and muscle.

INNERVATION OF THE MOTOR UNIT

The motor units of all postcranial skeletal muscles receive their innervation from motor neurones in lamina IX of the ventral grey columns of the spinal medulla. These cells have a bimodal size distribution, with mean diameters of 20 and 40–50 μm (Van Buren & Frank 1965), and the fibres to which they give rise show a similarly bimodal diameter distribution, both in the ventral spinal roots and in the distal branches close to the muscles supplied (Boyd & Davey 1968). Within the major nerve trunks these motor nerve fibres constitute only a minor proportion of the total fibre population, but this rises to more than 50% within the nerves to individual muscles. The large fibre population has diameters of between 12 and 20 μm, diminishing to 10–15 μm in the distal branches. This population consists of alpha fibres, which innervate fast motor units exclusively, and beta fibres which are distributed both to slow motor units and to some of the intrafusal myofibres of the muscle spindles. The tapering of individual fibres is associated with a substantial degree of branching within the major nerve trunks (Gilliatt 1966, Wray 1969) and further branching occurs within the muscle. As each motor end-plate in mature mammalian muscle receives only a single motor nerve terminal, each motor neurone is connected through its branching axon to several muscle fibres, the two elements constituting a single motor unit.

The nerves to individual limb muscles of mammals usually enter their deep surfaces in company with a major component of the arterial supply to that muscle and there divide into a number of minor branches which ramify and further subdivide within the central region of the muscle belly. The bundles of nerve fibres comprising each branch are enclosed by perineurial sheaths continuous with that of the parent nerve, the number of layers of perineurial cells diminishing progressively so that the finest branches consist of a single myelinated nerve fibre within a unilamellar sheath. At the neuromuscular junction the axon loses its myelin sheath and further divides into a small terminal arborisation in close contact with the surface membrane of the muscle cell, the region of contact being covered on its external surface by an extension of the Schwann cell sheath. This Schwann cell covering does not, however, provide an effective seal between the extracellular space at the interface between nerve and muscle and the endomysium and there is thus a potential portal of entry into the endoneurium of the parent nerve for extraneous materials of large molecular weight; this has been shown to be freely permeable to tracers such as horseradish peroxidase, which are excluded by the perineurial sheath.

THE NEUROMUSCULAR JUNCTION

The nerve axons of the motor unit terminate at specialised regions of the muscle fibres. The combination of the axon terminal (with its associated Schwann cell), with the postsynaptic membrane and postsynaptic sarcoplasm, constitutes the neuromuscular junction (Fig. 4.1). The physiology of electrical transmission at the junction will be covered in detail in Chapter 5 and we deal here only with its fine structure.

The most conspicuous components of the axon terminal are the synaptic vesicles and mitochondria, but there are also coated vesicles, dense-coated vesicles, vacuoles, microtubules, neurofilaments, lysosomes and glycogen granules (Fig. 4.2). The relative abundance of the different terminal constituents tends to vary within any one junction, from junction to junction, with the age of the junction and with its neural activity. Stereological studies have shown that in human and rat axon terminals the mitochondria generally occupy about 15% of the terminal volume and that there are on average 50–70 synaptic vesicle profiles per μm^2 of terminal (Engel & Santa 1971, Engel et al 1976). The diameter of the vesicles is 45–60 nm; they contain acetylcholine and ATP, and are coated with synapsin I, a synapse-specific phosphoprotein (Südhoferal 1989). The synaptic vesicles tend to cluster towards the side of the terminal facing the myofibre and concentrate in small groups close to the presynaptic membranes. These 'active zones' (Couteaux & Pecot-Dechauvassine 1970) are considered to be the sites of acetylcholine release from the synaptic vesicles and contain voltage-regulated calcium channels (Jones 1987). In the Lambert–Eaton myasthenic syndrome there is a marked decrease in the number of active zones and in the number of particles per zone (Engel 1987). Elegant time-resolved freeze-fracture studies of frog muscle have shown that the P face of the presynaptic membrane contains many exocytotic dimples 5 ms after being stimulated (Heuser et al 1979, Heuser & Reese 1981). The dimples, which appear immediately adjacent to the active zones,

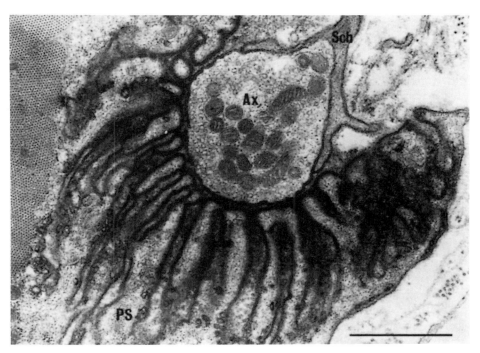

Fig. 4.1   Transverse section through a neuromuscular junction in a human quadriceps muscle which has been stained for acetylcholinesterase to highlight the membrane topography. Ax = axon terminal, Sch = Schwann cell process, PS = postsynaptic sarcoplasm (scale bar = 1 μm) (micrograph kindly donated by Dr Tim Walls).

are thought to represent the points of fusion of the synaptic vesicles with the presynaptic membrane. In fast-twitch frog muscle fibres the active zones are linear and are regularly spaced such that each zone is situated opposite the cleft between two folds of the postsynaptic membrane (see Ch. 5). In mammals where the neuromuscular junction is less elongated and more convoluted than in the frog, the active zones are shorter and less regularly dispersed.

The pre- and postsynaptic membranes at the neuromuscular junction are separated by a space 60–80 nm wide. It is into this synaptic space that acetylcholine is released when the nerve axon is stimulated. Within the synaptic space there is a basal lamina (Fig. 4.2) which is continuous at the edge of the junction with the basal laminae of both muscle fibre and the Schwann cell covering the axon terminal. It has become apparent over recent years that the basal lamina of the neuromuscular junction plays an important part in junction development and regeneration (Sanes & Chiu 1983).

This role must be dependent on unique properties of its molecular components, some of which are common to the remainder of the basal lamina and others not. Fibronectin, laminin and collagen IV are common to both junctional and extrajunctional basal lamina, but collagen V is found only in extrajunctional areas (Sanes 1982). Another unique component is a novel homologue of laminin, termed S-laminin, which is selectively associated with synaptic basal lamina and is recognised by regenerated motor axons (Hunter et al 1989). Agrin, a component of the junctional basal lamina, appears to direct the formation of acetylcholine receptor aggregates on the crests of the postsynaptic folds (Nitkin et al 1987, Reist et al 1987).

The postsynaptic membrane is deeply folded in such a way that the postsynaptic surface is considerably enlarged and the volume of the synaptic space is increased. Stereological measurements on human intercostal muscle and rat limb muscle show that the area ratio of the postsynaptic to

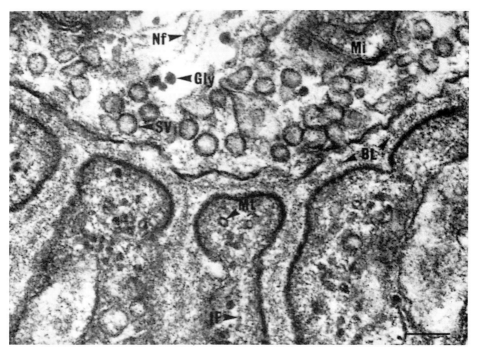

Fig. 4.2   Higher magnification view of a neuromuscular synapse. Note the clustering of the synaptic vesicles (SV) in zones facing the crests of the postsynaptic folds. The postsynaptic membrane is thickened at the crests and for a short distance into the clefts. Nf = neurofilament, Mi = mitochondrion, Gly = glycogen, BL = basal lamina, Mt = microtubule, IF = intermediate filament. Rat soleus muscle (scale bar = 0.1 μm).

presynaptic membranes is of the order of 10:1 (Engel & Santa 1971, Engel et al 1976). The clefts tend to be longer (~1.5 μm) in human end-plates than in rat end-plates (~1.0 μm), and in fast-twitch fibres than in slow-twitch fibres (Padykula & Gauthier 1970). In the end-plates of fast-twitch fibres, the junctional folds are numerous, deep and branched. In slow-twitch fibres they are fewer, shallower and less branched (Ogata 1988, Oki et al 1990). Figure 4.3 is a scanning electron micrograph showing the topography of the muscle surface at a mouse end-plate after removal of the nerve terminal. The synaptic clefts are variable in length and width and seem to have no preferred orientation. The complexity of the folding of the postsynaptic membrane is further displayed in Figure 4.4, where the membrane at a human neuromuscular junction has been sectioned face on.

The postsynaptic membrane appears thicker and more electron-dense at the crests of the folds and for a short distance into the clefts (Fig. 4.2). Electron microscopic autoradiography using labelled α-bungarotoxin has shown that these denser areas are the sites of highest concentration of the acetylcholine receptor (Fertuck & Salpeter 1974, Barnard et al 1975). The receptors are concentrated in these sites at a density of approximately 20 000 per μm^2 with relatively few elsewhere in the membrane (Fertuck & Salpeter 1976).

The shape and substructure of the acetylcholine receptor have been determined by a combination of electron microscopy and low-angle X-ray diffraction. Electrophysiological and recombinant DNA techniques have shown that mammalian muscle expresses two subtypes of end-plate channel: a low conductance fetal and a high conductance adult type. Both subtypes are comprised of α-, β and δ-subunits and either a γ- (fetal) or an ε- (adult) subunit (Mishina et al 1986, Gu & Hall 1988). The subunits span the

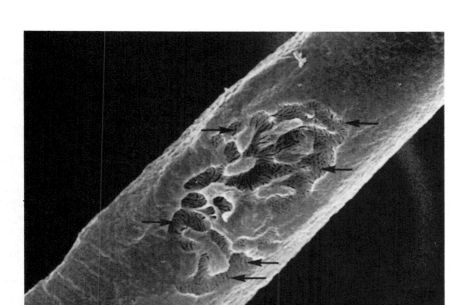

Fig. 4.3 The surface of a muscle fibre from which the axon terminal and basal lamina has been stripped by 6 N HCl, thus exposing the clefts (arrows) in the postsynaptic gutters. Fifteen-day-old mouse (scale bar = 5 μm) (scanning electron micrograph kindly donated by Dr K. Kitaoka, Ehime University, Japan).

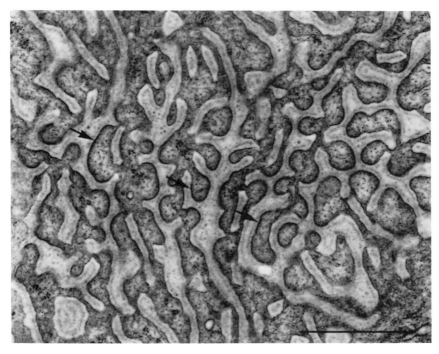

Fig. 4.4 A section which has passed through the clefts in the postsynaptic membrane in a human quadriceps muscle showing the complexity of the folding. Thickened membranes (arrows) correspond to the ACh-receptor-containing areas (scale bar = 1 μm).

postsynaptic membrane with most of the mass of the molecule in the extracellular space. Each subunit contains about 500 amino acid residues and the total mass of the receptor is about 300 000 daltons. When acetylcholine binds to the two subunits the channel opens and the end-plate current is initiated (see also Ch.1). The primary sequences of all four subunits have been elucidated by recombinant DNA techniques, and the structural basis of the difference between fetal and adult forms of the receptor has also been defined (Mishina et al 1986).

Microfilaments, microtubules, intermediate filaments and other cytoskeletal elements are found in the sarcoplasm adjacent to the postsynaptic membrane (Fig. 4.2) and are involved in maintaining the shape of the membrane and in determining the distribution of the membrane proteins. Dystrophin and β-spectrin, for example, are found throughout the muscle fibre surface but are most concentrated at the neuromuscular junction (Bloch & Morrow 1989). This dual localization is shared by a structurally unrelated protein, the 58 K protein, which has been shown to bind to dystrophin (Butler et al 1990). Within the junctional region, both dystrophin and the 58 K protein are located predominantly in the depths of the synaptic folds, thus occupying a different domain from that of the acetylcholine receptors (Byers et al 1991, Sealock et al 1991). Dystrophin-related protein (DRP) and the 43 K protein, in contrast, are located predominantly on the crests of the synaptic folds and appear to parallel the distribution of the acetylcholine receptors (Froehner et al 1987, Bewick et al 1992).

THE MYOFIBRE

Basal lamina

The basal lamina is the thin (20–30 nm) outermost coating of the muscle fibre; it ensheathes the entire muscle fibre, including its symphysis with the axon terminals at the neuromuscular junctions and its union with the tendons at the myotendinous junctions. The basal lamina is secreted by the muscle fibre itself, unlike the collagen fibrils immediately adjacent to it, which are of fibroblastic origin. This thin layer of collagen fibrils (the retic-

ular lamina), in combination with the basal lamina, constitutes the basement membrane described by nineteenth-century histologist and named the 'sarcolemma' by Bowman (1840), a term now often used wrongly as a synonym for the plasmalemma (plasma membrane).

The structural scaffolding of the basal lamina is formed by a polymerised network of type IV collagen. High-resolution electron microscopy has shown that the network is composed of monomolecular filaments (1.7 nm mean diameter) which twist around each other in a super helix and which have branch points that are spaced apart by an average of 45 nm (Yurchenco & Ruben 1987). Within the basal lamina there are also proteoglycans (primarily heparin sulphates) and the glycoproteins, laminin and entactin. Laminin is a large (850 000 Da) complex of three very long polypeptide chains arranged in the shape of a cross. It is located mainly on the plasma membrane side of the basal lamina. A single dumb-bell-shaped entactin molecule is thought to be bound to each laminin molecule where the short arms meet the long one. Fibronectin, a large adhesive glycoprotein, is usually present on the outer side of the basal lamina.

In conventionally fixed and embedded muscle tissue an electron-lucent layer, 10–15 nm wide (lamina lucida), can usually be seen separating the basal lamina from the underlying plasma membrane (Fig. 4.5) This gap is traversed by fine bridges. As it has now been found that the glycoprotein complex, to which dystrophin binds, is, on its external side, linked to laminin in the basal lamina (Ibraghimov-Beskrovnaya et al 1992), it might be expected that these glycoproteins cross the lamina lucida. The presence of these linked molecules must ensure that the plasma membrane and basal lamina move together during muscle contraction. (The existence of the lamina lucida as a real 'structure' has been questioned by Goldberg (1986) who prepared tongue muscle by rapid freezing and freeze substitution and found that, without aldehyde fixation, the basal lamina and plasma membrane were in tight contact with each other.)

The role of the basal lamina in the physiology of skeletal muscle is still only partly understood. Work on other tissues, in particular blood capil-

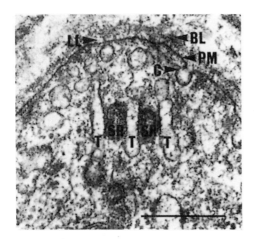

Fig. 4.5 Part of the periphery of a regenerating human muscle fibre. BL = basal lamina (lamina densa), LL = lamina lucida, PM = plasma membrane (plasmalemma), C = caveola, T = T tubule, SR = sarcoplasmic reticulum (scale bar = 0.5 μm).

laries and renal glomeruli, has attributed two functions to the basal lamina: as a semipermeable filter and as a supporting structure. The basal lamina of muscle allows the inward passage of 12 nm ferritin molecules but not a colloidal gold–horseradish peroxidase complex of 20–25 nm diameter, suggesting that it may act as a diffusion barrier for large molecules (Oldfors & Fardeau 1983). It does not, on the other hand, appear to prevent the passage of material expelled from pathological muscle into the extracellular space (Cullen & Mastaglia 1982).

In normal healthy muscle there is probably very little or no movement of cells across the basal lamina, in either direction. In diseased or traumatised muscle, however, this demarcation or barrier function is compromised. Macrophages and lymphocytes pass inwards into affected fibres (see Ch. 10) while satellite cells can be seen to pass outwards from normal fibres (perhaps to assist in the regeneration of necrotic fibres) (Maltin et al 1983). It is unclear how the basal lamina barrier is pierced but it is known that the cells can penetrate very small gaps (<2.0 μm) (Sesodia & Cullen 1991), so it is likely that only a very limited area of lamina has to be lysed.

The best evidence for the basal lamina as a supporting structure is seen in muscle which is regenerating. The basal lamina is remarkably resistant to noxious agents and persists as an 'empty tube' when the necrotic fibre debris is removed by phagocytes. Regeneration involves the fusion of satellite cell-derived myoblasts within the basal lamina tubes to form multinucleate myotubes. The myotubes are aligned in parallel with the longitudinal axis of the basal lamina tubes with which they make direct contact. While the myoblasts and myotubes appear to make use of the basal lamina as a support or guide when it is present (Vracko & Benditt 1972), regeneration can occur in its absence, e.g. in explanted muscle cultured in vivo in which new myotubes will grow out of, and away from, the original lamina (Bischoff 1975).

The basal lamina also appears to have an important influence in regeneration of the neuromuscular synapse, in guiding regrowth of axons of denervated fibres back to the original site of the end-plate, and in localising the accumulation of acetylcholine receptors on regenerated myofibres, also at the original site. Sanes et al (1978), using denervated frog cutaneous pectoralis muscle, damaged the myofibres so that they and their nerve terminals degenerated, and only the basal lamina sheath remained; muscle regeneration was prevented by X-irradiation. Axons regenerating into the region contacted the basal lamina almost exclusively at the original synaptic sites and, within the terminals, the synaptic organelles lined up opposite periodic specialisations in the basal lamina. When reinnervation was prevented while the myofibres were allowed to grow back, they developed accumulations of acetylcholine receptors selectively localised to the original synaptic site (Burden et al 1979). It seems from these two pieces of work that specific molecules within the junctional basal lamina attract the axon and also influence the differentiation of the postsynaptic membrane.

Plasmalemma

The outer surface of the muscle fibre is covered by a plasmalemma or cell membrane. This is itself related externally to the basal lamina component of the sarcolemma, from which it is separated by a 20 nm electron-lucent gap corresponding to the glycocalyx of the surface membrane which lacks contrast in conventionally stained electron micrographs (Fig. 4.5). Like other cell membranes, the muscle plasmalemma consists of a proteolipid bilayer, the latter component being comprised of neutral lipid, phospholipids, and cholesterol esters and cholesterol; the proportion of the last is reported to be highest in slow-twitch fibres (Fischbeck et al 1982). Apart from the proteins which contribute to its intrinsic structure, the plasmalemma also contains a number of particulate proteins serving a range of specialised functions: these include the acetylcholine receptor and other receptor molecules, transport channels for a range of ionic species, ATPases associated with metabolically driven ionic pumps, and transport proteins for glucose and amino acids.

Specialised regions of the plasmalemma occur at the neuromuscular junction and the myotendinous junction, and these will be discussed in detail elsewhere. Over the remainder of the fibre it possesses a relatively uniform ultrastructure and, at resting length, a smooth external contour indented at intervals by myosatellite cells (see p. 120), which on contraction is thrown into fine circumferential folds. This surface element of the plasmalemma is in direct continuity with an extensive system of subsurface caveolae via a series of 20–40 nm pores (Fig. 4.6), and many of these are in turn connected to the transverse tubular system. The pores are scattered in a semiregular fashion over the surface of the myofibre, and in human muscle number between 12 and 20 μm^2 (Schmalbruch 1979a, Bonilla et al 1981), but it has been reported that both their numbers and their distribution can be altered by hypoxia in vivo and by delayed fixation (Schmalbruch 1985, Lee et al 1986). The caveolae make a substantial contribution to the total plasmalemmal area, estimated to amount to 47% in sectioned (Mobley & Eisenberg 1975), and up to 80% in freeze-fractured frog muscle fibres (Dulhunty & Franzini-Armstrong 1975). The most superficial element of cytoplasm subjacent to the surface portions of the plasmalemma between the caveolae shows an increase in electron density in conventional sectioned preparations (Fig. 4.6) which in chicken slow-twitch fibres is associated with a peripheral layer of the structural protein, vinculin (Shear & Bloch 1985).

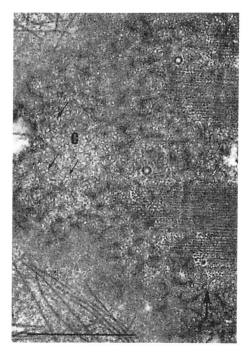

Fig. 4.6 A transmission micrograph of a longitudinal section which shaves the surface of a human myofibre. The superficial sarcoplasm is packed with lobulated subsurface caveolae (C). They are connected to the plasmalemma by small round pores (small arrows), and are continuous with the tubules of the T system (large arrow) (scale bar = 1 μm).

Freeze-fracture studies of skeletal muscle have revealed that the muscle-cell plasmalemma contains numerous intramembranous particles, occurring either singly or as aggregates (Ellisman et al 1976), the majority of the basic units having mean diameters of about either 6 or 10 nm. The 10 nm particles occur on both the P and E faces of the membrane and it has been claimed that in cultured chick myotubes up to 50% of these may represent sodium/potassium-ATPase molecules (Pumplin & Fambrough 1983). Change in the numbers and distribution of these 10 nm particles has been claimed to occur in both denervated and dystrophic muscle (Schotland et al 1981), but the values reported for normal muscle also vary widely (Yoshioka & Okuda 1977, Ketelsen 1980, Schotland et al 1981), and their numbers have also been reported to decrease during prolonged hypoxia (Schmalbruch 1980).

The 6 nm particles always occur on the P face of

the plasmalemma and characteristically form rect-angular arrays of up to 100 individual particles. In both human and animal muscle these 6 nm particle arrays are found almost exclusively on the type II, fast-twitch fibres (Rash & Ellisman 1974, Rash et al 1974, Schmalbruch 1979a, Shafiq et al 1979, Schotland et al 1981), with their highest incidence in a band 0.5–1 mm from the margin of the neuromuscular junction. 6 nm particle arrays are absent from the majority of slow-twitch fibres and from human fetal muscle (Schmalbruch 1979a), and appear relatively late in the development of fast-twitch fibres (Hudson et al 1982). Experimental denervation of fast fibres does not appear to affect either the numbers or sizes of their particle arrays, at least in the short term (Ellisman & Rash 1977, Tachikawa & Clementi 1979), but in the rat innervation is required for the development of square arrays up to 30 days postnatal (Sirken & Fischbeck 1985), and experimental reinnervation of slow muscle by a fast-muscle nerve has been shown to induce development of 6 nm particle arrays with a similar density and distribution to those found in normal fast-twitch fibres (Ellisman et al 1978). Neonatal tenotomy, in which function is impaired without loss of innervation, also slows the development of square arrays (Sirken & Fischbeck 1985). Square arrays are reported to be greatly reduced or absent in the plasmalemmae of myofibres in Duchenne dystrophy (Peluchetti et al 1985, Wakayama et al 1985) (see Ch. 9).

Myofibril

Some 80% of the mass of striated muscle fibres is composed of the myofilaments, and these are organised into compact longitudinally orientated bands, the myofibrils. The latter are usually described to be polygonal in cross-section with a maximum diameter of 1–2 μm, and to be unbranched with a length equivalent to that of the myofibre as a whole. Each myofibril is composed of serially repeating segments of identical struc-ture known as sarcomeres, and the fairly exact lateral alignment of these with their neighbours in adjacent myofibrils is responsible for the charac-teristic transverse striations of the myofibre as a whole. This generalised image of the myofibril is

subject to considerable variations between fibre types in individual species, and between species and phyla. These relate not only to the degree to which individual myofibrils can be distinguished as separate entities, a function of the extent to which they are enveloped by SR, the myofibrils of fast-twitch fibres being more clearly defined than those of slow fibres, particularly in the region of the A band (see below), a difference which permits fibres to be differentiated into Fibrillenstruktur and Felderstruktur fibres respec-tively by light microscopy (Kruger 1952, Gray 1958), but also to their geometry, the transverse sections of many myofibrils deviating widely from the normal polygonal shape to form flat ribbons 1–2 μm thick and many tens of microns wide. Myofibrils are also not infrequently branched, a tendency which increases in muscle disease.

Each sarcomere along the length of the myofibrils consists of a dense central 'A' (anisotropic) band 1.5–1.6 μm long, flanked by two paler 'I' (isotropic) bands of variable longitu-dinal dimension, depending upon the state of shortening of the fibre (Fig. 4.7). The A band is crossed at its mid-point by a dark narrow transverse line, the 'M' line (Mittelschreibe), bordered by a paler band of variable width, the 'H' zone (Hellerband). The A band is composed of a regular hexagonal array of filaments 15–18 nm in diameter and tapering gently at either end (Fig. 4.8a,b), the principal constituent of which is the protein 'myosin'. The pale I bands on either side of the A band are divided at their mid-point by a narrow dense line, the Z line (Zwischenscheibe) or Z disc. The I band is also constructed of parallel filaments which vary in length from 1.0 to 1.35 μm in different vertebrate species: they are considerably more slender, with a diameter of 7 nm, and are less regular in their arrangement than those of the A band. Each I filament consists of paired α-helices of chains of a globular protein 'actin' in combina-tion with a second globular protein 'troponin', and a long-chain protein 'tropomyosin'. At the Z line the I filaments of the two halves of one I band form regular square lattices and have a common attach-ment to the dense matrix material of the Z line (Fig. 4.8a,b). The Z lines mark the longitudinal boundaries of the individual sarcomeres, each of which consist of one A band and two half I bands

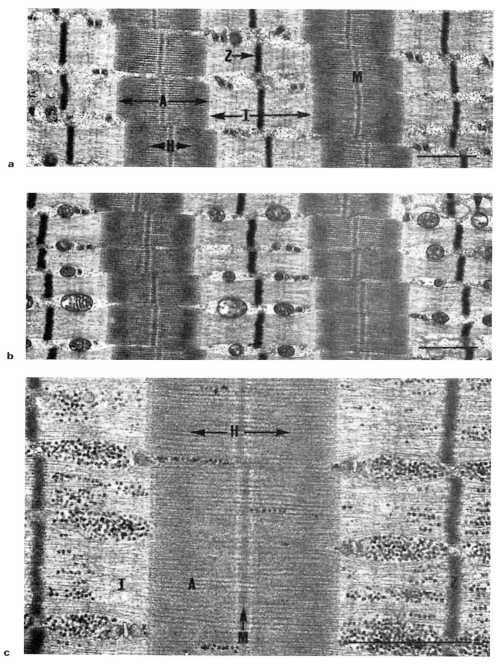

Fig. 4.7   Longitudinal sections through myofibrils from fast-twitch **a** and slow-twitch **b** human myofibres. Dark A bands (A) alternate with pale I bands (I), the latter bisected at their mid-points by dense narrow Z lines (Z). The parallel thick filaments which compose the A band are linked at their mid-points by a narrow transverse stripe, the M line (M). The thin I filaments interdigitate with the thick A-band filaments, and their central ends are marked by the presence of a central paler region of the A band, the H zone (H). Note the broader M and Z lines and more numerous mitochondria in the slow-twitch fibre. A detailed view of a single fast-twitch sarcomere is shown in **c**. The dense granules within and between the myofibrils are glycogen (scale bar = 1 μm).

(Fig. 4.7). The free ends of the I filaments interdigitate between the elements of the hexagonal A-band lattice, each I filament occupying the centre of a triangular space between three adjacent A filaments (Fig. 4.8b). Contraction of the myofibre is brought about by shortening of the sarcomeres that make up its constituent myofibrils, and this is accomplished by a sliding movement of the I filaments towards the centre of the A band: at its physiological limit this process results in the extinction of the I and H bands, the latter representing the portion of the A-filament lattice unoccupied by I filaments, and apposition of the Z discs to the ends of the A bands. During relaxation following a contraction this sliding movement is reversed until the normal resting length of the sarcomere of between 2.5 and 3.0 μm has been restored. The possible mechanisms responsible for the generation of force required to produce the inward movement of the I filaments are discussed below.

A band. The A filaments which compose the anisotropic band of the sarcomere have a remarkably constant length of between 1.5 and 1.6 μm in a wide range of vertebrate species, the precise value depending upon the method of tissue preparation employed, and a value of 1.57 μm has been obtained from frozen sections of human muscle (Sjostrom & Squire 1977). Each filament carries a series of regularly arranged side projections, cross-bridges, from their tapered tips to approximately 80 nm from their mid-points to leave a smooth 160 nm long central zone spanning the M line: this has become known as the pseudo H zone or bare zone. The individual myosin molecules which compose the A filaments are rod-shaped, 170 nm long, two-stranded alpha helices 2 nm in diameter bearing two pear-shaped heads 19 nm by 4.5 nm at one end (Fig. 4.8c) (Elliott & Offer 1978). Each myosin molecule is a hexamer comprised of two 'heavy' chains of about 200 000 daltons, and four 'light' chains of 20 000 daltons each. The two heavy chains wind around each other in a coiled coil of α-helices to form the tail of the molecule, and then fold separately to produce the two heads. The light chains are of two chemically distinct classes and one of each class is associated with each head (Craig & Knight 1983), and those of fast muscle appear to differ from those of slow muscle, a difference which is reflected in their actomyosin ATPase activities. The shaft of this molecule can be dissected into two components by tryptic digestion to yield: (1) a straight length of two chain alpha helices approximately 90 nm long with a molecular weight of 150 000 known as light meromyosin (LMM); (2) a shorter, more massive portion consisting of the remaining part of the shaft and its two attached heads, heavy meromyosin (HMM), having a molecular weight of around 350 000. The heads, which alone possess actin binding and ATPase activity, may be separated from the helical component by papain digestion (Lowey et al 1969) to give the S_1 (heads) and S_2 (shaft) subunits of HMM (Fig. 4.8c). The shafts of the individual myosin molecules have been shown by Huxley (1963) to stack together to form the shaft of the A filament, and in such a manner that the paired heads lie on its surface, with the myosin molecules in each half of one A filament arrayed with opposite polarities, the heads pointing towards the two ends of the filament. The region of overlap of the two arrays of LMM tails from each half gives rise to the central bare zone (Fig. 4.8d). X-ray diffraction studies have demonstrated that the myosin heads are arranged round the A filaments in a semi-regular helix (Craig & Offer 1976a), with pairs of heads on opposite sides of the shaft at intervals of 14.3 nm, each successive pair being rotated by 120 degrees about the axis of the shaft relative to its nearest neighbours, to give an overall axial repeat of 43.0 nm (Huxley & Brown 1967). It has been suggested that the HMM component of the molecule interacts only weakly with the shafts of adjacent myosin molecules, and that its junction with LMM may act as a flexible joint, permitting the HMM component of each myosin molecule to lie at a variable angle to the shaft (Huxley 1969, Lowey et al 1969, Trinick & Elliott 1979).

The pseudo-H zone of the A band shows a number of transverse striations, of which a central dense band and a pair flanking it at 22 nm to either side are the most prominent, and together constitute the histological M line (Fig. 4.8a). With some methods of preparation the A bands of slow-twitch fibres show an additional pair of less dense lines at 43.7 nm from the centre of the A filament, to give a

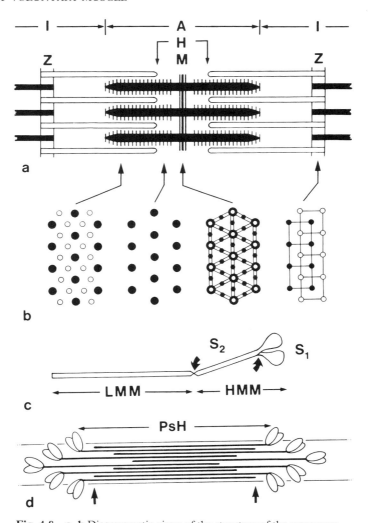

Fig. 4.8   a, b Diagrammatic views of the structure of the sarcomere. The A band (A) is composed of a hexagonal lattice of thick filaments with tapered ends, linked together by M-line bridges (M) at their midpoints. The central bare zone of each filament is flanked by longer terminal regions which carry a regular series of lateral projections. The I filaments of each half I band (I) are attached to the Z discs (Z) in a regular square array, and interdigitate with the A-band filaments to form a second hexagonal lattice. The interval between the central ends of the two sets of I filaments constitutes the H zone (H). Representative cross-sectional appearances are illustrated in b. **c** A schematic view of the myosin molecule. The rod-shaped shaft of the light meromyosin (LMM) component is joined by a more flexible section to heavy meromyosin (HMM), which consists of a straight shaft (the S_2 subunit) and two pear-shaped heads (the S_1 subunits). The sites on the molecule susceptible to enzymic attack are indicated by curved arrows. **d** A diagram of the antiparallel packing of the individual myosin molecules at the centre of an I filament. The heads project from the surface of the filament, and the smooth region between the most central pair of heads is the 'pseudo-H zone'. The somewhat shorter region of overlap of the shafts of the molecules is marked by arrows (reproduced from Landon (1982) with permission from the editors and publishers).

five-banded M line (Sjostrom & Squire 1977). Studies of the three-dimensional structure of the M line have shown that its constituent bands represent the positions of substantial cross-bridges which link each A filament to its six nearest neighbours in a hexagonal array (Fig. 4.8b). When the M-line region of the A band is viewed in transverse section each of these bridges shows a thickening at its mid-point, and these have been interpreted to indicate the existence of a set of short small-diameter (4–5 nm) longitudinally orientated 'M filaments' midway between each A filament (Fig. 4.8b). A model structure of a three-banded M line incorporating these components has been described by Knappeis & Carlsen (1968), the main features of which have been confirmed by Luther & Squire (1978). The M line is presumed to stabilise the transverse and longitudinal order of the thick filament lattice of the A band, and in muscles which do not have M lines the thick filaments are in general in less good register (Page 1965). Several non-myosin M proteins have been isolated, but their locations and function within the intact M line are at present unknown: examples are a 150 000 Da component which has been ascribed a structural role in the M cross-bridges (Chowrashi & Pepe 1979); myomesin, a 185 000 Da protein also associated with M-line cross-bridges (Grove et al 1984, 1989), and the MM isoenzyme of creatine kinase which co-migrates with a 42 000 Da M-line component (Walliman et al 1979).

A number of other non-myosin proteins are now known to be located in the A band, and the most abundant and the best characterised of these is C protein. It is an elongated monomer lacking any helical component, 35 nm in length, with a molecular weight of 140 000 Da (Offer et al 1973). It has been shown to bind tightly to both the LMM and S2 portions of myosin at physiological ionic strength, but not to the myosin heads, and thus does not interfere with either its ATPase or actin-binding properties. Antibody-staining studies have shown that C protein is bound strongly and solely to seven narrow stripes in the mid-zone of the cross-bridge region of the A band, and that these have the same 43 nm repeat as the underlying myosin backbone of the thick filament (Pepe & Drucker 1975, Craig & Offer 1976b).

The function of the C protein is not known, but it has been suggested to have a role in regulating the assembly of the myosin molecules into thick filaments. Another non-myosin protein, H protein, has been isolated from crude preparations of C protein, and has been found to be restricted to a narrow band in the inner region of the cross-bridge zone, two 43 nm repeats central to the inner edge of the region containing C protein (Craig & Megerman 1979); other proteins, so far uncharacterised, are thought to be located in the distal (D) cross-bridge zone.

I band. The major component of the thin myofilaments which characterise the I bands of the sarcomeres is the protein 'actin'. Its monomeric form (G actin) is an asymmetrical ellipsoid, consisting of two distinct and roughly globular domains separated by a cleft, with overall dimensions of $6.7 \times 4.0 \times 3.7$ nm and a molecular weight of about 45 000. The actin monomers are assembled into a filamentous polymer (F actin), which is a right-handed, two-stranded helix of the filament (Milligan et al 1990). The centre-to-centre spacing of the monomers along each chain is 5.46 nm, with the units of the two chains staggered relative to one another by one half period (Fig. 4.9a). The pitch of the helix in vertebrate striated muscle is 3.60 nm (Huxley & Brown 1967). The grooves on either side of the twin chains of actin molecules are occupied by a second I-filament protein, 'tropomyosin'. This is a rod-shaped molecule 38.5 nm long containing a left-handed alpha helix with a molecular weight of 66 000 daltons. These units are assembled end to end to form a pair of continous spiral strands running the length of the I filament (Cohen et al 1971, Ebashi 1980). Each tropomyosin molecule is attached to exactly seven actin monomers, and it is this relationship rather than the more variable pitch of the actin helix which defines the functional unit of the I filament. I filaments vary in length from 1.0 to 1.35 μm in various animal species, but within any one species have a constant and well-defined length (Huxley 1963, Sjöstrom & Squire 1977). At the distal ends of the sarcomere the I filaments end in the Z line in a regular square 22 nm array, and at their central ends penetrate the hexagonal lattice of the A band where each occupies a trigonal point between

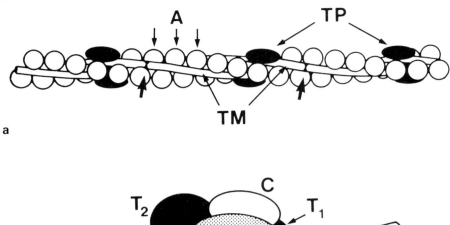

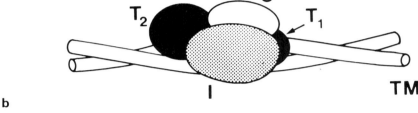

Fig. 4.9 a A diagrammatic representation of a portion of an I filament. Two chains of actin molecules represented as spheres (A) are wound in a right-handed helix, the two grooves between them containing rod-shaped molecules of tropomyosin (TM) assembled end-to-end to produce a second double helix. A third, more or less globular protein troponin (TP), is attached to a specific binding site on each tropomyosin molecule and is thus located at regular intervals along the I filament. Broad arrows indicate the points of contact of individual tropomyosin molecules. **b** An enlarged view of the subcomponents of the troponin complex attached to the tropomyosin double helix stripped of its actin helices. T_1 binds the complex to the tropomyosin molecule; T_2 links it to the C and I subunits, which have calcium-binding and inhibitory functions respectively (redrawn after Ebashi (1980), and reproduced from Landon (1982) with permission from the editors and publishers).

three adjacent thick filaments to form a second interlocking hexagonal lattice. The affinity of the I filaments for myosin has been demonstrated by treating I bands isolated from homogenised muscle with the S_1 subfragments of HMM (Huxley 1963): the individual filaments become 'decorated' with regularly arranged arrowheads of S_1 subunits at intervals of 35–37 nm. These arrowheads are always directed towards the free ends of the filaments, demonstrating that they are structurally polarised, with the polarity reversing on the two sides of the Z line.

The I bands of longitudinally sectioned muscle often show regular transverse striations with a period of approximately 40 nm (Huxley 1967), and a similar periodicity has been detected in X-ray diffraction images of unfixed muscle (Huxley & Brown 1967). Studies using antibody staining (Pepe 1966, Ohtsuki et al 1967) have shown that these cross-striations represent the location of a third I-filament protein, 'troponin' (Ebashi et al

1968). This has a molecular weight of around 80 000 Da and a roughly globular structure composed of three major subunits: 'troponin C', the Ca^{2+}-binding component which confers Ca^{2+} sensitivity to the actomyosin complex; 'troponin I' with an inhibitory function, and 'troponin T', responsible for binding the complex to a specific point on each tropomyosin molecule in the grooves of the actin helix (Fig. 4.9), to give the observed periodicity of 38.5 nm along the I filaments (Ohtsuki 1975, 1979). Each of the subcomponents of troponin is polymorphic with specific variants related to myofibre type (Perry & Dhoot 1980). The properties of troponin have been reviewed by Ebashi (1980) and its role in the regulation of muscular contraction is outlined below. The molecular structures of the principal A and I-band proteins, and their interactions during muscle contraction and relaxation, are described and discussed in greater detail in Chapter 6.

In addition to the fine cross-banding attributable to the regular attachments of the troponin complexes, the I band also usually shows one or more broader transverse bands, the N lines. The most constant is the N_1 line which lies close to the Z disc at the point at which the I filaments become organised into a regular square array (see below). A second N_2 line may also be visible some 0.2–0.3 μm further into the I band (Page 1968, Franzini-Armstrong 1970). Both N lines are sites of concentration of a high molecular weight (600–900 kDa) polypeptide, nebulin, which accounts for 3% of myofibrillar mass and binds strongly to alpha actinin (Nave et al 1990). Nebulin is believed to be present throughout the greater part of the I band as a set of inextensible filaments anchored to the Z disc by their C-terminals, and attached by a regular series of interactions with the I-filaments corresponding to the repeat period of the actin–tropomyosin helix. It has been proposed that it may act as a precise regulator of I-filament assembly and determinant of thin filament length (Jin & Wang 1991, Labeit et al 1991). The functional significance of the regions of its concentration at the N lines is unknown. A further high molecular weight ($1–2.8 \times 10^6$ Da) protein for which there is good evidence within the I-band is titin (connectin). Individual molecules consist of a slender 900 nm rod attached to a single globular head, which associate as dimers or higher oligomers by their head regions (Nave et al 1989), and contribute a major component to a set of fine (4 nm) elastic filaments which traverse the I band in parallel with the I filaments; these appear to connect the A filaments to the Z disc (Maruyama 1986, Wang 1982), with the C-terminal end of the titin molecule located near the Z disc and the N-terminal in the M-band region (Wang et al 1991a), through binding sites to LMM and C-protein (Labeit et al 1992). It has been proposed that these titin-containing filaments are responsible for a significant proportion of the resting tension of muscle fibres (Wang et al 1991b) and play an important part in maintaining the mechanical continuity of the sarcomeres under stretch (Maruyama et al 1989, Fulton & Isaacs 1991). They have been identified with the 'gap filaments' which become visible between the ends of the I and A filaments when sarcomeres are stretched beyond the point of thick/thin filament overlap (Trombitas et al 1991).

Z disc. The Z line or disc is an optically and electron-dense transverse structure which divides each I band at its mid-point, and constitutes the boundary between adjacent sarcomeres. Electron micrographs of sections cut at a shallow angle to the plane of the disc show that the filaments of each half I band lose their apparently haphazard arrangement immediately adjacent to the disc, and become organised into a regular 22 nm^2 array, the square lattices so formed on the two surfaces of the disc being offset one from another by 50% along each axis (Fig. 4.8a). Each individual I filament is therefore positioned opposite the centre of a square formed by the ends of four filaments from the I band of the opposite side of the disc. In the plane of the disc itself the two lattices combine to create a small regular square lattice of half the period (Fig. 4.10a). Longitudinal sections show that the terminal 20–30 nm portions of the I filaments thicken as they approach the disc, and acquire increased electron density which merges with that of the amorphous dense material of the Z disc itself. Within the thickness of the disc the ends of the I filament interdigitate (Fig. 4.10b); the extent of the overlap varies with myofibre type, slow-twitch fibres having Z discs of approximately twice the thickness (90–100 nm) of those of fast-twitch fibres (40–50 nm).

The appearances described above are those usually seen following conventional aldehyde fixation, but where the primary fixative is osmium tetroxide, as was almost invariably the case before the introduction of glutaraldehyde, the fine structure of the disc shows certain consistent differences (Fardeau 1969a,b, Landon 1969, 1970b, MacDonald & Engel 1971). The lattice period of the disc is increased to 15.5 nm and its axes are rotated so that they lie at 45 degrees to those of the I-filament arrays of the adjacent I bands and also present a characteristic 'woven' appearance (Reedy 1964). In longitudinal sections the I filaments of the opposed sarcomeres no longer interdigitate, and appear to be linked by short oblique Z filaments to their nearest neighbours in the next sarcomere (Fig. 4.11). A number of models of Z-disc structure have been proposed.

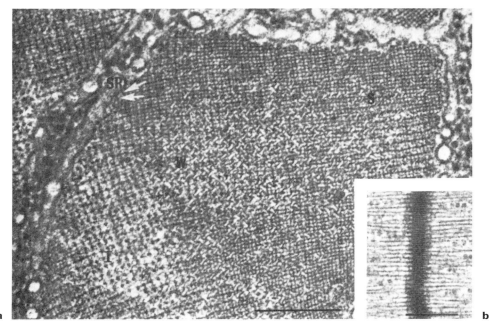

Fig. 4.10   a A transverse section through the Z-line region of a rat myofibre fixed with glutaraldehyde during the course of a tetanic contraction. The plane of section passes through the end of the I band (I), where the I filaments form a regular square array with a 22 nm period, and also through the Z-disc lattice, part of which (S) shows the small square 11 nm lattice characteristic of unstimulated glutaraldehyde-fixed tissue, and part of the larger woven lattice (W) with its axes at 45 degrees to those of the small and large square lattices, usually associated with primary fixation in osmium tetroxide (see text). Note the short filaments (arrows) connecting the Z disc to the sarcoplasmic reticulum (SR). **b** The appearance of a glutaraldehyde-fixed, fast-twitch Z line in longitudinal section (scale bar = 0.25 μm).

The earliest of these were necessarily based upon observations of osmium tetroxide-fixed tissue, and invoked the existence of 'Z filaments' (Knappeis & Carlsen 1962), a 'Z membrane' (Franzini-Armstrong & Porter 1964), and looping actin filaments (Kelly 1967) to account for the linking elements between the I filaments of adjacent sarcomeres seen in longitudinal sections. These models are not readily compatible with the Z-disc structure found in glutaraldehyde-fixed tissue and various alternative models have been proposed (Landon 1970b, MacDonald & Engel 1971, Rowe 1971, 1973, Kelly & Cahill 1972, Ullrick et al 1977), some of which have placed more emphasis on the non-filamentous components of the disc, while others invoke more ingenious looping configurations. The merits and weaknesses of these various proposals have been reviewed elsewhere (Squire 1981, Landon 1982, O'Brien & Dickins 1983).

Most explanations of the mechanisms underlying the process of muscular contraction assign the Z disc an entirely passive role as an anchor upon which the I filaments of adjacent sarcomeres may pull, and through which the tension they generate is transmitted to the attachments of the myofibre. In the intact fibre each sarcomere acts as a closed-volume system and it is well established that shortening is accompanied by an appropriate increase in the transverse diameter of the A band, brought about by an increase in the inter-A-filament spacing (Elliott et al 1963, Brandt et al 1967). There is also evidence from fine structural studies of fixed tissue (Reedy 1967, Franzini-Armstrong 1973), and X-ray diffraction studies on living muscle (Elliott et al 1967, Yu et al 1977), that the I-filament spacing in the zone of the ordered square array adjacent to the Z disc also increases with sarcomere shortening. Experiments in which rat muscles were fixed with glutaralde-

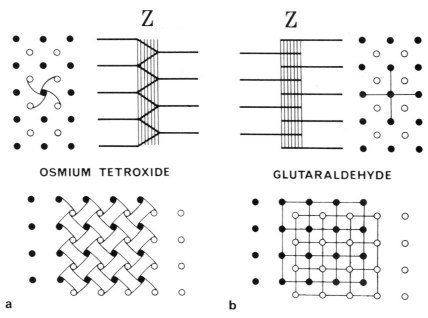

OSMIUM TETROXIDE   GLUTARALDEHYDE

a   b

Fig. 4.11 A diagrammatic view of the internal structure of the Z disc seen in longitudinal and transverse section following osmium tetroxide (**a**) and glutaraldehyde (**b**) primary fixation. Transected I filaments arising from one side of the disc are represented by open circles, those from the other by closed circles. The dense matrix is indicated by vertical hatching (reproduced from Landon (1982) with permission from the editors and the publishers).

hyde during the course of a tetanic contraction (Landon 1970c) have confirmed that the I-filament spacing increases in contracted muscles, and have shown that the fine square lattice characteristic of muscles fixed with aldehydes is converted wholly or in part to the larger woven form normally seen during primary osmium tetroxide fixation (Fig. 4.10a). The observations suggest that the Z disc undergoes transitory and reversible changes in both its radial dimensions and internal structure during the course of muscular contraction in vivo, and it has been proposed that the fine square and coarse woven lattices represent alternative and interconvertible forms of Z-disc structure which correspond to the relaxed and contracted states of the sarcomere respectively (Landon 1970c). It is not known whether these changes are active components of the contractile process, as envisaged in the theory of contraction proposed by Ullrick (1967), or whether they are a passive corollary of the process of sarcomere shortening as has been suggested by Davey (1976), enabling the I filaments to maintain

optimal geometrical alignment for the transmission of tension as the sarcomere shortens.

The close similarity of the appearance of the 40 nm orthorhombic lattice of negatively stained isolated tropomyosin crystals to the large woven lattice of the Z disc prompted suggestions that tropomyosin in a somewhat similar crystalline form could constitute the backbone of the disc, the I filaments being attached to the corners of each square by means of their individual tropomyosin double helices (Huxley 1963). It was subsequently demonstrated that none of the polymorphic forms of tropomyosin was known to have a symmetry that could be manipulated to fit the Z lattice without distorting the basic pattern of their internal connections (Caspar et al 1969), and that only minor amounts of tropomyosin can be demonstrated within the disc by immunostaining (Endo et al 1966), or by chemical extraction (Stromer et al 1967, 1969). The protein α-actinin (Ebashi et al 1964), which has a strong cross-linking affinity for actin (Briskey et al 1967), has since been shown to be localised to the lattice region of the Z disc

(Masaki et al 1967, Schollmeyer et al 1974), and to contribute approximately 50% of its mass (Suzuki et al 1976). It is an asymmetrical rod-shaped molecule, 4×40 nm, which appears to be a homodimer of a 100 000 Da polypeptide chain (Suzuki et al 1976, Singh et al 1977): it is believed to cross-link the interpenetrating ends of the I filaments within the disc, and it has been suggested that it may also be responsible for imposing consistent 'polarity' on the I filaments emerging from the two faces of the disc. Several other proteins have been extracted from Z lines, including a 55 000 Da protein isolated from chicken muscle by Ohashi & Maruyama (1980). This is distinguishable both immunologically and in its amino acid composition from both α-actinin and desmin; it is located exclusively in the Z discs and, when precipitated from solution, yields crystals having a square lattice structure of similar dimensions to the fine square Z lattice. It is yet to be determined whether it has a structural role within the disc. Abnormalities of Z-disc structure, including the Z-line 'streaming' and 'nemaline bodies', are described in Chapter 9.

Leptomeres

The myofibres of a number of vertebrate species have been reported to contain transversely banded fibrous bodies which have been variously termed 'leptomeres', 'leptomeric fibrils', 'striated bodies' and 'microladders' (Ruska & Edwards 1957, Mair & Tomé 1972). They appear to consist of bundles of fine filaments bound together at regular intervals by cross bands of dense matrix material, with a periodicity reported to range from 120 to 200 nm. They may occur anywhere within the myofibre, and with any orientation, but are chiefly found within the cytoplasm immediately beneath the plasmalemma and are often, but by no means always, associated with the margin of a Z disc of a superficial myofibril. Leptomeres are most abundant in skeletal or cardiac muscle fibres which have become modified for special functions, e.g. the intrafusal myofibres of the muscle spindles (Katz 1961, Gruner 1961, Landon 1966, Scalzi & Price 1971), and the fibres of cardiac conducting tissue (Page et al 1969, Viragh & Challice 1969, Bogusch 1975). The function and significance of leptomeres is not known, although they have been

ascribed a mechanical role in some situations (Thornell et al 1976). They occur in large numbers in the rare Zebra Body myopathy (Lake & Wilson 1975).

Muscle contraction

Certain of the links in the chain of events which lead to the contraction of the myofibrils and the generation of force are well understood, but others have still to be elucidated. Events at the neuromuscular junction are discussed in preceding and subsequent chapters. After generation of the action potential at the end-plate and its spread across the surface membrane, depolarisation enters and passes along the T tubules to trigger release of calcium ions from the SR. Various proposals have been made as to how this electrical signal initiates the release of chemical energy, but the issue is still not resolved. In contrast, much more is known about how chemical energy is transformed into mechanical work when a muscle contracts, and some theories of muscle contraction are outlined below.

The sliding filament model of muscle contraction was suggested independently by H. E. Huxley & Hanson (1954) and by A. F. Huxley & Niedergerke (1954) on the basis of electron microscopy and the results of X-ray diffraction. It was proposed that contraction was the result of two sets of filaments sliding between each other, with an increase in their overlap but no change in the length of the individual filaments. During the last 40 years the sliding-filament model has become generally accepted but it does not, by itself, reveal how the force to move the filaments is generated. A possible explanation for this was suggested by the observations by H. E. Huxley (1957) of cross-bridges projecting from the surface of the A filaments towards the I filaments. It was subsequently proposed that these cross-bridges could provide the necessary physical link between the two sets of filament and that the sliding force was produced by a change in conformation of the cross-bridges while they were attached to the I filament. Since 1957 enormous effort has been put into attempts to test the validity of the 'cross-bridge theory' and to clarify the molecular details of the mechanism. Various schemes have been proposed (A. F. Huxley 1957, 1974, H. E. Huxley 1969, A. F. Huxley & Simmons 1971); for details of these and other models the reader is referred to the reviews by Squire (1981) and Craig (1986).

In the A. F. Huxley & Simmons (1971) model, itself a development of H. E. Huxley's (1957) hypothesis, the attachment of the cross-bridges (myosin heads) to the I-filament (actin) sites is considered to be a transient event resulting in cooperative hydrolysis of ATP, to be followed by detachment of the myosin heads, the energy released powering a force-generating movement of the cross-bridges. Serial repetition of this process, each cross-bridge engaging a succession of actin monomers along an adjacent I filament in a ratchet-like manner, would drive the I-filament array deeper into the A band and thereby cause the sarcomere to shorten.

The key role of the calcium ions, released from the SR when the muscle fibre is stimulated, is to remove the block which prevents interaction between the A and I filaments in relaxed muscle. During activation troponin C responds to the local rise in calcium ion concentration by changing its tertiary structure and, via troponin T, causes tropomyosin to move in the groove between the paired actin helices, thereby removing the obstacle which has previously prevented interaction between the cross-bridges and the active sites on the thin filaments. This hypothesis is known as the 'steric blocking' model, and has gained wide acceptance in recent years. During relaxation, calcium ions are actively sequestered by the SR, thus reducing their concentration within the myofibril lattice; this results in a reverse shift of the troponin and tropomyosin molecules, and thus inactivation, by reblocking, of the cross-bridge binding sites. The regulation of muscle contraction by calcium and the roles of the non-actin and non-myosin proteins have been reviewed by Ebashi (1980).

The cross-bridge theory of muscle contraction has not gone unchallenged; e.g. McClare (1971) attacked it on thermodynamic principles and formulated an alternative 'molecular machine' in which the myosin molecules exist in a long-lived excited state after hydrolysing ATP. The existence of such a state has not been verified but it has proved to be unnecessary, as working thermodynamic cross-bridge models have since been formulated (Tregear & Marston 1979). Another alternative model suggested that electrostatic repulsive forces between the thick and thin filaments caused the sarcomeres to expand laterally and thus to shorten in order to maintain constant volume (Spencer & Worthington 1960, Elliott et al 1970). A variant of this idea invokes dynamic outward expansion of the Z discs as the driving force responsible for fibre shortening (Ullrick 1967). These theories are, however, incompatible with the observation that in skinned fibres the myofibrils are contractile although the interfilament distance does not appear to increase with shortening (Matsubara & Elliott 1972). Another alternative hypothesis proposes that during contraction the thick filaments shorten in a step-wise way as the myosin rods undergo a transition from a helix to a random coil (summarised in Pollack 1990). This 'melting' is supposedly triggered by phosphorylation. However the hypothesis ignores the fact that myosin subfragment 1, which lacks the rod portion, supports motility. A hint of the academic 'heat' generated when the cross-bridge theory is debated can be obtained from reading Simmons (1991).

Mitochondria

The mitochondria of skeletal muscle are irregularly shaped closed sacs, with walls composed of two proteolipid membranes; the outer provides the organelle with a continuous smooth external contour, while the inner is thrown into a series of flat folds, the cristae, which partly subdivide the central cavity. In skeletal muscle the cristae usually have the shape of flat plates, but zig-zag forms can be found occasionally in normal muscle, and concentric and branched cristae may occur in a number of myopathic conditions. The space enclosed by the inner membrane contains a moderately electron-dense finely granular matrix, within which are scattered small dense calcium-containing granules and occasional larger spherical osmiophilic lipid droplets.

The inner and outer mitochondrial membranes differ substantially in both their chemical composition and biological properties. The outer membrane closely resembles other cellular membranes in structure, consisting of protein and lipid in approximately equal proportions, and shows little specific enzyme or transport activity; the inner membrane possesses a greatly increased proportion of protein, reflecting the presence of enzymes responsible for electron transport and oxidative phosphorylation, as well as numerous transport systems involved in the movement of substrates, metabolic intermediates and adenine nucleotides between the cytoplasm and the mitochondrial matrix, which itself contains a further battery of enzymes.

The space between the membranes, often called the intramembrane space, is the site of some enzymic activity and may also contain organic paracrystalline inclusions. Two varieties of these have been identified (Hammersen et al 1980, Stadhouders 1981): the more common is the 'parking lot' or type 1 inclusion which has a distinctive and complex structure (Fig. 4.12a) with a highly variable appearance in micrographs dependent upon its orientation relative to the plane of section (Schmalbruch 1983); the other, type 2, crystals are dense rectangular or elongated rhomboidal bodies (Fig. 4.12b) with an internal structure which is a fine regular lattice (Morgan-Hughes et al 1977). The type 1 crystals tend to occupy and distend that part of the intramembrane space which forms the core of the mitochondrial cristae, whereas the type 2 crystals usually lie between the inner and outer membranes, often in chains which displace the matrix and cristae to the ends of the mitochondrion, and to short segments between adjacent crystals (Fig. 4.12b); however, type 1 crystals can also on occasion be found in an intramural position and small type 2 crystals within the cristae.

The composition and functional significance of the paracrystalline inclusions are unknown, and although there appear to be structural similarities between the type 1 crystals and isolated cytochrome *c* oxidase crystals (Maniloff et al 1973, Landon 1982), Bonilla et al (1975) and Sato et al (1990) were unable to obtain electron histochemical evidence that they possess cytochrome oxidase activity. Smeitik et al (1992) have recently reported immunocytochemical evidence of mitochondrial creatine kinase in both type 1 and type 2 crystals obtained from patients suffering from chronic progressive external ophthalmoplegia. There appears to be no relationship between either type of crystalloid and any particular class of myofibre; both may be found within a single fibre and, rarely, within a single mitochondrion (D. N. Landon, unpublished observations).

Paracrystalline inclusions may be found occasionally in normal human muscle of all ages (Hammersen et al 1980) and they are a regular feature of the myopathology of a number of disease states (DiMauro 1979, Carafoli & Roman 1980, Stadhouders 1981, Morgan-Hughes 1982), not all of which may involve a primary disturbance of mitochondrial function (Engel & Dale 1968, Chou 1969, Fardeau 1970). They may also be induced experimentally by ischaemia (Hanzlikova & Schiaffino 1977, Heine & Schaeg 1979), and by the administration of mitochondrial poisons including the uncoupling agent 2,4-dinitrophenol (Melmed et al 1975, Sahgal et al 1979), and the respiratory chain inhibitor diphenyleneiodonium (Byrne et al 1982).

The mitochondria of skeletal muscle are situated both between the myofibrils and as aggregations beneath the plasmalemma. The latter are more prominent in type I, slow-twitch fibres, particularly in small rodents, and are greatly accentuated in certain human metabolic disorders, to give rise to the 'ragged-red' fibres seen in frozen sections stained with the Gomori trichrome technique. In mammalian muscles in general, mitochondrial content is inversely related to body size (Gauthier & Padykula 1966), and in human muscle the fibres of children contain, on average, a higher mitochondrial volume fraction (4.5%) than do those of adults (3.4%) (Jerusalem et al 1975), and those of men (5.2%) more than those of women (4.1%) (Hoppeler et al 1973). The majority of the intermyofibrillar mitochondria are located adjacent to the Z lines of the sarcomeres, appearing in longitudinal sections as relatively inconspicuous, paired profiles at the level of each half I band, with the remainder orientated longitudinally between the myofibrils. Transverse sections taken close to the plane of the Z line show that the paired profiles represent mitochondria

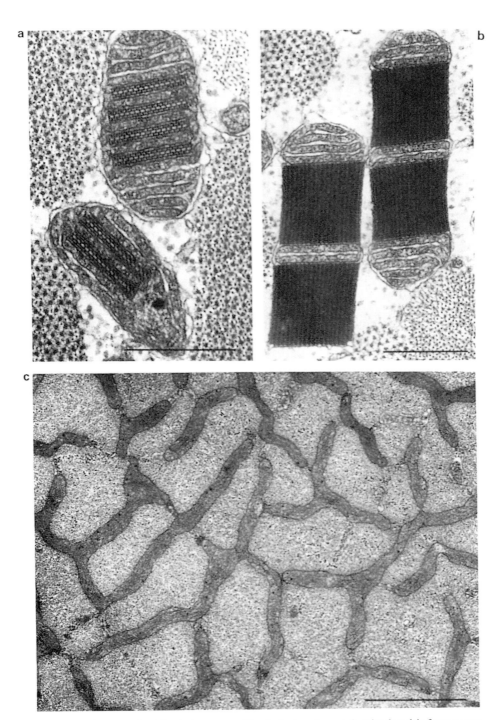

Fig. 4.12   a Type 1 or 'parking lot' paracrystalline inclusions in muscle mitochondria from a case of mitochondrial myopathy. The crystals lie within the cristae in the intramembrane space. **b** Type 2 paracrystalline inclusions from the same case. They are more dense, with a fine regular internal structure always distinguishable from that of the type 1 crystals, and usually, as in this example, lie between the inner and outer membranes of the mitochondrion, displacing the matrix and cristae to its ends, and to small segments between adjacent crystals. **c** A transverse section through the I-band region of a myofibre from the soleus muscle of a rat, illustrating the massive and extensively branched mitochondria characteristic of slow red muscle fibres (scale bars = 5 μm).

which partly or completely encircle each myofibril like a bracelet. In several mammalian species the mitochondria which surround individual myofibrils, particularly those in type I and type IIA fibres, can be shown to be parts of extensively branched 'mega' mitochondria which form continuous networks across the transverse dimension of the fibre (Fig. 4.12c) (Gauthier & Padykula 1966, Gauthier 1969, Schiaffino et al 1970, Rambourg & Segretain 1980), and are also connected to the longitudinal chains of intermyofibrillar mitochondria.

Quantitative studies of animal muscle have demonstrated substantial and consistent differences in the volume fractions of mitochondria in different myofibre types. The mitochondrial volume fractions of guinea pig red (soleus) and white (vastus) fibres are 5% and 1.9% respectively (Eisenberg et al 1974, Eisenberg & Kuda 1975), and similar figures have been obtained in studies of the rat soleus (6.6%) and medial gastrocnemius (2.1%) muscles (Stonnington & Engel 1973, Davey & Wong 1980), and for the red (4.9%) and white (1.6%) fibres of the cat gastrocnemius (Kamieniecka & Schmalbruch 1980). Fast red (type IIA) fibres generally possess larger individual mitochondrial profiles than either slow (type I) or fast glycolytic (type IIB) fibres, but their orientation is predominantly longitudinal in contrast with the transverse orientation of the majority of the mitochondria in the slow type I fibres (Eisenberg & Kuda 1976). Quantitative fine structural studies of human muscle have confirmed the histochemical observation that there are greater numbers of mitochondria in type I than in type II fibres (Shafiq et al 1966, Ogata & Murata 1969, Eisenberg 1983), and differences in the numbers and sizes of mitochondrial profiles have been used to identify myofibre types in human biopsies (Payne et al 1975).

Mitochondrial volume fraction has been shown to increase in the muscle of trained human subjects (orienteers) by Hoppeler et al (1973), and in long-distance runners when compared with untrained controls (Fridén et al 1984). Comparisons of distance runners with weight lifters have shown opposing trends in mitochondrial volume fraction when compared with controls, runners showing a generalised increase in all fibre types, but greatest in type I fibres, and weight lifters a loss of mitochondrial volume fraction in all except type IIA fibres (Prince et al 1981). In a study of the effects of training on sedentary middle-aged men, mitochondrial fraction increase was shown to be restricted to fibre types I and IIA (Sjöstrom et al 1982b).

Internal membrane systems

Sarcoplasmic reticulum. The sarcoplasmic reticulum (SR) is a meshwork of membrane-bound tubules and cisternae which ensheath the myofibrils and abut upon the T-system tubules. There is, however, no membrane continuity with the T system, nor any communication with the extracellular space. The greater part of the SR is in the form of tubules which are organised roughly parallel to the longitudinal axis of the muscle fibre and which, in mammalian muscle, are divided by the T tubules into two intercommunicating systems, one lying over the A band and the other over the I band (Fig. 4.13). The longitudinal tubules over the I band are less regularly organised than those over the A band, probably because they share the space between the myofibrils with mitochondria and also have to withstand longitudinal compression during contraction of the muscle fibres. Where the SR tubules approach the T tubules they fuse circumferentially to form two transversely orientated terminal cisternae, one on either side of each T tubule (Fig. 4.14). This arrangement of two elements of the SR sandwiching one T-system tubule is known as a 'triad'.

For convenience of nomenclature the SR is commonly divided into the longitudinal tubules and the terminal cisternae. An alternative more functional division is into free SR and junctional SR, the latter being the part of the terminal cisterna which faces the T tubule. The free SR is highly specialised as a calcium pump, while the junctional SR is in some way adapted to receive signals from the T system which control its capacity to accumulate calcium. The SR is the main calcium storage and release site in the muscle fibre. When the fibre is relaxed the SR maintains a Ca^{2+} concentration gradient of at least 1 : 1000 across its membrane (Hasselbach 1979).

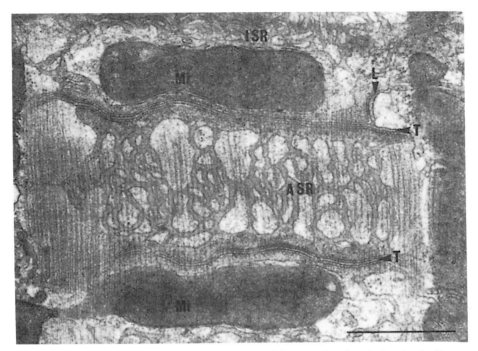

Fig. 4.13 Longitudinal section showing the division of the sarcoplasmic reticulum by the T tubules (T) into elements adjacent to the A band (ASR) and those adjacent to the I band (ISR). Note the longitudinal branch (L) to the T tubule. Mi = Mitochondrion. Mouse diaphragm muscle (scale bar = 1 μm).

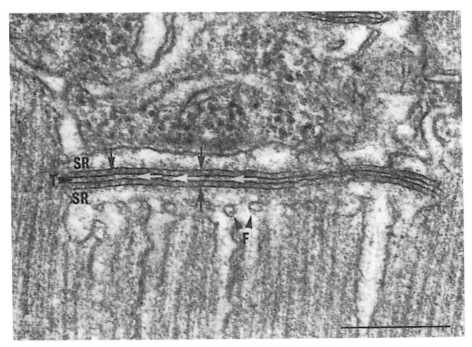

Fig. 4.14 Longitudinal section of a triad made up of a T tubule (T) and two terminal cisternae of the sarcoplasmic reticulum (SR). Note the feet (black arrows) which can appear as blocks, pillars or laminae. Note also the lamina (white arrows) in the lumen of the T tubule. F = fenestrations in the SR. Rat EDL muscle (scale bar = 0.5 μm).

It is able to achieve this because the free SR membrane is very richly endowed with Ca^{2+} transport ATPase, which in rabbit muscle makes up 50–70% of all the SR membrane protein (Meissner & Fleischer 1971, Sarzala et al 1975). The ATPase molecules are concentrated in the cytoplasmic leaflet of the SR membrane, making the membrane highly asymmetrical. The P faces of freeze-fracture replicas of SR membranes contain abundant 8.5 nm intramembranous particles, and on the outer surface there are equally numerous particles 4 nm high which are the extramembranous tails of the intramembranous particles. Their packing is irregular (Franzini-Armstrong 1983) but they have an overall density of about 16 000 per μm^2 (Jilka et al 1975). It is thought that these particles represent a major portion of the ATPase molecule which projects from the membrane into the water phase of the sarcoplasm (Martonosi 1982). Using the technique of site-specific mutagenesis the Ca^{2+}-binding sites of the ATPase molecule have been localised to its transmembrane domain (Clarke et al 1989).

As well as being composed of a membrane which is highly specialised as a calcium pump, the interior of the SR contains large quantities of a calcium-binding protein, calsequestrin. Calsequestrin is confined to the terminal cisternae of the SR where it sometimes appears as a granular electron-dense material in electron micrographs (MacLennan & Holland 1975). Isolated SR forms a heterogeneous mixture of 'light' and 'heavy' SR, of which the heavy fraction is derived from the terminal cisternae: it contains the calsequestrin and is composed of both free and junctional SR; the light fraction is composed entirely of free SR.

The amount of SR contained by a muscle fibre varies from muscle to muscle and from species to species. Published figures for the volume fraction range from <1.0% in the cat soleus and gastrocnemius (Schmalbruch 1979b) to >9% in the rat EDL (Davey & Wong 1980). In general, within any one species the fast-twitch glycolytic fibres contain approximately twice the volume of SR found in the slow-twitch oxidative fibres. The minimum interval after which a muscle contraction can be repeated is dependent upon the speed with which the free calcium ions can be sequestered by the SR following their release; the membrane surface area is therefore probably a more physiologically significant parameter than the contained volume. Published figures for the surface density of SR in mammalian muscle range from 0.09 μm^2 per μm^3 fibre in human slow-twitch fibres (Eisenberg 1983) to 4.59 μm^2 per μm^3 fibre in the fast-twitch fibres of the rat gastrocnemius (Stonnington & Engel 1973). Within any one species the fine structural parameter that correlates most strongly with the myofibre type is the surface density of the terminal cisternae (Eisenberg 1983).

There is a small subcomponent of the SR which is usually overlooked in the standard texts. This forms a tight band around the Z lines of the myofibrils: the tubules are narrower (30–50 nm) than other SR tubules, and can be difficult to identify in longitudinal sections, but show up clearly in transverse sections which pass through the plane of the Z line (Fig. 4.15). Short filamentous bridges link the SR to the Z line (Fig. 4.10a) to give the appearance of a mechanically stable structure. One may speculate that this part of the SR constitutes an anchor for the whole meshwork and prevents any major longitudinal displacement during contraction of the myofibrils. It is of interest that this association between the Z line and SR is present from a very early stage of

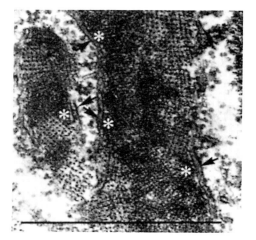

Fig. 4.15 Transverse section through the Z line of human triceps muscle showing the close apposition of a narrow SR tubule (arrows) to those areas corresponding to the exact centre of the Z line (asterisks) (scale bar = 1.0 μm).

myofibril development (Walker et al 1975), implying that the SR collar must grow in conjunction with the myofibril as new filaments are added to its periphery. Whether this band of SR is linked to the intermediate filaments of desmin which link adjacent Z lines is not clear.

T system. The transverse tubular system or T system is a network of fine extensions of the plasma membrane which penetrates the muscle fibre and acts as a pathway for the inward propagation of the action potential. In man and other mammals the tubules of the T system skirt the myofibrils at the level of the A- and I-band junctions, two per sarcomere (Fig. 4.13). Although the greater part of the T system follows a transverse course, there are also occasional longitudinal elements linking these transverse tubules (Fig. 4.13). The peripheral connections of the T tubules to the plasma membrane may be direct or via caveolae. Although the T tubules are continuous with the plasmalemma the protein composition of the two types of membrane is quite distinct (Jorgensen et al 1990).

T tubules are flattened in profile and, at their outer surfaces, measure 25–35 nm in the direction of the fibre axis and 90–130 nm perpendicular to it (Cullen et al 1984). The dimensions of the tubules seem to be fairly constant, although experimental modification of the tonicity of the extracellular fluid can cause swelling or shrinkage (Davey & O'Brien 1978). The volume of the muscle fibre occupied by the T system is extremely small: it varies with the type of myofibre but generally falls within the range 0.1–0.5% (Eisenberg 1983), the volume in fast glycolytic fibres being approximately twice that of slow oxidative fibres; this is due to a difference in the relative spacing of the tubules, not in their dimensions (Cullen et al 1984). More physiologically significant is the surface area of the T system per unit volume of the myofibre (surface density). This has a range in value of approximately 0.06–0.4 μm^2 per μm^3 muscle fibre, with the value for the fast glycolytic fibres being again approximately twice that of the slow oxidative fibres.

The T tubule is usually considered to be hollow and in diagrammatic representations is normally depicted as an empty tube (e.g. Fig. 55 in Schmalbruch 1985). However, in glutaraldehyde-fixed material a thin central lamina can often be resolved within the tubule lumen (Fig. 4.14). The significance of this structure and whether it corresponds to the tannic-acid-binding material described by Bonilla (1977) is uncertain. It is unusual to observe any larger structures within the T tubules of healthy muscle but, in stressed or diseased muscle, cellular debris can sometimes be seen in expanded tubules (Libelius et al 1979, Kelly et al 1986) as though they are acting as channels or gutters through which intracellular debris can escape to the extracellular space. This housekeeping role of the T system is probably of minor significance in healthy muscle where exocytosis appears to occur mainly via the plasma membrane.

The triad. The three-component complex formed by a transverse tubule flanked by two SR terminal cisternae is termed a triad (Fig. 4.14). The triads are inconspicuous elements of the muscle fibre but their fine structure has received considerable attention, as the site at which the electrical signal propagated along the T tubule is converted into a signal for Ca^{2+} release from the SR, thus occupying a central role in the contractile function of skeletal muscle — so central, in fact, that it would not be exaggerating to describe the question of transmission from the T tubules to the SR as an obsession with many groups of researchers (see review by Rios et al 1991).

At the triad the apposed membranes of the T tubule and terminal cisterna are separated by a junctional gap of 11–14 nm. This gap is spanned by a double row of periodic densities or 'feet' (Franzini-Armstrong 1980). These originate on the SR side of the gap and in some views appear to make contact with the membrane of the T tubule. In a study of the three-dimensional structure of the feet on freeze-dried heavy SR vesicles, Ferguson et al (1984) found that they are composed of four identical subunits.

Further details of the feet and their role in excitation–contraction (EC) coupling has come from research on the 'ryanodine receptor'. When heavy SR membranes are fused into planar bilayers, a multi-state cationic channel is observed which is highly conductive to Ca^{2+} and is locked into a conducting substate by ryanodine. Thus the ryanodine receptor, exclusively associated with the terminal cisternae, seems to be an outstanding candidate for the Ca^{2+} release channel. Remarkably, when this receptor was examined under the electron microscope, investigators found themselves looking at the SR foot (Lai et al 1988, Saito et al 1988). The ryanodine receptor/foot protein/calcium release channel has now been purified by several groups (Smith et al 1988, Anderson et al 1989, Lindsay & Williams 1991) and complementary DNAs encoding full-length sequences have been cloned (Takeshima et al 1989, Zorzato et al 1990).

The foot process is formed from four copies of a large 560 K polypeptide and displays an elaborate four-fold symmetry (Wagenknecht et al 1989). Each peptide subunit contributes to a single central calcium channel. The foot extends at least 10 nm into the luminal space towards the T-tubule membrane and has a base plate inserted approximately 4 nm into the SR terminal membrane. The calcium release channels in the feet are in some way opened when depolarisation of the T tubules activates 'voltage sensors' in the T-tubule membrane. The voltage sensors have been identified as dihydropyridine (DHP) receptors (Rios & Brum 1987). (DHP is a Ca-channel blocker, the receptors for which can be isolated as proteins and are very abundant in T tubules.) DHP receptors comprise a large peptide of molecular mass 135–175 K and one or two smaller subunits of 32–34 K and 50 K (Leung et al 1988). Like the ryanodine receptor the DHP receptor has been cloned (Tanabe et al 1990), which opens the possibility that at some point the entire triadic complex will be reconstructed from the cloned component cDNAs.

The exact mechanism of EC coupling at the triad is still largely unresolved (Lamb 1992). The most favoured mechanisms have all been under consideration for several years and include: (1) Ca^{2+}-induced Ca^{2+} release; (2) release of inositol (1, 4, 5) triphosphate ($InsP_3$) near the SR channels, which causes their opening; and (3) a direct action of the DHP receptor on the SR channel by contact ('mechanical coupling'). The first mechanism has been largely ruled out because it is known that skeletal muscle can work in the absence of external calcium (Armstrong et al 1972), showing that an actual translocation of Ca^{2+} from the outside to the inside of the muscle cell is not needed (Rios et al 1991). However a modification of this hypothesis, i.e. that Ca^{2+} might be released from the inside of the T membrane to act as a trigger, is more difficult to dismiss. The second mechanism was first proposed by Vergara and his colleagues (1985) but despite a wealth of interesting observations there is no consensus on a central role of $InsP_3$ in transmission. However research on $InsP_3$ in skeletal muscle is a dynamic area (reviewed by Jaimovich 1991) and important new information may be gained when the molecular structure of the $InsP_3$ receptor is revealed. According to the third mechanism, depolarisation of the T tubules causes a slight outward movement of the voltage sensors (probably the DHP receptors, arranged in quartets opposite each foot) which in turn causes a slight outward movement of the luminal segments of the feet which has the effect of 'unplugging' the outlets to the Ca^{2+} channels, thus allowing release of Ca^{2+} from the SR. Which mechanism will eventually prove to be correct is still unclear but the third scheme (summarised in Rios et al 1991) perhaps correlates best with the ultrastructural data.

Although the triad is the most common form of association between the T system and SR in mammalian muscle, other combinations are also seen. Dyads, where the T tubule is flanked by the SR on only one side, often occur in slow-twitch fibres; for example, about 10% of associations in the rat soleus muscle are dyads (Cullen et al 1984). In contrast, pentads (two T tubules, three terminal cisternae) are the commonest naturally occurring associations seen in some particularly fast-contracting muscles (Revel 1962). Pentads and other multiple complexes are also common in atrophic, immature and regenerating fibres (Fig. 4.5). Peripheral couplings, where the SR receives its trigger directly from the plasma membrane, are often seen in immature muscle and also in the primitive chordate, *Amphioxus*, which has no T system.

Cytoskeleton

There has been a rapid expansion of interest in the cytoskeleton during the last decade as its central role in such complex cellular functions as motility, trans-membrane signalling and growth regulation has become appreciated. This increase in knowledge has been largely driven by advances in molecular biology, immunology and microscopy. At the electron microscope level three major classes of filamentous structures make up the cytoskeleton in muscle, as in other cell types: actin filaments (6–10 nm in diameter), intermediate filaments (7–11 nm) and microtubules (25 nm).

In mature skeletal muscle by far the greatest part of the F-actin resides in the I filaments of the myofibrils but there is also a layer on the cytoplasmic surface of the plasma membrane, known as the cortical layer, which seems to be a universal feature of eukaryotic cells. Organelles are normally excluded from the cortical layer but during secretion by exocytosis, or uptake by endocytosis, the layer is probably signalled to move aside by contraction or disassembly.

The major intermediate filament protein of mature skeletal muscle is desmin (Lazarides 1980, Tokuyasu et al 1983). Desmin is an alpha-helical polypeptide (mass 53 kDa) that pairs into a coiled-coil arrangement. Being a long rod-shaped molecule it is ideal for contributing tensile strength to the cytoskeleton. In skeletal muscle desmin is found linking the Z lines of adjacent myofibrils (Fig. 4.16) and linking the Z lines of peripheral myofibrils to the plasma membrane. During early development and during the early stages of muscle regeneration the position of desmin is occupied by vimentin (mass 55 kDa), a closely related intermediate filament protein (Tokuyasu et al 1985) which is found in a wide range of cell types.

The microtubules, composed of α- and β-tubulin, are in general aligned parallel with the longitudinal axis of the muscle fibres, but others spiral around the myofibrils. They are prominent in immature myotubes where they closely surround the growing myofibrils (Fig. 4.17), but become less conspicuous in mature fibres. Experiments in which interdigitating microtubule and myosin arrays were observed following the addition of taxol to chick myoblast cultures, have led to the suggestion that, during myofibrillogenesis, microtubules provide a scaffolding or substrate along which myosin monomers poly-

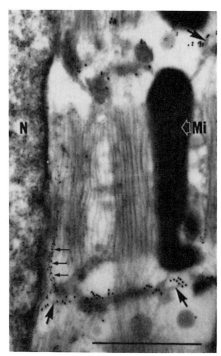

Fig. 4.16 Longitudinal cryosection which has been double-stained with 15 nm immunogold conjugated anti-desmin to identify the intermediate filaments (large arrows) and 5 nm immunogold conjugated anti-tubulin to identify the microtubules (small arrows). Mi = mitochondrion, N = myonucleus (scale bar = 1.0 μm) (micrograph kindly donated by Dr Simon Watkins, Harvard University, Boston).

merise and are delivered as myosin filaments to the myofibril periphery (Antin et al 1981). Other evidence that microtubules play a part in the development of the myofibrils has come from experiments on cultured myotubes in which the microtubules were depolymerised by the addition of colcemide or cytochalasin and the myofibrils became greatly distorted (Holtzer et al 1975). As well as acting as structural supports, microtubules have a major role in functioning as tracts for the transport of organelles in a variety of cell types. Cell components transported include mitochondria, lysosomes, pigment granules, endosomes and phagosomes. Slow (0.02–0.1 μm/s) and fast (2.3–4.6 μm/s) axonal transport are also microtubule-dependent. Readers interested in knowing more about these transport mechanisms are referred to the review by Amos & Amos (1991).

Besides the three main classes of protein

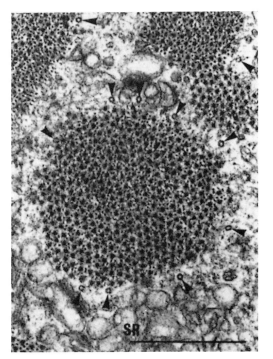

Fig. 4.17 Transverse section through an immature myofibril in regenerating rat muscle. Note the microtubules (arrowheads) closely surrounding the myofibril. SR = sarcoplasmic reticulum. (scale bar = 0.6 μm) (micrograph kindly donated by Dr Sanjay Sesodia, Pasteur Institute, Paris).

components of the cytoskeleton there are numerous other proteins that co-purify with them and are known as associated proteins. (Some can be resolved by EM; others are undetectable without suitable labels). It is probable for example that almost all cells contain dozens of proteins that interact with actin, often competitively. These include proteins that control: (1) assembly and disassembly of actin filaments (e.g. α-actinin, spectrin); (2) bundling of filaments (e.g. aldolase); (3) force generation by filament movement (e.g. myosin), and (4) actin activity modulation by calcium binding (e.g. calmodulin). Less is known at present about intermediate filament-associated proteins which, compared with the above, tend to be more cell and tissue specific. Paranemin and synemin, for example, are large polypeptides which associate with desmin in muscle, while epinemin associates with vimentin (Lawson 1983). There are probably as many proteins involved in controlling the interactions of micro-

tubules in cells as there are for actin. These include motor proteins (e.g. dynein, kinesin), bundling proteins (e.g. brain spectrin), proteins that crosslink to other structures (e.g. synapsin l) and assembly-promoting proteins (MAPs 1A, 1B, 2 and Tau group).

Among the cytoskeleton-associated proteins is one which in the context of muscle and muscle disease has been assigned great importance: dystrophin (see also Chs 7, 8 and 14).

Dystrophin. Dystrophin is the protein product of the Duchenne muscular dystrophy (DMD) gene, and its absence due to mutation of the gene leads to development of this fatal disorder. A milder form of the disease, Becker muscular dystrophy (BMD), is associated with a reduced size and/or abundance of dystrophin. Dystrophin, first described in 1987 (Hoffman et al 1987), was identified by reverse genetics, i.e. its gene and cDNA were isolated and its amino acid sequence then deduced from the DNA sequence. The gene at approximately 2500 kb is the largest yet discovered, which may account for the high mutation rate of DMD at roughly 35% of new cases.

Dystrophin has a molecular weight of 427 K and shares some structural features with spectrin and α-actinin. On the basis of these structural homologies it can be divided into four domains: the N-terminal with sequence homologies to the F-actin binding domain of α-actinin, a major rod-like domain comprising 25 repeating elements similar to those in spectrin, a cysteine-rich domain with a weak homology to α-actinin, and finally a unique and highly conserved C-terminal domain that shows similarity to an autosomal analogue of dystrophin (Love et al 1989).

Dystrophin is localized at the periphery of the muscle fibre where ultrastructural immunogold labelling has shown it to lie close to the cytoplasmic face of the plasma membrane. It is associated with a large oligomeric complex of glycoproteins which span the membrane and link with laminin in the extracellular matrix (Ibraghimov-Beskrovnaya et al 1992). The glycoprotein-binding site of dystrophin is confined to the cysteine-rich domain and the first half of the carboxy-terminal domain. At the opposite end of the molecule, at the N-terminal domain, dystrophin binds to F-actin.

The exact cellular function of dystrophin is not yet clear but its proposed roles roughly fall into three categories: (1) it may contribute mechanical strength to the membrane; (2) it may anchor an integral membrane protein (part of the glycoprotein complex) to the cytoskeleton; or (3) it may act as a link between the cell cytoskeleton and the extracellular matrix. At present there is evidence for each of these functions. Because of its importance in understanding the mechanism of muscular dystrophy, this is an extremely active and ongoing area of research.

Ultrastructure and histochemical fibre type

Attempts have been made by several groups of workers to correlate ultrastructural differences between muscle fibres with their histochemically defined fibre type: types I, IIA and IIB (slow-twitch oxidative, fast-twitch oxidative/glycolytic and fast-twitch glycolytic respectively). Electron-microscopic identification of defined fibre types would have potential use in obtaining ultra-structural correlates of known physiological or biochemical differences. This has been achieved quite successfully in animal muscles (Eisenberg et al 1974, Eisenberg & Kuda 1975, 1976, Schmalbruch 1979b), but the results obtained from human muscle have been more equivocal.

The features which have been most often measured are the Z-line and M-line widths, and mitochondrial and sarcotubular volume fractions. Reports of Z-line widths have varied widely between different studies, from values of 69 nm (type I), 58 nm (IIA) and 56 nm (IIB) obtained by Prince et al (1981), to 128 nm (type I), 104 nm (IIA) and 88 nm (IIB) obtained by Sjöstrom et al (1982b). The differences reflect the problems of measuring Z-line widths in thin sections due to the difficulty of defining the physical limits of the structure. There is, however, general agreement that Z lines are broadest in type I fibres and narrowest in type IIB fibres.

The M line (Fig. 4.7) consists of three or five parallel lines of transverse M bridges (Knappeis & Carlsen 1968), the outer pair of which show considerable variation in staining intensity (Cullen & Weightman 1975). Using ultrathin frozen sections Sjöstrom & his colleagues (1982a,

b) have shown that only type I fibres display all five lines strongly; type IIA fibres have three strong central and two weak outer lines, and IIB fibres have only three central lines.

More recent results from the same laboratory however, have reported that the type I fibres have a four-line M-line pattern while the IIA and IIB fibres have a three- or five-line pattern depending on the muscle under examination (Thornell et al 1987).

The mitochondrial content of muscles differs in men and women, and also varies with the extent to which a muscle is exercised (Hoppeler et al 1973). In general, however, oxidative fibres have a higher content than glycolytic fibres. Sjöstrom's group (Angquist & Sjöstrom 1980, Sjöstrom et al 1982b) obtained volume fraction values of 5.6% (type I), 4.0% (IIA) and 2.8% (IIB) in the vastus lateralis muscle. In contrast Eisenberg (1983) measured only 1.14% in the fast fibres in the same muscle, with 3.03% in the slow fibres.

Several animal studies have shown an up to two-fold difference in the volume of SR (Eisenberg & Kuda 1975, 1976, Schmalbruch 1979b) and of the T system (Luff & Atwood 1971, Cullen et al 1984) in fast fibres compared with slow. This relationship also seems to hold in man where Eisenberg (1983) has obtained values of 1.22% and 1.94% for the volume of SR in slow and fast fibres respectively in the quadriceps muscle, and values of 0.13% and 0.28% for the volumes of the T system in the same muscle. Franzini-Armstrong & her coworkers (1988), by contrast, found approximately equal surface densities of the T system in slow and fast guinea pig fibres, but calculated that the fast fibres had a much higher proportion of junctional T system giving rise to a two-fold difference in foot density.

To date, no single ultrastructural feature has been found which can be used reliably to distinguish muscle fibre type. The difficulty stems from the fact that features such as Z-line width, and mitochondrial and SR volume, show continuous variation with overlap between values for defined fibre types (Schmalbruch 1985). Accuracy may be improved by using more than one feature but, whereas the identification may be reliable at either end of the continuum, fibres showing intermediate values are still difficult to type. Sjöstrom and his colleagues (1982b) examined the human anterior tibialis and vastus lateralis muscles, using the M-line structure as the criterion of fibre type, and found that 83% of fibres were identified correctly using Z-line width, but that mitochondrial content was a much less reliable indicator, correlating with M-line width in only 37% of fibres.

Other myofibre constituents

In mature adult muscle the myofibrils, mitochondria, SR and T systems occupy most of the visible space in the myofibres. However, there are other constituents of the cytoplasm, minor in terms of space occupied but nevertheless having important roles in its metabolism: the fuels (glycogen and neutral lipid) and the organelles involved in synthesis and breakdown of the cell's various components (ribosomes, rough endoplasmic reticulum, Golgi apparatus and lysosomes).

Particles of *glycogen* can be seen in most muscle fibres, although they are scarce in a muscle which has just undergone prolonged exercise. The particles are 25–30 nm in diameter and are usually located around the I band (Fig. 4.18) but, in fibres in which they are plentiful, they may form regularly spaced rows in parallel with the A filaments. Fast-twitch fibres usually contain more glycogen particles than the slow-twitch fibres, but there is great variation in glycogen content among fibre types, and also within the same fibre type, and Essen & Henriksson (1974) reported a seven-fold variation in both slow-twitch and fast-twitch fibres in man.

Droplets of neutral *lipid* are usually found in close association with mitochondria. They represent approximately one-quarter of the total lipid in human muscle, most of the remainder being the phospholipid of the various membrane systems (Waku 1977). Stereological measurements of the volume fraction occupied by lipid droplets in human muscle fibres have yielded a range of values from 0.12% (Jerusalem et al 1975) to 0.36% (Cullen & Weightman 1975). Lipid droplets are more common in slow-twitch oxidative fibres, but probably never constitute more than 1% of their volume in healthy muscle. Prince and his co-workers (1981) measured the lipid

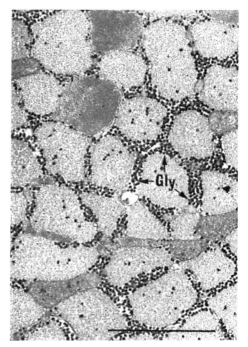

Fig. 4.18 Transverse section through the I band of a human fast-twitch fibre showing the accumulation of glycogen (Gly) between the myofibrils (scale bar = 1 μm).

volume of slow-twitch oxidative, fast-twitch oxidative glycolytic and fast-twitch glycolytic fibres separately and reported values of 0.66%, 0.22% and 0.15% respectively.

The organelles involved in protein synthesis are, not surprisingly, most conspicuous in developing or regenerating muscle fibres. *Ribosomes*, on which the events of protein synthesis are catalysed, are distributed throughout the cytoplasm (Fig. 4.19a). They are composed of a complex of RNA and protein and are slightly smaller (15–20 nm) than glycogen particles. *Polyribosomes* consist of a set of ribosomes spaced along a single messenger RNA molecule (Fig. 4.19a).

The endoplasmic reticulum, which is in continuity with the outer membrane of the nuclear envelope (Fig. 4.19a), is a complex system of interconnecting tubules and cisternae. In skeletal muscle the smooth endoplasmic reticulum, the sarcoplasmic reticulum, has become specialised for the binding and release of calcium ions. In *rough endoplasmic reticulum* (RER) the cytoplasmic surface of the membrane is studded with ribosomes and polyribosomes (Fig. 4.19a) with

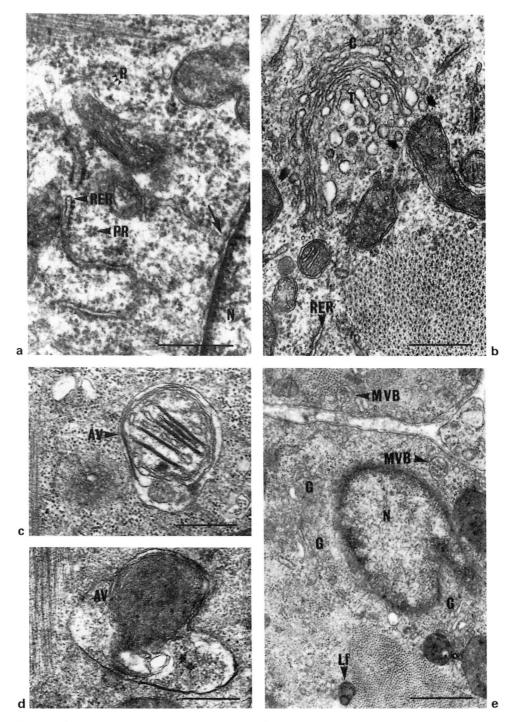

Fig. 4.19 **a** Part of an immature muscle fibre showing ribosomes (R), polyribosomes (PR) and rough endoplasmic reticulum (RER). Note the continuity of the membranes of the endoplasmic reticulum and nuclear envelope (arrow). N = nucleus. **b** Golgi apparatus in an immature myofibre showing cis (C) and trans (T) faces, with Golgi vesicles (arrows) being shed at the periphery. RER = rough endoplasmic reticulum. **c** An autophagic vacuole (AV) containing a degenerate mitochondrion in a mouse soleus muscle. **d**. An autophagic vacuole (AV) containing a mitochondrion and cytoplasmic debris in a case of motor neurone disease (scale bar (**a–d**) = 0.5 μm). **e** The perinuclear area of an immature myofibre showing Golgi apparatus (G), multivesicular bodies (MVB) and a small lipofuscin granule (Lf). N = nucleus (scale bar = 1.0 μm).

the larger (60s) subunit attached to the membrane and the smaller (40s) subunit distal to it. It is a major site of protein synthesis. Some of the proteins synthesised by the RER are moved via transfer vesicles to the *Golgi apparatus*, a stack of membrane-bound flattened cisternae (Fig. 4.19b). Each stack has two distinct sides: a usually convex 'cis' or forming face, and a usually concave 'trans' or maturing face. Within the Golgi apparatus macromolecules are modified, sorted and packaged for secretion or for delivery to other organelles. Golgi vesicles (~50 nm diameter) are shed from the periphery of the flattened cisternae. Golgi membrane systems are rare in mature muscle, being occasionally seen subsarcolemmally close to the nuclei, but like the ribosomes and RER are more conspicuous in developing muscle.

In liver parenchymal cells, and other metabolically active tissues, acid phosphatase and other lysosomal enzymes are concentrated in the most superficial cisternae of the 'trans' face, and in coated vesicles nearby. This suggests that primary *lysosomes* originate from the Golgi apparatus. It is not clear whether this is also the case in skeletal muscle where structures indistinguishable from the SR have been found to stain for lysosomal enzymes. For a summary of the evidence for an SR origin for primary lysosomes in muscle, the reader is referred to the review by Bird & Roisen (1986). Whatever the source of the primary lysosomes, their fate is to form secondary lysosomes by fusion with a membrane-bound substrate: this may be extracellular material in an endosome or intracellular material which has been wrapped prior to digestion. The autophagic vacuoles (Fig. 4.19c, d) thus formed are heterogeneous in size and appearance but can frequently be seen to contain mitochondrial remains or glycogen. Multivesicular bodies (Fig. 4.19e) are secondary lysosomes which are thought to be involved in membrane recycling. Myelin figures and lipofuscin granules are late-stage products of lysosomal digestion. Each of these various types of lysosome is comparatively rare in healthy muscle where the turnover of organelles is low, but they become much more common in diseased muscle and in old age (see Ch. 9). The cellular source of the membranes which wrap and isolate the contents of the secondary lysosomes is controversial: they may be derived from the T

system (Libelius et al 1979, Engel & Banker 1986) or, by homology with other classes of cell, from the SR (Christie & Stoward 1977, Cullen & Mastaglia 1982).

Myonuclei

The myofibre is a multinucleate syncytium which arises during ontogeny from the fusion of successive generations of mononuclear myoblasts/satellite cells. Each individual myofibre contains between 40 and 120 nuclei per mm of length, slow-twitch red fibres containing on average three times the nuclear population of white fast-twitch fibres (Burleigh 1977, Schmalbruch & Hellhammer 1977), and a 10cm fibre may therefore contain upwards of 4000 nuclei in total. All intrinsic nuclei of skeletal muscle are diploid (Lash et al 1957, Strehler et al 1963, Bischoff & Holtzer 1969), with the corollary that they are incapable of synthesising DNA or of mitosis once incorporated into the myofibre. The mass of sarcoplasm which each nucleus is able to sustain appears to have a finite upper limit (Moss 1968), and work-induced hypertrophy of mature muscle is accompanied by an increase in the total content of nuclei within each fibre, obtained from the proliferation and fusion of its associated satellite cells (see p. 120), and not by a shift towards polyploidy of existing nuclei, as has been reported to be the case in hypertrophied human cardiac myocytes (Adler & Costabel 1975).

Most of the nuclei of normal mature myofibres are located superficially immediately beneath the plasmalemma. In relaxed muscle they are smooth ellipsoidal structures, approximately 10 μm long and 2.5 μm wide, with their long axis parallel to that of the fibre. In contracted muscle they develop an undulant profile with a series of ridges and grooves at right angles to the fibre axis. They therefore appear to have a defined location within the superficial zone of the myofibre, and are there surrounded by a small aggregation of sarcoplasm which normally contains one or two small stacks of Golgi membranes, some small elements of rough endoplasmic reticulum and a few mitochondria, and glycogen. Granules of lipofuscin, when present, are also usually located in the perinuclear cytoplasm.

In normal active skeletal muscle the intrinsic myonuclei usually show well-dispersed chromatin and have two nucleoli (Fig. 4.20a). In fibres which have undergone long-term denervation atrophy the nuclei become smaller, spherical and accumulate in small groups, and these changes are accompanied by disappearance of the nucleoli and condensation of their nucleoplasm into conspic-

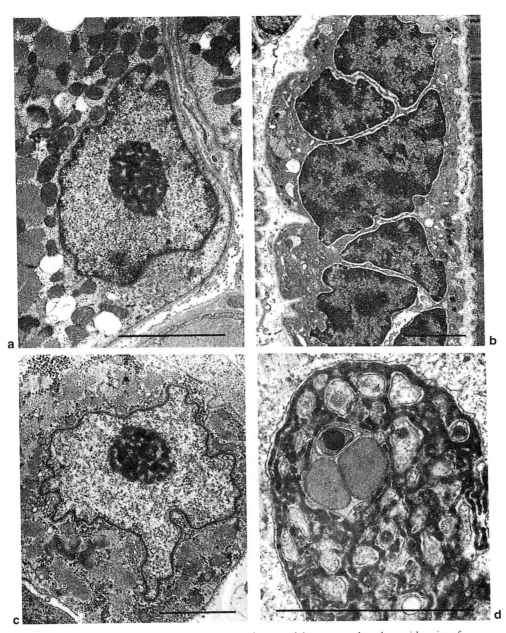

Fig. 4.20 Examples of the differing appearances of myonuclei: **a** a normal nucleus with a rim of heterochromatin and a prominent nucleolus, lying in the superficial sarcoplasm beneath the plasmalemma; **b** the nuclei of an atrophied fibre with condensed 'tigroid' heterochromatin; **c** a nucleus in a developing myofibre having an irregular profile, dispersed chromatin and a massive nucleolus with conspicuous nucleonemata; **d** part of a collapsed pyknotic nucleus from a denervated atrophying fibre (scale bar = 3 μm).

uous dense clumps of heterochromatin attached to the nuclear envelope (Fig. 4.20b). The nuclei of growing or regenerating myofibres, on the other hand, are characterised by increase in size, an overall irregularity of outline in transverse section, and have fully dispersed chromatin and one or more large nucleoli containing prominent nucleonemata (Fig. 4.20c). In the more acute stages of fibre atrophy or degeneration from any cause, numbers of nuclei may undergo pyknosis, which is characterised by loss of volume, with condensation of the chromatin and collapse of the nuclear envelope, to produce a shrunken convoluted structure (Fig. 4.20d and Ch. 9). Further degeneration results in fragmentation of the collapsed nuclear envelope and its destruction by lysosomal activity.

Satellite cells

Myosatellite cells are a population of small, flattened mononucleate cells found in close apposition to the surface membrane of striated muscle fibres and beneath their basal laminae (Mauro 1961, Muir et al 1965, Campion 1984). They appear to be evenly distributed along the length of the myofibres (Muir 1970, Schultz 1979), but not necessarily entirely at random, as they are found more frequently in close associa-

tion with intrinsic myonuclei than would occur by chance (Teravainen 1970, Ontell 1974), and they also commonly occur in increased numbers adjacent to the sole plates of neuromuscular junctions (perisynaptic satellite cells, Kelly 1978). Increased numbers of myosatellite cells are also found in association with the polar intracapsular regions of intrafusal myofibres in muscle spindles (Landon 1966). Myosatellite cells are considered to be a persisting population of myoblastic stem cells, the source of additional myofibre nuclei during the hypertrophic phase of muscle growth (Ishikawa 1966, Church 1969, Moss & Leblond 1971), and the source of the cells responsible for the regenerative repair of damaged muscle fibres in situ (Reznik 1969, 1970), in reimplanted minced muscle (Snow 1979), and in muscle cells cultured in vitro (Bischoff 1979).

The myosatellite cells lie beneath the myofibre basal lamina in a matching depression in the fibre surface (Fig. 4.21), and this close relationship, and the inclusion of the cell within the overall contour of the fibre, ensures that myosatellite cells can be identified with confidence only by the use of electron microscopy (Mauro 1961). They have, however, been identified in living frog muscle fibres by means of interference contrast optics (Lawrence & Mauro 1979), and their distinctive nuclear morphology allows a proportion to be

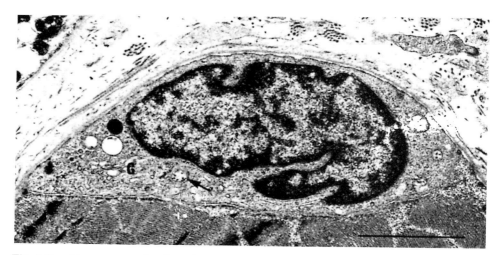

Fig. 4.21   A transverse section through a myosatellite cell lying beneath the basal lamina of a human muscle fibre. The nucleus is indented, and contains conspicuous clumped heterochromatin. The cytoplasm is characterised by numerous free ribosomes, Golgi vesicles (G) and contains the shaft of a cilium (arrow) (scale bar = 2 μm).

identified in stained plastic sections (Ontell 1974). The numbers of myosatellite cells associated with each fibre decline with increase in age in mammals, including man (Allbrook et al 1971, Gibson & Schultz 1983); 10% of the 'myonuclei' are satellite cells in young human subjects, with the numbers failling to 2–3% in the normal muscle of adults. Myosatellite cell numbers increase in denervated muscle (Hess & Rosner 1970, Aloisi et al 1973, Ontell 1975, McGeatchie & Allbrook 1978, Schultz 1978, Murray & Robbins 1982, Snow 1983), in mildly traumatised muscle (Teravainen 1970) and in many muscle diseases (Shafiq et al 1967, Mair & Tomé 1972, Chou & Nonaka 1977, Lipton 1979, Wakayama & Schotland 1979). Myosatellite cells can be liberated from mature animal muscle fibres for study in vitro by enzymatic destruction of the basal laminae (Bischoff 1974); a quantitative method for obtaining myogenic cells from adult human muscle has been described by Yasin et al (1977).

The fine structure of myosatellite cells reflects their supposed stem-cell function (Fig. 4.21). Their nuclei contain conspicuous masses of clumped peripheral heterochromatin (Conen & Bell 1970, Schmalbruch 1985), lack nucleoli and are usually asymmetrically placed towards one pole of their fusiform cytoplasm (Franzini-Armstrong 1979). The perinuclear cytoplasm contains a few small mitochondria, and occasional stacks of RER and Golgi membrane systems; they may also contain glycogen, collections of phospholipid and lipofuscin granules in older human subjects. Paired centrioles also occur in this region, and one is occasionally associated with a longitudinal cilium lying embedded within the adjacent cytoplasm (Muir 1970, Conen & Bell 1970, Mair & Tomé 1972). The apposed plasma membranes of the myosatellite cell and the myofibre are characteristically marked by numbers of attached pinocytotic vesicles, and over most of their region of apposition have a uniform separation of around 15 nm; this is occasionally increased by the presence of lamellated phospholipid material between the two cells, and narrowed by the presence of adherens-type junctions. Myosatellite cells seldom, if ever, contain organised arrays of myofilaments, and cells containing myofibrils in a similar satellite position can be shown by serial sectioning to be developing satellite myotubes (Landon 1970a, Ontell 1977).

THE MYOTENDINOUS JUNCTION

Muscle fibres usually taper as they approach their associated tendon and in the tapered zone become folded and ridged (Fig. 4.22a). In the area of attachment, finger-like projections of the fibres overlap and attach to collagenous projections of the tendon. The complex subdivision of the fibres results in a greatly increased surface area for attachment, and this extra membrane has been calculated to be 32 times that of the fibre cross-sectional area in the frog sartorius muscle (Eisenberg & Milton 1984). The observation that, in the chick, fast fibres have approximately 40% more membrane at the myotendinous junction than have the slow fibres is consistent with the idea that the amount of cell surface specialised for force transmission is related to the functional properties of the muscle fibre (Trotter & Baca 1987).

At the myotendinous junction the myofibrils terminate in a Z-line-like material which may occupy the length of a sarcomere or more. This dense material is filamentous and closely approaches the cytoplasmic face of the plasma membrane which itself appears thickened. Immunoperoxidase labelling has suggested that α-actinin is a component of the dense structures (Trotter et al 1981) but this has been disputed by Tidball (1987). Fine filaments project from the outer face of the plasma membrane across the lamina lucida and insert into the basal lamina (lamina densa). It has been suggested that these 'spines' transmit force from the muscle fibre to the basal lamina and thence to the closely attached collagen fibrils (Fig. 4.22b) of the tendon (Korneliussen 1973). Force transmission at the myotendinous junction is unimpaired after detergent extraction of the plasma membrane. The fine filaments running from the cytoplasmic dense material to the basal lamina persist after the detergent treatment, suggesting that in intact fibres they run through the hydrophobic centre of the plasma membrane which in itself plays no significant part in the transmission of tension (Trotter et al 1981).

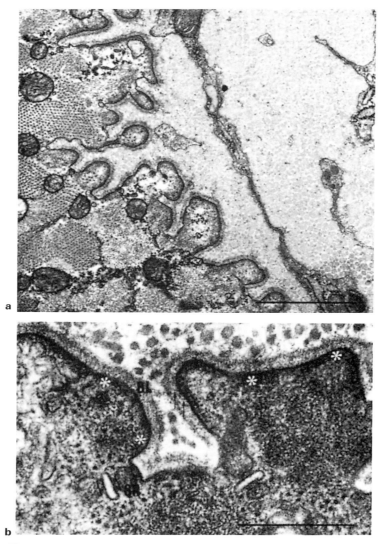

Fig. 4.22   a Transverse section through the myotendinous junction region of a rat myofibre. The surface area of the fibre is greatly increased by irregular folds and ridges. The adjacent collagen fibrils have a wide range of diameters typical of a tendon (scale bar = 1 μm). **b** The plasma membrane at a myotendinous junction. Note the electron-dense plaques (asterisks) below the membrane and the filaments (arrows) crossing the lamina lucida to the basal lamina (BL). Note also the sarcoplasmic reticulum cisterna (SR) extending feet to the plasma membrane (scale bar = 0.5 μm).

The collagen fibrils close to the myotendinous junction are more ordered than those in the endomysium away from the junction, although their mean diameter of 30 nm is unchanged (Fig. 4.22b). This contrasts with the tendon itself in which the fibrils range in diameter from 20 to 250 nm (Moore 1983, Matthew & Moore 1991).

An unexplained feature of myotendinous junctions is that they display acetylcholinesterase (AChE) activity (Couteaux 1953, Zelena 1965). Nishikawa (1981) stained several different rat muscles for AChE activity at the light and electron microscopy level, and found that the activity was in the basal lamina, that it was higher in newborn than adult animals, and in slow fibres than fast fibres, and that it persisted for a time when a muscle was denervated but later declined as the fibres atrophied.

An elevated concentration of dystrophin has also been described at the myotendinous junction (Samitt & Bonilla 1990, Byers et al 1991). This seems to be a real increase in density at the membrane (Byers et al 1991) and not just an apparent elevation due to the increased folding of the membrane. Its increased concentration at this site, where tension is transmitted from the muscle to the tendon, suggests that dystrophin may be involved in the transmission of tension from the muscle cytoskeleton to the extracellular matrix (Samitt & Bonilla 1990, Tidball & Law 1991). Perhaps arguing against this is the report that, in the limb muscles of the mdx mouse which lack dystrophin, there is no reduction in tension development (Dangain & Vrbova 1984).

MUSCLE DEVELOPMENT

Mammalian striated muscle arises from cells in the metamerically segmented paraxial myotomes of the embryonic somatic mesoderm, differentiation following a proximo-distal and cephalo-caudal progression. The cells of the more medial parts of the myotomes differentiate in situ to give rise to the axial muscles of the trunk, while the more lateral and ventral migrate outwards into the somatopleuric mesoderm to form the muscles of the limbs and body wall. In the human embryo, condensations of mesenchyme are detectable at the sites of future muscle masses in the limb buds at the sixth week of gestation, and by the eighth week the primordia of the majority of the individual muscles are clearly defined. These anlage are composed of groups of small myotubes, multinucleate syncytia consisting of a central chain of rounded nuclei enclosed by a peripheral shell of amphiphilic cytoplasm bearing the first traces of cross-striation, lying within a loose stroma of connective tissue. Ultrastructurally the myotubes are characterised by central columns of nuclei containing prominent nucleoli, and syncytial cytoplasm rich in ribosomes, sarcotubular

membranes, glycogen granules, lipid droplets and small myofibrils. The myotubes occur in small clusters separated by a reticulum of angular mesenchymal fibroblasts in a structureless matrix, and each is closely related to a number of less differentiated myogenic cells (Kelly & Zacks 1969). These consist of true mononucleate myoblasts — rounded cells containing small dense nuclei lacking nucleoli, and with cytoplasm rich in free ribosomes and large undulating cisterns of rough endoplasmic reticulum — and multinucleated myofilament-containing cells which represent the initial stage in the formation of the next generation of myotubes (see below); both varieties lie within the basal lamina of the established myotube, against which they abut. Only the mononucleate cells show evidence of mitosis, and it has been proposed that a proportion of myoblast divisions is 'critical' or 'quantal' (Holtzer 1970), in that one or both of the daughter cells are thereafter irrevocably committed to differentiation and fusion, either with other post-mitotic myoblasts to form a new myotube, or with an existing myotube to add to its complement of nuclei and cytoplasm (see below). Studies of muscle regeneration in vitro have shown that the switch from proliferation to fusion requires a minimal density of cells, and appears to be promoted by the accumulation of a high-molecular-weight diffusible polypeptide within the culture medium (Konigsberg 1971). The shift into the post-mitotic phase is signalled by a prolongation of the G1 portion of the mitotic cycle (Konigsberg et al 1978), and initiation of the synthesis of muscle-specific proteins (Stockdale & Holtzer 1961). A few of the mononucleate cells associated with the myotubes show evidence of proliferation of rough endoplasmic reticulum from the nuclear envelope and the presence of a rudimentary nucleolus attached to the peripheral heterochromatin, and these structural modifications may be associated with the onset of perfusion differentiation in 'postquantal' cells.

Myoblast fusion has been observed by light-microscopic time-lapse photography (Cooper & Konigsberg 1961), but convincing fine structural images of the process are rare. Focal breakdown of the adjacent membranes of laterally aligned chick myoblasts in tissue culture has been observed by Shimada (1971), and this appeared to lead to the formation of cytoplasmic bridges between the cells which subsequently coalesced by breakdown of the residual portions of the membranes into vesicles. Lipton & Konigsberg (1972) described fusion in tissue-cultured quail muscle in which a single initial pore created by a small focal area of membrane fusion expanded by lateral extension without further membrane breakdown until fusion was complete. Discontinuous lengths of paired membranes between areas of cytoplasm containing differing patterns of myofibril content can be seen in transverse sections of muscle fibres regenerating in vivo: such appearances presumably represent incomplete stages of fusion. The individual contributions of fused myogenic cells to their joint cytoplasm have been identified by Ross et al (1970) on the basis of their differing content of ribosomes.

Once myotube formation has been initiated at the site of a future muscle their numbers increase rapidly: in the small mammals most studied experimentally, this continues until the second or third postnatal week (Kelly & Zacks 1969), and in man until at least the fourth postnatal month (Montgomery 1962) and possibly until the fifth decade (Adams & DeReuck 1973). This process of myotube hyperplasia is accompanied, and eventually succeeded, by a more prolonged phase of fibre hypertrophy extending throughout the growing period of the animal, in which the individual fibres increase in diameter and nuclear content and also in length to keep pace with the increasing dimensions of the trunk and limb segments within which they lie. The source of the additional myotubes which appear during the hyperplastic phase of muscle growth has been the subject of controversy in the past, some histologists favouring the idea that the increase in numbers is obtained from the splitting of pre-existing myotubes (MacCallum 1898, Cuajunco 1942), others that the new myotubes arise from the fusion of a continuously proliferating population of myogenic stem cells (Schwann 1839). Modern studies of the fine structure of muscle development, both in vivo and in vitro, have clearly demonstrated that the latter view is correct. Rows of mononucleate myoblasts become aligned along the length of pre-existing myotubes, and there fuse to form slender flattened multi-nucleated bands closely adherent to their more developed neighbour (Fig. 4.23a). Their nuclei possess prominent nucleoli, and the cytoplasm contains numerous free polysomes, Golgi membrane systems, some rough endoplasmic reticulum and thin bundles of thick and thin myofilaments organised into myofibrils. A striking feature of the interface between the new myotube and its more mature neighbour is the presence of finger or keel-like projections from the surface of the former, which lie within reciprocal invaginations of the cell membrane and cytoplasm of the older myotube (Kelly & Zacks 1969, Landon 1970a, 1971). The projections extend deep into the substance of the established myotube and are frequently found in close proximity to its nuclei (Fig. 4.23a), and the surfaces of both the invading and invaded cells bear 'coated' uptake vesicles. Quantitative studies (Landon 1971) have shown that these contacts achieve their greatest morphological complexity at the earliest stages of differentiation of the new myotubes, as judged by their content of myofibrils. It has been suggested that the phenomenon may be associated with the transfer of morphogenetic information (Landon 1982) or provide a transient insertion of the secondary myotubes into the primary myotubes until their longitudinal growth has extended to the myotendinous junctions (Duxson & Usson 1989). More subtle sites of intercellular contact in the form of 'gap junctions' have been reported to be widespread among the myogenic cells at early stages of muscle differentiation (Kelly & Zacks 1969, Rash & Staehelin 1974) and Rash & Fambrough (1973) have proposed that the appearance of gap junctions, and the concomitant increase in the electrical coupling of the cells in contact, are a normal prelude to cell fusion. The initial development and formation of the primary myotubes precedes and is independent of motor innervation of the muscle, whereas the secondary and subsequent generations of myotubes seem to have an absolute requirement for both innervation and contractile activity for their maturation and maintenance (Harris 1981), and possibly also for their initial formation, in that new secondary myotubes make their first appearance exclusively within the innervation zone of the primary myotube (Duxson et al 1989).

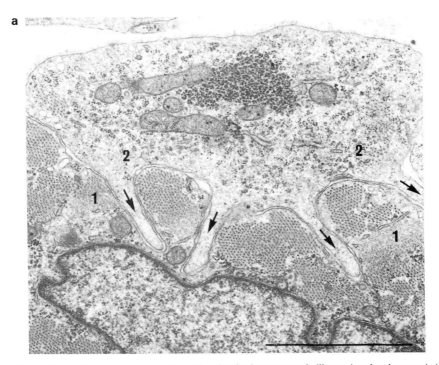

Fig. 4.23 **a** A transverse section through a developing rat muscle illustrating the characteristic contacts between two generations of developing myotubes. The younger myotube (2) possesses numerous processes on its deep surface (arrows) which penetrate matching clefts into the substance of its more mature neighbour (1) (scale bar = 2 μm). **b** (overleaf) A schematic illustration of the events associated with the production of new myotubes during the hyperplastic phase of myogenesis. Mononucleate myoblasts (1) adherent to the surface of pre-existing myotubes proliferate and differentiate to form chains of overlapping spindle-shaped cells (2). These then fuse, and the resulting nascent myotube (3) starts to synthesise contractile proteins and develops a close morphological relationship with the surface of its more mature neighbour. This contact is lost with further differentiation (4), and the two myotubes becomes separated by proliferation of myoblasts between their opposed surfaces. Repetition of these processes (5) gives rise to successive generations of new myotubes (reproduced from Landon (1982) with permission from the editors and publishers).

Continued differentiation of the secondary myotubes is associated with increase in their diameter, nuclear number and myofilament content, and with their separation from the primary myotubes (Landon 1971, Ontell 1979). The last is frequently accompanied by the appearance of columns of myoblasts interposed between the adjacent primary and secondary myotubes, and within their common basal lamina; these are the progenitors of the tertiary and later generations of myotubes, and there is evidence that such cells preferentially associate with the smallest, and thus by inference the least mature, of the existing myotube pair (Kelly & Zacks 1969). The new myotube resulting from their fusion will thus lie alongside, and differentiate in association with a secondary myotube in a similar manner to that described for the primary and secondary generations (Fig. 4.23b). Proliferation of new myotubes is accompanied by the concurrent maturation of established myotubes to myofibres, with migration of the nuclei to a peripheral subplasmalemmal position, synthesis of contractile proteins and their assembly into larger and more numerous myofibrils, maturation of the sarcotubular system and the establishment of a neuromuscular synapse.

Primitive myofibrils make an early appearance

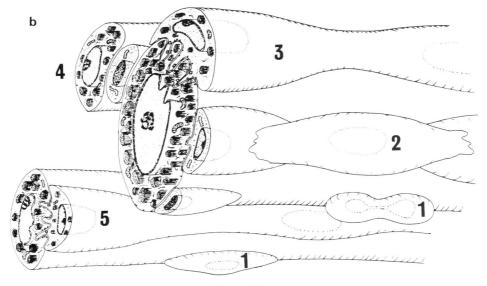

Fig. 4.23 b

in the postfusion development of mammalian myotubes and have been reported to be present in prefusion myoblasts in chicken muscle (Stockdale & Holtzer 1961). Slender organised bundles of I filaments attached to small dense bodies occur first in the more superficial parts of the myotube cytoplasm (Heuson-Stiennon 1965), coincidentally with the appearance of the first small regular arrays of A filaments (Dessouky & Hibbs 1965, Fischman 1967); the latter are apparently synthesised in situ by long spiral polysomes which are closely associated with the peripheral filaments of each nascent A band (Allen & Pepe 1965, Larson et al 1973). Titin (connectin) filaments form synchronously with the A filaments and appear to play a role in integrating the nascent A bands with the I-Z-I primordia (Komiyama et al 1990). Other filamentous components of the early developing myotube are the actin filaments of stress fibres which form a discontinuous feltwork beneath the plasmalemma, and randomly orientated 10 nm filaments (Ishikawa et al 1968), composed of 'desmin' (Lazarides & Balzer 1978); these diminish as the myofibrils increase in size and density (Bennett et al 1979) but some persist in the vicinity of the Z disc of the mature fibre and may assist in controlling the transverse alignment of the myofibrils (Thornell et al 1980).

The two components of the sarcotubular system, the transverse tubules and the sarcoplasmic reticulum, can be identified from the earliest stages of myotube differentiation, and appear to develop simultaneously (Ezerman & Ishikawa 1967, Schiaffino & Margreth 1969), the T tubules from invaginations of the surface membrane, and the sarcoplasmic reticulum from outgrowths of the rough endoplasmic reticulum of the early myotube. An extensive branched system of T tubules develops within the subplasmalemmal cytoplasm, from which branches penetrate between the myofibrils where they make triadic contacts with elements of the sarcoplasmic reticulum (Walker & Schrodt 1968, Kelly 1971, 1980). In the rat the sarcoplasmic reticulum has become organised into cylindrical segments by the second postnatal week, alternately in register with the A and I bands of successive sarcomeres, and triadic junctions have developed between the T tubules and the terminal cisterns of the reticulum at their interfaces opposite the junction of each A and I band. The differences in the extent and arrangement of the sarcoplasmic reticulum in fast- and slow-twitch fibres visible in adult muscle develops rather later in postnatal life (Luff & Atwood 1971), concurrently with their acquisition of mature contractile properties.

The hypertrophic phase of muscle growth,

during which established fibres increase in both diameter and length, is associated with an increase in the numbers of their contained nuclei. It is now clear that this increase is brought about by the fusion of mononucleate cells with the growing fibres, and that this population of stem cells can be identified with the satellite cells (see p. 120). Satellite cells divide continuously throughout the period of active myogenesis (Hellmuth & Allbrook 1973) and it has been shown by radioautography (Moss & Leblond 1970, 1971) that a substantial proportion of the labelled daughter nuclei become incorporated into the myofibres as true muscle nuclei. Similar results have been obtained by implanting clonal cultures of labelled myoblasts into normal muscles of the original donor (Lipton & Schultz 1979). During the most active phase of myogenesis approximately 50% of the products of satellite cell divisions failed to fuse with myofibres (Hellmuth & Allbrook 1973) thereby maintaining a constant satellite cell population equivalent to approximately one-third of the numbers of true myonuclei (Schultz 1974). With cessation of growth, satellite cell numbers decline to about 5% of the total number of myofibre nuclei in small animals and to 2% in man.

The increase in fibre diameter associated with postnatal growth of the myofibres is largely attributable to an increase in the numbers of their contained myofibrils. These have a bimodal diameter distribution in growing muscle, and it has been suggested that myofibrils may have an optimum maximum diameter of 1–1.2 μm, and that when this value is exceeded they proliferate by subdivision (Goldspink 1970). Fine structural appearances compatible with this hypothesis are common, both during postnatal growth (Goldspink 1970) and in muscles responding to release from immobilisation (Shear 1975) or undergoing work hypertrophy (Goldspink & Ward 1979). These take the form of longitudinal clefts partly subdividing large myofibrils in the regions of their A and I bands, and areas of disorganisation at the Z disc; Goldspink (1970, 1971) has suggested that such division may be caused by an imbalance of mechanical forces during contraction.

Growth in length of individual myofibres is achieved by the addition of extra sarcomeres (Close 1964, 1972), with a small contribution from a reduction in the extent of the overlap of the thick and thin myofilaments at resting length as growth proceeds (Goldspink 1968), resulting in an increase in mean sarcomere length. Studies in which markers have been inserted into growing muscles (Kitiyakara & Angevine 1963) and autoradiographic experiments using isotope-labelled precursors of myofilament proteins (Williams & Goldspink 1971), have shown that the additional sarcomeres are incorporated into the ends of the growing myofibre at its osseous or tendinous insertions. Other workers have failed to confirm these findings (Crawford 1954, MacKay & Harrop 1969), and Schmalbruch (1985) has proposed an alternative mechanism in which sarcomere formation occurs along the length of the myofibril at foci of Z-disc damage of the kind observed in human muscle fibres subject to excessive 'eccentric' contraction (Fridén 1984). Immobilisation of growing mouse muscle at shortened length has been shown to result in a decrease in the rate of addition of sarcomeres (Williams & Goldspink 1971, 1973), normal numbers being recovered when the restriction to movement is removed. A similar adjustment of sarcomere numbers to functional length has been shown by Tabary et al (1972) to occur in the adult cat.

The histochemical and immunocytochemical differentiation of human muscle is described in Chapter 8.

ACKNOWLEDGEMENTS

The authors are grateful to Mr B. C. Young and Mr J. M. Walsh for their expert technical assistance in preparing material used to illustrate this chapter, to Mrs J. P. Humphreys for preparing the typescript, and to the editors and publishers referred to in figure captions for their permission to include material from previous publications in this chapter.

REFERENCES

Adams R D, DeReuck J 1973 Metrics of muscle. In: Kakulas B A (ed) Basic research in myology. Excerpta Medica, Amsterdam, vol I, p 3

Adler C-P, Costabel U 1975 Cell number in human heart in atrophy, hypertrophy, and under the influence of cytostatics. In: Fleckenstein A, Rona G (eds) Recent advances in studies on cardiac structure and metabolism, Vol 6. Pathophysiology and morphology of myocardial cell alteration. University Park Press, Baltimore, p 343–355

Allbrook D B, Han M F, Hellmuth A E 1971 Population of muscle satellite cells in relation to age and mitotic activity. Pathology 3: 233

Allen E R, Pepe F A 1965 Ultrastructure of developing muscle cells in the chick embryo. American Journal of Anatomy 116: 115

Aloisi M, Mussini I, Schiaffino S 1973 Activation of muscle nuclei in denervation and hypertrophy. In: Kakulas B A (ed) Basic research in myology, vol I. Excerpta Medica, Amsterdam, pp 338–342

Amos L A, Amos W B 1991 Molecules of the cytoskeleton. Macmillan, Basingstoke.

Anderson K, Lai F A, Liu Q Y, Rousseau E, Erickson H P, Meissner G 1989 Structural and functional characterization of the purified cardiac ryanodine receptor–Ca^{2+} release channel complex. Journal of Biological Chemistry 264: 1329

Angquist K-A, Sjostrom M 1980 Intermittent claudication and muscle fibre fine structure. Morphometric data on mitochondrial volumes. Ultrastructural Pathology 1: 461

Antin P B, Forry-Schandies S, Friedman T M, Tapscott S J, Holtzer H 1981 Taxol induces postmitotic myoblasts to assemble interdigitating microtubule-myosin arrays that exclude actin filaments. Journal of Cell Biology 90: 300

Armstrong C M, Bezanilla F, Horowicz P 1972 Twitches in the presence of ethylene glycol bis (β-aminoethylether)-N,N^1-tetracetic acid. Biochimica Biophysica Acta 267: 605

Barnard E A, Dolly J O, Porter C W, Albuquerque E 1975 The acetylcholine receptor and the tonic conductance modulation system of skeletal muscle. Experimental Neurology 48: 1

Bennett G S, Fellini S A, Toyama Y, Holtzer H 1979 Redistribution of intermediate filament subunits during skeletal myogenesis and maturation in vitro. Journal of Cell Biology 82: 577

Bewick G S, Nicholson L V B, Young C, O'Donnel E, Slater C R 1992 Different distributions of dystrophins and related proteins at nerve–muscle junctions. Neuroreport 3: 857

Bird J W C, Rolisen F J 1986 Lysosomes in muscle: developmental aspects, enzyme activities, and role in protein turnover. In: Engel A G, Banker B Q (eds) Myology. McGraw-Hill, New York, p 745

Bischoff R 1974 Enzymatic liberation of myogenic cells from adult rat muscle. Anatomical Record 180: 645

Bischoff R 1975 Regeneration of single skeletal muscle fibers in vitro. Anatomical Record 182: 215

Bischoff R 1979 Tissue culture studies on the origin of myogenic cells during muscle regeneration in the rat. In: Mauro A (ed) Muscle regeneration. Raven Press, New York, pp 13–29

Bischoff R, Holtzer H 1969 Mitosis and the processes of differentiation of myogenic cells in vitro. Journal of Cell Biology 41: 188

Bloch R J, Morrow J S 1989 An unusual β-spectrin associated with clustered acetylcholine receptors. Journal of Cell Biology 108: 481

Bogusch G 1975 Electron microscopic observations on leptomeric fibrils and leptomeric complexes in the hen and pigeon heart. Journal of Molecular and Cellular Cardiology 7: 733

Bonilla E 1977 Staining of transverse tubular system of skeletal muscles by tannic acid-glutaraldehyde fixation. Journal of Ultrastructure Research 58: 162

Bonilla E, Schotland D L, DiMauro S, Aldover B 1975 Electron cytochemistry of crystalline inclusions in human skeletal muscle mitochondria. Journal of Ultrastructure Research 51: 404

Bonilla E, Fischbeck K, Schotland D L 1981 Freeze-fracture studies of muscle caveolae in human muscular dystrophy. American Journal of Pathology 104: 167

Bowman W 1840 On the minute structure and movements of voluntary muscle. Philosophical Transactions of the Royal Society of London, pp 457–501

Boyd I A, Davey M R 1968 Composition of peripheral nerves. Livingstone, Edinburgh

Brandt P W, Lopez E, Reuben J P, Grundfest H 1967 The relationship between myofilament packing density and sarcomere length in frog striated muscle. Journal of Cell Biology 33: 255

Briskey E J, Seraydarian K, Mommaerts W F H M 1967 The modification of actomyosin by α actinin. II. The interaction between α actinin and actin. Biochimica et Biophysica Acta 133: 424

Burden S J, Sargent P B, McMahan U J 1979 Acetylcholine receptors in regenerating muscle accumulate at original synaptic sites in the absence of the nerve. Journal of Cell Biology 82: 412

Burleigh I G 1974 On the cellular regulation of growth and development in skeletal muscle. Biological Reviews 49: 267

Burleigh I G 1977 Observations on the number of nuclei within the fibres of some red and white muscles. Journal of Cell Science 23: 269

Butler M H, Douville K, Murnane A A, Sealock R, Froehner C 1990 Association of the cytoskeletal postsynaptic 58 K protein with dystrophin. Journal of Cell Biology 111:165a

Byers T J, Kunkel L M, Watkins S C 1991 The subcellular distribution of dystrophin in mouse skeletal, cardiac, and smooth muscle. Journal of Cell Biology 115: 411

Byrne E, Hayes D J, Morgan-Hughes J A, Clark J B 1982 Some effects of experimentally induced mitochondrial lesions on the function and metabolic content of rat muscle. Proceedings of the Vth International Congress on Neuromuscular Diseases, Marseille 1982, (Abst) 35: 3

Campion D R 1984 The muscle satellite cell: a review. International Review of Cytology 87: 225

Carafoli E, Roman I 1980 Mitochondria and disease. Molecular Aspects of Medicine 3: 295

Caspar D L D, Cohen C, Longley W 1969 Tropomyosin: crystal structure, polymorphism and molecular interactions. Journal of Molecular Biology 41: 87

Chou S M 1969 'Megaconial' mitochondria observed in a case of chronic polymyositis. Acta Neuropathologica (Berlin) 12: 68

Chou S M, Nonaka I 1977 Satellite cells and muscle

regeneration in diseased human skeletal muscle. Journal of the Neurological Sciences 34: 131

Chowrashi P K, Pepe F A 1979 M-band proteins: evidence for more than one component. In: Pepe F A, Sanger J W, Nachmias V T (eds) Motility in cell function. Academic Press, New York, pp 419–422

Christie K N, Stoward P J 1977 A cytochemical study of acid phosphatases in dystrophic hamster muscle. Journal of Ultrastructure Research 58: 219

Church J C T 1969 Satellite cells and myogenesis; a study in the fruit bat web. Journal of Anatomy 105: 419

Clarke D M, Loo T W, Inesi G, MacLennan D H 1989 Location of high affinity Ca^{2+}-binding sites within the predicted transmembrane domain of the sarcoplasmic reticulum Ca^{2+}-ATPase. Nature 339: 476

Close R I 1964 Dynamic properties of fast and slow skeletal muscles of the rat during development. Journal of Physiology (London) 173: 74

Close R I 1972 Dynamic properties of mammalian skeletal muscles. Physiological Reviews 52: 129

Cohen C, Caspar D L D, Parry D A D, Lucas R M 1971 Tropomyosin crystal dynamics. Cold Spring Harbor Symposium on Quantitative Biology 36: 205

Conen P E, Bell C D 1970 Study of satellite cells in mature and fetal human muscle and rhabdomyosarcoma. In: Mauro A, Shafiq S A, Milhorat A T (eds) Regeneration of striated muscle and myogenesis. Excerpta Medica, Amsterdam, pp 194–217

Cooper W G, Konigsberg I R 1961 Dynamics of myogenesis in vitro. Anatomical Record 140: 195

Couteaux R 1953 Particularités histochimique des zones d'insertion du muscle strié. Comptes rendus des séances de la Société de Biologie 147: 1974

Couteaux R, Pecot-Dechauvassine M 1970 Vesicules synaptiques et poches au niveau des 'zones actives' de la junction neuromusculaire. Comptes rendus hebdomadaires des séances de l'Académie des sciences D 271: 2346

Craig R 1986 The structure of the contractile filaments. In: Engel A G, Banker B Q (eds) Myology. McGraw-Hill, New York, pp 73

Craig R, Offer G 1976a Axial arrangement of crossbridges in thick filaments of vertebrate skeletal muscle. Journal of Molecular Biology 102: 325

Craig R, Offer G 1976b The location of C-protein in rabbit skeletal muscle. Proceedings of the Royal Society of London B 192: 451

Craig R, Megerman J 1979 Electron microscope studies on muscle thick filaments. In: Pepe F A, Sanger J W, Nachmias V T (eds) Motility in cell function. Academic Press, New York, pp 91–102

Craig R, Knight P 1983 Myosin molecules, thick filaments and the actin-myosin complex. In: Harris J R (ed) Electron microscopy of proteins. Macromolecular structure and function, vol 4, pp 97–203

Crawford G N C 1954 An experimental study of muscle growth in the rabbit. Journal of Bone and Joint Surgery 36: 294

Cuajunco F 1942 Development of the human motor end plate. Carnegie Institute, Washington publications 541. Contributions to Embryology 30: 127

Cullen M J, Weightman D 1975 The ultrastructure of normal human muscle in relation to fibre type. Journal of the Neurological Sciences 25: 43

Cullen M J, Mastaglia F L 1982 Pathological reactions of skeletal muscle. In: Mastaglia F L, Walton J N (eds)

Skeletal muscle pathology. Churchill Livingstone, Edinburgh, pp 88–139

Cullen M J, Hollingworth S, Marshall M W 1984 A comparative study of the transverse tubular system of the rat extensor digitorum longus and soleus muscles. Journal of Anatomy 138: 297

Dangain J, Vrbova G 1984 Muscle development in mdx mutant mice. Muscle and Nerve 7: 700

Davey D F 1976 The relation between Z-disk lattice spacing and sarcomere length in sartorius muscle fibres from *Hyla cerulea*. Australian Journal of Experimental Biological and Medical Science 54: 441

Davey D F, O'Brien G M 1978 The sarcoplasmic reticulum and T-system of rat extensor digitorum longus muscles exposed to hypertonic solutions. Australian Journal of Experimental Biology and Medical Science 56: 409

Davey D F, Wong S Y P 1980 Morphometric analysis of rat extensor digitorum longus and soleus muscles. Australian Journal of Experimental Biology and Medical Science 58: 213

Dessouky D A, Hibbs R G 1965 An electron microscope study of the development of the somatic muscle of the chick embryo. American Journal of Anatomy 116: 523

DiMauro S 1979 Metabolic myopathies. In: Vinken P J, Bruyn G W (eds) Handbook of clinical neurology, vol. 41. North Holland, Amsterdam, pp 175–234

Dulhunty A F, Franzini-Armstrong C 1975 The relative contribution of folds and caveolae to the surface membrane of frog skeletal muscle fibres at different sarcomere lengths. Journal of Physiology (London) 250: 513

Duxson M J, Usson Y 1989 Cellular insertion of primary and secondary myotubes in embryonic rat muscles. Development 107: 243

Duxson M J, Usson Y, Harris A J 1989 The origin of secondary myotubes in mammalian skeletal muscle: ultrastructural studies. Development 107: 743

Ebashi S 1980 Regulation of muscle contraction. Proceedings of the Royal Soceity of London B 207: 259

Ebashi S, Ebashi F, Maruyama K 1964 A new protein factor promoting contraction of actomyosin. Nature 203: 645–646

Ebashi S, Kodama A, Ebashi F 1968 Troponin. I. Preparation and physiological function. Journal of Biochemistry (Tokyo) 64: 465

Eisenberg B R 1983 Quantitative ultrastructure of mammalian skeletal muscle. In: Peachey L D, Adrian R H (eds) Handbook of physiology, section 10: Skeletal muscle. American Physiological Society, Bethesda, p 73

Eisenberg B R, Kuda A M, Peter J B 1974 Stereological analysis of mammalian skeletal muscle. I Soleus muscle of the adult guinea pig. Journal of Cell Biology 60: 732

Eisenberg B R, Kuda A M 1975 Stereological analysis of mammalian skeletal muscle. II White vastus muscle of the adult guinea pig. Journal of Ultrastructure Research 51: 176

Eisenberg B R, Kuda A M 1976 Discrimination between fiber populations in mammalian skeletal muscle by using ultrastructural parameters. Journal of Ultrastructure Research 54: 76

Eisenberg B R, Milton R L 1984 Muscle fiber termination at the tendon in the frog's sartorius: a stereological study. American Journal of Anatomy 171: 273

Elliott A, Offer G 1978 Shape and flexibility of the myosin molecule. Journal of Molecular Biology 123: 505

Elliott G F, Lowy J, Worthington C R 1963 An X-ray and

light diffraction study of the filament lattice of striated muscle in the living state and rigor. Journal of Molecular Biology 6: 295

Elliott G F, Lowy J, Millman B M 1967 Low angle X-ray diffraction studies of living striated muscle during contraction. Journal of Molecular Biology 25: 31

Elliott G F, Rome E M, Spencer M 1970 A type of contraction hypothesis applicable to all muscle. Nature 226: 400

Ellisman M H, Rash J E, Staehelin L A, Porter K R 1976 Studies of excitable membranes — II. A comparison of specializations at neuromuscular junctions and nonjunctional sarcolemmas of mammalian fast and slow twitch muscle fibers. Journal of Cell Biology 68: 752

Ellisman M H, Rash J E 1977 Studies of excitable membranes. III. Freeze-fracture examination of the membrane specializations at the neuromuscular junction and in the non-junctional sarcolemma after denervation. Brain Research 137: 197

Ellisman M H, Brooke M H, Kaiser K K, Rash J E 1978 Appearance in slow muscle sarcolemma of specializations characteristic of fast muscle after reinnervation by a fast muscle nerve. Experimental Neurology 58: 59

Endo M, Nonomura Y, Mosaki T, Ohtsuki I, Ebashi S 1966 Localization of native tropomyosin in relation to striation patterns. Journal of Biochemistry (Tokyo) 60: 605

Engel A G 1987 The molecular biology of end-plate diseases. In: Salpeter M M (ed) The vertebrate neuromuscular junction. Alan Liss, New York, p 361

Engel A G, Dale A J D 1968 Autophagic glycogenosis of late onset with mitochondrial abnormalities: light and electronmicroscopic observations. Proceedings of the Mayo Clinic 43: 233

Engel A G, Santa T 1971 Histometric analysis of the ultrastructure of the neuromuscular junction in myasthenia gravis and in the myasthenic syndrome. Annals of the New York Academy of Sciences 183: 46

Engel A G, Tsujihata M, Lindstrom J M, Lennon V A 1976 The motor end-plate in myasthenia gravis and in experimental autoimmune myasthenia gravis. A quantitative ultrastructural study. Annals of the New York Academy of Sciences 274: 60

Engel A G, Banker B Q 1986 Ultrastructural changes in diseased muscle. In: Engel A G, Banker B Q (eds) Myology. McGraw-Hill, New York, p 909

Essen B, Henriksson J 1974 Glycogen content of individual muscle fibers in man. Acta Physiologica Scandinavica 90: 645

Ezerman E B, Ishikawa H 1967 Differentiation of the sarcoplasmic reticulum and the T-system in developing chick skeletal muscle. Journal of Cell Biology 35: 405

Fardeau M 1969a Ultrastructure des fibres musculaires squelettiques. La Presse Médicale 77: 1341

Fardeau M 1969b Etude d'une nouvelle observation de 'nemaline myopathy'. II. Données ultrastructurales. Acta Neuropathologica (Berlin) 13: 250

Fardeau M 1970 Ultrastructural lesions in progressive muscular dystrophies: a critical study of their specificity. In: Canal N, Scarlato G, Walton J N (eds) Muscle diseases. Excerpta Medica, Amsterdam, pp 98–108

Ferguson D G, Schwartz H W, Franzini-Armstrong C 1984 Subunit structure of junctional feet in triads of skeletal muscle. A freeze-drying rotary shadowing study. Journal of Cell Biology 99: 1735

Fertuck H C, Salpeter M M 1974 Localization of acetylcholine receptor by ^{125}I-labelled, α-bungarotoxin binding at mouse motor endplates. Proceedings of the National Academy of Sciences USA 71: 1376

Fertuck H C, Salpeter M M 1976 Quantitation of junctional and extrajunctional acetylcholine receptors by electron microscope autoradiography after ^{125}I-α-bungarotoxin binding at mouse neuromuscular junctions. Journal of Cell Biology 69: 144

Fischbeck K H, Bonilla E, Schotland D L 1982 Freeze-fracture analysis of plasma membrane cholesterol in fast- and slow-twitch muscles. Journal of Ultrastructure Research 81: 117

Fischman D A 1967 An electron microscope study of myofibril formation in embryonic chick skeletal muscle. Journal of Cell Biology 32: 557

Franzini-Armstrong C 1970 Details of the I-band structure as revealed by the location of Ferritin. Tissue and Cell 2: 327

Franzini-Armstrong C 1973 The structure of a simple Z line. Journal of Cell Biology 58: 630

Franzini-Armstrong C 1979 A description of satellite and invasive cells in frog sartorius. In: Mauro A (ed) Muscle regeneration. Raven Press, New York, pp 233–238

Franzini-Armstrong C 1980 Structure of sarcoplasmic reticulum. Federation Proceedings 39: 2403

Franzini-Armstrong C 1983 Disposition of Ca ATPase in SR membrane from skeletal muscle. Journal of Cell Biology 97: 260a

Franzini-Armstrong C, Porter K R 1964 The Z disc of skeletal muscle fibrils. Zeitschrift für Zellforschung und mikroskopische Anatomie 61: 661

Franzini-Armstrong C, Ferguson D G, Champ C 1988 Discrimination between fast- and slow-twitch fibres of guinea pig skeletal muscle using the relative surface density of junctional transverse tubule membrane. Journal of Muscle Research and Cell Motility 9: 403

Fridén J 1984 Changes in human skeletal muscle induced by long-term eccentric exercise. Cell and Tissue Research 236: 365

Fridén J, Sjostrom M, Ekblom B 1984 Muscle fibre type characteristics in endurance trained and untrained individuals. European Journal of Applied Physiology 52: 266

Froehner S C, Murnane A A, Tobler M, Peng H B, Sealock R 1987 A postsynaptic M_r 58,000 (58 K) protein concentrated at acetylcholine receptor-rich sites in Torpedo electroplaques and skeletal muscle. Journal of Cell Biology 104: 1633

Fulton A B, Isaacs W B 1991 Titin, a huge, elastic sarcomeric protein with a probable role in morphogenesis. Bioessays 13: 157

Gauthier G F 1969 On the relationship of ultrastructural and cytochemical features to colour in mammalian skeletal muscle. Zeitschrift für Zellforschung und mikroskopische Anatomie 95: 462

Gauthier G F, Padykula H A 1966 Cytological studies of fiber types in skeletal muscle. Journal of Cell Biology 28: 333

Gibson M C, Schultz E 1983 Age-related differences in absolute numbers of skeletal muscle satellite cells. Muscle and Nerve 6: 574

Gilliatt R W 1966 Axon branching in motor nerves. In: Andrew B L (ed) Control and innervation of skeletal muscle. Thomson, Dundee, pp 53–60

Goldberg M 1986 Is the lamina lucida of the basement

membrane a fixation artefact? European Journal of Cell Biology 42: 365

Goldspink G 1968 Sarcomere length during postnatal growth of mammalian muscle fibres. Journal of Cell Science 3: 539

Goldspink G 1970 The proliferation of myofibrils during muscle fibre growth. Journal of Cell Science 6: 593

Goldspink G 1971 Changes in striated muscle fibres during contraction and growth with particular reference to myofibril splitting. Journal of Cell Science 9: 123

Goldspink G, Ward P S 1979 Changes in rodent muscle fibre types during post-natal growth, undernutrition and exercise. Journal of Physiology 296: 453

Goldstein M A, Schroeter J P, Sass R L 1990 Two structural states of the vertebrate Z band. Electron Microscopy Review 3: 227

Gray E G 1958 The structures of fast and slow muscle fibres in the frog. Journal of Anatomy 92: 559

Grove B K, Kurer V, Lehrer C L, Doetchman T C, Perriard J-C, Eppenberger H M 1984 A new 185 000 dalton skeletal muscle protein detected by monoclonal antibodies. Journal of Cell Biology 98: 518

Grove B K, Cerny L, Perriard C-J, Eppenberger H M, Thornell L E 1989 Fiber type-specific distribution of M-band proteins in chick–muscle. Journal of Histochemistry and Cytochemistry 37: 447

Gruner J-E 1961 La structure fine du fuseau neuromusculaire humain. Revue Neurologique 104: 490

Gu Y, Hall Z W 1988 Immunological evidence for a change in subunits of the acetylcholine receptor in developing and denervated rat muscle. Neuron 1: 117

Hammersen F, Gidlof A, Larsson J, Lewis D H 1980 The occurrence of paracrystalline mitochondrial inclusions in normal human skeletal muscle. Acta Neuropathologica (Berlin) 49: 35

Hanzlikova V, Schiaffino S 1977 Mitochondrial changes in ischaemic skeletal muscle. Journal of Ultrastructure Research 60: 121

Harris A J, 1981 Embryonic growth and innervation of rat skeletal muscle. 1. Neural regulation of muscle fibre numbers. Philosophical Transactions of the Royal Society of London B 293: 257

Hasselbach W 1979 The sarcoplasmic calcium pump. A model of energy transmission in biological membranes. Topics in Current Chemistry 78: 1

Heine H, Schaeg G 1979 Origin and function of 'rod-like' structures in mitochondria. Acta Anatomica (Basel) 103: 1

Hellmuth A E, Allbrook D 1973 Satellite cells as the stem cells of skeletal muscle. In: Kakulas B A (ed) Basic research in myology. Excerpta Medica, Amsterdam, pp 343–345

Hess A, Rosner S 1970 The satellite cell bud and myoblast in denervated mammalian muscle fibers. American Journal of Anatomy 129: 21

Heuser J E, Reese T S, Dennis M J, Jan Y, Jan L, Evans L 1979 Synaptic vesicle exocytosis captured by quick freezing and correlated with quantal transmitter release. Journal of Cell Biology 81: 275

Heuser J E, Reese T S 1981 Structural changes after transmitter release at the frog neuromuscular junction. Journal of Cell Biology 88: 564

Heuson-Stiennon J A 1965 Morphogenése de la cellule musculaire striée, etudiée au microscope électronique. I Formation des structures fibrillaires. Journal de Microscopie 4: 657

Hoffman E P, Brown R H, Kunkel L M 1987 Dystrophin: the protein product on the Duchenne muscular dystrophy locus. Cell 51: 919

Holtzer H 1970 Proliferation and quantal cell cycles in the differentiation of muscle, cartilage and red blood cells. In: Padykula H A (ed) Gene expression in somatic cells. Academic Press, New York, pp 69–88

Holtzer H, Croop J, Dienstman S, Ishikawa H, Somlyo A P 1975 Effects of cytochalasin B and colcemide on myogenic cultures. Proceedings of the National Academy of Sciences USA 72: 513

Hoppeler H, Luthi P, Claassen H, Weibel E R, Howald H 1973 The ultrastructure of the normal human skeletal muscle: a morphometric analysis on untrained men, women and well trained orienteers. Pfluegers Archiv für die gesamte Physiologie des Menschen und der Tiere 344: 217

Hudson C S, Dyas B K, Rash J E 1982 Changes in number and distribution of orthogonal arrays during postnatal muscle development. Developmental Brain Research 4: 91

Hunter D D, Shah V, Merlie J P, Sanes J R 1989 A laminin-like adhesive protein concentrated in the synaptic cleft of the neuromuscular junction. Nature 338: 229

Huxley A F 1957 Muscle structure and theories of contraction. Progress in Biophysical Chemistry 7: 255

Huxley A F 1974 Muscular contraction. Journal of Physiology 243: 1

Huxley A F, Niedergerke R 1954 Interference microscopy of living muscle fibres. Nature 173: 971

Huxley A F, Simmons R M 1971 Proposed mechanism of force generation in striated muscle. Nature 233: 533

Huxley H E 1957 The double array of filaments in cross-striated muscle. Journal of Biophysical and Biochemical Cytology 3: 631

Huxley H E 1963 Electron microscopic studies on the structure of natural and synthetic protein filaments from striated muscle. Journal of Molecular Biology 7: 281

Huxley H E 1967 Recent X-ray diffraction and electron microscope studies of striated muscle. Journal of General Physiology 50: 71

Huxley H E 1969 The mechanism of muscle contraction. Science 164: 1356

Huxley H E, Hanson J 1954 Changes in the cross striations of muscle during contraction and stretch and their structural interpretation. Nature 173: 973

Huxley H E, Brown W 1967 The low-angle X-ray diagram of vertebrate striated muscle and its behaviour during contraction and rigor. Journal of Molecular Biology 30: 383

Ibraghimov-Beskrovnaya O, Ervasti JM, Leveille C J, Slaughter C A, Sernett S W, Campbell K P 1992 Primary structure of dystrophin-associated glycoproteins linking dystrophin to the extra-cellular matrix. Nature 355: 696

Ishikawa H 1966 Electron microscopic observations of satellite cells with special reference to the development of mammalian skeletal muscle. Zeitschrift für Anatomie und Entwicklungsgeschichte 125: 43

Ishikawa H, Bischoff R, Holtzer H 1968 Mitosis and intermediate sized filaments in developing skeletal muscle. Journal of Cell Biology 38: 538

Jaimovich E 1991 Chemical transmission at the triad. Journal of Muscle Research and Cell Motility 12: 316

Jerusalem F, Engel A G, Peterson H A 1975 Human muscle fiber fine structure: morphometric data on controls. Neurology (Minneapolis) 25: 127

Jilka R L, Martonosi A N, Tillack T W 1975 Effect of purified $(Mg^{2+} + Ca^{2+})$ activated ATPase of sarcoplasmic reticulum upon the passive Ca^{2+} permeability and ultrastructure of phospholipid vesicles. Journal of Biological Chemistry 250: 7511

Jin J P, Wang K 1991 Nebulin as a giant actin-building template protein in skeletal muscle sarcomere. Interaction of actin and cloned human nebulin fragments. FEBS Letters 281: 93

Jones S W 1987 Presynaptic mechanisms at vertebrate neuromuscular junctions. In: Salpeter M M (ed) The vertebrate neuromuscular junction. Alan Liss, New York, p 187

Jorgensen A O, Arnold W, Shen A C-Y, Yuan S, Gaver M, Campbell K P 1990 Identification of novel proteins unique to either transverse tubules (TS28) or the sarcolemma (SL50) in rabbit skeletal muscle. Journal of Cell Biology 110: 1173

Kamieniecka Z, Schmalbruch H 1980 Neuromuscular disorders with abnormal mitochondria. In: Bourne G H, Danielli J F (eds) International Review of Cytology, vol 65. Academic Press, New York, pp 321–357

Katz B 1961 The terminations of the afferent nerve fibre in the muscle spindle of the frog. Philosphical Transactions of the Royal Society of London B 243: 221

Kelly A M 1971 Sarcoplasmic reticulum and T tubules in differentiating rat skeletal muscle. Journal of Cell Biology 49: 335

Kelly A M 1978 Perisynaptic satellite cells in the developing and mature rat soleus muscle. Anatomical Record 190: 891

Kelly A M 1980 T tubules in neonatal rat soleus and extensor digitorum longus muscles. Developmental Biology 80: 501

Kelly A M, Zacks S I 1969 The histogenesis of rat intercostal muscle. Journal of Cell Biology 42: 135

Kelly D E 1967 Models of muscle Z-band fine structure based on a looping filament configuration. Journal of Cell Biology 34: 827

Kelly D E, Cahill M A 1972 Filamentous and matrix components of skeletal muscle Z-disks. Anatomical Record 172: 623

Kelly F J, McGrath J A, Goldspink D F, Cullen M J 1986 A morphological/biochemical study on the actions of corticosteroids on rat skeletal muscle. Muscle and Nerve 9: 1

Ketelsen U-P 1980 Quantitative freeze-fracture studies of human skeletal muscle cell membranes under normal and pathological conditions. In: Angelini C, Danieli G A, Fontanari A (eds) Muscular dystrophy research: advances and trends. Excerpta Medica, Amsterdam, pp 79–87

Kitiyakara A, Angevine D M 1963 A study of the pattern of post embryonic growth of *m. gracilis* in mice. Developmental Biology 8: 322

Knappeis G G, Carlsen F 1962 The ultrastructure of the Z disc in skeletal muscle. Journal of Cell Biology 13: 323

Knappeis G G, Carlsen F 1968 The ultrastructure of the M-line in skeletal muscle. Journal of Cell Biology 38: 202

Komiyama M, Maruyama K, Shimada Y 1990 Assembly of connectin (titin) in relation to myosin and alpha-actinin in cultured cardiac myocytes. Journal of Muscle Research and Cell Motility 11: 419

Konigsberg I R 1971 Diffusion-mediated control of myoblast fusion. Developmental Biology 26: 133

Konigsberg I R, Sollman P A, Mixter L O 1978 The duration of the terminal G^1 of fusing myoblasts. Developmental Biology 63: 11

Korneliussen H 1973 Ultrastructure of myotendinous junctions in myxine and rat. Specializations between the plasma membrane and the lamina densa. Zietschrift für Anatomie und Entwicklungsgeschichte 142: 91

Kruger P 1952 Tetanus und Tonus der quergestriefften Skelettmuskeln der Wirbeltiere und des Menschen. Akademischer Verlag, Liepzig

Labeit S, Gautel M, Lakey A, Trinick J 1992 Towards a molecular understanding of titin. EMBO Journal 11: 1711

Labeit S, Gibson R, Lakey A, Leonard K, Zeviani M, Knight P, Wardale J, Trinick J 1991 Evidence that nebulin is a protein-ruler in muscle thick filaments. FEBS Letters 295: 232

Lai F A, Erickson H P, Rousseau E, Liu Q-Y, Meissner G 1988 Purification and reconstitution of the calcium release channel from skeletal muscle. Nature 331: 315

Lake B D, Wilson J 1975 Zebra Body myopathy. Clinical, histochemical and ultrastructural studies. Journal of the Neurological Sciences 24: 437

Lamb G D 1992 DHP receptors and excitation–contraction coupling. Journal of Muscle Research and Cell Motility 13: 394

Landon D N 1966 Electron microscopy of muscle spindles. In: Andrew B L (ed) Control and innervation of skeletal muscle. Thomson, Dundee, pp 96–111

Landon D N 1969 The fine structure of the Z disc of rat striated muscle. Journal of Anatomy 106: 172p

Landon D N 1970a Observations on the morphogenesis of rat skeletal muscle. Journal of Anatomy 107: 385

Landon D N 1970b The influence of fixation upon the fine structure of the Z-disk of rat striated muscle. Journal of Cell Science 6: 257–276

Landon D N 1970c Change in Z-disk structure with muscular contraction. Journal of Physiology 211: 44

Landon D N 1971 A quantitative study of some of the fine structural features of developing myotubes in the rat. Journal of Anatomy 110: 170

Landon D N 1982 Skeletal muscle — normal morphology, development and innervation. In: Mastaglia F L, Walton J N (eds) Skeletal muscle pathology. Churchill Livingstone, Edinburgh, pp 1–87

Larson P F, Fulthorpe J J, Hudgson P 1973 The alignment of polysomes along myosin filaments in developing myofibrils. Journal of Anatomy 116: 327

Lash J W, Holtzer H, Swift H 1957 Regeneration of mature skeletal muscle. Anatomical Record 128: 679

Lawrence T, Mauro A 1979 Identification of satellite cells in vitro in frog muscle fibers by Nomarski optics. In: Mauro A (ed) Muscle regeneration. Raven Press, New York, p 275

Lawson D 1983 Epinemin: a new protein associated with vimentin filaments in non-neural cells. Journal of Cell Biology 97: 1891

Lazarides E 1980 Intermediate filaments as mechanical integrators of cellular space. Nature 283: 249

Lazarides E, Balzer D R 1978 Specificity of desmin to avian and mammalian muscle cells. Cell 14: 429

Lee R E, Poulos A C, Mayer R F, Rash J E 1986 Caveolae preservation in the characterization of human neuromuscular disease. Muscle and Nerve 9: 127

Leung A T, Imagawa T, Block B, Franzini-Armstrong C, Campbell K P 1988 Biochemical and ultrastructural characterization of the 1,4-dihydropyridine receptor from rabbit skeletal muscle. Journal of Biological Chemistry 263: 994

Libelius R, Jirmanova I, Lundquist, I, Thesleff S, Barnard E A 1979 T-tubule endocytosis in dystrophic chicken muscle and its relation to muscle fiber degeneration. Acta Neuropathologica (Berlin) 48: 31

Lindsay A R G, Williams A J 1991 Functional characterisation of the ryanodine receptor purified from sheep cardiac muscle sarcoplasmic reticulum. Biochimica et Biophysica Acta 1064: 89

Lipton B H 1979 Skeletal muscle regeneration in muscular dystrophy. In: Mauro A (ed) Muscle regeneration. Raven Press, New York, pp 31–40

Lipton B H, Konigsberg I R 1972 A fine structural analysis of the fusion of myogenic cells. Journal of Cell Biology 53: 348

Lipton B H, Schultz E 1979 Developmental fate of skeletal muscle satellite cells. Science 205: 1292

Love D R, Hill D F, Dickson G et al 1989 An autosomal transcript in skeletal muscle with homology to dystrophin. Nature 339: 55

Lowey S, Slayter H S, Weeds A G, Baker H 1969 Structure of the myosin molecule. I Subfragments of myosin by enzymic degradation. Journal of Molecular Biology 42: 1

Luff A R, Atwood H L 1971 Changes in the sarcoplasmic reticulum and transverse tubular system of fast and slow skeletal muscles of the mouse during post-natal development. Journal of Cell Biology 51: 369

Luther P, Squire S 1978 Three-dimensional structure of the vertebrate muscle M-region. Journal of Molecular Biology 125: 313

MacCallum J B 1898 On the histogenesis of the striated muscle fibre and the growth of the human sartorius muscle. Johns Hopkins Hospital Bullettin 9: 208

McClare C W F 1971 Biochemical machines. Maxwell's demon and living organisms. Journal of Theoretical Biology 30: 1

MacDonald R D, Engel A G 1971 Observations on organization of Z-disk components and on rod-bodies of Z-disk origin. Journal of Cell Biology 48: 431

McGeatchie J, Allbrook D 1978 Cell proliferation in skeletal muscle following denervation or tenotomy. Cell and Tissue Research 193: 259

MacKay B, Harrop T J 1969 An experimental study of the longitudinal growth of skeletal muscle in the rat. Acta Anatomica (Basel) 72: 38

MacLennan D H, Holland P C 1975 Calcium transport in sarcoplasmic reticulum. Annual Review of Biophysics and Bioengineering 4: 377

Mair W G P, Tomé F M S 1972 Atlas of the ultrastructure of diseased human muscle. Churchill Livingstone, Edinburgh

Maltin C A, Harris J B, Cullen M J 1983 Regeneration of mammalian skeletal muscle following the injection of the snake venom toxin, taipoxin. Cell and Tissue Research 232: 565

Maniloff J, Vanderkooi G, Hayashi H, Capaldi R A 1973 Optical analysis of electron micrographs of cytochrome oxidase membranes. Biochimica et Biophysica Acta 298: 180

Martonosi A N 1982 Regulation of cytoplasmic calcium concentration by sarcoplasmic reticulum. In: Schotland D L (ed) Disorders of the motor unit. John Wiley, New York, pp 565–583

Maruyama K 1986 Connectin: an elastic filamentous protein of striated muscle. International Review of Cytology 104: 81

Maruyama K, Matsuno A, Higuchi H, Shimoaka S, Kimura S, Shimizue T 1989 Behaviour of connectin (titin) and nebulin in skinned muscle fibres released after external stretch as revealed by immunoelectron microscopy. Journal of Muscle Research and Cell Motility 10: 350

Masaki T, Endo M, Ebashi S 1967 Localization of 6s component of alpha actinin at the Z-band. Journal of Biochemistry (Tokyo) 62: 630

Matsubara I, Elliott G F 1972 X-ray diffraction studies on skinned single fibres of frog skeletal muscle. Journal of Molecular Biology 72: 657

Matthew C A, Moore M J 1991 Collagen fibril morphometry in transected rat extensor tendons. Journal of Anatomy 175: 263

Mauro A 1961 Satellite cell of skeletal muscle fibres. Journal of Biophysical and Biochemical Cytology 9: 493

Meissner G, Fleischer S 1971 Characterization of sarcoplasmic reticulum from skeletal muscle. Biochimica et Biophysica Acta 241: 356

Melmed C, Karpati G, Carpenter S 1975 Experimental mitochondrial myopathy produced by in vivo uncoupling of oxidative phosphorylation. Journal of the Neurological Sciences 26: 305

Milligan R A, Whittaker M, Safer D 1990 Molecular structure of F-actin and location of surface binding sites. Nature 348: 217

Mishina M, Takai T, Imoto K, Noda M, Takahashi T, Numa S, Methfessel C, Sakmann B 1986 Molecular distinction between fetal and adult forms of muscle acetylcholine receptor. Nature 321: 406

Mobley B A, Eisenberg B R 1975 Sizes of components in frog skeletal muscle measured by methods of stereology. Journal of General Physiology 66: 31

Montgomery R D 1962 Growth of human striated muscle. Nature 195: 194

Moore M J 1983 The dual connective tissue system of rat soleus muscle. Muscle and Nerve 6: 416

Morgan-Hughes J A 1982 Mitochondrial myopathies. In: Mastaglia F L, Walton J N (eds) Skeletal muscle pathology. Churchill Livingstone, Edinburgh, pp 309–339

Morgan-Hughes J A, Darveniza P, Kahn S N, Landon D N, Sherratt R M, Land J M, Clark J B 1977 A mitochondrial myopathy characterized by a deficiency in reducible cytochrome b. Brain 100: 617

Moss F P 1968 The relationship between the dimensions of the fibres and the number of nuclei during normal growth of skeletal muscle in the domestic fowl. American Journal of Anatomy 122: 555

Moss F P, Leblond C P 1970 Nature of dividing nuclei in skeletal muscle of growing rats. Journal of Cell Biology 44: 459

Moss F P, Leblond C P 1971 Satellite cells as the source of nuclei in muscles of growing rats. Anatomical Record 170: 421

Muir A R 1970 The structure and distibution of satellite cells. In: Mauro A, Shafiq S A, Milhorat A T (eds) Regeneration of striated muscle and myogenesis. Excerpta Medica, Amsterdam, pp 91–100

Muir A R, Kanji A H M, Allbrook D B 1965 The structure of satellite cells in skeletal muscle. Journal of Anatomy 99: 435

Murray M A, Robbins N 1982 Cell proliferation in denervated muscle: identity and origin of the dividing cells. Neuroscience 7: 1823

Nave R, Furst D O, Weber K 1989 Visualization of the polarity of isolated titin molecules: a single globular head on a long thin rod as the M band anchoring domain? Journal of Cell Biology 109: 2177

Nave R, Furst D O, Weber K 1990 Interaction of nebulin and alpha-actinin *in vitro*. Support for the existence of a fourth filament system in skeletal muscle. FEBS Letters 269: 163

Nishikawa M 1981 Histo- and cytochemistry of acetylcholinesterase activity at the myotendinous junctions in skeletal muscles of rats. Acta Histochemica et Cytochemica 14: 670

Nitkin R M, Smith M A, Magil C, Fallon J R, Yao Y-M M, Wallace B G, McMahan U J 1987 Identification of agrin, a synaptic organizing protein from Torpedo electric organ. Journal of Cell Biology 105: 2471

O'Brien E J, Dickens M J 1983 Actin and thin filaments. In: Harris J R (ed) Electron microscopy of proteins. Macromolecular structure and function, vol 4, pp 1–95

Offer G, Moss C, Starr R 1973 A new protein of the thick filaments of vertebrate skeletal myofibrils. Extraction purification and characterization. Journal of Molecular Biology 74: 653

Ogata T 1988 Structure of motor endplates in the different fiber types of vetebrate skeletal muscles. Archives of Histology and Cytology 51: 385

Ogata T, Murata F 1969 Cytological features of three fiber types in human striated muscle. Tohoko Journal of Experimental Medicine 99: 225

Ohashi K, Maruyama K 1980 A new structural protein located in the Z-line of chicken skeletal muscle. In: Ebashi S, Maruyama K, Endo M (eds) Muscle contraction its regulatory mechanisms. Japanese Scientific Societies Press, Tokyo, pp 497–505

Ohtsuki I 1975 Distribution of troponin components in the thin filament studied by immunoelectron microscopy. Journal of Biochemistry (Tokyo) 77: 633

Ohtsuki I 1979 Molecular arrangement of troponin-T in the thin filament. Journal of Biochemistry (Tokyo) 86: 491

Ohtsuki I, Masaki T, Nonomura Y, Ebashi S 1967 Periodic distribution of troponin along the thin filament. Journal of Biochemistry (Tokyo) 61: 817

Oki S, Matsuda Y, Kitaoka K, Nagano Y, Nojima M, Desaki J 1990 Scanning electron microscope study of neuromuscular junctions in different muscle fiber types in the zebra finch and rat. Archives of Histology and Cytology 53: 327

Oldfors A, Fardeau M 1983 The permeability of the basal lamina at the neuromuscular junction. An ultrastructural study of rat skeletal muscle using particulate tracers. Neuropathology and Applied Neurobiology 9: 419

Ontell M 1974 Muscle satellite cells. Anatomical Record 178: 211

Ontell M 1975 Evidence of myoblastic potential of satellite cells in denervated muscles. Cell and Tissue Research 160: 345

Ontell M 1977 Neonatal muscle: an electron microscopic study. Anatomical Record 189: 669

Ontell M 1979 The source of 'new' muscle fibers in neonatal muscle. In: Mauro A (ed) Muscle regeneration. Raven Press, New York, pp 137–146

Padykula H A, Gauthier G F 1970 The ultrastructure of the neuromuscular junctions of mammalian red, white, and intermediate skeletal muscle fibers. Journal of Cell Biology 46: 27

Page E, Power B, Fozzard H A, Meddoff D A 1969 Sarcolemmal evaginations with knob-like or stalked projections in purkinje fibers of the sheep's heart. Journal of Ultrastructure Research 28: 288

Page S G 1965 A comparison of the fine structure of frog slow and twitch muscle fibres. Journal of Cell Biology 26: 477

Page S G 1968 Fine structure of tortoise skeletal muscle. Journal of Physiology 197: 709

Payne C M, Stern L Z, Curless R G, Hannapel L K 1975 Ultrastructural fiber typing in normal and diseased human muscle. Journal of the Neurological Sciences 25: 99

Peluchetti D, Mora M, Protti A, Cornelio F 1985 Freeze-fracture analysis of the muscle fiber plasma membrane in Duchenne dystrophy. Neurology 35: 928

Pepe F A 1966 Some aspects of the structural organization of the myofibril as revealed by antibody-staining methods. Journal of Cell Biology 28: 505

Pepe F A, Drucker B 1975 The myosin filament. III. C-protein. Journal of Molecular Biology 99: 609

Perry S V, Dhoot G K 1980 Biochemical aspects of muscle development and differentiation. In: Goldspink D F (ed) Development and specialization of skeletal muscle. Cambridge University Press, Cambridge, pp 51–64

Pollack G H 1990 Muscles and molecules. Uncovering the principles of biological motion. Ebner & Sons, Seattle

Prince F P, Hikida R S, Hagerman F C, Staron R S, Allen W H 1981 A morphometric analysis of human muscle fibers with relation to fiber types and adaptations to exercise. Journal of the Neurological Sciences 49: 165

Pumplin D W, Fambrough D M 1983 $(Na^+ + K^+)$-ATPase correlated with a major group of intramembrane particles in freeze-fracture replicas of cultured chick myotubes. Journal of Cell Biology 97: 1214

Rambourg A, Segretain D 1980 Three-dimensional electron microscopy of mitochondria and endoplasmic reticulum in the red muscle fiber of the rat diaphragm. Anatomical Record 197: 33

Rash J E, Fambrough D 1973 Ultrastructural and electrophysiological correlates of cell coupling and cytoplasmic fusion during myogenesis in vitro. Developmental Biology 30: 166

Rash J E, Ellisman M H 1974 Studies of excitable membranes. I. Macromolecular specializations of the neuromuscular junction and the nonjunctional sarcolemma. Journal of Cell Biology 63: 567

Rash J E, Staehelin L A 1974 Freeze-cleave demonstration of gap junctions between skeletal myogenic cells in vitro. Developmental Biology 36: 455

Rash J E, Ellisman M H, Staehelin L A, Porter K R 1974 Molecular specializations of excitable membranes in normal, chronically denervated, and dystrophic muscle fibers. In: Milhorat A T (ed) Exploratory concepts in muscular dystrophy II. Excerpta Medica, Amsterdam, pp 271–291

Reedy M K 1964 The structure of actin filaments and the origin of the axial periodicity in the I substance of vertebrate striated muscle. Proceedings of the Royal Society of London B 160: 458

Reedy M K 1967 Personal communication, quoted by Elliott, Lowy and Millman 1967

Reist N E, Magill C, McMahan U J 1987 Agrin-like molecules at synaptic sites in normal, denervated, and damaged skeletal muscles. Journal of Cell Biology 105: 2457

Revel J P 1962 The sarcoplasmic reticulum of the bat cricothyroid muscle. Journal of Cell Biology 12: 571

Reznik M 1969 Thymidine ^{3}H uptake by satellite cells of regenerating skeletal muscle. Journal of Cell Biology 40: 568

Reznik M 1970 Satellite cells, myoblasts and skeletal muscle regeneration. In: Mauro A, Shafiq S A, Milhorat A T (eds)

Regeneration of skeletal muscle, and myogenesis. Excerpta Medica, Amsterdam, pp 133–156

Rios E, Brum G 1987 Involvement of dihydropyridine receptors in excitation–contraction (EC) coupling in skeletal muscle. Nature 325: 717

Rios E, Ma J, Gonzalez A 1991 The mechanical hypothesis of excitation–contraction (EC) coupling in skeletal muscle. Journal of Muscle Research and Cell Motility 12: 127

Ross K F A, Jans D E, Larson P F et al 1970 Distribution of ribosomal RNA in fusing myoblasts. Nature 226: 545

Rowe R W 1971 Ultrastructure of the Z-line of skeletal muscle fibers. Journal of Cell Biology 51: 674

Rowe R W 1973 The ultrastructure of Z-disks from white, intermediate, and red fibers of mammalian striated muscle. Journal of Cell Biology 57: 261

Ruska H A, Edwards G A 1957 A new cytoplasmic pattern in striated muscle fibres and its possible relation to growth. Growth 21: 73

Sahgal V, Subramani V, Hughes R, Shah H, Singh H 1979 On the pathogenesis of mitochondrial myopathies: an experimental study. Acta Neuropathologica (Berlin) 46: 177

Saito A, Inui M, Radermacher M, Frank J, Fleischer S 1988 Ultrastructure of the calcium release channel of sarcoplasmic reticulum. Journal of Cell Biology 107: 211

Samitt C E, Bonilla E 1990 Immunocytochemical study of dystrophin at the myotendinous junction. Muscle and Nerve 13: 493

Sanes J R 1982 Laminin, fibronectin and collagen in synaptic and extrasynaptic portions of muscle fiber basement membrane. Journal of Cell Biology 93: 442

Sanes J R, Marshall L M, McMahan U J 1978 Reinnervation of muscle fiber basal lamina after removal of myofibers. Differentiation of regenerating axons at original synaptic sites. Journal of Cell Biology 78: 176

Sanes J R, Chiu A Y 1983 The basal lamina of the neuromuscular junction. Cold Spring Harbor Symposium on Quantitative Biology 48: 667

Sarzala M G, Pilarska M, Zubrzycka E, Michalak M 1975 Changes in the structure, composition and function of sarcoplasmic reticulum membrane during development. European Journal of Biochemistry 57: 25

Sato T, Seki K, Hirawake H, Nakamura S, Horais S, Ozawa T 1990 Immunocytochemistry of mitochondria. Journal of the Neurological Sciences 98: 58

Scalzi H A, Price H M 1971 The arrangement and sensory innervation of the intrafusal fibers in the feline muscle spindle. Journal of Ultrastructure Research 36: 375

Schiaffino S, Margreth A 1969 Coordinated development of the sarcoplasmic reticulum and T-system during postnatal differentiation of rat skeletal muscle. Journal of Cell Biology 41: 855

Schiaffino S, Hanzlikova V, Pierobon S 1970 Relations between structure and function in rat skeletal muscle fibers. Journal of Cell Biology 47: 107

Schmalbruch H 1979a 'Square arrays' in the sarcolemma of human skeletal muscle fibres. Nature 281: 145

Schmalbruch H 1979b The membrane systems in different fibre types of the triceps surae muscle of cat. Cell and Tissue Research 204: 187

Schmalbruch H 1980 Delayed fixation alters the pattern of intramembrane particles in mammalian muscle fibers. Journal of Ultrastructure Research 70: 15

Schmalbruch H 1983 The fine structure of mitochondrial abnormalities in muscle diseases. In: Scarlatto G, Cerri C

(eds) Mitochondrial pathology in muscle diseases. Piccin, Padua, pp 41–56

Schmalbruch H 1985 Skeletal muscle. Handbook of microscopic anatomy, vol 2, Pt 6. Springer-Verlag, Berlin

Schmalbruch H, Hellhammer U 1977 The number of nuclei in adult rat muscles with special reference to satellite cells. Anatomical Record 189: 169

Schollmeyer J V, Goll D E, Stromer M H, Dayton W, Singh I, Robson R 1974 Studies on the composition of the Z-disk. Journal of Cell Biology 63: 303a

Schotland D L, Bonilla E, Wakayama Y 1981 Freeze-fracture studies of muscle plasma membrane in human muscular dystrophy. Acta Neuropathologica (Berlin) 54: 189

Schultz E 1974 A quantitative study of the satellite cell population in post-natal mouse lumbrical muscle. Anatomical Record 180: 589

Schultz E 1978 Changes in satellite cells of growing muscle following denervation. Anatomical Record 190: 299

Schultz E 1979 Quantification of satellite cells in growing muscle using electron microscopy and fiber whole mounts. In: Mauro A (ed) Muscle regeneration. Raven Press, New York, pp 131–135

Schwann T 1839 Mikroskopische Untersuchungen uber die Uebereinstimmung in der Struktur und dem Wachsthum der Thiere und Pflanzen. Reimer, Berlin

Sealock R, Butler M H, Kramarcy N R et al 1991 Localization of dystrophin relative to acetylcholine receptor domains in electric tissue and adult and cultured skeletal muscle. Journal of Cell Biology 113: 1133

Sesodia S, Cullen M J 1991 The effect of denervation on the morphology of regenerating rat soleus muscle. Acta Neuropathologica 82: 21

Shafiq S A, Gorycki M A, Goldstone L, Milhorat A T 1966 Fine structure of fiber types in normal human muscle. Anatomical Record 156: 283

Shafiq S A, Gorycki M, Milhorat A T 1967 An electron microscopic study of regeneration and satellite cells in human muscle. Neurology (Minneapolis) 17: 567

Shafiq S A, Leung B, Schutta H S 1979 A freeze-fracture study of fibre types in normal human muscle. Journal of the Neurological Sciences 42: 129

Shear C R 1975 Myofibril proliferation in developing skeletal muscle. In: Bradley W G, Gardner-Medwin D, Walton J N (eds) Recent advances in myology. Excerpta Medica, Amsterdam, pp 364–373

Shear C R, Bloch R J 1985 Vinculin in subsarcolemmal densities in chicken skeletal muscle: localization and relationship to intracellular and extracellular structures. Journal of Cell Biology 101: 240

Shimada Y 1971 Electron microscope observations on the fusion of chick myoblasts in vitro. Journal of Cell Biology 48: 128

Simmons R 1991 Moving story. Review of 'muscles and molecules: uncovering the principles of biological motion', by G Pollack. Nature 351: 452

Singh I, Goll D E, Robson R M, Stromer M H 1977 N- and C-terminal amino acids of purified alpha actinin. Biochimica et Biophysica Acta 491: 29

Sirken S M, Fischbeck K H 1985 Freeze-fracture studies of denervated and tenotomized rat muscle. Journal of Neuropathology and Experimental Neurology 44: 147

Sjöstrom M, Squire J M 1977 The fine structure of the A-band in cryo-sections. Journal of Molecular Biology 109: 49

Sjöstrom M, Kidman S, Henriksson-Larsen K, Angquist K-A

1982a Z- and M-band appearance in different histochemically defined types of human skeletal muscle fibres. Journal of Histochemistry and Cytochemistry 30: 1

Sjöstrom M, Angqvist K-A, Bylund A-C, Friden J, Gustavsson L, Shersten T 1982b Morphometric analysis of human muscle fiber types. Muscle and Nerve 5: 538

Smeitik J, Stadhouders A, Sengers R et al 1992 Mitochondrial creatine kinase containing crystals, creatine content and mitochondrial creatine kinase activity in chronic progressive external ophthalmoplegia. Neuromuscular Disorders 2: 35

Smith J S, Imagawa T, Ma J, Fill M, Campbell K P, Coronado R 1988 Purified ryanodine receptor from rabbit skeletal muscle is the calcium release channel of sarcoplasmic reticulum. Journal of General Physiology 92: 1

Snow M H 1979 Origin of regenerating myoblasts in mammalian skeletal muscle. In: Mauro A (ed) Muscle regeneration. Raven Press, New York, pp 91–100

Snow M H 1983 A quantitative ultrastructural analysis of satellite cells in denervated fast and slow muscles of the mouse. Anatomical Record 207: 593

Spencer M, Worthington C R 1960 A hypothesis of contraction in striated muscle. Nature 187: 388

Squire J 1981 The structural basis of muscular contraction. Plenum, New York

Stadhouders A M 1981 Mitochondrial ultrastructural changes in muscular diseases. In: Busch H F M, Jennekens F G I, Scholte H R (eds) Mitochondria and muscular diseases. Mefar, Netherlands, pp 113–132

Stockdale F E, Holtzer H 1961 DNA synthesis and myogenesis. Experimental Cell Research 24: 508

Stonnington H H, Engel A G 1973 Normal and denervated muscle. A morphometric study of fine structure. Neurology (New York) 23: 714

Strehler B L, Konigsberg I R, Kelley J E T 1963 Ploidy of myotube nuclei developing in vitro as determined with a recording double beam micro-spectrophotometer. Experimental Cell Research 32: 232

Stromer M H, Hartshorne D J, Rice R V 1967 Removal and reconstruction of Z-line material in striated muscle. Journal of Cell Biology 35: 623

Stromer M H, Hartshorne D J, Mueller H, Rice R V 1969 The effects of various protein fractions on Z- and M- line reconstruction. Journal of Cell Biology 40: 167

Südhof T C, Czernick A J, Kao H et al 1989 The synapsins: mosaics of shared and unique domains in a family of synaptic vesicle phosphoproteins. Science 245: 1474

Suzuki A, Goll D E, Singh I, Allen R E, Robson R M, Stromer M H 1976 Some properties of purified skeletal muscle alpha actinin. Journal of Biological Chemistry 251: 6860

Tabary J C, Tabart C, Tardieu C, Tardieu G, Goldspink G 1972 Physiological and structural changes in the cat's soleus muscle due to immobilization at different lengths by plaster casts. Journal of Physiology 224: 231

Tachikawa T, Clementi F 1979 Early effects of denervation on the morphology of junctional and extrajunctional sarcolemma. Neuroscience 4: 437

Takeshima H, Nishimura S, Matsumoto T et al 1989 Primary structure and expression from complementary DNA of skeletal muscle ryanodine receptor. Nature 339: 439

Tanabe T, Beam K G, Adams B A, Niidome T, Numa S 1990 Regions of the skeletal muscle dihydropyridine receptor critical for excitation–contraction coupling. Nature 346: 567

Teravainen H 1970 Satellite cells of striated muscle after

compression injury so slight as not to cause degeneration of the muscle fibres. Zeitschrift für Zellforschung und Mikroskopische Anatomie 103: 320

Thornell L-E, Sjostrom M, Andersson K-E 1976 The relationship between mechanical stress and myofibrillar organization in heart purkinje fibres. Journal of Molecular and Cellular Cardiology 8: 689

Thornell L-E, Edstrom L, Eriksson A, Henrikson K-G, Angquist K-A 1980 The distribution of intermediate filament protein (skeletin) in normal and diseased human skeletal muscle. Journal of the Neurological Sciences 47: 153

Thornell L-E, Carlsson E, Kugelberg E, Grove B K 1987 Myofibrillar M-band structure and composition of physiologically defined rat motor units. American Journal of Physiology 253: C456

Tidball J G 1987 Alpha-actinin is absent from the terminal segments of myofibrils and from subsarcolemmal densities in frog skeletal muscle. Experimental Cell Research 170: 469

Tidball J G, Law D J 1991 Dystrophin is required for normal thin filament-membrane associations at myotendinous junctions. American Journal of Pathology 138: 17

Tokuyasu K T, Dutton A H, Singer S J 1983 Immunoelectromicroscopic studies of desmin (skeletin) localization and intermediate filament organization in chicken skeletal muscle. Journal of Cell Biology 96: 1727

Tokuyasu K T, Maher P A, Singer S J 1985 Distributions of vimentin and desmin in developing chick myotubes in vivo. II. Immunoelectronmicroscopic study. Journal of Cell Biology 100: 1157

Tregear R T, Marston S B 1979 The crossbridge theory. Annual Reviews of Physiology 41: 723

Trinick J, Elliott A 1979 Electron microscopic studies of thick filaments from vertebrate skeletal muscle. Journal of Molecular Biology 131: 133

Trombitas K, Baasten P H, Kellermayer M S, Pollack G H 1991 Nature and origin of gap filaments in striated muscle. Journal of Cell Science 100: 809

Trotter J A, Baca J M 1987 A stereological comparison of the muscle-tendon junction of fast and slow fibers in the chicken. Anatomical Record 218: 256

Trotter J A, Corbett K, Avner B P 1981 Structure and function of the murine muscle–tendon junction. Anatomical Record 201: 293

Trotter J A, Eberhard S, Samora A 1983 Structural connections of the muscle–tendon junction. Cell Motility 3: 431

Ullrick W C 1967 A theory of contraction for striated muscle. Journal of Theoretical Biology 15: 53

Ullrick W C, Toselli P A, Saide J D, Phear W P C 1977 Fine structure of the vertebrate Z-disc. Journal of Molecular Biology 115: 61

Van Buren J M, Frank K 1965 Correlation between the morphology and potential field of a spinal motor nucleus in the cat. Electroencephalography and Clinical Neurophysiology 19: 112

Vergara J, Tsien R Y, Delay M 1985 Inositol 1,4,5-triphosphate: a possible chemical link in excitation contraction coupling in muscle. Proceedings of the National Academy of Science USA 82: 6352

Viragh S Z, Challice C E 1969 Variation in filamentous and fibrillar organization and associated sarcolemmal structures in cells of the normal mammalian heart. Journal of Ultrastructure Research 28: 321

Vracko R, Benditt E P 1972 Basal lamina: the scaffold for

orderly cell replacement. Observations on regeneration of injured skeletal muscle fibres and capillaries. Journal of Cell Biology 55: 406

Wagenknecht T, Gassucci R, Frank J, DeSaito A, Inui M, Fleischer S 1989 Three-dimensional architecture of the calcium channel/foot structure of sarcoplasmic reticulum. Nature 338: 167

Wakayama Y, Schotland D L 1979 Muscle satellite cell populations in Duchenne dystrophy. In: Mauro A (ed) Muscle regeneration. Raven Press, New York, pp 121–130

Wakayama Y, Okayasu H, Shibuya A, Kumagai T 1985 Duchenne dystrophy: reduced density of orthogonal array subunit particles in muscle plasma membrane. Neurology 34: 1313

Waku K 1977 Skeletal muscle. In: Snyder F (ed) Lipid metabolism in mammals. Plenum, New York, p 189

Walker S M, Schrodt G R 1968 Triads in skeletal muscle fibers of 19-day fetal rats. Journal of Cell Biology 37: 564

Walker S M, Schrodt G R, Currier F J, Turner E V 1975 Relationship of the sarcoplasmic reticulum to fibril and triadic junction development in skeletal muscle fibers of fetal monkeys and humans. Journal of Morphology 146: 97

Wallimann T, Pelloni G, Turner D C, Eppenberger H M 1979 Removal of the M-line by treatment with Fab' fragments of antibodies against MM creatine kinase. In: Pepe F A, Sanger J W, Nachmias V T (eds) Motility in cell function. Academic Press, New York, pp 415–417

Wang K 1982 Myofilamentous and myofibrillar connections: role of titin, nebulin and intermediate filaments. In: Pearson M L, Epstein H F (eds) Muscle development. Cold Spring Harbor Laboratory, pp 439–452

Wang S M, Sun M C, Jeng C J 1991a Location of the C-terminus of titin at the Z-line region in the sarcomere. Biochemical and Biophysical Research Communications 176: 189

Wang K, McCarter R, Wright J, Beverly J, Ramirez-Mitchell R 1991b Regulation of skeletal muscle stiffness and elasticity by titin isoforms: a test of the segmental extension model of resting tension. Proceedings of the National Academy of Sciences of the USA 88: 7101

Williams P E, Goldspink G 1971 Longitudinal growth of striated muscle fibres. Journal of Cell Science 9: 751

Williams P E, Goldspink G 1973 The effect of immobilization on the longitudinal growth of striated muscle fibres. Journal of Anatomy 116: 45

Wray S H 1969 Innervation ratios for large and small limb muscles in the baboon. Journal of Comparative Neurology 137: 227

Yasin R, Van Beers G, Nurse K C E, Al-Ani S, Landon D N, Thompson E J 1977 A quantitative technique for growing human skeletal muscle in culture starting from mononucleated cells. Journal of the Neurological Sciences 32: 347

Yoshioka M, Okuda R 1977 Human skeletal muscle fibers in normal and pathological states; freeze-etch replica observations. Journal of Electron Microscopy (Tokyo) 26: 103

Yu L C, Lymn R W, Podolsky R J 1977 Characterization of a non-indexible equatorial X-ray reflection from frog sartorius muscle. Journal of Molecular Biology 115: 455

Yurchenco P D, Ruben G C 1987 Basement membrane structure in situ: evidence for lateral associations in the type IV collagen network. Journal of Cell Biology 105: 2559

Zelena J 1965 Development of acetylcholinesterose activity at muscle junctions. Nature 205: 295

Zorzato F, Fujii J, Otsu K et al 1990 Molecular cloning of cDNA encoding human and rabbit forms of the Ca^{2+} release channel (ryanodine receptor) of skeletal muscle sarcoplasmic reticulum. Journal of Biological Chemistry 265: 2244

5. Neuromuscular transmission

D. Wray

INTRODUCTION

Many of the processes involved in neuromuscular transmission are well understood (for a recent textbook review see Vincent & Wray 1992). When the motor nerve is stimulated, an action potential travels along the nerve as far as the nerve terminal where the transmitter, acetylcholine (ACh), is released. ACh then travels across the synaptic cleft to the postsynaptic membrane causing a local depolarisation in the muscle fibre. This in turn triggers a propagated action potential in the muscle fibre, leading to muscle contraction. ACh is meanwhile hydrolysed to choline by the enzyme acetylcholinesterase (EC 3.1.1.7). Choline is taken up by nerve terminals and used to resynthesise ACh via the enzyme choline acetyltransferase (EC 2.3.1.6) (MacIntosh & Collier 1976).

Concerning the release process, depolarisation associated with the nerve terminal action potential causes voltage-dependent calcium channels in the nerve membrane to open briefly. This allows calcium ions to enter nerve terminals, leading to ACh release in distinct multimolecular packets (for review see Baker 1977, Ginsborg & Jenkinson, 1976).

ACh released by nerve stimulation combines with specific acetylcholine receptors on the postsynaptic membrane. This causes end-plate channels to open transiently, leading to a large brief ionic current via the channels and consequent depolarisation in the muscle fibre (for reviews see e.g. Wray 1980, Hille 1992). The ACh receptor (AChR) and its associated channel is a protein the amino acid sequence of which has been determined (e.g. Noda et al 1983b).

Nerve endings are found in surface depressions

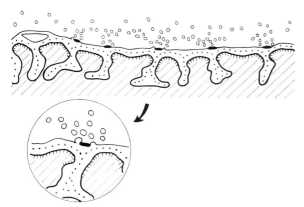

Fig. 5.1 Schematic diagram of frog neuromuscular junction (Porter & Barnard 1975) traced from micrographs by Couteaux & Pecot-Dechavassine (1968). Vesicles can be seen in the nerve terminal aligned in stacks near the thickenings (dense bars) in the presynaptic membrane (Birks et al 1960a,b, Heuser et al 1974). The striations on the postsynaptic membrane represent its 'thickened' zone, rich in AChRs. Dotted lines show the acetylcholinesterase present throughout the cleft. The inset shows fusion of vesicles with the presynaptic membrane at either side of the presynaptic thickening. After being released from the nerve terminal, ACh binds first to receptors located conveniently at the crests of the folds, and then probably diffuses into the fold depths where it is hydrolysed.

of the muscle membrane (synaptic 'gutters' or 'troughs'). The nerve terminal is separated by a gap of around 50 nm from the postsynaptic membrane which is highly folded (Fig. 5.1). Specific histochemical staining (reviewed by e.g. Bowden & Duchen 1976) has shown that the acetylcholinesterase enzyme is present throughout the cleft, including the folds. This location of the enzyme was confirmed by autoradiographic studies using radiolabelled disopropylfluorophosphate, DFP (see e.g. Barnard 1974).

The aim of this chapter is to provide an up-to-date summary of present understanding of neuromuscular transmission, without trying to replace accounts in standard textbooks or more detailed technical reviews. The above mechanisms will be discussed, especially where relevant to known neuromuscular disorders.

PRESYNAPTIC EVENTS

Active zones

Thickenings of the nerve terminal membrane usually occur opposite the mouths of the post-synaptic folds. Membrane-bound vesicles (around 50 nm in diameter) are aligned in stacks around these thickenings (Fig. 5.1). Vesicles appear to touch or fuse with the axolemma on either side of the thickenings. These observations led to the suggestion that ACh is released at such areas: 'active zones' (e.g. Heuser, 1976). The active zone membrane, when examined by freeze-fracture electron microscopy, consists of particles (each of width around 11 nm) arranged in parallel double rows (Fig. 5.2). For frog neuromuscular junctions, which have elongated nerve terminals, rows of active zone particles are located at right angles to the longitudinal axis of the terminal, opposite the sites of the postsynaptic folds (e.g. Heuser et al 1974). For mammalian muscles, which have less elongated nerve terminals, active zones continue to follow the sites of postsynaptic

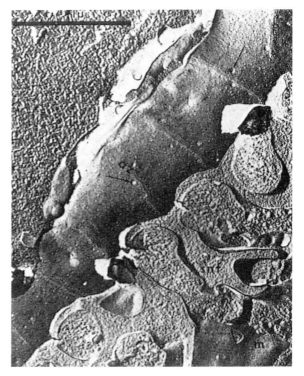

Fig. 5.2 Freeze-fracture view of a frog nerve terminal membrane fixed during nerve stimulation (Heuser et al 1974). Parallel rows of particles are seen at active zones. Circular dimples beside the active zones probably represent vesicles fusing with membrane, presumably to discharge ACh by exocytosis.

folds, but they are shorter and less regularly spaced (e.g. Fukunaga et al 1982, 1983).

Since ACh release appears to occur close to the active zone particles (circular dimples in Fig. 5.2), it has been suggested that these membrane-spanning particles are the voltage-dependent calcium channels which open when the nerve terminal is depolarised (Heuser et al 1974, Pumplin et al 1981).

End-plate potentials and miniature end-plate potentials

Much useful insight into neuromuscular transmission has been gained by recording voltages intracellularly with fine-tipped glass microelectrodes inserted into single muscle cells. Many of the classic papers are collected in the source book by Cooke & Lipkin (1972). The potential difference between inside and outside the muscle cell ('membrane potential') is usually about –70 mV in resting muscle. In unstimulated muscle fibres, if the microelectrode is placed in an end-plate region, small potential changes are observed (Fatt & Katz, 1952) — the miniature end-plate potential (mepp) (Fig. 5.3A). These mepps occur spontaneously and at random (around one per second), each mepp having a small amplitude (0.5–1 mV), which is insufficient to trigger action potentials in muscle fibres. The mepp comes about by the release of a single multimolecular packet of ACh from the nerve terminal. The ACh then acts postsynaptically to produce the observed electrical changes in the muscle fibre.

When the nerve is stimulated, many such packets of ACh are released almost simultaneously from the nerve terminal (Katz 1966). The depolarisation produced in the muscle fibre at the end-plate by this ACh is known as the end-plate potential (epp) (Fig. 5.3B). The number of packets released for each single nerve stimulus is usually called the quantal content, *m*. As *each* packet produces a response of magnitude corresponding to the mepp amplitude, the epp amplitude is, therefore, the quantal content times the mepp amplitude. Thus if the mepp and epp amplitudes are measured, the quantal content can be found (for corrections to this method of calculation, and for other methods of obtaining quantal

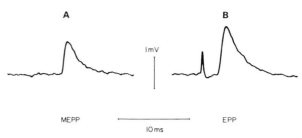

Fig. 5.3 Intracellular recordings using microelectrodes at end-plate regions of mouse diaphragm muscle (23°C) (Peers & Wray, unpublished data). **A** Spontaneously occurring miniature end-plate potential (MEPP) **B** End-plate potential (EPP) evoked by nerve stimulation. The narrow spike preceding the epp is caused by the brief pulse used to stimulate the nerve. The epp is normally much larger in amplitude then the mepp, and so the epp would normally trigger an action potential in the muscle fibre causing muscle contraction and the expulsion of the microelectrode. Therefore, in B, the epp has been reduced in amplitude by tubocurarine so that it is below threshold for stimulating an action potential.

content, see e.g. Martin 1966). Quantal content for human muscle is around 60 (Lambert & Elmqvist 1971).

Detailed statistical analysis has shown that the *single* packet of ACh released spontaneously to produce a mepp contains on average the same number of ACh molecules as are found in *each* of the packets released almost simultaneously by nerve stimulation to form an epp (del Castillo & Katz 1954a, Martin 1966).

A mepp and an epp differ in the number of packets of ACh involved, but otherwise have many features in common. Thus both mepps and epps follow a similar time-course (Fig. 5.3) and both respond similarly to drugs such as neostigmine and tubocurarine (Fatt & Katz 1952).

The number of ACh molecules released in a single packet is remarkably constant and unaffected by most drugs, by changes in ionic environment or by osmotic changes. The *amplitude* of the mepp is determined mainly by the number of ACh molecules in a packet and by the postsynaptic action of the ACh. As the former is relatively constant, the mepp amplitude is largely determined by the postsynaptic action of ACh, which can be readily varied by postsynaptically acting drugs such as tubocurarine. On the other hand, the *frequency* of random release of packets of ACh can be easily and markedly affected by factors which change the presynaptic conditions.

So, for instance, mepp frequency is increased by a rise in the osmolarity of the bathing solution (for further discussion see Ginsborg & Jenkinson 1976).

Calcium ion influx

In solutions containing low Ca^{2+} concentrations, epp amplitudes are reduced. Analysis of such epps to find the number of packets released per nerve stimulus (i.e. the quantal content) shows that epp amplitudes are reduced because the quantal content is reduced (del Castillo & Katz 1954a). In other words, Ca^{2+} ions act presynaptically to affect the number of packets of ACh released.

Provided Ca^{2+} ions are present in the bathing solution, depolarisation of nerve terminals, *however caused*, is effective in inducing Ca^{2+} entry and release of ACh. So, for instance, increasing the K^+ ion concentration of the bathing solution will depolarise cells. This depolarisation at the nerve terminal leads to an increase in release of packets of ACh which can be recorded as an increase in mepp frequency (Liley 1956). Alternatively, nerve terminals can be depolarised by passing current pulses from a nearby extracellular electrode and this again leads to ACh release (Liley 1956). Sodium ions themselves are not responsible for release, since ACh is also released using such current pulses in the absence of sodium ions (Katz & Miledi 1969a).

For ACh release to occur, Ca^{2+} ions must be present externally during nerve terminal depolarisation. Thus nerve stimulation in Ca^{2+}-free solution completely abolishes ACh release. In such Ca^{2+}-free solutions, short pulses of Ca^{2+} ions can be applied externally via a microelectrode at different times in relation to the time of a depolarising pulse. In this way it was shown that ACh release occurs only when Ca^{2+} ions are present externally during the period of the depolarisation and for a very short time afterwards (Katz & Miledi 1967a). During the period of depolarisation, the nerve terminal membrane becomes transiently more permeable to Ca^{2+} ions, allowing Ca^{2+} entry into the nerve terminal. Intracellular free Ca^{2+} concentration is normally very low (around 0.1 μM) (Baker 1977), while the physiological concentration of extracellular *free* Ca^{2+} is around 2 mM.

Intracellular presynaptic recordings cannot be made at the small terminals of the skeletal neuromuscular junction. However, Ca^{2+} currents can be studied extracellularly (from under the perineural sheath), especially when K^+ currents are eliminated by suitable drugs (Penner & Dreyer 1986). Regenerative Ca^{2+} action potentials can be produced in skeletal muscle nerve terminals, particularly when solutions containing high Ca^{2+} concentrations are used (Katz & Miledi 1969a). The squid giant synapse has large presynaptic terminals and this allows the direct intracellular presynaptic recording of such Ca^{2+} action potentials (Katz & Miledi 1969b). It has to be emphasised that Ca^{2+} action potentials do not occur under normal physiological conditions.

It might be expected that, as the Ca^{2+} ion is positively charged, making the inside of the nerve terminal very positive would electrostatically repel Ca^{2+} entry. This is in fact found to be the case: very large experimentally induced presynaptic depolarisations in the squid giant synapse (about 200 mV) prevent Ca^{2+} entry, even though the depolarisation itself has made the presynaptic membrane permeable to Ca^{2+} ions (Katz & Miledi 1967b, Llinas et al 1981). Similar results are found at frog (Katz & Miledi 1977a, Dudel 1983) and crayfish (Dudel et al 1983) neuromuscular junctions. These experiments shed light on the process of Ca^{2+} ion entry. However, presynaptic depolarisation under *normal* physiological conditions at nerve terminals is not large enough to cause electrostatic repulsion of Ca^{2+} ions.

Direct recording of Ca^{2+} currents is possible at the squid giant synapse (Llinas et al 1976, 1981, Augustine et al 1985b). From such recordings it was shown that the Ca^{2+} permeability rises at the beginning of a depolarising pulse, and falls back to normal after the pulse. These Ca^{2+} permeability changes do not take place instantaneously, but rather have time constants of the order of milliseconds.

Furthermore, increase in Ca^{2+} concentration inside presynaptic terminals during nerve depolarisation has been detected for the squid giant synapse. For this, compounds sensitive to Ca^{2+} ions (aequorin or arsenazo III) were injected into nerve terminals. Aequorin emits light in the presence of Ca^{2+} ions (Llinas et al 1972, Llinas &

Nicholson 1975), while Ca^{2+} ions also affect light transmission through preparations containing arsenazo III (Miledi & Parker 1981, Charlton et al 1982, Augustine et al 1985a).

Current through *individual* Ca^{2+} channels has not been observed electrophysiologically at the small presynaptic terminals of the skeletal neuromuscular junction. However, currents produced by single voltage-dependent Ca^{2+} channels have now been observed in other neurones and in heart muscle membranes using the 'patch-clamp' technique (see below) (e.g. Tsien 1983, Reuter 1983, Reuter et al 1985). In heart muscle, for instance, each Ca^{2+} channel opens for about 1 ms. The frequency of Ca^{2+} channel opening increases when the membrane is suddenly depolarised, leading to an increase in overall Ca^{2+} current.

Studies on a wide range of tissues (e.g. heart, smooth muscle and neurones) indicate that there appear to be several types of voltage-dependent Ca^{2+} channels (e.g. Nilius et al 1985, Nowycky et al 1985, Penner & Dreyer 1986, Llinas et al 1992, Spedding & Paoletti 1992). These have been classified as e.g. 'N', 'L', 'T' and 'P' type channels on the basis of their electrophysiological (activation and inactivation) characteristics and pharmacological properties. Furthermore, biochemical investigations have led to the isolation of Ca^{2+} channels from, for example, skeletal muscle transverse tubules (Borsotto et al 1984, Curtis & Catterall 1984, Catterall 1991) and the subunit structure is known (α_1, α_2, δ, β and γ subunits). The α_1 subunit forms the channel pore; all the subunits have been cloned and the amino acid sequence determined (Catterall 1991).

However, none of these detailed characterisations have yet been carried out on nerve terminal calcium channels at the mature skeletal neuromuscular junction; the types of calcium channel present at the motor nerve terminal are still unclear. This channel would not be identified as L type because the characteristic blocker of this channel type (the dihydropyridines) has little or no effect (Burges & Wray 1989). Furthermore, ω-conotoxin (a blocker of N-type channels) has no effect on the mammalian (mouse) motor nerve terminal (Sano et al 1987), suggesting that this channel is not N type either. However, there may be some degree of resemblance to L- or N-type channels since antibodies can cross-react between motor nerve calcium channels and L-, N-type channels (see discussion of Lambert–Eaton myasthenic syndrome below). Furthermore, ω-conotoxin blocks motor nerve terminal calcium channels at frog nerve terminals (Sano et al 1987). A comparison of potencies of various divalent ions also suggests some resemblance with L and N (but not T type) channels (Wray & Porter 1993). The nerve terminal calcium channel may in fact be closer to a P-type channel since funnel web spider toxin (a characteristic P-type blocker) interferes with transmitter release (Uchitel et al 1992).

Acetylcholine release

Intracellular action of calcium ions. The fact that Ca^{2+} ions cause release of transmitter has been shown directly for the squid giant synapse. A pulse of Ca^{2+} ions injected via a microelectrode into the nerve terminal of the synapse causes transmitter release (Miledi 1973, Miledi & Parker 1981, Charlton et al 1982).

Following a brief depolarisation of motor nerve terminals, there is a time interval ('synaptic delay') of at least 0.5 ms (20°C) before the epp appears (Katz & Miledi 1965). This delay does not arise because of the time taken for the ACh to diffuse across the synaptic cleft to the postsynaptic membrane, nor because of the time taken for the ACh to act on the postsynaptic membrane (see 'End-plate response', below). Thus the synaptic delay occurs presynaptically by a delay in the release of ACh following the brief depolarisation of the nerve terminal.

This presynaptic delay is made up from two steps, at least in the squid giant synapse. Firstly, following presynaptic depolarisation, there is a delay before Ca^{2+} channels open and Ca^{2+} current starts to flow into the nerve. Secondly, once Ca^{2+} current has started to flow, there is a further delay (approximately 0.2 ms) before transmitter is released (Llinas et al 1981). During the latter very short delay, Ca^{2+} ions which enter the nerve terminal via Ca^{2+} channels must travel to an intracellular binding site and then cause release. Therefore the Ca^{2+} channels (active zone particles) must be situated very near to intracellular

Ca^{2+} binding sites and to release sites (see 'Active zones' above).

The number of packets of ACh released by nerve stimulation increases steeply and non-linearly ($\alpha[Ca]^n$, $n=3$ to 4) with increasing extra-cellular calcium concentration, [Ca] (Fig. 5.4), before eventually reaching a plateau (see e.g. Cull-Candy et al 1980, Lang et al 1987a). The entry of Ca^{2+} into the nerve terminal during the epp is proportional to the extracellular Ca^{2+} concentration (see e.g. Silinsky, 1985): a graph of ACh release against intracellular Ca^{2+} concentration during the epp might therefore also be expected to have a similar shape to that of Figure 5.4. The non-linear release curve has been interpreted to imply 'co-operation' between 3 or 4 Ca^{2+} ions to cause release (Dodge & Rahamimoff 1967), and such co-operation probably occurs intracellularly.

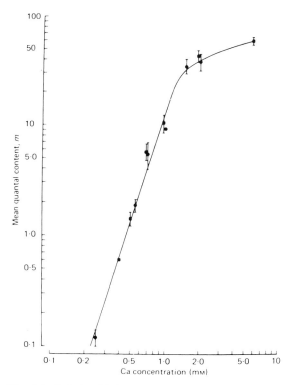

Fig. 5.4 Relationship between nerve-evoked release of ACh (quantal content) and extracellular Ca^{2+} concentration in normal human intercostal muscle ($24°C$). The initial part of the curve is steep and non-linear (release proportional to $[Ca]^{3.3}$) with increasing calcium concentration, [Ca], and only appears linear in this figure because logarithmic scales have been used for the axes (after Cull-Candy et al 1980).

When the release versus Ca^{2+} concentration curve (Fig. 5.4) reaches an eventual plateau, this probably comes about by saturation of the intra-cellular action of Ca^{2+}, not by a saturation of Ca^{2+} entry via the channels (Silinsky 1985, Lang et al 1987a).

The curve of electrically stimulated ACh release versus Ca^{2+} concentration is shifted to the right by Mg^{2+} ions (Jenkinson 1957, Silinsky 1985, Lang et al 1987a). Mg^{2+} ions act as a competitive antagonist to Ca^{2+} ions in causing release of ACh following electrical stimulation. The site of competition is probably at the external surface of the Ca^{2+} channel, because if Mg^{2+} is delivered intracellularly, it does not inhibit release (Kharasch et al 1981). In addition, large ($2-3$ mM) concentrations of ionised Mg^{2+} are normally found intracellularly (Baker 1972), and this would probably have produced a block of release if the Mg^{2+} ions had acted inside the nerve terminal. However, under conditions where release is triggered by high potassium solutions, Mg^{2+} ions act by a non-competitive mechanism (Pearson & Wray 1993).

Although Ca^{2+} is necessary for initiating trans-mitter release, the actual level of release may also be independently modulated by the potential of the presynaptic membrane (Llinas et al 1981, Dudel 1983, Dudel et al 1983). It appears that entry of a fixed amount of Ca^{2+} ions might become more effective in producing transmitter release as the nerve terminal is depolarised, although the effect may be small (Augustine et al 1985b). Potential-sensitive proteins in the membrane may be involved. Further evidence for potential-dependent effects comes from studies of the time-course of release. After a nerve impulse, packets of ACh are not released simultaneously, but are distributed in time (Fig. 5.5) after a minimum delay. It appears that the minimum delay is also controlled directly by the potential of the presynaptic membrane (Datyner & Gage 1980, Dudel, 1984a, 1984b).

For unstimulated spontaneous release (mepps), it is likely that intracellular free Ca^{2+} is also involved in causing release of packets of ACh (e.g. Hubbard 1973). Under resting conditions, where voltage-dependent Ca^{2+} channels in the membrane are not open, the mepp frequency is not very dependent on extracellular Ca^{2+} concentra-

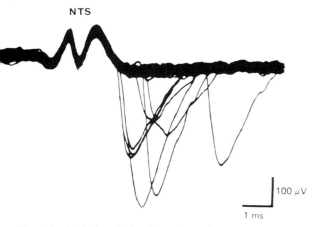

NTS

100 μV

1 ms

Fig. 5.5 Variations in the delay when release occurs following nerve stimulation. Responses were detected by an extracellular microelectrode placed very near to the end-plate in a mouse diaphragm muscle. Recordings were made in solutions containing high Mg^{2+} and low Ca^{2+} concentrations to reduce release. Usually, stimulation of the nerve under these conditions gave either a failure to release ACh, or the release of one packet of ACh. The release of a single packet of ACh occurs with a variable delay and this has been shown by superimposing the results of many nerve stimuli. Downward deflections = end-plate responses, NTS = nerve terminal action potential (Datyner & Gage 1980).

tion. Since intracellular Ca^{2+} concentration is low, the resting frequency of release is also low. Intracellular free Ca^{2+} can be increased by agents causing the release of Ca^{2+} from bound intracellular stores, such as mitochondria. Poisoning the mitochondria with agents such as ruthenium red, 2-4-dinitrophenol or hypoxia causes the release of free Ca^{2+} and, as expected, a marked increase in mepp frequency (Alnaes & Rahamimoff 1975, Lande 1987).

Vesicular release. The vesicles found in nerve terminals (see 'Active zones' above and Fig. 5.1) contain ACh and are roughly constant in size. Electrophysiological recordings have shown that ACh is released in 'packets' (see 'End-plate potentials and miniature end-plate potentials'), each apparently of a fairly constant number of ACh molecules, leading to constant mepp amplitudes. It was natural to suggest that a 'packet' of ACh is released when a vesicle fuses with the cytoplasmic membrane, rapidly discharging its contents by exocytosis (del Castillo & Katz 1955, Hubbard & Kwanbunbumpen 1968, Katz 1978). Constancy of the amount of ACh released in a packet would

arise because of constancy of size of the vesicles. Convincing evidence for exocytosis is available from electron microscopy of freeze-fractured membranes. The presynaptic membrane becomes marked with circular dimples if terminals are fixed while packets of ACh are being secreted (Heuser et al 1974) (Fig. 5.2). The dimples usually occur alongside the rows of particles forming the active zones, and may be caused by the exocytosis of vesicles of ACh. Further support for the vesicular release theory (see e.g. Ceccarelli & Hurlbut 1980) comes from studies using black widow spider venom and lanthanum ions. Both these agents cause a large release of ACh followed by virtually complete depletion of vesicles, at which point secretion of ACh is almost completely abolished.

Approximately 10^4 ACh molecules are *released* into the synaptic cleft during the action of a single 'packet' of transmitter at the skeletal neuromuscular junction (Fletcher & Forrester 1975, Kuffler & Yoshikami 1975, Miledi et al 1983). Synaptic vesicles probably *contain* around this number of ACh molecules (e.g. Miledi et al 1980, 1982), suggesting that the whole content of a vesicle is released as a packet.

Vesicles are filled with ACh in an energy-dependent way as follows. It appears that there is an ATPase in the vesicle membrane which acts to pump H^+ ions into the vesicle; ACh is then transported into the vesicle in exchange for H^+ ions by a separate exchange mechanism (Marshall & Parsons 1987).

The processes linking calcium influx to vesicle mobilisation and vesicle fusion with the presynaptic membrane followed by exocytosis are not well understood. However, recently there has been much progress in the study of proteins associated with the synaptic vesicle membranes (for review see Südhof & Jahn 1991). For many of these proteins, the amino acid sequence is known and there are reasonable indications as to their function. For instance, synapsin 1 links synaptic vesicles to cytoskeletal elements such as actin or microtubules, and these vesicles may act as a reservoir which is not immediately available for release (Südhof & Jahn 1991). Phosphorylation of synapsin 1 by Ca/calmodulin-dependent kinase seems to detach the synaptic vesicles from the cytoskeleton (Benfenati et al 1989). Calcium influx could therefore trigger the mobilisation of some of this reservoir, vesicles could become free to move to the presynaptic membrane and so become available for release following subsequent nerve stimulation (Hirokawa et al 1989).

Synaptic vesicles need to be docked to pre-existing sites on the presynaptic membrane before they can undergo exocytosis in response to a nerve stimulus. This docking may occur by another synaptic vesicle protein: synaptotagmin (Südhof & Jahn 1991). It is a transmembrane protein in vesicles and could readily link the vesicles to the presynaptic membrane because of its affinity for acidic phospholipids. It has an internally repeated sequence homologous to the regulatory region of protein kinase C (Perin et al 1991, Südhof & Jahn 1991); this sequence may bind calcium which in turn could trigger exocytosis. Further support for this comes from the close association of synapto-tagmin with calcium channels located close to active zones where release is known to occur. It also binds to (and may therefore dock with) the α-latrotoxin receptor (located on the nerve membrane) (Petrenko et al 1991), stimulation of which by black widow venom leads to vesicle exocy-tosis and transmitter release. The precise docking of vesicles at the active zones may also be guided by small GTP-binding proteins (G proteins) (Mizoguchi et al 1992).

Once the vesicles have been docked at active zones, another important synaptic vesicle trans-membrane protein, synaptophysin, seems to come into play (Südhof & Jahn 1991). This protein has been shown to be necessary for transmitter release (Alder et al 1992), and it may participate in the formation of a fusion pore which has been shown to form during synaptic vesicle exocytosis (Breckenridge & Almers 1987). Indeed it is known to form channels in artificial lipid bilayer membranes.

Although much is now known about vesicular release it is worth mentioning that the theory of vesicular release continues to be under attack by some workers. An alternative theory suggests that ACh is released directly from the cytoplasm via some membrane gate (Tauc 1982, Tauc & Poulain 1991). It is known that free ACh is found in the cytoplasm, where it is synthesised from choline using the enzyme choline acetyltransferase (MacIntosh & Collier 1976). However, it is probably fair to say that vesicular exocytosis is now widely regarded as the established mecha-nism.

Facilitation and depression

Transmitter release depends on the frequency of nerve stimulation (see e.g. del Castillo & Katz 1954b, Ginsborg & Jenkinson 1976, Silinsky 1985). In normal Ca^{2+} solutions (where many packets of ACh are released per nerve impulse), if the nerve is repetitively stimulated, successive epps generally decline in amplitude (in the presence of tubocurarine, Fig. 5.6, top trace). This 'depression' comes about because succes-sively fewer packets of ACh are released per nerve impulse. On the other hand, under conditions

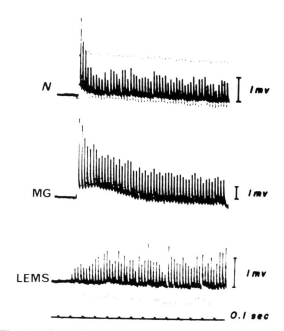

Fig. 5.6 Intracellular recordings of epps evoked by 40 Hz nerve stimulation for human intercostal muscle in vitro. N = normal muscle with tubocurarine (2 μg/ml) in the bath, MG = myasthenia gravis patient, no tubocurarine, LEMS = Lambert–Eaton myasthenic syndrome patient with tubocurarine (0.2 μg/ml). Approximate equality of epp amplitudes in this figure comes about because a relatively high concentration of tubocurarine was used in normals (N) for which transmission was not already clinically impaired (Lambert & Elmqvist 1971).

where only a small number of packets of ACh are released (for instance in low Ca^{2+} solutions or in the Lambert–Eaton myasthenic syndrome, see below), successive epps generally increase in size during a train of nerve stimuli ('facilitation') (Fig. 5.6, lower trace). Again, the mechanism is a presynaptic effect; there is a progressive increase in the number of packets of ACh released.

During both facilitation and depression, the amount of Ca^{2+} ion entry into the nerve terminal *per nerve impulse* does not change — at least in the squid giant synapse where such Ca^{2+} currents can be measured (Miledi & Parker 1981, Charlton et al 1982). Similarly, intracellular Ca^{2+} concentration (as detected by Ca^{2+}-sensitive dyes) increases by the same amount each time the nerve is stimulated in the train. There is an increase in intracellular Ca^{2+} concentration lasting for several seconds even after a single nerve stimulation. Since ACh release is a highly non-linear function of intracellular Ca^{2+} concentration (see above), a fixed increase in intracellular Ca^{2+} concentration produced by a nerve impulse would be more effective in releasing ACh when added to residual intracellular Ca^{2+} from an earlier nerve impulse (Katz & Miledi 1968, Rahamimoff 1968). Therefore, summation of intracellular Ca^{2+} levels in the nerve terminal during a train may produce facilitation.

Facilitation is short-lasting: the interval between successive nerve stimuli must be less than a few milliseconds for the effect to be seen. Facilitation occurs after a single stimulus as well as immediately following a high-frequency train of nerve stimuli. Two further stimulus-induced processes are seen after such a high-frequency train (though not after a single stimulus): these are termed augmentation and potentiation. Both are again characterised by increases in transmitter release, and are most easily differentiated on the basis of their time-course of decay. Augmentation typically lasts approx. 10 s while potentiation lasts for several minutes after the train of stimuli. (Hubbard 1963, Magleby, 1973a,b, Magleby & Zengel 1975a,b, Zucker 1989, Bain & Quastel 1992, Tanabe & Kijima 1992). As well as the increase in epp amplitudes, the resting frequency of mepps is also increased during these periods following high-frequency nerve stimulation

(Miledi & Thies 1971, Lev-Tov & Rahamimoff 1980, Zengel & Magleby 1981).

The mechanisms underlying augmentation and potentiation are not well understood, in contrast to the residual calcium theory for facilitation (see above). In contrast to facilitation, calcium entry via channels during high-frequency nerve stimulation is not necessary: potentiation still occurs after nerve stimulation in calcium-free solutions (Misler & Hurlbut 1983). Longer-term changes may be induced in the terminal (perhaps by intraterminal release of calcium or consequent upon increases in intracellular sodium), affecting proteins concerned with secretion (Magleby & Zengel 1976a,b,c, 1982, Silinsky 1985).

For normal Ca^{2+} concentrations where quantal release is high, during high-frequency nerve stimulation, there is probably a depletion of ACh available for release (e.g. Martin 1966, Ginsborg & Jenkinson 1976). Therefore ACh release decreases throughout the train (even though there is an underlying increase in intracellular residual Ca^{2+}) and depression of epp amplitude is seen. When quantal content is low, ACh depletion does not occur and then facilitation can be observed as described above.

Presynaptic receptors

Electrophysiologists usually record epps either in low Ca^{2+} solutions without tubocurarine or in normal solutions with tubocurarine to prevent triggering of action potentials which would expel the electrode. It now seems clear that although the phenomenon of ACh depletion can lead to depression, tubocurarine itself can also produce depression (Bowman 1980, Magleby et al 1981, Gibb & Marshall 1984). The drug does this by acting presynaptically, causing a reduction in quantal release during the high-frequency nerve stimulation. It seems likely that this effect is mediated via a block of presynaptic nicotinic receptors. These receptors can be stimulated by ACh itself (i.e. positive feedback) to cause mobilisation of the ACh store and hence maintain release without waning, especially at high stimulation rates (Bowman et al 1988). This situation is, however, complicated by the presence of presynaptic muscarinic receptors which may have an inhibitory role (see Bowman et al 1990 for a more detailed review).

Another way of studying neuromuscular transmission is by the use of μ-conotoxin instead of tubocurarine to paralyse the muscle and so prevent expulsion of the microelectrode. This toxin acts by preferentially blocking muscle (rather than nerve) sodium channels, so allowing the nerve to be stimulated while still preventing muscle contraction. Indeed, high-frequency trains of epps do not show depression in the presence of this toxin rather than tubocurarine (Hong & Chang 1989). An added bonus to the use of this toxin is that both mepps and epps can be simultaneously recorded.

Lambert–Eaton myasthenic syndrome

The Lambert–Eaton myasthenic syndrome (LEMS) is a presynaptic disorder of the neuromuscular junction characterised by muscle weakness (for a review see Wray 1992). In biopsied muscle from LEMS patients, there is a reduced release of ACh following a single nerve stimulation: the quantal content of the epp is reduced to a few packets (Lambert & Elmqvist 1971, Cull-Candy et al 1980). This can lead to failure to trigger muscle action potentials; hence muscle twitch tension is reduced. High-frequency nerve stimulation leads to a progressive increase in ACh release; this is the phenomenon of facilitation associated with a low initial quantal content (Fig. 5.6, see above). Along with the progressive increase in epp amplitudes at high-frequency nerve stimulation, action potentials can be triggered progressively in more muscle fibres and so muscle tension increases during the high-frequency train. As a result, the patient's strength improves during continuous exercise.

The disorder is due to the presence of autoantibodies against nerve terminal calcium channels. To show the autoimmune nature of the syndrome, the IgG fraction was taken from plasma of LEMS patients and injected daily into mice (Lang et al 1981, 1983, Prior et al 1985). The epps produced in these mice were then measured and the quantal content determined. It was found that such injections of LEMS IgG caused a reduction in quantal content in the mice. Furthermore, measurements

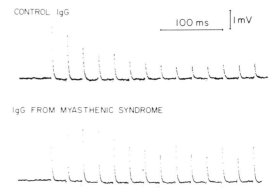

Fig. 5.7 Intracellular recordings of epps evoked by 40 Hz nerve stimulation for mouse diaphragm muscle in vitro. Upper trace = mouse injected with control IgG, lower trace = mouse injected with LEMS IgG. Tubocurarine was present in the bath at concentrations of 3.3 and 2.4 μg/ml respectively. As for Figure 5.6, approximate equality of amplitudes arises because a higher tubocurarine concentration was used for controls (Newsom-Davis et al 1982).

of high-frequency trains of epps in mice showed either facilitation or less marked depression than usual (Fig 5.7). This showed that the main electrophysiological features of the syndrome could be transferred to mice via the IgG fraction, strongly suggesting an autoimmune basis for the disorder (Lang et al 1981, 1983, 1984a, Prior et al 1985). Consistent with this, immunosuppressive therapy (using azathioprine and prednisolone) and plasma exchange (which should reduce antibody levels) have both proved effective in the treatment of LEMS patients (Newsom-Davis & Murray 1984).

As mentioned above, the site of action of the IgG antibody is the voltage-dependent Ca^{2+} channel at the motor nerve terminal. LEMS IgG probably causes the loss of function of these channels, leading to decreased Ca^{2+} entry following nerve terminal depolarisation, thereby reducing quantal ACh release. Evidence that LEMS antibody acts on calcium channels has been inferred indirectly at the neuromuscular junction (Fukunaga et al 1982, 1983, Lang et al 1984b, 1985, 1987a, Wray et al 1984, 1987) and has been shown directly by block of calcium currents in neuroblastoma, small cell carcinoma, thyroid and chromaffin cells (Roberts et al 1985, Lang et al 1987b, Kim & Neher 1988, Peers et al 1990, Kim et al 1992, 1993), though not cardiac calcium channels (Lang et al 1988). Following binding of the LEMS antibody at the active zones of the motor nerve terminal (shown by immunolocalisation studies — Engel et al 1987), loss of function occurs because these divalent antibodies cross-link calcium channels so causing their internalisation and degradation (Fukuoka et al 1987, Nagel et al 1988, Peers et al 1993). In around 60% of patients, LEMS is associated with small cell lung cancer, and the antibodies may be initially directed against calcium channels in the tumour (O'Neill et al 1988).

The presence of autoantibodies in LEMS patients now forms the basis of a diagnostic test. For this, calcium channels bound to ω-conotoxin (selective for N-type channels, see above) are solubilised from human neuroblastoma or small cell lung carcinoma cells and shown to bind LEMS antibody by immunoprecipitation (Sher et al 1989, 1990, Lennon & Lambert 1989, Leys et al 1991). The LEMS antibody seems to interact with more than one channel type. For instance, it inhibits both N- and L-type currents in a range of cells (thyroid cancer cells, chromaffin cells, small cell carcinoma cells and neuroblastoma cells (Peers et al 1990, Kim et al 1992, Hulsizer et al 1991, Blandino & Kim 1993, Viglione et al 1993)), but does not seem to inhibit T-type channels (in neuroblastoma and thyroid cells (Peers et al 1990, Kim et al 1993)). However, surprisingly, in Western blots, LEMS antibody did not seem to bind in a consistent way to any of the known subunits of the calcium channel (Chester et al 1988, Leveque et al 1992, Viglione et al 1992, but see Rosenfeld et al 1993 for possible binding to the β subunit). It has recently been suggested that LEMS antibody may also bind to synaptotagmin, a protein present in vesicular membranes (see above) and which can be tightly bound to calcium channels (Leveque et al 1992). Presumably this protein would become exposed to the surface of the nerve terminal after exocytosis and available to bind antibody.

Other sites of presynaptic drug action

Aminopyridines. The duration of the nerve terminal action potential is prolonged by 4-aminopyridine (4-AP) or 3,4-diaminopyridine (3,4-DAP) (Lundh & Thesleff 1977, Lundh et al 1977a, Meves & Pichon 1977, Molgo et al 1977, 1979, 1980, Illes & Thesleff 1978, Kenyon & Gibbons 1979, Thesleff 1980). These drugs probably act mainly by blocking voltage-operated K^+ channels involved in the action potential. The prolongation in depolarisation thereby produced at the nerve terminal allows more Ca^{2+} ions to enter the terminal than normal, leading to an increased quantal ACh release following nerve stimulation; correspondingly, the epp amplitude is greatly increased. Spontaneous quantal release (i.e. mepps) is in general not affected by 4-AP or 3,4-DAP, as action potentials are not involved in the generation of mepps. Both drugs have proved of some limited use in the treatment of LEMS (see above) (Lambert & Elmqvist 1971, Lundh et al 1977b, Murray & Newsom-Davis 1981, Murray et al 1984). However, both drugs can also act on the central nervous system to produce convulsions, but 3,4-DAP is less convulsant and is therefore preferred.

Botulinum neurotoxin. Several types of neurotoxin are produced by strains of *Clostridium botulinum* and can lead to fatal poisoning when present in foodstuffs. This class of toxins consists of a large molecular weight protein composed of a light chain (~50 kDa) and a heavy chain (~100 kDa) joined by a disulphide bond. Botulinum neurotoxin acts at nerve terminals of the skeletal neuromuscular junction to block transmitter release and hence cause paralysis (Sellin 1985). The neurotoxin produces this effect by binding to receptors (Middlebrook 1989) on the nerve terminal membrane and then travelling to the inside of the nerve terminal where it produces its action (Simpson 1980, Dolly et al 1984). The toxin does not affect Ca^{2+} entry into nerve terminals (Gundersen et al, 1982), but acts intraterminally to reduce the effect of Ca^{2+} in promoting release. Following nerve stimulation, the quantal content of the epp is therefore reduced (Harris & Miledi 1971, Cull-Candy et al 1976) so that action potentials cannot be triggered resulting in paralysis. Probably because of this reduced quantal content, facilitation of epp amplitudes occurs in high-frequency trains of epps; however this increase is not usually enough to trigger action potentials. Quantal spontaneous release (i.e.

mepps) is determined by intraterminal processes and this form of release is also reduced by the toxin: there is a marked reduction in mepp frequency (Thesleff 1982, Tse et al 1982, 1986, Kim et al 1984). Interestingly, the toxin does not totally block all the mepps, but leaves some mepps unaffected; these are rarely occurring slow rise-time mepps also found in controls at low frequency, and the only mepps observed after poisoning with the toxin (Dolly et al 1987). However, it is still not understood where precisely the toxin acts inside the nerve terminal to produce these effects. The process of vesicle exocytosis itself may be directly impaired by the toxin, leading to reduction in quantal content. Once internalised, the light chain of the toxin may mediate the toxin's action (De Paiva & Dolly 1990). The effect on vesicles seems to come about by an endopeptidase action of the toxin on a synaptic vesicle protein (synaptobrevin) (Schiavo et al 1992). Although the function of some other synaptic vesicle proteins, e.g. synaptotagmin, synaptophysin, in the release process is beginning to be understood (see above), the role of synapto-brevin in release is still unclear; however, the latter may be involved in vesicle fusion which is consequently blocked by the toxin.

Hemicholinium-3. As mentioned in the Introduction, choline is used for the resynthesis of ACh within the nerve terminal by choline acetyltransferase (MacIntosh & Collier 1976). Choline is found in the extracellular fluid and is transported into the nerve terminal by a specific carrier mechanism in the membrane. Hemicholinium-3 (HC-3) inhibits this choline transport system, leading to a decrease in ACh synthesis and hence a decrease in total and 'bound' (vesicular) ACh levels (Potter 1970, Gundersen et al 1981, Dolezal & Tucek 1983, Veldesema-Currie et al 1984). Continuous nerve stimulation at high frequency or continuous exposure to high [K+] solutions leads to a gradual decrease in the rate of release of ACh (Elmqvist & Quastel 1965). This decrease in ACh release occurs by a reduction in the number of ACh molecules per packet released. Hemicholinium-3 is one of the few drugs to affect the size of the packet. On the other hand the quantal content of the epp is unchanged by HC-3. The overall result is a gradual decrease in both

mepp and epp amplitudes during continuous high-frequency nerve stimulation. At high concentrations, there is in addition an immediate postsynaptic action of HC-3 to decrease ACh sensitivity (Martin & Orkand 1961, Thies & Brooks 1961).

POSTSYNAPTIC EVENTS

End-plate response

The postsynaptic events generating epps following nerve stimulation are as follows (see e.g. Katz 1966, Ginsborg & Jenkinson 1976). As mentioned in the Introduction, ACh causes channels to open briefly and current flows via these channels. This 'end-plate current' (epc) flowing into the muscle cell causes a depolarisation, so initiating the epp at the end-plate region (Fig. 5.8). When the epc has subsided, the remaining depolarisation of the epp then decays more slowly by a purely passive process determined by the passive electrical properties of the membrane.

The spontaneous release of a single packet of ACh leads to a similar but smaller event, the miniature end-plate potential (mepp). A correspondingly smaller current flows via the post-

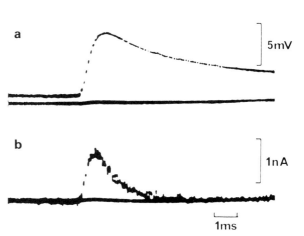

Fig. 5.8 Intracellular recordings at frog end-plate. Upper trace = end-plate potential, lower trace = end-plate current in the same fibre. The end-plate current normally leads to depolarisation, producing the end-plate potential. In the lower recording, potential changes have been eliminated experimentally using the voltage-clamp technique (see Fig. 5.9) (after Takeuchi & Takeuchi 1959).

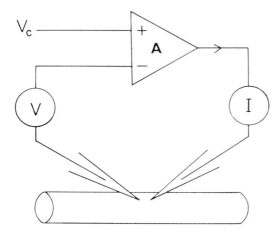

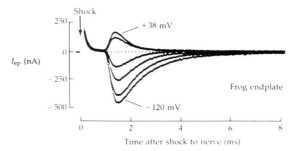

Fig. 5.10 End-plate currents measured by the voltage-clamp technique. Recordings of current (I_{ep}) were made at various membrane potentials from −120 mV (bottom trace) in steps to +38 mV (top trace). The end-plate current is reduced to zero at around 0 mV (Magleby & Stevens 1972, Hille 1992).

Fig. 5.9 Voltage-clamp technique. Two microelectrodes are inserted into the muscle fibre near each other at the end-plate region. One microelectrode records the intracellular voltage (V) while the other passes current (I) into or out of the muscle fibre. Electronic circuitry (amplifier, A) controls the current passed by the latter electrode so that the intracellular voltage is held constant ('clamped') at voltage V_c. Postsynaptic currents induced by ACh can be measured under these clamped conditions since such currents are then equal to the current passed into the fibre by one of the microelectrodes. Passive changes involving charging the capacitance of the membrane cannot occur under these conditions.

synaptic channels: the 'miniature end-plate current' (mepc). The mepc has a similar time-course to the epc. The current flowing across the end-plate membrane during the action of ACh (the epc or mepc) can be measured experimentally by the voltage-clamp technique (Fig. 5.9).

During the time that end-plate channels are open, ions flow down their concentration and electrical gradients. Clamping the inside of the muscle fibre at less negative voltages (i.e. depolarisation) decreases the electrical gradient and hence the epc is also decreased in amplitude (Fig. 5.10). Further depolarisation eventually reduces the epc amplitude to zero. The membrane potential where this happens is known as the reversal potential and is usually in the range −15 to 0 mV. The actual value of the reversal potential is determined by concentration gradients and permeabilities of only those ions which flow through the channels. The concentrations of Na⁺ and K⁺ ions were found to affect the reversal potential while the concentration of Cl⁻ ions did not (Takeuchi & Takeuchi 1960). Therefore, the

end-plate channels are permeable to Na⁺ ions (usually flowing inwards) and K⁺ ions (usually flowing outwards) but not to Cl⁻ ions.

There are important differences between the epp and the muscle action potential triggered by the epp. The epp can only be recorded locally in a region around the end-plate with an amplitude falling off passively within a millimetre or so from the postsynaptic region (Fatt & Katz 1951). This is unlike the action potential, which is a propagated response throughout the whole fibre. Secondly, the epp is continuously graded: the amplitude varies with the amount of ACh liberated by the nerve terminal or with a change in the postsynaptic sensitivity to the depolarising action of ACh. This is in contrast to the action potential which is an all-or-nothing regenerative event. Thirdly, channels are opened chemically (i.e. by ACh) at the end-plate (Anderson & Stevens 1973), while the channels producing the action potential are opened by electrical changes in membrane potential (Hodgkin & Huxley 1952a,b,c,d, Hille, 1992). Action potentials involve the opening firstly of channels specific for Na⁺ ions, and these channels can be blocked selectively by tetrodotoxin (Narahashi et al 1964) which has no effect at the end-plate channels. During the action potential, after a delay, channels specific for K⁺ ions open, and these channels can be blocked with 4-aminopyridine or tetraethylammonium (see e.g. Hille 1992). An individual channel at the end-plate, when opened by ACh, becomes permeable to *both* Na⁺ and K⁺ ions. Thus the chemically operated channels at the end-plate are different from the Na⁺ and K⁺ channels involved in the action potential (Kordas 1969, Dionne & Ruff 1977, Wray 1980).

The effects of ACh released by the nerve impulse can be mimicked fairly well by applying a short pulse of ACh locally. This can be done by the iontophoretic technique. For this, ACh is electrically ejected from an ACh-filled micropipette placed near the postsynaptic membrane (Krnjevic & Miledi 1958). The end-plate response to nerve stimulation is fairly similar to that for iontophoretically applied ACh (Fig. 5.11). Unlike nerve-stimulated release there is almost no appreciable delay in the onset of the response after suitable iontophoretic application (Katz & Miledi 1965). This lack of delay for iontophoretic application comes about because ACh reacts rapidly with postsynaptic receptors while the delay for nerve-stimulated release occurs presynaptically (see 'Acetylcholine release' above).

Sensitivity to iontophoretically applied ACh is limited to around the end-plate region in nomal muscle fibres (Miledi 1960a). However, some days after denervation, muscle fibres develop sensitivity to iontophoretically applied ACh over their whole length (Axelsson & Thesleff 1959, Miledi 1960b). This is because 'extrajunctional' receptors and their associated channels appear

throughout the length of the muscle fibre after denervation.

Single channels

Patch-clamp recording. It is possible to record directly the tiny current flowing through a single ion channel (Neher & Sakmann 1976a, Sakmann & Neher 1983, Hille 1992). For this technique, a rather blunt glass microelectrode or 'pipette' (tip diameter around 1 μm) filled with an agonist such as ACh is placed in contact with a small patch of membrane (Fig. 5.12). The current flowing through this very small patch of membrane can then be recorded. It is found that ACh and other depolarising drugs produce tiny rectangular pulses of current.

The amplitude, i, of each pulse is fairly constant (Fig. 5.12) and equal to a few pA. The conductance of the channel can be found by applying Ohm's Law, knowing the voltage V_m, across the membrane: conductance, $\gamma = i/V_m$. With i in amps and V_m in volts, the units of conductance are Siemens (S) (1 pS=10^{-12} Siemens).

Channels appear to have at least two states: an open conducting state and a closed state. Under constant experimental conditions, the duration of the open state (i.e. the duration of each current pulse) varies (Fig. 5.12). Channels in the open state appear to 'decay' to the closed state under much the same physical laws as those governing radioactive decays. To be precise, there is a constant probability per unit time for *each* single channel open state to 'decay' to the closed state, independent of when the channel opened in the first place (see e.g. Colquhoun & Hawkes 1983). For radioactive decay, this law leads to the well-known exponential loss of radioactivity. Analogously to this, channel open times also follow an exponential distribution (Fig. 5.13), at least as a first approximation (in some cases several exponential components are present representing the presence of several open or closed states). The *mean* open time at approximately 22°C and at normal resting potentials is found to be about 1 ms for muscle end-plate channels when ACh is the agonist. A form of congenital myasthenia, known as the 'slow-channel syndrome', has been described (See Ch. 21) in which channels are open

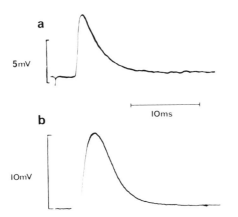

Fig. 5.11 Intracellular recordings from rat diaphragm muscle (24–25°C). **a** End-plate potential following nerve stimulation. Initial small deflection: nerve stimulation. **b** End-plate response following a 1 ms application of ACh by the iontophoretic technique. Break in trace immediately before the response corresponds to the iontophoretic pulse (after Krnjevic & Miledi 1958).

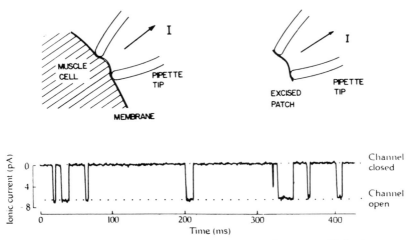

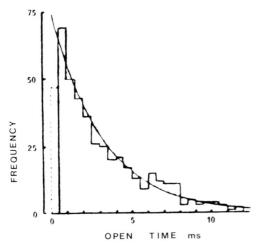

Fig. 5.12 Upper left: the patch clamp method of recording current (I) flowing through a small area (about 1 μm in diameter) of membrane of a cell. The pipette tip is tightly sealed against the outer face of the membrane. Upper right: withdrawal of pipette from the cell can result in a patch of membrane continuing to be attached to the pipette. Currents can be recorded across this excised patch of membrane. The effects on the excised membrane of known changes in ionic and drug concentration can therefore be investigated. Lower trace (Hille 1992): current flowing across an excised patch of membrane (cultured rat myotube, 23°C) showing brief openings of single channels in response to ACh. Note the constant amplitude of each current pulse but the variable open time.

for a longer time (Oosterhuis et al 1987, Engel 1992).

The patch-clamp technique has found wide applications for studies of a range of different channels (e.g. voltage-sensitive Na^+, K^+ and Ca^+ channels — Hille 1992). The noise levels in this type of recording depend on how well the membrane is sealed to the rim of the glass pipette: the better the seal the lower the noise. Applying suction to the electrode improves the seal, producing a high leakage resistance or 'gigaseal' (Horn & Patlak 1980, Hamill et al 1981, Sakmann & Neher 1984). The patch-clamp method finds immediate application to cultured cells, where good membrane–pipette seals can be formed. For non-cultured muscle cells, pretreatment with collagenase and other enzymes has been used to improve the seal.

Noise analysis. Direct recording of the individual pulses of current produced by single channel opening is not possible by classical *intra-cellular* microelectrode techniques, because such individual current pulses are too small to detect by this method; instead the patch-clamp method is normally used (see above). However, before the advent of patch recording, much had already been learnt *indirectly* about the properties of channels by intracellular recording methods using the technique of noise analysis (Katz & Miledi 1970,

Fig. 5.13 Distribution of channel open time durations. Recordings were made from the frog neuromuscular junction in the presence of 50 nM ACh (membrane potential –80 mV, temperature 8°C). The distribution is fitted with a single exponential curve (after Colquhoun & Hawkes 1983).

1972, 1977b, Anderson & Stevens 1973, Colquhoun 1975, 1979, 1981, Rang 1975, Neher & Stevens 1977, Wray 1980). For this technique, ACh is applied continuously at an end-plate, either in the bath or iontophoretically, while current flowing at the end-plate is measured by the voltage-clamp technique using intracellular microelectrodes. The collision of ACh molecules with receptors is a random process leading in turn to random opening of channels. Therefore the number of channels open at any one time is not a constant. This creates fluctuations in the current flowing across the end-plate membrane. These current fluctuations produced by ACh (or other agonists) can be detected: the current recording at high amplification becomes more 'noisy' in the presence of ACh (Fig. 5.14). This noise can be analysed to give indirect information about the underlying single channel currents (see e.g. Wray 1980). Besides information on single channel properties, noise analysis also gives information on the frequency of channel opening; for instance when 1-2 μM ACh is applied to cat muscle at 37°C it leads to the opening of around 3×10^8 channels per second (Wray 1981b).

Single channel properties. Open time and conductance of the end-plate channel activated by ACh have been extensively measured by both noise analysis and patch recording (Katz & Miledi 1972, Anderson & Stevens 1973, Ben-Haim et al 1975, Dreyer & Peper 1975, Dreyer et al 1976a, Colquhoun et al 1977, Cull-Candy et al 1979, Wray 1980, 1981b, Sakmann & Neher 1983, Hille 1992). The open time depends strongly on

temperature; e.g. the normal mean open time of about 1 ms at 22°C is increased to about 3 ms when the temperature is lowered by 10°C (at a membrane potential of –75 mV). The open time also depends strongly on membrane potential; as the membrane potential is hyperpolarised by 50 mV, channel open time increases by about 50% (at 19°C). On the other hand, the conductance of the channel opened by ACh varies little with temperature or membrane potential, having values usually in the range 20–40 pS for normal end-plates.

From the above values of channel conductance and open time (at room temperature and normal membrane potential), one finds that each channel, while open, passes a quantity of charge equal to around 2×10^{-15} coulombs, equivalent to the passage of about 10^4 univalent ions.

Useful information can be obtained from knowing the size of the depolarisation produced by a single channel opening, a. Thus for cat muscle (37°C) a is 0.1 μV (Wray 1981b), which compares with a mepp amplitude of about 0.5 mV. Therefore the single channel depolarisation is some three orders of magnitude smaller than the mepp. This suggests that a mepp is produced by the synchronous opening of several thousand ion channels, implicating the simultaneous action of several thousand ACh molecules on the postsynaptic receptors.

An important discovery by Anderson & Stevens (1973) was that, at 8°C, the open time of a single channel was found to be identical to the decay constant of mepcs or epcs, even at different membrane potentials. Therefore the decay of both mepcs and epcs is determined by the rate of closing of the channel. Thus, after the nerve is stimulated, any ACh which has not bound to receptors must disappear (i.e. by hydrolysis and diffusion) from the synaptic cleft in a time much less than the channel open time. At higher temperatures (22°C), epc decay is somewhat slower than the channel open time (by a factor of 1.4) (Katz & Miledi 1973a, Colquhoun et al 1977). At higher temperatures, therefore, some ACh remains in the cleft after some channels have closed, and continues to open channels, so prolonging the epc slightly.

Improvements in patch clamp recording techni-

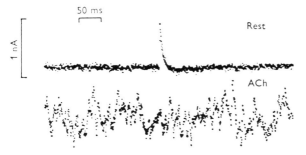

Fig. 5.14 Currents measured at a frog end-plate in a voltage clamped fibre (–100 mV, 8°C). The upper trace shows control current, including a spontaneously occurring mepc. The lower trace shows the increase in noise produced by the application of ACh (Anderson & Stevens 1973).

ques have shown further that ACh is normally removed from the synaptic cleft by rapid hydrolysis via the enzyme acetylcholinesterase which is present in the cleft. The effect of acetylcholinesterase is made clear after it has been inhibited with a drug such as neostigmine. Then one finds that epcs and mepcs are prolonged by two to six times, while the channel open time, from noise analysis, is unchanged (Katz & Miledi 1973a). In this case, ACh molecules persist in the synaptic cleft, and so can act repeatedly, causing channels to open. The prolongation of epcs by acetylcholinesterase inhibitors leads in turn to the well-known increase in amplitude and prolongation of epps and mepps.

For the extrajunctional channels found in denervated muscle (see 'End-plate response'), noise analysis and patch recording show that the open time of the channels is three to five times longer than that of normal end-plate channels, while the conductance of the channels is about 70% of normal (Dreyer et al 1976a,b, Neher & Sakmann 1976b). Channel open time and conductance for denervated muscle have similar temperature and membrane-potential dependence to that for normal end-plate channels.

During the open state of the end-plate channel, there are *brief* interruptions of shut periods (Fig. 5.15a): the channel appears to 'flicker' briefly to a shut state (Colquhoun & Sakmann 1981, Sakmann & Neher 1984, Colquhoun & Sakmann 1985, Jaramillo & Schuetze 1988, Colquhoun 1992). During the flicker, both agonist molecules appear to remain bound to the receptor. When the channel eventually closes at the end of the current pulse, the agonist then finally dissociates. There then follows a much longer shut state before agonist again binds to the receptor to re-open the channel. These observations allow estimates (albeit approximate — Lingle et al 1992) to be made of the rate constants for channel opening and closing and of the rates for dissociation/ association of agonist at the receptor. Thus it is known that the opening rate constant (once agonist has bound) is very fast, which ensures that mepcs reach their peak in less than 0.1 ms. On the other hand, the rate of channel closing is much slower (by a factor of about 1/50 times). Once bound, ACh can dissociate rapidly following an opening.

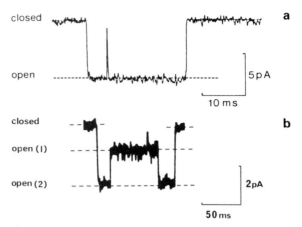

Fig. 5.15 Single channel patch-clamp recordings during applications of ACh. **a** The open channel current is interrupted by a brief flicker to the closed state (frog end-plate) (Sakmann & Neher 1984). **b** The open channel current has at least two different open conductance levels or 'states', (1) and (2) (cultured rat myoballs) (after Hamill & Sakmann, 1981)

Another finding (at least for channels in cultured muscle cells) is the discovery that there is more than one open state of the channel, each state having a different conductance (Fig. 5.15b) (Hamill & Sakmann 1981, Trautmann 1982, Auerbach & Sachs 1983, Sachs 1983, Takeda & Trautmann 1984, Jaramillo & Schuetze 1988). The same channel appears to exhibit transitions between at least two open conductance states. Multiple conductance states also occur rarely at normal muscle end-plate channels (Colquhoun & Sakmann 1985).

Conductances obtained by the patch-clamp method are about 40% higher than values found by noise analysis in the same cells. This could be because noise analysis gives *mean* results, thereby averaging over flickerings and any multiple conductance states (Fenwick et al 1982).

The acetylcholine receptor

Considerable progress in understanding the acetylcholine receptor (AChR) has come about by the use of neurotoxins found in certain snake venoms (Lee 1972). These neurotoxins bind specifically and almost irreversibly to the AChR, preventing its reaction with ACh. This action accounts for the paralysing effect resulting from the venom of such snakes. One of the most useful toxins is α-bungarotoxin (α-BuTX) obtained from the snake *Bungarus multicinctus*. The toxin can be labelled with a radioactive, fluorescent or enzyme marker without appreciable loss of activity. When such labelled toxin is bound to receptors, the resulting complex then leads to ready detection of AChR (Barnard 1979, Dolly 1979, Dolly & Barnard 1984). Much work has been carried out on the receptor-rich electric organs of the fish *Electrophorus* and *Torpedo*. Mammalian muscle has also been investigated, although this is more difficult experimentally owing to the less rich distribution of receptors.

Localisation. Electron-microscope autoradiography of muscles pretreated with radioactively labelled α-BuTX has shown that AChR is mainly found on the crests of the postsynaptic folds of the motor end-plate (Fig. 5.1) at a density of around 25 000 receptors per μm^2 (Barnard et al 1975, Porter & Barnard 1975, 1976, Fertuck & Salpeter 1976, Matthews-Bellinger & Salpeter 1978). The total number of α-BuTX binding sites per muscle end-plate is in the range $3–9\times10^7$.

Labelling by a peroxidase conjugate of α-BuTX has shown that some binding sites also appear to exist on the presynaptic membrane (Bender et al 1976, Engel et al 1977b, Lentz et al 1977). Thus AChRs could also be present presynaptically (see above). The *quantitative* extent of these binding sites cannot be readily assessed by peroxidase-labelled α-BuTX. However, the extent of presynaptic binding must be quite small, as the more quantitative (but less sensitive) technique using radiolabelled α-BuTX does not lead to detection of presynaptic binding. Indeed removal of the nerve terminal before binding with [³H]α-BuTX did not measurably affect binding. Therefore, any presynaptic AChR sites were below the error limit of the radiolabelled technique, and numbers of AChR (if present) are likely to be less than 10% of the number of postsynaptic receptors.

Isolation. The AChR has been isolated from muscles by the following technique (Dolly 1979, Dolly & Barnard 1984). Membrane proteins, including the AChR, are brought into solution with a detergent (in the presence of protease

inhibitors to prevent AChR degradation). For purification, the AChR is then absorbed on to α-toxin immobilised on a gel. The AChR can then be eluted from the column by application of a high concentration of, for example, carbachol. Variations in these methods exist, for example monoclonal antibodies directed against the AChR may be used in the column instead of the α-toxin (Lennon et al 1980, Momoi & Lennon 1982).

After purification, the AChR retains its ability to bind nicotinic cholinoceptor agonists and antagonists. This binding can be detected and made quantitative as the rate of binding of [³H]α-BuTX to the isolated AChR is, as expected, found to be retarded by the presence of such agonists or antagonists (Barnard et al 1977, Dolly 1979).

Molecular structure. Muscle AChR is an acidic glycoprotein, composed of subunits which can be dissociated using sodium dodecyl sulphate gel electrophoresis. The molecular weights of these dissociated subunits, termed α, β, γ, δ are approximately 40–45, 49–53, 53–56, 57–68 kDa respectively in muscle (Dolly & Barnard 1984, Beeson & Barnard 1992), and rather similar for fish (Raftery et al 1980). The AChR exists normally as a pentamer, $\alpha_2\beta\gamma\delta$, and the α-subunit contains the ACh binding site: thus the pentameric AChR has two ACh binding sites (Karlin 1980, Changeux 1981, Conti-Tronconi & Raftery 1982). Recently it has been suggested that ligands may bind at the interface of αγ and αδ, thus implicating the γ and δ subunits in the ligand binding domain (Pedersen & Cohen 1990). There is a difference between fetal (or denervated) AChR, with structure as above, and adult AChR which has the γ subunit replaced by an isoform termed ε (Takai et al 1985, Mishina et al 1986).

The pentameric receptor/channel complex spans the membrane with the five subunits comprising a 'rosette' around the central pore/channel which is formed between them (Fig. 5.16) (e.g. Kistler et al 1982, Brisson & Unwin 1985, Unwin et al 1988, Mitra et al 1989). The channel protein protrudes out of the membrane a considerable distance (about 60 Å) on the extracellular side. Following binding of ACh molecules to the two recognition sites, the whole AChR pentamer undergoes a conformational change causing the channel to open.

a SIDE VIEW

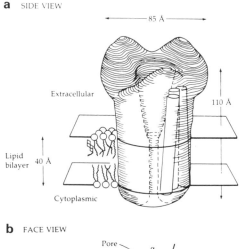

b FACE VIEW

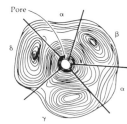

Fig. 5.16 Three-dimensional structure of the acetylcholine receptor, based on electron microscopy and X-ray diffraction. **a** Side view of receptor in relation to the lipid bilayer of the plasma membrane. Cylinders represent helices of the peptide chains. **b** Face view of AChR with arrangement of subunits around the central pore (from Kistler et al 1982, Kubalek et al 1987, Hille 1992).

Subunits consist of around 430–500 amino acids and there is considerable amino acid sequence homology between subunits in the same species, and also between different species. Knowing the amino acid structure, reasonable predictions can be made concerning the secondary structure. For each subunit there are probably four hydrophobic membrane-spanning helices, referred to as M1, M2, M3 and M4 (Fig. 5.17) (Beeson & Barnard 1992). The long extracellular region from the N-terminus end contains the ACh and toxin binding sites as well as the binding sites

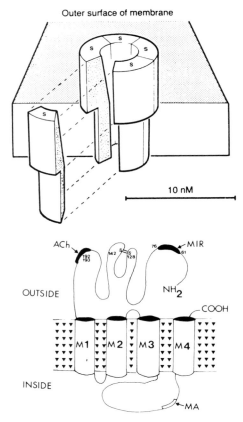

Fig. 5.17 Tentative model of secondary structure. Each subunit (s) consists of a single polypeptide chain composed of transmembrane helices (M1–M4) spanning the membrane. The subunits fit together as shown in the figure to form the receptor channel complex (after Stevens 1985). The ACh binding site, main immunogenic region (MIR) and a possible fifth helix (MA) are also shown (Beeson & Barnard 1992). Other tentative models have the polypeptide chain spanning the membrane three, five or seven times instead of four so that the C-terminus is intracellular (e.g. Criado et al 1985, Ratnam et al 1986b, McCrea et al 1987).

Complete amino acid sequences have been obtained for each subunit of the AChR obtained from fish electric organ and muscle (Noda et al 1982, 1983a–c, Sumikawa et al 1982, Claudio et al 1983, Devilliers-Thiery et al 1983, Takai et al 1984, 1985, Tanabe et al 1984, Kubo et al 1985, Mishina et al 1985, Shibahara et al 1985. To obtain these sequences, mRNA was taken from muscle or electric organs and used to produce cDNA corresponding to that responsible for the synthesis of AChR subunit protein. The screening of cDNA libraries was initially carried out using oligonucleotide probes devised from a knowledge of short amino acid sequences of subunit N-termini. The sequence of the cDNA was then found and hence the full amino acid sequence of the corresponding subunit proteins could be deduced.

for many antibodies. With four membrane-spanning helices, the C-terminus would also be placed extracellularly; however there is still some doubt about this as the tertiary structure is still somewhat uncertain (see below). Each subunit probably has a similar structure, spanning the membrane and fitting together to form a pore down the middle (Figs 5.16, 5.17). From a knowledge of the size of ions able to pass through the channel, it seems that the central pore has an internal diameter of about 0.65 nm at its narrowest, during its open state (Adams et al 1980, Dwyer et al 1980).

A further use of cDNA for AChR subunits has been to measure specific mRNA levels in muscle fibres. This assay is based on the fact that specific mRNA for an AChR subunit binds to the corresponding cDNA. In this way it was found that denervation causes a large increase in AChR subunit mRNA in the muscle fibre. This reflects an increase in synthesis of AChR which underlies the increase in number of receptors throughout the membrane of denervated muscle (see 'End-plate response' above) (Merlie et al 1984, Klarsfeld & Changeux, 1985). Similar techniques have been applied to show that AChR-subunit mRNA in innervated fibres is more abundant near synapses, corresponding to synthesis of receptors there (Merlie & Sanes 1985). In general, expression of AChRs appears to be regulated by steady-state levels of corresponding mRNA, which in turn is mainly dependent on the rate of gene transcription (Moss et al 1989, Buonanno & Merlie 1986, Goldman et al 1988, Beeson & Barnard 1992). The nature of control during development of the AChR from embryonic muscle to adult muscle (i.e. corresponding to the switch from γ to ε) has been studied. It seems likely that gene transcription of the ε subunit at the end-plate is initially triggered by neuronal humoral factors; such transcription then becomes independent of this or other signals. On the other hand, gene transcription of the γ subunit (occurring throughout the embryonic muscle fibre) is controlled both by muscle mechanical/electrical activity (which suppresses mRNA transcription outside the end-plate region present in e.g. denervated muscle) as well as by an inhibitory neural signal (Witzemann et al 1991).

Function. Progress in understanding the function of the AChR has been made by using the cDNA for the receptor subunits. Corresponding mRNA specific for each subunit can be injected into *Xenopus* oocytes, which translate the mRNA into functional protein (Mishina et al 1984, 1985, Sakmann et al 1985, Takai et al 1985, Barnard & Bilbe 1987). Functional AChR is expressed in the oocyte membrane when mRNA corresponding to all four subunits is injected into the same oocyte. In support of this, the oocyte then binds α-BuTX and, when ACh is applied, a rapid depolarisation is produced which is blocked by tubocurarine. The underlying ion channels also have the expected reversal potential, open time and conductance. Furthermore, isolation of this expressed AChR shows a similar subunit structure as for native AChR. This expression system has proved a convenient tool in the study of the relation between the structure and function of the AChR by making changes in subunit composition or sequence (by appropriate mutations), and observing their functional effects.

For instance, experiments have been carried out using chimaeric forms of the δ subunit (Imoto et al 1986). It is known that calf AChR has a lower single channel conductance (in low divalent cation solutions) than *Torpedo* AChR. Chimaeric forms of the δ subunit cDNA were constructed and the corresponding RNA expressed in oocytes (together with the α, β and γ subunits). The chimaeric forms were constructed by replacing sections of the amino acid sequence of the *Torpedo* subunit with corresponding sections from the calf subunit (and vice versa). The conductance of the channel was found to be determined by whether the M2 helix and the M2/M3 loop region was calf or *Torpedo* in origin, implying that this region is important in determining the rate of ion flux through the channel.

These studies have been taken further by Imoto et al (1988), who made a series of mutations for all four subunits. They showed that point mutations of charged amino acids in the regions bordering the M2 transmembrane region (i.e. the M1/M2 and M2/M3 loops) alter single channel conductance. This implies that the conductance is determined in an important way by these charged residues. These data suggest that the M2 helices from each subunit line the pore (see also review by Dani 1989). This is further supported by other investigations using channel-blocking drugs (see below), which bind within the channel pore. These drugs can be attached covalently at their site of action by photoactivation. Subsequent enzymatic digestion and sequencing of fragments of *Torpedo* AChR have shown that these channel blockers bind to a serine residue at a homologous position within the M2 region of the α, β, γ and δ subunits (Giraudat et al 1986, 1987, Hucho et al 1986, Oberthür et al 1986, Revah et al 1990), and similarly for a nearby leucine residue. Furthermore, mutations of these sites of the M2 helix affect single channel conductance and binding of channel blocker and have therefore further confirmed the location of these sites within the channel pore (Leonard et al 1988, Revah et al 1991, Bertrand et al 1992). It therefore seems likely that five M2 helices line the pore (i.e. one helix from each subunit), and this has allowed molecular models to be proposed as to how the amino acids lining the pore move when the channel opens or closes (Akabos et al 1992); for instance there may be a twisting movement of these five helices (Unwin 1989, Fairclough et al 1993).

Experiments similar in spirit to the above have been carried out in order to locate the ACh and toxin binding regions on the α subunit. These experiments have involved either amino acid mutations and measurements of ligand binding (Mishina et al 1985, Ohana & Gershoni 1990, Tzartos & Remoundos 1990), the use of covalently bound (affinity labelled) ligands together with amino acid analysis of peptide fragments (Kao et al 1984, Kao & Karlin 1986, Pedersen et al 1986, Ohana & Gershoni 1990, Tzartos & Remoundos 1990) and the study of binding to synthetic and recombinant peptides (Wilson et al 1985, Fuchs et al 1986, Mulac-Jericevic & Atassi 1986, Neumann et al 1986a,b, Barkas et al 1987, Gershoni 1987, Gotti et al 1987, Ralston et al 1987). These binding regions are located on the long extracellular chain at the N-terminal region (see Fig. 5.17). The ACh binding site is located at cysteine residues 192, 193, while α-bungarotoxin binds to the surrounding region (amino acids 185–197). Within this region, toxin binding is particularly determined by residues 187, 189 and

194, because variations at these residues can confer insensitivity to α-bungarotoxin, as happens for snake, mongoose and mammalian neuronal acetylcholine receptors (Boulter et al 1986, Fuchs et al 1993). These changes in amino acids can therefore explain why the mongoose (and indeed snakes themselves) do not fall victim to this snake venom.

Antibodies against acetylcholine receptor

Studies using antibodies against the AChR have proved valuable for two main reasons. Firstly, they have provided an understanding of the muscle weakness disorder myasthenia gravis (MG) and, secondly, they have led to a better understanding of the structure and function of the AChR itself.

Approximately 90% of patients with MG possess antibodies against the AChR (see e.g. Lindstrom et al 1976b). The fact that such antibodies can lead to the symptoms of MG was first shown by injecting purified AChR into rabbits (Patrick & Lindstrom 1973, Newsom-Davis 1982, Vincent 1983, Lindstrom 1985, De Baets 1992). In these animals, production of antibody directed against the receptor led to muscle weakness. This 'animal model' of the disorder is usually referred to as experimental autoimmune myasthenia gravis (EAMG). Furthermore, passive transfer to animals of AChR antibody (from MG patients or EAMG animals) also leads to muscle weakness (Lindstrom et al 1976a, Toyka et al 1977, 1978). Interestingly, monoclonal antibodies against the AChR can also transfer impairment of neuromuscular transmission to animals (see e.g. Dwyer et al 1981, Lennon & Lambert 1980, Burres et al 1981, Tzartos 1984).

For both MG patients and EAMG animals there is decreased binding of α-bungarotoxin at end-plates, indicative of loss of receptors from the postsynaptic membrane (Fambrough et al 1973, Heinemann et al 1978, Ito et al 1978, Reiness & Weinberg 1978, Stanley & Drachman 1978, Drachman 1983). This loss of receptors comes about, both in MG and chronically in EAMG, by antibodies cross-linking the receptors. Receptors are then internalised and hence degraded faster than normal (the half-life of normal AChR is about 1 week). Another mechanism by which antibodies cause receptor loss is by complement-mediated lysis of the postsynaptic membrane (Engel et al 1977a, Sahashi et al 1978).

The loss of AChRs caused by antibodies leads to reductions in epp and mepp amplitudes in MG and EAMG (e.g. Elmqvist et al 1964, Green et al 1975, Rash et al 1976). These decreases in epp amplitudes lead to failure of many muscle fibres to trigger an action potential and therefore muscle weakness is produced. Such decreases in epp amplitudes can be reversed by anticholinesterase drugs (see above). Indeed anticholinesterases are used in both diagnosis of MG using short-acting drugs such as edrophonium ('tensilon test') and in its symptomatic treatment using longer-acting drugs (e.g. pyridostigmine, neostigmine).

For MG patients and for EAMG animals, the channel open time and channel conductance are similar to normal values (Cull-Candy et al 1979, Alema et al 1981). Therefore those channels which remain functional in MG and EAMG appear to have normal properties, at least in this respect (but see Albuquerque et al 1981).

Polyclonal and especially monoclonal antibodies have provided useful information about the normal ACh receptor (Lindstrom 1992). For instance, antibodies have assisted in understanding the orientation of the chain of amino acids in the membrane. The binding sites for antibodies on the amino acid chain have been mapped using subunit fragments (Ratnam et al 1986a, Pedersen et al 1990) and synthetic peptides (Atassi et al 1987, Tzartos et al 1988, Barkas et al 1988, Bellone et al 1989, Conti-Tronconi et al 1990). The finding of antibodies against the region between M3 and M4 bound on the intracellular side of the membrane supports the model of the AChR subunit shown in Figure 5.17 (Ratnam et al 1986a,b). However discussion still continues as to whether the C terminal should be placed intra-cellularly (based on the intracellular location for binding of antibodies against the C terminal (Lindstrom et al 1984, Ratnam & Lindstrom 1984, Young et al 1985)), or whether the C-terminal should be extracellularly located (based on experiments studying the accessibility to reducing agents of a disulphide bond at the C-terminal (McCrea et al 1987)). Subunit-specific antibodies have also been used to study

the arrangement of the subunits around the pore in conjunction with electron-image analysis. The arrangement is probably as shown in Figure 5.16, i.e. with the β subunit located between the two α subunits, and the γ and δ located as indicated (Kubalek et al 1987). This interpretation has been generally supported (Kistler et al 1982, Zingsheim et al 1982, Fairclough et al 1983, Hamilton et al 1985, Fairclough et al 1993), although there is conflicting evidence that the γ subunit instead of β may lie between the two α subunits (Karlin et al 1983, Blount & Merlie 1989, Pedersen & Cohen 1990). Monoclonal antibody (against the ligand-binding site) has also been used in related studies to show that the ACh binding sites seem to be located high up on the extracellular protrusion of the AChR protein out of the membrane (Fairclough et al 1993).

Antibody preparations (raised in the laboratory against the receptor as well as found in MG patients' sera) have been tested for their effects on channel function (Albuquerque et al 1976, Bevan et al 1977, 1978, Harvey et al 1978, Lindstrom et al 1981, 1983, Dolly et al 1982, 1983, 1988, Lerrick et al 1983, Donnelly et al 1984, Lacey et al 1985, Wan & Lindstrom 1985, Blatt et al 1986, Mihovilovic & Richman 1987, Burges et al 1990) and for their effects on interference with agonist/antagonist toxin binding (Lindstrom 1976, Fulpius et al 1980, James et al 1980, Gomez et al 1981, Lennon & Lambert 1981, Mochly-Rosen & Fuchs 1981, Donnelly et al 1984, Whiting et al 1985a,b, Mihovilovic & Richman 1987, Burges et al 1990). A wide range of specificities was found when applied acutely (i.e. before degradation has time to occur) — antibodies either: (i) block the binding of ACh and/or α-BuTX to their binding sites on the AChR; or (ii) prevent channels opening by binding away from the ACh binding site; or (iii) bind away from the ACh binding site without loss of function. The majority of antibodies against the AChR fall into category (iii). Many of these latter antibodies compete amongst themselves for a well-defined conformationally dependent structural region of the AChR — the 'main immunogenic region' (MIR) — which is located on the α subunit between residues 67 and 76 (Fig. 5.17) (Tzartos & Lindstrom 1980, Tzartos et al 1981, 1992, Lindstrom 1985,

Bellone et al 1989, Das & Lindstrom 1989, Papadouli et al 1990, Saedi et al 1990, Marraud et al 1992). Thus the vast majority of antibodies found in MG patients do not cause direct, acute block of receptors. The antibodies in category (ii) above are especially interesting because they may be interfering with the step(s) between ACh binding and subsequent channel opening, possibly by binding to the channel itself. In the few instances where acute functional block occurs, channels continue to have normal open time and conductance, indicating that block occurs via reduction in channel opening frequency rather than by a change in single channel properties (Dolly et al 1982, 1988, Lacey et al 1985, Blatt et al 1986).

Channel-blocking drugs

As described above, agonists such as ACh cause channels to open. Certain drugs, such as local anaesthetics, appear to block these open channels (Katz & Miledi 1975, Adams 1977, Ruff 1977, Neher & Steinbach 1978, Wray 1980, Ogden et al 1981, Dreyer 1982, Colquhoun 1992). They interact with the open channel, causing the channel conductance to fall to zero. When the channel-blocking drug leaves its binding site, the channel is thought to revert back to its open state with agonist still bound. The open channel may then either shut as agonist dissociates or it may first encounter repeated blockings by the drug (Fig. 5.18).

Channel-blocking drugs lead to characteristic changes in for example end-plate currents (Kordas 1970, Beam 1976). Following initial opening of the channel by nerve-released ACh, channels become rapidly blocked by such drugs. This rapid initial block of channels in turn causes epcs initially to decay more rapidly than normal. Later dissociation of blocking drug from the channel causes channels to re-open transiently, producing a slower tail of epc decay: a two-component epc is produced (Fig. 5.19b). For certain channel-blocking drugs, the dissociation rate is so slow that the 'tail' cannot be detected: the epc then consists of a single component decay which is more rapid than normal (Fig. 5.19c).

Although the rate of dissociation of different channel-blocking drugs varies widely, the rate of

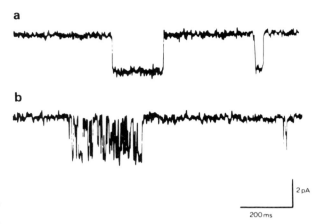

Fig. 5.18   The effect of the channel-blocking drug benzocaine. Patch-clamp recordings were made of single channel currents induced by ACh in denervated frog muscle (9°C). **a** In the absence of benzocaine. **b** In the presence of benzocaine. Repeated channel blockings can be seen in the lower trace. (Ogden et al 1981).

binding of these drugs to the channel is usually rather similar. One possibility is a simple plugging of the open channel by the drug molecule. The extent of channel block increases with the concentration of channel blocking drug and with the number of open channels available for block.

Besides local anaesthetics, a wide range of drugs has been found which block open channels. Some examples are histrionicotoxin (Albuquerque et al 1974), atropine (Adler et al 1978), mecamylamine (Wray 1981a, Varanda et al 1985), tubocurarine (Katz & Miledi 1978, Colquhoun et al 1979), gallamine (Colquhoun & Sheridan 1981), certain antibiotics (e.g. clindamycin and lincomycin) (Fiekers et al 1979, 1983), some barbiturates (Adams 1976) as well as agonists themselves (Adams & Sakmann 1978, Sine & Steinbach 1984, Ogden & Colquhoun 1985).

Neuromuscular blocking drugs

Neuromuscular blocking drugs in use by anaesthetists to obtain muscle relaxation during surgical operations are of two types: competitive antagonists and depolarising agonists.

Competitive antagonists. Drugs in the category of competitive antagonist, of which tubocurarine is the classic example (Jenkinson

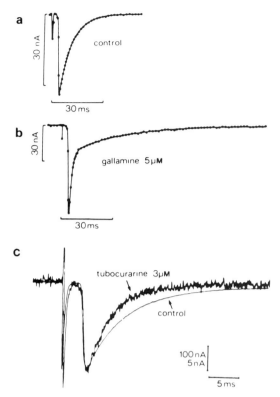

Fig. 5.19 Action of channel-blocking drugs on the epc. Besides their competitive action, gallamine and tubocurarine also block open channels. The figure (Dreyer 1982) shows epcs at frog end-plates (11–12°C). Epcs normally decay exponentially, shown in **a**. Gallamine induces a two-component decay, shown in **b** (Colquhoun & Sheridan 1981). Tubocurarine produces a single component epc with a faster exponential decay, shown in **c** (Colquhoun et al 1979).

1960), act by combining reversibly with the ACh binding site on the receptor. They do not themselves cause channels to open at the neuro-muscular junction, but prevent ACh from triggering channel opening. Increasing the concentration of ACh in the cleft (e.g. by using an anticholinesterase such as neostigmine) can overcome the competitive block. Relatively rapidly acting competitive antagonists such as vecuronium (Marshall et al 1980, 1983) and atracurium (Hughes & Chapple 1981, Payne & Hughes 1981) have been introduced for use during anaesthesia.

Besides the action of tubocurarine as a competitive antagonist, the drug can also block open channels (see above). However, the main effect of

the drug under conditions encountered clinically is mainly competitive. So, for instance, tubocurarine at micromolar concentrations does not markedly affect the channel open time and epc decay rate at normal resting potentials, but simply reduces the frequency of channel opening induced by agonists such as ACh (Katz & Miledi 1972, Colquhoun et al 1979). This competitive mechanism underlies the well-known shift in dose–response curves produced by tubocurarine. On the other hand, channel block becomes more important at hyperpolarised potentials and at higher agonist concentrations.

Agonists. Depolarising blocking drugs (such as suxamethonium and decamethonium) are agonists at the neuromuscular junction. They act at AChRs to cause channels to open, and this in turn produces a depolarisation at the end-plate region (Zaimis & Head 1976, Zaimis & Wray 1981). The action is similar to that of ACh in the presence of inhibitors of acetylcholinesterase to prevent ACh breakdown (Burns & Paton 1951, Wray 1981b) (Fig. 5.20). At drug concentrations found clinically (around 1 μM) and for many minutes, depolarisation is well maintained, at least for cat and man. This maintained depolarisation causes inactivation of the electrically operated Na^+ channels (not the AChR channels) responsible for action potentials (see 'End-plate response'). Hence no action potentials can be triggered and paralysis results.

During the application of depolarising drugs at micromolar concentrations, the depolarisation wanes rather slowly (Fig. 5.20). Throughout this period, channels continue to be opened by the agonist. The frequency of opening of channels can be followed by noise analysis and this is also shown in Fig. 5.20. The number of channels opened per second by the agonist also falls quite slowly. The process of inactivation of receptor function during prolonged agonist application is known as desensitisation (e.g. Elmqvist & Thesleff 1962, Nastuk et al 1966, Rang 1975, Ginsborg & Jenkinson 1976), which is a little-understood process whereby the receptor/channel complex appears to revert to inactive conformational states (e.g. by a movement of the M2 helices which line the pore, Fairclough et al 1993). At *low* concentrations, it can be seen from Figure 5.20, for example, that desensitisation occurs slowly. Similar slow desensitisation is

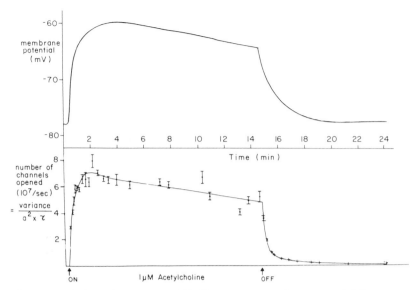

Fig. 5.20 Prolonged exposure to ACh. Upper trace: membrane potential. Lower trace: frequency of opening of channels obtained from the analysis of voltage noise. Recordings were made during application of ACh (1 μM) to cat tenuissimus muscle (38°C) in the presence of physostigmine to prevent hydrolysis of ACh (Wray 1978b, 1981b).

also seen with suberyldicholine, suxamethonium and decamethonium at a concentration of 1 μM. Therefore the end-plate remains sensitive to agonists for many minutes: blockade of neuromuscular transmission does not occur by this slow process of desensitisation of ACh receptors at these concentrations. The maintained depolarisation itself will normally be sufficient to produce neuromuscular blockade by inactivating action potentials.

The fact that some desensitisation does occur (albeit slowly) during exposure to depolarising drugs is indicated also by the fact that repeated applications of decamethonium produce progressively smaller depolarisations (Burns & Paton 1951). Furthermore, desensitisation proceeds at a faster rate for higher agonist concentrations (e.g. Katz & Thesleff 1957, Wray 1981b). Such concentrations are probably found when ACh is applied locally by iontophoresis, leading to more rapid desensitisation (Axelsson & Thesleff 1958). Of course, if the ACh receptors are inactivated (desensitised) by depolarising drugs, they will also be unable to respond to nerve-released ACh and block of transmission would again be produced. During *prolonged* doses of depolarising drugs,

sufficient desensitisation may occur for the mechanism of the block to change from that due to depolarisation to that due to desensitisation and this is probably the mechanism of the so-called 'dual block' (Zaimis 1953). For certain species (e.g. rat, see Zaimis & Head 1976), the end-plate is normally rather insensitive to depolarising drugs so that small depolarisations are produced and higher concentrations of blocking drug are needed to produce neuromuscular blockade. The mechanism of blockade at such higher concentrations may then be due throughout to desensitisation for such species.

Noise analysis and patch-clamp recording have shown that channel open time differs markedly for different agonists (Katz & Miledi 1973b, Colquhoun et al 1975, 1977, Dreyer et al 1976b, Neher & Sakmann 1976a,b). The mean channel open times are: suberyldicholine, 1.6–3.3 ms; ACh, 1.1 ms; acetylmonoethylcholine, 0.66 ms; carbachol, 0.3–0.4 ms; decamethonium, 0.5 ms; nicotine, 0.22 ms; acetylthiocholine 0.12 ms (20°C, –75 mV). On the other hand, the single channel conductance is approximately the same value as that for ACh for each of these agonists. The variation in channel open time suggests that agonist remains attached to the receptor while the channel is open. At concentrations which produce neuromuscular block (about 1 μM), the depolarising drugs ACh, suberyldicholine, suxamethonium and decamethonium all produce large depolarisations of about 20 mV for cat muscle (37°C) (Wray 1978a). Such a depolarisation is large enough to cause depolarisation block. As mentioned, channel open time (and hence the depolarisation produced by a single channel opening, a), varies widely between these agonists. The overall depolarisation of 20 mV produced in cat muscle is similar for each of these drugs because the smaller the single channel depolarisation, a, the larger the channel opening frequency turns out to be, at least for this muscle at this concentration.

Besides acting at the ACh binding site to cause channels to open, agonists can also block open channels (see 'Channel blocking drugs'). However, since channel block occurs at high concentrations it is unlikely to be important in experiments and clinical procedures carried out to produce neuromuscular blockade at about 1 μM. Furthermore, channel block by ACh itself is unlikely to contribute during the action of ACh released by nerve stimulation.

Finally, it is interesting to note that the phenomenon of desensitisation discussed above can actually be turned to experimental advantage in the study of mechanisms of agonist action at high concentration using the patch clamp technique (Colquhoun & Ogden 1988, Sakmann et al 1980, Sine & Steinbach 1987, Mulrine & Ogden 1988, Colquhoun 1992, Lingle et al 1992). In the presence of an agonist, after an initial high rate of channel openings, activity subsides due to channels becoming desensitised. At high agonist concentrations, activity disappears completely except for the occasional appearance of a cluster of channel openings (see Fig. 5.21). This cluster has been interpreted as due to openings of a *single* channel (with normal opening and closing kinetics) which has emerged from desensitisation before lapsing back into silence. By restricting analysis to the events within a cluster, this has allowed the analysis of single channel kinetic parameters and dose–response behaviour even at high concentrations. If it were not for the

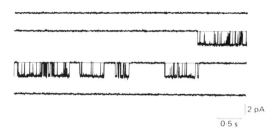

Fig. 5.21   A cluster of openings of a *single* channel preceded and followed by long silent periods corresponding to a desensitised state of the receptor. Each cluster of openings is usually from a different single channel found in the patch and which emerges from desensitisation. The cluster consists of several groups of openings; within each group the channel is assumed to function normally, i.e. as it would in the absence of desensitisation, allowing study of normal channel kinetics. Between groups within the cluster there are short silent periods, which probably represent another desensitised state of the single channel with a much shorter lifetime than for that occurring between clusters. The recording was made from a cell line (BC3H1) by the patch-clamp technique using 130 μM ACh (11°C) (Sine & Steinbach 1987).

phenomenon of desensitisation, patch-clamp recordings at high concentrations would involve the simultaneous activation of very many channels under the pipette, rendering single channel analysis impossible.

ACETYLCHOLINESTERASE

As mentioned above, acetylcholinesterase hydrolyses ACh released from the nerve. This enzyme (AChE, EC 3.1.1.7) is present in the cleft in roughly equal molecular numbers (approximately 3×10^7) to the number of AChRs (Barnard et al 1971, Porter et al 1973), but the AChR and the acetylcholinesterase enzyme are distinct molecules (Changeux 1975). The enzyme is extremely rapid in hydrolysing ACh; the substrate turnover is 25 000 molecules per second, equivalent to 40 μs per molecule. The high activity and suitable location of the enzyme guarantees that an ACh molecule is normally hydrolysed almost immediately after it has opened an AChR channel, so preventing interaction with a second AChR.

There are two main structural classes of the enzyme: asymmetric (A_4, A_8, and A_{12}) and globular (G_1, G_2 and G_4) (for reviews see Taylor et al 1986, Massoulié & Toutant 1988). All forms are composed of between 1 and 12 catalytic subunits (as detailed by the subscripts), while the asymmetrical forms are associated with structural subunits (Fig. 5.22). The structural subunit is usually collagen-like in composition and consists of three strands to each of which a tetramer of catalytic subunits may attach (Krejci et al 1991). The strands form a helical tail which attaches the assembly to the extracellular basal lamina (located in the cleft) rather than the cell membrane. Such asymmetrical forms of the enzyme are usually found at the neuromuscular junction. On the other hand, the globular forms of the enzyme are widely distributed throughout tissues, ranging from the CNS to erythrocytes to the neuro-muscular junction. Some of the globular forms are hydrophobic and may attach to plasma membranes via a glycophospholipid (or other small tail) which is sometimes part of their struc-ture; other globular forms are water soluble and occur in the serum of most vertebrates (Massoulie & Toutant 1988). Both asymmetrical and globular forms are held together by disulphide bonds between catalytic subunits and between the tail (Fig. 5.22).

The catalytic subunits have molecular weights in the range 66–110 kDa, and show some immunological variability between species. Interestingly, in the adult chick, the asymmetrical A_{12} enzyme consists of 12 identical catalytic subunits (mol. wt 110 kDa) with AChE activity; on the other hand, in the newborn chick the A_{12} enzyme consists of six catalytic subunits of mol wt 110 kDa (with AChE activity) and six subunits of mol. wt 72 kDa (Tsim et al 1988). The latter subunits have a rather different specificity characteristic of butyrylcholinesterase enzyme (EC 3.1.1.8, BuChE, pseudocholinesterase, cholinesterase).

The amino acid sequence of the catalytic subunit is now known from cloning studies for several species (MacPhee-Quigley et al 1985, Schumacher et al 1986, Maelicke 1991). There is considerable sequence homology between species and indeed between AChE and BuChE; the subunit is around 600 amino acids long. The enzyme acts as a 'serine hydrolase'; it acts via an intermediate step involving the splitting of the substrate, releasing choline and acylating the

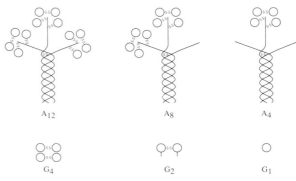

Fig. 5.22 Schematic representation of the quaternary structure of the polymorphic forms of the acetylcholinesterase enzyme. The molecular forms can be divided into two categories: asymmetrical (A_{12}, A_8, A_4) and globular (G_4, G_2, G_1). The catalytic subunits of the asymmetrical form are attached in tetramers to a collagen-like structural component. The catalytic tetramers can be attached by disulphide bridges to one or more of three collagen strands which come together to form a triple helical tail unit. The globular type can form monomers, dimers and tetramers. Sometimes the globular form can attach to membranes, by means of the addition of a glycophospholipid tail (shown for G_2). (adapted from Massoulie & Toutant 1988).

enzyme via covalent attachment of the acyl group to a serine residue of the enzyme. This bond is subsequently hydrolysed and acetate or butyrate is released. The active serine has been localised to residue 200 in *Torpedo* AChE (Hucho et al 1991). The purified catalytic subunit from *Torpedo* has now been crystallised and its tertiary structure determined by X-ray techniques (Sussman et al 1991). The substrate binds to a site at the bottom of a gorge in the subunit and a triad of amino acids (glutamate, histidine and the serine residue itself) are of key importance in catalytic activity. Interestingly the active site within the gorge is not adjacent to an anionic region, as had previously been thought. However, substrate molecules may queue up at an anionic rim of the gorge before reaching the active triad; this ready supply of substrate assists in promoting the high turnover of substrate by the enzyme (for review see Soreq et al 1992).

The increase in amplitude and prolongation of epps by inhibitors of AChE is of great value in the treatment of myasthenia gravis (see above). The mechanism of action of such anticholinesterases on the enzyme is now better understood. For instance, organophosphorous compounds and carbamates (such as neostigmine) mimic ACh as a substrate for the enzyme, forming a phosphorylated or carbamylated enzyme which is hydrolysed at a far slower rate.

CONCLUSION

The cohesive picture of neuromuscular transmission described in this chapter has been built up over several decades. This picture provides a sound basis for understanding disorders of human neuromuscular transmission, such as myasthenia gravis and the Lambert–Eaton myasthenic syndrome.

Much still remains, however, to be clarified at normal neuromuscular junctions. For instance, the amino acid sequence and structure/function relationships of voltage-dependent Ca^{2+} channels

on the presynaptic membrane remain to be determined. The intracellular mechanisms as to how Ca^{2+} causes release of ACh are still poorly understood. On the postsynaptic side, although much is now known about the acetylcholine receptor, it is still not yet clear at the molecular level how ACh binding causes the conformational change leading to channel opening. Exciting progress on these questions can be anticipated over the coming years, and this should prove useful both scientifically and clinically.

ACKNOWLEDGEMENTS

I am most grateful to V. Porter for unfailing help and for useful criticism and comments throughout the preparation of this chapter.

REFERENCES

Adams D J, Dwyer T M, Hille B 1980 The permeability of end plate channels to monovalent and divalent cations. Journal of General Physiology 75: 493

Adams P R 1976 Drug blockade of open end-plate channels. Journal of Physiology 260: 531

Adams P R 1977 Voltage jump analysis of procaine action at frog end plates. Journal of Physiology 268: 291

Adams P R, Sakmann B 1978 Decamethonium both opens and blocks endplate channels. Proceedings of the National Academy of Sciences USA 75: 2994

Adler M, Albuquerque E X, Lebeda F J 1978 Kinetic analysis of end-plate currents altered by atropine and scopolamine. Molecular Pharmacology 14: 514

Akabas M H, Stauffer D A, XuM, Karlim A 1992 Acetylcholine receptor channel structure probed in cysteine – substitution mutants. Science 258: 307

Albuquerque E X, Kuba K, Daly J 1974 Effect of histrionicotoxin on the ionic conductance modulator of the cholinergic receptor: a quantitative analysis of the end-plate current. Journal of Pharmacological and Experimental Therapeutics 189: 513

Albuquerque E X, Lebeda F J, Appel S H, Almon R, Kauffmann F C, Mayer R F, Narahashi T, Yeh J Z 1976 Effects of normal and myasthenic serum factors on innervated and chronically denervated mammalian muscles. Annals of the New York Academy of Sciences 274: 475

Albuquerque E X, Warnick J E, Mayer R F, Eldefrawi A T, Eldefrawi M E 1981 Recent advances in the molecular mechanisms of human and animal models of myasthenia gravis. In: Myasthenia gravis. Annals of the New York Academy of Sciences 377: 496

Alder J, Lu B, Valtorta F, Greengard P, Poo M 1992 Calcium-dependent transmitter secretion reconstituted in Xenopus oocytes: requirement for synaptophysin. Science 257: 657

Alema S, Cull-Candy S G, Miledi R, Trautmann A 1981 Properties of end-plate channels in rats immunized against acetylcholine receptors. Journal of Physiology 311: 251

Alnaes E, Rahamimoff R 1975 On the role of mitochondria in transmitter release from motor nerve terminals. Journal of Physiology 248: 285

Anderson C R, Stevens C F 1973 Voltage clamp analysis of acetylcholine produced end-plate current fluctuations at frog neuromuscular junction. Journal of Physiology 235: 655

Atassi M Z, Mulac-Jericevic B, Yokoi T, Manshouri T 1987 Localisation of the functional sites on the α-chain of acetylcholine receptor. Federation Proceedings 46: 3538

Auerbach A, Sachs F 1983 Flickering of a nicotinic ion channel to a subconductance state. Biophysical Journal 42: 1

Augustine G J, Charlton M P, Smith S J 1985a Calcium entry into voltage-clamped presynaptic terminals of squid. Journal of Physiology 367: 143

Augustine G J, Charlton M P, Smith S J 1985b Calcium entry and transmitter release at voltage-clamped nerve terminals of squid. Journal of Physiology 369: 163

Axelsson J, Thesleff S 1958 The desensitizing effect of acetylcholine on mammalian motor end-plate. Acta Physiologica Scandinavica 43: 15

Axelsson J, Thesleff S 1959 A study of supersensitivity in denervated mammalian skeletal muscle. Journal of Physiology 147: 178

Baker P F 1972 Transport and metabolism of calcium ions in nerves. Progress in Biophysical and Molecular Biology 24: 177

Baker P F 1977 Calcium and the control of neurosecretion. Scientific Progress, Oxford 64: 95

Bain A I, Quastel D M J 1992 Multiplicative and additive Ca^{2+}-dependent components of facilitation at mouse endplates. Journal of Physiology 455: 383

Barkas T, Gabriel J-M, Mauron A, Hughes G J, Roth B, Alliod C, Tzartos S J, Ballivet M 1988 Monoclonal antibodies to the main immunogenic region of the nicotinic acetylcholine receptor bind to residues 61–76 of the α-subunit. Journal of Biological Chemistry 263: 5916

Barkas T, Mauron A, Roth B, Alliod C, Tzartos S J,

Ballivet M 1987 Mapping the main immunogenic region and toxin binding site of the nicotinic acetylcholine receptor. Science 235: 77

Barnard E A 1974 Neuromuscular junction – enzymatic destruction of acetylcholine. In: Hubbard J I (ed) The peripheral nervous system. Plenum, New York, p 201

Barnard E A 1979 Visualization and counting of receptors at the light and electron microscope levels. In: O'Brien R D (ed) The receptors, a comprehensive treatise, vol 1. Plenum, New York, p 247

Barnard E A, Bilbe G 1987 Functional expression in the *Xenopus* oocyte of mRNA for receptors and ion channels. In: Turner A J, Bachelard H (eds) Neurochemistry: a practical approach. IRL Press, Oxford, p 243

Barnard E A, Dolly J O, Porter C W, Albuquerque E X 1975 The acetylcholine receptor and the ionic conductance modulation system of skeletal muscle. Experimental Neurobiology 48: 1

Barnard E A, Coates V, Dolly J O, Mallick B 1977 Binding of α-bungarotoxin and cholinergic ligands to acetylcholine receptors in the membrane of skeletal muscle. Cell Biology International Reports 1: 99

Barnard E A, Miledi R, Sumikawa K 1982 Translation of exogenous messenger RNA coding for nicotinic acetylcholine receptors produces functioning receptors in *Xenopus* oocytes. Proceedings of the Royal Society B215: 241

Barnard E A, Wieckowski J, Chiu T H 1971 Cholinergic receptor molecules and cholinesterase molecules at mouse skeletal muscle junction. Nature 234: 207

Beam K G 1976 A quantitative description of end-plate currents in the presence of two lidocaine derivatives. Journal of Physiology 258: 301

Beeson D, Barnard E 1992 Acetylcholine receptors at the neuromuscular junction. In: Vincent A, Wray D (eds) Neuromuscular transmission: basic and applied aspects. Pergamon, Oxford, p 157

Bellone M, Tang F, Milius R, Conti-Tronconi B M 1989 The main immunogenic region of the nicotinic acetylcholine receptor, identification of amino acid residues interacting with different antibodies. Journal of Immunology 143: 3568

Bender A N, Ringel S P, Engel W K, Vogel Z, Daniels M P 1976 Immunoperoxidase localization of α bungarotoxin: a new approach to myasthenia gravis. Annals of the New York Academy of Sciences 274: 20

Benfenati F, Valtorta F, Bähler M, Greengard P 1989 Synapsin 1, a neuron-specific phosphoprotein interacting with small synaptic vesicles and F-actin. Cell Biology International Reports 13: 1007

Ben-Haim D, Dreyer F, Peper K 1975 Acetylcholine receptor: modification of synaptic gating mechanism after treatment with a disulphide bond reducing agent. Pflugers Achives 355: 19

Bertrand D, Ballivet M, Changeux J P 1992 Unconventional pharmacology of a neuronal nicotinic receptor mutated in the channel domain. Proceedings of the National Academy of Sciences USA 89: 1261

Bevan S, Kullberg R W, Heinemann S F 1977 Human myasthenic sera reduce acetylcholine sensitivity of human muscle cells in tissue culture. Nature 267: 263

Bevan S, Kullberg R W, Rice J 1978 Acetylcholine induced conductance fluctuations in cultured human myotubes. Nature 273: 469

Birks R, Huxley H E, Katz B 1960a The fine structure of the neuromuscular junction of the frog. Journal of Physiology 150: 134

Birks R, Katz B, Miledi R 1960b Physiological and structural changes at the amphibian myoneural junction in the course of nerve degeneration. Journal of Physiology 150: 145

Blandino J K W, Kim Y I 1993 Lambert–Eaton syndrome IgG reacts with dihydropyridine-sensitive, slowly-inactivating (L-type) calcium channels in bovine adrenal chromaffin cells. New York Academy of Sciences 681: 394

Blatt Y, Montal M S, Lindstrom J M, Montal M 1986 Monoclonal antibodies specific to the β and γ subunits of the *Torpedo* acetylcholine receptor inhibit single-channel activity. Journal of Neuroscience 6: 481

Blount P, Merlie J P 1989 Molecular basis of the two nonequivalent ligand binding sites of the muscle nicotinic acetylcholine receptor. Neuron 3: 349

Borsotto M, Barhanin J, Norman R I, Lazdunski M 1984 Purification of the dihydropyridine receptor of the voltage-dependent Ca^{2+} channel from skeletal muscle transverse tubules using (+) [^{3}H] PN200-110. Biochemical and Biophysical Research Communications 122: 1357

Boulter J, Evens K, Goldman D, Martin G, Treco D, Heinemann S, Patrick J 1986 Isolation of a cDNA clone coding for a possible neural nicotinic acetylcholine receptor α-subunit. Nature 319: 368

Bowden R E M, Duchen L W 1976 The anatomy and pathology of the neuromuscular junction. In: Zaimis E (ed) Handbook of experimental pharmacology XLII Neuromuscular junction. Springer, Berlin, p 23

Bowman W C 1980 Prejunctional and postjunctional cholinoceptors at the neuromuscular junction. Anaesthesia and Analgesia 59: 935

Bowman W C, Marshall I G, Gibb A J, Harborne A J 1988 Feedback control of transmitter release at the neuromuscular junction. Trends in Pharmacological Sciences 9: 16

Bowman W C, Prior C, Marshall I G 1990 Presynaptic receptors in the neuromuscular junction. Annals of the New York Academy of Sciences 604: 69

Breckenridge L J, Almers W 1987 Currents through the fusion pore that forms during exocytosis of a secretory vesicle. Nature 328: 814

Brisson A, Unwin P N T 1985 Quaternary structure of the acetylcholine receptor. Nature 315: 474

Buonanno A, Merlie J P 1986 Transcriptional regulation of nicotinic acetylcholine receptor genes during muscle development. Journal of Biological Chemistry 261: 11452

Burges J, Wray D W 1989 Effect of the calcium-channel agonist CGP 28392 on transmitter release at mouse neuromuscular junctions. Annals of the New York Academy of Sciences 560: 297

Burges J, Wray D W, Pizzighella S, Hall Z, Vincent A 1990 A myasthenia gravis plasma immunogobulin reduces miniature endplate potentials at human endplates in vitro. Muscle & Nerve 13: 407

Burns B D, Paton W D M 1951 Depolarization of the motor end-plate by decamethonium and acetylcholine. Journal of Physiology 115: 41

Burres S A, Crayton J W, Gomez C M, Richman D P 1981 Myasthenia induced by monoclonal anti-acetylcholine receptor antibodies: clinical and electrophysiological aspects. Annals of Neurology 9: 563

Catterall W A 1991 Structure and function of voltage-gated sodium and calcium channels. Current Opinion in Neurobiology 1: 5

Ceccarelli B, Hurlbut W P 1980 Vesicle hypothesis of the release of quanta of acetylcholine. Pharmacological Reviews 60: 396

Changeux J P 1975 The cholinergic receptor protein from fish electric organ. In: Iversen L L, Iversen S D, Snyder S H (eds) Handbook of psychopharmacology, vol. 6. Plenum, New York, p 235

Changeux J P 1981 The acetylcholine receptor: an 'allosteric' membrane protein. Harvey Lectures 75: 85

Charlton M P, Smith S J, Zucker R S 1982 Role of presynaptic calcium ions and channels in synaptic facilitation and depression at the squid giant synapse. Journal of Physiology 323: 173

Chester K A, Lang B, Gill J, Vincent A, Newsom-Davis J 1988 Lambert–Eaton syndrome antibodies: reaction with membranes from small cell lung cancer xenograft. Journal of Neuroimmunology 18: 97

Claudio T, Ballivet M, Patrick J, Heinemann S 1983 Nucleotide and deduced amino acid sequences of *Torpedo californica* acetylcholine receptor γ subunit. Proceedings of the National Academy of Sciences USA 80: 1111

Colquhoun D 1975 Mechanisms of drug action at the voluntary muscle endplate. Annual Review of Pharmacology 15: 307

Colquhoun D 1979 The link between drug binding and response: theories and observations. In: O'Brien R D (ed) The receptors: a comprehensive treatise, vol 1. Plenum, New York, p 93

Colquhoun D 1981 How fast do drugs work? Trends in Pharmacological Sciences 2: 212

Colquhoun D 1992 Agonists, antagonists and synaptic transmission at the neuromuscular junction. In: Vincent A, Wray D (eds) Neuromuscular transmission: basic and applied aspects. Pergamon, Oxford, p 132

Colquhoun D, Dionne V E, Steinbach J H, Stevens C F 1975 Conductance of channels opened by acetylcholine-type drugs in muscle end-plate. Nature 253: 204

Colquhoun D, Dreyer F, Sheridan R E 1979 The actions of tubocurarine at the frog neuromuscular junction. Journal of Physiology 293: 247

Colquhoun D, Hawkes A G 1983 The principles of the stochastic interpretation of ion-channel mechanisms. In: Sakmann B, Neher E (eds) Single channel recording. Plenum, New York, ch 9, p 135

Colquhoun D, Large W A, Rang H P 1977 An analysis of the action of false transmitter at the neuromuscular junction. Journal of Physiology 266: 361

Colquhoun D, Ogden D C 1988 Activation of ion channels in the frog end-plate by high concentrations of acetylcholine. Journal of Physiology 395: 131

Colquhoun D, Sakmann B 1981 Fluctuations in the microsecond time range of the current through single acetylcholine receptor ion channels. Nature 294: 464

Colquhoun D, Sakmann B 1985 Fast events in single-channel currents activated by acetylcholine and its analogues at the frog muscle end-plate. Journal of Physiology 369: 501

Colquhoun D, Sheridan R E 1981 The modes of action of gallamine. Proceedings of the Royal Society B211: 181

Conti-Tronconi B M, Raftery M A 1982 The nicotinic cholinergic receptor: correlation of molecular structure with functional properties. Annual Review of Biochemistry 51: 491

Conti-Tronconi B M, Tang F, Diethelm B M, Spencer S R, Reinhar D T, Maelicke S, Maelicke A 1990 Mapping of a cholinergic binding site by means of synthetic peptides, monoclonal antibodies and α-bungarotoxin. Biochemistry 29: 6221

Cooke I, Lipkin Jr M 1972 Cellular neurophysiology: a source book. Holt, Rinehart and Winston, New York

Couteaux R, Pecot-Dechavassine M 1968 Particularities structurales de sarcoplasme sous-neural. Comptes rendues hebdomadaires des séances de l'Académie des Sciences 266: 8

Criado M, Sarin V, Fox J L, Lindstrom J 1985 Structural localization of the sequence 235–242 of the nicotinic acetylcholine receptor. Biochemical and Biophysical Research Communications 128: 864

Cull-Candy S G, Lundh H, Thesleff S 1976 Effects of botulinum toxin on neuromuscular transmission in the rat. Journal of Physiology 260: 177

Cull-Candy S G, Miledi R, Trautmann A 1979 End-plate currents and acetylcholine noise at normal and myasthenic human end-plates. Journal of Physiology 287: 247

Cull-Candy S G, Miledi R, Trautmann A, Uchitel O D 1980 On the release of transmitter at normal, myasthenia gravis and myasthenic syndrome affected human end-plates. Journal of Physiology 299: 621

Curtis B M, Catterall W A 1984 Purification of the calcium antagonist receptor of the voltage-sensitive calcium channel from skeletal muscle transverse tubules. Biochemistry 23: 2113

Dani J A 1989 Site-directed mutagenesis and single-channel currents define the ionic channel of the nicotinic acetylcholine receptor. Trends in Neurosciences 12: 125

Das M R, Lindstrom J 1989 The main immunogenic region of the nicotinic acetylcholine receptor: interaction of monoclonal antibodies with synthetic peptides. Biochemical and Biophysical Research Communications 165: 865

Datyner N B, Gage P W 1980 Phasic secretion of acetylcholine at a mammalian neuromuscular junction. Journal of Physiology 303: 299

De Baets M 1992 Experimental autoimmune myasthenia gravis. In Vincent A, Wray D (eds) Neuromuscular transmission: basic and applied aspects. Pergamon, Oxford, p 268

De Paiva A, Dolly J O 1990 Light chain botulinum neurotoxin is active in mammalian motor nerve terminals when delivered via liposomes. FEBS Letters 277: 171

Del Castillo J, Katz B 1954a Quantal components of the end-plate potential. Journal of Physiology 124: 560

Del Castillo J, Katz B 1954b Statistical factors involved in neuromuscular facilitation and depression. Journal of Physiology 124: 574

Del Castillo J, Katz B 1955 Local activity at a depolarized nerve–muscle junction. Journal of Physiology 128: 396

Devilliers-Thiery A, Giraudat J, Bentaboulet M, Changeux J P 1983 Complete mRNA coding sequence of the acetylcholine binding α-subunit of *Torpedo marmorata* acetylcholine receptor: a model for the transmembrane organization of the polypeptide chain. Proceedings of the National Academy of Sciences USA 80: 2067

Dionne V E, Ruff R L 1977 Endplate current fluctuations reveal only one channel type at frog neuromuscular junction. Nature 266: 263

Dodge Jr F A, Rahamimoff R 1967 Co-operative action of Ca^{2+} ions in the transmitter release at the neuromuscular junction. Journal of Physiology 193: 419

Dolezal V, Tucek S 1983 The synthesis and release of acetylcholine in normal and denervated rat diaphragms during incubation in vitro. Journal of Physiology 334: 461

Dolly J O 1979 Biochemistry of acetylcholine receptors from skeletal muscle. In: Tipton K F (ed) Physiological and pharmacological biochemistry, vol 26. University Park Press, Baltimore, ch 6, p 257

Dolly J O, Barnard E A 1984 Nicotinic acetylcholine receptors: an overview. Biochemical Pharmacology 33: 841

Dolly J O, Black J, Williams R S, Melling J 1984 Acceptors for botulinum neurotoxin reside on motor nerve terminals and mediate its internalization. Nature 307: 457

Dolly J O, Gwilt M, Lacey G et al 1988 Action of antibodies directed against the acetylcholine receptor on channel function at mouse and rat end-plates. Journal of Physiology 399: 577

Dolly J O, Gwilt M, Mehraban F, Wray D 1982 Action on end-plate channels of antibodies against pure acetylcholine receptors from muscle. Journal of Physiology 336: 56P

Dolly J O, Lande S, Wray D W 1987 The effects of in vitro application of purified botulinum neurotoxin at mouse motor nerve terminals. Journal of Physiology 386: 475

Dolly J O, Mehraban F, Gwilt M, Wray D 1983 Biochemical and electrophysiological properties of antibodies against pure acetylcholine receptor from vertebrate muscles and its subunits from Torpedo in relation to experimental myasthenia. Neurochemistry International 5: 455

Donnelly D, Mihovilovic M, Gonzalez-Ros J M, Ferragut J A, Richman D, Martinez-Carrion M 1984 A non-cholinergic site directed monoclonal antibody can impair agonist-induced ion flux in Torpedo californica acetylcholine receptor. Proceedings of the National Academy of Sciences USA 81: 7999

Drachman D B 1983 Myasthenia gravis: immunobiology of a receptor disorder. Trends in Neurosciences 6: 446

Dreyer F 1982 Acetylcholine receptor. British Journal of Anaesthesia 54: 115

Dreyer F, Muller K-D, Peper K, Stertz R 1976a The M. omohyoideus of the mouse as a convenient mammalian muscle preparation. Pflugers Achives 367: 115

Dreyer F, Peper K 1975 Density and dose-response curve of acetylcholine receptors in frog neuromuscular junction. Nature 253: 641

Dreyer F, Walther Chr, Peper K 1976b Junctional and extrajunctional acetylcholine receptors in normal and denervated frog muscle fibres: noise analysis experiments with different agonists. Pflugers Archives 366: 1

Dudel J 1983 Transmitter release triggered by a local depolarization in motor nerve terminals of the frog: role of calcium entry and of depolarization. Neuroscience Letters 41: 133

Dudel J 1984a Control of transmitter release at frog's motor nerve terminals I. Dependence on amplitude and duration of depolarization. Pflugers Archives 402: 225

Dudel J 1984b Control of quantal transmitter release at frog's motor nerve terminals II. Modulation by de- or hyperpolarizing pulses. Pflugers Archives 402: 235

Dudel J, Parnas I, Parnas H 1983 Neurotransmitter release and its facilitation in crayfish muscle VI. Release determined by both intracellular calcium concentration and depolarization of the nerve terminal. Pflugers Archives 399: 1

Dwyer T M, Adams D J, Hille B 1980 The permeability of the endplate channel to organic cations in frog muscle. Journal of General Physiology 75: 469

Dwyer D S, Kearney J F, Bradley R J, Kemp G E, Oh S J 1981 Interaction of human antibody and murine monoclonal antibody with muscle acetylcholine receptor. Annals of the New York Academy of Science 377: 143

Elmqvist D, Hoffman W W, Kugelberg J, Quastel D M J 1964 An electrophysiological investigation of neuromuscular transmission in myasthenia gravis. Journal of Physiology 174: 417

Elmqvist D, Quastel D M J 1965 Presynaptic action of hemicholinium at the neuromuscular junction. Journal of Physiology 177: 463

Elmqvist D, Thesleff S 1962 Ideas regarding receptor desensitization at the motor end-plate. Revue Canadienne de Biologie 21: 229

Engel A G 1992 Congenital myasthenic syndromes. In: Vincent A, Wray D (eds) Neuromuscular transmission: basic and applied aspects. Pergamon, Oxford, p 200

Engel A G, Fukuoka T, Lang B, Newsom-Davis J, Vincent A, Wray D W 1987 Lambert–Eaton myasthenic syndrome. IgG: early morphological effects and immunolocalization at the motor end-plate. Annals of the New York Academy of Sciences 505: 333

Engel A G, Lambert E H, Howard F M 1977a Immune complexes (IgG and C3) at the motor end-plate in myasthenia gravis. Ultrastructural and light microscopic localization and electrophysiologic correlations. Mayo Clinic Proceedings 52: 267

Engel A G, Lindstrom J M, Lambert E H, Lennon V A 1977b Ultrastructural localization of the acetylcholine receptor in myasthenia gravis and in its experimental autoimmune model. Neurology (Minneapolis) 27: 307

Fairclough R H, Finer-Moore J, Love R A, Kristofferson D, Desmeules P J, Stroud R M 1983 Subunit organization and structure of an acetylcholine receptor. Cold Spring Harbor Symposium 48: 9

Fairclough R H, Josephs R, Richman D P 1993 Imaging ligand binding sites on the Torpedo acetylcholine receptor. Annals of the New York Academy of Sciences 681: 113

Fambrough D M, Drachmann D B, Satyamurti S 1973 Neuromuscular junction in myasthenia gravis: decreased acetylcholine receptors. Science 182: 293

Fatt P, Katz B 1951 An analysis of the end-plate potential recorded with an intracellular electrode. Journal of Physiology 115: 320

Fatt P, Katz B 1952 Spontaneous subthreshold activity at motor nerve endings. Journal of Physiology 117: 109

Fenwick E M, Marty A, Neher E 1982 Sodium and calcium channels in bovine chromaffin cells. Journal of Physiology 331: 599

Fertuck H C, Salpeter M M 1976 Quantitation of junctional and extrajunctional acetylcholine receptors by electron microscope autoradiography after ^{125}I-α-bungarotoxin binding at mouse neuromuscular junctions. Journal of Cell Biology 69: 144

Fiekers J F, Henderson F, Marshall I G, Parsons R L 1983 An electrophysiological study of lincomycin and clindamycin at the neuromuscular junction. Comparative effects on endplate currents and quantal content. Journal of Pharmacological and Experimental Therapeutics 227: 308

Fiekers J F, Marshall I G, Parsons R L 1979 Clindamycin and lincomycin alter miniature end-plate current decay. Nature 281: 680

Fletcher P, Forrester T 1975 The effect of curare on the release of acetylcholine from mammalian motor nerve terminals and an estimate of quantum content. Journal of Physiology 251: 131

Fuchs S, Barchan D, Kachalski S, Neumann D, Aladjem M, Vogel Z, Ovadia M, Kochva E 1993 Molecular evolution of the binding size of the acetylcholine receptor. Annals of the New York Academy of Sciences 681: 126

Fuchs S, Neumann D, Safran A, Souroujon M, Barchan D, Fridkin M, Gershoni J M, Mantegazza R, Pizzighella S 1986 Synthetic peptides and their antibodies in the analysis of the acetylcholine receptor. Annals of the New York Academy of Sciences 505: 256

Fukunaga H, Engel A G, Lang B, Newsom-Davis J, Vincent A 1983 Passive transfer of Lambert–Eaton myasthenic syndrome with IgG from man to mouse depletes the presynaptic active zones. Proceedings of the National Academy of Sciences USA 80: 7636

Fukunaga H, Engel A G, Osame M, Lambert E H 1982 Paucity and disorganization of presynaptic membrane active zones in the Lambert–Eaton myasthenic syndrome. Muscle and Nerve 5: 686

Fukuoka T, Engel A G, Lang B, Newsom-Davis J, Prior C, Wray D W 1987 Lambert–Eaton myasthenic syndrome. I. Early morphological effects of IgG on the presynaptic membrane active zones. Annals of Neurology 22: 193

Fulpius B W, Miskin R, Reich E 1980 Antibodies from myasthenic patients that compete with cholinergic agents for binding to nicotinic receptors. Proceedings of the National Academy of Sciences USA 77: 4326

Gershoni J M 1987 Expression of the α-bungarotoxin binding site of the nicotinic acetylcholine receptor by *Escherichia coli* transformants. Proceedings of the National Academy of Sciences USA 84: 4318

Gibb A J, Marshall I G 1984 Pre- and post-junctional effects of tubocurarine and other nicotinic antagonists during repetitive stimulation in the rat. Journal of Physiology 351: 275

Ginsborg B L, Jenkinson D H 1976 Transmission of impulses from nerve to muscle. In: Zaimis E (ed) Handbook of experimental pharmacology, XLII Neuromuscular junction. Springer, Berlin, p 229

Giraudat J, Dennis M, Heidmann T, Chang J-Y, Changeux J-P 1986 Structure of the high-affinity binding site for noncompetitive blockers of the acetylcholine receptor: serine-262 of the δ subunit is labeled by [³H]chlorpromazine. Proceedings of the National Academy of Sciences USA 83: 2719

Giraudat J, Dennis M, Heidmann T, Haumont P Y, Lederer F, Changeux J P 1987 Structure of the high-affinity binding site for non-competitive blockers of the acetylcholine receptor: [³H]chlorpromazine labels homologous residues in the β and δ chains. Biochemistry 26: 2410

Goldman D, Brenner H, Heinemann S 1988 Acetylcholine receptor α, β, γ and δ subunit mRNA levels are regulated by muscle activity. Neuron 1: 329

Gomez C M, Richman D P, Burres S A, Arnason B G W, Berman P W, Fitch F W 1981 Monoclonal hybridoma anti-acetylcholine receptor antibodies: antibody specificity and effect of passive transfer. Annals of the New York Academy of Sciences 377: 96

Gotti C, Mazzola G, Longhi R, Fornasari D, Clementi F 1987 The binding site for α-bungarotoxin residues in the sequence 188–201 of the α-subunit of acetylcholine receptor: structure conformation and binding characteristics of peptide [lys] 188–201. Neuroscience Letters 82: 113

Gundersen C B, Jenden D J, Newton M W 1981

β-Bungarotoxin stimulates the synthesis and accumulation of acetylcholine in rat phrenic nerve diaphragm preparations. Journal of Physiology 310: 13

Gundersen C B, Katz B, Miledi R 1982 The antagonism between botulinum toxin and calcium in motor nerve terminals. Proceedings of the Royal Society B216: 369

Green D P L, Miledi R, Perez de la Mora M, Vincent A 1975 Acetylcholine receptors. Philosophical Transactions of the Royal Society B270: 551

Hamill O P, Marty A, Neher E, Sakmann B, Sigworth F J 1981 Improved patch-clamp techniques for high resolution current recording from cells and cell-free membrane patches. Pflugers Archives 391: 85

Hamill O P, Sakmann B 1981 Multiple conductance states of single acetylcholine receptor channels in embryonic muscle cells. Nature 294: 462

Hamilton S L, Pratt D R, Eaton D C 1985 Arrangement of the subunits of the nicotinic acetylcholine receptor of *Torpedo californica* as determined by α-neurotoxin cross-linking. Biochemistry 24: 2210

Harris A J, Miledi R 1971 The effect of type D botulinum toxin on frog neuromuscular junction. Journal of Physiology 217: 497

Harvey A L, Robertson J G, Barkas T, Harrison R, Lunt G G, Stephenson F A, Cambel M J, Teague R H 1978 Reduction of acetylcholine sensitivity of chick muscle in culture by myasthenia gravis serum. Clinical and Experimental Immunology 34: 411

Heinemann S, Merlie J, Lindstrom J 1978 Modulation of acetylcholine receptor in rat diaphragm by anti-receptor sera. Nature 274: 65

Heuser J 1976 Morphology of synaptic vesicle discharge and reformation at the frog neuromuscular junction. In: Thesleff S (ed) Motor innervation of muscle. Academic Press, London, p 51

Heuser J E, Reese T S, Landis D M D 1974 Functional changes in frog neuromuscular junctions studied with freeze fracture. Journal of Neurocytology 3: 109

Hille B 1992 Ionic channels of excitable membranes. 2nd Edn Sinauer Associates Inc, Massachusetts

Hirokawa N, Sobue K, Kanda K, Harada A, Yorifuji H 1989 The cytoskeletal architecture of the presynaptic terminal and molecular structure of synapsin 1. Journal of Cell Biology 108: 111

Hodgkin A L, Huxley A F 1952a Currents carried by sodium and potassium ions through the membrane of the giant axon of loligo. Journal of Physiology 116: 449

Hodgkin A L, Huxley A F 1952b The components of membrane conductance in the giant axon of loligo. Journal of Physiology 116: 473

Hodgkin A L, Huxley A F 1952c The dual effect of membrane potential on sodium conductance in the giant axon of loligo. Journal of Physiology 116: 497

Hodgkin A L, Huxley A F 1952d A quantitative description of membrane current and its application to conductance and excitation in nerve. Journal of Physiology 117: 500

Hong S J, Chang C C 1989 Use of geographutoxin II (μ-conotoxin) for the study of neuromuscular transmission in mouse. British Journal of Pharmacology 97: 934

Horn R, Patlak J 1980 Single channel currents from excised patches of muscle membrane. Proceedings of the National Academy of Sciences USA 77: 6930

Hubbard J I 1963 Repetitive stimulation at the mammalian neuromuscular junction, and the mobilization of transmitter. Journal of Physiology 169: 641

Hubbard J I 1973 Microphysiology of vertebrate neuromuscular transmission. Physiological Reviews 53: 674

Hubbard J I, Kwanbunbumpen S 1968 Evidence for the vesicle hypothesis. Journal of Physiology 194: 407

Hucho F, Järv J, Weise C 1991 Substrate-binding sites in acetylcholinesterase. Trends in Pharmacological Sciences 12: 422

Hucho F, Oberthür W, Lottspeich F 1986 The ion channel of the nicotinic acetylcholine receptor is formed by the homologous helices M II of the receptor subunits. FEBS Letters 205: 137

Hughes R, Chapple D J 1981 Pharmacology of atracurium: a new competitive neuromuscular blocking drug. British Journal of Anaesthesia 53: 31

Hulsizer S C, Meriney S D, Grinnell A D, Lennon V A 1991 'N'- and 'L'-like calcium currents in lung cancer cells are blocked by Lambert–Eaton IgG. Society of Neuroscience Abstracts 17: 1159

Illes P, Thesleff S 1978 4-Aminopyridine and evoked transmitter release from motor nerve endings. British Journal of Pharmacology 64: 623

Imoto K, Busch C, Sakmann B et al 1988 Rings of negatively charged amino acids determine the acetylcholine receptor channel conductance. Nature 335: 645

Imoto K, Methfessel C, Sakmann B et al 1986 Location of a δ-subunit region determining ion transport through the acetylcholine receptor channel. Nature 324: 670

Ito Y, Miledi R, Vincent A, Newsom-Davis J 1978 Acetylcholine receptors and end-plate electrophysiology in myasthenia gravis. Brain 101: 345

James R W, Kato A C, Rey M J, Fulpius B W 1980 Monoclonal antibodies directed against the neurotransmitter binding site of nicotinic acetylcholine receptor. FEBS Letters 120: 145

Jaramillo F, Schuetze S 1988 Kinetic differences between embryonic- and adult-type acetylcholine receptors in rat myotubes. Journal of Physiology 396: 267

Jenkinson D H 1957 The nature of the antagonism between calcium and magnesium ions at the neuromuscular junction. Journal of Physiology 138: 434

Jenkinson D H 1960 The antagonism between tubocurarine and substances which depolarize the motor end plate. Journal of Physiology 152: 309

Kao P, Dwork A, Kaldany R, Silver M, Weideman J, Stein S, Karlin A 1984 Identification of the α-subunit half cystine specifically labeled by an affinity reagent for the acetylcholine receptor binding site. Journal of Biological Chemistry 259: 11662

Kao P N, Karlin A 1986 Acetylcholine receptor binding site contains a disulfide cross-link between adjacent half-cystinyl residues. Journal of Biological Chemistry 261: 8085

Karlin A 1980 Molecular properties of nicotinic acetylcholine receptors. In: Cotman C W, Poste G, Nicolson G (eds) Cell surface reviews, vol 6, North-Holland Publishing Co. Amsterdam p 191

Karlin A, Holtzman E, Yodh N, Lobel P, Wall J, Hainfield J 1983 The arrangement of the subunits of the acetylcholine receptor of the Torpedo californica. Journal of Biological Chemistry 258: 6678

Katz B 1966 Nerve, muscle and synapse. New York: McGraw-Hill

Katz B 1978 The release of the neuromuscular transmitter and the present state of the vesicular hypothesis. In: Porter R (ed) Studies in neurophysiology. Cambridge: Cambridge University Press

Katz B, Miledi R 1965 The measurement of synaptic delay, and the time course of acetylcholine release at the neuromuscular junction. Proceedings of the Royal Society B161: 483

Katz B, Miledi R 1967a The timing of calcium action during neuromuscular transmission. Journal of Physiology 189: 535

Katz B, Miledi R 1967b A study of synaptic transmission in the absence of nerve impulses. Journal of Physiology 192: 407

Katz B, Miledi R 1968 The role of calcium in neuromuscular facilitation. Journal of Physiology 195: 481

Katz B, Miledi R 1969a Spontaneous and evoked activity of motor nerve endings in calcium ringer. Journal of Physiology 203: 689

Katz B, Miledi R 1969b Tetrodotoxin-resistant electrical activity in presynaptic terminals. Journal of Physiology 203: 459

Katz B, Miledi R 1970 Membrane noise produced by acetylcholine. Nature 226: 962

Katz B, Miledi R 1972 The statistical nature of the acetylcholine potential and its molecular components. Journal of Physiology 224: 665

Katz B, Miledi R 1973a The binding of acetylcholine to receptors and its removal from the synaptic cleft. Journal of Physiology 231: 549

Katz B, Miledi R 1973b The characteristics of 'end-plate noise' produced by different depolarizing drugs. Journal of Physiology 230: 707

Katz B, Miledi R 1975 The effect of procaine on the action of acetylcholine at the neuromuscular junction. Journal of Physiology 249: 269

Katz B, Miledi R 1977a Suppression of transmitter release at the neuromuscular junction. Proceedings of the Royal Society B196: 465

Katz B, Miledi R 1977b The analysis of end-plate noise—a new approach to the study of acetylcholine/receptor interaction. In: Thesleff S (ed) Motor innervation of muscle. Academic, New York, p 31

Katz B, Miledi R 1978 A re-examination of curare action at the motor end-plate. Proceedings of the Royal Society B203: 119

Katz B, Thesleff S 1957 A study of the 'desensitization' produced by acetylcholine at the motor end-plate. Journal of Physiology 138: 63

Kenyon J L, Gibbons W R 1979 4-Aminopyridine and the early outward current of sheep cardiac purkinje fibres. Journal of General Physiology 73: 139

Kharasch E D, Mellow A M, Silinsky 1981 Intracellular magnesium does not antagonize calcium-dependent acetylcholine secretion. Journal of Physiology 314: 255

Kim Y I, Blandino J K W, O'Shaughnessy T J 1993 Inhibitory action of Lambert–Eaton syndrome IgG on N- and L-type calcium currents in a thyroid C-cell line. Annals of the New York Academy of Sciences 681: 398

Kim Y I, Lomo T, Lupa M T, Thesleff S 1984 Miniature end-plate potentials in rat skeletal muscle poisoned with botulinum toxin. Journal of Physiology 356: 587

Kim Y I, Neher E 1988 IgG from patients with Lambert–Eaton syndrome blocks voltage-dependent calcium channels. Science 239: 405

Kim J, Viglione M P, Bradly W A, Kim Y I 1992 Action of Lambert–Eaton syndrome antibodies on voltage-dependent calcium currents and exocytosis in human small-cell lung cancer cells and bovine adrenal chromaffin cells. Journal of Physiology 446: 245P

Kistler J, Stroud R M, Klymkowsky M W, Lalancette R A, Fairclough R H 1982 Structure and function of an acetylcholine receptor. Biophysical Journal 37: 371

Klarsfeld A, Changeux J-P 1985 Activity regulates the levels of acetylcholine receptor α-subunit mRNA in cultured chicken myotubes. Proceedings of the National Academy of Science USA 82: 4558

Kordas M 1969 The effect of membrane polarization on the time course of the end plate current in frog sartorius muscle. Journal of Physiology 204: 493

Kordas M 1970 The effect of procaine on neuromuscular transmission. Journal of Physiology 209: 689

Krejci E, Coussen F, Duval N, Chatel J M, Legay C, Puype M, Vandekerckhove J, Cartaud J, Bon S, Massoulié J 1991 Primary structure of a collagenic tail peptide of *Torpedo* acetylcholinesterase: co-expression with catalytic subunit induces the production of collagen-tailed forms in transfected cells. EMBO Journal 10: 1285

Krnjevic K, Miledi R 1958 Acetylcholine in mammalian neuromuscular transmission. Nature 182: 805

Kubalek E, Ralston S, Lindstrom J, Unwin N 1987 Location of subunits within the acetylcholine receptor by electron image analysis of tubular crystals from *Torpedo marmorata*. Journal of Cell Biology 105: 9

Kubo T, Noda M, Takai T et al 1985 Primary structure of δ subunit precursor of calf muscle acetylcholine receptor deduced from cDNA sequence. European Journal of Biochemistry 149: 5

Kuffler S W, Yoshikami D 1975 The number of transmitter molecules in a quantum: an estimate from iontophoretic application of acetylcholine at the neuromuscular synapse. Journal of Physiology 251: 465

Lacey G, Newsom-Davis J, Vincent A, Whiting P, Wray D 1985 The effect of monoclonal antibodies on the function of mouse acetylcholine receptor. British Journal of Pharmacology 85: 214P

Lambert E H, Elmqvist D 1971 Quantal components of end-plate potentials in the myasthenic syndrome. Annals of the New York Academy of Sciences 183: 183

Lande S 1987 PhD Thesis, University of London

Lang B, Newsom-Davis J, Vincent A 1981 Autoimmune aetiology for myasthenic (Eaton-Lambert) syndrome. The Lancet ii: 224

Lang B, Newsom-Davis J, Prior C, Wray D 1983 Antibodies to nerve terminals: an electrophysiological study of a human myasthenic syndrome transferred to mouse. Journal of Physiology 344: 335

Lang B, Molenaar P C, Newsom-Davis J, Vincent A 1984a Passive transfer of Lambert–Eaton myasthenic syndrome in mice: decreased rates of resting and evoked release of acetylcholine from skeletal muscle. Journal of Neurochemistry 42: 658

Lang B, Newsom-Davis J, Prior C, Wray D 1984b Effect of passively transferred Lambert-Eaton myasthenic syndrome antibodies on the calcium sensitivity of transmitter release in the mouse. Journal of Physiology 357: 28P

Lang B, Newsom-Davis J, Peers C, Wray D 1985 Mechanism of action of human autoantibodies interfering with acetylcholine release in the mouse. Journal of Physiology 365: 79P

Lang B, Newsom-Davis J, Peers C, Prior C, Wray D 1987 The effect of myasthenic syndrome antibody on presynaptic calcium channels in the mouse. Journal of Physiology 390: 257

Lang B, Newsom–Davis J, Peers C, Wray D W 1987b Selective action of Lambert–Eaton myasthenic syndrome antibodies on Ca^{2+} channels in the neuroblastoma × glioma hybrid cell line NG108 15. Journal of Physiology 394: 43p

Lang B, Newsom-Davis J, Wray D 1988 The effect of Lambert–Eaton myasthenic syndrome antibody on slow action potentials in mouse cardiac ventricle. Proceedings of the Royal Society 235: 103

Lee C Y 1972 Chemistry and pharmacology of polypeptide toxins in snake venoms. Annual Review of Pharmacology 12: 265

Lennon V A, Lambert E H 1980 Myasthenia gravis induced by monoclonal antibodies to acetylcholine receptors. Nature 285: 238

Lennon V A, Lambert E H 1981 Monoclonal autoantibodies to acetylcholine receptors: evidence for a dominant idiotype and requirement of complement for pathogenicity. Annals of the New York Academy of Sciences 377: 77

Lennon V A, Lambert E H 1989 Autoantibodies bind solubilized calcium channel-ω-conotoxin complexes from small cell lung carcinoma: a diagnostic aid for Lambert–Eaton myasthenic syndrome. Mayo Clinic Proceedings 64: 1498

Lennon V A, Thompson M, Chen J 1980 Properties of nicotinic acetylcholine receptors isolated by affinity chromatography on monoclonal antibodies. Journal of Biological Chemistry 255: 4395

Lentz T L, Mazurkiewicz J E, Rosenthal J 1977 Cytochemical localization of acetylcholine receptors at the neuromuscular junction by means of horseradish peroxidase-labelled bungarotoxin. Brain Research 132: 423

Leonard R, Labarca C, Charnet P, Davidson N, Lester H 1988 Evidence that the M2 membrane-spanning region lines the ion-channel pore of the nicotinic receptor. Science 242: 1578

Lerrick A J, Wray D, Vincent A, Newsom-Davis J 1983 Electrophysiological effects of myasthenic serum factors studied in mouse muscle. Annals of Neurology 13: 186

Leveque C, Hoshino T, David P et al 1992 The synaptic vesicle protein synaptotagmin associates with calcium channels and is a putative Lambert–Eaton myasthenic syndrome antigen. Proceedings of the National Academy USA 89: 3625

Lev-Tov A, Rahamimoff R 1980 A study of tetanic and post-tetanic potentiation of miniature end-plate potentials at the frog neuromuscular junction. Journal of Physiology 309: 247

Leys K, Lang B, Johnston I, Newsom-Davis J 1991 Calcium channel autoantibodies in the Lambert–Eaton myasthenic syndrome. Annals of Neurology 29: 307

Liley A W 1956 The effects of presynaptic polarization on the spontaneous activity at the mammalian neuromuscular junction. Journal of Physiology 134: 427

Lindstrom J M 1976 Immunological studies of acetylcholine receptors. Journal of Supramolecular Structures 4: 389

Lindstrom J M 1985 Immunobiology of myasthenia gravis, experimental autoimmune myasthenia gravis and Lambert–Eaton syndrome. Annual Review of Immunology 3: 109

Lindstrom J M 1992 Monoclonal antibodies in the study of acetylcholine receptors. In: Vincent A, Wray D (eds) Neuromuscular transmission: basic and applied aspects. Pergamon, Oxford, p 182

Lindstrom J M, Criado M, Hochschwender S, Fox J L, Sarlin V 1984 Immunochemical tests of acetylcholine receptor subunit models. Nature 311: 573

Lindstrom J M, Engel A G, Seybold M E, Lennon V A, Lambert E H 1976a Pathological mechanisms in experimental autoimmune myasthenia gravis. II Passive transfer of experimental autoimmune myasthenia gravis in rats with antiacetylcholine receptor antibodies. Journal of Experimental Medicine 144: 739

Lindstrom J M, Seybold M E, Lennon V A, Whittingham S, Duane D D 1976b Antibody to acetylcholine receptor in myasthenia gravis. Neurology 26: 1054

Lindstrom J M, Tzartos S, Gullick W 1981 Structure and function of the acetylcholine receptor molecule studied using monoclonal antibodies. Annals of the New York Academy of Sciences 377: 1

Lindstrom J M, Tzartos S J, Gullick W et al 1983 Use of monoclonal antibodies to study acetylcholine receptors from electric organs, muscle and brain, and the autoimmune response to receptors in myasthenia gravis. Cold Spring Harbor Symposium in Quantitative Biology 48: 89

Lingle C J, Maconochie D, Steinbach J H 1992 Activation of skeletal muscle nicotinic acetylcholine receptors. Journal of Membrane Biology 126: 195

Llinas R, Blinks J R, Nicholson C 1972 Calcium transient in presynaptic terminal of squid giant synapse: detection with aequorin. Science, New York 176: 1127

Llinas R, Nicholson C 1975 Calcium role in depolarization–secretion coupling: an aequorin study in squid giant synapse. Proceedings of the National Academy of Sciences USA 72: 187

Llinas R, Steinberg I Z, Walton K 1976 Presynaptic calcium currents and their relation to synaptic transmission: voltage clamp study in squid giant synapse and theoretical model for the calcium gate. Proceedings of the National Academy of Sciences USA 73: 2918

Llinas R, Steinberg I Z, Walton K 1981 Relationship between presynaptic calcium current and postsynaptic potential in squid giant synapse. Biophysical Journal 33: 323

Llinas R, Sugimori M, Hillman D E, Cherksey B 1992 Distribution and functional significance of the P-type, voltage-dependent Ca^{2+} channels in the mammalian central nervous system. Trends in Neurosciences 15: 351

Lundh H, Leander S, Thesleff S 1977a Antagonism of the paralysis produced by botulinum toxin in the rat. Journal of Neurobiology 32: 29

Lundh H, Nilsson O, Rosen I 1977b 4-Aminopyridine—a new drug tested in the treatment of Eaton–Lambert syndrome. Journal of Neurology, Neurosurgery and Psychiatry 40: 1109

Lundh H, Thesleff S 1977 The mode of action of 4-aminopyridine and guanidine on transmitter release from motor nerve terminals. European Journal of Pharmacology 42: 411

MacIntosh F C, Collier B 1976 Neurochemistry of cholinergic terminals. In: Zaimis E (ed) Handbook of experimental pharmacology. XLII Neuromuscular junction. Springer, Berlin, p 99

McCrea P D, Popot J-L, Engelman D M 1987 Transmembrane topography of the nicotinic acetylcholine receptor δ subunit. EMBO Journal 6: 3619

MacPhee-Quigley K, Taylor P, Taylor S 1985 Primary structures of the catalytic subunits from two molecular forms of acetylcholinesterase. A comparison of NH2-terminal and active centre sequences. Journal of Biological Chemistry 260: 12185

Maelicke A 1991 Acetylcholine esterase: the structure. Trends in Biochemical Sciences 16: 355

Magleby K L 1973a The effect of repetitive stimulation on facilitation of transmitter release at the frog neuromuscular junction. Journal of Physiology 234: 327

Magleby K L 1973b The effect of tetanic and post-tetanic potentiation on facilitation of transmitter release at the frog neuromuscular junction. Journal of Physiology 234: 353

Magleby K L, Pallotta B S, Terrar D A 1981 The effect of (+)-tubocurarine on neuromuscular transmission during repetitive stimulation in the rat, mouse and frog. Journal of Physiology 312: 97

Magleby K L, Stevens C F 1972 The effect of voltage on the time course of end-plate currents. Journal of Physiology 223: 151

Magleby K L, Zengel J E 1975a A dual effect of repetitive stimulation on post-tetanic potentiation of transmitter release at the frog neuromuscular junction. Journal of Physiology 245: 163

Magleby K L, Zengel J E 1975b A quantitative description of tetanic and post-tetanic potentiation of transmitter release at the frog neuromuscular junction. Journal of Physiology 245: 183

Magleby K L, Zengel J E 1976a Augmentation: a process that acts to increase transmitter release at the frog neuromuscular junction. Journal of Physiology 257: 449

Magleby K L, Zengel J E 1976b Long term changes in augmentation, potentiation and depression of transmitter release as a function of repeated synaptic activity at the frog neuromuscular junction. Journal of Physiology 257: 471

Magleby K L, Zengel J E 1976c Stimulation-induced factors which affect augmentation and potentiation of transmitter release at the neuromuscular junction. Journal of Physiology 260: 687

Magleby K L, Zengel J E 1982 A quantitative description of stimulation-induced changes in transmitter release at the frog neuromuscular junction. Journal of General Physiology 80: 613

Marraud M, Demange P, Cung M-T, Tsikaris V, Sakarellos C, Vazaki E, Tzartos S J 1992 Sequence-specific peptides for probing receptors and ion-channel functions. Biochemical Society Transactions 20: 837

Marshall I G, Agoston S, Booij L H D J, Durant N N, Foldes F F 1980 Pharmacology of Org NC45 compared with other non-depolarizing blocking drugs. British Journal of Anaesthesia 52: 113

Marshall I G, Gibb A J, Durant N N 1983 Neuromuscular and vagal blocking actions of pancuronium bromide, its metabolites, and vecuronium bromide (Org NC45) and its potential metabolites in the anaesthetized cat. British Journal of Anaesthesia 55: 703

Marshall L G, Parsons S M 1987 The vesicular acetylcholine transport system. Trends in Neurosciences 10: 174

Martin A R 1966 Quantal nature of synaptic transmission. Physiological Reviews 46: 51

Martin A R, Orkand R K 1961 Postsynaptic action of HC-3 on neuromuscular transmission. Federation Proceedings 20: 579

Massoulié J, Toutant J-P 1988 Vertebrate cholinesterases: structure and types of interaction. In Whittaker V P (ed) Handbook of experimental pharmacology. The cholinergic synapse. Springer, Berlin, p 167

Matthews-Bellinger J, Salpeter M M 1978 Distribution of acetylcholine receptors at frog neuromuscular junctions with a discussion of some physiological implications. Journal of Physiology 279: 197

Merlie J P, Isenberg K E, Russel S D, Sanes J R 1984

Denervation supersensitivity in skeletal muscle: analysis with a cloned cDNA probe. Journal of Cell Biology 99: 332

Merlie J P, Sanes J R 1985 Concentration of acetylcholine receptor mRNA in synaptic regions of adult muscle fibres. Nature 317: 66

Meves H, Pichon Y 1977 The effects of internal and external 4-aminopyridine on the potassium-currents in intracellularly perfused squid giant axons. Journal of Physiology 268: 511

Middlebrook J L 1989 Cell surface receptors for protein toxins. In Simpson L L (ed) Botulinum neurotoxin and tetanus toxin. Academic, San Diego, p 95

Mihovilovic M, Richman D P 1987 Monoclonal antibodies as probes of the α-bungarotoxin and cholinergic binding regions of the acetylcholine receptor. Journal of Biological Chemistry 262: 4978

Miledi R 1960a Junctional and extra-junctional acetylcholine receptors in skeletal muscle fibres. Journal of Physiology 151: 24

Miledi R 1960b The acetylcholine sensitivity of frog muscle fibres after complete or partial denervation. Journal of Physiology 151: 1

Miledi R 1973 Transmitter release induced by injection of calcium ions into nerve terminals. Proceedings of the Royal Society B183: 421

Miledi R, Molenaar P C, Polak R L 1980 The effect of lanthanum ions on acetylcholine in frog muscles. Journal of Physiology 309: 199

Miledi R, Molenaar P C, Polak R L 1982 Free and bound acetylcholine in frog muscle. Journal of Physiology 333: 189

Miledi R, Molenaar P C, Polak R L 1983 Electrophysiological and chemical determination of acetylcholine release at the frog neuromuscular junction. Journal of Physiology 334: 245

Miledi R, Parker I 1981 Calcium transients recorded with arsenazo III in the presynaptic terminal of the squid giant synapse. Proceedings of the Royal Society B212: 197

Miledi R, Thies R 1971 Tetanic and post-tetanic rise in frequency of miniature end-plate potentials in low-calcium solutions. Journal of Physiology 212: 245

Mishina M, Kurosaki T, Tobimatsu T et al 1984 Expression of functional acetylcholine receptor from cloned cDNAs. Nature 307: 604

Mishina M, Takai T, Imoto K et al 1986 Molecular distinction between foetal and adult forms of muscle acetylcholine receptor. Nature 321: 406

Mishina M, Tobimatsu T, Imoto K et al 1985 Location of functional regions of acetylcholine receptor α subunit by site-directed mutagenesis. Nature 313: 364

Misler S, Hurlbut W P 1983 Post-tetanic potentiation of acetylcholine release at the frog neuromuscular junction develops after stimulation in Ca^{2+}-free solutions. Proceedings of the National Academy of Sciences USA 80: 315

Mitra A K, McCarthy M P, Stroud R M 1989 Three-dimensional structure of the nicotinic acetylcholine receptor and localisation of the major associated 43 KD cytoskeletal protein determined at 22 Å by low dose electron microscopy and X-ray diffraction to 12.5 Å. Journal of Cell Biology 109: 755

Mizoguchi A, Arakawa M, Masutani M et al 1992 Localization of smg p25A/rab3A p25, a small GTP-binding protein, at the active zone of the rat neuromuscular junction. Biochemical and Biophysical Research Communications 186: 1345

Mochly-Rosen D, Fuchs S 1981 Monoclonal anti-acetylcholine-receptor antibodies directed against the cholinergic binding site. Biochemistry 20: 5920

Molgo J, Lemeignan J, Lechat P 1977 Effects of 4-aminopyridine at the frog neuromuscular junction. Journal of Pharmacology and Experimental Therapeutics 203: 653

Molgo J, Lemeignan M, Lechat P 1979 Analysis of the action of 4-aminopyridine during repetitive stimulation at the neuromuscular junction. European Journal of Pharmacology 53: 307

Molgo J E, Lundh H, Thesleff S 1980 Potency of 3,4 diaminopyridine and 4-aminopyridine on mammalian neuromuscular transmission and the effect of pH changes. European Journal of Pharmacology 61: 25

Momoi M Y, Lennon V A 1982 Purification and biochemical characterization of nicotinic acetylcholine receptors of human muscle. Journal of Biological Chemistry 257: 12757

Moss S J, Darlison M G, Beeson D M W, Barnard E A 1989 Developmental expression of the genes encoding the four subunits of the chicken muscle acetylcholine receptor. Journal of Biological Chemistry 264: 20199

Mulac-Jericevic B, Atassi M Z 1986 Segment α182-198 of Torpedo californica acetylcholine receptor contains a second toxin-binding region and binds anti-receptor antibodies. FEBS Letters 199: 68

Mulrine N K, Ogden D C 1988 The equilibrium open probability of nicotinic ion channels at the rat neuromuscular junction. Journal of Physiology 401: 95P

Murray N M F, Newsom-Davis J 1981 Treatment with oral 4-aminopyridine in disorders of neuromuscular transmission. Neurology (NY) 31: 256

Murray N M F, Newsom-Davis J, Karni Y, Wiles C M 1984 Oral 3,4 diaminopyridine in the treatment of the Lambert–Eaton myasthenic syndrome. Journal of Neurology, Neurosurgery and Psychiatry 47: 1052

Nagel A, Engel A G, Lang B, Newsom-Davis J, Fukuoka T 1988 Lambert–Eaton syndrome IgG depletes presynaptic active zone particles by antigenic modulation. Annals of Neurology 24: 552

Narahashi T, Moore J W, Scott W R 1964 Tetrodotoxin blockage of sodium conductance increase in lobster giant axons. Journal of General Physiology 47: 965

Nastuk W L, Manthey A A, Gissen A J 1966 Activation and inactivation of postjunctional membrane receptors. Annals of the New York Academy of Sciences 137: 999

Neher E, Sakmann B 1976a Single channel currents recorded from membrane of denervated frog muscle fibres. Nature 260: 799

Neher E, Sakmann B 1976b Noise analysis of drug induced voltage clamp currents in denervated frog muscle fibres. Journal of Physiology 258: 705

Neher E, Steinbach J H 1978 Local anaesthetics transiently block currents through single acetylcholine-receptor channels. Journal of Physiology 277: 153

Neher E, Stevens C F 1977 Conductance fluctuations and ionic pores in membranes. Annual Review of Biophysics and Bioengineering 6: 345

Neumann D, Barchan D, Safran A, Gershoni J M, Fuchs S 1986a Mapping of the α-bungarotoxin binding site within the α-subunit on the acetylcholine receptor. Proceedings of the National Academy of Sciences USA 83: 3008

Neumann D, Barchan D, Fridkin M, Fuchs S 1986b Analysis of ligand binding to the synthetic dodecapeptide 185–196 of the acetylcholine receptor α-subunit.

Proceedings of the National Academy of Sciences USA 83: 9250

Newsom-Davis J 1982 Autoimmune diseases of neuromuscular transmission. Clinics in Immunology and Allergy 2: 405

Newsom-Davis J, Murray N M F 1984 Plasma exchange and immunosuppressive drug treatment in the Lambert–Eaton myasthenic syndrome. Neurology 34: 480

Newsom-Davis J, Murray N, Wray D et al 1982 Lambert–Eaton myasthenic syndrome: electrophysiological evidence for a humoral factor. Muscle and Nerve 5: S17

Nilius B, Hess P, Lansman J B, Tsien R W 1985 A novel type of cardiac calcium channel in ventricular cells. Nature 316: 433

Noda M, Furutani Y, Takahashi H et al 1983c Cloning and sequence analysis of calf cDNA and human genoic DNA encoding α-subunit precursor of muscle acetylcholine receptor. Nature 305: 818

Noda M, Takahashi H, Tanake T et al 1982 Primary structure of α-subunit precursor of Torpedo californica acetylcholine receptor deduced from cDNA sequence. Nature 299: 793

Noda M, Takahashi H, Tanake T et al 1983a Primary structures of β- and δ-subunit precursors of Torpedo californica acetylcholine receptor deduced from cDNA sequences. Nature 301: 251

Noda M, Takahashi H, Tanabe T et al 1983b Structural homology of Torpedo californica acetylcholine receptor subunits. Nature 302: 528

Nowycky M C, Fox A P, Tsien R W 1985 Three types of neuronal calcium channel with different calcium agonist selectivity. Nature 316: 440

Oberthür W, Muhn P, Baumann H, Lottspeich F, Wittmann-Liebold B, Hucho F 1986 The reaction site of a non-competitive antagonist in the δ-subunit of the nicotinic acetylcholine receptor. EMBO Journal 5: 1815

Ogden D C, Colquhoun D 1985 Ion channel block by acetylcholine, carbachol and suberyldicholine at the frog neuromuscular junction. Proceedings of the Royal Society B225: 329

Ogden D C, Siegelbaum S A, Colquhoun D 1981 Block of acetylcholine-activated ion channels by an uncharged local anaesthetic. Nature 289: 596

Ohana B, Gershoni J M 1990 Comparison of the toxin binding sites of the nicotinic acetylcholine receptor from Drosophila to human. Biochemistry 29: 6409

O'Neill J H, Murray N M F, Newsom-Davis J 1988 The Lambert–Eaton myasthenic syndrome, a review of 50 cases. Brain 111: 577

Oosterhuis H J, Newsom–Davis J, Wokke J H et al 1987. The slow channel syndrome. Two new cases. Brain 110: 1061

Papadouli I, Potamianos S, Hadjidakis I et al 1990 Antigenic role of single residues within the main immunogenic region of the nicotinic acetylcholine receptor. Biochemical Journal 269: 239

Patrick J, Lindstrom J 1973 Autoimmune response to acetylcholine receptor. Science 180: 871

Payne J P, Hughes R 1981 Evaluation of atracurium in anaesthetized man. British Journal of Anaesthesia 53: 45

Pearson H A, Wray D 1993 Non-competitive antagonism of calcium by magnesium ions at the K+-depolarised mouse neuromuscular junction. European Journal of Pharmacology 236: 323

Pedersen S E, Brigman P C, Sharp S D, Cohen J B 1990 Identification of a cytoplasmic region of the Torpedo nicotinic acetylcholine receptor α subunit by epitope mapping. Journal of Biological Chemistry 265: 569

Pedersen S E, Cohen J B 1990 d-Tubocurarine binding sites are localised at α-γ and α-δ subunit interfaces of the nicotinic acetylcholine receptor. Proceedings of the National Academy of Sciences USA 87: 2785

Pedersen S E, Dreyer E B, Cohen J B 1986 Location of ligand binding sites on the nicotinic acetylcholine receptor α-subunit. Journal of Biological Chemistry 261: 13735

Peers C, Johnston I, Lang B, Wray D 1993 Cross-linking of presynaptic calcium channels: a mechanism of action for Lambert–Eaton myasthenic syndrome antibodies at the mouse neuromuscular junction. Neuroscience Letters 153: 45

Peers C, Lang B, Newsom-Davis J, Wray D W 1990 Selective action of myasthenic syndrome antibodies on calcium channels in a rodent neuroblastoma × glioma cell line. Journal of Physiology 421: 293

Penner R, Dreyer F 1986 Two different presynaptic calcium currents in mouse motor nerve terminals. Pflügers Archives 406: 190

Perin M S, Brose N, Jahn R, Südhof T C 1991 Domain structure of synaptotagmin (p65). Journal of Biological Chemistry 266: 623

Petrenko A G, Perin M S, Davletov B A, Ushkaryov Y A, Geppert M, Südhof T C 1991 Binding of synaptotagmin to the α-latrotoxin receptor implicates both in synaptic vesicle exocytosis. Nature 353: 65

Porter C W, Barnard E A 1975 The density of cholinergic receptors at the end-plate postsynaptic membrane: ultrastructural studies in two mammalian species. Journal of Membrane Biology 20: 31

Porter C W, Barnard E A 1976 Ultrastructural studies on the acetylcholine receptor at the motor end plates of normal and pathologic muscles. Annals of the New York Academy of Sciences 274: 85

Porter C W, Barnard E A, Chiu T H 1973 The ultrastructural localization and quantitation of cholinergic receptors at the mouse end-plate. Journal of Membrane Biology 14: 383

Potter L T 1970 Synthesis, storage and release of [14C] acetylcholine in isolated rat diaphragm muscles. Journal of Physiology 206: 145

Prior C, Lang B, Wray D, Newsom-Davis J 1985 Action of Lambert–Eaton myasthenic syndrome IgG at mouse motor nerve terminals. Annals of Neurology 17: 587

Pumplin D W, Reese T S, Llinas R 1981 Are the presynaptic membrane particles the calcium channels? Proceedings of the National Academy of Sciences USA 78: 7210

Raftery M A, Hunkapiller M W, Strader C D, Hood L E 1980 Acetylcholine receptor: complex of homologous subunits. Science 208: 1454

Rahamimoff R 1968 A dual effect of calcium ions on neuromuscular facilitation. Journal of Physiology 195: 471

Ralston S, Sarin V, Thanh H L, Rivier J, Fox L, Lindstrom J 1987 Synthetic peptides used to locate the α-bungarotoxin binding site and immunogenic regions on α subunits of the nicotinic acetylcholine receptor. Biochemistry 26: 3261

Rang H P 1975 Acetylcholine receptors. Quarterly Reviews of Biophysics 7: 283

Rash J E, Albuquerque E X, Hudson C S, Mayer R F, Sattersfield 1976 Studies on human myasthenia gravis: electrophysiological and ultrastructural evidence compatible with antibody attachment to acetylcholine receptor complex. Proceedings of the National Academy of Sciences USA 73: 4584

Ratnam M, Lindstrom J 1984 Structural features of the nicotinic acetylcholine receptor revealed by autoantibodies to synthetic peptides. Biochemical and Biophysical Research Communications 122: 1225

Ratnam M, Sargent P B, Sarin V, Fox J L, Le Nguyen D, Rivier J, Criado M, Lindstrom J 1986a Location of antigenic determinants on primary sequences of subunits of nicotinic acetylcholine receptor by peptide mapping. Biochemistry 25: 2621

Ratnam M, Le Nguyen D, Rivier J, Sargent P B, Lindstrom J 1986b Transmembrane topography of nicotinic acetylcholine receptor: immunochemical tests contradict theoretical predictions based on hydrophobicity profiles. Biochemistry 25: 2633

Reiness C G, Weinberg C B 1978 Antibody to acetylcholine receptor increases degradation of junctional and extrajunctional receptors in adult muscle. Nature 274: 68

Reuter H 1983 Calcium channel modulation by neurotransmitters, enzymes and drugs. Nature 301: 569

Reuter H, Porzig H, Kokubun S, Prod'hom B 1985 1,4-Dihydropyridines as tools in the study of Ca^{2+} channels. Trends in Neurosciences 8: 396

Revah F, Bertrand D, Galazi J L et al 1991 Mutations in the channel domain alter desensitization of a neuronal nicotinic receptor. Nature 353: 846

Revah F, Galazi J L, Giraudat J, Haumont P Y, Lederer F, Changeux J P 1990 The noncompetitive blocker [³H] chlorpromazine labels three amino acids of the acetylcholine receptor γ-subunit: implications for the α-helical organisation of regions MII and for the structure of the ion channel. Proceedings of the National Academy of Sciences USA 87: 4675

Roberts A, Perera S, Lang B, Vincent A, Newsom-Davis J 1985 Paraneoplastic myasthenic syndrome IgG inhibits $^{45}Ca^{2+}$ flux in a human small cell carcinoma line. Nature 317: 737

Rosenfeld M R, Wong E, Dalmau J, Manley G, Egan D, Posner J B, Sher E, Furneaux H M 1993 Sera from patients with Lambert–Eaton myasthenic syndrome recognize the β-subunit of Ca^{2+} channel complexes. Annals of the New York Academy of Sciences 681: 408

Ruff R L 1977 A quantitative analysis of local anaesthetic alteration of miniature end-plate currents and end-plate current fluctuations. Journal of Physiology 264: 89

Sachs F 1983 Is the acetylcholine receptor a unit-conductance channel? In: Sakmann B, Neher E (eds) Single channel recording. Plenum, New York, p 365

Saedi M S, Anand R, Conroy W G, Lindstrom J 1990 Determination of amino acids critical to the main immunogenic region of intact acetylcholine receptor by in vitro mutagenesis. FEBS Letters 267: 55

Sahashi K, Engel A G, Lindstrom J M, Lambert E H, Lennon V A 1978 Ultrastructural localization of immune complexes (IgG and C3) at the end plate in experimental autoimmune myasthenia gravis. Journal of Neuropathology and Experimental Neurology 37: 212

Sakmann B, Methfessel C, Mishina M et al 1985 Role of acetylcholine receptor subunits in gating of the channel. Nature 318: 538

Sakmann B, Neher E 1983 Single channel recording. Plenum, New York

Sakmann B, Neher E 1984 Patch clamp techniques for studying ionic channels in excitable membranes. Annual Review of Physiology 46: 455

Sakmann B, Patlak J, Neher E 1980 Single acetylcholine-activated channels show burst-kinetics in presence of desensitizing concentrations of agonist. Nature 286: 71

Sano K, Enomoto K, Maeno T 1987 Effects of synthetic ω-conotoxin, a new type Ca^{2+} antagonist, on frog and mouse neuromuscular transmission. European Journal of Pharmacology 141: 235

Schiavo G, Benfenati F, Poulain B et al 1992 Tetanus and botulinum-B neurotoxins block neurotransmitter release by proteolytic cleavage of synaptobrevin. Nature 359: 832

Schumacher M, Camp S, Maulet Y et al 1986 Primary structure of *Torpedo californica* acetylcholinesterase deduced from its cDNA sequence. Nature 319: 407

Sellin L C 1985 The pharmacological mechanism of botulism. Trends in Pharmacological Sciences 6: 80

Sher E, Carbone E, Clementi F 1993 Neuronal calcium channels as a target for Lambert–Eaton myasthenic syndrome autoantibodies. Annals of the New York Academy of Sciences 681: 373

Sher E, Gotti C, Canal N, Scoppetta C, Piccolo G, Evoli A, Clementi F 1989 Specificity of calcium channel autoantibodies in Lambert–Eaton myasthenic syndrome. Lancet (ii): 640

Sher E, Pandiella A, Clementi F 1990 Voltage operated calcium channels in small cell lung carcinoma cell lines: pharmacological, functional and immunological properties. Cancer Research 50: 3892

Shibahara S, Kubo T, Perski H, Takahashi M, Noda M, Numa S 1985 Cloning and sequence analysis of human genomic DNA encoding γ subunit precursor of muscle acetylcholine receptor. European Journal of Biochemistry 146: 15

Silinsky E M 1985 The biophysical pharmacology of calcium-dependent acetylcholine secretion. Pharmacological Reviews 37: 81

Simpson L L 1980 Kinetic studies on the interaction between botulinum toxin type A and the cholinergic neuromuscular junction. Journal of Pharmacological and Experimental Therapeutics 212: 16

Sine S M, Steinbach J H 1984 Agonists block currents through acetylcholine receptor channels. Biophysics Journal 46: 277

Sine S M, Steinbach J H 1987 Activation of acetylcholine receptors on clonal mammalian BC3H-1 cells by high concentrations of agonist. Journal of Physiology 385: 325

Soreq H, Gnatt A, Loewenstein Y, Neville L F 1992 Excavations into the active-site gorge of cholinesterases. Trends in Biochemical Sciences 17: 353

Spedding M, Paoletti R 1992 Classification of calcium channels and the sites of action of drugs modifying channel function. Pharmacological Reviews 44: 363

Stanley E F, Drachman D B 1978 Effect of myasthenic immunoglobulin on acetylcholine receptors on intact mammalian neuromuscular junctions. Science 200: 1285

Stevens C F 1985 AChR structure: a new twist in the story. Trends in Neurosciences 79: 1

Südhof T C, Jahn R 1991 Proteins of synaptic vesicles involved in exocytosis and membrane recycling. Neuron 6: 665

Sumikawa K, Houghton M, Smith J C, Richards B M, Barnard E A 1982 The molecular cloning and characterization of cDNA coding for the α-subunit of the acetylcholine receptor. Nucleic Acids Research 10: 5809

Sussman J L, Harel M, Frolow F et al 1991 Atomic structure of acetylcholinesterase from *Torpedo californica*; a prototypic acetylcholine-binding protein. Science 253: 872

Takai T, Noda M, Furutani Y et al 1984 Primary structure of γ subunit precursor of calf-muscle acetylcholine receptor deduced from the cDNA sequence. European Journal of Biochemistry 143: 109

Takai T, Noda M, Mishina M et al 1985 Cloning, sequencing and expression of cDNA for a novel subunit of acetylcholine receptor from calf muscle. Nature 315: 761

Takeda K, Trautmann A 1984 A patch clamp study of the partial agonist actions of tubocurarine on rat myotubes. Journal of Physiology 349: 353

Takeuchi A, Takeuchi N 1959 Active phase of frog's end-plate potential. Journal of Neurophysiology 22: 395

Takeuchi A, Takeuchi N 1960 On the permeability of end-plate membrane during the action of transmitter. Journal of Physiology 154: 52

Tanabe N, Kijima H 1992 Ca^{2+}-dependent and independent components of transmitter release at the frog neuromuscular junction. Journal of Physiology 455: 271

Tanabe T, Noda M, Furutani Y et al 1984 Primary structure of β subunit precursor of calf muscle acetylcholine receptor deduced from cDNA sequence. European Journal of Biochemistry 144: 11

Tauc L 1983 Nonvesicular release of neurotransmitter. Physiological Reviews 62: 857

Tauc L, Poulain B 1991 Vesigate hypothesis of neurotransmitter release explains the formation of quanta by a non-vesicular mechanism. Physiological Research 40: 279

Taylor P, Schumacher M, Maulet Y, Newton M 1986 A molecular perspective on the polymorphism of acetylcholinesterase. Trends in Pharmacological Sciences 7: 321

Thesleff S 1980 Aminopyridines and synaptic transmission. Neuroscience 5: 1413

Thesleff S 1982 Spontaneous transmitter release in experimental neuromuscular disorders of the rat. Muscle and Nerve 5: S12

Thies R E, Brooks V B 1961 Postsynaptic neuromuscular block produced by hemicholinium no. 3 Federation Proceedings 20: 569

Toyka K V, Birnberger K L, Anzil A P, Schlegel C, Besinger U, Struppler A 1978 Myasthenia gravis: further electrophysiological and ultrastructural analysis of transmission failure in the mouse passive transfer model. Journal of Neurology, Neurosurgery and Psychiatry 41: 746

Toyka K V, Drachman D B, Griffin D E et al 1977 Myasthenia gravis. Study of humoral immune mechanisms by passive transfer to mice. New England Journal of Medicine 296: 125

Trautmann A 1982 Curare can open and block ion channels associated with cholinergic receptors. Nature 298: 272

Tse C K, Dolly J O, Hambleton P, Wray D, Melling J 1982 Preparation and characterization of homogeneous neurotoxin type A from Clostridium botulinum. Its inhibitory action on neuronal release of acetylcholine in the absence and presence of β-bungarotoxin. European Journal of Biochemistry 122: 493

Tse C K, Wray D, Melling J, Dolly J O 1986 Actions of β-bungarotoxin on spontaneous release of transmitter at muscle end-plates treated with botulinum toxin. Toxicon 24: 123

Tsien R W 1983 Calcium channels in excitable cell membranes. Annual Reviews of Physiology 45: 351

Tsim K W K, Randall W R, Barnard E A 1988 Synaptic acetylcholinesterase of chicken muscle changes during development from a hybrid to a homogeneous enzyme. EMBO Journal 7: 2451

Tzartos S J 1984 Monoclonal antibodies as probes of the acetylcholine receptor and myasthenia gravis. Trends in Biochemical Sciences 9: 63

Tzartos S J, Cung M T, Demange P et al 1991 The main immunogenic region (MIR) of the nicotinic acetylcholine receptor and the anti-MIR antibodies. Molecular Neurobiology 5: 1

Tzartos S J, Kokla A, Walgrave S L, Conti-Tronconi B M 1988 Localisation of the main immunogenic region of human muscle acetylcholine receptor to residues 67–76 of the α subunit. Proceedings of the National Academy of Sciences USA 85: 2899

Tzartos S J, Lindstrom J M 1980 Monoclonal antibodies used to probe acetylcholine receptor structure: localization of the main immunogenic region and detection of similarities between subunits. Proceedings of the National Academy of Sciences USA 77: 755

Tzartos S J, Rand D E, Einarson B L, Lindstrom J M 1981 Mapping of surface structures of electrophorus acetylcholine receptor using monoclonal antibodies. Journal of Biological Chemistry 256: 8635

Tzartos S J, Remoundos M S 1990 Fine localisation of the major α-bungarotoxin binding site to residues α 189–195 of the Torpedo acetylcholine receptor. Journal of Biological Chemistry 265: 21462

Uchitel O D, Protti D A, Sanchez V, Cherksey B D, Sugimori M, Llinas R 1992 P-type voltage-dependent calcium channel mediates presynaptic calcium influx and transmitter release in mammalian synapses. Proceedings of the National Academy of Sciences USA 89: 3330

Unwin N 1989 The structure of ion channels in membranes of excitable cells. Neuron 3: 665

Unwin N, Toyoshima C, Kubalek E 1988 Arrangement of the acetylcholine receptor subunits in the resting and desensitized states, determined by cryoelectron microscopy of crystallised Torpedo post-synaptic membranes. Journal of Cell Biology 107: 1123

Varanda W A, Aracava Y, Sherby S M, VanMeter W G, Eldefrawi M E, Albuquerque E X 1985 The acetylcholine receptor of the neuromuscular junction recognizes mecamylamine as a noncompetitive antagonist. Molecular Pharmacology 28: 128

Veldesema-Currie R D, Labruyere W T, Langmeuer M W E 1984 Depletion of total acetylcholine by hemicholinium-3 in isolated rat diaphragm is less in the presence of dexamethasone. Brain Research 324: 305

Viglione M P, Creutz C E, Kim Y I 1992 Lambert–Eaton syndrome: antigen–antibody interaction and calcium current inhibition in chromaffin cells. Muscle and Nerve 15: 1325

Viglione M P, Blandino J K W, Kim S J, Kim Y I 1993 Effects of Lambert–Eaton syndrome serum and IgG on calcium and sodium currents in small-cell lung cancer cells. Annals of the New York Academy of Sciences 681: 418

Vincent A 1983 Acetylcholine receptors and myasthenia gravis. Clinics in Endocrinology and Metabolism 12: 57

Vincent A, Wray D (eds) 1992 Neuromuscular transmission: basic and applied aspects. Pergamon, Oxford

Wan K K, Lindstrom J M 1985 Effects of monoclonal antibodies on the function of acetylcholine receptors purified from Torpedo californica and reconstituted into vesicles. Biochemistry 24: 1212

Whiting P, Vincent A, Newsom-Davis J 1985a Monoclonal antibodies to Torpedo acetylcholine receptor.

Characterization of antigenic determinants within the cholinergic binding site. European Journal of Biochemistry 150: 533

Whiting P J, Vincent A, Newsom-Davis J 1985b Monoclonal antibodies to the human acetylcholine receptor. Biochemical Society Transactions 13: 116

Wilson P T, Lenz T L, Hawrot E 1985 Determination of the primary amino acid sequence specifying the α-bungarotoxin binding site on the α-subunit of the acetylcholine receptor from *Torpedo californica*. Proceedings of the National Academy of Sciences USA 82: 8790

Witzemann V, Brenner H R, Sakmann B 1991 Neural factors regulate AChR subunit mRNAs at rat neuromuscular synapses. Journal of Cell Biology 114: 125

Wray D 1978a Frequency of opening of channels by depolarizing drugs. Journal of Physiology 284: 149P

Wray D 1978b End-plate voltage noise during prolonged application of acetylcholine in cat tenuissimus muscle. Journal of Physiology 278: 4P

Wray D 1980 Noise analysis and channels at the postsynaptic membrane of skeletal muscle. Progress in Drug Research 24: 9

Wray D 1981a The action of mecamylamine at the postsynaptic channels of cat skeletal muscle: noise analysis. British Journal of Pharmacology 74: 248P

Wray D 1981b Prolonged exposure to acetylcholine: noise analysis and channel inactivation in cat tenuissimus muscle. Journal of Physiology 310: 37

Wray D 1992 The Lambert–Eaton myasthenic syndrome. In: Vincent A, Wray D (eds) Neuromuscular transmission: basic and applied aspects. Pergamon, Oxford, p 249

Wray D, Peers C, Lang B, Lande S, Newsom-Davis J 1987 Interference with calcium channels in the Lambert–Eaton myasthenic syndrome. Annals of the New York Academy of Sciences 505: 368

Wray D, Prior C, Newsom-Davis J, Lang B 1984 Site of action of Lambert–Eaton myasthenic syndrome antibodies at mouse nerve terminals. IUPHAR 9th International Congress of Pharmacology Proceedings 2: 349

Wray D, Porter V 1993 Calcium channel types at the neuromuscular junction. Annals of the New York Academy of Sciences 681: 356

Young E F, Ralston E, Blake J, Ramachandran J, Hall Z W, Stroud R M 1985 Topological mapping of acetylcholine receptor: evidence for a model with five transmembrane segments and a cytoplasmic COOH-terminal peptide. Proceedings of the National Academy of Sciences USA 82: 626

Zaimis E 1953 Motor end plate differences as a determining factor in the mode of action of neuromuscular blocking substances. Journal of Physiology 122: 238

Zaimis E, Head S 1976 Depolarizing neuromuscular blocking drugs. In: Zaimis E (ed) Handbook of experimental pharmacology XLII. Neuromuscular junction. Springer, Berlin, p 365

Zaimis E, Wray D 1981 General physiology and pharmacology of neuromuscular transmission. In: Walton J (ed) Disorders of voluntary muscle, 4th edn. Churchill Livingstone, Edinburgh, p 76

Zengel J E, Magleby K L 1981 Changes in miniature end-plate potential frequency during repetitive nerve stimulation in the presence of Ca^{2+}, Ba^{2+} and Sr^{2+} at the frog neuromuscular junction. Journal of General Physiology 77: 503

Zingsheim H P, Barrantes F J, Frank F, Hanike W, Nehgebauer D C 1982 Direct structural localization of two toxin recognition sites on an ACh receptor protein. Nature 299: 81

Zucker R S 1989 Short-term synaptic plasticity. Annual Review of Neuroscience 12: 13

6. Biochemical aspects of muscular structure and function

J. Gergely

INTRODUCTION*

All cells of the organism utilise more or less the same metabolic pathways to use chemical energy — more precisely, free energy as discussed below — that is available in foodstuff to produce adenosine triphosphate (ATP) which then serves as the immediate energy source for various cell functions. What distinguishes muscle from many other tissues is the close relationship between the energy transducing and energy utilising systems; we have known for about 50 years that one component of the contractile machinery — myosin — is also the enzyme (myosin ATPase, EC 3.6.1.32) that hydrolyses ATP and that in the process the transduction of chemical into mechanical energy is achieved.

In this chapter the emphasis is on those structures, components and processes that are characteristic of muscle and relate to contraction, relaxation and their control. Some structural and physiological aspects are covered in Chapters 1 and 3, and features of the cell membrane in Chapter 10. Many excellent textbooks of biochemistry provide a general background to metabolic pathways, protein structure and membrane architecture. Two recent texts (Alberts et al 1989, Darnell et al 1990) orientated towards cell biology may be especially useful for readers interested in obtaining, or as the case may be, brushing up on, an integrated picture.

---

* Readers interested in obtaining more information on topics covered in this chapter and on related matters may wish to consult the following reviews: Needham 1971, Jolesz & Sreter 1981, Squire 1981, 1986, Small et al 1992, Sweeney et al 1993, Strynadka & James 1991, Holmes & Kabsch 1991, Grabarek et al 1992, El-Saleh et al 1986, Pette & Staron 1990, Pette & Vrbova 1992, Zot & Potter 1987, Ashley et al 1991, Geeves 1991, Engel & Banker 1993.

ENERGY METABOLISM

Carbohydrate metabolism

General. Glucose entering the muscle cell is either used immediately or is stored in the form of glycogen which is broken down according to the energy requirements of the muscle. The breakdown may occur, depending on the conditions, either essentially anaerobically — i.e. without oxygen — going as far as lactic acid, or it may continue with the participation of oxygen to complete the breakdown to CO_2 and water. In muscles where sudden demands on energy may arise, the anaerobic pathway is predominant and the lactic acid formed is carried by the blood stream to the liver where it is partly oxidised, partly resynthesised to glycogen (Cori 1941). In other muscles, such as cardiac muscle, where there is a slower but steady activity, the complete oxidative breakdown plays a greater part.

Anaerobic glycogen metabolism. The breakdown of glycogen involves the enzyme phosphorylase, the reaction being:

Glycogen + phosphate → glucose-1-phosphate

Phosphorylase is itself a complex enzyme system, the structure, function and regulation of which have been clarified through extensive research taking its origin in the work of the Coris (Cori & Cori 1945). As it now appears, phosphorylase can exist in an inactive form, phosphorylase *b*, and an active form, phosphorylase *a* (see e.g. Fischer et al 1971, Krebs 1972) (Fig. 6.1). The *b* → *a* transformation is effected by ATP-dependent phosphorylation catalysed by phosphorylase kinase (EC 2.7.1.38), while the reconversion of phosphorylase *a* to *b* is catalysed by phosphorylase phosphatase (EC 3.1.3.17). Phosphorylase kinase contains four different subunits, one of which has been identified (Cohen et al 1978) with the ubiquitous Ca^{2+}-binding protein, calmodulin, which participates in the regulation of numerous cellular processes (for a review see Klee & Vanaman 1982). The calmodulin subunit of phosphorylase kinase is presumably the site of binding of the activating Ca^{2+} which is released from the sarcoplasmic reticulum (see below) when muscle contraction is initiated. Phosphorylase kinase also exists in an active and an inactive form, and, again, inactivation is brought about by phosphorylation, catalysed in this case by a cyclic adenosine monophosphatase-(AMP)-dependent protein kinase. The production from ATP of cyclic AMP — now recognised as a key mediator in many regulatory processes — is catalysed by an enzyme, adenylate cyclase (EC 4.6.1.1), which is under the influence of hormones (glucagon) and neurohumoral agents (e.g. adrenaline).

The conversion of glucose into glycogen depends on a distinct enzyme system — glycogen synthase (or glycogen (starch) synthase, EC 2.4.1.11) — involving UTP and the coenzyme

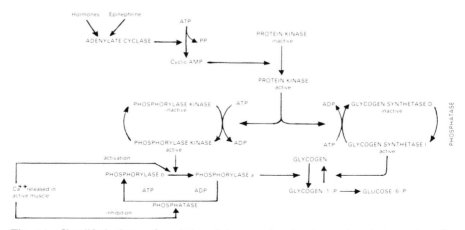

Fig. 6.1 Simplified scheme of regulation of glycogen phosphorylase and synthetase system. For details see text.

uridine diphosphate glucose (UDPG). Glycogen synthetase also exists in two interconvertible forms of differing activity, D and I. In the case of both the glycogen phosphorylase and synthase the state of phosphorylation is regulated by phosphatases, which in turn are controlled in a complex way by inhibitor proteins that are also affected by cAMP-dependent enzymatic phosphorylation and by dephosphorylation. In contrast to phosphorylase, in this case the phosphorylated form is inhibited (see Cohen 1978, 1988, 1989).

ATP synthesis. The reaction involving glyceraldehyde-3-phosphate oxidation and NAD* in the breakdown scheme of glycogen leads to the esterification of a phosphate residue; eventually it is transferred to adenosine diphosphate (ADP) to form ATP. The phosphate residue that participated in the phosphorolytic breakdown of glycogen also ends up as ATP, through the pyruvate kinase (EC 2.7.1.40) reaction. Thus in the anaerobic breakdown of one glucose unit of glycogen there is a net formation of three molecules of ATP. If glucose were the starting material, only two moles of ATP would be formed from glucose because of the ATP requirement in the formation of glucose-1-phosphate via the hexokinase (EC 2.7.1.1.) reaction.

Glyceraldehyde phosphate, as already mentioned, reduces NAD. Under anaerobic conditions the reduction of NAD has to be reversed through its reaction with pyruvic acid resulting in the formation of lactic acid and the reoxidised form of NAD. The glycolytic process, therefore, does not involve a net change in the state of oxidation or reduction.

Aerobic metabolism. The anaerobic path of the breakdown of carbohydrates is linked to the oxidative pathway at the point of pyruvate. If there is oxidative breakdown of pyruvate the NADH formed in the reduction of glyceraldehyde phosphate is not used to form lactate by reducing pyruvate but reacts with dihydroxyacetone phosphate to form glycerol-3-phosphate (G3P) or with oxaloacetate to form malate. The latter or

G3P can enter the mitochondria to regenerate dihydroxyacetone phosphate and NADH (G3P or malate shuttle).

Krebs cycle. The reaction sequence — catalysed by enzymes located in the mitochondria — leading to the complete breakdown of pyruvic acid to CO_2 and H_2O is known as the Krebs cycle or tricarboxylic acid cycle, the latter name taking its origin from the organic acids, containing three carboxyl groups, that participate in the cycle. Pyruvate is oxidised to acetate, forming a derivative with coenzyme A (CoA), acetyl-CoA. The latter interacts with an intermediate of the Krebs cycle, oxaloacetic acid, to form citric acid. In the complex sequence of reactions following this condensation both NAD and flavin-containing coenzymes are reduced and the removal of two molecules of CO_2 and water results in the complete breakdown of the acetate residue that entered the cycle, and in the regeneration of the oxaloacetic acid.

Terminal electron transport and oxidative phosphorylation. Coenzymes reduced in the operation of the citric acid cycle are finally reoxidised through a long chain of reactions catalysed by a chain of enzymes whose active groups are flavins, coenzyme Q, and iron-containing compounds, the cytochromes. In addition, non-haem Fe and Cu are involved. These enzymes form what is known as the respiratory chain and are localised in the mitochondria. They undergo cyclic reduction and reoxidation, with the formation of three ATPs for each pair of electrons. It is now clear that the energy derived from the flow of electrons is converted to a proton gradient between the matrix of the mitochondrion and the space between the external and internal mitochondrial membrane. The osmotic and electric energy of the proton gradient is then channelled into the formation of ATP from ADP and inorganic phosphate (Mitchell 1977). The detailed mechanism of the formation of osmotic into chemical energy is still being debated (see also Hill 1977 (energy transduction), Jencks 1980, 1983). There are indications that the energy is required to release tightly bound ATP which would be spontaneously formed from P_i and ADP (Boyer 1977). The energy derived from electron flow can also be used — instead of synthesising ATP — either to drive electrons backwards or for the transport of various ions. Interaction between

---

* NAD, nicotinamide adenine dinucleotide, is the name of the coenzyme related to the vitamin nicotinic acid.

oxidative phosphorylation and muscle contraction is established by virtue of the fact that with a tightly coupled physiologically operating oxidation–phosphorylation system, the formation of ADP in muscle contraction, by furnishing an acceptor for phosphorylation, may serve as a regulating link between the energy-conserving and energy-producing process.

Fatty acid oxidation

The oxidation of fatty acids is an important source of energy in both skeletal and cardiac muscle (Fritz et al 1958). Detailed enzymatic studies of the breakdown of fatty acids (Lynen & Ochoa 1953, Green 1954), the hydrolytic product of neutral fats, have fully confirmed the ideas expressed by Knoop as early as 1904 on the basis of results obtained on whole animals. Accordingly, fatty acids are broken down by the repeated pair-wise removal of carbon residues starting at the COOH end of the fatty acid molecule and leading to the formation of an acetate residue or propionic acid residue, in even or odd-numbered fatty acids, respectively. Actually, both the acetate and propionate residue appear to be linked to the coenzyme CoA mentioned earlier in connection with the operation of a citric acid cycle. Acetyl-CoA enters the citric acid cycle in exactly the same way as that formed from the oxidation of pyruvic acid and originating in glucose. Propionyl-CoA is converted into succinate, another intermediate in the citric acid cycle, by a path involving an ATP-dependent carboxylation (Flavin & Ochoa 1957). It should be added that the further flow of electrons involved in the reoxidation of the reduced NAD and NADP is the same as that in the metabolism of carbohydrates discussed above.

High-energy compounds

General. ATP belongs to a class of phosphate compounds known as high-energy phosphates. This statement means that in the reaction of ATP with water, which is catalysed by various enzymes, a relatively large amount of free energy is liberated. Free energy is the type of energy that is available for doing useful work or driving a reaction that would not occur spontaneously. The various phosphate compounds can, broadly speaking, be grouped into two classes, high- and low-energy compounds, depending on the amount of energy that becomes available for work upon cleaving the phosphate bond. The concept that phosphate bonds are carriers in energy transformation and biosynthesis was originally proposed by Lipmann (1941). In the class of high-energy compounds we have ATP, acetyl phosphate, 1-phosphoglycerol-3-phosphate, phosphoenolpyruvate, creatine phosphate; low-energy phosphates are glycerol-1-phosphate, glucose-6-phosphate, fructose-6 phosphate, glucose-1-phosphate.

The difference between the two classes of compounds is often somewhat blurred because the actual amount of free energy available depends on the concentration of the reactants and products of the reaction, and the so-called standard free energy of reaction ($\Delta F°$), usually listed in tables, refers to a hypothetical state when all the reactants are present in the concentration of 1 mole per litre. A useful way of thinking about this so-called standard free-energy change of a reaction is in terms of the relationship of standard free-energy change with the equilibrium constant (K) of the reaction, given by

$$\Delta G° = -RT \ln K$$

Typical $\Delta G°$ values for high-energy compounds are about 40 kJ/mol and for low-energy compounds 10–20 kJ/mol. The actual free energy available, ΔG, depends on the concentration (or more precisely activity) of the reactants and products; it is related to $\Delta G°$ by the following equation

$$\Delta G = \Delta G° + RT \ln$$

$$\frac{\text{(product of concentrations of products)}}{\text{(product of concentrations of reactants)}}$$

Thus for the hydrolysis of ATP,

$$\Delta G = \Delta G° + RT \ln \frac{(ADP)(P_i)}{(ATP)},$$

where

$$\Delta G° = -RT \ln \frac{(ADP)_{eq}(P_i)_{eq}}{(ATP)_{eq}} = -RT \ln K,$$

the subscript 'eq' referring to the concentrations at equilibrium.

In considering biological energy transduction involving macromolecular systems, as in the case of muscle, some useful distinctions can and should be made among various types of free-energy definitions. The papers by Hill and his colleagues (Hill & Simmons 1976, Eisenberg & Hill 1985) as well as Tanford (1983) and Jencks (1980, 1983) should be consulted in this context.

Reactions of ATP. Both the bond between the terminal and the middle phosphate and that between the middle phosphate and that nearest to the ribose ring of ATP are of a high-energy character. There are several enzyme systems, phosphotransferases, in the cell which provide essentially equi-energetic transfer of phosphate from one compound to another. One is the so-called creatine kinase (EC 2.7.3.2), which catalyses the reaction:

$$CrP + ADP \rightleftharpoons Cr + ATP$$

Another enzyme present in muscle, myokinase or adenylate kinase (EC 2.7.4.3), catalyses the transfer of phosphate from ATP to AMP resulting in the formation of two ADP molecules, thus making, by the reverse reaction, further utilisation of energy available.

In addition to the reactions of ATP involving transfer of phosphates, there are enzymes in muscle that lead to the deamination of the purine ring. No evidence exists that ATP itself can be deaminated, but both ADP and AMP can serve as substrates of deaminase. Furthermore, in vivo it seems that the NH_2 group attached to the purine ring of the ATP molecule undergoes rapid exchange. This exchange, however, is not a simple reversal of the deamination reaction but seems to proceed by a pathway involving adenylosuccinate (Newton & Perry 1960).

Energetics of muscle contraction

Views on the ultimate source of the energy released by muscle in the course of contraction have undergone considerable changes over the years. The lactic acid era gave way to phosphagen, as creatine phosphate was originally called, particularly under the weight of evidence adduced by

Lundsgaard (1930) showing the disappearance of creatine phosphate from exhausted muscle, even under conditions when no lactic acid appeared (for an historical review see Needham 1971). In the middle 1950s, doubts were cast on the immediate participation of ATP and CrP in the elementary event of muscle contraction (Mommaerts 1954, 1955, Fleckenstein et al 1954), but it has now been shown quite convincingly that 0.5–0.6 μmol of ATP are hydrolysed per gram of muscle during a single contraction (Cain et al 1962). Fenn (1923, 1924) showed 70 years ago that the total energy output of the muscle is increased as it shortens to do work (see also Mommaerts 1970). Hill (1949) originally partitioned the energy released by muscle during contraction into three terms, one corresponding to activation, another to shortening, and a third to mechanical work. The existence of a heat term which is dependent only on shortening appears doubtful in the light of subsequent work (Hill, 1964a–d, Wilkie 1966).

There is good evidence for extra breakdown of CrP and ATP corresponding to work done (see e.g. Kushmerick & Davies 1969). The precise relationship between chemical change, activation heat and shortening heat has yet to be established. Comparison of mechanical work and thermal and chemical changes has been complicated by the fact that different investigators use different experimental material. In a stimulated muscle the sum of work done and heat liberated (enthalpy) can be accounted for in terms of the enthalpy changes of known chemical reactions if the contraction phase, relaxation and recovery are included. Over shorter periods, however, at the beginning of contraction there may be discrepancies between thermal, mechanical and chemical measurements. This has led to the concept of unexplained energy or enthalpy. The shift between chemical change and energy liberation may involve redistribution among various cross-bridge states (see below) and energy changes associated with calcium release from, and binding to, the sarcoplasmic reticulum, troponin and parvalbumin. (For a detailed discussion see Kushmerick 1983, Woledge et al 1985, Homsher 1986, 1987). The application of NMR techniques (see below) to whole isolated muscles, or whole limbs in vivo, or the use of single fibres combined with sophisticated recording techniques, caged ATP, i.e. ATP releasable by laser illumination and isotopic compounds (see Hibberd & Trentham 1986), will undoubtedly bring further clarification to the problem.

Metabolism and activity. As discussed above, the immediate source of energy for muscle contraction is ATP. The major moiety in equilibrium with it in striated muscle is creatine phosphate. The various pathways that produce ATP, anaerobic or aerobic in character and utilising substrates are determined by the nature of the muscle and its activity. Fast muscle fibres are predominant in 'white muscles'; they are characterised by predominantly anaerobic metabolism and contain only a small number of mitochondria (see Ch. 8). Fibres rich in mitochondria are in the majority in slow 'red muscles' and also account for some fibres of fast-twitch muscle. These fibres can carry out oxidative metabolism utilising either carbohydrates or fats.

High-speed contraction requiring considerable amounts of energy depends first on the use of the preformed high-energy phosphate stores, viz. creatine phosphate; when they are exhausted, anaerobic breakdown of glycogen becomes the main source of energy. Extended medium-level activity depends on oxidative metabolism of either carbohydrates or fats. After the disappearance of the muscle glycogen store, the carbohydrate substrate would be glucose, carried to the muscles by the circulation, or fatty acids also derived from plasma (Hultman et al 1986). The use of glycogen or glucose is more efficient than that of fatty acids in terms of the number of ATPs produced per oxygen molecule consumed. Other factors that determine the choice of the substrate include the rate of their uptake and, in the case of fatty acids, the rate of triglyceride hydrolysis. (For a review on the integration of anaerobic and aerobic pathways as well as of various fuel systems see Hochachka 1985.)

Whereas early work on the metabolism of muscles relied on muscle biopsies and the biochemical analysis of samples so obtained, more recently ^{31}P NMR studies have opened up new ways of analysing muscle metabolism, permitting continuous monitoring of the metabolic state of the muscle. The use of NMR for imaging, for which ^{1}H nuclei are important, is outside the scope of this chapter.

For metabolic studies on muscle — particularly in man — most of the NMR work has been done with ^{31}P and to some extent with ^{13}C spectroscopy. Two-dimensional ^{1}H magnetic resonance for the study of human muscle extracts is also promising for distinguishing metabolites in normal and diseased muscles (Venkatasubramanian et al 1986). Topical magnetic resonance studies permit the detection of signals over a well-defined muscle area with the use of ^{31}P. Changes in ATP, phosphocreatine and other phosphorylated compounds can be detected as muscles contract and, utilising the change in the position of some peaks, information can be obtained about the intracellular pH of muscle. NMR is useful, not only for detecting changes in concentration of metabolites but, with the use of so-called saturation transfer, the rate of exchange of phosphorus between two compounds, e.g. phosphocreatine and ATP, can be measured. For details on these topics see earlier reviews (Dawson & Wilkie 1984, Edwards et al 1985, Dawson 1986, Radda 1986, Sapega et al 1993 as well as Chapter 2.)

Fatigue. The study of muscle metabolism, both in its conventional form utilising muscle biopsy, as well as the more recent technique of NMR including the topical magnetic resonance version, have thrown new light on this problem, for a more recent review see Fitts 1994. The decline in force associated with fatigue is regarded as being dependent on metabolic changes in muscle as well as on alterations in the activation of contraction. In the intact organism a central component has also to be considered: i.e. alterations of stimuli originating in the brain. The biochemical approach is particularly suited to studying the first two factors. For recent work on neural mechanisms of fatiguability, see Enoka & Stuart (1992). Fatigue is clearly correlated with decrease in phosphocreatine and pH and an increase in inorganic phosphate (Dawson et al 1978). These changes can be readily studied with the use of topical magnetic resonance instruments on human volunteers. Decreases in ATP and increases in ADP occur only in extreme exhaustion of muscle which could be produced only by electrical stimulation. According to Dawson (1986) (see also Wilkie 1986), the accumulation of phosphate and particularly its mono-anionic form is most closely correlated with the decline of force. It should be borne in mind that, as the products of creatine phosphate and ATP accumulate, the free energy available from the hydrolysis of the ATP which is available for contraction also decreases (cf. Wilkie 1986). Recent work on isolated skinned muscle fibres (Hibberd et al 1985), to be discussed below, suggests that inorganic phosphate is able to decrease force development by shifting some of the equilibria involving intermediates in the myosin- or actomyosin-catalysed ATPase cycle. In relating work on animal models to human muscle and in comparing different muscles in the same species the fibre type composition has to be kept in mind because of type-dependent differences (Kushmerick et al 1992, McKenzie et al 1992, Soderlund et al 1992).

More recent ^{31}P NMR work (Bertocci et al 1992) indicates that skeletal muscle fatigue can occur without decreased pH or increased $H_2PO_4^-$, but it confirms the significance of increased ADP concentration. Studies using the photogeneration of P_i from so-called caged form on the mechanism by which inorganic phosphate reduces force may throw new light on processes that could play a role in bringing about fatigue (Dantzig et al 1992, Millar & Homsher 1992). The interaction between oxidative and glycolytic metabolism during exercise, its variation from individual to individual and its dependence on training is illustrated by the work of Chance and his colleagues (Chance et al 1986).

Repeated stimulation of muscle not only affects changes in metabolites but also shows changes in membrane properties resulting in reduced velocity of propagation of depolarisation and changes in the frequency dependence in the response to stimulation (Bigland-Ritchie & Woods 1984, Edwards 1984, Milner-Brown & Miller 1986, Metzger & Fitts 1986). It has been suggested that a reactive mechanism is at work in the intact organism resulting in a lower firing frequency of neurones just high enough to obtain maximum force development relaxation (Bigland-Ritchie et al 1986). Details of the biochemical mechanisms underlying these processes are yet to be fully explored, but failure of T-tubule depolarization may lead to inadequate Ca^{2+} release and consequently impaired muscle activation (see Westerblad et al 1991).

MYOFIBRILLAR PROTEINS

Myosin

Extraction, solubility. Myosin accounts for about half of the myofibrillar proteins (Hanson & Huxley 1957, Yates & Greaser 1983). It can be extracted from muscle at about pH 6.5 with minimal contamination by actin. Raising the pH and prolonging the time of extraction leads to the extraction of both actin and myosin in the form of actomyosin, which is discussed in more detail below. The solubility of myosin increases with ionic strength: about 0.6 M is the ionic strength used for extraction. Myosin is insoluble at ionic strengths less than 0.2 M when formation of aggregates occurs. This property is used for the precipitation or, as it is often somewhat loosely termed, crystallisation, of myosin (Szent-Györgyi 1945).

Structure, subunits. Myosin, a highly asymmetrical hexameric molecule, is among the largest proteins that have been well characterised. It contains two heavy chains, $M_r \sim 220\,000$, and four light chains, $M_r \sim 20\,000$. The carboxyl-terminal portions of the two heavy chains form an α-helical coiled rod while the N-terminal portions of each chain appear as separate globular structures clearly shown by electron microscopy following rotary shadowing (Lowey et al 1969); these are the so-called heads of the myosin molecule (Fig. 6.2). Each head contains an ATP binding site, where

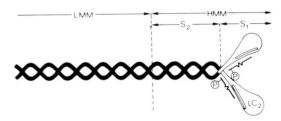

Fig. 6.2 Schematic representation of a myosin molecule showing points (broken lines) at which limited proteolysis results in formation of stable fragments. The head regions contain two kinds of light chains, one phosphorylatable. Heavy lines are intertwined α-helices. The model is not drawn to scale. For details see text (copied with permission from Kendrick-Jones & Scholey 1981).

the hydrolysis of ATP to ADP and phosphate takes place to yield the energy for muscle contraction, and an actin binding site.

Early work (Gergely 1950, 1953, Perry 1951, Mihalyi & Szent-Györgyi 1953, Gergely et al 1955) has shown that myosin can be cleaved into smaller fragments without loss of ATPase activity and the ability to interact with actin (Fig. 6.2). Cleavage of the heavy chains by trypsin or chymotrypsin produces a two-headed N-terminal fragment: heavy meromyosin (HMM), that contains part of the rod, and light meromyosin (LMM) (Szent-Györgyi 1953), representing about two-thirds of the rod including its C-terminus. Further digestion of HMM yields the smaller subfragment 1 (S-1) (Mueller & Perry 1962) corresponding to single myosin heads and a coiled-coil fragment (S-2) (Lowey 1964, Lowey et al 1966) linking the myosin head with the LMM portion. S-2, obtainable in a long and short form (Highsmith et al 1977, Weeds & Pope 1977, Sutoh et al 1978), corresponds to the part of the cross-bridge that connects the body of the thick filament with the myosin head and plays a role in transmitting the force generated at the head–actin interface or within the head itself (see Rayment et al 1993a,b). On the basis of experiments probing the properties of the S-2 segment under conditions corresponding to activation of muscle contraction, Harrington and his colleagues (Harrington 1979, Ueno & Harrington 1981, Harrington & Rodgers 1984) have argued for the view that the S-2 segment itself may play a role in force generation. The success of obtaining movement of actin filaments and force development in motility assay systems containing only myosin heads as motors makes it seem more likely that the role of S-2 is passive (Sugi et al 1992). Some recent experiments with antibodies against S-2 or against the hinge joining S-2 and S-1 (Margossian et al 1991) still argue in favour of a more active role for S-2.

Under carefully controlled conditions of digestion, S-1 can be further broken down into smaller fragments that remain non-covalently held together without loss of ATPase activity. The main fragments of the heavy chain obtained by tryptic or chymotryptic digestion starting at the N-terminus have been referred to as the 25 kDa, 50 kDa and 20 kDa peptides (Balint et al 1978).

Separation of these fragments on sodium dodecyl-sulphate- (SDS)-containing polyacrylamide gels has made it possible to locate binding sites for ATP and actin and to locate various residues of functional significance within the myosin head (see below).

Light chains. The two light chains associated with each myosin head belong to two different chemically distinguishable classes.

In fast skeletal muscle, the light chains have originally been named 'DTNB light chains' and 'alkali light chains'. The nomenclature is based on the fact that one light chain of MW 18 000 can be dissociated by treatment with Ellman's thiol reagent (5,5′-dithio bis-2-nitrobenzoic acid (DTNB or Nbs_2 according to the new nomenclature)) without significant loss of ATPase activity (Gazith et al 1970, Weeds & Lowey 1971). Further alkali treatment liberates two light chains, which have apparent molecular weights on SDS gels of about 25 000 and 16 000, and which are termed A1 and A2. The three chains have distinctive chemical features, although there are common sequences in the alkali light chains (Weeds 1969, Weeds & Frank 1972). Early studies of the amino acid sequence of the light chains established that there are many similarities with, however, significant differences. In particular, A1 has an additional stretch of 40 residues at its N-terminus compared to A2. As the sequence work progressed it became clear that light chains belong to a superfamily of proteins that include calmodulin, troponin C and parvalbumin (the prototype) among its members. Whereas parvalbumin, calmodulin and troponin C bind Ca^{2+} with rather high affinity and have Ca^{2+}-binding sites of characteristic sequences, the light chains of myosin have what one might call defective Ca^{2+}-binding sites (for a detailed review see Collins 1991). Light chains similar to the alkali light chains have become known as essential light chains, based on the difficulty in early experiments of removing them from the heavy chain without destroying the activity of myosin. The recently completed X-ray crystallographic structure of the myosin head (S-1) (Rayment et al 1993a) shows that light chains are bound to the distal part of the S-1 portion, the essential light chain being closer to the compact N-terminal half of S-1, while the regulatory light chain is close to the junction of S-1 and S-2. This is in good agreement with results obtained by electron-microscopic localization of antibodies against the light chains (Yamamoto et al 1985, Winkelmann & Lowey 1985, Katoh & Lowey 1989). Based on the electrophoretic mobility on SDS-containing polyacrylamide gels, the three light chains have also been designated LC_1, LC_2 and LC_3, in order of increasing rates of mobility. LC_2 is the DTNB light chain and LC_1 and LC_3 correspond to A1 and A2, respectively. Myosin slow-twitch muscle contains only two main types of light chains, the mobilities of which are similar to, but distinguishable from, those of LC_1 and LC_2 respectively, of fast-muscle myosin (Lowey & Risby 1971, Sarkar et al 1971, Frank & Weeds 1974). Cardiac muscle myosin also contains light chains corresponding to LC_1 and LC_2 but there are differences between those found in atria and those in the ventricles. The latter seem to be identical with those of slow skeletal myosin; the atrial light chains differ in mobility from both fast and slow skeletal muscle light chains (Bandman 1985, Barton & Buckingham 1985).

Light chains in the LC_2 mobility class (fast and slow skeletal, cardiac) seem to be related in their ability to undergo phosphorylation by a kinase (Pires et al 1974, Yagi et al 1978), the activator of which is the ubiquitous Ca-binding protein calmodulin (see Klee & Vanaman 1982). These light chains are also known as P or regulatory chains.

The term 'regulatory' was first applied to the light chains involved in the regulation of smooth muscle and in molluscan muscle (Kendrick-Jones et al 1970), the regulation occurring by phosphorylation of light chains and Ca^{2+}-binding to the light chain–heavy chain complex, respectively. Phosphorylation of the light chain catalysed by a kinase (Pires et al 1974, Yagi et al 1978), the activator of which is the ubiquitous Ca-binding protein calmodulin (see Klee & Vanaman 1982), is now well established as a key event in the regulation of smooth muscle contraction (Sherry et al 1978, Hartshorne & Siemankowski 1981; for a recent overview on smooth muscle see Somlyo & Somlyo 1992). Phosphorylation and dephosphorylation in vivo during contraction and relaxation respectively,

have been reported (Bárány & Bárány 1980), and in vitro the effect on the mechanical properties of fibres has been observed (see e.g. Cooke & Stull 1981, Persechini et al 1985). The mechanism of the post-tetanic potentiation of force production, which involves phosphorylation of the light chain, appears to be sarcomere length-dependent (Levine et al 1993). There is evidence that phosphorylation by myosin light chain kinase of the regulatory light chain produces movement of the myosin heads away from the filament backbone in vertebrate striated muscle, an observation similar to those previously reported for smooth muscle.

Myosin isozymes. In the broadest sense all myosins exhibiting different functional and structural features may be regarded as isozymes. Thus various forms found in fast and slow skeletal, cardiac and smooth muscles are isozymes. In a narrower sense, myosin molecules differing in their subunit composition but found in the same type of muscle have been regarded as isozymes. The fact that in fast-muscle myosin the sum of A1 + A2 is two per molecule although they occur in a ratio of about 1.4 : 0.6 suggests that some myosin molecules contain pairs of either A1 or A2 (Sarkar 1972). The existence of such homodimers has been shown by Holt & Lowey (1977) with the use of antibodies specific for one or the other light chain. Evidence for heterodimer molecules containing one A1 and one A2 has been obtained with the use of electrophoresis under non-dissociating conditions in pyrophosphate-containing gels where myosin separates into three bands corresponding to the $(A1)_2$, A1A2 and $(A2)_2$ species, in order of increasing mobility (Hoh 1978, d'Albis et al 1979, Lowey et al 1979). Electrophoresis under non-dissociating conditions has also shown the existence of myosin isozymes in cardiac muscle; here, however, the differences reside in the heavy chains. Two heavy chains, referred to as α and β, have been identified as giving rise to $\beta\beta$, $\alpha\beta$ and $\alpha\alpha$ moieties, in order of increasing mobility, also known as V_3, V_2 and V_1 isozymes, respectively (Hoh et al 1978, Lompre et al 1981).

Recent studies have revealed the presence of subtypes among the heavy chains and the combination of various heavy and light chain isoforms in a single fibre gives rise to a more complex pattern of fibre types than the early I, IIA and IIB classification (see Ch. 8).

Genetic basis of myosin isoforms. The identification of various isoforms of myosin subunits and the clarification of their relationship has been greatly aided by advances both in protein and DNA sequencing, as well as immunological and DNA cloning techniques. Thus the β-chain of cardiac muscle myosin appears to be identical with the heavy chain of slow skeletal muscle myosin, being the products of the same gene (Lompre et al 1984, Sinha et al 1984). Distinct genes code for the fast myosin heavy chains found in IIA and IIB type fibres (Nadal-Ginard et al 1982). The DTNB-light chain is coded for by a gene distinct from that coding for both alkali-light chains; in the latter case the transcription of a single gene leads by alternative initiating sites and splicing to two messenger RNAs, the translation of which produces two distinct light chains (Nabeshima et al 1984, Periasamy et al 1984, Robert et al 1984, 1986). Alternative splicing mechanisms (for a general reference see Leff et al 1986, Padgett et al 1986) have an important role in the production of a number of isoforms of various muscle proteins (e.g. troponin T — Medford et al 1984, tropomyosin — Ruiz-Opazo et al 1985). Differences in proteins may also arise from post-translational modifications of the peptide chain, e.g. methylation of lysine and histidine residues in fast adult myosin heavy chains (Kuehl & Adelstein 1970, Huszar 1975). For a comprehensive review of multiple forms of myosin and other muscle proteins, see Pette & Staron (1990).

ATPase activity. Myosin is not only a structural component of muscle but also an enzyme able to hydrolyse the terminal phosphate of ATP, producing ADP and inorganic phosphate, as first shown by Engelhardt & Ljubimova (1939). This reaction is greatly stimulated by Ca^{2+} and much less by Mg^{2+} ions (Szent-Györgyi 1945). Actin greatly increases the ATPase activity of myosin in the presence of Mg^{2+}. As discussed above, ATPase activity is entirely restricted to the heavy meromyosin fraction (Szent-Györgyi 1953, Gergely et al 1955) and can be recovered in the even smaller HMM-S-1 fragments.

The ATPase activity of myosin in fast muscle is considerably higher than that of myosin in slow muscles (Bárány et al 1965, Sreter et al 1966). Bárány (1967) has shown that, in general, good correlation exists between the ATPase activity of myosin and the speed of shortening of the muscle from which it has been isolated, independently of the species or the type of muscle (smooth or striated). Myosin of slow muscles shows considerable lability at pH 9, not present in myosin of fast muscles (Sreter et al 1966, Seidel 1967). Differences in ATPase activity between various myosins are mainly attributable to the differences in the heavy chains, as shown by experiments with hybrid myosins containing subunits from cardiac and fast skeletal myosins (Wagner 1981). Kinetic analysis of the ATPase reaction led to attribution of rate differences to the ADP dissociation step (Marston & Taylor 1980, Siemankowski & White 1984, Rosenfeld & Taylor 1984). Native fast-type myosin isozymes (Pastra-Landis et al 1983) and S-1 isozymes containing either A1 or A2 light chains (Wagner et al 1979) also showed only small differences at ionic strengths below the physiological level.

The work of Lymn & Taylor (1970, 1971) laid the foundations for our current views of the mechanisms of myosin-catalysed ATP hydrolysis and its acceleration by actin. They showed that the hydrolysis of ATP involves a rapid step resulting in the formation of tightly, but non-covalently bound products which are in equilibrium with bound ATP.

$$M + ATP \rightleftharpoons MATP \rightleftharpoons M^{\star}ATP \rightleftharpoons M^{\star\star}ADP.P_i \xrightarrow{slow} M^{\star}ADP.P_i \rightarrow product.$$

One or two asterisks indicate different conformations of myosin or states in the complexes, some detectable by optical or electron spin resonance spectroscopy (see Gergely & Seidel 1983, Webb & Trentham 1983). The equilibrium between the bound forms of ATP and ADP + P_i is shifted by a factor of 10^5–10^6 towards ATP, compared with the equilibrium between free ATP and ADP + P_i. This is a simplified scheme — more details will be added below in discussing the hydrolytic cycle in the presence of actin and its relation to the mechanical cross-bridge cycle and energetic coupling of ATP hydrolysis to mechanical work in muscle.

Functionally important regions. During the

past few years there has been considerable interest in assigning various functional aspects of the myosin head to the peptides derived from it by limited proteolysis and in attempting to locate them in the three-dimensional structure. Thus the 25 kDa N-terminal portion has been shown to be involved in interaction with ATP, as is the 50 kDa central peptide of S1. Chemical cross-linking has led to the identification of actin-binding regions in the 50 kDa and 20 kDa region. The sulphydryl groups, whose modification by thiol reagents affects the ATPase activity of myosin and whose reactivity is in turn influenced by the nucleotide–protein interaction, have been localised in the 20 kDa segment (Elzinga & Collins 1977, Balint et al 1978). The so-called SH1 thiol has been useful as a site for binding optical and magnetic probes to myosin; these will be referred to below. While earlier studies (Reisler et al 1974, Wells & Yount 1979) suggested that the two thiol groups are in close proximity to the nucleotide binding site, subsequent work (Tao & Lamkin 1981, Perkins et al 1984) has furnished evidence that there is a considerable distance between the thiol groups and the nucleotide binding site. Thus the trapping of the nucleotide at its binding site (Wells & Yount 1979) resulting from cross-linking of the two thiol groups, cannot, in view of the distance between thiols and the binding site, be due to direct immobilisation of the nucleotide by closing a cavity by the disulphide bridge at its mouth but would rather have to be attributable to a conformational change induced at some distance from the site of cross-linking. Conversely, the conformational change induced by the binding of ATP or its hydrolytic products at their binding sites may play an important role in the force-generating process as recently emphasised by Rayment et al (1993a). A review by Mornet et al (1989) provides a useful summary of various recent results concerning chemically identifiable functional sequences in the myosin head.

Domains and myosin head structure. The fact that a number of proteolytic enzymes produce similar fragments within the myosin head has led to the idea that these fragments are not merely segments of the primary structure separated by regions of high proteolytic susceptibility but, rather, are more or less independently folded regions, so-called domains, within the three-dimensional structure of the myosin head (Harrington & Rodgers 1984). The domain concept (see Applegate & Reisler 1983, Mornet et al 1981, 1984) has gained some support from partial renaturation of isolated fragments of the head (Muhlrad & Morales 1984, Muhlrad et al 1986). The idea of truly independent domains in the myosin head does not appear to be supported by its recently established atomic structure (Rayment et al 1993a), a culmination of studies started some 10 years ago (Rayment & Winkelmann 1984, Winkelmann et al 1985, 1991). It appears that the relation of the primary and secondary structure to the tertiary structure of the myosin head is such that various functionally important regions may involve interactions among stretches of the polypeptide chain that are separated from each other by a considerable distance in the primary structure. It also appears that, while the overall shape of the myosin head is similar to that derived from electron-microscopic studies, there is an unusually long single helical region forming a link between the N-terminal globular portion of S1 with the alpha helical S2 segment. It is this long helical region that interacts with the light chains in a way perhaps similar to that described for the helical fragment of myosin light-chain kinase with calmodulin (Ikura et al 1992, Meador et al 1992). When all the details of the structure of the myosin head are available a great deal of work will be stimulated with a view to relating already-established and yet-to-be established biochemical information to the structure and to producing a better molecular understanding of the interaction between actin and myosin and the mechanism of force production.

If independently folding domains exist, they are rather close to each other so that the formation of cross-linking between side-chains located in different putative domains is possible (Mornet et al 1985, Chaussepied et al 1986, Lu et al 1986, Bertrand et al 1992). Moreover, both ATP binding (Szilagyi et al 1979, Mahmood & Yount 1984, Okamoto & Yount 1985, Yount et al 1992) and actin binding (Mornet et al 1981, Chen et al 1985) may involve sites in more than one domain. Studies of this nature will produce useful information on the interaction of various regions within the myosin head. Data have also been accumulating on distances between a number of points in the myosin molecule utilising energy transfer between chromophores attached to residues whose location is known in the primary structure. On the basis of such data tentative three-dimensional maps of the myosin head and its relation to actin have been suggested and have been used to interpret the mechanism of energy transduction in the myosin head (Morales et al 1982, Botts et al 1984). The combination of electron microscopy and labelling of chemically identifiable residues on the myosin head with avidin appears to hold promise for visualising topographical relations (Sutoh et al 1984, 1986, Yamamoto et al 1985, Wakabayashi et al 1986).

Relation of myosin to myofilaments. As shown in Chapter 2, the electron-microscope picture of a myofibril shows that myosin filaments have a diameter of about 10 nm. A myosin filament is a bundle of many myosin molecules per cross-section; the rigid rod-like part of the myosin molecules makes up the body of these filaments and the enzymatically active globular end would correspond to the bridges seen in electron-micrographs between myosin and actin filaments. (For details of thick filament structure see Squire 1981, 1986.) At low ionic strength, myosin forms regular aggregates with the sidewise apposition of the rod-like part of the myosin molecules, and the globular ends appear on the side of the aggregates. The formation of the aggregates proceeds in two directions leaving a central zone free of lateral projections quite reminiscent of the appearance of the thick filaments of myofibrils seen in electron-micrographs of muscle itself (Huxley 1963).

Electron-microscopic and X-ray data suggest that the cross-bridges on the myosin aggregates and thick filaments are arranged on the surface in a helical fashion, the rod portions forming the core at levels separated by 14.3 nm (Huxley & Brown 1967, Huxley 1969). The amino-acid sequence of the rod portion of the myosin heavy chain exhibits a pattern of hydrophobic and polar residues characteristic of α-helical coiled structures first suggested by Crick (1953). There is a seven-residue repeat and hydrophobic residues are flanked by two and three polar ones in the sequence. This kind of sequence was first detected in tropomyosin (Sodek et al 1972). There is also a 28-residue repeat pattern (see McLachlan & Karn 1982, McLachlan 1984) producing alternate clusters of positive and negative charges. The spatial separation of these charges in the helix is 14.3 nm, making it possible to stabilise the interacting adjacent rods shifted by 14.3 nm. This interaction would thus play an important part in the assembly of the thick filaments, where a 14.3 nm axial repeat with helix repeats of 42.9 nm in vertebrate striated muscle has long been established (Huxley & Brown 1967). These spacings give rise to the X-ray diffraction pattern of muscle which has recently been studied with techniques capable of resolving changes on a millisecond time-scale (Huxley & Faruqi 1983). The original estimate of the number of cross-bridges on each level was two, and it was suggested that the two are diametrically opposed (Huxley & Brown 1967). However, evidence has been accumulating in favour of a thick filament structure in which there are three myosin cross-bridges on successive levels separated by 14.3 nm (Fig. 6.3) (Ip & Heuser 1983, Kensler & Stewart 1983, Varriano-Marston et al 1984).

The idea that the myosin molecule contains hinges permitting segmental flexibility (Huxley 1969) has played an important part in relating information on the molecular structure of myosin, and thick filament ultrastructure, to theories of contraction. Electron-microscopic and physicochemical evidence and the loci of proteolytic susceptibility suggest regions of flexibility at the junction of the globular heads and the rod (S-1/S-2) and within the rod itself at the junction of S-2 and light meromyosin (cf.

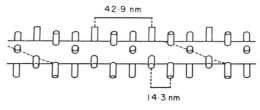

Fig. 6.3 Schematic representation of a three-stranded myosin thick filament, the model currently favoured for vertebrate muscle (see text). The helically arranged projections represent myosin heads (copied with permission from Offer 1974).

Fig. 6.2) (Mendelson et al 1973, Thomas et al 1975, Highsmith et al 1977, Elliott & Offer 1978, Sutoh et al 1978, for reviews see Gergely & Seidel 1983, Harrington & Rodgers 1984). However, alternative views on overall flexibility rather than localised hinges have also been proposed (Hvidt et al 1982, 1984).

Actin

The discovery of actin by Straub (1942) in Szent-Györgyi's laboratory showed that what in the early literature had been described as myosin was actually a complex of two proteins, myosin and actin. Actin itself can be extracted from acetone-dried muscle powder with distilled water. It is present in this extract as a globular protein — G-actin. Its molecular weight on the basis of its amino-acid sequence is 41 785 (Elzinga et al 1973).

Although G-actin was originally thought of as a spherical protein, three-dimensional reconstructions of electron micrographs of actin filaments combined with myosin subfragment-1 (decorated filaments) suggested over two decades ago (Moore et al 1970) that actin monomers are somewhat asymmetrical. More details of the actin structure emerged from electron-microscopic studies of actin sheets (Aebi et al 1981, Smith et al 1983) and from X-ray diffraction studies of crystals of the actin-DNase I complex (Suck et al 1981, Kabsch et al 1985). These eventually led to solution of the atomic structure of G-actin (Kabsch et al 1990). Before turning to details of the structure we shall discuss some well-established properties of actin, viz polymerisation and nucleotide and metal interactions.

Polymerisability. On addition of various salts, conventionally about 0.1 M for monovalent cations and about 1 mM for divalent cations, a G-actin solution undergoes a drastic change: its viscosity increases and it exhibits birefringence of flow, suggesting the presence of large asymmetrical molecules. There are so-called F-actin (for fibrous actin) particles produced through polymerisation of the globular units (Straub 1942). Polymerisation is probably of importance in the process by which actin filaments are laid down in vivo, but it is unlikely (Martonosi et al 1960b) that the polymerisation–depolymerisation cycle plays a significant part in the mechanism of muscle contraction. Structural and chemical aspects of polymerisation are discussed below. F-actin forms filaments in vitro for vertebrate muscle 10 μm or longer, in contrast to actin filaments in vivo which have a length of 1 μm per half sarcomere (Page & Huxley 1963). The factors that limit the length of actin filaments in vivo have not been identified, although the involvement of other proteins associated with the filament, e.g. tropomyosin and β-actinin, has been suggested (Maruyama 1965 a, b).

G-actin contains tightly bound Ca^{2+} or Mg^{2+}, $K_{ass} \sim 10^5 M^{-1}$ (Strzelecka-Golaszewska 1973, Strzelecka-Golaszewska et al 1978, Frieden et al 1980), or even $10^8 M^{-1}$ (Konno & Morales 1985) and ATP, $K_{ass} \sim 10^8-10^{10} M^{-1}$ (Waechter & Engel 1977, Niedl & Engel 1979), 1 mol of each per mole of actin. In the G, but not in the F, form both the metal and nucleotide can undergo rapid exchange with added divalent cations or nucleotides respectively (Martonosi et al 1960a, Bárány et al 1962, Martonosi 1962, Drabikowski & Strzelecka-Golaszewska 1963, Iyengar & Weber 1964). It appears likely that both the bound metal and nucleotide are necessary in G-actin to stabilise its tertiary structure — removal of either leads to the irreversible denaturation of the protein and the loss of polymerisability (Nagy & Jencks 1962, Lehrer & Kerwar 1972, Frieden et al 1980), although under special conditions polymerisability and binding to myosin can be preserved (Kasai et al 1964).

Mechanism of polymerisation. The polymerisation of actin is accompanied by the hydrolysis of the bound ATP (Straub & Feuer 1950, Mommaerts 1952) and ADP remains tightly bound while the phosphate is released. Polymerisation stops when the actin monomer concentration drops below the so-called critical concentration, as first shown by Oosawa and colleagues (Oosawa et al 1959, Asakura et al 1960, Oosawa & Asakura 1975). ATP hydrolysis continues after polymerisation has stopped, and the rate of this steady-state hydrolysis, which involves the exchange of G-ADP units in the filament for G-ATP units in solution, depends upon the ionic conditions (Wegner & Engel 1975, Hill 1980, Pollard & Mooseker 1981, Wegner &

Neuhaus 1981, Wegner 1982a). It has now been established that actin monomers attach and detach at the ends of the filaments, which exhibit polarity as shown by the formation of arrowheads on addition of myosin subfragment 1 or HMM. Although attachment and detachment occur at both ends of the filaments, monomers attach preferentially to the barbed end of the filament, while detachment is favoured at the pointed end (Woodrum et al 1975, Hayashi & Ip 1976, Kondo & Ishiwata 1976).

The first step in the polymerisation process is the formation of nuclei consisting of three to four monomers (see Frieden 1985, Pollard & Cooper 1986). Several recent studies have addressed the possibility of G-actin undergoing changes before formation of nuclei. Rich & Estes (1976), in studying the susceptibility of actin to enzymatic proteolysis, discovered a new monomer form that was generated by the addition of KC1 to subcritical concentrations of G-actin. The new form, although clearly monomeric and containing bound ATP, showed a decreased susceptibility to digestion, which is characteristic of F-actin. They concluded that this novel actin represented a conformationally distinct form of monomer that precedes nucleation. A conformational change preceding nucleation is also associated with polymerisation induced by Mg binding (Frieden et al 1980, Gershman et al 1984, Selden et al 1986) and is distinguishable by spectroscopic techniques (see Frieden & Patane 1985, Carlier et al 1986, 1991).

Whereas earlier models of polymerisation implied a tight coupling between ATP hydrolysis and incorporation of a monomeric actin into the filament, newer models consider the existence of ATP–actin subunits in the filament with either random hydrolysis of ATP or hydrolysis at the boundary between the central portion of the actin filament containing ADP–actin subunits and a terminal region containing ATP–actin (also referred to as a 'cap', Carlier et al 1984). As ATP–G-actin polymerises the ratio of ATP, ADP+P_i and ADP containing subunits changes gradually from those containing ATP through ADP+P_i to ADP (Carlier 1991). In vitro actin filaments polymerised from ATP–G-actin are more rigid than those started with ADP–G-actin (Janmey

et al 1990) possibly because of the presence of some ADP.P_i containing subunits in the former. The continuous addition of monomers at one end and the removal at the other requires steady hydrolysis of ATP (treadmilling) (Wegner & Engel 1975, Hill 1980, Hill & Kirschner 1982, Wegner 1982a, Selve & Wegner 1986) in the steady state too. For a more detailed discussion of this problem see Pollard & Cooper (1986) and references therein.

A variety of factors indigenous to muscle tissue have a regulatory role in actin polymerisation and depolymerisation. Thus, in addition to the above-mentioned mono- and divalent cation-induced (Estes et al 1992) actin polymerisation, several other muscle proteins including myosin (Kikuchi et al 1969), tropomyosin (Wegner 1982b), and β-actinin (Hama et al 1965, Maruyama 1971, Kawamura & Maruyama 1972) can affect the rate or extent of polymerisation. In addition to these muscle proteins, the recent interest in non-muscle actins has led to the discovery of an ever-increasing list of intracellular proteins involved in actin assembly and disassembly. These include proteins that affect either the nucleation (e.g. profilin) (Carlsson et al 1977) or the elongation stage (e.g. capping protein) (Isenberg et al 1980) of filament formation and may or may not be sensitive to intracellular Ca^{2+} concentrations. Several recent reviews have provided descriptions of these agents and the mechanisms of their actions on actin. In many instances, a variety of effects may be understood in terms of a factor's preferential binding to the pointed or barbed end of the filaments (see Hitchcock-DeGregori 1980, Schliwa 1981, Craig & Pollard 1982, Korn 1982).

Functionally important amino-acid residues in actin. A considerable body of information is accumulating that identifies individual amino-acid residues likely to be involved in various functional roles. Of the five Cys residues in actin (Elzinga & Collins 1972), three can be labelled in the native molecule (Lusty & Fasold 1969) without affecting its polymerisability or ATP-binding characteristics. Cys 374, which is adjacent to the COOH-terminal phenylalanyl residue, is the most reactive. In addition to its selective reaction with Cu^{2+} (Lehrer et al 1972), it can be labelled with a variety of SH-directed optical (Cheung et al 1971, Leavis & Lehrer 1974, Ando & Asai 1979, Tao & Cho 1979, Taylor et al 1981) or spin probes (Stone et al 1970, Burley et al 1971, 1972, Thomas et al 1979). The work of Tao & Cho (1979), for example, in which acrylamide was used to quench the fluorescence of Cys-374-bound AEDANS*, has provided evidence that this thiol group is located in a region of the molecule that is partly covered in the F-form of actin. Taylor et al (1981) utilised donor and acceptor molecules attached to this residue to study intersubunit energy transfer in actin filaments. The reactivity of Cys 374 increases upon the combination of actin with HMM subfragment 1, suggesting either the proximity of the group to the myosin heads or at least some coupling between the region of actin containing Cys 374 and that directly involved in myosin binding (Duke et al 1976). Chemical cross-linking experiments have also provided indications for the participation of Cys 374 and Lys 191 in actin–actin interactions that may be involved in polymerisation (Elzinga & Phelan 1984, Sutoh 1984). Hegyi et al (1986) have identified, using a photo-activatable analogue of ATP, residues (Lys 336, Trp-356) likely to be involved in — or close to — the nucleotide binding site. The fact that cross-linking to the Trp residue takes place in G- but not in F-actin suggests that a conformational change in this region takes place upon polymerisation.

Another residue in actin that functions as an internal probe is Tyr 69, located near the single N-methylhistidine residue in the protein. Tyr 69 is selectively nitrated by tetranitromethane, and changes in the absorption of light at 425 nm by the resulting nitrotyrosyl residue suggest that it may be somehow involved in the polymerisation process (Elzinga & Collins 1972).

A study by Lu & Szilagyi (1981) has provided insight into the surfaces of the protein involved in polymerisation. They measured differences in the reactivities of the various lysines on the protein surface in F- vs. G-actin and found that polymerisation reduced the reactivities of several, viz. Lys 61, 68, 113 and 283. The decrease in reactivity can be explained if the affected residues are located in the area of contact between monomers, although one cannot rule out conformational changes in the protein. An intriguing observation in this work was that Lys 335 exhibited a substantial increase in reactivity in the polymerised form of actin, although it decreased again if actin was complexed with either myosin subfragment 1 of tropomyosin, suggesting possible conformational change in actin induced by tropomyosin incorporated into the filament. Modification of another lysine residue — 237 — (El-Saleh et al 1986) leads to changes in the Ca^{2+}-sensitivity of the actin–myosin interaction (see below).

Isoforms. Actins isolated from various sources including non-muscular contractile systems (Korn 1982, Vanderkerckhove & Weber 1984, Robert et al 1986) have similar chemical structures. Different actins, even in the same organism, are encoded by distinct members of a multigene family. Amino-acid replacements in actin are of a very conservative nature, i.e. preserving the character (charge, hydrophobicity) of the residue, even if species far from each other on the evolutionary scale are compared. Differences in the amino-acid sequence of actins in different cell types, skeletal muscle, cardiac muscle, brain and platelets, have been found in the same organisms. Gel electrophoretic differences among actins depend on a few residues at the N terminus; although the differences correlate with certain broad groupings, the full genetic variety is not revealed by this technique, but it is reflected in the sequence at the protein, DNA or RNA level.

Atomic structure of the actin monomer. The crystallisation of G-actin complexed to an unrelated enzyme, DNAse I, and the subsequent determination of the structure by X-ray diffraction studies has led to a detailed picture of the actin monomer. The three-dimensional structure of G-actin reveals two major lobes separated by a cleft into which ATP-Me^{2+} or ADP-Me^{2+} fits, Me^{2+} being Ca^{2+} or Mg^{2+}. Each lobe is divided into two subdomains. The N- and C-termini are close to each other in the first subdomain which contains the main myosin binding site. A secondary binding site appears to be present in the second subdomain, but two different myosin heads may be attached to each actin monomer.

---

* (acetamidoethyl) aminonaphthalene-1-sulphonate.

Actin–actin contact regions have also been identified (see below, 'Actin filament structure and relation to myofilaments'). The identification of those regions in actin that interact with tropomyosin and a number of other actin-binding proteins, e.g. gelsolin, caldesmon, profilin, is currently in progress in various laboratories (for reviews see Holmes & Kabsch (1991), Kabsch & Vandekerckhove (1992).

Actin filament structure and relation to myofilaments. Electron-microscopic studies by Hanson & Lowy (1963) revealed that F-actin is a helical structure made up of subunits. Actin filaments directly isolated from muscle also have the same basic structure. Different actins, even in the same organism, are coded for by members of a multigene family. The participation of other proteins in the thin filaments found in muscle, including tropomyosin and troponin, is discussed below. The original model envisaged a twisted two-strand structure of spherical subunits.

Earlier efforts to model F-actin involved aligning the monomers with their own axis approximately at right angles to the helix axis (Egelman 1985, Trinick et al 1986) (Fig. 6.4). An alternative model with the actin monomer being orientated nearly parallel to the filament axis has also been proposed (Fowler & Aebi

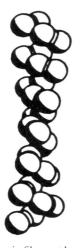

Fig. 6.4 Model of actin filament based on a preliminary bilobar structure of G-actin monomers (copied with permission from Egelman et al 1983). For atomic level details see Holmes et al (1990).

1983, Smith et al 1983, 1984). In the light of the shape of G-actin revealed by X-ray diffraction, the previously made distinction between a long and short axis in the monomer has become a moot issue. By optimally fitting the actin monomers into the X-ray diffraction pattern of filamentous actin, Holmes et al (1990) have obtained an atomic model of the actin filament. Mapping of interacting regions of actin with myosin and tropomyosin, combining the knowledge derived from X-ray diffraction of actin filaments with electron-microscopic studies (Holmes et al 1990, Milligan et al 1990; for reviews see Holmes & Kabsch 1991, Kabsch & Vandekerckhove 1992, Rayment et al 1993b), will resolve still outstanding questions of the mechanism of contraction and regulation. These include the precise nature of the change in the position of tropomyosin on the actin filament that takes place in the course of the calcium-induced triggering of muscle contraction and the still unresolved question of the kind of movement that may take place within the myosin head or at the interface between myosin and actin (see below).

The F-actin filament, once formed, exhibits considerable flexibility; bending motions were first demonstrated by the quasi-elastic laser light-scattering experiments (Fujime & Ishiwata 1972, Ishiwata & Fujime 1972), and later by electron microscopy (Takebayashi et al 1977), fluorescence polarisation of labelled filaments (Yanagida & Oosawa 1978), saturation transfer EPR of spin-labelled filaments (Thomas et al 1979), and by direct dark-field microscopic visualisation of filaments labelled with a fluorescent probe (Nagashima & Asakura 1980). The correlation times characterising these motions range from seconds to nanoseconds; the motions may involve whole filaments, subunits within filaments, or segments within subunits. In the case of labels, particularly for faster motions, it becomes difficult to distinguish between motions attributable to the protein and those of the probe itself relative to its attachment site. Addition of tropomyosin and troponin in the absence of Ca^{2+} results in a more rigid filament; however, the addition of Ca^{2+} restores the flexibility to the level of the pure actin filament (Fujime & Ishiwata 1972, Ishiwata & Fujime 1972). In addition to the bending motions along the filament, fluctuations also appear to occur in the twist of the actin helix up to 10 degrees in the azimuthal angle between adjacent monomer units (Egelman et al 1982).

Actomyosin

Natural actomyosin-reaction with ATP. As mentioned above, the early work on fibrous muscle proteins was done on solutions which according to our present knowledge would be considered to be the combination of actin and myosin, viz. actomyosin. The striking physical changes that took place on adding ATP to what then was still called myosin (Needham et al 1941) became interpreted in the light of subsequent discoveries as a dissociation of actomyosin by ATP into actin and myosin (Szent-Györgyi 1945). The discovery and isolation of the pure proteins, myosin and actin, made it possible to study their combination.

Reconstituted actomyosin. On mixing myosin and actin there is a considerable increase in viscosity and birefringence of flow, both being reversed on addition of ATP. This was interpreted as the dissociation of actomyosin into actin and myosin (Szent-Györgyi 1945) and could be confirmed on the basis of light-scattering measurements and ultracentrifuge experiments (Gergely 1956, Weber 1956).

Most of the physicochemical studies on actomyosin were carried out at high ionic strength (0.6) because of the problems of solubility. On the other hand, it is at lower ionic strength (of the order of 0.05–0.15), more closely corresponding to that prevailing in the muscle cell itself, that the most interesting properties of the actin–myosin interaction come to light. Under these conditions myosin ATPase (EC 3.6.1.32) is changed into what we might call the actomyosin enzyme characterised by a high rate even in the presence of Mg in contrast to the inhibition of the myosin enzyme (Szent-Györgyi 1945). Thus actin acts as a powerful modifier of the ATPase activity of myosin, immediately suggesting interesting possibilities from the point of view of physiological regulation of energy release. It should be noted that, for quantitative studies on myosin–actin interaction, active fragments of myosin (HMM and HMM-S-1) have been widely used because

complications arising out of the aggregation of myosin molecules are thereby avoided.

Until recently it was generally accepted that in actin-activated myosin ATPase activity the hydrolysis of ATP occurs following the dissociation of actomyosin and results in the formation of an $ADP.P_i$–myosin complex (Lymn & Taylor 1970, 1971, Taylor 1979). The high rate of reaction would be due to the rapid dissociation of the products upon reassociation of myosin with actin. Subsequently, Eisenberg and his colleagues have produced evidence to show that hydrolysis of ATP also takes place on undissociated actin–myosin complexes and that myosin complexes with ATP and $ADP.P_i$ are in rapid equilibrium with the corresponding actomyosin complexes (Chalovich & Eisenberg 1982, Stein et al 1984, 1985). No consensus has been reached on the precise number of intermediate complexes. This has led to a distinction between a four-state model — with one ATP complex and one $ADP.P_i$ complex for myosin and similar complexes for actomyosin — and a six-state model containing two more $ADP.P_i$ complexes, one for myosin and one for actomyosin (see Rosenfeld & Taylor 1984, Stein et al 1985).

Another problem of interest is the identification of the chemical complex that corresponds to the tension-generating — or strong-binding — state. It appears that tension generation requires the dissociation of P_i. Studies on single fibres utilising 'caged' ATP, i.e. a form of inactive ATP that can be activated by laser irradiation (for a review see Hibberd & Trentham 1986), suggest that following dissociation a short-lived ADP complex is released which is capable of reversible binding of P_i. Studies of this type also show that the P_i interferes with tension development (Hibberd et al 1985, Webb et al 1986).

Myofibrils, glycerol-extracted, and skinned fibres. In addition to the study of actomyosin after reconstitution, studies on systems of somewhat higher complexity have also yielded interesting results. Glycerol-extracted muscle fibres or fibre bundles (Szent-Györgyi 1949) or myofibrils contain actomyosin in their essentially undisturbed configuration. However, these preparations do not contain the excitatory mechanism of the intact cells, nor do they contain the energy supply necessary for contraction. It was found, however, that on the addition of ATP single glycerinated fibres contract, or, depending on the experimental conditions, develop tension. Another useful system was introduced by Natori (1954): the skinned fibre, the sarcolemma of which is mechanically removed. Myofibrils exhibit ATPase activity that has the characteristic feature of Mg^{2+} activation observed on reconstituted and natural actomyosin, and their contraction results in a readily observable syneresis.

Regulatory proteins: Ca^{2+} dependence

Ca^{2+} requirement of actin–myosin interaction. Bozler (1954) and, independently, Watanabe (1955) found that ethylenediaminotetra-acetic acid (EDTA), a chelating agent, inhibits the ATP-induced contraction of glycerinated fibres; the Mg-ATPase activity of myofibrils was also found to be inhibited by EDTA (Perry & Grey 1956). The basis of the action of EDTA on myofibrils and actomyosin at low ionic strength (Weber & Winicur 1961) as well as of the inhibitory effect of higher concentrations of ATP on actomyosin superprecipitation (Weber 1959) is the removal of free Ca^{2+} ions which appear to be essential for the interaction of actin and myosin. Particularly helpful in this area was the introduction of the use of EDTA analogues (Ebashi et al 1960). One of these analogues, EGTA*, has a higher affinity to Ca^{2+} than to Mg^{2+}, thus eliminating the complications arising from the simultaneous binding of both divalent cations present in most of the systems under study.

It was first shown by Ebashi & Ebashi (1964) that the Ca^{2+} (or EGTA) sensitivity depends on the presence of protein factors other than actin and myosin. Natural actomyosin from striated muscle, unless subjected to special purification procedures (Schaub et al 1967), contains these sensitising factors whereas reconstituted actomyosin made with highly purified actin is insensitive to EGTA. The EGTA-sensitising factors have been resolved into several components and are usually referred to as the regulatory

proteins of the myofibril. They consist of tropomyosin — a protein that has been known and characterised for many years but which until recently has lacked a role — and troponin (discovered later), a term coined by Ebashi and his colleagues (Ebashi et al 1964, Ebashi & Kodama 1965, 1966, Ebashi et al 1969). Troponin is now recognised to be a complex of three protein components (Greaser & Gergely 1971, 1973). These proteins, as discussed below, are components of the thin actin filaments. Details of regulatory mechanisms that primarily depend on myosin, viz. the already-mentioned mechanism based on Ca^{2+}-dependent myosin phosphorylation in smooth muscle and that prevalent in various lower species (e.g. molluscs) involving a regulatory light chain and direct Ca^{2+} binding to myosin (see Lehman & Szent-Györgyi 1975, Kendrick-Jones & Scholey 1981), are beyond the scope of this chapter.

Tropomyosin. Tropomyosin can be extracted from an ethanol-treated muscle preparation (Bailey 1948). It shows a very strong tendency to aggregation at lower ionic strength and its true physical characteristics can be obtained only by increasing the ionic strength. Tropomyosin consists of two subunits, each having a molecular weight of about 33 000, which can be separated under denaturing conditions (Woods 1967). Tropomyosin is notable for its high α-helical content. In this respect it is very similar to the light meromyosin fraction of myosin (Cohen & Szent-Györgyi 1957), and the two subunits are arranged in a coiled-coil fashion (Cohen & Holmes 1963). Tropomyosin is characterised by a very high proportion of polar amino-acid residues, which may account for its tendency to be a stubborn contaminant of actin preparations. Various methods have been developed to obtain actin free of tropomyosin (Drabikowski & Gergely 1962, Spudich & Watt 1971). Vertebrate striated muscle tropomyosin preparations contain two different subunits (α and β) distinguishable by their electrophoretic mobility on SDS-polyacrylamide gels that form $\alpha\alpha$ and $\alpha\beta$ dimers (Yamaguchi et al 1974). The ratio of the two kinds of subunits differs in different types of muscle (e.g. only α is found in heart muscle, and the ratio of $\alpha : \beta$ also varies according to the fibre type (Cummins &

---

* EGTA: 1,2-bis (2-dicarboxymethylaminoethoxy)-ethane

Perry 1978) or the stage of ontological development (Roy et al 1979). The aggregation of tropomyosin at low ionic strength can occur both in the form of true three-dimensional crystals and so-called paracrystalline aggregates (Caspar et al 1971, Cohen et al 1971). Various forms are observed in the electron microscope that greatly contribute to our understanding of the size and shape of the molecules and the factors responsible for the interaction among the molecules. The amino-acid sequence of the tropomyosin subunits has been established (Stone et al 1974, Stone & Smillie 1978). The hydrophobic (non-polar) residues are alternately separated by three and two polar residues. This pattern, as discussed above for the myosin rod, results in the formation of the hydrophobic ridges on each of the two helices and the interaction of these hydrophobic regions forms the basis of the coiled-coil structure. Crick (1953) originally proposed such a 'knobs-into-holes' pattern for interacting α-helices. The helix–helix interaction in tropomyosin is further stabilised by ionic interactions among polar residues (Stone et al 1974, Parry 1975).

A wealth of detailed information has accumulated about tropomyosin (see Leavis & Gergely 1984) which cannot be discussed in full detail. A few important points, however, that contribute to our understanding of structural and functional features of tropomyosin are worth singling out. Notwithstanding the apparently uniform helical structure, there are variations in the stability of the molecule along its length. This differing flexibility (see Privalov 1982, Phillips et al 1986) may play an important part in the structural changes that tropomyosin may undergo in its regulatory role (see below). The region around the single SH group of β-tropomyosin (Cys 190) shows greater temperature dependence than the rest of the molecule, which is reflected in the behaviour of fluorescent pyrene derivatives attached to its Cys 190 (Betcher-Lange & Lehrer 1978, Lehrer et al 1981).

The availability of the amino-acid sequence has made it possible to interpret the postulated end-to-end interaction of TM molecules, which may be the structural basis for some of the co-operative effects in the thin filament. Equally important is a seven-fold repeat of pairs of regions of acidic residues in the primary structure of tropomyosin which may correspond to seven pairs of actin binding sites (McLachlan & Stewart 1976). The zones in each pair would be turned by 90 degrees relative to each other, representing on and off states in vivo (see below), and switching would involve a quarter turn of tropomyosin. Phillips et al (1986) find evidence for seven single sites and offer a different interpretation, discussed below. Important new insights on the nature and number of actin binding sites have been gained by Hitchcock-DeGregori & Varnell (1990) using bacterial expression of the protein. This work is consistent with there being seven pairs of actin-binding sites on tropomyosin with non-equivalent sites within each pair.

Finally, mention should be made of the genetic basis, already alluded to earlier, of variety in forms of tropomyosin, both from one species to another and also within the same organism. Some of the diversity is due to the presence of distinct genes encoding different chains, viz. α and β, and to multiple products derived from the same gene by means of alternative splicing (Ruiz-Opazo et al 1985, Flach et al 1986, Nadal-Ginard et al 1986).

Troponin. Tropomyosin alone does not account for the Ca^{2+} requirement of actomyosin ATPase activity. Ebashi & Ebashi (1964) initially assumed that a 'native tropomyosin' did exist, but now it is well established that another moiety, troponin, is also involved (Ebashi & Kodama 1965, 1966, Ebashi & Endo 1968).

Subunits. Troponin was at first considered to be a single protein and various molecular weights have been suggested (see e.g. Hartshorne & Dreizen 1972). The work of Hartshorne and his colleagues (Hartshorne & Mueller 1968, Hartshorne et al 1969) and Schaub & Perry (1969) has shown that troponin can be separated into at least two components. Greaser & Gergely (1971), by applying SDS-polyacrylamide gel electrophoresis, have shown that three components, with molecular weights of 37 000, 24 000 and 20 000, are necessary for reconstruction of troponin activity. This activity is defined as the conferring of Ca^{2+} sensitivity on actomyosin in the presence of tropomyosin. The three troponin components are referred to in decreasing order of molecular weight as TnT, TnI and TnC (Greaser et al 1972), the letters indicating that the three separate components have the ability to combine with tropomyosin, inhibit actomyosin ATPase regardless of the presence of Ca^{2+} (cf. Wilkinson et al 1972), and bind Ca^{2+}, respectively. The three troponin subunits occur in a 1 : 1 : 1 ratio, there being one troponin complex for each tropomyosin molecule. The amino-acid sequence of the subunits has been determined (TnC: Collins et al 1973, 1977; TnI: Wilkinson & Grand 1975; TnT: Pearlstone et al 1976); and the molecular weights are 18 000, 21 000 and 30 503 for TnC, TnI and TnT, respectively.

Ca^{2+} binding. When Ca^{2+} activates the actin–myosin interaction it binds to troponin via the TnC subunit. There are four Ca-binding sites in a TnC molecule, falling into two classes differing in their binding constants (Potter & Gergely 1974): about $2.5 \times 10^7 M^{-1}$ and $4 \times 10^5 M^{-1}$. The higher affinity sites competitively bind Mg^{2+} ($K = 5 \times 10^3 M^{-1}$); the other two are specific for Ca^{2+}. The affinity of TnC for Ca^{2+} is enhanced upon interaction with TnI, either in the TnC–TnI complex or in whole troponin. Effects of this interaction are also reflected in other physicochemical properties that have been studied in various laboratories, suggesting conformational changes induced in TnC by other subunits and vice versa. (For details see Leavis & Gergely 1984.)

An important relationship between TnC and the family of proteins first found in fish muscle able to bind Ca^{2+} — parvalbumin or muscle Ca^{2+}-binding proteins — and more recently discovered in muscles of higher species (Lehky et al 1974) has emerged. Parvalbumin differs from the myofibril-bound TnC in that it is free in the cytoplasm; its molecular weight is about half that of TnC. X-ray diffraction and amino-acid sequence studies have suggested certain repeating features within the parvalbumin molecules, attributable to gene duplication or triplication (Kretsinger 1972). Two Ca^{2+}-binding sites have been identified, each involving a 'loop' flanked by a pair of α-helices (Kretsinger & Nockolds 1973). Kretsinger and his colleagues predicted that there would be similarities between parvalbumin and TnC, and Collins and his colleagues (Collins et al 1973) showed that extensive homologies exist between the amino-acid sequences of TnC and parvalbumin. By comparison with the parvalbumin sequence there are four regions that would be probable candidates for the four Ca^{2+}-binding sites in TnC referred to above. Structural homologies between the light chains of myosin and parvalbumin and TnC have also been found (Collins 1974, Weeds & McLachlan 1974). Interestingly, with the exception of the regulatory light chain in molluscan muscle (see below), none of the other light chains contains a specific Ca^{2+}-binding site (see e.g. Bagshaw & Kendrick-Jones 1979).

From studies of the interaction of Ca^{2+} with enzymatically and chemically (cyanogen Br) produced fragments of TnC (Drabikowski et al 1977, Leavis et al 1978, Weeks & Perry 1978), it appears that the high-affinity sites are in the C-terminal half of the molecule (sites III and IV) while the low-affinity Ca^{2+}-specific sites (I and II) are in the α-terminal half. Ca^{2+}-binding to sites III and IV produces major conformational changes in the structure of TnC, while the changes occurring upon binding to sites I and II are more subtle (Potter et al 1976, Levine et al 1977, Seamon et al 1977, Johnson et al 1978). Yet it appears that the binding of Ca^{2+} to the latter (Ca^{2+}-specific) sites plays a crucial part in the regulation of actin–myosin interaction (Potter & Gergely 1974) which is also reflected in the kinetics of Ca^{2+} exchange (Johnson et al 1979). One of the important developments concerning the regulatory system of striated muscle has been the crystallisation of TnC and the determination of its structure by X-ray diffraction (Herzberg & James 1985, Sundaralingam et al 1985). TnC turns out to be a dumb-bell-shaped molecule: two globular regions, each containing two Ca^{2+}-binding sites, are connected by a nine-turn single α-helix; it is much more extended than the models previously considered with an overall length of 7 nm (see Kretsinger & Barry 1975, Leavis & Gergely 1984). The crystallisation of troponin C — the calcium receptor of the regulatory complex in striated muscle — has opened up new vistas of the molecular mechanism of switching on and off the interaction between actin and myosin. The fact that crystallisation was carried out under conditions in which only the two C-terminal calcium-binding sites that bind either Mg^{2+} or Ca^{2+} were occupied while the putative triggering binding sites in the N-terminal domain were vacant, combined with the differences in structure in the two domains, led James and his colleagues (Herzberg & James 1985, Herzberg et al 1986, Strynadka & James 1990, 1991) to propose that the switch in troponin C involves movement of a pair of α-helices with respect to the rest of the structure. This proposal has received experimental confirmation by establishing that cross-linking between two molecular-genetically introduced cysteine residues (Grabarek et al 1990) or changes in the charged nature of certain residues that were expected to undergo a distance change on Ca^{2+}-binding (Fujimori et al 1990) were accompanied by changes in the regulatory activity. Under conditions where movement was either prevented or made less likely by the engineered changes, inhibition of Ca^{2+} activation of actomyosin inter-action occurred. In some experiments changes in charges that would be expected to facilitate movement within the troponin C structure led to enhanced calcium binding and activation. Whether the connection between the two globular domains of the TnC molecule is as extended as in the crystals is at present an undecided question. Studies on calmodulin which — already referred to above — has a structure similar to that of TnC, indicates that the overall shape changes consider-ably on interaction with other proteins, particu-larly a fragment of the enzyme myosin light chain kinase which is activated by calmodulin (Ikura et al 1992, Meador et al 1992).

Other subunits. Structural information available on the other two subunits is of a less direct nature. Studies on the interaction among the subunits, actin and tropomyosin, utilising electron-microscopy, antibodies and fragments involved in protein–protein interactions, however, shed some light on the structures of the proteins involved while also furnishing data of potential importance for understanding their function. Suggestions for the structure of troponin T have been derived from electron-micrographs of troponin in combi-nation with tropomyosin (Ohtsuki 1979, Flicker et al 1982, Phillips et al 1986). These studies have suggested that troponin T is a rather elongated structure; its C-terminus forms a globular head with TnC and TnI which in its

complex with tropomyosin is close to the cysteine 190 of the latter. The C-terminal portion of TnT appears as a tail that extends somewhat beyond the C-terminus of tropomyosin. Thus in the thin filament troponin T would interact with the N-terminus of the adjacent tropomyosin as well (Fig. 6.5). In view of the fact that the regions of TnC that interact with TnI are 4–5 nm apart according to the new structural information, it is likely that troponin I also has a rather elongated shape. An answer to these questions will have to await more detailed structural studies on troponin I and troponin T.

Structural change and subunit interactions. In the meantime, information about distances within subunits and between subunits can be obtained from energy-transfer measurements utilising various acceptor and donor groups (Wang & Cheung 1986). Such studies also afford insight into changes that occur when Ca^{2+} binds to troponin C. A variety of studies utilising optical probes as well as nuclear magnetic resonance, electron paramagnetic resonance and cross-linking techniques have led to the conclusion that the first event in the chain that triggers muscle contraction is the conformational change in the N-terminal part that contains the Ca^{2+}-specific sites of troponin C. Studies with proteolytic fragments of TnC (Leavis et al 1978) have shown that a stretch of the primary structure of Tn encompassing residues 89–100 is of crucial importance in the activation of actomyosin ATPase (Grabarek et al 1981) and exhibits Ca^{2+}-dependent binding to TnI. Optical and paramag-netic probes attached to the -SH group in this region show a response to Ca^{2+}-binding at the triggering sites (Grabarek et al 1983, Wang et al

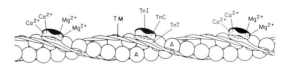

Fig. 6.5 Schematic representation of regulated thin filament. Note that actin monomers are represented as simple globular units. (For a more realistic actin structure, see Fig. 6.4.) Tropomyosin molecules are shown as coiled-coil helices; troponin subunits are drawn to suggest currently accepted structural features (see text) (copied with permission from Moss et al 1986).

1983, Rosenfeld & Taylor 1985). Changes also occur in the subunits interacting with troponin C. This is well documented for troponin I (see e.g. Strasburg et al 1985), whereas changes in troponin T are less easily demonstrable. (For details of interactions among the subunits see Leavis & Gergely 1984, Zot & Potter 1987, El-Saleh et al 1986, Grabarek et al 1992).

The second switch in the tropomyosin system involves changes in troponin I following the structural changes that take place in troponin C. Changes in troponin I have been detected by spectroscopic techniques (Strasburg et al 1985). It has also been established that a portion of troponin I moves away from actin and becomes more closely associated with troponin C in the course of activation (Tao et al 1990). The question whether the changes so far detected in the actin–tropomyosin–troponin system require the direct blocking by tropomyosin of the interaction of actin with myosin in the relaxed state and subsequent unblocking by a movement of the tropomysin molecule, or whether more subtle indirect changes in actin are involved in the inhibition and activation of contraction, remains to be resolved.

Phosphorylation. Phosphorylation of the TnI and TnT subunits has been reported (Cole & Perry 1975, England 1976, Moir et al 1977). Their functional role is at present not clear except that in the cardiac system, phosphorylation of TnI in vitro (Ray & England 1976) and in the perfused heart (Solaro et al 1976) decreases Ca^{2+} sensitivity and could act as part of a negative feedback system. No functional role has been assigned to the phosphorylation of tropomyosin (Mak et al 1978).

Additional myofibrillar and cytoskeletal proteins

A number of proteins in the muscle fibre play a structural role in addition to those directly involved in force generation and its control. Some of these represent a scaffolding that orders the arrangements of parts of the contractile machinery. Others are part of the Z discs linking actin filaments in abutting sarcomeres. Finally, there are those proteins that link myofibils to the

cell membranes or those that provide structural support for the membrane itself. Many of these so-called cytoskeletal proteins contain common motifs recognisable by their amino acid sequence. These include a triple helical structural motif found in spectrin, the chief submembrane cytoskeletal protein in the red blood cell; others show features found in immunoglobulins. We shall briefly discuss some of these proteins, among which are dystrophin and its associated proteins. Two excellent reviews provide a wealth of information for the interested reader (Luna & Hitt 1992, Small et al 1992).

α-Actinin, desmin, and β-actinin. These proteins have amino-acid compositions similar to that of actin (Ebashi et al 1964, Ebashi & Ebashi 1965, Maruyama 1965b). α-Actinin, which appears to be a highly asymmetrical rod-like molecule (Suzuki et al 1976, see also Pollard & Cooper 1986), is located in the Z band as shown by antibody labelling (Masaki et al 1967). The ability of α-actinin to cross-link F-actin (Maruyama & Ebashi 1965) may play a part in linking the actin filaments in the Z band. Since immunochemical techniques have revealed the presence of tropomyosin in the I band but not in the Z band (Pepe 1966), the disease of muscle — nemaline myopathy — in which rod-like bodies appear to be connected with the Z bands (Shy et al 1963, Price et al 1965), requires reinterpretation in molecular terms. Originally the rod-like bodies were thought to consist of tropomyosin but this now seems unlikely and the presence of α-actinin in these structures has been demonstrated (Sugita et al 1974).

Desmin (M_r 50 000), another constituent of the Z band, has been identified as the subunit of the so-called 10 nm filaments (Granger & Lazarides 1978). Filaments in the 10 nm class have been found in a variety of cells and are considered part of the so-called cytoskeleton (see Goldman et al 1979). For additional proteins, including vimentin, vinculin, spectrin and ankyrin, involved in anchoring actin filaments and the Z band to the muscle cell membrane see Lazarides & Capetanaki (1986) and Pollard & Cooper (1986).

β-Actinin may be a capping protein of actin (cf Maruyama 1965a,b, Pollard & Cooper 1986) suppressing the elongation of actin filaments at their pointed end (Maruyama et al 1977, Funatsu & Ishiwata 1985).

Thick filament proteins.

M-line constituents. The identity of the M-line protein (Morimoto & Harrington 1972), which would play a part in linking the thick filaments in the middle of the sarcomere (Pepe 1972), has been considerably clarified. The presence of creatine kinase in the M line has been demonstrated (Turner et al 1973). In addition to a 165 kDa M protein (Masaki & Takaiti 1974, Trinick & Lowey 1977) there is also a 185 kDA protein, myomesin (Grove et al 1984), forming part of connecting bridges between thick filaments (Strehler et al 1983, Wallimann et al 1983). The functional role of the presence of creatine kinase — separating a small fraction of the total creatine content — remains to be elucidated. For a review see Wallimann & Eppenberger (1985).

Other thick filament proteins. The C protein plays a structural role in the architecture of the thick filaments (Offer 1972, Offer et al 1973), which exhibits homology to immunoglobulins (Einheber & Fischman 1990, Epstein & Fischman 1991), and in regulating the interaction of myosin cross-bridges with actin (Starr & Offer 1978). Additional components associated with thick filaments are X and H proteins (Starr & Offer 1983, Bennett et al 1985) which, together with the C protein, are associated with distinct transverse structures identifiable with specific antibodies. Their function remains to be established.

Continuous filaments.

It has been suggested that fibrillin and connectin filaments are running from Z band to Z band across the entire sarcomere (Guba et al 1968). Such filaments have also been described by Hoyle and his colleagues (Hoyle 1967, Hoyle et al 1973). Connectin (Maruyama et al 1977), the main constituent of elastic protein filaments in muscle, appears to be identical with titin, a large myofibrillar protein (Wang et al 1983). A related protein is nebulin (for reviews see Wang 1982, Maruyama 1986, Trinick 1992). X-irradiation of a skinned rabbit fibre selectively destroys nebulin and titin, leading to disorganisation of sarcomeres, and interferes with force development (Horowits et al 1986).

Dystrophin and associated proteins.

Dystrophin, the product of the gene that is deleted or otherwise defective in Duchenne muscular dystrophy, is another important membrane-associated cytoskeletal protein of striated muscle (for reviews see Monaco 1989, Anderson & Kunkel 1992). Dystrophin is a rod-shaped protein of high molecular mass (427 kDa). It contains four distinct domains. The N-terminal domain has features found in various actin-binding proteins including α-actinin (c.f. Way et al 1992); the central portion has 24 repeats resembling those found in spectrin, the chief membrane-associated protein of red cells; a cysteine-rich portion similar to one found in α-actinin; and there is a 420 amino acid unique C-terminal segment (Koenig et al 1988, Koenig & Kunkel 1990). Campbell and his colleagues have recently shown that dystrophin interacts with the membrane via a multicomponent glycoprotein complex, including a transmembrane component, thus providing a means for interaction with extracellular matrix elements such as laminin (Ervasti et al 1991, Ervasti & Campbell 1991, Ibraghimov-Beskrovnaya et al 1992; for a review see Matsumura & Campbell 1994) (Fig. 6.6). Current models envisage a dimeric dystrophin structure with the two molecules in an antiparallel arrangement and suggest that the N-terminus interacts with actin and the C-terminus with the membrane-bound glycoprotein. The existence of dimeric dystrophin molecules has been shown in electron-microscopic studies along with monomeric and tetrameric forms (Sato et al 1992). Studies using specific antibodies in combination with electron-microscopy have shown that dystrophin co-localizes with various cytoskeletal proteins along the plasma membrane forming costameric structures or longitudinal strands as well as showing a distribution related to sarcomeric segments (Lakonishok et al 1992, Minetti et al 1992, Porter et al 1992, Straub et al 1992).

A protein encoded by an autosomal gene in human chromosome 6 and mouse chromosome 10 (Love et al 1989) has been shown to exhibit a high degree of overall similarity to dystrophin in its structure, with a particularly highly conserved C-terminal region (Khurana et al 1990, Tinsley et al 1992). This protein, first named dystrophin-

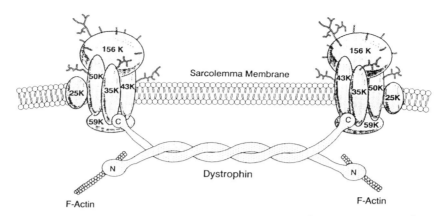

Fig. 6.6 Model of the dystrophin-glycoprotein complex. Numbers on components of membrane-imbedded complex indicate mass in kDa. Branched structures on complex indicate carbohydrate moiety. (Reproduced with permission from Ervasti and Campbell, and Cell Press, Cell 66: 1121, 1991)

related protein (DRP) and subsequently *utrophin*, is expressed in all muscles, as well as in other tissues (Love et al 1991, Nguyen thi Man et al 1992). Its level of expression is especially high in fetal muscle. In normal adult muscles it is localised at the neuromuscular junction, whereas in fetal muscles and in Duchenne muscular dystrophy and in muscles of the mdx mouse there is wide distribution along the plasma membrane. The high level of expression of utrophin in muscles that lack dystrophin has led to the suggestion that utrophin may in some cases conpensate for it. The direct demonstration of the interaction of utrophin with the dystrophin-associated membrane proteins (Matsumura et al 1992) is further evidence for the functional similarity between dystrophin and utrophin and lends support for possible therapeutic interventions involving utrophin (Matsumura et al 1992, Karpati et al 1993, Takemitsu et al 1993).

SARCOPLASMIC RETICULUM

Introduction

The key role of the free Ca^{2+} concentration in regulating the state of muscle contraction or relaxation is well established (for a comprehensive review see Ashley et al 1991). $[Ca^{2+}]$ itself is controlled by the transverse tubule (T tubule)/sarcoplasmic reticulum (SR) system, the

anatomy of which is discussed in Chapter 2. In relaxed muscle $[Ca^{2+}]$ is kept at ~ 0.01 μM, ~ 10^5 times lower than that in blood plasma, while activation requires $[Ca^{2+}]$ between 1 and 10 μM. The abrupt increase in free $[Ca^{2+}]$ at the onset of contraction is accomplished by release from the Ca store within the SR and the return to the resting value is attributable to the ATP-dependent Ca^{2+} pump located in the SR. It should be noted that the low intracellular $[Ca^{2+}]$ in a resting muscle could not be maintained solely by the SR which has a finite capacity, in view of the influx of Ca^{2+} due to the large gradient between the extracellular and intracellular space. An ATP-dependent Ca^{2+}-pump is also located in the plasma membrane and the T tubules (Brandt et al 1980, Hidalgo et al 1983, Mickelson et al 1985), which may fulfil the role of similar enzymes in other types of cells, including those in cardiac muscle. (For a review see Carafoli 1991).

Work on the biochemistry of the mechanism of control of contraction and relaxation started with the studies of Marsh (1951, 1952) and Bendall (1952). This led to the discovery of the so-called relaxing factor, the relation of which to intracellular membranes was first recognised by Ebashi and his colleagues (Kumagai et al 1955, Ebashi 1957). They also identified ATPase activity with the so-called Kielley–Meyerhof enzyme (Kielley & Meyerhof 1948, 1950). These particulate preparations contain fragments of the sarcoplasmic reticulum that form closed vesicles. For a review of the early work see Weber (1966), Tada et al (1978), Hasselbach (1979).

Ca²⁺-uptake, ATPase and phosphorylation

The Ca^{2+} uptake by fragments of the sarcoplasmic reticulum in the presence of ATP is promoted by a number of anions such as oxalate, phosphate and pyrophosphate (Ebashi 1961, Hasselbach & Makinose 1961, Ebashi & Lipmann 1962, Martonosi & Feretos 1964). The splitting of ATP is the energy source for the active transport of Ca^{2+} into the interior of the SR. Ca^{2+}-accumulation in the presence of a precipitant anion, oxalate, has been demonstrated electron-microscopically in situ in the terminal cisternae of the reticulum (Costantin et al 1965, Pease et al 1965) and in vesicles of fragmented SR (Ikemoto et al 1968). A value of 2.0 for the $\Delta Ca/\Delta ATP$ ratio is most likely under physiological conditions (see Hasselbach 1979). A change in the Ca^{2+} affinity of the protein appears to be correlated with the translocation of Ca^{2+} from the low-concentration outside compartment into the high-concentration interior (Ikemoto 1976). This is an important feature of current models of Ca^{2+} transport (Jencks 1980, 1983, Tanford 1983, 1984, Eisenberg & Hill 1985).

Demonstration of the Ca^{2+}-dependent formation of an acid-stable phosphorylated enzyme from ATP (Yamamoto & Tonomura 1967) implied in the ADP–ATP exchange described earlier (Ebashi & Lipmann 1962, Haselbach & Makinose 1963) has opened up the way to the elucidation of the mechanism of an ATPase-coupled Ca^{2+}-transport process. The calcium pump can run in reverse, i.e. ATP is synthesised on the efflux of calcium from a Ca^{2+}-loaded vesicle (Makinose 1971, Makinose & Hasselbach 1971). This synthesis of ATP involves the formation of the phosphoprotein intermediate from inorganic phosphate.

Proteins

Ca²⁺-pumping ATPase. The ATPase moiety has a molecular weight of about 100 000 and contains the sites at which phosphorylation occurs (Martonosi 1969). The spherical particles seen in electron micrographs of negatively stained preparations have been attributed to this component (Migala et al 1973, Thorley-Lawson & Green 1973, Stewart & MacLennan 1974). It also contains three types of Ca^{2+}-binding sites (Ikemoto 1975). Phosphorylation occurs at an aspartic acid residue (Bastide et al 1973). The state of some of the -SH groups of the ATPase protein appears to be influencing the activity. Conversely, the -SH groups fall into certain classes on the basis of their reactivity to thiol reagents; moreover, these reactivities change depending on the occupancy of various Ca^{2+}-binding sites (Ikemoto et al 1978, see also Tada et al 1978).

The amino-acid sequence of the Ca-ATPase of the SR, on which work was started many years ago by protein sequencing techniques, has now been deduced from the nucleotide sequence of the ATPase gene. There seem to be two distinct genes encoding the Ca^{2+}-ATPases of fast- and slow-twitch muscle SR; the highly homologous cardiac and slow-twitch muscle SR Ca^{2+}-ATPase may be products of the same gene resulting from alternative splices (Brandl et al 1986). The first reported sequence (MacLennan et al 1985) that led to a proposed three-dimensional structure embedded in the membrane appears to have been that of the skeletal slow-twitch muscle enzyme (Brandl et al 1986). The sequences are largely consistent with previous partial sequence studies and tentative connectivities established on the basis of accessibility of the SR ATPase to proteolytic enzymes. The expression of the Ca^{2+}-pump cDNA in COS-cells permitted a series of important studies utilizing site-directed mutagenesis for putting previous conjectures on structure–function relations on a firm basis (MacLennan 1990). It appears that ATP-binding, phosphorylation of an aspartic acid residue, and energy transduction functions can be assigned to three distinct domains on the cytoplasmic surface of the SR membrane. Of the 10 transmembrane α-helical segments, four (4, 5, 6 and 8) seem to be intimately involved in Ca^{2+}-binding. In the primary structure the energy-transducing region links helices 2 and 3 via the putative cytoplasmic stalks attached to them, while the phosphorylation domain and the ATP-binding domain form the link between helices 4 and 5 (Inesi et al 1992, MacLennan et al 1992).

Clarification of the details of the mechanism by which energy transduction between the phosphorylated Asp residue and the Ca^{2+}-binding region occurs requires further investigation, although models involving rotation or tilting of transmembrane segments have been proposed. The use of spectroscopic techniques involving resonance energy transfer among various sites provides information on distances among landmarks on the pump protein and may be useful in the evaluation of structural and functional models. Progress has been achieved in studies on a two-dimensional crystalline array of the Ca^{2+}-pump protein both in situ and in isolated vesicles (Castellani & Hardwicke 1983, Dux & Martonosi 1983). Three-dimensional image reconstruction of electron-micrographs of these crystalline structures has led to the delineation of the overall shape of the transport enzyme and to renewed interest in, and speculation about, the possible existence of dimers that may form a functional unit of the transport enzyme (Castellani et al 1985, Franzini-Armstrong & Ferguson 1985, Taylor et al 1986). Anti-ATPase antibodies against well-defined segments of protein provide further information on the disposition of regions within the protein with respect to their relation to the membrane in conjunction with these two-dimensional crystals (Martonosi et al 1990). Studies on three-dimensional crystals of the Ca-ATPase (Stokes & Green 1990a,b) have now yielded cryo-electron microscopic images at 14 Å resolution (Toyoshima et al 1993). The detailed three-dimensional structure will eventually have to be based on X-ray crystallography.

Studies on the two-dimensional crystals also afford support for the generally held view that the mechanism of Ca^{2+}-transport involves cyclic alternation between two main states of the enzyme, usually referred to as E1 and E2 or E and E*. Chemically, these states are characterised by differing affinities for Ca^{2+} and differing reactivities with respect to phosphorylation by ATP on the one hand and inorganic phosphate on the other. Conditions that lead to the stabilisation of

putative states, E1 and E2 respectively, result in changes detectable in the pattern of interaction among monomeric units in the two-dimensional lattice (Dux et al 1985). A somewhat simplified scheme incorporating the essential features of the ATP-dependent Ca^{2+}-transport system (DeMeis & Vianna 1979) is given below. For additional details see Inesi (1985).

$$E_1 \rightleftharpoons \quad Ca_2.E_1 \rightleftharpoons \quad Ca_2.E_1.ATP \rightleftharpoons \quad Ca_2.E{\sim}P$$
$$\updownarrow \qquad\qquad\qquad\qquad\qquad\qquad\qquad \updownarrow$$
$$E_2 \hookleftarrow \quad E_2.P_i \hookleftarrow \quad E_2{-}P \hookleftarrow \quad Ca_2.E_2{\sim}P$$

The provisional nature of this scheme should be appreciated. Jencks (1989) has proposed a simpler model.

Calsequestrin is another protein capable of binding Ca^{2+} (MacLennan & Wong 1971, Ikemoto et al 1971, 1972). It possesses numerous (~ 50) but rather low-affinity ($K \sim 10^3 M^{-1}$) Ca^{1+}-binding sites per molecule ($M_r \sim 41$–45 K depending on the species). Its role in Ca^{2+}-storage is supported by recent evidence showing its localisation in the terminal cisternae of the sarcoplasmic reticulum. These are the regions that are in close contact with the T-tubule system which, as discussed below, is involved in transmission of the depolarisation of the plasma membrane to the interior of the muscle, resulting in the release of Ca^{2+} from the sarcoplasmic reticulum on excitation.

Comparison of the time-course of Ca^{2+}-release with changes in the free $[Ca^{2+}]$ inside SR vesicles shows a rise in $[Ca^{2+}]_i$ before the release, thus suggesting a more active role for calsequestrin in the regulation of cytoplasmic Ca^{2+} than that of a passive Ca^{2+}-store (Ikemoto et al 1991).

Other proteins include a proteolipid and a high-affinity Ca^{2+}-binding protein (Ostwald & MacLennan 1974), but their functional and structural role has yet to be determined. Phospholamban was originally described as a protein with a molecular weight of 22 000 present in cardiac sarcoplasmic reticulum (Tada et al 1974, 1975). The true molecular weight of phospholamban is 6000 based on amino acid sequence data (Fujii et al 1986, Simmerman et al 1986). It appears to be present in the SR membrane as a pentamer; a preliminary model (Simmerman et al 1986) places the C-termini inside the membrane with the N-termini disposed on the cytoplasmic side of the membrane. Phospholamban has also been found in slow twitch skeletal muscle fibres (Jorgensen & Jones 1986). It can be phosphorylated by a cyclic AMP-dependent or a calmodulin-dependent protein kinase, and in view of the reported stimulation of calcium transport by the kinase (Tada et al 1974) a regulatory role for phospholamban as a mediator of the effect of catecholamines in cardiac muscle has been suggested; calmodulin-dependent phosphorylation has also been reported (LePeuch et al 1979, for a detailed discussion see Tada & Inui 1983).

Lipid–protein interaction. Early experiments showing that phospholipase destroys the ATPase and relaxing activity of elements of the SR (Ebashi 1957) pointed to the involvement of phospholipids in its structure and function. Phospholipase-C-treated fragments of the sarcoplasmic reticulum that have lost their ATPase and Ca^{2+}-accumulating ability again become active on the addition of phospholipids (Martonosi 1963, Martonosi et al 1968). It is now clear that the sarcoplasmic reticulum represents a membrane-bound enzyme system carrying out the ATPase-linked Ca^{2+}-transport function.

Although many details of the protein–lipid interaction remain to be elucidated, it is apparent that replacement of SR lipids with another lipid moiety determines some properties of the ATPase-transport protein. The ATPase activity depends on certain properties of the lipid moiety (Warren et al 1974) and temperature-induced changes in the motion of the ATPase reflect changes in the fluidity of the lipid (Inesi et al 1973, Hidalgo et al 1976, 1978). A variety of studies indicate that there is a correlation between the Ca^{2+}-dependent dephosphorylation of the phosphoprotein, the mobility of the protein, and the fluidity of the membrane (see Martonosi 1984).

Excitation–contraction coupling

The first step in the physiological mechanism of Ca^{2+} release, it is generally believed, involves some change in the T-tubule/SR junctional region related to the charge movement demonstrated some years ago (Schneider & Chandler 1973, Kovacs et al 1979; for a review see Schneider 1981). The link between this charge movement to

the induction of changes in the SR membrane may, according to various suggestions (Volpe et al 1986), be mediated by the actual movements of proteins, by electrical currents, or by some chemical process involving either Ca^{2+} — more likely in cardiac than in skeletal muscle (Fabiato & Fabiato 1979) — or, as more recent evidence suggests, phosphorylated inositol derivatives. The latter have been implicated as chemical messengers in various cellular processes (Berridge & Irvine 1984) and in smooth muscle (Somlyo & Somlyo 1992).

The difficulty of studying Ca^{2+}-release in vitro has been partly ascribable to the lack of systems that can be safely regarded as in vitro models of the triggering in situ of the intact T–SR complex. One criterion should be whether or not the speed at which Ca^{2+} is released in vitro is comparable with that involved in the physiological process, viz. $60–140 \ s^{-1}$. Various methods used in vitro for the induction of Ca^{2+} release — drugs (caffeine, halothane) — interact extravesicularly and depolarisation is achieved by ion replacement under conditions that minimise osmotic effects (Ikemoto et al 1984). The T tubule plays an important part in the Ca^{2+} release from the SR induced by ionic replacement (depolarisation). This has been shown in vitro on vesicular preparations from which the T-tubular elements were or were not removed (Ikemoto et al 1984) and on single fibres devoid of the plasma membrane and in which the T system had been inactivated (Donaldson 1986, Lamb & Stephenson 1990). In contrast, Ca^{2+} release induced by increased Ca^{2+} or by drugs such as caffeine or quercitin does not involve the T system.

Molecular components. The components of the molecular machinery of the excitation–contraction mechanism have now been characterized to a great extent by a combination of biochemical, biophysical, molecular-genetic and electron-microscopic techniques (for extensive reviews see Fleischer & Inui 1989, Rios & Pizarro 1991, MacLennan 1990, Lamb 1992, Rios et al 1992). One of the proteins involved has a mass of 565 kDa protein — established by cloning of the full-length cDNA (Fleischer & Inui 1989). This protein is also referred to as the ryanodine receptor (RR) in view of its ability to bind ryanodine, a plant alkaloid that also modulates the receptor's function in reconstituted membranes. Earlier electron-microscopic work (Franzini-Armstrong & Nunzi 1983) has revealed structures connecting the T-tubule and SR membrane; the so-called feet (Fig. 6.7). Each foot has been shown to represent a homotetrameric complex of the ryanodine receptor. Electron-micrographs suggest that most of the cytoplasmic bulk of the RR lies between the SR and T-tubule membrane, and chemical features of the amino acid sequence deduced from that of cDNA indicate that the C-terminal is embedded in the SR membrane (Takeshima et al 1989, Otsu et al 1990, Zorzato et al 1990). Electron-micrographs of the RR tetramer also suggest the presence of a channel in the centre of the complex as well as a radial channel in each of the subunits. The former would be the release channel from the SR, opening into

the radial channels leading into the sarcoplasm (Wagenknecht et al 1989). The feet form a tetragonal array and every other foot appears opposite a tetrad of proteins embedded in the T-tubule membrane (Block et al 1988).

The protein facing the ryanodine receptor (the tetrad in the T-tubule) has been identified as the so-called dihydropyridine (DHP) receptor, characterized in cardiac and skeletal muscle as a Ca^{2+}-channel that can be inhibited by dihydropyridine (DHP)-channel blockers (Coronado & Affolter 1986, Catterall et al 1988, Leung et al 1988). The role of the DHP-receptor in skeletal muscle excitation–contraction (EC) has emerged from the work of Lamb (1986) and Rios & Brum (1987); however, there is no evidence that in skeletal muscle the DHP receptor's Ca^{2+}-channel plays a functional role. Nevertheless, the DHP

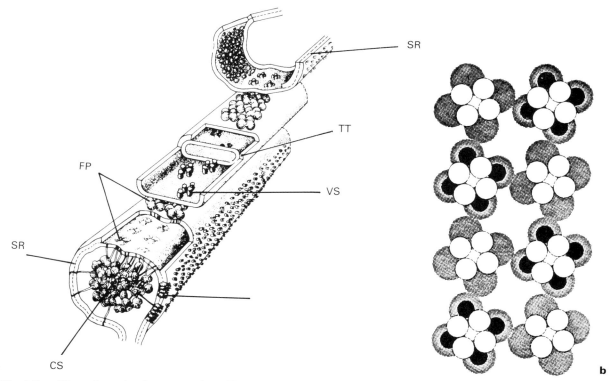

Fig. 6.7   a Three-dimensional reconstruction of T-tubule-sarcoplasmic reticulum junction. Key to figure: SR sarcoplasmic reticulum junctional membrane (bilayer); TT t-tubule membrane (bilayer); FP foot-protein (4 subunits) with 'bumps' on inner layer of SR; VS voltage sensor (dihydropyridine receptor) tetrad; CS calsequestrin.
b Diagram of the spatial relationships between the junctional complex components. Four large shaded spheres represent each foot; small white spheres are the intramembranous portion of the foot protein (bumps); black discs represent the position (but not necessarily the size) of the tubule tetrads. In this diagram tetrads interact with alternate feet. (Reproduced with permission from Block et al., Journal of Cell Biology 107: 2587, 1988)

receptor has a key role, as shown by the fact that in mice with muscle dysgenesis there is no EC coupling and the α_1 subunit of the DHP receptor is missing (Sharp et al 1989). Expression of the α_1 subunit following injection of the appropriate cDNA restores EC coupling (Tanabe et al 1988). The DHP receptor is a multi-subunit heteromeric complex; the precise role played by the different subunits is still under study. The α_1 subunit of the receptor complex is regarded as the sensor of voltage change in the T-tubule membrane, while the β subunit plays a modulatory role (Beam et al 1992, Lamb 1992). The importance of electric charge movement in the T-tubule membrane is well established but the A_3 mechanism of signal transmission from voltage sensor to RR is not finally settled (Brandt et al 1990, Kim et al 1990).

A 95 kDA protein component of the junctional SR, triadin (Kim et al 1990, Caswell et al 1991), may be identical to the 94 kDA glycoprotein recently characterized by Campbell and colleagues (Knudson et al, 1993a,b). In earlier work (Caswell et al 1991) it was suggested that triadin may bind to both the ryanodine receptor and the DHP receptor (voltage sensor), representing a link between the two. In light of recent work (McPherson & Campbell 1993) it seems that most of the glycoprotein (or triadin) is inside the reticulum, supported by, triadin's primary structure deduced from cloned cDNA, suggesting only a 47-residue cytoplasmic portion. These results would be consistent with direct triadin calsequestrin interaction, possibly affecting calcium binding to, or release from, the latter.

EFFECT OF CHANGES IN ACTIVITY AND INNERVATION

Starting with the work of Eccles and his colleagues (Eccles et al 1958, Buller et al 1960), several authors have reported that when a fast muscle is cross-reinnervated by a nerve that originally supplied a slow muscle, it acquires properties characteristic of a slow muscle; reciprocal changes take place in a slow muscle that has been cross-reinnervated by a fast muscle nerve. Changes in contractile speed are accompanied by corresponding changes in both the myosin ATPase activity (Buller et al 1969, Bárány & Close 1971)

and the protein subunit pattern (Sreter et al 1974, Weeds et al 1974). Changes have also been observed in the pattern of metabolic enzymes (Dubowitz 1967, Romanul & Van Der Meulen 1967, Guth et al 1968, Weeds et al 1974) and in the activity of the sarcoplasmic reticulum.

The work of Salmons & Vrbová (1969) shows that, even with undisturbed nerve–muscle connections, changes in physiological parameters can be brought about if the pattern of neural activity reaching the muscle is changed. When the motor nerve is stimulated continuously over a period of weeks, imposing on the fast muscle a pattern of activity similar to that normally reaching a slow muscle, a marked slowing of the time-course of isometric contraction and relaxation ensues. Such stimulation also produces changes in the subunit pattern of myosin, the ATPase activity of myosin, the staining pattern of LMM paracrystals, and the Ca^{2+} uptake of the sarcoplasmic reticulum. The changes correspond to an essentially complete fast–slow transformation. The biochemical changes in myosin are paralleled by changes in the histochemical ATPase reaction, as well as by changes in the glycolytic oxidative enzyme pattern (Sreter et al 1973, Pette et al 1973, Romanul et al 1974, Salmons & Sreter 1976, Heilmann & Pette 1979).

Changes in various components on chronic stimulation do not take place synchronously (see Jolesz & Sreter 1981, Pette 1984, Swynghedauw 1986). This has been documented in many studies. Changes in metabolic enzymes and in components of the sarcoplasmic reticulum occur rather early and changes in myosin light chains precede those in the heavy chains. The latter process has been documented in detail (Brown et al 1983). Perhaps the earliest changes, within the first few days (Klug et al 1983, Leberer & Pette 1986), occur in the cytoplasmic Ca^{2+}-binding protein, parvalbumin, found in fast muscle (see Celio & Heizmann 1982). Studies on changes in the RNA level and their products suggest involvement of translational control in fibre transformation (Heilig & Pette 1983, Pluskal & Sreter 1983).

The change-over in the muscle type is attributable to the transformation of the existing fibres by the switching on of normally inactive genes and the switching off of those that had been active, rather than to the destruction of the original fibre population and its replacement by new fibres. Depending on the actual conditions of stimulation, degeneration–regeneration processes involving the formation of new fibres may also contribute to fast-to-slow muscle conversion (Maier et al 1986). Early in the course of the transformation of fast muscle, antibodies against both fast and slow myosins react with the same fibre (Rubinstein et al 1978), while in normal fast muscle only the antibody against fast myosin reacts (Arndt & Pepe 1975, Weeds et al 1975). After complete transformation, again only one type of antibody reacts — that reacting with slow myosin. The same conclusion has been reached from SDS-gel electrophoretic studies on single fibres showing the transient presence of both fast- and slow-type myosin light chains (Pette & Schnez 1977). As has recently been shown, myosin transitions in chronic stimulation do not involve embryonic isozymes (Hoffman et al 1985). Low-frequency (10 Hz) intermittent stimulation has been shown to lead to Type IIB to IIA fibre transformation (Mabuchi et al 1982), suggesting that IIB fibres undergoing fast-to-slow transformation may go through a transitional IIA stage (see also Pette 1984). Other interventions leaving the nerve–muscle connection intact are also able to change the muscle type, as judged by histochemical and biochemical criteria. Thus, sectioning of the peroneal nerve caused changes in the ipsilateral soleus from slow to fast type (Guth & Wells 1976). Removal of the gastrocnemius and soleus muscle in the rat caused the ipsilateral plantaris to change from the relatively fast to the slow type (Samaha & Theis 1976).

During the past few years studies on fibre transformation have not only relied on the protein pattern for following the process but started to rely increasingly on complementary information derived from mRNA work. The nature of the signal(s) that may be involved in activating the expression of certain genes while turning off those of the others is still unknown. Important new investigations on the development of muscle and the emergence of a family of regulatory factors controlling differentiation of muscle tissue are likely to provide clues for progress in this field (Hoh 1991, Weintraub et al 1991, Bandman 1992, Blau 1992, Hughes & Blau 1992, Olson 1992, Stockdale 1992).

THEORIES OF CONTRACTION AND RELAXATION

Sliding model

It is well established that myosin and actin are localised in distinct filaments in the myofibril. Furthermore, during contraction the length of the individual filaments does not change, but rather their relative position, which leads to what is summed up in the term 'sliding' or 'interdigitating' model of muscle contraction (Hanson & Huxley 1955, Huxley 1960). The classic experiments of Gordon et al (1966) on single fibres, establishing a direct relationship between overlap speed of shortening independent of overlap, not only support the sliding filament model but also the concept of independent force generators (see the thoughtful analysis of A. F. Huxley 1974, 1979) identifiable with actin–myosin links in the overlap zone.

Molecular mechanisms

The question arises, how does the interaction between actin and myosin located in different structural elements lead to tension development and to shortening of the sarcomere? X-ray work on living muscle points to the movement of the bridges projecting from the myosin filaments as the molecular event underlying contraction (Huxley & Brown 1967). Pepe's work (1966, 1967a,b) with the use of antibody staining techniques has revealed considerable changes within the thick filament structure during shortening, indicative of flexibility in some part — presumably the rod portion — of the myosin molecule. Flexibility of the rod portion would also account for the fact that the interaction between myosin and actin filaments results in the production of constant force per cross-bridge and the separation among filaments increases with decreasing sarcomere length (see Huxley 1968, 1969). As mentioned above, various lines of experimental evidence support such flexibility in myosin. While most authors consider a direct interaction between the nearly globular portions (subfragment-1) of myosin and actin as the key to contraction, a less direct type — perhaps longer range — interaction involving electrostatic and Van der Waals forces has also been suggested (Pollack 1983). The arrowhead structures resulting from the interaction of HMM or S-1 with actin (Huxley 1963) can be explained in terms of a regular attachment of the individual myosin heads to the actin globules, each head making a precise angle with the actin filament axis (Moore et al 1970). It appeared reasonable to assume that the tendency of the myosin heads to align themselves on actin in this fashion represents an important driving force in the mechanism of muscle contraction.

It has generally been assumed that the basis of force development and contraction is a rotation of the myosin heads attached to actin with respect to the filament axis. Force development would — at the molecular level — be due to the stretching of an elastic structure, forming part either of myosin or of the myosin–actin interface (Huxley 1974, 1979). Many current models place the elastic element in the S-2 portion of myosin, which is the connecting link between the rod portion and the myosin heads.

The rotating-head model implies that attachment of the head occurs in a specific orientation and that force development is associated with a rotation into another orientation, the latter being the thermodynamically favoured one also to be found in rigor. A difficulty, not fully resolved, has arisen owing to the fact that many attempts to detect intermediate orientations of probes rigidly attached to the myosin heads in fibres devoid of sarcolemma (skinned fibres) have failed. With some fluorescent dyes (Yanagida 1981, Nagano & Yanagida 1984, Yanagida 1985) as probes, and with paramagnetic spin labels on myosin (Thomas & Cooke 1980, Cooke et al 1982b), only one attached state with rigor-like orientation could be detected. On the other hand, a rhodamine probe, also on the same thiol group on the myosin head, did reveal a state other than rigor or detached (relaxed) in the presence of ADP or under conditions corresponding to activation of a fibre (Borejdo et al 1982, Burghardt et al 1984). However, a time-resolved study (Tanner et al

1992) using the probe employed by Borejdo et al (1982) showed no temporal correlation between force development and optical changes. This suggests that the latter cannot be attributed to a molecular process underlying force generation but may show a local change occurring subsequently. Energy-transfer measurements leading to an estimate of the distance between a point (thiol group of light chain 1) on the myosin head attached to actin and another point on actin (Cys 374) also show two attached states in a system simulating contraction (Bhandari et al 1985). X-ray diffraction studies (see Huxley & Faruqi 1983) on contracting intact muscles show that under isometric conditions up to 90% of the myosin heads are close to the actin filaments, but the so-called layer line pattern indicates azimuthal disorder.

The use of time-resolved cryo-electron-microscopy on frozen hydrated samples appears most promising for direct observations of the myosin cross-bridges and their interaction with actin. Pollard et al (1993) have recently reported that no detectable angular change takes place in the cross-bridge population, underlying its cyclic interaction with actin. On the other hand Funatsu et al (1993), by using a cryo-electron-microscope in combination with photogenerated liberation of ATP from a caged compound, do report some change in attachment angle. Clearly, more work is needed to resolve the question. The difficulty may be that movement may occur within the myosin head in such a way that the bulk of the mass remains attached without change in angle while the moving part may not always be detectable at the relatively low resolution of electron-microscopy. This view would be consistent with the structural changes revealed by X-ray scattering of the myosin head in solution (Wakabayashi et al 1992), with earlier interpretations of electric birefringence results (Highsmith & Eden 1990), and with recent suggestions derived from X-ray diffraction studies (cf Rayment et al 1993a).

Time-resolved (on the millisecond time-scale) diffraction patterns show that on activation the first changes are attributable to structural changes in the thin filaments, followed in about 15 ms by changes indicative of myosin-head attachment and, after a further similar lag period, tension development takes place. The earliest changes have been interpreted (Huxley et al 1982) as being related to the activation process; they suggest that the lag between changes indicative of myosin attachment to actin and tension development is due to the formation of cross-bridges that at first do not develop tension — i.e. weak attachment. Tension appears as these bridges enter a strongly attached state capable of tension development. Huxley & Kress (1985) have proposed a model of the attached cross-bridge that would develop tension over only about 4 nm of its 12 nm total excursion. This model may reconcile some apparent discrepancies between EPR and X-ray measurements with regard to the fraction of rigidly attached cross-bridges in an active muscle. It would also provide some explanation for the apparent lack of intermediate orientations in attached states. (For details see Huxley & Kress 1985, Cooke 1986.)

The precise mode of the force generation by muscle has not been settled (Fig. 6.8). A. F. Huxley (1957) originally proposed a mechanism in which thermal energy stored in some portion of

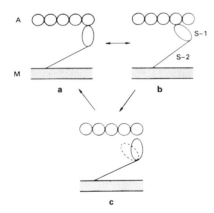

Fig. 6.8 Model of interaction of the myosin head with actin based on Huxley (1969) and Huxley & Simmons (1971). **a** Attachment of myosin to actin. **b** Tilting of myosin head. **c** Detachment produced by ATP followed by its hydrolysis. On the basis of in vitro kinetic studies the myosin species present in **a** + **b** carries the ADP-P product complex. The attached head may oscillate between positions **a** and **b**. Whether the dissociated myosin head can oscillate between the perpendicular or tilted position or whether it is locked in the perpendicular position is not finally settled. For details see text.

the connecting bridges played an important part. A later proposal (Huxley & Simmons 1971) based on very rapid mechanical transients involved attachment of myosin heads to actin via elastic connections, with the possibility of a tension-dependent equilibrium among several stable positions. Eisenberg & Hill (1978) located the elasticity in the bond between the myosin head and actin and assumed a rigid connecting link. The details of the way in which various intermediate stages in the hydrolysis of ATP can be correlated with configurational states on the myosin head with respect to actin are currently under investigation in several laboratories. Recent studies using a photoactivatable ATP (caged ATP) appear promising (see Hibberd & Trentham 1986). The original mathematical analysis given by Huxley (1957) accounted for a number of mechanical and energetic features of muscle. More recent developments in muscle energetics and mechanics and our knowledge of the details of the molecular apparatus have prompted refinements in the theoretical models, such as those by T. L. Hill and his colleagues (Hill 1977, Eisenberg & Hill 1985) describing in terms of statistical mechanics, thermodynamics and kinetics the actin–myosin nucleotide system and serving as a framework for future theoretical and experimental interpretations.

Harrington and his colleagues have been concerned, over the years, with the possible role of the S-2 portion of myosin in force generation rather than serving as a passive string. They have proposed an α-helix random coil phase-change-like transformation as the basis of contractile force generation. These views are backed by experiments showing increased proteolytic sensitivity in the putative hinge region of S-2 under conditions of fibre activation by ATP (see Harrington 1979, Harrington & Rodgers 1984, Ueno & Harrington 1981, 1986a,b and references in the later two papers). If S-2 is the site of force generation, the path of energy transduction from ATP hydrolysis in the remote head region remains to be elucidated.

The work of Yanagida et al (1985) has raised some problems for the conventional view that the free energy of ATP is transduced into mechanical work within the span of the stretch of a single cross-bridge. These authors calculate a distance of >60 nm over which movement occurs as a result of the hydrolysis of a single ATP molecule. In these experiments unloaded relative movement of thick and thin filaments takes place, so that direct conversion of energy could not be determined.

Yanagida and his colleagues (Harada et al 1990, Ishiyima et al 1991) have continued to produce evidence for a long interaction distance between myosin heads and actin, while others (Uyeda et al 1990, Pate et al 1993) arrive at distances more consistant with step-sizes corresponding to single myosin head/actin interactions. All investigators in the field are aware of the importance of identifying possible experimental problems and sorting out assumptions that may be involved in the interpretation of the results. Increasingly sophisticated techniques (e.g. the use of so-called optical tweezers), making it possible to measure forces exerted by and movement of single molecules, are likely to bring about a solution of the problem (for comprehensive reviews see Huxley 1990, Burton 1992).

Study of the kinetics of tension recovery following repeated quick releases while the muscle was shortening, led Lombardi and his colleagues (Lombardi et al 1992, see also Huxley 1992) to the conclusion that the free energy of hydrolysis of one ATP molecule can be distributed for work performance over several cycles of tension recovery. Tension recovery occurred on the same time-scale as that of the recovery of the intensity of the 14.3 nm line in the X-ray diffraction pattern of the fibre (Irving et al 1992), suggesting that the myosin heads underwent movement — power stroke — as tension developed, rather than as a result of rapid shortening itself. These results — if the interpretations are correct — have important implications for our understanding of the molecular events underlying force development and may require revision concerning the mechanism of energy transduction.

Regulation

The key role of Ca^{2+} in the regulation of the actin–myosin in vitro interaction has been discussed above, together with the role of the sarcoplasmic reticulum in the modulation of the free sarcoplasmic Ca^{2+}-concentration during contraction and relaxation. The question remains of how the in vivo interaction of Ca^{2+} with the contractile apparatus fits the picture. There is the (by now classic) physiological evidence that injection of Ca^{2+} into muscle cells produces contraction (Heilbrunn & Wiercinski 1947). Podolsky & Constantin (1964), working on muscle stripped of its outer membrane, could by local application of Ca^{2+} elicit contraction which, owing to the presence of Ca-accumulating reticular elements, spontaneously gave way to relaxation.

Activation by Ca^{2+} would correspond to the removal of the inhibitory effect of the tropomyosin–troponin system in the interaction of actin and myosin observed in vitro. The molecular basis of this process appears to lie in a movement, deduced from X-ray and combined electron-microscopic and optical diffraction studies, of the tropomyosin molecules located in the grooves of the actin filaments into positions where they would not interfere with the attachment of myosin heads (Haselgrove 1972, Huxley 1972, Spudich et al 1972, Parry & Squire 1973). Although questions raised by Seymour & O'Brien (1980) concerning the possibility of direct contact between myosin and tropomyosin, which is essential in a straightforward steric blocking model, have in part been answered (Taylor & Amos 1981, O'Brien et al 1983), the precise details of the structure of the thin filament, including the spatial relation between tropomyosin-binding and myosin-binding sites, has not been fully resolved (Toyoshima & Wakabayashi 1984a,b, Amos 1985). The importance of movement in the activation process of tropomyosin or some equivalent structural change in the thin filament has received further support by X-ray diffraction studies mentioned above (Kress et al 1986). Biochemical studies have raised some challenges to the simple steric blocking model in that there is considerable evidence to show that the switch from relaxation to contraction, which in vitro is brought about by adding Ca^{2+}, is not accompanied by a drastic change in the binding of myosin or active myosin fragments to actin (Chalovich et al 1981, Chalovich & Eisenberg 1982), leading to the view that the regulation of contraction involves a change in one of the kinetic steps of the actin–myosin cycle rather than a simple shift in the equilibrium. The biochemical data have been interpreted in terms of the existence of weakly and strongly attached cross-bridges and regulation would involve a shift in distribution among these (see Hill 1983, Eisenberg & Hill 1985). Brenner and his colleagues (Brenner et al 1982) found evidence for the existence of cross-bridges in relaxed muscle at low ionic strength from high-velocity stretch. Brenner et al (1984) noted differences in the X-ray diffraction pattern between relaxed muscle at low ionic strength and muscle in rigor. As mentioned above, Huxley and his colleagues (Huxley & Kress 1985, Kress et al 1986) also postulated weakly attached cross-bridges that do not generate tension and it remains to be seen whether these correspond to those deduced from in vitro studies and from stretch–velocity dependent stiffness measurements (for a discussion see Irving 1985).

Although early work has shown that phosphorylation and dephosphorylation of the regulatory light chain of myosin takes place in association with contraction and relaxation, respectively (Bárány & Bárány 1980), attempts to find in vitro correlates in terms of ATPase activity of actomyosin or maximal tension-force development in isolated muscle have failed (see Sweeney et al 1993). However, evidence for phosphorylation-dependent post-tetanic potentiation of development in fast-twitch muscles (see e.g. Cooke & Stull 1981, Persechini et al 1985) stimulated interest in the problem. Metzger et al (1989) have shown that phosphorylation of myosin increases the Ca^{2+}-sensitivity of the rate constant of force development at intermediate levels of activation. They suggested that this was related to facilitation of the release of cross-bridges from the thick filaments. More recently Levine et al (1993) have produced evidence that movement of cross-bridges away from the thick filaments takes place on phosphorylation as previously found for smooth and invertebrate muscle (for more details on the role of the light chain see Sweeney et al 1993). The possibility that other components of the thick filament, e.g. C protein, play a regulatory role has emerged from experiments involving solution extraction from and replacement in permeabilized fibres (see Moss 1992). This technique is also applicable to the identification of other functionally important moieties.

The idea of co-operativity in the thin filament was first expressed by A. Weber and her colleagues some 15 years ago. The original co-operative model involved seven actins attached to one tropomyosin molecule and envisaged spreading of the effects of myosin binding within one tropomyosin–actin heptamer as well as providing a basis for the ability of Ca^{2+} bound to the troponin complex to affect more than one actin. More recently, Hill and his colleagues introduced a co-operative model involving nearest-neighbour interactions between tropomyosin molecules in the thin filament using the Ising formalism (Hill et al 1980). This model is capable of explaining the high degree of co-operativity observed in studies on binding of myosin S-1 to actin in the absence of Ca^{2+} (Greene & Eisenberg 1980), which could not be accounted for by assuming only the co-operativity based on the seven-fold interaction within a tropomyosin domain. For an alternative model see Geeves (1991). Tropomyosin–tropomyosin interactions have also been used to explain the variation of actin-activated S-1 ATPase as a function of S-1 concentration (Lehrer & Morris 1984). Studies with optical probes attached to troponin have not been fully interpretable in a simple manner based on the Hill–Ising model (Trybus & Taylor 1981, Greene 1986). Electron-microscopy and X-ray diffraction on muscle fibres suggest tropomyosin movement in the course of activation. Correspondingly two groups of residues have been identified in the actin structure as possible interaction sites with tropomyosin in the 'on' and 'off' states of the thin filament (see Kabsch & Vandekerckhove 1992). In terms of the ATPase activity of regulated actin-activated myosin there are three states: inhibited, low activity, and high, or potentiated, activity. The relationship of these states to structurally distinguishable states is not fully understood.

CONCLUSION

This brief survey of the biochemical features of muscle and their relation to structural problems is of necessity incomplete, but it should give an impression of the complexity of the processes involved. It clearly shows that a large number of sites exist at which defects may lead to serious disturbances of muscle function. However, the continued application of techniques of molecular genetics, X-ray diffraction, electron-microscopy, and other tools of physical chemistry promise a rapid filling in of the gaps in our knowledge of normal muscle structure and function. Future studies of this nature are, therefore, of crucial importance for the understanding of the manifold disorders that are the subject of this volume.

ACKNOWLEDGEMENT

The preparation of this chapter was supported by grants from the NIH (HL-5949) and the Muscular Dystrophy Association.

REFERENCES

Aebi U, Fowler W E, Isenberg G, Pollard T D, Smith P R 1981 Crystalline actin sheets: their structure and polymorphism. Journal of Cell Biology 91: 340

Alberts B, Bray D, Lewis J, Raff M, Roberts K, Watson J D 1989 Molecular biology of Ca^{++}, 2nd edn. Garland Publishing, New York

Amos L A 1985 Structure of muscle filaments studied by electron microscopy. Annual Review of Biophysics and Biophysical Chemistry 14: 291

Anderson M S, Kunkel L M 1992 The molecular and biochemical basis of Duchenne muscular dystrophy. Trends in Biomedical Sciences 17: 289

Ando T, Asai H 1979 Conformational change in actin filament induced by the interaction with heavy meromyosin: effects of pH, tropomyosin and deoxy-ATP. Journal of Molecular Biology 129: 265

Applegate D, Reisler E 1983 Protease-sensitive regions in myosin subfragment 1. Proceedings of the National Academy of Sciences (USA) 80: 7109

Arndt I, Pepe F 1975 Antigenic specificity of red and white muscle myosin. Journal of Histochemistry and Cytochemistry 23: 159

Asakura S, Kasai M, Oosawa F 1960 The effect of temperature on the equilibrium state of actin solutions. Journal of Polymer Science 44: 35

Ashley C C, Mulligan I P, Lea T J 1991 Ca^{2+} and activation mechanisms in skeletal muscle. Quarterly Reviews of Biophysics 24: 1

Bagshaw C R, Kendrick-Jones J 1979 Characterization of homologous divalent metal ion binding sites of vertebrate and molluscan myosins using electron paramagnetic resonance spectroscopy. Journal of Molecular Biology 130: 317

Bailey K 1948 Tropomyosin: A new asymmetric protein component of the muscle fibril. Biochemical Journal 43: 271

Balint M, Wolf I, Tarcsafvi A, Gergely J, Sreter F 1978 Location of SH-1 and SH-2 in the heavy chain segment of heavy meromyosin. Archives of Biochemistry and Biophysics 190: 793

Bandman E 1985 Myosin isoenzyme transitions in muscle development, maturation and disease. International Review of Cytology 97: 97

Bandman E 1992 Contractile protein isoforms in muscle development. Developmental Biology 154: 273

Bárány M 1967 Activity of myosin correlated with speed of muscle shortening. Journal of General Physiology 50: 197

Bárány M, Finkelman F, Therattil-Antony T 1962 Studies on the bound calcium of actin. Archives of Biochemistry and Biophysics 98: 28

Bárány M, Bárány K, Reckard T, Volpe A 1965 Myosin of fast and slow muscles of the rabbit. Archives of Biochemistry and Biophysics 109: 185

Bárány M, Close R I 1971 The transformation of myosin in cross-reinnervated rat muscle. Journal of Physiology 213: 458

Bárány M, Bárány K 1980 Phosphorylation of the myofibrillar proteins. Annual Review of Physiology 42: 275

Barton J R, Buckingham M E 1985 The myosin alkali light chain proteins and their genes. Biochemical Journal 231: 249

Bastide F, Meissner G, Fleischer S, Post R L 1973 Similarity of the active site of phosphorylation of the ATPase for transport of sodium and potassium ions in kidney to that for transport of calcium ions in the sarcoplasmic reticulum of muscle. Journal of Biological Chemistry 248: 8385

Beam K G, Adams B A, Niidome T, Numa S, Tanabe T 1992 Function of a truncated dihydropyridine receptor as both voltage sensor and calcium channel. Nature 360: 169

Bendall J R 1952 Effect of the 'Marsh Factor' on the shortening of muscle fibre models in the presence of adenosine triphosphate. Nature 170: 1058

Bennett P, Starr R, Elliott A, Offer G 1985 The structure of C-protein and X-protein molecules and a polymer of X-protein. Journal of Molecular Biology 184: 297

Berridge M J, Irvine R F 1984 Inositol triphosphate, a novel second messenger in cellular signal transduction. Nature (London) 312: 315

Bertocci L A, Fleckenstein J L, Antoniu J 1992 Human muscle fatigue after glycogen depletion. A ^{31}P magnetic resonance study. Journal of Applied Physiology 73: 75

Bertrand R, Derancourt J, Kassab R 1992 Molecular movements in the actomyosin complex: F-actin-promoted internal crosslinking of the 25- and 20-kDa heavy chain fragments of skeletal myosin subfragment 1. Biochemistry 31: 12219

Betcher-Lange S, Lehrer S S 1978 Pyrene excimer fluorescence in rabbit skeletal αα tropomyosin labelled with N-(1-pyrene) maleimide. Journal of Biological Chemistry 253: 3757

Bhandari D G, Trayer H R, Trayer I P 1985 Resonance energy transfer evidence for two attached states of the actomyosin complex. Federation of European Biochemical Societies 187: 160

Bigland-Ritchie B, Woods J J 1984 Changes in muscle

contractile properties and neural control during human muscle fatigue. Muscle and Nerve 7: 691

Bigland-Ritchie B R, Dawson N J, Johansson R S, Lippold O C J 1986 Reflex origin for the slowing of motoneurone firing rates in fatigue of human voluntary contractions. Journal of Physiology 379: 451

Blau H M 1992 Differentiation requires continuous active control. Annual Review of Biochemistry 61: 1213

Block B A, Imagawa T, Campbell K P, Franzini-Armstrong C 1988. Structural evidence for direct interaction between the molecular components of the transverse tubule/sarcoplasmic reticulum in skeletal muscle. Journal of Cell Biology 107: 2587

Borejdo J, Assulin O, Ando T, Putnam S 1982 Crossbridge orientation in skeletal muscle measured by linear dichroism of an extrinsic chromophore. Journal of Molecular Biology 158: 391

Botts J, Takashi R, Torgerson P, Hozumi T, Muhlrad A, Mornet D 1984 On the mechanism of energy transduction in myosin subfragment 1. Proceedings of the National Academy of Sciences USA 81: 2060

Boyer P F 1977 Oxidative phosphorylation and photophosphorylation. Annual Review of Biochemistry 46: 955

Bozler E 1954 Relaxation in extracted muscle fibers. Journal of General Physiology 38: 149

Brandl C J, Green N M, Korczak B, MacLennan D H 1986 Two Ca^{2+} ATPase genes: homologies and mechanistic implications of deduced amino acid sequences. Cell 44: 597

Brandt N R, Caswell A H, Brunschwig J-P 1980 ATP-energized Ca^{2+} pump in isolated transverse tubules of skeletal muscle. Journal of Biological Chemistry 255: 6290

Brandt N R, Caswell A H, Brunschwig J P, Kang J J, Antoniu B, Ikemoto N 1992 Effects of anti-triadin antibody on Ca^{++} release from sarcoplasmic reticulum FEBS Letters 299: 57

Brandt N R, Caswell A H, Wen S-R, Talvenheimo J A 1990 Molecular interactions of the junctional foot protein and dihydropyridine receptor in skeletal muscle triads. Journal of Membrane Biology 113: 237

Brenner B, Schoenberg M, Chalovich J M, Green L E, Eisenberg E 1982 Evidence for cross-bridge attachment in relaxed muscle at low ionic strength. Proceedings of the National Academy of Sciences USA 79: 7288

Brenner B, Yu L C, Podolsky R J 1984 X-ray diffraction evidence for cross-bridge formation in relaxed muscle fibers at various ionic strengths. Biophysical Journal 46: 299

Brown W E, Salmons S, Whalen R G 1983 The sequential replacement of myosin subunit isoforms during muscle type transformation induced by long term electrical stimulation. Journal of Biological Chemistry 258: 14686

Buller A J, Eccles J C, Eccles R M 1960 Interactions between motor neurones and muscles in respect of the characteristic speeds of their responses. Journal of Physiology 150: 417

Buller A J, Mommaerts W F H M, Seraydarian K 1969 Enzymatic properties of myosin in fast and slow twitch muscles of the cat following cross-innervation. Journal of Physiology 205: 581

Burghardt T P, Tidswell M, Borejdo J 1984 Crossbridge order and orientation in resting single diglycerinated muscle fibres studied by linear dichroism of bound rhodamine labels. Journal of Muscle Research and Cell Motility 5: 657

Burley R, Seidel J C, Gergely J 1971 The stoichiometry of the reaction of the spin labeling of F actin and the effect of orientation of spin labeled F actin filaments. Archives of Biochemistry and Biophysics 146: 597

Burley R, Seidel J C, Gergely J 1972 The effect of divalent metal binding on the electron spin resonance spectra of spin labeled actin. Evidence for a spin–spin interaction involving Mn^{2+}. Archives of Biochemistry and Biophysics 150: 792

Burton K 1992 Myosin step size: estimates from motility assays and shortening muscle. Journal of Muscle Research and Cell Motility 13: 590

Cain D F, Infante A A, Davies R E 1962 Chemistry of muscle contraction. Nature 196: 214

Carafoli E 1991 The calcium pumping ATPase of the plasma membrane. Annual Review of Physiology 53: 531

Carlier, M-F 1991 Actin: protein structure and filament dynamics. Journal of Biological Chemistry 266: 1

Carlier M F, Pantaloni D, Korn E D 1984 Steady state length distribution of F-actin under controlled fragmentation and mechanism of length redistribution following fragmentation. Journal of Biological Chemistry 259: 9987

Carlier M, Pantaloni D, Korn E D 1986 The effects of Mg^{2-} at the high affinity and low affinity sites on the polymerization of actin and associated ATP hydrolysis. Journal of Biological Chemistry 261: 10785

Carlsson L, Nystrom L-E, Sundkvist I, Markey F, Lindberg J 1977 Actin polymerizability is influenced by profilin, a low molecular weight protein in non-muscle cells. Journal of Molecular Biology 115: 465

Caspar D L D, Cohen C, Longley W 1971 Tropomyosin: crystal structure polymorphism and molecular interactions. Journal of Molecular Biology 41: 87

Castellani L, Hardwicke P 1983 Crystalline structure of sarcoplasmic reticulum from scallop. Journal of Cell Biology 97: 557

Castellani L, Hardwicke P M D, Vibert P 1985 Dimer ribbons in the three-dimensional structure of sarcoplasmic reticulum. Journal of Molecular Biology 185: 579

Caswell A H, Brandt N R, Burnschwig J-P, Purkerson S 1991 Localisation and partial characterisation of the oligomeric disulfide-linked molecular weight 95 000 protein (triadin) which binds the ryanodine and dihydropyridine receptors in skeletal muscle triadic vesicles. Biochemistry 30: 1507

Catterall W A, Seagar M J, Takahashi M 1988 Molecular properties of dihydropyridine-sensitive calcium channels in skeletal muscle. Journal of Biological Chemistry 263: 3535

Celio M R, Heizmann C W 1982 Calcium-binding protein parvalbumin is associated with fast contracting muscle fibres. Nature 297: 504

Chalovich J M, Chock P B, Eisenberg E 1981 Mechanism of action of troponin-tropomyosin inhibition of actomyosin ATPase activity without inhibition of myosin binding to actin. Journal of Biological Chemistry 256: 575

Chalovich J M, Eisenberg E 1982 Inhibition of actomyosin ATPase activity by troponin-tropomyosin without blocking the binding of myosin to actin. Journal of Biological Chemistry 257: 2432

Chance B, Leigh J S Jr, Kent J, McCully K 1986 Metabolic control principles and ^{31}P NMR. Federation Proceedings 45: 2915

Chaussepied P, Mornet E, Kassab R 1986 Nucleotide trapping at the ATPase site of myosin subfragment 1 by a new interthiol crosslinking. Proceedings of the National Academy of Sciences (USA) 83: 2037

Chen T, Applegate D, Reisler E 1985 Crosslinking of actin to myosin subfragment 1 in the presence of nucleotides. Biochemistry 24: 5620

Cheung H, Cooke R, Smith L 1971 The G-actin–F-actin transformation as studied by the fluorescence of bound dansyl cysteine. Archives of Biochemistry and Biophysics 142: 333

Cohen C 1985 Hormones, second messengers and the reversible phosphorylation of proteins: an overview. BioEssays 2: 63

Cohen P 1988 Protein-phosphorylation and hormone action. Proceedings of the Royal Society of London Series B 234: 115

Cohen P 1989 The structure and regulation of phosphatases. Annual Review of Biochemistry 58: 453

Cohen C, Szent-Györgyi A G 1957 Optical rotation and helical polypeptide chain configuration in α proteins. Journal of the American Chemical Society 79: 248

Cohen C, Holmes K C 1963 X-ray diffraction evidence for α helical coiled coils in native myosins. Journal of Molecular Biology 6: 423

Cohen C, Caspar D L D, Parry D A D, Lucas R M 1971 Tropomyosin crystal dynamics. Cold Spring Harbor Symposia on Quantitative Biology 36: 205

Cohen P 1978 The role of cyclic AMP-dependent protein kinase in the regulation of glycose metabolism in mammalian skeletal muscle. In: Horecker B L, Stadtman E R (eds) Current topics in cell regulation. 1. Academic Press, New York, p 117

Cohen P, Burchell A, Foulkes G, Cohen P T W, Vanaman T C, Nairn A C 1978 Identification of the Ca^{2+}-dependent modulator protein of the fourth sub-unit of rabbit skeletal phosphorylase kinase. Federation of European Biochemical Society: Letters, 92: 287

Cole H A, Perry S V 1975 The phosphorylation of troponin 1 from cardiac muscle. Biochemical Journal 149: 525

Collins J H 1974 Homology of myosin light chains, troponin C and parvalbumin deduced from comparison of their amino acid sequences. Biochemical and Biophysical Research Communications 58: 301

Collins J H 1991 Myosin light chains and troponin C: structural and evolutionary relationships revealed by amino acid sequence comparisons. Journal of Muscle Research and Cell Motility 12: 3

Collins J H, Potter J D, Horn M, Wilshire G, Jackman N 1973 Structural studies on rabbit skeletal muscle troponin C: evidence for gene replications and homology with calcium binding proteins from carp and hake muscle. Federation of European Biochemical Society Letters 36: 268

Collins J H, Greaser M, Potter J D, Horn M 1977 Determination of the amino acid sequence of troponin C from rabbit skeletal muscle. Journal of Biological Chemistry 252: 6356

Cooke R 1986 The mechanism of muscle contraction. CRC Critical Reviews in Biochemistry 21: 53

Cooke R, Stull J T 1981 Myosin phosphorylation: a biochemical mechanism for regulating contractility. In: Dowben R M, Shay J W (eds) Cell and muscle motility, vol 1. Plenum Press, New York, p 99

Cooke R, Crowder M S, Thomas D D 1982a Orientation of spin labels attached to cross-bridges in contracting muscle fibers. Nature (London) 300: 776

Cooke R, Franks K, Stull J T 1982b Myosin phosphorylation regulates the ATPase activity of permeable skeletal muscle fibers. Federation of European Biochemical Societies 144: 33

Coronado R, Affolter H 1986 Characterization of dihydropyridine-sensitive calcium channels from purified skeletal muscle tranverse tubules. In: Miller C (ed) Ion channel reconstitution. Plenum, New York, p 403

Cori C F 1941 Phosphorylation of glycogen and glucose. Biological Symposia 5: 131

Cori G T, Cori C F 1945 The enzymatic conversion of phosphorylase a to b. Journal of Biological Chemistry 158: 321

Constantin L, Franzini-Armstrong C, Podolsky R 1965 Localization of calcium accumulating structures in striated muscle fibers. Science 147: 158

Craig S W, Pollard T D 1982 Actin binding proteins. Trends in Biochemical Sciences 7: 88

Crick F H C 1953 The packing of α helices: simple coiled coils. Acta Crystallographica 6: 689

Cummins P, Perry S V 1978 Troponin I from human skeletal and cardiac muscles. Biochemical Journal 171: 251

d'Albis A, Pantaloni C, Bechett J J 1979 An electrophoretic study of native myosin isozymes and their subunit content. European Journal of Biochemistry 99: 297

Dantzig J A, Goldman Y E, Millar N C, Lacktis J, Homsher E 1992 Reversal of the cross-bridge force-generating transition by photogeneration of phosphate in rabbit psoas muscle fibres. Journal of Physiology 451: 247

Darnell J E, Lodish H, Baltimore D 1990 Molecular cell biology, 2nd edn. Scientific American Books, New York

Dawson M J 1986 The relation between muscle function and metabolism studied by ^{31}P NMR spectroscopy. In: Chen S, Ho C (eds) NMR in biology and medicine. Raven Press, New York, p 185

Dawson M J, Gadian D G, Wilkie D R 1978 Muscular fatigue investigated by phosphorus nuclear magnetic resonance. Nature (London) 274: 861

Dawson M J, Wilkie D R 1984 Muscle and brain metabolism studied by ^{31}P nuclear magnetic resonance. In: Baker P (ed) Recent advances in physiology. Churchill Livingstone, Edinburgh, p 247

DeMeis L, Vianna A L 1979 Energy interconversion by the Ca^{2+}-dependent ATPase of the sarcoplasmic reticulum. Annual Review of Biochemistry 48: 275

Donaldson S K B 1986 Peeled mammalian skeletal muscle fibers. Journal of General Physiology 86: 501

Drabikowski W, Gergely J 1962 The effect of the temperature of extraction on the tropomyosin content in actin. Journal of Biological Chemistry 237: 3412

Drabikowski W, Strzelecka-Golaszewska H 1963 The exchange of actin-bound calcium with various bivalent cations. Biochimica et Biophysica Acta 71: 486

Drabikowski W, Grabarek Z, Barylko B 1977 Degradation of the TnC component of troponin by trypsin. Biochimica et Biophysica Acta 490: 216

Dubowitz V 1967 Cross-innervated mammalian skeletal muscle. Histochemical, physiological and biochemical observations. Journal of Physiology 193: 481

Duke J, Takashi R, Eu K, Morales M F 1976 Reciprocal reactivities of specific thiols when actin binds to myosin. Proceedings of the National Academy of Sciences (USA) 73: 302

Dux L, Martonosi A 1983 Two dimensional arrays of proteins in sarcoplasmic reticulum and purified Ca^{2+}–ATPase vesicles treated with vanadate. Journal of Biological Chemistry 258: 2599

Dux L, Taylor K A, Ting-Beall H P, Martonosi A 1985 Crystallization of the Ca^{2+}-ATPase of sarcoplasmic reticulum by calcium and lanthanide ions. Journal of Biological Chemistry 260: 11730

Ebashi S 1957 Kielley-Meyerhof's granules and the relaxation of glycerinated muscle fibers. In: Conference on the Chemistry of Muscle Contraction. Igaku Shoin, Tokyo, p 89

Ebashi S, 1972 Separation of troponin into three components. Journal of Biochemistry 72: 787

Ebashi S, Ebashi F, Fujie Y 1960 The effect of EDTA and its analogues on glycerinated muscle fibers and myosin adenosine triphosphatase. Journal of Biochemistry 47: 54

Ebashi S, Lipmann F 1962 Adenosine triphosphate linked concentration of calcium ions in a particulate fraction of rabbit muscle. Journal of Cell Biology 14: 389

Ebashi S, Ebashi F 1964 A new protein component participating in the superprecipitation of myosin B. Journal of Biochemistry 55: 604

Ebashi S, Ebashi F, Maruyama K 1964 A new protein factor promoting contraction of actomyosin. Nature 203: 645

Ebashi S, Ebashi F 1965 α-actinin: a new structural protein from striated muscle I. Preparation and action on actomyosin ATP interactions. Journal of Biochemistry 58: 7

Ebashi S, Kodama A 1965 A new protein factor promoting aggregation of tropomyosin. Journal of Biochemistry 58: 107

Ebashi S, Kodama A 1966 Interaction of troponin with F actin in the presence of tropomyosin. Journal of Biochemistry 59: 425

Ebashi S, Endo M, 1968 Calcium ion and muscle contraction. Progress in Biophysics and Molecular Biology 18: 123

Ebashi S, Endo M, Ohtsuki I 1969 Control of muscle contraction. Quarterly Review of Biophysics 2: 351

Eccles J C, Eccles R M, Lundberg A 1958 The action potentials of the α motor neurones supplying fast and slow muscle. Journal of Physiology 142: 275

Edwards R H T 1984 New techniques for studying human muscle function, metabolism and fatigue. Muscle and Nerve 7: 599

Edwards R H T, Griffiths R D, Cady E B 1985 Topical magnetic resonance for the study of muscle metabolism in human myopathy. Clinical Physiology 5: 95

Egelman E H, Francis N, DeRosier D 1982 F-actin is a helix with a random variable twist. Nature (London) 298: 131

Egelman E H, Francis N, DeRosier D 1983 Helical disorder and the filament structure of F-actin are elucidated by the angle-layered aggregate. Journal of Molecular Biology 166: 605

Einheber S, Fischman D A 1990 Isolation and characterization of a cDNA clone encoding avian skeletal muscle C-protein: an intracellular member of the immunoglobulin superfamily. Proceedings of the National Academy of Sciences of the USA 87: 2157

Eisenberg E, Hill T L 1978 A crossbridge model of muscle contraction. Progress in Biophysics and Molecular Biology 13: 55

Eisenberg E, Hill T L 1985 Muscle contraction and free energy transduction in biological systems. Science 227: 999

Elliott A, Offer G 1978 Shape and flexibility of the myosin molecule. Journal of Molecular Biology 123: 505

El-Saleh S C, Potter J D, Solaro R J 1986 Alteration of actin-tropomyosin interaction in 2,4-pentanedione-treated rabbit skeletal myofibrils. Journal of Biological Chemistry 261: 14646

Elzinga M, Collins J H 1972 The amino acid sequence of rabbit skeletal muscle actin. Cold Spring Harbor Symposia on Quantitative Biology 37: 1

Elzinga M, Collins J H, Kuehl W M, Adelstein R S 1973 The complete amino acid sequence of rabbit skeletal muscle actin. Proceedings of the National Academy of Sciences (USA) 70: 2687

Elzinga M, Collins J H 1977 Amino acid sequence of a myosin fragment that contains SH-1, SH-2 and N$^\tau$-methylhistidine. Proceedings of the National Academy of Sciences (USA) 74: 4281

Elzinga M, Phelan J J 1984 F-actin is intermolecularly crosslinked by N,N'-p-phenylenedimaleimide through lysine-191 and cysteine-374. Proceedings of the National Academy of Sciences (USA) 812: 6599

Engel A G, Banker B Q 1993 Myology, 2nd ed. McGraw Hill, New York

Engelhardt W A, Ljubimova M N 1939 Myosins and adenosinetriphosphatase. Nature 144: 668

England P 1976 Studies on the phosphorylation of the inhibitory sub-unit of troponin during modification of contraction in perfused heart. Biochemical Journal 160: 295

Enoka R M, Stuart D G 1992 Neurobiology of muscle fatigue. Journal of Applied Physiology 72: 1631

El-Saleh S C, Warber K D, Potter J D 1986 The role of tropomyosin–troponin in the regulation of skeletal muscle contraction. Journal of Muscle Research and Cell Motility 7: 387

Epstein H F, Fischman D A 1991 Molecular analysis of protein assembly in muscle development. Science 251: 1039

Ervasti J M, Campbell K P 1991 Membrane organization of the dystrophin–glycoprotein complex. Cell 66: 1121

Ervasti J M, Kahl S D, Campbell K P 1991 Purification of dystrophin from skeletal muscle. Journal of Biological Chemistry 266: 9161

Estes, J E, Selden L A, Kinosian H J, Gershman L C 1992 Tightly-bound divalent cation of actin. Journal of Muscle Research and Cell Motility 13: 272

Fabiato A, Fabiato F 1979 Calcium and cardiac excitation–contraction coupling. Annual Review of Physiology 41: 473

Fenn W O 1923 A quantitative comparison between the energy liberated and the work performed by isolated sartorius muscle. Journal of Physiology 58: 175

Fenn W O 1924 The relation between the work performed and the energy liberated in muscular contraction. Journal of Physiology 58: 373

Fischer E H, Heilmeyer L M G Jr, Haschke R H 1971 Phosphorylase and the control of glycogen degradation. In: Horecker B L, Stadtman E R (eds) Current topics in cell regulation, vol IV. Academic Press, New York, p 211

Fitts R H 1994 Cellular mechanisms of muscle fatigue. Physiological Reviews 74: 49

Flach J, Lindquester G, Berish S, Hickman K, Devlin R 1986 Analysis of tropomyosin cDNAs isolated from skeletal and smooth muscle mRNA. Nucleic Acids Research 14: 9193

Flavin M, Ochoa S 1957 Metabolism of propionic acid in animal tissues I. Enzymatic conversion of propionate to succinate. Journal of Biological Chemistry 229: 965

Fleckenstein A, Janke J, Davies R E, Krebs H A 1954 Chemistry of muscle contraction. Nature 174: 1081

Fleischer S, Inui M 1989 Biochemistry and biophysics of excitation-contraction coupling. Annual Review of Biophysics and Biomolecular structure 18: 333

Flicker P F, Phillips G N Jr, Cohen C 1982 Troponin and its interactions with tropomyosin. Journal of Molecular Biology 162: 495

Fowler W E, Aebi U 1983 A consistent picture of the actin filament related to the orientation of the actin molecule. Journal of Cell Biology 97: 264

Frank G, Weeds A G 1974 The amino acid sequence of some alkali light chains of rabbit skeletal muscle myosin. European Journal of Biochemistry 44: 317

Franzini-Armstrong C, Nunzi G 1983 Junctional feet and particles in the triads of a fast-twitch muscle fibre. Journal of Muscle Research and Cell Motility 4: 233

Franzini-Armstrong C, Ferguson D G 1985 Density and disposition of Ca^{2+}-ATPase in sarcoplasmic reticulum membrane as determined by shadowing techniques. Biophysical Journal 48: 607

Frieden C 1985 Actin and tubulin polymerisation: the use of kinetic methods to determine mechanism. Annual Review of Biophysics and Biophysical Chemistry 14: 189

Frieden C, Lieberman D, Gilbert H R 1980 A fluorescent probe for conformational changes in skeletal muscle G-actin. Journal of Biological Chemistry 255: 8991

Frieden C, Patane K 1985 Differences on G-actin containing bound ATP or ADP: The Mg^{2+}-induced conformational change requires ATP. Biochemistry 24: 4192

Fritz I B, Davis D G, Holtrop R H, Dundee H 1958 Fatty acid oxidation by skeletal muscle during rest and activity. American Journal of Physiology 194: 379

Fujii J, Kodama M, Tada M, Toda H, Sakiyama F 1986 Characterization of structural unit of phospholamban by amino acid sequencing and electrophoretic analysis. Biochemical and Biophysical Research Communications 138: 1044

Fujime S, Ishiwata S 1972 Dynamic study of F-actin by quasielastic scattering of laser light. Journal of Molecular Biology 62: 251

Fujimori K, Sorenson M, Herzberg O, Moult J, Reinach F C 1990 Probing the calcium-induced conformational transition of troponin C with site directed mutants. Nature 344: 182

Funatsu T, Ishiwata S 1985 Characterization of β-actinin: A suppressor of the elongation at the pointed end of thin filaments in skeletal muscle. Journal of Biochemistry (Japan) 98: 535

Funatsu T, Kono E, Tsukita S 1993 Time-resolved electron microscopic analysis of the behavior of myosin heads on actin filaments after photolysis of caged ATP. Journal of Cell Biology 121: 1053

Gazith J S, Himmelfarb S, Harrington W F 1970 Studies on the sub-unit structure of myosin. Journal of Biological Chemistry 245: 15

Geeves M A 1991 The dynamics of actin and myosin association and the crossbridge model of muscle contraction. Biochemical Journal 274: 1

Gergely J 1950 Relation of ATPase and myosin. Federation Proceedings. Federation of American Societies for Experimental Biology 9: 176

Gergely J 1953 Studies on myosin-adenosine triphosphatase. Journal of Biological Chemistry 200: 543

Gergely J 1956 The interaction between actomyosin and adenosine triphosphate. Light scattering studies. Journal of Biological Chemistry 220: 917

Gergely J, Gouvea M A, Karibian D 1955 Fragmentation of myosin by chymotrypsin. Journal of Biological Chemistry 212: 165

Gergely J, Seidel J 1983 Conformational change and molecular dynamics of myosin. In: Peachey L E, Adrian R H (eds) Skeletal muscle, Handbook of Physiology. American Physiological Society, Bethesda, p 257

Gershman L C, Newman J, Seldon L A, Estes J E 1984 Bound cation exchange affects true lag phase in actin polymerisation. Biochemistry 23: 2199

Goldman R D, Milsted A, Schloss J A, Starger J, Yerna M J 1979 Cytoplasmic fibers in mammalian cells: cytoskeletal and contractile elements. Annual Review of Physiology 41: 703

Gordon A M, Huxley A F, Julian F J 1966 The variation in isometric tension with sarcomere lengths in vertebrate muscle fibers. Journal of Physiology 184: 170

Grabarek A, Drabikowski W, Leavis P C, Rosenfeld S S, Gergely J 1981 Proteolytic fragments of troponin C. Journal of Biological Chemistry 256: 13121

Grabarek Z, Grabarek J, Leavis P C, Gergely J 1983 Cooperative binding to the Ca^{2+}-specific sites of troponin C in regulated actin and actomyosin. Journal of Biological Chemistry 258: 14098

Grabarek Z, Tan R-Y, Wang J, Tao T, Gergely J 1990 Inhibition of mutant troponin C activity by an interdomain disulfide bond. Nature 345: 132

Grabarek Z, Tao T, Gergely J 1992 Molecular mechanism of troponin C function. J Muscle Res. Cell Motility 13: 383

Granger D L, Lazarides E 1978 The existence of an insoluble Z disc scaffold in chicken skeletal muscle. Cell 15: 1253

Greaser M, Gergely J 1971 Reconstitution of troponin activity from three protein components. Journal of Biological Chemistry 244: 4226

Greaser M, Gergely J 1973 Purification and properties of the components from troponin. Journal of Biological Chemistry 248: 2125

Greaser M, Yamaguchi M, Brekke C, Potter J, Gergely J 1972 Troponin subunits and their interactions. Cold Spring Harbor Symposia on Quantitative Biology 37: 235

Green D E 1954 Fatty acid oxidation in soluble systems of animal tissues. Biological Reviews 29: 330

Green N M, Stokes D L 1992 Structural modelling of P-type ion pumps. Acta Physiol. Scand. 146: 59

Greene L E 1986 Cooperative binding of myosin subfragment one to regulated actin as measured by fluorescence changes of troponin I modified with different fluorophores. Journal of Biological Chemistry 26: 1279

Greene L E, Eisenberg E 1980 Cooperative binding of myosin subfragment-1 to the actin-troponin-tropomyosin complex. Proceedings of the National Academy of Sciences (USA) 77: 2616

Grove B K, Kurer V, Lehner Ch, Doetschman T C, Perriard J-C, Eppenberger H M 1984 A new 185 000 dalton skeletal muscle protein detected by monoclonal antibodies. Journal of Cell Biology 98: 518

Guba F, Harsanyi V, Vajda E 1968 The muscle protein fibrillin. Acta Biochimica et Biophysica Acadamica Scientiarum Hungaricae 3: 353

Guth L, Watson P K, Brown W C 1968 Effects of cross reinnervation on some chemical properties of red and white muscles of rat and cat. Experimental Neurology 20: 52

Guth L, Wells J B 1976 Physiological and histochemical properties of the soleus muscle after denervation of its antagonists. Experimental Neurology 51: 310

Hama H, Maruyama K, Noda H 1965 Direct isolation of F actin from myofibrils and its physiochemical properties. Biochimica et Biophysica Acta 102: 149

Hanson J, Huxley H E 1955 The structural basis of contraction in striated muscle. Symposium of the Society of Experimental Biology 9: 228

Hanson J, Huxley H E 1957 Quantitative studies on the structure of cross-striated myofibrils II. Investigations by biochemical techniques. Biochimica et Biophysica Acta 23: 250

Hanson J, Lowy J 1963 The structure of F actin and of elements isolated from muscle. Journal of Molecular Biology 6: 46

Harada Y, Sakurada K, Aoki T, Thomas D D, Yanagida T 1990 Mechanochemical coupling in actomyosin energy transduction studied by in vitro movement assay. Journal of Molecular Biology 216: 49

Harrington W F 1979 Origin of the contractile force in skeletal muscle. Proceedings of the National Academy of Sciences (USA) 76: 5066

Harrington W F, Rodgers M E 1984 Myosin. Annual Review of Biochemistry 53: 35

Hartshorne D J, Mueller H 1968 Fractionation of troponin into two distinct proteins. Biochemical and Biophysical Research Communications 31: 647

Hartshorne D J, Theiner M, Mueller H 1969 Studies on troponin. Biochimica et Biophysica Acta 175: 320

Hartshorne D J, Dreizen P 1972 Studies on the subunit composition of troponin. Cold Spring Harbor Symposia on Quantitative Biology 37: 255

Hartshorne D J, Siemankowski R F 1981 Regulation of smooth muscle actomyosin. Annual Review of Physiology 43: 519

Haselgrove J C 1972 X-ray evidence for a conformational change in the actin-containing filaments of vertebrate striated muscle. Cold Spring Harbor Symposia on Quantitative Biology 37: 341

Hasselbach W 1979 The sarcoplasmic calcium pump. A model of energy transduction. In: Biological membranes. Current Topics in Chemistry 78: 1

Hasselbach W, Makinose M 1961 Die calciumpumpe der erschlaffungs grana des muskels und ihre abhangigheit von der ATP spaltung. Biochemische Zeitschrift 333: 518

Hasselbach W, Makinose M 1963 Uber den mechanismus des calcium transportes durch die membranen des sarkoplasmiatchen reticulums. Biochemische Zeitschrift 339: 94

Hayashi T, Ip W 1976 Polymerization polarity of actin. Journal of Mechanochemistry and Cell Motility 3: 163

Hegyi G, Szilagyi L, Elzinga H 1986 Photoaffinity labeling of the nucleotide binding site of actin. Biochemistry 25: 5793

Heilbrunn L V, Wiercinski F J 1947 The action of various cations on muscle protoplasm. Journal of Cellular and Comparative Physiology 29: 15

Heilig A, Pette D 1983 Changes in transcriptional activity of chronically stimulated fast twitch muscle. Federation of European Biochemical Societies 51: 211

Heilmann C, Pette D 1979 Molecular transformations in sarcoplasmic reticulum of fast twitch muscle by electro-stimulation. European Journal of Biochemistry 93: 437

Herzberg O, James M N G 1985 Structure of the calcium regulatory muscle protein troponin-C at 2.8A resolution. Nature (London) 313: 653

Herzberg O, Moult J, James M N G 1986 A model for the Ca^{2+}-induced conformational transition of troponin C. Journal of Biological Chemistry 261: 2638

Hibberd M G, Dantzig J A, Trentham D R, Goldman Y E 1985 Phosphate release and force generation in skeletal muscle fibers. Science 228: 1317

Hibberd M G, Trentham D R 1986 Relationships between chemical and mechanical events during muscular contraction. Annual Review of Biophysics and Biophysical Chemistry 15: 119

Hidalgo C, Ikemoto N, Gergely J 1976 Role of phospholipids in the Ca-dependent ATPase of the sarcoplasmic reticulum. Enzymatic and electron spin resonance studies with phospholipid replaced membrane. Journal of Biological Chemistry 250: 7219

Hidalgo C, Thomas D D, Ikemoto N 1978 Effect of the lipid environment on protein motion and enzymatic activity of the sarcoplasmic reticulum Ca ATPase. Journal of Biological Chemistry 253: 6879

Hidalgo C, Gonzalez M E, Lagos R 1983 Characterization of the Ca^{2+} or Mg^{2+} ATPase of transverse tubule membranes isolated from rabbit skeletal muscle. Journal of Biological Chemistry 258: 13937

Highsmith S, Eden D 1990 Ligand-induced myosin subfragment 1 global conformational change. Biochemistry 29: 4087

Highsmith S, Kretzchmar K M, O'Konski C T, Morales M F 1977 Flexibility of the myosin rod, light meromyosin and myosin subfragment 2 in solution. Proceedings of the National Academy of Sciences (USA) 74: 4986

Hill A V 1949 Work and heat in a muscle twitch. Proceedings of the Royal Society, Series B, 136: 220

Hill A V 1964a The effect of load on the heat of shortening of muscle. Proceedings of the Royal Society, Series B, 159: 297

Hill A V 1964b The efficiency of mechanical power development during muscular shortening and its relation to load. Proceedings of the Royal Society, Series B, 159: 319

Hill A V 1964c The effect of tension in prolonging the active state in a twitch. Proceedings of the Royal Society, Series B, 159: 589

Hill A V 1964d The variation of total heat production in a twitch with velocity of shortening. Proceedings of the Royal Society, Series B, 159: 596

Hill T L 1977 Free energy transduction in biology. The steady-state kinetic and thermodynamic formalism. Academic Press, New York

Hill T L 1980 Bioenergetic aspects and polymer length distribution in steady state head to tail polymerization of actin or microtubules. Proceedings of the National Academy of Sciences (USA) 77: 4803

Hill T L 1983 Two elementary models for the regulation of skeletal muscle contraction by calcium. Biophysical Journal 44: 383

Hill T L, Simmons R M 1976 Free energy levels and entropy production in muscle contraction and in related solution systems. Proceedings of the National Academy of Sciences (USA) 73: 336

Hill T L, Eisenberg E, Greene L 1980 Theoretical model for the cooperative equilibrium binding of myosin subfragment 1 to the actin-troponin-tropomyosin complex. Proceedings of the National Academy of Sciences (USA) 77: 3186

Hill T L, Kirschner M W 1982 Bioenergetics and kinetics of microtubule and actin filament assembly-disassembly. International Review of Cytology 78: 1

Hitchcock-DeGregori S E 1980 Actin assembly. Nature (London) 288: 437

Hitchcock-DeGregori S E, Varnell T A 1990 Tropomyosin has discrete actin-binding sites with sevenfold and fourteen-fold predictions. Journal of Molecular Biology 214: 805

Hochachka P W 1985 Fuels and pathways as designed systems for support of muscle work. Journal of Experimental Biology 115: 149

Hoffman R K, Gambke B, Stephenson L W, Rubinstein N A 1985 Myosin transitions in chronic stimulation do not involve embryonic isozymes. Muscle and Nerve 8: 796

Hoh J F Y 1978 Light chain distribution of chicken skeletal muscle myosin isoenzymes. Federation of European Biochemical Society Letters 90: 297

Hoh J F Y 1991 Myogenic regulation of mammalian skeletal muscle fibres. NIPS 6: 1

Hoh J F Y, McGrath P A, Hale P T 1978 Electrophoretic analysis of multiple forms of rat cardiac myosin: Effects of hypophysectomy and thyroxine replacement. Journal of Molecular and Cellular Cardiology 10: 1053

Holmes K C, Kabsch W 1991 Muscle proteins: actin. Current Opinion in Structural Biology 1: 270

Holmes K C, Popp D, Gebhard W, Kabsch W 1990 Atomic model of the actin filament. Nature 237: 44

Holt J C, Lowey S 1977 Distribution of alkali light chains in myosin: isolation of isozymes. Biochemistry 16: 4398

Homsher E 1986 The energetics of contraction. In: Engel A G, Banker B Q (eds) Myology. McGraw-Hill, New York, p 497

Homsher E 1987 Muscle enthalpy production and its relationship to actomyosin ATPase. Annual Review of Physiology 49: 673

Horowits R, Kempner E S, Bisher M E, Podolsky R J 1986 A physiological role for titin and nebulin in skeletal muscle. Nature (London) 323: 160

Hoyle G 1967 Diversity of striated muscle. American Zoologist 7: 435

Hoyle G, McNeil P A, Selverston A I 1973 Ultrastructure of barnacle giant muscle fibers. Journal of Cell Biology 56: 74

Hughes S M, Blau H M 1992 Muscle fiber pattern is independent of cell lineage in postnatal rodent development. Cell 68: 659

Hultman E, Spriet L L, Soderlund K 1986 Biochemistry of muscle fatigue. Biomedica et Biochimica Acta 45: S-97

Huszar G 1975 Tissue-specific biosynthesis of ε-N-monomethyllysine and ε-N-trimethyllysine in skeletal and cardiac muscle myosin. A model for the cell-free study of post-translational amino acid modifications in proteins. Journal of Molecular Biology 94: 311

Huxley A 1992 A fine time for contractual alterations. Nature 357: 110

Huxley A F 1957 Muscle structure and theories of contraction. Progress in Biophysics 7: 255

Huxley A F 1974 Muscular contraction: review lecture. Journal of Physiology 243: 1

Huxley A F 1979 Reflections on muscle. University of Liverpool Press, Liverpool

Huxley A F, Simmons R M 1971 Proposed mechanism of force generation in striated muscle. Nature 233: 533

Huxley H E 1960 Muscle cells. In: Brachet J, Mirsky A E (eds) The cell, vol. IV. Academic Press, New York, p. 365

Huxley H E 1963 Electron microscope studies on the structure of natural and synthetic protein filaments from striated muscle. Journal of Molecular Biology 7: 281

Huxley H E 1968 Structural difference between resting and rigor muscle. Evidence from intensity changes in the low angle equatorial X-ray diagram. Journal of Molecular Biology 37: 3542

Huxley H E 1969 The mechanism of muscle contraction. Science 164: 1356

Huxley H E 1972 Structural changes in the actin- and myosin-containing filaments during contraction. Cold Spring Harbor Symposia on Quantitative Biology 37: 361

Huxley H E 1990 Sliding filaments and molecular motile systems. Journal of Biological Chemistry 265: 8347

Huxley H E, Brown W 1967 The low angle X-ray diagram of vertebrate striated muscle and its behaviour during contraction and rigor. Journal of Molecular Biology 1: 30

Huxley H E, Faruqi A R, Kress M, Bordas J, Koch M H J 1982 Time resolved X-ray diffraction studies of the myosin layer-line reflections during muscle contraction. Journal of Molecular Biology 158: 637

Huxley H E, Faruqi A R 1983 Time-resolved x-ray diffraction studies on vertebrate striated muscle. Annual Review of Biophysics and Bioengineering 12: 381

Huxley H E, Kress M 1985 Crossbridge behaviour during muscle contraction. Journal of Muscle Research and Cell Motility 6: 163

Hvidt S, Neatler F H M, Greaser M L, Ferry J D 1982 Flexibility of myosin rod determined from dilute solution viscoelastic measurements. Biochemistry 21: 4064

Hvidt S, Chang T, Yu H 1984 Rigidity of myosin and myosin rod by electric birefringence. Biopolymers 23: 1283

Ibraghimov-Beskrovnaya O, Ervasti J M, Leveille C J, Slaughter C A, Sernett W, Campbell K P 1992 Primary structure of dystrophin-associated glycoproteins linking dystrophin to the extracellular matrix. Nature 355: 696

Ikemoto N 1975 Transporting and inhibitory Ca^{2+}-binding sites on the ATPase enzyme isolated from sarcoplasmic reticulum. Journal of Biological Chemistry 250: 7219

Ikemoto N 1976 Behaviour of the Ca^{2+}-transport sites linked with the phosphorylation reaction of ATPase purified from the sarcoplasmic reticulum. Journal of Biological Chemistry 251: 7275

Ikemoto N, Sreter F A, Nakamura A, Gergely J 1968 Tryptic digestion and localization of Ca-uptake and ATPase activity in fragments of sarcoplasmic reticulum. Journal of Ultrastructure Research 23: 216

Ikemoto N, Bhatnagar G, Gergely J 1971 Fractionation of solubilized sarcoplasmic reticulum. Biochemical and Biophysical Research Communications 44: 1510

Ikemoto N, Bhatnagar G, Nagy B, Gergely J 1972 Interaction of divalent cations with the 55 000 dalton protein component of the sarcoplasmic reticulum. Studies of fluorescence and circular dichroism. Journal of Biological Chemistry 247: 7835

Ikemoto N, Morgan J, Yamada S 1978 Controlled conformational states of the Ca^{2+}-transport enzyme of sarcoplasmic reticulum. Journal of Biological Chemistry 253: 8027

Ikemoto N, Antoniu B, Kim D H 1984 Rapid calcium release from the isolated sarcoplasmic reticulum is triggered via the attached transverse tubular system. Journal of Biological Chemistry 259: 13151

Ikemoto N, Antoniu B, Kang J J 1992 Characterization of 'depolarization'-induced calcium release from sarcoplasmic reticulum in vitro with the use of membrane potential probe. Biochemical and Biophysical Research Communications 184: 538

Ikemoto N, Antoniu B, Kang J-J, Meszaros L G, Ronjat M 1991 Intravesicular calcium transient during calcium release from sarcoplasmic reticulum. Biochemistry 30: 5230

Ikura M, Clore G M, Gronenborn A M, Zhu G, Klee C B, Bax A 1992 Solution structure of a calmodulin-target peptide complex by multidimensional NMR. Science 256: 632

Inesi G 1985 Mechanism of calcium transport. Annual Review of Physiology 47: 573

Inesi G, Millman M, Eletr S 1973 Temperature induced transitions of function structure in sarcoplasmic reticulum membranes. Journal of Molecular Biology 81: 483

Inesi G, Kirtley M R 1992 Structural features of cation transport ATPases. J. Bioenergetics Biomembranes 24: 271

Inesi G, Lewis D, Nikic D, Hussain A, Kirtley M E 1992 Long-range intramolecular linked functions in the calcium transport ATPase. In: Meister A (ed) Advances in enzymology and related areas of molecular biology. John Wiley, Chichester, p 185

Ip W, Heuser J 1983 Direct visualization of the myosin crossbridge helices on relaxed rabbit psoas thick filaments. Journal of Molecular Biology 171: 105

Irving M 1985 Weak and strong crossbridges. Nature (London) 316: 292

Irving M, Lombardi V, Piazzesi G, Ferenczi M A 1992 Myosin head movements are synchronous with the elementary force-generating process in muscle. Nature 357: 156

Isenberg G, Aebi U, Pollard T D 1980 An actin-binding protein from regulated actin filament polymerization and interactions from Acanthamoeba regulates actin filament polymerization and interactions. Nature (London) 288: 455

Ishijima A, Doi T, Sakurada K, Yanagida T 1991 Sub-piconewton force fluctuations of actomyosin in vitro. Nature 352: 301

Ishiwata S, Fujime S 1972 Effect of calcium ions on the flexibility of reconstituted thin filaments of muscle studied by quasi-elastic scattering of laser light. Journal of Molecular Biology 68: 511

Iyengar M R, Weber H H 1964 The relative affinities of nucleotides to G actin and their effects. Biochimica et Biophysica Acta 86: 543

Janmey P A, Hvidt S, Oster G F, Lamb J, Stossel T P, Hartwig J N 1990 Effect of ATP on actin filament stiffening. Nature 347: 95

Jencks W P 1980 The utilization of binding energy in coupled vectorial processes. Advances in Enzymology 51: 75

Jencks W P 1983 What is a coupled vectorial process? Current Topics in Membrane and Transport 19: 1

Jencks W P 1989 How does a calcium pump pump calcium. Journal of Biological Chemistry 264: 18855

Johnson J D, Collins J H, Potter J D 1978 Dansylaziridine-labelled troponin C. A fluorescent probe of Ca^{2+}-binding for the Ca^{2+}-specific regulatory sites. Journal of Biological Chemistry 253: 6451

Johnson J D, Charlton S C, Potter J D 1979 A fluorescence stopped-flow analysis of Ca^{2+}-exchange with troponin C. Journal of Biological Chemistry 254: 3497

Jolesz F, Sreter F A 1981 Development, innervation and activity pattern induced changes in skeletal muscle. Annual Review of Physiology 43: 531

Jorgensen A O, Jones J R 1986 Localization of phospholamban in slow but not fast canine skeletal muscle fibers. An immunocytochemical and biochemical study. Journal of Biological Chemistry 261: 3775

Kabsch W, Mannherz H G, Suck D 1985 Three-dimensional structure of the complex of actin and DNAse I at 4.5 A resolution. European Molecular Biology Organization Journal 4: 2113

Kabsch W, Mannherz H G, Suck D, Pai E F, Holmes K C 1990 Atomic structure of the actin : DNase I complex. Nature 347: 37

Kabsch W, Vandekerckhove J 1992 Structure and function of actin. Annual Review of Biophysics and Biomolecular Structure 21: 49

Karpati G, Carpenter S, Morris G E, Davies K E, Guerin C, Holland P 1993 Localization and quantitation of the chromosome 6-encoded dystrophin-related protein in normal and pathological human muscle. Journal of Neuropathology and Experimental Neurology 52: 119

Kasai M, Nakano F, Oosawa F 1964 Polymerization of actin free from nucleotides and divalent cations. Biochimica et Biophysica Acta 94: 494

Katoh T, Lowey S 1989 Mapping myosin light chains by immunoelectron microscopy. Journal of Cell Biology 109: 1549

Kawamura M, Maruyama K 1972 Length distribution of F-actin transformed from Mg-polymer. Biochimica et Biophysica Acta 267: 422

Kendrick-Jones J, Lehman W, Szent-Gyorgyi A G 1970. Regulation in molluscan muscle. Journal of Molecular Biology 54: 313

Kendrick-Jones J, Scholey J M 1981 Myosin linked regulatory systems. Journal of Muscle Research and Cell Motility 2: 347

Kensler R W, Stewart M 1983 Frog skeletal muscle thick filaments are three-stranded. Journal of Molecular Biology 96: 1797

Khurana T S, Hoffman E P, Kunkel L M 1990 Identification of a chromosome 6-encoded dystrophin-related protein. Journal of Biological Chemistry 265: 16767

Kielley W W, Meyerhof O 1948 Studies on adenosinetriphosphate of muscle. II. A new magnesium-activated adenosinetriphosphatase. Journal of Biological Chemistry 176: 591

Kielley W W, Meyerhof O 1950 Studies on adenosinetriphosphatase of muscle III. The lipoprotein nature of the magnesium-activated adenosine triphosphatase. Journal of Biological Chemistry 183: 391

Kikuchi M, Noda H, Maruyama K 1969 Interaction of actin within H-meromyosin at low ionic strength. Journal of Biochemistry (Japan) 65: 945

Kim K C, Caswell A H, Talvenheimo J A, Brandt N R 1990 Isolation of a terminal cisterna protein which may link the dihydropyridine receptor to the junctional foot protein in skeletal muscle. Biochemistry 29: 9281

Klee C B, Vanaman T C 1982 Calmodulin. Advances in Protein Chemistry 35: 213

Klug G, Wiehrer W, Reichmann H, Leberer E, Pette D 1983 Relationships between early alterations in parvalbumins, sarcoplasmic reticulum and metabolic enzymes in chronically stimulated fast twitch muscle. Pflugers Archives 399: 280

Knudson C C, Stang K K, Moomaw C R, Slaughter C A and Campbell K P 1993 Primary structure and topological analysis of a skeletal muscle-specific junctional sarcoplasmic reticulum glycoprotein (triadin). Journal of Biological Chemistry 268: 12646

Knudson C M, Stang K K, Jorgensen A O, Campbell K P 1993 Biochemical characterization and ultrastructural localization of a major junctional sarcoplasmic reticulum glycoprotein (triadin). Journal of Biological Chemistry 268: 12637

Koenig M, Kunkel L M 1990 Detailed analysis of the repeat domain of dystrophin reveals four potential hinge segments that may confer flexibility. Journal of Biological Chemistry 265: 4560

Koenig M, Monaco A P, Kunkel L M 1988 The complete sequence of dystrophin predicts a rod-shaped cytoskeletal protein. Cell 53: 219

Kondo H, Ishiwata S 1976 Uni-directional growth of F-actin. Journal of Biochemistry (Japan) 79: 159

Konno K, Morales M F 1985 Exposure of actin thiols by the

removal of tightly held calcium ions. Proceedings of the National Academy of Sciences (USA) 82: 7904

Korn E D 1982 Actin polymerization and its regulation by proteins from nonmuscle cells. Physiological Reviews 62: 672

Kovacs L, Rios E, Schneider M E 1979 Calcium transients and intra-membrane charge movement in skeletal muscle fibers. Nature 279: 391

Krebs E G 1972 Protein kinases. In: Horecker B L, Stadtman E R (eds) Current Topics in Cell Regulation. Academic Press, New York, p 99

Kress M, Huxley H E, Faruqi A R, Hendrix J 1986 Structural changes during activation of frog muscle studied by time-resolved X-ray diffraction. Journal of Molecular Biology 188: 325

Kretsinger R H 1972 Gene triplication deduced from the tertiary structure of a muscle calcium binding protein. Nature 85: 240

Kretsinger R H, Nockolds C E 1973 Carp muscle calcium binding protein II. Structure determination and general description. Journal of Biological Chemistry 248: 3313

Kretsinger R H, Barry C D 1975 The predicted structure of the calcium-binding component of troponin. Biochimica et Biophysica Acta 405: 40

Kuehl W M, Adelstein R S 1970 The absence of 3-methylhistidine in red, cardiac and fetal myosins. Biochemical and Biophysical Research Communications 39: 956

Kumagai H, Ebashi S, Takeda F 1955 Essential relaxing factor in muscle other than myokinase and creatine phosphokinase. Nature 176: 166

Kushmerick M J, Davies R E 1969 The chemical energetics of muscle contraction II. The chemistry, efficiency and power of maximally working sartorius muscles with an appendix-free energy and enthalpy of ATP hydrolysis in the sarcoplasm. Proceedings of the Royal Society, Series B, 174: 315

Kushmerick M J 1983 Energetics of muscle contraction. In: Peachey L D, Adrian R H, Geiger S R (eds) Handbook of physiology. American Physiological Society, Bethesda, p 189

Kushmerick M J, Moerland T S, Wiseman R W 1992 Mammalian skeletal muscle fibers distinguished by contents of phosphocreatine, ATP and Pi. Proceedings of the National Academy of Sciences USA 89: 7521

Lakonishok M, Muschler J, Horwitz A F 1992 The a5b1 integrin associates with a dystrophin-containing lattice during muscle development. Developmental Biology 152: 209

Lamb G D 1986 Components of charge movement in rabbit muscle: the effect of tetracaine and nifedipine. Journal of Physiology 376: 85

Lamb G D 1992 DHP receptors and excitation–contraction coupling. Journal of Muscle Research and Cell Motility 13: 394

Lamb G D, Stephenson D G 1990 Calcium release in skinned muscle fibers of the toad by transverse tubule depolarization or by direct stimulation. Journal of Physiology 495: 517

Lazarides E, Capetanaki Y G 1986 The striated muscle cytoskeleton: expression and assembly in development. In: Emerson C, Fischman D, Nadal-Ginard B, Siddiqui M A Q (eds) Muscular biology of muscle development. Alan R Liss, New York, p 749

Leavis P C, Lehrer S S 1974 A sulfhydryl-specific fluorescent label, S-mercuric-N-dansylcysteine. Titrations of glutathione and muscle proteins. Biochemistry 13: 3042

Leavis P C, Rosenfeld S, Gergely J, Grabarek Z, Drabikowski W 1978 Proteolytic fragments of troponin C. Localization of high and low affinity Ca^{2+}-binding sites and interactions with troponin I and troponin T. Journal of Biological Chemistry 253: 5452

Leavis P C, Gergely J 1984 Thin filament proteins and thin filament-linked regulation of vertebrate muscle contraction. CRC Critical Reviews in Biochemistry 16: 235

Leberer E, Pette D 1986 Neural regulation of parvalbumin expression in mammalian skeletal muscle. Biochemical Journal 235: 67

Leff S E, Rosenfeld M G, Evans R M 1986 Complex transcriptional units: diversity in gene expression by alternative RNA processing. Annual Reviews of Biochemistry 55: 1091

Lehky P L, Blum H E, Stein E A, Fischer E H 1974 Isolation and characterization of parvalbumins from the skeletal muscle of higher vertebrates. Journal of Biological Chemistry 249: 4332

Lehman W, Szent-Györgyi A G 1975 Regulation of muscle contraction. Distribution of actin control and myosin control in the animal kingdom. Journal of General Physiology 66: 1

Lehrer S S, Kerwar G 1972 The intrinsic fluorescence of actin. Biochemistry 11: 1211

Lehrer S S, Nagy B, Gergely J 1972 The binding of copper to actin without loss of polymerizability. The involvement of the rapidly reacting SH groups. Archives of Biochemistry and Biophysics 150: 164

Lehrer S S, Graceffa P, Betteridge D 1981 Conformational dynamics of tropomyosin in solution: evidence for two conformational states. Annals of the New York Academy of Sciences 366: 285

Lehrer S S, Morris E 1984 Comparison of the effects of smooth and skeletal tropomyosin on skeletal actomyosin subfragment 1 ATPase. Journal of Biological Chemistry 259: 2070

LePeuch C J, Halech J, Demaille J G 1979 Concerted regulation of cardiac sarcoplasmic reticulum calcium transport by cyclic adenosine monophosphate dependent and calcium-calmodulin-dependent phosphorylations. Biochemistry 18: 5150

Leung A T, Imagawa T, Block B, Franzini-Armstrong C, Campbell K P 1988 Biochemical and ultrastructural characterization of the 1,4-dihydropyridine receptor from rabbit skeletal muscle. Journal of Biological Chemistry 263: 994

Levine B A, Mercola D, Coffman D, Thornton J M 1977 Calcium binding by TnC. A proton magnetic resonance study. Journal of Molecular Biology 115: 743

Levine R J C, Sweeney H L, Kensler R W, Yang Z 1993 Myosin heads moving out: myosin phosphorylation in mammalian striated muscle. Biophysical Journal 64: A142

Lipmann F 1941 Metabolic generation and utilization of phosphate bound energy. Advances in Enzymology 1: 99

Lombardi V, Piazzesi G, Linari M 1992 Rapid regeneration of the actin–myosin powerstroke in contracting muscle. Nature 355: 638

Lompre A M, Mercadier J J, Wismewsky C, Bouveret P, Pantaloni C, d'Albis A, Schwartz K 1981 Species and age dependent changes in the relative amount of cardiac myosin isoenzymes in mammals. Developmental Biology 84: 286

Lompre A M, Nadal-Ginard B, Mahdavi B 1984 Expression

of the cardiac ventricular α and β myosin heavy chain gene is developmentally and hormonally regulated. Journal of Biological Chemistry 259: 6437

Love D R, Hill D F, Dickson G, Spurr N K, Blyth B C, Marsden R F, Walsh F S, Edwards Y H, Davies K E 1989 An autosomal transcript in skeletal muscle with homology to dystrophin. Nature 339: 55

Love D R, Morris G E, Ellis J M, Fairbrother U, Marsden R F, Bloomfield J F, Edwards Y H, Slater C P, Parry D J, Davies K E 1991 Tissue distribution of the dystrophin-related gene product and expression in the mdx and dy mouse. Proceedings of the National Academy of Sciences USA 88: 3243

Lowey S 1964 Meromyosin substructure: isolation of a helical sub-unit from heavy meromyosin. Science 145: 597

Lowey S, Goldstein L, Luck S 1966 Isolation and characterization of a helical sub-unit from heavy meromyosin. Biochemische Zeitschrift 345: 248

Lowey S, Risby D 1971 Light chains from fast and slow muscle myosin. Nature 234: 81

Lowey S, Slayter H S, Weeds A G, Baker H 1969 Substructure of the myosin molecule I. Subfragments of myosin by enzymic degradation. Journal of Molecular Biology 42: 1

Lowey S, Benfield P A, Silberstein L, Lang L M 1979 Distribution of light chains in fast skeletal myosin. Nature (London) 282: 522

Lu R C, Szilagyi L 1981 Change of reactivity of lysine residues upon actin polymerization. Biochemistry 20: 5914

Lu R C, Moo L, Wong A G 1986 Both the 25-kDa and 50-kDa domains in myosin subfragment 1 are close to the reactive thiols. Proceedings of the National Academy of Sciences USA 83: 6392

Luna E J, Hitt A L 1992 Cytoskeleton–plasma membrane interaction. Science 258: 955

Lundsgaard E 1930 Untersuchungen uber Muskelkontraktionen ohne Milchsaurebildung, Biochemische Zeitschrift 217: 162

Lusty C J, Fasold H 1969 Characterisation of sulfhydryl groups of actin. Biochemistry 8: 2933

Lymn R W, Taylor E W 1970 Transient state phosphate production in the hydrolysis of nucleoside triphosphates by myosin. Biochemistry 9: 2975

Lymn R W, Taylor E W 1971 Mechanism of adenosine triphosphate hydrolysis by actomyosin. Biochemistry 10: 4617

Lynen F, Ochoa S 1953 Enzymes of fatty acid metabolism. Biochimica et Biophysica Acta 12: 299

Lymn R W, Taylor E W 1970 Transient state phosphate production in the hydrolysis of nucleoside triphosphates by myosin. Biochemistry 9: 2975

Mabuchi K, Szvetko D, Pinter K, Sreter F A 1982 Type 2B to 2A fiber transformation in intermittently stimulated rabbit muscle. American Journal of Physiology 242: C373

McKenzie D K, Bigland-Ritchie B, Gorman R B, Gandevia S C 1992 Central and peripheral fatigue of human diaphragm and limb muscles assessed by twitch interpolation. Journal of Physiology 454: 643

McLachlan A D 1984 Structural implications of the myosin amino acid sequence. Annual Review of Biophysics and Bioengineering 13: 167

McLachlan A D, Stewart M 1976 The 14-fold periodicity in α-tropomyosin and the interaction with actin. Journal of Molecular Biology 103: 271

McLachlan A D, Karn J 1982 Periodic charge distributions in the myosin rod amino acid sequence match cross-bridge spacings in muscle. Nature (London) 299: 226

MacLennan D H 1990 Molecular tools to elucidate problems in excitation–contraction coupling. Biophysical Journal 54: 1355

MacLennan D H, Wong P T S 1971 Isolation of a calcium-sequestering protein from sarcoplasmic reticulum. Proceedings of the National Academy of Sciences (USA) 68: 1231

MacLennan D H, Brandl C J, Korczak B, Green N M 1985 Amino acid sequence of a $Ca^{2+} + Mg^{2+}$-dependent ATPase from rabbit muscle sarcoplasmic reticulum deduced from its complementary DNA sequence. Nature 316: 6030

MacLennan D H, Clarke D M, Loo T W, Skerjianc I S 1992 Site-directed mutagenesis of the Ca^{2+} ATPase of sarcoplasmic reticulum. Acta Physiologica Scandinavica 146: 141

MacLennan D H, Duff C, Zorzato F, Fujii J, Phillips M, Korneluk R G, Frodis W, Britt B A, Worton R G 1990 Ryanodine receptor gene is a candidate for predisposition to malignant hyperthermia. Nature 343: 559

McPherson P S, Campbell K P 1993 The ryanodine receptor/Ca^{2+} release channel. Journal of Biological Chemistry 268: 13765

Mahmood R, Yount R G 1984 Photochemical probes of the active site of myosin. Irradiation of trapped 3'-0-(4-benzoyl) benzoyl-adenosine 5'-triphosphate labels the 50-kilodalton heavy chain tryptic peptide. Journal of Biological Chemistry 259: 12956

Maier A, Gambke B, Pette D 1986 Degeneration–regeneration as a mechanism contributing to the fast to slow conversion of chronically stimulated fast-twitch rabbit muscle. Cell and Tissue Research 244: 635

Mak A, Smillie L B, Barany M 1978 Specific phosphorylation at serine 283 of a tropomyosin from rabbit skeletal and cardiac muscle. Proceedings of the National Academy of Sciences USA 75: 3588

Makinose M 1971 Calcium efflux-dependent formation of ATP from ADP and orthophosphate by the membranes of the sarcoplasmic reticulum vesicles. Federation of European Biochemical Society Letters 12: 269

Makinose M, Hasselbach W 1971 ATP synthesis by the reverse of the sarcoplasmic reticulum pump. Federation of European Biochemical Society Letters 12: 271

Margossian S S, Krueger J W, Sellers J R, Cuda G, Caulfield J B, Norton P, Slayter H S 1991 Influence of the cardiac myosin hinge region on contractile activity. Proceedings of the National Academy of Sciences USA 88: 4941

Marsh B B 1951 A factor modifying muscle syneresis. Nature 167: 1065

Marsh B B 1952 The effects of adenosine triphosphate on the fibre volume of a muscle homogenate. Biochimica et Biophysica Acta 9: 247

Marston S B, Taylor E W 1980 Comparison of the myosin and actomysoin ATPase mechanisms of the four types of vertebrate muscles. Journal of Molecular Biology 139: 573

Martonosi A 1962 The specificity of the interaction of ATP with G actin. Biochimica et Biophysica Acta 57: 163

Martonosi A 1963 The activating effect of phospholipids on the ATPase activity and calcium uptake of fragmented sarcoplasmic reticulum. Biochemical and Biophysical Research Communications 13: 273

Martonosi A 1969 The protein composition of sarcoplasmic reticulum membranes. Biochemical and Biophysical Research Communications 36: 1039

Martonosi A 1984 Mechanisms of Ca^{2+}-release from sarcoplasmic reticulum of skeletal muscle. Physiological Reviews 64: 1240

Martonosi A, Feretos R 1964 Sarcoplasmic reticulum I. The uptake of calcium by sarcoplasmic reticulum fragments. Journal of Biological Chemistry 239: 648

Martonosi A, Gouvea M A, Gergely J 1960a The interaction of C-labelled adenine nucleotides with actin. Journal of Biological Chemistry 235: 1700

Martonosi A, Molino C, Gergely J 1960b The binding of divalent cations to actin. Journal of Biological Chemistry 235: 1700

Martonosi A, Donley J, Halpin R A 1968 Sarcoplasmic reticulum III. The role of phospholipids in the adenosine triphosphatase activity of Ca^{2+} transport. Journal of Biological Chemistry 243: 61

Martonosi A N, Jona I, Molnar E, Seidler N W, Buchet R, Varga S 1990 Emerging views on the structure and dynamics of the Ca^{2+}-ATPase in sarcoplasmic reticulum. Federation of European Biochemical Societies 268: 365

Maruyama K 1965a A new protein factor hindering network formation of F actin in solution. Biochimica et Biophysica Acta 94: 208

Maruyama K 1965b Some physico-chemical properties of β-actinin. Actin factor isolated from striated muscle. Biochimica et Biophysica Acta 102: 542

Maruyama K 1971 A study of β-actinin, myofibrillar protein from rabbit skeletal muscle. Journal of Biochemistry (Japan) 69: 369

Maruyama K 1986 Connectin, an elastic filamentous protein of striated muscle. International Review of Cytology 104: 81

Maruyama K, Ebashi S 1965 α-actinin. A new structural protein from striated muscle. II. Action on actin. Journal of Biochemistry 58: 13

Maruyama K, Matsubara S, Natori R et al 1977 Connectin, an elastic protein of muscle, characterization and function. Journal of Biochemistry 82: 317

Masaki T, Endo M, Ebashi S 1967 Localization of 6S component of α-actinin at Z-band. Journal of Biochemistry (Tokyo) 62: 630

Masaki T, Takaiti O 1974 M-protein. Journal of Biochemistry (Tokyo) 75: 367

Matsumura K, Ervasti J M, Ohlendieck K, Kahl S D, Campbell K P 1992 Association of dystrophin-related protein with dystrophin-associated proteins in mdx mouse muscle. Nature 360: 588

Matsumura K, Campbell K P 1994 Dystrophin–glycoprotein complex: its role in the molecular pathogenesis of muscular dystrophies. Muscle and Nerve 17: 2

Meador W E, Means A R, Quiocho F A 1992 Target enzyme recognition by calmodulin: 2.4. A structure of a calmodulin–peptide complex. Science 257: 1251

Medford R M, Nguyen H T, Destree A T, Summers E, Nadal-Ginard B 1984 A novel mechanism of alternative RNA splicing for the developmentally regulated generation of troponin T isoforms from a single gene. Cell 38: 409

Mendelson R A, Morales M F, Botts J 1973 Segmental flexibility of the S-1 moiety of myosin. Biochemistry 12: 2250

Metzger J M, Fitts R H 1986 Fatigue from high- and low-frequency muscle stimulation: role of sarcolemma action potentials. Experimental Neurology 93: 320

Metzger J M, Greaser M L, Moss R L 1989 Variations in cross-bridge attachment rate and tension with phosphorylation of myosin in mammalian skinned skeletal muscle fibers. Journal of General Physiology 93: 855

Mickelson J R, Beaudry T M, Louis C F 1985 Regulation of skeletal muscle sarcolemmal ATP-dependent calcium transport by calmodulin and cAMP-dependent protein kinase. Archives of Biochemistry and Biophysics 242: 127

Migala A, Agostini B, Hasselbach W 1973 Tryptic fragmentation of the calcium transport system in the sarcoplasmic reticulum. Zeitschrift für Naturforschung 28: 178

Mihalyi E, Szent-Györgyi A G 1953 Trypsin digestion of muscle proteins III. Adenosinetriphosphatase activity and actin-binding capacity of the digested myosin. Journal of Biological Chemistry 201: 211

Millar N C, Homsher E 1992 Kinetics of force generation and phosphate release in skinned rabbit psoas muscle fibers. American Journal of Physiology 262: C1239

Milligan R A, Whittaker M, Safer D 1990 Myosin structure of F-actin and location of surface binding sites. Nature (London) 348: 217

Milner-Brown H S, Miller R G 1986 Muscle membrane excitation and impulse propagation velocity are reduced during muscle fatigue. Muscle and Nerve 9: 367

Minetti C, Beltrame F, Marcenaro G, Bonilla E 1992 Dystrophin at the plasma membrane of human muscle fibers shows a costameric localization. Neurological Disorders 2: 99

Mitchell P 1977 Vectorial chemiosmotic processes. Annual Review of Biochemistry 46: 966

Moir A J G, Cole H A, Perry S V 1977 The phosphorylation sites of troponin T from white skeletal muscle and the effects of interaction with troponin C on their phosphorylation by phosphorylase kinase. Biochemical Journal 161: 371

Mommaerts W F H M 1952 The molecular transformation of actin. III. The participation of nucleotides. Journal of Biological Chemistry 198: 469

Mommaerts W F H M 1954 Is adenosine triphosphate broken down during a single muscle twitch? Nature 174: 1081

Mommaerts W F H M 1955 Investigation of the presumed breakdown of adenosine triphosphate and phosphocreatine during a single muscle twitch. American Journal of Physiology 182: 585

Mommaerts W F H M 1970 What is the Fenn effect? Naturwissenschaften 57: 326

Monaco A P 1989 Dystrophin, the protein product of the Duchenne/Becker muscular dystrophy gene. Trends in Biochemical Sciences 14: 412

Moore P B, Huxley H E, DeRosier D J 1970 Three dimensional reconstruction of F actin, thin filaments and decorated thin filaments. Journal of Molecular Biology 50: 279

Morales M F, Borejdo J, Botts J, Cooke R, Mendelson R A, Takashi R 1982 Some physical studies of the contractile mechanism in muscle. Annual Review of Physical Chemistry 33: 319

Morimoto K, Harrington W F 1972 Isolation and physical chemical properties of an M-line protein from skeletal muscle. Journal of Biological Chemistry 247: 3052

Mornet D R, Bertrand P, Pantel E, Aüdemard E, Kassab R 1981 Structure of the actin-myosin interface. Nature (London) 292: 301

Mornet D, Bonet A, Audemard E, Bonicel J 1989 Functional sequences of the myosin head. Journal of Muscle Research and Cell Motility 10: 10

Mornet D, Ue K, Morales M F 1984 Proteolysis and the domain organization of myosin subfragment 1. Proceedings of the National Academy of Sciences (USA) 1: 736

Mornet D, Ue K, Morales M F 1985 Stabilization of a primary loop in myosin subfragment 1 with a fluorescent crosslinker. Proceedings of the National Academy of Sciences USA 82: 1658

Moss R L 1992 Ca^{2+} regulation of mechanical properties of striated muscle. Mechanistic studies using extraction and replacement of regulatory proteins. Circulation Research 70: 865

Moss R L, Allen J D, Greaser M L 1986 Effects of partial extraction of troponin complex upon the tension-pCa relation in rabbit skeletal muscle. Further evidence that tension development involves cooperative effects within the thin filament. Journal of General Physiology 87: 751

Mueller H, Perry S V 1962 The degradation of heavy meromyosin by trypsin. Biochemical Journal 85: 431

Muhlrad A, Morales M F 1984 Isolation and partial renaturation of proteolytic fragments of the myosin head. Proceedings of the National Academy of Sciences (USA) 81: 1003

Muhlrad A, Kasprzak A A, Ue K, Ajtai K, Burghardt T P 1986 Characterization of the isolated 20 kDa and 50 kDa fragments of the myosin head. Biochimica et Biophysica Acta 869: 128

Nabeshima Y, Kurajama-Fuji Y, Muramatsu M, Ogata K 1984 Alternative transcription and two modes of splicing result in two myosin light chains from one gene. Nature (London) 308: 1984

Nadal-Ginard B, Medford R M, Nguyen H T et al 1982 Structure and regulation of a mammalian sarcomeric myosin heavy chain gene. In: Pearson M L, Epstein H F (eds) Muscle development. Cold Spring Harbor Laboratories, Cold Spring Harbor, p 143

Nadal-Ginard B, Breitbart R E, Strehler E E, Ruiz-Opazo N, Periasamy M, Mahdavi V 1986 Alternative splicing: a common mechanism for the generation of contractile protein diversity from single genes. In: Emerson C, Fischman D, Nadal-Ginard B, Siddiqui M A Q (eds) Molecular biology of muscle development. UCLA Symposium on Molecular and Cellular Biology, vol 29. Alan R. Liss, New York, p 387

Nagashima H, Asakura S 1980 Dark-field light microscopic study of the flexibility of F-actin complexes. Journal of Molecular Biology 136: 169

Nagano H, Yanagida T 1984 Predominant attached state of myosin cross-bridges during contraction and relaxation at low ionic strength. Journal of Molecular Biology 177: 769

Nagy B, Jencks W P 1962 Optical rotatory dispersion of G-actin. Biochemistry 1: 987

Natori R 1954 The property and contraction process of isolated myofibrils. Jikei Medical Journal 1: 119

Needham D M 1971 Machina carnis. University of Cambridge Press, Cambridge

Needham J, Chen S L, Needham D M, Lawrence A S G 1941 Myosin birefringence and adenylpyrophosphate. Nature 147: 766

Newton A A, Perry S V 1960 The incorporation of ^{15}N into adenine nucleotides and their formation from inosine monophosphate by skeletal muscle preparations. Biochemical Journal 74: 127

Nguyen thi Main, Le Thiet Thanh, Blake D J, Davies K E, Morris G E 1992 Utrophin, the autosomal homologue of dystrophin, is widely-expressed and membrane-associated in cultured cell lines. Federation of European Biochemical Societies 313: 19

Niedl C, Engel J 1979 Exchange of ADP, ATP and $1:N^6$-ethenoadenosine 5'-triphosphate at G-actin. European Journal of Biochemistry 101: 163

O'Brien E J, Couch J, Johnson G R P, Morris E P 1983 In: dos Remedios C, Barden J A (eds) Structure of actin and the thin filament, In actin. Academic Press, Sydney, p 3

Ochs R S 1986 Inositol trisphosphate and muscle. Trends in Biochemical Sciences 11: 388

Offer G 1972 C-protein and the periodicity in the thick filaments of vertebrate skeletal muscle. Cold Spring Harbor Symposia on Quantitative Biology 37: 87

Offer G 1974 The molecular basis of muscular contraction. In: Bull A T, Lagnado J R, Thomas J O, Tipton K F (eds) Companion to biochemistry. Longmans, London, p 623

Offer G, Moos C, Starr R 1973 A new protein of the thick filaments of vertebrate skeletal myofibrils. Journal of Molecular Biology 74: 653

Ohtsuki I 1979 Molecular arrangement of troponin T in the thin filament. Journal of Biochemistry (Tokyo) 86: 491

Okamoto Y, Yount R G 1985 Identification of an active site peptide of skeletal myosin after photoaffinity labelling with N-(4-azido-2-nitrophenyl)-2-aminoethyl diphosphate. Proceedings of the National Academy of Sciences (USA) 82: 1575

Olson E N 1992 Interplay between proliferation and differentiation within the myogenic lineage. Developmental Biology 154: 261

Oosawa F, Asakura S, Hotta K, Imai N, Ooi T 1959 G-F transformation of actin as a fibrous condensation. Journal of Polymer Science 37: 323

Oosawa F, Asakura S 1975 Thermodynamics of the polymerization of protein. Academic Press, London

Ostwald T J, MacLennan D H 1974 Isolation of a high affinity calcium-binding protein from sarcoplasmic reticulum. Journal of Biological Chemistry 249: 974

Otsu K, Willard R F, Khanna V K, Zorzato F, Green N M, MacLennan D H 1990 Molecular cloning of cDNA encoding the Ca^{2+} release channel (ryanodine receptor) of rabbit cardiac muscle sarcoplasmic reticulum. Journal of Biological Chemistry 265: 13472

Padgett R, Grabowski P J, Konarska M M, Seiler S, Sharp P A 1986 Splicing of messenger RNA precursors. Annual Review of Biochemistry 55: 1119

Page S, Huxley H E 1963 Filament lengths in striated muscle. Journal of Cell Biology 19: 369

Parry D A D 1975 Analysis of the primary sequence of α-tropomyosin from rabbit skeletal muscle. Journal of Molecular Biology 98: 519

Parry D A D, Squire J M 1973 Structural role of tropomyosin in muscle regulation. Analysis of X-ray diffraction patterns from relaxed and contracting muscles. Journal of Molecular Biology 75: 33

Pastra-Landis S C, Huiatt T, Lowey S 1983 Assembly and kinetic properties of myosin light chain isozymes from fast skeletal muscle. Journal of Molecular Biology 170: 403

Pate E, White H, Cooke R 1993 Determination of the myosin step size from mechanical and kinetic data. Proceedings of the National Academy of Sciences of the USA 90: 2451

Pearlstone J R, Carpenter M R, Johnson P, Smillie L B 1976 Amino acid sequence of tropomyosin binding component of rabbit skeletal muscle troponin. Proceedings of the National Academy of Sciences (USA) 73: 1902

Pease D C, Jenden D J, Howell J N 1965 Calcium uptake in glycerol-extracted rabbit psoas muscle fibres. Journal of Cellular and Comparative Physiology 65: 141

Pepe F A 1966 Some aspects of the structural organisation of the myofibril as revealed by antibody-staining methods. Journal of Cell Biology 28: 505

Pepe F A 1967a The myosin filament. I. Structural organisation from antibody staining observed in electron microscopy. Journal of Molecular Biology 27: 203

Pepe F A 1967b The myosin filament II. Interaction between myosin and actin filaments observed during antibody staining in fluorescent and electron microscopy. Journal of Molecular Biology 27: 227

Pepe F A 1972 The myosin filament: immunochemical and ultrastructural approaches to molecular organisation. Cold Spring Harbor Symposia on Quantitative Biology 37: 97

Periasamy M, Strehler E E, Garfinkel L I, Gubits R M, Ruiz-Opazo N, Nadal-Ginard B 1984 Fast skeletal muscle myosin light chains 1 and 3 are produced from a single gene by a combined process of differential RNA transcription and splicing. Journal of Biological Chemistry 259: 13595

Perkins W J, Weiel J, Grammer J, Yount R G 1984 Introduction of a donor-acceptor pair by a single protein modification. Journal of Biological Chemistry 259: 8786

Perry S V 1951 The adenosinetriphosphatase activity of myofibrils isolated from skeletal muscle. Biochemical Journal 48: 257

Perry S V, Grey T C 1956 A study of the effects of substrate concentration and certain relaxing factors on magnesium-activated myofibrillar adenosine triphosphatase. Biochemical Journal 64: 184

Persechini A, Stull J T, Cooke R 1985 The effect of myosin phosphorylation on the contractile properties of skinned rabbit skeletal muscle fibers. Journal of Biological Chemistry 260: 7951

Pette D 1984 Activity induced fast to slow transition in mammalian muscle. Medicine and Science in Sports and Exercise 16: 517

Pette D, Smith M E, Staudte H W, Vrbová G 1973 Effects of long-term electrical stimulation on some contractile and metabolic characteristics of fast rabbit muscle. Pflügers Archiv für die gesamte Physiologie des Menschen und der Tiere 338: 257

Pette D, Schnez U 1977 Co-existence of fast and slow type myosin light chains in single muscle fibers during transformation as induced by long-term stimulation. Federation of European Biochemical Society Letters 83: 128

Pette D, Staron R S 1990 Cellular and molecular diversities of mammalian skeletal muscle fibers. Reviews Physiology, Biochemistry and Pharmacology 116: 1

Pette D, Vrbová G 1992 Adaptation of mammalian skeletal muscle fibers to chronic electrical stimulation. Reviews Physiology, Biochemistry and Pharmacology 120: 115

Phillips G N, Fillers J P, Cohen C 1986 Tropomyosin crystal structure and muscle regulation. Journal of Molecular Biology 192: 111

Pires E, Perry S V, Thomas M A W 1974 Myosin light chain kinase. A new enzyme from striated muscle. Federation of European Biochemical Society Letters 41: 292

Pluskal M, Sreter F A 1983 Correlation between protein phenotype and gene expression in adult rabbit fast twitch muscles undergoing a fast to slow fiber type transformation in response to electrical stimulation in vivo. Biochemical and Biophysical Research Communications 113: 325

Podolsky R J, Costantin L L 1964 Regulation by calcium of the contraction and relaxation of muscle fibres. Federation Proceedings. Federation of American Societies for Experimental Biology 23: 933

Pollack G H 1983 The cross-bridge theory. Physiological Reviews 63: 1049

Pollard T D, Bhandari D, Maupin P, Wachsstock D, Weeds A G, Zot H G 1993 Direct visualization by electron microscopy of the weakly bound intermediates in the actomyosin adenosine triphosphatase cycle. Biophysical Journal 64: 454

Pollard T D, Mooseker M S 1981 Direct measurement of actin polymerization rate constants by electron microscopy of actin filaments nucleated by isolated microvillus cores. Journal of Cell Biology 80: 654

Pollard T D, Cooper J A 1986 Actin and actin binding protein. A critical evaluation of mechanism and function. Annual Review of Biochemistry 55: 987

Porter G A, Dmytrenko G M, Winkelman J C, Bloch R J 1992 Dystrophin colocalizes with β spectrin in distinct subsarcolemmal domains in mammalian skeletal muscle. Journal of Cell Biology 117: 997

Potter J D, Gergely J 1974 Troponin, tropomyosin and actin interactions in the Ca^{2+} regulation of muscle contraction. Biochemistry 13: 2697

Potter J D, Seidel J C, Leavis P, Lehrer S S, Gergely J 1976 The effect of Ca^{2+}-binding on troponin C. Changes in spin label mobility, extrinsic fluorescence and SH reactivity. Journal of Biological Chemistry 251: 7551

Price H M, Gordon J M, Pearson C M, Munsat T C, Blumberg J M 1965 New evidence for excessive accumulation of Z band material in nemaline myopathy. Proceedings of the National Academy of Sciences (USA) 54: 1398

Privalov P L 1982 Stability of proteins. Proteins which do not present a single cooperative system. Advances in Protein Chemistry 35: 1

Radda G K 1986 The use of NMR spectroscopy for the understanding of disease. Science 233: 640

Ray K P, England P J 1976 Phosphorylation of the inhibitory subunit of troponin and its effect on the calcium dependence of cardiac myofibril adenosine triphosphatase. Federation of European Biochemical Societies 70: 11

Rayment I, Rypniewski W R, Schmidt-Base K et al 1993a The three-dimensional structure of myosin subfragment 1– a molecular model, Science 261: 50

Rayment I, Holden H M, Whittaker M et al 1993b Structure of the actin-myosin complex and its implications for muscle contraction. Science 261: 58

Reisler E, Burke M, Himmelfarb S, Harrington W F 1974 Spacial proximity of two essential SH groups of myosin. Biochemistry 13: 3837

Rich S A, Estes J E 1976 Detection of conformational changes in actin by proteolytic digestion: evidence for a new monomeric species. Journal of Molecular Biology 104: 777.

Rios E, Brum G 1987 Involvement of dihydropyridine receptors in excitation–contraction coupling in skeletal muscle. Nature (London) 325: 717

Rios E, Pizarro G 1991 Voltage sensor of excitation–contraction coupling in skeletal muscle. Physiological Reviews 71: 849

Rios E, Pizarro G, Stefani E 1992 Charge movement and the nature of signal transduction in skeletal muscle excitation–contraction coupling. Annual Review of Physiology 54: 109

Robert B, Barton P, Alonso S et al 1986 The structure and

organization of actin and myosin genes and their expression in mouse striated muscle. In: Emerson C, Fischman D, Nadal-Ginard B, Siddiqui M A Q (eds) Molecular biology of muscle development. Alan Liss, New York, p 487

Robert B, Daubas P, Akimenko M A, Cohen A, Garner I, Guenet J L, Buckingham M E 1984 A single locus in the mouse encodes both myosin light chains 1 and 3; a second locus corresponds to a related pseudogene. Cell 39: 129

Romanul F C, Van der Meulen J P 1967 Slow and fast muscles after cross innervation. Archives of Neurology 17: 387

Romanul F C A, Sreter F A, Salmons S, Gergely J 1974 The effect of a changed pattern of activity on histochemical characteristics of muscle fibers. In: Milhorat A T (ed) Exploratory concepts in muscular dystrophy. Elsevier, Amsterdam, p 344

Rosenfeld S S, Taylor E W 1984 The ATPase mechanism of skeletal and smooth muscle acto-subfragment 1. Journal of Biological Chemistry 259: 11908

Rosenfeld S S, Taylor E W 1985 Kinetic studies of calcium binding to regulatory complexes from skeletal muscle. Journal of Biological Chemistry 260: 252

Roy R, Sreter F A, Sarkar S 1979 Changes in tropomyosin sub-units and myosin light chains during development of chicken and rabbit striated muscle. Developmental Biology 69: 15

Rubinstein N, Mabuchi K, Pepe F, Salmons S, Sreter F 1978 Use of type-specific antimyosins to demonstrate the transformation of individual fibers in chronically stimulated rabbit fast muscles. Journal of Cell Biology 79: 252

Ruiz-Opazo, N, Weinberger J, Nadal-Ginard B 1985 Comparison of α tropomyosin sequences from smooth and striated muscle. Nature (London) 315: 67

Salmons S, Sreter F A 1976 Impulse activity in the transformation of skeletal muscle type. Nature 263: 30

Salmons S, Vrbová G 1969 The influence of activity on some contractile characteristics of mammalian fast and slow muscle. Journal of Physiology 201: 535

Samaha F J, Theis W H 1976 Actomyosin changes in muscle with altered function. Experimental Neurology 51: 310

Sapega A A, Sokolow D P, Graham T J, Chance B 1993 Phosphorus nuclear magnetic resonance—a non-invasive technique for the study of muscle bioenergetics during exercise. Medical Science of Sports and Exercise 25: 410

Sarkar S 1972 Stoichiometry and sequential removal of light chains of myosin. Cold Spring Harbor Symposia on Quantitative Biology 37: 14

Sarkar S, Sreter F A, Gergely J 1971 Light chains of myosins from fast, slow and cardiac muscles. Proceedings of the National Academy of Sciences (USA) 68: 946

Sato O, Nonomura Y, Kimura S, Maruyama K 1992 Molecular shaping of dystrophin. Journal of Biochemistry (Japan) 112: 631

Schaub M C, Hartshorne D J, Perry S V 1967 The adenosine triphosphatase activity of desensitised actomyosin. Biochemical Journal 104: 263

Schaub M C, Perry S V 1969 The relaxing protein system of striated muscle. Resolution of the troponin complex into inhibitory and calcium ion sensitising factors and their relationship to tropomyosin. Biochemical Journal 115: 993

Schliwa M 1981 Proteins associated with cytoplasmic actin. Cell 25: 57

Schneider M F 1981 Membrane charge movement and depolarization-contraction coupling. Annual Review of Physiology 43: 507

Schneider M F, Chandler W K 1973 Voltage dependent charge movement in skeletal muscle: a possible step in excitation-contraction coupling. Nature 242: 244

Seamon K B, Hartshorne D J, Bothnerby A A 1977 Ca^{2+} and Mg^{2+} conformations of TnC as determined by ^1H and ^{19}F nuclear magnetic resonance. Biochemistry 16: 4039

Seidel J C 1967 Studies on myosin from red and white skeletal muscles of the rabbit. II. Inactivation of myosin from red muscle under mild alkaline conditions. Journal of Biological Chemistry 242: 5623

Selden L A, Gershman L C, Estees J E 1986 A kinetic comparison between Mg-actin and Ca-actin. Journal of Muscle Research and Cell Motility 7: 215

Selve N, Wegner A 1986 Rate of treadmilling of actin filaments in vitro. Journal of Molecular Biology 187: 627

Seymour J, O'Brien E J 1980 The position of tropomyosin in muscle thin filaments. Nature 283: 680

Sharp A H, Piwell J A, Beam K G, Campbell K P 1989 Specific absence of the α subunit of the DHP receptor in mice with muscular dysgenesis. Journal of Biological Chemistry 264: 1345

Sherry J M F, Gorecka A, Aksoy M O, Dabrowska R, Hartshorne D J 1978 Roles of calcium and phosphorylation in the regulation of the activity of gizzard myosin. Biochemistry 17: 4411

Shy G M, Engel W K, Somers J E, Wanko T 1963 Nemaline myopathy: new congenital myopathy. Brain 86: 793

Siemankowski R F, White H D 1984 Kinetics of the interaction between actin, ADP, and cardiac myosin-S1. Journal of Biological Chemistry 259: 5045

Simmerman H K B, Collins J H, Theibert J L, Wegener L R, Jones R L 1986 Sequence analysis of phospholamban. Identification of phosphorylation sites and two major structural domains. Journal of Biological Chemistry 261: 13333

Sinha A M, Friedman D J, Nigro J M, Jakovcic S, Rabinowitz M, Umeda P K 1984 Expression of rabbit ventricular α-myosin heavy chain messenger RNA sequences in atrial muscle. Journal of Biological Chemistry 259: 6674

Smith P R, Fowler W E, Pollard T E, Aebi U 1983 Structure of the actin molecule determined from the electron micrographs of crystalline actin sheets with a tentative alignment of the molecule in the actin filament. Journal of Molecular Biology 167: 641

Smith P R, Fowler W E, Aebi U 1984 Towards an alignment of the actin molecule within the actin filament. Ultramicroscopy 13: 113

Small J M, Furst D O, Thornell L-E 1992 The cytoskeletal lattice of muscle cells. European Journal of Biochemistry 208: 559

Sodek J, Hodges R S, Smillie L B, Jurasek L 1972 Amino-acid sequence of rabbit skeletal tropomyosin and its coiled-coil structure. Proceedings of the National Academy of Sciences (USA) 69: 3800

Soderlund K, Greenhoff P L, Hultman E 1992 Energy metabolism in type I and type II human muscle fibers during short term electrical stimulation at different frequencies. Acta Physiologica Scandinavia 144: 15

Solaro R J, Moir A J G, Perry S V 1976 Phosphorylation of troponin I and the inotropic effect of adrenalin in the perfused rabbit heart. Nature (London) 262: 615

Somlyo A P, Somlyo A V 1992 Smooth muscle structure and function. In: Fozzard H A et al (eds) The heart and cardiovascular system. Raven Press, New York, p 1295

Somlyo A V, Bond M, Somlyo A P, Scarpa A 1985 Inositol-triphosphate InsP$_3$-induced calcium release and contraction in vascular smooth muscle. Proceedings of the National Academy of Sciences (USA) 82: 5231

Spudich J A, Huxley H E, Finch J T 1972 Regulation of skeletal muscle contraction II. Structural studies of the interaction of the tropomyosin-troponin complex with actin. Journal of Molecular Biology 72: 619

Spudich J A, Watt S 1971 The regulation of rabbit skeletal muscle contraction I. Biochemical studies of the interaction of the tropomyosin-troponin complex with actin and the proteolytic fragments of myosin. Journal of Biological Chemistry 246: 4866

Squire J 1981 The structural basis of muscle contraction. Plenum Press, New York

Squire J M 1986 Muscle: design, diversity and disease. The Benjamin/Cummings Publishing Company, Menlo Park, CA

Sreter F A, Gergely J, Luff A L 1974 The effect of cross reinnervation on the synthesis of myosin light chains. Biochemical and Biophysical Research Communications 56: 84

Sreter F A, Gergely J, Salmons S, Romanul F 1973 Synthesis by fast muscle of myosin light chains characteristic of slow muscle in response to long-term stimulation. Nature 241: 17

Sreter F A, Seidel J C, Gergely J 1966 Studies on myosin from red and white skeletal muscle of the rabbit. I. adenosine triphosphate activity. Journal of Biological Chemistry 241: 5772

Starr R, Offer G 1978 Interaction of C protein with heavy meromyosin and subfragment 2. Biochemical Journal 71: 813

Starr R, Offer G 1983 H-protein and X-protein. Two new components of the thick filaments of vertebrate skeletal muscle. Journal of Molecular Biology 170: 675

Stein L A, Chock P B, Eisenberg E 1984 The rate limiting step in the actomyosin adenosinetriphosphatase cycle. Biochemistry 23: 1555

Stein L A, Greene L E, Chock P B, Eisenberg E 1985 Rate-limiting step in the actomyosin adenosinetriphosphatase cycle: studies with myosin subfragment 1 crosslinked to actin. Biochemistry 24: 1357

Stewart P S, MacLennan D H 1974 Surface particles of sarcoplasmic reticulum membranes. Structural features of the ATPase. Journal of Biological Chemistry 249: 985

Stockdale F E 1992 Myogenic cell lineages. Developmental Biology 154: 284

Stokes D L, Green N M 1990a Three dimensional crystals of Ca-ATPase from sarcoplasmic reticulum; symmetry and molecular packing. Biophysical Journal 57: 1

Stokes D L, Green N M 1990b Structure of Ca-ATPase: electron microscopy of frozen hydrated crystals at 6 A resolution in projection. Journal of Molecular Biology 213: 529

Stone D B, Prevost S C, Botts J 1970 Studies on spin labeled actin. Biochemistry 9: 3937

Stone D, Smillie L B 1978 The amino acid sequence of rabbit skeletal α-tropomyosin. The NH$_2$– terminal half and complete sequence. Journal of Biological Chemistry 253: 1137

Stone D, Sodek J, Johnson P, Smillie L B 1974 Tropomyosin: Correlation of amino acid sequence and structure. In:

Biro N A (ed) Proteins of the contractile system vol. 31. Proceedings of the IX Federation of European Biochemical Society Meeting. Akad. Kiado, Budapest, p 125

Strasburg G M, Leavis P C, Gergely J 1985 Troponin C mediated calcium sensitive changes in the conformation of troponin I detected by pyrene excimer fluorescence. Journal of Biological Chemistry 260: 366

Straub F B, 1942 Actin. In: Studies for the Institute of Medical Chemistry. University of Szeged, Vol. II, p 3

Straub F B, Feuer G 1950 Adenoinetriphosphate: the functional group of actin. Biochimica et Biophysica Acta 4: 455

Straub V, Bittner R E, Leger J J, Voit T 1992b Direct visualization of the dystrophin network on skeletal muscle fiber membrane. Journal of Cell Biology 119: 1183

Strehler E E, Carlsson E, Eppenberger H M, Thornell L E 1983 Ultrastructural localization of M-band proteins in chicken breast muscle as revealed by combined immunochemistry and ultramicrotomy. Journal of Molecular Biology 166: 141

Strynadka N C J, James M N G 1990 Model for the interaction of amphiphilic helices with troponin C and calmodulin. Proteins 7: 234

Strynadka N C J, James M N G 1991 Towards an understanding of the effect of calcium on protein structure and function. Current Opinions in Structural Biology 1: 905

Strzelecka-Golaszewska H 1973 Relative affinities of divalent cations to the site of the tight Ca-binding in G-actin. Biochimica et Biophysica Acta 310: 60

Strzelecka-Golaszewska H, Prochniewicz E, Drabikowski W 1978 Interaction of actin with divalent cations II. Characterization of protein metal complexes. European Journal of Biochemistry 88: 229

Suck D, Kabsch W, Mannherz H G 1981 Three dimensional structure of the complex of skeletal muscle actin and bovine pancreatic DNase I at 6 A resolution. Proceedings of the National Academy of Sciences (USA) 78: 4319

Sugi H, Kobayashi T, Gross T, Noguchi K, Karr T, Harrington W F 1992 Contraction characteristics and ATPase activity of skeletal muscle fibers in the presence of antibody to myosin subfragment 2. Proceedings of the National Academy of Sciences USA 89: 6134

Sugita H, Masaki T, Ebashi S, Pearson C 1974 Staining of nemaline rod by fluorescent antibody against 10s-actin. Proceedings of the Japan Academy 50: 237

Sundaralingam M, Bergstrom R, Strasburg G, Rao S T, Roychowdhury P 1985 Molecular structure of troponin C from chicken skeletal muscle at 3-angstrom resolution. Science 227: 945

Sutoh K 1984 Actin-actin and actin-deoxyribonuclease I contact sites in the actin sequence. Biochemistry 23: 1942

Sutoh K, Sutoh K, Karr T, Harrington W F 1978 Isolation and physicochemical properties of a high molecular weight subfragment 2 of myosin. Journal of Molecular Biology 126: 1

Sutoh K, Yamamoto K, Wakabayashi T 1984 Electron microscopic visualization of the SH 1 thiol of myosin by the use of an avidin-biotin system. Journal of Molecular Biology 178: 323

Sutoh K, Yamamoto K, Wakabayashi T 1986 Electron microscopic visualization of the ATPase site of myosin by photoaffinity labeling with a biotinylated photoreactive ADP analog. Proceedings of the National Academy of Sciences (USA) 83: 212

Suzuki A, Goll D E, Singh I, Allen R E, Robson R M, Stromer M H 1976 Some properties of purified skeletal α-actinin. Journal of Biological Chemistry 251: 6860

Sweeney H L, Bowman B F, Stull J T 1993 Myosin light chain phosphorylation in vertebrate striated muscle; regulation and function. American Journal of Physiology 264: 93

Swynghedauw B 1986 Developmental and functional adaptation of contractile proteins in cardiac and skeletal muscles. Physiological Reviews 66: 710

Szent-Györgyi A 1945 Studies on muscle. Acta Physiologica Scandinavica, Suppl XXV

Szent-Györgyi A 1949 Free energy relations and contraction of actomyosin. Biological Bulletin, Marine Biological Laboratory, Woods Hole, Mass 96: 140

Szent-Györgyi A G 1953 Meromyosins, the sub-units of myosin. Archives of Biochemistry 42: 305

Szilagyi L, Balint M, Sreter F A, Gergely J 1979 Photoaffinity labelling with an ATP analog of the N-terminal peptide of myosin. Biochemical and Biophysical Research Communications 87: 936

Tada M, Kirchenberger M A, Repke D I, Katz A M 1974 The stimulation of calcium transport in cardiac sarcoplasmic reticulum by adenosine 3'–5' monophosphate dependent protein kinase. Journal of Biological Chemistry 249: 6174

Tada M, Kirchenberger M A, Katz A 1975 Phosphorylation of a 22 000 dalton component of the cardiac sarcoplasmic reticulum by adenosine 3':5'-monophosphate dependent protein kinase. Journal of Biological Chemistry 250: 2640

Tada M, Inui M 1983 Regulation of calcium transport by the ATPase-phospholamban system. Journal of Molecular and Cellular Cardiology 15: 565

Tada M, Yamamoto T, Tonomura Y 1978 Molecular mechanism of active calcium transport by sarcoplasmic reticulum. Physiological Reviews 58: 1

Takebayashi T, Morita T, Oosawa F 1977 Electron microscopic investigation of the flexibility of F-actin. Biochimica et Biophysica Acta 492: 357

Takemitsu M, Nonaka I, Sugita H 1993 Dystrophin-related protein in skeletal muscles in neuromuscular disorders: immunohistochemical study. Acta Neuropathologica 85: 256

Takeshima H, Nishimura S, Matsumoto T, Ishida H, Kangawa K, Minamino N, Matsuo H, Ueda M, Hanaoka M, Hirose T, Numa S 1989 Primary structure and expression from complementary DNA of skeletal muscle ryanodine receptor. Nature 339: 439

Tanabe T, Beam K G, Powell J A, Numa S 1988 Restoration of excitation–contraction coupling and slow calcium current in dysgenic muscle by dihydropyridine receptor complementary DNA. Nature 336: 134

Tanabe T, Takeshima H, Mikami A, Flockerzi V, Takahashi H, Kangawa K, Kojima M, Matsuo H, Hirose T, Numa S 1987 Primary structure of the receptor for calcium channel blockers from skeletal muscle. Nature 328: 313

Tanford C 1983 Mechanism of free energy coupling in active transport. Annual Review of Biochemistry 52: 379

Tanford C 1984 Twenty questions concerning the reaction cycle of the sarcoplasmic reticulum calcium pump. CRC Critical Reviews in Biochemistry 17: 123

Tanner J W, Thomas D D, Goldman Y E 1992 Transients in orientation of a fluorescent cross-bridge probe following photolysis of caged nucleotides in skeletal muscle fibres. Journal of Molecular Biology 223: 185

Tao T, Cho J 1979 Fluorescence lifetime quenching studies on the accessibilities of actin sulfhyldryl sites. Biochemistry 18: 2759

Tao T, Lamkin M 1981 Excitation energy transfer studies on the proximity between Sh1 and the adenosine-triphosphatase site in myosin subfragment 1. Biochemistry 20: 5051

Tao T, Gong B-J, Leavis P C 1990 Calcium-induced movement of troponin I relative to actin in skeletal muscle thin filaments. Science 247: 1339

Taylor D L, Reidler J, Spudich J A, Stryer L 1981 Detection of actin assembly by fluorescence energy transfer. Journal of Cell Biology 89: 362

Taylor E W 1979 Mechanism of actomyosin ATPase and the problem of muscle contraction. Critical Reviews in Biochemistry 6: 103

Taylor K A, Amos L A 1981 A new model for the geometry of the binding of myosin crossbridges to muscle thin filaments. Journal of Molecular Biology 147: 297

Taylor K A, Dux L, Martonosi A 1986 Three-dimensional reconstruction of negatively stained crystals of the Ca^{2+}-ATPase from muscle sarcoplasmic reticulum. Journal of Molecular Biology 187: 417

Thomas D D, Cooke R 1980 Orientation of spin labeled myosin heads in glycerinated muscle fibers. Biophysical Journal 32: 981

Thomas D D, Seidel J C, Hyde J S, Gergely J 1975 Motion of the S-1 segment in myosin: Its proteolytic fragments and its supramolecular complexes: saturation transfer electron spin resonance. Proceedings of the National Academy of Sciences (USA) 72: 1729

Thomas D D, Seidel J C, Gergely J 1979 Rotational dynamics of spin labelled F actin in the submillisecond time range. Journal of Molecular Biology 132: 257

Thorley-Lawson D A, Green N M 1973 Studies on the location and orientation of proteins on the sarcoplasmic reticulum. European Journal of Biochemistry 40: 403

Tinsley J M, Blake D J, Roche A, Fairbrother U, Riss J, Blyth B C, Knight A E, Kendrick-Jones J, Suthers G K, Love D R, Edwards Y H, Davies K E 1992 Primary structure of dystrophin-related protein. Nature 360: 591

Toyoshima C, Wakabayashi T 1984a Three-dimensional image analysis of the complex of thin filaments and myosin molecules from skeletal muscle. IV. Reconstitution from minimal- and high-dose images of the actin–tropomyosin–myosin subfragment-I complex. Journal of Biochemistry (Japan) 97: 219

Toyoshima C, Wakabayashi T 1984b Three-dimensional image analysis of the complex of thin filaments and myosin molecules from skeletal muscle. V. Assignment of actin in the actin–tropomyosin–myosin subfragment-1 complex. Journal of Biochemistry (Japan) 97: 245

Toyoshima Y Y, Kron S J, Spudich J A 1990 The myosin step size: measurement of the unit displacement per ATP hydrolyzed in an in vitro assay. Proceedings of the National Academy of Sciences USA 87: 7130

Toyoshima C, Sasabe H, Stokes D L 1993 3-dimensional cryo-electron microscopy of the calcium ion pump in the sarcoplasmic reticulum membrane. Nature 363: 286

Trinick J 1992 Understanding the functions of titin and nebulin. FEBS Letters 307: 44

Trinick J, Lowey S 1977 M-protein from chicken pectoralis muscle: isolation and characterization. Journal of Molecular Biology 113: 343

Trinick J, Cooper J, Seymour J, Egelman E H 1986 Cryo-electron microscopy and three dimensional reconstruction of actin filaments. Journal of Microscopy 86: 349

Trybus K M, Taylor E W 1981 Kinetic studies of the cooperative binding of subfragment 1 to regulated actin. Proceedings of the National Academy of Sciences USA 77: 7209

Turner D C, Walliman T, Eppenberger H 1973 A protein that binds specifically to the M-line of skeletal muscle is identified as the muscle form of creatine kinase. Proceedings of the National Academy of Sciences USA 70: 702

Ueno H, Harrington W F 1981 Conformational transition in the myosin hinges upon activation of muscle. Proceedings of the National Academy of Sciences USA 78: 6101

Ueno H, Harrington W F 1986a Temperature dependence of local melting in the myosin subfragment 2 region of the rigor crossbridge. Journal of Molecular Biology 190: 59

Ueno H, Harrington W F 1986b Local melting in the subfragment 2 region of myosin in activated muscle and its correlation with contractile force. Journal of Molecular Biology 190: 69

Uyeda T Q P, Kron S J, Spudich J A 1990 Myosin step size. Estimation from slow sliding movement of actin over low densities of heavy meromyosin. Journal of Molecular Biology 214: 699

Vanderkerckhove J, Weber K 1984 Chordate muscle actins differ distinctly from invertebrate muscle actins. Journal of Molecular Biology 179: 391

Varriano-Marston E, Franzini-Armstrong C, Haselgrove J C 1984 The structure and disposition of crossbridges in deep-etched fish muscle. Journal of Muscle Research and Cell Motility 5: 351

Venkatasubramanian P N, Arus C, Bárány M 1986 Two-dimensional protein magnetic resonance of human muscle extracts. Clinical Physiology and Biochemistry 4: 285

Volpe P, DiVirgilio F, Pozzan T, Salviati G 1986 Role of inositol 1,4,5-trisphosphate in excitation–contraction coupling in skeletal muscle. Federation of European Biochemical Societies 197: 1

Waechter F, Engel J 1977 Association kinetics and binding constants of nucleoside triphosphates with G actin. European Journal of Biochemistry 74: 227

Wagenknecht T, Grassucci R, Frank A, Saito M, Innui M, Fleischer S 1989 Three dimensional architecture of the calcium channel foot structure of sarcoplasmic reticulum. Nature 338: 167

Wagner P D 1981 Formation and characterization of myosin hybrids containing essential light chains and heavy chains from different muscle myosins. Journal of Biological Chemistry 256: 2493

Wagner P D, Slater C S, Pope B, Weeds A G 1979 Studies on the actin activation of myosin subfragment 1 isoenzymes and the role of myosin light chains. European Journal of Biochemistry 99: 385

Wakabayashi K, Kotunaga M, Kohno I, Sugimoto Y, Hamanaka T, Takezaawa Y, Wakabayashi T, Amemiya Y 1992 Small angle synchroton X-ray scattering reveals distinct shape changes of the myosin head during hydrolysis of ATP. Science 258: 443

Wakabayashi T, Tomioka A, Toyoshima C, Tokunaga M, Sutoh K, Yamamoto K 1986 Three dimensional structure of the thin filament and its complex with myosin subfragment: Location of functional sites of actin and myosin. Proceedings of the XIth International Congress on Electron Microscopy, Kyoto, p 1813

Walliman T, Doetschman T C, Eppenberger H M 1983 Novel staining pattern of skeletal muscle M-lines upon incubation with antibodies against MM-creatine kinase. Journal of Cell Biology 96: 1772

Wallimann T, Eppenberger H M 1985 Localization and function of M-line-bound creatine kinase. In: Shay J W (ed) Cell and muscle motility, vol 6. Plenum Press, New York, p 239

Wang C-K, Cheung H C 1986 Proximity relationship in the binary complex formed between troponin I and troponin C. Journal of Molecular Biology 191: 509

Wang C-L, Leavis P C, Gergely J 1983 Kinetics of Ca^{2+} interactions between the two classes of sites of troponin C. Journal of Biological Chemistry 258: 9195

Wang K 1982 Myofilamentous and myofibrillar connections: role of titin, nebulin and intermediate filaments. In: Pearson M L, Epstein H F (ed) Muscle development: Molecular and cellular control. Cold Spring Harbor Laboratories, Cold Spring Harbor, p 439

Warren G B, Toon P A, Birdshall N J M, Lee A G, Metcalfe J C 1974 Reconstitution of a calcium pump using defined membrane components. Proceedings of the National Academy of Sciences (USA) 71: 622

Watanabe S 1955 Relaxing effects of EDTA on glycerol treated muscle fibers. Archives of Biochemistry and Biophysics 45: 559

Way M, Pope B, Cross R A, Kendrick-Jones J, Weeds A G 1992 Expression of the N-terminal domain of dystrophin in E. coli and demonstration of binding to F-actin. Federation of European Biochemical Societies 301: 243

Webb M R, Trentham D R 1983 Chemical mechanism of myosin catalyzed ATP hydrolysis. In: Peachey L E, Adrian R H (eds) Skeletal muscle. Handbook of physiology. American Physiological Society, Bethesda, p 173

Webb M R, Hibberd M G, Goldman Y E, Trentham D R 1986 Oxygen exchange between P_i in the medium and water during ATP hydrolysis mediated by skinned fibers from rabbit skeletal muscle. Evidence for P_i binding to a force-generating state. Journal of Biological Chemistry 261: 15557

Weber A 1956 The ultracentrifugal separation of L-myosin and actin in an actomyosin sol under the influence of ATP. Biochimica et Biophysica Acta 19: 345

Weber A 1959 On the role of calcium in the activity of adenosine 5′-triphosphate hydrolysis by actomyosin. Journal of Biological Chemistry 234: 2764

Weber A 1966 Energized calcium transport and relaxing factors. In: Sanadi D R (ed) Current topics in bioenergetics Vol 1. Academic Press, New York, p 203

Weber A, Winicur S 1961 The role of calcium in the superprecipitation of actomyosin. Journal of Biological Chemistry 236: 3198

Weeds A G 1969 Light chains of myosin. Nature 223: 1362

Weeds A G, Frank G 1972 Structural studies on the light chains of myosin. Cold Spring Harbor Symposia on Quantitative Biology 37: 9

Weeds A G, Lowey S 1971 Substructure of the myosin molecule II. The light chains of myosin. Journal of Molecular Biology 61: 701

Weeds A G, McLachlan A D 1974 Structural homology of myosin alkali light chains, troponin C and carp calcium binding protein. Nature 252: 646

Weeds A G, Pope B 1977 Studies on the chymotryptic digestion of myosin. Effects of divalent cations on proteolytic susceptibility. Journal of Molecular Biology 111: 129

Weeds A G, Hall R, Spurway N C S 1975 Characterisation of myosin light chains from histochemically identified fibers of rabbit psoas muscle. FEBS Letters 49: 320

Weeds A G, Trentham D R, Kean C J C, Buller A J 1974 Myosin from cross-reinnervated cat muscles. Nature 247: 135

Weeks R A, Perry S V 1978 Characterisation of a region of the primary sequence of troponin C involved in calcium ion dependent interaction with troponin I. Biochemical Journal 173: 449

Wegner A, Engel J 1975 Kinetics of the cooperative association of actin to actin filament. Biophysical Chemistry 3: 215

Wegner A, Neuhaus J-M 1981 Requirement of divalent cations for fast exchange of actin monomers and actin filament subunits. Journal of Molecular Biology 153: 681

Wegner A 1982a Treadmilling of actin at physiological salt concentration. Journal of Molecular Biology 161: 607

Wegner A 1982b Kinetic analysis of actin assembly suggests that tropomyosin inhibits spontaneous fragmentation of actin filaments. Journal of Molecular Biology 161: 217

Wells J A, Yount R G 1979 Active site trapping of nucleotide by crosslinking 2 sulfhydryls in myosin subfragment 1. Proceedings of the National Academy of Sciences (USA) 76: 4966

Weintraub H, Davis R, Tapscott S, Thayer M, Krause M, Benezra R, Blackwell T K, Turner D, Rulpp R, Hollenberg S, Zhuang Y, Lassar A 1991 The myoD gene family: nodal point during specification of the muscle cell lineage. Science 251: 761

Westerblad H, Lee J A, Lannergren J, Allen D G 1991 Cellular mechanisms of fatigue in skeletal muscle. American Journal of Physiology 261: C195

Wilkie D R 1966 Muscle. Annual Review of Physiology 28: 17

Wilkie D R 1986 Muscular fatigue: effects of hydrogen ions and inorganic phosphate. Federation Proceedings 45: 2921

Wilkinson J M, Grand R J A 1975 The amino acid sequence of TnI from rabbit skeletal muscle. Biochemical Journal 149: 493

Wilkinson J M, Perry S V, Cole H A, Trayer I P 1972 The regulatory proteins of the myofibril. Separation and biological activity of the components of inhibitory factor preparations. Biochemical Journal 127: 215

Winkelman D A, Lowey S 1985 Probing myosin head structure with monoclonal antibodies. Journal of Molecular Biology 188: 595

Winkelmann D A, Mekeel H, Rayment I 1985 Packing analysis of crystalline myosin subfragment-1. Implications for the size and shape of the myosin head. Journal of Molecular Biology 181: 487

Winkelmann D A, Baker T S, Rayment I 1991 Three-dimensional structure of myosin subfragment-1 from electron microscopy of sectioned cryostats. Journal of Cell Biology 114: 701

Woledge R C, Curtin N A, Homsher E 1985 Energetic aspects of muscle contraction. Monograph of the Biological Society No. 49. Academic Press, Orlando

Woods E F 1967 Molecular weight and sub-unit structure of tropomyosin B. Journal of Biological Chemistry 242: 2859

Woodrum D T, Rich S A, Pollard T D 1975 Evidence for biased bidirectional polymerization of actin filaments using heavy meromyosin prepared by an improved method. Journal of Cell Biology 67: 231

Yagi K, Yazawa M, Kakiuchi S, Ohshima M, Uenishi K 1978 Identification of an activator protein for myosin light chain kinase as the Ca^{2+}-dependent modulator protein. Journal of Biological Chemistry 253: 1338

Yamaguchi M, Greaser M, Cassens R G 1974 Interactions of troponin sub-units with different forms of tropomyosin. Journal of Ultrastructure Research 33: 48

Yamamoto T, Tonomura Y 1967 Reaction mechanism of the Ca^{2+}-dependent ATPase of sarcoplasmic reticulum from skeletal muscle. Journal of Biochemistry 62: 558

Yamamoto K, Tokunaga M, Sutoh K, Wakabayashi T, Sekine T 1985 Location of the SH group of the alkali light chain on the myosin head as revealed by electron microscopy. Journal of Molecular Biology 183: 287

Yanagida T 1981 Angles of nucleotides bound to cross-bridges in glycerinated muscle fiber at various concentrations of ε-ATP, ε-ADP and ε-AMPPNP detected by polarized fluorescence. Journal of Molecular Biology 146: 539

Yanagida T 1985 Angle of active site of myosin heads in contracting muscle during sudden length changes. Journal of Muscle Research and Cell Motility 6: 43

Yanagida T, Oosawa F 1978 Polarized fluorescence from ε-ADP incorporated into F-actin in a myosin-free single fiber: conformation of F-actin and changes induced in it by heavy meromyosin. Journal of Molecular Biology 126: 507

Yanagida T, Arata T, Oosawa F 1985 Sliding distance of actin filament induced by a myosin crossbridge during one ATP hydrolysis cycle. Nature 316: 366

Yates L D, Greaser M L 1983 Quantitative determination of myosin and actin in rabbit skeletal muscle. Journal of Molecular Biology 168: 123

Yount R G, Cremo C R, Grammer J C, Kerwin B A 1992 Photochemical mapping of the active site of myosin. Philosophical Transactions of the Royal Society London B 336: 55

Zorzato F, Fuji J, Otsu K, Phillips M, Green N M, Lai F A, Meissner G, MacLennan D H 1990 Molecular cloning of cDNA encoding human and rabbit forms of the Ca^{2+} release channel (ryanodine receptor) of skeletal muscle sarcoplasmic reticulum. Journal of Biological Chemistry 265: 2244

Zot H G, Potter J D 1987 Structural aspects of troponin-tropomyosin regulation of skeletal muscle contraction. Annual Review of Biophysics and Biophysical Chemistry 16: 535

Pathology

7. Light-microscopic pathology of skeletal muscle

S. Carpenter

INTRODUCTION

This chapter discusses light-microscopic morpho-logical features of skeletal muscle disease, with minimal reference to histochemistry, immuno-cytochemistry and electron microscopy. This is a somewhat artificial procedure, since much of our knowledge has come from correlation of methods. Nevertheless as an exercise it can be stimulating. The emphasis will be on semithin epoxy resin sections, since resin sections offer the most exact morphology. Despite this, they are often neglected, considered only as a stage in processing for electron-microscopy, and not considered useful enough to send to a consultant along with the cryostat sections and the electron-micrographs. Nevertheless they offer a view analogous to very low power electron-microscopy with the advan-tage of a much larger sampling area (Fig. 7.1a).

For good semithin sections the muscle specimen should be removed in an isometric clamp and promptly placed, still clamped, in the fixative, preferably 2% buffered glutaraldehyde. After 2–6 hours of fixation, the specimen is moved to refrigerated buffer without the clamp. Well-oriented cross and longitudinal sections can then be obtained as thin but comparatively wide slices. Both views are informative. Cutting the muscle into small cubes is counter-productive since it randomises orientation.

GENERAL REACTIONS OF MUSCLE FIBRES

Necrosis and regeneration

Important general pathological reactions of skeletal muscle cells occur in the sequence of

233

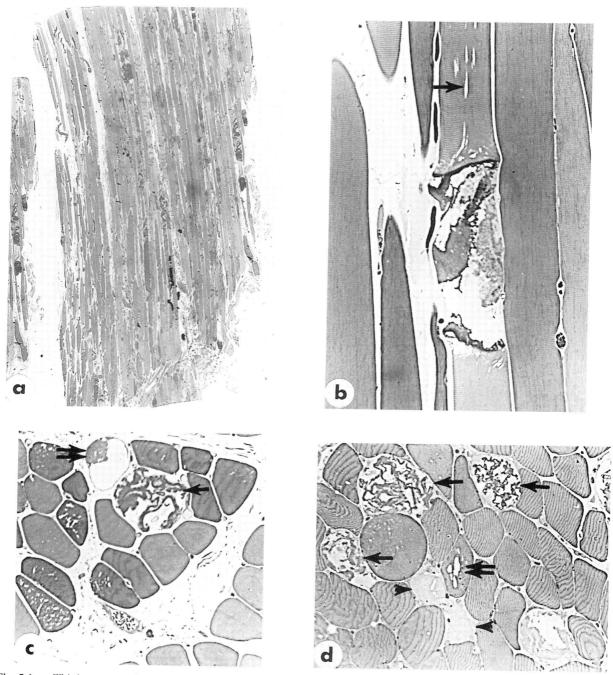

Fig. 7.1 **a** This low-power photomicrograph shows the extent of sampling possible in a semithin section. The muscle fibres are straight, because the sample was removed in an isometric clamp. This and other resin sections illustrated are stained with paraphenylenediamine and photographed through phase optics. Duchenne dystrophy (× 32). **b** Segmental necrosis in a single muscle fibre 2 hours after puncture by a fine wire. The width of the necrotic segment may be exaggerated by retraction of the stumps. Elongated vacuoles (arrow) result from swelling of T-tubules (× 550). **c** Experimental micropuncture, 2 hours. The section passes through the middle of a necrotic segment in one fibre (arrow) and grazes the stump in an adjoining one (double arrow). Other fibres which show T-tubule swelling are cut deep in stumps (× 320). **d** Adult dermatomyositis. Fibres in which the myofibrillar material is contracted into a ragged net (arrows) resemble those of acute micropuncture. Others (arrowheads) are pale and have been necrotic for a longer time. Vacuoles (double arrows) in another fibre have presumably arisen from T-tubules (× 320).

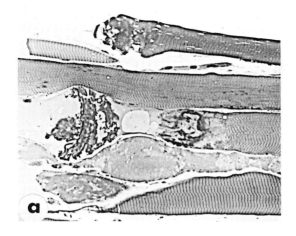

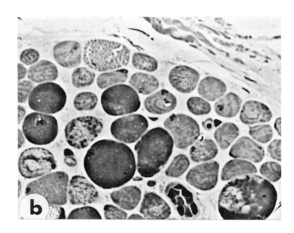

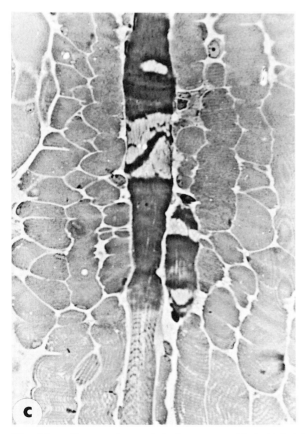

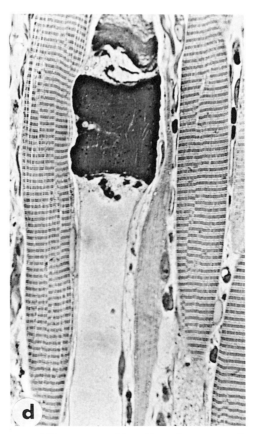

Fig. 7.2   a Segmental necrosis in dermatomyositis ($\times$ 320). **b** Hypercontracted fibres, presumably artifactual, are present in an otherwise normal biopsy from a child with CNS disease ($\times$ 550). **c** Longitudinal view of hypercontraction from the same normal biopsy. Note that hypercontraction in one segment will result in stretching or tearing of sarcomeres in other segments. **d** Hypercontracted fibre in Duchenne dystrophy ($\times$ 550)

necrosis, phagocytosis and regeneration. Necrosis means the death of a cell, its inability to maintain homeostasis, and its inevitable transition to debris. Necrosis occurs in many, but by no means all, muscle diseases. Many reactions of muscle cells do not promote necrosis, and in many diseases necrosis occurs at such a low rate that it is rarely seen in biopsies. In Duchenne dystrophy it is usually prominent until late in the disease, when few fibres are left.

In Duchenne dystrophy, necrotic fibres often appear to be clustered, while by contrast in polymyositis, necrotic fibres tend to be single and apparently random. Necrosis is less commonly seen in dermatomyositis, where it may follow one of two patterns: occasional fibres at the periphery of fascicles, or many adjacent fibres comprising the larger part of a fascicle, that is, an infarct.

As muscle cells are elongated and multinucleated, their necrosis is often segmental, though this is seldom visualised. Necrosis, when initiated in one small segment of a muscle fibre, spreads in both directions along the fibre for a variable distance and for a time which is generally less than 6 hours, until the surviving stumps become covered by a protective membrane (Carpenter & Karpati 1989).

What are the changes that take place after necrosis is initiated, and by which necrosis can be recognized? Our data come primarily from Duchenne dystrophy, polymyositis, dermatomyositis, and the experimental model of micropuncture (Carpenter & Karpati 1989).

Early stages of experimental necrosis, at the point where it begins, tend to show marked hypercontraction and tearing of myofibrils, giving a reticulated net-like appearance (Fig. 7.1b, c). A similar appearance tends to be found in dermatomyositis (Fig. 7.1d, 7.2a) (but not in Duchenne dystrophy). It must be distinguished from hypercontraction which occurs as a reaction to the biopsy procedure, in which relatively long segments tend to contract as a whole, while on their ends they stretch or tear the rest of the fibre. Fibres severed on the edges of the biopsy contract, and, particularly in children's biopsies, isolated normal fibres in the centre of fascicles sometimes also contract excessively and tear themselves (Fig. 7.2b, c). Such fibres can be indistinguishable

from the hypercontracted fibres that are particularly common in biopsies from Duchenne dystrophy (Fig. 7.2d). This suggests that Duchenne fibres may be unusually fragile.

In early necrotic fibre segments where hypercontraction has not occurred, the Z disc can be seen to have disappeared within 2 hours (Fig. 7.3a). The best examples of this tend to occur in ischaemic necrosis. In more contracted segments only homogenisation of the myofibrils is evident. Mitochondria lose their laterally elongated shape and become round and dark, often forming chains. While hypercontraction can cause the myofibrillar material of necrotic fibres to appear darker than normal, with time the fibres lose density until they are paler than normal (Fig. 7.3b). This can happen without phagocytosis. The nuclei of necrotic fibres disappear rapidly; thus nuclei seen within necrotic fibres are generally those of phagocytes or regenerative cells.

Invasion of necrotic fibres by mononuclear phagocytes is probably rare before 10 hours have passed. In Duchenne dystrophy, where monocytes are already present in the interstitial tissue, it may occur faster. Polymorphonuclear leucocytes are almost never a factor in human muscle biopsies except in acute infections or infestations, such as trichinosis. Phagocytic invasion is dependent on blood supply (Hansen-Smith & Carlson 1979). So is proliferation of regenerative cells, but less so. In conditions like dermatomyositis where blood supply is curtailed, phagocytosis is often delayed, so that regenerative cells may be seen forming a thick ring around a centre of necrotic debris (Fig. 7.3c). In the centre of infarcts, necrotic fibres may persist for some time with neither phagocytosis nor regeneration.

Regeneration comes from the migration and proliferation of satellite cells as regenerative myoblasts (Bischoff 1979). These appear first on sections as thin cells on the periphery of the old fibre. They divide, grow fatter, and fuse (Fig. 7.3d). Ribosomes make their cytoplasm bluish on haematoxylin-eosin. After they have fused, myofibrils develop, at first separated by considerable cytoplasmic space (Fig. 7.4a). On cross-section a regenerated but not yet mature segment appears somewhat pale (Fig. 7.4b). The myofibrils are still slightly separated. Glycogen is

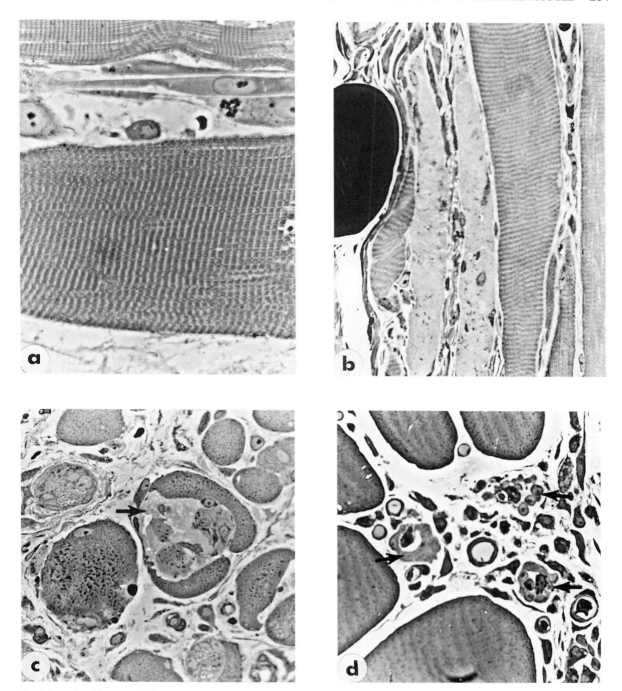

Fig. 7.3   a In this necrotic fibre segment the Z disc has disappeared although thick filaments are well preserved and well ordered. Acute ischaemic myopathy secondary to pitressin therapy (× 1370). **b** The two very pale muscle fibres are in a stage of necrosis that takes several hours to develop. Small clusters of dark granules on their periphery indicate early phagocytosis. Polymyositis (× 550). **c** In this infarcted tissue regeneration has occurred before the necrotic material of the dead fibre was completely phagocytosed. The regenerating fibres thus form a ring more or less surrounding the necrotic debris (arrow) (× 550). **d** Experimental micropuncture, 72 hours. Three muscle fibre segments (arrows) are regenerating. Lateral fusion of the myoblasts or myotubes has not yet obliterated the space in the centre of each fibre (× 1350).

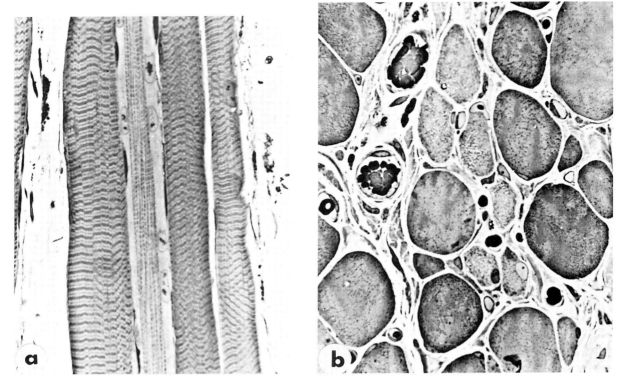

Fig. 7.4 **a** A typical regenerating fibre from a case of polymyositis shows a band of slightly separated myofibrils in the centre of its cytoplasm and myofibril-free zones on the periphery in which large vesicular nuclei with prominent nuclei can be seen (× 577). **b** In the centre of the picture is a group of six muscle fibres in a relatively late stage of regeneration. Their cytoplasm is still paler than that of the surrounding mature fibres, and most of their nuclei are still quite pale. Duchenne dystrophy (× 577).

abundant and sometimes forms subsarcolemmal collections. Mitochondria are rounded or extended in the long axis of the fibre. Nuclei are large and pale with large nucleoli, and are often at a distance from the sarcolemma.

Regeneration is not always a success. It may fail completely if satellite cells fail to proliferate, or, if proliferation is meagre, may result in thin rounded fibres. Incomplete lateral fusion of myoblasts will show up as forked or split fibres. If myoblasts fail to proliferate adequately, fibres will stay small and end prematurely. Myoblasts and regenerating fibres in general appear to be immune, until they mature, to whatever agent originally caused necrosis.

Fibre smallness

Smallness may mean shrinkage or failure to grow,

either primarily or after regeneration. Shrinkage is exemplified by the angular atrophic fibres of denervation, which tend to occur in groups. Their angular shape on cross-section may reflect pressure on them from their working neighbours. Bizarre spidery shapes are sometimes seen at high power on resin sections (Fig. 7.5a). When denervation involves whole fascicles, as in juvenile spinal muscular atrophy, angularity is much less pronounced. As denervated fibres shrink, they retain their nuclei. A far-gone denervated fibre thus will often appear as a small bag of nuclei. These nuclear clump fibres are usually rounded (Fig. 7.5b). In Werdnig–Hoffmann disease atrophic fibres tend to be very numerous, and all tend to be round (Fig. 7.5c). Diagnosis is made easier by finding groups of hypertrophied fibres. Probably many of the fibres are denervated before birth.

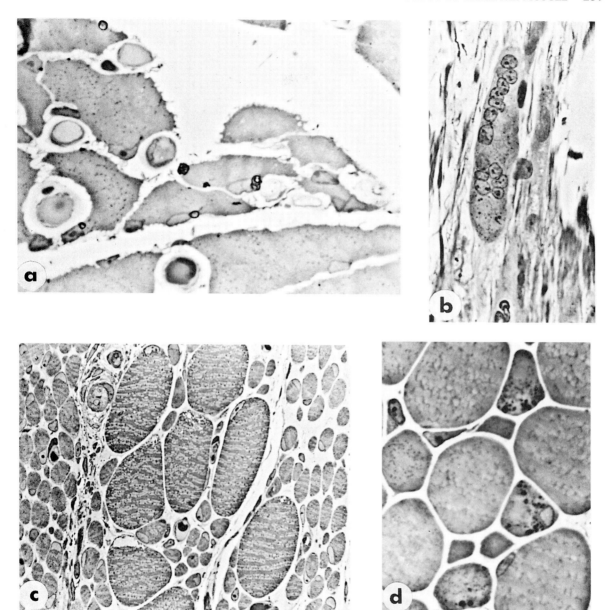

Fig. 7.5 a Denervated fibres in adult muscle are usually angular. When viewed at high power, like those here, extreme irregularity of the surface with thin branches can be seen (× 1350). **b** As denervated fibres shrink, their nuclei are retained, so that very small fibres may appear as nuclear clumps (× 1350). **c** In Werdnig–Hoffmann disease the numerous small fibres are rounded. Diagnosis is made more easy by finding grouped hypertrophied fibres as illustrated here (× 550). **d** This biopsy from a 15-year-old boy with nemaline myopathy diagnosed in the first year of life shows a mixture of normal-sized fibres and small fibres. Rods are present only in small fibres which have not been able to grow (× 1350).

Type II fibre atrophy, as seen in disuse, cachexia, and steroid treatment, obviously calls for histochemistry for its identification. Here the atrophic fibres, though angular, are scattered, and atrophy does not go as far as when it is from denervation.

Angular atrophic fibres, tending to be grouped, are seen in most cases of inclusion body myositis.

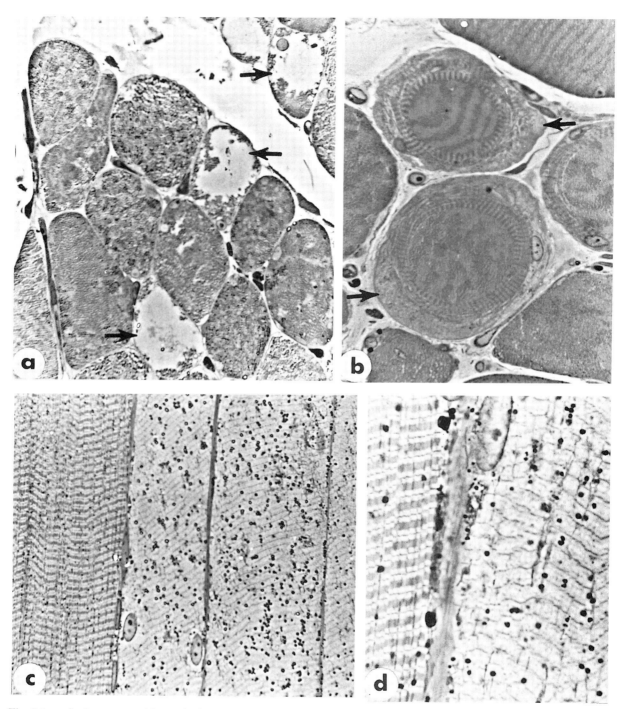

Fig. 7.6 **a** In dermatomyositis punched-out areas of myofibrillar loss may be found within muscle fibres (arrows). The space from which myofibrils have disappeared is largely filled with glycogen. Reduction in fibre volume is a subsequent event (× 577). **b** In this biopsy from a patient with myotonic dystrophy, sarcoplasmic masses (arrows) are present between the sarcolemma and ring myofibrils. They appear paler than the normal myofibrillar areas (× 577). **c** This biopsy is from a patient who was paralysed with vecuronium while on a respirator and given high doses of steroids. While the fibre on the left has normal myofibrils, those on the right show no trace of A-band density, although Z discs are present and the fibres are in no sense necrotic. There has been selective loss of thick filaments (× 577). **d** This high-power view of the preceding biopsy shows bands of pallor in the fibre where the A bands should be. The small dark rounded densities are lipid droplets, which are excessive here (× 1417).

They have been interpreted as evidence that there is a component of denervation in the disease, although they tend to be more miscellaneous in size than typical denervated fibres. Perhaps they are merely damaged fibres in a multifocal disease which have shrunk following loss of nuclei.

In diseases where necrosis is prevalent, as in Duchenne dystrophy, small rounded fibres represent regenerants which have not been able to grow larger because they lack enough nuclei (Schmalbruch 1984). There is no lack of satellite cells in Duchenne dystrophy, but with repeated cycles of necrosis and regeneration, their mitotic potential is progressively reduced. Fewer and fewer regenerative myoblasts are then available to fill long necrotic segments. The resultant new fibre segments are slender and rounded and may end prematurely. They usually have surprisingly regular myofibrils.

In congenital myopathies, small rounded fibres, for obscure reasons, have remained small (Fig. 7.5d). This may not, however, protect them from further injury and loss.

REACTIONS AND ALTERATIONS OF COMPONENTS OF MUSCLE FIBRES

Myofibrils

Loss of myofibrils in many conditions occurs concurrently with loss of cell volume, so that myofibrillar loss per se is not evident. This occurs with type II fibre atrophy and with denervation atrophy until its advanced stage. When denervated fibres have shrunk to the diameter of three or four nuclei, the myofibrillar material frequently appears pale. In dermatomyositis, punched-out areas of myofibrillar loss are often seen in damaged fibres (Fig. 7.6a). Sometimes myofibrils disappear from most of the cross-sectional area. The zones from which myofibrils are lost tend to be filled with glycogen. Loss of cell volume appears to be a subsequent event.

Sarcoplasmic masses, seen in some biopsies from myotonic dystrophy, seem to be zones not of myofibrillar loss but of aberrant organisation, in which myofilaments do not join into normal myofibrils but remain mixed with other cytoplasmic components (Fig. 7.6b).

Selective loss of thick filaments (myosin), or of the A band, is best appreciated on longitudinal sections. It is encountered in ischaemic conditions, in particular in some cases of dermatomyositis, in the vicinity of infarcts. It is also seen in rather pure form in biopsies from patients treated with high doses of corticosteroids when they have been given a neuromuscular blocking agent to facilitate artificial respiration (Fig. 7.6c, d). Most of these patients have been in status asthmaticus. When weaned from the respirator after a few days the patient may be unable to walk and only recovers strength in weeks or months. The loss of the A band may be limited to the centre of fibres in a 'core-like' pattern (Danon & Carpenter 1991). Similar A-band loss has been produced in rats by the combination of high-dose steroids and denervation. Myofibrils were promptly renewed when reinnervation was allowed (Masson et al 1992). The experimental lesions produced in the soleus muscle by Achilles tendon section also go through a stage where there is predominantly loss of thick filaments, but the lesion progresses to total zonal myofibrillar loss (Karpati et al 1972). Occasional muscle fibres in other myopathies (e.g. cytochrome oxidase deficiency) may show fairly selective myosin loss. Some very atrophic denervated fibres with very pale myofibrils but preserved Z discs may have predominant thick filament loss.

Selective loss of thin filaments is rarely seen, but it can occur focally in large fibres in denervation.

Z-disc reactions. Z-disc streaming is a common pathological change in muscle fibres. In particular it occurs in zones where mitochondria are lacking. The target and targetoid fibres associated with denervation are circumscribed zones of mitochondrial lack within which there is Z-disc streaming (Fig. 7.7a–c). This may be a feature of reinnervation rather than of denervation per se. In one study it was limited to reinnervated fibres (Massa et al 1992). It tends to be rare in biopsies from motor neurone disease. Careful inspection of normal muscle sections will show small zones free of mitochondria wherever vessels cross a muscle fibre transversely. Within these zones there is occasionally Z-disc streaming. A lack of mitochondria is characteristic of the cores of central core disease and the minicores of multi-

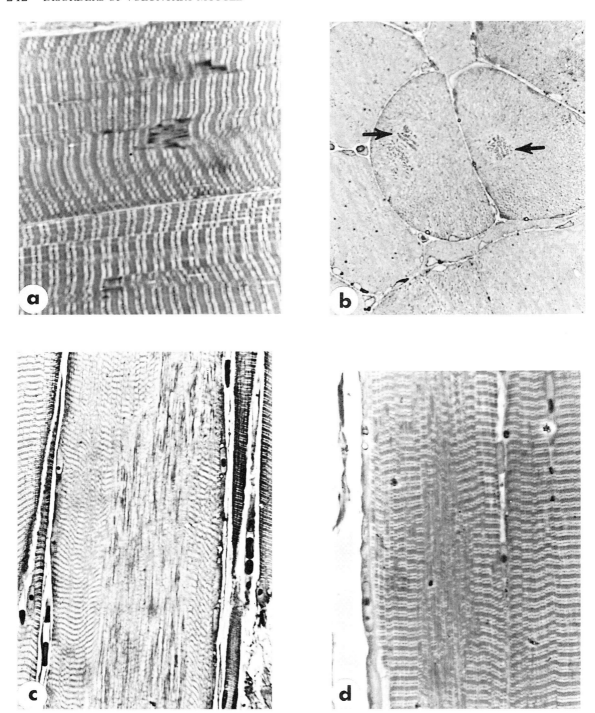

Fig. 7.7   **a** Very small foci of Z-disc streaming, some involving only one sarcomere, can be seen in these fibres from a partially denervated muscle (× 1350). **b** On transverse section foci of Z-disc streaming, as in this field from a partially denervated muscle, appear as irregular areas with stippled dark density (arrows) (× 550). **c** This fibre, from the same biopsy, contains a large central focus of Z-disc streaming that would make it appear as a target fibre on cryostat sections (× 550). **d** In dermatomyositis there is often untidy multifocal Z-disc streaming as shown here (× 550).

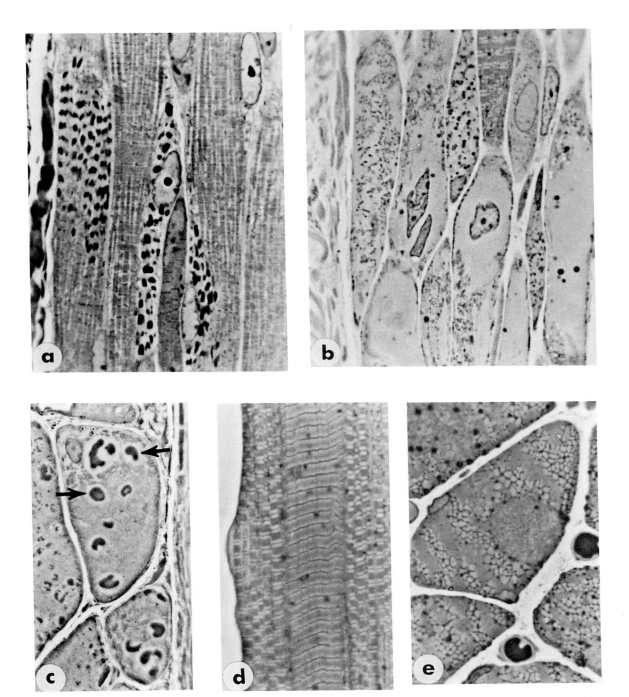

Fig. 7.8 **a** Nemaline bodies are very dense on resin sections. They appear to form within myofibrils from enlargement of the lattice of the Z disc. Their spacing can then be seen to approximate that of Z discs. When myofibrils break down, the nemaline bodies tend to accumulate under the sarcolemma (× 550). **b** In nemaline myopathy which is symptomatic in the newborn, there may be large areas in the muscle fibres which lack myofibrillar structure. By phase microscopy these areas look as if they might contain glycogen, but electron-microscopy shows them to be filled with thin filaments. The number of actual nemaline bodies is not particularly large (× 550). **c** Cytoplasmic bodies are dense oval to c-shaped structures within fibres, usually surrounded by a halo (arrows). They are non-specific. This is a case of multicore disease with desmin accumulations (× 550). **d** Central cores tend to show a different state of contraction from the surrounding normal myofibrillar areas in the same fibre (× 550). **e** Central cores, as seen here, are not always central. They lack mitochondria, and thus the mitochondrial grid as seen in normal I bands is missing (× 550).

core disease, and it may be accompanied in both by Z-disc streaming. Streaming is also common in ischaemia (Karpati et al 1974). It is often seen in inflammatory myopathies, but it is most common and characteristic in dermatomyositis, where it tends to be multifocal within fibres (Fig. 7.7d). The above are the most characteristic settings for Z-disc streaming, but it occurs occasionally in others.

Nemaline bodies or rods appear on transverse sections as very black flecks within fibres (Fig. 7.8a). Their shape and the spacing which relates them to Z-discs is best seen on longitudinal sections. They are more easily seen on resin sections than on cryostat or paraffin sections. When nemaline myopathy is symptomatic in the neonatal period, it tends to have a bad prognosis unlike later-onset cases, and the muscle cells tend to show more marked myofibrillar changes (Schmalbruch et al 1987). Large segments without evident substructure may be filled with masses of thin filaments which can be mistaken for glycogen lakes (Fig. 7.8b). Outside of cases of nemaline myopathy, formation of rods can probably occur as a secondary phenomenon. Tenotomy of the rat soleus, which usually produces zones of myofibrillar loss, will sometimes lead to rod formation (Karpati et al 1972). When there is A-band loss, some enlargement of Z-discs tends to occur, even reaching the size of small rods.

Cytoplasmic bodies appear as dense rounded structures with a clear halo (Fig. 7.8c). Occasionally they are seen with tail-like connections to a line of Z-discs. They are brightly eosinophilic on cryostat sections. They may be numerous in inclusion body myositis, but they should not be confused with the rather specific eosinophilic inclusion surrounded by basophilic granules. Cytoplasmic bodies are highly non-specific, although a plethora might suggest a specific syndrome described as cytoplasmic body myopathy (Jerusalem et al 1979).

In central core disease, cytoplasmic organisation is abnormal; in particular, myofibrils are affected. Cores are a circumscribed cytoplasmic area which extends from end to end of the muscle fibre, and in which myofibrils are not distinct from one another, intermyofibrillar mitochondria are lacking, Z discs are not quite straight, and the degree of contraction is independent from that of the rest of the fibre (Fig. 7.8d, e). Since they lack mitochondria, cores often show Z-disc streaming.

Loss of Z-discs occurs in early necrotic fibres, sometimes affecting long segments.

Mitochondria

Individual mitochondria can be seen on longitudinal sections of nicely relaxed muscle fibres as small blips on either side of the Z-disc (Fig. 7.9a). On transverse sections they constitute the main density of the intermyofibrillar lattice in the I band, reflecting the fact that they are elongated transversely to the myofibrillar axis. Normally mitochondria do not project into the A band in relaxed muscle; when they do, it is a subtle, sensitive, and non-specific sign of abnormality. On good sections one can detect the focal absence of mitochondria that normally occurs where a vessel crosses transversely a muscle fibre. Absence of mitochondria in and around minicores and targets can also be seen (Fig. 7.9b).

In muscle from children, subsarcolemmal collections of crowded mitochondria can normally occur along one or even two sides of several fibres, appearing as dark crescents in which individual mitochondria cannot be distinguished (Fig. 7.9c). These crescents are much rarer in normal adult muscle. The point at which they become clearly excessive may be difficult to decide. Fibres that correspond to ragged red fibres show subsarcolemmal dark mitochondria collections on all sides, as well as a focal increase between myofibrils (Fig. 7.9d). Crystals in mitochondria can be distinguished under oil immersion if large and numerous (Fig. 7.10a). The tendency of ragged red fibres to be wreathed by numerous capillaries is clearly seen (Fig. 7.10b).

Vacuolation of mitochondria is a common artefact resulting from slowness of fixation (Fig. 7.11a). The contraction of muscle that has not been fixed in an isometric clamp slows penetration of fixative. Likewise, too generous a muscle sample compressed in a clamp will be poorly fixed in its centre.

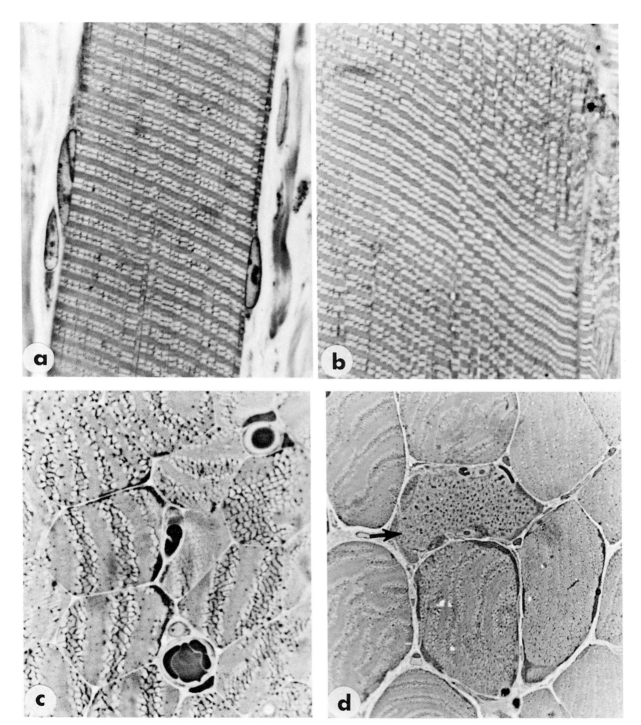

Fig. 7.9 **a** In well-relaxed muscle fibres, mitochondria can be seen as small bars next to the Z disc (× 1417). **b** This fibre from a partly denervated muscle contains a large area in which mitochondria are virtually lacking from sarcomeres (× 1417). **c** In normal biopsies from children, and to some extent from adults, subsarcolemmal dark accumulations of mitochondria, as here, are a normal finding. Note the normal grid of mitochondria in the I band and their absence from the A band (× 1417). **d** In a ragged red fibre, dark subsarcolemmal mitochondrial accumulations tend to be present on all sides of a fibre, and excess mitochondria are also present between myofibrils, but all degrees of abnormality can be seen, as here, where one fibre (arrow) has marked abnormality in its centre, while two adjacent fibres only appear to have increased subsarcolemmal mitochondria (× 577).

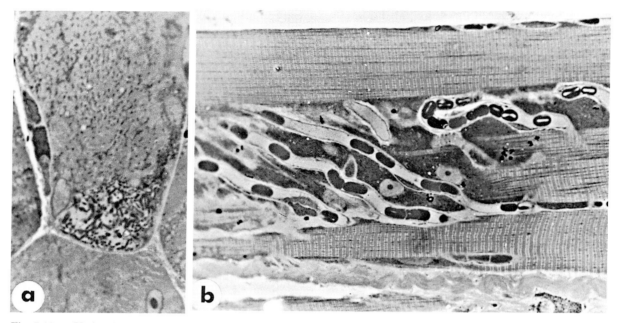

Fig. 7.10   a Under oil immersion, elongated subsarcolemmal mitochondria can sometimes be demonstrated. These abnormal forms would be shown by electron-microscopy to contain crystals (× 1417). **b** This section is cut tangentially to a fibre which is passing out of the plane of section to the left. Its cytoplasm is packed with mitochondria. A surprising number of capillaries are present next to the fibre (× 577).

Glycogen

Some degree of leaching of glycogen from muscle fibres is often seen, depending on whether the stabilising effect of the fixative predominates or the solubilising effect of its water vehicle. Roughly treated muscle that has been allowed to contract may squeeze glycogen into blebs that might raise a question of glycogen storage. Regenerating fibres often contain enough glycogen to form visible accumulations.

In almost all glycogen storage diseases, whatever excess of glycogen there may be will be found free in the cytoplasm. An excess is not always detectable even with periodic-acid-Schiff (PAS) staining. The largest amounts probably occur in debranching enzyme deficiency (Fig. 7.11b). In acid maltase deficiency, both free cytoplasmic and membrane-bound lysosomal glycogen are present (Fig. 7.11c). The latter tends to form clearly rounded masses or vacuoles. In the infantile form these are quite characteristic in interstitial cells. A PAS stain can be easily done on resin sections for further demonstration of glycogen.

Fat

Neutral lipid globules may appear on resin sections as clear vacuoles or as dark droplets which lack the refractility of lipofuscin granules. The neutral lipid content of skeletal muscle is normally relatively labile and reflects levels of serum fatty acids. Significant lipid storage, such as occurs in carnitine deficiency, is generally easy to distinguish from non-significant excess (Fig. 7.11d).

Motor end-plates

Motor end-plates will not be encountered in most biopsies unless special techniques are used such as motor point or intercostal muscle biopsy with parallel histochemical and resin sections. Motor end-plates when present are fairly easy to recognise on resin sections (Fig. 7.12a). If individual myelinated fibres circled by perineurium are present, motor end-plates generally will be too. On the other hand the pathology of motor end-plates is best studied with immunocytochemistry, bungarotoxin binding, or electron-microscopy.

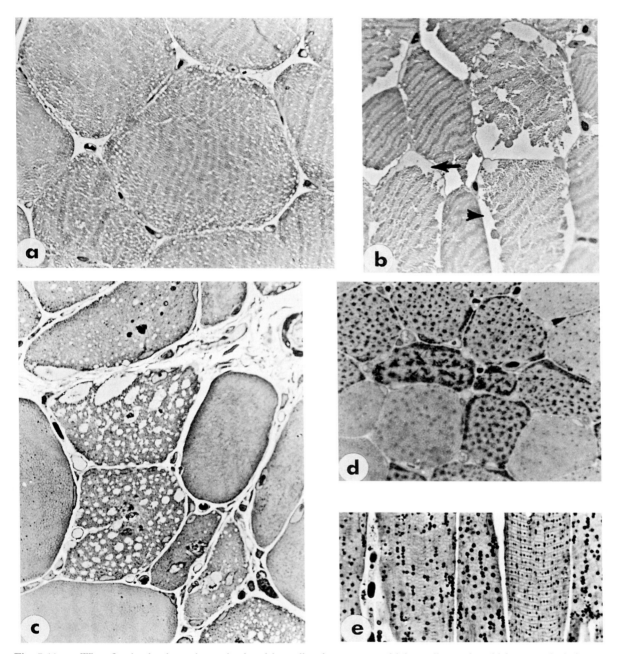

Fig. 7.11   a When fixation has been slow, mitochondria swell and appear as multiple small vacuoles which are particularly numerous close to the sarcolemma. This can often be related to the deeper portions of the biopsy. The fibres may also appear somewhat pale from loss of glycogen ($\times$ 550). **b** Glycogen in excess amounts forms areas with a ground-glass density (arrow), from which other organelles tend to be excluded. Glycogen may, however, be leached out from certain fibres, leaving only empty areas (arrowhead). This biopsy is from type 3 glycogenosis ($\times$ 550). **c** In acid maltase deficiency, muscle fibres contain multiple small vacuoles from which glycogen may or may not have been leached out. Dense material is also seen within some vacuoles. This biopsy is from the adult-onset variety, in which there may be sparing of many fibres or of many areas of some muscles ($\times$ 550). **d** In carnitine deficiency very numerous lipid globules are seen within muscle fibres, with the relative amount depending on fibre type. Some fibres also contain an excess of mitochondria ($\times$ 550). **e** In dermatomyositis in the vicinity of fresh infarcts there may be a large increase of lipid globules in muscle fibres ($\times$ 550).

Nuclei

Displacement of nuclei from their normal sub-sarcolemmal position is the commonest abnormality involving nuclei. Since semithin sections are much thinner than cryostat sections, they will reveal far fewer central nuclei. In some cases of infantile centronuclear myopathy, this may make the diagnosis problematical if only resin sections are used. The nuclei tend to be in the precise geometric centre of the fibre, although some sarcolemmal nuclei are usually also present. In late-onset centronuclear myopathy, tight clusters of nuclei may occur in the geometrical centre, as well as some which seem to be lifting away from the sarcolemma (Fig. 7.12b). In adult myotonic dystrophy by contrast, the numerous central nuclei tend to be scattered randomly in the interior of fibres on cross-section (Fig. 7.12c).

Nuclei in regenerating fibres are pale and large with prominent nucleoli. Similar active nuclei are seen in injured fibres in dermatomyositis in which reparative processes are active. Likewise some vacuolated fibres in periodic paralysis have large pale nuclei with prominent nucleoli. Pyknotic nuclei are not often seen in muscle disease, aside from artefact. They occur in infantile polymyositis (Fig. 7.12d) (Carpenter & Karpati 1984), and reducing body myopathy (Carpenter et al 1985), occasionally in myotonic dystrophy and in inclusion body myositis. They also occur in rare unclassified myopathies. We have seen two such cases associated with respiratory failure.

Intranuclear inclusions in inclusion body myositis are almost never apparent in semithin sections, although egg-shaped spaces with a ground-glass density, a little larger than nuclei, may represent a stage of nuclear breakdown when almost all nuclear contents are replaced by filaments. In oculopharyngeal dystrophy, the relatively rare nuclei which, by electron-microscopy, contain the pathognomonic fine tubular inclusions, by light microscopy have very pale contents (Tomé & Fardeau 1980). Intranuclear nemaline bodies have been seen in a small number of cases of nemaline myopathy, some with neonatal (Jenis et al 1969), others with adult onset (Engel & Oberc 1975). On cryostat sections they are red with trichrome stains and surrounded by a halo.

Clumps of nuclei in markedly atrophic fibres are suggestive of denervation atrophy. Nuclei are apparently not lost as denervated fibres shrink. This seems not to be true in dermatomyositis, though disintegrating nuclei are rarely seen. Nuclear clumps occur in some cases designated as limb-girdle dystrophy, where they have been interpreted as evidence of a neurogenic component. They occur also in myotonic dystrophy and in some familial cases of inclusion body myositis.

Vacuoles

Vacuoles in skeletal muscle fibres can be of many sorts. Division into clear vacuoles and those with visible contents is helpful.

An important source of clear vacuoles is the T-tubules, which can undergo marked acute swelling when there is massive ingress of sodium into a fibre. This was first shown by in vitro experiments with transected normal fibres (Casademont et al 1988); dilatation of T-tubules extended with time progressively further and further from the cut end, provided that the incubation medium contained levels of sodium like those in the extracellular space (Fig. 7.13a). It was postulated that increased cytoplasmic sodium stimulates the Na^+-K^+ ATPase in the T-tubules, which expel three Na^+ ions while taking in two of K^+. The increased ionic concentration in the T-tubular lumen draws water into it from the cytoplasm. Similar T-tubular swelling in the stumps of necrotic fibres was found in an in vivo model of focal necrosis (micropuncture). When these vacuoles became large, their connection to T-tubules was difficult to demonstrate. Similar vacuoles are seen in human muscle fibres in many conditions where focal necrosis has recently occurred. We may call them 'stump vacuoles', since they occur in the stumps of necrotic fibres. The fact that they are not seen in Duchenne dystrophy, where necrosis is almost always present, is unexplained.

Some biopsies from Duchenne dystrophy on electron microscopy show fibres that lack a plasma

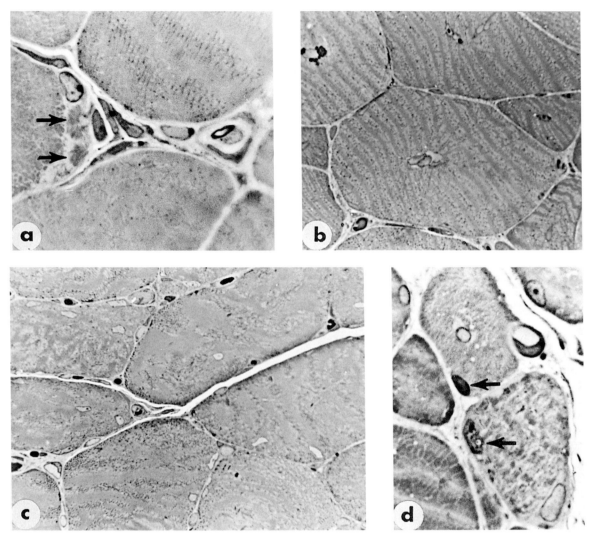

Fig. 7.12   a Motor end-plates are easy to recognise on resin sections. The secondary clefts (arrows) appear like narrow petals radiating from the primary cleft. One of the sole plate nuclei can be seen. The nucleus just outside the fibre next to the motor end-plate is a Schwann cell nucleus. To the right is a single myelinated fibre enclosed in its perineurial chamber. When such terminal nerves are visible in a biopsy, end-plates can almost always be found (× 1350). **b** In centronuclear myopathies, nuclei accumulate at the geometrical centre of muscle fibres. In the adult-onset type, pictured here, the central nuclei may form clumps and be accompanied by lipofuscin granules (× 550). **c** In myotonic dystrophy central nuclei are typically numerous but random in their location inside fibres (× 550). **d** There is a type of polymyositis in infants in which abnormal nuclei are found in muscle cells. Two such nuclei are seen here (arrows). One is pyknotic, and the other contains vacuoles (× 1350).

membrane and also lack other signs of necrosis. It is not clear whether this indicates retraction or dissolution. These fibres do show small rounded vacuoles of T-tubular origin, which can be seen by light-microscopy, although they are difficult to distinguish from swollen mitochondria. They are not seen in stumps.

Some biopsies from patients with periodic paralysis have widely scattered vacuolated fibres (Fig. 7.13b). A fibre may contain a single gigantic vacuole or many small ones. They are elongated on longitudinal sections. They connect to the extracellular space through T-tubules. The mechanism of their formation may be related to that of stump

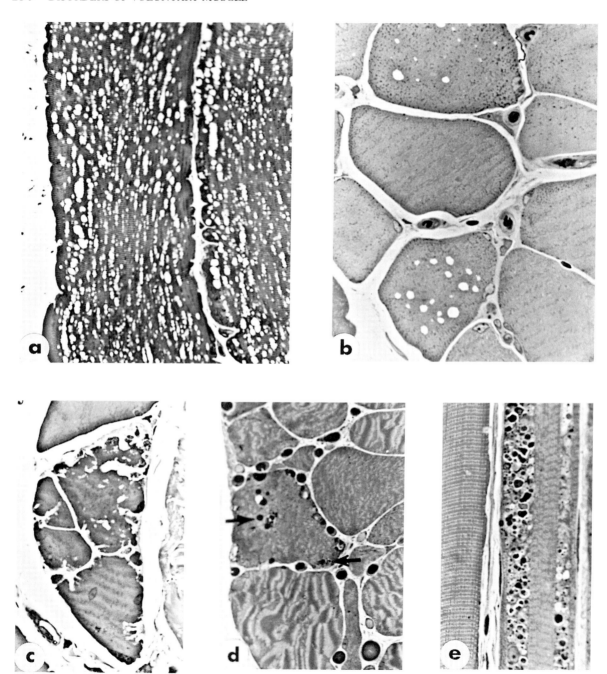

Fig 7.13   **a** These muscle fibres from a rat were cut and incubated for 20 min in oxygenated glucose-containing isotonic medium. The marked vacuolation seen here is produced by T-tubule dilatation. It was absent in fibre regions distant from the cut end. In similar incubations it could be prevented when sodium was omitted from the bathing medium (× 550). **b** In some cases of periodic paralysis, particularly those with permanent weakness, fibres with vacuoles of various sizes can be found (× 550). **c** At normal myotendinous junctions muscle fibres show splits and vacuole-like extensions of the extracellular space in their interior (× 550). **d** In inclusion body myositis, dark granules (arrows) in scattered muscle fibres are membranous whorls. There is a focal increase in capillaries (× 550). e Membranous whorls in inclusion body myositis sometimes form extended linear accumulations (× 550).

vacuoles, although it has been suggested that they are the end-stage of autophagic vacuoles following breakdown of masses of dilated sarcoplasmic reticulum vesicles (Engel & Oberc 1975).

Dilatation of sarcoplasmic reticulum to the point of forming light-microscopic vacuoles is probably rare. A single case reported as sarcotubular myopathy would be an example (Jerusalem et al 1973). Mild degrees of SR dilatation where the fine granular content is not lost are occasionally encountered. The significance is uncertain.

At myotendinous junctions, muscle fibres become deeply invaginated by the extracellular space. In some sections this can give the appearance of vacuoles inside fibres (Fig. 7.13c).

Lysosomal vacuoles are the mark of acid maltase deficiency. They may have the ground-glass density of glycogen or appear empty, if glycogen has been leached out, or may contain lipofuscin-like material or some membranous whorls. Non-membrane-bound glycogen lakes, present in the infantile form, probably result from rupture of lysosomes. In rare cases of Batten's disease, the storage lysosomes in muscle become distended to the point of forming vacuoles.

Rimmed vacuoles are an expected finding in inclusion body myositis. The designation arises from their appearance on cryostat sections. With haematoxylin-eosin, they appear as collections of blue granules separated by an irregular fissure. Occasionally a red inclusion appears among the granules. On resin sections the granules (which are membranous whorls) usually do not appear to be within vacuoles but to be free in the cytoplasm, which may retract slightly from them. In large accumulations, which may extend for inordinate lengths along muscle fibres (Fig. 7.13d), electron-microscopy shows numerous vacuoles of various sizes accompanying the membranous whorls. Membranous whorls are highly osmiophilic but tend to lack the refractility of lipofuscin granules. This distinction is inapparent on very thick sections. Membranous whorls are dissolved out of paraffin sections. If membranous whorls are not present on semi-thin sections, there is virtually no chance that electron-microscopy on thin sections from those blocks will show the characteristic filaments of inclusion body myositis. The membranes of these whorls by electron-microscopy never show any consistent periodicity, suggesting that they are not derived from preformed membranous organelles.

Membranous whorls occur in other situations, for example in some fibres in periodic paralysis (Fig. 7.14a) and in rare cases of Batten's disease (Fig. 7.14b). Some seem to be a broken-down form of cylindrical-spiral-like structures. Others occur in autophagic vacuoles, as in acid maltase deficiency. Colchicine myopathy is characterised by small groups of membranous whorls (Fig. 7.14c). Chloroquine, which inhibits lysosomal function, can produce clinically and experimentally membranous whorls in muscle (Macdonald & Engel 1970, Benke 1976), but they tend to be scattered rather than grouped into 'rimmed vacuoles' (Fig. 7.14d).

Autophagic vacuoles occur in occasional cases of myopathy, usually of obscure origin. In one such case, seen recently (Carpenter et al 1992), some fibres contained masses of tubules, probably of T-tubular origin, which appear to undergo breakdown, calcify, and become incorporated into autophagic vacuoles which contain various sorts of dark material (Fig. 7.14e). This process ended with the formation of fissures or lacunae lined with basal lamina in the centre of muscle fibres.

Abnormal organelles

Abnormal organelles lend some excitement to the study of a biopsy, but most are disappointingly non-specific in significance.

Cylindrical spirals. These complicated membranous structures are mostly seen in a subset of patients with cramps (Carpenter et al 1979). On transverse resin sections, they appear as groups of small regular dark circles, usually near the sarcolemma (Fig. 7.15a). They are easier to recognise on longitudinal sections, where they look like small piles of logs (Fig. 7.15b). They are red with the modified trichrome, though sometimes surrounded by blue-purple granules. Less regular cylindrical membranous structures are sometimes associated with tubular aggregates. Cylindrical spirals seem to be derived from sarcoplasmic reticulum (SR) membranes.

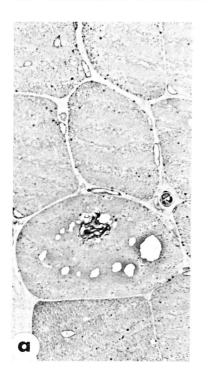
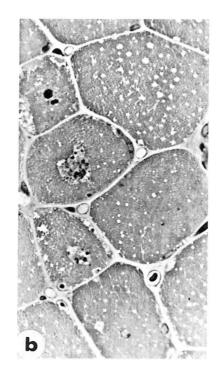
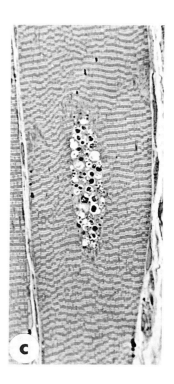
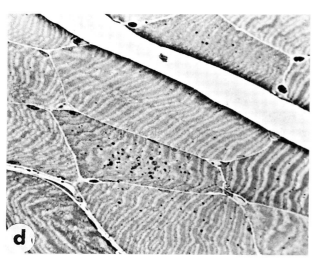
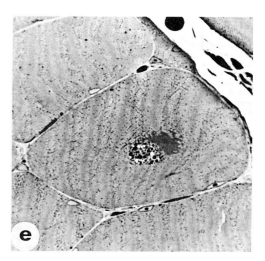

Fig. 7.14 **a** In periodic paralyses, occasional fibres may contain collections of membranous whorls (× 550). **b** In some cases of juvenile Batten's disease, storage cytosomes in muscle cells may be quite large and contain some membranous whorls within them. The multiple empty vacuoles seen here in many of the fibres are lipid droplets from which the lipid has been extracted in processing (× 550). **c** In myopathy secondary to colchicine treatment, collections of membranous whorls may be found (× 550). **d** Chloroquine treatment may result in accumulation of lysosomal inclusions, which may include membranous whorls and be visible by phase microscopy. They tend not to coalesce into so-called rimmed vacuoles (× 550). **e** In the centre of this muscle fibre, there is accumulation of dense material which extends between myofibrils on its edges. This area is filled with tubules derived from T-tubules. Next to it is an accumulation of membranous whorls and calcium which probably represents a stage in breakdown of the tubules. From a chronic myopathy (× 550).

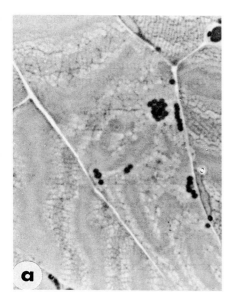

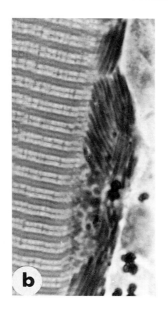

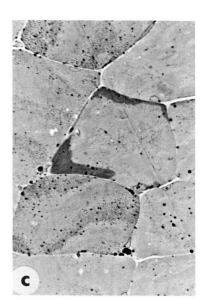

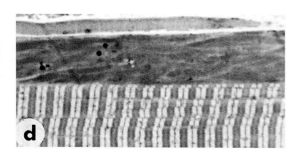

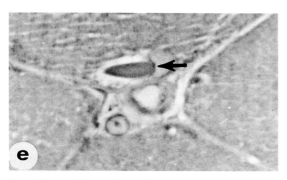

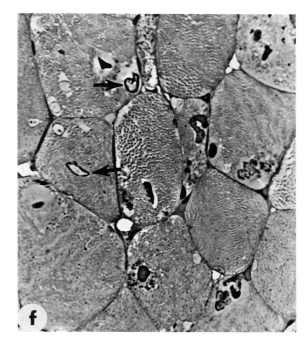

Fig. 7.15 **a** Cylindrical spirals on cross-section appear as small dark very uniform circles, usually grouped (× 1350).
b Cylindrical spirals are much easier to recognise on the longitudinal sections (× 1350). **c** Tubular aggegates form moderately
dense geographical areas, generally on the periphery of muscle fibres (× 550). **d** On longitudinal sections tubular aggregates
frequently appear subdivided into blocks (× 1350). **e** A fingerprint body (arrow) is the moderately dense inclusion seen here next
to a nucleus beneath the sarcolemma of a muscle fibre (× 1350). **f** Numerous very dense reducing bodies are present in this biopsy.
Two nuclei (arrows) are surrounded by a thin layer of reducing body filaments (× 550).

Tubular aggregates. Tubular aggregates are seen in some cramp syndromes, but also occur non-specifically in various myopathies, in particular periodic paralysis (Engel et al 1970). On resin sections they are relatively dark, tending to fill geographical areas next to the sarcolemma (Fig. 7.15c). On longitudinal sections, subdivisions may be visible within them, corresponding to blocks of parallel tubules (Fig. 7.15d). Definitive identification requires electron-microscopy, although their positivity with NADH tetrazolium reductase and negativity with succinic dehydrogenase is highly suggestive (Engel et al 1970).

Fingerprint bodies. These moderately rare structures are rather non-specific, although in some childhood cases of mild myopathy they are the most prominent abnormality (Engel et al 1972). On resin sections they appear as small, usually lens-shaped homogeneous, moderately pale, sharply demarcated structures, usually near the sarcolemma (Fig. 7.15e). On the modified trichrome stain they are red.

Reducing bodies. Reducing bodies are rare. They are specific for the disease of reducing body myopathy, although reported cases are clinically somewhat miscellaneous (Carpenter et al 1985). With haematoxylin-eosin they are eosinophilic on cryostat or paraffin sections. On resin sections they are very dark, especially on their periphery (Fig. 7.15f). Often they have a characteristic shape like a broken egg. Sometimes the dark material can be seen to surround nuclei. Precise identification depends on histochemistry to show their reducing capacity. Electron-microscopy shows their basic composition of tubular filaments, which may be so crowded that they are interpreted as granules.

OTHER STRUCTURES THAN MUSCLE CELLS

Connective tissue

Normally so little collagen is present between muscle fibres that it is only visible by electron-microscopy. An exception is in the neighbourhood of neuromuscular junctions, where a small amount of collagen tends to encircle muscle fibres. Muscle that has been severely damaged from a variety of causes tends to show increased endomysial connective tissue, usually in the form of rather loose, randomly orientated collagen. This is particularly well seen in polymyositis and inclusion body myositis. Fibrosis in end-stage denervation tends to show a proliferation of elastic fibres (black on resin sections, purple on the trichrome stain) along with the collagen.

In Duchenne and Becker dystrophy, the connective tissue proliferation, which begins to occur early, is distinctive, consisting of discrete collagen bundles laid down parallel to the muscle fibres (Fig. 7.16a). This pattern is also seen in some biopsies from patients without dystrophin deficiency but with a limb-girdle syndrome. Fibrosis in other conditions, such as polymyositis and inclusion body myositis, tends to be less discrete, less organised, and more obviously related to cell loss (Fig. 7.16b).

When muscle cells have been lost and replaced by fat cells, no matter what the cause, collagen also tends to be lost.

Vessels

Paraffin sections, because of their relatively large sample size, find their greatest scope in the diagnosis of arteritis.

Lymphatics are best seen on resin sections. They occur in septa close to arteries (Fig. 7.17a). Because of the thinness of their walls, they tend to collapse and become indistinguishable from the connective tissue unless they are filled with inflammatory cells.

Capillaries can be well visualised on resin sections, provided the muscle fibres have not been tightly squashed together. General tissue stains on cryostat or paraffin sections tend only to show part of the capillary population, but good selective staining of all capillaries is achieved by use of lectin staining or immunocytochemistry for major histocompatibility products.

In normal adult muscle the lumen of a capillary is seen in most intersections of the interstitial space among muscle fibres. Roughly 1.5 capillary lumina accompany each muscle cell, and there are about 400–500 lumina per mm^2 of transverse muscle fibre area. In newborn infants the

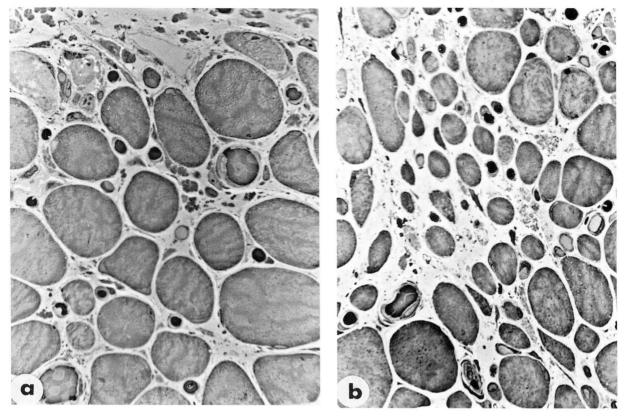

Fig. 7.16 a Connective tissue proliferation in Duchenne dystrophy characteristically takes the form of dense discrete bundles of collagen directed parallel to the muscle fibres (× 577). **b** Connective tissue proliferation in polymyositis tends to be looser, more randomly orientated, and more obviously associated with areas of fibre damage than in Duchenne dystrophy (× 577).

number of capillaries per muscle fibre is far lower.

There is some lability in the capillary network. In denervation atrophy, as muscle fibres shrink, the capillaries surrounding them come closer together, causing an increase in the number of capillaries per unit of transverse muscle fibre area (Carpenter & Karpati 1982). The muscle appears over-vascularised; at the same time, certain capillary lines become necrotic (Fig. 7.17b). In denervated muscle one can often see an occasional capillary which is represented only by a basal lamina circle without endothelium. Loss of capillaries is also seen in dermatomyositis, but the picture is very different (Emslie-Smith & Engel 1990). Perifascicular areas are most often involved. The number of capillaries per unit of transverse muscle fibre area drops (Fig. 7.17c).

Endothelial thickening and proliferation are usually seen, resulting in an increase of nuclei in surviving capillaries. Cells containing dark granules at the site of a capillary suggest active necrosis, as do single isolated red cells among the muscle fibres. Proliferation of thin-walled venules is sometimes present next to an area of capillary loss. Necrosis of larger vessels is seen in a few cases, where it tends to be associated with infarcts.

Thickening of the basal lamina of capillaries, appearing as a pale grey ground-glass density, is seen most commonly in diabetic patients (Fig. 7.17b). Occasionally it occurs without any obvious causal association. In an extreme form ('pipe-stem capillaries') it has been reported with connective tissue disease (Emslie-Smith & Engel 1991). Amyloid, which may be difficult to distinguish from a thick basal lamina on resin sections,

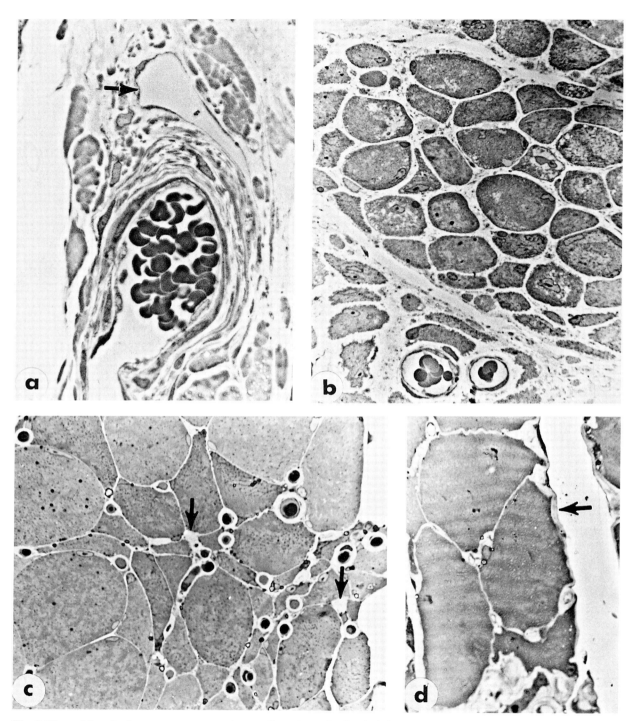

Fig. 7.17 **a** A lymphatic appears as a space whose wall consists only of endothelium (arrow). Lymphatics are seen in septa close to large vessels (× 913). **b** In dermatomyositis there is a loss of capillaries which can reach the extreme stage seen here, where a subfascicle contains no intact capillaries. Remaining vessels like those below tend to be dilated (× 577). **c** In this sample of partially denervated muscle from a diabetic, there is marked thickening of the basal lamina of capillaries. Some masses of basal lamina material can be seen (arrows) where a capillary has disappeared (× 577). **d** Amyloid may form collars around small intramuscular vessels, but this can be mimicked by non-specific basal lamina thickening. More characteristic is a tendency of amyloid to coat the surface of muscle fibres on the periphery of fascicles (arrow) (× 577).

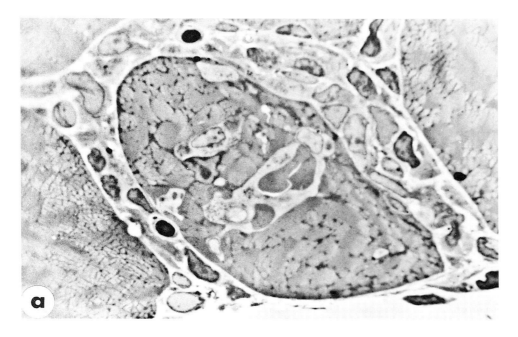

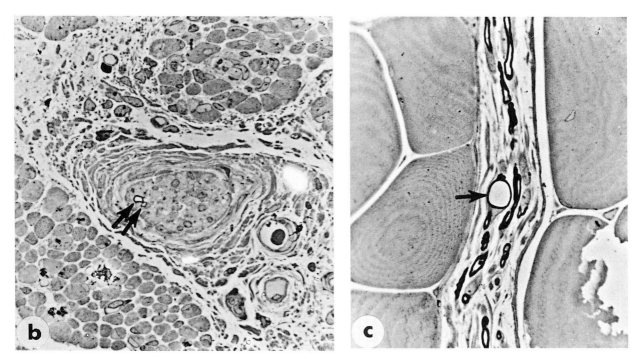

Fig. 7.18   a In inclusion body myositis, seen here, and in polymyositis, lymphocytes and macrophages are seen invading non-necrotic muscle fibres (× 1350). **b** In Werdnig–Hoffman disease, there tends to be marked loss of motor axons from intramuscular nerves. This nerve only contains two residual myelinated fibres (arrows); several other nerves of the same size contained none (× 550). **c** A polyglucosan body (arrow) distends one myelin sheath in an intramuscular nerve. In this 45-year-old man with motor neurone disease it was considered an incidental finding (× 550).

characteristically coats the surface of muscle fibres on the outside of fascicles (Fig. 7.17d).

An excess of capillaries is seen in some cases of inclusion body myositis and in cases of marked histochemical type I fibre predominance. Ragged red fibres are often surrounded, and even indented, by an excess number of capillary lumina.

Inflammatory cells

In polymyositis, inflammatory infiltrates tend to be conspicuous within muscle fascicles, where they are often associated with the phenomenon of partial invasion of non-necrotic fibres by lymphocytes and macrophages (Engel & Arahata 1982). Partial invasion is also commonly seen in inclusion body myositis (Fig. 7.18a), although sizeable inflammatory infiltrates are rare and may be absent from a biopsy. In dermatomyositis infiltrates are confined to septa, although separate cells, in particular macrophages, may be found between muscle fibres in involved regions.

Intramuscular nerves

Specific changes in intramuscular nerves can rarely be seen. In denervating conditions, a decrease in myelinated axons is frequently visible in intramuscular nerves. Wallerian ovoids are not often visible. In Werdnig–Hofmann disease, intramuscular nerves usually show extreme depletion of myelinated fibres (Fig. 7.18b). This can be diagnostically useful if the characteristic groups of hypertrophied muscle fibres are not present among the sea of round atrophic fibres. In chronic demyelinating diseases, onion bulbs are rarely and perhaps never seen in small intramuscular nerves. Polyglucosan bodies occur non-specifically in intramuscular axons of patients over the age of 40 (Robitaille et al 1980). If they are particularly numerous and the clinical data are suggestive, the possibility of adult polyglucosan disease must be considered, and the sural nerve, a more specific site, should be scrutinised (Fig. 7.18c). In giant axonal disease, focal distension of axons with neurofilaments occurs in intramuscular nerves, although the greater sample of the sural nerve is preferable for diagnosis (Carpenter et al 1974). In infantile neuroaxonal dystrophy, changes occur predominantly in the most distal parts of axons, and abnormalities may be detectable, even before electron-microscopy, in the large axons in muscle spindles, although electron-microscopy on a skin sample is the optimal diagnostic procedure.

REFERENCES

Benke B 1976 Mass occurrence of multilamellar bodies in myopathy. Virchows Archiv B Cell Pathology 20: 77

Bischoff R 1979 Tissue culture studies on the origin of myogenic cells during muscle regeneration in the rat. In: Mauro A (ed) Muscle regeneration. Raven, New York, p 493

Carpenter S, Karpati G 1982 Necrosis of capillaries in denervation atrophy of human skeletal muscle. Muscle and Nerve 5: 250

Carpenter S, Karpati G 1984 Pathology of skeletal muscle, 1st edn. Churchill Livingstone, New York, p 581

Carpenter S, Karpati G 1989 Segmental necrosis and its demarcation in experimental micropuncture injury of skeletal muscle fibers. Journal of Neuropathology and Experimental Neurology 48: 154

Carpenter S, Karpati G, Robitaille Y, Melmed C 1979 Cylindrical spirals in human skeletal muscle. Muscle and Nerve 2: 282

Carpenter S, Karpati G, Holland P 1985 New observations in reducing body myopathy. Neurology 35: 818

Carpenter S, Karpati G, Holland P 1992 A chronic myopathy with coated vesicles and tubular masses. Neuromuscular Disorders 2: 209

Carpenter S, Karpati G, Andermann F, Gold R 1974 Giant axonal neuropathy: a clinically and morphologically distinct neurological disease. Archives of Neurology 31: 312

Casademont J, Carpenter S, Karpati G 1988 Vacuolation of muscle fibres near sarcolemmal breaks represents T-tubule dilatation secondary to enhanced sodium pump activity. Journal of Neuropathology and Experimental Neurology 47: 618

Danon M J, Carpenter S 1991 Myopathy with thick filament (myosin) loss following prolonged paralysis with vecuronium during steroid treatment. Muscle and Nerve 14: 1131

Emslie-Smith A M, Engel A G 1990 Microvascular changes in early and advanced dermatomyositis: a quantitative study. Annals of Neurology 27: 343

Emslie-Smith A M, Engel A G 1991 Necrotizing myopathy with pipestem capillaries, microvascular deposition of the complement membrane attack complex (MAC), and minimal cellular infiltration. Neurology 41: 936

Engel A G, Angelini C, Gomez M R 1972 Fingerprint body myopathy: a newly recognized congenital muscle disease. Mayo Clinic Proceedings 47: 377

Engel A G, Arahata K 1982 Monoclonal analysis of mononuclear cells in myopathies. II: Phenotypes of autoinvasive cells in polymyositis and inclusion body myositis. Annals of Neurology 16: 209

Engel W K, Bishop D W, Cunningham G G 1970 Tubular aggregates in type II muscle fibers: ultrastructural and histochemical correlation. Journal of Ultrastructural Research 31: 507

Engel W K, Oberc M A 1975 Abundant nuclear rods in adult-onset rod disease. Journal of Neuropathology and Experimental Neurology 34: 119

Hansen-Smith F M, Carlson B M 1979 Cellular responses to free grafting of the extensor digitorum longus muscle of the rat. Journal of the Neurological Sciences 41: 149

Jenis E H, Lindquist R R, Lister R C 1969 New congenital myopathy with crystalline intranuclear inclusions. Archives of Neurology 20: 281

Jerusalem F, Engel A G, Gomez M R 1973 Sarcotubular myopathy: a newly recognized benign congenital, familial muscle disease. Neurology 23: 897

Jerusalem F, Ludin H, Bischoff A, Hartmann G 1979 Cytoplasmic body neuromyopathy presenting as respiratory failure and weight loss. Journal of the Neurological Sciences 41: 1

Karpati G, Carpenter S, Eisen A A 1972 Experimental core-like lesions and nemaline rods: a correlative morphological and physiological study. Archives of Neurology 27: 237

Karpati G, Carpenter S, Melmed C, Eisen A A 1974 Experimental ischemic myopathy. Journal of the Neurological Sciences 23: 129

Macdonald R D, Engel A G 1970 Experimental chloroquine myopathy. Journal of Neuropathology and Experimental Neurology 29: 479

Massa R, Carpenter S, Holland P, Karpati G 1992 Loss and renewal of thick myofilaments in glucocorticoid treated rat soleus after denervation and reinnervation. Muscle and Nerve 15: 1290

Robitaille Y, Carpenter S, Karpati G, DiMauro S 1980 A distinct form of adult polyglucosan body disease with massive involvement of central and peripheral neuronal processes and astrocytes: a report of four cases and a review of the occurrence of polyglucosan bodies in other conditions such as Lafora's disease and normal ageing. Brain 103: 315

Rouleau G, Karpati G, Carpenter S, Soza M, Prescott S, Holland P 1987 Glucocorticoid excess induces preferential depletion of myosin in denervated skeletal muscle fibres. Muscle and Nerve 10: 428

Schmalbruch H 1984 Regenerated muscle fibers in Duchenne muscular dystrophy: a serial section study. Neurology 34: 60

Schmalbruch H, Kamieniecka Z, Arrøe M 1987 Early fatal nemaline myopathy: case report and review. Developmental Medicine and Child Neurology 29: 784

Tomé F M S, Fardeau M 1980 Nuclear inclusions in oculopharyngeal dystrophy. Acta Neuropathologica (Berlin) 49: 85

8. Histochemical and immunocytochemical studies in neuromuscular diseases

Caroline A. Sewry   V. Dubowitz

INTRODUCTION

Histochemistry is the combination of morphology and biochemistry. It provides precise localisation of specific chemical moieties and aids the characterisation of a cell. The past few decades have seen an increase in the application of histochemical techniques to many biological problems and they now have an essential diagnostic and research role in the study of neuromuscular disorders.

The main contributions of histochemistry in the study of muscle are: (1) the recognition of fibre types and their response to disease, and to neural, hormonal and other influences; (2) the demonstration of structural defects in muscle fibres; (3) the detection of enzyme deficiencies and the storage of metabolic compounds. Histochemistry has exposed many abnormalities not detected by routine histological stains and with the advances in molecular biology, immunocytochemistry is now proving to be of equal importance in the assessment of some disorders.

Recent advances have identified the gene locations of a wide variety of neuromuscular disorders (see the Journal *Neuromuscular Disorders* 1994) and the characterisation of specific genes and their products is developing rapidly. This has paved the way for improved diagnosis and genetic counselling. The most notable advances have been in the field of Duchenne and Becker muscular dystrophy and the advent of antibodies to the gene product, dystrophin, has provided a valuable diagnostic tool and emphasised the importance of immunocytochemical techniques. The full potential of other affinity cytochemical techniques, such as lectin binding, receptor binding and in situ hybridization have yet to be fulfilled.

This review aims to cover the application of the

most relevant histochemical and immunocyto-chemical techniques to the study of normal and diseased human muscle, and to illustrate their diagnostic value.

Histochemistry and immunocytochemistry have had a wide application to both human and animal muscle. As it is not possible to cover all aspects, this review is confined to the histochemical and immunocytochemical aspects of human muscle. The application of these techniques is discussed with regard to normal and diseased muscle.

METHODS

Choice of biopsy material

In humans, as in animals, there may be differences between muscles, particularly with regard to fibre-type proportions (Johnson et al 1973). It is thus desirable to confine studies to the same anatomical groups of muscle so as to become familiar with the normal pattern of that group.

Selection of the muscle for biopsy should be based on clinical assessment of muscle weakness. It is important not to select a muscle that is so severely involved that the tissue has degenerated so much that no trace of the underlying disease remains; nor, on the other hand, to choose a muscle which is pathologically unaffected. In general, the rectus femoris or vastus lateralis muscles are easily accessible and suitable for the study of most proximal muscle syndromes. Even within the quadriceps, however, selective involvement of the vasti and relative sparing of the rectus femoris can occur in some diseases (Heckmatt & Dubowitz 1985). In some circumstances the gastrocnemius, deltoid or biceps may also be suitable for biopsy. Ultrasound has proved useful in routine screening to assess the differential involvement of individual muscles and can help to decide which muscle to biopsy.

The choice of biopsy site must also take into account previous invasive techniques, such as electromyography or any form of injection. Trauma of this kind can produce pathological changes in muscle (Engel 1967).

Biopsy techniques

All muscle biopsies from both adult and paediatric

patients can be performed under local anaes-thesia. Premedication of children is often desirable. There is no advantage in the use of general anaesthesia and it may at times be hazardous in patients with neuromuscular disease because of poor respiratory function. To avoid artefacts in the biopsy it is essential that the local anaesthetic infiltrates the skin and subcutaneous tissue only and does not penetrate the muscle itself.

Biopsies can be obtained by an open surgical technique or by using several commercially available needles (Edwards & Maunder 1977). The needle we favour is that developed by Bergström and it has now been used extensively in both adults and children (Edwards et al 1973, 1983, Heckmatt et al 1984). The samples obtained with such needles are approximately 3–4 mm in diameter and may contain 1000 or more fibres in transverse section. These small pieces must be properly orientated under a dissecting micro-scope before processing. Although this requires some expertise, is it readily acquired by technical staff.

The Bergström needle biopsy technique has the advantage of providing adequate samples by a rapid, simple and less traumatic procedure than open biopsy. In addition, the risk of infection is reduced as the incision is small, no stitches are required and the residual mark is only a few millimetres in length; multiple samples can be made through the same incision; and samples for biochemical studies can be taken rapidly.

Open biopsy procedures provide larger quantities of muscle which may still be needed for some biochemical techniques not yet adapted to small samples. With open biopsy it is also possible to avoid contraction artefacts in the sample by taking the muscle at resting length. This can be achieved either with clamps or by suturing the sample and tying it to a strip of wood before removal. For light microscopy this offers no special advantage as samples are usually transversely orientated and contraction does not adversely affect the appearance. For electron-microscopy, contraction may cause distortion and samples stretched before fixation best reveal sarcomeric regularity. Needle biopsies, however, can provide adequate samples for electron microscopy even if the results may not be quite as pleasing as those derived from open biopsies (Sewry 1985).

Specimen preparation

All muscle biopsies must be frozen rapidly. If this is done correctly, very little ice crystal damage or other artefact is detectable at the light-microscopical level. All histological and histochemical studies can be carried out on cryostat sections and for some enzyme techniques this is essential. Ideally, samples should be frozen as soon as possible after removal but delays of up to 30 minutes have no deleterious effect on the pathological interpretation of biopsies. Some enzymes, e.g. the myosin ATPases, will withstand considerable delays in freezing. It is therefore still possible to do meaningful histochemical studies on some post-mortem samples or those that may have to travel from another hospital.

Immunocytochemical studies at both light- and electron-microscopic levels can also be performed on cryostat sections from the same blocks of tissue (Fitzsimons & Sewry 1985, Sewry et al 1985). It is often an advantage to prepare serial sections for both histochemical and immunocytochemical investigations for detailed comparisons. As with histochemical techniques, the localisation of many muscle antigens does not require fixation and in some instances it may have a deleterious effect on antigenicity; some antigens, in contrast, benefit from mild fixation. Most immunocytochemical methods applied to muscle use an indirect technique and utilise a secondary antibody directed against the primary antibody of interest. Amplification of antibody labelling can be obtained using the biotin–avidin technique (Hsu et al 1981). This method, particularly with streptococcal avidin, has the additional benefit of overcoming some problems of non-specific binding to the sarcolemma, connective tissue and necrotic fibres (Fitzsimons & Sewry 1985, Sewry et al 1985). The antibody is visualised by the use of conjugates of enzymes, such as peroxidase or alkaline phosphatase, or fluorochromes, such as fluorescein isothiocyanate (FITC) or Texas Red, or metals, such as gold.

Ultrastructural localisation of muscle antigens is usually achieved using electron-dense markers such as ferritin, colloidal gold or enzymes which produce electron-dense end products (Polak & Varndell 1984).

Histochemical techniques

Histochemical techniques are not performed in isolation and reference is always made to histological preparations. In particular, haematoxylin and eosin, Verhoeff–van Gieson and the modified Gomori trichrome stains (Engel & Cunningham 1963) clearly demonstrate the size and shape of the fibres, the position of nuclei, the presence of interstitial cells, blood vessels, nerves, connective tissue and adipose tissue. In addition, abnormal structures such as rods in nemaline myopathy and abnormal mitochondria can be demonstrated with the trichrome technique (Dubowitz 1985). Other stains are useful in particular circumstances such as periodic acid-Schiff for glycogen, Sudan black B or oil red O for lipids, techniques for nucleic acids (DNA and RNA), cresyl fast violet or toluidine blue for metachromatic material and alizarin red for calcium.

Enzyme histochemistry adds an extra dimension to the study of muscle. In the early days many enzymes were examined in muscle biopsies (Dubowitz & Pearse 1961) but now assessment of diseased muscle is easily made using a few selected procedures. Additional methods are of research interest and necessary only in specific circumstances. Details of techniques can be found in manuals by Lojda et al (1979), Bancroft & Stevens (1982), Pearse (1980, 1985) and Filipe & Lake (1990). The following sections will cover studies of the most important enzyme groups and chemical radicals in muscle and will illustrate their pathological value.

Immunocytochemical techniques

Several immunocytochemical studies of human muscle have now been reported and these have provided alternative methods for localising specific enzymes and have expanded our understanding of the precise nature of intracellular and extracellular muscle components. Some of the cellular components and the antibodies localised in human muscle are summarised in Table 8.1.

A variety of lectins have also been studied in human muscle and as similar techniques to those of immunocytochemistry are used to localise them, they are often considered with antibody localisation studies. Lectins are glycoproteins isolated from plants and animals that bind to specific glycoside groups. They have an important role in the characterisation of muscle membranes.

With a variety of techniques, therefore, many properties of normal muscle have been established and deviations from the normal pattern can be used as markers for disease and an aid to the diagnosis of neuromuscular disorders.

Table 8.1   Immunocytochemical studies of human muscle

Antigen	Localisation in normal and/or diseased muscle*
Collagen types I, II, III, IV	Extracellular matrix
Laminin	Extracellular matrix
Fibronectin	Extracellular matrix
HLA class I	Blood vessels, sarcolemma
HLA class II	Blood vessels
β_2 microglobulin	Sarcolemma, blood vessels
Immunoglobulin and complement	Sarcolemma, blood vessels
Neural cell adhesion molecules	Neuromuscular junction, sarcolemma
Dystrophin	Subsarcolemmal
Dystrophin-associated glycoprotein complex	Sarcolemma
Dystrophin-related protein (utrophin)	Sarcolemma, blood vessels, nerves
β-spectrin	Subsarcolemmal cytoskeleton
Desmin (skeletin)	Cytoskeleton
Vimentin	Cytosketeton, blood vessels
Vinculin	Cytoskeleton
α-actinin	Cytoskeleton, Z lines, rods
Fast, slow, fetal myosins	Myofibrils of specific fibre types
Titin (connectin)	Myofilaments
Nebulin	Myofilaments
Ubiquitin	Neuromuscular junction, filamentous inclusions
Protein kinase C	Sarcolemma, nerves
Mitochondrial enzymes	Mitochondria
Carbonic anhydrase III	Specific fibre types
Myoglobin	Specific fibre types
Cathepsins	Interstitial cells, some fibres
B- and T-cell subsets	Interstitial cells
Heat shock protein	Capillaries, inflammatory cells, sarcolemma, cytoplasm

* See text for details.

MUSCLE ENZYMES COMMONLY STUDIED HISTOCHEMICALLY

Oxidoreductases

The oxidoreductases include a large number of enzymes that catalyse the oxidation of various substrates and provide energy for cell metabolism.

They are divided into oxidases, which oxidise by catalysing the reaction between the substrate and oxygen, and the dehydrogenases that oxidise by the transfer of hydrogen from the substrate along a hydrogen acceptor pathway. Histochemical localisation of these enzymes provides information on muscle fibre types, mitochondrial function and distribution, and disturbances in fibre architecture.

Cytochrome c oxidase (EC 1.9.3.1) is a haem–copper enzyme and is part of the succinic oxidase system. It is composed of 13 subunits (Kadenbach et al 1983, Takamiya et al 1987), some of which are nuclear-encoded whilst others are mitochondrially coded, and it is entirely mitochondrial in its localisation. Muscle is rich in cytochrome oxidase and it demonstrates a distinction between the darker type I fibres and the less intensely stained type II fibres, because of their varying mitochondrial content. In disease situations cytochrome oxidase is associated with the abnormal mitochondria in 'ragged red' fibres, seen with Gomori's trichrome, and with the tubular aggregates that characterise periodic paralysis. The latter led to the suggestion that tubular aggregates originate from mitochondria (Lewis et al 1971) rather than the sarcoplasmic reticulum (Engel et al 1970a). Fibres deficient, or partially deficient, in cytochrome oxidase can be detected in several mitochondrial myopathies and encephalomyopathies (Capaldi 1988, Holt et al 1989, Oldfors et al 1992). Evidence that cytochrome oxidase activity may be reduced secondarily in various neuromuscular conditions has been reported by Ohtaki (1990), who also suggested that denervation may result in a reduction in activity.

Peroxidases (EC 1.11.1) are haem–copper oxidases that require peroxide as catalyst. Endogenous peroxidases are present in small amounts in muscle and are found in leucocytes, some erythrocytes and occasionally in some abnormal fibres (Dunn et al 1982). This is of relevance to immunocytochemical studies when peroxidase-labelled antisera are applied and it may then be necessary to remove endogenous peroxidase before proceeding with immuno-labelling.

Dehydrogenases. The dehydrogenases oxidise specific substrates anaerobically and the hydrogen removed is usually accepted by the coenzyme nicotinamide adenine dinucleotide (NAD) or nicotinamide adenine dinucleotide phosphate (NADH). Some dehydrogenases, such as succinate and glycerol-3-phosphate (SDH, EC 1.3.99.1; GPDH, EC 1.1.99.5), do not require a coenzyme and can act as hydrogen acceptors themselves. Oxidation of reduced coenzymes (NADH and NADPH) can be catalysed by flavin enzymes, which can transfer hydrogen to various acceptors, including tetrazolium salts. The flavin enzymes are then known as tetrazolium reductases (TR) (NADH-tetrazolium and NADPH-tetrazolium reductases). Tetrazolium salts are used to demonstrate dehydrogenases histochemically. These are soluble, almost colourless, salts which yield a coloured insoluble formazan on reduction. The most commonly studied enzymes are NADH-TR and SDH.

Dehydrogenases, in common with oxidases, clearly distinguish between the different fibre types. In normal muscle the NADH-TR and NADPH-TR reactions stain type I fibres more intensely than type II fibres (Fig. 8.1). The fibres showing the least reaction are IIB fibres and those with intermediate activity are IIA fibres. The myofibrils are unstained but the intermyofibrillar network comprising the mitochondria and sarcoplasmic reticulum is well demonstrated. Succinate dehydrogenase (EC 1.3.9.9.1) is entirely mitochondrial and gives similar differentiation of fibre types. In longitudinal section a striated appearance is seen with a series of paired dots located at the A–I junction. Lactate dehydrogenase differentiates fibre types less well with a more uniform intermyofibrillar network, possibly because of the sarcoplasmic LDH. Type I fibres, however, are still more intensely stained than type II. Coenzyme-linked GPDH also gives a strong reaction in type I fibres but the coenzyme-independent menadione-linked GPDH is seen

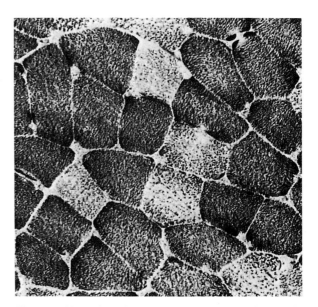

Fig. 8.1 Normal quadriceps muscle showing checkerboard pattern of dark (type I) and light (type II) fibres (NADH-TR × 330).

predominately in type II fibres. In addition to the differentiation of fibre types, oxidative enzymes often show increased concentration of stain at the periphery of fibres and in areas adjacent to nuclei. If central nuclei are present, areas of increased stain may be seen within the fibre; these probably represent focal aggregates of mitochondria.

In diseased muscle, oxidative enzymes not only reveal alterations in fibre-type proportions and distribution but they also reveal structural changes in the fibre architecture. Many of these are not apparent with routine histological stains. Some changes reflect a specific pathological change and characterise a disorder, whereas others are non-specific and are common pathological features.

Oxidative enzyme staining is the best method to demonstrate the presence of cores. *Cores* are unstained regions of the fibre (Fig. 8.2). The presence of large central cores in most fibres is pathognomonic of central core disease (see p. 299) but sporadic cores also occur in other disorders and these fibres are difficult to distinguish from target fibres associated with denervation (see below).

Minicores are also easily recognised with oxidative enzymes and are small, focal areas of disruption (Fig. 8.3). The myofibrillar material is

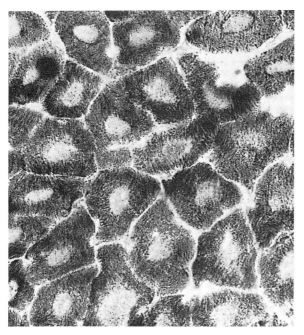

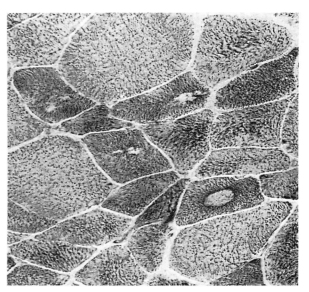

Fig. 8.4   Target fibres with an unreactive core and surrounded by a darker-staining rim or intermediate zone (NADH-TR × 380).

Fig. 8.2   Biopsy from quadriceps of a 29-year-old woman showing central cores in most fibres and uniformity of enzyme pattern (type I) (NADH-TR × 330).

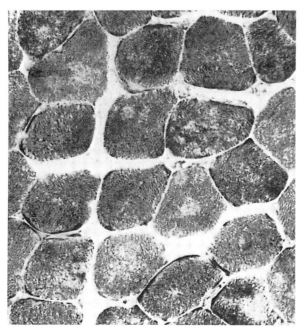

Fig. 8.3   Deltoid muscle from a 10-year-old child showing minicores (multicores) in many fibres (NADH-TR × 330).

disrupted in these regions and shows up as a weaker staining area with the ATPase reactions.

Target fibres resemble central core fibres but are characterised by three distinct zones (Fig. 8.4). The central zone is devoid of enzyme activity and is circumscribed by an intermediate zone with increased oxidative enzyme activity; peripheral to this is a relatively normal zone. Most target fibres are of type I and they are usually associated with denervating disorders.

Common changes, occurring particularly in type I fibres, are disruption and disorientation of the intermyofibrillar network. This may result in patchy staining giving rise to a 'moth-eaten' appearance (Fig. 8.5) or bizarre patterning of the myofibrils in whorled fibres (Fig. 8.6). Oxidative enzyme stains also reveal alterations in the distribution of mitochondria. This is particularly striking in *lobulated fibres*, which have small subsarcolemmal aggregates of stain that project into the fibre (Fig. 8.7). They occur in a variety of disorders but we have not observed them in our extensive studies of paediatric cases (Guerard et al 1985). Suspected structural changes in mitochondria are seen with oxidative enzyme staining as

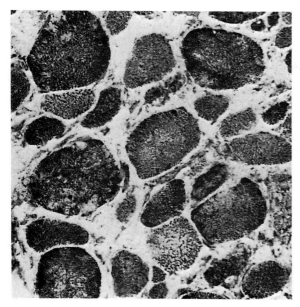

Fig. 8.5 Disruption of intermyofibrillar network in moth-eaten fibres in a 9-year-old boy with congenital muscular dystrophy (NADH-TR × 330).

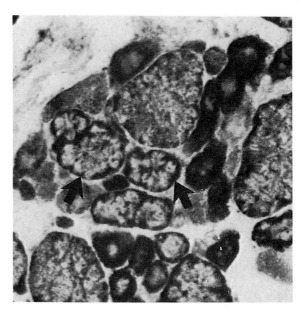

Fig. 8.7 Lobulated fibres (arrows) with marked aggregation of stain at the periphery of the fibre (NADH-TR × 270).

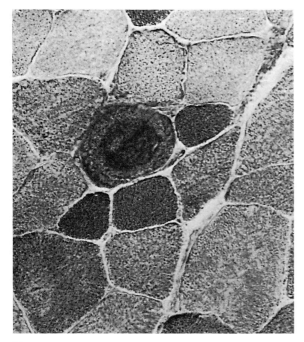

Fig. 8.6 Disorganised pattern in a whorled fibre from a 13-year-old girl with limb girdle dystrophy (NADH-TR × 330).

excessively intense regions (Fig. 8.8). They are often granular in appearance and the formazan colour may differ slightly from normal. These regions correspond to the 'ragged red' areas seen with the Gomori trichrome stain. Electron-microscopy is needed to confirm the presence of the structural defect.

Transferases

Phosphorylase (EC 2.4.1.1) This cytoplasmic enzyme has an essential role in the utilisation and synthesis of glycogen in muscle. It catalyses a reversible reaction that transfers glucosyl residues from combination with phosphate to a long-chain polysaccharide. A large proportion of phosphorylase in muscle is present in an inactive form, phosphorylase *b*, and the histochemical demonstration of phosphorylase is dependent on the conversion of this to the active form, phosphorylase *a* (Takeuchi 1956). Enzyme activity is assessed by the resulting glycogen production which is visualised with iodine or the periodic acid-Schiff reaction.

Histochemical staining for phosphorylase shows a variation in activity of individual fibres. There is a

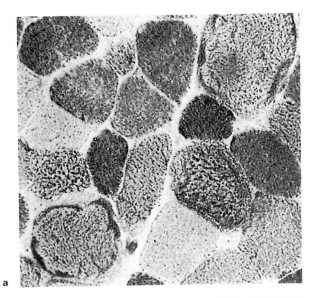

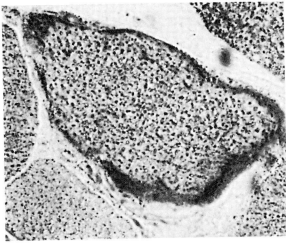

Fig. 8.8 Biopsy from biceps muscle of an 11-year-old boy with 'ophthalmoplegia plus' syndrome showing: **a** increased oxidative enzyme activity in individual fibres with abnormal mitochondria (NADH-TR × 330); **b** higher power showing increased activity at the periphery of the fibre (NADH-TR × 830).

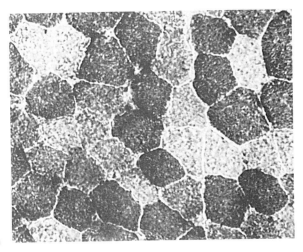

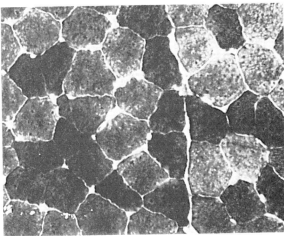

Fig. 8.9 Normal muscle showing **a** reciprocal activity between oxidative enzyme activity and **b** phosphorylase activity in individual fibres. Quadriceps (a, NADH-TR × 330; phosphorylase × 330).

reciprocal relationship between phosphorylase and oxidative enzymes in human muscle (Fig. 8.9). The main application of the phosphorylase technique is in the study of glycogen storage diseases, in particular type V (McArdle's disease): this is characterised by a total absence of phosphorylase from all fibres.

Deficiencies of 1-phosphofructokinase (EC 2.7.1.56) (Bonilla & Schotland 1970) and the hydrolase myoadenylate deaminase (AMP deaminase, EC 3.5.4.6) (Fishbein et al 1978) can also be revealed histochemically and are useful techniques for the differential diagnosis of the glycogenoses.

Hydrolases

Phosphatases catalyse the hydrolysis of organic esters. They are classified into alkaline or acid phosphatases according to their optimal pH. Most phosphatases catalyse the hydrolysis of a wide range of substrates but some, such as glucose-6-phosphatase (EC 3.1.3.9) and 5'-nucleotidase (EC 3.1.3.5), are substrate-specific. Phosphatases are usually demonstrated either by metal chelation of the released phosphate or by coupling the alcoholic residue to an azo dye. A method using metachromatic dyes has also been reported (Doriguzzi et al 1983).

Alkaline phosphatase (EC 3.1.3.1) has an optimum pH of 9–10 and is found primarily in cell membranes where active transport occurs, such as endothelium of arteries, endoplasmic reticulum and Golgi apparatus. Normal human muscle fibres appear negative when stained for alkaline phosphatase but arterioles 15–35 μm in diameter are clearly depicted. Large blood vessels and capillaries in human muscle do not stain, unlike those in animal muscle (Engel & Cunningham 1970). In diseased human muscle alkaline phosphatase identifies certain abnormal fibres (Engel & Cunningham 1970). These fibres are usually small, often contain internal nuclei and most, but not all, have basophilia. Necrotic fibres, however, are negative. Fibres positive for alkaline phosphatase are common in X-linked dystrophies and active myositic conditions. They are also seen in carriers of Duchenne dystrophy and in neurogenic disorders. Occasional positive fibres occur in other conditions. In dermatomyositis, polymyositis and some acute inflammatory situations there is prominent staining of the endomysial and perimysial connective tissue (Engel 1977). This is thought to be a diagnostic feature of these inflammatory disorders, as it is rarely seen in the dystrophies.

Acid phosphatase (EC 3.1.3.2) has an optimum pH of 4–5; its main localisation is believed to be in lysosomes. Very little acid phosphatase activity is seen in normal muscle and morphologically identifiable lysosomes are rarely observed ultrastructurally. Using azo dye coupling techniques, acid phosphatase activity is seen in muscle spindles and interstitial cells and in small discrete subsarcolemmal areas. This activity is often adjacent to nuclei and is probably associated with lipofuscin (Cullen et al 1979). In vitamin E deficiency lipoprotein accumulates and is identified in punctate areas with the acid phosphatase technique. The lipoprotein is also autofluorescent. The curvilinear bodies typical of Batten's disease, and inducible by chloroquine (Neville et al 1979), are also seen with this enzyme technique, and are autofluorescent. The colour of the autofluorescence, however, is orange-yellow in the case of lipopigment and yellow in Batten's disease. In diseased muscle, acid phosphatase activity is increased. Basophilic fibres show high diffuse activity (Neerunjun & Dubowitz 1977) and such activity is prominent in necrotic areas, both in the fibres and in the associated cellular infiltrate. In type II glycogenosis, acid phosphatase staining is also intense.

Adenosine triphosphatase (ATPase) (EC 3.6.1.3) There are several ATPases in animal tissues that differ in their localisation and biochemical properties in relation to activators and inhibitors. One of the most important histochemically is calcium-activated myosin-ATPase. This enzyme is responsible for the hydrolysis of ATP which results in the release of energy required for muscle contraction. Histochemical demonstration of myosin ATPase is usually by the metal chelation method at pH 9.4 as applied by Padykula & Hermann (1955). The end result of this reaction is the deposition of cobalt sulphide which is localised to the A band. It gives a clear differentiation into muscle fibre types and distinguishes the lightly stained type I fibres from the heavily stained type II fibres (Fig. 8.10). The ATPase technique forms the basis for the identification of fibre types in diagnostic pathology. In addition to the two main fibre types, Brooke & Kaiser (1970) defined three fibre types in human muscle by utilising a pre-incubation at varying pH (9.4, 4.6 and 4.3). With acid pre-incubation at 4.3 the pattern seen at 9.4 is reversed and type I fibres are heavily stained in contrast to the pale type II fibres. Pre-incubation at pH 4.6 demonstrates three populations of fibres, with the type I fibres being heavily stained and the type II fibres subdivided into pale type IIA fibres and darkly stained IIB fibres (Fig. 8.10); in addition, a few fibres, type IIC fibres, stain darkly at pH 9.4 and show some residual staining at pH 4.3 (Fig. 8.11).

In normal muscle, the myosin ATPase reaction reveals a checkerboard pattern of fibre types. The three fibre types I, IIA and IIB, are randomly distributed, present in more or less equal propor-

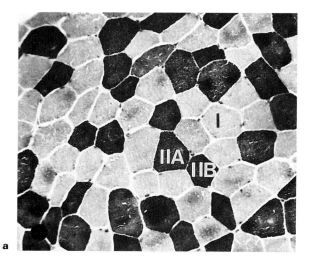

a

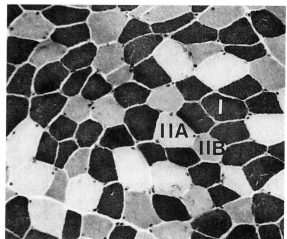

b

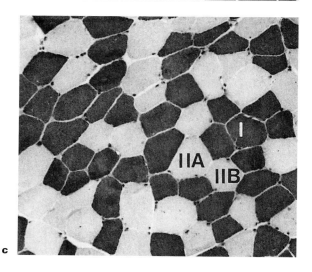

c

Fig. 8.10 Serial sections from quadriceps muscle showing the three main fibre types (I, IIA, IIB) stained for: **a** myosin ATPase, pH 9.4; **b** ATPase after pre-incubation at pH 4.6; **c** ATPase after pre-incubation at pH 4.3 (counterstained with haematoxylin and eosin, × 335).

HISTOCHEMICAL REACTIONS IN HUMAN MUSCLE

MUSCLE FIBRE TYPE	I	IIA	IIB	IIC
Routine ATP-ase	1+	3+	3+	3+
ATP-ase pre-incubated pH 4.6	3+	0	2+	3+
ATP-ase pre-incubated pH 4.3	3+	0	0	2+
NADH-TR	3+	2+	1+	2+
SDH	3+	2+	1+	2+
α glycerophosphate - menadione linked	0	2+	2+	1+
PAS	1+ & 2+	3+	2+	2+
Phosphorylase	1+ & 0	3+	3+	3+

$\bigcirc$ = 0 $\oslash$ = 1+ $\otimes$ = 2+ $\bullet$ = 3+

Fig. 8.11 Histochemical reactions of the different fibre types in human muscle (from Dubowitz & Brooke 1973).

tions, and show a similar small variation in size. The normal pattern can be influenced by exercise, nerve stimulation, hormones and disease (see Dubowitz 1985). In diseased muscle the changes include selective alteration in size of one fibre type, alterations in the distribution of fibre types (fibre-type grouping) and predominance of one fibre type.

Selective atrophy of type II fibres (Fig. 8.12) is one of the commonest abnormalities associated with muscle pathology. The commonest form of type II atrophy selectively involves type IIB fibres. Although atrophy of type IIA and IIB fibres may occur concomitantly, it is unusual to see selective atrophy of type IIA fibres. Type II atrophy occurs in a wide variety of disorders and in situations where muscle strength is secondarily impaired or when the muscle is not used. It is also a common feature associated with steroid therapy. Although disuse resulting from bedrest is commonly thought to induce type II atrophy, other forms of disuse such as immobilisation following fractures involve type I fibres (Sargeant et al 1977). Selective involvement of type I fibres is less common but may occur in myotonic dystrophy

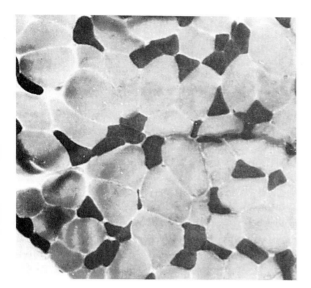

Fig. 8.12 Quadriceps muscle biopsy showing marked type II fibre atrophy (ATPase pH 9.4 × 160).

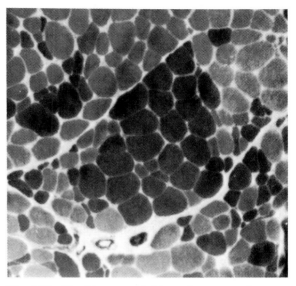

Fig. 8.13 Quadriceps muscle biopsy from a case of peripheral neuropathy showing fibre-type grouping in association with small group atrophy of both fibre types (ATPase pH 9.4 × 230).

(Engel & Brooke 1966) and in some congenital myopathies, such as centronuclear myopathy and nemaline myopathy (see below).

Alterations in the distribution of fibre types are most clearly seen in denervating disorders such as peripheral neuropathies and spinal muscular atrophy. In these situations it is common to find large groups of fibres of one type, in association with groups of atrophic fibres of mixed types (Fig. 8.13). This fibre-type grouping is associated with collateral sprouting of terminal axons (Morris & Raybould 1971) and reinnervation.

Predominance of either fibre type may occur but it is essential that normal limits for the muscle in question are clearly defined. Predominance of type I in the rectus femoris is defined as meaning that more than 55% of the fibres are type I (Dubowitz & Brooke 1973). Type II predominance occurs when more than 80% of the fibres are of type II. Type I predominance tends to be associated with myopathic conditions, particularly the genetically determined dystrophies (Fig. 8.14). It is also commonly associated with hormonal imbalance as in hypothyroidism. Type II predominance is associated with motor neurone diseases.

Esterases. Carboxylic ester hydrolases (EC 3.1.1) hydrolyse carboxylic acids and are classified into three closely related groups —

lipases, non-specific esterases and specific esterases. Of particular interest to muscle are the non-specific esterases and the specific cholinesterase, acetylcholinesterase (EC 3.1.1.7). Normal

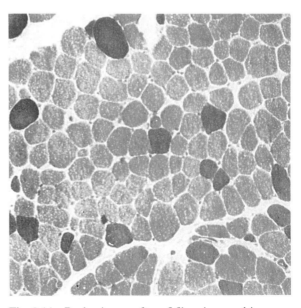

Fig. 8.14 Predominance of type I fibres in a quadriceps biopsy from a boy with Duchenne muscular dystrophy (ATPase pH 9.4 × 170).

muscle fibres show no non-specific esterase staining but the small basophilic fibres, seen in some dystrophies and often referred to as regenerating fibres, show a high activity (Engel 1979). The high activity of this and other hydrolytic enzymes in regenerating fibres has led to the term regenerate–degenerate (regen–degen) fibres (Engel 1979).

Acetylcholinesterase in normal fibres is restricted to the motor end-plate. Denervated fibres, basophilic fibres and cultured myotubes, however, show extrajunctional acetylcholine receptors (Engel 1979).

Proteases (peptide hydrolases, EC 3.4) are a group of hydrolytic enzymes classified into endopeptidases and exopeptidases according to the position of the peptide bond they attack (McDonald 1985). Interest in proteases from both classes arose because of their involvement in the metabolic turnover of myofibrillar proteins (Bird et al 1978, Kar & Pearson 1978, 1979). In diseased muscle, myofibrillar degradation is increased and is thought to result from increased activities of proteases (Kar & Pearson 1978, Warnes et al 1981). Many of the studies of muscle proteases have been biochemical estimates from homogenates. Investigations using fluorescent histochemical methods (Stauber et al 1985), semipermeable techniques (White et al 1985) or immunocytochemical methods (Whitaker et al 1983), however, have localised several proteolytic enzymes in diseased human muscle. Cathepsins have been demonstrated in muscle fibres in many neuromuscular disorders (Whitaker et al 1983, Stauber et al 1985) and cathepsin D (EC 3.4.23.5) is particularly prominent in basophilic fibres. It is not associated with necrotic fibres and the authors therefore suggested that it may have a role in repair processes (Whitaker et al 1983). Aminopeptidases (L-amino acyl peptide hydrolases, EC. 3.4.11) and dipeptidyl peptide hydrolases (EC 3.4.14) show low activity in muscle fibres from normal and diseased muscle, but higher activity in the interstitial tissue, particularly in relation to mast cells and macrophages (White et al 1985).

Lyases

Adenylate cyclase (AC, EC 4.6.1.1) regulates the synthesis of cyclic adenosine monophosphate (cAMP) from Mg-adenosine triphosphate (MgATP). Its precise localisation in muscle is still uncertain but biochemical studies of sarcolemma derived from dystrophic patients and of cultured myotubes have shown differences in AC activity and its response to inhibitors (Willner et al 1982). Few histochemical studies of AC have been reported but a technique using an artificial substrate was thought to demonstrate it specifically (Dubrovsky & Engel 1976, Engel 1977). In normal human muscle AC was localised to blood vessels and to the sarcolemma and intermyofibrillar network. Diseased muscle showed high AC activity in basophilic (regenerating) fibres. In Duchenne dystrophy not only were basophilic fibres strongly stained but so too were fibres that otherwise seemed normal. Denervating disorders showed slight to moderate staining in atrophic fibres.

GLYCOGEN

Glycogen is stored to a varying degree in all muscle fibres. Historically, the periodic acid–Schiff (PAS) stain has been used to demonstrate glycogen but the specificity of the reaction for glycogen has to be checked with α-amylase digestion. In normal human muscle the PAS reaction stains type II fibres more intensely than type I (Fig. 8.11). Intermediate fibres are also demonstrated and correspond to IIB fibres. Excessive quantities of glycogen are a characteristic feature of glycogenoses. In some dystrophies, fibres with no detectable PAS staining are often seen.

In addition to demonstrating glycogen, the PAS stain is also useful for recognising ring fibres (Fig. 8.15). These abnormal fibres have a peripheral band of myofibrils at right angles to the central myofibrils. This gives the appearance of a striated annulet around the fibre. Although they are non-specific such fibres often occur in myotonic and limb-girdle dystrophy.

The PAS stain demonstrates not only glycogen but also other polysaccharides, mucopolysaccharides and glycoproteins. After α-amylase digestion, PAS is a simple method for revealing the sarcolemma and the position of capillaries.

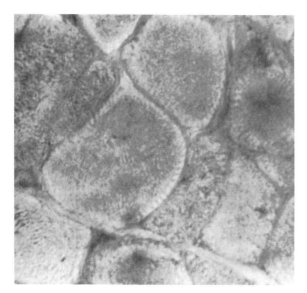

Fig. 8.15 Ring fibres in a quadriceps biopsy from a child with myotonic dystrophy (PAS × 740).

Capillaries can be counted easily using this method (Hermansen & Wachtlova 1971) and numbers can be related to fibre type by comparison with serial ATPase sections (Andersen 1975).

LIPID

Neutral lipids in normal muscle fibres appear as small droplets distributed throughout the fibre. Their concentration and size is related to fibre type. Excessive lipid accumulation in muscle fibres occurs in some disorders of lipid metabolism. In other disorders, e.g. polymyositis, fibres with excess lipid occur occasionally. The proliferation of adipose tissue that occurs in muscular dystrophies and to some extent in other conditions is shown clearly by lipid stains.

NUCLEIC ACIDS

The demonstration of nuclei acids is sometimes of value, particularly with respect to RNA. The methyl green pyronine reaction and the fluorescent acridine orange technique differentiate DNA from RNA. Accumulations of RNA are seen in basophilic fibres in diseased muscle suggesting that these are regenerating fibres.

QUANTITATION

It is notoriously difficult to judge the size of fibres in a muscle biopsy by simple inspection. A more objective assessment is often necessary for the interpretation of pathological changes and to this end various measurements of fibres have been applied: these include orthogonal diameters, fibre circumference, fibre area and lesser diameter, and fibre-type proportions. Measurement of the lesser fibre diameter has had wide acceptance as a simple, reproducible measurement of fibre size (Dubowitz & Brooke 1973, Dubowitz 1985). Sections stained for myosin ATPase are usually studied and the data are used to construct a histogram showing the variations in each fibre type. In addition, the number of fibres outside the normal range (atrophy and hypertrophy factors) and the degree of variability can be assessed.

Although measurements of fibre diameter can be made easily using an eye-piece micrometer, a variety of computer-assisted systems is now commercially available. These have been applied to several studies of human muscle (see Dubowitz 1985) and demonstrate the importance of quantitation in the objective assessment of biopsies, particularly those with minor pathological changes.

IMMUNOCYTOCHEMISTRY

Immunocytochemistry is proving to have as dramatic an impact on the study of muscle as histochemistry did a few decades ago. A wide variety of antibodies have been applied to human muscle (see Table 8.1) and as more genes, both normal and abnormal, are characterised, the availability of informative antibodies is rapidly expanding. Immunocytochemistry has an essential diagnostic role in the study of a growing number of neuromuscular disorders and classical pathological features of muscle are now being reinterpreted.

Extracellular matrix

Immunolocalisation of collagen types has shown that in normal muscle types I and III collagen are localised to the perimysial connective tissue. The endomysium also stains strongly with antibodies to type III collagen but anti-type I staining is relatively weak (Fig. 8.16). Collagen type IV is localised to the basement membrane of muscle fibres, major blood vessels and capillaries (Duance et al 1980, Stephens et al 1982, Dunn et al 1984). In muscle from dystrophic patients, collagen antibodies reflect the increase in connective tissue seen histologically with a marked increase in perimysial and endomysial type III collagen (Fig. 8.16). The distribution of collagen

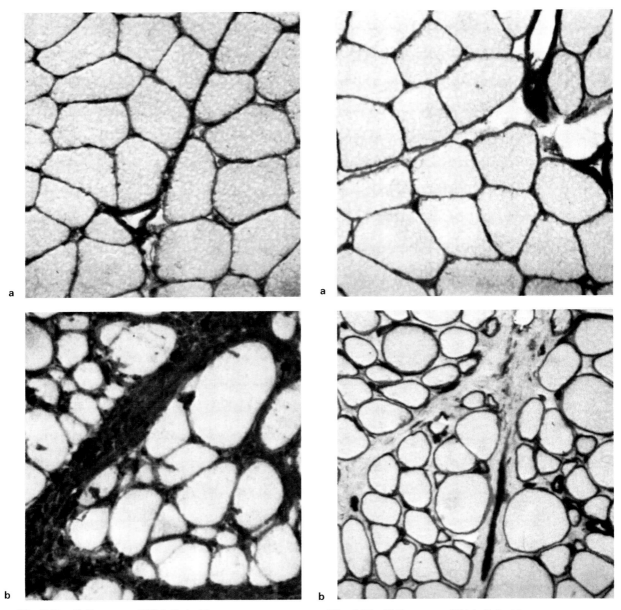

Fig. 8.16 Collagen type III labelled with an avidin–biotin–peroxidase immunotechnique in: **a** normal muscle; **b** muscle from a boy with Duchenne muscular dystrophy. There is a marked increase in staining of the perimysial and endomysial connective tissue in dystrophic muscle ($\times 230$).

Fig. 8.17 Collagen type IV labelled with an avidin–biotin–peroxidase immunotechnique in: **a** normal muscle; **b** muscle from a boy with Duchenne muscular dystrophy. Staining is confined to the basement membrane of the fibres and blood vessels ($\times 230$).

type IV appears to be unaltered but is sometimes intense around small fibres (Fig. 8.17). Fibres that are split or whorled show collagen types I, III and IV, associated with the abnormal membrane features, mentioned above (Fig. 8.18). Neurogenic disorders such as spinal muscular atrophy show an

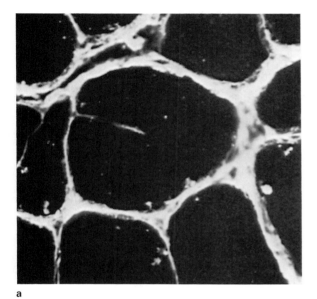

a

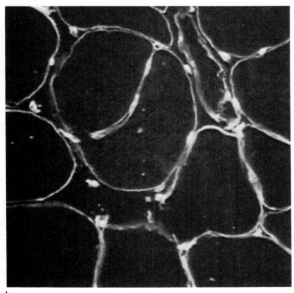

b

Fig. 8.18 Split fibres in dystrophic muscle stained by an indirect immunofluorescent technique showing **a** type III collagen and **b** type IV collagen associated with the membrane abnormality (× 360).

increase in perimysial connective tissue and a concomitant increase in type III collagen. Isoforms of various extracellular components have been identified and differences in their distribution have been found between synaptic and extrasynaptic sites in human and animal muscle (Sanes et al 1990). Isoform distributions, however, have not been extensively studied in diseased human muscle.

In normal and diseased muscle, staining with antibodies to fibronectin parallels that with collagen type III antibodies whereas antibodies to laminin show a similar distribution to that of type IV collagen (Bertolotto et al 1983, Dunn et al 1984, Sewry et al 1985).

Membrane-associated proteins

Membrane-associated proteins that have been studied immunocytochemically include HLA class I and II antigens, β_2-microglobulin, immunoglobulins and components of the complement pathway, cell adhesion molecules, and a glycoprotein complex associated with dystrophin.

HLA antigens are polymorphic surface glycoproteins involved in the immune response. HLA class I antigens are required for the recognition of antigens by cytotoxic T-cells and class II for the presentation of antigen to helper T-cells (Roitt 1988). Normal mature muscle fibres express minimal or no class I or class II antigens or β_2-microglobulin, but all are detectable on endothelial cells of blood vessels, including capillaries (Appleyard et al 1985, Isenberg et al 1986, Karpati et al 1988, Emslie-Smith et al 1989, McDouall et al 1989). HLA class I antigens and β_2-microglobulin are expressed, however, by regenerating fibres in a variety of disorders, and by a proportion of fibres in inflammatory myopathies and Xp21 dystrophies (Figs 8.19, 8.36). Class II antigens, in contrast, are not expressed by muscle fibres in any disorder studied (Appleyard et al 1985, Karpati et al 1988, Emslie-Smith et al 1989, McDouall et al 1989), although there has been a report of class II expression in some inflammatory situations (Zuk & Fletcher 1988). Myoblasts in culture also express HLA class I antigens (Karpati et al 1988, Hohlfeld & Engel 1990), but the expression of class II is dependent

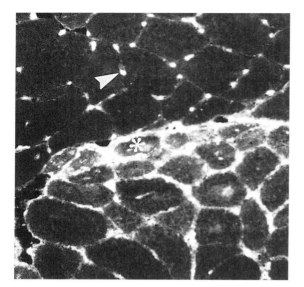

Fig. 8.19 HLA class I antigens in a case of dermatomyositis localised with a biotin–streptavidin–Texas Red technique showing labelling of perifascicular fibres in one area (*) but only of the capillaries in the adjacent area (arrow head) (× 200).

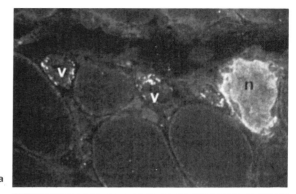

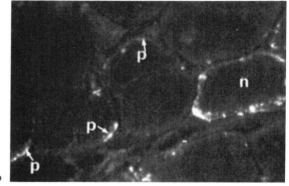

Fig. 8.20 Complement C9 in a case of polymyositis localised with an avidin–biotin–Texas Red immunofluorescent technique showing: **a** a necrotic fibre (n) with internal staining and two vacuolated fibres (v) with C9 localised to the periphery of the fibres; **b** a necrotic fibre (n) with a bright peripheral rim and non-necrotic fibres with small localised patches of C9 (p) (× 300).

on culture conditions, in particular the presence of gamma-interferon (Bao et al 1990, Hohlfeld & Engel 1990, Goebels et al 1992). This expression of HLA antigens on myoblasts has important implications for myoblast transfer therapy.

Immunoglobulin and complement deposition occur in inflammatory disorders, the muscular dystrophies and myasthenia gravis (Engel & Biesecker 1982, Isenberg 1983, Morgan et al 1984). Immunoglobins and complement have been localised to the sarcolemma, blood vessel endothelium and whole muscle fibres. Isenberg (1983) also suggested that immunoglobulin deposition can be used to distinguish myopathic from neuropathic disorders.

The formation of the membrane-attack complex (C5b-9,MAC) on a cell surface is associated with events leading to lysis. Thus antibodies to MAC and to the terminal component C9 are found in necrotic fibres in several diseases (Engel & Biesecker 1982, Cornelio & Dones 1984). Using a monoclonal antibody to C9 we have shown that MAC is also present as discrete patches on the surface of non-necrotic fibres (Morgan et al 1984) (Fig. 8.20). This suggests a more primary role for complement in muscle necrosis.

Studies of myasthenia gravis have shown immunoglobulin and complement (C3 and C9) at motor end-plates (Engel et al 1977, Sahashi et al 1980). This provides evidence for antibody-dependent complement-mediated injury at the postsynaptic membrane.

Antibodies to the *neural cell adhesion molecule* (N-CAM) and its isoforms have been used to demonstrate that N-CAM is confined to the neuromuscular junction in innervated fibres but is extrajunctional in denervated and immature fibres (Hurko & Walsh 1983, Covault & Sanes 1985, Moore & Walsh 1985, 1986, Covault & Sanes 1986, Cashman et al 1987, Figarella-Branger et al 1990, 1992a). Normal mature fibres therefore do not express N-CAM but it is detected on regenerating fibres (Fig. 8.21), non-innervated fetal

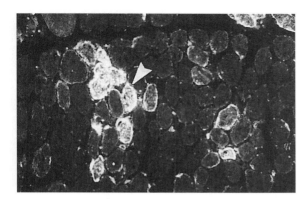

Fig. 8.21 Regenerating fibres (arrowhead) in a case of Duchenne muscular dystrophy labelled with antibodies to N-CAM (Leu 19), using a biotin–streptavidin–Texas Red technique, showing sarcolemmal and internal staining but no staining of the larger fibres ($\times$ 200).

fibres, myotubes in culture and denervated fibres in neurogenic disorders. The expression of N-CAM on myoblasts has been used to purify both human and mouse myogenic cells by fluorescence-activated cell sorting (Webster et al 1988a), panning techniques (Jones et al 1990, Watt & Sewry, unpublished results) and by magnetic beads (Murphy et al 1992). Antibodies to the differentiation determinant CD56 (Leu 19, NKH-1), have been shown to recognise N-CAM (Lanier et al 1989). These antibodies have demonstrated N-CAM on cultured myoblasts and myotubes, satellite cells, regenerating fibres and denervated fibres in a variety of neuromuscular disorders (Fig. 8.21; Illa et al 1992).

The *glycoprotein complex associated with dystrophin* consists of a cytoskeletal, four-transmembrane and an extracellular component and has been shown to interact with dystrophin and laminin (Campbell & Kahl 1989, Ervasti et al 1990, Ervasti & Campbell 1991, Ohlendieck et al 1991b, Ibraghimov-Beskrovnaya et al 1992). It has been proposed that the complex spans the sarcolemma and provides a structural link between the subsarcolemmal cytoskeleton and the extracellular matrix (Ibraghimov-Beskrovnaya et al 1992). Antibodies raised to the complex have shown that all components localise to the sarcolemma but are absent or markedly reduced in Duchenne muscular dystrophy. The expression of all components is normal in a range of neuro-

muscular disorders where dystrophin is normal, with the notable exceptions of severe childhood autosomal recessive muscular dystrophy (SCARMD) (Matsumura et al 1992) and Fukuyama-type congenital muscular dystrophy (Matsumura et al 1993). In the severe childhood autosomal dystrophy, which has clinical features in common with Duchenne dystrophy, the 50 kDa transmembrane component of the glycoprotein is absent, whilst in Fukuyama-type congenital dystrophy there is a reduction of all the dystrophin-associated proteins, particularly the 43 kDa component. As a result of these findings, it has been proposed that the loss of components of the glycoprotein complex may cause the cascade of events leading to muscle necrosis in several muscle disorders (Matsumura et al 1992).

Cytoskeleton

The cytoskeleton forms a filamentous network that links the myofibrils to each other and to the sarcolemma and nucleus. The number of proteins believed to be involved in the cytoskeleton is increasing and those that have been studied in human muscle include β-spectrin, vinculin and the intermediate filament proteins, desmin and vimentin. It has been suggested that dystrophin and a dystrophin-related protein are also cytoskeletal proteins because of their structural homology to other cytoskeletal proteins and their localisation. Alpha-actinin is also part of the same family of cytoskeletal proteins but most studies in human muscle have been on the myofibrillar form. Several cytoskeletal proteins have a periodic distribution at the sarcolemma and are prominent at areas termed costameres, overlying the Z line or I bands (Pardoe et al 1983, Thornell & Price 1991, Minetti et al 1992, Porter et al 1992, Straub et al 1992). Several cytoskeletal proteins are also localised to the neuromuscular junction (see below).

Subsarcolemmal proteins. The sarcolemma of human skeletal muscle fibres expresses a β-spectrin-like protein (Appleyard et al 1984). The periphery of fibres is clearly delineated (Fig. 8.22) and in some neuromuscular disorders there appears to be enhancement of antibody binding to some fibres. Basophilic, regenerating fibres, in

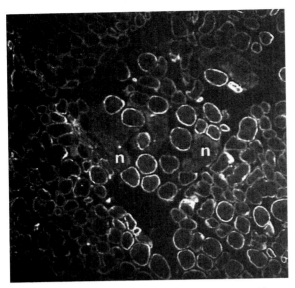

Fig. 8.22   Localisation of β-spectrin in a quadriceps biopsy from a case of Duchenne muscular dystrophy using an avidin–biotin–Texas Red immunofluorescent technique. All fibres have a brightly stained sarcolemma except the necrotic fibres (n) (× 90).

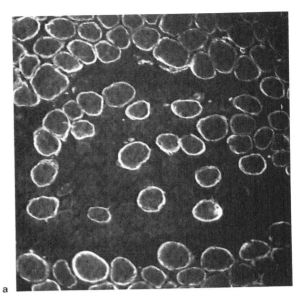

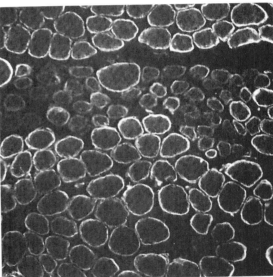

Fig. 8.23   Basophilic fibres in a quadriceps biopsy from a 2-year-old boy with Duchenne muscular dystrophy stained for β spectrin with an avidin–biotin–Texas Red immunofluorescent technique showing: **a** absence of β-spectrin labelling in one group of basophilic fibres, and **b** reduced labelling in another group of basophilic fibres in the same biopsy (× 230).

contrast, show reduced labelling with antibodies to β-spectrin (Fig. 8.23) and in Duchenne dystrophy some basophilic fibres have no detectable β-spectrin (Fig. 8.23) (Sewry et al 1986). Normal regenerating fibres gradually acquire β-spectrin (Sewry et al 1992a) and some fetal myotubes at early stages of development also have reduced expression (Clerk et al 1991b). Necrotic fibres do not label with antibodies to β-spectrin (Fig. 8.22), as they lose their plasma membrane. Similarly, focal regions where the plasma membrane is lost also appear negative. Antibodies to β-spectrin are therefore a useful way of assessing the integrity of the plasma membrane and of avoiding false-negative results with antibodies to other sarcolemmal proteins such as dystrophin.

In normal human muscle antibodies to vinculin label the sarcolemma continuously and also arteries (Minetti et al 1992). A reduction in expression has been shown in Duchenne but not Becker muscular dystrophy.

Dystrophin is a high molecular weight protein (approx. 427 kDa) encoded by a large gene on the short arm of the X chromosome (Xp21). It has been identified as the defective gene product in Duchenne and Becker muscular dystrophy (Hoffman et al 1987, Kunkel & Hoffman 1989). The gene encompasses at least 2.3 Mb of DNA and the full-length transcript of mRNA is about 14 kb (Koenig et al 1987, Hoffman et al 1987,

Kunkel & Hoffman 1989, Monaco & Kunkel 1988, Worton & Thompson 1988, Hoffman & Kunkel 1989). It is now known that several transcripts with different promotors are coded by the dystrophin gene, giving rise to isoforms in skeletal, cardiac and smooth muscle, fetal muscle and neural tissue (Chamberlain et al 1988, Dickson et al 1988, Hoffman et al 1988, Feener et al 1989, Nudel et al 1989, Bar et al 1990, Barnea et al 1990, Chelly et al 1990b, Byers et al 1991, Geng et al 1991, Blake et al 1992). Dystrophin is thought to have a cytoskeletal function because of its structural homology to members of the spectrin family (Hoffman & Kunkel 1989). It has an N-terminal region that resembles α-actinin, a central rod region with spectrin-like repeats, a cysteine-rich region with EF-hand calcium binding sites and a unique C-terminal domain. Antibodies corresponding to various regions have been raised using synthetic peptides or fusion protein constructs, and all show dystrophin uniformly localised to the sarcolemma of fibres in normal muscle and in non-Xp21 disorders (see Fig. 8.38; Arahata et al 1988, Bonilla et al 1988b, Patel et al 1988, Zubrzycka-Gaarn et al 1988). Ultra-structural studies show that dystrophin is on the cytoplasmic face of the sarcolemma (Watkins et al 1988, Cullen et al 1990) and suggest that the C-terminus may insert into the plasma membrane (Cullen et al 1991). Recent studies have shown that it has a costameric distribution at the sarcolemma, in common with spectrin and vinculin (Porter et al 1992), and α-actinin (Straub et al 1992). Immunolabelling of dystrophin is enhanced at the myotendinous junction (Samitt & Bonilla 1990) and at the neuromuscular junction (Miike et al 1989, Shimizu et al 1989). In Duchenne dystrophy dystrophin is usually absent or greatly reduced, whilst in Becker dystrophy it is abnormal in size and/or amount (Arahata et al 1988, Bonilla et al 1988b, Hoffman & Kunkel 1989). Abnormalities also occur in carriers of Duchenne dystrophy (see Fig. 8.38 and 'The muscular dystrophies' below). Initial studies with antibodies to dystrophin indicated that abnormalites were only seen in Xp21 disorders (Hoffman et al 1987, Patel et al 1988), but it is now apparent that secondary changes in dystrophin expression can occur. Abnormalities in the membrane glycopro-

tein complex associated with dystrophin result in a reduction of dystrophin in some cases of severe childhood autosomal recessive muscular dystrophy (Matsumura et al 1992), and changes in the Fukuyama-type congenital muscular dystrophy (Arikawa et al 1991) and inflammatory myopathies (Sewry et al 1991) have been reported. Nevertheless, the advances that have been made in diagnostic muscle pathology, as a result of the application of dystrophin antibodies, are substantial and they play a major role in differential diagnosis.

An autosomal protein, coded by human chromosome 6, has considerable homology to dystrophin (Love et al 1989, Khurana et al 1990, Tinsley et al 1992). This dystrophin-like protein or dystrophin-related protein is expressed in a variety of tissues, as well as muscle (Love et al 1991), and its ubiquitous distribution has led to the name utrophin (Blake et al 1992). In normal mature muscle utrophin/dystrophin-related protein is expressed in the vasculature, capillaries and peripheral nerves but is absent from fibres, except at the neuromuscular junction (see Fig. 8.37; Nguyen thi Man et al 1991, Ohlendieck et al 1991a, Pons et al 1991, Tanaka et al 1991, Augier et al 1992). In regenerating fibres in a variety of disorders, however, it is expressed on the sarcolemma and internally (Khurana et al 1991, Helliwell et al 1992b). Additional staining of other fibres also occurs in Duchenne and Becker muscular dystrophy (see Fig. 8.37; Voit et al 1991, Helliwell et al 1992b).

Intermediate filaments. Intermediate filaments are a group of immunologically related proteins approximately 10 nm in diameter that have a characteristic, tissue-specific distribution. Desmin (skeletin) (Thornell et al 1983), vimentin (Lazarides 1980), synemin (Granger & Lazarides 1980) and a neural filament-associated polypeptide (Wang et al 1980) have been identified in muscle fibres and cultured myotubes. Only desmin and vimentin, however, have been extensively studied in human muscle.

Desmin (52 kDa) occurs exclusively in muscle cells of all types and in skeletal muscle forms a three-dimensional lattice encircling and linking the myofibrils to each other at the Z lines, to maintain alignment (Lazarides & Hubbard 1976,

Thornell et al 1980, 1983, Osborn et al 1982, Cullen et al 1992). Desmin filaments are also involved in linking the myofibrils to the sarcolemma and to the nuclear membrane (Tokuyasu et al 1983, Cullen et al 1992). Desmin filaments are abundant in immature and regenerating muscle fibres (Fig. 8.24) and in rhabdomyosarcomas (Battifora 1988), but in normal mature muscle their concentration is low (Thornell et al 1980, 1983, Bornemann & Schmalbruch 1992, Sarnat 1992). Desmin persists in smooth muscle but is not detected in capillaries. In diseased muscle changes in desmin distribution accompany the myofibrillar disruption and disorientation seen in cores, mini-cores and ring fibres and with Z-line streaming (Thornell et al 1983). Abnormal structures such as rods, cytoplasmic bodies and Mallory bodies have been shown to have desmin associated with them (Jockusch et al 1980, Thornell et al 1980, Fidzianska et al 1983, Osborn & Goebel 1983). A variety of myopathies are also characterised by inclusions associated with desmin (Edström et al 1980, Pellissier et al 1989, Telerman-Toppet et al 1991, Sabatelli et al 1992), whilst other disorders show increased levels in certain fibres, including X-linked myotubular myopathy, myotonic dystrophy, congenital fibre type disproportion (Sarnat 1990, 1991), spinal

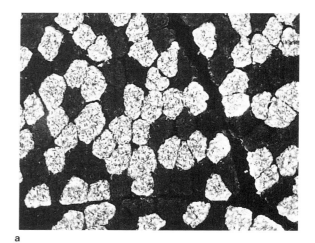

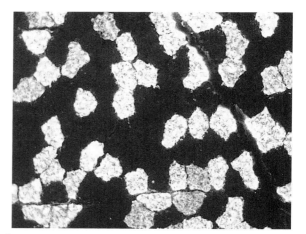

b

Fig. 8.25   Serial sections of normal quadriceps muscle immunolabelled with monoclonal antibodies to **a** slow and **b** fast myosin heavy chains showing a reciprocal pattern (× 200).

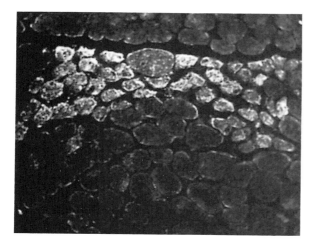

Fig. 8.24   Basophilic fibres in a 2-year-old boy with Duchenne muscular dystrophy labelled with anti-desmin monoclonal antibody using an avidin–biotin–Texas Red immunofluorescent technique (× 200).

muscular atrophy and neuropathies (Helliwell et al 1989, Sewry 1989, Sarnat 1991). In necrotic fibres the peripheral immunostaining for desmin is lost (Helliwell et al 1989).

Vimentin is also highly expressed in developing and regenerating skeletal muscle fibres but it declines to an undetectable level in mature fibres (Sarnat 1991, Bornemann & Schmalbruch 1992). It persists, however, in the endothelial cells of capillaries. Abnormalities in the distribution of vimentin parallel those of desmin (Sarnat 1990, 1991).

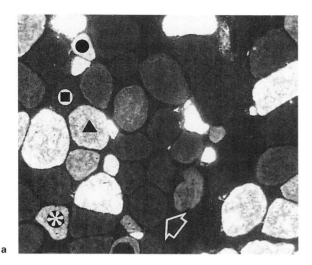

a

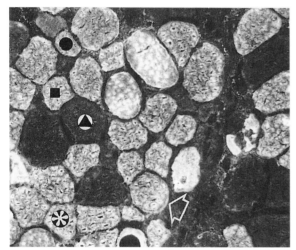

b

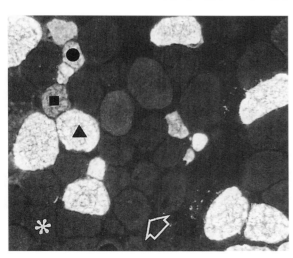

c

Fig. 8.26 Serial sections of the quadriceps from a case of limb-girdle dystrophy immunolabelled with monoclonal antibodies to **a** fetal, **b** slow, **c** fast myosin heavy chains showing co-expression of all isoforms in some fibres (●), or co-expression of fetal and fast (▲), fetal and slow (*), fast and slow (■) myosin in others. Several fibres only express slow myosin (open arrow) (× 250).

Myofibrillar proteins

In addition to the well-established myofibrillar components such as actin and myosin, immuno-cytochemistry has helped to identify and localise several other proteins associated with the myofibrils (Fitzsimons & Sewry 1985). A growing number of these proteins has been studied in human muscle, a knowledge of which is advancing our understanding of myofibrillar structure, whilst studies in diseased muscle are providing an important contribution to the interpretation of pathological changes. The myofibrillar proteins studied immunocytochemically in normal and diseased human muscle include myosin heavy chain isoforms, troponin isoforms, α-actinin, titin and nebulin.

Myosin heavy chains are encoded by a multigene family and exist in several isoforms which are regulated in a tissue- and developmental-specific manner (Whalen et al 1981, Nguyen et al 1982, Buckingham 1985, Izumo et al 1986). In addition, hormones such as the thyroid hormone, activity and innervation can influence and induce isoform transitions (see Evered & Whealan 1988). During development, embryonic and fetal (neonatal) isoforms are replaced by the adult fast and slow forms (Whalen et al 1981, Fitzsimons & Hoh 1981, Pons et al 1986, Draeger et al 1987, Butler-Browne et al 1990). Most mature fibres express either the slow or fast isoform (Fig. 8.25), corresponding to the histochemical fibre types I and II respectively (Billeter et al 1980), although occasional fibres may express both. In diseased muscle co-expression of one or more isoforms in the same fibre is common (Fig. 8.26) and can be used as an indicator of abnormality (Sewry et al 1988, Sawchak et al 1989, Sewry 1989, Sewry et al 1990, Marini et al 1991).

Embryonic and fetal myosin are not expressed in adult skeletal muscle and indicate the immaturity of fibres. The stage at which fetal myosin is no longer detected in normal human muscle has not been fully established. Muscles develop at different rates and the normal controls used for many studies have either been premature births or neonates who were biopsied because of a suspected neuromuscular problem. Traces of fetal myosin have been found at up to 4 weeks of postnatal life (Fitzsimons & Hoh 1981), but our own experience suggests that fetal myosin is not expressed in neonatal quadriceps from 12 days of age. Embryonic and fetal myosin are abundant in regenerating fibres (Fig. 8.27; Schiaffino et al 1986) and fetal myosin is also expressed in an appreciable proportion of non-basophilic fibres in the muscular dystrophies (Figs 8.26, 8.34; Sewry et al 1988, Marini et al 1991). Small fibres in several disorders including spinal muscular atrophy, congenital muscular dystrophy and many of the perifascicular fibres in dermatomyositis also express fetal myosin. Such fibres, therefore, may not be atrophic, as is commonly thought, but may be immature fibres. Fetal myosin is frequently co-expressed with fast and/or slow isoforms in a variety of disorders. This co-expression accounts for the poor differentiation of fibre types that is sometimes seen in the muscular dystrophies with the myosin ATPase technique at pH 9.4, as the method cannot distinguish between the enzymes associated with each myosin isoform (Thornell et al 1984).

The investigation of myosin isoforms in diseased muscle has shed new light on the interpretation of classical pathological features and further work will lead to a better understanding of fibre-type distributions, fibre-type conversions and the maturation of muscle.

Immunochemically distinct slow and fast forms of *troponin I and II* also exist and are segregated into type I and type II fibres. In muscular dystrophies and spinal muscular atrophy, intermediate fibres occur which bind antibodies to fast and to slow troponin I (Dhoot & Pearce 1984a, b).

The major component of the Z line is α-*actinin*; antibodies to α-actinin have been shown to bind in large quantities to the rod-like structures that characterise nemaline myopathy (Jockusch et al 1980, Jennekens et al 1983) (Fig. 8.28). This supports the origin of rods from the Z line.

Titin and nebulin. Titin (connectin) and nebulin are two of the largest proteins yet described (1000–3000 kDa and 500–800 kDa respectively) (Wang 1985, Maruyama 1986). They are believed to have a role in maintaining myofibrillar alignment and contribute to the elastic properties of the myofibrils (Horowits et al 1986). Interest arose in nebulin after a report by

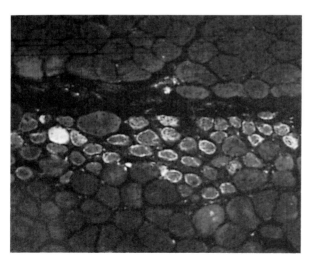

Fig. 8.27   Basophilic fibres from a case of Duchenne muscular dystrophy labelled with monoclonal antibody to embryonic myosin by an avidin–biotin–Texas Red immunofluorescent technique (× 220).

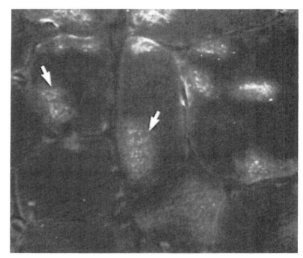

Fig. 8.28   Quadriceps biopsy from a case of nemaline myopathy showing α-actinin antibodies localised to the rods (arrows) using an indirect fluorescent technique (× 400).

Wood et al (1987) that nebulin was absent or reduced in Duchenne muscular dystrophy. Prior to the identification of the dystrophin gene, they suggested that nebulin was the defective gene product. Later immunocytochemical studies, however, showed that nebulin and titin are both expressed in Duchenne dystrophy (Fürst et al 1987, Bonilla et al 1988a) but that some degradation occurs (Sugita et al 1987, Patel et al 1988, Matsumura et al 1989, Cullen et al 1992).

Inflammation

Cellular infiltrates are a feature of inflammatory myopathies and other myopathies, including the muscular dystrophies. Cathepsin D has been identified immunocytochemically in interstitial cells and in invading phagocytes (Whitaker et al 1983) but most interest has centred around T-cell subsets, B-cells and macrophages. Commercially available monoclonal antibodies have been used to examine the distribution and proportion of each cell type in muscle biopsies (Arahata & Engel 1984, Engel & Arahata 1984, Giorno et al 1984, Arahata & Engel 1988a, b). No differences have been found in the proportion of T-cell subsets in peripheral blood (Iyer et al 1983), but in muscle the proportion of suppressor/cytotoxic and helper/inducer phenotypes and B-cells varies between endomysial and perivascular areas. The data show that T-cells are more prevalent in the endomysial than in perivascular areas (Fig. 8.29), but the reverse occurs with B-cells. There are more T8+-cells in the endomysium than perivascular areas, whereas T4+-cells are more common in perivascular regions. In polymyositis and inclusion body myositis, but not in dermatomyositis, T8+-cells accompanied by macrophages invade apparently non-necrotic fibres and the cytotoxic phenotype is predominant (Arahata & Engel 1988a). This has been put forward as evidence of cell-mediated muscle fibre injury in polymyositis and inclusion body myositis. The identification of non-necrotic fibres, however, was based on the appearance with the Gomori trichrome stain and absence of the membrane-attack complex, but fibre damage prior to necrosis may have gone undetected. The possibility that fibre injury could be caused by another mechanism prior to invasion

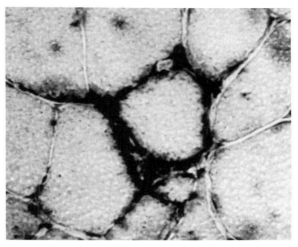

Fig. 8.29   T lymphocytes in a case of polymyositis labelled with an avidin–biotin–peroxidase technique. Counterstained with haematoxylin (× 300).

by T-cells has not been excluded. Many of the infiltrating cells are HLA-DR positive and therefore considered to be activated. In Duchenne dystrophy, where cellular infiltrates are also observed, the suppressor/cytotoxic T-cell phenotype is predominant (Arahata & Engel 1984) and these authors suggested that T-cell-mediated fibre damage may also occur in inherited disorders. Most T8+-cells use the α/β receptor for antigen recognition but a second T-cell type that expresses a γ/σ receptor has been identified. These two populations of T-cells can be distinguished immunocytochemically but the γ/σ type has only been seen in a rare case of polymyositis (Hohlfeld et al 1991).

Necrosis

Muscle fibre necrosis plays an important role in several neuromuscular disorders, in particular the muscular dystrophies and the inflammatory disorders. Acute muscle necrosis may be accompanied by myoglobinuria and can occur in malignant hyperthermia, muscular dystrophies, and a number of metabolic myopathies including those due to deficiencies of phosphorylase, phosphorylase kinase, phosphoglycerate kinase, myoadenylate deaminase and carnitine palmitoyl transferase (Tonin et al 1990). The cause of necrosis and the events leading to the final destruction of the fibre are, however, incompletely understood. Calcium has been implicated as an important factor in necrosis but calcium overload is probably a secondary event (Sewry & Dubowitz 1984).

Necrotic fibres are usually identified by abnormalities in intensity with histological stains such as Gomori's trichrome. These fibres have already reached the terminal stage but little is known about the intermediate steps between the initial damage to the fibre and the 'point of no return'. Immunocytochemistry is revealing new information on the properties of necrotic fibres and may help to elucidate some of the events involved. Necrotic fibres contain C3, C9 (Fig. 8.21) and the membrane-attack complex C5b-9 (Engel & Biesecker 1982, Morgan et al 1984). The same necrotic fibres also contain excess calcium and are penetrated by albumin (Cornelio & Dones 1984). The peroxidase methods used in these studies did not reveal any complement binding to non-necrotic fibres in contrast to our own fluorescent studies with monoclonal antibodies to C9 (Morgan et al 1984) (see 'Membrane-associated proteins' above).

Necrotic fibres do not bind antibodies to β-spectrin because the plasma membrane is lost from these fibres. Antibodies to β-spectrin should therefore be used as a control for dystrophin immunolabelling to avoid false-negative results caused by loss of the plasma membrane. Basement membrane proteins such as laminin and collagen type IV, however, are preserved around necrotic fibres. Other antibodies also bind to necrotic fibres, such as those to HLA class I and complement components (Sewry et al 1987) and some dystrophin antibodies (Sewry et al 1992a), but care in interpretation is required as degradation may result in the exposure of a variety of epitopes that bind several antibodies. Hypercontracted and necrotic fibres do not bind cathepsin D antibodies, suggesting that this lysosomal enzyme is not a marker for necrosis (Whitaker et al 1983).

Immunoglobulin (IgG) is deposited in necrotic fibres and blood vessels in some muscle disorders (Engel & Biesecker 1982, Isenberg 1983) but caution in interpretation is needed when fluorescein-conjugated secondary antibodies are used, as these may bind non-specifically to necrotic fibres.

In addition, IgG is present in the extracellular fluid and immunostaining will reveal binding of IgG to the sarcolemma and to connective tissue (Garlepp & Dawkins 1984). Some IgG may also diffuse from the extracellular fluid into necrotic fluids (Engel & Biesecker 1982).

Lectins

Lectins are proteins or glycoproteins of non-immune origin which bind to specific carbohydrate residues. They can be conjugated to biotin, enzymes or fluorochromes and their binding sites can be localised in tissue sections by similar detection systems to those used for conjugated antibodies (Ponder 1983).

Several lectins with various sugar specificities have been used to stain human muscle at both light-microscopic (Pena et al 1981, Dunn et al 1982, Capaldi et al 1985) and electron-microscopic levels (Bonilla et al 1978, Capaldi et al 1984a, b, Helliwell et al 1989). Perimysial and endomysial connective tissue is stained by several lectins and parallels the distribution of extracellular matrix antibodies. Split fibres and whorled fibres also bind several lectins (Dunn et al 1982). An increase in staining intensity of the perimysial and endomysial connective tissue in X-linked muscular dystrophies has been reported with peanut agglutinin and wheat-germ agglutinin (Paljarvi et al 1984).

Fibre peripheries are clearly delineated with several lectins (Fig. 8.30) (Capaldi et al 1985). Electron-microscopy, however, has revealed an absence of binding of *Ricinus communis* I agglutinin (RCA I) to the plasma membrane of muscle fibres from cases of Duchenne muscular dystrophy in contrast to its presence in normal muscle (Capaldi 1984a). Blood vessels and capillaries are also positively stained with several lectins. The lectin *Bandeiraea simplicifolia* agglutinin I (BSA I) is unusual in not staining the capillaries in muscle specimens from patients with blood group O; however, larger blood vessels are positive. The fucose-binding lectin *Ulex euxopaeus* 1 binds to human endothelial cells and is a useful marker for capillaries (Holthofer et al 1982, Emslie-Smith & Engel 1990).

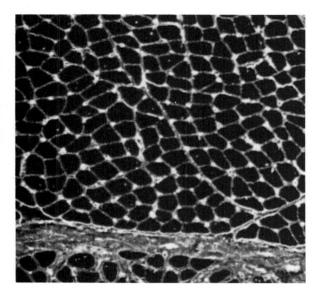

Fig. 8.30 Localisation of *Ricinus communis* I agglutinin in a quadriceps biopsy from a case of dermatomyositis using an avidin–biotin–Texas Red fluorescent technique. The sarcolemma and connective tissue are both heavily labelled (× 150).

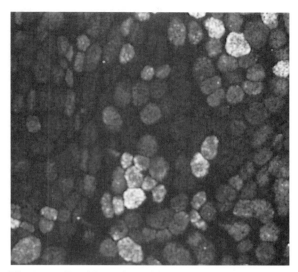

Fig. 8.31 *Bandeiraea simplicifolia* agglutinin I localisation in a quadriceps biopsy from a case of Duchenne muscular dystrophy using an avidin–biotin fluorescent technique. Several fibres are positively stained (× 120).

Internal staining of muscle fibres with lectins is not observed in normal muscle but in diseased muscle necrotic fibres are often positive (Helliwell et al 1989). In Duchenne muscular dystrophy some fibres that do not appear to be necrotic stain with BSA I and some of the same fibres also bind C9 antibodies peripherally (Fig. 8.31).

Studies with lectins have shown that, although their binding is not solely governed by monosaccharide specificity, they are useful probes for identifying tissue glycoconjugates and can be used to reveal abnormalities in diseased muscle.

Histochemistry and immunocytochemistry of the neuromuscular junction

The neuromuscular junction is the highly specialised interface between peripheral nerve and the muscle fibre. Membranes of the presynaptic, postsynaptic and non-junctional regions are distinct and express different proteins. The most characterised features of the neuromuscular junction are acetylcholinesterase (AChE) and the postsynaptic acetylcholine receptor (AChR). In mature muscle these are localised to the motor end-plate but in immature, non-innervated or denervated fibres they occur extrajunctionally. AChE activity can be

demonstrated histochemically (Stoward & Everson Pearse 1991) and antibodies are also available. Both the junctional and extrajunctional enzyme have been detected in human muscle and in neuromuscular disorders the latter is observed on basophilic fibres, on some larger fibres in Duchenne dystrophy (Fig. 8.32) and on some small fibres in neurogenic disorders, such as spinal muscular atrophy. The distribution of AChRs is

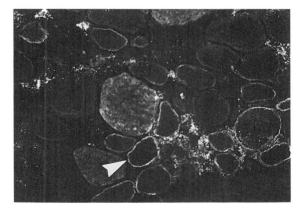

Fig. 8.32 Muscle fibres in a case of Duchenne muscular dystrophy immunolabelled with a monoclonal antibody to acetylcholinesterase showing extrajunctional labelling on regenerating/non-innervated fibres (arrowhead) (× 200).

similar to that of AChE and they can be demonstrated by the irreversible binding of labelled α-bungarotoxin and by antibody binding (see Garabedian & Morel 1983, Dolly & Barnard 1984). Five subunits of the AChR have been characterised but the majority of antibodies are directed against the α-subunit (Tzartos & Lindstrom 1980). Extrajunctional receptors differ from those at the neuromuscular junction and their number is significantly lower, making them difficult to detect with bungarotoxin. Antibodies can distinguish between normal junctional receptors and those in denervated and embryonic muscle (Whiting et al 1986). Morphological differences in motor end-plates and alterations in the distribution of AChR occur in a variety of neuromuscular disorders. In myasthenia gravis anti-AChR antibodies are present in the sera (Vincent 1980) and both immunoglobulins and complement components have been demonstrated at the neuromuscular junction, suggesting an autoimmune aetiology (Engel et al 1977, Sahashi et al 1980).

Several non-AChR proteins have been localised to the postsynaptic membrane of neuromuscular junctions in animals (Bloch & Pumplin 1988) and in human muscle. These include desmin (Askanas et al 1990), β-spectrin, dystrophin (Miike et al 1989, Shimizu et al 1989), dystrophin-related protein (Nguyen thi Man et al 1991, Pons et al 1991) and ubiquitin (Serdaroglu et al 1992). The role of these proteins at the neuromuscular junction is still to be determined.

HISTOCHEMICAL AND IMMUNOCYTOCHEMICAL CHANGES IN SPECIFIC DISEASES

The muscular dystrophies

Clinical assessment of patients with muscle disorders is often insufficient for accurate diagnosis. Histochemical and immunocytochemical techniques have an essential role in the differential diagnosis of neuromuscular disorders and they are now extensively applied to the study of the muscular dystrophies, diseases of the lower motor neurone, congenital myopathies and the glycogenoses as well as other, unclassified disorders.

Many of the histochemical abnormalities already referred to are non-specific and may occur in more than one clinical condition but experience has shown that consistent patterns of change can be attributed to certain diseases.

X-linked muscular dystrophies

Duchenne muscular dystrophy. This is the commonest and most severe form of muscular dystrophy. Histology and histochemistry reveal a diffuse pattern of pathology characterised by degeneration, loss of fibres with replacement by adipose and connective tissue, variation in fibre size and increased cellularity.

Both major fibre types show an abnormally wide variation in fibre size with hypertrophy of some and atrophy of others (Fig. 8.33). Some of the variation observed in cross-section is also due to branching of several fibres (Schmalbruch 1984). Mean diameter values, however, are not markedly altered.

Alterations in fibre-type proportions occur and a predominance of type I fibres is common (Fig. 8.33). The differentiation into type I and

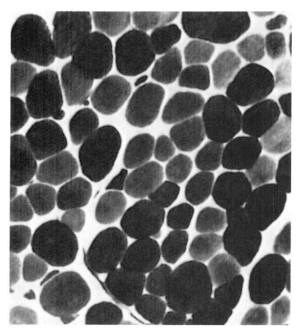

Fig. 8.33 Duchenne muscular dystrophy showing variability in fibre size with hypertrophy and atrophy of both fibre types (ATPase pH 9.4 × 200).

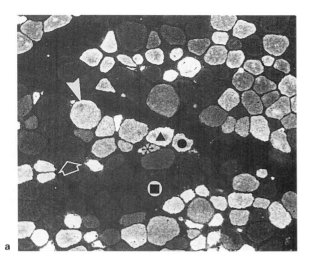

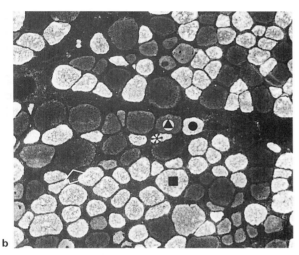

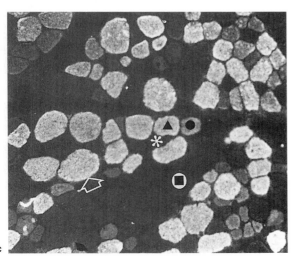

Fig. 8.34 Serial sections of the quadriceps from a case of Duchenne muscular dystrophy immunolabelled with monoclonal antibodies to **a** fetal, **b** slow and **c** fast myosin heavy chains. Note the fetal myosin in several non-basophilic fibres (**a**, arrowhead), co-expression of all isoforms in some fibres (●) and co-expression of fetal and fast (▲), or fetal and slow myosin in others (*). Several fibres only express slow myosin (■) but only occasional fibres express fast myosin alone (open arrow) (× 200).

type II fibres with the routine pH 9.4 ATPase, however, is not always clear. Type IIC fibres, which are rare in normal muscle, frequently occur (Johnson & Kucukyalcin 1978, Nonaka et al 1981) and type IIB deficiency is also common.

Immunocytochemical studies of myosin isoforms in Duchenne dystrophy have shown that co-expression of more than one isoform in an individual fibre is common (Fig. 8.34; Sewry et al 1988, Webster et al 1988b, Marini et al 1991). The co-expression of the ATPases associated with these isoforms probably accounts for the unclear differentiation pattern obtained with the routine pH 9.4 enzyme method. Fibres expressing slow myosin, either alone or in combination with the fast and/or fetal isoforms, are often predominant (Fig. 8.34) and Webster et al (1988b) have shown that fast type IIB fibres may be preferentially affected in Duchenne dystrophy. Fetal myosin is expressed not only in the basophilic regenerating fibres (Schiaffino et al 1986) but also in non-basophilic fibres of varying size and number (Fig. 8.34; Sewry et al 1986, 1988, Marini et al 1991). The presence of fetal myosin is thought to be the result of regeneration, and its presence in several small fibres suggests that some fibres defined as atrophic by morphological criteria may in fact be regenerating fibres.

Architectural changes in the intermyofibrillar network are relatively uncommon compared with other forms of dystrophy. Slight granularity or patchiness of stain are seen on occasion but moth-eaten and whorled fibres are less common than in other dystrophies (Fig. 8.35).

Degeneration, necrosis and phagocytosis are marked in Duchenne dystrophy. Necrotic fibres frequently occur in groups and they appear pale with the routine histological stains. Their histochemical fibre-type properties, however, are often retained.

Basophilic fibres also commonly occur in small groups and characterise biopsies of early cases.

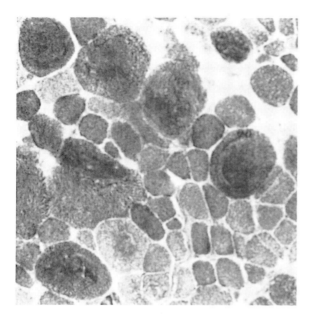

Fig. 8.35 Duchenne muscular dystrophy showing variation in fibre size, predominance of strongly reactive (type I) fibres and presence of whorled fibres (NADH-TR × 200).

Basophilic fibres are considered to be regenerating fibres because of their high RNA content and the presence of a prominent nucleolus in the nucleus. The nucleus is often centrally placed. Basophilic fibres also contain increased activity of acid and alkaline phosphatases, cathepsin D, non-specific esterases and acetylcholinesterase. Histochemically, they usually correspond to the fetal IIC fibres and immunolabelling shows that they contain developmental isoforms of myosin and express prominent amounts of various proteins, including desmin, vimentin, neural cell adhesion proteins and HLA class I antigens (Figs 8.21 & 8.36; Thornell et al 1980, Hurko & Walsh 1983, Appleyard et al 1985, Karpati et al 1988, Figarella-Branger et al 1990, Sarnat 1991). Antibodies to β-spectrin often show weak labelling of basophilic fibres (see Fig. 8.23) and our studies of fetal muscle (Clerk et al 1992) and regenerating muscle (Sewry et al 1986, 1992a) have shown that this is a feature of developing fibres. An absence of β-spectrin on basophilic fibres, however, has only been observed in Duchenne dystrophy. Some basophilic fibres bind antibodies to complement (Sewry et al 1987) suggesting that they may be damaged. Regenerating fibres also bind antibodies

to the dystrophin-related protein, utrophin, but labelling is not confined to these fibres and occurs to a varying extent on other fibres (Fig. 8.37; Khurana et al 1991, Voit et al 1991, Helliwell et al 1992b). Similarly, HLA class I antigens are also expressed on non-basophilic fibres (Fig. 8.36b; Appleyard et al 1985) but no direct correlation in

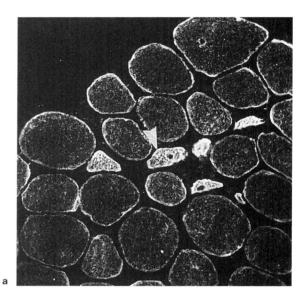

a

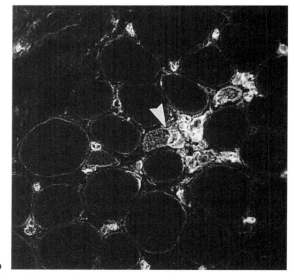

b

Fig. 8.36 Serial sections of the quadriceps from a case immunolabelled with antibodies to **a** desmin and **b** HLA class I antigens showing high levels of both in regenerating fibres (arrow), and additional labelling of HLA I on most of the other fibres as well as capillaries (× 280).

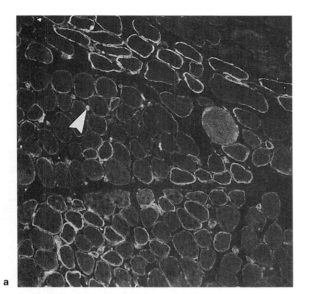

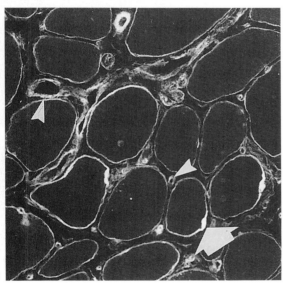

Fig. 8.37 Immunolabelling of quadriceps muscle with a monoclonal antibody to the dystrophin-related protein utrophin (Mancho 7) from two cases of Duchenne dystrophy aged **a** 1 year and **b** 8 years showing a variable number of labelled fibres and labelling of the capillaries and blood vessels (arrowheads). Note also the thickened sarcolemmal regions in b (large arrow) which parallel studies with antibodies to acetylcholinesterase showing neuromuscular junctions ($\times 200$).

expression has been found between these proteins (Helliwell et al 1992b).

Becker muscular dystrophy. This form of X-linked dystrophy is similar in clinical distribution

to the Duchenne type but milder in severity (Becker & Kiener 1955).

Muscle biopsies show similar changes to those of Duchenne dystrophy in many cases (Ringel et al 1977, Dubowitz 1985) with a wide variation in the size of both fibre types. Type IIB fibres, however, are not deficient in contrast to Duchenne dystrophy. Some workers (Bradley et al 1978, ten Houten & De Visser 1984) have reported neurogenic changes in Becker dystrophy based on the finding of angular atrophic fibres, small groups of atrophic fibres, slight fibre-type grouping and clumps of pyknotic nuclei. There is no evidence, however, of primary involvement of the nervous system.

Dystrophin expression in Duchenne and Becker muscular dystrophy. Identification of dystrophin as the defective gene product responsible for Duchenne and Becker dystrophy, and the availability of antibodies to it, have revolutionised the diagnosis of neuromuscular disorders (Hoffman et al 1987). In normal muscle dystrophin appears evenly distributed at the periphery of all fibres (Fig. 8.38), although recent studies have shown it has a costameric distribution (Porter et al 1992, Straub et al 1992). In Duchenne dystrophy, in contrast, dystrophin is absent, or very reduced, on the majority of fibres, and in Becker dystrophy the labelling is usually reduced or discontinuous (Fig. 8.38; Arahata et al 1988, 1989, Bonilla et al 1988b, Zubrzycka-Gaarn et al 1988, Bushby et al 1991, Slater & Nicholson 1991). Immunolabelling results are supported by Western blot analysis and in Becker dystrophy the abnormal size of the protein can be detected in cases where the deletion is of significant size (Hoffman et al 1988, Hoffman & Kunkel 1989, Patel et al 1988, Nicholson et al 1989a,b, 1990). The difference in dystrophin expression between Duchenne and Becker patients is believed to be the result of deletions that disrupt the translational reading frame in Duchenne dystrophy but maintain it in Becker dystrophy, allowing a smaller protein to be formed (Monaco et al 1988). Exceptions to this rule are found (Malhotra et al 1988, Baumbach et al 1989, Gangopadhyay et al 1992), notably patients with a frame-shift deletion affecting exons 3–7, who have a reduced amount of dystrophin

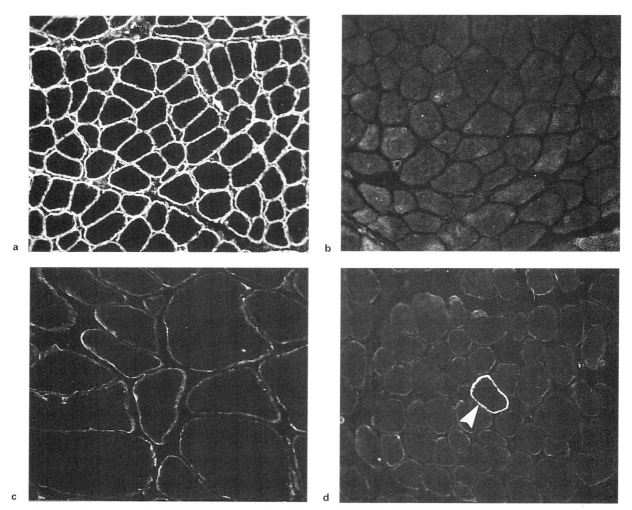

Fig. 8.38   Immunolabelling with a polyclonal antibody to dystrophin (P6) corresponding to a C-terminal region of the rod domain in **a** control muscle **b, d**, cases of Duchenne dystrophy **c** a case of Becker dystrophy. Note the uniform sarcolemmal staining in control muscle, the absence of dystrophin in Duchenne dystrophy **b** and the reduced and discontinuous labelling in Becker dystrophy **c**. In **d** a revertant fibre is intensely labelled (arrow) and low levels of dystrophin are detected on several fibres (× 200).

that is localised to the sarcolemma (Gangopadhyay et al 1992). It is interesting to note that several patients with this deletion have a milder phenotype and are intermediate in severity between Duchenne and Becker dystrophy patients. Low levels of dystrophin expression can be detected both on immunoblots and immunocytochemically in some Duchenne patients (Nicholson et al 1989a, b, 1990). This is believed to result from exon skipping that restores the reading frame and leads to the coding of transcripts of smaller size

(Chelly et al 1990a, Nicholson et al 1992). Restoration of the reading frame also occurs in the positive fibres, known as 'revertant' fibres, that are seen in small clusters or as isolated fibres in at least 40% of cases of Duchenne dystrophy (Fig. 8.38; Shimizu et al 1988, Nicholson et al 1989b, Gold et al 1990, Vainzof et al 1990, Burrow et al 1991). This has been supported by recent evidence that revertant fibres are not labelled with antibodies corresponding to the deleted region of dystrophin but are labelled by C-terminal

antibodies (Klein et al 1992), and by the identification of specific splicing events across deletions
that restore the reading-frame (Sherratt et al
1993). In addition, there is a good correlation
between the predicted size of dystrophin if the
reading was restored and that actually detected on
immunoblots (Nicholson et al 1992). Fanin et al
(1992) have reported no correlation between the
degree of phenotype and the number of revertant
fibres. Others, however, have shown that small
amounts of dystrophin on immunoblots show a
good correlation between phenotype and the
presence of 'revertant' fibres and weakly labelled
fibres immunocytochemically (Nicholson et al
1990, 1992).

Antibodies corresponding to different domains
of dystrophin have shown that most Duchenne
dystrophy patients lack the C-terminus, whilst in
Becker dystrophy it is usually preserved (Arahata
et al 1991). This has been put forward as evidence
for the importance of the C-terminus for localisation but cases in which the dystrophin lacks the C-
terminus or cysteine-rich domain, and yet is
correctly localised to the sarcolemma, have been
reported (Clemens et al 1992, Helliwell et al
1992a, Recan et al 1992).

Dystrophin can be detected in fetal muscle from
at least 9 weeks of gestation (Clerk et al 1991b)
and a significant reduction or absence is found in
fetuses at high risk for Duchenne dystrophy (Clerk
et al 1992). Analysis of selectively aborted fetal
samples can therefore be useful in counselling a
female with a risk of being a carrier of Duchenne
dystrophy, in the absence of linkage studies or a
detectable deletion in the proband case.

Dystrophin is associated with a glycoprotein
complex which is believed to span the sarcolemma
and act as a link between laminin in the extracellular matrix and the cytoskeleton (Ibraghimov-
Beskrovnaya et al 1992). In Duchenne dystrophy
the absence of dystrophin is accompanied by a
reduction in all components of the glycoprotein
complex (Ervasti et al 1990, Ibraghimov-
Beskrovnaya et al 1992).

Emery–Dreifuss muscular dystrophy. This is clinically distinct from both the other X-linked dystrophies (Emery & Dreifuss 1966). Muscle biopsies
usually show only mild changes with variation in
fibre size, an increase in internal nuclei, occasional

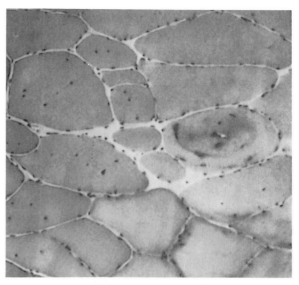

Fig. 8.39 Emery–Dreifuss dystrophy showing variation in
fibre size, an increase in internal nuclei, a split fibre and a
whorled fibre (haematoxylin and eosin × 140).

necrotic fibres and focal proliferation of connective tissue. Whorled, split and moth-eaten fibres
may also occur (Figs 8.39, 8.40). Studies with
DNA probes have shown that the gene is separate

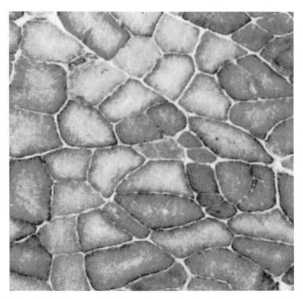

Fig. 8.40 Emery–Dreifuss dystrophy showing a normal fibre
type distribution and only minor disruptions of the
intermyofibrillar network (NADH-TR × 90).

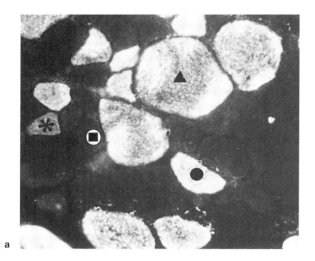

a

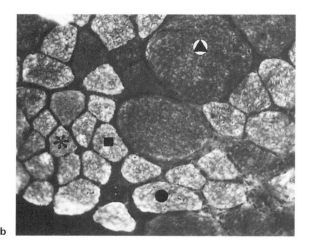

b

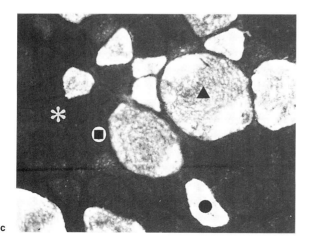

c

Fig. 8.41 Serial sections of quadriceps muscle from a manifesting carrier of Duchenne dystrophy labelled with monoclonal antibodies to **a** fetal, **b** slow and **c** fast myosin heavy chains showing predominance of slow fibres and co-expression of all isoforms in some fibres (●), or fetal and fast (▲), fetal and slow (*), or slow myosin alone (■) in others (× 200).

from that of Duchenne or Becker dystrophy and is located near the end of the long arm of the X-chromosome at position Xq28 (Hodgson et al 1986).

Carriers of X-linked dystrophies. Muscle biopsies from known carriers of Duchenne and Becker muscular dystrophy may show changes (Dubowitz 1985). Changes may occur when creatine kinase activity is normal but not all carriers have pathologically abnormal biopsies. The abnormalities are mild and include variation in fibre size, increase in internal nuclei and patchiness or moth-eaten fibres with oxidative enzyme techniques. Some biopsies from carriers are unequivocally abnormal but in others the significance of minor deviations is difficult to assess. Quantitative assessment provides a basis for evaluating these changes (Maunder-Sewry & Dubowitz 1981, Dubowitz 1985).

Immunocytochemical studies of carriers of Duchenne and Becker dystrophy have been confined to studies of the expression of myosin (Marini et al 1991) and dystrophin (Bonilla et al 1988c, Arahata et al 1989, Clerk et al 1991a, Hoffman et al 1992). Fibres expressing slow myosin are often predominant and cases with marked pathological changes have fibres that co-express the fast and slow, and/or fetal isoforms (Fig. 8.41).

Dystrophin analysis has an essential role in differentiating between a manifesting carrier of Duchenne dystrophy and autosomal forms of muscular dystrophy in which dystrophin expression is normal. Manifesting carriers show a mosaic pattern of dystrophin-positive and dystrophin-negative or deficient fibres (Fig. 8.42; Bonilla et al 1988, Arahata et al 1989), although the pattern of dystrophin expression may vary along the length of the fibre. The degree of weakness is variable in symptomatic carriers and in some cases this has been reported to correlate with the number of dystrophin-negative fibres (Hoffman et al 1992), whilst in others it does not (Sewry et al 1993). The

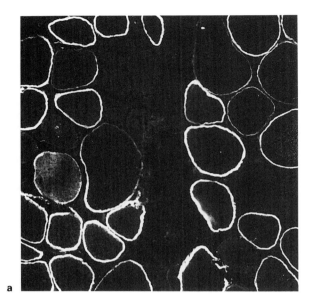

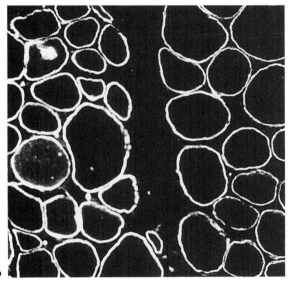

Fig. 8.42 Serial sections of quadriceps muscle of a manifesting carrier immunolabelled with: **a** a polyclonal antibody corresponding to the C-terminal region of the rod domain of dystrophin; **b** a monoclonal antibody to β-spectrin showing dystrophin-positive and dystrophin-deficient fibres but uniform β-spectrin labelling of all fibres (× 200).

Changes in the number of dystrophin-negative fibres with age have been shown in heterozygote *mdx* mice (Karpati et al 1990) and dystrophic dogs (Cooper et al 1990) and studies in human Duchenne muscular dystrophy carriers also suggest this. There is also evidence to suggest that the number of dystrophin-negative fibres may vary between muscles (Muntoni et al 1992). Asymptomatic carriers, in contrast, generally show more uniform immunolabelling, with only minor changes and occasional dystrophin-negative fibres, but a reduced abundance on immunoblots is often seen (Clerk et al 1991a).

Other dystrophies. A number of histochemical and structural changes appear to be more characteristic of other dystrophic syndromes. The following are some of the more distinctive changes that occur in addition to the 'myopathic' changes in the biopsies.

Limb-girdle dystrophy. The clinical presentation of limb-girdle dystrophy is variable and several genetically distinct forms have been identified. Both autosomal recessive and dominant forms (Marconi et al 1991) with either early or late onset have been reported and the chromosome locations of some are now known (see Bushby 1992). Fibre typing with the ATPase pH 9.4 technique is often more distinct than in Duchenne dystrophy and oxidative enzyme staining may show more abundant moth-eaten and whorled fibres. Fibre size variation is often very great with many extremely large fibres. Fibre splitting is common and the number of internal nuclei is increased. Ring fibres also occur in several cases and are easily seen with the PAS stain and oxidative enzyme stains. Other features that have been reported include lobulated, floccular fibres, inclusion bodies and vacuoles (Guerard et al 1985, Nonaka et al 1985, Marconi et al 1991). Autosomal dystrophies can be distinguished from Xp21 dystrophies by their normal expression of dystrophin.

Severe childhood autosomal recessive dystrophy. Interest has recently been aroused in this form of muscular dystrophy (SCARMD) that occurs in Tunisia and other parts of North Africa (Ben Hamida et al 1983). These patients lack expression of the 50 kDa component of the dystrophin glycoprotein complex (Matsumura et al 1992) but dystrophin is usually normal (Ben Jelloun-Dellagi

number (Sewry et al 1993) and distribution (Hoffman et al 1992) of dystrophin-negative fibres may be influenced by age at biopsy (Sewry et al 1993), with younger cases showing a higher number and a more random distribution.

1990). SCARMD has many clinical and pathological features in common with Duchenne dystrophy, including variation in the size of both fibre types, fibre necrosis, regeneration, an increase in internal nuclei and endomysial connective tissue. Some cases map to chromosome 13q (Ben Othmane et al 1992).

Facioscapulohumeral dystrophy. This slowly progressive form of dystrophy shows variable degrees of pathological change. Some biopsies show good retention of architecture and are characterised by scattered, very atrophic fibres and several hypertrophied fibres. Others are overtly dystrophic and moth-eaten and whorled fibres also occur. An inflammatory response may be a predominant feature in some biopsies. Clusters of small fibres are seen in some cases and this has been put forward as evidence of neurogenic atrophy. Many of the small fibres, and the characteristic scattered small fibres, however, are type IIC fibres (Lin & Nonaka 1991) and express fetal myosin suggesting that some may be regenerating fibres (Fig. 8.43).

Congenital muscular dystrophy. The pathological picture in this disorder is often very striking and may be disproportionate to the relatively static or slowly progressive nature of the disease; neither severity nor prognosis can therefore be assessed from the biopsy. There is usually marked proliferation of connective tissue and replacement of muscle by adipose tissue (Fig. 8.44). The residual

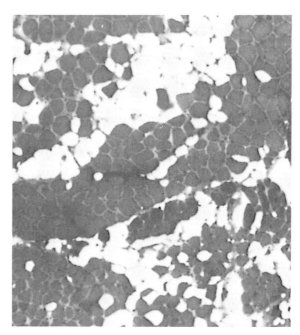

Fig. 8.44 Congenital muscular dystrophy showing replacement of large areas of muscle by adipose tissue and marked variation in fibre size (haematoxylin and eosin × 75).

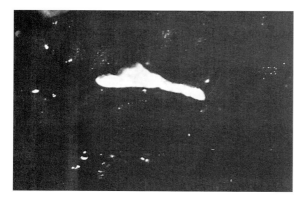

Fig. 8.43 Quadriceps biopsy from a case of facioscapulohumeral dystrophy immunolabelled with a monoclonal antibody to fetal myosin showing a small characteristic fibre that is positive. (The punctate areas are autofluorescent lipofuscin) (× 200).

fibres show some variation in fibre size but degenerative changes are mild. Type I fibres are often predominant and there is a high incidence of moth-eaten fibres. Fetal myosin is expressed in a high proportion of fibres (Sewry et al 1992b), which cannot be accounted for by regeneration, and suggests that there may be an abnormality in fibre maturation. Dystrophin expression is normal in congenital muscular dystrophy, but studies of the Japanese Fukuyama type, with central nervous system involvement, have shown abnormally labelled fibres (Arikawa et al 1991). Spectrin immunolabelling was also reported to be abnormal. A few unusual cases of Fukuyama congenital dystrophy have been reported that lack expression of dystrophin (Arikawa et al 1991, Beggs et al 1992). These patients have detectable deletions to account for the absence of dystrophin and it has been proposed that their unusual clinical presentation results from their being heterozygous for the Fukuyama mutation in addition to being hemizygous for the Duchenne mutation (Beggs et al 1992). This genotype is predicted to occur in 1/175 000 Japanese males. Recent studies

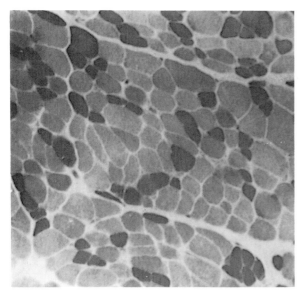

Fig. 8.45   Myotonic dystrophy in a boy aged 7 showing atrophy of type I fibres (darkly stained) and hypertrophy of type II fibres (pale) (ATPase pH 4.3 × 200).

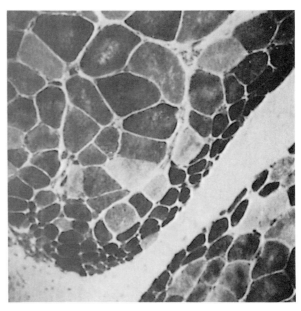

Fig. 8.46   Dermatomyositis showing perifascicular atrophy and the presence of 'moth-eaten' fibres (NADH-TR × 330).

of the dystrophin-associated glycoproteins in the Fukuyama type of congenital muscular dystrophy have shown a reduction, particularly of the 43 kDa component (Matsumura et al 1993).

Myotonic dystrophy. The distinctive features of this condition are selective atrophy of type I fibres and hypertrophy of type II fibres, particularly in the early stages of the disease (Fig. 8.45). Excessive numbers of internal nuclei occur and structural changes such as moth-eaten fibres, ring fibres and sarcoplasmic masses are common (Harper 1979).

Inflammatory myopathies

In dermatomyositis and polymyositis the classic feature is the marked inflammatory response (see section on inflammation). This, however, may be absent, particularly in acute childhood dermatomyositis. Atrophy of both fibre types occurs and in dermatomyositis this has a characteristic perifascicular distribution (Fig. 8.46). These perifascicular fibres have decreased cytochrome oxidase activity

and a proportion have the characteristics of IIC fibres (Comola et al 1987, Woo et al 1988). Hypertrophy is rare and can be used as a distinguishing feature. Oxidative enzyme staining may show dark-centred fibres, in addition to moth-eaten fibres (Whitaker 1982, Mastaglia & Ojeda 1985a,b, Dubowitz 1985). Vacuolar degeneration is frequently seen and in inclusion body myositis the vacuoles have a basophilic rim and contain basophilic inclusions (Carpenter et al 1978). In dermatomyositis the connective tissue is reactive for alkaline phosphatase (Engel 1977). Immunocytochemical studies show that the expression of fetal myosin, particularly in the small perifascicular fibres in dermatomyositis, is common. These fibres also have other properties of regenerating fibres, including desmin, utrophin and HLA class I expression (Helliwell et al 1992b). This suggests that some of the pathological features of dermatomyositis are associated with regeneration. HLA class I antigens are also detected on fibres not expressing fetal myosin (Appleyard et al 1985) and in some cases of polymyositis this may be the only detectable abnormality. HLA class I expression is not a universal feature of inflammatory myopathies but it is often a useful diagnostic marker. In inclusion body myositis vacuolated fibres and the filaments are labelled with antibodies to ubiquitin and β-amyloid protein (Askanas et al 1991, 1992). The 65 kDa heat-shock protein has been studied in a variety of inflammatory myopathies and is localised to blood vessels, inflammatory cells, regenerating fibres and some non-necrotic fibres (Hohlfeld et al 1991). Viruses have been implicated in the aetiology of polymyositis, dermatomyositis (Coxsackie B) and inclusion body myositis (mumps) (Chou 1986, Bowles et al 1987), but results have been inconsistent and in situ hybridization studies have failed to localise them in muscle biopsies. Components of the complement pathway can be detected in necrotic muscle fibres (Engel & Biesecker 1982) and on the surface of non-necrotic fibres (Sewry et al 1987). In dermatomyositis complement components are also observed in capillaries, and the number of capillaries is reduced (Emslie-Smith & Engel 1990).

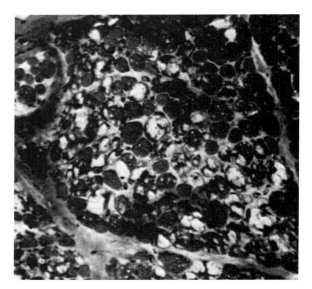

Fig. 8.47   Type II glycogenosis (Pompe's disease) showing marked vacuolation (haematoxylin and eosin × 390).

Metabolic myopathies

Glycogenoses. The inborn errors of glycogen metabolism have been categorised into seven types (Cori 1958); four of these affect muscle and a fifth (type IV) may also do so. Type II glycogenosis (acid maltase deficiency) — the severest form (Pompe's disease) — affects infants and is usually fatal but there is also a milder myopathy of late onset presenting as a mild proximal weakness. Biopsies characteristically show vacuolation and excess glycogen (Fig. 8.47). The vacuolated fibres also show high activity of acid phosphatase. Vacuolation and glycogen storage can also be demonstrated in lymphocytes (Trend et al 1985). Type III glycogenosis (debranching enzyme deficiency) is characterised by an abnormal form of glycogen in cardiac and skeletal muscle and the liver (Illingworth & Cori 1952, Forbes 1953, Krivit et al 1953) due to the absence of amylo-1, 6-glucosidase. Changes in biopsies are not marked and the overall architecture is retained. The PAS stain shows a moderately strong reaction but differentiation of fibre types is retained.

Type V glycogenosis (myophosphorylase deficiency). In 1951 McArdle described a myopathy due to a defect in the breakdown of muscle glycogen. It was later shown that this was due to an absence of myophosphorylase (Schmid & Mahler 1959). Pathological changes in muscle biopsies are mild in type V glycogenosis although occasional necrotic fibres may be present. The consistent findings are an absence of phosphorylase and excess glycogen on PAS staining. Different isomeric forms of phosphorylase exist in fetal and cultured muscle compared with mature muscle (Sato et al 1977, DiMauro et al 1978). Thus phosphorylase activity can be demonstrated histochemically in regenerating muscle fibres and cultured myotubes from patients with type V glycogenosis (Roelofs et al 1972, Mitsumoto 1979). There is also an infantile form of phosphorylase deficiency which presents as a floppy infant syndrome in the neonatal period.

Type VII glycogenosis. The histological changes are similar to those of McArdle's disease and the absence of phosphofructokinase can be demonstrated histochemically (Bonilla & Schotland 1970).

A number of additional glycogenoses affecting

muscle have been identified over the past few years, including lactic dehydrogenase deficiency (Kanno et al 1980), phosphoglycerate kinase deficiency (Rosa et al 1982, DiMauro et al 1983) and phosphoglycerate mutase deficiency (DiMauro et al 1981).

Mitochondrial myopathies. Several myopathies, cardiomyopathies, encephalopathies and multisystem disorders are caused by mutations, deletions, depletion or duplication in the maternally inherited mitochondrial DNA or in related nuclear-derived factors (Holt et al 1988, Zeviani & DiDonato 1991, Nonaka 1992) (also see Ch. 18). The ultrastructural changes in mitochondria are varied and non-specific (Sewry 1985) and no specific abnormality has been associated with a particular disorder (Morgan-Hughes 1982). Mitochondrial abnormalities may be overlooked on routine histological staining, although some increased granularity may be seen with haematoxylin and eosin, and Verhoeff–van Gieson stains. Their presence becomes obvious when disrupted, red-staining fibres ('ragged-red' fibres) are seen with the Gomori trichrome stain and the oxidative enzyme preparations show strongly reactive fibres (Fig. 8.48). Sometimes this increased activity may be restricted to the periphery of the fibre (Fig. 8.49) and the term 'ragged-red' is now frequently used to describe these fibres too (Hammans et al 1992). Normal muscle fibres often show accumulations of peripheral mitochondria which consequently stain red with the trichrome technique, but these should not be confused with 'ragged-red' fibres. Electron-microscopy confirms the presence of an abnormality in the number, size and structure of the mitochondria. 'Ragged-red' fibres are not a consistent feature of mitochondrial myopathies, similarly ultrastructural abnormalities may be absent.

Cytochrome oxidase deficiency occurs in most patients with mitochondrial encephalopathies and mitochondrial DNA deletions, although this may not necessarily be a primary effect (Johnson et al 1988, Holt et al 1989, DiMauro et al 1990, Nonaka 1992, Oldfors et al 1992). Fibres with low cytochrome oxidase staining have high succinic dehydrogenase enzyme activity and often, but not always, correspond to the 'ragged-red' fibres. In a high proportion of patients with mitochondrial

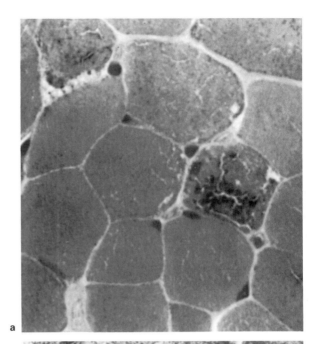

a

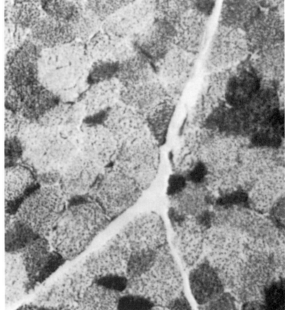

b

Fig. 8.48 Mitochondrial myopathy showing: **a** 'ragged-red' fibres with the Gomori trichrome stain ($\times$ 560); **b** several fibres with intense oxidative activity (NADH-TR $\times$ 330).

encephalopathy, lactic acidosis and stroke-like episodes (MELAS), blood vessels in the muscle frequently react strongly for succinate dehydroge-

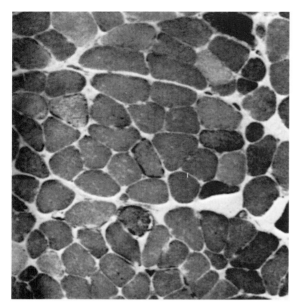

Fig. 8.49 Mitochondrial myopathy showing a population of fibres with intense oxidative activity at the periphery of the fibres (NADH-TR × 120).

nase (Hasegawa et al 1991). Cytochrome oxidase activity in the blood vessels, however, is normal, suggesting that a deficiency of cytochrome oxidase in MELAS, when present, is a secondary effect.

Deficiencies in cytochrome oxidase can be demonstrated immunocytochemically with antibodies to both the mitochondrial (I-III) and nuclear (IV-VIII) encoded subunits of cytochrome oxidase (Johnson et al 1988, DiMauro et al 1990). Antibodies can distinguish between the fatal, infantile form of cytochrome oxidase deficiency and the benign, spontaneously remitting myopathy (Tritschler et al 1991). The fatal infantile form is characterised by an absence of the nuclear-encoded VIIa,b subunits in all fibres, whilst in early stages of the benign form both VIIa,b and the mitochondrially encoded subunit II are absent. Later, however, when the patients show a clinical improvement, 50–60% of fibres show the presence of both the VIIa,b and II subunits. In cases of mitochondrial DNA deletions, in situ hybridization studies show that transcription of the mutated mitochondrial DNA occurs, and that the expression of nuclear-encoded subunits can also be reduced (Oldfors et al 1992). Depletion of mitochonrial DNA can also

be demonstrated with anti-DNA antibodies and in situ hybridisation (Andreetta et al 1991, Tritschler et al 1992).

Lipid storage myopathies. In 1970 Engel et al (1970b) reported excess lipid droplets in muscle biopsies from identical twin sisters who had muscle cramps and myoglobinuria some hours after exercise; they postulated a defect in the utilisation of long-chain fatty acids. Bressler (1970) predicted that a deficiency of carnitine or carnitine palmitoyl transferase (EC 2.3.1.21; CPT) could account for this lipid storage myopathy. Since then many cases of carnitine or CPT deficiency have been described (Pleasure & Bonilla 1982). In carnitine deficiency lipid accumulation is more striking in type I fibres than type II. CPT deficiency, however, is not usually associated with marked lipid storage in the muscle fibres. A recent study, however, reported lipid accumulation in a few cases, as well as elevated glycogen, abnormal mitochondria and atrophic fibres (Vladutiu et al 1992).

Other metabolic myopathies. Pathological changes can be found in a variety of other metabolic myopathies including malignant hyperpyrexia (Harriman 1982), periodic paralysis (Tomé 1982) and endocrine myopathies (Hudgson & Hall 1982, Dubowitz 1985). Most histochemical features are non-specific and include selective type II atrophy, moth-eaten fibres, core-targetoid fibres and vacuolar changes. In periodic paralysis there is a characteristic vacuolar myopathy, especially during attacks of weakness, and an additional feature is the presence of tubular aggregates (Engel et al 1970a, Pearse & Johnson 1970, Lewis et al 1971). These are confined to type II fibres and show an intense reaction with oxidative enzymes but lack ATPase staining. On electron microscopy they have a typical tubular appearance.

Congenital myopathies

The congenital myopathies are a heterogeneous group of disorders delineated by specific structural abnormalities in the muscle (Bodensteiner 1988, Tomé & Fardeau 1988, Goebel 1991). Many of these abnormalities are not apparent with routine histological stains and are only identified by histochemical or immunocytochemical techniques.

Several congenital myopathies present in infancy with a floppy infant syndrome, but juvenile and adult clinical subtypes are also now recognised.

Central core disease. In 1956 Shy & Magee described a non-progressive congenital myopathy characterised by amorphous central cores in the muscle fibres. It was later named central core disease (Greenfield et al 1958) and several cases have been reported since (see Dubowitz 1985). It is an autosomal dominant disorder that is linked to chromosome 19q13.1 (Kausch et al 1991). The cores can be distinguished with the Gomori trichrome stain but are seen more easily with oxidative enzyme techniques, which show them to be devoid of activity. Characteristically, the cores are single and central, but they may also be multiple or eccentric. In longitudinal section they are seen to run the length of the fibre. Cases have also been reported with an apparent evolution of cores with time (Dubowitz 1985). A 4-year-old boy, whose mother had centrally placed cores in all type I fibres, showed eccentric cores in only a small proportion of fibres (Fig. 8.50a) but at 12 years of age he showed an identical picture to that of his mother with single, or occasional multiple, central cores in most fibres (Fig. 8.50b).

The cores consistently affect type I fibres and in some cases the muscle appears undifferentiated, being composed entirely, or almost entirely, of type I fibres (see Dubowitz 1985). Staining for ATPase activity and electron-microscopy can distinguish two types of core based on the degree of myofibrillar disruption (Neville & Brooke 1973, Sewry 1985). All cores show an absence of mitochondria but in 'structured' cores the myofibrils are contracted and retain their striation pattern and ATPase activity. 'Unstructured' cores, in contrast, show severe disruption of the myofibrils, an excess of Z-line material and are devoid of ATPase activity. Cases showing both structured and unstructured cores have been reported (Telerman-Toppet et al 1973, Isaacs et al 1975), but this is considered unusual (Neville 1979) and it is more common to find one or other type.

'Target' fibres resemble central core fibres and may occur in long-standing neurogenic atrophies (Fig. 8.4), suggesting that both may result from denervation (Engel 1961). Core-like structures have also been observed in experimental animals

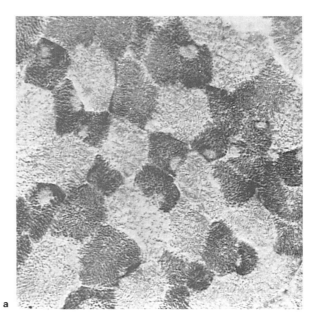

a

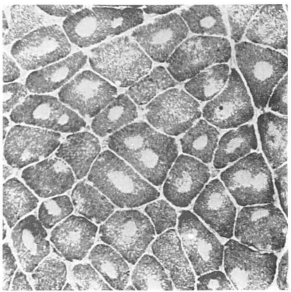

b

Fig. 8.50 Central core disease. **a** Biopsy from quadriceps of 4-year-old boy showing a normal distribution of fibre types and the presence of eccentric cores in several type I fibres (NADH-TR × 330). **b** Biopsy from the same child as in **a** at 16 years of age showing evolution of the disease with uniformity of fibre type and centrally placed cores in almost all fibres (NADH-TR × 200).

during reinnervation (Dubowitz 1967) and following tenotomy (Shafiq et al 1969). Occasional core-like areas can be observed in a variety of myopathic situations but these are less defined and less frequent than those occurring in central core disease. Cases in which cores occur in conjunction with rod bodies have also been reported (see Dubowitz 1985) but in most situations one feature predominates.

Minicore disease (multicore disease). In 1971 Engel et al documented two unrelated children with a non-progressive myopathy associated with multifocal areas of degeneration in the muscle fibres. As in central core disease, these areas are devoid of oxidative enzyme activity and show marked myofibrillar disruption (see Fig. 8.3). The number of affected sarcomeres may vary but, unlike central cores, minicores do not run the length of the fibre. There is a tendency for the muscle to show a predominance of type I fibres and for the minicores to have a predilection for type I fibres (Dubowitz 1985). On routine histological staining the muscle may show only variability in fibre size and the presence of internal nuclei. The condition is genetically distinct from central core disease and most cases have an autosomal recessive inheritance. Occasional cases with a dominant mode of heritance have, however, been reported (Paljarvi et al 1987). Age of onset is usually in early childhood but later presentation can occur and most cases show little or no progression of symptoms (Penegyres & Kakulas 1991).

Nemaline myopathy. This is another non-progressive congenital myopathy. The characteristic rod bodies or nemaline rods were first recognised by Conen et al (1963) and Shy et al (1963). The nemaline rods are devoid of enzyme activity and stain red with the Gomori trichrome. They have been shown in electron microscopy to be in continuity with the Z bands (Price et al 1965, Sewry 1985). Recent studies have shown that rods resemble Z lines in several respects. Their lattice structure is similar and both rods and Z lines contain α-actinin and tropomyosin (Schollmeyer et al 1974, Jockusch et al 1980). Desmin is also located at their periphery and they may contain actin (Thornell et al 1980, Yamaguchi et al 1978, 1982).

Nienhuis et al (1967) noted in their cases of nemaline myopathy that all fibres were uniform in enzyme activity and showed no differentiation into fibre types. Other cases may show fibre typing

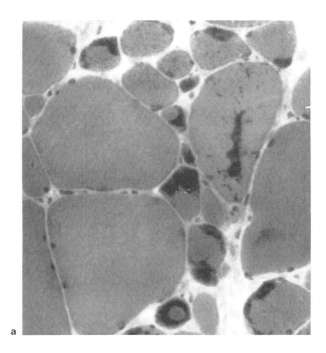

a

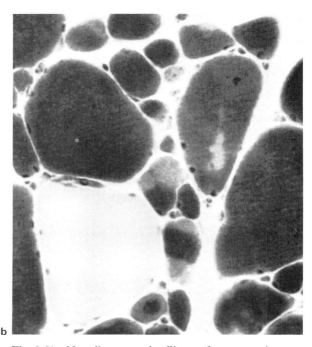

b

Fig. 8.51 Nemaline myopathy. Biopsy of gastrocnemius from 12-year-old boy showing: **a** variation in fibre size and presence of dark (red) stained rods (Gomori trichrome × 330); **b** absence of staining in the rods with the ATPase reaction. (ATPase pH 4.3 × 330).

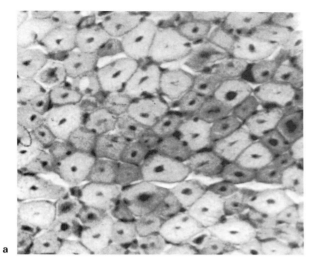

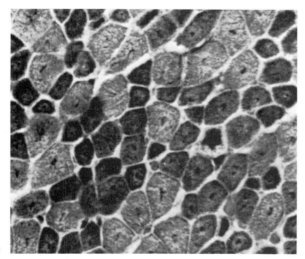

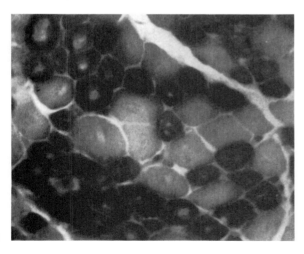

Fig. 8.52 Myotubular myopathy. Biopsy from rectus femoris of a 14-year-old boy. **a** Striking internal nuclei (VVG × 330). **b** Focal aggregation of oxidative activity at site of nuclei (NADH-TR × 330). **c** 'Holes' in fibres at site of nuclei due to absence of myofibrillar structure (ATPase × 330).

and a tendency towards a bimodal distribution of small and large fibres with the type I fibres being atrophic. In these cases the rods tend to be confined to the atrophic type I fibres (Gonatas et al 1966, Dubowitz 1978) but other cases show involvement of both fibre types (Shafiq et al 1967) or selective involvement of type II fibres (Shy et al 1963) (Fig. 8.51). In the majority of cases rods are exclusively sarcoplasmic, although their distribution within a fibre may vary. A few unusual cases have been reported with intranuclear as well as myofibrillar rods (Paulus et al 1988). Immunocytochemically, intranuclear rods differ from myofibrillar rods in that they lack α-actinin.

Studies of the distribution of rods in several muscles from autopsied cases have shown variation in the proportion of affected fibres between muscles and also in different parts of the same muscle (Shafiq et al 1967). There is no correlation between the number of rods, or affected fibres, and clinical severity in the severe neonatal, congenital or adult-onset forms (Nienhuis et al 1967, Shimomura & Nonaka 1989).

Although rods are the characteristic feature of nemaline myopathy, they have been observed in a variety of other conditions, in normal human extraocular muscle (Mukuno 1969) and in myotendinous regions.

Centronuclear myopathy (myotubular myopathy). In 1966 Spiro et al reported the first case of a disorder characterised by prominent central nuclei in several fibres. The similarity of these fibres to fetal myotubes led to the authors naming this disorder myotubular myopathy. Later Sher et al (1967) proposed the more descriptive term of centronuclear myopathy. Since these early reports several cases have been published (De Angelis et al 1991) and it is now clear that there are genetically, clinically and pathologically distinct types of centronuclear myopathy (Dubowitz 1980, Fardeau 1982, Heckmatt et al 1985, Sasaki et al 1989, van der Ven et al 1991). The common feature of all types is the presence of a population of fibres with central nuclei (Fig. 8.52).

In longitudinal sections central nuclei are seen down the length of the fibre and are often separated by sarcoplasm. The number of central nuclei observed in transverse section is thus dependent on the plane of section. The central region shows striking aggregation of oxidative enzyme activity, often with a clear halo, and an absence of ATPase activity (Fig. 8.52). Oxidative enzyme techniques sometimes show a radial deposition of the intermyofibrillar network and type I fibre predominance is common. Central nuclei are usually seen at the time of clinical presentation, but a case with generalised weakness from birth showing no central nuclei until re-biopsied at 11 months of age has been reported (van der Ven et al 1991).

Genetically, most cases fall into three main types: (1) severe neonatal X-linked; (2) neonatal autosomal recessive; (3) autosomal dominant with onset in childhood or adult life. A survey by de Angelis et al (1991) showed that the X-linked and autosomal dominant forms are the most common.

The X-linked form is severe and usually fatal. Muscle biopsies show uniform small fibres with only a few large fibres. Female carriers show no clinical signs of the disorder but the muscle may show mild pathological changes with central nuclei in a few small fibres (Heckmatt et al 1985).

Immunocytochemistry has shown accumulations of the cytoskeletal proteins desmin and vimentin and it has been suggested that this may reflect a defect in the development of the cytoskeleton and a delay in maturation (Sarnat 1990, Figarella-Branger et al 1992b, van der Ven 1991). There does not appear to be a generalised arrest in development in any form of centro-nuclear myopathy, and the expression of myo-fibrillar proteins and N-CAM is normal (Soussi-Yanicostas et al 1991, Figarella-Branger et al 1992b). In particular, embryonic and fetal myosin do not persist in the fibres with central nuclei and they therefore differ from fetal myotubes (Fig. 8.53, Sewry et al 1990, van der Ven et al 1991). In most disorders no abnormalities in the basement membrane constituents laminin and collagen type IV have been observed (Dunn et al 1984, Hantai et al 1985), but thickening of the basement membrane has been reported in centronuclear myopathy (van der Ven et al 1991).

Centronuclear myopathy with type I fibre hypotrophy. Engel et al (1968) reported an 11-month-old child with severe and progressive weakness, whose muscle had profuse central nuclei, restricted to type I fibres, which were also small in diameter. They suggested that this might represent a maturational arrest, or 'hypotrophy' of the type I fibres rather than an atrophy. Further cases with milder clinical involvement but a similar biopsy picture have been reported by Bethlem et al (1969), Karpati et al (1970) and Dubowitz (1985).

Congenital fibre-type disproportion. In their histographic analysis of muscle biopsies, Brooke & Engel (1969) suggested classifying children's biopsies according to the relative size of type I and type II fibres. Normally the fibre types are of approximately equal diameter. In some cases with a relatively non-progressive weakness, type I fibres were noted to be smaller than type II. Brooke (1973) subsequently delineated a fairly consistent clinical picture, usually presenting with hypotonia at birth or in early infancy and having a benign course. The only abnormality on biopsy is the disproportion in size of the fibre types, with striking and uniform atrophy of the type I fibres and normal-sized or enlarged type II fibres (Fig. 8.54). Type I fibres are frequently predominant.

This condition has to be distinguished from dystrophia myotonica and myotubular myopathy with type I fibre atrophy, which also present with hypotonia and weakness in early infancy (Dubowitz & Brooke 1973) and from the early stage of infantile spinal muscular atrophy (Werdnig-Hoffmann disease) (Dubowitz 1980), where all the fibres may be small with type I smaller than type II.

Infantile hypotonia. There are many causes of the floppy infant syndrome and this has been the subject of a separate monograph (Dubowitz 1980). From a practical point of view it is important to separate those cases with weakness and involvement of the lower motor neurone from the floppy infants with hypotonia of 'central' nervous origin or related to more remote disorders. In addition to electrodiagnostic investigations, which offer a useful screening test for identifying a myopathic, neurogenic or normal pattern of muscle activity, muscle biopsy with detailed histochemical study is essential in this group of disorders in order to

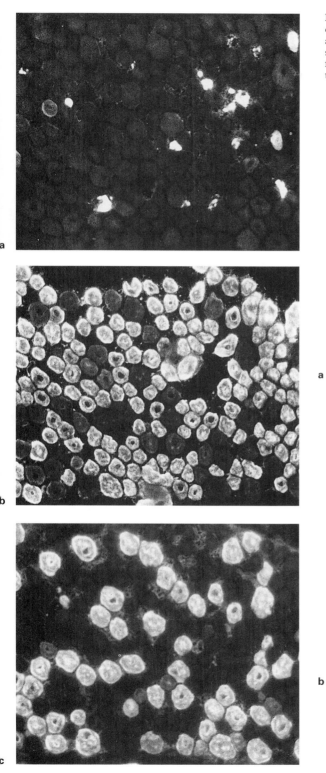

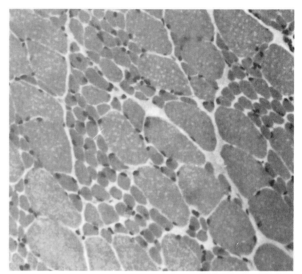

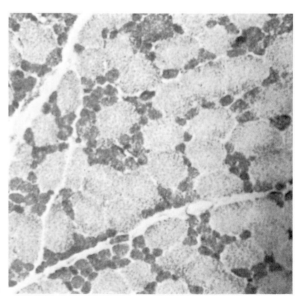

Fig. 8.53 Serial sections from a case of X-linked centronuclear myopathy immunolabelled with monoclonal antibodies to **a** fetal, **b** slow and **c** fast myosin heavy chains showing a predominance of slow myosin and an absence of fetal myosin in most fibres with central nuclei (position of these corresponds to the central holes) ($\times$ 200).

Fig. 8.54 Congenital fibre type disproportion in a 4¹/₂-year-old floppy weak child, showing: **a** presence of two populations of fibres on routine staining (haematoxylin and eosin x 200); **b** strikingly uniform atrophy (hypotrophy) of type I fibres (dark) in contrast to normal-sized or enlarged type II fibres (NADH-TR $\times$ 200).

differentiate between spinal muscular atrophy and congenital muscular dystrophy, or to identify one of the rarer forms of congenital myopathy with a specific structural abnormality. In the congenital form of myotonic dystrophy, the muscle may be essentially normal apart from a tendency to atrophy of type I fibres, and the diagnosis is more readily confirmed by clinical and electrodiagnostic assessment of the mother, who invariably has the dominantly inherited condition. In the Prader–Willi syndrome (Prader et al 1956, Prader & Willi 1963) the infant presents with profound hypotonia and associated sucking and swallowing difficulty at birth, but with relatively good muscle power and a gradual resolution of the hypotonia. Muscle biopsy is unlikely to be of diagnostic help as the histological and histochemical patterns are usually normal. The diagnosis then has to rest on the typical clinical features and identifying the deletion in chromosome 15, which is present in about 50% of cases.

Congenital myopathies with abnormal ultrastructural inclusions. The occurrence of certain ultrastructural features has been shown to characterise some congenital myopathies (see Tomé & Fardeau 1988, Goebel 1991). These include fingerprint body myopathy (Engel et al 1972, Fardeau et al 1976), sarcotubular myopathy (Jerusalem et al 1973), zebra body myopathy (Lake & Wilson 1975), reducing body myopathy (Jerusalem et al 1979) and trilaminar muscle fibre disease (Ringel et al 1978). These disorders may show disturbances in fibre size and fibre typing, in particular a predominance of type I fibres. Occasionally more than one structural defect may occur, such as cytoplasmic bodies and reducing bodies (Goebel 1991), or tubular aggregates with central cores (Castro et al 1990). Few immunocytochemical studies have been performed on patients with congenital myopathies but desmin has been shown to be associated with some structural defects such as cytoplasmic bodies and Mallory-like bodies (Fidzianska et al 1983, Osborn & Goebel 1983).

Neurogenic disorders

Many clinical disorders affect the lower motor neurone, some having a proximal distribution of weakness (e.g. spinal muscular atrophy), whilst in others, weakness is distal (e.g. peroneal muscular atrophy). The denervation process is reflected in muscle biopsies and histochemical studies reveal distinctive patterns associated with these syndromes.

The characteristic features of denervated muscle are the presence of atrophic fibres associated with fibres of normal or enlarged size (Fig. 8.55), and fibre-type grouping, where large groups of fibres of one histochemical type occur alongside groups of

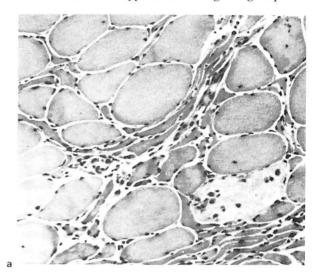

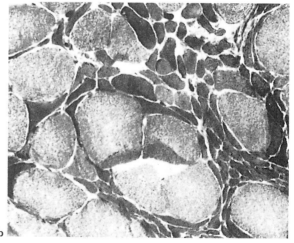

Fig. 8.55 Neurogenic atrophy. Biopsy from quadriceps of a 35-year-old man with rapidly progressive motor neurone disease showing: **a** large groups of atrophic fibres and also 'myopathic changes' in some large fibres with internal nuclei and presence of necrotic (pale) fibres (haematoxylin and eosin × 120); **b** mixed fibre-type pattern in atrophic fibres and uniformity of enzyme reaction in large fibres (NADH-TR × 120).

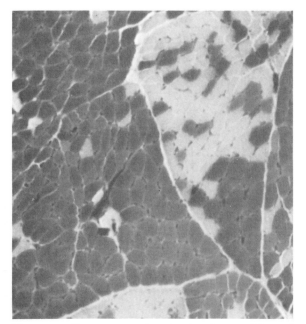

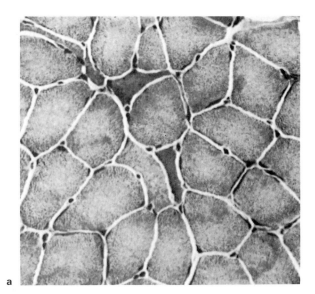

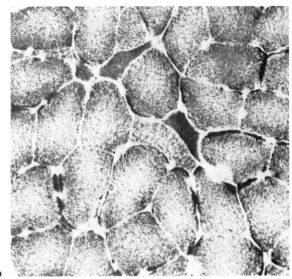

Fig. 8.56 Fibre type-grouping, showing clusters of fibres of uniform fibre type, characteristic of reinnervation. Biopsy of gastrocnemius of 5-year-old girl with mild almost non-progressive neurogenic weakness (?spinal muscular atrophy, ?peripheral neuropathy) (ATPase × 120).

the other type (Fig. 8.56). The atrophic fibres may be present in large or small groups and are of both histochemical fibre types. The larger fibres are often uniform in type, which, like fibre-type grouping, is thought to result from reinnervation of previously denervated fibres by surviving terminal axons that have sprouted. Small angulated fibres that are intensely stained with oxidative enzymes are also a feature of denervated muscle (Fig. 8.57). These fibres vary in their ATPase activity and may be of either type.

Other pathological features of neurogenic disorders include split fibres, moth-eaten fibres and 'target' fibres (see Fig. 8.4; Engel 1961, Froes et al 1987). In motor neurone disease the degree of pathological change is variable and there is no correlation with age or severity (Froes et al 1987). The study by Froes et al (1987) also suggested that changes in females may be more severe.

Studies of myosin heavy chain expression in chronic neuropathies and motor neurone disease have shown that fast and slow isoforms can occur together in some fibres (Sawchak et al 1989). This

Fig. 8.57 Biopsy from rectus femoris of a 12-year-old boy with mild slowly progressive motor neurone disease showing focal angulated atrophic fibres which have intense activity with oxidative enzyme reaction, while remaining fibres are uniform in enzyme activity, suggesting a reinnervation process (**a** VVG × 330; **b**, NADH-TR × 330).

was thought to be the result of neurally directed fibre type transformations, but there is no conclusive evidence of this and it is a common feature in most neuromuscular disorders. In addition, Sawchak et al (1989) observed a small population of fibres that expressed fetal myosin and considered

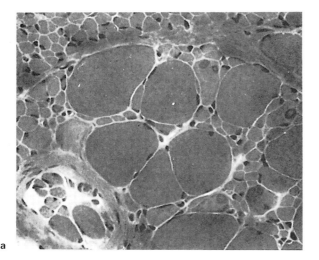

a

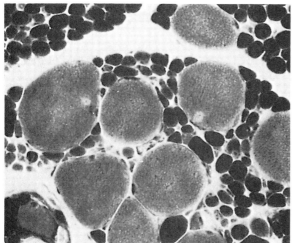

b

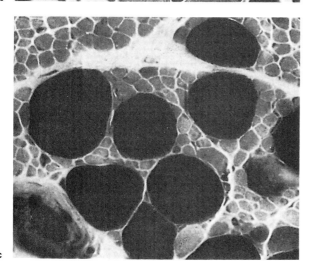

c

Fig. 8.58 Spinal muscular atrophy of intermediate severity in a 21-month-old child. Rectus femoris shows atrophy of large groups of mixed fibre type together with enlarged fibres of uniform enzyme type. Note muscle spindle (bottom left) with intrafusal fibres of size comparable with the atrophic fibres. Serial sections. (**a**, Haematoxylin-eosin × 330; **b**, ATPase pH 9.4 × 330; **c**, ATPase pH 4.6. × 330).

these to be regenerating. We have also observed fibres expressing fetal myosin in a few cases of motor neurone disease (unpublished results).

Spinal muscular atrophy. Spinal muscular atrophy is a genetically determined condition in which there is degeneration of the anterior horn cells of the spinal cord and sometimes of the cranial nerve nuclei. Three groups of patients have been defined on the basis of clinical severity and current evidence has mapped the defect in all forms to chromosome 5q11–q13 (Gilliam et al 1990). The severity ranges from severe in the fatal infantile form (Werdnig–Hoffman disease) to mild proximal weakness in Kugelberg–Welander disease, and an intermediate group spanning these two extremes. Overlap in severity may occasionally occur within a family (Dubowitz 1964).

The pathology in cases of the severe infantile form is similar to that in cases of the intermediate type, irrespective of the degree of weakness (Fig. 8.58). It is usual to see large group atrophy of fibres; occasionally a section may show universal atrophy. The small fibres are rounded and of both fibre types, although many often stain as type II fibres at pH 9.4 (Saito 1985, Biral et al 1989, Soussi-Yanicostas et al 1992). The larger fibres may occur singly, or in groups, and are often hypertrophic. They usually have a uniform enzyme activity and stain as type I fibres, although occasional larger type II fibres may be present (Fig. 8.58).

Our immunocytochemical studies have shown that the larger fibres usually exclusively express slow myosin, but that the small fibres co-express fast, slow and fetal myosin in various combinations (Fig. 8.59; Sewry 1989). This has been confirmed by others (Biral et al 1989, Soussi-Yanicostas et al 1992) and similar results have been obtained with antibodies to troponin I isoforms (Dhoot & Pearce 1984a). It is in agreement with the hypothesis that type I slow-twitch motor units persist but type II phasic motor units

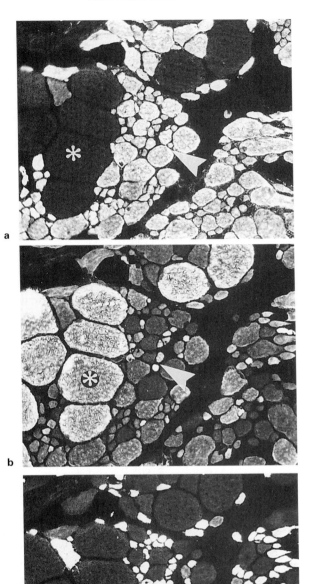

Fig. 8.59 Serial sections of quadriceps muscle from a case of intermediate spinal muscular atrophy immunolabelled with monoclonal antibodies to: **a** fetal, **b** slow and **c** fast myosin heavy chains showing fetal myosin co-expressed with slow and/or fast myosin in the small fibres (arrowheads), and only slow myosin in the large fibres (*) (× 200).

are lost. The presence of fetal myosin suggests that these fibres may be denervated before they are fully mature but there does not seem to be a general arrest in maturation as other developmentally regulated proteins such as desmin, vimentin and titin are only detected in some atrophic fibres (Sewry 1989, Soussi-Yanicostas et al 1992). The expression of these proteins may be the result of regeneration. It is interesting to note that N-CAM, which is usually extrajunctional on non-innervated fibres, is not uniformily expressed on all the atrophic fibres and is only observed on the fibres with higher levels of desmin (Sewry 1989). The factors that control protein expression in muscle are complex and varied, and there are differences between species as well as between muscles in the same species. The mechanisms that produce the characteristic pathology in spinal muscular atrophy therefore remain to be fully elucidated.

In milder cases of spinal muscular atrophy (Kugelberg–Welander) there may be less atrophy and fibre-type grouping. The extent of the atrophy varies and it is not possible to prognosticate on the basis of the findings in the muscle biopsy. In longer-standing cases of Kugelberg–Welander type structural changes in the larger fibres may occur, such as whorled fibres or disruption of the myofibrillar network. Internal nuclei may also be a feature of the larger fibres and sometimes connective tissue may be increased. The similarity of these features to those in muscular dystrophies may be misleading when interpreting a biopsy.

CONCLUSION

Histochemistry has made a considerable contribution to the understanding of normal and diseased muscle. Its various techniques are essential for the investigation of muscle biopsies and they have now become routine procedures. Immunocytochemistry is now of equal importance and not only provides further insight into the structure of muscle and the changes associated with disease, but also has an essential role in differential diagnosis, particularly in the muscular dystrophies. As the number of gene products associated with specific disorders grows, immunocytochemistry will become increasingly important.

ACKNOWLEDGEMENTS

The financial support of the Muscular Dystrophy Group for the work reported in this chapter is gratefully acknowledged.

We are grateful to Dr M. H. Brooke and Baillière Tindall for permission to reproduce Figure 8.11 and to Baillière Tindall for permission to reproduce Figures 8.3, 8.4, 8.5, 8.6, 8.7, 8.15, 8.16, 8.17, 8.20b, 8.39, 8.40, 8.44, 8.45, 8.47, 8.48, 8.49, 8.50, 8.51, 8.52, 8.54, 8.57b, 8.58b and 8.57c. We thank Mrs Karen Davidson for photographic assistance.

We are also grateful to collaborators who have generously donated the antibodies shown in this chapter: Dr W. Brown (fetal myosin), Dr R. Fitzsimons (slow and fast myosin), Dr G. Morris (dystrophin-related protein/utrophin), Mr T. Sherratt (dystrophin P6) and Dr D. Shotton (β-spectrin).

REFERENCES

Andersen P 1975 Capillary density in skeletal muscle of man. Acta Physiologica Scandinavica 95: 203

Andreetta F, Tritschler H J, Schon E A, DiMauro S, Bonilla E 1991 Localization of mitochondrial DNA in normal and pathological muscle using immunological probes: a new approach to the study of mitochondrial myopathies. Journal of the Neurological Sciences 105: 88

Appleyard S T, Dunn M J, Dubowitz V, Scott M L, Pittman S J, Shotton D M 1984 Monoclonal antibodies detect a spectrin-like protein in normal and dystrophic human skeletal muscle. Proceedings of the National Academy of Sciences USA 81: 776

Appleyard S T, Dunn M J, Dubowitz V, Rose M L 1985 Increased expression of HLA ABC class I antigens by muscle fibres in Duchenne muscular dystrophy, inflammatory myopathy and other neuromuscular disorders. Lancet i: 361

Arahata K, Engel A G 1984 Monoclonal antibody analysis of mononuclear cells in myopathies. I Quantitation of subsets according to diagnosis and sites of accumulation and demonstration and counts of muscle fibers invaded by T cells. Annals of Neurology 16: 193

Arahata K, Engel A G 1988a Monoclonal antibody analysis of mononuclear cells in myopathies. IV: Cell-mediated cytotoxicity and muscle fibre necrosis. Annals of Neurology 23: 168

Arahata K, Engel A G 1988b Monoclonal antibody analysis of mononuclear cells in myopathies. V: Identification and quantitation of T8+ cytotoxic and T8+ suppressor cells. Annals of Neurology 23: 493

Arahata K, Ishiura S, Ishiguro T et al 1988 Immunostaining of skeletal and cardiac muscle surface membrane with antibody against Duchenne muscular dystrophy peptide. Nature 333: 861

Arahata K, Ishihara T, Kamakura K et al 1989 Mosaic expression of dystrophin in symptomatic carriers of Duchenne's muscular dystrophy. New England Journal of Medicine 320: 138

Arahata K, Beggs A, Honda H et al 1991 Preservation of the C-terminus of dystrophin molecule in the skeletal muscle from Becker muscular dystrophy. Journal of the Neurological Sciences 101: 148

Arikawa E, Ishihara T, Nonaka I, Sugita H, Arahata K 1991 Immunocytochemical analysis of dystrophin in congenital muscular dystrophy. Journal of the Neurological Sciences 105: 79

Askanas V, Bornemann A, Engel W K 1990 Immuno-cytochemical localization of desmin at human neuromuscular junctions. Neurology 40: 949

Askanas V, Serdaroglu P, Engel W K, Alvarez R B 1991 Immunolocalisation of ubiquitin in muscle biopsies of patients with inclusion body myositis and oculopharyngeal muscular dystrophy. Neuroscience Letters 130: 73

Askanas V, Engel W K, Alvarez R B 1992 Light and electron microscopic localisation of β-amyloid protein in muscle biopsies of patients with inclusion body myositis. American Journal of Pathology 141: 31

Augier N, Boucraut J, Leger J et al 1992 A homologue of dystrophin is expressed at the blood vessel membrane of DMD and BMD patients: immunological evidence. Journal of the Neurological Sciences 107: 233

Bancroft J D, Stevens A (eds) 1982 Theory and practice of histological techniques, 2nd edn. Churchill Livingstone, Edinburgh

Bao S, King N J C, dos Remedios C G 1990 Elevated MHC class I and II antigens in cultured human embryonic myoblasts following stimulation with γ-interferon. Immunology and Cell Biology 68: 235

Bar S, Barnea E, Levy Z, Neumann S, Yaffe D, Nudel U 1990 A novel product of the DMD gene which greatly differs from the known isoforms in its structure and tissue distribution. Biochemical Journal 272: 557

Barnea E, Zuk D, Simantov R, Nudel U, Yaffe D 1990 Specificity of expression of the muscle and brain dystrophin gene promoters in muscle and brain cells. Neuron 5: 881

Battifora H 1988 Desmin and sarcomeric myosin in the diagnosis of rhabdomyosarcoma. In: De Lellis R A (ed) Advances in immunohistochemistry. Raven Press, New York, p 223

Baumbach L L, Chamberlain J S, Ward P A, Farwell N J, Caskey C T 1989 Molecular and clinical correlations of deletions leading to Duchenne and Becker muscular dystrophies. Neurology 39: 465

Becker P E, Kiener F 1955 Eine neue X-chromosomale Muskeldystrophie. Archiv für Psychiatrie und Nervenkrankenheiten 193: 427

Beggs A H, Neumann P E, Arahata K et al 1992 Possible influences on the expression of X chromosome-linked dystrophin abnormalities by heterozygosity for autosomal recessive Fukuyama congenital muscular dystrophy. Proceedings of the National Academy of Sciences USA 89: 623

Ben Hamida M, Fardeau M, Attia N 1983 Severe childhood

muscular dystrophy affecting both sexes and frequent in Tunisia. Muscle and Nerve 6: 469

Ben Jelloun-Dellagi S, Chaffey P, Hentati F et al 1990 Presence of normal dystrophin in Tunisian severe childhood autosomal recessive muscular dystrophy. Neurology 40: 1903

Ben Othmane K, Ben Hamida M, Pericak-Vance M et al 1992 Linkage of Tunisian autosomal recessive Duchenne-like muscular dystrophy to the pericentromeric region of chromosome 13q. Nature Genetics 2: 315

Bertolotto A, Palmucci L, Doriguzzi C et al 1983 Laminin and fibronectin distribution in normal and pathological human muscle. Journal of the Neurological Sciences 60: 377

Bethlem J, van Wijngaarden G K, Meijer A E F H, Hülsmann W C 1969 Neuromuscular disease with type 1 fiber atrophy, central nuclei, and myotube-like structures. Neurology 19: 705

Billeter R, Weber H, Lutz H, Howald H, Eppenberger H M, Jenny E 1980 Myosin types in human skeletal muscle fibers. Histochemistry 65: 249

Biral D, Scarpini E, Angelini C, Salviati G, Margreth A 1989 Myosin heavy chain composition of fibers in spinal muscular atrophy. Muscle and Nerve 12: 43

Bird J W C, Spanier A M, Schwartz W N 1978 Cathepsin B and D: proteolytic activity and ultrastructural localisation in skeletal muscle. In: Segal H L, Doyl D J (eds) Protein turnover and lysosome function. Academic, New York, p 589

Blake D J, Love D R, Tinsley J et al 1992 Characterisation of a 4.8 kb transcript from the Duchenne muscular dystrophy locus expressed in Schwannoma cells. Human Molecular Genetics 1: 103

Bloch R J, Pumplin D W 1988 Molecular events in synaptogenesis: nerve-muscle adhesion and postsynaptic differentiation. American Journal of Physiology 254: C364

Bodensteiner J 1988 Congenital myopathies. Neurologic Clinics 6: 499

Bonilla E, Schotland D L 1970 Histochemical diagnosis of muscle phosphofructokinase deficiency. Archives of Neurology (Chicago) 22: 8

Bonilla E, Schotland D L, Wakayama Y 1978 Duchenne dystrophy: focal alterations in the distribution of Concanavalin A binding sites at the muscle cell surface. Annals of Neurology 4: 117

Bonilla E, Miranda A F, Prelle A et al 1988a Immunocytochemical study of nebulin in Duchenne muscular dystrophy. Neurology 38: 1600

Bonilla E, Samitt C E, Miranda A F et al 1988b Duchenne muscular dystrophy: deficiency of dystrophin at the muscle cell surface. Cell 54: 447

Bonilla E, Samitt C E, Miranda A F et al 1988c Normal and dystrophin-deficient muscle fibers in carriers of the gene for Duchenne muscular dystrophy. American Journal of Pathology 133: 440

Bornemann A, Schmalbruch H 1992 Desmin and vimentin in regenerating fibres. Muscle and Nerve 15: 14

Bowles N E, Dubowitz V, Sewry C A, Archard L C 1987 Dermatomyositis, polymyositis, and coxsackie B virus infection. Lancet i: 1004

Bradley W G, Jones M Z, Mussini J-M, Fawcett P R W 1978 Becker-type muscular dystrophy. Muscle and Nerve 1: 111

Bressler R 1970 Carnitine and the twins (editorial). New England Journal of Medicine 282: 745

Brooke M H 1973 A neuromuscular disease characterized by fiber type disproportion. In: Kakulas B A (ed) Proceedings of II International Congress on Muscle Disease, ICS No 237. Excerpta Medica, Amsterdam

Brooke M H, Engel W K 1969 The histographic analysis of human muscle biopsies with regard to fibre types. 4. Children's biopsies. Neurology (Minneapolis) 19: 591

Brooke M H, Kaiser K K 1970 Muscle fiber types: how many and what kind? Archives of Neurology 23: 369

Buckingham M E 1985 Actin and myosin multigene family: their expression during the formation of skeletal muscle. Essays in Biochemistry 20: 77

Burrow K L, Coovert D D, Klein C J et al 1991 Dystrophin expression and somatic reversion in prednisone-treated and untreated Duchenne muscular dystrophy. Neurology 41: 661

Bushby K 1992 Report on the 12th ENMC sponsored international workshop — the 'limb-girdle' muscular dystrophies. Neuromuscular Disorders 2: 3

Bushby K M D, Cleghorn N J, Curtis A et al 1991 Identification of a mutation in the promoter region of the dystrophin gene in a patient with atypical Becker muscular dystrophy. Human Genetics 88: 195

Butler-Browne G S, Barbet J P, Thornell L E 1990 Myosin heavy and light chain expression during human skeletal muscle development and the precocious accumulation of the adult heavy chain isoforms by thyroid hormone. Anatomy and Embryology 181: 513

Byers T J, Kunkel L M, Watkins S C 1991 The subcellular distribution of dystrophin in mouse skeletal, cardiac, and smooth muscle. Journal of Cell Biology 115: 411

Campbell K P, Kahl S D 1989 Association of dystrophin and an integral membrane glycoprotein. Nature 338: 259

Capaldi M J, Dunn M J, Sewry C A, Dubowitz V 1984a Altered binding of *Ricinus communis* I lectin by muscle membranes in Duchenne muscular dystrophy. Journal of the Neurological Sciences 63: 129

Capaldi M J, Dunn M J, Sewry C A, Dubowitz V 1984b Binding of *Ricinus communis* I lectin to the muscle cell plasma membrane in diseased muscle. Journal of the Neurological Sciences 64: 315

Capaldi M J, Dunn M J, Sewry C A, Dubowitz V 1985 Lectin binding in human skeletal muscle: a comparison of 15 different lectins. Histochemical Journal 17: 81

Capaldi R 1988 Mitochondrial myopathies and respiratory chain proteins. Trends in Biological Sciences 13: 144

Carpenter S, Karpati G, Heller I, Eisen A 1978 Inclusion body myositis: a distinct variety of idiopathic inflammatory myopathy. Neurology 28: 8

Cashman N R, Covault J, Wollman R L, Sanes J R 1987 Neural cell adhesion molecule in normal, denervated, and myopathic muscle. Annals of Neurology 21: 481

Castro L, Coelho T, Pinheiro A V, Guimaraes A 1990 Tubular aggregates in a case of central core disease. Journal of the Neurological Sciences 98: 337

Chamberlain J S, Pearlman J A, Muzny D M et al 1988 Expression of the murine Duchenne muscular dystrophy gene in muscle and brain. Science 239: 1416

Chelly J, Gilgencrantz H, Lambert M et al 1990a Effect of dystrophin gene deletions on mRNA levels and processing in Duchenne and Becker muscular dystrophies. Cell 63: 1239

Chelly J, Hamard G, Koulakoff A, Kaplan J-C, Kahn A, Berwald-Netter Y 1990b Dystrophin gene transcribed from different promoters in neuronal and glial cells. Nature 344: 64

Chou S M 1986 Inclusion body myositis: a chronic persistent mumps myositis? Human Pathology 17: 765

Clemens P R, Ward P A, Caskey C T, Bulman D E, Fenwick R G 1992 Premature chain termination causing Duchenne muscular dystrophy. Neurology 42: 1755

Clerk A, Rodillo E, Heckmatt J Z, Dubowitz V, Strong P N, Sewry C A 1991a Characterisation of dystrophin in carriers of Duchenne muscular dystrophy. Journal of the Neurological Sciences 102: 197

Clerk A, Strong P N, Sewry C A 1991b Characterisation of dystrophin during development of human skeletal muscle. Development 114: 395

Clerk A, Dubowitz V, Sewry C A, Strong P N 1992 Characterisation of dystrophin in foetuses at risk for Duchenne muscular dystrophy. Journal of the Neurological Sciences 111: 82

Comola M, Johnson M A, Howel D, Brunsdon C 1987 Spatial distribution of muscle necrosis in biopsies from patients with inflammatory muscle disorders. Journal of the Neurological Sciences 82: 229

Conen P E, Murphy E G, Donohue W L 1963 Light and electron microscopic studies of 'myogranules' in a child with hypotonia and muscle weakness. Canadian Medical Association Journal 89: 983

Cooper B J, Gallagher E A, Smith C A, Valentine B A, Winand N J 1990 Mosaic expression of dystrophin in carriers of canine X-linked muscular dystrophy. Laboratory Investigation 62: 171

Cori G T 1958 Biochemical aspects of glycogen deposition diseases. Modern Problems in Pediatrics 3: 344

Cornelio F, Dones I 1984 Muscle fiber degeneration and necrosis in muscular dystrophy and other muscle diseases. Annals of Neurology 6: 694

Covault J, Sanes J R 1985 Neural cell adhesion molecule (N-CAM) accumulates in denervated and paralyzed skeletal muscles. Proceedings of the National Academy of Sciences USA 82: 4544

Covault J, Sanes J R 1986 Distribution of N-CAM in synaptic and extrasynaptic portions of adult and developing skeletal muscles. Journal of Cell Biology 102: 716

Cullen M J, Appleyard S T, Bindoff L 1979 Morphological aspects of muscle breakdown and lysosomal activation. Annals of the New York Academy of Sciences 317: 440

Cullen M J, Walsh J, Nicholson L V B, Harris J B 1990 Ultrastructural localisation of dystrophin in human muscle by gold immunolabelling. Proceedings of the Royal Society of Medicine London B 240: 197

Cullen M J, Walsh F, Nicholson L V B, Harris J B, Zubrzycka-Gaarn E E, Ray P N, Worton R G 1991 Immunogold labelling of dystrophin in human muscle using an antibody to the last 17 amino acids of the C-terminus. Neuromuscular Disorders 1: 113

Cullen M J, Fulthorpe J J, Harris J B 1992 The distribution of desmin and titin in normal and dystrophic human muscle. Acta Neuropathologica 83: 158

De Angelis M S, Palmucci L, Leone M, Doriguzzi C 1991 Centronuclear myopathy: clinical, morphological and genetic characters. A review of 288 cases. Journal of Neurological Sciences 103: 2

Dhoot G K, Pearce G W 1984a Changes in the distribution of fast and slow forms of troponin I in some neuromuscular disorders. Journal of the Neurological Sciences 65: 1

Dhoot G K, Pearce G W 1984b Transformation of fibre types in muscular dystrophies. Journal of the Neurological Sciences 65: 17

Dickson G, Pizzey J A, Elsom V E, Love D, Davies K E, Walsh F S 1988 Distinct dystrophin mRNA species are expressed in embryonic and adult mouse skeletal muscle. FEBS Letters 242: 47

DiMauro S, Arnold S, Miranda A, Rowland L P 1978 McArdle disease; the mystery of reappearing phosphorylase activity in muscle culture — a fetal isoenzyme. Annals of Neurology 3: 60

DiMauro S, Miranda A F, Khan S, Gitlin K, Friedman R 1981 Human muscle phosphoglycerate mutase deficiency: newly discovered metabolic myopathy. Science 212: 1277

DiMauro S, Dalakas M, Miranda A F 1983 Phosphoglycerate kinase deficiency: another cause of recurrent myoglobinuria. Annals of Neurology 13: 11

DiMauro S, Lombes A, Nakase H et al 1990 Cytochrome c oxidase deficiency. Pediatric Research 28: 536

Dolly O J, Barnard E A 1984 Nicotinic acetylcholine receptors: an overview. Biochemical Pharmacology 33: 841

Doriguzzi C, Mongini T, Palmucci L, Schiffer D 1983 A new method for myofibrillar Ca^{++}-ATPase reaction based on the use of metachromatic dyes: its advantages in muscle fibre typing. Histochemistry 79: 289

Draeger A, Weeds A, Fitzsimons R B 1987 Primary, secondary and tertiary myotubes in developing skeletal muscle: a new approach to the analysis of human myogenesis. Journal of the Neurological Sciences 81: 19

Duance V C, Stephens H R, Dunn M J, Bailey A J, Dubowitz V 1980 A role for collagen in the pathogenesis of muscular dystrophy? Nature (London) 284: 470

Dubowitz V 1964 Infantile muscular atrophy. A prospective study with particular reference to a slowly progressive variety. Brain 87: 707

Dubowitz V 1967 Pathology of experimentally re-innervated skeletal muscle. Journal of Neurology, Neurosurgery and Psychiatry 30: 99

Dubowitz V 1978 Muscle disorders in childhood. Saunders, London

Dubowitz V 1980 The floppy infant, 2nd edn. Clinics in Developmental Medicine No 76. Spastics International Medical Publications, Blackwell Scientific Publications, Oxford

Dubowitz V 1985 Muscle biopsy: a practical approach, 2nd edn. Baillière Tindall, London

Dubowitz V, Brooke M H 1973 Muscle biopsy: A modern approach. Saunders, London

Dubowitz V, Pearse A G E 1961 Enzymic activity of normal and diseased human muscle: a histochemical study. Journal of Pathology and Bacteriology 81: 365

Dubrovsky A L, Engel W K 1976 New histochemical technique for demonstrating adenyl cyclase in nervous tissue and muscle. Archives of Neurology 33: 386

Dunn M J, Sewry C A, Dubowitz V 1982 Cytochemical studies of lectin binding by diseased human muscle. Journal of the Neurological Sciences 55: 147

Dunn M J, Sewry C A, Statham H E, Dubowitz V 1984 Studies on the extracellular matrix in diseased human muscle. In: Kemp R B, Hinchcliffe J R (eds) Matrices and cell differentiation. Alan R Liss, New York, p 213

Edström L, Thornell L-E, Eriksson L 1980 A new type of hereditary distal myopathy with characteristic sarcoplasmic bodies and intermediate (skeletin) filaments. Journal of the Neurological Sciences 47: 171

Edwards R H T, Maunder C, Lewis P D, Pearse A G E 1973 Percutaneous needle biopsy in the diagnosis of muscle diseases. Lancet ii: 1070

Edwards R H T, Maunder C A 1977 Muscle biopsy. Hospital Update, October: 569

Edwards R H T, Round J M, Jones D A 1983 Needle biopsy of skeletal muscle: a review of 10 years' experience. Muscle and Nerve 6: 676

Emery A E H, Dreifuss F E 1966 Unusual type of benign X-linked muscular dystrophy. Journal of Neurology, Neurosurgery and Psychiatry 29: 338

Emslie-Smith A, Arahata K, Engel A G 1989 Major histocompatibility complex class I antigen expression, immunolocalization of interfon subtypes, and T cell-mediated cytotoxicity in myopathies. Human Pathology 20: 224

Emslie-Smith A M, Engel A G 1990 Microvascular changes in early and advanced dermatomyositis: a quantitative study. Annals of Neurology 27: 343

Engel A G, Gomez M R, Groover R V 1971 Multicore disease. Mayo Clinic Proceedings 10: 666

Engel A G, Angelini C, Gomez M R 1972 Fingerprint body myopathy. Mayo Clinic Proceedings 47: 377

Engel A G, Lambert E H, Howard F M 1977 Immune complexes (IgG and C3) at the motor end-plate in myasthenia gravis. Ultrastructural and light microscopic localization and electrophysiologic correlations. Mayo Clinic Proceedings 52: 267

Engel A G, Biesecker G 1982 Complement activation in muscle fiber necrosis: demonstration of the membrane attack complex of complement in necrotic fibers. Annals of Neurology 12: 289

Engel A G, Arahata K 1984 Monoclonal antibody analysis of mononuclear cells in myopathies. II Phenotypes of autoinvasive cells in polymyositis and inclusion body myositis. Annals of Neurology 16: 209

Engel W K 1961 Muscle target fibres, a newly recognized sign of denervation. Nature (London) 191: 389

Engel W K 1967 Focal myopathic changes produced by electromyographic and hypodermic needles. Archives of Neurology 16: 509

Engel W K 1977 Integrative histochemical approach to the defect of Duchenne muscular dystrophy. In: Rowland L P (ed) Pathogenesis of human muscular dystrophies. Excerpta Medica, Amsterdam, p 277

Engel W K 1979 Muscle fiber regeneration in human neuromuscular disease. In: Mauro A (ed) Muscle regeneration. Raven, New York, p 285

Engel W K, Cunningham G C 1963 Rapid examination of muscle tissue. An improved trichrome method for fresh-frozen biopsy sections. Neurology (Minneapolis) 13: 919

Engel W K, Brooke M H 1966 Histochemistry of the myotonic disorders. In: Kuhn E (ed) Progressive muskeldystrophie, myotonie, myasthenie. Springer, Stuttgart, p 203

Engel W K, Gold G N, Karpati G 1968 Type I fibre hypotrophy and central nuclei. A rare congenital muscle abnormality with a possible experimental model. Archives of Neurology (Chicago) 18: 435

Engel W K, Cunningham G G 1970 Alkaline phosphatase-positive abnormal muscle fibers of humans. Journal of Histochemistry and Cytochemistry 18: 55

Engel W K, Bishop D W, Cunningham G G 1970a Tubular aggregates in type II muscle fibers: ultrastructural and histochemical correlation. Journal of Ultrastructural Research 31: 507

Engel W K, Vick N A, Glueck C J, Levy R I 1970b A skeletal muscle disorder associated with intermittent symptoms and a possible defect of lipid metabolism. New England Journal of Medicine 282: 697

Ervasti J M, Campbell K P 1991 Membrane organisation of the dystrophin–glycoprotein complex. Cell 66: 1121

Ervasti J M, Ohlendieck K, Kahl S D, Gaver M G, Campbell K P 1990 Deficiency of a glycoprotein component of the dystrophin complex in dystrophic muscle. Nature 345: 315

Evered D, Whealan J (eds) 1988 Plasticity of the neuromuscular system. Ciba Foundation Symposium 138. Wiley, Chichester

Fanin M, Danieli G A, Vitiello L, Senter L, Angelini C 1992 Prevelance of dystrophin positive fibers in 85 Duchenne muscular dystrophy patients. Neuromuscular Disorders 2: 41

Fardeau M 1982 Congenital myopathies. In: Mastaglia F L, Walton J (eds) Skeletal muscle pathology. Churchill Livingstone, Edinburgh, p 161

Fardeau M, Tomé F M S, Derambure S 1976 Familial fingerprint body myopathy. Archives of Neurology 33: 724

Feener C A, Koenig M, Kunkel L M 1989 Alternative splicing of human dystrophin mRNA generates isoforms at the carboxy terminus. Nature 338: 509

Fidzianska A, Goebel M, Osborn M et al 1983 Mallory body-like inclusions in a hereditary congenital neuromuscular disease. Muscle and Nerve 6: 195

Figarella-Branger D, Nedelec J, Pellisier J F, Boucraut J, Bianco N, Rougon G 1990 Expression of various isoforms of neural cell adhesive molecules and their highly polysialylated counterparts in diseased human muscles. Journal of the Neurological Sciences 98: 21

Figarella-Branger D, Calore E E, Boucraut J, Bianco N, Rougon G, Pellisier J F 1992a Expression of cell surface and cytoskeleton developmentally regulated proteins in adult centronuclear myopathies. Journal of the Neurological Sciences 109: 69

Figarella-Branger D, Pellissier J F, Bianco N, Pons F, Leger J J, Rougon G 1992b Expression of various NCAM isoforms in human embryonic muscles: correlation with myosin heavy chain phenotypes. Journal of Neuropathology and Experimental Neurology 51: 12

Filipe M I, Lake B D (eds) 1990 Histochemistry in pathology, 2nd edn. Churchill Livingstone, Edinburgh

Fishbein W N, Armbrustmacher V W, Griffin J L 1978 Myoadenylate deaminase deficiency — a new disease of muscle. Science 200: 545

Fitzsimons R B, Hoh J F Y 1981 Embryonic and foetal myosins in human skeletal muscle. The presence of foetal myosins in Duchenne muscular dystrophy and infantile spinal muscular atrophy. Journal of the Neurological Sciences 52: 367

Fitzsimons R B, Sewry C A 1985 Immunocytochemistry of muscle. In: Dubowitz V (ed) Muscle biopsy: a practical approach, 2nd edn. Baillière Tindall, London, p 184

Forbes G B 1953 Glycogen disease. Report of a case with abnormal glycogen storage structure in liver and skeletal muscle. Journal of Pediatrics 42: 645

Froes M M Q, Kristmundsdottir F, Mahon M, Cumming W J K 1987 Muscle morphometry in motor neurone disease. Neuropathology and Applied Neurobiology 13: 405

Fürst D, Nave R, Osborn M et al 1987 Nebulin and titin expression in Duchenne muscular dystrophy appears normal. FEBS Letters 224: 49

Gangopadhyay S B, Sherratt T G, Heckmatt J Z et al 1992 Dystrophin frame shift deletion in patients with Becker muscular dystrophy. American Journal of Human Genetics 51: 562

Garabedian B, Morel E 1983 Monoclonal antibodies against the human acetylcholine receptor. Biochemical and Biophysical Research Communications 113: 1

Garlepp M J, Dawkins R L 1984 Immunological aspects. In: Ansell B (ed) Clinics in rheumatic diseases, vol 10. Saunders, London, p 35

Geng Y, Sicinski P, Gorecki D, Barnard P J 1991 Developmental and tissue-specific regulation of mouse dystrophin: the embryonic isoform in muscular dystrophy. Neuromuscular Disorders 1: 125

Gilliam T, Brzustowicz L, Casilla L et al 1990 Genetic homogeneity between acute and chronic forms of spinal muscular atrophy. Nature 345: 823

Giorno R, Barden M T, Kohler P F, Ringel S P 1984 Immunohistochemical characterization of the mononuclear cells infiltrating muscle of patients with inflammatory and non-inflammatory myopathies. Clinical Immunology and Immunopathology 30: 405

Goebel H H 1991 Congenital myopathies. Acta Paediatrica Japonica 33: 247

Goebels N, Michaelis D, Wekerle H, Hohlfeld R 1992 Human myoblasts as antigen presenting cells. Journal of Immunology 149: 661

Gold R, Meurers B, Reichmann H, Kress W, Mueller C R 1990 Duchenne muscular dystrophy: evidence of somatic reversion of the mutation in man. Journal of the Neurological Sciences 237: 494

Gonatas N K, Shy G M, Godfrey E H 1966 Nemaline myopathy. The origin of nemaline structures. New England Journal of Medicine 274: 535

Granger B L, Lazarides E 1980 Synemin: a new high molecular weight protein associated with desmin and vimentin filaments in muscle. Cell 22: 727

Greenfield J G, Cornman T, Shy G M 1958 The prognostic value of the muscle biopsy in the floppy infant. Brain 81: 461

Guerard M J, Sewry C A, Dubowitz V 1985 Lobulated fibres in neuromuscular diseases. Journal of the Neurological Sciences 69: 345

Hammans S R, Sweeney M G, Holt I J et al 1992 Evidence for intramitochondrial complementation between deleted and normal mitochondrial DNA in some patients with mitochondrial myopathy. Journal of the Neurological Sciences 107: 87

Hantaï D, Labat-Robert J, Grimaud J A, Fardeau M 1985 Fibronectin, laminin, type I, III and IV collagens in Duchenne's muscular dystrophy, congenital muscular dystrophies and congenital myopathies: an immunocytochemical study. Connective Tissue Research 13: 273

Harper P S 1979 Muscle pathology in myotonic dystrophy. In: Harper P S (ed) Myotonic dystrophy. Saunders, Philadelphia, p 250

Harriman D G F 1982 The pathology of malignant hyperpyrexia. In: Mastaglia F L, Walton J (eds) Skeletal muscle pathology. Churchill Livingstone, Edinburgh, p 575

Hasegawa H, Matsuoka T, Goto Y, Nonaka I 1991 Strongly succinate dehydrogenase-reactive blood vessels in muscles from patients with mitochondrial myopathy, encephalopathy, lactic acidosis, and stroke-like episodes. Annals of Neurology 29: 601

Heckmatt J Z, Moosa A, Hutson C, Maunder-Sewry C A, Dubowitz V 1984 Diagnostic needle muscle biopsy: a practical and reliable alternative to open biopsy. Archives of Disease in Childhood 59: 528

Heckmatt J Z, Dubowitz V 1985 Diagnostic advantage of needle biopsy and ultrasound imaging in the detection of focal pathology in a girl with limb girdle dystrophy. Muscle and Nerve 8: 705

Heckmatt J Z, Sewry C A, Hodes D, Dubowitz V 1985 Congenital centronuclear (myotubular) myopathy. A clinical, pathological and genetic study in eight children. Brain 18: 941

Helliwell T R, Gunhan O, Edwards R H T 1989 Lectin binding and desmin necrosis, regeneration, and neurogenic atrophy of human skeletal muscle. Journal of Pathology 159: 43

Helliwell T R, Ellis J M, Mountford R C, Appleton R E, Morris G E 1992a A truncated dystrophin lacking the C-terminal domain is localized at the muscle membrane. American Journal of Human Genetics 50: 508

Helliwell T R, Nguyen thi Man, Morris G E, Davies K E 1992b The dystrophin-related protein, utrophin, is expressed on the sarcolemma of regenerating human skeletal muscle fibres in dystrophies and inflammatory myopathies. Neuromuscular Disorders 2: 177

Hermansen L, Wachtlova M 1971 Capillary density of skeletal muscle in well-trained and untrained men. Journal of Applied Physiology 30: 860

Hodgson S V, Boswinkel E, Cole C et al 1986 A linkage study of Emery–Dreifuss muscular dystrophy. Human Medical Genetics 74: 409

Hoffman E P, Brown R H, Kunkel L M 1987 Dystrophin: the protein product of the Duchenne muscular dystrophy locus. Cell 51: 919

Hoffman E P, Fischbeck K H, Brown R H et al 1988 Dystrophin analysis in muscle biopsies from Duchenne and Becker muscular dystrophy. New England Journal of Medicine 318: 1363

Hoffman E P, Kunkel L M 1989 Dystrophin abnormalities in Duchenne/Becker muscular dystrophy. Neuron 2: 1019

Hoffman E P, Arahata K, Minetti C et al 1992 Dystrophinopathy in isolated cases of myopathy in females. Neurology 42: 967

Hohlfeld R, Engel A G 1990 Induction of HLA-DR expression on human myoblasts with interferon-gamma. American Journal of Pathology 136: 503

Hohlfeld R, Engel A G, Kunio I, Harper M C 1991 Polymyositis mediated by lymphocytes that express the γ/σ receptor. New England Journal of Medicine 324: 877

Holt I J, Harding A E, Morgan-Hughes J A 1988 Deletions of muscle mitochondrial DNA in patients with mitochondrial myopathies. Nature 331: 717

Holt I J, Harding A E, Cooper J M et al 1989 Mitochondrial myopathies: clinical and biochemical features of 30 patients with major deletions of muscle mitochondrial DNA. Annals of Neurology 26: 699

Holthofer H, Virtanen I, Karniemi A L et al 1982 Ulex europaeus I lectin as a marker for vascular endothelium in human tissues. Laboratory Investigation 47: 60

Horowits R, Kempner E S, Bisher E, Podolsky R J 1986 A physiological role for titin and nebulin in skeletal muscle. Nature 323: 160

Hsu S-M, Raine L, Fanger H 1981 Use of avidin–biotin–peroxidase complex (ABC) in immunoperoxidase techniques. Journal of Histochemistry and Cytochemistry 29: 577

Hudgson P, Hall R 1982 Endocrine myopathies. In: Mastaglia F L, Walton J (eds) Skeletal muscle pathology. Churchill Livingstone, Edinburgh, p 393

Hurko O, Walsh F S 1983 Human fetal muscle-specific antigen is restricted to regenerating myofibres in diseased adult muscle. Neurology 33: 737

Ibraghimov-Beskrovnaya O, Ervasti J M, Leveille C J, Slaughter C A, Sernett S W, Campbell K P 1992 Primary structure of dystrophin-associated glycoproteins linking dystrophin to the extracellular matrix. Nature 355: 696

Illa I, Leon-Monzon M, Dalakas C 1992 Regenerating and denervated human muscle fibres and satellite cells express neural cell adhesion molecule recognized by monoclonal antibodies to natural killer cells. Annals of Neurology 31: 46

Illingworth B, Cori G T 1952 Structure of glycogens and amylopectins. III Normal and abnormal human glycogen. Journal of Biological Chemistry 199: 653

Isaacs H, Heffron J J A, Badenhorst M 1975 Central core disease: a correlated genetic, histochemical, ultrastructural and biochemical study. Journal of Neurology, Neurosurgery and Psychiatry 38: 1177

Isenberg D A 1983 Immunoglobulin deposition in skeletal muscle in primary muscle disease. Quarterly Journal of Medicine 207: 297

Isenberg D A, Rowe D, Shearer M, Novick D M, Beverley P C L 1986 Localisation of interferons and interleukin 2 in polymyositis and muscular dystrophy. Clinical and Experimental Immunology 63: 450

Iyer V, Lawton A R, Fenichel G M 1983 T-cell subsets in polymyositis. Annals of Neurology 13: 452

Izumo S, Nadal-Ginard B, Mahdavi V 1986 All members of the MHC multigene family respond to thyroid hormone in a highly tissue-specific manner. Science 231: 597

Jennekens F G I, Roord J J, Veldman H, Willemse J, Jockusch B M 1983 Congenital nemaline myopathy. I Defective organization of α-actinin is restricted to muscle. Muscle and Nerve 6: 61

Jerusalem F, Engel A G, Gomez M R 1973 Sarcotubular myopathy; a newly recognized benign, congenital, familial muscle disease. Neurology 23: 897

Jerusalem F, Ludin H, Bischoff A, Hartmann G 1979 Cytoplasmic body neuromyopathy presenting as respiratory failure and weight loss. Journal of the Neurological Sciences 41: 1

Jockusch B M, Veldman H, Griffiths G W, van Oost B A, Jennekens F G I 1980 Immunofluorescence microscopy of a myopathy. α-Actinin is a major constituent of nemaline rods. Experimental Cell Research 127: 409

Johnson M A, Polgar J, Weightman D, Appleton D 1973 Data on the distribution of fibre types in 36 human muscles. An autopsy study. Journal of the Neurological Sciences 18: 111

Johnson M A, Kucukyalcin D K 1978 Patterns of abnormal histochemical fibre type differentiation in human muscle biopsies. Journal of the Neurological Sciences 37: 159

Johnson M A, Kadenback B, Droste M, Old S L, Turnbull D M 1988 Immunocytochemical studies of cytochrome oxidase subunits in skeletal muscle of patients with partial cytochrome oxidase deficiency. Journal of the Neurological Sciences 87: 75

Jones G E, Murphy S, Watt D J 1990 Segregation of the myogenic cell lineage in mouse muscle development. Journal of Cell Science 97: 659

Kadenbach B, Jarausch J, Hatmann R, Merle P 1983 Separation of mammalian cytochrome c oxidase into 13 polypeptides by a sodium dodecyl sulfate-gel electrophoretic procedure. Annals of Biochemistry 129: 113

Kanno T, Sudok Takeuchi I, Kanda S, Honda N, Nishimura Y, Oyamak et al 1980 Hereditary deficiency of lactate dehydrogenase M-subunit. Clinica Chimica Acta 108: 267

Kar N C, Pearson C M 1978 Muscular dystrophy and activation of proteinases. Muscle and Nerve 1: 308

Kar N C, Pearson C M 1979 Activity of some proteolytic enzymes in normal and dystrophic human muscle. Clinical Biochemistry 12: 37

Karpati G, Carpenter S, Nelson R F 1970 Type I muscle fibre atrophy and central nuclei. A rare familial neuromuscular disease. Journal of the Neurological Sciences 10: 489

Karpati G, Pouliot Y, Carpenter S 1988 Expression of immunoreactive major histocompatibility complex products in human skeletal muscles. Annals of Neurology 23: 64

Karpati G, Zubrzycka-Gaarn E E, Carpenter S, Bulman D E, Ray P N, Worton R G 1990 Age-related conversion of dystrophin-negative to positive fiber segments of skeletal but not cardiac muscle fibres in heterozygote mdx mice. Journal of Neuropathology and Experimental Neurology 49: 96

Kausch K, Lehmann-Horn F, Janka M, Wieringa B, Grimm T, Müller C 1991 Evidence for linkage of the central core disease locus to the proximal long arm of human chromosome 19. Genomics 10: 765

Khurana T S, Hoffman E P, Kunkel L M 1990 Identification of a chromosome 6 encoded dystrophin related protein. Journal of Biological Chemistry 265: 16717

Khurana T S, Watkins S C, Chafey P et al 1991 Immunolocalization and development of dystrophin related protein in skeletal muscle. Neuromuscular Disorders 1: 185

Klein C J, Coovert D D, Bulman D E, Ray P N, Mendell J R, Burghes A H M 1992 Somatic reversion/suppression in Duchenne muscular dystrophy (DMD): evidence supporting a frame-restoring mechanism in rare dystrophin-positive fibers. American Journal of Human Genetics 50: 950

Koenig M, Hoffman E P, Bertelson C J, Monaco A P, Feener C, Kunkel L M 1987 Complete cloning of the Duchenne muscular dystrophy (DMD) cDNA and preliminary genomic organisation of the DMD gene in normal and affected individuals. Cell 50: 509

Krivit W, Polglase W J, Gunn F D, Tyler F H 1953 Studies in disorders of muscle. IX Glycogen storage disease primarily affecting skeletal muscle and clinically resembling amyotonia congenita. Pediatrics 12: 165

Kunkel L M, Hoffman E P 1989 Duchenne/Becker muscular dystrophy: a short overview of the gene, the protein, and current diagnostics. British Medical Bulletin 45: 630

Lake B D, Wilson J 1975 Zebra body myopathy: clinical, histochemical and ultrastructural studies. Journal of the Neurological Sciences 24: 437

Lanier L L, Testi R, Bindl J, Phillips J H 1989 Idenity of Leu-19 (CD56) leukocyte differentiation antigen and neural cell adhesion molecule. Journal of Experimental Medicine 169: 2233

Lazarides E 1980 Intermediate filaments as mechanical integrators of cellular space. Nature (London) 283: 249

Lazarides E, Hubbard R D 1976 Immunological characterization of the subunit of the 100 A-filaments from muscle cells. Proceedings of the National Academy of Sciences USA 73: 4344

Lewis P D, Pallis C, Pearse A G E 1971 'Myopathy' with tubular aggregates. Journal of the Neurological Sciences 13: 381

Lin M-Y, Nonaka I 1991 Facioscapulohumeral muscular dystrophy: muscle fiber type analysis with particular reference to small angular fibres. Brain and Development 13: 331

Lojda Z, Gossrau R, Schiebler T H 1979 Enzyme histochemistry: a laboratory manual. Springer, Berlin

Love D R, Hill D F, Dickson G et al 1989 An autosomal transcript in skeletal muscle with homology to dystrophin. Nature 339: 55

Love D R, Morris G E, Ellis J M et al 1991 Tissue distribution of the dystrophin-related gene product and expression in the mdx and dy mouse. Proceedings of the National Academy of Sciences USA 88: 3243

Malhotra S B, Hart K A, Thomas N S T et al 1988 Frame-shift deletions in patients with Duchenne and Becker muscular dystrophy. Science 242: 755

Marconi G, Pizzi A, Arimondi C G, Vannelli B 1991 Limb girdle muscular dystrophy with autosomal dominant inheritance. Acta Neurologica Scandinavica 83: 234

Marini J-F, Pons F, Léger J et al 1991 Expression of myosin heavy chain isoforms in Duchenne muscular dystrophy patients and carriers. Neuromuscular Disorders 1: 397

Maruyama K 1986 Connectin, an elastic filamentous protein of striated muscle. International Review of Cytology 104: 81

Mastaglia F L, Ojeda V J 1985a Inflammatory myopathies. Part I. Annals of Neurology 17: 215

Mastaglia F L, Ojeda V J 1985b Inflammatory myopathies. Part II. Annals of Neurology 17: 317

Matsumura K, Shimizu T, Nonaka I, Mannen T 1989 Immunocytochemical study of connectin (titin) in neuromuscular diseases using a monoclonal antibody: connectin is degraded extensively in Duchenne muscular dystrophy. Journal of the Neurological Sciences 93: 147

Matsumura K, Tomé F M S, Collin H et al 1992 Deficiency of the 50 K dystrophin-associated glycoprotein in severe childhood autosomal recessive muscular dystrophy. Nature 359: 320

Matsumara K, Nonaka I, Campbell K P 1993 Abnormal expression of dystrophin-associated proteins in Fukuyama-type congenital muscular dystrophy. Lancet 341: 521

Maunder-Sewry C A, Dubowitz V 1981 Needle muscle biopsy for carrier detection in Duchenne muscular dystrophy. I Light microscopy — histology, histochemistry and quantitation. Journal of the Neurological Sciences 49: 305

McArdle B 1951 Myopathy due to a defect in muscle glycogen breakdown. Clinical Science 10: 13

McDonald J K 1985 An overview of protease specificity and catalytic mechanisms: aspects related to nomenclature and classification. Histochemical Journal 17: 773

McDouall R M, Dunn M J, Dubowitz V 1989 Expression of class I and II MHC antigens in neuromuscular diseases. Journal of the Neurological Sciences 89: 213

Miike T, Miyatake M, Zhao J E, Yoshioka K, Uchino M 1989 Immunohistochemical dystrophin reaction in synaptic regions. Brain and Development 11: 344

Minetti C, Tanji K, Bonilla E 1992 Immunologic study of vinculin in Duchenne muscular dystrophy. Neurology 42: 1751

Mitsumoto H 1979 McArdle disease: phosphorylase activity in regenerating muscle fibres. Neurology 29: 258

Monaco A P, Kunkel L M 1988. Cloning of the Duchenne/Becker muscular dystrophy locus. Advances in Human Genetics 17: 61

Monaco A P, Bertelson C J, Liechti-Gallati S, Moser H, Kunkel L M 1988 An explanation for the phenotypic differences between patients bearing partial deletions of the DMD locus. Genomics 2: 90

Moore S E, Walsh F S 1985 Specific regulation of N-CAM/D2-CAM cell adhesion molecule during skeletal muscle development. EMBO Journal 4: 623

Moore S E, Walsh F S 1986 Nerve dependent regulation of neural cell adhesion molecule expression in skeletal muscle. Neuroscience 18: 499

Morgan B P, Sewry C A, Siddle K, Luzio J P, Campbell A K 1984 Immunolocalization of complement component C9 on necrotic and non-necrotic muscle fibres in myositis using monoclonal antibodies: a primary role of complement in autoimmune cell damage. Immunology 52: 181

Morgan-Hughes J A 1982 Mitochondrial myopathies. In: Mastaglia F L, Walton J (eds) Skeletal muscle pathology. Churchill Livingstone, Edinburgh, p 309

Morris C J, Raybould J A 1971 Fiber type grouping and end-plate diameter in human skeletal muscle. Journal of the Neurological Sciences 13: 181

Mukuno K 1969 Electron microscopic studies on human extraocular muscles under pathologic conditions. I. Rod formation in normal and diseased muscles (polymyositis and ocular myasthenia). Japanese Journal of Ophthalmology 13: 35

Muntoni F, Mateddu A, Marrosu M G et al 1992 Variable dystrophin expression in different muscles of a Duchenne muscular dystrophy carrier. Clinical Genetics 42: 35

Murphy S, Watt G E, Jones G E 1992 An evaluation of cell separation techniques in a model mixed cell population. Journal of Cell Science 102: 789

Neerunjun J S, Dubowitz V 1977 Concomitance of basophilia, ribonucleic acid and acid phosphatase activity in regenerating muscle fibres. Journal of the Neurological Sciences 33: 95

Neville H E 1979 Ultrastructural changes in diseases of human skeletal muscle. In: Vinken P J, Bruyn G W (eds) Handbook of clinical neurology, vol 40. Diseases of muscle, Part 1. North-Holland, Amsterdam, p 63

Neville H E, Brooke M H 1973 Central core fibers: structured and unstructured. In: Kakulas B (ed) Basic research in myology. Proceedings of International Congress on Muscle Diseases, Part I, ICS No 294. Excerpta Medica, Amsterdam, p 497

Neville H E, Maunder-Sewry C A, McDougall J, Sewell J R, Dubowitz V 1979 Chloroquine-induced cytosomes with curvilinear profiles in muscle. Muscle and Nerve 2: 376

Nguyen H T, Gubis R M, Wydro R M, Nadal-Ginard B 1982 Sarcomeric myosin heavy chain is coded by a highly conserved multigene family. Proceedings of the National Academy of Sciences USA 79: 5230

Nguyen thi Man, Ellis J M, Love D R, Davies K E, Gatter K C, Dickson G, Morris G E 1991 Localisation of the DMDL gene-encoded dystrophin-related protein using a panel of nineteen monoclonal antibodies: presence at neuromuscular junctions, in the sarcolemma of dystrophic skeletal muscle, in vascular and other smooth muscles, and in proliferating brain cell lines. Journal of Cell Biology 115: 1695

Nicholson L V B, Davison K, Falkous G et al 1989a Dystrophin in skeletal muscle. I Western blot analysis using a monoclonal antibody. Journal of the Neurological Sciences 94: 125

Nicholson L V B, Davison K, Johnson M A 1989b

Dystrophin in skeletal muscle. II Immunoreactivity in patients with Xp21 muscular dystrophy. Journal of the Neurological Sciences 94: 137

Nicholson L V B, Johnson M A, Gardner-Medwin D, Bhattacharya S, Harris J B 1990 Heterogeneity of dystrophin expression in patients with Duchenne and Becker muscular dystrophy. Acta Neuropathologica 80: 239

Nicholson L V B, Bushby K M D, Johnson M A, den Dunnen J T, Ginjaar L B, van Ommen G-J B 1992 Predicted and observed sizes of dystrophin in some patients with gene deletions that disrupt the open reading frame. Journal of Medical Genetics 29: 892

Nienhuis A W, Coleman R F, Jann Brown W, Munsat T L, Pearson C M 1967 Nemaline myopathy. A histopathologic and histochemical study. American Journal of Clincial Pathology 48: 1

Nonaka I 1992 Mitochondrial disease. Current Opinion in Neurology and Neurosurgery 5: 622

Nonaka I, Takagi A, Sugita H 1981 The significance of type 2C muscle fibres in Duchenne muscular dystrophy. Muscle and Nerve 4: 326

Nonaka I, Sunahara N, Satoyoshi E et al 1985 Autosomal recessive distal muscular dystrophy: a comparative study with distal myopathy with rimmed vacuoles. Annals of Neurology 17: 51

Nudel U, Zuk D, Einat P, Zeelon P, Levy Z, Neumann S, Yaffe D 1989. Duchenne muscular dystrophy gene product in brain is not identical to its product in muscle. Nature 337: 76

Ohlendieck K, Ervasti J M, Matsumara K, Kahl S D, Leveille C J, Campbell K P 1991a Dystrophin-related protein is localised to neuromuscular junctions of adult skeletal muscle. Neuron 7: 499

Ohlendieck K, Ervasti J M, Snook J B, Campbell K P 1991b Dystrophin–glycoprotein complex is highly enriched in isolated skeletal muscle sarcolemma. Journal of Cell Biology 112: 135

Ohtaki E 1990 Secondarily reduced cytochrome c oxidase activity in various neuromuscular disorders. Brain and Development 12: 326

Oldfors A, Larsson N-G, Holme E, Tulinius M, Kadenbach B, Droste M 1992 Mitochondrial DNA deletions and cytochrome c oxidase deficiency in muscle fibres. Journal of the Neurological Sciences 110: 169

Osborn M, Geisler N, Shaw G, Sharp G, Weber K 1982 Intermediate filaments. Cold Spring Harbor Symposia on Quantitative Biology 46: 413

Osborn M, Goebel H H 1983 The cytoplasmic bodies in a congenital myopathy can be stained with antibodies to desmin, the muscle-specific intermediate filament protein. Acta Neuropathologica (Berlin) 62: 149

Padykula H A, Hermann E 1955 The specificity of the histochemical method for adenosine triphosphate. Journal of Histochemistry and Cytochemistry 3: 170

Paljarvi L, Karjalainen K, Kalimo H 1984 Altered muscle saccharide pattern in X-linked muscular dystrophy. Archives of Neurology 41: 39

Paljarvi L, Kalimo H, Lang H, Savontaus M-L, Sonninen V 1987 Minicore myopathy with dominant inheritance. Journal of Neurological Sciences 77: 11

Pardoe J V, D'Angelo Siliciano J, Craig S W 1983 A vinculin-containing cortical lattice in skeletal muscle: transverse lattice elements ('costameres') mark sites of attachment between myofibrils and sarcolemma. Proceedings of the National Academy of Sciences USA 80: 1008

Patel K, Voit T, Dunn M J, Strong P N, Dubowitz V 1988 Dystrophin and nebulin in muscular dystrophies. Journal of the Neurological Sciences 87: 315

Paulus W, Peiffer J, Becker I, Roggendorf W, Schumm F 1988 Adult-onset disease with abundant intranuclear rods. Journal of Neurology 235: 343

Pearse A G E 1980 Histochemistry: theoretical and applied, vol 1, 4th edn. Churchill Livingstone, Edinburgh

Pearse A G E 1985 Histochemistry: theoretical and applied, vol 2, 4th edn. Churchill Livingstone, Edinburgh

Pearse A G, Johnson M 1970 Histochemistry in the study of normal and diseased muscle with special reference to myopathy with tubular aggregates. In: Walton J N, Canal N, Scarlato G (eds) Muscle diseases, ICS No 199. Excerpta Medica, Amsterdam, p 25

Pellissier J F, Pouget J, Charpin C, Figarella D 1989 Myopathy associated with desmin type intermediate filaments. An immunoelectron microscopic study. Journal of the Neurological Sciences 89: 49

Pena S D J, Gordon B B, Karpati G, Carpenter S 1981 Lectin histochemistry of human skeletal muscle. Journal of Histochemistry and Cytochemistry 29: 542

Penegyres P K, Kakulas B A 1991 The natural history of minicore-multicore myopathy. Muscle and Nerve 14: 411

Pleasure D, Bonilla E 1982 Skeletal muscle storage diseases: myopathies resulting from errors in carbohydrate and fatty acid metabolism. In: Mastaglia F L, Walton J (eds) Skeletal muscle pathology. Churchill Livingstone, Edinburgh, p 340

Polak J M, Varndell I M (eds) 1984 Immunolabelling for electron microscopy. Elsevier, Amsterdam

Ponder B A J 1983 Lectin histochemistry. In: Polak J M, van Noorden S (eds) Immunocytochemistry: practical applications in pathology and biology. Wright, Bristol, p 129

Pons F, Augier N, Léger J O C et al 1991 A homologue of dystrophin is expressed at the neuromuscular junctions of normal individuals and DMD patients, and of normal and mdx mice: immunological evidence. FEBS Letters 282: 161

Porter G A, Dmytrenko G M, Winkelmann J C, Bloch R J 1992 Dystrophin co-localizes with β-spectrin in distinct subsarcolemma domains in mammalian skeletal muscle. Journal of Cell Biology 117: 997

Prader A, Labhart A, Willi H 1956 Ein Syndrom von Adipositas, Kleinwuchs, Kryptorchismus und Oligophrenie nach myotonieartigem Zustand im Neugeborenenalter. Schweizerische medizinische Wochenschrift 86: 1260

Prader A, Willi H 1963 Das Syndrom von Imbezillitat, Adipositas, Muskelhypotonie, Hypogenitalismus, Hypogonadismus, und Diabetes Mellitus mit 'Myatonie'-anamnese, Verh 2 Int Kong Psych EntwStor Kindes-Alt Vienne 1961, pt 1, p 353

Price H M, Gordon G B, Pearson C M, Munsat T L, Blumberg J M 1965 New evidence for excessive accumulation of Z-band material in nemaline myopathy. Proceedings of the American Academy of Sciences 54: 1398

Récan D, Chafey P, Leturcq F et al 1992 Are cysteine and COOH-terminal domains critical for sarcolemmal localisation? Journal of Clinical Investigation 89: 712

Ringel S P, Carroll J E, Schold C 1977 The spectrum of mild X-linked recessive muscular dystrophy. Archives of Neurology (Chicago) 34: 408

Ringel S P, Neville H E, Duster M C, Carroll J E 1978 A new congenital neuromuscular disease with trilaminar fibers. Neurology 28: 282

Roelofs R I, Engel W K, Chauvin P B 1972 Histochemical

demonstration of phosphorylase activity in regenerating skeletal muscle fibers from myophosphorylase deficency patients. Science 177: 795

Roitt I M 1988 Essential Immunology 6th edition. Blackwell Scientific Publications, Oxford

Rosa R, George C, Fardeau M, Calvin M-C, Rapin M, Rosa J 1982 A new case of phosphoglycerate kinase deficiency: PGK creteil associated with rhabdomyolysis and lacking hemolytic anemia. Blood 60: 84

Sabatelli M, Bertini E, Ricci E et al 1992 Peripheral neuropathy with giant axons and cardiomyopathy associated with desmin type intermediate filaments in skeletal muscle. Journal of the Neurological Sciences 109: 1

Sahashi K, Engel A G, Lambert E H, Howard F M 1980 Ultrastructural localization of the terminal component (C9) at the motor end-plate in myasthenia gravis. Journal of Neuropathology and Experimental Neurology 39: 160

Saito Y 1985 Muscle fiber type differentiation and satellite cell population in W–H disease. Journal of the Neurological Sciences 68: 75

Samitt C E, Bonilla E 1990 Immunocytochemical study of dystrophin at the myotendinous junction. Muscle and Nerve 13: 493

Sanes J R, Engvall E, Butkowski R, Hunter D D 1990 Molecular heterogeneity of basal laminae: isoforms of laminin and collagen IV at the neuromuscular junction and elsewhere. Journal of Cell Biology 111: 1685

Sargeant A S, Davis C T M, Young A, Maunder C A, Edwards R H T 1977 Functional and structural changes after disuse of human muscle. Clinical Science and Molecular Medicine 52: 337

Sarnat H B 1990 Myotubular myopathy: arrest of myofibres associated with persistence of fetal vimentin and desmin. Four cases compared with fetal and neonatal muscle. Canadian Journal of Neurological Sciences 17: 109

Sarnat H B 1991 Vimentin/desmin immunoreactivity of myofibres in developmental myopathies. Acta Paediatrica Japonica 33: 238

Sarnat H B 1992 Vimentin and desmin in maturing skeletal muscle and developing myopathies. Neurology 42: 1616

Sasaki T, Shikura K, Sugai K, Nonaka I, Kumagai K 1989 Muscle histochemistry in myotubular (centronuclear) myopathy. Brain and Development 1: 26

Sato K et al 1977 Characterization of glycogen phosphorylase isoenzymes present in cultured skeletal muscle from patients with McArdle's disease. Biochemical and Biophysical Research Communications 78: 663

Sawchak J A, Lewis S, Shafiq S A 1989 Coexpression of myosin isoforms in muscle of patients with neurogenic disease. Muscle and Nerve 12: 679

Schiaffino S, Gorza L, Dones I, Cornelio F, Sartore S 1986 Fetal myosin immunoreactivity in human dystrophic muscle. Muscle and Nerve 9: 51

Schmalbruch H 1984 Regenerated muscle fibers in Duchenne muscular dystrophy: a serial section study. Neurology (Cleveland) 34: 60

Schmid R, Mahler R 1959 Chronic progressive myopathy with myoglobinuria. Demonstration of a glycogenolytic defect in the muscle. Journal of Clinical Investigation 38: 2044

Schollmeyer J V, Goll D, Stromer M H, Dayton W, Singh I, Robson R M 1974 Studies on the composition of the Z disk. Journal of Cell Biology 63: 303a

Serdaroglu P, Askanas V, Engel W K 1992 Immunocytochemical localisation of ubiquitin at human neuromuscular junctions. Neuropathology and Applied Neurobiology 18: 232

Sewry C A 1985 Ultrastructural changes in diseased muscle. In: Dubowitz V (ed) Muscle biopsy: a practical approach, 2nd edn. Baillière Tindall, London, p 129

Sewry C A 1989 Contribution of immunocytochemistry to the pathogenesis of spinal muscular atrophy. In: Merlini L, Granata C, Dubowitz V (eds) Current concepts in childhood spinal muscular atrophy. Springer, Berlin, p 57

Sewry C A, Dubowitz V 1984 Calcium and necrosis. In: Serratrice G et al (eds) Neuromuscular diseases. Raven, New York, p 131

Sewry C A, Dubowitz V, Abraha A, Luzio P, Campbell A K 1987 Immunocytochemical localisation of complement components C8 and C9 in human diseased muscle; the role of complement in muscle fibre damage. Journal of the Neurological Sciences 81: 141

Sewry C A, Appleyard S T, Dunn M J, Capaldi M J 1985 Immunocytochemistry of human skeletal muscle diseases. In: Polak J, van Noorden S (eds) Immunocytochemistry, practical applications in pathology and biology, 2nd edn. Wright, Bristol, p 664

Sewry C A, Lovegrove C, Dubowitz V 1986 Immunocytochemistry of basophilic fibres in Duchenne muscular dystrophy. Journal of Neuropathology and Neurobiology 12: 429

Sewry C A, Banati R, Fitzsimons R, Dubowitz V 1988 Immunocytochemical characterisation of 2C fibres in dystrophic muscle. Neuropathology and Applied Neuropathology 14: 257

Sewry C A, Rodillo E, Heckmatt J Z, Dubowitz V 1990 Immunocytochemical studies of congenital centronuclear and nemaline myopathies. Journal of the Neurological Sciences 98: 100

Sewry C A, Clerk A, Heckmatt J Z, Vyse T, Dubowitz V 1991 Dystrophin abnormalities in polymyositis and dermatomyositis. Neuromuscular Disorders 1: 333

Sewry C A, Wilson L A, Dux L, Dubowitz V, Cooper B J 1992a Experimental regeneration in canine muscular dystrophy. 1. Immunocytochemical evaluation of dystrophin and β-spectrin expression. Neuromuscular Disorders 2: 131

Sewry C A, Topuloglu H, Dubowitz V 1992b Myosin isoforms in congenital muscular dystrophy. 6th Congress of the International Child Neurology Association, Argentina

Sewry C A, Sansome A, Clerk A, Sherratt T, Strong P N, Dubowitz V 1993 Manifesting carriers of Xp21 muscular dystrophy: lack of correlation between dystrophin expression and clinical weakness. Neuromuscular Disorders 3: 141

Shafiq S A, Dubowitz V, Peterson H de C, Milhorat A T 1967 Nemaline myopathy: report of a fatal case with histochemical and electron microscopic studies. Brain 90: 817

Shafiq S A, Gorycki M A, Asiedu S A, Milhorat A T 1969 Tenotomy. Effects on the fine structure of the soleus of the rat. Archives of Neurology (Chicago) 20: 625

Sher J H, Rimalovski A B, Athanassiades T J, Aronson S M 1967 Familial centronuclear myopathy: a clinical and pathological study. Neurology 17: 727

Sherratt T G, Vulliamy T, Dubowitz V, Sewry C A, Strong P N 1993 Exon skipping and translation in patients with a frameshift deletion in the dystrophin gene. American Journal of Human Genetics 53: 1007

Shimizu T, Matsumura K, Hashimoto K et al 1988 A

monoclonal antibody against a synthetic polypeptide fragment of dystrophin (amino acid sequence from position 215 to 264). Proceedings of the Japan Academy 64: 205

Shimizu T, Matsumura K, Sunada Y, Mannen T 1989 Dense immunostaining on both neuromuscular and myotendinous junctions with an antidystrophin monoclonal antibody. Biomedical Research 10: 405

Shimomura C, Nonaka I 1989 Nemaline myopathy: comparative muscle histochemistry in the severe neonatal, moderate congenital and adult-onset forms. Paediatric Neurology 5: 25

Shy G M, Magee K R 1956 A new congenital non-progressive myopathy. Brain 79: 610

Shy G M, Engel W K, Somers J E, Wanko T 1963 Nemaline myopathy. A new congenital myopathy. Brain 86: 793

Slater C R, Nicholson L V B 1991 Is dystrophin labelling always discontinuous in Becker muscular dystrophy? Journal of the Neurological Sciences 101: 187

Soussi-Yanicostas N, Chevallay M, Laurent-Winter C, Tomé F M S, Fardeau M, Butler-Browne G 1991 Distinct contractile protein profile in congenital myotonic dystrophy and X-linked myotubular myopathy. Neuromuscular Disorders 1: 103

Soussi-Yanicostas N, Ben Hamida C, Bejaoui K, Hentati F, Ben Hamida M, Butler-Browne G S 1992 Evolution of muscle specific proteins in Werdnig–Hoffman disease. Journal of the Neurological Sciences 109: 111

Spiro A J, Shy G M, Gonatas N K 1966 Myotubular myopathy. Archives of Neurology (Chicago) 14: 1

Stauber W, Fritz V, Dahlmann B, Gauthier F, Kirschke H, Ulrich R 1985 Fluorescence methods of localizing proteinases and proteinase inhibitors in skeletal muscle. Histochemical Journal 17: 787

Stephens H R, Duance V C, Dunn M J, Bailey A J, Dubowitz V 1982 Collagen types in neuromuscular diseases. Journal of the Neurological Sciences 53: 45

Stoward P J, Everson Pearse A G 1991 Histochemistry, 4th edn., vol. 3. Churchill Livingstone, Edinburgh

Straub V, Bittner R E, Leger J J, Voit T 1992 Direct visualisation of the dystrophin network on skeletal muscle fiber membrane. Journal of Cell Biology 119: 1183

Sugita H, Nonaka I, Itoh Y et al 1987 Is nebulin the product of the muscular dystrophy gene? Proceedings of the Japan Academy Series B 63: 107

Takamiya S, Lindorfer M A, Capaldi R A 1987 Purification of all 13 polypeptides of bovine heart cytochrome c oxidase from one aliquot of enzyme: characteristics of bovine fetal heart cytochrome c oxidase. FEBS Letters 218: 277

Takeuchi T 1956 Histochemical demonstration of phosphorylase. Journal of Histochemistry and Cytochemistry 4: 84

Tanaka H, Ishiguro T, Eguchi C, Saito K, Ozawa E 1991 Expression of dystrophin-related protein associated with the skeletal muscle cell membrane. Histochemistry 96: 1

Telerman-Toppet N, Gerard J M, Coërs C 1973 Central core disease; a study of clinically unaffected muscle. Journal of the Neurological Sciences 19: 207

Telerman-Toppet N, Bauherz G, Noel S 1991 Auriculo-ventricular block and distal myopathy with rimmed vacuoles and desmin storage. Clinical Neuropathology 10: 61

Ten Houten R, De Visser M 1984 Histopathological findings in Becker-type muscular dystrophy. Archives of Neurology (Chicago) 41: 729

Thornell L-E, Edström L, Eriksson A, Henriksson K-G, Angqvist K A 1980 The distribution of intermediate

filament protein (skeletin) in normal and diseased human skeletal muscle. Journal of the Neurological Sciences 47: 153

Thornell L-E, Eriksson A, Edström L 1983 Intermediate filaments in human myopathies. In: Dowben R M, Shay J W (eds) Cell and muscle motility, vol 4. Plenum, New York, p 84

Thornell L-E, Billeter R, Butler-Browne G S, Erickson P-O, Ringqvist M, Whalen R G 1984 Development of fiber types in human fetal muscle; an immunocytochemical study. Journal of the Neurological Sciences 66: 107

Thornell L-E, Price M G 1991 The cytoskeleton in muscle cells in relation to function. Biochemical Society Transactions 19: 1990

Tinsley J M, Blake D J, Roche A et al 1992 Primary structure of dystrophin-related protein. Nature 360: 591

Tokuyasu K T, Dutton A H, Singer S J 1983 Immunoelectron microscopic studies of desmin (skeletin) localization and intermediate filament organization in chicken skeletal muscle. Journal of Cell Biology 96: 1727

Tomé F M S 1982 Periodic paralysis and electrolyte disorders. In: Mastaglia F L, Walton J (eds) Skeletal muscle pathology. Churchill Livingstone, London, p 287

Tomé F M S, Fardeau M 1988 Congenital myopathies. Current Opinion in Neurology and Neurosurgery 1: 782

Tonin P, Lewis P, Servidei S, DiMauro S 1990 Metabolic causes of myoglobinuria. Annals of Neurology 27: 181

Trend P St J, Wiles C M, Spencer G T, Morgan-Hughes J A, Lake B D, Patrick A D 1985 Acid maltase deficiency in adults: diagnosis and management in five cases. Brain 109: 845

Tritschler H J, Bonilla E, Lombes A et al 1991 Differential diagnosis of fatal and benign cytochrome c oxidase-deficient myopathies of infancy: an immunohistochemical approach. Neurology 41: 300

Tritschler H J, Andreetta F, Moraes C T 1992 Mitochondrial myopathy of childhood associated with depletion of mitochondrial DNA. Neurology 42: 209

Tzartos S, Lindstrom J 1980 Monoclonal antibodies used to probe acetylcholine receptor structure: localisation of the main immunogenic region and detection of similarities between subunits. Proceedings of the National Academy of Sciences USA 77: 755

Vainzof M, Pavanello R C, Pavanello-Filho I et al 1990 Dystrophin immunostaining in muscles from patients with different types of muscular dystrophies: a Brazilian study. Journal of the Neurological Sciences 98: 221

Vladutiu G D, Saponara I, Conroy J M, Grier R E, Brady L, Brady P 1992 Immunoquantitation of carnitine palmitoyl transferase in skeletal muscle of 31 patients. Neuromuscular Disorders 2: 249

van der Ven P F M, Jap P H K, Wetzels R H W et al 1991 Postnatal centralization of muscle fibre nuclei in centronuclear myopathy. Neuromuscular Disorders 1: 211

Vincent A 1980 Immunology of acetylcholine receptors in relation to myasthenia gravis. Physiological Reviews 60: 757

Voit T, Haas K, Leger J O C, Pons F, Leger J J 1991 Xp21 dystrophin and 6q dystrophin-related protein. Comparative immunolocalisation using multiple antibodies. American Journal of Pathology 139: 969

Wang C, Asai D J, Lazarides E 1980 The 68 000 dalton neurofilament-associated polypeptide is a component of non-neuronal cells and skeletal myofibrils. Proceedings of the National Academy of Sciences USA 77: 1541

Wang K 1985 Sarcomere-associated cytoskeletal lattices in striated muscle. Cell and Muscle Motility 6: 315

Warnes D M, Tomas F M, Ballard J F 1981 Increased rates of myofibrillar protein breakdown in muscle-wasting diseases. Muscle and Nerve 4: 62

Watkins S C, Hoffman E P, Slayter H S, Kunkel L M 1988 Immunoelectron microscopic localization of dystrophin in myofibres. Nature 333: 863

Webster C, Pavlath G K, Parks D R, Walsh F S, Blau H 1988a Isolation of human myoblasts with the fluorescent-activated cell sorter. Experimental Cell Research 174: 252

Webster C, Silberstein L, Hays A P, Blau H 1988b Fast muscle fibers are preferentially affected in Duchenne muscular dystrophy. Cell 52: 530

Whalen R G, Snell S M, Butler-Browne G S, Schwartz K, Bouveret P, Pinset-Harstrom I 1981 Three myosin heavy chain isozymes appear sequentially in rat muscle development. Nature 292: 805

Whitaker J N 1982 Inflammatory myopathy: a review of etiologic and pathogenetic factors. Muscle and Nerve 5: 573

Whitaker J N, Bertorini T E, Mendell J R 1983 Immunocytochemical studies of cathepsin D in human skeletal muscle. Annals of Neurology 13: 133

White M G, Stoward P J, Christie K N, Anderson J M 1985 Proteases in normal and diseased human skeletal muscle; a preliminary histochemical survey. Histochemical Journal 17: 819

Whiting P J, Vincent A, Schluep M, Newsom-Davies J 1986 Monoclonal antibodies that distinguish between normal and denervated human acetylcholine receptors. Journal of Neuroimmunology 11: 223

Willner J H, Cerri C, Wood D S 1982 Adenylate cyclase in human genetic myopathies. In: Schotland D S (ed) Disorders of the motor unit. Wiley, New York, p 423

Woo M, Chung S J, Nonaka I 1988 Perifascicular atrophy of fibers in childhood dermatomyositis with particular reference to mitochondrial changes. Journal of the Neurological Sciences 88: 133

Wood D S, Zeviani M, Prelle A 1987 Is nebulin the defective gene product in Duchenne muscular dystrophy? New England Journal of Medicine 316: 107

Worton R G, Thompson M W 1988 Genetics of Duchenne muscular dystrophy. Annual Review of Genetics 22: 601

Yamaguchi M, Robson R M, Stromer M H, Dahl D S, Oda T 1978 Actin filaments form the backbone of nemaline myopathy rods. Nature (London) 271: 265

Yamaguchi M, Robson R M, Stromer M H, Dahl D S, Oda T 1982 Nemaline myopathy rod bodies: structure and composition. Journal of the Neurological Sciences 56: 35

Zeviani M, DiDonato S 1991 Neurological disorders due to mutations of the mitochondrial genome. Neuromuscular Disorders 1: 165

Zubrzycka-Gaarn E, Bulman D E, Karpati G et al 1988 The Duchenne muscular dystrophy gene product is localised in sarcolemma of human skeletal muscle. Nature 333: 466

Zuk J A, Fletcher A 1988 Skeletal muscle expression of class II histocompatibility antigens (HLA-DR) in polymyositis and other muscle diseases with an inflammatory infiltrate. Journal of Clinical Pathology 41: 410

9. Ultrastructural studies of diseased muscle

M. J. Cullen   P. Hudgson   F. L. Mastaglia

INTRODUCTION

Advances in our knowledge of the ultrastructure of diseased muscle have depended upon advances in techniques which disclose previously inaccessible morphological information. Since the fifth edition of this book was published several powerful new procedures have become established and are referred to in this chapter.

Freeze fracture is a technique which has wide applications in cell biology and which has now been applied to the study of muscle pathology and immunopathology. Freeze fracture permits the electron microscopist an en face view of the internal structure of cell membranes and their components and has therefore been employed to study the plasma membrane of dystrophic muscle. However it is still clear that there are problems with interpretation of freeze-fracture images because of variability induced by fixation and freezing (Lee et al 1986). This type of work will be further discussed in the section 'Duchenne muscular dystrophy' (see below).

Another technique, the accuracy of which depends crucially on the preparatory freezing procedures, is X-ray microanalysis which can be used to determine the concentration of individual elements in a section. As the probe size is usually smaller than most organelles, the elemental concentrations from one compartment to another can be compared. Thus Somlyo and her colleagues (Somlyo et al 1981) were able to measure the concentrations of sodium, magnesium, phosphorus, sulphur, chlorine, potassium and calcium in different parts of the sarcotubular system and to examine how these changed during tetanus. Edström's group in Sweden (see below) have applied X-ray microanalysis to human muscle biopsies (Wróblewski et al 1978a,b, 1982, Edström et al 1986) but, thus far, the potential of this very powerful technique has not been fully realised in the examination of diseased muscle.

A third technique which has considerable potential for adding an extra dimension to our understanding of cell ultrastructure is that of electron-microscopic (EM) immunocytochemistry. For this a label (peroxidase, ferritin or gold) is conjugated to an antibody against the antigen of interest or, more usually, to a secondary antibody to the primary IgG. By using colloidal gold particles of different sizes, different antigens can be labelled on the same section. An example of dual labelling of tubulin and desmin in skeletal muscle is illustrated in Chapter 4. Examples where peroxidase labelling has been used include the demonstration of the membrane-attack complex of complement in necrotic muscle fibres (Engel & Biesecker 1982), the localisation of cathepsin D in human skeletal muscle (Whitaker et al 1983) and the detection of a spectrin-like protein in normal and dystrophic human skeletal muscle (Appleyard et al 1984).

Ferritin-labelled antibodies have been used for the precise localisation of collagen types III and IV, laminin and fibronectin in Duchenne muscular dystrophy (Dunn et al 1984). Immunogold labelling has been used increasingly to localise a wide range of muscle proteins including dystrophin, desmin, titin and creatine kinase (Watkins et al, 1988, Byers et al 1991, Eppenberger-Eberhardt et al 1991, Cullen et al 1991).

In terms of scientific chronology these techniques have just emerged from their infancy, yet used singly or in combination with other techniques, such as computer-aided image analysis, they represent advances in approach which are beginning to yield important information in our understanding of muscle disease.

ULTRASTRUCTURAL REACTIONS OF THE MUSCLE FIBRE

During the past 20 years, electron-microscopists have become increasingly aware of the fact that few ultrastructural reactions are specific for partic-

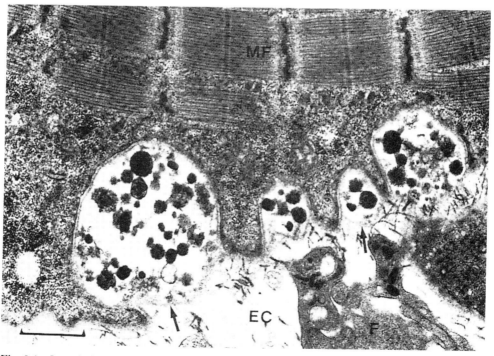

Fig. 9.1 Irregularity of the surface of a muscle fibre due to the presence of exocytotic vacuoles which contain granular and membranous debris enclosed by the basal lamina (arrows). MF = myofibrils, EC = extracellular space; F = fibroblast. Myopathy due to ϵ-aminocaproic acid (Scale bar = 1.0 μm).

ular disease entities. Despite this lack of specificity, certain combinations or sequences of changes (reaction patterns) seen in some disorders are sufficiently distinctive to be of diagnostic value. The more important ultrastructural reactions of the muscle fibre components and the ultrastructural correlates of some of the well-known light-microscopic reactions of the muscle fibre are considered below.

Reactions of muscle fibre components

Surface membrane changes. The muscle fibre surface is usually relatively smooth and under normal circumstances the plasma membrane and basal lamina run parallel with each other (see Ch. 2). Irregular projections of the surface may be due to the fibre being fixed while contracted but these have also been noted frequently in various neuromuscular disorders (Neville 1973). Papillary projections from the surface of diseased muscle fibres may be seen in fibres which are undergoing atrophy or in fibres of normal size, and either may be due to loss of fibre bulk or else may be a sequel to extrusion of degradation products from the surface of the fibre (exocytosis) (Fig. 9.1) (Engel & MacDonald 1970). Deep infoldings of the sarcolemma are seen in fibres which are undergoing longitudinal splitting, and are particularly prominent in dystrophia myotonica (Schröder 1970, Casanova & Jerusalem 1979).

In atrophying fibres the basal lamina may separate from the plasma membrane forming redundant folds which may remain even after the

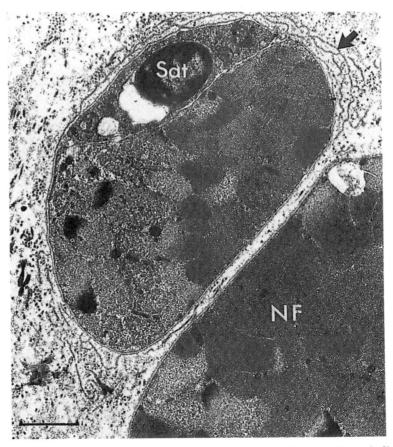

Fig. 9.2 Redundant folds of basal lamina (arrow) surrounding a small muscle fibre. An inactive satellite cell (Sat) is situated internal to the basal lamina. NF = normal muscle fibre. Congenital myotonic dystrophy (scale bar = 1.0 μm).

rest of the fibre has broken down (Fig. 9.2). Duplication of the basal lamina is a common finding in the muscular dystrophies and other necrotising myopathies and is a result of the regenerating fibre producing a new basal lamina while underlying the 'parental' basal lamina. Thickening of the basal lamina is a non-specific finding in a variety of situations (Mastaglia et al 1970).

Focal or more extensive deficits in the plasma membrane are frequently observed in fibres undergoing necrosis. Focal defects have also been described in otherwise normal fibres in carefully prepared material from patients with Duchenne muscular dystrophy (see below). Increased numbers of pinocytotic vesicles associated with the plasma membrane are also found in a variety of situations (Engel & MacDonald 1970).

Nuclear reactions. Changes in the myonuclei are sometimes found in fibres that otherwise appear morphologically normal (Cullen & Mastaglia 1982) but are usually seen in fibres that are atrophic, necrotic or sublethally injured. In a recent review Tomé & Fardeau (1986) have categorised the changes as changes in location, number, shape, size, internal structure or envelope structure. Localisation of all or some of the nuclei in a central or internal position is usually an indication of a chronic myopathic or neurogenic disorder. Central nuclei are particularly prominent in dystrophia myotonica and centronuclear myopathy. Why the nuclei do not move to the periphery, as they do during normal myogenesis, and why some peripheral nuclei should be displaced centrally, is not understood, although changes in the mechanical constraints imposed by the myofibrils are probably involved (Cullen & Mastaglia 1982, Tomé & Fardeau 1986).

Changes in the numbers of nuclei may be caused by the degeneration of individual nuclei prior to fibre necrosis in myopathic conditions. Numbers of myonuclei have been reported to be decreased in children with acquired hypothyroidism (Cheek et al 1971) and in Down's syndrome (Landing & Shankle 1982). In neurogenic atrophy the nuclei tend to aggregate into clumps, where they persist with intact nuclear membranes when most of the other fibre components have been lost. This may give the false impression that numbers have increased.

The myonuclei of diseased muscle fibres often become extremely irregular in shape and deep indentations of the nuclear membrane can give rise to the appearance of 'pseudo-inclusions'. These can be distinguished from real inclusions by being bound by the double nuclear membrane. The indentations of the nucleus can be so extensive that it takes on a spongiform appearance (Fig. 9.3). Irregularly shaped nuclei have been described in polymyositis (Mastaglia & Walton 1971b), distal myopathy (Markesbery et al 1977), inclusion body myositis (Carpenter et al 1978) and dystrophia myotonica (Tomé & Fardeau 1986) and are totally non-specific.

The nuclei of diseased muscle sometimes contain aggregations of filaments of various types. Actin-like 6 nm filaments have been described in polymyositis (Chou 1973, Cullen & Mastaglia 1982). Larger 8.5 nm tubular filaments have been

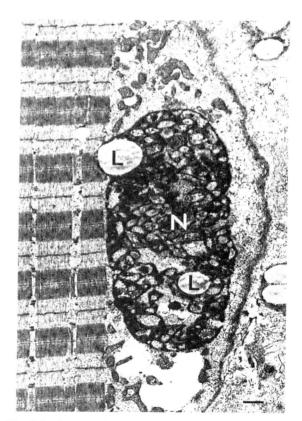

Fig. 9.3 A myonucleus (N) with numerous complex indentations giving 'spongiform' structure. Lipid storage myopathy. L = lipid (Scale bar = 1 μm).

observed in oculopharyngeal muscular dystrophy (Tomé & Fardeau 1986), and 16–18 nm tubular filaments in reducing body myopathy (Carpenter et al 1985), inclusion body myositis (Tomé & Fardeau 1986, Verma et al 1991) and distal myopathy (Welander-type) (Borg et al 1991). In this laboratory we have seen 25 nm filaments in a case of dermatomyositis (Cullen & Mastaglia 1982). The chemical identity of none of these filament types has yet been elucidated, although Carpenter and his colleagues (1985) give a thorough account of the staining properties of the 17 nm filaments found in reducing body myopathy.

Wröblewski and his colleagues (1982) were able to distinguish between two myopathies exhibiting central nuclei on the basis of the elementary spectra produced when subjected to X-ray microanalysis. One of the myopathies (myotubular) exhibited spectra with high sodium and chlorine and low potassium signals which is an indication of immature properties. In the other myopathy the elemental spectra conformed to the adult state. It was concluded that there was an arrest in development in the first but not in the second myopathy.

Reactions of myofibrils. The orderly sarcomere pattern and regular alignment of myofibrils seen in normal muscle may be disorganised in a number of different ways in disease. Focal areas of disruption involving a single or a few adjoining sarcomeres are commonly found in a variety of disorders and their significance is uncertain. In a number of children with a congenital myopathy this was found to be the principal change in the muscle fibres and the terms *multicore* and *minicore* disease were applied (Engel et al 1971). Typically there is Z-line streaming and loss of mitochondria, sarcoplasmic reticulum (SR) and glycogen within the minicores (Fig. 9.4) (Swash & Schwartz 1981, Pagès et al 1985, Martin et al 1986, Halbig et al 1988).

More extensive disorganisation of the myofibrils is found in *central cores* and in *target fibres*. Central cores were first described 30 years ago (Shy & Magee 1956). Ultrastructurally they display a variable amount of myofibril disorganisation (Fig. 9.5); Z-line streaming is common (Palmucci et al 1978) and there may be extensive rod formation (Bethlem et al 1978); there is also marked

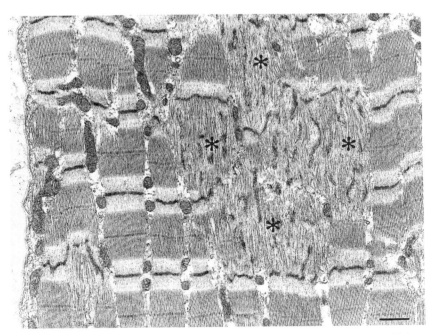

Fig. 9.4 Minicore disease. In this example the area of myofibril disruption (asterisks) encompasses the width of approximately four myofibrils and the length of three sarcomeres (scale bar = 1 μm).

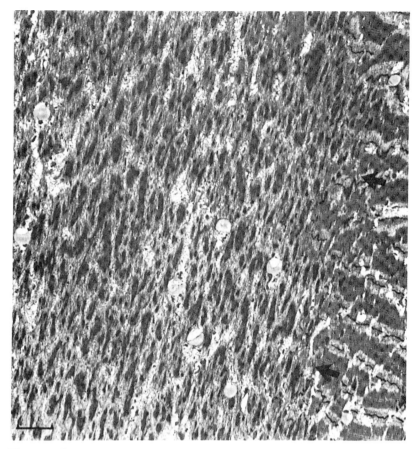

Fig. 9.5 Central core-like area (arrows) showing marked disorganisation of the sarcomere pattern of myofibrils in a muscle fibre. Mitochondrial myopathy (scale bar = 2.0 μm).

reduction or absence of mitochondria and a lack of intermediate filaments (Thornell et al 1983, Lacomis et al 1993).

Neville & Brooke (1973) subdivided central cores into structured and unstructured types according to whether the cross-striations and myofibrillar ATPase staining were retained or lost. However both types of core have been reported in the same biopsy (Telerman-Toppet et al 1973, Isaacs et al 1975), although Neville (1979) considers this to be unusual. Sewry (1985) has pointed out that some cores can have both structured and unstructured features.

Target fibres are found in denervating conditions, after reinnervation, and in some myopathies including familial periodic paralysis and polymyositis. Within such fibres, a central zone of marked myofibrillar disorganisation is separated from an outer zone of normal myofibrils by an intermediate zone in which the degree of myofibrillar disarray is relatively mild. Within the central zone there is disruption of the myofibril pattern, spreading of Z-band material, loss of mitochondria and disorganisation of the SR (Schotland 1969). Autophagic vacuoles and honeycomb structures have also been observed in the target centres with mitochondrial disintegration in the intermediate area (Mrak et al 1982). In so-called *targetoid* fibres, which may be found in both myopathic and neurogenic conditions, the intermediate zone is lacking (Dubowitz & Brooke 1973, Dubowitz 1985). Another unusual myofibrillar rearrangement is where they take up a largely radial orientation with the Z-lines closely abutting the plasma membrane (Fig. 9.6).

Z-Line streaming is probably the commonest

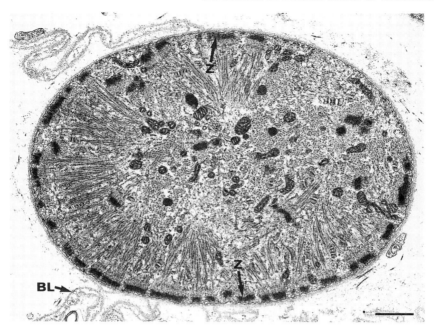

Fig. 9.6   A bizarre fibre with radial myofibrils in a patient with myasthenic features and severe fibre atrophy. Z = Z lines; BL = redundant basal lamina (scale bar = 1 μm).

alteration in myofibril structure seen in diseased muscle. It is commonly seen in the areas of disorganisation mentioned above and in a variety of other disorders. At its simplest it appears as an extension of the electron-dense component of the Z line into the adjacent I band. More commonly the density extends throughout the length of the sarcomere and into neighbouring sarcomeres and, at its most severe, zones of Z-line streaming can occupy large areas of a fibre (Fig. 9.7). Z-line streaming should not always be regarded as pathological; a certain amount of Z-line streaming can be detected in normal muscle, especially where there is a 'mismatch' between the Z lines of adjacent myofibrils. Less common changes include splitting (Edström et al 1990) or doubling (Jakobsson et al 1990) of the Z lines (Fig. 9.8).

Rod-body formation is the central feature of nemaline myopathy (Shy et al 1963, Hudgson et al 1967) but has now been described in a variety of conditions (Cullen & Mastaglia 1982, Konno et al 1987, Schmalbruch et al 1987, Kristmundsdottir et al 1990, Hantai et al 1991). The rods are highly electron-dense, usually about the width of a myofibril and up to 7–8 μm in length (Fig. 9.9).

Biochemical and immunocytochemical evidence indicates that the electron-dense material is α-actinin (Ebashi 1967, Yamaguchi et al 1978a). Longitudinal filaments within the rods may be composed of actin. Desmin is found around the margins of the rods (Jockusch et al 1980, Thornell et al 1980). These observations seem to support suggestions that the rods can be regarded as a lateral polymer of the Z-line subunit (MacDonald & Engel 1971, Stromer et al 1976). Stauber and his colleagues (1986) recently found an apparent absence of dipeptidyl peptidase 1 in two cases of nemaline myopathy and speculate whether this protease might be involved in the post-translational modification of proteins that are to be assembled into the Z line.

Another structure probably derived from the myofibrils is the *cytoplasmic body* (MacDonald & Engel 1969). These are usually round or oval in profile and have a dense core and a peripheral zone of radially arranged filaments which in some case connect with adjoining myofibrils (Fig. 9.10). The dense core contains tightly packed randomly arranged filaments. Its biochemical nature is unknown but it is sometimes linked to an

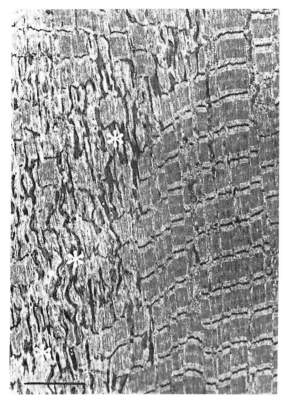

Fig. 9.7 Widespread Z-line streaming (asterisks). Emetine-induced myopathy (scale bar = 5 μm) (from Bindoff & Cullen 1978. Journal of the Neurological Sciences 39: 1, with permission from Elsevier, North-Holland Biomedical Press).

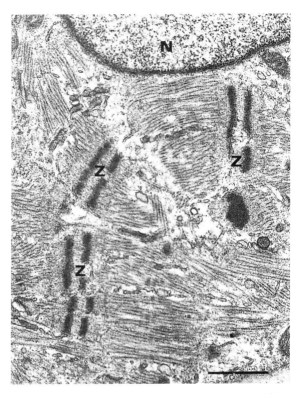

Fig. 9.8 Double Z lines in an abnormally regenerating fibre in a case of Becker muscular dystrophy. Z = Z-lines; N = Myonucleus (scale bar = 1 μm).

adjoining Z line. The radiating filaments resemble actin although cases have been reported in which they contain desmin (Osborn & Goebel 1983, Schröder et al 1990). Cytoplasmic bodies have been found in a number of conditions and seem to be non-specific (Cullen & Mastaglia 1982). They have, however, represented a major change in two cases of an unusual form of chronic progressive neuromyopathy which has been termed 'cytoplasmic body neuromyopathy' (Jerusalem et al 1979).

Filamentous bodies are another class of filamentous structure thought to be derived from the myofibrils. They usually consist of tightly packed masses of 6 nm actin-like filaments and are frequently subsarcolemmal in location (Fig. 9.11). They have been observed in muscular dystrophy (Hurwitz et al 1967), hypokalaemic periodic paralysis (Odor et al 1967, MacDonald et al

1969), intermittent claudication (Teräväinen & Mäkitie 1977) and centronuclear myopathy (van der Ven et al 1991). They have also been seen in healthy human muscle (Shafiq et al 1966, Schmalbruch 1968). A similar, but probably unrelated, structure consisting of 10 nm intermediate filaments has been described by Cullen & Mastaglia (1982) and by Thornell and his co-workers (1983).

Ring fibres are fibres in which one or more myofibrils are arranged circumferentially instead of longitudinally (Fig. 9.12). The disorientated myofibrils may be situated in the immediate subsarcolemmal region or, in some instances, are separated from the plasma membrane by an area of sarcoplasm containing disorganised myofilaments, nuclei and other organelles (Coulter et al 1991). These peripheral areas are termed sarcoplasmic masses. Ring fibres have been found in a variety of

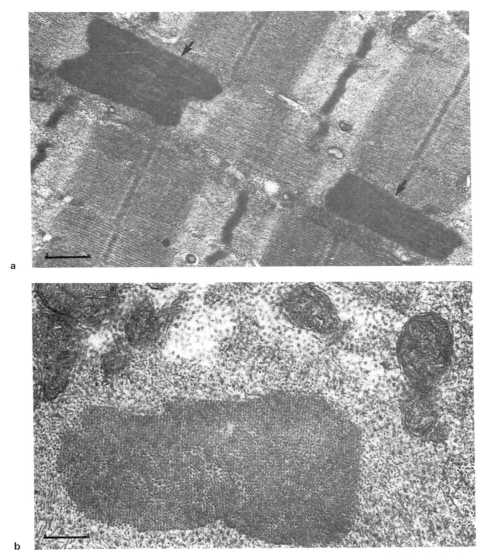

Fig. 9.9 Nemaline myopathy. **a** Two small rod bodies are present in a myofibril at the level of the Z lines (arrows), (scale bar = 0.5 μm). **b** Higher magnification of a transversely sectioned rod body showing the characteristic lattice-like appearance (scale bar = 0.25 μm)

situations including myotonic dystrophy, Becker dystrophy, limb-girdle syndrome and some cases of hypothyroid myopathy (Fardeau 1970).

Reactions of the SR and T system. The main morphological changes seen in the SR in diseased muscle are dilatation and proliferation. Dilatation of the SR appears to be the first ultrastructural change that can be identified in Duchenne muscular dystrophy (Hudgson & Pearce 1969, Cullen & Fulthorpe 1975)

(Fig. 9.13). Other conditions in which it has been reported include chronic alcoholism (Rubin et al 1976), distal myopathy (Markesbery et al 1977), myopathy with hyperaldosteronism (Gallai 1977), myotonic dystrophy (Casanova & Jerusalem 1979), perhexiline maleate-induced polyneuropathy (Fardeau et al 1979) and oculopharyngeal muscular dystrophy (Tomé et al 1989). Somlyo and her colleagues (1981), using X-ray microanalysis, have shown the dilatation of the SR in

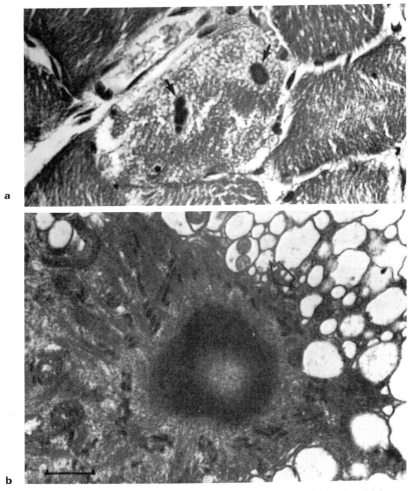

Fig. 9.10   Cytoplasmic bodies in muscle fibres in two cases of mitochondrial myopathy (arrows). **a** Haematoxylin and eosin (× 640). **b** Electron-micrograph showing electron-dense centre surrounded by radially orientated myofibrils and triads (scale bar = 1.0 μm).

frog muscle is associated with calcium over-loading, although there is no direct evidence to suggest that this is the case in the human conditions mentioned above.

Proliferation of the SR is frequently seen in atrophic fibres. In denervated muscle the amount of SR appears to increase but this is relative as the sarcotubular reticulum seems to remain longer after the myofibrils and mitochondria have begun to break down (Cullen & Pluskal 1977). After denervation, the SR appears to revert to an immature configuration with frequent duplication or stacking at the triads (Fig. 9.14). This configuration of the sarcotubular system is also seen in regenerating fibres (see Ch. 4). In certain patients localised proliferation of the SR gives rise to tubular aggregates (see below).

Three types of changes to the T tubules are quite commonly seen in diseased muscle: they may become receptacles for cell debris; they may change their orientation, or they may form 'honeycomb' or labyrinthine structures. In healthy muscle the lamina of the tubules usually appear empty but, where the fibres are breaking

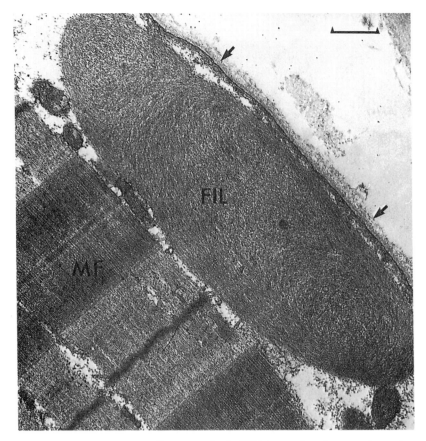

Fig. 9.11 Sub-sarcolemmal filamentous body (FIL) in an otherwise normal muscle fibre. Arrows = basal lamina; MF = myofibrils (scale bar = 0.5 μm).

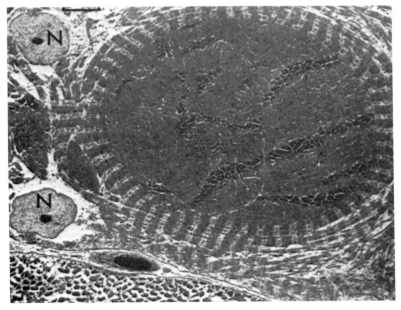

Fig. 9.12 Ring fibre from a case of hypothyroid myopathy. N = nuclei (scale bar = 5.0 μm).

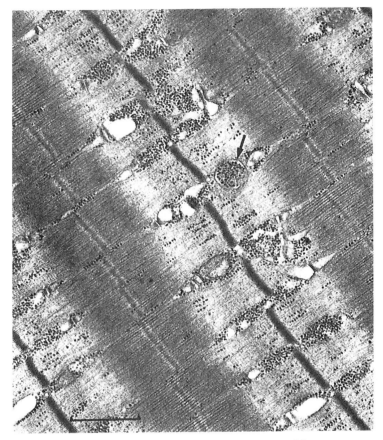

Fig. 9.13 Dilatation of transverse tubules and lateral sacs of the sarcoplasmic reticulum. Arrow = small area of autophagia. Duchenne muscular dystrophy (scale bar = 1.0 μm).

down, material may be exocytosed into them, resulting in their dilatation. The T tubules open to the outside of the fibres; they may therefore, in effect, be acting as gutters for the disposal of cellular debris (Kelly et al 1986).

In diseased muscle the T tubules often change their orientation from transverse to longitudinal (Martin et al 1986, Rouleau et al 1987, Salvatori et al 1989), which is the configuration usually seen in developing and regenerating muscle. This change in orientation is most commonly seen in conditions producing denervation and in other forms of muscle fibre atrophy. At the same time there is often duplication of the tubules and the adherent cisternae of the SR so that complex associations of the T system and SR are formed (Fig. 9.14) (Martin et al 1986, Mizusawa et al

1987, Salvatori et al 1989). Massive dilatation of these tubules is commonly seen in surviving stumps of muscle fibres adjacent to necrotic segments, being therefore a probable indication of early regenerative activity.

'Honeycomb' structures, first described in denervated rat muscle (Pellegrino & Franzini 1963), take the form of a regular three-dimensional array of interconnecting tubules (Fig. 9.15). They are connected to elements of the T system and their intercommunication with the T tubules has been demonstrated by tracer experiments (Engel & MacDonald 1970, Schotland 1970). They are a non-specific phenomenon and have been described in a large range of unrelated neuromuscular diseases (Halbig et al 1988, Tomé et al 1989, Jakobsson et al 1990, Fidzianska & Goebel 1991).

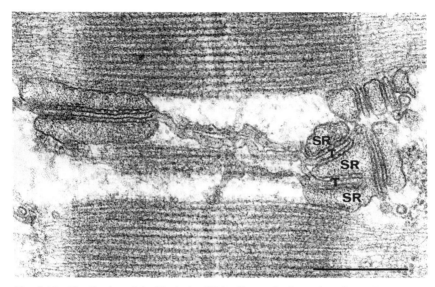

Fig. 9.14 Duplication of the T tubules (T) leading to the formation of complex associations with the terminal cisternae of the sarcoplasmic reticulum (SR). Werdnig–Hoffman disease (scale bar = 0.5 μm).

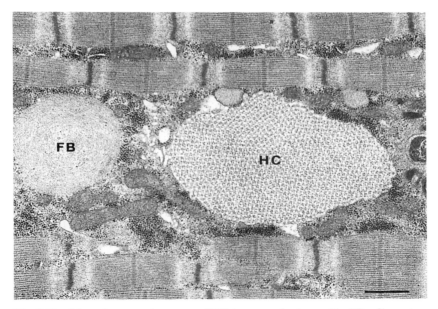

Fig. 9.15 A large honeycomb structure (HC) in a case of polymyositis. FB = filamentous body (scale bar = 1.0 μm).

Mitochondrial reactions. The number and size of mitochondria in muscle fibres vary considerably. Focal loss of mitochondria is a common accompaniment of myofibrillar disorganisation or breakdown in various myopathies (Engel & MacDonald 1970). Focal increases in mitochon-drial numbers have been noted in a variety of myopathies. Peripheral aggregates of morphologically normal mitochondria (Fig. 9.16) have been found to be particularly prominent in corticosteroid myopathy (Engel 1966) and in hypokalaemic periodic paralysis (MacDonald et al

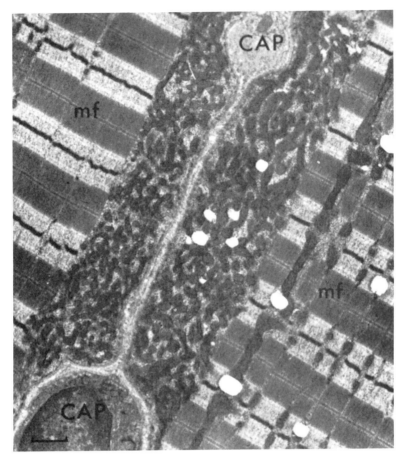

Fig. 9.16 Large sub-sarcolemmal aggregates of morphologically normal mitochondria in two muscle fibres (mf) in a case of mitochondrial myopathy. Two capillaries (CAP) indent the surface of the muscle fibres (scale bar = 1.0 μm).

1969). Triangular subsarcolemmal aggregates of normal mitochondria are found in the lobulated fibres which occur in facioscapulohumeral dystrophy and a number of other neuromuscular disorders, and account for the characteristic histochemical appearances of these fibres in oxidative enzyme preparations (Bethlem et al 1973).

Cases in which mitochondria are not only abundant but also show bizarre abnormalities such as increases in size, abnormal cristae and the presence of amorphous, tubular or paracrystalline inclusions are in a separate category (Fig. 9.17) (Koga et al 1988, Nonaka et al 1988, Takeda et al 1990, Chalmers et al 1991, Fidzianska & Goebel 1991, Mhiri et al 1991, Pauzner et al 1991, Riggs

et al 1992). Such changes have been found in various forms of inherited or acquired myopathy but are especially prominent in the group of so-called 'mitochondrial' myopathies in which they represent the most prominent and earliest morphological change seen in muscle fibres (see below, p. 362). The structure of the mitochondrial inclusions has been considered in detail by a number of authors (Chou 1969, Neville 1973, Morgan-Hughes & Landon 1983, Rowland et al 1983, Schmalbruch 1983). Electron-probe X-ray microanalysis of the paracrystalline inclusions has revealed an excess of phosphorus, sulphur, chlorine, potassium and calcium ions over those in control mitochondria (Baruah et al 1983). The

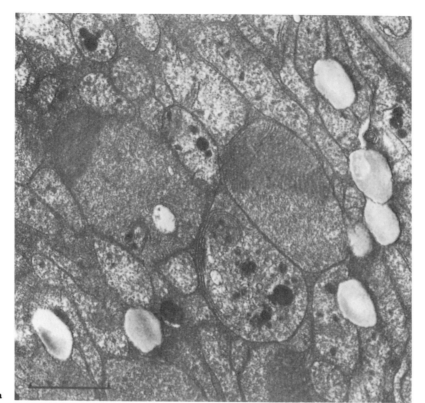

Fig. 9.17a

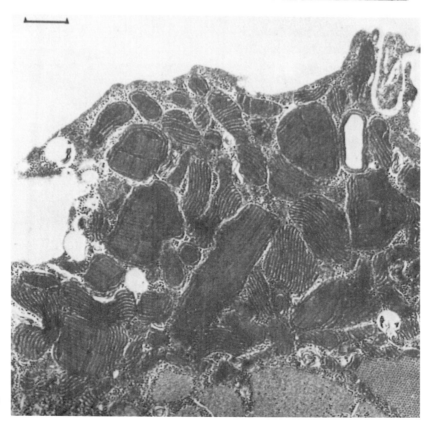

Fig. 9.17b

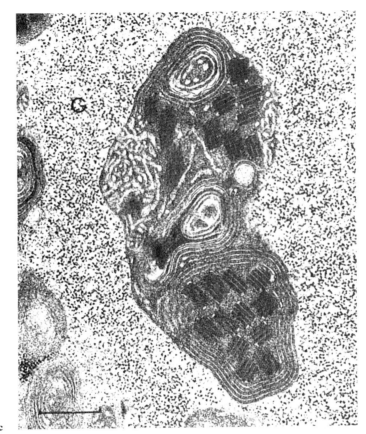

Fig. 9.17c

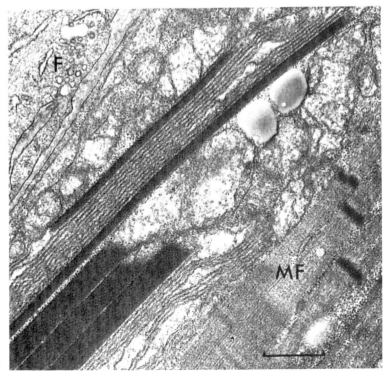

Fig. 9.17d

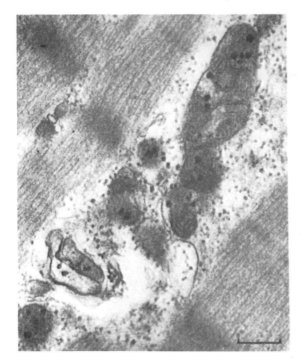

Fig. 9.18 Unduly prominent electron-dense granules of probable calcific nature within mitochondria. Hypothyroid myopathy (scale bar = 0.25 μm).

relative excess of phosphorus and sulphur suggests that the inclusions are proteinaceous in nature. More recently immunogold labelling experiments have shown that the paracrystalline inclusions are composed of mitochondrial creatine kinase (Eppenberger-Eberhardt et al 1991). Electron-dense granules (Fig. 9.18) thought to be calcific, have been noted in a number of situations including glycogen storage disease (Engel & Dale 1968) and hypothyroid myopathy (F. L. Mastaglia, unpublished observations).

Other distinctive changes

Tubular aggregates. These are collections of parallel tubules 60–80 nm in diameter, usually found at the edges of type II fibres in a number of unrelated clinical and experimental conditions (Gilchrist et al 1991, Martin et al 1991), the only definite disease connection apparently being with periodic paralysis (Bradley 1969, Meyers et al 1972, Rosenberg et al 1985, Roullet et al 1985, Gold & Reichman 1992). On morphological criteria there are at least three types of aggregate occurring in the literature: in the first, the commonest, the tubules contain a co-axial non-membranous inner tubule (Fig. 9.19); in the second the tubules have a more densely staining granular core, and in the third the tubules have filaments, approximately 10 nm in diameter, attached around their outer edge. It is clear that the first type, at least, is derived from elements of the SR.

Concentric laminated bodies. Concentric laminated bodies are hollow cylindrical structures of characteristic form which occur principally in type II fibres (Payne & Curless 1976). Concentric laminae approximately 7 nm thick, with centre-to-centre spacing of 8.5 nm, make up the walls of the cylinders. The laminae consist of parallel double bands approximately 12 nm wide running circumferentially and projecting about 7 nm at the outside edge with a repeat of 16 nm (Fig. 9.20). There may be up to 25 laminae to each cylinder. Their origin is uncertain. Luft et al (1962) considered that they arise from mitochondria, whereas Toga et al (1970) and Payne & Curless (1976) thought that they derive from myofilaments. However they are not membranous and the subunit dimensions do not correspond to those of the thick or thin filaments. They were first described in hypermetabolism of non-thyroid origin (Luft et al 1962) and have since been described in many types of condition, although these do not offer any clue to their origin (Cullen & Mastaglia 1982).

Fingerprint bodies. These consist of short lamellae spaced approximately 30 nm apart and arranged in patterns resembling fingerprints. They are non-specific, having been described in benign congenital myopathy (Engel et al 1972),

Fig. 9.17 Mitochondrial myopathy. **a** Sub-sarcolemmal collection of pleomorphic mitochondria some of which have electron-dense inclusions and abnormal cristal configurations (scale bar = 1.0 μm). **b** Peripheral aggregate of mitochondria with paracrystalline inclusions of various types and abnormal cristal patterns (scale bar = 0.5 μm). **c** Abnormal mitochondrion with rectangular 'parking-lot' inclusions and coiled cristae. G = glycogen granules (scale bar = 0.5 μm). **d** Electron-dense elongated crystalline mitochondrial inclusions. MF = myofibrils; F = fibroblast (scale bar = 0.5 μm).

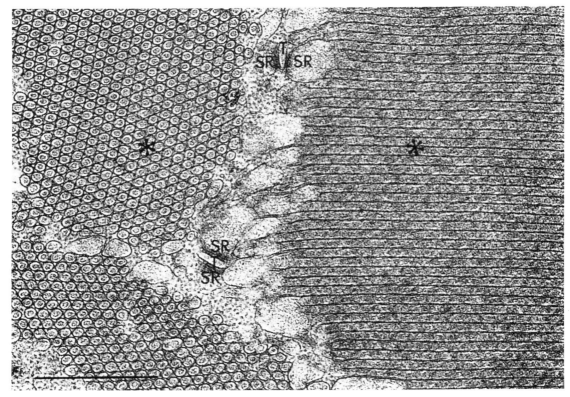

Fig. 9.19 Tubular aggregates (asterisks) sectioned transversely on the left and longitudinally on the right. Two triads show that the sacs from which the tubules are derived are SR. T = T tubule (scale bar = 1 μm). (Electron micrograph kindly provided by Dr D. N. Landon).

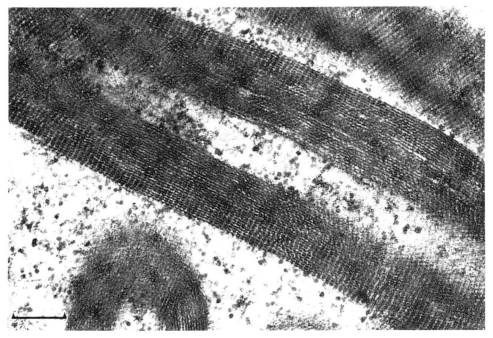

Fig. 9.20 Concentric laminated bodies in an otherwise normal muscle fibre in a patient with acromegaly (scale bar = 0.25 μm).

dystrophia myotonica (Tomé & Fardeau 1973), oculopharyngeal muscular dystrophy (Julien et al 1974), distal myopathy (Borg et al 1991) and in normal fetal muscle (Ambler et al 1987). Their origin is obscure.

Zebra bodies or leptomeres. These are filamentous structures with light bands alternating with thinner darker bands with a repeat of about 150 nm (Fig. 9.21). They are found at normal myotendinous junctions, in normal extraocular muscle and in intrafusal muscle fibres as well as in diseased muscle. They were a frequent finding in a patient with an unusual form of slowly progressive congenital myopathy (Lake & Wilson 1975) and we have observed them in a case of hypothyroid myopathy.

Curvilinear bodies. These structures, which appear to be basically membranous in nature, have been observed in association with lipofuscin bodies in chloroquine myopathy (Mastaglia et al 1977, Neville et al 1979) and are identical to the curvilinear bodies described in cerebral glial cells and the neurones in neuronal ceroid-lipofuscinosis (Rapola & Haltia 1973).

Reactions of satellite cells. Several studies have shown that there is a two- to three-fold increase in satellite cell numbers in Duchenne muscular dystrophy (DMD) (Wakayama & Schotland 1979, Wakayama et al 1979, Cullen & Watkins 1981, Ishimoto et al 1983), distal muscular dystrophy (Nonaka et al 1985), dermatomyositis (Chou & Nonaka 1977) and polymyositis (Ishimoto et al 1983). This holds true whether the numbers are expressed in relation to the number of myonuclei or the numbers of myofibres. Despite the abundance of satellite cells, regeneration eventually fails in dystrophic muscles: it would seem, therefore, that the events causing this failure occur later than the satellite cell or myoblast stage (Watkins & Cullen 1986).

Satellite cell numbers have also been reported to increase after experimental denervation of animal muscle (Hess & Rosner 1970, Aloisi et al 1973, Ontell 1974, Hanzlikova et al 1975, Schultz 1978, Snow 1983). However, in all these studies the satellite cell numbers were expressed in relation to myonuclear number which can also vary after denervation; the data are therefore difficult to interpret. Normally, growth after reinnervation is by regrowth of existing atrophic myofibres, not by regeneration, sensu stricto, of new fibres derived from the progeny of satellite cells. The role, if any, of satellite cells in denervated and reinnervated muscle has not yet been thoroughly examined and remains an interesting area of investigation.

It is widely believed that satellite cells adopt a resting conformation in healthy mature muscle (see Ch. 4, p. 120) and that when they become activated their structure changes as the amount of cytoplasm and the number of cytoplasmic organelles increases. Figure 9.22 shows a profile of such an 'activated' cell in a case of DMD (compare with the resting cell in Fig. 9.23). However, to describe satellite cells as either 'resting' or 'activated' on ultrastructural grounds alone is unjustifiable. In a detailed comparison of

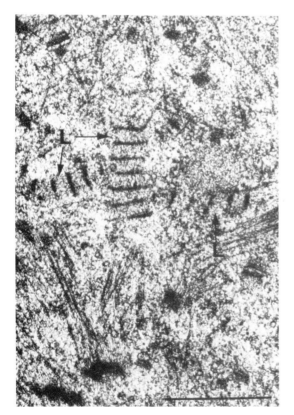

Fig. 9.21 Leptomeres (L) in a disorganised fibre in a patient with hypothyroid myopathy (scale bar = 1 μm).

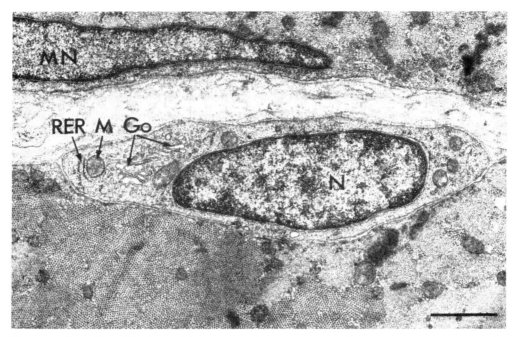

Fig. 9.22 A satellite cell in the quadriceps muscle of a 6-year-old boy with Duchenne muscular dystrophy. The section has passed through an area of cytoplasm containing rough endoplasmic reticulum (RER), mitochondria (M) and Golgi apparatus (Go). N = nucleus (scale bar = 1 μm) (from Watkins & Cullen 1986, with permission from John Wiley).

satellite cell profiles in DMD, polymyositis and normal controls, Watkins & Cullen (1986) found that the nuclear-to-cytoplasmic area ratios were the same in each sample, i.e. one was as likely to find an 'activated' cell in the control muscle as in the diseased. The cellular constituents were also similar in all three samples; the only detectable difference was that the satellite cells in the DMD sample contained on average more micropinocytotic vesicles or caveolae than those in the normal sample. This was attributed to a generalised cell response to a physiologically altered environment in the dystrophic muscle.

Blood vessel reactions. Ultrastructural observations have been made on the muscle capillaries and other small blood vessels in a variety of neuromuscular disorders. Thickening of the capillary basal lamina is a common finding which is particularly prominent in diabetes (Zacks et al 1962), polymyositis (Vick 1971, Mastaglia & Walton 1971b) and a variety of other disorders. Lamellation of the capillary basal lamina is also seen in a number of conditions including DMD,

periodic paralysis (Koehler 1977) and polymyositis (Mastaglia & Walton 1971b).

An increase in size of the endothelial cells and increased numbers of pinocytotic vesicles in such cells have been found in polymyositis (Mastaglia & Walton 1971b), DMD (Jerusalem et al 1974b) and in various other situations and is clearly a non-specific reaction. Degenerative changes in the endothelial cells of small vessels, such as the finding of myelin-like bodies, are also non-specific and have been noted in hypothyroid myopathy and in chloroquine neuromyopathy (Mastaglia et al 1977).

Basic pathological reactions

Atrophy. The most obvious indication of atrophy, whether it results from disuse (Mendell & Engel 1971), denervation (Recondo et al 1966, Mastaglia & Walton 1971a) or any other cause, is a reduction in the cross-sectional area of the fibres. This is often accompanied by a change in shape of the fibres: they may become angular in

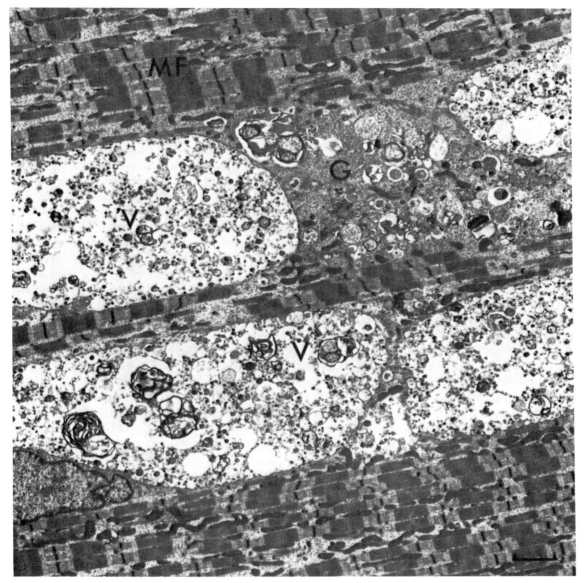

Fig. 9.23 Large autophagic vacuoles (V) containing granular and membranous material. The vacuoles have led to wide separation of the myofibrils (MF). G = glycogen. Acid maltase deficiency (scale bar = 2.0 μm).

profile and sometimes become heavily indented at the periphery. The main loss of material in the fibres is from the myofibrils which gradually decline in diameter, although this may not become clear until intermyofibrillar spaces develop. The myofibrillar atrophy usually begins at the periphery of the fibres and moves centrally. In longitudinal section there may be clear disorgani-

sation of myofilament and myofibril alignment, although in some situations well-organised myofibrils persist until very late stages of atrophy. Z-line streaming is common in atrophying muscle (Fig. 9.7).

The amount of SR and T system appears to increase in atrophic fibres, although this is probably relative (to the volume of myofibrils) and not a real increase (Stonnington & Engel 1973, Cullen & Pluskal 1977). The T tubules and triads lose their transverse alignment and take up a random or nearly longitudinal orientation. Honeycomb structures are formed in association with the T tubules (Fig. 9.15). The sarcoplasm of atrophic fibres is usually well endowed with Golgi apparatus, rough endoplasmic reticulum and ribosomes (Stonnington & Engel 1973, Cullen et al 1978), suggesting that active synthesis as well as breakdown occurs. As the fibres atrophy their edges can become deeply invaginated. The basal lamina follows these invaginations but can also get thrown into redundant empty folds (Fig. 9.2).

The cellular mechanisms controlling myofibre atrophy are still poorly understood. Little is known about how the different myofibrillar proteins are broken down but there is widespread evidence for lysosomal participation (Bird & Roisen 1986). The degradation of purified myofibrillar proteins by cathepsins B and D has been demonstrated using SDS-polyacrylamide-gel electrophoresis (Schwartz & Bird 1977) and immunofluorescence studies have shown an intra-cellular localisation of cathepsins B and H in developing myoblasts (Bird et al 1982). A major area of uncertainty is the role of non-lysosomal proteinases, such as calpain, which, it has been suggested, may be involved in the release of polypeptides from myofilaments prior to being taken up by lysosomes for digestion (Dayton et al 1976). Recently developed techniques using antibodies against specific enzymes for their ultra-structural localisation should provide information on the intracellular sites of activity of these enzymes and greatly enhance our understanding of the mechanism of protein turnover in muscle.

Hypertrophy. Muscle fibre hypertrophy may occur physiologically as a response to an increased workload in individuals with a high level of physical activity and may also occur in certain disease states. In muscle pathology it is found most markedly in myotonia congenita and in the more slowly progressive muscular dystrophies such as the Becker and limb-girdle varieties. Myofibre hypertrophy is also found in long-standing hypothyroidism and acromegaly where both fibre types are affected (Mastaglia 1973). Muscle fibre hypertrophy, which is presumably

of a compensatory nature, is also encountered in states of chronic partial denervation such as the slowly progressive forms of spinal muscle atrophy.

The increased cross-sectional area of the muscle fibres has been shown to be due mainly to an increase in the number of myofibrils (Miledi & Slater 1969). The basic mechanisms involved in the laying down of new myofibrils are still incompletely understood. Longitudinal splitting of myofibrils, once they reach a critical size, may be one of the ways in which they increase their numbers (Goldspink 1972). Hypertrophied fibres contain an increased number of myonuclei, with the new nuclei presumably being incorporated following division of the satellite cells.

Autophagy. Autophagy or self-digestion is a normal cellular activity of living tissues and is a mechanism for the turnover of cytoplasmic components, for the disposal of redundant components and for the use of cell constituents as emergency sources of energy. The process becomes stimulated and especially important when the tissue is exposed to unfavourable conditions such as starvation, dietary deficiency or inhibition of protein synthesis. When the stress is prolonged, autophagy may be followed by death and necrosis of the cells.

Autophagic vacuoles can be found in small numbers in normal muscle but increase in numbers in both myopathic (Nonaka et al 1985, Koga et al 1988, Goto et al 1990, Borg et al 1991, Himmelman & Schröder 1992) and neurogenic (Mrak et al 1982) neuromuscular diseases. They are particularly prominent in vincristine and chloroquine myopathies (Rewcastle & Humphrey 1965, Tagerud er al 1986). They contain sarcoplasm, glycogen, mitochondria and other organelles undergoing degradation (Fig. 9.23) but to the authors' knowledge have not been found to contain myofibrillar material. The turnover of myofilaments is thought to occur by non-lysosomal pathways, at least in the early stages (Cullen et al 1978).

Autophagic vacuoles are bounded by single, double or multiple membranes, the source of which is still controversial. For discussion of this question the reader is referred to the article by Cullen & Mastaglia (1982). Some of the conflicting observations could be explained if the initial enveloping membrane were derived from the SR and if the digested debris were, under certain circumstances, exocytosed into the (expanded) T tubules, which thus would act as a gutter to the fibre periphery (Kelly et al 1986). Normally, exocytosis of the cell debris is through the plasma membrane (Fig. 9.1) but, as the T system is continuous with the plasma membrane, it could act as a channel from the interior to the exterior of the muscle fibre. Cell debris is usually in the form of myeloid figures or membrane whorls. If these are not expelled they accumulate in the myofibres where they can form large aggregations (Goto et al 1990, Borg et al 1991).

Necrosis. Although necrosis of a cell may result from a variety of exogenous or endogenous stresses, the immediate cause is the loss by the cell of the ability to maintain physiological homeostasis. The plasma membrane, separating the cell cytoplasm from the extracellular space, ceases to act as an ionic barrier and the cytosol becomes isosmotic with the extracellular fluid. Whereas cell death can usually be recognised without great difficulty in mononuclear cells, it can be much more difficult to distinguish in skeletal muscle because of the multinucleate nature of the myofibres. Part of a fibre may appear healthy, while another part of the same fibre may be clearly necrotic. This segmental necrosis can be observed only in longitudinal sections and has been most commonly observed in DMD (Adams et al 1962, Schmalbruch 1975, Cullen & Mastaglia 1980). There is often a longitudinal gradient of events from a normal to a necrotic segment of the fibre, but the line of demarcation between the living and the dead part of the fibre can be extremely difficult to identify because conventional electron-microscopy can tell us little about the biochemical status of the cell. Thus, one can sometimes be very certain that an area is necrotic (e.g. if phagocytosis is taking place) and can be confident that another area is normal; but the intermediate areas of prenecrosis and early necrosis have to be interpreted with considerable caution. The components of a muscle fibre may appear extremely bizarre without the fibre being necessarily necrotic.

Certain features, however, can be reliable indicators of necrosis. Nuclei can undergo a variety of changes in diseased muscle (see above, p. 322) but in necrotic muscle the changes are terminal: e.g. loss of the membranes of the nuclear envelope (Fig. 9.24) must preclude any normal nuclear function. An intact plasma membrane is also a requisite for normal cell function and a necrotic fibre will usually demonstrate either partial or complete loss of this membrane (Fig. 9.24). In DMD an apparent loss of the plasma membrane may also be a feature of prenecrosis (see below).

The changes to the myofibrils may conveniently be grouped into three main forms. First, there may be severe hypercontraction of the myofibrils. As this can also be caused by mechanical damage to muscle fibres in contact with calcium-containing media (Karpati & Carpenter 1982,

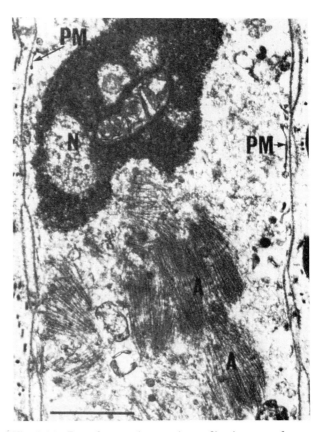

Fig. 9.24 Part of a severely necrotic myofibre in a case of polymyositis showing loss of the nuclear membrane and plasma membrane (PM). A = A band. N = nucleus (scale bar = 1 μm) (from Cullen & Fulthorpe 1982).

Lotz & Engel 1987), it seems likely that it is initiated in vivo by a massive, perhaps rapid, influx of calcium from the extracellular fluid which overwhelms the buffering capacity of the SR and mitochondria. Secondly, there can be preferential loss of different segments of the myofibrils. Loss of the Z line and I band (Fig. 9.25) has been described in a variety of diseases and conditions (Gonatas et al 1965, Johnson 1969, Afifi 1972, Cullen & Fulthorpe 1982). It is also one of the characteristics of ischaemic (Karpati et al 1974) and post-mortem muscle. This suggests that it is caused by a more spatially uniform and gradual rise of cytosol calcium concentrations. The dissolution of the Z lines may be mediated by calpain, the calcium-activated neutral protease which is able to extract Z lines, at least in vitro (Busch et al 1972, Dayton et al 1976). A-band loss (Fig. 9.26) is less common than Z-line and I-band loss, but has been described in childhood dermatomyositis,

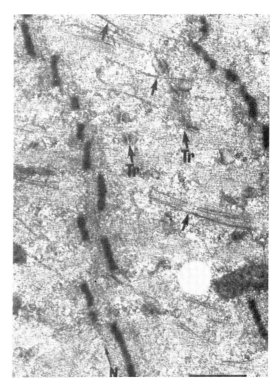

Fig. 9.26 Part of a myofibre in a case of dermatomyositis in which the A bands are absent. There is a small number of individual A filaments (arrows). The triads (Tr) are prominent and are still in their normal position. N = N line. (scale bar = 1 μm) (from Cullen & Mastaglia 1982).

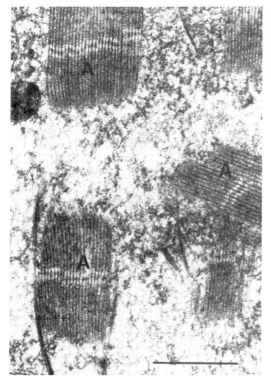

Fig. 9.25 Part of a myofibre in which the Z lines and I bands have been lost. Polymyositis. A = A band (scale bar = 1 μm) (from Cullen & Mastaglia 1982).

adult dermatomyositis (Carpenter et al 1976), polymyositis (Cullen & Mastaglia 1982), congenital hypotonia (Yarom & Shapira 1977), polyradiculopathy (Yarom & Reches 1980) and a case of steroid-induced quadriplegic myopathy (Hirano et al 1992). The third type of myofibrillar breakdown seen in necrotic fibres involves the reduction of the myofibrils to a homogeneous mixture of filamentous fragments (Fig. 9.27). The mitochondria of necrotic fibres usually round off and the cristae become indistinct or condensed and plate-like. The tubules of the SR break up into small vesicles which, in hypercontracted fibres, often accumulate between the contraction bands.

Death of the fibres is followed by their phagocytosis by invasive cells which enter through the basal lamina and move through the basal lamina tube. There may be some specialisation by the cells in what they phagocytose and digest. In those fibres in which the Z line and I band are lost it is

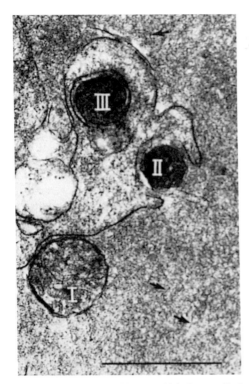

Fig. 9.27   Part of a necrotic fibre on which the myofibrils are reduced to a near-homogeneous pool of filament and fragments of filaments (arrows). The part of the macrophage shown appears to be actively engaged in ingesting muscle mitochondria (successive steps I, II and III). Duchenne muscular dystrophy (scale bar = 1 μm) (from Cullen & Mastaglia 1982).

muscle fibre occurs, regeneration is brought about by myoblasts which arise internal to the basal lamina of the fibre while its degenerate contents are undergoing phagocytosis (Fig. 9.29). The cytoplasm of these cells contains many ribosomes, polyribosomes and rough endoplasmic reticulum and the nuclei are usually large with prominent nucleoli.

Until quite recently the site of origin of the new myoblasts had been the source of considerable argument. A major impetus to answering this question came with the discovery 25 years ago of the muscle satellite cell (see Ch. 4). A combination of electron-microscopic, tissue-culture (Bischoff 1975, Konigsberg et al 1975) and autoradiographic techniques (Snow 1977, 1978, Hsu et al 1979, Trupin & Hsu 1979) has now shown beyond doubt that the satellite cells are the major, and probably the only, source of new myoblasts in regenerating skeletal muscle. Interestingly,

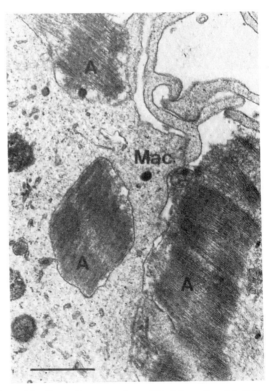

Fig. 9.28   Part of a macrophage (Mac) ingesting A bands (A). Note the near-intact structure of the A band in the early phagosome. Polymyositis (scale bar = 1 μm) (from Cullen & Fulthorpe 1982).

often possible to see cells which are filled with phagosomes which contain only A bands (Cullen & Fulthorpe 1982). Figure 9.28 shows part of a macrophage ingesting A bands which are nearly intact when they are first taken up; later they become increasingly condensed as they are broken down. Figure 9.27, in contrast, shows part of a macrophage, in a necrotic fibre, which is specialising in ingesting mitochondria.

Regeneration. After mild forms of injury that do not lead to necrosis, degradation and repair of the injured portion occur together and new myofibrils are formed to replace those which have been broken down. The ultrastructural signs of such synthetic activity are the presence of many ribosomes and polyribosomes, and prominent Golgi apparatus and rough endoplasmic reticulum within the sarcoplasm. When necrosis of the

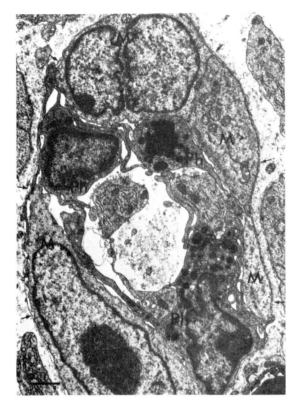

Fig. 9.29 A myofibre at an early stage of regeneration. Four myoblasts (M) or myotubes surround a central area that still contains phagocytic cells (Ph). The boundary of the fibre is delimited by the basal lamina (arrows). X-linked mouse dystrophy (scale bar = 1 μm).

cardiac muscle, which does not possess satellite cells, is unable to regenerate.

The satellite cells undergo mitotic division and generate the population of myoblasts which, in turn, fuse to form multinucleate myotubes. (The normal ratio of myonuclei to satellite cells is approximately 10:1 so the satellite cells need only undergo three or four divisions on average to restore the myonuclear population completely.) Myofilaments and nascent myofibrils appear first in the early myotubes. The first myofibrils usually develop in close conjunction with the plasma membrane, although later they form throughout the body of the myotube. The future positions of the Z lines are marked by ill-defined dense bodies which are linked to narrow bundles of actin filaments (Fig. 9.30). As well as numerous polyribosomes and abundant RER, the developing myotubes contain many

microtubules which lie closely parallel with the myofibrils and may be involved in guiding the assembly of the new myofilaments at the myofibril periphery (Antin et al 1981).

Several myotubes may form in parallel in the original basal lamina and normally these will fuse to replace the original myofibre. If, as frequently happens in diseased muscle, the fusion is incomplete, this gives rise to branched fibres which in transverse section can appear as splits (Schmalbruch 1976, 1984, Chou & Nonaka 1977). During regeneration the persisting basal lamina of the parent fibre acts as a scaffolding for the developing myotubes. The myotubes later form new basal laminae so a regenerated myofibre usually shows duplication of this outer sheath.

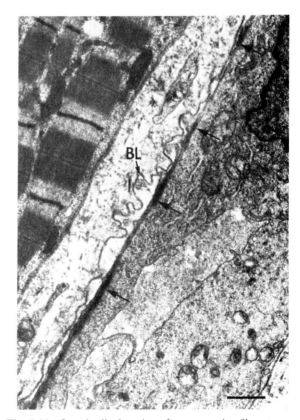

Fig. 9.30 Longitudinal section of a regenerating fibre at about the same stage as that in Fig. 9.29. A nascent myofibril is forming in association with the plasma membrane. The dense bodies (arrows) are Z-line precursors. The young fibre can be distinguished from a capillary by the near absence of pinocytotic vesicles. Duchenne muscular dystrophy (scale bar = 1 μm).

THE MUSCULAR DYSTROPHIES

At the time of our involvement in the fifth edition of this book there was some doubt about the status of certain disorders normally included under the heading of muscular dystrophy. However the great advances made in molecular genetics during the past 5 years have considerably clarified the situation in many cases. As well as the renowned work on the Xp21 dystrophies, separate gene locations have now been defined for Emery–Dreifuss dystrophy, facioscapulohumeral dystrophy, recessive limb-girdle dystrophy, dominant limb-girdle dystrophy, severe autosomal recessive muscular dystrophy and myotonic dystrophy. The nosological integrity of these disorders is therefore well established on genetic grounds. The gene location of all the neuromuscular disorders is regularly published and updated in the journal of that name.

In this section attention is focused on Duchenne muscular dystrophy because the considerable work carried out on the ultrastructure of this disorder has been found to be very relevant to what is now known to be the molecular abnormality.

Duchenne muscular dystrophy

Dystrophin. At the time of writing of the fifth edition of this book, researchers were on the brink of identifying the gene for Duchenne muscular dystrophy (DMD). Success in this, in particular by Kunkel's laboratory (Koenig et al 1987), was followed by the rapid application of reverse genetics in sequencing the protein, named dystrophin (Hoffman et al 1987a), encoded by the gene (Koenig et al 1988). The molecular biology of the gene and the protein are fully described by Dr Nicholson in Chapter 3.

From its amino acid sequence certain features of the structure and properties of the dystrophin molecule could be deduced (Koenig et al 1988). The molecule, with a calculated molecular weight of 427 K, was predicted to have four domains: a globular amino terminal domain, a central rod-like domain of triple helical repeats, a short cysteine-rich domain and a globular carboxy terminal domain. The central rod-like domain

was calculated to have a length of 100–125 nm (Koenig et al 1988, Cross et al 1990). This prediction of a roughly dumbbell-shaped molecule approximately 110 nm long has been confirmed by electron-microscopy employing rotary-shadowed images of isolated molecules from rabbit skeletal muscle (Murayama et al 1990, Sato et al 1992), although a longer length of 175 nm was found for dystrophin from chicken gizzard (Pons et al 1990).

Knowledge of the cDNA sequence of the gene and the amino acid sequence of the protein has allowed the generation of a rapidly growing number of antibodies to different epitopes within the dystrophin molecule. These have been used in immunolocalisation experiments to identify the normal position of dystrophin in the cell as a necessary step in attempting to understand its function. A series of immunofluorescence and immunoperoxidase studies from several different laboratories showed that dystrophin is situated close to the 'sarcolemma' (Zubrzycka-Gaarn et al 1988, Arahata et al 1988, Bonilla et al 1988, Nicholson et al 1990) and not at the triads as had been inferred from earlier cell fractionation studies (Hoffman et al 1987b, Knudson et al 1988). In DMD dystrophin is wholly or nearly wholly absent (see Fig. 3.2) while in Becker muscular dystrophy (BMD) it is either quantitatively or qualitatively reduced.

While the immunofluorescence and immunoperoxidase studies showed that dystrophin is located peripherally in the fibres at the sarcolemma, they were unable to show which particular component of the sarcolemma contained it. The sarcolemma, first described over a century and a half ago (Bowman 1840), is essentially a histological term for a structure which ultrastructurally can be divided into four distinct components. There is: (1) the plasma membrane; peripheral to which lie (2) the basal lamina; and (3) the reticular lamina. Internal to the plasma membrane and closely associated with it is (4) the membrane cytoskeleton. To be able to distinguish which of these components dystrophin is associated with, immunolabelling at the ultrastructural level is required.

This can be achieved using the immunoperoxidase technique because the reaction product is electron-dense (Carpenter et al 1990, Samitt &

Bonilla 1990) but it also tends to smear in the section so that the exact labelling site is poorly defined. A better alternative is colloidal gold which has several advantages as an ultrastructural marker: it is highly electron-dense, it is discrete and so can be quantified, and it can be prepared in different sizes thus allowing the possibility of labelling more than one antigen concomitantly. When antibodies to the rod portion of dystrophin are used the immunogold particles are found mostly in the cortical cytoskeleton, very close to the cytoplasmic face of the plasma membrane (Fig. 9.31a) (Watkins et al 1988, Cullen et al 1990, 1991, Cullen & Watkins 1993). When antibodies to the last 17 amino acids of the C-terminus are used the average position of the labelling sites is over the membrane itself (Fig. 9.31b,c) (Cullen et al 1991). It can be concluded from these results that the greater part of the dystrophin molecule lies in the membrane cytoskeleton while the C-terminus in some way interacts with a component of the membrane.

Costameres. The relatively even distribution of labelling sites at the plasma membrane seen under the electron microscope suggests that dystrophin is arranged as a uniform lattice work at the surface of the muscle fibre. Under the light microscope, however, dystrophin labelling, whether by fluorescence or peroxidase, can sometimes appear discontinuous with a periodicity corresponding to one sarcomere length. Recently several papers have been published which describe this 'costameric' distribution of dystrophin in some detail (Masuda et al 1992, Minetti et al 1992, Porter et al 1992, Straub et al 1992). The term costamere was introduced by Pardo et al (1983) approximately 10 years ago to describe vinculin-rich bands which encircled the muscle fibres at the level of the I bands and which were thought to mark sites of attachment between the myofibrils and the sarcolemma. Subsequently, spectrin and α-actinin have also been shown to be components of costameres. In the recent descriptions of dystrophin in costameres it has been described as co-localising with vinculin (Minetti et al 1992), spectrin (Porter et al 1992) and α-actinin (Straub et al 1992), although one report noted inconsistencies in the co-localisation with vinculin (Masuda et al 1992). Each of the papers describes an increased concentration of dystrophin opposite the I band but with a reduction exactly opposite the Z line. Interestingly, a recent immunofluorescence and immunogold study of dystrophin and vinculin has shown that in smooth muscle these two proteins are situated in separate and distinct domains (North et al 1993). While, in skeletal muscle, an association with costameres cannot be refuted, it is intriguing that in none of the ultrastructural immunogold studies of dystrophin (Watkins et al 1988, Cullen et al 1990, Byers et al 1991, Cullen et al 1991, Squarzoni et al 1992, Cullen & Watkins 1993) has such a discontinuous distribution been observed. Labelling is as dense opposite the A band as opposite the I band and there is no visible reduction opposite the Z line or elevation opposite the M line. It is suggested by Porter et al (1992) that immunogold labelling is too sparse for a costameric pattern to be detected, but we would maintain that the density is indeed sufficient for any differences to be detectable. If the distribution of dystrophin is indeed costameric (in vivo), it implies that there is some redistribution of the antigen before the sections are viewed under the electron microscope. As the tissue is fixed prior to processing, this seems unlikely. At the moment we are unable to explain the discrepancy between the light-microscopic and electron-microscopic results, but expect that, with increasing knowledge of the tissue and techniques employed, these differences will be resolvable.

The membrane hypothesis. Electron-microscopy first made positive contributions to our understanding of the pathogenesis of muscular dystrophy during the 1970s. For about 20 years researchers had speculated about a 'leaky membrane' following the discovery of increased aldolase activity in the serum of boys with DMD (Dreyfus et al 1954, Zieler 1958). This finding, together with subsequent findings of raised serum levels of creatine kinase and other muscle enzymes remained, until recently, one of the strongest sources of evidence for membrane lesions. Electron-microscopic evidence for lesions in the plasma membrane was first published in 1975 (Mokri & Engel 1975, Schmalbruch 1975) and subsequently supported by work in other laboratories (Carpenter & Karpati 1979, Cullen & Mastaglia 1980) (Figs 9.32, 9.33). Although the

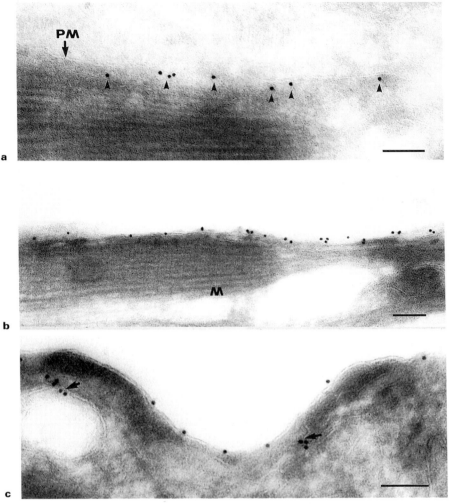

Fig. 9.31   **a** An example of 10 nm immunogold labelling using a monoclonal antibody (Dy4/6D3) directed against part of the rod domain of dystrophin. The labelling sites (arrowheads) are mostly immediately internal to the plasma membrane (PM) (scale bar = 100 nm). **b** Immunogold labelling using a monoclonal antibody (Dy8/6C5) directed against the last 17 amino acids of the C-terminus domain. M = myofibril (scale bar = 100 nm). **c** Immunogold labelling using Dy8/6C5. Note that some of the gold particles are associated with internal membrane (arrows) (scale bar = 100 nm).

cause of these visible lesions is still not wholly understood, the evidence of recent years that a protein of the membrane cytoskeleton, i.e. dystrophin, is absent in DMD imparts a new importance to the membrane hypothesis. Moreover the finding that dystrophin is bound to a complex of glycoproteins that span the plasma membrane and which are also lost in DMD (Ervasti et al 1990, Ibraghimov-Beskrovnaya et al 1991) lends a physical basis to the hypothesis.

At the time of writing the cellular function of neither dystrophin nor the glycoprotein complex have been established. The suggested cellular roles for dystrophin can be conveniently divided into three categories: (1) it may contribute mechanical strength to the membrane, important during length changes of the muscle; (2) it may anchor an integral membrane protein to the cytoskeleton; or (3) it may act as a link between the cell cytoskeleton and the extracellular matrix

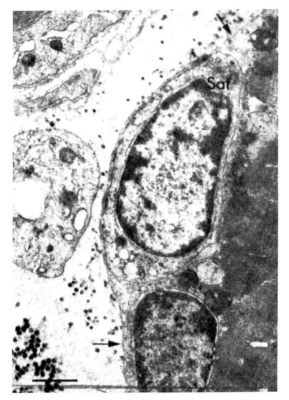

Fig. 9.32   The edge of a fibre in a 3-year-old DMD patient showing the absence of plasma membrane beneath the basal lamina (arrows). In contrast the membranes of the myonucleus, mitochondria, satellite cell (Sat) and surrounding cells seem well preserved (scale bar = 1 μm).

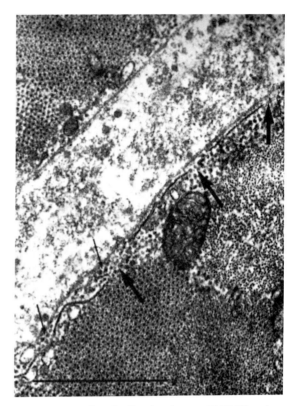

Fig. 9.33   The edge of a fibre in a 4-year-old DMD patient showing perforations (large arrows) in the plasma membrane. Glycogen (small arrows) has passed through the perforations (scale bar = 1 μm).

(see also Chs 3 and 4). It may of course fulfil more than one of these functions. Carpenter et al (1990), on the basis of earlier observations that the plasma membrane was sometimes seen to separate from the basal lamina in DMD (Carpenter & Karpati 1979), suggested that dystrophin linked the cytoskeleton to the basal lamina via the plasma membrane. This proposal has been given considerable support by the work of Campbell's group on the dystrophin–glycoprotein complex, a major component of which lies on the extracellular side of the plasma membrane and binds to laminin in the basal lamina (Campbell & Kahl 1989, Ibraghimov-Beskrovnaya et al 1991). While binding to the integral membrane glycoproteins at one of its ends (through the cysteine-rich domain and first half of the C-terminal domain) (Suzuki et al 1992), dystrophin binds to actin at

the other (amino terminal domain). It is thus uniquely situated to carry out both the second and third functions enumerated above.

Freeze-fracture of plasma membranes. Freeze-fracture has been used for comparing three features in normal and dystrophic muscle: integral membrane proteins (IMPs), orthogonal arrays (OAs) and caveolae. Schotland's group found a significant diminution of IMPs in DMD at both protoplasmic and exoplasmic faces (Schotland et al 1981a,b, Bonilla et al 1982). They also reported a significant diminution in the number of OAs from a median of 13.2 per μm^2 to almost none and an increase in the number of caveolae by 50%. Wakayama and his coworkers (1984, 1989) similarly reported a large reduction in the number of OAs (Fig. 9.34) and also found that the number of subunit particles per array was reduced from a

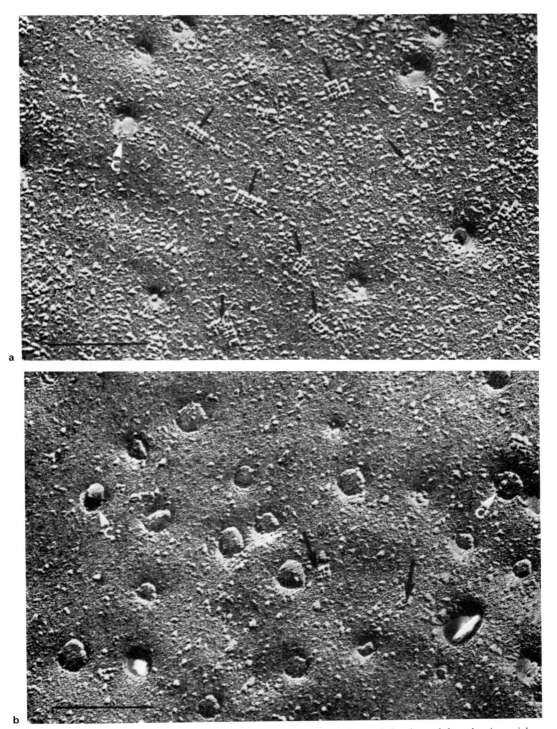

Fig. 9.34 Freeze-fracture images illustrating the differences in orthogonal array (arrows) density and the subunit particle number per array in normal and Duchenne muscle plasma membrane. **a** Normal P face. **b** Duchenne P face. Note also the increased number of caveolae (C) in the Duchenne (scale bar = 1 μm) (electron micrographs kindly provided by Dr Y. Wakayama, Showa University; from Wakayama et al 1984).

mean of 21.4 in the controls to 15.2 in the DMD patients.

It might be speculated, as both are lost in DMD, that there is a close association between the OAs and dystrophin. There are, however, several pieces of evidence that argue against this. First, OAs are depleted in Fukuyama muscular dystrophy (Wakayama et al 1985) but Fukuyama dystrophy stains normally for dystrophin (Arahata et al 1988). Conversely, mdx mice do not have dystrophin but show only a small reduction in the number of OAs. Secondly, OAs are reported to have a greater density in type II than type I fibres (Schmalbruch 1979) whereas no type-associated differences have been found in dystrophin labelling. Thirdly, OAs are only in the cytoplasmic half of the plasma membranes whereas the glyco-protein complex, with which dystrophin is tightly associated, has a transmembrane location (Ervasti & Campbell 1991). Lastly, based on a lateral

spacing of 120 nm, the density of dystrophin molecules at 69.4 per μm^2 (Cullen et al 1990) is approximately one order higher than the density of OAs (4.8 per μm^2) in adult human muscle (Wakayama et al 1989).

Regeneration in DMD. One of the unexplained features of DMD is that regeneration does not compensate for the wasting that occurs. In contrast to many other conditions and to regen-eration following trauma, where there is extensive repair of the muscle, regeneration in DMD fails to keep pace with the breakdown of the muscle fibres. This is crucial because restoration of useful muscle function and strength is the major aim of myoblast transfer therapy which has been tested at various centres (Karpati 1991, Law et al 1991, Tremblay et al 1991, Gussoni et al 1992).

The inadequacy of the regenerative response is not due simply to a reduced population of satellite cells. Satellite cell numbers are in fact increased

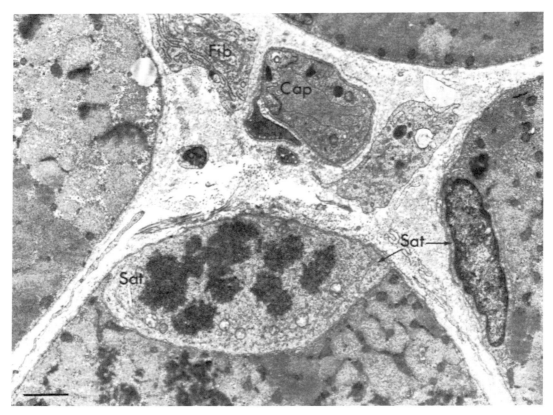

Fig. 9.35   Two satellite cells (Sat) in adjoining fibres in a 2-year-old patient with Duchenne dystrophy. The left-hand cell is in mitosis. Fib = fibroblast, Cap = capillary (scale bar = 1 μm).

two- to three-fold in DMD (Wakayama & Schotland 1979, Cullen & Watkins 1981, Ishimoto et al 1983). The cells are able to undergo mitosis (Fig. 9.35) and the resulting myoblasts are able to fuse as indicated by the presence of multinucleate myotubes in the DMD biopsies (Fig. 9.36). The restriction to regeneration thus appears to operate after myoblast fusion.

Many of the regenerating fibres show ultrastructural abnormalities. The myofibrils are frequently ill-defined and poorly orientated (Fig. 9.37), and the SR and T system are often poorly differentiated and are sometimes dilated. Two more features, perhaps aspects of the same phenomenon, seem particularly relevant to the impaired regeneration. First, many of the fibres are extremely small, down to 1–2 μm in diameter (Fig. 9.38), and secondly the edges of the fibres are often indented and fragmented (Fig. 9.39a).

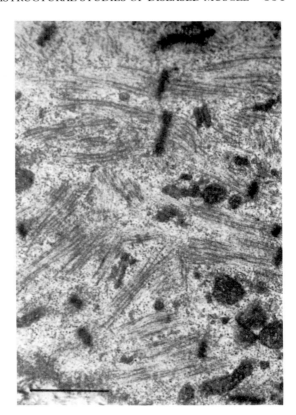

Fig. 9.37 Poorly orientated myofibrils in a regenerating fibre in Duchenne muscular dystrophy (scale bar = 1 μm).

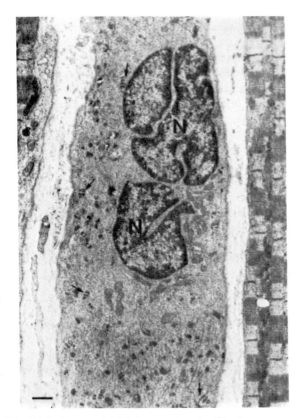

Fig. 9.36 Two nuclei (N) in a regenerating fibre in Duchenne muscular dystrophy. Note the immature triads and pentads (arrows) (scale bar = 1 μm).

At higher magnification it can be seen that in these areas there is an electron-dense 20–40 nm coating to the cytoplasmic face of the plasma membrane (Fig. 9.39b) and fine hook-like bridges extend from the plasma membrane towards the basal lamina. This appearance is exactly like that of the myofibre periphery at a myotendinous junction (see Ch. 4, Fig. 4.22). It suggests that the growing regenerating fibres react to the proliferating fibrous connective tissue (a striking feature of DMD, see below) by forming pseudo-myotendinous junctions with it. One can thus envisage growth being restricted by the connective tissue and effectively ceasing once the junctions are formed (Watkins & Cullen 1985). In support of this suggestion, Schmalbruch (1984) has reported the formation of myotendinous junctions when branching fibres end blindly in the connective tissue in DMD.

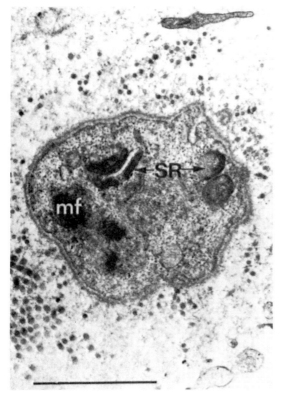

Fig. 9.38 An extremely small myofibre, approximately 1.5 μm in diameter, in a 2-year-old patient with Duchenne dystrophy. SR = sarcoplasmic reticulum, mf = myofibril (scale bar = 1 μm).

The marked growth in amount of fibrous connective tissue in DMD patients is usually interpreted as a natural secondary response to the wasting of the muscle tissue. The alternative interpretation suggested here is that the wasting of the muscle is partly or wholly caused by the connective tissue having a restricting effect on the regeneration of the myofibres. The interaction between muscle fibres and the surrounding endomysium and perimysium is poorly understood, although in DMD it appears to be a very close one (Fig. 9.40). In the fifth edition of this book we suggested that there might be an abnormality at the interface between the plasma membrane and basal lamina (both of muscle origin) on one side and the very closely associated collagen fibrils (of fibroblast origin) on the other. Although we have found that dystrophin does not itself connect with the basal

lamina, the linkage of the dystrophin-associated glycoproteins to the extracellular matrix (Ibraghimov-Beskrovnaya et al 1991) lends some substance to this suggestion.

Myotonic dystrophy (Steinert's disease)

Myotonic dystrophy is the most prevalent inherited neuromuscular disease in adults and is a multisystem disorder involving many tissues and organs. It is characterised by progressive weakness and myotonia of skeletal muscle but abnormalities may also be seen in smooth muscle, heart, lungs, peripheral nerve, brain, endocrine system, eyes and skin. The skeletal muscles most usually involved are the facial muscles, sternomastoids, foot dorsiflexors and distal forearm muscles.

Histologically the most characteristic features of myotonic dystrophy are the selective atrophy of type I fibres and the hypertrophy of type II fibres. Excessive numbers of internal nuclei occur, often seen in chains in longitudinal sections, and ring fibres and sarcoplasmic masses are also common. The ultrastructural changes tend to be non-specific. As in DMD, dilatation of the sarcoplasmic reticulum is often seen, but the plasma membrane lesions, characteristic of Duchenne dystrophy, do not occur. Myotonic dystrophy is described in greater detail in Chapter 15.

Very recently there have been considerable advances in understanding the molecular genetics of myotonic dystrophy. The genetic defect in myotonic dystrophy is thought to be any abnormal expansion of a trinucleotide (CTG) repeat located in the 3' untranslated region of a gene which encodes a serine-threonine protein kinase (Harley et al 1992, Buxton et al 1992, Mahadevan et al 1992, Yu et al 1992). The defect in the protein kinase may be expected to be the indirect cause of the variety of abnormalities seen in myotonic dystrophy. The number of CTG repeats in normal individuals (5–30) is both mitotically and meiotically stable within a lineage. In contrast the number of CTG repeats on the myotonic dystrophy chromosome can be unstable and extremely large. Mildly affected patients have 50–80 CTG repeats whereas severely affected individuals have 2000 or more copies. A case has recently been reported in which a delay in the

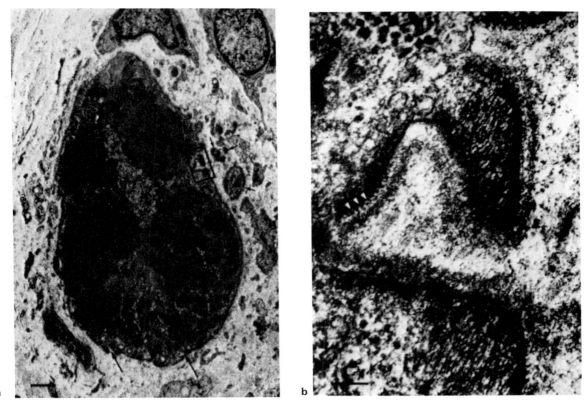

Fig. 9.39 **a** A small regenerated fibre in a 3-year-old patient with Duchenne muscular dystrophy. The fibre outline is indented (large arrows) and fragmented (small arrows) and there is increased electron density associated with the plasma membrane in these areas (scale bar = 1 μm). **b** The boxed area of **a** at higher magnification. Electron-dense material lies inside the plasma membrane and bridges (arrow) extend out towards the basal lamina (scale bar = 0.1 μm) (from Watkins & Cullen 1985, with permission from Blackwell Scientific Publications).

onset of clinical signs of myotonic dystrophy correlated with a reduction in the number of CTG repeats to within the normal range during transmission of the myotonic dystrophy allele (O'Hoy et al 1993).

INFLAMMATORY MYOPATHY

Electron-microscopic studies have provided information on the ultrastructural changes in muscle and have contributed to our understanding of the pathogenesis of inflammatory myopathies.

Muscle fibre changes

A variety of degenerative changes has been described in muscle fibres (Shafiq et al 1967c,d, Rose et al 1967, Chou 1967, 1968, 1969, Mintz et al 1968, Mastaglia & Walton 1971b). The most severe of these is the myofibrillar contracture which occurs in segments of muscle fibres undergoing necrosis and which is followed by progressive disruption of the contractile elements and phagocytosis (Fig. 9.28). Less severe changes include areas of focal myofibrillar disorganisation which may take the form of cytoplasmic bodies (Fig. 9.10) or of targetoid areas and the formation of myeloid bodies and autophagic vacuoles. The relationship between these latter changes and the segmental necrosis which appears to be the fundamental lesion both at light- and electron-microscopic levels is uncertain. The mechanism of breakdown of the myofibrillar apparatus in degenerating fibres has been discussed in detail by

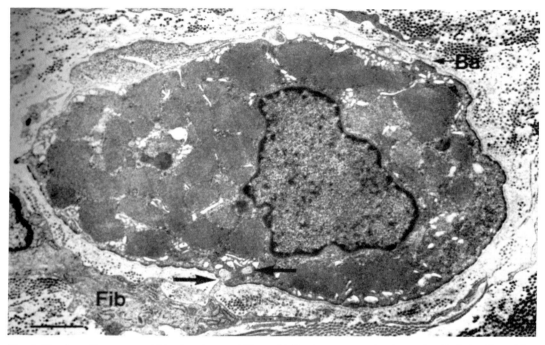

Fig. 9.40   A small regenerated fibre in a 4-year-old boy with Duchenne muscular dystrophy. Both the SR and T system are dilated. An adjacent fibroblast-like cell (Fib) has penetrated the myofibre by extending a cell process (arrows) into a dilated T tubule. Ba = basal lamina (scale bar = 1 μm) (from Watkins & Cullen 1985, with permission from Blackwell Scientific Publications).

Cullen & Fulthorpe (1982). The regenerative changes in necrotic muscle fibres have also been well described by a number of authors (Shafiq et al 1967b, Engel & MacDonald 1970, Mastaglia & Walton 1971b).

Blood vessel changes

Numerous changes have been described in the small intramuscular blood vessels in polymyositis and dermatomyositis. These include thickening and reduplication of the basement membrane and swelling of endothelial cells which may contain autophagic vacuoles, multivesicular bodies (Shafiq et al 1967c, Gonzalez-Angulo et al 1968, Mastaglia & Currie 1971) and tubuloreticular inclusions within the endoplasmic reticulum (Jerusalem et al 1974a, Carpenter et al 1976). Such inclusions are found most characteristically in the childhood form of dermatomyositis (Banker 1975, Carpenter et al 1976, Oshima et al 1979). They have also been described in the endothelium

of cutaneous blood vessels (Landry & Winkelmann 1972) and in lymphocytes in some cases of dermatomyositis; and identical structures are found in the lymphocytes of some normal subjects (White 1972) and in endothelial cells in a variety of other conditions (Györkey et al 1969, Baringer 1971). The original view that they are viral in nature is now regarded as unlikely.

Attention has been drawn to the occurrence of capillary necrosis and other microvascular changes (Banker 1975, Crowe et al 1992), particularly in the form of dermatomyositis which occurs in children and young adults (Jerusalem et al 1974a, Carpenter et al 1976). Depletion of capillaries is an early change (Emslie-Smith & Engel 1990) and is thought to be responsible for the muscle fibre damage by causing ischaemia. Immune complex deposition has been demonstrated in childhood dermatomyositis by Whitaker & Engel (1972) and by Kissel et al (1986) and has been demonstrated ultrastructurally in the walls of intramuscular blood vessels in a case of polymyositis associated with Waldenström's macroglobulinaemia (Ringel et al 1979). Deposits of the C5b−9 complement membrane attack complex have been found to be present in capillaries and other small vessels in dermatomyositis (Kissel et al 1991). These observations suggest that a complement-mediated vasculopathy is the primary immunopathogenic process in dermatomyositis (Griggs & Karpati 1991).

Inflammatory cells

Electron-microscopic and immunocytochemical observations on the inflammatory cells in the muscle lesions have provided strong evidence for the involvement of cell-mediated immune mechanisms in the pathogenesis of the muscle damage in polymyositis and inclusion body myositis. Mastaglia & Currie (1971) found 'activated', 'transformed' and dividing lymphoid cells among the perivascular and interstitial inflammatory cells in two cases of polymyositis as well as lymphoid cells situated internal to the basement membrane of some non-necrotic muscle fibres and in some instances actually lying within the fibre, having invaginated the plasma membrane (Fig. 9.41). Similar observations were also made by Cullen & Fulthorpe (1982). Invasion of muscle fibres by lymphocytes has also been seen in allogeneic muscle grafts undergoing rejection (Mastaglia et al 1975). The recent elegant immunocytochemical studies by Arahata & Engel (1986) have shown that the majority of invading mononuclear cells in polymyositis and inclusion body myositis are lymphocytes with the CD8+ phenotype or macrophages. In a recent exceptional case of polymyositis the predominant invading cells were γ-δ lymphocytes (Hohfeld et al 1991).

An interesting change found in the region of contact between lymphoid cells and the muscle fibres is the formation of tubular arrays, probably arising from the T system and identical to the honeycomb arrays found within muscle fibres in a variety of conditions. Whether some form of physical contact between activated lymphoid cells and muscle fibres is integral to the mechanism of cell-mediated myotoxicity or whether muscle fibre damage may be effected by lymphoid cells at a distance remains to be determined.

Inclusions

Several types of intranuclear or cytoplasmic inclusion bodies may be seen in muscle fibres or capillary endothelial cells in different types of inflammatory myopathy.

In inclusion body myositis (Fig. 9.42a,b) one of the hallmarks of the condition is the presence within myonuclei and in the sarcoplasm of eosinophilic inclusions which are made up of aggregates of tubular filaments with a diameter of 14–18 nm in the sarcoplasm and 10–14 nm in nuclei (Carpenter et al 1978, Lotz et al 1989). Although these were originally thought to represent myxo- or paramyxovirus nucleocapsids (Chou 1967, 1968), this now seems unlikely. These inclusions are distinct from *cytoplasmic bodies* (see p. 325), which are also commonly found in some cases. The recently described deposits of β-amyloid in muscle fibres in this condition are also separate from the tubular filamentous inclusions (Askanas et al 1992).

A second variety of virus-like inclusions has been described in a heterogeneous group of cases of inflammatory myopathy. These were confined to the sarcoplasm and consisted of paracrystalline arrays resembling viruses of the picorna group (Chou & Gutmann 1970, Ben-Bassat & Machtey 1972, Tang et al 1975, De Reuck et al 1977a, Fukuyama et al 1977, Györkey et al 1978), or in one case, of non-crystalline aggregates of 16–24 nm particles resembling viral ribonucleoprotein (Mastaglia & Walton 1970). Attempts at viral isolation from muscle have usually been unsuccessful in such cases. The finding of identical structures, often without accompanying pathological changes, in cases of malignant hyperpyrexia (Schiller & Mair 1974), Reye's syndrome (Alvira & Mendoza 1975, Hanson & Urizar 1975), idiopathic scoliosis (Webb & Gillespie 1976, Papadimitriou & Mastaglia 1982) and various other situations (Schmalbruch 1967, Caulfield et al 1968) suggested that these structures may not be viral in nature but that the paracrystalline arrays may represent one of the forms in which glycogen may be present in muscle fibres. However, Fukuhara (1979), using the cis-platinum (II) technique, showed that they contain nucleic acids and concluded that they may, after all, represent an RNA virus.

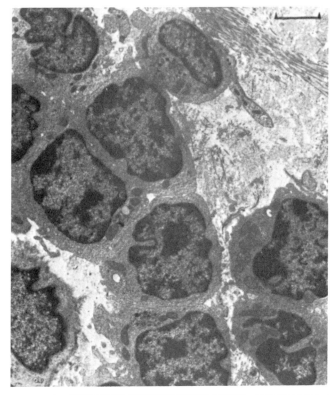

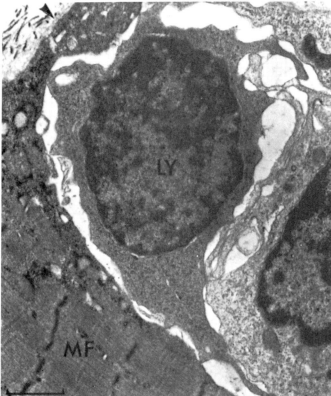

Fig. 9.41 Sub-acute polymyositis. **a**
Interstitial lymphoid cells (scale bar = 2.0 μm).
b Lymphoid cells (LY) which have penetrated
the basement membrane (arrowhead) of a
muscle fibre (MF) (scale bar = 1.0 μm).

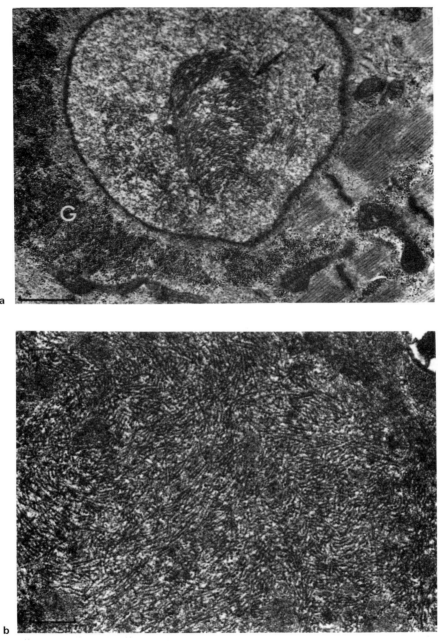

Fig. 9.42   Inclusion body myositis. Intranuclear (arrow) (**a**) and cytoplasmic (**b**) aggregates of virus-like filamentous tubules. G = glycogen granules (scale bars: **a** = 1.0 μm; **b** = 0.5 μm).

Cytoplasmic aggregates of larger (87 nm) spherical particles of possible viral origin were also described in muscle fibres in a young woman with rapidly progressive fatal polymyositis (Martinez et al 1974). However, attempts at virus isolation from muscle in this case were also unsuccessful.

METABOLIC MYOPATHIES

An increasing number of genetically determined or acquired systemic metabolic diseases, in which myopathy forms a major part of the clinical syndrome, have been recognised. These include the periodic paralyses and other electrolyte disturbances, the glycogen storage disorders and a number of endocrine disturbances, the most important of which are thyrotoxicosis, hypothyroidism, disturbances of adrenal cortical function and acromegaly. In addition to these disorders, we have included in this section those myopathies in which there is a primary abnormality of mitochondrial structure and function or of lipid metabolism in muscle.

Periodic paralysis syndromes

These rare disorders, which are usually familial, are associated with abrupt rises or falls in the serum potassium level. Hypokalaemic periodic paralysis is also a well-recognised but uncommon feature of thyrotoxicosis, particularly among Cantonese, Chinese and Thais, and may be the presenting manifestation of the disorder.

Electron-microscopic studies of muscle have been carried out in the hypokalaemic (Shy et al 1961, Pearce 1964, MacDonald et al 1969), the hyperkalaemic (adynamia episodica hereditaria) and so-called normokalaemic forms (Bradley 1969), and in the thyrotoxic form of periodic paralysis (Engel 1966, Norris et al 1968, Takagi et al 1973). The most characteristic ultrastructural change found in muscle fibres in each of these disorders has been a marked dilatation of the sarcotubular system which leads to the formation of the vacuoles (Fig. 9.43) which are seen with the light microscope during paralytic attacks (Pearson 1964). This dilatation is thought to arise in the terminal cisternae of the SR (Bradley 1969) and comparable observations have been made in experimental studies of the effects of chronic hypokalaemia in the rat (Kao & Gordon 1977, De Coster 1979). It is known from light-microscopic observations (Pearson 1964) that the vacuolation of muscle fibres is most striking during attacks of paralysis and that little, if any, abnormality may be seen in biopsies obtained in the interval between attacks. In contrast, dilatation of the SR and other ultrastructural changes may be found even between attacks, although these changes are more marked during an attack, or when weakness becomes established in the later stages of the disease. In one particular study of the hypokalaemic form of periodic paralysis, it was found that the numbers and sizes of vacuoles did not appear to vary appreciably during or between attacks (Gordon et al 1970). That the function of the SR is significantly disturbed during attacks of paralysis is shown by the finding of impaired Ca^{2+}-binding and Mg^{2+}-ATPase activity in SR membranes from cases of thyrotoxic periodic paralysis (Takagi et al 1973).

Several other ultrastructural changes have been prominent in cases of periodic paralysis. These include tubular aggregates (see p. 335), which have been found in cases of hypo- and hyperkalaemic periodic paralysis (Grüner 1966, Odor et al 1967, Engel & MacDonald 1970) and in thyrotoxic periodic paralysis (Bergman et al 1970). As mentioned previously, these structures appear to be derived from the SR (Schiaffino et al 1977). Other types of tubular proliferation that probably are also derived from the SR have been described in cases of hypokalaemic periodic paralysis (MacDonald et al 1969). The presence of apparently increased quantities of glycogen lying free in the SR in the subsarcolemmal region and between myofibrils has been noted in the hypokalaemic (Howes et al 1966, Odor et al 1967), the hyperkalaemic and normokalaemic forms (Bradley 1969) and in thyrotoxic periodic paralysis (Takagi et al 1973) and is in accord with the finding of granular PAS-positive material in the sub-sarcolemmal region in some cases (Engel et al 1967, Brody & Dudley 1969). In some cases this observation was supported by the finding of an increased content of glycogen measured quantitatively (Takagi et al 1973), whereas in others the glycogen content has been found to be within the normal range (Engel et al 1967).

Weller & McArdle (1971) have drawn attention to the finding of a characteristic type of basophilic granular degeneration in muscle fibres in various types of periodic paralysis, which they

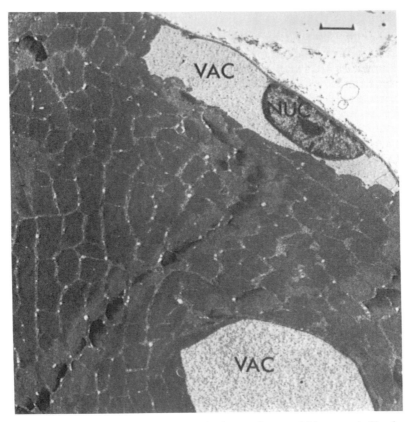

Fig. 9.43 Vacuoles (VAC) containing finely granular material in a muscle fibre in a case of hypokalaemic periodic paralysis. NUC = nucleus (scale bar = 2.0 μm).

consider to be caused by the deposition of calcium salts (in a form resembling hydroxy-apatite crystals) in association with acid mucopolysaccharide. They postulate that this intracellular deposition of calcium salts occurs initially in the SR, but have also found evidence of calcium deposition in the extracellular space.

Glycogen storage disease

Children with skeletal muscle glycogenosis usually present with infantile hypotonia; adult patients with glycogen storage disease presenting exclusively or predominantly with myopathy are rare. In the relatively few cases of this kind reported to date, a number of different deficiencies of enzymes of the glycolytic pathway have been reported. These have included muscle phosphorylase (Engel et al 1963), acid maltase (α-1, 4-glucosidase)

(Courtecuisse et al 1965, Zellweger et al 1965, Cardiff 1966, Smith et al 1966, Isch et al 1966, Hudgson et al 1968, Engel 1970, Martin et al 1973, 1976, Hudgson & Fulthorpe 1975, Schlenska et al 1976, Karpati et al 1977), amylo-1,6-glucosidase (Oliner et al 1961, Murase et al 1973) and possibly phosphoglucomutase (Thomson et al 1963). In addition, a number of familial cases have been reported in which the disorder presented with symptoms indistinguishable from those due to muscle phosphorylase deficiency and in which there were no demonstrable clinical abnormalities at rest. In two families the symptoms were shown to be due to phosphofructokinase deficiency (Tarui et al 1965, Layzer et al 1967) and in one to a possible disturbance of hexosephosphate isomerase activity (Satoyoshi & Kowa 1967).

The light-microscopic changes found in muscle

obtained at biopsy in these patients have been essentially similar: a vacuolar myopathy of greater or lesser severity, with accumulation of glycogen granules within the vacuoles, particularly in those lying immediately under the sarcolemma. Electron-microscopic studies have been performed in a number of these conditions. In the case of acid maltase deficiency, Hudgson et al (1968) and Engel (1970) emphasised the sequestration of glycogen within vacuoles lined by a unit membrane, believing this to be a hallmark of a lysosomal storage disorder (Fig. 9.44a, b). They also described vacuoles containing osmiophilic material and complex lipid structures, regarding these as autophagic vacuoles or secondary lysosomes, their contents being the degradation products of phospholipid membranes within the muscle cell. Engel (1970) classified the deposits of glycogen within the muscle according to the abnormal spaces in which they were stored, calling these Types 1–4 on the basis of their ultra-structural appearance.

Type 1 spaces. These are sarcoplasmic intermyofibrillar deposits of glycogen which displace other subcellular organelles and which appear to occupy whole segments of affected fibres in some areas. The facile explanation for these deposits has been the rupture of overdistended 'lysosomes' and Hudgson & Fulthorpe (1975) adduced some ultrastructural evidence in support of this (see below). However, it has to be conceded that most of the glycogen appears to be sarcoplasmic in location in both the infantile and late-onset forms of acid maltase deficiency and this has led Cardiff (1966) to question its status as a single-enzyme-defect disease.

Type 2 spaces. Engel (1970) defined these as smooth-contoured sacs lined by a continuous unit or double membranes and containing only glycogen (Fig. 9.44a,b). Many of these were quite small (<0.5 μm in diameter) and, in some instances, appeared to be the only abnormality in the muscle cell. Hudgson & Fulthorpe (1975) were able to demonstrate these structures within a satellite cell.

Type 3 spaces. Engel (1970) and Hudgson & Fulthorpe (1975) all described numerous autophagic vacuoles in material from infantile and adult cases (Type 3 spaces). These contained a variety of structures including small dense osmiophilic bodies, lipid droplets and complex membranous structures (Fig. 9.44c). Using Barka's technique (Barka 1964), Engel was able to demonstrate acid phosphatase activity within these spaces in material from three of his cases, supporting the concept that these structures were lysosomal in nature. In contrast, he found no evidence of acid phosphatase activity within the Type 2 spaces or on their membranes, concluding that they may have been abnormal lysosomes deficient in acid hydrolases.

Type 4 spaces. Engel defined these as transitional regions in which admixtures of two or more of the other categories could be seen.

Essentially similar abnormalities to those described above have been reported in a series of subsequent reports on cases of acid maltase deficiency by Martin et al (1973, 1976), Schlenska et al (1976) and Karpati et al (1977). In addition, Martin et al (1973) adduced histological and ultrastructural evidence of glycogen storage within the central and peripheral nervous systems in their infantile case, and Karpati et al (1977) found electrophysiological and histochemical abnormalities suggesting denervation in material from their case, an adult male. Interestingly, Askanas et al (1976) were able to demonstrate identical changes in muscle grown in tissue cultures established from the biopsy.

In McArdle's disease, glycogen accumulates mainly in the sub-sarcolemmal region (Fig. 8.42d) (Korenyi-Both et al 1977) and in debrancher enzyme deficiency in the intermyofibrillar spaces (Murase et al 1973, DiMauro et al 1979).

In addition to these 'cardinal' ultrastructural features, Engel & Dale (1968), Hudgson et al (1968), Engel (1970) and Hudgson & Fulthorpe (1975) all reported increased numbers of lipid droplets within the muscle fibres of their patients with adult acid maltase deficiency. Hudgson & Fulthorpe were impressed particularly by the number of lipid droplets in the material from their infantile cases and speculated that this may have been due to increased mobilisation of fat stores because of impaired glycogen breakdown. Certainly, hyperlipidaemia is well recognised in other forms of glycogenosis (Types I, III and VI), possibly because of the chronic hypoglycaemia

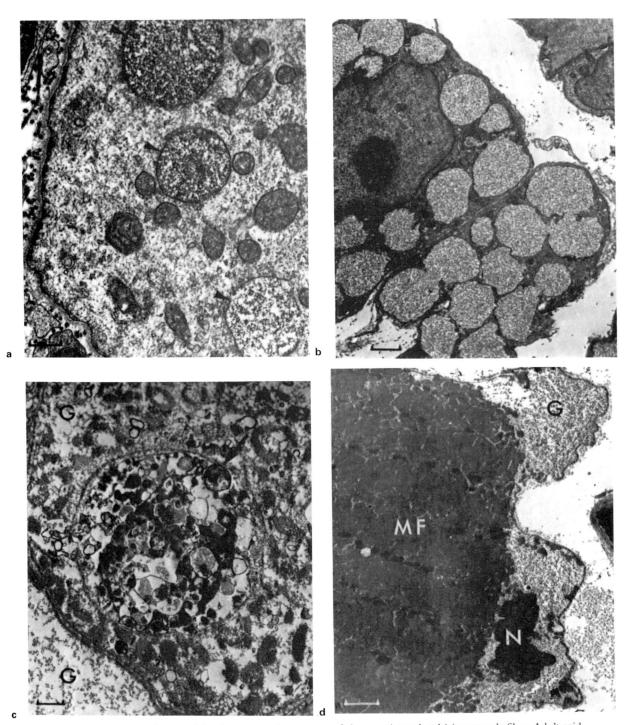

Fig. 9.44 Glycogen storage disease. a Membrane-bound aggregates of glycogen (arrowheads) in a muscle fibre. Adult acid-maltase deficiency (scale bar = 0.5 μm). **b** Large membrane-bound collections of glycogen in two interstitial cells. Infantile acid-maltase deficiency (Pompe's disease) (scale bar = 1 μm). **c** Autophagic vacuole (arrow) containing sequestered glycogen and other granular and membranous debris in a muscle fibre in which there is also excessive accumulation of free glycogen (G) in the sarcoplasm (some of which has been lost during preparation of the section) leading to separation of the myofibrils. Adult acid-maltase deficiency (scale bar = 1.0 μm). **d** Sub-sarcolemmal and perinuclear accumulation of glycogen (G) in a case of McArdle's disease. N = nucleus; MF = myofibrils (scale bar = 2.0 μm).

associated with these conditions (Jakovics et al 1966), and this mechanism was suggested as a causal factor for the lipid storage myopathy developing in Type I glycogenosis (von Gierke's disease) (Yamaguchi et al 1978b). In this context it is also of interest that mixed glycogen and lipid storage in the presence of structurally abnormal mitochondria has been reported in a child with an improving congenital myopathy (Jerusalem et al 1973a), and in glycogen storage disease associated with structurally and functionally abnormal mitochondria in a patient with progressive external ophthalmoplegia (DiMauro et al 1973).

Engel & Dale (1968) described a coiled inclusion in one muscle fibre in their case of late onset adult muscular dystrophy and Engel (1970) found giant mitochondria with crystalloid inclusions in one of his four cases. Hudgson & Fulthorpe (1975) and Korenyi-Both et al (1977) described concentrically laminated inclusions in material from patients with the adult form of acid maltase deficiency and McArdle's disease respectively. The former authors likened these to the inclusions in the muscle fibres of patients with abnormal carbohydrate tolerance, described by Fisher et al (1972), and of a patient with mucopolysaccharidosis (Afifi et al 1974a).

Myopathies associated with abnormalities of oxidative metabolism

The history of the mitochondrial myopathies or cytopathies is so well known that it scarcely bears repetition. The reader is referred to the previous edition (Mastaglia & Hudgson 1981), to the comprehensive review by Morgan-Hughes (1982) and to Chapter 18, for detailed references to earlier reports in this area. However it is worth recording that it was an electron-microscopic study (Shy et al 1966) which first established the concept of mitochondrial muscle disease.

Although some early papers questioned the specificity of mitochondrial abnormalities (Shafiq et al 1967d, Fardeau 1970), there is no reasonable doubt that the stereotyped and quite spectacular abnormalities observed histologically, histochemically (see Chs 4 and 8) and ultrastructurally are

virtually pathognomonic of mitochondrial myopathy (see Fig. 4.12). It has to be conceded, however, that it is impossible to predict the clinical presentation of the affected patient on the one hand and the probable metabolic error on the other on the basis of the morphological abnormalities described. The clinical syndromes associated with these abnormalities and their related metabolic errors (mainly involving the respiratory chain) are discussed in Chapter 18.

Disorders of lipid metabolism

In the last decade it has become clear that there is a group of 'storage' disorders affecting muscle in which neutral lipid accumulates within the muscle fibre, in most cases as a result of defective transport of free fatty acids (FFA) across the mitochondrial membrane to participate in β-oxidation. There appear to be two modes of presentation, one with a relapsing and remitting myopathy and the second with exercise-induced muscle cramps, sometimes accompanied by myoglobinuria (cf. disorders of glycolytic metabolism in muscle). In the first instance, the patients usually present in early adult life with clinical features not unlike those of polymyositis (Bradley et al 1969, Engel & Siekert 1972) and they may even show a partial response to treatment with corticosteroids (Engel & Siekert 1972, Johnson et al 1973). Engel & Angelini (1973) demonstrated deficiency of carnitine, a base with which FFAs combine before crossing the mitochondrial membrane, in one of their cases and this observation has been confirmed in a number of other cases with similar presentations. It has been suggested in the past that carnitine deficiency may be restricted to the skeletal muscle cell in some cases and generalised in others (Engel 1981). However, it has become clear that this distinction is apparent rather than real (Angelini et al 1986); furthermore, recent biochemical studies have shown that carnitine deficiency is likely to be epiphenomenal in many cases, the fundamental metabolic error being acyl CoA dehydrogenase deficiencies with fatty aciduria (Turnbull et al 1984). In addition, the sub-sarcolemmal mitochondrial aggregates are usually larger than normal and the individual organelles may contain inclusions. In general terms, however, their appearance is less bizarre than in the 'mitochondrial' myopathies.

Deficiency of the transferase enzyme systems, notably CPT, responsible for transporting the acyl-carnitine complex across the mitochondrial membrane, may also lead to lipid accumulation within the muscle fibre (Fig. 9.45) and causes recurrent episodes of exertional muscle pain, cramps and myoglobinuria. In these patients, lipid storage may be demonstrable only while the patient has symptoms, the abnormal accumulations disappearing after a period of rest (Cumming et al 1976).

Myopathies associated with hyperthyroidism and hypothyroidism

Hyperthyroidism. The few electron-microscopic studies of muscle from patients with thyrotoxicosis have shown only relatively minor changes and have not contributed significantly to our understanding of the mechanism of muscle dysfunction in such patients. In a study of biopsy material from two cases of thyrotoxic myopathy, Engel (1966) found prominent papillary projections from the sarcolemma of muscle fibres, large sub-sarcolemmal accumulations of glycogen in some fibres, focal dilatations of transverse tubules and degenerative changes in mitochondria, but no abnormality of the contractile elements. He

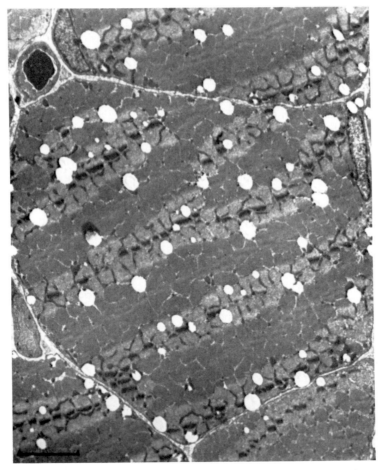

Fig. 9.45   Increased numbers of lipid droplets in muscle fibres in a case of CPT deficiency (scale bar = 0.5 μm).

suggested that the last two changes may have been relevant to the pathogenesis of thyrotoxic myopathy, the mitochondrial abnormalities suggesting the possibility of a disturbance of oxidative metabolism, and the T-tubule changes a possible disturbance of electrical excitation of muscle fibres. Similar changes were found by Gruener et al (1975) who also noted atrophy of both type I and type II fibres.

In thyrotoxic periodic paralysis, glycogen accumulation and distension of the lateral sacs of the SR have been described both during and between attacks of paralysis (Engel 1966, Bergman et al 1970, Takagi et al 1973).

Hypothyroidism. There have been few ultrastructural studies of muscle in patients with hypothyroid myopathy. In general, the changes found have been more striking than those in thyrotoxic myopathy. Norris & Panner (1966) found focal areas of mitochondrial disorganisation, paracrystalline and other types of mitochondrial inclusion, and excessive amounts of glycogen in an adult with a hypertrophic myopathy associated with severe myxoedema. They also noted occasional necrotic fibres but commented that the majority of muscle fibres showed no ultrastructural abnormality. The electron-microscopic findings in the hypertrophic form of myopathy associated with congenital hypothyroidism (Kocher–Debré–Semelaigne syndrome) have been described in a number of cases (Spiro et al 1970, Afifi et al 1974b). Spiro et al (1970) found focal accumulations of glycogen, distension of the SR, and sub-sarcolemmal areas devoid of myofibrils and other organelles in one patient. Afifi et al (1974b), in a study of 10 such children, found very variable ultrastructural changes and commented upon dilatation of the SR, sub-sarcolemmal crescents which in some cases were very large, focal areas of myofibrillar disruption, ring fibres, and the presence of honeycomb-like tubular arrays which were striking in some cases. In a study of a patient with an atrophic form of hypothyroid myopathy, Godet-Guillain & Fardeau (1970) also commented upon the frequency of inclusions and other structural changes in mitochondria, the presence of focal areas of myofibrillar damage which were at times associated with autophagic vacuole formation, dilatation and proliferation of the SR, and

abnormal sub-sarcolemmal areas filled with disorganised filaments (sarcoplasmic masses) and often associated with annular myofibrils. They commented upon the similarity of these changes to those found in myotonic dystrophy.

We have confirmed the above observations in a study of four cases of hypothyroid myopathy (unpublished observations). Degenerative changes in mitochondria, and the presence of small myeloid bodies in muscle fibres and in endothelial cells, were the most frequent findings. In addition, in two cases core-like areas of variable size, which were devoid of enzyme activity in histochemical preparations, were prominent and were found to contain finely granular material which bore a superficial resemblance to glycogen but showed unusual staining properties (Fig. 9.46). Mitochondria contained unduly prominent calcific granules (Fig. 9.18) and, in some instances, paracrystalline inclusions.

The ultrastructural findings therefore suggest that the principal effects of prolonged hypothyroidism are on mitochondria and on carbohydrate metabolism, with the accumulation of glycogen and possibly of some abnormal form of polysaccharide. These findings are in accord with experimental studies which have shown defective oxidative phosphorylation, with changes in mitochondrial morphology and numbers, in thyroidectomised animals (Meijer 1972), and with the impairment of glycogenolysis which has been reported in patients with hypothyroid myopathy (Hurwitz et al 1970, McDaniel et al 1977).

Myopathies associated with disturbances of ACTH and adrenal corticosteroid metabolism

Proximal muscle weakness is commonly found in cases both of Cushing's syndrome and of Addison's disease and is a relatively common finding in patients on long-term corticosteroid therapy, particularly with the fluorinated steroids (see Ch. 28). There have been few studies of the ultrastructural changes in muscle in such cases (Pearce 1964, Engel 1966, Afifi et al 1968). These have not shown any specific changes and have not contributed materially to our understanding of the

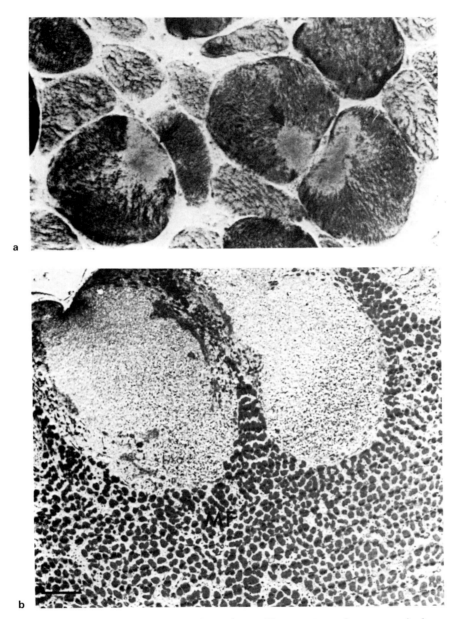

Fig. 9.46 Hypothyroid myopathy. **a** Eccentric core-like areas (arrows) are present in three muscle fibres. Succinic dehydrogenase preparation (× 400). **b** Electron-micrograph of core-like areas showing that they consist of finely granular material with varying staining properties. Similar material separates the myofibrils (MF) (scale bar = 5.0 μm).

pathogenesis of the muscle dysfunction. Focal accumulations of mitochondria, and vacuolation and degeneration of these organelles, have been noted in some cases (Pearce 1964, Engel 1966) but it is not clear to what extent these changes were artefactual. Enlargement of muscle mitochondria and similar changes to those found in some of the human cases have also been found in experimental steroid myopathy in the rat and in the rabbit (D'Agostino & Chiga 1966, Ritter

1967, Afifi & Bergman 1969, Freund-Mölbert et al 1973).

Other changes which have been described in the human and experimental myopathy include an increase in intermyofibrillar sarcoplasm, an apparent increase in glycogen (Pearce 1964, D'Agostino & Chiga 1966, Ritter 1967) and neutral lipid droplets (D'Agostino & Chiga 1966, Harriman & Reed 1972, Freund-Mölbert et al 1973) and thickening of the basement membrane of muscle fibres (Afifi et al 1968, Mastaglia et al 1970). The accumulation of glycogen is in accord with the finding of increased glycogen synthetase activity in muscle in experimental steroid myopathy (Shoji et al 1974). Necrosis and calcification of muscle fibres has been found in some of the short-term high-dose experimental animal studies (Afifi & Bergman 1969, Freund-Molbert et al 1973). An acute necrotising myopathy has been reported in human subjects treated with high doses of hydrocortisone for status asthmaticus (MacFarlane & Rosenthal 1977, Van Marle & Woods 1980, Knox et al 1986). Presumably this is analogous to the experimental models referred to above, although no ultrastructural studies have been carried out on the human material, as far as the authors are aware.

The question of the differential involvement of the type II (glycolytic) fibres in human steroid myopathy and of fast-twitch (white) muscles in animals has not been adequately explored in ultrastructural studies.

It is also appropriate to include in this section a reference to the myopathy which develops in patients who have undergone bilateral adrenalectomy for Cushing's syndrome (Prineas et al 1968). A proportion of such patients develop very high serum ACTH levels with generalised skin pigmentation (Nelson's syndrome) and, subsequently, proximal limb muscle weakness. The presence of myopathy was confirmed in these patients electromyographically and Prineas and his colleagues showed histochemically and electron-microscopically that the type I fibres contained excessive amounts of neutral lipid droplets, which were almost exclusively situated beneath the sarcolemma, usually in association with sentinel mitochondria.

CONGENITAL MYOPATHIES

The difficulties encountered in the clinical classification of this heterogeneous group of disorders are discussed in detail in Chapter 21. Unfortunately, the ultrastructural study of biopsy material from 'floppy' infants and other patients with congenital myopathies has not contributed as much as was expected to the clarification of their nosology. However electron-microscopic studies have provided the morphological substrate for the provisional designation of a number of pathological entities since the mid-1950s, although some of their supposedly 'characteristic' structural abnormalities are not entirely specific. Nevertheless, some of these have stood the test of time and are discussed in detail below. In addition, brief accounts are given of the numerous descriptions of single cases of families in which infantile hypotonia or congenital myopathy has been associated with unusual ultrastructural findings in muscle. These disorders will be discussed under the following headings:

1. Abnormalities of the contractile apparatus,
2. Abnormalities of other sarcoplasmic organelles
3. Myopathies with intracellular inclusions of various types.

Abnormalities of the contractile apparatus

The first account of a congenital myopathy with a 'specific' pathological basis was given by Shy & Magee (1956) in their description of central core disease, a benign condition usually presenting with infantile hypotonia and with a family history suggesting autosomal dominant inheritance. In this disorder, the type I muscle fibres in particular contain cores in which there are variable degrees of disruption of the normal myofibrillar architecture, the cores being termed 'structured' or 'unstructured', depending upon the degree of abnormality (Neville 1973). In the most severely affected fibres, the cores contain no normal cytoplasmic organelles such as SR or mitochondria. Absence of the latter is reflected in the failure of the appropriate histochemical stains to demonstrate any evidence of oxidative enzyme activity within the cores (Dubowitz & Pearce 1960, Engel et al 1961). Since then a number of variations on the original description have been reported. Afifi et al (1965) described two members of a family in which central cores were demonstrated in biopsy specimens, but in which foci of Z-band degeneration resembling that seen in nemaline myopathy were also found. Engel & MacDonald (1970) described congenital myopathies characterised by the presence of multiple and/or miniature cores (multi- and mini-core disease respectively). In addition Radu et al (1977) described two cases in which the muscle fibres contained structured, unstructured and 'reversed' cores, the latter containing central agglomerations of mitochondria.

Loss of the normal ultrastructure of the contractile elements and reduction in the mitochondrial population occurs also in target and targetoid fibres. These are seen most often in denervated muscle, and focal lesions of a similar nature have been described in patients with progressive congenital muscle weakness (Van Wijngaarden et al 1977, Yarom & Shapira 1977). This curious abnormality is accompanied by type I fibre predominance, the individual fibres being significantly reduced in diameter. The pathogenetic basis for this condition is unknown, although Van Wijngaarden and colleagues suggested that delayed development of motor nerves may have been involved on the basis of abnormalities demonstrated by supravital staining of the motor end-plates. Van Wijngaarden and colleagues (1977), in a comprehensive review of the literature, considered that several other reported cases were either identical or very similar to their own.

The next disease 'entity' to be described was nemaline myopathy, first reported by Conen et al (1963) under the name 'myogranular' myopathy. Subsequently, sporadic cases, or families with members suffering from the disease, were described by Shy et al (1963), Engel et al (1964), Spiro & Kennedy (1964), Price et al (1965), Gonatas (1966), Gonatas et al (1966), Engel & Gomez (1967), Hudgson et al (1967) and Shafiq et al (1967a). Autopsy confirmation of the widespread distribution of nemaline rods in a patient with adult-onset symptoms diagnosed on biopsy in life has recently been provided by Brownell et al (1978). Bender & Willner (1978), in a histochemical study of a biopsy specimen of muscle obtained from the mother of a patient with myopathy who had been diagnosed on ultrastruc-

tural grounds as having nemaline myopathy, found abnormalities closely resembling those seen in the child's biopsy, although the mother's muscle contained no rod bodies. They suggested that this established her status as the gene carrier.

Nemaline myopathy is characterised pathologically by the presence of tiny rod-like bodies (up to 5 μm in length and 1.5 μm in diameter) which lie within the muscle fibre; most of these bodies are concentrated in aggregates at the poles of the muscle nuclei. At the light-microscopic level these 'rod' bodies are usually brilliantly refractile with phase-contrast and interference illumination (Gonatas 1966, Hudgson et al 1967) and stain intensely with the modified Gomori trichrome, picro-Mallory and PTAH stains. Ultrastructurally the rod bodies are electron-dense and the larger ones correspond roughly in size to those seen in light-microscopic sections. These larger bodies may occupy a space in the affected fibres up to two sarcomeres in length and, as in the light-microscopic sections, appear to be concentrated near the poles of the muscle nuclei. Moving away from the nuclei, the bodies steadily decrease in number and it becomes increasingly obvious that they are intimately related to the Z bands (Fig. 9.9a).

In many illustrations, the rods appear 'cross-hatched' due to the presence of transverse and axial striae (Fig. 9.9b). In various reports the transverse striae have had a periodicity of approximately 14.5 nm and the axial ones a periodicity ranging from 12 to 18 nm. The measurements quoted by Price et al (1965) differed significantly from those in most other descriptions, and led them to propose that the rod bodies might be composed of an altered form of tropomyosin B. Engel & Gomez (1967) found that the periodicity of the striae in the rod bodies in their material did not correspond with that of the crystal lattice of the Z bands. On the basis of experiments involving glycerination of the biopsy and extraction of the filaments with Guba-Straub-ATP solution, followed by treatment of the residue with Szent-Gyorgyi's actin-extracting solution, they suggested that the rods might contain actin, tropomyosin B, a combination of the two, or another protein with solubility properties common to both. However, most recent evidence suggests that the rods are composed of α-actinin on a skeleton of actin (Ebashi 1967, Yamaguchi et al 1978a).

As we have pointed out above, many so-called specific ultrastructural anomalies, previously identified with discrete clinical syndromes, can occur in a variety of naturally occurring and experimental myopathies. This is certainly the case with nemaline-like degeneration in the Z bands, which can be produced by experimental denervation or tenotomy in animals (Engel et al 1966). Fardeau (1970) has described a similar change in myotonic dystrophy; Cape et al (1970) found rod bodies in material from a patient with polymyositis and we have seen them in various other disorders including muscular dystrophy, mitochondrial myopathy, the myopathy associated with chronic renal failure and in spinal muscular atrophy and glycogen storage disease (Hudgson & Fulthorpe 1975). However, we believe that rod-body formation is still the most important single structural abnormality in some congenital myopathies, particularly those associated with dysmorphogenetic states such as Marfan's syndrome (Hudgson et al 1967).

The last entity to be considered in this section is the 'new' congenital neuromuscular disease with trilaminar fibres described by Ringel et al (1978). In what was clearly an unusual clinical situation, the authors described an infant born with a marked increase in muscle tone, paucity of spontaneous movements and increased serum creatine kinase (CK) activity. Biopsy of muscle at 7 weeks of age demonstrated numerous 'trilaminar' fibres containing three concentric zones (see their figures 2 & 3). Electron microscopy showed that the central zone contained densely packed mitochondria, glycogen, electron-dense material and single myofilaments; the middle zone consisted of deranged myofibrils with Z-band streaming, and the outer zone resembled a sarcoplasmic mass (see their figures 4–7). Appropriate cytochemical techniques demonstrated extrajunctional AChR between the middle and outer zones in the trilaminar fibres. The authors considered that this finding, together with the child's rigidity, was in keeping with abnormal neural influences. It is, however, a little difficult to reconcile this with the grossly elevated serum CK activities (2240 i.u./l at birth and 2290 at 14 days) and the gross disruption of the cyto-architecture of the muscle fibres.

Abnormalities of other sarcoplasmic organelles

The first condition to be described under this heading was myotubular myopathy (Spiro et al 1966), now better known as centronuclear myopathy (Sher et al 1967). There are now approximately 50 cases recorded in the literature, although Palmucci et al (1978) have questioned the validity of some of these cases, pointing out that the mere presence of internal nuclei in fibres otherwise resembling myotubes is not sufficient to justify the diagnosis. Nevertheless, there does appear to be a substantial measure of agreement about the histochemical and ultrastructural characteristics of the disease.

In this condition, which appears to be genetically determined (with a variable mode of inheritance) and slowly progressive, the majority of the muscle fibres (up to 85% in the cases described by Spiro and colleagues) resemble fetal muscle fibres, being of small diameter and containing central nuclei. Histochemical studies (Sher et al 1967, Kinoshita & Cadman 1968) have shown that oxidative enzyme activity may be either increased or decreased in the central region of the fibres, and that myofibrillar adenosine triphosphatase activity is usually absent centrally (Sher et al 1967). Electron-microscopic studies (Spiro et al 1966, Sher et al 1967, Kinoshita & Cadman 1968) have demonstrated that, in addition to the presence of central nuclei, the central region of the fibres is usually devoid of myofibrils. Sher and her co-workers also found a small number (less than 1%) of centrally situated mitochondria which were vacuolated and contained myelin whorls. In contrast, Campbell et al (1969) found large numbers of similarly placed mitochondria in material from a case of myotubular myopathy studied in this department.

The aetiology and pathogenesis of this condition is unknown, although Spiro and associates (1966) suggested that it may develop as a result of 'maturation arrest' because of the structural resemblances between the myopathic fibres and those seen in fetal skeletal muscle. Bethlem and co-workers (1969) suggested a neurogenic basis for the condition in their discussion of the fourth reported case and Serratrice et al (1978) supported this suggestion. They considered that their histo-chemical evidence particularly favoured a neurogenic aetiology, their material showing a type I fibre preponderance and atrophy. The authors likened the latter feature to the appearance of type I fibre hypotrophy with internal nuclei (Engel et al 1968) in which a neurogenic basis has also been suggested. In this context, it may also be relevant that De Reuck et al (1977b) described type I fibre atrophy, particularly in respiratory muscle, in a child with severe neonatal respiratory distress. They considered that a neurogenic basis for the muscle disorder was the most attractive of the possible hypotheses. However, Palmucci et al (1978) claimed that centronuclear myopathy is likely to be a histopathological syndrome produced by several unrelated disease entities, a suggestion mooted previously by Bradley et al (1970).

In 1973, Jerusalem and co-workers described a new, benign congenital disorder in two brothers born of a consanguineous marriage. They called this condition sarcotubular myopathy and reported that it was characterised histopathologically by microvacuolar degeneration affecting the type II more than the type I fibres (see their figures 3 & 4), and which was segmental in distribution in longitudinal sections. Electron micrographs of the affected fibres showed that they contained rows of membrane-bound spaces, some of which were coalescing and some of which were in close relationship to tubular profiles (see their figure 7). Appropriate electron-cytochemical techniques showed that the vacuoles probably originated from the SR rather than the T system. The authors concluded that segmental vacuolation of the SR with selective affection of type II fibres was the characteristic morphological abnormality and they differentiated this from the non-specific dilatation of the SR which occurs in many necrobiotic myopathies and in the periodic paralyses.

Myopathies with intracellular inclusions

The presence of inclusion bodies of various kinds within mitochondria in patients with mitochondrial myopathy and other conditions has already been discussed. In this section, we propose to consider a number of congenital myopathies with inclusions in other compartments of the muscle cell.

Jenis et al (1969) described a fatal congenital myopathy in which they were able to demonstrate eosinophilic crystalline inclusions within the myonuclei, with similar smaller bodies within the sarcoplasm and arising from the Z bands of the muscle fibres. Multiple passage of material from this case through suckling mice and rhesus monkey and human embryonal kidney in tissue culture failed to adduce any evidence of viral infection, but electron microscopy of the intranuclear and sarcoplasmic inclusions indicated that they possessed a crystal lattice not unlike that of nemaline rods (see, in particular, their figure 7). The authors were unable to reach any definite conclusions about the fundamental nature of this condition and particularly about its relationship to other congenital myopathies. As far as we are aware, no similar case has been described subsequently.

Brooke & Neville (1972) reported two unrelated cases of a progressive congenital myopathy which also had a fatal termination. In each case, light-microscopy of muscle biopsies revealed scattered sub-sarcolemmal inclusions which were eosinophilic with haematoxylin and eosin, and red in the modified trichrome preparation. Further histochemical studies demonstrated that the bodies contained both RNA and sulphydryl groups in high concentration, the latter observation prompting the authors to call them 'reducing bodies'. Electron microscopy showed that these bodies were densely osmiophilic, porous structures up to about 10 μm in length. They were not membrane-bound, contained beaded fibrillar material in places and the pores often contained glycogen (see their figures 10 & 13). Speculating on the possible origin of these structures, the authors considered the possibility that they were derived from an RNA virus. They noted, in addition, that the presence of sulphydryl groups in high concentration in skeletal muscle is most unusual, although the sulphydryl-containing amino acid, homocysteine, is produced during the transmethylation of guanidoacetate to creatine.

As far as we know, no other cases of this kind have been reported, although Sahgal & Sahgal (1977) described a non-progressive congenital myopathy characterised by the presence of sub-sarcolemmal inclusions reacting strongly for sulphydryl groups, particularly in type I fibres.

However, these inclusions contained granular and filamentous material only at the ultrastructural level and did not resemble the 'reducing bodies' of Brooke & Neville (1972) in any other respect.

At about the same time as the description of reducing-body myopathy appeared, Engel et al (1972) described another curious inclusion in a child with non-progressive weakness since infancy. These inclusions were observed first by phase-contrast microscopy of semithin Epon sections, and were described as being oval or irregularly circular in shape, invariably sub-sarcolemmal in situation, often near the muscle nuclei and from 7 to 10 μm in length. Ultrastructurally they were composed of complex convoluted lamellae arranged in 'fingerprint' patterns (see their figure 5). In each inclusion the lamellae were spaced 30 nm apart and were studded with sawtooth-like projections 6.5 nm wide and 16 nm high, with a period varying from 14.5 to 16 nm. Predigestion of the muscle with RNase and amylase, disruption of the membranous components of the muscle fibres by glycerination and selective extraction of the myosin and actin filaments, M bands and Z bands, did not alter the appearance of these structures. 'Fingerprint' inclusions have been reported in several other cases of congenital myopathy (Fardeau et al 1976), dystrophia myotonica (Tomé & Fardeau 1973) and oculopharyngeal dystrophy (Julien et al 1974). In addition, we have seen a similar structure in material from a patient with uraemic myopathy.

Fardeau's group (Fardeau et al 1978) reported a family with a genetically determined myopathy (autosomal dominant inheritance) with affection of skeletal, pharyngeal and respiratory musculature, cardiomyopathy and lens opacities. The biopsies from affected members of the family revealed what the authors described as 'rubbing out' of the intermyofibrillar network in the type I fibres, electron microscopy showing that this was associated with the deposition of electron-dense granular and filamentous material in the sarcoplasm of the fibres. In some areas, this material was arranged in a meshwork around the myofibrils, although it did not appear to have any structural relationship with the Z band or indeed with any of the other components of the contractile apparatus.

The final condition cited in this section is the recently reported myofibrillar inclusion-body myopathy or cytoplasmic-body neuromyopathy presenting with respiratory insufficiency and weight loss (Clark et al 1978, Jerusalem et al 1979). In this condition the type I fibres contain numerous typical cytoplasmic bodies (Jerusalem et al 1979, see their figure 4). The nature of this condition remains obscure, although some cases are familial with an autosomal dominant form of inheritance.

CONCLUSIONS

The role of electron-microscopy in the investigation of diseased muscle has changed since the first edition of this book was published nearly a quarter of a century ago. Then, the electron-microscope was used principally to acquire basic morphological information about the many different neuromuscular disorders. This cataloguing role is now relatively less important because it has been realised that conventional electron-microscopy by itself is unlikely to reveal the basic defect in any one disease. Accordingly, it is being used increasingly in combination with other techniques and the electron-microscopic specimen itself is being manipulated, probed, fractured and labelled in a variety of ways, some referred to in this chapter. Ultrastructural studies have therefore become less descriptive and more analytical. Increasingly they are being used to pinpoint the location in the specimen of chemical elements (by electron-probe microanalysis), enzymes (by electron-microscopic cytochemistry) and other proteins (by electron-microscopic immunolabelling). Already the last-mentioned technique, in particular, is transforming our view of muscle and thereby providing new insights into the pathogenesis of those muscular disorders which continue to confound medical science.

ACKNOWLEDGEMENTS

The work discussed in this chapter was carried out with the aid of grants from the Muscular Dystrophy Group of Great Britain. We wish to acknowledge the invaluable technical assistance of Mr John Walsh and Mr John Fulthorpe.

The manuscript was typed by Miss Carol Atkinson whose efficient services are greatly appreciated.

REFERENCES

Adams R D, Denny-Brown D, Pearson C M 1962 Diseases of muscle: A study in pathology, 2nd edn. Hoeber, New York

Afifi A K 1972 The myopathology of the prune belly syndrome. Journal of the Neurological Sciences 15: 153

Afifi A K, Smith J W, Zellweger H 1965 Congenital non-progressive myopathy. Central core disease and nemaline myopathy in one family. Neurology (Minneapolis) 15: 371

Afifi A K, Bergman R A, Harvey J C 1968 Steroid myopathy. Clinical, histologic and cytologic observation. Johns Hopkins Medical Journal 123: 158

Afifi A K, Bergman R A 1969 Steroid myopathy. A study of the evolution of the muscle lesion in rabbits. Johns Hopkins Medical Journal 124: 66

Afifi A K, der Kaloustian V M, Bahuth W B, Mire-Salman J 1974a Concentrically-laminated membranous inclusions in myofibres of Dyggve-Melchior-Clausen syndrome. Journal of the Neurological Sciences 21: 335

Afifi A K, Najjar S S, Mire-Salman J, Bergman R A 1974b The myopathology of the Kocher-Debré-Semelaigne syndrome. Journal of the Neurological Sciences 22: 445

Aloisi M, Mussini I, Schiaffino S 1973 Activation of nuclei in denervation and hypertrophy. In: Kakulas B A (ed) Basic research in myology. Excerpta Medica, Amsterdam, p 338

Alvira M M, Mendoza M 1975 Reye's syndrome: A viral myopathy? New England Journal of Medicine 292: 1297

Anand R 1983 Cellular membranes in Duchenne muscular dystrophy. European Journal of Biochemistry 15: 1211

Ambler M W, Neave C, Entwistle R 1987 Fingerprint inclusions in normal fetal muscle. Acta Neuropathologica 73: 185

Angelini C, Trevisan C, Vergani L 1986 Disorders of lipid metabolism. Muscle & Nerve 9: 6 (53/Suppl)

Antin P B, Forry-Schandies S, Friedman T M, Tapscott S J, Holtzer H 1981 Taxol induces postmitotic myoblasts to assemble interdigitating microtubule-myosin arrays that exclude actin filaments. Journal of Cell Biology 90: 300

Appleyard S T, Dunn M J, Dubowitz V, Scott M L, Pittman S J, Shotton D M 1984 Monoclonal antibodies detect a spectrin-like protein in normal and dystrophic human skeletal muscle. Proceedings of the National Academy of Science 81: 767

Arahata K, Engel A G 1986 Monoclonal antibody analysis of mononuclear cells in myopathies. III: Immunoelectron microscopy aspects of cell-mediated muscle fiber injury. Annals of Neurology 19: 112

Arahata K, Ishiura S, Ishiguro T et al 1988 Immunostaining of skeletal and cardiac muscle cell surface membrane with antibody against Duchenne muscular dystrophy peptide. Nature (London) 33: 861

Askanas V, Engel W K, Di Mauro S, Brooks B R, Mehler M 1976 Adult onset acid maltase deficiency. New England Journal of Medicine 294: 573

Askanas V, Engel W K, Alvarez R 1992 Light and electronmicroscopic localisation of β-amyloid protein in muscle biopsies of patients with inclusion body myositis. American Journal of Pathology 141: 31

Banker B Q 1975 Dermatomyositis of childhood. Ultrastructural observations of muscle and intramuscular blood vessels. Journal of Neuropathology and Experimental Neurology 34: 46

Banker B Q 1986 The ultrastructural features of dermatomyositis. Muscle and Nerve 9: 34 (59/Suppl)

Baringer J R 1971 Tubular aggregates in endoplasmic reticulum in herpes-simplex encephalitis. New England Journal of Medicine 285: 943

Barka T 1964 Electron histochemical localization of acid phosphatase activity in the small intestine of mouse. Journal of Histochemistry and Cytochemistry 12: 229

Baruah J K, Sulaiman A R, Kinder D, Murtha T 1983 Electron probe, X-ray microanalysis of mitochondrial paracrystalline inclusions. In: Scarlato G, Cerri C (eds) Mitochondrial pathology in muscle disease. Piccin, Padua, p 159

Ben-Bassat M, Machtey I 1972 Picornavirus-like structures in acute dermatomyositis. American Journal of Clinical Pathology 58: 245

Bender A N, Willner J P 1978 Nemaline (rod) myopathy: the need for histochemical evaluation of affected families. Annals of Neurology 4: 37

Bergman R A, Afifi A K, Dunke L M, Johns R T 1970 Muscle pathology in hypokalaemic periodic paralysis with hyperthyroidism. Annals of the New York Academy of Sciences 126: 100

Bethlem J, Van Wijngaarden G K, Meijer AEFH, Hülsmann W C 1969 Neuromuscular disease with type I fiber atrophy, central nuclei and myotube-like structures. Neurology (Minneapolis) 19: 705

Bethlem J, Van Wijngaarden G K, De Jong J 1973 The incidence of lobulated fibres in the FSH type of muscular dystrophy and the limb-girdle syndrome. Journal of the Neurological Sciences 18: 351

Bethlem J, Arts W F, Dingemans K F 1978 Common origin of rods, cores, miniature cores and focal loss of cross-striations. Archives of Neurology 35: 555

Bird J W C, Kirschke H, Wood L 1982 Proteolytic enzyme activities in differentiating muscle cells. Federation Proceedings 41: 507

Bird J W C, Roisen F J 1986 Lysosomes in muscle: developmental aspects, enzyme activities, and role in protein turnover. In: Engel A G, Banker B Q (eds) Myology. McGraw-Hill, New York, p 745

Bischoff R 1975 Regeneration of single skeletal muscle fibers in vitro. Anatomical Record 182: 215

Bonilla E, Schotland D L, Wakayama Y 1982 Freeze-fracture studies in human muscular dystrophy. In: Schotland D L (ed) Disorders of the motor unit. John Wiley, New York, p 475

Bonilla E, Samitt C E, Miranda A F et al 1988 Duchenne muscular dystrophy: deficiency of dystrophin at the muscle cell surface. Cell 54: 447

Borg K, Tomé F M S, Edstrom L 1991 Intranuclear and cytoplasmic filamentous inclusions in distal myopathy (Welander). Acta Neuropathologica 82: 102

Bowman W 1840. On the minute structure and movements of voluntary muscle. Philosophical Transactions of the Royal Society of London, series B 130: 457

Bradley W G 1969 Ultrastructural changes in adynamia episodica hereditaria and normokalaemic familial periodic paralysis. Brain 92: 379

Bradley W G, Hudgson P, Gardner-Medwin D, Walton J N 1969 Myopathy with abnormal lipid metabolism in skeletal muscle. Lancet 1: 495

Bradley W G, Price D L, Watanabe C K 1970 Familial centronuclear myopathy. Journal of Neurology, Neurosurgery and Psychiatry 33: 687

Brody I A, Dudley A W 1969 Thyrotoxic hypokalemic periodic paralysis. Muscle morphology and functional assay of sarcoplasmic reticulum. Archives of Neurology 21: 1

Brownell A K W, Gilbert J J, Shaw D T, Garcia B, Wenkeback G F, Lam A K S 1978 Adult onset nemaline myopathy. Neurology (Minneapolis) 28: 1306

Brooke M H, Neville H E 1972 Reducing body myopathy. Neurology (Minneapolis) 22: 829

Busch W A, Stromer M H, Goll D E, Suzuki A 1972 Ca^{2+}-specific removal of Z lines from rabbit skeletal muscle. Journal of Cell Biology 52: 367

Buxton J, Shelbourne P, Davies J et al 1992 Detection of an unstable fragment of DNA specific to individuals with myotonic dystrophy. Nature 355: 547

Byers T J, Kunkel L M, Watkins S C 1991 The subcellular distribution of dystrophin in mouse skeletal, cardiac, and smooth muscle. Journal of Cell Biology 115: 411

Campbell K P, Kahl S D 1989 Association of dystrophin and an integral membrane glycoprotein. Nature 338: 259

Campbell M, Rebeiz J J, Walton J N 1969 Myotubular, centronuclear or pericentrinuclear myopathy. Journal of the Neurological Sciences 8: 425

Cape C A, Johnson W M, Pitner S E 1970 Nemaline structures in polymyositis. Neurology (Minneapolis) 20: 494

Cardiff D R 1966 A histochemical and electron microscopic study of skeletal muscle in a case of Pompe's disease (glycogenosis II). Pediatrics 37: 249

Carpenter S, Karpati G, Wolfe L 1970 Virus-like filaments and phospholipid accumulation in skeletal muscle. Neurology (Minneapolis) 20: 889

Carpenter S, Karpati G, Rothman S, Watters G 1976 The childhood type of dermatomyositis. Neurology (Minneapolis) 26: 952

Carpenter S, Karpati G, Heller I, Eisen A 1978 Inclusion body myositis: a distinct variety of idiopathic inflammatory myopathy. Neurology (Minneapolis) 28: 78

Carpenter S, Karpati G 1979 Duchenne muscular dystrophy. Plasma membrane loss initiates muscle cell necrosis unless it is repaired. Brain 102: 147

Carpenter S, Karpati G, Holland P 1985 New observations in reducing body myopathy. Neurology (Cleveland) 35: 818

Carpenter S, Karpati G, Zubrzycka-Gaarn E E, Bulman D E, Ray P N, Worton R G 1990 Dystrophin is localized to the plasma membrane of human skeletal muscle fibers by electron-microscopic cytochemical study. Muscle and Nerve 13: 376

Casanova G, Jerusalem F 1979 Myopathology of myotonic dystrophy. Acta Neuropathologica (Berlin) 45: 231

Caulfield J B, Rebeiz J J, Adams R D 1968 Viral involvement of human muscle. Journal of Pathology and Bacteriology 96: 232

Chalmers A C, Greco C M, Miller R G 1991 Prognosis in AZT myopathy. Neurology 41: 1181

Cheek D B, Holt A B, Hill D E, Talbert J L 1971 Skeletal muscle cell mass and growth: the concept of the deoxyribonuclei acid unit. Paediatric Research 5: 312

Chou S M 1967 Myxovirus-like structures in a case of human chronic polymyositis. Science 158: 1453

Chou S M 1968 Mxovirus-like structures and accompanying nuclear changes in chronic polymyositis. Archives of Pathology 86: 649

Chou S M 1969 'Megaconial' mitochondria in a case of chronic polymyositis. Acta Neuropathologica (Berlin) 12: 68

Chou S M 1973 Prospects of viral etiology in polymyositis. In: Kakulas B A (ed), Clinical studies in myology, Part 2. p 17

Chou S M, Gutmann L 1970 Picornavirus-like crystals in subacute polymyositis. Neurology (Minneapolis) 20: 205

Chou S M, Nonaka I 1977 Satellite cells and muscle regeneration in diseased human skeletal muscles. Journal of the Neurological Sciences 34: 131

Clark J R, D'Agostino A N, Wilson J, Brooks R R, Cole G C 1978 Autosomal dominant myofibrillar inclusion body myopathy — clinical, histologic histochemical and ultrastructural characteristics. Neurology (Minneapolis) 28: 399

Conen P E, Murphy E G, Donohue W L 1963 Light and electron microscopic studies of 'myogranules' in a child with hypotonia and weakness. Canadian Medical Association Journal 89: 983

Coulter C L, Marks W A, Bodensteiner J B et al 1991 An adult-onset myopathy characterized by a double ring appearance of muscle fibers. Neuromuscular Disorders 1: 205

Courtecuisse V, Royer P, Habib R, Monnier C, Demos J 1965 Glycogenose musculaire per deficit d'alpha-1,4-glucosidase simulant une dystrophie musculaire progressive. Archives françaises de pédiatrie 22: 1153

Cross R A, Stewart M, Kendrick-Jones J 1990 Structural predictions for the central domain of dystrophin. FEBS Letters 262: 87

Crowe W E, Bove K E, Levinson J E, Hilton P K 1992 Clinical and pathogenetic implications of histopathology in childhood polydermatomyositis. Arthritis and Rheumatism 25: 126

Cullen M J, Fulthorpe J J 1975 Stages in fibre breakdown in Duchenne muscular dystrophy. Journal of the Neurological Sciences 24: 179

Cullen M J, Pluskal M J 1977 Early changes in the ultrastructure of denervated rat skeletal muscle. Experimental Neurology 56: 115

Cullen M J, Appleyard S T, Bindoff L 1978 Morphologic aspects of muscle breakdown and lysosomal activation. Annals of the New York Academy of Sciences 317: 440

Cullen M J, Mastaglia F L 1980 Morphological changes in dystrophic muscle. British Medical Bulletin 36: 143

Cullen M J, Watkins S C 1981 The role of satellite cells in regeneration in diseased muscle. Advances in the Physiological Sciences 24: 341

Cullen M J, Fulthorpe J J 1982 Phagocytosis of the A band following Z line and I band loss. Its significance in skeletal muscle breakdown. Journal of Pathology 138: 129

Cullen M J, Mastaglia F L 1982 Pathological reactions of skeletal muscle. In: Mastaglia F L, Walton J N (eds) Skeletal muscle pathology. Churchill Livingstone, Edinburgh, p 88

Cullen M J, Walsh J, Nicholson L V B, Harris J B 1990 Ultrastructural localization of dystrophin in human muscle using gold immunolabelling. Proceedings of the Royal Society (London) B 240: 197

Cullen M J, Walsh J, Nicholson L V B et al 1991 Immunogold labelling of dystrophin in human muscle, using an antibody to the last 17 amino acids of the C-terminus. Neuromuscular Disorders 1: 113

Cullen M J, Watkins S C 1993 Ultrastructure of muscular dystrophy: new aspects. Micron 24: 287

Cumming W J K, Hardy M, Hudgson P, Walls J 1976 Carnitine palmityl transferase deficiency. Journal of the Neurological Sciences 30: 347

D'Agostino A N, Chiga M 1966 Corticosteroid myopathy in rabbits: A light and electron microscopic study. Neurology (Minneapolis) 16: 257

Dayton W R, Reville W J, Goll D E, Stromer M H 1976 A Ca^{2+}-activated protease possibly involved in myofibrillar protein turnover. Partial characterization of the purified enzyme. Biochemistry 15: 2159

De Coster W J P 1979 Experimental hypokalaemia: ultrastructural changes in rat gastrocnemius muscle. Archives of Neurology 45: 79

De Reuck J, De Coster W, Inderadjaja N 1977a Acute viral polymyositis with predominant diaphragm involvement. Journal of the Neurological Sciences 33: 453

De Reuck J, Hooft C, De Coster W, Van den Bossche H, Cuvelier C 1977b A progressive congenital myopathy. European Neurology 15: 217

Dreyfus J C, Schapira G, Schapira F 1954 Biochemical study of muscle in progressive muscular dystrophy. Journal of Clinical Investigation 33: 794

DiMauro S, Schotland D L, Bonilla E, Lee C-P, Gambetti P, Rowland L P 1973 Progressive ophthalmoplegia, glycogen storage and abnormal mitochondria. Archives of Neurology 29: 170

DiMauro S, Hartwig G B, Hays A et al 1979 Debrancher deficiency: neuromuscular disorder in 5 adults. Annals of Neurology 5: 422

Dubowitz V 1985 Muscle biopsy. A practical approach. Baillière Tindall, London

Dubowitz V, Pearse A G E 1960 Oxidative enzymes and phosphorylase in central core disease of muscle. Lancet 2: 23

Dubowitz V, Brooke M H 1973 Muscle biopsy: a modern approach. W B Saunders, London

Dunn M J, Sewry C A, Statham H E, Dubowitz V 1984 Studies on the extracellular matrix in diseased human muscle. In: Demp R B, Hinchcliffe J R, Matrices and cell differentiation. Alan Liss, New York, p 213

Ebashi S 1967 Quoted by C M Pearson. In: Skeletal muscle. Basic and clinical aspects and illustrative new diseases. Annals of Internal Medicine 67: 614

Edström L, Thornell L-E, Albo J, Landin S, Samuelsson M 1990 Myopathy with respiratory failure and typical myofibrillar lesions. Journal of the Neurological Sciences 96: 211

Edström L, Mair W G P, Wroblewski R, Hovmoller M, Malm G 1986 Type distribution of muscle fibres and their ultrastructure related to ultracellular elemental composition as revealed by energy dispersive X-ray microanalysis. Journal of the Neurological Sciences 76: 31

Emslie-Smith A M, Engel A G 1990 Microvascular changes in early and advanced dermatomyositis: a quantitative study. Annals of Neurology

Engel A G 1966 Thyrotoxic and corticosteroid-induced myopathies. Mayo Clinic Proceedings 41: 785

Engel A G 1970 Acid maltase deficiency in adult life. Brain 93: 599

Engel A G 1981 Metabolic and endocrine myopathies. In: Walton J N (ed) Disorders of Voluntary Muscle 4th edn. Churchill Livingstone, Edinburgh, p 664

Engel A G, Gomez M R 1967 Nemaline (Z disc) myopathy: Observations of the origin, structure and solubility properties of the nemaline structures. Journal of Neuropathology and Experimental Neurology 26: 601

Engel A G, Potter C S, Rosevear J W 1967 Studies on carbohydrate metabolism and mitochondrial respiratory activities in primary hypokalemic periodic paralysis. Neurology (Minneapolis) 17: 329

Engel A G, Dale A J D 1968 Autophagic glycogenosis of late onset with mitochondrial abnormalities; light and electron microscopic observations. Mayo Clinic Proceedings 43: 233

Engel A G, MacDonald R D 1970 Ultrastructural reactions in muscle disease and their light-microscopic correlates. In: Walton J N, Canal N, Scarlato G (eds) Muscle diseases. Excerpta Medica, Amsterdam

Engel A G, Gomez M R, Groover R V 1971 Multicore disease: a recently recognized congenital myopathy associated with multifocal degeneration of muscle fibres. Mayo Clinic Proceedings 46: 666

Engel A G, Siekert R G 1972 Lipid storage myopathy responsive to prednisone. Archives of Neurology 27: 174

Engel A G, Angelini C, Gomez M R 1972 Fingerprint body myopathy. Mayo Clinic Proceedings 47: 377

Engel A G, Angelini C 1973 Carnitine deficiency of human skeletal muscle with associated lipid storage. Science 179: 899

Engel A G, Biesecker G 1982 Complement activation in muscle fiber necrosis: demonstration of the membrane attack complex of complement in necrotic fibers. Annals of Neurology 12: 289

Engel W K, Foster J B, Hughes B P, Huxley H E, Mahler R 1961 Central core disease: An investigation of a rare muscle cell abnormality. Brain 84: 167

Engel W K, Eyerman E L, Williams H E 1963 Late onset type of skeletal muscle phosphorylase deficiency: A new familial variety with completely and partly affected subjects. New England Journal of Medicine 268: 135

Engel W K, Wanko T, Fenichel G M 1964 Nemaline myopathy: A second case. Archives of Neurology 11: 22

Engel W K, Brooke M H, Nelson P G 1966 Histochemical studies of denervated or tenotomized muscle. Annals of the New York Academy of Sciences 138: 160

Engel W K, Gold N, Karpati G 1968 Type I fiber hypotrophy and central nuclei. Archives of Neurology 18: 435

Eppenberger-Eberhardt M, Riesinger I, Messerli et al 1991 Adult rat cardiomyocytes cultured in creatine-deficient medium display large mitochondria with paracrystalline inclusions, enriched for creatine kinase. Journal of Cell Biology 113: 289

Ervasti J M, Ohlendieck K, Kahl S D, Gaver M G, Campbell K P 1990 Deficiency of a glycoprotein component of the dystrophin complex in dystrophic muscle. Nature 345: 315

Ervasti J M, Campbell K P 1991 Membrane organization of the dystrophin–glycoprotein complex. Cell 66: 1121

Fardeau M 1970 Ultrastructural lesions in progressive muscular dystrophies. A critical study of their specificity. In: Muscle diseases. Proceedings of an International Congress. Excerpta Medica, Amsterdam

Fardeau M, Tomé F M S, Derambure S 1976 Familial fingerprint body myopathy. Archives of Neurology 33: 724

Fardeau M, Godet-Guillain J, Tomé F M S, Collin H, Gaudeau S, Boffety Cl, L, Vernant P 1978 Une nouvelle affection musculaire. Revue Neurologique 131: 411

Fardeau M, Tomé F M S, Simon P 1979 Muscle and nerve changes induced by perhexiline maleate in man and mice. Muscle and Nerve 2: 24

Fidzianska A, Goebel H H 1991 Human ontogenesis. 3. Cell death in fetal muscle. Acta Neuropathological 81: 572

Fidzianska A, Goebel H H, Warlo I 1990 Acute infantile spinal muscular atrophy. Muscle apoptosis as a proposed pathogenetic mechanism. Brain 113: 433

Fisher E R, Gonzalez A R, Khurana R C, Danowski T S 1972 Unique, concentrically laminated, membranous, inclusions in myofibers. American Journal of Clinical Pathology 48: 239

Freund-Mölbert E, Ketelsen U-P, Beckmann R 1973 Ultrastructural study of experimental steroid myopathy. In: Kakulas B A (ed), Basic research in myology. Excerpta Medica, Amsterdam, p 595

Fukuhara N 1979 Electron microscopical demonstration of nucleic acids in virus-like particles in the skeletal muscle of a traffic accident victim. Acta Neuropathologica (Berlin) 47: 55

Fukuyama Y, Ando J T, Yokota J 1977 Acute fulminant myoglobinuric polymyositis with picornavirus-like crystals. Journal of Neurology, Neurosurgery and Psychiatry 40: 755

Gallai M 1977 Myopathy with hyperaldosteronism — An electron microscopic study. Journal of the Neurological Sciences 32: 337

Gilchrist J M, Ambler M, Agtiello P 1991 Steroid-responsive tubular aggregate myopathy. Muscle and Nerve 14: 233

Godet-Guillain J, Fardeau M 1970 Hypothyroid myopathy. Histological and ultrastructural study of an atrophic form. In: J N Walton, N Canal, G Scarlato (eds) Muscle disease. Excerpta Medica, Amsterdam, p 512

Gold R, Reichman H 1992 Muscle pathology correlates with permanent weakness in hypokalemic periodic paralysis: a case report. Acta Neuropathologica 84: 202

Goldspink D 1972 Postembryonic growth and differentiation of striated muscle. In: Bourne G H (ed) Function of muscle. Academic Press, New York, vol 1, p 179

Gonatas N K 1966 The fine structure of the rod-like bodies in nemaline myopathy and their relation to the Z discs. Journal of Neuropathology and Experimental Neurology 25: 409

Gonatas N K, Perez M C, Shy G M, Evangelista I 1965 Central 'core' disease of skeletal muscle. Ultrastructural and cytochemical observations in two cases. American Journal of Pathology 47: 503

Gonatas N K, Shy G M, Godfrey E H 1966 The origin of nemaline structures. New England Journal of Medicine 274: 535

Gonzalez-Angulo A, Fraga A, Mintz G, Zavala B 1968 Sub-microscopic alterations in capillaries of skeletal muscle in polymyositis. American Journal of Medicine 45: 873

Gordon A M, Green J R, Lagunoff D 1970 Studies on a patient with hypokalaemic familial periodic paralysis. American Journal of Medicine 48: 185

Goto Y, Komiyama A, Tanabe Y, Katafuchi Y, Ohtaki E, Nonaka I 1990 Myopathy in Marinesco–Sjögren syndrome: an ultrastructural study. Acta Neuropathologica 80: 123

Griggs R C, Karpati G G 1991 The pathogenesis of dermatomyositis. Archives of Neurology 48: 21

Gruener R, Stern L Z, Payne C, Hannapel L 1975 Hyperthyroid myopathy. Journal of the Neurological Sciences 24: 339

Grüner J E 1966 Anomalies du reticulum sarcoplasmique et prolifération des tubules dans le muscle d'une paralysie périodique familiale. Comptes rendus des seances de la Societé de biologie et des filiales 26: 555

Gussoni E, Pavlath G K, Lanctot A M et al 1992 Normal dystrophin transcripts detected in Duchenne muscular dystrophy patients after myoblast transplantation. Nature 356: 435

Györkey F, Min F-W, Sinkovics J G, Györkey P 1969 Systemic lupus erythematosus and myxovirus. New England Journal of Medicine 280: 333

Györkey F, Labral G A, Györkey P, Uribe-Botero G, Dressman G-R, Melnick J L 1978 Coxsackie virus aggregates in muscle cells of a polymyositis patient. Intervirology 10: 69

Halbig L, Gutmann L, Goebel H H, Brick J F, Schochet S 1988 Ultrastructural pathology in emetine-induced myopathy. Acta Neuropathologica 75: 577

Hanson P A, Urizar R E 1975 Reye's syndrome — virus or artifact in muscle. New England Journal of Medicine 293: 505

Hantai D, Founier J-G, Vazeux R, Collin H, Baudrimont M, Fardeau M 1991 Skeletal muscle involvement in human immunodeficiency virus infection. Acta Neuropathologica 81: 496

Hanzlikova V, Makova E V, Hnik P 1975 Satellite cells of rat soleus in the process of compensatory hypertrophy combined with denervation. Cell and Tissue Research 160: 411

Harley H, Brook J D, Rundle S A et al 1992 Expansion of an unstable DNA region and phenotypic variation in myotonic dystrophy. Nature 355: 545

Harriman D G F, Reed R 1972 The incidence of lipid droplets in human skeletal muscle in neuromuscular disorders. Journal of Pathology 106: 1

Hashimoto K, Robinson L, Velayos E, Niizuma K 1971 Dermatomyositis. Electron microscopic, immunological, and tissue culture studies of paramyxovirus-like inclusions. Archives of Dermatology 103: 120

Hess A, Rosner S 1970 The satellite cell bud and myoblast in denervated mammalian muscle. American Journal of Anatomy 129: 21

Himmelman F, Schröder J M 1992 Colchicine myopathy in a case of familial mediterranean fever: immunohistochemical and ultrastructural study of accumulated tubulin-immunoreactive material. Acta Neuropathologica 83: 440

Hirano M, Ott B R, Raps E C et al 1992 Acute quadriplegic myopathy: a complication of treatment with steroids, nondepolarizing blocking agents or both. Neurology 42: 2082

Ho K-L 1987 Crystalloid bodies in skeletal muscle of hypothyroid myopathy. Ultrastructural and histochemical studies. Acta Neuropathologica 74: 22

Hoffman E P, Brown R H, Kunkel L M 1987a Dystrophin: the protein product of the Duchenne muscular dystrophy locus. Cell 51: 919

Hoffman E P, Knudson C M, Campbell K P, Kunkel L M 1987b Subcellular fractionation of dystrophin to the triads of skeletal muscle. Nature 330: 754

Hohlfeld R, Engel A G, Il K, Harper M C 1991 Polymyositis mediated by T lymphocytes that express the γ/δ receptor. New England Journal of Medicine 324: 877

Howes E L, Price H M, Pearson C M, Blumberg J M 1966 Hypokalemic periodic paralysis: electron microscopic changes in the sarcoplasm. Neurology (Minneapolis) 16: 242

Hsu L, Trupin G L, Roisen F J 1979 The role of satellite cells and myonuclei during myogenesis in vitro. In: Mauro A (ed) Muscle regeneration. Raven Press, New York, p 115

Hudgson P, Fulthorpe J J 1975 The pathology of type II skeletal muscle glycogenosis. A light and electronmicroscopic study. Journal of Pathology 116:139

Hudgson P, Gardner-Medwin D, Fulthorpe J J, Walton J N 1967 Nemaline myopathy. Neurology (Minneapolis) 17: 1125

Hudgson P, Gardner-Medwin D, Worsfold M, Pennington R J T, Walton J N 1968 Adult myopathy from glycogen storage disease due to acid maltase deficiency. Brain 91: 435

Hudgson P, Pearce G W 1969 Ultramicroscopic studies of

diseased muscle. In: Walton J N (ed) Disorders of voluntary muscle. 1st edn. Churchill, London, p 277

Hughes J T, Esiri M M 1978 Ultrastructural studies in human polymyositis. Journal of the Neurological Sciences 25: 347

Hurwitz L J, Carson N A, Allen I V, Fannin T F, Lyttle J A, Neill D W 1967 Clinical, biochemical and histopathological findings in a family with muscular dystrophy. Brain 90: 799

Hurwtiz L, McCormick D, Allen V I 1970 Reduced muscle α-glucosidase (acid maltase) activity in hypothyroid myopathy. Lancet 1:67

Ibraghimov-Beskrovnaya O, Ervasti J M, Leveille C J, Slaughter C A, Sernett S W, Campbell K P 1991 Primary structure of dystrophin-associated glycoproteins linking dystrophin to the extracellular matrix. Nature (London) 355: 696

Isaacs H, Heffron J J A, Badenhorst M 1975 Central core disease: a correlated genetic, histochemical, ultramicroscopic and biochemical study. Journal of Neurology, Neurosurgery and Psychiatry 38: 1177

Isch F, Juif J-G, Sacrez R, Thiebaut F 1966 Glycogénose musculaire; forme myopathique par déficit en maltase acide. Pédiatrie 21: 71

Ishimoto S, Goto I, Ohta M, Kuroiwa Y 1983 A quantitative study of the muscle satellite cells in various neuromuscular disorders. Journal of the Neurological Sciences 62: 303

Jakobsson F, Borg K, Edstrom L 1990 Fibre-type composition, structure and cytoskeletal protein location of fibres in anterior tibial muscle. Comparison between young adults and physically active aged humans. Acta Neuropathologica 80: 459

Jakovics S, Khachadurian A K, Tsia D Y Y 1966 The hyperlipidemia in glycogen storage disease. Journal of Clinical Laboratory Medicine 68: 769

Jenis E H, Lindquist R R, Lister R C 1969 New congenital myopathy with crystalline intramuscular inclusions. Archives of Neurology 20: 281

Jerusalem F, Angelini C, Engel A G, Groover R V 1973a Mitochondria-lipid-glycogen (MLG) disease of muscle. Archives of Neurology 29: 162

Jerusalem F, Engel A G, Gomez M R 1973b Sarcotubular myopathy. Neurology (Minneapolis) 23: 897

Jerusalem F, Engel A G, Gomez M R 1974a Duchenne dystrophy. I. Morphometric study of the muscle microvasculature. Brain 97: 115

Jerusalem F, Engel A G, Gomez M R 1974b Duchenne dystrophy. II Morphological study of motor end-plate fine structure. Brain 97: 123

Jerusalem F, Ludin H, Bischoff A, Bartmann G 1979 Cytoplasmic body neuromyopathy presenting as respiratory failure and weight loss. Journal of the Neurological Sciences 41: 1

Jockusch B M, Veldman H, Griffiths G W, van Oot B A, Jennekens F G T 1980 Immunofluorescence microscopy of a myopathy. α-Actinin is a major constituent of nemaline rods. Experimental Cellular Research 127: 409

Johnson A G 1969 Alterations of the Z-lines and I-band myofilaments in human skeletal muscle. Acta Neuropathologica 12: 218

Johnson M A, Fulthorpe J J, Hudgson P 1973 Lipid storage myopathy. A clinicopathologically recognizable entity. Acta Neuropathologica (Berlin) 24: 97

Jones K W, Kinross J, Maitland N, Norval M 1979 Normal human tissues contain RNA and antigens related to infectious adenovirus Type 2. Nature 277: 274

Julien J, Vital C L, Vallat J-M, Vallat M, Le Blanc M 1974 Oculopharyngeal muscular dystrophy — a case with abnormal mitochondria and 'fingerprint' inclusions. Journal of the Neurological Sciences 21: 165

Kao I, Gordon A M 1977 Alteration of skeletal muscle cellular structures by potassium depletion. Neurology (Minneapolis) 27: 855

Karpati G 1991 Myoblast transfer in Duchenne muscular dystrophy. A perspective. In: Angelini C, Danieli G A, Fontanari D (eds) Muscular dystrophy research: from molecular diagnosis towards therapy. Excerpta Medica, Amsterdam, p 101

Karpati G, Carpenter S, Eisen A, Aube M, DiMauro S 1977 The adult form of acid maltase (-1,4-glucosidase) deficiency. Annals of Neurology 1: 276

Karpati G, Carpenter S, Melmed C, Eisen A A 1974 Experimental ischaemic myopathy. Journal of the Neurological Sciences 23: 129

Karpati G, Carpenter S 1982 Micropuncture lesions of skeletal muscle cells: a new experimental model for the study of muscle cell damage, repair and regeneration. In: Schotland D L (ed) Disorders of the motor unit. John Wiley, New York, p 517

Kelly F J, McGrath J A, Goldspink D F, Cullen M J 1986 A morphological/biochemical study of the actions of corticosteroids on rat skeletal muscle. Muscle and Nerve 9: 1

Ketelsen U P, Beckmann R, Zimmerman H, Sauer M 1977 Inclusion body myositis. A 'slow virus' infection of skeletal musculature? Klinische Wochenschrift 55: 1063

Kinoshita M, Cadman T E 1968 Myotubular myopathy. Archives of Neurology 18: 265

Kissel J T, Mendell J R, Rammohan K W 1986 Microvascular deposition of complement membrane attack complex in dermatomyositis. New England Journal of Medicine 314: 329

Kissel J T, Halterman R K, Rammohan K W, Mendell J R 1991 The relationship of complement-mediated microvasculopathy to the histological features and clinical duration of disease in dermatomyositis. Archives of Neurology 48: 26

Klinkerfuss G H 1967 An electron microscopic study of myotonic dystrophy. Archives of Neurology 16:181

Knox A J, Mascie-Taylor B H, Muers M F 1986 Acute hydrocortisone myopathy in acute severe asthma. Thorax 41: 411

Knudson C M, Hoffman E P, Kahl S D, Kunkel L M, Campbell K P 1988 Characterization of dystrophin in skeletal muscle triads. Journal of Biological Chemistry 163: 8480

Koehler J 1977 Blood vessel structure in Duchenne muscular dystrophy. 1. Light and electron microscopic observations in resting muscle. Neurology (Minneapolis) 27: 861

Koenig M, Hoffman E P, Bertelson C J, Monaco A P, Feener C, Kunkel L M 1987 Complete cloning of the Duchenne muscular dystrophy (DMD) cDNA and preliminary genomic organization of the DMD gene in normal and affected individuals. Cell 50: 509

Koenig M, Monaco A P, Kunkel L M 1988 The complete sequence of dystrophin predicts a rod-shaped cytoskeletal protein. Cell 53: 219

Koga Y, Nonaka I, Kobayashi M, Tojyo M, Nihei K 1988 Findings in muscle in complex I (NADH coenzyme Q reductase) deficiency. Annals of Neurology 24: 749

Konigsberg U R, Lipton B H, Konigsberg I R 1975 The regenerative response of single mature muscle fibres isolated in vitro. Developmental Biology 45: 260

Konno H, Iwasaki Y, Yamamoto T, Inosaka T 1987 Nemaline bodies in spinal muscular atrophy. An autopsy case. Acta Neuropathologica 74: 84

Korenyi-Both A, Smith B H, Baruah J K 1977 McArdle's syndrome. Fine structural changes in muscle. Acta Neuropathologica 40: 11

Kristmundsdottir F, Mahon M, Froes M M Q, Cumming W J K 1990 Histomorphometric and histopathological study of the human cricopharyngeus muscle: in health and in motor neuron disease. Neuropathology and Applied Neurobiology 16: 461

Lacomis D, Smith T W, Chad D 1993 Acute myopathy and neuropathy in status asthmaticus: case report and literature review. Muscle and Nerve 16: 34

Lake B D, Wilson J 1975 Zebra body myopathy. Clinical, histochemical and ultrastructural studies. Journal of the Neurological Sciences 24: 437

Landing B H, Shankle W R 1982 Reduced number of skeletal muscle fiber nuclei in Down's syndrome: speculation on a 'shut off' of chromosome 21 in control of DNA and nuclear replication rates, possibly via determination of cell surface area per nucleus. Birth Defects 18: 81

Landry M, Winkelmann R K 1972 Tubular cytoplasmic inclusion in dermatomyositis. Mayo Clinic Proceedings 47: 479

Lane R J M, Fulthorpe J J, Hudson P 1985 Inclusion body myositis: a case with associated collagen vascular disease responding to treatment. Journal of Neurology, Neurosurgery and Psychiatry 48: 270

Law P, Goodwin T, Fang Q et al 1991 Pioneering development of myoblast transfer therapy. In: Angelini C, Danielli G A, Fonenari D (eds) Muscular dystrophy research: from molecular diagnosis towards therapy. Excerpta Medica, Amsterdam, p 109

Layzer R B, Rowland L P, Ranney H M 1967 Muscle phosphofructokinase deficiency. Archives of Neurology 17: 512

Lee R E, Poulos A C, Mayer R F, Rash J E 1986 Caveolae preservation in the characterization of human neuromuscular disease. Muscle and Nerve 9: 127

Lotz B P, Engel A G 1987 Are hypercontracted muscle fibers artifacts and do they cause rupture of the plasma membrane? Neurology 37: 1466

Lotz B P, Engel A G, Nishino H, Stevens J C, Litchy W J 1989 Inclusion body myositis. Brain 112: 727

Luft R, Ikkos D, Palmieri G, Ernster L, Afzelius B 1962 A case of severe hypermetabolism of non-thyroid origin with a defect in the maintenance of mitochondrial respiratory control: a correlated clinical, biochemical and morphological study. Journal of Clinical Investigation 41: 1776

McDaniel H G, Pitman C S, Oh S J, DiMauro S 1977 Carbohydrate metabolism in hypothyroid myopathy. Metabolism 26: 867

MacDonald R D, Engel A G 1969 The cytoplasmic body: another structural anomaly of the Z discs. Acta Neuropathologica (Berlin) 14: 99

MacDonald R D, Rewcastle N B, Humphrey J G 1969 Myopathy of hypokalaemic periodic paralysis. Archives of Neurology 20: 565

MacDonald R D, Engel A G 1971 Observations on organization of Z-disk components and on rod-bodies of Z-disk origin. Journal of Cell Biology 48: 431

MacFarlane I A, Rosenthal F D 1977 Severe myopathy after status asthmaticus. Lancet 2: 615

Mahadevan M, Tsilfidis C, Sabourin L et al 1992 Myotonic dystrophy mutation: an unstable CTG repeat in the 3' untranslated region of the gene. Science 255: 1253

Markesbery W R, Griggs R C, Herr B 1977 Distal myopathy: electron microscopic and histochemical studies. Neurology 27: 727

Martin J J, De Barsy Th, Van Hoof F, Palladini G 1973 Pompe's disease: an inborn lysosomal disorder with storage of glycogen. Acta Neuropathologica (Berlin) 23: 229

Martin J J, De Barsy Th, De Schrijver F, Leroy J G, Palladini G 1976 Acid maltase deficiency (Type II glycogenosis). Journal of the Neurological Sciences 30: 155

Martin J J, Bruyland M, Busch H F M, Farriaux J P, Krivosic I, Ceuterick C 1986 Pleocore disease. Multi-minicore disease and focal loss of cross striations. Acta Neuropathologica 72: 142

Martin J E, Mather K, Swash M, Gray A B 1991 Expression of heat shock protein epitopes in tubular aggregates. Muscle and Nerve 14: 219

Masuda T, Fujimaki N, Oxawa E, Ishikawa H 1992 Confocal laser microscopy of dystrophin localization in guinea pig skeletal muscle fibers. Journal of Cell Biology 119: 543

Martinez A J, Hooshmand H, Indolos Mendoza G, Winston Y E 1974 Fatal polymyositis: Morphogenesis and ultrastructural features. Acta Neuropathologica (Berlin) 29: 251

Mastaglia F L 1973 Pathological changes in skeletal muscle in acromegaly. Acta Neuropathologica (Berlin) 24: 273

Mastaglia F L, Walton J N 1970 Coxsackie virus-like particles in skeletal muscle from a case of polymyositis. Journal of the Neurological Sciences 11: 593

Mastaglia F L, McCollum J P K, Larson P F, Hudson P 1970 Steroid myopathy complicating McArdle's disease. Journal of Neurology, Neurosurgery and Psychiatry 33: 111

Mastaglia F L, Currie S 1971 Immunological and ultrastructural observations on the role of lymphoid cells in the pathogenesis of polymyositis. Acta Neuropathologica (Berlin) 18: 1

Mastaglia F L, Walton J N 1971a An electron microscopic study of skeletal muscle from cases of the Kugelberg–Welander syndrome. Acta Neuropathologica (Berlin) 17: 201

Mastaglia F L, Walton J N 1971b An ultrastructural study of skeletal muscle in polymyositis. Journal of the Neurological Sciences 12: 473

Mastaglia F L, Papadimitriou J M, Dawkins R L 1975 Mechanisms of cell-mediated myotoxicity. Morphological observations in muscle grafts and in muscle exposed to sensitized spleen cells in vivo. Journal of the Neurological Sciences 25: 26

Mastaglia F L, Papadimitriou J M, Dawkins R L, Beveridge B 1977 Vacuolar myopathy associated with chloroquine, lupus erythematosus and thymoma. Journal of the Neurological Sciences 34: 315

Mastaglia F L, Hudson P 1981 Ultrastructure of diseased muscle In: Walton J N (ed) Disorders of voluntary muscle 4th edn. Churchill Livingstone, Edinburgh, ch 9, p 327

Meijer A E F H 1972 Mitochondria with defective respiratory control of oxidative phosphorylation isolated from muscle tissues of thyroidectomised rabbits. Journal of the Neurological Sciences 16: 445

Mendell J R, Engel W K 1971 The fine structure of type II muscle fibre atrophy. Neurology (Minneapolis) 21: 358

Meyers K R, Gilden D H, Rinaldi C F 1972 Periodic muscle weakness, normokalemia and tubular aggregates. Neurology 22: 269

Mhiri C, Baudrimont M, Bonne G et al 1991 Zidovudine myopathy: a distinctive disorder associated with mitochondrial dysfunction. Annals of Neurology 29: 606

Miledi R, Slater C R 1969 Electron microscopic structure of denervated skeletal muscle. Proceedings of the Royal Society of London, Series B 174: 253

Minetti C, Beltrame F, Marcenaro G, Bonilla E 1992 Dystrophin at the plasma membrane of human muscle fibers shows a costameric localization. Neuromuscular Disorders 2: 99

Mintz G, Gonzalez-Angulo A, Graga A, Zavala B 1968 Ultrastructure of muscle in polymyositis. American Journal of Medicine 44: 216

Mizusawa H, Kurisaki H, Takatsu M et al 1987 Rimmed vacuolar distal myopathy. An ultrastructural study. Journal of Neurology 234: 137

Mokri B, Engel A G 1975 Duchenne dystrophy: electron microscopic findings pointing to a basic or early abnormality in the plasma membrane of the muscle fibre. Neurology (Minneapolis) 25: 1111

Morgan-Hughes J A 1982 Defects of the energy pathways of skeletal muscle. In: Matthews W B, Glaser G H (eds) Recent advances in clinical neurology 3. Churchill Livingstone, Edinburgh, ch 7, p 1

Morgan-Hughes J A, Landon D N 1983 Mitochondrial respiratory chain deficiencies in man. Some histochemical and fine-structure observations. In: Scarlato G, Cerri C (eds) Mitochondrial pathology in muscle diseases. Piccin, Padua, p 19

Mrak R E, Saito A, Evans O B, Fleischer S 1982 Autophagic degradation in human skeletal muscle target fibers. Muscle and Nerve 5: 745

Murase T, Ikeda H, Muro T, Nakao K, Sugita H 1973 Myopathy associated with Type III glycogenosis. Journal of the Neurological Sciences 20: 287

Murayama T, Sato O, Kimura S, Shimizu T, Sawada H, Maruyama K 1990 Molecular shape of dystrophin purified from rabbit skeletal muscle myofibrils. Proceedings of the Japanese Academy 66: 96

Neville H E 1973 Ultrastructural changes in muscle disease. In: Dubowitz V, Brooke M (eds) Muscle biopsy. Saunders, London, p 383

Neville H E 1979 Ultrastructural changes in diseases of human skeletal muscle. In: Vinken P J, Bruyn G W (eds) Handbook of Clinical Neurology. North Holland, Amsterdam, vol 40, p 63

Neville H E, Brooke M H 1973 Central core fibres: structured and unstructured. In: Kakulas B (ed) Basic research in myology. Excerpta Medica, Amsterdam, p 497

Neville H E, Maunder-Sewry C A, McDougall J, Sewell J R, Dubowitz V 1979 Chloroquine-induced cytosomes with curvilinear profiles in muscle. Muscle and Nerve 2: 376

Nicholson L V B, Johnson M A, Gardner-Medwin D, Bhattacharya S, Harris J B 1990 Heterogeneity of dystrophin expression in patients with Duchenne and Becker muscular dystrophy. Acta Neuropathologica 80: 239

Nonaka I, Sunohara N, Satoyoshi E, Teerasawa K, Yonemoto K 1985 Autosomal recessive distal muscular dystrophy: a comparative study of distal myopathy with rimmed vacuole formation. Annals of Neurology 17: 51

Nonaka I, Koga Y, Shikura K et al 1988 Muscle pathology in cytochrome c oxidase deficiency. Acta Neuropathologica 77: 152

Norris F H, Panner B J 1966 Hypothyroid myopathy: Clinical, electromyographical and ultrastructural observations. Archives of Neurology 14: 574

Norris F H, Panner B J, Stormont J M 1968 Thyrotoxic periodic paralysis. Metabolic and ultrastructural studies. Archives of Neurology 19: 88

North A J, Galazkiewicz B, Byers T J, Glenney J R, Small J V 1993 Complementary distributions of vinculin and dystrophin define two distinct sarcolemma domains in smooth muscle. Journal of Cell Biology 120: 1159

Odor D L, Patel A N, Pearce L A 1967 Familial hypokalemic periodic paralysis with permanent myopathy. Journal of Neuropathology and Experimental Neurology 26: 98

O'Hoy K L, Tsilfidis C, Hahadevan M M et al 1993 Reduction in size of the myotonic dystrophy trinucleotide repeat mutation during transmission. Science 259: 809

Oliner L, Schulman X, Larner J 1961 Myopathy associated with glycogen deposition resulting from generalised lack of amylo -1,6-glucosidase. Clinical Research 243

Ontell M 1974 Muscle satellite cells: a validated technique for light microscopic identification and a quantitative study of changes in their population following denervation. The Anatomical Record 178: 211

Osborn M, Goebel H H 1983 The cytoplasmic bodies in a congenital myopathy can be stained with antibodies to desmin, the muscle-specific intermediate filament protein. Acta Neuropathologica (Berlin) 62: 149

Oshima Y, Becker L E, Armstrong D L 1979 An electron microscopic study of childhood dermatomyositis. Acta Neuropathologica (Berlin) 47: 189

Pagès M, Echenne B, Pages A-M, Dimeglio A, Sires A 1985 Multicore disease and Marfan's syndrome: a case report. European Neurology 24: 170

Palmucci L, Bertolotto A, Monga G, Ardizzone G, Schiffer D 1978 Histochemical and ultrastructural findings in a case of centronuclear myopathy. European Neurology 17: 327

Papadimitriou J M, Mastaglia F L 1982 Ultrastructural changes in human muscle fibres in disease. Journal of Submicroscopic Cytology 14: 525

Pardo J V, Siliciano J D, Craig S W 1983 A vinculin-containing cortical lattice in skeletal muscle: transverse lattice elements ('costameres') mark sites of attachment between myofibrils and sarcolemma. Proceedings of the National Academy of Sciences USA 80: 1008

Pauzner R, Blatt I, Mouallem M, Ben-David E, Farfel Z, Sadeh M 1991 Mitochondrial abnormalities in oculopharyngeal muscular dystrophy. Muscle and Nerve 14: 947

Payne C M, Curless R G 1976 Concentric laminated bodies — ultrastructural demonstration of fibre type specificity. Journal of the Neurological Sciences 29: 311

Pearce G W 1964 Tissue culture and electron microscopy in muscle disease. In: Walton J N (ed) Disorders of voluntary muscle. 1st edn. Churchill, London

Pearson C M 1964 The periodic paralyses: Differential features and pathological observations in permanent myopathic weakness. Brain 87: 341

Pellegrino C, Franzini C 1963 An electron microscopic study of denervation atrophy in red and white skeletal muscle fibers. Journal of Cell Biology 17: 327

Pons F, Augier H, Heilig R, Leger J, Mornet D, Leger J J 1990 Isolated dystrophin molecules as seen by electron microscopy. Proceedings of the National Academy of Sciences USA 87: 7851

Porter G A, Dymtrenko G M, Winkelmann J C, Bloch R J 1992 Dystrophin colocalizes with β-spectrin in distinct subsarcolemmal domains in mammalian skeletal muscle. Journal of Cell Biology 117: 997

Price H M, Gordon G B, Pearson C M, Munsat T L, Blumberg J M 1965 New evidence for accumulation of excessive Z band material in nemaline myopathy. Proceedings of the National Academy of Sciences USA 64: 1398

Prineas J W, Hall R, Barwick D D, Watson A J 1968 Myopathy associated with pigmentation following adrenalectomy for Cushing's syndrome. Quarterly Journal of Medicine 37: 63

Radu H, Rosu-Serbu A M, Ionescu V, Radu A 1977 Focal abnormalities in mitochondrial distribution in muscle. Acta Neuropathologica (Berlin) 39: 25

Rapola J, Haltia M 1973 Cytoplasmic inclusions in the vermiform appendix and skeletal muscle in two types of so-called neuronal ceroid-lipofuscinosis. Brain 96: 833

Recondo J de, Fardeau M, Lapresle J 1966 Étude au microscope electronique des lesions musculaires d'atrophie neurogène par atteinte de la corne anterieure (observées dans huit cas de sclerose lateral amyotrophique). Revue Neurologique 114: 169

Rewcastle N B, Humphrey J G 1965 Vacuolar myopathy: clinical, histochemical and microscopic study. Archives of Neurology (Chicago) 12: 570

Riggs J E, Klingberg W G, Flink E B, Schochet S S, Balian A A, Jenkins J J 1992 Cardioskeletal mitochondrial myopathy associated with chronic magnesium deficiency. Neurology 42: 128

Ringel S P, Kenny C, Neville H, Gilden D 1986 Spectrum of inclusion body myositis. Muscle and Nerve 9: 218

Ringel S P, Neville H E, Duster M C, Carroll J E 1978 A new congenital neuromuscular disease with trilaminar muscle fibers. Neurology (Minneapolis) 28: 282

Ringel S P, Thorne E G, Phanuphak P, Lava N S, Kohler P S 1979 Immune complex vasculitis, polymyositis and hyperglobulinaemic purpura. Neurology (Minneapolis) 29: 682

Ritter R A 1967 The effect of cortisone on the structure and strength of skeletal muscle. Archives of Neurology 17: 493

Rose A L, Walton J N, Pearce G W 1967 Polymyositis: An ultramicroscopic study of muscle biopsy material. Journal of the Neurological Sciences 5: 457

Rosenberg N L, Neville H E, Ringel S P 1985 Tubular aggregates. Their association with neuromuscular diseases, including the syndrome of myalgias/cramps. Archives of Neurology 42: 973

Rouleau G, Karpati G, Carpenter S, Soza M, Prescott S, Holland P 1987 Glucocorticoid excess induces preferential depletion of myosin in denervated skeletal muscle fibers. Muscle and Nerve 10: 428

Roullet E, Fardeau M, Collin H, Marteau R 1985 Myopathie avec agrégates tubulaires. Étude clinique biologique et histologique de deux cas. Revue Neurologique 141: 655

Rowland L P, Hays A P, DiMauro S, De Vivo D C, Behrens M 1983 Diverse clinical disorders associated with morphological abnormalities of mitochondria. In: Scarlato G, Cerri C (eds) Mitochondrial pathology in muscle diseases. Piccin, Padua, p 141

Rubin E, Katz A M, Lieber C S, Stein E, Purzkin S 1976 Muscle damage caused by chronic alcohol consumption. American Journal of Pathology 83: 499

Sahgal V, Sahgal S 1977 A new congenital myopathy. Acta Neuropathologica (Berlin) 37: 225

Salvatori S, Damiani E, Zorzato F et al 1989 Denervation-induced proliferative changes of triads in rabbit skeletal muscle. Muscle and Nerve 11: 1246

Samitt C E, Bonilla E 1990 Immunocytochemical study of dystrophin at the myotendinous junction. Muscle and Nerve 13: 493

Sato O, Nonomura Y, Kimura S, Maruyama K 1992 Molecular shape of dystrophin. Journal of Biochemistry 112: 631

Satoyoshi E, Kowa H 1967 A myopathy due to a glycolytic abnormality. Archives of Neurology 17: 248

Schiaffino S, Severin E, Cautini M, Sartore S 1977 Tubular aggregates induced by anoxia in isolated rat skeletal muscle. Laboratory Investigation 37: 228

Schiller H H, Mair W G P 1974 Ultrastructural changes of muscle in malignant hyperthermia. Journal of the Neurological Sciences 21: 93

Schlenska G K, Heene R, Spalke G, Seiler D 1976 The symptomatology, morphology and biochemistry of glycogenosis type II (Pompe) in the adult. Journal of Neurology 212: 237

Schmalbruch H 1967 Kristalloide in menschlichen skelett-muskelfasern. Naturwissenschaften 54: 519

Schmalbruch H 1968 Lyse und regeneration von fibrillen in der normalen menschlichen skelettmuskulatur. Virchows Archiv für pathologische Anatomie und physiologie und für Klinische Medizin 344: 159

Schmalbruch H 1975 Segmental fibre breakdown and defects of the plasmalemma in diseased human muscle. Acta Neuropathologica (Berlin) 33: 129

Schmalbruch H 1976 Muscle fibre splitting and regeneration in diseased human muscle. Neuropathology and Applied Neurobiology 2: 3

Schmalbruch H 1979 'Square arrays' in the sarcolemma of human skeletal muscle fibres. Nature (London) 281: 145

Schmalbruch H 1983 The fine structure of mitochondrial abnormalities in muscle diseases. In: Scarlato G, Cerri C (eds) Mitochondrial pathology in muscle disease. Piccin, Padua, p 39

Schmalbruch H 1984 Regenerated muscle fibres in Duchenne muscular dystrophy: a serial section study. Neurology (Cleveland) 34: 60

Schmalbruch H, Kamieniecka Z, Arroe M 1987 Early fatal nemaline myopathy: case report and review. Developmental Medicine and Child Neurology 29: 784

Schotland D L 1969 An electron microscopic study of target fibers, target-like fibers and related abnormalities in human muscle. Journal of Neuropathology and Experimental Neurology 28: 214

Schotland D L 1970 An electron microscopic investigation of myotonic dystrophy. Journal of Neuropathology and Experimental Neurology 29: 241

Schotland D L, Bonilla E and Wakayama Y 1981a Application of freeze-fracture technique to the study of human neuromuscular disease. Muscle and Nerve 3: 21

Schotland D L, Bonilla E, Wakayama Y 1981b Freeze-fracture studies of muscle plasma membrane in human muscular dystrophy. Acta Neuropathologica 54: 189

Schröder J M 1970 Sarcolemmal indentations resembling junctional folds in myotonic dystrophy. In: Walton J N, Canal N, Scarlato G (eds) Muscle diseases. Excerpta Medica, Amsterdam, p 109

Schröder J M, Sommer C, Schmidt B 1990 Desmin and actin associated with cytoplasmic bodies in skeletal muscle fibres: immunocytochemical and fine structural studies, with a note on unusual 18- to 20-mm filaments. Acta Neuropathologica 80: 406

Schultz E 1978 Changes in the satellite cells of growing muscle following denervation. Anatomical Record 190: 299

Schwartz W N, Bird J W C 1977 Degradation of myofibrillar proteins by cathepsins B and D. Biochemical Journal 167: 811

Serratrice G, Pellissier J F, Faugère M C, Gastaut J L 1978 Centronuclear myopathy: possible central nervous system origin. Muscle and Nerve 1: 62

Sewry C A 1985 Ultrastructural changes in diseased muscle. In: Dubowitz V (ed) Muscle biopsy. A practical approach. Baillière Tindall, London, p 129

Shafiq S A, Gorycki M, Goldstone L, Milhorat A T 1966 Fine structure of fiber types in normal human muscle. Anatomical Record 156: 283

Shafiq S A, Dubowitz V, Peterson H de C, Milhorat A T 1967a Nemaline myopathy: Report of a fatal case with histochemical and electronmicroscopic studies. Brain 90: 817

Shafiq S A, Gorycki M A, Milhorat A T 1967b An electron microscopic study of regeneration and satellite cells in human muscle. Neurology (Minneapolis) 17: 507

Shafiq S A, Milhorat A T, Gorycki M A 1967c An electron microscopic study of muscle degeneration and changes in blood vessels in polymyositis. Journal of Pathology and Bacteriology 94: 139

Shafiq S A, Milhorat A T, Gorycki M A 1967d Giant mitochondria in human muscle with inclusions. Archives of Neurology 17: 666

Sher J H, Rimalovski A B, Athanassiades T J, Aronson S M 1967 Familial centronuclear myopathy. Neurology (Minneapolis) 17: 721

Shoji S, Takagi A, Sugita H, Toyokura Y 1974 Muscle glycogen metabolism in steroid-induced myopathy in rabbits. Experimental Neurology 45: 1

Shy G M, Magee K R 1956 A new non-progressive myopathy. Brain 79: 610

Shy G M, Wanko T, Rowley P T, Engel A G 1961 Studies in familial periodic paralysis. Experimental Neurology 3: 53

Shy G M, Engel W K, Somers J E, Wanko T 1963 Nemaline myopathy: a new congenital myopathy. Brain 86: 739

Shy G M, Gonatas N K, Perez M 1966 Two childhood myopathies with abnormal mitochondria. I. Megaconial myopathy. II. Pleoconial myopathy. Brain 89: 133

Smith H L, Amick L D, Sidbury J B 1966 Type II glycogenosis: report of a case with 4 year survival and absence of acid maltase associated with an abnormal glycogen. American Journal of Diseases of Children 111: 475

Snow M H 1977 Myogenic cell formation in regenerating rat skeletal muscle injured by mincing. II An autoradiographic Study. Anatomical Record 188: 201

Snow M H 1978 An autoradiographic study of satellite cell differentiation into regenerating myotubes following transplantation of muscle in young rats. Cell Tissue Research 186: 537

Snow M H 1983 A quantitative ultrastructural analysis of satellite cells in denervated fast and slow muscles of the mouse. Anatomical Record 207: 593

Somlyo A V, Gonzalez-Serratos H, Shuman H, McClellan G, Somlyo A P 1981 Calcium release and ionic changes in the sarcoplasmic reticulum of tetanized muscle — an electron-probe study. Journal of Cell Biology 90: 577

Spiro A J, Kennedy C 1964 Hereditary occurrence of nemaline myopathy. Transactions of the American Neurological Association 89: 62

Spiro A J, Shy G M, Gonatas N K 1966 Myotubular myopathy. Archives of Neurology 14: 1

Spiro A J, Hirano A, Beilin R L, Finkelstein J W 1970 Cretinism with muscular hypertrophy (Kocher-Debré-Semelaigne syndrome). Archives of Neurology 23: 340

Squarzoni S, Sabatelli P, Maltarello M C, Cataldi A, DiPrimio R, Maraldi N M 1992 Localization of dystrophin COOH-terminal domain by the fracture-label technique. Journal of Cell Biology 118: 1401

Stauber W T, Riggs J E, Schochet S S, Gutmann L, Crosby T W 1986 Nemaline myopathy. Evidence of dipeptidyl peptidase 1 deficiency. Archives of Neurology 43: 39

Stonnington H H, Engel A G 1973 Normal and denervated muscle. Neurology (Minneapolis) 23: 714

Straub V, Bittner R E, Leger J J, Voit T 1992 Direct visualization of the dystrophin network on skeletal muscle fiber membrane. Journal of Cell Biology 119: 1183

Stromer M H, Tabatabai L B, Robson R M, Goll D E, Zeece M G 1976 Nemaline myopathy, an integrated study: selective extraction. Experimental Neurology 50: 402

Suzuki A, Yoshida M, Yamamoto H, Ozawa E 1992 Glycoprotein-binding site of dystrophin is confined to the cysteine-rich domain and the first half of the carboxy-terminal domain. FEBS Letters 308: 154

Swash M, Schwartz M S 1981 Familial multicore disease with focal loss of cross-striations and ophthalmoplegia. Journal of the Neurological Sciences 52: 1

Tagerud S, Jirmanova I, Libelius R 1986 Biochemical and ultrastructural effects of chloroquine on horseradish peroxidase uptake and lysosomal enzyme activities in innervated and denervated mouse skeletal muscle. Journal of the Neurological Sciences 75: 159

Takagi A, Schotland D L, Di Mauro S, Rowland L P 1973 Thyrotoxic periodic paralysis. Function of sarcoplasmic reticulum and muscle glycogen. Neurology (Minneapolis) 23: 1008

Takeda S, Ohama E, Ikuta F 1990 Involvement of extraocular muscle in mitochondrial encephalomyopathy. Acta Neuropathologica 80: 118

Tang T T, Sedmak G V, Siegesmund K A, McCreadie S R 1975 Chronic myopathy associated with Coxsackie virus type A9. A combined electron microscopical and viral isolation study. New England Journal of Medicine 292: 608

Tarui S, Okuno G, Ikura Y, Suda M 1965 Phosphofructokinase deficiency in skeletal muscle: A new type of glycogenosis. Biochemical and Biophysical Research Communications 19: 517

Telerman-Toppet N, Gerrard J M, Cöers C 1973 Central core disease: a study of clinically unaffected muscle. Journal of the Neurological Sciences 19: 207

Teräväinen H, Mäkitie J 1977 Striated muscle ultrastructure in intermittent claudication. Archives of Pathological Laboratory Medicine 101: 230

Thomson W H S, Maclaurin J C, Prineas J W 1963 Skeletal muscle glycogenosis: An investigation of two dissimilar cases. Journal of Neurology, Neurosurgery and Psychiatry 26: 60

Thornell L-E, Edström L, Eriksson A, Henriksson K-G, Ängqvist K-A 1980 The distribution of intermediate filament protein (skeletin) in normal and diseased human skeletal muscle: an immunohistochemical and electron-microscopic study. Journal of the Neurological Sciences 47: 153

Thornell L-E, Eriksson A, Edström L 1983 Intermediate filaments in human myopathies. In: Dowben R M, Shay J W (eds) Cell and muscle motility. Plenum, New York, vol. 4, p 85

Toga M, Berard-Badier M, Gambarelli D, Pinsard N 1970 Ultrastructure des lesions neuromusculaires dans un cas de dystrophie neuroaxonale infantile ou maladie de Seitelberger. Communication to II Journées Internationales de Pathologie Neuromusculaire, Marseilles

Tomé F M S, Fardeau M 1973 'Fingerprint inclusions' in muscle fibres in dystrophia myotonica. Acta Neuropathologica (Berlin) 24: 62

Tomé F M S, Fardeau M 1986 Nuclear changes in muscle disorders. Methods and Achievements in Experimental Pathology 12: 261

Tomé F M S, Askanas V, Engel W K, Alvarez R B, Lee C-S 1989 Nuclear inclusions in innervated cultured muscle fibers from patients with oculopharyngeal muscular dystrophy. Neurology 39: 926

Tremblay J P, Roy R, Bouchard J-P et al 1991 Human myoblast transplantation. In: Angelini C, Danieli G A, Fontanari D (eds) Muscular dystrophy research: from molecular diagnosis towards therapy. Excerpta Medica, Amsterdam, pp 123–132

Trupin G L, Hsu L 1979 The identification of myogenic cells in regenerating skeletal muscle. Developmental Biology 68: 72

Turnbull D M, Bartlett K, Steven D L, Alberti K G M M, Gibson G J, Johnson M A, McCulloch A J, Sherratt H S A 1984 Lipid storage myopathy and secondary carnitine deficiency due to short acyl-CoA dehydrogenase deficiency. New England Journal of Medicine 311: 1232

van der Ven P F M, Jap P H K, Wetzels R H W et al 1991 Postnatal centralization of muscle fibre nuclei in centronuclear myopathy. Neuromuscular Disorders 1: 211

Van Marle W, Woods K L 1980 Acute hydrocortisone myopathy. British Medical Journal 3: 271

Van Wijngaarden G K, Bethlem J, Dingemans K P, Cöers C, Telerman-Toppet N, Gerard J M 1977 Familial focal loss of striations. Journal of Neurology 216: 163

Verma A, Bradley W G, Adesina A M, Sofferman R, Pendelbury W W 1991 Inclusion body myositis with cricopharyngeus muscle involvement and severe dysphagia. Muscle and Nerve 14: 470

Vick N A 1971 Skeletal muscle capillary basement membranes in humans. Acta Neuropathologica (Berlin) 17: 1

Wakayama Y, Schotland D L 1979 Muscle satellite cell populations in Duchenne dystrophy. In: Mauro A (ed) Muscle regeneration. Raven Press, New York, p 212

Wakayama Y, Schotland D L, Bonilla E, Orecchio E 1979 Quantitative ultrastructural study of muscle satellite cells in Duchenne dystrophy. Neurology (Minneapolis) 29: 401

Wakayama Y, Okayasu H, Shibuya S, Kumagai T 1984 Duchenne dystrophy: reduced density of orthogonal array sub-unit particles in muscle plasma membrane. Neurology (Cleveland) 34: 1313

Wakayama Y, Kumagai T, Shibuya S 1985 Freeze-fracture studies of muscle plasma membrane in Fukuyama-type congenital muscular dystrophy. Neurology 35: 1587

Wakayama Y, Jimi T, Misugi N et al 1989 Dystrophin immunostaining and freeze-fracture studies of muscles of patients with early stage amyotrophic lateral sclerosis and Duchenne muscular dystrophy. Journal of the Neurological Sciences 91: 191

Watkins S C, Cullen M J 1985 Histochemical fibre typing and ultrastructure of the small fibres in Duchenne muscular dystrophy. Neuropathology and Applied Neurobiology 11: 447

Watkins S C, Cullen M J 1986 A quantitative comparison of satellite cell ultrastructure in Duchenne muscular dystrophy, polymyositis and normal controls. Muscle and Nerve 9: 724

Watkins S C, Hoffman E P, Slayter H S, Kunkel L M 1988 Immunoelectron microscopic localization of dystrophin in myofibres. Nature 333: 863

Webb J N, Gillespie W J 1976 Virus-like particles in paraspinal muscle in scoliosis. British Medical Journal 4: 912

Weller R O, McArdle B 1971 Calcification within muscle fibres in the periodic paralyses. Brain 94: 263

Whitaker J N, Engel W K 1972 Vascular deposits of immunoglobulin and complement in idiopathic inflammatory myopathy. New England Journal of Medicine 286: 333

Whitaker J N, Bertorini T E, Mendell J R 1983 Immunocytochemical studies of cathepsin D in human skeletal muscle. Annals of Neurology 13: 133

White J G 1972 Lymphocyte inclusions. Annals of Internal Medicine 76: 1042

Wróblewski R, Gremski W, Nordemar R, Edström L 1978a Electron probe X-ray microanalysis of human skeletal muscles involved in rheumatoid arthritis. Histochemistry 57: 1–8

Wróblewski R, Roomans G, Jansson E, Edström L 1978b Electron probe X-ray microanalysis of human biopsies. Histochemistry 55: 281–292

Wróblewski R, Edström L, Mair W G P 1982 Five different types of centrally nucleated muscle fibres in man: elemental composition and morphological criteria. Journal of Submicroscopic Cytology 14: 377

Yamaguchi M, Robson R M, Stromer M H, Dahl D S, Oda T 1978a Actin filaments form the backbone of nemaline myopathy rods. Nature (London) 271: 265

Yamaguchi K, Santa T, Inoue K, Omae T 1978b Lipid storage in Von Gierke's disease. Journal of the Neurological Sciences 38: 195

Yarom R, Shapira Y 1977 Myosin degeneration in a congenital myopathy. Archives of Neurology 34: 114

Yarom R, Reches A 1980 Thick filament degeneration in a case of acute quadriplegia. Journal of the Neurological Sciences 45: 13

Yu Y-H, Pizzuti A, Fenwick R G et al 1992 An unstable triplet repeat in a gene related to myotonic muscular dystrophy. Science 255: 1256

Yunis E J, Samaha F J 1971 Inclusion body myositis. Laboratory Investigation 25: 240

Zacks S I, Pegues J J, Elliott F A 1962 Interstitial muscle capillaries in patients with diabetes mellitus: A light and electron microscope study. Metabolism II: 381

Zellweger H, Brown B I, McCormick W F, Tu J-B 1965 A mild form of muscular glycogenosis in two brothers with alpha-1,4-glucosidase deficiency. Annals of Paediatrics 205: 413

Zierler K L 1958 Muscle membrane as a dynamic structure and its permeability to aldolase. Annals of the New York Academy of Sciences 75: 227

Zubrzycka-Gaarn E E, Bulman D E, Karpati G et al 1988 The Duchenne muscular dystrophy gene product is localized in sarcolemma of human skeletal muscle. Nature 333: 466

therefore, that it has been difficult to provide simple explanations as to the role of the immune system in the aetiology and pathogenesis of many putative immunopathologically mediated disorders.

Lymphocytes were at first simply divided into T-cells (thymic-dependent), B-cells (thymic-independent and bursal-equivalent) and null cells, based originally on the presence or absence of particular cell-surface characteristics (antigens or receptors). It is clear that the T-cells can be further classified by functional characteristics such as helper-inducer, cytotoxic/suppressor, memory-cells or naive, etc. It is also clear that T-cells have different phenotypes (markers) that represent their state of activation and maturation. In addition they can also bear markers that affect their circulation and trafficking and act as ligands for interactions with vascular endothelial adhesion molecules on activated endothelium. T-cells may exert their function in a non-specific fashion upon stimulation by non-antigen-specific polyclonal stimulators or in response to specific antigen (Cantor 1984) The interaction of a T-cell with a specific antigen for each T lymphocyte is controlled by a T-cell specific receptor (TCR) for that antigenic determinant. The specificity and tremendous diversity of T-cell reactivity resides in the ability of the peptide chains of the TCR to undergo somatic rearrangement. There are two types of TCR. One has two chains called α and β and the other two chains called γ and δ. The latter is a less mature type of receptor. T-cells with the $\gamma\delta$ configuration may be important in response to the heat-shock proteins. These proteins are up-regulated in cells undergoing heat or other stress reactions and may cross-react with microbial antigens. Like immunoglobulins, which both bind antibody and serve as the antigen receptors for individual B-cells, TCR peptides have non-variable and variable regions and it is the variable and hypervariable region rearrangements that confer the exquisite antigen specificity of T-cells (Hedrick 1989). The T-cell 'sees' and reacts to its specific antigen through the so-called trimolecular complex. This complex consists of the TCR, the antigenic determinant and the major histocompatibility complex (MHC) molecule which is on the antigen-presenting cell (APC). The APC is

capable of internalizing and processing the antigen to present the specific peptide determinant in the cleft of the MHC molecule. In addition the CD8 and CD4 molecules, as well as the CD3 and other activation antigens, serve accessory functions in the interaction between the T-cell and the APC (Unanue 1989). It is also clear that much of the interaction of T-cells with other T-cells, B-cells and other cells of the organism is mediated by products of these cells, called lymphokines (Gillis 1989).

Each B-cell also reacts with a specific antigen by the nature of the specific immunoglobulin (Ig) on its surface. In addition, B-cells undergo phenotypic changes with maturation and activation. For B-cells to respond by secreting appropriately the specific immunoglobulin (antibody), interaction with products of T-cells is generally necessary (DeFranco 1987, Kishimoto & Hirano 1989). This is especially true for production of IgG, IgA and IgE. It is, therefore, clear that normal antibody responses depend not only on B-cells but on regulatory T-cells, APCs and their products.

We have learned a great deal about those non-T, non-B lymphocytes previously called null cells. Many of these cells mediate cytotoxic effects against tumour cells (in vitro) although little is known about the mechanisms of cell recognition or killing: these cells are called natural killer (NK) cells (Heberman 1982). Cells of this lineage are also able to participate in specific killing of immune targets. Although these cells themselves do not specifically recognise antigens, they interact with the Fc portion (crystallisable fragment of proteolytic digest of Ig) of immunoglobulins (antibodies) that have bound to the specific antigen. The binding to the antigen is mediated by the specific antibody (idiotype) portion of the molecule contained in the FAb fragment (Ziegler & Henney 1977).

The monocyte (circulating phase)–macrophages and related accessory cells of the immune system (dendritic cells and Langerhans cells of the skin) are extremely important in the normal function of the immune system. These cells are involved in the afferent phase (antigen processing and induction of specific sensitised cells), being important in the processing of antigen activation of T-cells and presentation of antigen to the specific lymphocyte. They are also highly important in the efferent phase. (Sensitised cells and products interact with non-specific factors to mediate the functions of the immune system.) They may be activated by lymphokines, attracted to inflammatory sites by chemotactic factors and interact with antigen–antibody reactions by nature of the presence of receptors for the Fc portion of IgG and components of the complement system (Shevach 1984). In addition to participating in immune phagocytosis, macrophages also participate in non-immune phagocytosis. Products of macrophages, such as prostaglandins, may have regulatory as well as direct effector actions (Dore-Duffy et al 1985). In addition, cells of the monocyte–macrophage lineage secrete proteins, called monokines, which interact with T-cells, B-cells, and other non-immune system cells, to modulate the function of these target cells (Durum & Oppenheim 1989).

IMMUNOPATHOLOGICAL REACTIONS

The immune system is capable of many complex and interrelated immunological reactions which are necessary for the maintenance of the health of the organism. When these reactions or immune mechanisms are excessive, prolonged, misdirected or inappropriate, they are capable of causing damage to the host and are termed immunopathological reactions. There were originally thought to be four types of reaction (Coombs & Gell 1968) but it has become clear that many more exist, or at least that there are several subtypes. There has been considerable progress in determining the reactants amd mediators of these reactions and in determining which of them are likely to be important in several human diseases (Table 10.1). One can also consider diseases associated with auto-antibodies to receptors on cell surfaces as an entirely separate immunopathological group of disorders; these antibodies may have inhibitory or stimulatory effects. These diseases include myasthenia gravis, type B insulin-resistant diabetes mellitus with acanthocytosis, Graves' disease and perhaps some forms of hay fever (asthma). In the discussion to follow of different neuromuscular diseases of man and experimental animals of immunopathological origin, an attempt

is made to review the evidence for the possible role of such reactions in these disorders.

TOLERANCE

The immune system normally does not react to self (autoantigens) but, in true autoimmune diseases, the reaction by sensitised cells or antibody to a component of self represents a failure of maintenance of the normal state of self-tolerance. There are several mechanisms that have been proposed by which the immune system prevents the attack on self antigens. These include: (a) clonal deletion (or abortion); (b) suppressor T-cells (antigen-specific or non-specific cells); (c) sequestration of self antigens; (d) idiotype networks; and (e) antigen-specific antigen-induced tolerance. There is evidence for and against each of these theories. It is possible that each of these mechanisms may be important but none can completely explain the maintenance of tolerance (Cohen & Lisak 1987).

Burnet (1959) proposed that exposure to self-antigens during ontogeny renders the immune system unable to react to that antigen and that this tolerance results from deletion of clones of lymphoid cells that recognise that antigen. The presence of both antibodies and T-cells reactive to autoantigens in both experimental animals and man makes this hypothesis unlikely to be the major explanation for tolerance to self.

In the second scenario, suppressor cells, principally a subset of T lymphocytes, suppress the immune response of other T-cells and B-cells. Failure of these T-cells or a subset of them to suppress the activity of other cells that recognise self-antigens would result in the emergence of an autoimmune reaction (Miller & Schwartz 1982).

There is increasing interest in the possibility that the immune system is partly controlled by so-called idiotypic reactions (Jerne 1974). In this system every antibody molecule itself is an antigen which elicits a response by another immunoglobulin molecule: the reaction of the second antibody is to the portion of the first antibody that reacts with the antigen. That antigen-binding site is the idiotype and the antibody elicited by the first antibody is called the anti-idiotype. This second antibody (the anti-idiotype) can also elicit an

Table 10.1 Immunological effector mechanisms and immunopathological reactions in man and experimental animals

Immunological mechanism	Reactants	Mediators	Normal function	Diseases
Reaginic	IgE mast cell or basophil and antigen	Vasoactive amines (histamine) Arachidonic acid metabolites (leukotrienes, prostaglandins, platelet activating factor) Inflammatory cells (neutrophils, eosinophils, mononuclear leocoytes)	Parasite killing	Allergic respiratory diseases, anaphylaxis
Antibody to self-antigens Direct cytotoxic	IgG or IgM and antigen	Complement; inflammatory cells	Infections	Experimental autoimmune myasthenia gravis, certain haemolytic anaemias
Alteration of membranes and surface receptors (a) sequestration via cell surface activation		Immune complex between antigen on circulating cell and antibody; reacts with Fc receptor on reticuloendothelial cell	Infections	Certain haemolytic anaemias, idiopathic thrombocytopenic purpura
(b) block of ligand binding				Myasthenia gravis, experimental autoimmune myasthenia gravis, diabetes and acanthocytosis secondary to antibodies to insulin receptor
(c) receptor down-regulation				Myasthenia gravis, experimental autoimmune myasthenia gravis
(d) receptor stimulation				Autoimmune hyperthyroidism, anti-insulin receptor antibodies
Immune complex deposition	IgG or IgM + antigen (complement)	Complement; inflammatory cells	Antigen clearance	Serum sickness, vasculitides, lupus nephritis, rare haemolytic anaemias thrombocytopenias (drug-related)
Cell-mediated reactions T-cell mediated (a) delayed hypersensitivity	T-cells (helper-inducer) and antigen, Type II MHC dependent	Lymphocytes and lymphokines, monocyte-macrophages	Infections with obligate intracellular organisms	Experimental allergic encephalomyelitis, experimental allergic neuritis, acute disseminated encephalomyelitis (?), allograft rejection
(b) T-cell cytotoxic	T-cells (cytotoxic) and antigen, Type I MHC dependent	Lymphocytes and products, secondary phagocytosis	? Tumour necrosis, infection (with obligate intra-cellular organisms)	Certain forms of hepatitis, allograft rejection, graft versus host reaction
ADCC (see p. 389)	K-cells (lymphocytes) and macrophages, Fc and receptor	K-cell and macrophages	? Infections, tumour destruction	Allograft rejection
NK-cell reactions	NK lymphocytes	NK lymphocytes	? Tumour destruction and infections	?

antibody response called an anti-anti-idiotype. This network is called the idiotypic network. It is not clear if this system extends to antigen-specific cells. Ordinarily this network keeps the immune response in balance; a failure in the network allows the autoimmune antibody to emerge (Zanetti 1985). While there is considerable evidence for elements of this network in experimental animals and, to a lesser degree, in man, there is also considerable evidence that the hypothesis originally offered cannot be correct in its entirety. It is likely that under normal conditions at times of activation of immunoglobulin-producing cells the network becomes operative (Bona & Pernis 1984).

Another mechanism promoting tolerance is sequestration of antigen from the immune system during development. Nervous system antigens which are hidden behind the blood–brain or blood–nerve barrier are examples of such antigens. T-cells recognise antigen in the context of products of the major histocompatibility complex (MHC) expressed on the cell surface (Zinkernagel & Dougherty 1974). The normal nervous system is poor in MHC products (antigens). This MHC-dependent restriction may provide additional protection from the emergence of self-reactive clones (Cowing 1985). The later exposure of an immunologically appropriate cell, genetically programmed with the potential to react to that antigen in the context of MHC antigens, to that self antigen or an exogenous antigen that shares the epitope (molecular mimicry) would then result in an autoimmune response (Fujinami & Oldstone 1985). Normals have been shown to have T-cells which react to self-antigens that are components of organ systems which are relatively sequestered from the immune system and are components of organs that are relatively deficient in MHC-associated antigens, including the central and peripheral nervous systems and the eye (Burns et al 1983). Therefore, some other factors would be required to suppress these autoreactive T-cells.

A final mechanism is antigen-induced tolerance of autoantigen reactive clones (Nossal 1983). In this system the exposure of antigen-specific cells to that antigen, perhaps in the absence of MHC antigens (Cohn & Epstein 1978), causes suppression of the antigen-specific clones already present in the organism (Feldman et al 1985).

IMMUNOGENETICS

The immunological response of any particular organism is strongly influenced by the genetic make-up of that individual. Several allelic systems have been identified which determine the response of both humoral (antibody) and cellular elements of the immune response. These genes, therefore, in large part determine whether the host makes a response to a stimulus, be that response appropriate (protective) or inappropriate (failure to respond or an autoreactive response).

The structure of both the heavy and light chains of immunoglobulin molecules is controlled by many genetic elements which create a single gene that determines the structure of both variable and constant regions of the immunoglobulin molecule (Leder 1983, Tonegawa 1983). These regions respectively determine the antigenic specificity and biological properties of each immunoglobulin molecule. These genetic elements are not part of the MHC. In man, the haplotype in the Gm allotype system determines the allotypic nature of an individual's IgG (heavy chains). Similar allotypes have been identified for IgA heavy chains as well as kappa light chains. The genes of this system do not, of course, identify the fine specificity of the control exercised by the variable idiotype region of the heavy or light chains which determines the antigenic specificity of an antibody (immunoglobulin) molecule.

The MHC consists of several types of genes identified by gene products (these can be identified immunologically and are, therefore, themselves antigens) that are of great importance in the genetic control of the immune response. The ability of lymphocytes to react to an antigen requires co-recognition of that antigen with MHC type I (HLA, A, B and C molecules (antigens) in man for cytotoxic T-cells) or type II (HLA-DR and -DQ (DC) also called Ia in man) molecules for helper-inducer T-cells (Zinkernagel & Dougherty 1974, Unanue 1989). The MHC antigens control the response to transplantation (hence their name) and by a high degree of polymorphism and requirement for co-recognition with antigens, influence the capacity for a response of an individual organism to an antigen, be it exogenous or endogenous. It should be noted that the antigens identified to date do not seem to identify the entire repertoire of immune response genes. This need for co-recognition is true for soluble proteins as well as cell surface antigens. Moreover, genes that control other important components of the immune response include the second (C2) and fourth (C4) components of the complement system; and factor B (a component of the alternative complement pathway) (Alper 1981), maps to the MHC.

As noted, the genes have been shown to influence the immunological response of experimental animals, including the ability to develop several immunologically mediated diseases (McDevitt & Bodmer 1974). For these reasons, there have been many studies to see if there is an increased incidence of different MHC haplotypes and Gm allotypes in diseases believed to be of immunopathological origin. Among those diseases studied are several neuromuscular disor-

ders (Table 10.2). These MHC antigens may not themselves be the susceptibility determining gene products, but map near the appropriate gene, since these antigens appear in normals. It is also possible that patients may differ from normals who have the same serologically defined DR or DQ type in the pattern of the genes (DNA) that determine the different peptide chains controlling the fine specificity of the gene products (polymorphism) of the MHC II alleles. Alternatively, the MHC antigens might be the important gene product but other environmental factors determine whether a disease develops and which disease.

As described earlier the specificity of antigen recognition by T-cells is controlled by the TCR. The TCR consists of two peptide chains which undergo somatic gene rearrangement. This rearrangement accounts for the ability of the immune system of an organism to mount immune responses to the almost infinite number of potential antigens and epitopes. It has been suggested that certain families of both the α and β chains are

Table 10.2 Immunogenetic markers and neuromuscular disease associations

Disease	HLA associations	References
Polymyositis	B8; B8, DR3 (Caucasoids); B7, Dw6 (blacks)	Reviewed in Behan & Behan 1985 and Mastaglia & Ojeda 1985b
Dermatomyositis	B8, B14	Reviewed in Behan & Behan 1985, Mastaglia & Ojeda 1985b
Juvenile dermatomyositis	B6 or none	Reviewed in Behan & Behan 1985,
Myasthenia gravis		Mastaglia & Ojeda 1985b
No thymoma, <40 y.o. onset, females, probably males as well	A1, B8, DRw3 (B12 Japan); A1, B8, DR5 (blacks & other non-Caucasoids)	Compston et al 1980, reviewed in Behan & Shields 1982, Christiansen et al 1984, Engel 1984
No thymoma, >40 y.o. onset, males	A3, B7, DRw2 (B10 Japan)	
Thymoma, older onset	?A2, ? A3	
Lambert–Eaton myasthenic syndrome	B8 — idiopathic > carcinomatous	Willcox et al 1985
Guillain–Barré syndrome	None	Adams et al 1977, Stewart et al 1978, Kaslow et al 1984
Chronic demyelinating inflammatory neuropathy	A1, B8, DRw3	Stewart et al 1978, Adams et al 1979
Amyotrophic lateral sclerosis	A3 (classic) or none; B12 (slow progressive); BW35 (rapid progressive guamanian)	Reviewed in Cashman et al 1985
	Gm allotypes	
Myasthenia gravis	Gm[1,2,21] (Japan); none (Finland)	Nakao et al 1980, Smith et al 1984
Lambert–Eaton	Glm[(2)]	Willcox et al 1985
Amyotrophic lateral sclerosis	None	Reviewed in Cashman et al 1985

more frequently involved in the recognition of particular antigens including autoantigens but it is not clear that this is the case in human diseases such as multiple sclerosis or myasthenia gravis. In addition, because of rearrangements the TCRs for antigens can differ even in monozygotic twins which could serve as one explanation for the failure to see 100% concordance for autoimmune diseases in such twin pairs. Indeed it is likely that the tendency towards familial occurrence of immunopathologically mediated diseases, which do not in general follow simple Mendelian genetic patterns, represent examples of polygenetic inheritance.

IDIOPATHIC INFLAMMATORY MYOPATHIES

The term 'inflammatory myopathy' encompasses a large number of disorders. A group of these, of unknown aetiology, with certain clinical features in common, are generally referred to as idiopathic inflammatory myopathy or polymyositis and dermatomyositis (Whitaker 1982, Behan & Behan 1985, Mastaglia & Ojeda 1985a, b). There is now strong immunological and histopathological evidence to support the hypothesis that there are several subtypes of disease embraced by the terms polymyositis and dermatomyositis and that different immunopathological abnormalities and different aetiological factors are important in these different syndromes (Whitaker 1982, Behan & Behan 1985).

Experimental autoimmune myositis (EAM) and other models

Some investigators have reported successful production of experimental myositis; this has been a histological finding, while others have been unable to demonstrate reproducibly even histological myositis (Dawkins 1975, Smith et al 1979, Whitaker 1982, Behan & Behan 1985). SJL mice have been shown consistently to develop histological EAM (Rosenberg et al 1985, Kakulas 1988). The relative roles of cell-mediated and humoral (antibody) effector mechanisms in EAM are not clear. It is possible to induce inflammatory changes and necrosis in muscles of animals under-

going a graft-versus-host reaction (Mastaglia et al 1975, Kakulas 1988). Polymyositis has been reported in patients with graft-versus-host disease (Anderson et al 1982, Reyer et al 1983). It has not been possible to produce a disorder similar to childhood dermatomyositis by inducing the vascular lesions (Hathaway et al 1970). Polymyositis and both sporadic and familial canine dermatomyositis have been reported (Kornegay et al 1980, Hargis et al 1985).

Immunopathological mechanisms

There are no reported studies to suggest that the serum of patients with polymyositis or dermatomyositis contains IgE class antibodies to muscle. Basophils and mast cells are not prominent in muscle in idiopathic inflammatory myopathies. Eosinophils, which are important cells in reaginic immunity, are seen in eosinophilic polymyositis, a disorder that is part of the hypereosinophilic syndrome — a condition of unknown aetiology in which vasculitis (presumptive immune complex deposition) is frequently observed (Layzer et al 1977).

The possibility that the serum of patients with idiopathic inflammatory myopathies contains antibodies to one or more muscle antigens that are involved in Type II immunopathological reactions has been investigated. There have been reports of deposition of immunoglobulin and complement components at the site of muscle fibre necrosis (Heffner et al 1976, Engel & Biesecker 1982, Isenberg 1983, Morgan et al 1984), a finding that is certainly compatible with the hypothesis that antibodies to muscle are involved in the pathogenesis of these disorders. While the presence of components of the complement system seems to be reproducible, it should be noted that this is not proof that antimuscle antibodies are responsible for this deposition, activation and subsequent fibre necrosis. Immune complex deposition (see below) could also be responsible for complement activation and the alternate pathway of complement can be activated through non-antibody-related mechanisms. The demonstration of immunoglobulin deposition has suggested, to some, non-specific in vitro staining or in vivo deposition (Mastaglia & Ojeda 1985) as a result of changes in the vasculature. Studies of serum of patients with polymyositis and dermatomyositis have not revealed disease-specific increases in antibodies to muscle, muscle extracts or purified muscle antigens such as myoglobin, actin or myosin (Whitaker 1982, reviewed in Behan & Behan 1985, Mastaglia & Ojeda 1985b). One would expect that pathogenic antibodies would be directed at a surface component rather than at a component of the cytoplasm or nucleus. As noted later, an antibody-dependent cell-mediated cytotoxic reaction could be involved in disease pathogenesis.

The serum of patients with polymyositis frequently contains antibodies to nuclear and/or cytoplasmic antigens. It has been suggested that some of these are relatively specific for clinical subsets of the idiopathic inflammatory myopathies (Table 10.3) and that subsets of myositis may be classified on the basis of these antibodies (Love et al 1991). It is unlikely that these antibodies are responsible for muscle damage but they may be useful in defining subsets of these disorders and, more importantly, in helping to delineate the cause of some of these syndromes. For example, the Jo antigen is the enzyme that catalyses the charging of histidine to its transfer RNA. Picornaviruses have been shown to interact with the transfer RNA synthetase enzymes (Matthews & Bernstein 1983). If the antibodies were to cross-react with a membrane antigen they could then cause tissue damage directly or become internalised and cause damage by reacting with the cytoplasmic or nuclear antigen and interfering with its role in cell function.

There is considerable evidence to support the hypothesis that deposition of circulating immune complexes in vessels within muscle is critical in initiation in the pathogenesis of certain idiopathic inflammatory myopathies, specifically dermatomyositis. Frank vasculitis is found in the muscle and in other tissues, especially in patients with juvenile dermatomyositis (Banker 1975). Milder changes are also observed, including changes in capillary endothelial cells and basement membrane (Behan & Behan 1985). It should be noted that changes can be noted in vessels at the site of clear-cut cell mediated non-antibody reactions. Deposition of immunoglobulin and complement in the vessels were described by Whitaker & Engel (1972). The incidence was highest among patients with juvenile dermatomyositis. Indeed, in studies which did not include a significant number of patients of this subtype, immunoglobulin and complement deposition was seldom, if ever, observed in vessel walls. Evidence of complement activation was found in vessels of patients with dermatomyositis (Kissel et al 1986).

Table 10.3 Antinuclear and related antibodies in polymyositis/dermatomyositis

Antibody	Disease subset	Antigen	Reference
PM-1	60–70% PM; some childhood DM	Unknown	Wolfe et al 1977, Pachman & Cooke 1980
Jo-1	30–40% PM; 60–70% with pulmonary fibrosis	Histidyl-tRNA synthetase	Arnett et al 1981, Matthews & Bernstein 1983
Mi	Exclusively seen with dermatomyositis	Cathodic non-histone protein	Nishikai & Reichlin 1980, Targoff & Reichlin 1985
Ku	PM with scleroderma features	Acidic protein (80 and 70 kDa)	Mimori et al 1981
PM-Scl	PM with scleroderma features	Nucleus/nucleolar	Reichlin et al 1984
PL-7	Polymyositis	Threonyl-tRNA synthetase	Matthews et al 1984
RNP	Mixed connective tissue disease; some SLE	Small nuclear ribonuclear proteins	Sharp et al 1972, 1976
Sm	SLE	Small nuclear ribonuclear proteins	
DS-DNA	SLE-active	Native DNA	Zweiman & Lisak 1990, Behan & Behan 1985
Ro	Sjögren's syndrome; some SLE, polymyositis, mothers of infants with congenital heart block	Small cytoplasmic ribonuclear proteins (60 and 52 kDa)	Lisak 1992
La	Sjögren's syndrome	Small ribonuclear protein involved in termination of RNA polymerase transcription (48 kDa)	Moore & Lisak 1990

Emslie-Smith & Engel (1990) have convincingly shown that muscles of patients with adult-onset dermatomyositis have focal capillary depletion, reduced capillary density and immunohistological evidence of complement membrane attack complex (MAC) deposition in vessels in the muscle. The MAC neoantigen is involved in this process. The presence of elevated levels of immune complexes in the serum of patients with both polymyositis and dermatomyositis has been reported (Behan et al 1982). The nature of antigen in these complexes is not known.

There is longstanding interest in the possibility that some cases of polymyositis may be caused by cell-mediated reactivity to muscle antigens or conceivably to viral antigens in latently infected muscle fibres. Myositis has been described recently in patients with the acquired immune deficiency syndrome (AIDS) (Levy et al 1985). With the exception of two studies (Johnson et al 1972, Hohfeld & Engel 1991), in vitro experiments assessing cell-mediated cytotoxicity have not used HLA-matched or autologous human muscle as the target (Currie et al 1971, Dawkins & Mastaglia 1973, Haas & Arnason 1974, Haas 1980). As T-cell cytotoxic reactions apparently do not occur across histocompatibility barriers, the reported cytotoxic reactions may not represent in vitro evidence of T-cell cytotoxicity. These experiments could represent: (a) antibody-dependent cell-mediated cytotoxic (ADCC) reactions; (b) reactions of the blood cells to allogenic histocompatibility antigens on the muscle; or (c) increases in NK cell activity. It should be noted that only one of the studies examined the cytotoxic effect of patients' cells on non-muscle tissue so that muscle-specific cytotoxicity has not been demonstrated absolutely conclusively. In addition, only one study employed purified T-cells or cytotoxic (CD8+) T-cells in in vitro cytotoxicity assays, demonstrating some cytotoxicity to autologous myotubes in vitro (Hohfeld & Engel 1991). Disease-specific in vitro reactivity to muscle using proliferation of lymphocytes has not been demonstrated (Behan et al 1975, Lisak & Zweiman 1975).

It has been reported that a CD4+ line obtained from a patient with dermatomyositis showed MHC-restricted proliferation to muscle but the cytotoxicity to rat muscle in vitro was MHC-independent. A CD8+ line from the same patient proliferated to muscle that was MHC-non-restricted and failed to induce in vitro cytotoxicity for rat muscle (Rosenschein et al 1987). It should be remembered that T-cells reactive to autoantigens can be isolated from blood of normal individuals (Burns et al 1993).

There is very strong indirect evidence for an important and perhaps primary role for an immunopathological cell-mediated reaction in polymyositis as well as in inclusion body myositis. Graft-versus-host disease (Anderson et al 1982) and experimental autoimmune myositis, as noted, bear some resemblance to polymyositis and these are cell-mediated disorders. The strongest evidence, however, can be found in detailed analysis of the phenotypes of the inflammatory cells resident in the muscles. In both polymyositis and inclusion body myositis the predominant infiltrating cell is the T-cell and both CD4+ and CD8+ subtypes are present (Figs 10.1, 10.2), as are macrophages (Rowe et al 1981, Arahata & Engel 1984, Engel & Arahata 1984, Giorno et al 1984, Olsson et al 1985, Arahata & Engel 1986). Although analysis of TCR in these lesions has shown α and β chains, there are other cases in which $\gamma\delta$ configurations have been found (Hohfeld et al 1991). As previously mentioned, the latter may be in response to up-regulation in heat-shock proteins in the muscle cells. Activation markers are seen on many of the T-cells in the muscles of patients with polymyositis (Giorno et al 1984, Olsson et al 1985, Isenberg et al 1986, Nennesmo et al 1989). These is also evidence that some of the inclusions in inclusion body myositis are ubiquitin-like in their immunoreactivity (Askanas et al 1992). Others have identified amyloid or amyloid-like material in some of the fibres of patients with both acquired and familial inclusion body myositis (Mendell et al 1991, Mendell & Sahenk 1992, Neville et al 1992a,b). B-cells and cells associated with NK and ADCC reactions are not frequent. It seems likely that the earliest cells are the CD8+ cell which can be seen to invade muscle fibres. MHC class I molecules predominate on the muscle fibres themselves (Appleyard et al 1985, Karpati et al 1988, McDouall et al 1989), which would be compatible with a CD8+ T-cell mediated reaction. Serial studies of nerves in experimental allergic

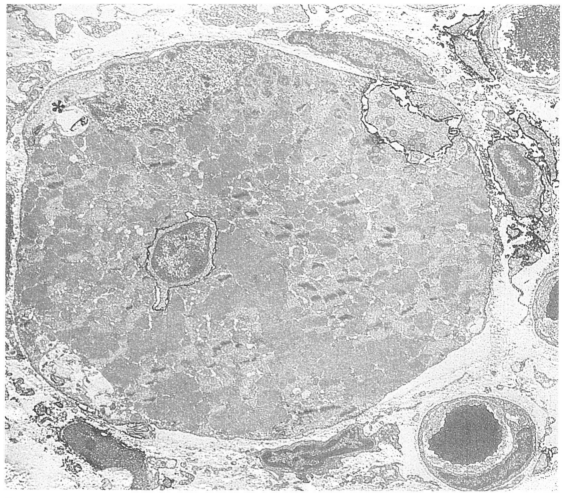

Fig. 10.1 A muscle fibre with surrounding and superficial and deeply placed T8+ invading cells. Small cavities in the fibre (asterisk) probably contained invading cells that retracted during fixation or dehydration, or indicate focal myofibrillar loss near invading cells. The plasma membrane of the fibre facing the invading cells, highlighted by diffusion artefact, shows no deletions (× 6000) (from Arahata & Engel 1986).

neuritis and spinal cords of animals with experimental allergic encephalomyelitis clearly demonstrate that there are differences in the proportion of different subtypes of T-cells during different phases of these T-cell-mediated experimental disorders. Unfortunately, true serial studies are not really feasible in patients. Analysis of muscle from patients with an HIV-associated myositis shows similar patterns to those of polymyositis (Illa et al 1991).

Thus, there is evidence for both cell-mediated and immune-complex-mediated immunopatho-logical mechanisms being involved in the pathogenesis of these disorders; there is less evidence for a pathogenic role for anti-muscle antibodies. It may be that more than one mechanism may be important and perhaps different mechanisms predominate in different subtypes of these disorders. It must be emphasised that the evidence is indirect and controversial.

Immunoregulation

If a disorder is immunopathogenic in origin or is

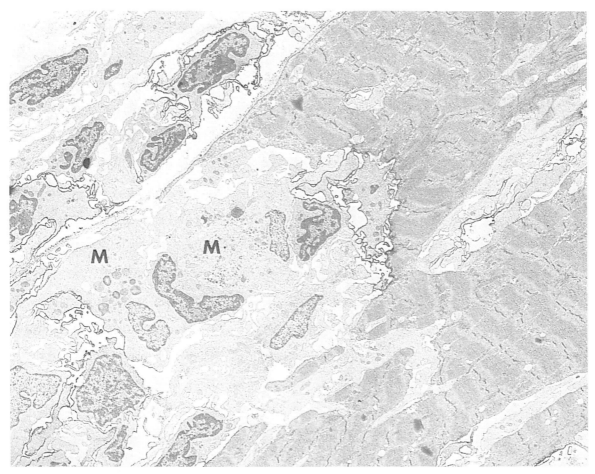

Fig. 10.2 More advanced fibre invasion. The T8 antigen is localised. The muscle fibre is honeycombed by cavities containing both T8+ and T8-negative invading cells and their spike-like extensions. Large invading cells with pale cytoplasm and multiple lysosomal structures are macrophages (M). The muscle fibre is depleted of mitochondria and shows focal myofibrillar degeneration beginning at the Z disk ($\times$ 4400) (from Arahata & Engel 1986).

the result of a persistent infection with a common virus, it is important to determine whether there is a defect in the normal regulatory mechanisms which would be permissive for such an abnormal state to develop and persist. Indeed, it has recently been noted that primates with an acquired immune deficiency (AIDS-like) illness have polymyositis-like lesions (Dalakas et al 1986) and similar lesions have recently been described in patients with AIDS (Levy et al 1985).

There have been several studies of the peripheral blood of patients with polymyositis and dermatomyositis which have assessed quantitatively the numbers of various lymphocyte subsets.

Some (Behan et al 1983, Lisak et al 1984b, Behan & Behan 1985) but not all (Iyer et al 1983) groups of investigators have found a reduction in the number of suppressor T-cells in the blood of such patients. Functional studies have also been performed to assess the immunoregulatory capacity of blood cells. A decrease in some but not other suppressor T-cell activities has been reported (Mastaglia & Ojeda 1985b) and an increase in B-cell activity, manifested by increased serum immunoglobulin levels, and increased spontaneous immunoglobulin-secreting cells (Lisak, Levinson & Zweimann, unpublished observations), which could be a consequence of decrease in suppressor activity, is also seen (Lisak & Zweiman 1976). The relationship between decreased T-cell suppressor activity and number and a reported decrease in the proliferative response of blood cells of patients with polymyositis to phytohaemagglutinin (Behan & Behan 1985) is not clear. One usually associates decreased proliferation of cells to this T-cell mitogen with defects in the number or function of helper rather than in suppressor T-cell defects.

MYASTHENIA GRAVIS

Myasthenia gravis has emerged as the prototypic autoimmune disease. Although its aetiology is unknown, in the past 20 years we have learned much about immunopathological mechanisms important at the end-plate, the nature of important antigenic sites of the acetylcholine (ACh) receptor (AChR), and a good deal about defects in normal immunological control which may have a role in the loss of tolerance and emergence of pathogenic autoantibodies.

Experimental autoimmune myasthenia gravis (EAMG) and other models

Sensitisation of experimental animals with material rich in AChR with the production of weakness and neuromuscular block responsive to acetylcholinesterase inhibitors, was a major development in our understanding of the immunopathogenesis of myasthenia gravis (Patrick & Lindstrom 1973, reviewed in Ashizawa & Appel 1985). It became clear that while T-cells and macrophages were important in the production of antibodies to AChR, the antibodies were responsible for the actual reduction of available AChR at the postsynaptic membrane (Sahashi et al 1978). The EAMG model has continued to be of use in investigation of pathogenic mechanisms by which the antibodies actually cause a decrease in available receptor, as well as in the study of interactions of cells of their immune system that bring about disease induction and, potentially, suppression of the autoimmune response (Christados et al 1981, Pachner & Cantor 1984, Lennon et al 1985). Experimental myasthenia and anti-AChR antibodies have been induced by immunising

animals either with antibodies to an agonist of AChR (Wasserman et al 1982) or with the agonist (Bis Q) itself (Cleveland et al 1983) via the idiotype network.

Monoclonal antibodies produced in rodents against AChR have also provided insight into the events at the end-plate. Because of the exquisite specificity of these immunoglobulins against defined epitopes (antigenic sites), it is possible to employ these monoclonal antibodies in in vitro and in vivo experiments to determine which epitopes serve as potentially pathogenic reactants and to investigate which immunopathological mechanisms involving anti-AChR antibodies are important (see below). Analysis with this degree of specificity is not possible in passive transfer experiments employing heteroantisera or human immunoglobulins (Toyka et al 1975).

Acquired autoimmune myasthenia gravis occurs in several breeds of dogs, as does congenital myasthenia gravis which is not immunologically mediated (Lennon et al 1978).

Immunopathological events at the end-plate

It has become clear that there are several mechanisms by which anti-AChR antibodies cause a reduction in AChR at the muscle end-plate (Lisak & Barchi 1982, Ashizawa & Appel 1985). The original demonstration of serum anti-AChR antibodies employed an assay that detected antibodies directed against the α-bungarotoxin binding site which is close to or perhaps identical to the ligand (ACh) binding site (Almon et al 1974). For some time it was felt that this was not an important mechanism for pathological manifestation in vivo, principally because most patients do not have detectable antibodies to this site and the proportion of antibodies blocking α-bungarotoxin binding is small in patients with such antibodies (Whiting et al 1983, Sterz et al 1986). However, it is possible that in some patients antibodies which block or alter the conformation of the ligand binding site may be important in certain stages of the disease. This is supported by the finding that monoclonal antibodies to the α-bungarotoxin binding site cause a rapidly evolving neuromuscular block when passively transferred to avian recipients

(Gomez & Richman 1983). Assays of serum from patients with MG employing a human tumour cell line bearing nicotinic AChR also support the importance of blocking antibodies (Pachner 1989).

A second mechanism is complement-mediated destruction of the end-plate. It is clear that some end-plates show evidence of necrosis with the presence of both the third and ninth components of the complement cascade (Fig. 10.3) (Engel et al 1977, Sahashi et al 1980) and the membrane complement attack complex (Engel & Arahata 1987). In vitro studies and passive transfer protocols with experimental antibodies and IgG from patients with myasthenia confirm the importance of antibody-determined complement-mediated membrane destruction.

The other important mechanism is antigen-specific antibody-mediated degradation, down-regulation of AChR. AChR, like other membrane constituents, is constantly degraded, resynthesised and inserted into the membrane. It has been shown that an antibody molecule can bind to antigenic sites on adjacent molecules of AChR by virtue of its two antigen-binding sites (bivalent). This results in a cross-linking of adjacent molecules which in turn causes a rearrangement of receptor molecules (Bursztajn et al 1983) and an increased rate of AChR degradation (Appel et al 1977, Kao & Drachman 1977, Drachmann et al 1978, Stanley & Drachman 1978). While eventually there is an increase in synthesis, it does not occur acutely and at any rate is insufficient to maintain a normal density of receptor in the membrane. If the immunoglobulin (antibody) binds to two sites in the same molecule, such as on each of the α-chains, there is no increase in receptor-specific degradation (Conti-Tronconi et al 1982).

Although cells can be found at the end-plate in acute stages of EAMG in some species, either in response to complement activation or as an antibody-dependent cell-mediated cytotoxic reaction (ADCC), there is little evidence for such mechanisms being of primary importance in man. It should be noted, however, that there are few, if any, studies of the human end-plate at an equivalent stage of the disease.

Several groups have reported increased in vitro reactivity to AChR by blood and thymic lymphocytes in patients with myasthenia gravis (Abramsky et al 1975, Richman et al 1976, McQuillen et al 1983, Sisley et al 1989). This reactivity, while significantly greater than that observed in controls, is

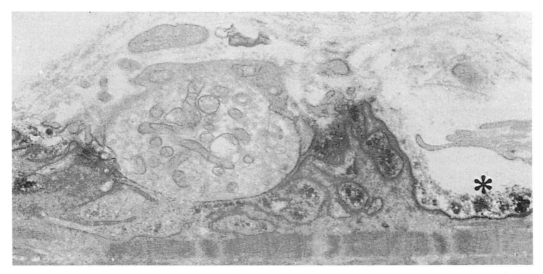

Fig. 10.3 C9 localisation in myasthenia gravis. The postsynaptic region is relatively simple. Reaction for C9 appears on debris in the synaptic space, over short segments of the junctional folds and on material to the right of the folds, and on the surface of the muscle fibre and positioned between layers of basal lamina (asterisk) (× 15 300) (from Sahashi et al 1980).

quite modest and does not approach the levels of reactivity observed in sensitised animals with EAMG. When one considers passive transfer studies in animals and the pathology of the end-plate in experimental models and in man, one is forced to conclude that a local delayed hypersensitivity reaction or cytotoxic T-cell reaction is not an important pathogenic mechanism in human myasthenia gravis (Lisak et al 1985a). There have also been studies demonstrating an increase in the frequency of γ-interferon-secreting AChR-reactive T-cells in the blood of patients with myasthenia gravis when compared to controls using an ELISPOT assay (Link et al 1991). It is likely that these cells are important in their interaction with B-cells in the synthesis of anti-AChR. It is also likely that autoimmune B-cells can be stimulated by the release of lymphokines by polyclonal-stimulated T-cells.

Antigenic determinants (epitopes)

Anti-AChR antibodies in the serum of patients with MG are not all directed against the same antigenic determinant on the molecule. Antibodies have been detected against all four subunits (α, β, γ, δ) of the protein, although the majority seem to be directed to a single region of the α subunits. The antigenic determinant (epitope) that comprises the so-called main immunogenic region (MIR) consists of amino acids 67–76 on the α-chain (Tzartos et al 1988). Monoclonal antibodies to this epitope transfer disease to naive animals. However, the concept of a single MIR in humans with myasthenia gravis who are 'outbred' has been challenged (Lennon & Griesman 1989).

Patients with myasthenia gravis also frequently have antibodies to other autoantigens, both organ-specific and non-organ-specific (Lisak & Barchi 1982). Among the most interesting are antibodies directed at a group of muscle proteins seen most often and in highest titre in patients with myasthenia associated with thymoma. These include antibodies to myosin, actin, α-actinin, titin and ryanodine (Williams & Lennon 1986, Aarli et al 1990, Ohta et al 1990, Mygland et al 1992a), as well as to sarcoplasmic reticulum (Mygland et al 1992b). The pathogenic role, if any, of those antibodies is not known.

Abnormalities of immunoregulation

As described earlier in this chapter, the emergence of significant levels of pathogenic antibodies to a self-antigen implies one or more abnormalities of normal immunological control and regulatory mechanisms (loss of tolerance). In addition, the occurrence of many autoantibodies in patients with myasthenia, which do not seem to be the result of cross-reactive epitopes in the different tissues and antigens (Gilhus et al 1984), suggests that in some patients there is a broad-based defect in immunoregulation. Indeed, there is evidence for abnormalities of broad-based and AChR-specific immune responses by both blood and thymic cells (Lisak & Barchi 1982, Levinson et al 1985, Lisak et al 1985a).

There have been quantitative analyses of levels of lymphocytes and lymphocyte subsets in the blood of patients with myasthenia gravis, most recently employing monoclonal antibodies that react with subsets with different functional characteristics. While there is no complete agreement, most have found significant, albeit modest, increases in the ratio of helper/suppressor cells, generally reflecting a decrease in suppressor cells (Bahir et al 1981, Skolnik et al 1982). Haynes et al (1983) found a decrease in helper cell numbers in a small number of patients with later onset of disease which was reversed after thymectomy. In vitro evidence for a decrease in T-cell suppressor function has been reported (Mishak & Dau 1981), as has evidence for an increase in in vivo B-cell activity (Levinson et al 1981). It has been reported that there is an increase in the percentage of cells that bear the CD5 antigen in the blood of patients with myasthenia gravis (Ragheb & Lisak 1990). This has also been reported in patients with Sjögren's syndrome, rheumatoid arthritis, insulin-dependent diabetes mellitus, recovery from bone marrow transplantation and auto-immune mice (these cells synthesise autoantibodies of the IgM and occasionally the IgG isotype). Thus, there is reason to believe that patients with myasthenia gravis have a mild decrease in some immunoregulatory capacity not limited to control of the response to AChR.

It is also clear that patients with myasthenia gravis differ from controls with regard to regulation of synthesis of antibodies to AChR. Culture of blood cells of patients with myasthenia in vitro results in detectable synthesis of anti-AChR antibodies in 50–60% of patients without any additional stimulation. The addition of pokeweed mitogen, a T-cell- and monocyte-dependent polyclonal stimulant of B-cell growth and differentiation, results in a dramatic increase in the amount of antibody synthesised, and detectable synthesis of antibody in 70–80% of patients. The amount of antibody correlates with the serum titres of anti-AChR antibodies. The peripheral blood cells of normal individuals rarely synthesise detectable levels of anti-AChR and even then in minimal amounts (Lisak et al 1983b, 1984b). Removal of CD8 suppressor lymphocytes from cultures of blood cells from normals does not result in an increase in detectable anti-AChR synthesis. Thus, the lack of anti-AChR synthesis by normals cannot be attributed simply to normal CD8 suppressor cell function (Lisak et al 1984b). The most likely explanation is the lack of sufficient numbers of the autoimmune B-cells to respond to non-specific T-cell helper factors. In contrast, the removal of CD8 positive cells from cultures of blood from myasthenics does result in an increase in both anti-AChR and total IgG synthesis (Lisak et al 1986a). Therefore, anti-AChR synthesis by abnormal B-cells and helper T-cells, including the AChR-specific helper T-cells reported to be present in the blood of myasthenics (Hohlfeld et al 1984, Harcaut et al 1989, Protti et al 1990), is subject to some normal immunoregulatory influences. Since we do not know what triggers anti-AChR synthesis in vivo, it is possible that increased numbers of antigen-specific helper T-cells may be important in the loss of immunological tolerance in myasthenics. As noted earlier, it has been reported that there is a higher frequency of T-cells reactive to AChR in the blood of patients with myasthenia gravis than in controls. There are several reports demonstrating reactivity of T-cells from patients with myasthenia gravis and controls to various sequences on the α, β, and δ chains. As yet there has been no demonstration of a specific sequence on any of the peptide chains that is reactive for T-cells of myasthenia gravis patients but not present in controls (reviewed in Ragheb & Lisak 1993).

It has also been found that the thymus, which is histologically abnormal in the majority of patients with myasthenia, is the site of abnormal immune responses. This is of special interest because of the central role of the thymus in the development of the immune response, the presence of myoid cells in the thymus and the reports of a beneficial effect of thymectomy.

The distribution of lymphocytes in the thymus of patients with myasthenia gravis has received considerable study. While earlier studies did not indicate any abnormality in the major subsets of T-cells (CD4+ and CD8+), more recent studies using double and triple labelling with monoclonal antibodies demonstrate that there is an increase in mature T-cells (CD3+ CD4+ CD8− and CD3+CD4−CD8+) in the thymus of patients with myasthenia gravis compared to controls (Durelli et al 1990, Fujii et al 1990). Histochemical studies of hyperplastic thymuses from patients with myasthenia gravis indicate that germinal follicles are organised identically to germinal follicles in reactive lymph nodes (Kornstein et al 1984).

Little is known about potential abnormalities in accessory cells in the myasthenic thymus including epithelial cells and dendritic cells. There seems to be an increase in the percentage of DR-positive lymphoid cells in suspensions obtained from thymuses of myasthenic subjects. Whether these are dendritic cells or B-cells that do not bear the other usual B-cell phenotypic markers is not known (Lisak et al 1983c).

Functional studies of thymic lymphocytes have also provided evidence of immunological abnormalities. Despite the fact that relatively few B-cells bear surface IgM, cell suspensions from myasthenic thymuses demonstrate increased spontaneous levels of immunoglobulin-secreting cells, an indicator of enhanced in vivo B-cell activity (Levinson et al 1984). This activity is frequently greater than that of autologous blood cells. It is not clear whether this activity is inherent in the B-cells or represents an abnormal milieu because of abnormal T-cell or accessory-cell function, or because of the presence of AChR itself in the thymus, perhaps in an immunogenetically susceptible subject. The potential for B-cell activation is probably present in the normal thymus, as mitogen stimulation of thymic lymphocytes in vitro results in an equivalent immunoglobulin-secreting cell response, often greater than that of blood cells in control and myasthenic thymic cell suspensions. Using CD20 as a marker of B-cells, Durelli and associates (1990) reported an increase in B-cells in cell suspensions of thymuses from patients with myasthenia gravis. Many of these CD20+ B-cells do not bear the usual IgM surface marker (Zweiman et al 1989). It has also been reported that B-cells in thymus cell suspensions from patients with myasthenia gravis secrete predominately IgG with in vitro polyclonal stimulation, whereas blood B-cells secrete equal amounts of IgG and IgM (Levinson et al 1990) and these same studies indicate that the difference resides in the thymic B-cells rather than in the nature of the T-cell help.

It has been shown that thymic lymphocytes secrete anti-AChR in vitro (Vincent et al 1978, McLachlan et al 1981, Newsom-Davis et al 1981, Fujii et al 1986, Lisak et al 1986b), although there is controversy over the response to mitogenic stimulation in vitro and the relative production of thymic and blood cell production of these antibodies. It seems unlikely that the thymus is the major site of in vivo anti-AChR production: normal thymus cells do not synthesise detectable anti-AChR with or without mitogen stimulation; cells from patients with myasthenia and thymoma either do not make anti-AChR or make less than those from patients with germinal centre hyperplasia (Vincent et al 1978, Fujii et al 1984). It is also clear that while much of the IgG synthesised by thymic lymphocytes may be anti-AChR (Fujii et al 1986), other antibodies are synthesised by these cells in vitro (Newsom-Davis et al 1981, Lisak et al 1986b).

It has been reported that thymic cells provide specific help to blood cells of patients with myasthenia gravis, in increasing the in vitro synthesis of anti-AChR but not of other antibodies by the blood cells (Newson-Davis et al 1981). The exact nature of this help or of the thymic cells involved is not known.

It has been suggested that the thymus may be the site of origin of the autoimmune response in myasthenia gravis (Lisak et al 1976, Werkele & Ketelsen 1977). The roles of accessory antigen-presenting cells and epithelial cells, and the possibility that AChR, perhaps in an altered form, might initiate some cases of myasthenia, requires further investigation. It has been postulated that a viral infection could trigger the autoimmune response (Datta & Schwartz 1974) but evidence for a viral trigger is lacking (Aoki et al 1985, Klavinskis et al 1985). However, it has been reported that monoclonal antibodies to AChR react with several Gram-negative bacteria, raising the possibility of stimulation of anti-AChR antibodies in susceptible subjects via molecular mimicry (Stephansson et al 1984).

Anti-idiotype control

There is interest in naturally occurring anti-idiotype antibodies to anti-AChR as possible immunoregulatory modulators in patients with myasthenia gravis, and Dwyer et al (1983) have described activity that they feel is compatible with such a possibility; others have failed to detect such activity (Heininger et al 1983). However, if this were important in patients, one would have expected an inverse relation with titre and/or clinical disease. If anti-idiotypic antibodies were important in preventing myasthenia gravis in normals, one might also have expected such activity in serum from normal individuals.

There is also interest in the production of anti-idiotype antibodies as potential therapeutic agents in patients with myasthenia gravis. To date, such antibodies raised to anti-AChR of one individual have not shown extensive cross-reactivity in other patients (Lefvert 1981, Lang et al 1985), a finding not limited to anti-AChR (Kahn 1985). Thus, if such reagents were used, they would have to be produced for individual patients. In addition, anti-idiotype antibodies have not been unequivocally useful in modifying clinical manifestations of disease in animals with EAMG (Fuchs et al 1981, Agius et al 1985), especially once the disease is clinically manifest.

Heterogeneity of myasthenia gravis

Most patients with acquired myasthenia gravis can be shown to have antibodies to AChR, as determined by assays that measure total binding to AChR and/or certain biological effects of such antibodies, such as modulation of AChR, complement-mediated lysis or ligand blocking (Howard et al 1986). It has been suggested that, in others, the autoimmune response is directed at another as yet uncharacterised postsynaptic neuromuscular component (Newsom-Davis et al 1987). One can also find a heterogeneity among patients with myasthenia with serum anti-AChR antibodies. Such heterogeneity may represent different defects in immunological control and different aetiologies, leading to similar or identical anti-AChR antibodies with a final common step of neuromuscular block. Such heterogeneity may be represented by differences in age of onset, HLA associations, thymic pathology (hyperplasia vs thymoma vs atrophy) and response to thymectomy (Lisak et al 1985a, Newsom-Davis et al 1987). These factors may not be totally independent variables (Compston et al 1980). In addition, the development of myasthenia gravis as a result of therapy with penicillamine and after bone marrow transplantation in the absence of graft-versus-host disease (Smith et al 1983, 1987, Cain et al 1986) may represent two other mechanisms allowing for the emergence of the pathogenic anti-AChR antibodies.

LAMBERT–EATON MYASTHENIC SYNDROME

The Eaton–Lambert (or Lambert–Eaton) myasthenic syndrome, a neuromuscular disease in which the muscular symptoms are due to a presynaptic deficit in the release of ACh, now seems to be established as an immunopathologically determined disorder (Newsom-Davis 1985). The syndrome is associated with carcinoma, almost always small (oat)-cell carcinoma of the lung, in approximately two-thirds of cases (O'Neill et al 1988). In idiopathic cases there is an increased incidence of other putative immunopathological diseases and of elevated serum titres of several autoantibodies directed at antigens not present in muscle or nerve (Lennon et al 1982). The presynaptic membrane has reduced and rearranged active zones (Fukunaga et al 1983). It has been shown that serum IgG of patients with both idiopathic and oat-cell carcinoma-associated Lambert–Eaton myasthenic syndrome can passively transfer the characteristic electrophysiological and pathological deficit to immunosuppressed mice (Lang et al 1981, Fukunaga et al 1983, Kim 1985, Newsom-Davis 1985, Engel et al 1987). Indirect supportive evidence for an autoimmune-immunopathological pathogenesis comes from the clinical observation that plasma exchange and immunosuppressive therapy (corticosteroids and cytotoxic agents) have a beneficial effect in many of these patients. There has been recent evidence that the target antigen in some patients is a presynaptic voltage-gated calcium channel associated with AChR release from somatic motor and autonomic nerve terminals (Kim 1987, Logan et al 1987, Wray et al 1987, Vincent et al 1989) and more recently the β-chain has been identified as a target antigen in some patients (Rosenfeld et al 1993). As with myasthenia gravis it is not unlikely that several different sequences on more than one chain of the calcium channel will be found to be antigenic. Elevated titres to voltage-gated calcium channels have been reported in serum from patients with Lambert–Eaton syndrome (Sher et al 1989, Lennon & Lambert 1990). There is very recent preliminary evidence that some of the antibodies directed at the presynaptic nerve terminal react with a protein called synaptotagmin which is asssociated with the presynaptic calcium channel.

The mechanisms responsible for this autoimmune disease are not clear. It has been suggested that the patients with the idiopathic disorder develop antibodies to a presynaptic antigen as part of a more generalised defect in immunoregulatory mechanisms, similar to the multiple autoantibodies frequently seen in patients with myasthenia gravis (Lennon et al 1982). Once the antigen has been identified we may indeed find that some patients with other immunopathologically determined disoders have an increased incidence of antibodies to the Lambert–Eaton antigen without necessarily having the clinical Lambert–Eaton syndrome.

The explanation for the association with oat-cell carcinoma is also uncertain. Patients with neoplasia frequently have abnormal immune function and it has recently been reported that patients with the Lambert–Eaton syndrome associated with oat-cell carcinoma, although not idiopathic cases, have depressed levels of T8 (suppressor/cytotoxic) cells in their blood (Robb et al 1985). Given the theoretical explanation for the emergence of autoimmunity in the idiopathic disorder, the lack of abnormalities in that group is rather surprising. As patients with many types of neoplasia have abnormal immune function we still need an explanation for the very high association with oat-cell carcinoma, which is not a very common tumour. Oat-cell tumours may be associated with other neurological and non-neurological disorders and have been reported to secrete various peptides. However, the increased association of oat-cell carcinoma with the Lambert–Eaton syndrome, and perhaps with other nervous system paraneoplastic syndromes, may lie in possible shared antigens between the nervous system and the Kulchitsky cell in the lung, which is thought to derive from neural crest (Tischler et al 1977, Newsom-Davis 1985). Indeed, patients with the Lambert–Eaton syndrome have prominent autonomic dysfunction, raising the possibility that the target antigen is not limited to the presynaptic region of peripheral motor neurones. Whether a patient develops a remote effect of an oat-cell tumour and, if so, which remote effect may be under immunogenetic control (Willcox et al 1985), is still not known.

ACQUIRED DEMYELINATING NEUROPATHIES

There are several disorders of the peripheral nervous system which are thought to be immuno-pathologically mediated. The evidence is best in the acute and chronic acquired demyelinating neuropathies, although some data suggest a role for the immune system in the pathogenesis of a small number of primarily axonal diseases.

Guillain–Barré syndrome

The Guillain–Barré syndrome (post-infectious, post-immunisation or idiopathic radiculopoly-neuritis) is an acquired inflammatory segmental demyelinating disease which develops acutely or subacutely. In approximately two-thirds of patients a preceding associated event (trigger) can be identified. These include infections (often short-lived and banal, involving the respiratory or gastrointestinal tracts or exanthems), immunisa-tions, surgery, or other diseases (lymphomas, systemic lupus erythematosus and acquired immune deficiency syndrome (AIDS) or AIDS-related complex). Recently it has become clear that there are cases of the Guillain–Barré syndrome that occur after gastroenteritis caused by one of several strains of *Campylobacter jejuni* (Kaldor & Speed 1984). It has been suggested that such patients tend to have a poorer prognosis than other cases of Guillain–Barré syndrome and may be associated with high titres against ganglio-sides, especially GM1. Others have found anti-GM1 antibodies in elevated titres in other patients with Guillain–Barré syndrome without agreement on the effect on prognosis (Ilyas et al 1988, Yuki et al 1990, Walsh et al 1992). There may be cross-reactivity between the microbe and myelin antigens leading to an immune reaction against PNS myelin/Schwann cells, making the pathogen-esis of Guillain–Barré syndrome in these cases an example of molecular mimicry. It has also been suggested that such antibodies may cause early axonal damage, thus leading to a poorer recovery. It has also been suggested that patients with the Miller-Fisher variant of Gullain–Barré syndrome tend to have elevated titres against another ganglioside, GQ1b (Chiba et al 1992, Willison et al 1993, Yuki et al 1993). It is not clear how these findings can be explained in the not infre-quent occurrence of ophthalmoplegia developing early or late in otherwise typical instances of the Guillain–Barré syndrome. Patients with Lyme disease have a predominately axonal polyradicu-lopathy but cases have been reported of what seems to be a demyelinating neuropathy in associ-ation with infection with the Lyme disease agent (Mancardi et al 1989).

The relationship between these events and the Guillain–Barré syndrome is not clear and may be different for different triggering events. The disease is generally self-limiting with varying degrees of recovery (often excellent) with remyeli-nation. The presence of inflammatory cells in the nerves and nerve roots which resemble those seen in certain immunopathological experimental and naturally occurring animal diseases, and the association with immunological preceding events in many patients, have naturally led to the view that immunological factors are important in the aetiology and pathogenesis of the Guillain–Barré syndrome (Asbury et al 1969, Steiner & Abramsky 1985).

Experimental and animal models

Experimental models. Experimental allergic neuritis (EAN) is the most widely accepted experimental model of the Guillain–Barré syndrome. It was originally produced by sensitisation of rodents with PNS tissue in adjuvant (Waksman & Adams 1955) and is characterised by perivascular infiltration by mononuclear inflammatory cells, stripping of myelin by monocyte-macrophages, and segmental demyelination (Waksman & Adams 1955, Asbury et al 1969, Steiner & Abramsky 1985); sensitisation with myelin produces the same disorder. More recently it has been possible to produce EAN by sensitisation with a cathodic PNS myelin protein called P2 (Kadlubowski & Hughes 1979), although it is not clear that P2-induced EAN reproduces all the clinical, electrophysiological, pathological and immunological features of whole-myelin-induced EAN; nevertheless, in general there seems to be little difference in all but serum abnormalities (Rostami et al 1984). It has also been possible to induce a demyelinating, relatively acellular neuropathy by sensitisation of animals with galactocerebroside, a major glycolipid component of myelin (T Saida et al 1979).

The relative roles of cell-mediated and antibody-mediated immune reactions and the number of antigens that serve as the target for these immune reactions in EAN is not certain. Serum from animals with disease induced by whole nerve, myelin or galactocerebroside have high levels of circulating antibodies to galactocerebroside and presumably to other myelin antigens. These sera are capable of mediating complement-mediated demyelination and cytotoxic reactions to Schwann cells in vitro (Armati-Gulson et al 1983) and in vivo (T Saida et al 1978, K Saida et al 1979). It has been possible to transfer EAN, with both inflammation and some degree of demyelination, with lines of helper T-cells specific for reactivity with P2 (Linnington et al 1984,

Rostami et al 1985). Whether such lines mediate the entire picture of EAN actively induced with myelin or even with P2 is not as yet known. Thus, in whole-myelin-induced EAN, both cell-mediated and several antibody-mediated reactions to more than one antigen may be involved in the immunopathogenesis of the disorder. When one studies patients with the Guillain–Barré syndrome, this complicated picture must be kept in mind.

Naturally occurring models of the Guillain–Barré syndrome. Several diseases of animals also have features in common with the Guillain–Barré syndrome. These include racoon hound paralysis (Cummings & Haas 1967), acute canine polyneuropathy (Northington & Brown 1982), cauda equina syndrome of horses (Kadlubowski & Ingram 1981) and Marek's disease of chickens (Stevens et al 1981; see also Ch. 12). Little is known about the immunopathogenesis or aetiology of these disorders. Serum from animals with acute canine polyneuropathy causes demyelination in vivo after endoneurial injection into rat sciatic nerve, although it is not known if this is mediated by antibodies (Brown et al 1985). The aetiological agent of Marek's disease is a herpes virus and affected chickens go on to develop lymphomas. Serum from these birds contains antibodies to myelin but it is not known if this is a cause or effect of the inflammatory polyneuropathy (Stevens et al 1981). Horses with the cauda equina syndrome have serum antibodies to P2 (Kadlubowski & Ingram 1981), but rats with P2-induced EAN have similar antibodies that seem not to be primarily pathogenic.

Immunopathogenic mechanisms in the Guillain–Barré syndrome. Although there has been a report of elevated serum IgE levels in patients with the Guillain–Barré syndrome, there are no studies showing that this IgE binds to PNS myelin. In addition, the pathology of the Guillain–Barré syndrome does not resemble a reaginic reaction although normal peripheral nerve does contain mast cells.

Much immunological investigation in the Guillain–Barré syndrome has centred on the possibility that antibodies to one or more components of PNS myelin/Schwann cells cause the disease. The evidence that such antibodies exist and are specific to patients with the Guillain–Barré syndrome (or the possibly related chronic or relapsing acquired demyelinating polyneuritis) is very controversial (Cook & Dowling 1981, Lisak et al 1983a, Steiner & Abramsky 1985). Although serum of patients with the Guillain–Barré syndrome has been reported to cause in vitro demyelination (Arnason 1971) and Schwann cell cytotoxicity (Lisak et al 1984a) as well as in vivo demyelination and cellular infiltration (Saida et al 1982, Sumner et al 1982, Feasby et al 1983), it is not clear that this effect is mediated by antibodies (immunoglobulins). In addition, there is little evidence that serum from these patients contains disease-specific antibodies to the three known autoantigens of PNS, P1, P2 and galactocerebroside or to myelin-associated glycoprotein (MAG). Even if antibodies to a myelin component were to be demonstrated, such an antibody might represent either an epiphenomenon (resulting from release of that substance from a nerve injured via another mechanism) or might represent evidence of a heightened immune response to that antigen but one in which another component of the response (cell-mediated immunity) is the primary or only effector mechanism. In addition, non-Ig acute phase reactants in the serum could contribute to demyelination initiated by other mechanisms (Tonnessen et al 1982). Koski and associates have published a series of papers demonstrating antibodies to myelin that seem to correlate with the course of disease employing a complement capture assay (Koski 1987). The target antigens seem to be one or more glycolipids, including Forssman antigen (Koski et al 1989). The antibodies are generally of the IgM isotype. Not all investigators agree on the nature of the glycolipid targets for serum antibodies in patients with the Guillain–Barré syndrome (Hughes 1990). Antibodies to GM1 and other gangliosides have been discussed earlier.

Several groups have reported the presence of circulating immune complexes in the serum of patients with the Guillain–Barré syndrome (Tachovsky et al 1976, Goust et al 1978, Cook & Dowling 1981). Such complexes may be deposited in the glomeruli and be responsible for the proteinuria and rare instances of clinical glomerulonephritis and nephrotic syndrome seen in association with the Guillain–Barré syndrome.

(Some have suggested that the Ig deposits represent shared antigens between the nerve and glomerular basement membrane.) There is, however, no evidence that the peripheral nerve is the site of deposition of such immune complexes. Although there are reports of IgG, IgM and complement components in nerves of patients with the Guillain–Barré syndrome, these are not clearly specific and could well represent antibodies to components of the PNS. There is no evidence of vasculitis in the PNS. It is conceivable that if the blood–nerve barrier was made more permeable by another immune process, complexes could then breach the barrier and contribute to the pathological process. Alternatively, it is conceivable that the complexes are responsible for opening the barrier, thus allowing other immune mechanisms to exert their effector role (Reik 1980). It is not clear whether immune complex deposition is involved in the pathogenesis of the Guillain–Barré syndrome (or chronic demyelinating polyneuritis) in patients with systemic lupus erythematosus. As the Guillain–Barré syndrome frequently occurs after other immunological stimuli, the complexes may simply represent part of that immune reaction. It is not known, for example, whether the antigen in the complexes consists of antigens of the virus that was the triggering event. The persistence of such immune complexes for a longer period than is usually seen with viral infections may represent defects in immunoregulation seen in some patients with the Guillain–Barré syndrome.

On the basis of the similarity in appearance between lesions of EAN and of the Guillain–Barré syndrome, and the clear-cut importance of cell-mediated immunity in EAN, many investigators feel that the Guillain–Barré syndrome is primarily the result of a T-cell mediated immunopathological mechanism directed against some component of myelin and/or Schwann cells (Arnason 1971, Steiner & Abramsky 1985). To date there has been no generally agreed demonstration of a single PNS myelin antigen that is the target of a pathogenic T-cell reaction (Zweiman et al 1983, Khalili-Shirazi et al 1992), although there is evidence of activation of T-cells in patients with Guillain–Barré syndrome (Hartung & Toyka 1990). Even the presence in the blood of antigen-specific T-cells of the helper and/or cytotoxic phenotype would not prove a direct causal relationship; specific demonstration of antigen-specific cells in an increased frequency in nerve and/or blood would be highly supportive, however. Macrophages are prominent in many EAN and Guillain–Barré lesions. Macrophages are important cells in immune phagocytosis because of the presence on their surface of receptors for the Fc portion of IgG and for certain components of complement. Thus, these cells could represent: (a) mediators of an ADCC reaction; (b) cells present in response to the release of lymphokines by antigen-specific T-cells (cell-mediated reaction); and/or (c), cells phagocytosing myelin injured by other mechanisms.

Immunoregulation. As noted earlier, the development of a disease due to immunopathological mechanisms suggests a failure of normal regulation of the immune response. There have been few systematic studies examining immune regulatory function in patients with the Guillain–Barré syndrome. There have been reports of a decrease in the number and function of suppressor T-cells in some patients as well as a decrease in the numbers of helper T-cells in others (Hughes et al 1983, Lisak et al 1985b). A typical Guillain–Barré syndrome has been reported in patients with immune deficiency in association with transplantation (Drachman et al 1970), Hodgkin's disease (Lisak et al 1977) and with AIDS and the AIDS-related complex (Levy et al 1985, Cornblath et al 1987). It is possible that different defects in immune regulation and loss of tolerance may lead to the same immunopathological mechanism and clinical syndrome. Alternatively, different abnormalities could lead to a different pathogenic mechanism, such as autoimmunity, or perhaps direct involvement of the PNS by a virus (Pepose 1982), in different patients.

Chronic inflammatory demyelinating polyneuropathy (CIDP)

Patients develop an acquired demyelinating neuropathy in either a chronic progressive pattern, a relapsing pattern, or a relapsing pattern superimposed on a chronic progressive pattern. In addition, a small number of patients with the Guillain–Barré syndrome experience one or, less commonly, more than one recurrence. As noted in Chapter 24, there are striking similarities, in acquired demyelinating neuropathies, to the pathological and physical findings seen in patients with the Guillain–Barré syndrome. There is considerable indirect evidence to support the view that these more chronic and recurrent demyelinating neuropathies result from an imunopathological reaction to PNS myelin and/or Schwann cells.

Much of the evidence for an immunopathogenic cause of the chronic demyelinating neuropathies is based on analogies to the Guillain–Barré syndrome and to acute and chronic forms of EAN (Wisniewski et al 1974, Pollard et al 1975). In addition, there are studies of serum of patients with CIDP suggesting that these patients have antibodies to myelin and/or Schwann cells which could serve in them as the effector mechanism (Nyland & Aarli 1978, Latov et al 1981). Unfortunately, as in the Guillain–Barré syndrome, the evidence is controversial as far as specificity is concerned. Moreover, evidence for an in vitro or systemic or local passive transfer in vivo demyelinating effect is not as strong as in the Guillain–Barré syndrome.

There have been several studies of patients with classic CIDP attempting to determine if there is a single target antigen in patients with this disorder but to date there is no agreement on such an antigen either for antibodies or T-cells (Zweiman et al 1983, Hughes et al 1984, Rostami et al 1987). Even in patients who have a serum paraprotein and classic CIDP there is no evidence that this group differs clinically or physiologically from patients with CIDP without a serum paraprotein. Pestronk and associates (Pestronk et al 1988a, Pestronk 1991) have recently suggested that there is another group of patients who have a multifocal conduction block (Lewis et al 1982) that have a particular profile of IgM antibodies to GM1 gangliosides and another protein termed NP9 and low antibodies to nuclear histone. They have termed this syndrome multifocal motor neuropathy. Previously some have considered this disorder to be a variant of CIDP but this has been challenged. Serum from patients with this disorder with elevated titres to GM1 ganglioside cause in vitro and in vivo conduction block in experimental animals (Arasaki et al 1993, Uncini et al 1993).

There is little known about the possible role of

immune complexes in the pathogenesis of CIDP (Dalakas & Engel 1980). The presence of inflammatory cells, including lymphocytes and monocyte-macrophages, in the nerves of patients with CIDP has also raised the possibility that cell-mediated immune processes, such as T-cell- specific delayed-type hypersensitivity or cytotoxicity or an ADCC reaction, are important in the pathogenesis of CIDP. Again, the evidence is indirect and controversial and a probable target antigen has not been clearly identified (Steiner & Abramsky 1985).

There are no systematic studies of immune regulation in CIDP. The occurrence of this syndrome in patients with other disorders associated with abnormalities of immunoregulatory mechanisms such as collagen-vascular diseases (Rechthand et al 1984, Steiner & Abramsky 1985), AIDS and the AIDS-related complex (Snider et al 1983, Cornblath et al 1987) — although other patterns of neuropathy are seen with HIV infection (Lipkin et al 1985) — lends credence to the hypothesis that, as in other putative and proven immunopathological disorders, abnormal immunoregulation is involved in the aetiology and pathogenesis of CIDP.

Paraproteinaemic neuropathies

Over the past 10 years there has been increasing recognition that there are patients with polyneuropathies that are associated with paraproteinaemias. For years it had been recognised that some of these patients with malignancies such as multiple myeloma and Waldenström's macroglobulinaemia had non-specific and generally axonal polyneuropathies with little evidence that they were immunologically mediated (Besinger et al 1981). It then became clear that there was another group of patients who had benign paraproteinaemia (monoclonal gammopathies) and neuropathies. These are sometimes referred to as monoclonal gammopathy of unknown significance (MGUS). A subset of patients was then identified who had predominately IgM kappa monoclonal gammopathy in which the IgM seemed to be an antibody directed at myelin-associated glycoprotein (MAG), a constituent of

CNS and PNS myelin (Braun et al 1982, Steck & Murray 1985). The neuropathy was slowly progressive, predominantly but not exclusively sensory, and demyelinating by electrophysiological and neuropathological criteria. Some of the patients did have Waldenström's disease but most did not. The target epitope is a carbohydrate that is also found on other glycoproteins including Po and on other glycolipids (Ilyas et al 1984, Quarles 1984, Ilyas et al 1985). This is probably the most homogeneous of the paraproteinaemic neuropathies but even here there is controversy.

Subsequently other antigens have been reported for other paraproteinaemic neuropathies, including GM1 ganglioside, GQ1b ganglioside, GD1b ganglioside, sulphatide and chondroitin sulphate (Sherman et al 1983, Ito & Latov 1988, Pestronk et al 1991, Duane et al 1992). There have been reports that antiganglioside antibodies from some patients can be shown to bind to the node of Ranvier which could cause conduction block (Santoro et al 1990, 1992), but this was in a patient who was reported to have amyotrophic lateral sclerosis. There is intense controversy in this entire area. It is not clear that there is a characteristic clinical picture associated with any of the paraproteinaemic neuropathies, except for the anti-MAG IgM kappa patients. There are patients who have neuropathies associated with antibodies to some of the same antigens without paraproteinaemias, and there have been reports of antibodies to gangliosides in patients with multifocal motor neuropathy, motor neurone disease and as previously noted some patients with the Gullain–Barré syndrome (Pestronk 1991). There is also controversy related to the methodology for determining titres to the different antigens as well as to the elevation of titres to be considered clinically significant. The nature of the isotype of the immunoglobulin may also be important in defining the clinical syndromes. There needs to be agreement on the methodology employed to test the antibodies, the sensitivity of methods to look for monoclonal immunoglobulins in the blood and urine, the thoroughness of the search for associated malignancy, the clinical characterisation of patients, electrophysiological studies and pathological studies in order to understand the role of antibodies in the paraproteinaemic and non-paraproteinaemic neuropathy patients as well as in motor neurone disease and the 'lower motor neurone syndrome'. It may also be that differences in the clinical syndromes associated with antibodies to the various glycoproteins and glycolipids may also vary with antibody isotypes and different epitopes on the same antigen.

MOTOR NEURONE DISEASE (MND) (AMYOTROPHIC LATERAL SCLEROSIS (ALS))

Classical motor neurone disease (amyotrophic lateral sclerosis) is generally not considered to be an immunopathologically mediated disease. In the past there has been evidence that immunopathological mechanisms and perhaps autoimmunity may be important in some instances of this disorder (Cashman et al 1985). The clues to an immunological and/or viral aetiology for amyotrophic lateral sclerosis in the past have included:

1. Naturally occurring viral disorders of man and animals and experimental animals limited to the motor neurone.
2. The late poliomyelitis syndrome somewhat resembles amyotrophic lateral sclerosis and has been postulated to be due to either an activation of the latent poliomyelitis virus (Dalakas et al 1986b, Sharief et al 1991) or an immunologically mediated reaction to that virus leading to damage of the motor neurones, although this view has been challenged.
3. Elevated levels of circulating immune complexes have been reported by some (Oldstone et al 1976) but not all groups of investigators (Tachovsky et al 1976, Bartfeld et al 1982) and Ig has been reported in the renal glomeruli in a 'lumpy-bumpy' pattern in some patients with motor neurone disease.
4. Serum from patients with motor neurone disease has been reported by some (Wolfgram & Myers 1973, Roisen et al 1982) but not others (Liveson et al 1975, Lerich & Couture 1978) to be toxic for motor neurones in vitro,

although even in those instances where toxicity has been detected it is not clear that the toxic factor is an immunoglobulin.

Others have reported IgG in upper and lower motor neurones and inflammatory cells (principally T-cells) are found in spinal cords of some of these patients (Engelhardt & Appel 1990). More recent interest has been triggered by reports of monoclonal gammopathies in some patients with amyotrophic lateral sclerosis and lower motor neurone syndromes (Rowland et al 1982, Freddo et al 1986, Latov et al 1988, Pestronk et al 1988b, Pestronk 1991, Sadiq et al 1990) as well as reports of increased titres to GM1 ganglioside in some patients with this disease and an association of lymphoma in others (Younger et al 1990). Some of the controversies relate to the exact clinical and electrophysiological classification of some patients in these studies. In addition it is not clear what percentage of patients with motor neurone disease have paraproteinaemias or elevated antibodies to GM1 or other neural antigens, although it seems likely that no more than 5–10% of patients with amyotrophic lateral sclerosis have these findings. It is also not clear that immunosuppressive therapy leads to any improvement or slowing of progression of the neurological disease. More recently there have been two additional findings to support the hypothesis of an autoimmune aetiology in amyotrophic lateral sclerosis. Sensitization of experimental animals against anterior horn cells leads to inflammation of the anterior horn cells as well as some clinical weakness (Engelhardt et al 1989, 1990). The exact nature of the antigen is not known. The same group has now reported that the majority of patients with amyotrophic lateral sclerosis have serum antibodies to some component of voltage-gated calcium channels (Smith et al 1992) and that serum from patients with motor neurone disease causes damage to neuromuscular junctions (Uchitel et al 1992). Patients with the Lambert–Eaton myasthenic syndrome, as might be expected from earlier reports, and other patients also had these antibodies. It is not clear how the same antibodies could have these different effects. Nor is it clear how antibodies to calcium channels would lead to the clinical syndrome of motor neurone disease.

PARANEOPLASTIC SYNDROMES

There is increasing evidence that some of the neurological syndromes seen in association with cancer are immunologically mediated (Posner & Furneaux 1990). Most of the neurological syndromes that are seen in association with malignancy, which is often occult, are also seen without malignancy and many of these seem to be immunopathologically mediated in the idiopathic form as well. Myasthenia gravis is clearly an autoimmune disease and is associated with thymoma in 10–15% (Lisak & Barchi 1982). Dermatomyositis is frequently associated with occult malignancy, especially in adult males (Dalakas 1988). There is a well-recognised if rare idiopathic dorsal root ganglioneuronopathy seen after viral illness (Asbury 1987). The majority of patients with the Lambert–Eaton myasthenic syndrome have an associated small-cell (oat-cell) carcinoma of the lung (O'Neill et al 1988). The Guillain–Barré syndrome has been reported in patients with Hodgkin's disease and other lymphomas (Lisak et al 1977).

Patients with small-cell carcinoma with several overlapping neurological syndromes, including pure sensory neuropathy (sensory ganglioneuronopathy), autonomic neuropathy, cerebellar degneration, limbic encephalitis, myelopathy and anterior horn cell disease are associated with inflammation, sometimes evident in the CSF, and elevated antibodies to a nuclear antigen found in neurones termed Hu (Horwich et al 1977, Graus et al 1985, Anderson et al 1988). Other antibodies have been reported with paraneoplastic syndromes including neuropathies, cerebellar degeneration in association with other tumours including gynaecological and breast tumours, non-Hodgkin's lymphoma and neuroblastoma. Whether these antibodies are pathogenic or merely markers of an immunological disorder is not known, since the best characterised of these antigens are not surface antigens and thus differ from the presynaptic calcium channel which is the target antigen in the Lambert–Eaton myasthenic syndrome. It is also clear that patients with paraneoplastic syndromes, including those affecting the peripheral nervous system, may not have detectable antibodies to any specific antigen or cell type but this may simply represent limitations in our current state of knowledge.

OTHER NEUROMUSCULAR SYNDROMES

Patients with the stiff-man (stiff-person's) syndrome have been reported to have antibodies directed against one of three antigens, glutamic acid decarboxylase with a molecular weight of 64 kDa (Solimena et al 1988, Gorin et al 1990), an as yet uncharacterised 80 kDa protein which may be another species of glutamic acid decarboxylase or a co-precipitating protein (Darnell et al 1993), or a 128 kDa protein concentrated in neurones/synapses (Folli et al 1993). To date antibodies to the latter protein have been limited to patients who have concomitant breast cancer. Since these also are not surface antigens it is not clear how they can cause neurological dysfunction. Most recently there has been a report to suggest that some aquired cases of neuromyotonia (Isaac's syndrome) may be immunologically mediated (Newsom-Davis & Mills 1993).

MYOBLAST TRANSFER THERAPY

There has been much interest in the prospect of treating patients with Duchenne dystrophy and other inherited myopathies by intramuscular injection (transplantation) of myoblasts. One of the factors impacting on the potential efficacy of such therapy is the possibility of immunological rejection of muscle tissue. To date this has not seemed to present a major problem owing to the low levels of Class I major histocompatibility complex (MHC) molecules present on cultured myoblasts and the absence of MHC Class II molecules in the absence of induction by interferon-gamma (IFN-γ) (Hohfeld & Engel 1990, Honda & Rostami 1989, Karpati 1990). In addition immunosuppression of transplanted dystrophic mice with one of several immunosuppressive regimens seems to increase the efficacy of transplantation as measured by the number of dystrophin-positive muscle fibre segments (Karpati 1990). In a recent study, patient recipients of allogenic myoblasts were found to have Class I MHC but no Class II MHC 8 weeks after transfer. One year after transplantation neither MHC Class I or II antigens were seen in the muscle biopsies (Karpati et al 1993). However, early rejection of muscle could not be ruled out and while there has been no systemic clinical immune response there is evidence of an antibody response to donor myoblasts in patients receiving non-allogenic cells that were MHC-matched in the absence of immunosuppression (reviewed in Engel 1993).

REFERENCES

Aarli J A, Stefansson K, Marton L S G, Wollmann R L 1990 Patients with myasthenia gravis and thymoma have in their sera IgG autoantibodies against titin. Clinical and Experimental Immunology 82: 284

Abramsky O, Aharonov A, Webb C, Fuchs S 1975 Cellular immune response to acetylcholine receptor-rich fraction in patients with myasthenia gravis. Clinical and Experimental Immunology 9: 11

Adams D, Gibson J D, Thomas P K, Batchelor J R, Hughes R A C, Kennedy L, Festenstein H, Sachs J 1977 HLA antigens in Guillain–Barré syndrome. Lancet 2: 504

Adams D, Festenstein H, Gibson J P, Hughes R A C, Jaraquemada J, Papasteriadis C, Sachs J, Thomas P K 1979 HLA antigens in chronic relapsing idiopathic inflammatory polyneuropathy. Journal of Neurology, Neurosurgery and Psychiatry 42: 184

Agius M A, Geannopoulos C G, Richman D P 1985 Anti-idiotypic modification of the immune response in experimental autoimmune myasthenia gravis. Society for Neuroscience 11: 139

Almon R R, Andrew C G, Appel S H 1974 Serum globulin in myasthenia gravis: inhibition of α-bungarotoxin binding to acetylcholine receptors. Science 186: 55

Alper C A 1981 Complement and the MHC. In: Dorf M E (ed) The role of the major histocompatibility complex in immunobiology. Garland, New York, p 173

Anderson B P, Young V, Kean W F, Ludwin S K, Galbraith P R, Anastassiades T P 1982 Polymyositis in chronic graft-versus-host disease. Archives of Neurology 39: 188

Anderson N E, Rosenbaum M K, Graus F et al 1988 Autoantibodies in paraneoplastic syndromes associated with small-cell lung cancer. Neurology 38: 1391

Aoki T, Drachman D M, Asher D M, Gibbs C J Jr, Bahmanyar S, Wolinsky J 1985 Attempts to implicate viruses in myasthenia gravis. Neurology 35: 185–192

Apatoff B, Antel J P, Gurney M 1984 Autoantibodies in amyotrophic lateral sclerosis. Annals of Neurology 16: 109

Appel S H, Anivyl R, McAdams M W, Elias S B 1977 Accelerated degradation of acetylcholine receptor of cultured rat myotubes with myasthenia gravis sera and globulins. Proceedings of the National Academy of Sciences USA 74: 2130

Appleyard S T, Dunn M J, Dubowitz V, Rose M L 1985 Increased expression of HLA ABC class I antigens by muscle fibers in Duchenne muscular dystrophy, inflammatory myopathy, and other neuromuscular disorders. Lancet i: 367

Arahata K, Engel A G 1984 Monoclonal antibody analysis of mononuclear cells in myopathies. I. Quantitation of subsets according to diagnosis and sites of accumulation and demonstrations and counts of muscle fibers invaded by T-cells. Annals of Neurology 16: 198

Arahata K, Engel A G 1986 Monoclonal antibody analysis of mononuclear cells in myopathies III. Immunoelectron microscopic aspects of cell-mediated muscle fiber injury. Annals of Neurology 19: 112

Arasaki K, Kusunoki S, Kudo N, Kanazawa I 1993 Acute conduction block in vitro following exposure to antiganglioside sera. Muscle and Nerve 16: 587

Armati-Gulson P, Lisak R P, Kuchmy D, Pollard J 1983 ^{51}Cr release cytotoxicity radioimmunoassay to detect immune cytotoxic reactions to rat Schwann cells in vitro. Neuroscience Letters 35: 321

Arnason B G W 1971 Idiopathic polyneuritis (Landry-Guillain-Barré-Stohl syndrome) and experimental allergic neuritis: A comparison. Research Publications of the Association for Research in Nervous and Mental Disorders. 49: 156

Arnett F C, Hirsch T J, Bias W B, Nishikai M, Reichlin M 1981 The Jo-1 antibody system in myositis: relationships to clinical features and HLA. Journal of Rheumatology 8: 925

Asbury A K 1987 Sensory neuropathy in: Brown M J (ed) Seminars in neurology. Neuropathy vol 7. Thieme Medical Publishers, New York, p 58

Asbury A K, Arnason B G W, Adams R D 1969 The inflammatory lesion in idiopathic polyneuritis. Its role in pathogenesis. Medicine 48: 173

Ashizawa T, Appel S H 1985 Immunopathologic events at the endplate in myasthenia gravis. In: Steck A J, Lisak R P (guest eds) Immunoneurology (II) Springer Seminars in Immunopathology 8: 177

Askanas V, Serdaroglu P, Engel W K, Alvarez R B 1992 Immunocytochemical localization of ubiquitin in inclusion body myositis allows its light microscopic distinction from polymyositis. Neurology 42: 460

Bahir S, Gaud C, Bach M-A, LeBrigand H, Binet J P, Bach J F 1981 Evaluation of T-cell subsets in myasthenia gravis using anti-T-cell monoclonal antibodies. Clinical and Experimental Immunology 45: 1

Banker B Q 1975 Dermatomyositis in childhood: Ultrastructural alterations of muscle and intramuscular blood vessels. Journal of Neuropathology and Experimental Neurology 34: 46

Bartfeld H, Dham C, Donnenfeld H, Jashnani L, Carp R, Kascsak R, Vilcek J, Rapport M, Wallenstein S 1982 Immunological profile of amyotrophic lateral sclerosis patients and their cell-mediated responses to viral and CNS antigens. Clinical and Experimental Immunology 48: 137

Behan P O, Shields J 1982 Genetics. In: Lisak R P, Barchi R L Myasthenia gravis. W B Saunders, Philadelphia, p 37

Behan W M H, Behan P O, Simpson J A 1975 Absence of cellular hypersensitivity to muscle and thymic antigens in myasthenia gravis. Journal of Neurology, Neurosurgery and Psychiatry 38: 1039

Behan W M H, Barkas T, Behan P O 1982 Detection of immune complexes in polymyositis. Acta Neurologica Scandinavia 65: 320

Behan W M H, Behan P O, Micklem H S, Durward W F 1983 Lymphocyte subset abnormalities in polymyositis. British Medical Journal 287: 181

Behan W M H, Behan P O 1985 Immunological features of polymyositis/dermatomyositis. in: Steck A J, Lisak R P (guest eds) Immunoneurology (II). Springer Seminars in Immunopathology 8: 267

Besinger U A, Toyka K V, Anzel A P, Neumeier D, Rauscher R, Heininger K 1981 Myeloma neuropathy: Passive transfer from man to mouse. Science 213: 1027

Bona C A, Pernis B 1984 Idiotypic networks. In: Paul W E (ed) Fundamental immunology. Raven, New York, p 577

Bornstein M B, Appel S H 1965 Tissue culture studies of demyelination. Annals of the New York Academy of Sciences 122: 280

Braun P E, Frail D E, Latov N 1982 Myelin-associated glycoprotein is the antigen for a monoclonal IgM in polyneuropathy. Journal of Neurochemistry 39: 1261

Brown M J, Northington J W, Rosen J L, Lisak R P 1985 Acute canine idiopathic polyneuropathy (ACIP) serum demyelinates peripheral nerve in vivo. Journal of Neuroimmunology 7: 239

Burnet F M 1959 The clonal selection theory of acquired immunity. Cambridge University Press, New York

Burns J B, Rosenzweig A, Zweiman B, Lisak R P 1983 Isolation of myelin basic protein-reactive T-cell lines from normal human blood. Cellular Immunology 81: 435

Burstajn S, McMassaman J L, Elias S B, Appel S H 1983 Myasthenia globulin enhances the loss of acetylcholine receptor cultures. Science 219: 195

Cain G R, Cardinet G H, Cuddon P A, Gale R P, Champlin R 1986 Myasthenia gravis and polymyositis in a dog following fetal hematopoetic cell transplantation. Transplantation 41: 21

Cantor H 1984 T lymphocytes. In: Paul W E (ed) Fundamental immunology. Raven, New York, p 57

Cashman N R, Gurney M E, Antel J P 1985 Immunology of amyotrophic lateral sclerosis. In: Steck A J, Lisak R P (guest eds) Immunoneurology (I). Springer Seminars in Immunopathology 8: 141

Chiba A, Kusunoki S, Shimizu T, Kanazawa I 1992 Serum IgG antibody to ganglioside GQ1b is a possible marker of Miller Fisher syndrome. Annals of Neurology 31: 677

Christados P, Lennon V A, Kroc C J, Lambert E H, David C S 1981 Genetic control of autoimmunity to acetylcholine receptors: Role of the Ia molecules. Annals of the New York Academy of Sciences 377: 258

Christiansen F T, Pollack M S, Garlepp M J, Dawkins R L 1984 Myasthenia gravis and HLA antigens in American blacks and other races. Journal of Neuroimmunology 7: 121

Cleveland W L, Wasserman N H, Sarangarajan R, Penn A S, Erlanger B F 1983 Monoclonal antibodies to the acetylcholine receptor by a normally functioning auto-anti-idiotypic mechanism. Nature 305: 56

Cohen J A, Lisak R P 1987 Acute disseminated encephalomyelitis In: Aarli J A, Behan W M H, Behan P O (eds) Clinical Neuroimmunology, Blacksmell Scientific Publications, Oxford p 192

Cohen M, Epstein R 1978 T-cell inhibition of humoral responsiveness. II. Theory on the role of restrictive recognition in immune regulation. Cellular Immunology 39: 125

Compston D A S, Vincent A, Newsom-Davis J, Batchelor J R 1980 Clinical, pathological, HLA antigen and immunological evidence for disease heterogeneity in myasthenia gravis. Brain 103: 579

Conti-Tronconi B M, Gotti C M, Hunkapeller M W, Rafferty M A 1982 Mammalian muscle acetylcholine receptor: a supramolecular structure formed by four related proteins. Science 218: 1227

Cook S D, Dowling P C 1981 The role of autoantibody and immune complexes in the pathogenesis of Guillain–Barré syndrome. Annals of Neurology 9 (Supplement): 70

Coombs R R A, Gell P G H 1968 Classification of allergic reactions responsible for clinical hypersensitivity and disease. In: Gell P G H, Coombs R R A (eds) Clinical aspects of immunity. FA Davis, Philadelphia, p 575

Cornblath D R, McArthur J C, Kennedy P G E, White A S, Griffin J W 1987 Inflammatory demyelinating peripheral neuropathies associated with human T-cell lymphotropic virus type III infection. Annals of Neurology 21: 32

Cowing C 1985 Does T-cell restriction to Ia limit the need for self-tolerance? Immunology Today 6: 72

Cummings J F, Hass D C 1967 Coonhound paralysis – an acute idiopathic polyneuritia in dogs resembling Landry–Guillain–Barré syndrome. Journal of the Neurological Sciences 4: 51

Currie S, Saunders M, Knowles M, Brown A E 1971 Immunologic aspects of polymyositis. The in vitro activity of lymphocytes on incubation with muscle antigen and with mouse cultures. Quarterly Journal of Medicine 60: 63–84

Dalakas M C 1988 A classification of polymyositis and dermatomyositis In: Dalakas M C (ed) Polymyositis and dermatomyositis. Butterworths, Boston, p 1

Dalakas M C, Engel W K 1980 Immunoglobulin and complement deposits in nerves of patients with chronic relapsing polyneuropathy. Archives of Neurology 37: 637

Dalakas M C, London W T, Gravell M, Sever J L 1986a Polymyositis in an immunodeficiency disease in monkeys induced by type D retrovirus. Neurology 36: 569

Dalakas M C, Elder G, Hallet M et al 1986b A long-term follow-up study of patients with post-poliomyelitis neuromuscular symptoms. New England Journal of Medicine 314: 959

Darnell R B, Victor J, Rubin M, Clouston P, Plum F 1993 A novel antineuronal antibody in stiff-man syndrome. Neurology 43: 114

Data S K, Schwartz R S 1974 Infectious (?) myasthenia. New England Journal of Medicine 291: 1304

Dawkins R L 1975 Experimental autoallergic polymyositis, polymyositis and myasthenia gravis. Clinical and Experimental Immunology 21: 185

Dawkins R L, Mastaglia F L 1973 Cell-mediated cytotoxicity to muscle in polymyositis. Effect of immunosuppression. New England Journal of Medicine 288: 434

DeFranco A L 1987 Molecular aspects of B-lymphocyte activation. Annual Review of Cell Biology 3: 143

Dore-Duffy P, Ho S-Y, Longo M 1985 The role of prostaglandins in altered leukocyte function in multiple sclerosis. In: Steck A J, Lisak R P (guest eds) Immunoneurology (II). Springer Seminars in Immunopathology 8: 305

Drachman D A, Paterson P Y, Berlin B S, Roguska J 1970 Immunosuppression and the Guillain-Barré syndrome. Archives of Neurology 23: 385

Drachman D B, Angus C W, Adams R N, Michelson J D, Hoffman G J 1978 Myasthenic antibodies cross-link acetylcholine receptors to accelerate degradation. New England Journal of Medicine 298: 1116

Duane G C, Farrer R G, Dalakas M C, Quarles R H 1992 Sensory neuropathy associated with monoclonal immunoglobulin M to GD1b ganglioside. Annals of Neurology 31: 683

Durelli L, Massazza U, Poccardi G et al 1990 Increased thymocyte differentiation in myasthenia gravis: a dual-color immunofluorescence phenotypic analysis. Annals of Neurology 27: 174

Durum S K, Oppenheim, J J 1989 Macrophage-derived mediators: interleukin 1, tumor necrosis factor, interleukin 6, interferons, and related cytokines. Raven, New York, p 639

Dwyer D S, Bradley R J, Urquhart C K, Kearney J F 1983 Naturally occurring anti-idiotypic antibodies in myasthenia gravis patients. Nature 301: 611

Emslie-Smith A, Engel A G 1990 Microvascular changes in early and advanced dermatomyositis: a quantitative study. Annals of Neurology 27: 343

Engel A G 1984 Myasthenia gravis and myasthenic syndromes. Annals of Neurology 16: 519

Engel A G 1993 Gene transfer therapy for Duchenne dystrophy. Annals of Neurology 34: 3

Engel A G, Lambert E H, Howard F M 1977 Immune complexes (IgG and C3) at the motor end-plate in myasthenia gravis: Ultrastructural and light microscopic localization and electrophysiologic correlations. Mayo Clinic Proceedings 52: 267

Engel A G, Biesicker G 1982 Complement activation in muscle fiber necrosis: Demonstration of the membrane attack complex of complement in necrotic fibers. Annals of Neurology 12: 289

Engel A G, Arahata K 1984 Monoclonal antibody analysis of mononuclear cells in myopathies. II. Phenotypes of autoinvasive cells in polymyositis and inclusion body myositis. Annals of Neurology 16: 209

Engel A G, Arahata K 1987 The membrane attacks complex of complement at the end plate in myasthenia gravis. Annals of the New York Academy of Sciences 505: 326

Engelhardt J I, Appel S H 1990 IgG reactivity in the spinal cord and motor cortex in amyotrophic lateral sclerosis. Archives of Neurology 47: 1210

Engelhardt J I, Appel S H, Killian J M 1989 Experimental autoimmune motor neuron disease. Annals of Neurology 26: 368

Engelhardt J I, Appel S H, Killian J M 1990 Motor neuron destruction in guinea pigs immunized with bovine spinal cord ventral horn homogenate: experimental autoimmune gray matter disease. Journal of Neuroimmunology 27: 21

Feasby T E, Hahn A F, Gilbert J J 1983 Passive transfer of demyelinating activity in Guillain–Barré polyneuropathy. Neurology 32: 1159

Feldmann M, Zanders E D, Lamb J R 1985 Tolerance in T-cell clones. Immunology Today 6: 58

Folli F, Solimena M, Cofiell R et al 1993 Autoantibodies to a 128-kD synaptic protein in three women with the stiff-man syndrome and breast cancer. New England Journal of Medicine 328: 546

Freddo L, Yu R, Latov N L et al 1986 Gangliosides GM1 and GD1b are antigens for IgM M-protein in a patient with motor neuron disease. Neurology 36: 454

Fuchs S, Bartfeld D, Mochly-Rosen D, Souroujon M, Feingold R 1981 Acetylcholine receptor: molecular dissection and monoclonal antibodies in the study of

myasthenia. Annals of the New York Academy of Sciences 377: 110

Fujii Y, Manden Y, Nakahara K, Hashimoto J, Kawashima Y 1984 Antibody to acetylcholine receptor in myasthenia gravis: Production by lymphocytes from thymus or thymoma. Neurology 34: 1182

Fujii Y, Hashimoto J, Monden Y, Ito T, Nakahara K, Kawashima Y 1986 Specific activation of lymphocytes against acetylcholine receptor in the thymus in myasthenia gravis. Journal of Immunology 136: 887

Fujii N, Itoyama Y, Goto I 1990 Increase in differentiated type of T lineage cells in the myasthenic thymus: two color fluorocytometric analysis. Annals of Neurology 27: 642

Fujinami R S, Oldstone M B 1985 Amino acid homology between the encephalitogenic site of myelin basic protein and virus: mechanism for autoimmunity. Science 230: 1043

Fukunaga H, Engel A G, Osame M, Lambert E H 1982 Paucity and disorganization of presynaptic membrane active zones in the Lambert–Eaton myasthenic syndrome. Muscle and Nerve 5: 686

Fukunaga H, Engel A G, Lang B, Newsom-Davis J, Vincent A 1983 Passive transfer of Lambert–Eaton myasthenic syndrome with IgG from man to mouse depletes the presynaptic membrane active zones. Proceedings of the National Academy of Sciences USA 80: 7636

Gilhus N E, Aarli J A, Matre R 1984 Myasthenia gravis: difference between thymoma-associated antibodies and cross-striational skeletal muscle antibodies. Neurology 34: 246

Gillis, S 1989 T-cell derived lymphokines. In: Paul W E (ed) Fundamental immunology, 2nd edn. Raven, New York, p 621

Giorno R, Barden M T, Kohler P F, Ringel S P 1984 Immunohistochemical characterization of the mononuclear cells infiltrating muscle of patients with inflammatory and noninflammatory myopathies. Immunology and Immunopathology 30: 405

Gomez C, Richman D P 1983 Anti-acetylcholine receptor antibodies directed against α-bungarotoxin binding site induce a unique form of experimental myasthenia. Proceedings of the National Academy of Sciences USA 80: 4089

Gorin F, Baldwin B, Tait R, Pathak R, Seyal M, Mugaini E. 1990 Stiff-man syndrome: a GABAergic autoimmune disorder with autoantigenic heterogeneity. Annals of Neurology 28: 711

Goust J-M, Chenais F, Carnes J E, Hames C G, Fudenberg H H, Hogan E L 1978 Abnormal T-cell subpopulations and circulating immune complexes in the Guillain–Barré syndrome and multiple sclerosis. Neurology 28: 421

Graus F, Cordon-Cardo C, Posner J B 1985 Neuronal antinuclear antibody in sensory neuronopathy from lung cancer. Neurology 35: 538

Guerney M E, Belton A C, Cashman N, Antel J P 1984 Inhibition of terminal axonal sprouting by serum from patients with amyotrophic lateral sclerosis. New England Journal of Medicine 311: 933

Haas D C 1980 Absence of cell-mediated cytotoxicity to muscle cultures in polymyositis. Journal of Rheumatology 7: 671

Haas D C, Arnason B G W 1974 Cell-mediated immunity in polymyositis: creatine phosphokinase release from muscle cultures. Archives of Neurology 31: 192

Hargis A M, Haupt K S, Prieur D J, Moore M P 1985 Animal

model of human disease. Dermatomyositis: familial canine dermatomyositis. American Journal of Pathology 120: 323

Hartung H-P, Toyka K V 1990 T-cell and macrophage activation in experimental autoimmune neuritis and Guillain–Barré syndrome. Annals of Neurology 27(suppl): S 57

Hathaway P W M, Engel W K, Zellweger H 1970 Experimental myopathy after microarterial embolization. Comparison with childhood X-linked pseudohypertrophic muscular dystrophy. Archives of Neurology 22: 365

Haynes B F, Harden E A, Olanow C W, Eisenborth G S, Wechsler A S, Hensley L L, Roses A D 1983 Effect of thymectomy on peripheral lymphocyte subsets in myasthenia gravis: selective effect on T-cells in patients with thymic atrophy. Journal of Immunology 131: 773

Heberman R E (ed) 1982 N K cells and other natural effector cells. Academic, New York

Hedrick S M 1989 T lymphocyte receptors. In: Paul W E (ed)s Fundamental immunology, 2nd edn. Raven, New York p 291

Heffner R R, Barron S A, Jenis F H, Valeski J C 1976 Skeletal muscle in polymyositis. Immunohistochemical study. Archives of Pathology and Laboratory Medicine 103: 310

Heininger K, Hendricks M, Toyka K V, Kalb H 1983 Myasthenia gravis remission not induced by blocking anti-idiotype antibodies. Muscle and Nerve 6: 386

Hohfeld R, Toyka K V, Heininger K, Grosse-Wilde H, Kalis I 1984 Autoimmune human T lymphocytes specific for acetylcholine receptor. Nature 310: 244

Hohfeld R, Engel A G 1990 Induction of HLA-DR expression on human myoblasts with interferon-gamma. American Journal of Pathology 136: 503

Hohlfeld R, Engel A G 1991 Coculture with autologous myotubes of cytotoxic T cells isolated from muscle in inflammatory myopathies. Annals of Neurology 29: 498

Hohfeld R, Engel A G, Ii K, Harper M C 1991 Polymyositis mediated by T lymphocytes that express the γ/δ receptor. New England Journal of Medicine 324: 877

Honda H, Rostami A 1989 Expression of major histocompatability complex Class I antigens in rat muscle cultures: the possible developmental role. Proceedings of the National Academy of Sciences USA 86: 7007

Horwich M S, Cho L, Porro R S, Posner J B 1977 Subacute sensory neuropathy: a remote effect of carcinoma. Annals of Neurology 2: 7

Howard F, Lennon V, Matsumato J, Finley J 1986 Clinical correlations of antibodies that bind, block and/or modulate human AChRs in myasthenia gravis. Annals of the New York Academy of Sciences (in press)

Hughes R A C 1990 Guillain-Barré Syndrome, Springer-Verlag, London, p183

Hughes R A C, Aslan S, Gray I A 1983 Lymphocyte subpopulations and suppressor cell activity in acute polyradiculoneuritis (Guillain–Barré syndrome). Clinical and Experimental Immunology 51: 448

Hughes R A C, Gray I A, Gregson N A et al 1984 Immune responses to myelin antigens in Guillain–Barré syndrome. Journal of Neuroimmunology 6: 303

Illa I, Nath A, Dalakas M 1991 Immunocytochemical and virological characteristics of HIV-associated inflammatory myopathies: similarities with seronegative polymyositis. Annals of Neurology 29: 474

Ilyas A A, Quarles R H, MacIntosh T D, Doberson M J, Trapp B D, Dalakas M C, Brady R O 1984 IgM in a

human neuropathy related to paraproteinemia binds to a carbohydrate determinant in the myelin-associated glycoprotein and to a ganglioside. Proceedings of the National Academy of Sciences USA 81: 1225

Ilyas A A, Quarles R H, Dalakas M C, Brady R O 1985 Polyneuropathy with monoclonal gammapathy: Glycolipids are frequently antigens for IgM paraproteins. Proceedings of the National Academy of Sciences USA 82: 6697

Ilyas A A, Willison H S, Quarles R H, Jungalwala K B, Cornblath D R 1988 Serum antibodies to gangliosides in Guillain–Barré syndrome. Annals of Neurology 23: 440

Isenberg D A 1983 Immunoglobulin deposition in skeletal muscle disease. Quarterly Journal of Medicine 52: 297

Isenberg D A, Rowe M, Shearer M, Novick D, Beverly P C L 1986 Localization of interferons and interleukin 2 in polymyositis and muscular dystrophy. Clinical and Experimental Immunology 63: 450

Ito H, Latov N 1988 Monoclonal IgM in two patients with MND bind to the carbohydrate antigens Gal(beta 1–3) GalNAc and Gal(beta 1–3)GlcNAc. Journal of Neuroimmunology 19: 245

Iyer V, Lawton A R, Finichel G M 1983 T-cell subsets in polymyositis. Annals of Neurology 13: 452–453

Jerne N K 1974 Towards a network theory of the immune system. Annals of the Immunologic Institute Pasteur (Paris) 125: 373

Johnson R L, Fink C W, Ziff M 1972 Lymphotoxin formation by lymphocytes and muscle in polymyositis. Journal of Clinical Investigation 51: 2435

Kadlubowski M, Hughes R A C 1979 Identification of the neuritogen for experimental allergic neuritis. Nature 277: 140

Kadlubowski M, Ingram P L 1981 Circulating antibodies to the neuritogenic myelin protein P2 in neuritis of the cauda equina of the horse. Nature 293: 299

Kahn S 1985 Human monoclonal IgM autoantibodies with restricted antigenic specificity for myelin express unrelated idiotypes. Journal of the Neurological Sciences 69: 161

Kakulas, B A 1988 Animal models of polymyositis and dermatomyositis. In: Dalakas M C (ed) Polymyositis and dermatomyositis. Butterworths, Boston, p 133

Kaldor J, Speed B R 1984 GBS and Campylobacter jejuni: a serologic study. British Medical Journal 288: 1867

Kao I, Drachman D B 1977 Myasthenic immunoglobulin accelerates acetylcholine receptor degradation. Science 196: 527

Karpati G 1990 Immunological aspects of histocompatible myoblast transfer into non-tolerant hosts. In: Griggs R C, Karpati G (eds) Myoblast transfer therapy. Advances in experimental medicine and biology, vol 280. Plenum, New York, p 31

Karpati G, Pouliot Y, Carpenter S 1988 Expression of immunoreactive major histocompatability complex products in human skeletal muscles. Annals of Neurology 23: 64

Karpati G, Ajdukovic D, Arnold D, Gledhill R B et al 1993 Myoblast transfer in Duchenne muscular dystrophy. Annals of Neurology 34: 8

Kaslow R A, Sullivan-Bolgai J Z, Hafken B et al 1984 HLA antigens in Guillain–Barré syndrome. Neurology 94: 240

Khalili-Shirazi A, Hughes R A C, Brostoff S W, Linington C, Gregson N 1992 T cell responses to myelin proteins in Guillain–Barré syndrome. Journal of Neurological Sciences 111: 200

Kim G I 1985 Passive transfer of the Lambert–Eaton

myasthenic syndrome: neuromuscular transmission in mice injected with plasma. Muscle and Nerve 8: 162

Kim Y I, 1987 Lambert–Eaton myasthenic syndrome: evidence for calcium channel blockade. Annals of New York Academy of Sciences 505: 377

Kishimoto T, Hirano T 1989 B lymphocyte activation, proliferation, and immunoglobulin secretion. In: Paul W E (ed) Fundamental immunology, 2nd edn. Raven, New York, p 385

Kissel J T, Mendell J R, Rammohan K W 1986 Microvascular deposition of complement membrane attack complex in dermatomyositis. New England Journal of Medicine 314: 329

Klavinskis L S, Willcox N, Oxford J S, Newsom-Davis J 1985 Antivirus antibodies in myasthenia gravis. Neurology 35: 1381

Kornegay J N, Gorgacz E J, Dawe D L, Bowen J M, White N A, DeBuysscher E V 1980 Polymyositis in dogs. Journal of the American Veterinary Medical Association 176: 431

Kornstein M J, Brooks J J, Anderson A O, Levinson A I, Lisak R P, Zweiman B 1984 The immunohistology of the thymus in myasthenia gravis. American Journal of Pathology 117: 184

Koski C L 1987 Complement-fixing antiperipheral myelin antibodies and C9 neoantigen in serum of patients with Guillain–Barré syndrome: quantitation, kinetics, and clinical correlation. Annals of the New York Academy of Sciences 505

Koski C L, Chou D K H, Jungalwala F B 1989 Anti-peripheral nerve myelin antibodies in Guillain–Barré syndrome bind a neutral glycolipid of peripheral myelin and cross-react with Forssman antigen. Journal of Clinical Investigation 84: 280

Lang B, Newsom-Davis J, Wray D, Vincent A, Murray N 1981 Autoimmune aetiology for myasthenic (Eaton-Lambert) syndrome. Lancet ii: 224

Lang B, Roberts A J, Vincent A, Newsom-Davis J 1985 Anti-acetylcholine receptor idiotypes in myasthenia gravis analyzed by rabbit antisera. Clinical and Experimental Immunology 60: 637

Latov N 1982 Plasma cell dyscrasias and motor neuron disease. In: Rowland L P (ed) Human motor neuron diseases. Raven, New York, p 273

Latov N, Gross R B, Kostelman J et al 1981 Complement-fixing anti-peripheral nerve myelin antibodies in patients with inflammatory polyneuritis and with polyneuropathy and paraproteinemia. Neurology 31: 1530

Latov N, Hays A P, Donofrio P D et al 1988 Monoclonal IgM with unique specificity to gangliosides GM1 and GD1b and to lacto-N-tetraose associated with human motor neuron disease. Neurology 38: 763

Layzer R B, Shearn M A, Satya-Murti S 1977 Eosinophilic polymyositis. Annals of Neurology 1: 65

Leder P 1983 Genetics of immunoglobulin production. In: Dixon F J, Fisher D W (eds) The biology of immunologic disease. Sinauer Associates, p 3

Lefvert A K 1981 Anti-idiotypic antibodies against the receptor antibodies in myasthenia gravis. Scandinavian Journal of Immunology 13: 493

Lennon V A, Palmer A C, Pflugfelder C, Indrieri R J 1978 Myasthenia gravis in dogs: acetylcholine receptor deficiency with and without autoantibodies. In: Rose N L, Bigzaai P E, Warner N L (eds) Genetic control of autoimmune disease. Elsevier North Holland, Amsterdam, p 295

Lennon V A, Lambert E H, Whittingham S, Fairbanks V 1982 Autoimmunity in the Lambert–Eaton myasthenic syndrome. Muscle and Nerve 5: 521

Lennon V A, McCormick D J, Lambert E H, Guesmann G E 1985 Region of peptide of acetylcholine receptor α subunit is exposed at neuromuscular junction and induces experimental autoimmune myasthenia gravis, T-cell immunity and modulating autoantibodies. Proceedings of the National Academy of Sciences USA 82: 8805

Lennon V A, Griesman G E 1989 Evidence against acetylcholine receptor having a main immunogenic region as target for autoantibodies in myasthenia gravis. Neurology 39: 1069

Lennon V A, Lambert E H 1990 Autoantibodies bind solubilized calcium channel ω-conotoxin complexes from small cell lung carcinoma: a diagnostic aid for Lambert–Eaton myasthenic syndrome. Proceedings of the Mayo Clinic 64: 1490

Lerich J R, Conture J 1978 Amyotrophic lateral sclerosis sera are not cytotoxic to neuroblastoma cells in tissue culture. Annals of Neurology 41: 384

Levinson A I, Dziarski A, Lisak R P, Zweiman B, Moskovitz A R, Brenner T, Abramsky O 1981 Comparative immunoglobulin synthesis by blood lymphocytes in myasthenics and normals. Annals of the New York Academy of Sciences 377: 385

Levinson A I, Zweiman B, Lisak R P, Dziarski A I, Moskovitz A R 1984 Thymic lymphocyte activation in myasthenia gravis. Neurology 34: 462

Levinson A I, Lisak R P, Zweiman B, Kornstein M J 1985 Phenotypic and functional analysis of lymphocytes in myasthenia gravis. In: Steck A J, Lisak R P (guest eds) Immunoneurology (II). Springer Seminars in Neuropathology 8: 209

Levinson A I, Zweiman B, Lisak R P 1990 Pokeweed mitogen-induced immunoglobulin secretory responses of thymic B cells in myasthenia gravis: selective secretion of IgG versus IgM cannot be explained by helper functions of thymic T cells. Clinical Immunology and Immunopathology 57: 211

Levy R M, Bredsen D E, Rosenblum M L 1985 Neurological manifestations of the acquired immunodeficiency syndrome (AIDS): Experience at UCSF and review of the literature. Journal of Neurosurgery 62: 475

Lewis R A, Sumner A J, Brown M J, Asbury A K 1982 Multifocal demyelinating neuropathy with persistent conduction block. Neurology 32: 958

Link H, Olsson O, Sun J et al 1991 Acetylcholine receptor-reactive T and B cells in myasthenia gravis and controls. Journal of Clinical Investigation 87: 2191

Linnington C, Izumo S, Suzuki M, Uyemura K, Meyermann R, Wekerle H 1984 A permanent rat T-cell line that mediates experimental allergic neuritis in the Lewis rat in vivo. Journal of Immunology 133: 1946

Lipkin I W, Parry G, Kiprov D, Abrams D 1985 Inflammatory neuropathy in homosexual men with lymphadenopathy. Neurology 35: 1479

Lisak R P 1992 Immunopathology of muscle disease. In: Mastaglia F L, Walton J N (eds) Skeletal muscle pathology. Churchill Livingstone, Edinburgh, p 187

Lisak R P, Zweiman B 1975 Mitogen and muscle extract induced in vitro proliferative responses in myasthenia gravis, dermatomyositis and polymyositis. Journal of Neurology, Neurosurgery and Psychiatry 38: 521

Lisak R P, Zweiman B 1976 Serum immunoglobulin levels in

myasthenia gravis, polymyositis and dermatomyositis. Journal of Neurology, Neurosurgery and Psychiatry 39: 34

Lisak R P, Abdou N I, Zweiman B, Zmijewski C, Penn A S 1976 Aspects of lymphocyte function in myasthenia gravis. Annals of the New York Academy of Science 274: 402

Lisak R P, Mitchell M, Zweiman B, Orrechio E, Asbury A K 1977 Guillain–Barré syndrome and Hodgkin's disease: three cases with immunological studies. Annals of Neurology 1: 72

Lisak R P, Barchi R L 1982 Myasthenia gravis. W B Saunders, Philadelphia

Lisak R P, Brown M J, Sumner A J 1983a Abnormal serum factors in Guillain–Barré syndrome. Italian Journal of Neurological Sciences 3: 265

Lisak R P, Laramore C, Levinson A I, Zweimann B, Moskovitz A R 1983b In vitro synthesis of antibodies to acetylcholine receptor by peripheral blood mononuclear cells of patients with myasthenia gravis. Neurology 33: 604

Lisak R P, Zweiman B, Skolnik P, Levinson A I, Moskovitz A R, Guerrero F 1983c Thymic lymphocyte subpopulations in myasthenia gravis. Neurology 33: 868

Lisak R P, Kuchmy D, Armati-Gulson P, Brown M J, Sumner A J 1984a Serum-mediated Schwann cell cytotoxicity in the Guillain–Barré syndrome. Neurology 34: 1240

Lisak R P, Laramore C, Levinson A I, Zweiman B, Moskovitz A R, Witte A 1984b In vitro synthesis of antibodies to acetylcholine receptor by peripheral blood cells: role of suppressor T-cells in normal subjects. Neurology 34: 802

Lisak R P, Levinson A I, Zweiman B 1985a Autoimmune aspects of myasthenia gravis. In: Cruse J M, Lewis R E Jr (eds) Concepts in immunopathology, vol 2. Karger, Basel, p 65

Lisak R P, Zweimann B, Guerrero F, Moskovitz A R 1985b Circulating T-cell subsets in Guillain–Barré syndrome. Journal of Neuroimmunology 8: 93

Lisak R P, Laramore C, Levinson A I, Zweiman B, Moskovitz A R 1986a Suppressor T-cells in myasthenia gravis and antibodies to acetylcholine receptor. Annals of Neurology 19: 87

Lisak R P, Levinson A I, Zweiman B, Kornstein M J 1986b Antibodies to acetylcholine receptor and tetanus toxoid: in vitro synthesis by thymic lymphocytes. Journal of Immunology 137: 1221

Liveson J, Fray H, Bornstein M B 1975 The effect of serum from ALS patients on organotypic nerve and muscle tissue cultures. Acta Neuropathologica (Berlin) 32: 127

Logan I S, Kim Y I, Judd A M, Spaneglo B L, MacLeod 1987 Immunoglobulins of Lambert-Eaton myasthenic syndrome inhibit rat pituitary hormone release. Annals of Neurology 22: 610

Love L A, Leff R L, Fraser D D et al 1991 A new approach to the classification of idiopathic inflammatory myopathy: myositis-specific autoantibodies define useful homogeneous patient groups: Medicine 70: 360

McDevitt H O, Bodmer W F 1974 HL-A, immune response genes and disease. Lancet 2: 1269

McDouall R M, Dunn M J, Dubowitz V 1989 Expression of class I and class II MHC antigens in neuromuscular diseases. Journal of the Neurological Sciences 89: 213

McLachlan S M, Nicholson L V B, Venables G et al 1981 Acetylcholine receptor antibody synthesis in lymphocyte cultures. Journal of Clinical and Laboratory Immunology 5: 137

McQuillen D P, Koethe S M, McQuillen M P 1983 Cellular response to human acetylcholine receptor in patients with myasthenia gravis. Journal of Neuroimmunology 5: 59

Mancardi G L, Del Sette M, Primavera A, Farinelli M, Fumarola D 1989 Borrelia burgdorferi infection and Guillain–Barré syndrome. Lancet ii: 485

Mastaglia F L, Papadimitriou J M, Dawkins R L 1975 Mechanisms of cell-mediated myotoxicity: morphological observations in muscle grafts and in muscle exposed to sensitized spleen cells in vivo. Journal of the Neurological Sciences 25: 269

Mastaglia F L, Ojeda V J 1985a Inflammatory myopathies: Part 1. Annals of Neurology 17: 215

Mastaglia F L, Ojeda V J 1985b Inflammatory myopathies: Part 2, Annals of Neurology 17: 317

Matthews M B, Bernstein R M 1983 Myositis autoantibody inhibits histidyl tRNA synthetase: a model for autoimmunity. Nature 304: 177

Matthews M B, Reichlin M, Hughes G R V, Bernstein R M 1984 Anti-threonyl-tRNA synthetase, a second myositis-related autoantibody. Journal of Experimental Medicine 160: 420

Mendell J R, Sahenk Z 1992 Inclusion body myositis. Neurology 42: 2231

Mendell J R, Sahenk Z, Gales T, Paul L 1991 Amyloid filaments in inclusion body myositis: novel findings provide insight into nature of filaments. Archives of Neurology 48: 1229

Miller K B, Schwartz R S 1982 Autoimmunity and suppressor T lymphocytes. Advances in Internal Medicine 27: 281

Mimori T, Akizu K, Yamagata H, Inada S, Yoshida S, Homma M 1981 Characterization of a high molecular weight acidic nuclear protein recognized by autoantibodies in sera from patients with polymyositis-scleroderma overlap. Journal of Clinical Investigation 68: 611

Mishak R P, Dau P C 1981 Lymphocyte binding antibodies and suppressor cell activity in myasthenia gravis. Annals of the New York Academy of Sciences 377: 436

Moore P M, Lisak R P 1990 Multiple sclerosis and Sjögren's syndrome: a problem in diagnosis or classification of two disorders of unknown etiology. Annals of Neurology 27: 585

Morgan B P, Sewry C A, Siddle K, Luzio J P, Campbell A K 1984 Immunolocalization of complement component C9 on necrotic and non-necrotic muscle fibers in myositis using monoclonal antibodies: a primary role for complement in autoimmune cell damage. Immunology 52: 181

Mygland A, Tynes O-B, Matre R, Volpe P, Aarli J A, Gilhus N E 1992a Ryanodine receptor autoantibodies in myasthenia gravis patients with a thymoma. Annals of Neurology 32: 589

Mygland A, Tynes O-B, Aarli J A et al 1992b Myasthenia gravis patients with a thymoma have antibodies against a high molecular weight protein in sarcoplasmic reticulum. Journal of Neuroimmunology 37: 1

Nakao Y, Matsumoto H, Miyazski T et al 1980 Gm allotypes in myasthenia gravis. Lancet 1: 677

Nennesmo I, Olsson T, Ljungdahl A, Kristensson K, van der Merde P H 1989 Interferon-gamma-like immunoreactivity and T-cell expression in rat skeletal muscle. Brain Research 504: 306

Neville H E, Baumbach L L, Ringel S P, Russo L S Jr, Sujanski E, Garcia C A 1992a Familial inclusion body myositis: evidence for autosomal dominant inheritance Neurology 42: 897

Neville H E, Ringel S P, Sujansky E, Bumbach L L, Russo L P, Garcia C 1992b Inclusion body myositis. Neurology 42: 2232

Newsom-Davis J 1985 Lambert-Eaton myasthenic syndrome. In: Steck A J, Lisak R P (guest eds) Immunoneurology (I). Springer Seminars in Immunopathology 8: 129

Newsom-Davis J, Mills K R 1993 Immunologic associations of acquired neuromyotonia (Isaac's syndrome). Report of five cases and literature review. Brain 116: 453

Newsom-Davis J, Wilcox N, Calder L 1981 Thymus cells in myasthenia gravis selectively enhance production of anti-acetylcholine receptor antibody by autologous blood lymphocytes. New England Journal of Medicine 305: 1313

Newsom-Davis J, Wilcox N, Schluep M et al 1987 Immunological heterogeneity and cellular mechanisms in myasthenia gravis. Annals of the New York Academy of Sciences 505: 12

Nishikai M, Reichlin M 1980 Purification and characterization of a nuclear non-histone basic protein (Mi-1) which reacts with anti-immunoglobulin sera and the sera of patients with dermatomyositis. Molecular Immunology 17: 1129

Nossal G J V 1983 Cellular mechanisms of immunologic tolerance. In: Paul W E, Fathman C G, Metzger H (eds) Annual Review of Immunology. Annual Reviews, Palo Alto, pp 33–62

Northington J W, Brown M J 1982 Acute canine idiopathic polyneuropathy: A Guillain–Barré-like syndrome in dogs. Journal of the Neurological Sciences 56: 259

Nyland H, Aarli J A 1978 Guillain–Barré syndrome: demonstration of antibodies to peripheral nerve tissue. Acta Neurologica Scandinavica 58: 35

Ohta M, Ohta K, Ohta N et al 1990 Anti-skeletal muscle antibodies in the sera from myasthenic patients with thymoma: identification of anti-myosin, actomyosin, actin, and α-actinin antibodies by a solid-phase radio-immunoassay and a Western blotting analysis. Clinica Chimica Acta 187: 255

Oldstone M B A, Wilson C B, Perrin L H, Norris F H 1976 Evidence for immune complex formation in patients with amyotrophic lateral sclerosis. Lancet 2: 168

Olsson T, Henriksson K G, Klareskog L, Farsum U 1985 HLA-DR expression, T lymphocyte phenotypes ILM1 and OKT9 reactive cells in inflammatory myopathy. Muscle and Nerve 8: 419

O'Neill J H, Murray J M, Newsom-Davis J 1988 The Lambert-Eaton myasthenic syndrome: a review of 50 cases. Brain 111: 577

Pachman L M, Cooke N 1980 Juvenile dermatomyositis: a clinical and immunologic study. Journal of Pediatrics 97: 226

Pachner A R 1989 Anti-acetylcholine receptor antibodies block bungarotoxin binding to native human acetylcholine receptor on the surface of TE 671 cells. Neurology 39: 1057

Pachner A R, Kantor F S 1984 In vitro and in vivo actions of acetylcholine receptor educated T-cell lines in murine experimental autoimmune myasthenia gravis. Clinical and Experimental Immunology 56: 659

Patrick J, Lindstrom J 1973 Autoimmune response to acetylcholine receptor. Science 180: 871

Patten B M 1984 Neuropathy and motor neuron syndromes associated with plasma cell disease. Acta Neurologica Scandinavica 69: 47

Perpose J S 1982 A theory of virus-induced demyelination in the Landry–Guillain–Barré syndrome. Journal of Neurology 227: 93

Pestronk A 1991 Invited review: Motor neuropathies, motor neuron disorders, and glycolipid antibodies. Muscle and Nerve 14: 927

Pestronk A, Cornblath D, Ilyas A A et al 1988a A treatable multifocal neuropathy with antibodies to GM1 ganglioside. Annals of Neurology 24: 73

Pestronk A, Adams R N, Clawson L et al 1988b Serum antibodies to GM1 ganglioside in amyotrophic lateral sclerosis. Neurology 38: 1457

Pestronk A, Li F, Griffin J et al 1991 Polyneuropathy syndromes associated with serum antibodies to sulfatide and myelin-associated glycoprotein. Neurology 41: 357

Pollard J D, King R H, Thomas P K 1975 Recurrent experimental allergic neuritis. An electron microscopic study. Journal of Neurological Sciences 24: 365

Posner J B, Furneaux H M 1990 Paraneoplastic syndromes in: Waksman B H (ed) Immunologic mechanisms. In: neurologic and psychiatric disease. Association for Research in Nervous and Mental Diseases, vol 68. Raven, New York p 187

Prior C, Lang B, Wray D, Newsom-Davis J 1985 Action of Lambert-Eaton myasthenic syndrome IgG at mouse motor nerve terminals. Annals of Neurology 17: 587

Quarles R H 1984 Myelin-associated glycoprotein in development and disease. Developmental Neuroscience 6: 285

Ragheb S, Lisak R P 1990 The frequency of CD5+ B lymphocytes in the peripheral blood of patients with myasthenia gravis. Neurology 40: 1120

Ragheb S, Lisak R P 1994 The immunopathogenesis of acquired (autoimmune) myasthenia gravis. In: Lisak R P (ed) Handbook of myasthenia gravis and myasthenic syndromes. Marcel Dekker, New York pp 239–276

Rechthand E, Cornblath D R, Stern B J, Meyerhoff J O 1984 Chronic demyelinating polyneuropathy in systemic lupus erythematosus. Neurology 34: 1375

Reichlin M, Madison P J, Targoff I et al 1984 Antibodies to a nuclear/nucleolar antigen in patients with polymyositis overlap syndromes. Journal of Clinical Immunology 4: 40

Reik L Jr 1980 Disseminated vasculomyelinopathy: an immune complex disease. Annals of Neurology 7: 191

Reyer M G, Norohna P, Thomas W, Hereda R 1983 Myositis of graft versus host disease. Neurology 33: 1222

Richman D P, Patrick J, Arnason B G W 1976 Cellular immunity in myasthenia gravis. New England Journal of Medicine 294: 694

Richman D P, Antel J P, Burns J B, Arnason B G W 1981 Nicotinic acetylcholine receptor on human lymphocytes. Annals of the New York Academy of Sciences 377: 427

Robb S A, Bowley T J, Willcox H N A, Newsom-Davis J 1985 Circulating T-cell subsets in the Lambert–Eaton myasthenic syndrome. Journal of Neurology, Neurosurgery and Psychiatry 48: 501

Roisen F J, Bartfeld H, Donnenfeld H, Baxter J 1982 Neuron specific cytotoxicity of sera from patients with amyotrophic lateral sclerosis. Muscle and Nerve 5: 48

Rosenberg N L, Ringel S P, Katzin B L 1985 Experimental

autoimmune myositis in SJL/J mice. Annals of Neurology 18: 161

Rosenfeld M R, Wong E, Dalmau J et al 1993 Cloning and characterization of a Lambert–Eaton myasthenic syndrome antigen. Annals of Neurology 33: 113

Rosenschein U, Radnay J, Shoham D, Shainberg A, Klajman A, Rosenszajn L A 1987 Human muscle-derived tissue specific, myotoxic T cell lines in dermatomyositis. Clinical and Experimental Immunology 67: 309

Rostami A, Brown M J, Lisak R P, Sumner A J, Zweiman B, Pleasure D E 1984 The role of myelin P_2 protein in the production of experimental allergic neuritis. Annals of Neurology 16: 680

Rostami A, Burns J B, Brown M J et al 1985 Transfer of experimental allergic neuritis with P_2-reactive T-cell lines. Cellular Immunology 91: 354

Rostami A M, Burns J B, Eccelston P A, Manning M C, Lisak R P, Silberg D H 1987 Search for antibodies to galactocerebroside in serum and cerebrospinal fluid in human demyelinating disorders. Annals of Neurology 22: 381

Rowe D J, Isenberg D A, McDougall J, Beverly P C L 1981 Characterization of polymyositis infiltrates using monoclonal antibodies to human leukocyte antigen. Clinical and Experimental Immunology 45: 290

Rowland L P, Defindini R, Sherman, W H et al 1982 Macroglobulinemia with peripheral neuropathy simulating motor neuron disease. Annals of Neurology 11: 532

Sadiq S A, Thomas F P, Kilidreas K et al 1990 The spectrum of neurologic disease associated with anti-GM1 antibodies. Neurology 40: 1067

Sahashi K, Engel A G, Lambert E H, Lennon V 1978 Ultrastructural localization of immune complexes (IgG and C3) at the endplate in experimental autoimmune myasthenia gravis. Journal of Neuropathology and Experimental Neurology 37: 212

Sahashi K, Engel A G, Lambert E H, Howard F M Jr 1980 Ultrastructural localization of the terminal and lytic ninth complement component (C9) at the motor endplate in myasthenia gravis. Journal of Neuropathology and Experimental Neurology 39: 160

Saida K, Saida T, Brown M J, Silberberg D H, Asbury A K 1979 In vivo demyelination induced by intraneural injection of antigalactocerebroside serum. A morphologic study. American Journal of Pathology 95: 99

Saida T, Saida K, Silberberg D H, Brown M J 1978 Transfer of demyelination with experimental neuritis serum. Nature 272: 639

Saida T, Saida K, Dorfman S H et al 1979 Experimental allergic neuritis induced by sensitization with galactocerebroside. Science 204: 1103

Saida T, Saida K, Lisak R P, Brown M J, Silberberg D H, Asbury A K 1982 In vivo demyelinating activity of sera from patients with Guillain–Barré syndrome. Annals of Neurology 11: 69

Santoro M, Thomas F P, Fink M E et al 1990 IgM deposits at nodes of Ranvier in a patient with amyotrophic lateral sclerosis, anti-GM1 antibodies, and multifocal conduction block. Annals of Neurology 28: 373

Santoro M, Uncini A, Corbo M, Staugaitis S M, Thomas F P, Hays A P, Latov N 1992 Experimental conduction block induced by serum from a patient with anti-GM1 antibodies. Annals of Neurology 31: 385

Sharief M K, Hentges R, Ciardi M 1991 Intrathecal immune response with the post-polio syndrome. New England Journal of Medicine 325: 749

Sharp G C, Irvin W S, Tan E M, Gould R C, Holman H R 1972 Mixed connective tissue disease — an apparently distinct rheumatic disease syndrome associated with specific antibody to an extractable nuclear antigen. American Journal of Medicine 52: 148

Sharp G C, Irvin W S, May C M et al 1976 Association of antibodies to ribonucleic protein and Sm antigens with mixed connective tissue disease, systemic lupus erythematosus and other rheumatic diseases. New England Journal of Medicine 295: 1149

Sher E, Gotti C, Canal N et al 1989 Specificity of calcium channel autoantibodies in Lambert–Eaton myasthenic syndrome. Lancet ii: 640

Sherman W H, Latov N, Hays A P 1983 Monoclonal IgM antibody precipitating with chondroitin sulfate C from patients with axonal polyneuropathy and epidermolysis. Neurology 33: 192

Shevach E M 1984 Macrophages and other accessory cells. In: Paul W E (ed) Fundamental immunology. Raven, New York, p 71

Sisley A, Lisak R P, Brenner T 1989 Proliferative response of blood cells of patients with myasthenia gravis to purified mammalian acetylcholine receptor. Pathobiology 8: 113

Skolnik P R, Lisak R P, Zweiman B 1982 Monoclonal antibody analysis of blood T-cell subsets in myasthenia gravis. Annals of Neurology 11: 170

Smith C I E, Aarli J A, Biberfeld P et al 1983 Myasthenia gravis after bone-marrow transplantation. Evidence for a donor origin. New England Journal of Medicine 309: 1565

Smith C I E, Grubb R, Hammarstrom L, Perskanen R 1984 Gm allotypes in Finnish myasthenia gravis patients. Neurology 34: 1604

Smith C I E, Hammarstrom L, Matell G, Perskanen R, Rabbitts T H 1987 Immunogenetics of myasthenia gravis. Annals of the New York Academy of Sciences 505: 388

Smith K A 1984 Lymphokine regulation of T-cell and B-cell function. In: Paul W E (ed) Fundamental immunology. Raven, New York, p 559

Smith P D, Butler R C, Partridge T S, Sloper J C 1979 the Current progress in the study of allergic polymyositis in the guinea pig and man. In: Rose F C (ed) Clinical neuroimmunology. Blackwell, Oxford, p 146

Smith R G, Hamilton S, Hofmann F et al 1992 Serum antibodies to L-type calcium channels in patients with amyotrophic lateral sclerosis. New England Journal of Medicine 327: 1721

Snider W D, Simpson D M, Nielsen S, Gold J W M, Metraka C E, Posner J B 1983 Neurological complications of acquired immune deficiency syndrome analysis of 50 patients. Annals of Neurology 14: 403

Solimena M, Folli F, Denis-Donni S et al 1988 Autoantibodies to glutamic acid decarboxylase in a patient with stiff-man syndrome, epilepsy, and type I diabetes mellitus. New England Journal of Medicine 318: 1012

Stanley E, Drachman D B 1978 Effect of myasthenic immunoglobulin on acetylcholine receptors of intact mammalian neuromuscular junctions. Science 200: 1285

Steck A J, Murray N, Meier C, Page N, Perruisseau G 1983 Demyelinating neuropathy and monoclonal IgM antibody to myelin-associated glycoprotein. Neurology 33: 19

Steck A J, Murray N 1985 Monoclonal antibodies to myelin-associated glycoprotein reveal antigenic structures and suggest pathogenic mechanisms. In: Steck A J, Lisak R P (guest eds) Immunoneurology (1). Springer Seminars in Immunopathology 8: 29

Steiner I, Abramsky O 1985 Immunology of Guillain–Barré syndrome. In: Steck A J, Lisak R P (guest eds) Immunoneurology (II) Springer Seminars in Immunopathology 8: 165

Stephansson K, Dieperink M E, Richman D P, Gomez C M, Marlton L S 1984 Sharing of antigenic determinants between the nicotinic acetylcholine receptor and proteins in *Escherichia coli*, *Proteus vulgaris*, and *Klebsiella pneumoniae*. New England Journal of Medicine 312: 221

Stevens J G, Pepose J S, Cook M L 1981 Marek's disease: a natural model for the Landry–Guillain–Barré syndrome. Annals of Neurology 9 (suppl): 102

Stewart G J, Pollard J D, McLeon J G, Wolnizer C M 1978 HLA antigens in the Landry-Guillain–Barré syndrome and chronic relapsing polyneuritis. Annals of Neurology 4: 285

Sumner A J, Said G, Idy I, Metral S 1982 Syndrome de Guillain–Barré: Effects electrophysiologiques et morphologiques du serum humain introduit dans l'espace endoneural du nerf sciatique du rat: résultats preliminaires. Revue Neurologique (Paris) 138: 17

Tachovsky T, Lisak R P, Koprowski H, Theofilopopoulus A N, Dixon F J 1976 Circulating immune complexes in multiple sclerosis and other neurological diseases. Lancet 2: 997

Targoff I N, Reichlin M 1985 The association between Mi-2 antibodies and dermatomyositis. Arthritis and Rheumatism 28: 796

Thomas J A, Wilcox H N A, Newsom-Davis J 1982 Immunohistological studies of the thymus in myasthenia gravis: Correlation with clinical state and thymocyte culture responses. Journal of Neuroimmunology 3: 319

Tischler A S, Dichter M, Beales B 1977 Electrical excitability of oat cell carcinoma. Journal of Pathology 122: 153

Tonegawa S 1983 Somatic generation of antibody diversity. Nature 302: 575

Tonnessen T I, Nyland H, Aarli J A 1982 Complement factors and acute phase reactants in the Guillain–Barré syndrome. European Neurology 21: 124

Toyka K V, Drachman D B, Pestronk A, Kao I 1975 Myasthenia gravis: passive transfer from man to mouse. Science 190: 397

Tzartos S J, Kokola A, Walgrave S L, Conti-Tronconi B M 1988 Localization of the main immunogenic region of human muscle acetylcholine receptor to residues 67–76 of the α subunit. Proceedings of the National Academy of Science USA 85: 2899

Uchitel O D, Scornik F, Protti D A, Fumhberg C G, Alvarez V, Appel S H 1992 Long-term neuromuscular dysfunction produced by passive transfer of amyotrophic lateral sclerosis immunoglobulins. Neurology 42: 2175

Unanue E 1989 Macrophages, antigen-presenting cells, and the phenomena of antigen handling and presentation. In: Paul W E (ed) Fundamental immunology, 2nd edn. Raven, New York, p 95

Uncini A, Santoro M, Corbo M, Lugaresi A, Latov N 1993 Conduction abnormalities induced by sera of patients with multifocal motor neuropathy and anti-GM1 antibodies. Muscle and Nerve 16: 610

Vincent A, Scadding G K, Thomas H C, Newsom-Davis J 1978 In vitro synthesis of antiacetylcholine receptor antibody by thymic lymphocytes in myasthenia gravis. Lancet i: 305

Vincent A, Lang B, Newsom-Davis J 1989 Autoimmunity to the voltage-gated calcium channel underlies the Lambert–Eaton myasthenic syndrome, a paraneoplastic disorder. Trends in Neurosciences 12: 17

Waksman B H, Adams R D 1955 Allergic neuritis: experimental disease of rabbits induced by peripheral nervous tissue and adjuvants. Journal of Experimental Medicine 102: 213

Walsh F S, Cronin M, Koblar S et al 1992 Association between glycoconjugate antibodies and Campylobacter infection in patients with Guillain–Barré syndrome. Journal of Neuroimmunology 34: 43

Wasserman N H, Penn A S, Freimuth P I et al 1982 Anti-idiotypic route to anti-acetylcholine receptor antibodies and experimental myasthenia gravis. Proceedings of the National Academy of Sciences USA 79: 4810

Werkele H, Ketelsen U-P 1977 Intrathymic pathogenesis and dual genetic control of myasthenia gravis. Lancet i: 678

Whitaker J N 1982 Inflammatory myopathy: a review of etiologic and pathogenetic factors. Muscle and Nerve 5: 573

Whitaker J N, Engel W K 1972 Vascular deposits of immunoglobulin and complement in idiopathic inflammatory myopathy. New England Journal of Medicine 286: 333

Whiting P J, Vincent A, Newsom-Davis J 1983 Acetylcholine receptor antibody characteristics in myasthenia gravis. Fractionation of alpha-bungarotoxin binding site antibodies and their relationship to IgG subclass. Journal of Neuroimmunology 5: 1

Willcox N A, Demaine A G, Newsom-Davis J, Welsh K I, Robb S A, Spiro S G 1985 Increased frequency of IgG heavy chain marker G1m(2) and of HLA-B8 in Lambert-Eaton myasthenic syndrome with and without associated lung carcinoma. Human Immunology 14: 29

Williams C L, Lennon V A 1986 B-lymphocyte clones from patients with myasthenia gravis secrete monoclonal striational autoantibodies reacting with myosin, actinin or actin. Journal of Experimental Medicine 164: 1043

Willison H J, Veitch J, Paterson G, Kennedy P G E 1993 Miller Fisher syndrome is associated with serum antibodies to GQ1b ganglioside. Journal of Neurology, Neurosurgery and Psychiatry 56: 204

Wisniewski H M, Brostoff S W, Carter H, Eylar E H 1974 Recurrent experimental allergic polyganglioradiculoneuritis. Multiple demyelinating episodes in the rhesus monkey sensitized with rabbit sciatic nerve myelin. Archives of Neurology 30: 347

Wolfe J F, Adelstein E, Sharp G C 1977 Antinuclear antibody with distinct specificity for polymyositis. Journal of Clinical Investigation 59: 176

Wolfgram F, Myers L 1973 Amyotrophic lateral sclerosis: effect of serum on anterior horn cells in tissue culture. Science 179: 579

Wray D W, Peers C, Lang B, Lande S, Newsom-Davis J 1987 Interference with calcium channels by Lambert–Eaton myasthenic syndrome antibody. Annals of the New York Academy of Sciences 505: 368

Younger D S, Rowland L P, Latov N et al 1990 Motor neuron disease and amyotrophic lateral sclerosis: relation of high CSF protein to paraproteinemia and clinical syndromes. Neurology 40: 595

Yuki N, Yoshino H, Sato S, Miyatake T 1990 Acute axonal

polyneuropathy associated with anti-GM1 antibodies following campylobacter enteritis. Neurology 40: 1900

Yuki N, Sato S, Tsuji S, Ohsawa T, Miyatake T 1993 Frequent presence of anti-GQ1b antibody in Fisher's syndrome. Neurology 43: 414

Zanetti M 1985 The idiotype network in autoimmune processes. Immunology Today 6: 299

Ziegler H K, Henney C S 1977 Studies on the cytotoxic activity of human lymphocytes. II. Interactions between IgG and Fc receptors leading to inhibition of K-cell function. Journal of Immunology 119: 1010

Zinkernagel R M, Dougherty P C 1974 Restriction of in vitro T-cell mediated cytotoxicity in lymphocytic

choriomeningitis within a syngeneic or semi-allogeneic system. Nature 248: 701

Zweiman B, Lisak R P 1984 Autoantibodies, autoimmunity and immune complexes. In: Henry J (ed) Clinical diagnosis and management by laboratory methods, 18th edn. WB Saunders, Philadelphia, pp 885, 924

Zweiman B, Rostami A, Lisak R P, Moskovits A R, Pleasure D E 1983 Immune reactions to P2 protein in human inflammatory demyelinative neuropathies. Neurology 33: 234

Zweiman B, Levinson A I, Lisak R P 1989 Phenotypic characteristics of thymic B lymphocytes in myasthenia gravis. Journal of Clinical Immunology 9: 942

11. The pathophysiology of excitation in skeletal muscle

R. L. Barchi

INTRODUCTION

Although the generation of force in skeletal muscle ultimately reflects the chemical interaction of actin and myosin, useful muscular activity can occur only when this chemical interaction is faithfully coupled to the electrical activity of a motor neurone. This coupling is provided by the propagation of regenerative spikes or action potentials along the muscle sarcolemma; these impulses originate in the region of the end-plate and subsequently spread across the entire muscle surface, eventually penetrating into the fibre interior along the elements of the T-tubular network. At membrane specialisations known as triads, the T-tubular elements interact closely with the terminal cisternae of the sarcoplasmic reticulum (SR); depolarisation here results in the release of calcium from the SR in a process known as excitation–contraction coupling (for review, see Fleischer & Inui 1989).

If the surface membrane of a muscle fibre fails to generate an action potential in response to end-plate depolarisation, contraction will not take place in spite of normal function in both the neuromuscular junction and the contractile proteins; inexcitable surface membranes result in muscle paralysis. Conversely, if the surface membrane generates multiple, uncontrolled action potentials in response to a normal stimulus at the neuromuscular junction, sustained contractions can occur where only a brief twitch was intended; hyperexcitable surface membranes are one cause of delayed relaxation in neuromuscular disease.

This chapter deals with the processes that control the action potential in normal skeletal muscle, and with membrane defects that can produce hypo- and hyperexcitable states of the sarcolemma. We then trace the relationship between these factors and the pathogenesis of the myotonic disorders and of the periodic paralyses.

NORMAL MEMBRANE EXCITATION IN SKELETAL MUSCLE

The resting membrane potential

A microelectrode inserted into a normal skeletal muscle fibre will record a potential of 70–90 mV with the inside of the cell negative relative to the extracellular space. This potential is developed across the thin barrier (50–75 Å) of the surface membrane. This membrane also marks the boundary across which concentration gradients are established for monovalent and divalent anions and cations between the cytoplasm and the external environment. It is the interrelationship between these concentration gradients and the selective permeability of the surface membrane to these ions that controls the sign and the magnitude of the membrane potential. This potential can be altered either through modification of the concentration gradients themselves or through modulation of the membrane's ionic conductances.

The interaction between membrane potential, ionic concentration gradients and membrane conductances can best be understood by considering first the simple case of a semipermeable membrane separating two chambers that contain different concentrations of a simple salt solution. Suppose such a membrane (Fig. 11.1), separating a 100 mM solution of KCl on the left-hand side from one of 5 mM on the right, is suddenly made selectively permeable to potassium only. Potassium ions (K+) will move down their concentration gradient from the side with the highest concentration (the left) to the side with the lowest (the right). However, as the membrane is not permeable to the counterion chloride (Cl−), any movement of K+ will produce an imbalance of charge, with more positive ions on the right side of the membrane and more negative ions on the left. This charge imbalance creates a membrane potential whose electrical field will retard the further

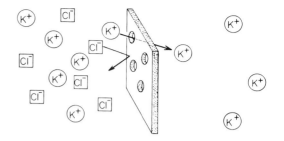

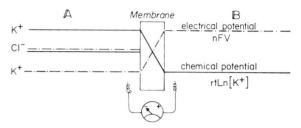

Fig. 11.1 A transmembrane potential develops when a semipermeable membrane separates two solutions with differing concentrations of a permeant ion. In this illustration, the membrane is permeable only to K+ ions. The electrical potential that results when K+ ions attempt to move down their concentration gradient will exactly balance the chemical potential produced by that concentration gradient, and the net force acting on a single K+ ion moving through the membrane will be zero. The membrane potential under these conditions, given by the Nernst equation, will vary as a function of the potassium concentration gradient (reproduced from Barchi 1980 with permission).

movements of K+ ions along their chemical gradient. Eventually an equilibrium will be reached where the driving force on a K+ ion due to the electrical field exactly balances the opposing drive of the concentration gradient and no further net movement of ions occurs. This potential, known as the Nernst potential after the nineteenth-century physiologist who first described it, is given by the simple equation:

$$V\text{m} = \frac{RT}{nF} \ln \left\{ \frac{[K_1^+]}{[K_2^+]} \right\} \tag{1}$$

where $V\text{m}$ is the membrane potential, $[K_1^+]$ is the concentration of potassium ions on side one, n is the charge on each ion (in this case, +1) and R, T, and F are physical constants. The equation predicts that increasing the concentration gradient increases the potential while decreasing the concentration gradient has the opposite effect.

Unfortunately, things are not as simple as this in the case of the muscle membrane. While the sarcolemma is very permeable to K^+, and the response of the membrane potential to changes in K^+ concentration does approximate to that predicted by the potassium Nernst potential, the membrane is measurably permeable to other ions as well, especially to Na^+ and to Cl^-. In normal muscle both the concentration gradients and the relative membrane permeabilities for each of these ions have a role in determining the actual membrane potential across the sarcolemma. Although the derivation of the equation describing this situation is complicated, the final result resembles in its general form the simple Nernst relationship:

$$Vm = \frac{RT}{nF} \ln \left\{ \frac{P_K[K_1^+] + P_{Na}[Na_1^+] + P_{Cl}[Cl_2^-]}{P_K[K_2^+] + P_{Na}[Na_2^+] + P_{Cl}[Cl_2^-]} \right\} \quad (2)$$

A new term, P, is now introduced that indicates the membrane's relative permeability to each ionic species. This equation, known as the Goldman–Hodgkin–Katz (GHK) relationship, predicts that the membrane potential will reflect both the concentration gradients for each of the permeant ion species and the relative permeability (P) of the membrane to each of those species. The dependence on relative permeabilities introduced by this equation is extremely important since it predicts that the membrane potential can be altered by modulating membrane permeability alone without any change in the concentration gradients themselves. With the typical concentration gradients for Na^+, K^+ and Cl^- found in mammalian skeletal muscle, the membrane potential can range between −90 mV or so when the permeability to K^+ predominates, and +50 mV when the membrane is made selectively permeable to Na^+. It is this relationship between permeability and potential that forms the basis for the generation of an action potential.

There is another fundamental difference between the situation described by the Nernst relationship and that quantitated by the GHK equation. With a perfectly selective membrane, the potential predicted by the Nernst equation will persist indefinitely; that is, the equation describes an equilibrium. This is not the case for a membrane permeable to multiple ions as described by the GHK equation. Here, for example, movement of K^+ in one direction can be electrically balanced by the movement of Na^+ ions along their concentration gradient in the opposite direction. Eventually these gradients will dissipate and the potential itself will disappear. To enable the membrane potential described by equation (2) to persist, there must be a mechanism for maintaining the underlying concentration gradients. Ideally, each ion that crosses the membrane passively must be pumped actively back across it. If this is done, a *steady state* results; the potential and the concentration gradients remain constant, but at the necessary cost of energy in the form of the ATP needed to run the pump.

In skeletal muscle the major membrane transport protein is Na^+-K^+-ATPase. This protein actively transports Na^+ against its concentration gradient from the inside of the cell to the extracellular space while simultaneously moving K^+ ions in the opposite direction (for a review, see Skou 1990). The coupling of Na^+ and K^+ in this energy-dependent pumping process is not 1:1, however; about three Na^+ ions move outwards for each two K^+ ions that are transported inwards. If negative counterions cannot keep up with the movement of their positive partners, this asymmetrical pumping will produce a small membrane potential of its own. In normal muscle, the activity of the Na^+-K^+-ATPase can generate 3–10 mV of hyperpolarisation, depending on the level of activity of the enzyme.

Active membrane properties

In muscle, small depolarising current pulses introduced through an intracellular microelectrode produce proportionate changes in the membrane potential as expected for a passive R-C circuit as long as the magnitude of the depolarisation does not exceed 10–15 mV. Larger depolarisations, however, trigger a unique all-or-none regenerative potential change which reflects highly non-linear changes in the underlying properties of the membrane itself. This regenerative spike or action potential is stereotyped in its form, and at its peak produces an internal potential that is actually positive with respect to the extracellular space.

Some insight into the mechanism by which the action potential arises can be gained by studying the relationship between the membrane potential at the peak of the spike and the external concentration of various cations. While the resting potential in muscle is sensitive to changes in external [K$^+$] but not to external [Na$^+$], the peak of the action potential demonstrates the reverse relationship; it is altered little by variations in [K$^+$] but varies with [Na$^+$] in a manner resembling a membrane that is permeable only to Na$^+$ ions.

Membrane currents during an action potential. The details of the conductance changes that underly the action potential in skeletal muscle have been defined mainly through the use of voltage clamp techniques. After its seminal application to the squid giant axon by Hodgkin & Huxley (1952), this technique was modified for single muscle fibres by Adrian and his colleagues (Adrian et al 1970). Their early findings confirmed that the basic mechanisms involved in producing action potentials in nerve and muscle were the same. The initial rising phase of the action potential is produced by a large, voltage-dependent increase in membrane conductance to sodium ions. The greater the depolarisation, the larger and more rapid is the conductance change; thus, once initiated, the action potential becomes its own stimulus. This increase in sodium conductance is transient, however, and reverts to its resting level within a few milliseconds. This conductance inactivation, in conjunction with a secondary delayed increase in membrane conductance to potassium ions, results in the return of the membrane potential to its normal resting value.

With the use of a voltage clamp, relationships between conductance, voltage and time have been detailed in muscle for both the sodium and the potassium systems (Adrian et al 1970, Adrian & Marshall 1977). Over the years, a number of points have become clear. First, the membrane proteins controlling these conductances represent two discrete populations of ion channels, each providing a separate time- and voltage-dependent aqueous pathway through the membrane for its selected cation. Secondly, the basic properties of these two channels differ little from comparable sodium and potassium channels involved in the production of action potentials in the nerves and muscles of virtually all multicellular organisms. Thirdly, the action potential is mainly the result of changes in *conductance* of the membrane to these cations; relatively little actual net movement of cations occurs and there is no significant change in the cation concentration gradients across the membrane during a single action potential.

Sodium channel inactivation. The kinetics of current flow through the sodium and potassium channels differ in a very fundamental way. When potassium channels are opened with depolarisation, they tend to stay in the opened state and potassium currents flow throughout the period of depolarisation, terminating only when the membrane repolarises. Sodium channels, on the other hand, open transiently in response to depolarisation and then revert to a non-conducting or inactivated state in spite of persistent depolarisation (for a review, see Hille 1986). The process of inactivation in the sodium channel is an extremely important one, and channel inactivation has a central role in the control of membrane excitability. This aspect of sodium channel function requires some additional comment.

The voltage-dependent sodium channel can exist in at least three states. In the normally closed state which predominates at the resting potential, the channel does not allow the movement of cations, but is available to be activated by depolarisation. With rapid depolarisation, a second, opened, state is seen in which sodium ions move freely through the channel pore. With continued depolarisation, the channel enters a third conformation known as the inactivated state; in this state the pore is closed but the channel is no longer able to be activated by depolarisation (Fig. 11.2). All three states appear to be interconvertible, and the inactivated state can be restored to the closed but activatable state simply by repolarising the membrane to its resting level.

In a population of sodium channels, the fraction that will be found in the inactivated state increases with depolarisation. The relationship between steady-state inactivation and membrane potential is sigmoidal, with the midpoint in skeletal muscle at about −50 mV. Prolonged depolarisation can thus paradoxically lead to inactivation of sodium channels and loss of membrane excitability rather than the increased excitability often expected.

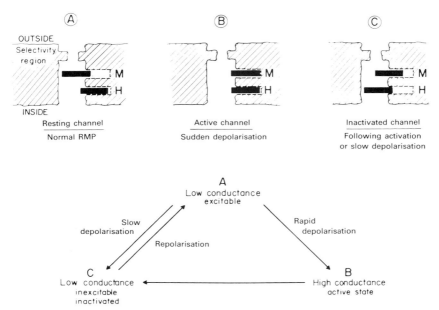

Fig. 11.2   Muscle action potentials are produced largely by transient changes in membrane conductance to sodium ions. Membrane sodium conductance is controlled by a voltage-sensitive sodium channel which provides a water-filled pathway across the muscle surface membrane. In the channel, ion movement is controlled by several 'gates' that switch open or closed as a function of membrane potential and time. At the normal membrane resting potential the channel is closed. Rapid depolarisation results in transient channel opening; during this interval, a Na^+ ion current can flow. Prolonged depolarisation causes a separate 'inactivation' gate to close; the channel no longer conducts Na^+ ions and cannot be opened again by further depolarisation. Repolarisation of the membrane restores the channel to its original closed but activatable state.

Although the actual kinetic interrelationships between the various conformations of the sodium channel are much more complex, this simple scheme is sufficient to explain many of the basic properties of channel behaviour.

Single channel properties

Our view of the behaviour of sodium and potassium channels as continuously modulated conductance pathways that open and close in a smooth, graded fashion in response to triggering stimuli was based on voltage-clamp measurements recording the response of large areas of surface membrane containing many thousands of channel molecules. This view has changed dramatically in recent years with the introduction of a technique known as patch clamping (Neher & Sakmann 1976) (Fig. 11.3a). In this method, very small patches of membrane (less than 1 μm² in

area) can be isolated at the tip of a fire-polished microelectrode and subjected to the same sort of analysis used with the traditional macroscopic voltage clamp. These patches are so small that they contain only one or two sodium or potassium channels each.

The response of these small membrane patches to abrupt depolarisation is quite different from that of whole fibres or squid axons. Instead of smoothly modulated changes in membrane current with depolarisation, sharp step-like transitions between discrete current levels are seen at a given driving voltage (Fig. 11.3b). The amplitude of these current steps is constant and the actual change in current occurs so rapidly that usually it cannot be accurately resolved (Horn & Patlack 1980). If the same depolarising step is repeated over and over again in the same patch, the characteristics of these current steps remain constant; only their duration and the time of their occur-

a

b

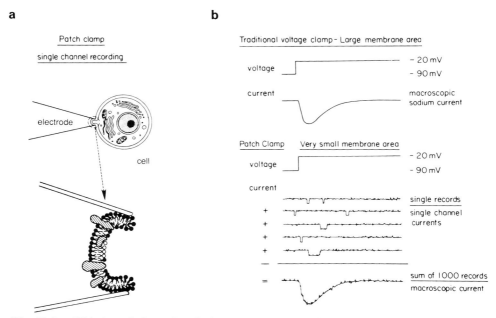

Fig. 11.3a With the technique of patch clamping, a small area of membrane can be sealed so tightly to the tip of a blunt glass microelectrode that it can be removed intact from the cell. The high resistance of the membrane-to-glass seal (usually tens of gigaohms) allows the investigator to resolve the tiny currents flowing through single ion channels in the membrane patch. **b** Classic macroscopic techniques for measuring membrane currents, such as voltage clamp, record the response of thousands of ion channels at a time. The current records often suggest a smoothly graded opening and closing of these channels with time, as shown in this record of membrane sodium currents flowing through the voltage-sensitive sodium channel. Using the patch clamp, the behaviour of single ion channels can be resolved. At this level, sodium channels are seen to open and close abruptly, moving rapidly between a zero conductance state and a characteristic open-channel conductance state. The smooth currents seen with macroscopic techniques really represent the statistical average of the stochastic behaviour of individual channels whose probabilities of opening and closing vary with voltage and time.

rence during the pulse vary, each in a statistically definable manner. If recordings of these current steps from thousands of such records are averaged, the smooth current increase and self-terminating inactivation characteristic of a traditional voltage-clamp record are reproduced.

These small current pulses represent the opening and closing of individual ion channels. Each channel opens very rapidly to a characteristic conductance level, remains opened for a period of time, and then closes again. The interval between the initiation of membrane depolarisation and channel opening varies in a statistical manner for a single channel on multiple trials. Following an abrupt depolarisation, the probability that a given single channel will be opened increases dramatically for a few milliseconds and then decreases again with time, reflecting the time-dependent

onset of inactivation. For skeletal muscle, single sodium channels have a conductance of about 20 pS, resulting in a current flow of several thousand ions through each channel during an average opened interval of 1 ms.

The response of the muscle membrane to depolarisation can no longer be considered as a smooth graded process; the currents recorded with macroscopic techniques such as the traditional voltage clamp actually represent the statistical average of the responses of many thousands of individual channels, each behaving in a stochastic manner in switching between its closed and opened state. The relationship between parameters such as the probability of channel opening and the duration of each channel opening, on the one hand, and the membrane potential and time after depolarisation, on the other, define the response characteristics of the channel in the membrane in a manner analogous to the time- and voltage-dependent rate constants of the classic Hodgkin–Huxley formulation.

Molecular characteristics of muscle ion channels

Voltage-dependent sodium channels. Along with an appreciation of single ion channel events at the biophysical level has come a greater understanding of the molecular properties of the channel proteins themselves. During the past 10 years, the voltage-dependent sodium channel protein has been purified, cloned, and sequenced from rat and human skeletal muscle as well as from mammalian brain and from eel and drosophila (for review, see Kallen et al 1993). All of these channel proteins are remarkably similar.

All voltage-dependent sodium channels contain one very large polypeptide of ~260 000 MW designated the alpha subunit. This subunit is a glycoprotein, with carbohydrate contributing about 24% by weight in skeletal muscle. The alpha subunit has within its structure all the elements necessary for a functioning voltage-dependent ion channel. While the alpha subunit is the only protein present in the eel sodium channel, the channel in mammalian skeletal muscle and brain is stoichiometrically associated with one or two additional small subunits of ~38 000 MW that are also heavily glycosylated (Hartshorne & Catterall 1984, Roberts & Barchi 1987). These beta subunits are capable of modifying the kinetics of channel activation and inactivation (Isom et al 1992).

The complete amino acid sequence for the alpha subunit of sodium channels from eel, drosophila, mammalian brain, and from skeletal and cardiac muscle, have all been deduced from their cloned cDNA (reviewed in Cohen & Barchi 1992). A number of interesting conclusions can be drawn from a comparison of these sequences. These channels are highly homologous, with more than 60% sequence identity at the amino acid level between channels in species as divergent as eel and rat. Each alpha subunit contains between 1800 and 2000 amino acids. Within this linear sequence are four large regions of internal homology, each encompassing 225–300 amino acids; sequence comparison indicates that these regions arose from duplication of the same primitive ancestral channel element. Within each of these regions are at least six areas predicted to be transmembrane alpha helices, and these regions are the most highly conserved areas when the domains are compared (Guy & Conti 1990). The fourth helix in each domain (S4) is particularly interesting in exhibiting a very highly conserved pattern of a positively charged arginine or lysine residue at every third position, separated by two non-polar amino acids.

Frog oocytes or mammalian cells in culture can be injected with RNA prepared from the cloned sodium channel cDNAs and induced to synthesise the channel protein and incorporate it into the surface membrane where it can be studied electrophysiologically. By modifying the cDNA, specific mutations can be introduced into the channel structure, and their effect on channel function assessed. Using this general approach, a considerable amount has been learned about the relationship between channel structure and function. For example, it is now clear that the positively charged S4 helix in each domain acts as part of the voltage-sensing elements of the channel (Stühmer et al 1989, Stühmer 1991, Auld et al 1990). The region connecting repeat domains 3 and 4 contributes to the inactivation of channel conductance after depolarization (Vassilev et al 1989). The ion channel itself is formed from elements contributed from each of the four repeat domains, with the regions between the S5 and S6 helices forming part of the channel lining and contributing to the specification of cation selectivity (Noda et al 1989, Heinemann et al 1992).

Potassium channels. The delayed rectifier potassium channel that contributes to repolarisation of the nerve and muscle membrane after activation has also been characterised at the molecular level during the past few years (reviewed in Kolb 1990). These channels are members of a larger superfamily of potassium channels that includes the A-current potassium channel in drosophila (Papazian et al 1987, Butler et al 1990) and related potassium channels in mammalian brain and muscle (Chandy et al 1990, Roberds &

Tankum 1991). Members of this family that have been cloned are smaller and more variable in size than sodium channels ranging in molecular weight between 60 000 and 75 000 Da.

Initially, potassium channel proteins appeared to be unrelated to sodium channels because of their much smaller size. However, when their primary sequence is carefully analysed, these two types of voltage-dependent ion channels are found to be clearly related (Papazian et al 1987). The sequence of these potassium channels resembles in its organisation one repeat domain of the larger sodium channel alpha subunit. Within this region are the familiar six trans-membrane helices, and the characteristic positive S4 helix. The region of amino acid sequence surrounding this S4 helix exhibits considerable homology with the analogous region of the sodium channel.

In the membrane, potassium channels are formed by tetramers of these smaller subunits (MacKinnon 1991). In their functional state, these potassium channels are comparable in organisation to the sodium channel. The individual subunits of the potassium channel play the same role as the repeat domains in the sodium channel. Virtually all the key functional elements documented by site-directed mutagenesis in potassium channels have been confirmed in analogous locations in the sodium channel (Stühmer 1991).

Chloride channels. The chloride conductance in muscle forms the dominant resting conductance in the sarcolemma (see below). The channel protein that controls this conductance has also been cloned, sequenced and functionally expressed from eel electroplax and from rat skeletal muscle (Jentsch et al 1990; Steinmeyer et al 1991b).

In rat skeletal muscle, the cDNA encoding this chloride channel contains a single open reading frame for a 994 amino acid protein that is identical in more than half of its residues with the comparable protein cloned from the eel electroplax. Structural analysis of the primary sequence predicts up to 13 trans-membrane helices in the central portion of the molecule, but shows no evidence of the internal organisational features characteristic of the voltage-dependent sodium and potassium channels discussed above. The chloride channel sequences show no homology to the sequences of any other known ion channel or transporter molecule, and do not contain the positively charged helix motif that is the hallmark of the voltage-dependent cation channels (Palade & Barchi 1977a, Steinmeyer et al 1991).

When expressed in vitro, cRNA from these clones produces functional chloride channels with the anion selectivity, voltage dependence and kinetics characteristic of the major chloride conductance pathway previously described in mammalian skeletal muscle.

MEMBRANES AND MUSCLE WEAKNESS IN PERIODIC PARALYSIS

The periodic paralyses are disorders of skeletal muscle characterised by transient episodes of muscle weakness or paralysis. During these episodes there are often profound shifts in the potassium concentration. These disorders usually occur as familial syndromes with autosomal dominant inheritance, although clinically indistinguishable sporadic cases do occur (see Ch. 17). The periodic paralyses have traditionally been classified according to the characteristic changes in serum potassium associated with the attacks of weakness, and hypokalaemic, normokalaemic and hyperkalaemic varieties are recognised. This classification is probably simplistic; e.g. it now appears that at least four different types of hyperkalaemic periodic paralysis can be identified (Rudel & Ricker 1985). The details of the clinical presentation of the various forms of periodic paralysis are considered in Chapter 17. We will discuss here some of the common aspects of the membrane events which lead to the development of muscle weakness.

Membrane potential and membrane excitability

Between attacks of paralysis, the resting membrane potential in skeletal muscle of patients with periodic paralysis is usually normal and excitation–contraction coupling proceeds without difficulty (Shy et al 1961, Creutzfeldt et al 1963, Riecker & Bolte 1966, McComas et al 1968). During the onset of an attack of weakness, muscle strength declines in direct proportion to the loss of muscle membrane excitability, as evidenced by the amplitude of the compound muscle action potential that can be elicited by either direct or indirect stimulation (Gordon et al 1970). At the peak of paralysis, individual muscle fibres exhibit abnormally low resting membrane potentials (Creutzfeldt et al 1963, Hofmann & Smith 1970) and cannot be stimulated to produce an action potential by the usual depolarising current stimuli. Hyperpolarisation of the membrane, on the other hand, will often produce an action potential when the stimulus is terminated — an 'anode break' potential. At the same time, motor nerve action potentials appear normal, processes at the end-plate are intact, and the underlying contractile apparatus responds normally to the direct application of calcium (Engel & Lambert 1969).

Although the details of this scenario vary from one type of periodic paralysis to another, the basic storyline is the same. Muscle paralysis is associated with failure of action potential generation in the fibre sarcolemma, and this in turn is correlated with a persistent depolarisation of the membrane resting potential. How can these facts be reconciled with our understanding of the molecular basis for action potential generation? We have seen above that prolonged depolarisation will shift the membrane voltage-sensitive sodium channels into an inactivated state. The percentage of the sodium channels in the membrane available for activation varies steeply with voltage near the resting potential. As an action potential can be generated only when the net inward sodium current through these channels exceeds the total outward current carried through all other channels in the membrane, the number of sodium channels available to be opened is critical for normal excitability.

At normal muscle resting potentials, about 70% of the membrane sodium channels are available for activation. With this number of channels, the inward sodium current needed for initiation of the action potential is easily achieved. A persistent depolarisation of only 10–20 mV, however, will increase the fraction of inactivated channels to nearly 50%, and the remaining channels are barely able to generate the needed inward current density of an action potential. A further small depolarisation renders the membrane totally incapable of generating an action potential even though the sodium channels themselves may be normal in number and in their molecular properties.

If the membrane is once again repolarised to its normal resting level, the equilibrium between closed but available channels and inactivated channels shifts back, the fraction of channels available for activation increases, and normal excitability is restored. When action potentials once again couple depolarisation of the neuro-muscular junction to calcium release from the sarcoplasmic reticulum, normal muscle function and strength return.

Pathophysiology of membrane depolarisation

This sequence of events appears to be shared by most, if not all, of the periodic paralyses during episodes of muscle weakness. The triggering factors which lead to the underlying membrane depolarisation, however, may be quite different in the various forms of this disease (Barchi & Furman 1991). If we recall the GHK equation (equation (2)) describing the origin of the muscle membrane potential, we can appreciate that persistent depolarisation can be produced by a variety of factors. These include an increase in external K^+ concentration, a decrease in external Na^+ concentration, or an increase in membrane permeability to Na^+ relative to that for K^+. Decreasing the contribution to the membrane potential from the electrogenic activity of the Na^+-K^+- ATPase will also depolarise the membrane.

In most of the familial periodic paralyses, membrane depolarisation is due mainly to an increase in the membrane permeability to Na^+ (see Rüdel & Ricker 1985, for review). In the toxic paralysis produced by barium ingestion or by experimental potassium deficiency in animals, on the other hand, depolarisation may be the result of a primary decrease in K^+ conductance, again with the ultimate effect to shifting the balance of membrane conductance to favour Na^+ (Kao & Gordon 1975, Gallant 1983). External factors, such as cooling, that lead to a further transient increase in Na^+ conductance or a decrease in electrogenic pump activity will tip the delicately balanced membrane into a more depolarised state, resulting in further inactivation of the voltage-sensitive sodium channel, failure of excitation, and paralysis.

In hypokalaemic periodic paralysis, the increased resting membrane sodium conductance does not involve the voltage-dependent sodium channel, but rather another sodium pathway which may be coupled in some way to the membrane actions of insulin (Rüdel et al 1984). In adynamia episodica hereditaria and paramyotonia congenita, the increased sodium conductance is mediated by the sodium channel itself, and can be prevented or reversed by the specific sodium-channel blocker tetrodotoxin (Lehmann-Horn et al 1981, 1983). Of particular interest is the defect in paramyotonia, where the sodium channel undergoes a temperature-dependent change, functioning normally at 37°C but becoming persistently opened when cooled to 27°C (Lehmann-Horn et al 1981).

Microelectrode measurements on isolated muscle fibres from patients with hyperkalaemic periodic paralysis have identified a non-inactivating, TTX-sensitive sodium current that is present only when the muscle fibre is exposed to elevated extracellular potassium (Lehmann-Horn et al 1987). This current represents a small percentage of the total membrane sodium current and is not present at normal potassium concentrations. Single channel recordings on myotubes formed from cultured muscle biopsy tissue obtained from patients with hyperkalaemic periodic paralysis demonstrate a class of sodium channels that undergo persistent re-openings during prolonged depolarisation, consistent with a failure of the inactivation process (Cannon et al 1991). When followed over time, single channels were seen to move into and out of this abnormal kinetic gating mode over a period of minutes. This intermittent failure of inactivation was observed only in the presence of elevated extracellular potassium. Abnormal inactivation of this type was not seen in control muscle and may be the molecular counterpart of the non-inactivating sodium current reported earlier with whole cell recording.

Sodium channel defects in periodic paralysis and paramyotonia congenita

The molecular cloning of the various mammalian skeletal muscle sodium channels (Trimmer et al 1989, Kallen et al 1990, George et al 1992) opened the way for the characterisation of defects in this channel protein in the periodic paralyses. Using information from the cloned human channel, the localisation of the gene encoding the adult muscle channel was determined to be at chromosome 17q23.1-25.5 (George et al 1991). This gene has been designated SCN4A. Using restriction fragment length polymorphisms (RFLPs) defined within this gene (Ebers et al 1991), a number of studies were carried out evaluating the potential linkage between the phenotypic expression of various forms of periodic paralysis and the skeletal muscle sodium channel SCN4A gene locus. Tight linkage was first shown between the SCN4A gene on chromosome 17 and hyperkalaemic periodic paralysis both with (Fountaine et al 1990, Koch et al 1991, Ptacek et al 1991b) and without (Ebers et al 1991) myotonic features. Shortly thereafter, linkage was confirmed for the SCN4A gene locus and paramyotonia congenita (Ebers et al 1991; Ptacek et al 1992a). The SCN4A gene was also found to be tightly linked to the expression of an atypical form of myotonia congenita with painful muscle contractions (Ptacek et al 1992b). Taken together, these studies indicate that hyperkalaemic periodic paralysis and paramyotonia congenita, as well as other familial disorders with related phenotypes, are allelic disorders at the same sodium channel gene locus (Fig. 11.4).

Using information about the gene structure of SCN4A (George et al 1993) to generate polymerase chain reaction (PCR) probes for the exon regions of this channel gene, Ptacek et al (1991c) analysed families with hyperkalaemic periodic paralysis for specific mutations within the protein's coding region. A unique mutation resulting in the substitution of a methionine for a conserved threonine in the S5 helix of domain 2 was identified that cosegregated with the disease phenotype in three separate families, but was not seen in any of 116 unrelated control individuals (Ptacek et al 1991c). This mutation is located at the predicted junction between the intramembrane S5 helix and the cytoplasmic extension linking S5 to S6. A second mutation was defined in several other families that introduced a valine

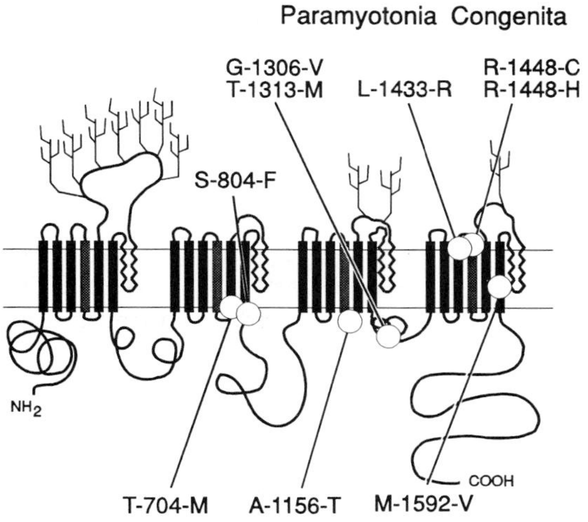

Paramyotonia Congenita

Fig. 11.4 Voltage-dependent sodium channel alpha subunits are encoded in mRNAs of ~8.5 kb. The mRNA contains an open reading frame for a protein of about 2000 amino acids; within this large protein are four regions, each encompassing 225–300 amino acids, that share extensive sequence homology and are derived by gene duplication from the same primitive channel element. Each internal repeat domain contains six predicted transmembrane helices, and these regions of sequence are the most highly conserved between domains. The fourth helix in each domain is particularly striking; it contains a positively charged lysine or arginine residue at every third position separated by two non-polar amino acids. This S4 helix forms part of the voltage-sensing element necessary for channel activation.

for a conserved methionine in the S6 helix of domain 4 (Rojas et al 1991). Families with the first mutation differed from those with the second in having persistent myopathic features in addition to the paralytic episodes and myotonic symptoms.

Families with paramyotonia congenita have also been analysed with similar methods. Two mutations in the cytoplasmic linker joining domains 3 and 4 (ID3–4), a region that is postulated to play a critical role in channel inactivation, were identified by one group in several families with the paramyotonia congenita phenotype (McClatchey et al 1992a). These mutations introduce a valine for a conserved glycine, or a methionine for a threonine within a short region near the amino-terminal end of the ID3–4 segment. Based on the experimental evidence associating this region with normal channel inactivation (Stühmer et al 1989, Vassilev et al 1989), these mutations

could easily interfere with the normal inactivation process, leading to persistent channel openings, prolonged currents, and depolarisation.

A second set of mutations in paramyotonia congenita are particularly interesting in that they involve one of the S4 helices that are thought to form the voltage-sensing elements of the channel (Ptacek et al 1992a). These two mutations both occur in the same codon, resulting in alterations to the same amino acid in the channel primary sequence. One alters an absolutely conserved arginine near the extracellular end of the S4 helix to a histidine, while the second substitutes a cysteine for the same arginine residue. In both cases, an uncharged amino acid replaces one of the critical positively charged residues in the helix. Again, none of these mutations is seen as a polymorphism in any of the control individuals examined.

In a separate paramyotonia congenita family, a T to G transversion was identified that introduces an arginine for a conserved leucine near the extracellular end of the S3 helix in D4 (Ptacek et al 1992c). This mutation will produce a major change in local charge and in side-chain packing at a region of the channel physically adjacent to the two S4 mutations.

Two additional mutations have been identified in hyperkalaemic periodic paralysis and paramyotonia congenita families with symptoms that overlap traditional diagnostic categories (McClatchey 1992b). One pedigree, with features of paramyotonia congenita and hyperkalaemic periodic paralysis, has an alanine to threonine amino acid change in the predicted intracellular loop between S4 and S5 in D3. The second pedigree exhibits features of paramyotonia congenita and myotonia congenita; this family expresses a serine to phenylalanine mutation near the cytoplasmic end of the S6 helix in D2.

It appears that abnormalities of sodium channel inactivation that can lead to the phenotype of periodic paralysis can be produced by a variety of mutations scattered throughout the channel structure. It is likely that more such mutations will come to light as other families with these disorders are studied in detail. These mutations could affect the specific portion of the channel involved in channel formation or occlusion, but more distant mutations which alter channels slightly have the real potential to alter the conformational energy of activated and inactivated states, thus shifting the state distribution toward an abnormal kinetic mode. Like the multiple mutations that can cause the various haemoglobinopathies, it is probable that many allelic mutations affecting the sodium channel structure will lead to disorders with similar phenotypes.

Serum K⁺, membrane potential and paralysis

The details of the interplay between serum potassium, membrane potential and paralysis in the individual disorders remain to be clarified, but shifts in serum K^+ probably reflect coupling to sodium movements through the Na^+-K^+-ATPase system rather than primary events directly responsible for paralysis (Fig. 11.5). This coupling can result clinically in either hypokalaemia or hyperkalaemia, depending upon the functional state of the Na^+-K^+-ATPase itself. For example, the increased inward Na^+ movement that would be associated with an abnormally large membrane Na^+ conductance will be a potent stimulus for pump activity. A sudden increase in Na^+ conductance from any specific triggering event will further stimulate this pump. As the Na^+-K^+-ATPase exchanges extracellular K^+ for intracellular Na^+, pumping activity can rapidly reduce the K^+ concentration in the small volume of the extracellular space and produce hypokalaemia. This sort of coupling accounts for the net K^+ movement into the cells of normal individuals that follows the administration of glucose and insulin.

In another setting, the Na^+-K^+-ATPase may not be able to increase its activity sufficiently to keep pace with an increased Na^+ leakage. In this case, progressive depolarisation will result, with inward Na^+ movement coupled electrically to outward movement of K^+ ions, leading to secondary hyperkalaemia. It is important to realise that either hyperkalaemia or hypokalaemia can result from the same fundamental defect in membrane sodium conductance depending on the magnitude of the conductance change and the capacity of the Na^+-K^+-ATPase to respond to the additional sodium load.

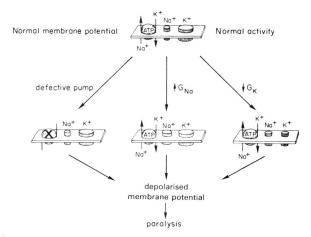

Fig. 11.5 Periodic paralysis is associated with depolarisation of the muscle fibre surface membrane. This depolarisation could result from an increase in membrane $Na;11+$ conductance, a decrease in membrane $K;11+$ conductance, or a reduction in the pumping activity of the membrane Na^+-K^+-ATPase. In the inherited periodic paralyses, an increase in membrane $Na;11+$ conductance appears to be the primary mechanism underlying membrane depolarisation (adapted with permission from Barchi & Furman 1991).

The Na^+-K^+-ATPase may also have a pivotal role in the onset of depolarisation. A muscle membrane in delicate balance as the result of an increased inward Na^+ leak just compensated by a maximally activated pump could be thrown out of balance by the selective slowing of pump activity. This can easily occur with cooling, as the change in activity of energy-dependent pumping with temperature is nearly three times as great as that for ion movement through an aqueous membrane channel.

HYPEREXCITABLE STATES OF THE MUSCLE MEMBRANE — MYOTONIA

The myotonic syndromes are easily identified among the disorders of the neuromuscular system by their characteristic mechanical and electrical features. Myotonia is expressed clinically as the delayed relaxation of skeletal muscle after a voluntary contraction or a contraction induced by an electrical or mechanical stimulus. This delayed relaxation is a cardinal finding in a number of

Table 11.1 Neuromuscular disorders associated with myotonia

Inherited disorders
Man   *Other mammals*
Mytonia congenita   Congenital myotonia:
  dominant and recessive forms   Goat
Myotonic dystrophy   Horse
Adynamica episodica   Dog
Paramyotonia congenita   Cattle
Chondrodystrophic myotonia

Acquired disorders
Drug-induced
Aromatic carboxylic acids
  2,4-D, anthracene-9-carboxylic acid, diuretics
Inhibitors of sterol synthesis
  20,25-Diazacholesterol
  Hypocholesterolaemic drugs
    Atromid-S, clofibrate, triparinol
Steroid administration in dogs.

Others
Iodine intoxication in birds

diseases that vary widely in their inheritance, pathology and prognosis (see Ch. 15); these include myotonia congenita, myotonic dystrophy, paramyotonia congenita, chondrodystrophic myotonia and even some forms of hyperkalaemic periodic paralysis. Myotonia indistinguishable from that found in these natural disorders may also be induced by several classes of drugs and chemicals and can be reproduced in laboratory animals (Table 11.1).

Patients with myotonia often report painless muscular stiffness that is worst at the beginning of movement and that slowly resolves with exercise. Brief muscular contractions are often not impaired, but forceful contractions can cause the muscles to lock in a contracted state, leading to functional disability and falls. Other factors that can aggravate myotonia include muscle cooling, fasting, menstruation, potassium ingestion and sudden emotional arousal.

When examined by electromyography, patients with myotonia exhibit a common picture of increased insertional activity and prolonged, repetitive discharges of motor unit potentials that wax and wane in frequency and amplitude (Fig. 11.6). This prolonged electrical activity correlates with the delay in muscular relaxation and in most of the myotonias is directly responsible for the abnormality of contraction. The waxing and waning

frequency of these discharges produce crescendo–decrescendo sound patterns on the audio monitor that early investigators referred to as 'dive bomber potentials'.

The remarkable similarity of the clinical and electrical appearance of myotonia in different muscle diseases initially suggested that a common underlying pathogenetic mechanism might explain this phenomenon at the membrane level in all diseases. Unfortunately, research over the past 20 years has shown that this is not the case (Rüdel & Lehmann-Horn 1985). Although one major group of myotonic disorders does share a common molecular mechanism, clinical myotonia is probably a common expression of a number of otherwise unrelated defects affecting the behaviour of membrane ion channels (Barchi 1982). In the following sections, some of the common themes relating to the appearance of repetitive electrical discharges in the various myotonic disorders will be discussed. The clinical aspects of these diseases are considered in Chapter 15.

Myotonia due to abnormal chloride conductance

Studies in animal models. Much of our knowledge of the pathophysiology of myotonia is based on the detailed electrophysiological and biophysical studies of a naturally occurring congenital myotonia in goats, carried out by Bryant and his colleagues (for a review, see Bryant 1979). This hereditary syndrome is very similar in its appearance to myotonia congenita in humans.

Classic experiments with nerve section and neuromuscular blockade localised the origin of the abnormal electrical activity to the muscle membrane itself (Brown & Harvey 1939). Subsequent measurements on single isolated intercostal muscle fibres demonstrated at the cellular level the correlate of the persistent electrical activity recorded by EMG (Adrian & Bryant 1974). When the surface membrane of a myotonic fibre is depolarised by a constant current, a repetitive series of driven action potentials is seen that is followed by a long, depolarising after-potential (Fig. 11.6). The amplitude of this depolarising after-potential is proportional to the number of action potentials produced during the current pulse. When the

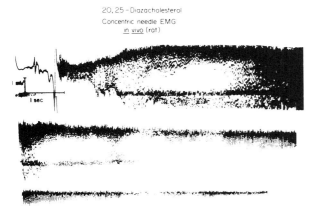

20, 25 – Diazacholesterol
Concentric needle EMG
in vivo (rat)

Fig. 11.6   Sustained membrane electrical activity that follows muscle activation or irritation is the electrical correlate of the delayed relaxation seen in myotonic skeletal muscle. In this example, a myotonic discharge was recorded in response to electrode movement from a rat treated with 20, 25-diazacholesterol, an agent that produces a toxic myotonic syndrome (reproduced with permission from Barchi & Furman 1981).

after-potential becomes large enough, long trains of self-sustaining, spontaneous action potentials are triggered. These events are not seen in normal fibres where depolarisation generates only a few driven potentials, much smaller after-depolarisations and no spontaneous activity.

Measurement of membrane conductance in these myotonic fibres reveals a remarkable increase in membrane resistance that is caused by the nearly complete absence of the normal membrane conductance to chloride ions (Bryant & Morales-Aguilera 1971). In myotonic goats, this is due to a reduced density of chloride channels rather than a normal number of channels having modified conductance properties, and probably represents the primary defect in this disorder (Bryant & Owenburg 1980).

The delayed relaxation of myotonic muscle fibres is believed to be the consequence of abnormal repetitive membrane firing that triggers a normal contractile activation process. Unfortunately, there have been few direct measurements of excitation–contraction coupling in myotonic goats. In one study, changes in voltage-dependent contractile activation were thought to indicate enhanced calcium re-uptake by the sarcoplasmic reticulum (Bryant 1979), and other findings on purified SR fragments also suggested an excitation–contraction abnormality (Swift et al 1979). A thorough study of SR function in chemically skinned single fibres from myotonic goats, however, found caffeine-induced contractions and other release and re-uptake parameters to be normal (Wood et al 1980).

Voltage-clamp techniques have been used to study the kinetics of sodium and potassium channel gating in myotonic goat intercostal fibres (Bryant & DeCoursey 1980). Although small changes were seen in the behaviour of both channels in myotonic muscle, these were not in themselves of sufficient magnitude to produce repetitive activity. They may play a part in the modulation of myotonic activity, however.

The mouse mutants designated *mto* or *adr* exhibit another syndrome that resembles human recessive generalised myotonia (Rüdel 1990). These and three other related mutants with similar phenotypes are thought to be allelic at a single site on mouse chromosome 6 (Heller et al 1982, Watkins & Watts 1984, Davisson et al 1989). When animals homozygous for the *adr* mutation start to walk, the hind legs become stiffly extended. The spasms of the hind limbs are especially prominent when the animal is startled. This stiffness causes problems in righting after an animal is placed on its back; this property accounts for the name given to the mutant: *arrested development of righting response (adr)*.

Animals homozygous for the *mto* allele exhibit delayed relaxation and myotonic discharges (Entriken et al 1987). The half-time for relaxation of skeletal muscle following tetanic stimulation was increased more than 25-fold over control. Work with the *adr* allele showed similar results (Reininghaus et al 1988). The electrical responses recorded intracellularly in both *mto* and *adr* mutants are identical to those found in goat myotonia or myotonia produced by aromatic carboxylic acids (Mehrke et al 1988). The membrane chloride conductance in skeletal muscle fibres is markedly reduced (Mehrke et al 1988).

Human myotonia congenita. Myotonia congenita is an inherited disorder in humans that closely resembles the hereditary myotonia of goats. Myotonia congenita can occur in either an autosomal dominant or a recessive form (see Ch. 15).

Generalised myotonia is usually noted in childhood at the onset of walking, but the severity of the symptoms does not increase with maturation. Membrane studies in human myotonia congenita indicate that here, too, the primary pathophysiological defect is a drastic reduction in muscle membrane chloride conductance. A specific reduction in sarcolemma chloride conductance has been found in intercostal muscle biopsies from these patients, through direct measurements using intracellular microelectrodes (Lipicky et al 1971, Lipicky & Bryant 1973).

Toxic myotonic syndromes. A number of acquired myotonias are also directly due to reduced Cl^- conductance in the sarcolemma. For example, carboxylic acids have long been known to induce myotonia. In 1946, the herbicide, 2,4-dichlorophenoxyacetic acid (2,4-D), was reported to produce a myotonic syndrome in man after accidental ingestion (Bucher 1946). Subsequently a group of 33 related hydrocarbon- and halogen-substituted benzoic acids were shown to induce similar symptoms after intraperitoneal injection in animals (Tang et al 1968).

These carboxylic acids produce myotonia by specific block of Cl^- conductance pathways. In one study on rat muscle, 19 substituted benzoic acid derivatives reduced membrane Cl^- conductance in vitro in a dose-dependent manner, and the inhibitory constant for chloride channel block correlated closely with each compound's ability to produce myotonia both in vivo and in vitro (Palade & Barchi 1977b, Furman & Barchi 1978). At the single-cell level, the electrophysiological features of this myotonia are indistinguishable from those found in hereditary myotonia (Bryant 1982).

The physiological basis of myotonia with reduced chloride conductance

The origin of repetitive electrical activity. The repetitive electrical discharges seen in each of the myotonic disorders can be explained by the marked reduction in membrane Cl^- conductance that they share. At the resting potential, muscle membranes are three to five times more permeable to Cl^- than to K^+, while Na^+ permeability

accounts for less than 1% of the total membrane permeability (Hutter & Nobel 1960, Palade & Barchi 1977a). As discussed above, the Na^+ and K^+ permeabilities undergo time- and voltage-dependent changes (in response to a depolarising stimulus) that result in the generation of an action potential, while Cl^- permeability remains relatively constant during the action potential and Cl^- fluxes passively follow cation movements.

During normal muscle activity, action potentials are propagated both longitudinally along the surface sarcolemma and radially into the fibre interior along elements of the T-tubular system. With each action potential, small amounts of K^+ move out of the cell while small amounts of Na^+ and Cl^- move inwards. The K^+ released into the large volume of the extracellular space has little effect on the overall K^+ concentration, but the situation is different in the limited 'extracellular' volume of the T-tubular system. Measurements indicate that the efflux of K^+ associated with a single action potential can increase its luminal concentration by 0.3 mM; this change could depolarise the T-tubular membrane by as much as 1.7 mV if the major conductance in the T-tubule were to K^+ (Adrian & Bryant 1974). With multiple action potentials, the cumulative effect of this intraluminal K^+ accumulation could be a membrane depolarisation of 10 mV or more.

Under normal conditions, this depolarisation is not reflected in the surface membrane potential because of the large stabilising Cl^- conductance that is present in the sarcolemma. In the absence of this Cl^- shunt, however, the K^+ accumulation in the T-tubular lumen produced by a series of action potentials can locally depolarise the surface membrane sufficiently to initiate self-sustaining action potentials (Fig. 11.7). The observed increase in the after-potential of 1 mV per impulse seen in myotonic fibres is compatible with this mechanism (Adrian & Bryant 1974). A study showing that potassium diffuses from the T-tubule with a time constant of 0.4 s (Almers 1972) compares favourably with the after-potential decay time of 0.5 s observed in intact muscle fibres.

The behaviour of myotonic fibres can be reproduced in normal skeletal muscle fibres by blocking Cl^- conductance through substitution of an impermeant anion for Cl^- (Rüdel & Senges 1972)

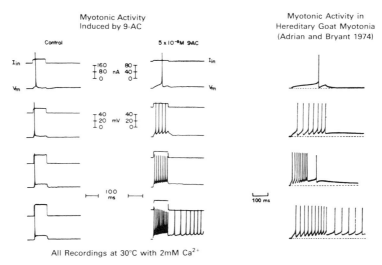

Fig. 11.7 Inherited and acquired myotonic syndromes associated with a reduction in membrane chloride conductance appear very similar at the single cell level. In normal muscle fibres, an intracellular microelectrode will record one or a small number of rapidly accommodating action potentials in response to a depolarising current pulse. In hereditary goat myotonia, or experimental myotonia produced with inhibitors of membrane chloride conductance, depolarisation produces multiple driven action potentials and a prolonged after-depolarisation. If this after-depolarisation exceeds a critical level, continuous self-sustaining action potentials will continue after the depolarising pulse is stopped; this represents myotonia at the single-cell level (reproduced with permission from Furman & Barchi 1986.)

or by specific Cl⁻ channel-blocking compounds (Furman & Barchi 1978). Disconnecting the T-tubular system from the surface membrane by glycerol shock abolishes the long-lasting, depolarising after-potential and sustained spontaneous activity produced by these compounds (Adrian & Bryant 1974), underscoring the importance of the T-tubular system in the generation of this repetitive activity. Figure 11.8 summarises several mechanisms that might lead to the reduced Cl⁻ conductance observed in the membranes of the above myotonic diseases.

The sequence of events in the low chloride-conductance myotonias appears to be as follows. Voluntary contraction of a skeletal muscle produces multiple action potentials which originate at the end-plate, propagate along the muscle fibre, and invade the T-tubular system. Each of these action potentials results in a small increase in the T-tubular K^+ concentration. Because of the markedly reduced Cl⁻ conductance, the effect of this increase in extracellular K^+ is a slight

depolarisation. This depolarisation is not large enough to force sodium channels into an inactivated state; rather, as they recover from the normal inactivation that occurs during the depolarisation of the action potential itself, some channels will begin to reopen as a result of this slight depolarisation. Because the sum of opposing currents is much reduced by the lack of a significant Cl⁻ conductance, the resultant small inward Na^+ current can again initiate depolarisation and recruitment of additional channels so that another action potential develops. The net result of this process is that each action potential creates a transient after depolarisation that in turn acts as a stimulus for the triggering of the next action potential in the sequence. As long as no channel kinetic parameters are altered, this repetitive chain of potentials can continue indefinitely.

Molecular pathology of chloride channel defects. The channel protein that controls membrane chloride conductance has been cloned,

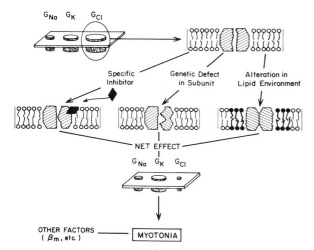

G_{Na} G_K G_{Cl}

Specific Inhibitor   Genetic Defect in Subunit   Alteration in Lipid Environment

NET EFFECT

G_{Na} G_K G_{Cl}

OTHER FACTORS
(β_m, etc.)   —————   MYOTONIA

Fig. 11.8 The best-studied group of myotonic disorders is characterised by a pathological reduction in membrane chloride conductance (see Table 11.1). Even within this group, however, there are multiple mechanisms that can ultimately lead to the same membrane abnormality. Chloride channels may be genetically abnormal, or may be specifically blocked by some exogenous or endogenous agent. Alternatively, normal channels might be induced to behave abnormally by an alteration in the membrane-lipid environment in which they reside. In each case the end result is membrane hyperexcitability and clinical myotonia (reproduced with permission from Furman & Barchi 1986).

sequenced and functionally expressed from both *Torpedo* electroplax and rat skeletal muscle (Jentsch et al 1990, Steinmeyer et al 1991b). Using the sequence for the rat chloride channel, oligonucleotide probes were developed that identify the homologous chloride channel gene in mice. These probes were then used to investigate the role of the chloride channel in the pathophysiology of the mouse ADR myotonic mutant. Through Southern blot analysis of DNA from affected and normal mice, Steinmeyer et al (1991a) demonstrated a consistent defect in the genomic DNA encoding the mouse skeletal muscle chloride channel on chromosome 6 that was present only in animals expressing the ADR phenotype. When this defective DNA was characterised, the normal gene was found to be interrupted at an exon–intron junction by the insertion of a transposable element or transposon. This insertion causes premature termination of transcription and loss of sequence encoding most of

the 3' end of the channel. No full-length chloride channel mRNA transcripts were found in the homozygous ADR mice. Conversely, the insertion was never seen in any of the normal mice examined. Analysis using interspecies backcrosses showed no evidence of recombination between the chloride channel gene and the ADR locus. Taken together, these data provide compelling evidence that the genetic defect in the mouse ADR model of recessive generalised myotonia is an insertional mutation in the muscle chloride channel gene.

Although some rare hereditary muscle diseases that clinically resemble myotonia congenita have been shown to be caused by mutations in the SCN4A sodium channel gene, recent studies in both dominant and recessive myotonia congenita confirm that, as in the *adr* mouse, these human myotonic disorders are usually caused by abnormalities in the skeletal muscle chloride channel. Single channel measurements carried out on muscle cells cultured from patients with recessive myotonia congenita have confirmed a reduction of at least 50% in the single channel conductance of the predominant chloride channel (Fahlke et al 1993). Linkage has been demonstrated between both the recessive and dominant forms of myotonia congenita and the gene encoding the human muscle chloride channel located at chromosome 7q32-qter (Koch et al 1992, Abdalla et al 1992). Two point mutations in the muscle chloride channel gene have been identified in separate families; one produces a phenylalanine to cysteine substitution in the proposed D8 transmembrane region of the channel while the second replaces a conserved glycine residue in the short loop connecting predicted helices 3 and 4 with glutamic acid (Koch et al 1992, George et al 1994). However, while neither of these mutations was found as a polymorphism in normal controls, proof of the causal relationship between the amino acid substitutions and the reduced chloride channel conductance still awaits functional expression of mutant channels in vitro.

Termination of the myotonic discharge. Results of computer modelling with skeletal muscles confirm the plausibility of this Cl⁻ hypothesis and indicate that repetitive activity can occur when the membrane Cl⁻ conductance is reduced to about 15% of normal, a value near the residual conductance found in these myotonic syndromes (Bretag 1973, Barchi 1975, Adrian & Marshall 1976). This modelling has been useful in demonstrating the sensitivity of the repetitive activity to minor changes in sodium channel kinetic parameters; e.g. a slight reduction in the rate of recovery from inactivation can completely abolish myotonic activity in spite of a very low Cl⁻ conductance. In addition, since the magnitude of the actual depolarisation which occurs depends on the K^+ equilibrium potential, small changes in the concentration of K^+ bathing the sarcolemma itself can prevent the appearance of repetitive activity. For example, a slight reduction in external K^+, of a magnitude expected with the activation of the Na^+-K^+-ATPase, will block repetitive firing, as well as the slight hyperpolarisation produced by the electrogenic activity of this pump.

Although the precise factors that alter the frequency of a myotonic discharge and ultimately cause it to stop in a given fibre are unknown, it is easy to speculate on how one or more of these factors could be involved. Continued muscular activity will certainly result in the influx of sufficient Na^+ to activate the Na^+-K^+-ATPase. This activation will have a hyperpolarising electrogenic component, and could equally well result in a transient decline in local K^+ concentration outside the sarcolemma. Both factors will slow down the frequency of, or stop, the myotonic discharge. Furthermore, the kinetic parameters of normal sodium channels vary over a considerable range and are probably modulated by cellular processes such as phosphorylation that remain to be completely elucidated. This sort of modulation could also play an important role in modifying myotonic activity.

Hyperactivity vs. paralysis. Why does the depolarisation following an action potential in a myotonic discharge produce hyperexcitability while the depolarisation associated with periodic paralysis results in the loss of all electrical excitability? Part of the answer lies in the magnitude of the depolarisation. In myotonia, the depolarisations are small; they are sufficient to cause some channel activation, yet not large enough to cause a significant increase in steady-state inactivation. A second component is the

time-scale on which the depolarisation takes place. The process of channel activation occurs much more rapidly than inactivation; if this were not so, sodium channels would never open during depolarisation, and an action potential could not be produced. With brief depolarisations, activation tends to predominate. Longer depolarisations will eventually lead to inactivation. In myotonia, these depolarising after-potentials last only for tens of milliseconds. In the periodic paralyses, the magnitude of depolarisation is greater and the duration is indefinite. Here steady-state effects predominate, and the influence of channel inactivation is the controlling factor. At the onset of membrane depolarisation in periodic paralysis, one might expect transient hyperexcitability if the critical criteria of rapidity and extent are satisfied. Indeed, in at least one form of hyperkalaemic periodic paralysis, hyperirritability and myotonic symptoms immediately precede the onset of paralysis. In several other of the periodic paralyses, symptoms of myotonia can be seen in the interictal stages.

Other mechanisms producing membrane hyperexcitability

Low membrane chloride conductance is a common factor that ties together a number of the myotonic disorders, but it certainly does not explain all of them. In myotonic dystrophy, the most common of the human muscle diseases in which myotonia is a major feature, membrane chloride conductance is normal or only slightly reduced (Lipicky 1977). In myotonia produced by 20,25-diazacholesterol, an inhibitor of cholesterol biosynthesis, repetitive electrical activity is again found, although the chloride conductance is reduced only slightly (Furman & Barchi 1981).

Although the exact defect that produces the myotonic activity in these disorders remains to be elucidated, it is clear that other factors in addition to alterations in Cl⁻ conductance can induce repetitive activity in skeletal muscle. One prominent mechanism which can produce repetitive activity is an alteration in the kinetics of channel inactivation. Several polypeptide neurotoxins that kill by interacting with the sodium channel do so by reducing or eliminating channel inactivation.

These toxins characteristically produce repetitive action potentials in excitable membranes exposed to them. Similar repetitive activity follows the application of alkaloid toxins such as veratridine or batrachotoxin to muscle; again, their principal effect is on sodium channel inactivation.

Any factor that delays the rate or extent of channel inactivation is a potential candidate for the production of repetitive electrical activity. With the failure of sodium inactivation, the repolarisation produced by the activation of potassium channels is incomplete, closed sodium channels are immediately available for activation, and opened, non-inactivated channels can contribute directly to the initiation of a new depolarisation phase. These factors could be exogenous, as with the neurotoxins, or could represent endogenous defects in the channel structure or its environment. It is the latter consideration which has made the concept of a generalised defect in the membrane lipid environment so attractive a hypothesis in myotonic muscular dystrophy.

Factors involving channels other than the sodium or chloride channel may also be implicated in the generation of repetitive electrical activity. For example, a common mechanism for periodic bursting activity in neurones and for rhythmical electrical discharges in cardiac pacemaking cells involves the modulation of calcium-dependent K^+ conductances. However, none of these potential mechanisms has yet been implicated in the production of human myotonic activity. Working out the mechanism of myotonia

in myotonic dystrophy remains an elusive yet fertile area for future research.

THE FUTURE

It is clear that several neuromuscular diseases involve either primary or secondary defects in membrane ion channels. These channels were once difficult to study, especially in human skeletal muscle. Most observations were indirect, and restricted to electrophysiological measurements of the transmembrane currents that the channels control.

That situation is changing rapidly. Biochemical approaches to the isolation and characterisation of a number of these channels have already been devised, and immunochemical techniques that allow channel isolation from small quantities of tissue are available. Details of channel structure can be derived through analysis of channel primary sequences, as deduced from the cloning of messenger RNA or analysis of the genomic DNA; again, such techniques are now applicable to small amounts of tissue. Patch-clamp methods allow individual ion channels to be studied directly in the muscle membrane, and in vitro expression techniques make it possible to measure the single-channel electrophysiological properties of these channels and their mutants.

The stage is now set for rapid advances in the study of disorders characterised by hyperexcitability or hypoexcitability of the muscle membrane and for direct analysis of the relationships between abnormal structure and function in the channel proteins themselves.

REFERENCES

Abdallah J A, Casley W L, Hudson A J et al 1992 Linkage analysis of candidate loci in autosomal dominant myotonia congenita, Neurology 42: 1561

Adrian R H, Chandler W K, Hodgkin A L 1970 Voltage clamp experiments in striated muscle fibres. Journal of Physiology (London) 208: 607

Adrian R H, Bryant S H 1974 On the repetitive discharge in myotonic muscle fibres. Journal of Physiology (London) 240: 505

Adrian R H, Marshall M W 1976 Action potentials reconstructed in normal and myotonic muscle fibres. Journal of Physiology (London) 258: 125

Adrian R H, Marshall M W 1977 Sodium currents in mammalian muscle. Journal of Physiology (London) 268: 233

Almers W 1972 Potassium conductance changes in skeletal muscle and the potassium concentration in the transverse tubules. Journal of Physiology (London) 225: 33

Auld V J, Goldin A L, Krafte D S, Catterall W A et al 1990 A neutral amino acid change in segment IIS4 dramatically alters the gating properties of the voltage-dependent sodium channel. Proceedings of the National Academy of Sciences USA 87: 323

Barchi R L 1975 Myotonia: an evaluation of the chloride hypothesis. Archives of Neurology 32: 175

Barchi R L 1980 Excitation and conduction in nerve. In: Sumner A J (ed) The physiology of peripheral nerve disease. W B Saunders, Philadelphia, pp 1–40

Barchi R L 1982 A mechanistic approach to the myotonic syndromes. Muscle and Nerve 5 (suppl 9): s60

Barchi R L, Furman R E 1991 Pathophysiology of myotonia and periodic paralysis. In: Asbury A K, McKhann G, McDonald W I (eds) Diseases of the nervous system. W B Saunders, Philadelphia, p 146

Bretag A H 1973 Mathematical modelling of the myotonic action potential. In: Desmedt J E (ed) New developments in electromyography and clinical neurophysiology, vol 1. Karger, Basel, p 464

Brown G L, Harvey A M 1939 Congenital myotonia in the goat. Brain 62: 341

Bryant S H, DeCoursey T E 1980 Sodium currents in cut skeletal muscle fibres from normal and myotonic goats (abstract). Journal of Physiology (London) 307: 31P

Bryant S H 1982 Abnormal repetitive impulse production in myotonic muscle. In: Culp W J, Ochoa J (eds) Abnormal nerves and muscles as impulse generators. Oxford University Press, New York, p 702

Bryant S H, Morales-Aguilera A 1971 Chloride conductance in normal and myotonic muscle fibres and the action of monocarboxylic aromatic acids. Journal of Physiology (London) 219: 367

Bryant S H 1979 Myotonia in the goat. Annals of the New York Academy of Sciences 317: 314

Bryant S H, Owenburg K 1980 Characteristics of the chloride channel in skeletal-muscle fibers from myotonic and normal goats. Federal Proceedings 39: 579

Bucher N L 1946 Effects of 2,4-dichlorophenoxyacetic acid on experimental animals. Proceedings of the Society for Experimental Biology and Medicine 63: 204

Butler A, Wei A, Salkoff L 1990 Shal, Shab, and Shaw: three genes encoding potassium channels in Drosophila. Nucleic Acids Research 18: 2173

Cannon S C, Brown R H, Corey D P 1991 A sodium channel defect in hyperkalemic periodic paralysis: potassium-induced failure of inactivation. Neuron 4: 619

Chandy K G, Williams C B, Spencer R H, Aguilar B A et al 1990 A family of three mouse potassium channel genes with intronless coding regions. Science 247: 973

Cohen S A, Barchi R L 1992 Voltage-dependent sodium channels. In: Friedlander M, Mueckler M (eds) Molecular biology of membrane transport. Academic Press, San Diego, in press

Creutzfeldt O D, Abbott B C, Fowler W M, Pearson C M 1963 Muscle membrane potentials in episodic adynamia. Electroencepholography and Clinical Neurophysiology 15: 508

Davisson M, Harris B, Lane P 1989 Chromosomal location of ADR. Mouse Newsletter 83: 167

Ebers G, George A L, Barchi R L, Ting-Passador S S et al 1991 Paramyotonia congenita and hyperkalemic periodic paralysis are linked to the adult muscle sodium channel gene. Annals of Neurology 30: 810

Engel A G, Lambert E H 1969 Calcium activation of electrically inexcitable muscle fibers in primary hypokalemic periodic paralysis. Neurology 19: 851

Entrikin R, Abresch R, Sharman R, Larson D, Levine N 1987 Contractile and EMG studies of murine myotonia (mto) and muscular dystrophy (dy/dy). Muscle and Nerve 10: 293

Fahlke C, Zachar E, Rudel R 1993 Chloride channels with reduced single-channel conductance in recessive myotonia congenita. Neuron 10: 225

Fleischer S, Inui M 1989 Biochemistry and biophysics of excitation–contraction coupling. Annual Review of Biophysics and Biophysical Chemistry 18: 333

Fontaine B, Khurana T S, Hoffman E P, Bruns G A et al 1990 Hyperkalemic periodic paralysis and the adult muscle sodium channel alpha-subunit gene. Science 250: 1000

Furman R E, Barchi R L 1978 The pathophysiology of myotonia produced by aromatic caboxylic acids. Annals of Neurology 4: 357

Furman R E, Barchi R L 1981 20,25-Diazacholesterol myotonia: an electrophysiological study. Annals of Neurology 10: 251

Gallant E M 1983 Barium-treated mammalian skeletal muscle: similarities to hypokalemic periodic paralysis. Journal of Physiology (London) 335: 577

George A L, Ledbetter D H, Kallen R G, Barchi R L 1991 Assignment of a human skeletal muscle sodium channel α-subunit gene (SCN4A) to 17q23.1–25.3. Genomics 9: 555

George A L, Komisarof J, Kallen R G, Barchi R L 1992 Primary structure of the adult skeletal muscle voltage-dependent sodium channel. Annals of Neurology 31: 131

George A L, Iyer G S, Kleinfield R, Kallen R G, Barchi R L 1993 Genomic organization of the adult skeletal muscle sodium channel gene. Genomics 15: 598

George A L, Crackower M A, Abdalla J A, Hudson A J, Ebers G C 1994 A mutation in the skeletal muscle chloride channel gene causes autosomal dominant myotonia congenita. In press

Gordon A M, Green J R, Lagunoff D 1970 Studies on a patient with hypokalemic familial periodic paralysis. American Journal of Medicine 48: 185

Guy H R, Conti F 1990 Pursuing the structure and function of voltage-gated ion channels. Trends in Neurological Sciences 13: 201

Hartshorne R P, Catterall W A 1984 The sodium channel from rat brain: purification and subunit composition. Journal of Biological Chemistry 159: 1667

Heinemann S H, Terlau H, Stühmer W, Imoto K, Numa S 1992 Calcium channel characteristics conferred on the sodium channel by single mutations. Nature 356: 441

Heller A, Eicher E, Hallett M, Sidman R 1982 Myotonia, a new inherited muscle disease in mice. Journal of Neuroscience 2: 924

Hille B 1986 Ionic channels: molecular pores of excitable membranes. Harvey Lectures 82: 47

Hodgkin A L, Huxley A F 1952 A quantitative description of membrane current and its application to conduction and excitation in nerve. Journal of Physiology (London) 117: 500

Hofmann W W, Smith R A 1970 Hypokalemic periodic paralysis studied in vitro. Brian 93: 445

Horn R, Patlack J 1980 Single channel currents from excised patches of muscle membrane. Proceedings of the National Academy of Sciences USA 11: 6930

Hutter O F, Noble D 1960 The chloride conductance of frog skeletal muscle. Journal of Physiology (London) 151: 89

Isom L L, De Jongh K S, Patton D E, Reber B F X et al 1992 Primary structure and functional expression of the β_1 subunit of the rat brain sodium channel. Science 256: 839

Jentsch T, Steinmeyer K, Schwarz G 1990 Primary structure of *Torpedo marmorata* chloride channel isolated by expression cloning in Xenopus oocytes. Nature 348: 510

Kallen R G, Sheng Z H, Yang J, Chen L, Rogart R B, Barchi R L 1990 Primary structure and expression of a sodium channel characteristic of denervated and immature rat skeletal muscle. Neuron 4: 233

Kallen R G, Cohen S A, Barchi R L 1993 Structure, function and expression of voltage-dependent sodium channels. Molecular Neurobiology 7: 383

Kao I, Gordon A M 1975 Mechanism of insulin produced paralysis of muscle from potassium-depleted rats. Science 188: 740

Koch M C, Ricker K, Otto M, Grimm T et al 1991 Confirmation of linkage of hyperkalemic periodic paralysis to chromosome 17. Journal of Medical Genetics 28: 583

Koch M C, Steinmeyer K, Lorenz C, Ricker K, Wolf F, Otto M, Zoll B, Lehmann-Horn F, Grzeschik K-H, Jentsch T 1992 The skeletal muscle chloride channel in dominant and recessive human myotonia. Science 7: 797

Kolb H A 1990 Potassium channels in excitable and nonexcitable cells. Review of Physiology, Biochemistry and Pharmacology 115: 93

Lehmann-Horn F, Rüdel R, Dengler R, Lorkovic H, Haas A, Ricker K 1981 Membrane defects in paramyotonia congenita with and without myotonia in a warm environment. Muscle and Nerve 4: 396

Lehmann-Horn F, Rüdel R, Ricker K, Lorkovic H, Dengler R, Hopf H C 1983 Two cases of adynamia episodica hereditaria: in vitro investigation of muscle cell membrane and contraction parameters. Muscle and Nerve 6: 113

Lehmann-Horn F, Küther G, Ricker K, Grafe P, Ballanyi K, Rüdel R 1987 Adynamia episodica hereditaria with myotonia: a non-inactivating sodium current and the effect of extracellular pH. Muscle and Nerve 10: 363

Lipicky R J 1977 Studies in human myotonic dystrophy. In: Rowland L P (ed) Pathogenesis of human muscular dystrophies. Excerpta Medica, Amsterdam, p 729

Lipicky R J, Bryant S H, Salmon J H 1971 Cable parameters, sodium, potassium, chloride and water content, and potassium efflux in isolated external intercostal muscles of normal volunteers and patients with myotonia congenita. Journal of Clinical Investigation 50: 2091

Lipicky R J, Bryant S H 1973 A biophysical study of human myotonias. In: Desmedt J E (ed) New developments in electromyography and clinical neurophysiology, vol 1. Karger, Basel, p 451

MacKinnon R 1991 Determination of the subunit stoichiometry of a voltage-activated potassium channel. Nature 350: 232

McClatchey A I, Van den Bergh P, Pericak-Vance M A, Rasking W et al 1992a Temperature-sensitive mutations in the III–IV cytoplasmic loop region of the skeletal muscle sodium channel gene in paramyotonia congenita. Cell 68: 769

McClatchey A I, McKenna-Yasek D, Cros D et al 1992b Novel mutations in families with unusual and variable disorders of the skeletal muscle sodium channel. Nature Genetics 2: 148

McComas A J, Mrozek K, Bradley W G 1968 The nature of the electrophysiological disorder in adynamia episodica. Journal of Neurology, Neurosurgery and Psychiatry 31: 448

Mehrke G, Brinkmeier H, Jockusch H 1988 The myotonic mouse mutant adr: electrophysiology of the muscle fiber. Muscle and Nerve 11: 440

Neher E, Sakmann B 1976 Single channel currents recorded from the membrane of denervated frog muscle fibers. Nature (London) 260: 799

Noda M, Suzuki H, Numa S, Stühmer W 1989 A single point mutation confers tetrodotoxin and saxitoxin insensitivity on the sodium channel II. FEBS Letters 259: 213

Palade P T, Barchi R L 1977a Characteristics of the chloride conductance in muscle fibers of the rat diaphragm. Journal of General Physiology 69: 325

Palade P T, Barchi R L 1977b On the inhibition of muscle membrane chloride conductances by aromatic carboxylic acids. Journal of General Physiology 69: 875

Papazian D M, Schwarz T L, Tempel B L, Jan Y N, Jan L Y 1987 Cloning of genomic and complementary DNA from Shaker, a putative potassium channel gene from Drosophila. Science 237: 749

Ptacek L J, Trimmer J S, Agnew W S, Roberts J W, Petajan J H, Leppert M 1991a Paramyotonia congenita and hyperkalemic periodic paralysis map to the same sodium channel gene locus. American Journal of Human Genetics 49: 851

Ptacek L J, Tyler F, Trimmer J S, Agnew W S, Leppert M 1991b Analysis in large hyperkalemic periodic paralysis pedigree supports tight linkage to a sodium channel locus. American Journal of Human Genetics 49: 378

Ptacek L J, George A L, Griggs R C, Tawil R et al 1991c Identification of a mutation in the gene causing hyperkalemic periodic paralysis. Cell 67: 1021

Ptacek L J, George A L, Barchi R L, Griggs R C et al 1992a Mutations in an S4 segment of the adult skeletal muscle sodium channel cause paramyotonia congenita. Neuron 8: 891

Ptacek L J, Tawil R, Griggs R C et al 1992b Linkage of atypical myotonia congenita to a sodium channel locus. Neurology 42: 431

Ptacek L J, Gouw L, Kwiecinski H et al 1992c Sodium channel mutations in paramyotonia and hyperkalemic periodic paralysis. Annals of Neurology 33: 300

Reininghaus J, Füchtbauer E-M, Bertran K, Jockusch H 1988 The myotonic mouse mutant adr: physiological and histochemical properties of muscle. Muscle and Nerve 11: 433

Riecker G, Bolte J D 1976 Membranpotentiale einzelner skeletmuskelzellen bei hypokalämischer periodischer muskelparalyse. Klinische Wochenschrift 44: 804

Roberds S, Tankum M 1991 Cloning and tissue-specific expression of five voltage-gated potassium channel cDNAs expressed in rat heart. Proceedings of the National Academy of Sciences USA 88: 1798

Roberts R, Barchi R L 1987 The voltage-sensitive sodium channel from rabbit skeletal muscle: chemical characterization of subunits. Journal of Biological Chemistry 262: 2298

Rojas C V, Wang J, Schwartz L S, Hoffman E P, Powel B R, Brown R H 1991 A Met-to-Val mutation in the skeletal muscle sodium channel α-subunit in hyperkalemic periodic paralysis. Nature 354: 387

Rüdel R 1990 The myotonic mouse — a realistic model for the study of human recessive generalized myotonia. Trends in Neuroscience 13: 1

Rüdel R, Senges J 1972 Experimental myotonia in mammalian skeletal muscle. Changes in membrane properties. Pfluegers Archives 331: 324

Rüdel R, Lehmann-Horn F, Ricker K, Kuther G 1984 Hypokalemic periodic paralysis: in vitro investigation of muscle fiber membrane parameters. Muscle and Nerve 7: 110

Rüdel R, Lehmann-Horn, F 1985 Membrane changes in cells from myotonia patients. Physiological Review 65: 310

Rüdel R, Ricker K 1985 The primary periodic paralyses. Trends in Neurosciences 8: 467

Shy G M, Wanko T, Rowley P T, Engel A G 1961 Studies in familial periodic paralysis. Experimental Neurology 3: 53

Skou J 1990 The energy-coupled exchange of Na^+ for K^+

across the cell membrane: the $Na^+ K^+$ pump. FEBS Letters 268: 314

Steinmeyer K, Klocke R, Ortland C et al 1991a Inactivation of muscle chloride channel by transposon insertion in myotonic mice. Nature 354: 304

Steinmeyer K, Ortland C, Jentsch T 1991b Primary structure and functional expression of a developmentally regulated skeletal muscle chloride channel. Nature 354: 301

Stühmer W 1991 Structure–function studies of voltage-gated ion channels. Annual Review of Biophysics and Biophysical Chemistry 20: 65

Stühmer W, Conti F, Suzuki H, Wang X et al 1989 Structural parts involved in activation and inactivation of the sodium channel. Nature 339: 597

Swift L L, Atkinson J B, Lequire V S 1979 Composition and calcium-transport activity of the sarcoplasmic-reticulum from goats with and without heritable myotonia. Laboratory Investigation 40: 384

Tang A H, Schroeder L A, Keasling H H 1968 U-23,223 (3-chloro-2,5,6-trimethylbenzoic acid), a veratrinic agent selective for the skeletal muscles. Archives of Internal Pharmacodynamics 175: 319

Trimmer J S, Cooperman S S, Tomiko S A, Zhou J et al 1989 Primary structure and functional expression of a mammalian skeletal muscle sodium channel. Neuron 3: 33

Vassilev P, Scheuer T, Catterall W A 1989 Inhibition of inactivation of single sodium channel by a site-directed antibody. Proceedings of the National Academy of Sciences USA 86: 8147

Watkins W, Watts D 1984 Developmental changes in lactate dehydrogenase and aldolase activity of the A2D-adr mouse with abnormal muscle function: further comparison with the 129Re-dy mutant. Journal of Neurochemistry 43: 517

Wood D S, Lipicky R J, Bryant S H 1980 Myotonic dystrophy: in vitro physiologic analysis of intact and skinned fibers. Neurology 30: 423

12. Experimental and animal models of human neuromuscular disease

B. A. Kakulas   B. J. Cooper

INTRODUCTION

In the past a fruitful source of information about the mechanisms underlying muscle damage in human disease has been by experiment. Thus the effects of ischaemia, infection, myotoxins and denervation have been thoroughly investigated in the laboratory. A further approach was the creation of animal models of the human counterpart using a variety of techniques, some immunological, others nutritional and so forth.

Another approach has been the study of naturally occurring, mostly inherited diseases in animals that have a human equivalent. In this way md 129 and dydy mice have been very useful. This aspect of research received a major impetus when exact homologues of Duchenne (DMD) and Becker muscular dystrophy (BMD) were identified in mutant animals. These include the mdx mouse with X-linked muscular dystrophy discovered by Bulfield et al (1984), followed by similar diseases being identified in the dog and cat. Notably the Golden Retriever muscular dystrophy (GRMD, or the xmd dog) is hailed as a very useful model for DMD. These animal homologues for DMD soon became known as the animal 'dystrophinopathies'.

This chapter reviews the experimentally induced and naturally occurring models of human muscle diseases, highlighting the insights which have been gained. Amongst the many neuromuscular diseases that occur in animals, those that are legitimate models of human disease are emphasised.

THE EFFECT OF TRAUMA

Simple section and crush are popular methods of investigating the reaction to injury of the muscle fibre. In both instances necrosis is soon followed by regeneration so that a model is produced for the histochemical and electron-microscopic evaluation of such reactions.

Following the classic studies of simple crush by Clark (1946) and Clark & Wajda (1947), regeneration after crush was investigated electron-microscopically by Allbrook (1962). These workers confirmed the classic observations of Volkmann (1893). The seminal observations of Clark (1946) were later greatly extended (Reznik 1973). The events which follow localised crush injury to muscle in the first few hours consist of altered morphology with obscured markings. Necrosis, evident as fragmentation and disintegration of sarcoplasm, is followed by phagocytosis of debris, spindle cell proliferation and 'isomorphic' regeneration.

Tongue-like myotubes are readily identified in massive trauma which is little studied experimentally. The experimental findings are similar to those which occur in accidental massive injury to muscle in man (Anastas & Kakulas 1968). Such lesions may be present clinically as tumorous masses and in this case they are the equivalent in muscle of the 'traumatic' neuroma of peripheral nerve.

Needle myopathy

These lesions are characterised initially by haemorrhagic focal destruction followed by cellular infiltration, local necrosis and single fibre degeneration, regeneration and dystrophy-like changes. After several weeks the muscle returns to normal (Mumenthaler & Paakkari 1974).

Muscle transplantation

This has attracted increasing attention in recent years and numerous reports have appeared (Mauro et al 1970). Factors which affect the success of transplantation of skeletal muscle in the rat were studied by Gutmann & Hanzlikova (1975). The 'morphogenetic effects of cross-transplantation of muscle upon the epimorphic regenerative process', were examined in detail by Carlson (1974). The host reaction of muscle grafts in mice was investigated by Mastaglia et al (1974). Partridge & Sloper (1977) were able to demonstrate a host contribution to the regeneration in muscle heterografts.

Sola et al (1985) have been successful in the transplantation of skeletal muscle grafted into the heart of dogs, a technique finding application in human myocardioplasty operations.

Physical methods

Temperature changes. Experimentally induced temperature changes are known to cause coagulative necrosis (Adams 1975). Gutmann & Guttmann (1942) studied the effect of electrical stimulation upon the prevention of changes secondary to denervation. Nageotte (1937) reported a shredding effect in muscle fibres produced by electrically induced severe contraction in vitro. Muscle changes caused by electrical stimulation have been described by a number of workers (Smith et al 1965). The lesions were produced by AC and DC electrical discharge through the fore- and hind-limbs of dogs. Skin and subcutaneous tissues were not injured but the skeletal muscle showed subsarcolemmal nuclear proliferation, loss of striations, vacuolisation and ultimately frank necrosis. Changes were indistinguishable, regardless of the type and polarity of the discharge. Ring fibres were not found, although these are reported to be easily produced by tendon-cutting (Bethlem & van Wijngaarden 1963), which also produced target fibres (De Reuck et al 1977). In addition to necrosis caused by burns, super-contraction of myofibrils and nuclear streaming result from electrical injury.

Examination of the ultrastructure of freeze-injured muscle fibres shows dissolution of organelles and rarefaction of myofibrils. Such injuries in partly affected muscle fibres result in the appearance of large numbers of ribosomes as a sign of early repair.

X-irradiation. Skeletal muscle is relatively resistant to X-irradiation as it is a highly differentiated tissue. The effects of massive experimental X-irradiation were described in the studies of Warren (1943) who considered the vascular changes to be primary. Aminoaciduria resulting from whole-body irradiation was reported (Goyer & Yin 1967). Khan (1974) studied radiation-induced changes in skeletal muscle under the electron microscope.

Nutritional disorders

As already indicated, there are many natural myopathies in animals deserving experimental enquiry, which are also the subject of therapeutic trials. Studies of these disorders have provided useful information in relation to the possible aetiology and pathogenesis of human muscle diseases. Many of these animal disorders are genetically determined and some are true muscular dystrophies; however, many others result from nutritional deficiencies or are caused by toxic agents. The most common nutritional disorder is vitamin E deficiency, which is sometimes associated with selenium deficiency. Otherwise electrolyte disturbances, such as hypokalaemia, are prominent. Other animal myopathies which can be induced by nutritional factors are the thiamine, choline, vitamin D (dogs) and vitamin C (guinea-pigs) deficiency disorders (Banker 1960).

Vitamin E deficiency is a very potent cause of muscle fibre necrosis and the resulting myopathic effects are well known (Hadlow 1962). Experimental vitamin E deficiency provides much useful information concerning the pathogenesis of muscle lesions in dystrophic states. In this regard the Rottnest Island quokka (*Setonix brachyurus*) has proved to be a most useful model (Kakulas & Adams 1966). Howell & Buxton (1975) described α-tocopherol-responsive muscular dystrophy in guinea-pigs. Muscle fibre necrosis, regeneration and cellular infiltrates were similar to those that were found in the Rottnest Island quokka with nutritional myopathy. Serum CK levels fell in the guinea-pigs and the animals revived after treatment with α-tocopherol.

Vitamin D deficiency results in defective calcium uptake in the sarcoplasmic reticulum and protein deficiency will cause pseudomyopathic changes (Francis et al 1974). Ward & Goldspink (1974) studied the response of different muscle fibre types to changes in the activity pattern in protein malnutrition in the mouse.

Rats placed on an iodine-deficient diet by Rosman et al (1978), in order to produce hypothyroidism, unexpectedly developed progressive muscle weakness. The myopathy was due to deficiency of a number of dietary constituents, only one of which was iodine. Necrosis and atrophy of cells were seen, as well as variability of muscle fibre size and shape.

SPECIAL LESIONS OF MUSCLE

Experimental disuse atrophy

Because reduced mobility is so common in muscle disease, disuse atrophy may be expected to have been the subject of extensive investigation. Myostatic contracture is a phenomenon closely associated with disuse and an understanding of both is essential basic knowledge for those involved in rehabilitation medicine. Joint fixation is rapidly followed by shortening of whole muscle as a result of myostatic contracture. The reduced length is due to the loss of sarcomeres from the muscle fibres, commensurate with the degree of shortening. Experimental studies also demonstrate the reverse effect, i.e. that lengthening of the muscle following a graduated exercise regimen, is due to the addition of more and more sarcomeres at each end of the muscle fibre.

The usual experimental methods utilised in the study of disuse atrophy are either section of a tendon or muscle or skeletal fixation. Such atrophy is also associated with a reduction in muscle fibre diameter and there is a tendency to darkening of the sarcoplasm by the accumulation of lipofuscin pigment ('brown atrophy' of general pathology).

Following division of the lumbosacral spinal cord segments, Eccles (1941) observed 40% loss of muscle bulk in 3 weeks as a result of inactivation of the leg muscles. Other workers such as Ferguson et al (1957) have employed casts. They also found that tension on a muscle, even though it is 'disused', would result in hypertrophy.

The effects of tenotomy have been extensively studied both by the pioneers (Eccles 1944) and more recently by others. Karpati et al (1972) showed that core-like lesions and nemaline rods were produced in type I fibres of the rat following Achilles tenotomy. They also reported that sciatic neurotomy or thoracic cordotomy prevented the development of the core-like lesions, so that intact innervation was a key factor in their formation.

Engel et al (1966) found that tenotomy in the cat resulted in greater atrophy of the soleus, which consists purely of type I fibres. In the gastrocnemius, which is a mixed muscle in the cat, there was greater atrophy of type I fibres and some hypertrophy of type II fibres. Target fibres, rods and sarcoplasmic masses were only observed in the soleus. They also found that tenotomy and denervation resulted in core targetoid fibres in their histochemical studies.

Sarnat and associates (1977) investigated the effects of tenotomy and denervation in the gastrocnemius muscle of the frog. The normal histochemical pattern persisted after denervation and they found that the small fibres of the gastrocnemius underwent further atrophy while the intermediate and large fibres were essentially unchanged 21–46 days after sciatic neurotomy.

Baker & Hall-Craggs (1980) found that the effects of tenotomy in the rat soleus were maximal 1 week postoperatively, after which a period of recovery occurred. Core targetoid fibres appeared within a few days of tenotomy and were maximal after 1 week when examined by electron-microscopy. Baker & Hall-Craggs (1980) reported a reduction in sarcomere length following tenotomy. They were also able to demonstrate the appearance of 'unstructured cores' in the tenotomised muscle after 1 week. Muscle histology returned to normal in 6 weeks.

In a further study by Baker (1983) it was found that, after tenotomy and within the first few days, the affected fibres of the soleus underwent a complete morphological reorganisation. Initially necrosis with phagocytosis occurred, especially near the tendon. He also found that, by the seventh day, the fibres with central core lesions were associated with regeneration of myofibrils at the periphery of the fibre and this regeneration continued to complete reconstruction. Chou (1984) extensively reviews the topic of the experimental and natural 'core-genic neuro-myopathies' in conjunction with his own experimental observations.

Central cores, targetoid changes, snake coils, Z-band streaming and necrosis, all induced by tenotomy, are illustrated in Figures 12.1 and 12.2.

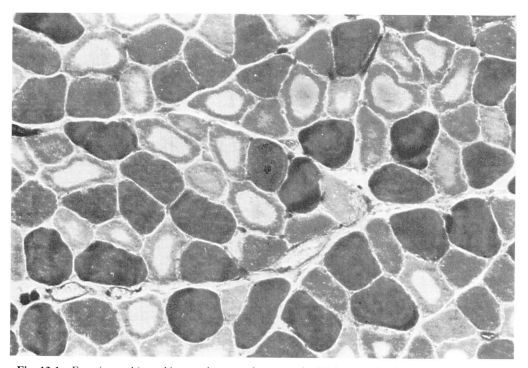

Fig. 12.1   Experimental 'cores' in rat soleus muscle tenotomised 7 days previously. The central zones of many muscle fibres fail to stain by the ATPase method at pH 4.6. The muscle fibres with central core-like lesions are probably histochemical type I (× 512).

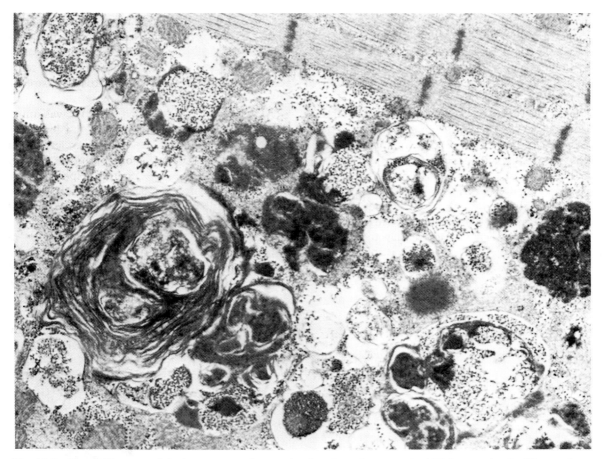

Fig. 12.2   Muscle fibre necrosis in the gastrocnemius muscle of a guinea-pig tenotomised 30 days previously. All normal organelles are lost, except for rarified sarcomeres (top right), and are replaced by myelin figures, dense bodies, lysosomes, and abundant glycogen granules (EM, × 25 300).

Bourne (1973) investigated the effect of zero gravity. In addition to the atrophic changes, he reported circulatory disturbances, redistribution of body fluids and other effects of weightlessness on muscle.

Mendell (1979) in his extensive review of the histochemistry of experimental myopathology, noted that in general disuse caused preferential type II fibre atrophy. He also described the histochemistry of increased muscle usage, joint fixation, cordotomy and tenotomy with or without nerve section.

Experimental hypertrophy

Experimental investigation has established that the stimulus for hypertrophy is simple use or work. Controlled exercise of the muscle of laboratory animals shows that hypertrophy occurs only when a muscle contracts with a force greater than that to which it is usually accustomed. For hypertrophy to occur, the contraction should be close to the maximum power generated. The stimulus is related more to the intensity than to the duration of the effort.

The classic work on exercise hypertrophy is that of Morpurgo (1897) who measured the sartorius muscles of dogs before and after exercising on running wheels for a 2-month period. He reported that the number of fibres increased very slightly in each muscle and that hypertrophy of the order of 55% occurred under these conditions. He found that the enlargement was due almost entirely to an increase in the diameter of the individual muscle fibres. He assumed that each enlarged fibre contained a greater number of myofibrils, an observation which was later confirmed by Denny-Brown in 1951.

Endocrine effects on muscle hypertrophy have been little studied. Papanicolaou & Falk (1938) showed that the temporal muscle of the male guinea-pig, which is normally larger than that of the female, remained small if the animal was castrated at puberty. On the other hand, androgenic hormones injected into females caused enlargement of their temporal muscles. Similar effects have been shown for somatotrophin by Bigland & Jehring (1952) who found the number of muscle fibres to be increased in rats treated with somatotrophin.

Experimental denervation atrophy

The close interaction of nerve and muscle has been the subject of investigation and conjecture from the beginning of the serious study of muscle disease. The dependence of muscle on an intact nerve supply, in order to maintain its size, is a longstanding clinical observation. Almost immediately, hypothetical trophic factors were postulated in the last century, as mediators of the phenomenon. The trophic factors which could theoretically exist number more than 15; however, perhaps only one such factor has really been identified, namely acetylcholine, and even this well-known neurotransmitter may not be the actual trophic factor itself (Kakulas & Adams 1985). Trophic factors are postulated for the maintenance of normal fibre size, membrane stability, reinnervation, end-plate production, hypertrophy, splitting, regeneration and histochemical specificity of muscle fibres. It has also been suggested that the human congenital myopathies, many of which show dysmorphic features, may reflect disturbances of a trophic nature (Engel 1979).

Numerous reports of the effects of denervation, as observed by light microscopy, histochemical studies and electron microscopy are in existence. The first experimental investigation which identified the functional and histochemical specificity of motor units was that of Eccles (1941, 1944). The work of Buller et al (1960) on the physiological relationship between motor nerve and muscle is now well known. Edstrom & Kugelberg (1968) elegantly confirmed Eccles' observation by histochemical means. It is now well established that the special functional qualities of a motor unit are dictated by the motor neurone to its muscle fibres; this fact is used in routine muscle biopsy diagnosis. The denervation studies of Kugelberg et al (1970) defined the histochemical specificity of muscle fibre types within individual motor units. Peter (1973), in a full review of this subject, concluded that the particular histochemical qualities of a fibre type are governed by the physiological function of the motor unit rather than by anterior horn cell 'trophic' specificity. The histochemical type is thus determined by physiological demand rather than by an 'immutable' motor unit-specific determinant.

There is considerable interest in the definition of trophic and developmental influences in fetal muscle under experimental conditions and denervation is employed in such studies (Margreth et al 1974). In the biochemistry of denervated muscle, attention was paid to protein synthesis and oxidation by Gauthier & Schaeffer (1975) and by Kark et al (1975).

Myographic and electroneurographic responses of leg muscles to cross-innervated sciatic nerves are reported to be normal in dystrophic mice united by parabiosis (Douglas 1974). The investigation of neurotrophic influences has extended to the investigation of intramuscular injection of spinal cord homogenate. Such studies demonstrate enhancement of protein synthesis (Crockett & Edgerton 1974).

The histochemistry of regenerating myofibres before and after reinnervation was studied to determine the role of 'trophic influences' in creating 'type specificity' of muscle fibres (Reznik 1973, Manolov 1974). It was found that differentiation of regenerated myofibres into several types begins 4–5 weeks after injury and is related to reinnervation. Unusual checkerboard distributions of type I and type II fibres and heterogeneous myofibres occur in the major part of a muscle which, before injury, contained type II fibres almost exclusively. Additionally, large and small regenerating myofibres had end-plates which were often abnormal. The results suggest that axons sprouting from different motor units proliferate in the same area and innervate new myofibres at random. Such modifications are quite different from the fibre type grouping described after spontaneous or experimentally induced reinnervation of normal myofibres.

Denervation caused the appearance of central nuclei and muscle fibre splitting with eventual loss of architecture in the experimental myopathy induced by paroxan and organophosphorus (Wecker & Dettbarn 1977).

The more recent histochemical and electron-microscopic studies of the effects of denervation are fully reviewed by Mendell (1979) and details of the observations of the pioneers of experimental denervation may be found in Kakulas & Adams (1985).

Post-denervation hypertrophy

The paradoxical phenomenon of 'denervation hypertrophy' is of considerable experimental interest. Formation of new muscle fibres, i.e. hyperplasia, as well as true hypertrophy (of 'intermediate' fibres) is produced in the diaphragm of most species and the anterior latissimus dorsi muscle of chickens (Sola et al 1973).

Experimental ischaemia

Experimentally induced muscle ischaemia has been studied in the past because of its relevance to human myopathology. Apart from circulatory disorders as such, an ischaemic component may occur as a result of polyarteritis nodosa or other vasculitides. A reduced capillary bed is found in dermatomyositis. Early experiments were conducted by Clark (1946) who produced necrosis by ligation of the vessels to the anterior tibial muscle or by excision and replacement of that muscle. He described absence of nuclei, fragmentation of sarcoplasm with generally intact membranes, followed by infiltration with neutrophils and macrophages in early ischaemic lesions. The process rapidly evolved with massive phagocytosis of the necrotic muscle. Regeneration appeared in the form of sprouts from intact muscle at the border of the ischaemic area and the new muscle fibres rapidly grew down the endomysial tubes. Fibrosis was proportional to the degree of haemorrhage. Clark & Wajda (1947) showed the rate of regeneration to be 1.5 mm per day becoming complete in about 3 months. The importance of the endomysial tubes in regeneration was thus demonstrated in their experiments, a consistent finding in other experimental myopathies.

Engel (1973) induced focal muscle fibre necrosis in rabbits using microembolisation. His interest was to compare such experimental lesions with those of Duchenne muscular dystrophy in which grouped muscle fibre necrosis is a feature. The contribution of ischaemia to the dystrophic lesion continues to be an open question.

Karpati et al (1974) also studied the effects of ischaemia on muscle. Ligation of the abdominal aorta in rats produced ischaemic lesions in the gastrocnemius muscles which were examined by histochemistry and electron-microscopy. The first lesions were observed in type IIC muscle fibres. Acid phosphatase activity increased prior to phagocytosis. ATPase activity was not lost until invasion by phagocytes. Electron-microscopic changes were observed within a few hours, consisting of vacuolation of mitochondria and disruption of the plasma membrane with streaming or loss of the Z discs. Grouped and focal necrosis was observed 4–7 days after ligation. Karpati et al (1974) reported in long-term experiments that no necrotic fibres were observed 1–4 months after the aortic occlusion; however central nuclei remained prominent.

Experimental myotoxicity

Skeletal muscles are prone to injury by drugs and toxins. As a result, numerous toxic chemicals have been investigated for their effects on the muscle fibre. There are also many 'iatrogenic' drug-induced myopathies known clinically and which are the subject of experimental investigation (Kakulas 1982, Kakulas & Adams 1985, also see Ch. 28).

The effect of metabolic poisons. Powerful metabolic poisons are commonly used in experimental myopathology; e.g. iodoacetate

(Lundsgaard 1930), which blocks lactate production by the inhibition of glyceraldehyde-3-phosphate dehydrogenase, causes massive rhabdomyolysis. A metabolic myopathy which may be induced in rabbits by hypoglycaemia following administration of insulin (Tannenberg 1939) is associated with single fibre necrosis in both cardiac and skeletal muscle. Another chemical agent investigated experimentally is imidazole, which accelerates the catabolism of cyclic AMP and is associated with myopathic changes in the gastrocnemius muscle of rats (Fenichel & Martin 1974).

Such chemical myopathies usually cause pure sarcoplasmic necrosis and spare the endomysial fibrous tissue sheaths. Because of this, in the recovery phase following withdrawal of the agent, connective tissue proliferation is minimal and the muscle regeneration is complete. These experimental conditions bear a resemblance to a number of natural and drug-induced metabolic myopathies in man. Again, regeneration is complete when the cause is removed.

Jasmin & Gareau (1961) studied with light microscopy the skeletal muscle lesions produced in rats injected with diphenylenediamine. Swelling and homogenisation were visible in 24 hours followed by coagulative necrosis. The necrotic muscle segments acted as foreign bodies and gave rise to a histiocytic reaction of multinucleated giant cells. Regenerative changes occurred parallel to the severity of the lesions with regeneration and integrity restored in less than 20 days. Mascres & Jasmin (1975) later used ρ-phenylenediamine (PPD) to investigate the inflammatory and degenerative patterns of muscle lesions in rats. Fifteen minutes after the injection of PPD, subsarcolemmal oedema was visible in the diaphragm under the electron-microscope. Enzymatic changes appeared in the first hour while pathological features were prominent after 24 hours. There was segmental necrosis adjacent to unaltered fibres and several particular types of abnormal fibres such as target, snake coils and core fibres were seen.

Uraemic myopathy may be produced in rats. In this disorder, atrophy of type I fibres occurs but there are no other structural changes (Bundschu et al 1974).

Graham et al (1976) reported that core forma-

tion was observed in the muscle of rats intoxicated by triethyltin sulphate (TET). The changes affected only the type I fibres and were observed in the thigh muscles of animals intoxicated with TET for up to 23 days. The development of core-like structures, which occur after tenotomy in association with nemaline body formation and vacuolar degeneration of muscle fibres, may be compared with those structures which are found after emetine intoxication and in which there are large lesions extending throughout the transverse axis of fibres, associated with loss of oxidative enzyme activity. In contrast, alkyltin intoxication differs in that in this case the central nervous system shows intramyelinic vacuolation.

Biological toxins are powerful myonecrotic agents. Morita (1926) studied the effect of clostridial toxin, such as that from *Clostridium welchii*, which usually destroys connective tissue as well as causing muscle fibre necrosis. The effects of *Clostridium botulinum* were recently studied, with denervation changes being reported by Johnston & Drachman (1974).

Adams (1975) reported fatty degeneration in cardiac muscle after the administration of diphtheria toxin to guinea-pigs. However, no consistent changes in skeletal muscle were observed, and he found that direct inoculation of diphtheria organisms into muscle caused lesions which did not differ from those produced by any bacterial necrosis.

Tiger snake toxin causes skeletal muscle degeneration and subsequent regeneration when injected into the rat (Pluskal et al 1974). The oriental hornet (*Vespa orientalis*) causes a lesion of the muscle transverse-tubular system (Ishay et al 1975). Light-microscopic examination showed that vacuoles appear in the sartorius muscle incubated in hornet venom-Ringer's solution. Under the electron-micsroscope it was observed that these vacuoles were accounted for by greatly distended T tubules and terminal cisternae.

Bacteria and viruses. Bacterial myositis has been studied in the laboratory and the subject was reviewed by Banker (1960) and by Adams (1975). As might be expected, pyogenic organisms cause acute abscesses and similar lesions result from injection of turpentine into muscle. Banker (1960) also discussed parasitic infections of the muscle.

Many viruses are capable of producing experimental myositis, including mouse encephalomyelitis (GD-VII and FA strains) and the Mitchell strain of lymphocytic choriomeningitis virus (Rustigan & Pappenheimer 1949). The Coxsackie viruses (Dalldorf 1950) are especially known to cause myositis and Type A (Field 1960) is more active in this regard.

Arboviruses also cause myositis. It has been demonstrated in this connection that myofibrils are severely damaged with accompanying dilatation of T tubules and of the sarcoplasmic reticulum (SR), with the accumulation of mature arbovirus particles within the cisternae and vacuoles (Sato et al 1974).

Miranda et al (1978) studied influenza virus infection of human skeletal muscle in tissue culture. Using scanning and transmission electron-microscopes they observed cytopathic changes, both in organelles and surface elements. Cell injury and death appear to be caused by massive accumulation of virus-induced products that alter cellular metabolism in vitro.

Alcohol. The adverse effect of alcohol on muscle has been well studied, both experimentally and in patients with alcoholic myopathy, and polyfocal muscle fibre necrosis is found in both situations. Cessation of exposure to ethanol is associated with rapid reversal of the process: necrosis ceases and regeneration proceeds. Electron-microscopic examination shows that all organelles are affected to some degree with changes in the mitochondria and dilatations of the SR occurring in the vicinity of the zones of total necrosis.

Extensive biochemical and morphological studies were carried out by Rubin et al (1976) in volunteers in relation to studies of human alcoholic myopathy. Ultrastructural changes consisted of deformation of mitochondria, dilatation of the SR and increased amounts of fat and glycogen.

Drugs. Drug-induced human myopathies are considered in Chapter 28. Suffice to say that experimental equivalents have been studied for the majority of such conditions.

EXPERIMENTAL MODELS OF HUMAN MYOPATHIES

Most of the induced models of muscle disease are concerned with three human conditions — progressive muscular dystrophy, myasthenia gravis and polymyositis. The human and animal dystrophies are the subject of intensive enquiry because of their devastating clinical effects. To help achieve an understanding of these conditions the natural dystrophies in animals are carefully investigated and attempts are made to reproduce similar myopathies in the laboratory. Some of this research examines simple chemical or physical injury to muscle, as shown above. Other methods, such as microembolisation (Engel 1973) and, more practically, the effects of controlled deprivation of vitamin E (Kakulas & Adams 1966) produce useful models.

Muscular dystrophy

Experimentally induced models for the study of muscular dystrophy have now been overshadowed by the investigation of the animal equivalents of DMD, i.e. the 'dystrophinopathies' and related diseases. These are considered in detail below.

Polymyositis

A variety of experimental methods are used to produce a 'polymyositis-like disorder' in animals. These observations began, indirectly, in 1937 with Kallos & Pagel who observed muscle lesions in rabbits with induced hypersensitivity and bronchial reactions. The suggestion that human polymyositis may be the result of disordered immune function was based on the presence of raised levels of serum globulins in the serum of many patients with the disease, on the sometimes dramatic response to steroid hormones given for therapeutic purposes, and on the known clinical association with disorders of presumed immunological aetiology, e.g. systemic lupus erythematosus (Walton & Adams 1958). An active immunological approach was employed by Pearson in 1956. Although noting that myositis was present, Pearson became more interested in the polyarthritis produced by Freund's adjuvant than in the myositis.

A 'polymyositis-like' condition, subsequently named experimental allergic myositis (EAM), can be produced in rats by immunological methods (Dawkins 1965, Kakulas 1966, 1973). Histological features include focal necrotic and inflammatory changes (Fig. 12.3). Electron-microscopy shows that the necrosis affects all ultrastructural elements, but especially the myofibrils with membranous bodies also prominent.

It has been shown that in vitro transfer of lymphocytes from animals with EAM produces cytotoxic effects in tissue cultures of fetal rat muscle (Kakulas 1966). Similar experiments with slight variations in technique or animal species give essentially similar results (Webb 1970, Currie et al 1971).

The close relationship of the experimental disease to human polymyositis is demonstrated by the presence of in vitro cytotoxic effects of human lymphocytes from patients with the disease, when these cells are applied to human fetal muscle in culture (Kakulas 1970, 1973). In muscle biopsies of patients with polymyositis, lymphocytes and plasma cells are mainly perivenular and appear to be closely related to necrotic foci (Adams 1973).

Experimental studies of EAM are also directed toward determining the nature of the antigen (Esiri & MacLennan 1975). Myofibrillar antigens appear to be more potent than those of other subcellular components of muscle (Manghani et al 1975). These workers established that lymphocytes from myositic animals are sensitised to the outer surface of muscle cells. The macrophage migration inhibition test was used to identify the components within the muscle fibres to which lymphocytes are also sensitised. Their studies indicate that there is lymphocyte sensitization against the myofibrillar fraction and especially against the proteins myosin and tropomyosin. Guinea-pigs injected with rabbit myofibrillar fractions and Freund's adjuvant regularly develop myositis. These animals show many more muscle

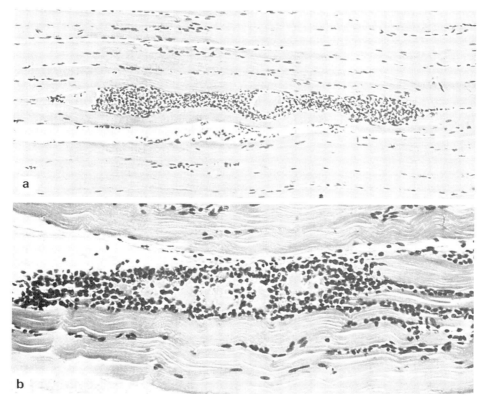

Fig. 12.3 **a** Immunologically induced muscle-fibre necrosis and leucocytic infiltration in guinea-pig following repeated injections of rabbit muscle and adjuvant (H & E, × 112). **b** Focal muscle-fibre necrosis and round-cell collections in rat, produced by similar means (H & E, × 208).

lesions, consisting of areas of round cell infiltration and muscle fibre necrosis, than do those animals given other subcellular fractions.

Penn (1977), in reviewing the pathogenesis of myasthenia gravis, polymyositis and dermato-myositis, concludes that the humoral arm of the defence apparatus appears to be directly responsible for the lesion in myasthenia gravis, but that cellular mechanisms at the thymic regulatory level are also involved. Cytotoxic T-cells seem to produce the lesion of experimental myositis, in which anti-muscle antibodies can be detected, and those cases of polymyositis and dermato-myositis in which antibodies have not been convincingly shown. Childhood dermatomyositis is considered to be a probable exception in which antibodies and complement contribute to under-lying vasculitis. Immunosuppressive measures can modify or prevent disease in experimental models and Penn (1977) believes that the evidence indicates a solid rationale for their use in the human diseases, although much more information is required concerning the site of action and appropriate therapeutic planning.

Animal models for polymyositis and dermato-myositis were recently reviewed (Kakulas 1988). In this survey the autoimmune diseases can be viewed as being the result of an excess in the number and ratio of T-4 helper cells compared to T-8 suppressor lymphocytes, whereas the immuno-depression syndromes are due to a relative excess of the T-8 suppressor cells. That is to say, autoim-mune disease and immunodeficiency syndromes may be regarded as being at opposite ends of a continuous spectrum, or even as mirror images of each other.

Experimental AIDS (acquired immune deficiency syndrome)

Animal models for the experimental study of AIDS are emerging, such as the naturally occur-ring simian AIDS, which is presumably due to virus infection (London et al 1983). In simian AIDS, focal necrosis of muscle fibres with inflammatory infiltrates and inclusion bodies are described. However, the changes are possibly due to an opportunistic infection rather than to the simian AIDS virus itself (Kakulas 1988).

Tumours

Experimentally induced muscle tumours are also the subject of study. In a biochemical report, muscle acid proteinase, alkaline proteinase arylamidase and cathepsin C were increased and cathepsin E 1 was decreased. Cathepsin A autolytic activity and trypsin inhibitory capacity were unchanged in the extensor digitorum muscle (Holmes et al 1974).

Congenital structural myopathies

It is now well known that the mitochondrial myopathies can be induced experimentally by drugs which block oxidative pathways. The best-known model is induced by the administration of 2,4-dinitrophenol: in this case the mitochondria are large, lack the normal cristae and may even contain crystalline inclusions. Mitochondrial abnormalities can also be induced by other agents which block oxidative metabolism (Melmed et al 1975, Sahgal et al 1979). Histochemical prepara-tions of oxidative enzymes provide an experi-mental counterpart for the 'ragged-red fibres' of the human mitochondrial myopathies.

As mentioned above, tenotomy and disuse may produce core-targetoid changes and rod bodies in type I muscle fibres which closely resemble the human central core and nemaline myopathies (Chou 1984) provided that the nerve supply re-mains intact.

Transgenic models

This chapter would be incomplete without some discussion of the potential of transgenic models of muscle disease. Such models, constructed in the laboratory, show great promise for the future exploration of the function of cellular proteins and the pathogenesis of various disease states. They will also allow the development of models of human disease that are as yet unavailable in naturally occurring form, which can be designed and used for the study of various therapeutic approaches.

It is beyond the scope of this chapter to discuss in detail the techniques used to produce trans-genic animals. Nevertheless, it is worth pointing out that several types of models can be made. These include models in which the function of a particular gene is disrupted ('gene knockouts'), models in which particular genes are over-expressed, and models in which the function of a defective gene has been replaced.

Gene knockout models are particularly suited to the engineering of models of human disease. For example, amongst others, murine models of cystic fibrosis have been developed by disruption of the cystic fibrosis transmembrane regulator (CFTR), and of atherosclerosis by disruption of apolipoprotein E (Smithies 1993). Not only are these models useful for the modelling of human diseases, but they often reveal and explain differences in the expression of genetic diseases between humans and animal models. This has been the case, for example, in cystic fibrosis, where the transgenic mice express severe intestinal disease but only mild pancreatic disease.

In the case of muscle disease, there are, so far, no published reports on the modelling of specific myopathies using this approach. However, reports have begun to appear in which the role of specific genes and gene products in muscle function and development are being explored. For example the function of the myogenic transcription factors myoD and myf-5 has been studied in transgenic knockout models by Rudnicki and co-workers. The results of some of these experiments are surprising. For example, inactivation of the myoD gene results in no apparent morphological or functional abnormalities of muscle (Rudnicki et al 1992). Homozygous mutant mice are viable and fertile. Expression of a variety of muscle-specific genes and proteins, as assessed by immunohisto-chemistry and northern blotting, was normal, as was the fibre type pattern, as assessed by ATPase staining. Interestingly, the expression of myf-5 in these mice was upregulated, suggesting that myoD might normally regulate negatively the expression of myf-5. These results suggest that myoD is not essential for normal development of skeletal muscle and that myf-5 might be able to compensate for the absence of myoD. The loss of myoD is not completely without effect, however, as homozygous mutant mice born to heterozygous parents show significant reduction in survival rate compared to those born to homozygous mutant parents. This suggests that homozygous mice lacking myoD compete poorly with wild-type or heterozygous siblings, but whether this effect is due to abnormalities of muscle function remains to be determined.

Similarly, the phenotype of transgenic mice in which myf-5 is inactivated is also surprising (Braun et al 1992). These animals die shortly after birth due to respiratory failure caused by the absence of the major distal part of the ribs but express no overt abnormalities of muscle morphology. Again, examination of the expression of muscle proteins and genes, including myoD, myogenin, and myf-6, revealed no abnormalities compared to controls. However, the appearance of myotomal cells in early somites is delayed. These results suggest that myf-5 may be important in the initiation of myogenesis, but that its absence can be compensated for in developing muscle, perhaps by substitution of other members of this family of myogenic factors. Furthermore, myf-5 appears to play an important role in the formation of lateral sclerotome derivatives, perhaps because of disruption of early tissue interactions.

More recently, mice bearing both mutant myoD and myf-5 genes have been produced (Rudnicki et al 1993). Such animals were born alive but died shortly after birth due to a complete lack of skeletal muscle development. No skeletal muscle-specific mRNAs were detectable and desmin-expressing myoblasts were apparently absent. It appears, therefore, that myoD and myf-5 may functionally substitute for one another in the development of skeletal muscle, but that one or the other must be present for determination and/or propagation of skeletal myoblasts.

Finally, two groups have recently reported on transgenic mice in which the myogenin gene has been inactivated (Hasty et al 1993, Nabeshima et al 1993). In both cases loss of the myogenin gene resulted in severe disruption of muscle development, both groups reporting a dramatic reduction in muscle tissue. In both cases some multinucleate muscle fibres were formed, but much of the tissue consisted of mononuclear cells. Furthermore, Nabeshima et al (1993) found that those muscle fibres that did form were ultrastructurally abnormal, with absence of Z lines. Hasty et al (1993) showed that in embryos these cells expressed myoD and Nabeshima et al (1993) demonstrated that they could generate fusion-competent muscle cells in culture. Together these results suggest that in animals lacking myogenin, myogenic cells form but are largely unable to differentiate appropriately. It is interesting to note that Hasty et al (1993) also reported defects in the development of the ribs and sternum, reminiscent of the findings in myf-5 deficient animals. These abnormalities were thought to be secondary to muscle defects.

In summary, the study of transgenic animals bearing targetted mutations in these myogenic regulatory genes has been of great value in understanding their function in vivo. Taking the results as a whole it appears that myoD and myf-5 are involved in the development of myogenic cells from cells in the somite, the presence of at least one being essential for this process, while myogenin is important for the normal development of myotubes from these cells (Rudnicki et al 1993). Additional studies using similar mutants are likely to contribute in the future to our knowledge of the function of many other muscle-specific genes and their products.

In the case of transgenic animals overexpressing particular genes, there are few examples relevant to understanding muscle disease. One example of this approach, however, is the finding that the overexpression of the c-ski oncogene results in dramatic muscle hypertrophy in homozygous mice (Sutrave et al 1990). Interestingly, although this gene was driven by a strong retroviral promoter and would be expected to be expressed widely, expression in the transgenic animals occurred only in muscle. Indeed, hypertrophy occurred only in type IIb and IIc fibres. The reasons for this are at present unknown, but such animals may be useful in the analysis of mechanisms of muscle hypertrophy. A second example is provided by the occurrence of rhabdomyosarcomas in transgenic mice expressing the SV40 T antigen (Tag) attached to the β-globin locus control region (LCR) (Teitz et al 1993). In this case the hope was to cause haematopoietic malignancies, but the result was to induce rhabdomyosarcomas and islet cell tumours. Both of these cases demonstrate a certain unpredictability to such transgenic experiments, but they nevertheless raise questions of interest to students of muscle disease.

The third type of transgenic model is of particular relevance to the development of gene therapy for human muscle disease. These are models in which the function of mutant genes is replaced using transgenic techniques. Of great interest, in the context of this chapter, are transgenic mdx mice in which the expression of dystrophin has been restored. Three such transgenic models have so far been described.

Wells et al (1992) have described the construction of transgenic mdx mice expressing a truncated dystrophin 'minigene' under the control of the Moloney murine leukaemia virus (MMLV) promoter. This 'minigene' is based on the Becker patient described by England et al (1990) in which deletion of a large portion of the dystrophin rod domain was accompanied by relatively mild clinical signs. In transgenic animals bearing multiple copies of the construct, serum creatine kinase activity was reduced when compared to untreated mdx animals, although not to normal levels. Furthermore, the predicted truncated form of dystrophin was expressed at low levels and localised to the sarcolemma. Finally, as assessed by the number of centrally nucleated fibres, muscle lesions in transgenic mdx mice were dramatically reduced. This study is of importance in relationship to possible gene therapy for DMD because the dystrophin gene, or even its cDNA, is too large to be accommodated by currently available viral vectors. The demonstration that the expression of the truncated form of dystrophin is beneficial is therefore particularly encouraging.

Transgenic mdx mice expressing full-length dystrophin under control of the muscle creatine kinase (MCK) regulatory regions have also been reported (Cox et al 1993). In these animals the expression of dystrophin was limited to skeletal and cardiac muscle and was located in the sarcolemma. Furthermore, the expression of dystrophin in these animals was accompanied by expression of dystrophin-associated proteins (DAPs), indicating that restoration of dystrophin can be expected to restore DAPs as well. Finally, skeletal muscle lesions were absent in these animals. An interesting finding in this study was that, although the level of expression of dystrophin was about 50 times that found in normal mouse muscle, this over-expression was apparently not deleterious. This is important in the context of gene therapy, where over-expression of the exogenous dystrophin may be unavoidable, or may even be desirable. Similar studies of transgenic mdx mice expressing full-length dystrophin under the control of MCK regulatory elements have also been reported by Matsumura et al (1993). Interestingly, in that study the expression of dystrophin varied between animals and between individual muscle fibres. As in the study by Cox et al (1993) those fibres expressing dystrophin also expressed DAPs, again suggesting that restoration of dystrophin expression should be accompanied by expression of DAPs. Thus these transgenic mdx mice have provided encouragement for the development of gene therapy techniques by which exogenous dystrophin constructs can be expressed, first in models of DMD, and eventually in human patients.

NATURALLY OCCURRING MODELS OF HUMAN MUSCLE DISEASE

A large number of neuromuscular diseases occur naturally in animals. Although many of these are inherently interesting, the following discussion is limited to those that are of direct relevance as animal models of human disease.

Animal models of muscular dystrophy

Over the years a number of inherited diseases in animals have been proposed as models of muscular dystrophy. These include the dy mouse, the myopathic hamster, and the dystrophic chicken. More recently X-linked myopathies in the mouse, the dog, and the cat have been described, and in each case, as described below, these have been shown to be due to defects in the gene for dystrophin. The latter diseases, therefore, are legitimate models for Duchenne and/or Becker muscular dystrophies in man. The dystrophic hamster has also been shown to be relevant to human disease. In this chapter, we will limit our discussion to these particular models.

The mdx mouse The mdx mouse was originally identified by Bulfield et al (1984) in a colony of inbred C57BL/10ScSn mice. Affected animals were identified by increased serum levels of pyruvate kinase and creatine kinase. The mutation was found to be inherited as an X-linked trait, and a preliminary linkage study using X-chromosomal markers was reported. In this original report it was proposed that the mdx mouse might serve as a model for Duchenne muscular dystrophy, based largely on the myopathic lesions that were found to be present.

Clinical signs. In their original report Bulfield et al reported mild clinical signs, in the form of muscular tremors and slight incoordination, in only a single 12-month-old affected animal. Subsequently, many other investigators have studied this mutant, and there is general agreement that the clinical signs are mild or absent (Dangain & Vrbova 1984, Tanabe et al 1986, Carnwath & Shotton 1987, Torres & Duchen 1987). Electromyographically, mdx mice exhibit prolonged insertional activity and complex repetitive discharges (CRDs), most obvious in older mice (Carter et al 1992). The minimal nature of clinical signs, and the failure of lesions in mdx mice to progress to fibrosis and fatty infiltration, led to considerable controversy regarding the suitability of this mutant as a model of Duchenne dystrophy. Since the identification of the mutant gene in Duchenne and Becker muscular dystrophies, however, the mdx mouse has been shown to be a biochemically accurate model of Duchenne muscular dystrophy.

A number of studies have been carried out in an attempt to document muscle weakness in the mdx mouse. Dangain & Vrbova (1984) found that anterior tibial muscles from adult affected mice developed somewhat greater tensions and weighed more than those of control mice. However, tensions developed in muscles from young mice, in the range of 2–5 weeks of age, were less than those of controls. As degenerative changes were reported to be at their peak at this age, this weakness can presumably be attributed to loss of functional muscle fibres. Similarly, Coulton et al (1988a) found that mdx mice were heavier than controls and that the soleus muscle was larger, both in weight and cross-sectional area, in affected mice than in controls, this difference being more pronounced in adult than in young animals. Soleus muscles from young affected mice were as strong as those of controls, while those of older mdx mice were stronger than controls. However, when these measurements were corrected for cross-sectional area of the muscle, young mdx muscles were weaker than controls, while those of older mice were similar to controls. Other studies (Anderson et al 1988, Quinlan et al 1992, Sacco et al 1992) have also found that anterior tibial and soleus muscles of mdx mice are weaker than those of controls. Finally, using a technique designed to measure whole-body tension, mdx mice have been found to have muscle weakness throughout their life (Carlson & Makiejus 1990). Therefore, although mdx mice demonstrate minimal signs on clinical examination, careful quantitative techniques can document muscle weakness.

Pathology. Since the original report by Bulfield et al, in which muscle necrosis was documented, several careful studies of muscle lesions in the mdx mouse have been published. There is general agreement that extensive muscle necrosis occurs early in the life of these animals. In most studies a dramatic onset of necrosis has been reported at about 3 weeks of age (Dangain & Vrbova 1984, Tanabe et al 1986, Carnwath & Shotton 1987, Coulton et al 1988b). A consistent finding is that necrotic fibres are usually found to occur in clusters (Tanabe et al 1986, Carnwath & Shotton 1987, Torres & Duchen 1987) (Fig. 12.4). Hyper-contracted fibres and fibres undergoing segmental necrosis and phagocytosis by macrophages are found, and calcification of fibres is sometimes reported (Coulton et al 1988b). It is important to note that, prior to the onset of necrosis, muscle fibre nuclei are peripherally located (Tanabe et al 1986). Following this wave of necrosis regeneration occurs, recognised by the usual criteria of cytoplasmic basophilia, and the presence of centrally placed, vesicular nuclei. A peculiar feature of the mouse is that centrally placed nuclei persist and, in fact, can be used as a marker for regenerated fibres (Tanabe et al 1986, Carnwath & Shotton 1987, Torres & Duchen 1987, Coulton et al 1988b) (Fig. 12.5). Most investigators agree that, in older mice, the great majority of muscle fibres have internalised nuclei, and therefore have undergone at least one round of necrosis and regeneration.

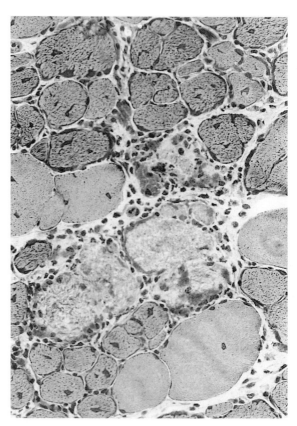

Fig. 12.4 Quadriceps muscle from a 3-month-old mdx mouse. There is a cluster of acutely necrotic fibres associated with infiltrating neutrophils and macrophages, and with adjacent small regenerated fibres with internal nuclei (frozen section, trichrome stain, × 228).

Torres & Duchen (1987) carried out a particularly detailed morphological study of the mdx mouse. They reported the occurrence of muscle lesions in younger animals than generally reported by other investigators. For example, they found scattered hyalinised fibres in 1-day-old animals, and full-fledged necrosis and phagocytosis by 5 days of age. These differences in age of onset of necrosis are most likely explained by the extensive sampling of several different muscles carried out by these authors, and they note that necrosis in very young animals was more common in the muscles of the head and shoulder girdle than in the limb muscles. As discussed below, similar muscle-specific variation in the age of onset of muscle lesions has also been clearly documented in dystrophic dogs. This variation in susceptibility

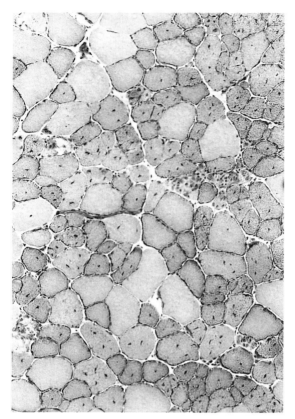

Fig. 12.5 Cranial tibial muscle from a 10-week-old mdx mouse. Many of the fibres have internal nuclei, indicating that they have undergone at least one round of necrosis and regeneration. A small cluster of necrotic fibres and some hypertrophied fibres containing peripheral nuclei are present (frozen section, trichrome stain, × 114).

of different muscles to necrosis may be due, in part, to differences in fibre size. It has been reported that small-calibre dystrophic muscle fibres are relatively resistant to injury (Karpati et al 1988). Torres and Duchen also reported that there is no preferential involvement of either type I or type II fibres.

Although some early studies reported that regeneration in muscles of mdx mice was complete, and that necrosis did not continue into later life (Dangain & Vrbova 1984), subsequent studies by other investigators have shown that some level of necrosis and regeneration occurs at all ages (Carnwath & Shotton 1987, Torres & Duchen 1987, Coulton et al 1988b). What is clear from these studies is that there is a peak incidence

of muscle necrosis at around 3 weeks of age, followed by accumulation of centrally nucleated muscle fibres and a progressive decline in the incidence of necrotic fibres, which nevertheless persist in low numbers in animals 1 year or more of age. In one study, for example, soleus and plantaris muscles of 3-week-old mdx mice contained more than 30% of fibres expressing the embryonic isoform of myosin heavy chain, a marker for regenerated fibres, while this number fell to 1–2% by 1 year of age (DiMario et al 1991). Thus, in limb muscles, regeneration seems to produce a population of centrally nucleated fibres that is relatively resistant to further bouts of necrosis. In the diaphragm, however, it appears likely that necrosis and regeneration continue, leading to fibre loss and fibrosis. The reasons for the resistance of limb muscles to repeated bouts of injury and for the discrepancies between limb muscles and diaphragm are unknown, but they may relate to differences in muscle work (Stedman et al 1991). Based on autoradiographic studies, muscle of mdx mice does not appear to have an inherently increased capacity for regeneration (Grounds & McGeachie 1992), although it is as capable of regeneration after experimental injury as normal muscle (Zacharias & Anderson 1991). It has also been suggested that regeneration following experimental injury is more effective in young (3-week) than in older (6-week) mdx mice. In mdx muscle regeneration results in the age-dependent accumulation of branching, or split fibres (Head et al 1992), which are more prevalent in muscles with long fibres than those with short. Both basic and acidic fibroblast growth factors have been reported to be increased in amount in mdx muscle (DiMario et al 1989, MacLennan & Edwards 1990, Anderson et al 1991). It has been proposed that they might be involved in the apparently more effective repair of mdx muscle, but their real role in altering the phenotype of this model is unclear.

The muscles of mdx mice also show consistently increased variation in fibre size (Torres & Duchen 1987, Coulton et al 1988b). This includes both abnormally large, as well as abnormally small fibres. Hypertrophied fibres are detectable as early as a few weeks of age (Torres & Duchen 1987) and become prominent in older mice (Fig. 12.5). This hypertrophy is presumably responsible for the increase in muscle weight noted by several investigators in mdx mice (Dangain & Vrbova 1984, Anderson et al 1987, Coulton et al 1988a). Fibre hypertrophy, as discussed below, is also a feature of muscular dystrophy in the dog and the cat. A progressive increase in the proportion of type I fibres has also been reported in mdx muscles (Carnwath & Shotton 1987, Stedman et al 1991).

A unique feature of the mdx mouse is that the dystrophic process, in most muscles, does not result in eventual fibrosis and loss of muscle fibres (Coulton et al 1988b). However, in a recent study, it has been reported that extensive fibrosis occurs in the diaphragm and intercostal muscles of older animals (Stedman et al 1991) (Fig. 12.6), the diaphragm showing an associated decrease in isometric strength and loss of tissue compliance (Stedman et al 1991, Dupont-Versteegden & McCarter 1992). Nevertheless, these changes in the diaphragm do not cause apparent respiratory compromise. In addition, irradiation of mdx muscle has been used to inhibit regeneration, which results in fibre loss and the accumulation of some endomysial connective tissue (Wakeford et al 1991, Weller et al 1991a). Although the irradiation model may be useful for some thera-peutic studies, it is difficult to argue that it mimics the profound fibrotic response that characterises advanced human (and canine) dystrophic muscle.

Ultrastructurally, necrosis in muscles of mdx mice is characterised by dilatation of the sarco-plasmic reticulum, hypercontraction, disorganisa-tion and lysis of myofibrils, and perforation of the sarcolemma. However, the latter is associated with necrosis of muscle fibres, unlike DMD, where it is reported to precede necrosis (Cullen & Jaros 1988). Although disruption of the basal lamina was reported by Bulfield in his original description of the mdx mouse (Bulfield et al 1984), this feature has not been observed in other studies (Torres & Duchen 1987, Cullen & Jaros 1988). Different studies have emphasised different early ultrastructural lesions, such as Z-band streaming (Torres & Duchen 1987) and the presence of vacuoles and pools of glycogen (Cullen & Jaros 1988). The significance of such findings in the light of the biochemical basis of the mdx mouse is unclear. The careful studies of Torres & Duchen (1987) failed to demonstrate lesions in the nervous system of mdx mice.

There has been considerable interest, over the years, in characterising alterations in the plasma membrane of dystrophic muscle cells using freeze-fracture techniques, and a number of changes

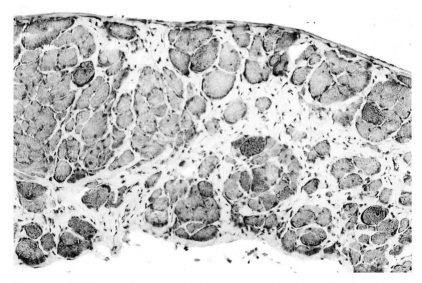

Fig. 12.6   Diaphragm of a 16-month-old mdx mouse. There is marked fibrosis and variation in fibre size (frozen section, trichrome stain, × 171).

have been reported in muscle of human patients with DMD (Bonilla et al 1981, Schotland et al 1981, Fischbeck et al 1984, Wakayama et al 1984, Peluchetti et al 1985). More recently, similar studies have been carried out in the mdx mouse. In adult mdx mice, ranging from 8 to 24 weeks of age, it was found that there was a reduction of P face intramembranous particles (IMPs) and ortho-gonal arrays (OAs), with a concurrent reduction in orthogonal array subunit particles (Shibuya & Wakayama 1988). There was an increase in density of caveolae. Because of the difficulty in interpreting such findings in adult muscle, in which there is a high proportion of regenerated fibres, these authors repeated these studies in mice 3, 7 and 14 days of age (Shibuya & Wakayama 1991). In the latter study it was found that P face IMPs were consistently reduced, a change already apparent by 3 days of age. OAs were similar in density in normal and mdx muscle at 3 days of age, but were reduced in the dystrophic at 7 and 14 days. It appears, therefore, that in the mdx mouse structural changes in the sarcolemma occur prior to the development of degenerative lesions. However, the significance of these changes, and the relationship of IMPs and OAs to dystrophin, remain unproven. Ultrastructural examination of the subsarcolemmal cytoskeleton using deep-etch, rotary-shadow replicas revealed no convincing differences between normal and mdx muscle (Wakayama & Shibuya 1990).

Dystrophin is expressed in cardiac muscle fibres and, in both DMD and the canine model, xmd cardiomyopathy is a consistent feature of the disease. Relatively little attention has been paid to the heart in the mdx mouse, and the literature, in terms of cardiac involvement, is inconsistent. Some investigators report having found no evidence of cardiomyopathy in mdx mice (Tanabe et al 1986, Torres & Duchen 1987), while others found cardiac lesions in at least some of the animals studied (Bridges 1986, Carnwath & Shotton 1987, Coulton et al 1988b). The cause of these inconsistencies is not clear, but may be related to the age of the animals studied. In the dog, for example, it is quite clear that the develop-ment of cardiac lesions is a relatively late event (see below).

Molecular basis. The mdx mouse has been shown to lack dystrophin, the protein product of the Duchenne locus (Hoffman et al 1987, Sugita et al 1988) and to have dramatically reduced levels of its message (Chamberlain et al 1988). Mapping studies have demonstrated that the responsible mutation lies within the murine homologue of the DMD locus (Cavanna et al 1988, Ryder-Cook et al 1988). Subsequently, the mutation responsible for the mdx mouse was shown to be a point mutation, substitution of a cytosine by thymine at nucleotide 3185 (Sicinski et al 1989), introducing a termination codon. Subsequently, three additional strains of mdx have been identified in mutagen-treated mice (Chapman et al 1989). Paradoxically, immuno-staining of mdx skeletal muscle shows occasional fibres, or small groups of fibres, that stain positively for dystrophin (Hoffman et al 1990). The frequency of such fibres, although always low, varies between strains of mdx mice (Hoffman et al 1990, Danko et al 1992) and tends to increase with age. Furthermore, mutagenic doses of X-irradiation cause an increase in the number of positive fibres, while doses sufficient to suppress muscle regeneration decrease them. Similar positive-staining fibres are also found in the heart of mdx mice, although the incidence is extremely low. Rare fibres staining for dystrophin have also been reported in muscle of humans with DMD (Nicholson et al 1989) and in dystrophic dogs (see below), suggesting that their occurrence is a general phenomenon. Although this process has been referred to as somatic reversion/suppression, its molecular basis is not proven. However, in one study (Tanaka et al 1991) it was shown that staining did not occur with DY4/6D3, a mono-clonal antibody recognising an epitope close to the mdx mutation. The latter result suggests that the protein responsible for positive staining is a truncated form of dystrophin.

Female mice heterozygous for the mdx mutation have been shown to express dystrophin in a mosaic pattern (Watkins et al 1989, Karpati et al 1990). However, the number of fibres negative for dystrophin, even in mice as young as 10 days, is considerably less than expected from the Lyon hypothesis, which would predict that 50% of myonuclei would be incompetent to synthesise dystrophin. Furthermore, the number of dystrophin-negative fibres declines progressively with age (Watkins et al 1989, Karpati et al 1990), such that by 60–90 days of age negative fibres are exceedingly rare. Inhibition of satellite cell proliferation by γ-irradiation does not alter the rate at which dystrophin-negative fibre segments are replaced by segments expressing dystrophin, indicating that this phenomenon is due to diffusion of dystrophin along the mosaic fibre, rather than incorporation of competent satellite cells during growth or regeneration (Weller et al 1991b). Necrotic and regenerate fibres are very rare in such mosaic heterozygote muscle (Watkins et al 1989, Karpati et al 1990) and serum CK levels are normal (Tanaka et al 1990), suggesting that expression of reduced levels of normal dystrophin is sufficient largely to protect the fibres from necrosis (Karpati et al 1990). In contrast to skeletal muscle, cardiac muscle of heterozygotes exhibits clear-cut mosaic staining for dystrophin (Karpati et al 1990). Again this is as predicted by the fact that cardiac myocytes are not multinucleate. Karpati et al (1990) estimated that about 30% of cardiac myocytes lacked dystrophin. This departure from the expected 50% is likely to be due to sampling error, given that dystrophin-positive and -negative cells occur in non-random clusters. In other studies, dystrophin-negative and -positive cardiac myocytes have been found to be present in about equal numbers (Tanaka et al 1990).

Pathogenesis. Despite the identification of defects in dystrophin as the molecular basis for muscular dystrophy in Duchenne-type muscular dystrophy, the events leading to muscle necrosis remain unclear. Nevertheless, the mdx mouse has proven useful in addressing a number of hypotheses relevant to the pathogenesis of the disease.

It seems clear from its sequence homology to spectrin and α-actinin that dystrophin is a cytoskeletal protein (Koenig et al 1988). Its localisation to the cytoplasmic face of the plasma membrane (Arahata et al 1988, Zubrzycka-Gaarn et al 1988), and interaction with a complex of membrane glycoproteins (Campbell & Kahl 1989, Ohlendieck et al 1991, Ervasti & Campbell 1991), have led several investigators to speculate that it plays a role in stabilising the sarcolemma,

protecting it from injury associated with contraction. Indeed, it has been shown that isolated mdx muscle fibres are abnormally sensitive to osmotic lysis (Menke & Jockusch 1991), suggesting that the dystrophic muscle membrane might be fragile. More direct studies of sarcolemmal membrane of mdx mice using the patch-clamp technique have shown small, but significant, differences in the tension required to rupture the membrane (Hutter et al 1991). However, the authors of the latter study argue that their technique does not necessarily assess cytoskeletal abnormalities, and that the tensile strength of the sarcolemma is too small to account for the differences in osmotic fragility described above. The interpretation of such studies is therefore open to debate. Nevertheless, it can be said that differences in physical behaviour of normal and dystrophic sarcolemma have been demonstrated.

If the lack of dystrophin does lead to contraction-associated injury, one might predict that dystrophic muscle would be abnormally sensitive to exercise-induced injury. In fact, it has been suggested that differences in the pattern of use may account for the relatively severe lesions that develop in mdx diaphragm compared to limb muscles (Stedman et al 1991). Experiments that address this question have been done in the mdx mouse. In one study it was found that both eccentric and concentric contractions produce more severe necrosis, measured by histochemical detection of bound IgG, in mdx muscle than in controls (Weller et al 1990). This result has been contradicted, however, in other studies. Sacco et al (1992) found that eccentric exercise produced no more necrosis in anterior tibial muscle of mdx mice than that of controls. Similarly, in experiments in vitro, mdx muscle released less CK into the medium than did controls, even though the whole muscle content of CK was similar (McArdle et al 1991), thus failing to support the idea that dystrophic muscle is abnormally susceptible to exercise-induced injury.

There has also been considerable interest in possible abnormalities of calcium handling in dystrophic muscle, stemming from studies in humans in which increased intracellular calcium levels have been demonstrated in affected muscle (Bodensteiner & Engel 1978). Total calcium content has also been shown to be elevated in skeletal and cardiac muscle at all ages in the mdx mouse (Dunn & Radda 1991). Using the fluorescent calcium chelator, fura-2, Turner et al demonstrated that resting intracellular Ca^{2+} concentration ($[Ca_i]$) is markedly increased in mdx muscle fibres compared to controls, and that calcium transients following stimulation were prolonged (Turner et al 1988). Furthermore, these investigators showed that increased $[Ca_i]$ was associated with increased rates of intracellular proteolysis. Increased rates of calcium-dependent proteolysis have also been implicated in mdx muscle by other investigators (MacLennan et al 1991). The reported differences in calcium transients were abolished when normal and dystrophic myotubes were studied under conditions of equal $[Ca_i]$ suggesting that calcium-buffering mechanisms are not altered in muscular dystrophy (Turner et al 1991). In addition, elevations of $[Ca_i]$ were more prominent adjacent to the sarcolemma than in the interior of the fibre (Turner et al 1991). Other studies have shown that similar increases in $[Ca_i]$ are present in both human and mdx cultured dystrophic myotubes (Fong et al 1990) and that dystrophic myotubes have impaired ability to regulate $[Ca_i]$ in response to changes in extracellular Ca^{2+} compared to control myotubes.

These alterations in calcium handling may be explained by increased activity of calcium-leak channels demonstrated by these investigators (Fong et al 1990). Such leak channels are selective for Ca^{2+} and the defect in ion handling appears to be specific for Ca^{2+}, since resting free sodium levels and sodium influx appear to be normal in dystrophic myotubes (Turner et al 1991). Studies by other investigators have implicated additional potential mechanisms that could result in increases in intracellular Ca^{2+}. Franco and Lansman have described stretch-activated channels in both normal and mdx myotubes, as well as stretch-inactivated, calcium-permeable channels that are open for long periods of time in mdx myotubes, but that are rarely observed in controls (Franco & Lansman 1990). Similar stretch-activated channels have been demonstrated in freshly dissociated normal and mdx flexor digitorum brevis muscles, although stretch-inactivated channels were not present in this preparation (Haws & Lansman 1991). Occasional patches from young mdx mice showed high levels of activity of stretch-activated channels. Activity of these channels decreased during development, but was higher in older mdx mice than in age-matched controls. Lastly, the membrane density of stretch-activated channels decreased during development of normal fibres, but remained relatively constant in mdx fibres.

The mdx mouse is also proving to be useful in studies of the molecular consequences of the absence of dystrophin. Studies by Campbell and his co-workers have identified a membrane complex of four glycoproteins and one non-glycosylated protein that interact with dystrophin (Campbell & Kahl 1989, Ervasti & Campbell 1991). In mdx muscle the components of this complex are greatly reduced (Ohlendieck & Campbell 1991). These findings suggest that, in the absence of dystrophin, these proteins cannot be maintained in the membrane, and that their reduction may be involved in the pathogenesis of the disease. Some credence is lent to this idea by the recent demonstration that a mutation affecting the 50GP can cause a severe autosomal recessive form of muscular dystrophy in man and the hamster (Matsumura et al 1992b, Roberds et al 1993). Campbell's group have shown that the autosomally encoded dystrophin analogue, utrophin, can also bind to components of this complex (Matsumura et al 1992a). These investigators speculate that the expression of utrophin in mdx muscle, particularly in small-calibre skeletal muscle fibres and cardiac myocytes, may be responsible for the resistance to degeneration of such fibres in this mutant. Although, as discussed above, reports are inconsistent, it should be pointed out that a number of investigators have found the heart to be involved in the mdx mouse.

Treatment. Animal models will also be important in developing and evaluating potential treatments for muscular dystrophy. The mdx mouse has already been useful in studying two approaches to therapy, namely myoblast transfer and gene therapy. In the first, normal myoblasts are transferred, or injected, into the muscle of the dystrophic patient or animal. These cells are predicted to fuse with host muscle during the cycle of degeneration and regeneration, thus incorporating nuclei competent to synthesise dystrophin into regenerated muscle fibres. The end-result of such therapy should, therefore, be to produce muscle fibres that are mosaic in their capacity to produce dystrophin. Observations in carrier muscle, described above, suggest that dystrophin might become disseminated throughout such mosaicised fibres.

Studies by Partridge and his colleagues have indicated that myoblast transfer can indeed result in the formation of mosaicised fibres and the expression of dystrophin in dystrophic muscle. In their experiments mdx/nude or tolerised recipient mice were used to avoid problems of immunorejection, and donors and recipients were homozygous for different glucose 6-phosphate isomerase (GPI) isoforms. Normal myoblasts, obtained by enzymatic dissociation of neonatal muscle, were injected into the EDL muscle of recipient mice. The formation of mosaic fibres was documented by the expression of hybrid GPI and the expression of dystrophin was demonstrated by both immunoblotting and immunohistochemistry (Partridge et al 1989). Muscles injected with normal myoblasts were found to contain many fibres expressing dystrophin at the sarcolemma, while control muscles injected with dystrophic myoblasts did not. Similar experiments, in which mdx myoblasts were injected into normal hosts, demonstrated that the regenerated grafted muscle recapitulated lesions characteristic of the mdx mouse, supporting the concept that muscular dystrophy is a primary myopathy caused by abnormalities of dystrophin (Morgan et al 1989). The injection of normal human myoblasts into mdx muscle has also been reported to result in the expression of dystrophin in a small percentage of fibres (Karpati et al 1989). In subsequent experiments, Partridge et al have shown that even more effective restoration of dystrophin-positive fibres occurs when normal myoblasts are injected into previously irradiated mdx muscle, in which endogenous satellite cell activity is inhibited (Morgan et al 1990). In those experiments up to 80% of muscle fibres expressed dystrophin, and the bulk and architecture of the treated muscle was restored to normal. Furthermore, injected myoblasts seemed to be able to migrate from the injection site throughout the treated tibialis anterior and EDL muscles, and even into the nearby, but uninjected, peroneus muscle. In summary, therefore, these results offer considerable encouragement for myoblast transfer as a form of therapy, and even for gene therapy, where transfected myoblasts from the patient might be injected back into dystrophic muscle.

A second approach to treatment that has aroused interest is gene therapy, where the aim is to introduce gene constructs into dystrophic muscle cells. Studies of gene therapy for muscular dystrophy are so far in their early stages, yet experiments in the mdx mouse have already yielded encouraging results. In particular, a truncated form of dystrophin has been expressed in cultured mdx myoblasts after retroviral-mediated transduction with a minigene (Dunckley et al 1992). The construct used in this case was derived from a patient with a very mild form of Becker muscular dystrophy. Furthermore, the expression of the same construct in transgenic mdx mice markedly reduced the occurrence of centrally nucleated fibres, indicating that the degree of fibre degeneration and regeneration had been reduced (Wells et al 1992). These encouraging results were obtained even though the level of expression of the truncated dystrophin was low. Recent studies using adenovirus constructs introduced into mdx muscle have shown significant expression of dystrophin (Ragot et al 1993). Finally, direct injection of either full-length or the truncated dystrophin cDNA into the muscles of mdx mice has been shown to result in the expression of the corresponding dystrophin protein in a small percentage of muscle fibres (Acsadi et al 1991). In these fibres the occurrence of centrally nucleated fibres was also reduced. Although the efficiency of this process is too low to be of clinical use, it is encouraging that the expression of introduced DNA can result in the synthesis and appropriate localisation of protein, and that there are demonstrable beneficial phenotypic effects.

Canine muscular dystrophy. In recent years it has become apparent that muscular dystrophy occurs sporadically in the dog. The best known canine model of muscular dystrophy is the Golden Retriever strain known as the xmd dog. The disease in the Golden Retriever was first described by de Lahunta (1983) as an inherited degenerative myopathy characterised by stiffness of gait, enlargement of the base of the tongue and prominent spontaneous activity on electromyography. The latter feature led to the condition being referred to as hereditary myotonic myopathy, although later studies have made it clear that this is a misnomer. In 1982 a litter of Golden Retrievers was initially studied at the College of Veterinary Medicine at North Carolina State University (Kornegay et al 1988) and a similar case was studied at Cornell University in 1983 (Valentine et al 1986). Subsequently, one of the dogs from North Carolina was transferred to Cornell where the first xmd colony was established.

Clinical signs. In contrast to the mouse, dogs with muscular dystrophy show marked clinical abnormalities, which are similar to those of humans with DMD (Kornegay et al 1988, Valentine et al 1988) (Fig. 12.7). In the typical form of the disease, as studied in the Cornell xmd colony (Valentine et al 1988), clinical signs first become obvious at 6–9 weeks of age. However, serum creatine kinase activity is consistently elevated from birth and dystrophic pups can be distinguished from normals at 2 days of age, based

on the levels of this enzyme in the serum. The growth rate of dystrophic pups is also depressed. One of the earliest clinical signs noted in xmd dogs is an inability to open the jaw fully. Affected dogs also tend to be less active than normal littermates and move with a stiff 'bunny-hopping' gait. By 3 months of age affected dogs may develop abduction of the elbows and adduction of the hocks, with overflexion of the tarsi and overextension of the carpi. Jaw mobility becomes further compromised, and the tongue is enlarged, particularly at its base. Muscle atrophy becomes apparent. The disease progresses until 6 months of age, when it tends to stabilise, at least in terms of clinical evidence of neuromuscular disease. By that age there is marked muscle atrophy, particularly involving the muscles of the head, trunk and limbs, with proximal limb muscles tending to be less severely affected. In fact, Kornegay reported enlargement of the proximal limb muscles in the litter that he studied (Kornegay et al 1988) (from one of which the xmd colony was established). Contracture associated with muscle fibrosis results in restricted extension of the shoulders and hips. Many of the affected muscles are firm to palpation. The base of the tongue is consistently

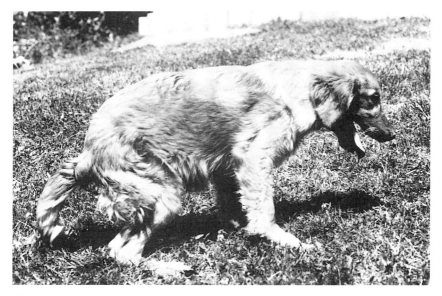

Fig. 12.7   A 6-month-old Retriever dog showing typical signs of muscular dystrophy. Note the overflexion of the limbs, due to muscle weakness, and the general loss of muscle mass (reproduced, with permission, from Cooper et al Proc. XIth Int. Congress of Neuropathol., Kyoto, 1990, Neuropathology Supplement 4, 1991).

enlarged, resulting in dysphagia and regurgitation. As the oesophagus of the dog contains skeletal muscle throughout its length, oesophageal dysfunction may contribute to dysphagia. Affected dogs tend to be reluctant to exercise, and have difficulty in such tasks as rising from recumbency and climbing stairs. Respiration is usually rapid and characterised by increased abdominal movement. Older dogs eventually develop lordosis and medial deviation of the ventrocaudal edge of the costal arch. The latter deformation is associated with severe contracture of the diaphragm.

In xmd dog colonies occasional dogs die in the first few days of life with a fulminant form of the disease (Valentine et al 1988). Such pups tend to be weak at birth, to have very high serum CK levels, and to be very weak sucklers. As described below these pups have very severe necrotising muscle lesions, including the diaphragm, which undoubtedly contribute to their early death.

Dystrophic dogs also have dramatic electromyographic abnormalities (Kornegay et al 1988, Valentine et al 1989). These consist of prominent spontaneous activity, predominantly complex repetitive discharges (pseudomyotonic discharges), which are found at all stages of the disease. Motor unit potentials are frequently brief and polyphasic. Nerve conduction velocities are normal.

Pathology. As in Duchenne muscular dystrophy, the essential lesion of muscular dystrophy in the xmd dog is necrosis (Valentine et al 1990b). In dogs showing early clinical signs, that is from about 2 to 4 months of age, the characteristic changes are the presence of numerous hypercontracted fibres, the so-called large dark fibres, active necrosis of muscle fibres, infiltration by macrophages, and active muscle regeneration (Fig. 12.8). Empty sarcolemmal outlines may also be present. Necrotic and regenerating fibres tend to appear in clusters. Histochemical staining shows increased levels of calcium in necrotic and large dark fibres (Valentine et al 1990b). Furthermore, occasional fibres that are normal by conventional histological criteria show subsarcolemmal rims or crescents of calcium staining reminiscent of the 'delta' lesions described in human muscle (Bodensteiner & Engel 1978) (Fig. 12.9). In young animals, particularly, the severity of lesions may vary from muscle to

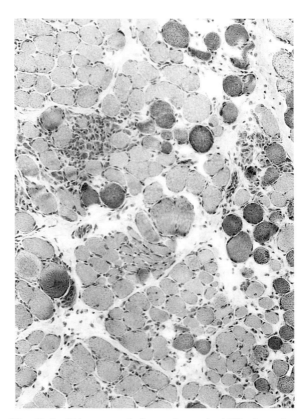

Fig. 12.8 Triceps muscle from a 4-month-old Retriever dog with muscular dystrophy. There are many large dark (hypercontracted) fibres, clusters of necrotic fibres infiltrated by macrophages, and clusters of small regenerating fibres (frozen section, trichrome stain, × 114).

muscle, although there is very predictable involvement of particular muscles, as described below. In the xmd dog, muscle necrosis and regeneration continue throughout life, although the degree of activity in the muscle of older animals is less marked. As the disease progresses, muscle fibrosis becomes apparent (Fig. 12.10), and there may be a modest degree of infiltration of the dystrophic muscle by adipose tissue. Chronic lesions are also characterised by marked fibre size variation, and a number of non-specific changes including the presence of occasional ragged-red fibres, cytoarchitectural alterations, such as whorls and moth-eaten appearance, and even the presence of nemaline rods. Fibre size variation is accounted for by the presence of both abnormally large and abnormally small fibres. Split fibres are also seen

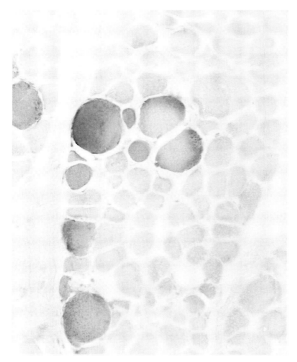

Fig. 12.9 Dystrophic canine muscle stained for calcium. There are several positive fibres some of which show subsarcolemmal staining reminiscent of delta lesions (frozen section, Aliziran red S stain, × 228).

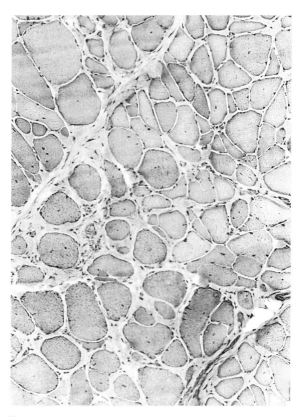

Fig. 12.10 Extensor carpi muscle from a 6-year-old dystrophic Retriever dog. There is extensive fibrosis with marked variation in fibre size, fibre splitting, and some internal nuclei. Some fibres are hypertrophied (frozen section, trichrome stain, × 114).

in chronically affected muscle. Although in the dog the majority of nuclei in regenerating muscle fibres quickly become subsarcolemmal, many muscle fibres in chronically affected dystrophic dogs contain a proportion of internalised nuclei. These are most common in hypertrophied fibres. Similar lesions also occur in the oesophagus of the dystrophic dog, due to the predominance of striated muscle in this organ in the dog (Watson 1973). There appears to be progressive emergence of type I fibre predominance in xmd muscle (Valentine et al 1990b) as is reported in both the mdx mouse and in human DMD patients (Carnwath & Shotton 1987). Fibre type grouping, a lesion usually associated with denervation and reinnervation, is also occasionally seen in the xmd dog (Kornegay et al 1988, Valentine et al 1990b), but the pathogenesis of this change is unknown.

Studies of lesion development in very young xmd dogs have revealed that the onset of necrosis is selective, with consistent involvement of particular muscles in the earliest stages of the disease (Valentine & Cooper 1991). As indicated above, occasional puppies die of a fulminant form of the disease in the first few days of life. These animals consistently show grossly apparent, severe necrotising lesions consistently involving the tongue, the diaphragm, and the trapezius, brachiocephalicus, omotransversarius, deltoideus, extensor carpi radialis, and sartorius muscles. Occasionally the medial head of the triceps, the insertion of the biceps femoris, the rectus femoris and the cranial tibial muscle also have lesions. Other muscles are grossly normal. Histological examination of a large number of muscles from affected pups (with typical progression of disease) from birth to 8 weeks of age has demonstrated that the same muscles were always involved early and severely in the xmd dog. Other muscles do not develop significant lesions until 6–8 weeks of age. In those muscles involved early in the disease process fibrosis is present by 4 weeks of age. In the tongue regeneration is present even at 1 day of age, indicating that lesions develop in utero. A striking observation in these young animals is that the average fibre diameter in those muscles developing early lesions is significantly larger than those in control muscles, or those involved late in the disease. Such differences appear to be due to marked hypertrophy of muscle fibres as an early component of the dystrophic disease process. This is reminiscent of the hypertrophy seen in the mdx mouse and in the dystrophic cat (see below), and suggests that fibre hypertrophy is a consistent abnormality in dystrophic muscle. The explanation of preferential susceptibility of these muscles is not entirely clear. It is apparent that those muscles that are susceptible at an early age are also developmentally advanced, having a more mature fibre typing pattern, and being of somewhat larger size than other muscles (Valentine & Cooper 1991). This suggests that fibre size may be a factor, as proposed by Karpati et al for the mdx mouse. However, at the stage at which marked degenerative lesions develop, susceptible muscles in control animals have fibre diameters considerably less than the 20–25 μm suggested by those authors to be the critical size. A more attractive hypothesis is that development of lesions in these muscles is associated with early demands for work (or exercise) (Valentine & Cooper 1991). Such an idea would be consistent with those discussed earlier for the mdx mouse. In fact, it has been shown in older xmd dogs that even mild exercise induces rapid, massive increases in serum CK levels, even though similar levels of exercise in controls produces little change (Valentine et al 1989). A requirement for muscle work in the pathogenesis of muscular dystrophy would also be consistent with the observation that cultured myotubes do not develop structural lesions, an observation true for both canine and human dystrophic cells (Witkowski, 1986a,b, Valentine et al 1990a).

Only limited ultrastructural studies have been done in the xmd dog. The majority of the findings reflect those described at the light-microscopic level (Valentine et al 1990b). At the ultrastructural level large dark fibres and empty sarcolemmal outlines are seen to be accounted for by hypercontraction of myofibrils. The earliest ultrastructural lesions appear to be dilatation of the sarcoplasmic reticulum, a feature noted in otherwise normal fibres, as well as hypercontracted fibres. Focal areas of subsarcolemmal degeneration, again reminiscent of 'delta' lesions, have also been seen and myelin figures are commonly present. Abnormalities of the Z-line, most commonly streaming and disorganisation, are found at all ages. Nemaline rods were present in one aged (6-year-old) dog studied. Aggregates of mitochondria and marked cytoarchitectural disorganisation can also be seen. In the xmd dog loss of the sarcolemma is seen in necrotic fibres, and focal loss of sarcolemma may be associated with delta lesions. However, no convincing evidence of primary defects in the sarcolemma has been found (Valentine et al 1990b). Although small breaks in the sarcolemma were observed in dystrophic canine muscle, similar breaks were seen in control muscle, making it impossible to distinguish such alterations from artefacts.

Like humans with DMD, xmd dogs consistently develop cardiomyopathy. Clinically this is characterised by ECG alterations resembling those reported in humans (Moise et al 1990). Specifically, affected dogs have increased Q/R ratios in leads II, III aVF, CV_6LL (V_2) and CV_6LU (V_4). PR intervals are also shorter in affected dogs than in controls, and older dogs may develop ventricular arrhythmias. Echocardiography shows hyperechoic areas, first seen in affected dogs at about 6 months of age. These lesions correspond to the fibrosis and mineralisation seen histologically. Echocardiography also reveals evidence of myocardial failure in older affected dogs, evidenced by low percent fractional shortening. One of the dogs used in this study died of heart failure at 6 years of age (Moise et al 1990).

Histological lesions, consisting of focal areas of mineralisation with accompanying macrophages and giant cells, first become apparent in affected dogs at about 6 months of age (Valentine et al 1989) (Fig. 12.11). These changes are most obvious in the left ventricular papillary muscles and the apical left ventricular free wall and correlate well with the initial observation by echocar-

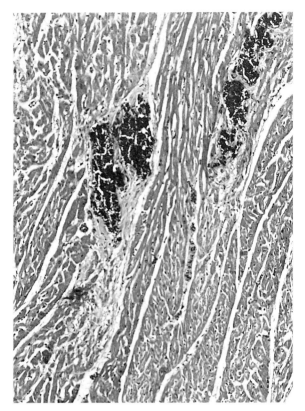

Fig. 12.11   Left ventricular myocardium from a 1-year-old dystrophic Retriever dog. Two foci of necrosis and mineralisation are present (H & E stain, × 114).

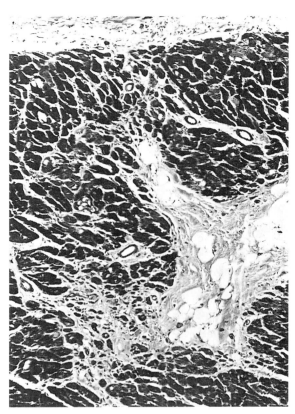

Fig. 12.12   Left ventricular myocardium from a 6-year-old dystrophic Retriever dog. The epicardium is shown at the top. There is marked fibrosis of the subepicardial myocardium (Trichrome stain, × 114).

diography of hyperechoic areas at this age. In dogs over 1 year of age, the most commonly observed lesion is fibrosis, most obvious in the subepicardial left ventricular free wall, the left ventricular papillary muscles, and in the right ventricular aspect of the interventricular septum (Fig. 12.12). In occasional dogs, especially in rare individuals that die acutely, active necrosis of myocardium may also be observed. The fibrotic myocardial lesions seen in older dogs are therefore virtually identical to those described in humans dying of Duchenne muscular dystrophy (Perloff et al 1966, Frankel & Rosser 1976, Hunter 1980). Studies in the dog suggest that cardiomyopathy develops as a consequence of myocardial necrosis with mineralisation, clearance by macrophages and giant cells, and subsequent fibrosis. No explanation is yet available for the relatively late onset of lesions in the heart compared to skeletal muscle, or for the restricted distribution of such lesions.

In canine dystrophic muscle there is abundant evidence of regenerative activity, particularly in young animals where lesions are active (Valentine et al 1990b). As in humans, however, the muscle eventually becomes fibrotic and regeneration fails in the sense that there is a net loss of muscle mass. Studies of necrotic lesions induced by the myotoxic venom, notexin, have shown that canine dystrophic muscle retains the capacity to mount a regenerative response. Even in 6-month-old dystrophic dogs, where advanced lesions of muscular dystrophy are already present, myotubes appeared 3–4 days after injury, and the membrane cytoskeletal protein β-spectrin appeared by about 7 days. These results are very similar to those for normal dogs (Sewry et al 1992). The long-term loss of muscle mass in dystrophic animals, therefore, does not appear to be due to the loss of the inherent capacity of satellite cells to respond. Interestingly, however, the maturation of newly formed muscle fibres appears to be delayed in canine dystrophic muscle, as judged by the prolonged expression of the neonatal isoform of myosin (Wilson et al 1993). These studies have also demonstrated the reappearance of immature fibres in experimentally regenerated muscle 6–8 weeks after the initial injury, suggesting that a second bout of degeneration and regeneration occurs within that time frame.

Molecular basis. Early observations on naturally occurring cases of muscular dystrophy in the Golden Retriever indicated that only male dogs were affected, suggesting that the disease was inherited as an X-linked recessive trait (de Lahunta 1983, Valentine et al 1986, Kornegay et al 1988). That hypothesis was supported by subsequent breeding trials (Cooper et al 1988a). Soon after it was shown that both dystrophin and its transcript were absent from xmd muscle (Cooper et al 1988b) (Fig. 12.13). Subsequent studies have shown that the xmd dog has a point mutation involving a single base change in the 3′ consensus splice site of intron 6 (Sharp et al 1992). This results in skipping of exon 7 and termination of the dystrophin reading frame in exon 8. These studies document the fact that the xmd dog is a genotypic homologue of DMD. Given its phenotypic resemblance to DMD, the xmd dog is therefore a potentially very useful model in which to investigate the pathogenesis of the disease and its treatment.

Canine carriers of the xmd trait have also been used to study the effects of X-inactivation on the expression and distribution of dystrophin, and descriptions of the heart and skeletal muscle of heterozygotes shortly preceded those in the mouse (Cooper et al 1990). In canine carriers, dystrophin is expressed in a mosaic pattern in skeletal muscle of very young animals, with about 10–12% of fibres in a particular cross-section being negative (Fig. 12.14). Many other fibres stain weakly. As the animals mature, dystrophin becomes more uniformly distributed and by 24 weeks of age fewer than 2% of fibres are negative. Serial sectioning shows that individual fibres are mosaic, with both dystrophin-positive and dystrophin-

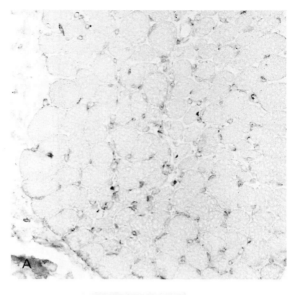

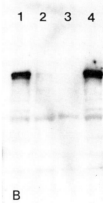

Fig. 12.13   **A** Muscle from a dystrophic Retriever dog immunostained for dystrophin. Muscle fibres lack dystrophin. Frozen section, ABC technique, polyclonal antibody (haematoxylin counterstain. × 228) **B** Immunoblot of control (lanes 1,4), dystrophic Retriever (lane 2), dystrophic Rottweiler (lane 3) muscle stained with Dy4/6D3 antibody. Dystrophin is absent from both dystrophic canine strains.

negative areas appearing along their length. Thus, in mosaic fibres of carrier dogs, as in the mdx mouse, dystrophin appears to be progressively redistributed as the animals mature. Clinically manifesting carriers have not been recognised in the dog, but carriers do have modest elevations of serum CK, and degenerate or, rarely, regenerate fibres can be seen in skeletal muscle (Cooper et al 1990).

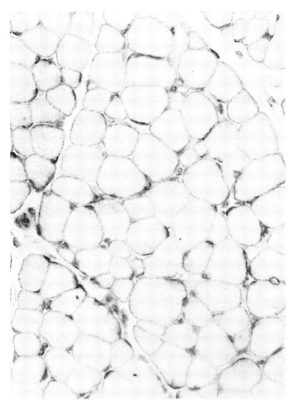

Fig. 12.14 Muscle from a 4-week-old canine muscular dystrophy carrier immunostained for dystrophin. There is variation in staining intensity and a number of fibres are negative. Frozen section, ABC technique, polyclonal antibody (haematoxylin counterstain, × 456).

In the heart there is absolute mosaicism, with fibres being either positive or negative, and with none of the intermediate or weakly staining fibres seen in skeletal muscle (Cooper et al 1990) (Fig. 12.15). This condition persists throughout the life of the carrier animal. Clinical studies of xmd carriers have shown that this persistent mosaicism results in the development of cardiomyopathy (Moise et al 1990), characterised by ECG changes and the presence of hyperechoic areas similar to, but less severe than, those seen in affected animals. Morphologically, myocardial fibrosis has been recognised in carriers (B.J.C, unpublished observations).

Since Duchenne-type muscular dystrophy was recognised in the Golden Retriever, it has become apparent that the disease occurs sporadically in the dog. In retrospect, an X-linked myopathy

reported in Irish Terriers almost certainly represented a dystrophin defect (Wentink et al 1972, 1974b), although the strain is no longer extant, and there remains no way to prove this. Suspected cases are also included in a description of animal myopathies published by Cardinet & Holliday (1979), including one of the original Golden Retrievers; the disease has been recognised in Miniature Schnauzers (Paola et al 1993) and suspected muscular dystrophy has been seen in the Samoyed (Presthus & Nordstoga 1989). One of us has recently studied cases in Rottweilers and in Dalmatians (B.J.C, unpublished observations). Both the Rottweilers and the Dalmatians have dystrophin defects, although the responsible mutations have not yet been characterised. Interestingly, the clinical phenotype in the Rottweiler, a large, heavily muscled breed, is very

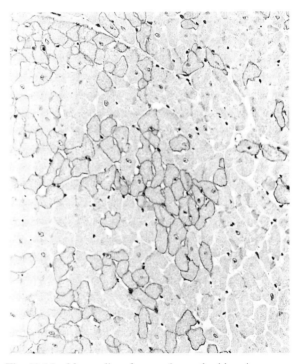

Fig. 12.15 Myocardium from an 8-month-old canine muscular dystrophy carrier immunostained for dystrophin. There are clusters of cardiac myocytes staining either positively or negatively for dystrophin. Frozen section, ABC technique, polyclonal antibody (haematoxylin counterstain, × 228).

severe, with affected animals not surviving beyond 1 year of age, while the disease in the Dalmatian is relatively mild. The reasons for these clinical differences are not entirely clear, although they may relate to growth rate and the differences in normal muscling between these breeds. Colonies of both strains are being established so that these and other questions can be addressed.

The dystrophic cat. Muscular dystrophy due to defects in dystrophin have also been reported in the cat. Two separate incidences have been reported involving a total of four males (Carpenter et al 1989, Gaschen et al 1992). In addition one of us (B.J.C., unpublished data) has studied an additional male that may be related to the cats described by Gaschen et al (1992). This assumption is based on the fact that all three animals originated from the same geographical area. However, the cats reported by Carpenter et al are assumed to be unrelated to these animals.

Clinical presentation. Interestingly, the major clinical manifestation of the disease in the cat is extreme muscle hypertrophy. Of the two siblings studied by Carpenter et al (1989), one developed signs at 21 months of age. The second was apparently abnormal as a young kitten. Both animals exhibited muscle hypertrophy, adduction of the hocks and muscle stiffness, which resulted in difficulty in lying down, curling up, and grooming. Serum levels of muscle-related enzymes were elevated. One of the cats had difficulty jumping on to chairs etc. and he developed a bunny-hopping gait. He also had an enlarged tongue. Neither cat appeared weak, but both tired easily and became dyspnoeic if stressed. Both cats had abnormal high-frequency discharges on electromyography. In the two animals studied by Gaschen et al (1992), marked muscle hypertrophy was again the prominent clinical finding. These animals had a stiff gait and they used a bunny-hopping gait. Both had enlargement of the tongue. They had elevated serum CK and aspartate aminotransferase (AST) activity. Both animals showed complex repetitive discharges on EMG. One of these animals developed severe dysphagia related to obstruction of the diaphragm by the hypertrophied diaphragm and was sacrificed. The second cat had difficulty drinking, but was still alive at 24 months of age. Clinical signs in the cat studied at

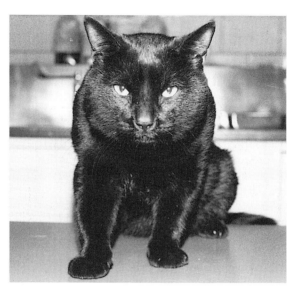

Fig. 12.16 One-year-old dystrophic cat showing the marked muscle hypertrophy characteristic of the feline disease.

Cornell were similar to those described here, with severe muscle hypertrophy (Fig. 12.16), stiff bunny-hopping gait, and enlargement of the tongue. Similar elevations of CK and EMG changes were also present.

Pathology. All of the dystrophic cats studied have had similar histopathological lesions. Carpenter et al described lesions from cats studied at about 2 years of age. These included muscle necrosis, with infiltration by macrophages, and regeneration. Hypercontracted fibres and a few mineralised fibres were also present. There was marked variation in muscle fibre size, with fibres ranging from very small to extremely large. Fibre splitting and internalised nuclei were common. There was mild endomysial fibrosis. Some fibre type grouping was present. Ultrastructurally there was dilatation of the SR and T-tubular system, with some swelling of mitochondria, some of which contained calcium granules. Some muscle fibres had disruption of the Z line and disarray of myofibrils. These authors described a few focal gaps in the sarcolemma, some in minimally altered muscle cells. Gaschen et al studied muscle samples at 5–6 months of age and at 2 years. They reported marked variation in fibre size with prominent hypertrophy, fibre splitting, and frequent central nuclei. Regenerating fibres were present and in some areas there was mild fibrosis. Mineralised fibres were also present. In the cat studied (at about 1 year of age) at Cornell there was marked variation in fibre size, scattered hyalinised or necrotic fibres, regenerated fibres and modest fibrosis (Fig. 12.17). Internalised nuclei were also commonly seen.

Cardiomyopathy also apparently occurs in dystrophic cats, with both cats reported by Carpenter et al having mineralisation and fibrosis of the left ventricular free wall, papillary muscle and septum (Carpenter et al 1989).

Molecular basis. Both groups of cats so far described, as well as the cat studied at Cornell, have had dystrophin defects. The cats described by Carpenter et al apparently lacked dystrophin completely (Carpenter et al 1989). Those

Fig. 12.18   Dystrophic feline muscle immunostained for dystrophin. In this particular cat there was weak expression of dystrophin in a mosaic pattern (frozen section, ABC technique, Dy4/6D3 monoclonal antibody, no counterstain, × 114).

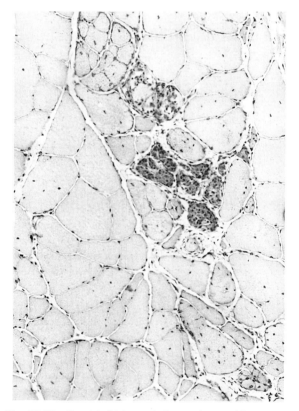

Fig. 12.17   Cranial tibial muscle from a 1-year-old dystrophic cat. There are clusters of necrotic fibres infiltrated by macrophages and a moderate degree of fibrosis. There is marked variation in muscle fibre size, many internal nuclei, and many of the fibres are hypertrophic (frozen section, trichrome stain, × 114).

described by Gaschen et al expressed dystrophin of apparently normal size at a greatly reduced level (about 5% of controls) (Gaschen et al 1992), with variable immunostaining of muscle fibres depending on the antibody used. The isolated positive fibres in this case were interpreted as revertant fibres. The cat studied at Cornell had a similar low level of expression of dystrophin of apparently normal size and a mosaic immunostaining pattern (Fig. 12.18). The defect in this animal has been characterised and shown to be due to a deletion of the muscle and the Purkinje promoters, while the cortical neuronal promoter is intact. This suggests that the low level of dystrophin present was accounted for by the expression of the cortical neuronal isoform.

It is likely that muscular dystrophy associated with dystrophin defects occurs sporadically in the cat. Cases of muscular dystrophy-like disease were reported in two male cats, one of which apparently had at least two affected littermates (Vos et al 1986). These animals had marked hypertrophy of the diaphragm, and histological muscle lesions consisting of muscle necrosis, mineralisation, regeneration, and marked variation in fibre size. These changes are consistent with those described in the proven cases of feline dystrophinopathy, and it is tempting to assume that they too had dystrophin defects.

The dystrophic hamster. Several strains of dystrophic hamster have been derived from the original mutants, which were first described in 1962 (Homburger & Bajusz 1970, Homburger 1979). All of these strains have a similar disease and will be reviewed here as a group. The dystrophic hamster has been studied as a model of both inherited muscle disease and cardiomyopathy, although it is fair to say that until recently the underlying pathogenesis of the disease, and its relationship to human disease remained obscure. Recent discoveries relating to the underlying defect in the dystrophic hamster are bound to renew interest in this model.

Clinically, the dystrophic hamster is characterised by signs of muscular weakness, often detected by subjecting the animals to exercise such as swimming (Homburger et al 1966), and cardiac failure. Onset of weakness can be detected at 60 days of age, or earlier. The longevity of the animals is reduced, depending to some degree on the strain studied (Homburger & Bajusz 1970, Homburger 1979). Serum CK levels are increased as early as 2 weeks of age (Homburger et al 1966, Bhattacharya et al 1987). The disease is inherited as an autosomal recessive trait (Homburger et al 1966).

Although a variety of early morphological changes have been described (Homburger 1979, Mendell et al 1979), the essential lesion in muscle of the dystrophic hamster appears to be necrosis (Homburger et al 1966, Homburger 1979, Mendell et al 1979) (Fig. 12.19a). Degenerative changes can be detected as early as 11 days of age (Mendell et al 1979). In well-developed lesions there is muscle necrosis, phagocytosis, marked variation in fibre diameter, fibre splitting, central nucleation, and basophilia (Homburger & Bajusz 1970, Bhattacharya et al 1987). Calcification of muscle fibres can be demonstrated histochemically (Homburger et al 1966, Mendell et al 1979), and calcium content of both skeletal and cardiac muscle is increased (Bhattacharya et al 1987). Lesions have been reported to be most severe in the musculature of the shoulder and to be exacerbated by exercise (Homburger et al 1966). Investigators differ on the effect of long-term training. Howells & Goldspink (1974) found that such training had a deleterious effect on the disease, while Elder (1992) found a beneficial effect, or at least no detrimental effect. There is also disagreement as to the degree to which fibrosis develops, with some investigators reporting none (Mendell et al 1979), while others report significant fibrosis and fatty infiltration (Homburger & Bajusz 1970, Bhattacharya et al 1987). These differences may depend on the strain and age of animals studied. Ultrastructural studies have shown early changes in dystrophic hamster muscle to consist of dilatation of the sarcotubular system, increase in lipid, cell swelling, destruction of myofibrils, and sarcolemmal defects (Caulfield 1966).

Cardiomyopathy is a prominent feature of muscular dystrophy in the hamster, to the extent that the animal is often used as a primary model of cardiac disease, and referred to as the cardiomyopathic hamster. Affected animals show electrocardiographic changes suggestive of cardiac hypertrophy, which are present from an early age (20–25 days) and are similar to those reported in human DMD patients (Bhattacharya et al 1987). Although the heart weights of normal and dystrophic hamster are similar, the heart weight relative to body weight is increased, due to the reduced body weight of affected animals. Histological changes in the myocardium include hyalinisation, necrosis and fragmentation of myocytes, phagocytosis and fibrosis (Bhattacharya et al 1987). Calcification is also present. Cardiac lesions are evident by 30–40 days of age (Jasmin & Eu 1979, Burbach 1987) and are essentially necrotising in nature. Early ultrastructural changes include cell swelling, hypercontraction of cardiac myocytes and contraction bands, dilatation of the sarcotubular network, myofibrillar lysis, the presence of perinuclear lysosomal bodies, and activation of perivascular fibroblasts (Jasmin & Eu 1979, Burbach 1987). Intercalated disks may also become disassociated and mitochondrial alterations and calcification may be present.

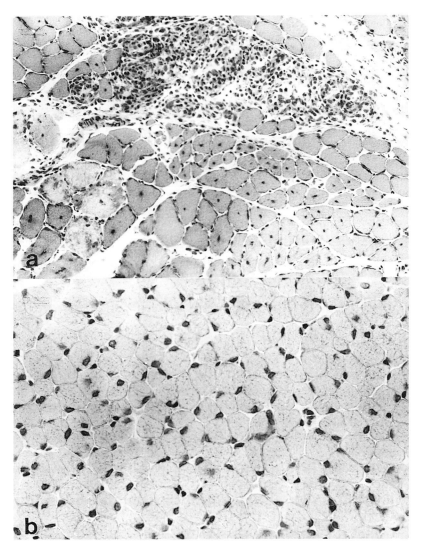

Fig. 12.19   **a** Cross-section of gastrocnemius muscle of a 45-day-old dystrophic hamster (UMX 7.1) showing a large cluster of necrotic fibres invaded by phagocytes (top) as well as a few early necrotic fibres (lower left). Other fibres are of variable calibre but all are centrally nucleated implying that they have undergone at least one cycle of necrosis and regeneration. **b** The contralateral muscle of the same animal, denervated by lumbosacral root avulsion at age 15 days. No necrosis, or significant central nucleation was present in the denervated muscle (H&E × 150; reproduced, with permission, from Karpati et al 1982).

There is a large literature describing biochemical, tissue culture and endocrine studies in the dystrophic hamster, aimed at elucidating the pathogenesis of this defect. These studies will have to be re-evaluated in the light of recent findings suggesting a defect in the dystrophin complex in this mutant, and are therefore not reviewed in detail here. However, some striking similarities to other models exists. For example, as in the mdx mouse, denervation of dystrophic hamster muscle largely prevents the expression of necrosis (Karpati et al 1982) (Fig. 12.19b). Whether such effects are due to reduced fibre size, to reduced usage, or to other reasons remains to be proven.

Iwata et al (1993) have shown reduced dystrophin content in dystrophic cardiac ventricular homogenates with increased extractability of dystrophin from dystrophic cardiac microsomes. From this data they infer an abnormality in the association of dystrophin with the sarcolemma. Studies in Campbell's laboratory (Roberds et al 1993) have demonstrated a specific deficiency of the 50-kDa dystrophin-associated glycoprotein (50GP) in both skeletal and cardiac muscle, leading to disruption of the link between dystrophin and the membrane complex of dystrophin-associated proteins. Thus it appears that the dystrophic hamster is a model for severe childhood autosomal recessive muscular dystrophy of humans (Matsumura et al 1992b). This discovery should reawaken interest in this model, and should lead to very interesting comparative pathogenetic studies.

Myotonic disorders

Several potential models of myotonic diseases have been described. Some, like myotonia congenita of humans (Thomsen's disease), are transmitted as autosomal dominant traits, while others resemble recessive generalised myotonia (Becker-type) in being autosomal recessive traits.

Caprine myotonia. Myotonia in the goat is the oldest recognised model of human muscle disease (Bryant 1979), and it has been extraordinarily useful in understanding the pathophysiological basis for myotonia. Affected goats show classical signs of myotonia and develop severe muscle spasms in response to sudden voluntary effort, particularly if startled. During an attack, which can last 5–20 seconds, they adopt a sawhorse stance and may fall over. After recovery, the animals move with a stiff gait, but become normal with continued movement. Affected goats also dimple in response to muscle percussion. Onset of myotonia is at about 2 weeks of age, and there is considerable variability in affected herds in the severity of signs. This is probably attributable to differences between heterozygotes and homozygous affected animals (Bryant et al 1968). Although there is some confusion in the literature, it seems clear that caprine myotonia is inherited as an autosomal dominant trait, and the disease is therefore a model for congenital myotonia of

humans (Thomsen's disease) (Harris & Mrak 1985).

Muscle from myotonic goats shows little in the way of morphological change (Atkinson et al 1981). Apart from moderate hypertrophy and a diffuse increase in staining for calcium, routine histological and histochemical methods show few changes (Bryant 1969, Atkinson et al 1981). Ultrastructurally, proliferation and dilatation of the T tubules and SR, as well as abnormalities of mitochondria have been reported, although the significance of these changes is unclear (Atkinson et al 1981). Finally, although changes in fibre type distribution have not been reported, Martin et al (1984) have demonstrated a consistent increase in fast myosin isoforms in myotonic goat muscle.

The myotonic goat has been the subject of detailed studies, chiefly by Bryant and colleagues, investigating the physiological abnormalities responsible for myotonia. Early studies showed that the major abnormality in myotonic muscle fibres was increased resting membrane resistance (or its converse, decreased membrane conductance), other cable properties being normal (Lipicky & Bryant 1966, Bryant 1969). Subsequent studies have implicated decreased chloride conductance as the cause of this phenomenon, even though subtle alterations of potassium conductance have also been demonstrated (Bryant & Morales-Aguilera 1971). The basis for repetitive firing of myotonic fibres has also been elucidated in the goat. It has been shown that myotonic fibres have a reduced rheobasic current (the minimum depolarising current required to produce an action potential) and a prolonged latency at rheobase (Adrian & Bryant 1974). This is associated with a prolonged after-depolarisation following a brief train of stimuli, which can become large enough to cause repetitive activity. Furthermore, this activity depends on the integrity of the transverse tubular system. These observations have led to the hypothesis that sustained activity in myotonic fibres is due to the accumulation of K^+ in the transverse tubules following normal activity. In normal muscle the majority of the surface membrane conductivity is attributable to Cl^-, which counters the depolarising action of the tubular K^+. Because myotonic fibres lack this conductance, accumulated K^+ leads to sustained trains of action potentials and myotonic activity (Adrian & Bryant 1974). Adrian & Marshall (1976), using computer modelling techniques, have shown that the absence of surface chloride conductance alone is sufficient to account for myotonic behaviour. Although abnormalities in calcium handling in the SR and mitochondria have been described in myotonic goats (Swift et al 1979, Harris & Mrak 1985), it is likely, given the findings described below for myotonic mice, that the molecular basis of this model involves a defect in the chloride channel itself. No abnormalities in the regulation of the chloride channel have been found (Bryant & Conte-Camerino 1991).

Murine models of myotonia: adr and mto.
Three strains of myotonic mice, adr (for arrested development of righting response), mto (for myotonic) and adr^k have been described. All are inherited as autosomal recessive traits (Watkins & Watts 1984) and all have been shown to be allelic. Thus the mto mouse is now generally designated as adr^{mto}. Onset of clinical signs in the adr strain is at 10–12 days of age (Watkins & Watts 1984). Signs are characterised by myotonic muscle contractions resulting in the inability of affected animals to right themselves when placed on their backs (hence the name of this mutant). Causing the animals to move results in myotonia-like muscle contractions, the hind-limbs being held in extension, until the muscles again relax. Older animals have difficulty in moving, although they never become paralysed, and exhibit thickening of the neck and fore-limbs. Growth rate in affected animals is also decreased and at maturity adr mice are considerably smaller than controls (Watkins & Watts 1984). Muscles of adr mice have been noted to be shorter and thicker, and more red than those of controls (Watkins & Watts 1984).

The adr^{mto} mutant shows similar myotonic signs characterised by slowness and stiffness of gait and extension of the hind-limbs when provoked (Heller et al 1982). Again, onset is at about 2 weeks of age, and signs are exacerbated by cold. Percussion of muscles can elicit sustained local contractions. Affected adr^{mto} also show reduced growth and are significantly smaller than controls at maturity, although older mice show increased bulk in the neck and shoulder girdle (Heller et al 1982).

Electrophysiological data support the hypothesis that these mice are models for myotonia. In the adr mouse stimulation of muscle leads to runs of action potentials and prolonged after-contractions, although the characteristic 'dive-bomber' patterns have not been observed. These effects are prolonged by cooling (Mehrke et al 1988, Reininghaus et al 1988). Blocking of neuromuscular transmission by curare does not prevent this behaviour, implying that the defect is inherent to the muscle rather than the nerve or nerve terminals (Költgen et al 1991). Based on measurements of muscle membrane time constants, chloride conductance in normal murine muscle accounts for more than 70% of the resting conductance, whereas in muscle of the adr mouse it represents less than 30%. Furthermore, myotonic characteristics can be induced in normal muscle by lowering the external concentration of chloride ions (Mehrke et al 1988). Thus, myotonia in this mutant can be accounted for by reduced chloride conductance. In addition, transplantation experiments have confirmed that myotonia is an inherent property of the mutant muscle (Füchtbauer et al 1988).

In the case of the adr^{mto} mouse, electromyography reveals characteristic myotonic discharges, with recurrent variation in frequency and amplitude (Heller et al 1982, Entrikin et al 1987). This behaviour can be elicited by insertion of the EMG needle, by percussion or stretching of the muscle or by stimulation of the motor nerve. Episodes can last several seconds and produce the characteristic 'dive-bomber' sounds from the EMG speaker. Neuromuscular block apparently does not block myotonia in the muscle (Heller et al 1982, Entrikin et al 1987, Költgen et al 1991), although there has been some controversy over this, arising from the observation that very high concentrations of curare in vitro can partially reverse the delayed relaxation that characterises myotonic muscle (Entrikin et al 1987). The latter observations probably result from non-specific effects of high levels of curare.

In both the adr and the adr^{mto} mutant there is apparently minimal necrosis of the muscle, and CK levels are normal (Heller et al 1982, Schimmelpfeng et al 1987, Jockusch et al 1990). However, a number of biochemical and histochemical alterations of the muscle have been described. These reflect a change to a red muscle phenotype (Watkins & Watts 1984). This is associated with an increase in oxidative enzyme activity (Reininghaus et al 1988), a decrease in content of parvalbumin (Stuhlfauth et al 1984, Jockusch et al 1988), and reduced phosphorylation of fast myosin light chain 2 (Jockusch et al 1988). These changes can be partially reversed by long-term treatment with tocainide (Jochusch et al 1988, Reininghaus et al 1988), a drug that can also reverse the electrophysiological features of myotonia in the adr mouse (Mehrke et al 1988, Reininghaus et al 1988). They are therefore considered to be secondary changes associated with the myotonic activity of the muscle.

The hypothesis that autosomal recessive myotonia in the mouse is due to a specific defect in chloride conductance has recently been confirmed by cloning and examination of the major muscle chloride channel, ClC-1 (Steinmeyer et al 1991). It has been shown that in the adr mutant a transposon of the ETn family has been inserted into the ClC-1 gene destroying its ability to encode several membrane-spanning domains (Steinmeyer et al 1991). This suggests that a lack of functional chloride channels is the primary cause of myotonia in the adr mouse. Southern blotting using probes for the ClC-1 channel also revealed aberrant fragments with one restriction enzyme in the adr[mto] mouse (Steinmeyer et al 1991). This and the fact that adr, adr[mto] and adr[k] are allelic, suggest that defects in the ClC-1 chloride are responsible for myotonia in all three mutants.

Canine myotonia. In the dog, myotonia can occur as either a primary disease or as a consequence of other muscle diseases, particularly hyperadrenocorticism (Griffiths & Duncan 1973, Duncan & Griffiths 1977). However, in the context of this chapter, most important is the inherited myotonia that occurs in the Chow Chow breed, a potentially useful model of myotonia congenita of humans.

Myotonia of the Chow Chow has been reported on a number of occasions (Wentink et al 1974a, Shores et al 1986, Duncan & Griffiths 1977b, Jones et al 1977, Farrow & Malik 1981, Shores et al 1986). Findings in all of these reports are similar. However, the most complete description of the clinical disease is that of Farrow & Malik (1981). Clinically, the disease is characterised by stiffness in the first movement after a period of rest, with the hind-limbs being most noticeably affected. Onset of signs in affected Chows is as early as 6 weeks of age. However, signs become more severe as the animals grow older. Affected animals move with splayed, stiff fore-limbs and often with a 'bunny-hopping' gait of the hind-limbs. Stiffness may become so severe that animals fall over, being unable to right themselves for as long as 30 seconds. These signs may be accompanied by dyspnoea. With exercise, signs become much less severe, although the gait may still be somewhat stiff. All voluntary muscles become dramatically hypertrophied. Percussion of the muscles produces a typical myotonic dimple lasting several seconds (Fig. 12.20). Histologically, there is marked variation in fibre size with occasional atrophic fibres (Fig. 12.21), and there may be mild muscle necrosis. Serum levels of CK are mildly elevated. Myotonic Chows show typical runs of myotonic discharges on electromyography. These are precipitated by insertion or movement of the EMG needle, or percussion of the muscle, and accompanied by the characteristic dive-bomber sounds in the EMG loudspeaker. Cooling the muscle prolongs the myotonic discharges. Nerve conduction is normal. In a therapeutic trial, Farrow & Malik (1981) found that quinidine, procainamide and phenytoin were all effective in relieving the signs of myotonia.

Myotonia in the Chow Chow is clearly an inherited disease (Wentink et al 1974, Farrow & Malik 1981), but the mode of inheritance has not been clearly established. Analysis of the cases in the literature, however, suggests that the disease is inherited as an autosomal recessive trait. This conclusion is supported by breeding experiments done by one of us (B.J.C., unpublished results). A similar myotonic disease has also been reported in the Staffordshire terrier (Shires et al 1983), although it has not been proven to be inherited.

Myotonia in the Chow Chow, therefore, is a potentially useful model of recessive generalised myotonia (Becker). It would be of interest to establish whether this disease is also caused by defects in the ClC-1 chloride channel.

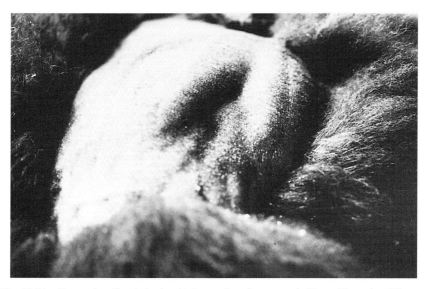

Fig. 12.20   Percussion dimple in the thigh muscles of a myotonic Chow Chow dog. The leg has been clipped to show the effect.

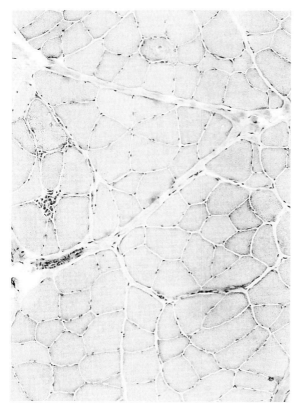

Fig. 12.21   Triceps muscle from a myotonic Chow Chow dog. There is generalised fibre hypertrophy and variation in fibre size. Scattered atrophic fibres and necrotic fibres are present (frozen section, trichrome stain, × 114).

Hyperkalaemic periodic paralysis

In recent years a condition resembling hyper-kalaemic periodic paralysis (HPP) has been recognised in American Quarterhorse lines. The syndrome is characterised by intermittent episodes of muscle fasciculation, weakness and, often, recumbency. It is usually recognised in young horses, 1–5 years old. However, signs may be seen in horses only a few months of age (Cox 1986). Although both sexes are involved, males are usually more severely affected (Cox 1986). The clinical characteristics of this disease have been well documented (Cox 1986, Steiss & Naylor 1986, Spier et al 1990). Clinical signs typically begin with transient muscle fascicula-tions or spasms that initially involve muscles of the neck and trunk and spread to involve most muscle groups. Severe weakness develops, leading to gait abnormalities or recumbency. The nictitating membrane (third eyelid) may be prolapsed, and horses usually sweat profusely during an attack. Muscle tone may be slightly increased and, during an attack, a percussion dimple may be elicited. Attacks typically last 15–90 minutes, but may be as long as 7 hours. Affected horses are sometimes found dead, presumably having succumbed during an attack (Cox 1986). Between attacks affected horses appear normal, although they are characteristically very heavily muscled. Factors causing clinical episodes cannot always be identified (Cox 1986, Spier et al 1990), but stress, or feeding material high in potassium (e.g. alfalfa hay) may be predisposing factors (Steiss & Naylor 1986). For diagnostic purposes attacks may be precipitated by oral administration of potassium chloride (Cox 1986, Spier et al 1990).

Laboratory investigation reveals that attacks are typically accompanied by haemoconcentration and hyperkalaemia (Cox 1986, Steiss & Naylor 1986, Spier et al 1990) but these return to normal as the animal recovers. Muscle-derived enzymes, CK and AST, may be elevated in the serum, probably due to recumbency, but are often normal (Cox 1986, Steiss & Naylor 1986, Spier et al 1990). Electromyographically, even during periods of clinical normality, affected horses show spontaneous activity, including complex repetitive discharges, and myotonic discharges, which produce typical dive-bomber sounds in the loudspeaker (Steiss & Naylor 1986, Robinson et al 1990, Spier et al 1990). Affected horses are also reported to have prolonged insertional activity (Steiss & Naylor 1986, Robinson et al 1990). In many cases muscle from affected horses is histopathologically normal (Steiss & Naylor 1986), but in some there may be central vacuoles in type IIb fibres (Spier et al 1990). Ultrastructurally, dilatation of the terminal cisternae of the SR has been reported (Spier et al 1990).

Only limited physiological studies have been done on equine HPP muscle. However, as in humans, muscle from affected horses shows lower than normal resting membrane potentials (Pickar et al 1991). These studies have shown also that muscle cell volume is increased and K^+ content is decreased in equine HPP muscle. Furthermore, the relative membrane permeability to Na^+ and K^+ (P_{Na}/P_k) is increased. This is thought to be due to an increase in P_{Na}, since tetrodotoxin hyperpolarises the membrane of HPP muscle, bringing the resting membrane potential closer to that of normal muscle. These studies therefore implicate an abnormality of sodium conductance in this disease.

It is clear that HPP in the horse is an inherited condition (Steiss & Naylor 1986, Spier et al 1990, Naylor et al 1992). In fact, it is known that all affected horses may be traced to a single sire, whose popularity stemmed from the heavy musculature of his progeny. This is an example, therefore, of a disease becoming concentrated in a line because of selection for an apparently desirable phenotypic characteristic. Because it has been difficult to identify all affected horses, specifically those that are affected but have not been observed to have clinical attacks (Spier et al 1990), the mode of inheritance has been difficult to analyse. However, the weight of evidence supports autosomal dominant inheritance (Naylor et al 1992). Linkage studies have identified the skeletal muscle sodium channel α-subunit as a candidate gene for HPP in horses (Rudolph et al 1992a). More recently it was shown that the equine disease, like that of the human, is due to a mutation in this gene. In the horse the mutation is a C to G change in domain IV, transmembrane region S_3 of the sodium channel (Rudolph et al 1992b). This results in the substitution of a leucine residue for a highly conserved phenylalanine, thought to lie in a transmembrane domain close to the cytoplasmic face of the membrane. Interestingly, amino acid substitutions in human cases of HPP also lie close to the cytoplasmic face of the membrane, although in different domains, suggesting that these domains are very important to the function of the channel.

In summary, HPP in horses is now known to be genetically analogous to HPP of humans and it should provide an excellent model in which to study functional alterations of the altered sodium channel. At present the horse provides the only model of this disease. Some confusion still exists in the literature about other myotonic syndromes in the horse, some of which have been likened to myotonic dystrophy (Jamison et al 1987, Beech et al 1988). The relationship of these to HPP needs to be established, but their relevance to myotonic dystrophy of humans is unconvincing. Finally, HPP has been reported in the dog (Jezyk 1982) but only a single case has been recognised and nothing is known about the possible inheritance or molecular basis of the disease.

Equine motor neurone disease

Motor neurone diseases have been reported on a

number of occasions in dogs, cats, pigs, mice, rabbits, cattle and other species (Sandefeldt et al 1973, Duchen 1978, Inada et al 1978, Shields & Vandevelde 1978, Leestma 1980, Mitsumoto & Bradley 1982, Miyata 1983, Shell et al 1987, Cummings et al 1989, El-Hamidi et al 1989, Montgomery et al 1989, Cork et al 1990, Nielsen et al 1990, Cork 1991, Schmalbruch et al 1991). Most of these are inherited diseases and, though of interest, their relationship to human motor neurone diseases is unclear. More recently, a sporadic, acquired form of motor neurone disease has been recognised in the horse. This disease bears close similarities to, and may serve as a model for, amyotrophic lateral sclerosis (ALS) of man, in particular the form known as progressive muscular atrophy.

The equine disease, known as equine motor neurone disease (EMND), has been recognised only since the early to mid 1980s, and probably represents a new disease (Divers et al 1992). Clinically, it is characterised by weakness with severe weight loss due to muscle atrophy, progressing over a period of one to several months (Fig. 12.22). Age of onset has varied from 1 to 16 years, and several breeds have been affected (Cummings et al 1991). The disease has been most commonly seen in the northeast of the USA, but cases have occurred in other parts of the country (Divers et al 1992), and in the UK (Hahn et al 1993). Affected horses show muscle fasciculations and tremors, shortened stride, a tendency to stand with the limbs held under the body, and weight-shifting (Cummings et al 1990). They may hang their head and spend unusual amounts of time in recumbency, often with the chin resting on the ground. They often sweat excessively. Ataxia is not present. The clinical course may progress for some months, then become static, or even improve somewhat (Cummings et al 1991, Divers et al 1992). However, affected horses never recover, and may occasionally relapse. CK and AST levels are often somewhat elevated in the serum, presumably due to muscle damage caused by recumbency, and there is often elevation of protein levels in the CSF without leukocytosis. Electromyography usually provides evidence of denervation in the form of positive sharp waves and fibrillation potentials.

Morphologically, major lesions consist of degen-

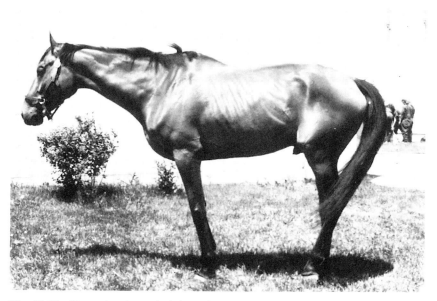

Fig. 12.22 Horse showing typical signs of equine motor neurone disease. Note the generalised muscle atrophy and the posture, with the feet held under the body for support, a manifestation of severe weakness (photograph courtesy of Dr John Cummings, Cornell University).

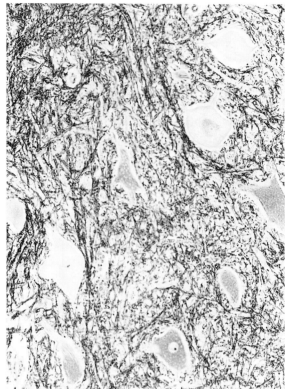

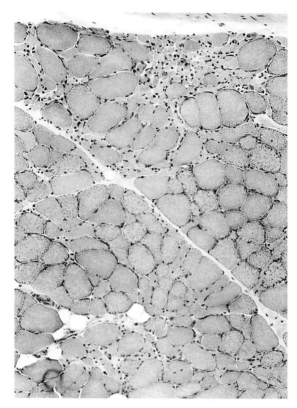

Fig. 12.23 Spinal cord ventral horn from a horse with motor neurone disease. Several motor neurones are swollen and chromatolytic (luxol fast blue/cresyl violet stain, × 114; material courtesy of Dr John Cummings, Cornell University).

Fig. 12.24 Vastus intermedius muscle from a horse with motor neurone disease. Clusters of atrophic denervated fibres are present (frozen section, trichrome stain, × 114; material courtesy of Dr Beth Valentine, Cornell University).

eration of motor neurones in the ventral horns of the spinal cord and, to a lesser degree, in the brainstem, and rarely in spinal ganglia (Cummings et al 1990) (Fig. 12.23). There is accompanying degeneration of axons in the ventral roots and peripheral nerves, and denervation atrophy of skeletal muscle affecting both fibre types (Fig. 12.24), although atrophic type I fibres predominate. Actively degenerating neurones are swollen and chromatolytic, with loss of Nissl substance such that they may appear as ghost cells. Such neurones often contain single or multiple inclusion bodies, which resemble Bunina bodies at the light-microscopic level. Swollen neurones are argyrophilic and stain strongly for neurofilament proteins, either diffusely or focally. More advanced lesions result in shrunken neurones containing lipofuscin. There is evidence

of neuronophagia and loss of neurones, with replacement by glial scars. Ultrastructural studies have confirmed the loss of ribosomes from degenerating neurones, the increased amounts of neurofilaments, and the degenerative changes in the peripheral nerves (Cummings et al 1990, 1993). Axonal regeneration is seen rarely. Several types of inclusion body have been recognised at the ultrastructural level (Cummings et al 1993). Two of these consist of aggregates of vesicular bodies, which appear to be derived from degenerate organelles, including mitochondria. The third type appears to be derived from the endoplasmic reticulum. None of these inclusions, therefore, exactly duplicate the appearance of Bunina bodies.

The aetiology of this disease is at present unknown. However, the fact that the disease seems to have appeared as a new entity in the early 1980s has focused the efforts of investigators on changes in the husbandry of horses that might have occurred around that time. It has been noted that affected horses come mostly from boarding or riding stables (Divers et al 1992), where access to pasture is limited. Furthermore, recent evidence is that most of the affected horses have low vitamin E levels (Divers, personal communication). Given this and the findings of Rosen et al (1993) that the inherited form of ALS in humans is associated with a defect in the gene for superoxide dismutase, it is tempting to speculate that acquired forms of motor neurone disease may be due to oxidant injury associated with deficiencies or defects in biological antioxidant systems. In this context EMND may be a useful model, and further study of the equine disease may contribute to an understanding of the pathogenesis of ALS.

Myasthenia gravis

Myasthenia gravis (MG) occurs in both the dog and the cat as either an acquired or a congenital disease. A relatively large number of dogs with acquired MG, now known to be immune mediated, have been documented in the literature (Zacks et al 1966, Fraser et al 1970, Lorenz et al 1972, Palmer & Barker 1974). From these cases and others cited below a description of the canine disease can be developed. The disease is most common in large breeds, especially the German Shepherd (Palmer 1980), and typically occurs in adult animals. Shelton et al (1988) have documented a bimodal age distribution with peaks at about 3 and 10.5 years of age. Both males and females are equally affected. As in humans, dogs with myasthenia gravis typically present with signs of weakness exacerbated by exercise, and alleviated by rest (Palmer 1980). In many cases the forelegs are affected before the hind legs, but sometimes the reverse is true. Reflexes are normal unless the animal is fatigued. The bark is often altered and is usually described as being high-pitched. Facial muscles and eyelids may also be weak. A very common clinical feature of MG in the dog is dysphagia, excessive salivation, and regurgitation of food. The latter is related to megaoesophagus, which is almost always present

in the dog and is attributed to the fact that the oesophagus in the dog contains striated muscle along its entire length. A localised form of the disease has also recently been described in the dog (Shelton et al 1990). In these cases, confirmed immunologically, the major presenting abnormality is megaoesophagus. The disease in the dog is often self-limiting with spontaneous remission after a period of treatment with anticholinesterases and/or corticosteroids being reported in many of the documented cases. Megaoesophagus has been reported to resolve in some cases (Lorenz et al 1972) but not in others (Palmer & Barker 1974, Darke et al 1975). Relapses have also been described occasionally (Garlepp et al 1984).

The diagnosis of MG in the dog can be confirmed pharmacologically and/or physiologically. Test doses of the short-acting anticholinesterase, edrophonium, usually produce a dramatic improvement in strength (Hall et al 1972, Palmer 1980) while repetitive nerve stimulation in most cases produces a decremental response in the muscle (Fraser et al 1970, Garlepp et al 1979). Morphological changes in muscle are usually unremarkable, although focal lymphocytic infiltrates have been described (Darke et al 1975). Almost no studies of alterations of the neuromuscular junction have been done in the dog. However, in one case widening of primary and secondary synaptic clefts was described (Zacks et al 1966), changes similar to the simplification of the end-plate seen in human cases. Thymoma has been reported to accompany MG in a number of dogs (Hall et al 1972, Palmer & Barker 1974, Darke et al 1975, Garlepp et al 1984).

As in human patients, the pathogenesis of MG in the dog is now known to involve the formation of antibodies to the acetylcholine receptor (AChR) (Dau et al 1979, Garlepp et al 1979, Palmer et al 1980, Garlepp et al 1984). These have been shown to be present in about 90% of dogs with the acquired disease, and there is some evidence that their titre is correlated with the presence or absence of clinical signs (Dau et al 1979, Palmer et al 1980, Garlepp et al 1984). The presence of antibody at the end-plate, complexing of receptor with antibody, and an associated reduction in the content of AChR in muscle have all been demonstrated (Palmer et al 1980,

Pflugfelder et al 1981). Incubation of normal muscle with canine MG sera accelerates the turnover of AChR in vitro, thus implicating antibody in the pathogenesis of receptor loss (Oda et al 1984b). Antibody from dogs with MG has been shown to be predominantly IgG, heterogeneous and, as in humans, to be most often directed against the main immunogenic region (MIR) located on the α-subunit of the AChR (Shelton et al 1988). Some antibodies are also directed against the β- and γ-subunits. Antibodies directed against the ACh-binding domain are rare. As mentioned above it has also been shown that antibodies to AChR may be present in a significant proportion of dogs with idiopathic megaoesophagus, and these cases therefore represent a form of localised MG (Shelton et al 1990). Antistriational antibodies have also been reported in some canine cases, sometimes associated with thymoma (Garlepp et al 1979, 1984).

Acquired MG has also been reported in the cat, although much less commonly than in the dog (Dawson 1970, Mason 1976, Indrieri et al 1983, Joseph et al 1988, Scott-Moncrieff et al 1990). Affected animals have ranged in age from 1 to 9 years and include both males and females. Clinical signs are similar, with weakness exacerbated by exercise, short-strided gait, muscle tremors, loss of palpebral reflexes, regurgitation of food and dysphonia. Megaoesophagus occurs in some cases. The disease is responsive to anticholinesterases, may show a typical decremental response on electrodiagnostic testing and the presence of antibodies to AChR has been reported in some cases (Indrieri et al 1983, Joseph et al 1988, Scott-Moncrieff et al 1990). One immunologically confirmed case also had a thymoma (Scott-Moncrieff et al 1990).

Congenital myasthenia gravis

Congenital MG has been reported in three breeds of dogs, the Jack Russell terrier, the Springer Spaniel, and the smooth-haired Fox Terrier (Palmer & Barker 1974, Johnson et al 1975, Jenkins et al 1976, Palmer 1980, Miller et al 1983). Onset of signs occurs at an early age, typically 6–8 weeks. Clinical signs are very similar to those occurring in acquired MG, with weakness

exacerbated by exercise, regurgitation, muscle tremors and dyspnoea. Muscle atrophy can occur (Miller et al 1983). Megaoesophagus is apparently an inconsistent finding, but has been reported in some cases (Miller et al 1983). Signs are responsive to anticholinesterases, which are useful for diagnosis. However, the disease is quite severe and persistent and is difficult to control with anticholinesterase treatment. In all three breeds congenital myasthenia gravis is inherited as an autosomal recessive trait with complete penetrance (Hartman & Standish 1974, Wallace & Palmer 1984).

Electrophysiological investigations of congenital MG in the dog suggest that the disease is similar in all three breeds, and reveal similarities to the acquired form of the disease. Repetitive nerve stimulation results in a typical decremental response (Johnson et al 1975, Miller et al 1983) and the amplitude of miniature end-plate potentials (mepps) is reduced even though quantal content, quantal stores and probability of release are apparently unaltered (Miller et al 1983, Oda et al 1984a). Onset of signs at about 6–8 weeks appears to be related to growth in muscle fibre size and consequent decrease in input resistance (Oda et al 1984a). No consistent alterations in end-plate morphology have been demonstrated by light-microscopic techniques (Oda et al 1984a). However, ultrastructural morphometry has revealed increased postsynaptic membrane density and reduced length of secondary synaptic folds (Wilkes et al 1987).

The amount of AChR in skeletal muscle is reduced, with end-plates from affected dogs having about 10–20% of the levels of AChR found in controls (Oda et al 1984a). Antibody to AChR is not present (Miller et al 1983, Oda et al 1984a). Interestingly, when muscle from dogs with congenital myasthenia gravis is denervated or cultured, extrajunctional AChR are normally synthesised and inserted diffusely into the muscle cell membrane (Oda et al 1984b). There is also no difference in turnover of receptors in normal and affected muscle. It therefore appears that the insertion of AChR into the postsynaptic membrane at the neuromuscular junction itself is defective. Elucidation of the gene defect in this disease might therefore be of particular relevance to understanding mechanisms of synaptogenesis. It should also be mentioned that, although congenital MG appears to be very similar, if not identical, in these three breeds, other forms of congenital myasthenia appear to occur in the dog. For example, Garlepp et al (1979) briefly reported a litter of Old English Sheepdogs with neostigmine-responsive, antibody-negative, weakness that developed at 12 weeks of age and spontaneously resolved over a period of 2 weeks, and Flagstad and Trojaborg have reported a distinct entity in the Gammel Dansk Honsehund (Flagstad 1982, Trojaborg & Flagstad 1982, Flagstad et al 1989). In addition, two cats have been reported with antibody-negative MG, thought to represent a congenital form of the disease (Joseph et al 1988, Indrieri et al 1983).

Malignant hyperthermia

Malignant hyperthermia (MH) occurs in a number of domestic animal species, but undoubtedly it is of most importance in the pig, which serves as a very important model of the human disease. There is a very large literature on the disease in this species, but in recent years considerable progress has been made in understanding the pathophysiology and the molecular genetic basis of MH, much information being derived from the porcine model.

MH occurs in several breeds and strains of pigs, including the Pietrain, Landrace, Yorkshire, Poland China and Duroc breeds. Susceptibility to the disease varies in incidence between breeds and between locations. In certain breeds in Europe the incidence approaches 100%. The high incidence of the disease is thought to be associated with selection for heavily muscled, lean carcasses. MH in the pig, therefore, is another example of selection for a desirable phenotypic trait resulting in the concentration of a genetic disease in an animal population. In the pig, the disease may be manifested as three different syndromes. These are classical MH following exposure to halothane and/or depolarising muscle relaxants such as succinylcholine; so-called porcine stress syndrome (PSS), in which environmental stresses precipitate signs similar to those of MH; and pale soft exudative pork (PSE). The latter is a problem of meat

production in which stress at slaughter leads to the MH reaction and results in degradation of much of the carcase. The disease in the pig is of importance both as a model of human MH and as a problem of production. Both PSS and PSE are causes of considerable economic loss in the swine industry.

Clinically, porcine MH resembles the human disease, in that precipitating factors, whether they be related to anaesthesia or to stress, result in a fulminant syndrome usually involving muscle rigidity, a hypermetabolic state, and hyperthermia. These signs are accompanied by initial muscle fasciculation, lactic acidaemia, hypercapnia, hyperkalaemia, tachycardia and elevated CK levels (Jones et al 1973, Richter et al 1992). Body temperature can reach 45°C, with the source of heat apparently being increased metabolic rate in skeletal muscle (Williams et al 1978). Increased heat production is compounded by intense peripheral vasoconstriction, resulting in blotchy cyanosis of the skin (Williams et al 1978). Attacks are commonly fatal.

Morphologically, most studies report little in the way of abnormalities in skeletal muscle prior to the onset of an MH episode (Venable 1973). In some cases isolated necrotic fibres and some variation in fibre size and an increase in internal nuclei have been reported (Palmer et al 1977, 1978). However, there appears to be no consistent alterations in fibre size or fibre type distribution (Gallant 1980, Heffron et al 1982). Variation in the degree of abnormality reported may be related to variations in age and strain of pig, and to what degree prior MH episodes had occurred. Immediately following attacks the essential lesion is acute necrosis characterised by hypercontraction of muscle fibres, which is consistent with the rise in serum CK levels associated with an MH episode.

There is an extensive literature pertaining to the pathophysiological basis of MH in the pig. The sensitivity of porcine MH muscle to contractures caused by halothane or caffeine in vitro has been used as a method to detect susceptible animals and has focused attention on the potential role of calcium in the pathogenesis of the disease. This work has been reviewed by others (O'Brien 1987, Marvasti & Williams 1988). However, it is now generally accepted that MH in the pig is associated with abnormal calcium homeostasis. López et al, using calcium-sensitive microelectrodes in intact muscle, have shown that the resting levels of Ca^{2+} are raised about four-fold in muscle fibres of MH-susceptible pigs. During an MH episode there is a large increase in Ca^{2+} to about 20 times the resting levels (López et al 1988). Treatment with dantrolene reduces Ca^{2+} to near normal levels and aborts the MH episode. Using the calcium-sensitive dye, Fura-2, to study intracellular Ca^{2+} in MH muscle fibres in vitro, Iaizzo et al found no difference between normal and MH-susceptible pigs, but intracellular Ca^{2+} did rise following treatment with halothane (Iaizzo et al 1988). Moreover, studies using isolated SR preparations have shown that calcium-induced calcium release is hypersensitive, requiring lower concentrations of Ca^{2+}, ATP or caffeine than normal preparations (O'Brien 1986). Mickelson et al, using a preparation highly enriched for the calcium-sensitive calcium channel, showed enhanced release of Ca^{2+} from MH SR following exposure to Ca^{2+}, ATP or caffeine (Mickelson et al 1986). Similar results were obtained by Ohta et al using skinned muscle fibres from MH-susceptible pigs (Ohta et al 1989). Taken together, these results suggest that MH involves a defect in the calcium-induced calcium release mechanism of the SR. Further evidence is provided by the finding that the calcium-sensitive calcium channel shows higher than normal affinity for ryanodine. As ryanodine is thought to bind when the channel is open this suggests that there is an increased open-state probability in porcine MH muscle (Mickelson et al 1990). Finally, ryanodine receptor (i.e. the calcium channel) from MH-susceptible pigs reconstituted in lipid bilayers shows increased open probability, prolonged mean open times, and shortened mean closed times compared to normal receptor. In addition, although the calcium-dependence of channel opening is essentially normal, the calcium concentration required for channel closure is increased (Shomer et al 1993). These results confirm that the function of the MH receptor is abnormal and provide a rational explanation for the pathogenesis of porcine MH.

There has been some confusion in the literature about the mode of inheritance of MH in pigs. However, recent studies have suggested that it is inherited as an autosomal recessive trait (Andresen & Jensen 1977, Smith & Bampton 1977). This is in contrast to the human syndrome, which is inherited as an autosomal dominant trait (MacLennan & Phillips 1992). These differences are explained by the fact that the clinical porcine stress syndromes, including classical MH, are fully expressed in pigs homozygous for the trait, whereas in humans heterozygotes are susceptible to the expression of MH when anaesthetised with halothane and succinylcholine. Nevertheless, abnormalities can be detected in vitro in heterozygous pigs (O'Brien 1986, Mickelson et al 1989) and there is evidence that heterozygotes can express clinical signs on exposure to halothane (Gallant et al 1989). In pigs, the halothane susceptibility locus has been shown to be part of a linkage group including glucosephosphate isomerase (GPI), phosphogluconate dehydrogenase (PGD), plasma post-albumin 2 (PO-2), and blood group loci S and H on chromosome 6 (Andresen & Jensen 1977, Davies et al 1988, Doizé et al 1990). The gene for the ryanodine receptor has also been mapped to chromosome 6 (6p11→q21)(Harbitz et al 1990). Finally, a point mutation has been identified in the gene for the skeletal muscle ryanodine receptor (ryr-1) of MH-susceptible pigs. The mutation involves replacement of C^{1843} by a T, which results in substitution of a cysteine for arginine[615] (Fujii et al 1991). This mutation is extremely tightly linked to the MH phenotype, providing convincing evidence that it is indeed the mutation responsible for MH in the pig (Otsu et al 1991). It is present in all breeds of MH-susceptible pigs that have been examined, and all preserve a common haplotype, based on the analysis of polymorphic sites in the ryr-1 gene. These data suggest that the MH mutation in all breeds of pigs originated in a common founder animal (Fujii et al 1991). The ryr-1 gene has also been implicated in MH in at least some human families (MacLennan & Phillips 1992). MH in the pig is therefore an excellent model of the human disease, both genetically and phenotypically, and it should continue to be useful for study of the pathogenesis of the disease. The identification of a common mutation in affected pigs will allow normal, heterozygous and homozygous affected animals to be identified with certainty. This will allow genetically defined animals to be used in research as well as allowing the elimination of the trait from breeding stock, if that proves to be economically desirable (MacLennan & Phillips 1992).

Malignant hyperthermia has also been reported in other species including the dog (Leary et al 1983, Kirmayer et al 1984, Rand & O'Brien 1987, Cribb 1988), the horse (Short & Paddleford 1973, Bagshaw et al 1978, Hildebrand 1988, Short & Matthews 1988) and the cat (De Jong et al 1974). In most cases these are sporadic reports. However, in the dog breeding colonies have been established. The disease appears to be inherited as an autosomal dominant trait (O'Brien et al 1983, Nelson 1991). Clinically, dogs suffering anaesthesia-related episodes of MH show hyperthermia, tachycardia and tachypnoea. There is hyperkalaemia, increased production of CO_2 and serum CK levels rise after an attack. According to these various reports, muscle contracture is not consistently present. In many cases susceptible animals are reported to be heavily muscled. Histologically, muscle from susceptible animals has been reported to show fibre size variation and increased numbers of internal nuclei. A stress syndrome, in which hyperthermic episodes are precipitated by exercise or other stresses, has also been reported. It is difficult to determine whether all of these cases represent a single syndrome. Nevertheless, where colonies have been established, MH-susceptible dogs should prove to be useful models in which to study the pathophysiology and comparative molecular genetics of the syndrome.

Myopathic glycogenoses

A number of glycogen storage diseases having the potential to serve as animal models of the corresponding human conditions have been described. Those that are well characterised include glycogenosis types II, III, IV, and VII.

Glycogenosis type II (Pompe's disease) has been described in two breeds of cattle. A herd of Shorthorn cattle segregating this trait has been intensively studied in Western Australia by Howell et al (1981). Two clinical syndromes have been described in this inbred herd in which calves die at a young age (3–7 months) or later (at 1–1.5 years of age)(Howell et al 1981). Animals with the early-onset form, which has been compared to the infantile-onset disease in humans, develop respiratory distress and have evidence of heart failure. Those with the late-onset form, comparable to the human childhood form, develop signs predominated by muscle weakness. Both groups show cardiac conduction abnormalities (Robinson et al 1983). There is lysosomal storage of glycogen in skeletal muscle (Fig. 12.25), cardiac muscle and smooth muscle, and in neurones of the central and autonomic nervous systems. There is evidence of muscle degeneration (Edwards & Richards 1979, Howell et al 1981), especially terminally, when CK levels may be markedly elevated. Breeding studies have indicated that the disease is inherited as an autosomal recessive trait (Howell et al 1981). Tissue activity of acid α-glucosidase is markedly depressed in affected animals and heterozygotes express intermediate levels of the enzyme (Howell et al 1981). Glycogenosis type II has also been described in Brahman cattle (O'Sullivan et al 1981). In this breed the disease is expressed early and results in poor growth and neurological signs. Glycogen storage is evident in neurones of the central nervous system, heart, muscle and other tissues. Activity of acid α-glucosidase is markedly reduced.

A number of studies aimed at treatment of glycogenosis type II have been done in the Shorthorn model. Glycogen has been shown to accumulate in lysosomes in cultured muscle cells (Di Marco et al 1984) and addition of purified acid α-glucosidase to the medium results in uptake of the enzyme and reduction of the levels of glycogen (Di Marco et al 1985). Furthermore, lymphoreticular chimerism, as occurs in twin calves, has been used as a model of naturally occurring bone marrow transplantation (Howell et al 1991). This chimerism results in increased levels of acid α-glucosidase in muscle and other tissues. In affected twin calves, glycogen levels were lowered in liver, spleen and lymph node, but not in muscle. Clinical signs and lesions in muscle were not altered. Thus the authors conclude that bone marrow transplantation is unlikely to be useful in the treatment of Pompe's disease.

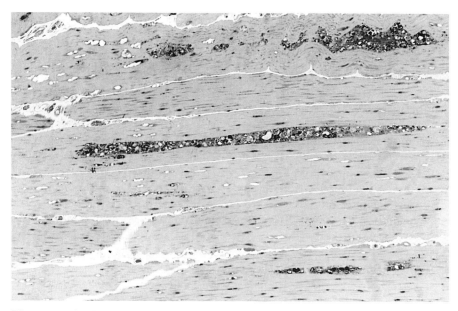

Fig. 12.25 Semitendinosus muscle from a 5-month-old calf with glycogenosis type II. Aggregates of glycogen are present throughout the muscle fibre. Damage to the central area is present in some fibres (Epon embedded, toluidine blue stain, × 306; micrograph courtesy of Dr John McC. Howell, Murdoch University).

Glycogenosis type II also has been described in the Lapland dog (Walvoort 1985). Clinically these animals show progressive muscle weakness from about 6 months of age and die by about 18 months. Because it is predominantly striated muscle, the oesophagus is involved, with mega-oesophagus and vomiting. There is generalised lysosomal glycogen storage, most severely involving skeletal, cardiac and smooth muscle. The disease is inherited as an autosomal recessive trait. Acid α-glucosidase activity is markedly reduced in affected dogs and is present at intermediate levels in heterozygotes (Walvoort et al 1982, 1985). However, the enzyme protein can be detected using immunological techniques, suggesting that the mutation interferes with the catalytic activity of the protein.

A third model of glycogenosis type II has been described in Japanese quail (Matsui et al 1983, Fujita 1991). The disease is manifested clinically as muscle weakness. There is glycogen storage in skeletal, cardiac and smooth muscle as well as in neurones and other tissues. In skeletal muscle there is also myofibrillar disorganisation (Higuchi et al 1987). Acid α-glucosidase activity

is reduced to about 10% of normal levels (Usuki et al 1986). Because of this residual activity the disease in quail has been compared to the adult-onset form in humans.

Glycogenosis type III has been reported in the German Shepherd dog. Clinical signs are apparently manifested from an early age and are dominated by muscle weakness and exercise intolerance (Rafiquzzaman et al 1976). The mode of inheritance has not been clearly established. The disease results in severe hepatomegaly. There is glycogen storage in hepatocytes, in skeletal, cardiac and smooth muscle, and in neurones of the central nervous system. Ultrastructurally, the glycogen lies free in the cytoplasm. Biochemical studies have shown that the activity of debranching enzyme (amylo-1,6-glucosidase) is markedly reduced (Ceh et al 1976). Furthermore, the stored glycogen has been shown to have abnormally short branches, as would be predicted.

Glycogenosis type IV has recently been reported in Norwegian forest cats (Fyfe et al 1992). Clinical signs are neuromuscular in nature, with muscle tremors, listlessness, and a 'bunny-hopping' gait. The disease is progressive, resulting in severe muscle atrophy and tetraplegia. Serum CK activity is increased. The EMG is abnormal with high-frequency discharges and fibrillation potentials. Nerve conduction is normal. There is generalised storage of glycogen in many tissues and cells, including skeletal, cardiac and smooth muscle (Fig. 12.26), hepatocytes, and neurones of the central and peripheral nervous systems. There is extensive atrophy and degeneration of skeletal muscle and axonal loss and demyelination in neural tissues. Ultrastructurally, stored glycogen is not membrane-bound. Pedigree analysis is consistent with autosomal recessive inheritance. The activity of branching enzyme is markedly reduced in liver and muscle of affected cats and intermediate enzyme activity is present in heterozygotes. Spectral analysis of the stored

glycogen has shown longer than normal average chain lengths, a finding consistent with a reduced number of branch points, as would be expected with a deficiency of branching enzyme. A colony of these cats has been established and they should be useful for further studies of the disease.

Phosphofructokinase (PFK) deficiency occurs in the English Springer Spaniel dog (Vora et al 1985). Myopathy with storage of amylopectin-like polysaccharide in muscle fibres has been reported in one animal (Harvey et al 1990), suggesting that this disease might serve as a model of glycogen storage disease type VII. However, muscle disease is usually absent in these animals, apparently due to the expression of the liver isoenzyme in muscle (Vora et al 1985). Thus, although the dog may be useful as a model of haemolysis due to PFK deficiency, it probably has little applicability to the study of muscle disease.

Other myopathies of interest

Many other neuromuscular diseases occur in animal species. These have not been discussed in detail here either because of non-availability or non-applicability as specific models of human disease. A few deserve passing mention, however.

In many domestic animals nutritional myopathy, due to vitamin E and/or selenium deficiencies, are relatively common (Ruth & Van Vleet 1974, Rice et al 1981, McMurray et al 1983, Allen 1986, Kennedy et al 1987). Like the quokka discussed elsewhere in this chapter, these animals may serve as models in which to study muscle degeneration and regeneration.

Polymyositis occurs sporadically in the dog (Krum et al 1977, Kornegay et al 1980). In a number of cases studied by one of us (B.J.C), and in some published cases, there has been evidence of an autoimmune basis, in particular positive ANA titres. The disease is typically characterised by muscle degeneration and regeneration accompanied by a variable inflammatory infiltrate (Fig. 12.27). The latter typically consists of lymphocytes and plasma cells and may include neutrophils and eosinophils. Clinical signs usually include weakness, which may be exacerbated by exercise, and pain on palpation of muscles. The main limitation of this disease as a model is its

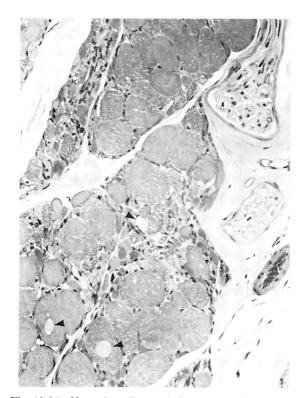

Fig. 12.26 Vastus lateralis muscle from a cat with glycogenosis type IV. Storage product is present in several otherwise normal muscle fibres (arrows). There are clusters of severely atrophic fibres, and two intramuscular nerve twigs showing degenerative changes are present (plastic-embedded tissue, toluidine blue stain, × 110; original material courtesy of Dr John Fyfe, University of Pennsylvania).

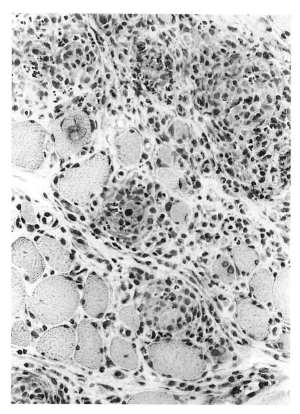

Fig. 12.27 Canine polymyositis. Triceps muscle showing extensive necrosis associated with an inflammatory infiltrate of neutrophils, eosinophils, lymphoid cells and macrophages. Remaining fibres are of variable size and some are regenerate (frozen section, H&E stain, × 228).

sporadic nature. However, it may be useful in comparative studies of the immunopathogenesis of polymyositis. Little such work has been done so far. Nevertheless, as suitable reagents emerge, it will become feasible to study the nature of the cells participating in the attack on muscle fibres.

One example of probable mitochondrial myopathy has been reported in two Old English Sheepdog littermates (Breitschwerdt et al 1992). These animals presented with severe exercise intolerance. They had lactic acidaemia and moderate elevations in serum CK and pyruvate, which were exacerbated by exercise. EMG revealed complex repetitive discharges and muscle biopsies revealed some necrosis. One dog had some ragged-red fibres, both had increased peripheral staining with oxidative enzyme stains and one had accumulations of glycogen in some fibres. Although it is likely that this was an inherited condition, neither the mode of inheritance nor the enzyme defect were established. One of us (B.J.C.) has recently studied a case of suspected mitochondrial myopathy in a Welsh terrier dog presenting with intermittent signs suggestive of muscle cramping. This animal had consistently elevated serum CK levels, which were exacerbated by exercise. Muscle biopsy revealed myopathic changes including the presence of ragged-red fibres. Ultrastructurally, many muscle mitochondria were greatly enlarged and had abnormal cristae. The enzymatic defect in this animal has not yet been determined. Repeat breedings of the parents are currently being made in an attempt to reproduce the disease for further study.

A form of nemaline rod myopathy has been reported in a family of related cats (Cooper et al 1986). These animals presented with gait abnormalities and progressive muscle wasting. Histologically, there was marked muscle fibre size variation with selective atrophy of type I and type IIa fibres. In advanced cases many fibres were severely atrophied. There was extensive fibre splitting, and some muscle necrosis. Nemaline rods were prominent in many muscle fibres on trichrome-stained frozen sections and in Epon-embedded sections. Ultrastructurally these had the characteristic lattice-like appearance and appeared to represent expansions of the Z line. The inheritance of this disease has not been formally established, but all affected animals were from a single dam, and pedigree analysis suggested an autosomal recessive trait.

CONCLUSIONS

The reaction of skeletal muscle to injury of various types is now reasonably well understood as a result of the increasing number of experimental studies and the wider range of techniques applied to the subject in recent years. In this respect, histochemical and electron-microscopic contributions, and more recently molecular genetic analyses, have been especially relevant.

Nevertheless it can still be said that the most notable aspect of the pathology of injured muscle is the remarkably stereotyped character of the resulting changes, a fact which is demonstrated by the many diverse agents producing similar results. The elementary lesion in the majority of these conditions is focal necrosis of the muscle fibre with preservation of the endomysial sheath. Focal or segmental necrosis is always followed by a series of reparative changes, leading to regeneration which is considered to be an inherent property of skeletal muscle. The sequence of regenerative events is the same regardless of whether the cause is physical, chemical, drug-induced or immunological provided that the duration of action of the noxious influence is finite.

Within the necrobiotic group of myopathies the variability in the microscopic appearance is related more to the severity of the noxious influence rather than to its specificity. This fact, together with the topographic distribution of the lesions and the time over which it acts, determines the morphology of the eventual architectural derangement.

However, because the regenerative potential of skeletal muscle is ultimately limited, continuous necrosis will eventually lead to the exhaustion of regeneration and outfall of muscle fibres, with fat and fibrous tissue taking up the dead space. This is known as end-stage disease.

If the term 'focal' is used to represent the anatomical aspect of the lesion and if the term 'phasic' refers to the time factor, and the prefixes 'mono' and 'poly' are added, the full spectrum of histopathological changes may be predicted and precisely described (Kakulas 1975). Examples are easily found for each of these possibilities.

The most important of these combinations occurs when the myopathological change is both polyfocal and polyphasic. This common lesion is observed in the muscular dystrophies and is also found in polymyositis and the other necrobiotic myopathies. The changes are therefore similar in the metabolic and nutritional myopathies, human, animal and experimental, and whenever necrosis continues over a long period of time.

The characteristic architectural disorganisation of muscle, the common feature of these states, results from the polyfocal and polyphasic necrosis occurring over an extended period. Initially, regenerative changes are prominent but, because the newly formed muscle fibres undergo further necrosis, regeneration is eventually exhausted so

that muscle fibres are lost altogether. The non-specific 'myopathic' features of the reduced number of muscle fibres which may remain, such as irregularity in size and shape, central location of nuclei and muscle fibre splitting, are largely due to compensatory hypertrophy and incomplete regeneration.

These principles emphasise that simple morphological similarity of lesions is not an indication of similarity of primary cause. Muscle fibre necrosis is the common denominator in many diverse conditions, whether they are infectious, toxic, immunological, metabolic, drug-induced, hormonal or genetically determined. The lesions may differ morphologically only because of variability in the severity, anatomical distribution and temporal action of these noxious agents.

It is axiomatic that when the cause of focal muscle fibre necrosis is corrected, removed or neutralised, regeneration will ensue as an inherent biological property of voluntary muscle. This principle applies as much to the (at present) incurable disorders such as muscular dystrophy as it does to the toxic myopathies or polymyositis.

It is evident from the above that experimental myopathology encompasses a very broad field of investigation. A loose definition would include all experimental investigations on skeletal muscle and thus much of laboratory myology. However, because most of these basic data relate only indirectly to disease processes, they are not considered in detail. Nevertheless, the more disease-orientated aspects of the subject have contributed significantly to the understanding of human myopathies.

A particularly impressive achievement in the field of pure experiment is understanding the experimental model (EAMG) which has contributed to the elucidation of the mechanisms which underlie human myasthenia gravis. Other significant advances are as follows.

Membrane instabilities due to nutritional or chemically induced abnormalities provide avenues for the investigation of muscle disease characterised by defects of electrolyte transfer such as the periodic paralyses, myotonia congenita and dystrophia myotonica.

As reviewed in this chapter, the experimental manipulation of hereditary muscular dystrophy in animals has also helped to elucidate the natural history of the lesions in human muscular dystrophy (Manda & Kakulas 1986).

The production of rods, target fibres and cores and other histochemical or structural changes similar to those encountered in the congenital group of myopathies is also a useful recent contribution of experimental myopathology. The laboratory production of mitochondrial abnormalities using chemical poisons which act within the oxidative pathways provides useful models for the study of those disorders.

The experimental investigation of the mode of action of myotoxic drugs and toxins in animals gives insight into these unwanted side-effects, within the enlarging field of iatrogenic disorders.

Experimental myopathology has shed some light on the basic processes of reaction of the muscle fibre encountered in human diseases and the analytical approach has led to the recognition of the essential elements which account for the muscle lesions in many of these myopathies. Most importantly, the ability of modern molecular genetic techniques to identify animal models that are molecular homologues of human diseases has, in recent years, revitalized the study of comparative myology. Investigators now await, with some excitement, the application of recombinant DNA technology to these and other issues.

However, while prospects of effective treatment for inherited myopathies in animals and man now seem bright, whether by means of myoblast transfer or gene therapy, it is important to realise that advances achieved in animal models cannot invariably or immediately be extrapolated to the comparable human conditions.

REFERENCES

Acsadi G, Dickson G, Love D R et al 1991 Human dystrophin expression in mdx mice after intramuscular injection of dDNA constructs. Nature 352: 815

Adams R D 1973 In: Kakulas B A (ed) Clinical studies in myology. Excerpta Medica, Amsterdam, p 40

Adams R D 1975 Diseases of muscle. A study of pathology, 3rd edn. Harper and Row, New York

Adrian R H, Bryant S H 1974 On the repetitive discharge in myotonic muscle fibres. Journal of Physiology 240: 505

Adrian R H, Marshall M W 1976 Action potentials reconstructed in normal and myotonic muscle fibres. Journal of Physiology 258: 125

Allbrook D 1962 An electron microscopic study of regenerative skeletal muscle. Journal of Anatomy 96: 137

Allen J G, Steele P, Masters H G, D'Antuono M F 1986 A study of nutritional myopathy in weaner sheep. Australian Veterinary Journal 63: 8

Anastas N C, Kakulas B A 1968 Muscle lesions associated with bone injuries. Proceedings of the Australian Association of Neurologists 5: 553

Anderson J E, Bressler B H, Ovalle W K 1988 Functional regeneration in the hindlimb skeletal muscle of the mdx mouse. Journal of Muscle Research and Cell Motility 9: 499

Anderson J E, Liu L, Kardami E 1991 Distinctive pattern of basic fibroblast growth factor (bFGF) distribution in degenerating and regenerating areas of dystrophic (mdx) striated muscles. Developmental Biology 147: 96

Anderson J E, Ovalle W K, Bressler B H 1987 Electron microscopic and autoradiographic characterization of hindlimb muscle regeneration in the mdx mouse. Anatomical Record 219: 243

Anderson P H, Bradley R, Berrett S, Patterson D S 1977 The sequence of myodegeneration in nutritional myopathy of the older calf. British Veterinary Journal 133: 160

Andresen E, Jensen P 1977 Close linkage established between the HAL locus for halothane sensitivity and the PHI (phosphohexose isomerase) locus in pigs of the Danish Landrace Breed. Nordisk Veterinaermedicin 29: 502

Arahata K, Ishiura S, Ishiguro T et al 1988 Immunostaining of skeletal and cardiac muscle surface membrane with antibody against Duchenne muscular dystrophy peptide. Nature 333: 861

Atkinson J B, Swift L L, Lequire V S 1981 Myotonia congenita. A histochemical and ultrastructural study in the goat: comparison with abnormalities found in human myotonia dystrophica. American Journal of Pathology 102: 324

Bagshaw R J, Cox R H, Knight D H, Detweiler D K 1978 Malignant hyperthermia in a greyhound. Journal of the American Veterinary Medical Association 172: 61

Baker J H 1983 Segmental necrosis in tenotomized muscle fibres. Muscle and Nerve 6: 29

Baker J H, Hall-Craggs E C G 1980 Recovery from central core degeneration of the tenotomized rat soleus muscle. Muscle and Nerve 3: 151

Banker B Q 1960 The experimental myopathies In: Research Publications, Association for Research in Nervous and Mental Diseases (ch VII) 38: 197

Beech J, Fletcher J E, Lisso F, Johnston J 1988 Effect of phenytoin on the clinical signs and in vitro muscle twitch characteristics in horses with chronic intermittent rhabdomyolysis and myotonia. American Journal of Veterinary Research 49: 2130

Bethlem J, van Wijngaarden G K 1963 The incidence of ringed fibres and sarcoplasmic masses in normal and diseased muscle. Journal of Neurology, Neurosurgery and Psychiatry 26: 326

Bhattacharya S K, Crawford A J, Pate J W 1987 Electrocardiographic, biochemical, and morphologic abnormalities in dystrophic hamster with cardiomyopathy. Muscle and Nerve 10: 168

Bigland B, Jehring B 1952 Muscle performance in rats— normal and treated with growth hormone. Journal of Physiology 116: 129

Bodensteiner J B, Engel A G 1978 Intracellular calcium accumulation in Duchenne dystrophy and other myopathies: a study of 567,000 muscle fibres in 114 biopsies. Neurology 28: 439

Bonilla E, Fischbeck K, Schotland D L 1981 Freeze-fracture studies of muscle caveolae in human muscular dystrophy. American Journal of Pathology 104: 167

Bourne G H 1973 The effects of weightlessness on muscle. In: Kakulas B A (ed) Clinical studies in myology Part 2. Proceedings of the Second International Congress on Muscle Diseases, International Congress Series, No 295, Perth, Western Australia. Excerpta Medica, Amsterdam, pp 115–123

Braun T, Rudnicki M A, Arnold H H, Jaenisch R 1992 Targeted inactivation of the muscle regulatory gene Myf-5 results in abnormal rib development and perinatal death. Cell 71: 369

Breitschwerdt E B, Kornegay J N, Wheeler S J, Stevens J B, Baty C J 1992 Episodic weakness associated with exertional lactic acidosis and myopathy in Old English Sheepdog littermates. Journal of the American Veterinary Medical Association 201: 731

Bridges L R 1986 The association of cardiac muscle necrosis and inflammation with the degenerative and persistent myopathy of MDX mice. Journal of the Neurological Sciences 72: 147

Bryant S H 1969 Cable properties of external intercostal muscle fibres from myotonic and nonmyotonic goats. Journal of Physiology 204: 539

Bryant S H 1979 Myotonia in the goat. Annals of the New York Academy of Sciences 317: 314

Bryant S H, Morales-Aguilera A 1971 Chloride conductance in normal and myotonic muscle fibres and the action of monocarboxylic aromatic acids. Journal of Physiology 219: 367

Bryant S H, Conte-Camerino D 1991 Chloride channel regulation in the skeletal muscle of normal and myotonic goats. Pflugers Archiv. European Journal of Physiology 417: 605

Bryant S H, Lipicky R J, Herzog W H 1968 Variability of myotonic signs in myotonic goats. American Journal of Veterinary Research 29: 2371

Bulfield G, Siller W G, Wight P A, Moore K J 1984 X chromosome-linked muscular dystrophy (mdx) in the mouse. Proceedings of the National Academy of Sciences USA 181: 1189

Buller A J, Eccles J C, Eccles R M 1960 Interactions between motor neurons and muscles in respect of the characteristic speeds of their response. Journal of Physiology 150: 417

Bundschu H D, Pfeilsticker H, Suchenwirth R, Matthews C, Ritz E 1974 Experimental uremic myopathy. In: IIIrd International Congress of Muscle Diseases, International Congress Series No 334, Abstract 3030 Excerpta Medica, Amsterdam

Burbach J A 1987 Ultrastructure of cardiocyte degeneration and myocardial calcification in the dystrophic hamster. American Journal of Anatomy 179: 291

Campbell K P, Kahl S D 1989 Association of dystrophin and an integral membrane glycoprotein. Nature 338: 259

Cardinet G H, Holliday T A 1979 Neuromuscular diseases of domestic animals: a summary of muscle biopsies from 159 cases. Annals of the New York Academy of Sciences 317: 290

Carlson B M 1974 Morphogenetic effects of cross-transplanted muscles upon an epimorphic regenerative process. In IIIrd International Congress on Muscle Diseases. International Congress Series No 334, Abstract 273. Excerpta Medica, Amsterdam

Carlson C G, Makiejus R V 1990 A noninvasive procedure to detect muscle weakness in the mdx mouse. Muscle and Nerve 13: 480

Carnwath J W, Shotton D M 1987 Muscular dystrophy in the mdx mouse: histopathology of the soleus and extensor digitorum longus muscles. Journal of the Neurological Sciences 80: 39

Carpenter J L, Hoffman E P, Romanul F C A et al 1989 Feline muscular dystrophy with dystrophin deficiency. American Journal of Pathology 135: 909

Carter G T, Longley K J, Entrikin R K 1992 Electromyographic and nerve conduction studies in the mdx mouse. American Journal of Physical Medicine and Rehabilitation 71: 2

Caulfield J B 1966 Electron microscopic observations on the dystrophic hamster muscle. Annals of the New York Academy of Sciences 138: 151

Cavanna J S, Coulton G, Morgan J E et al 1988 Molecular and genetic mapping of the mouse mdx locus. Genomics 3: 337

Ceh L, Hauge J G, Svenkerud R, Strande A 1976 Glycogenosis type III in the dog. Acta Veterinaria Scandinavica 17: 210

Chamberlain J S, Pearlman J A, Muzny D M et al 1988 Expression of the murine Duchenne muscular dystrophy gene in muscle and brain. Science 239: 1416

Chapman V M, Miller D R, Armstrong D, Caskey C T 1989 Recovery of induced mutations for X chromosome-linked muscular dystrophy in mice. Proceedings of the National Academy of Sciences USA 86: 1292

Chou S M 1984 Core-genic neuromyopathies. In: Heffner R R Jr (ed) Muscle pathology. Churchill Livingstone, New York, ch 7, pp 83–107

Clark W L 1946 An experimental study of the regeneration of mammalian striped muscle. Journal of Anatomy 80: 24

Clark W L, Wajda H S 1947 The growth and maturation of regenerating striated muscle fibers. Journal of Anatomy 81: 56

Cooper B J, de Lahunta A, Gallagher E A, Valentine B A 1986 Nemaline myopathy of cats. Muscle and Nerve 9: 618

Cooper B J, Gallagher E A, Smith C A, Valentine B A, Winand N J 1990 Mosaic expression of dystrophin in carriers of canine X-linked muscular dystrophy. Laboratory Investigation 62: 171

Cooper B J, Valentine B A, Wilson S, Patterson D F, Concannon P W 1988a Canine muscular dystrophy: confirmation of X-linked inheritance. Journal of Heredity 79: 405

Cooper B J, Winand N J, Stedman H et al 1988b The homologue of the Duchenne locus is defective in X-linked muscular dystrophy of dogs. Nature 334: 154

Cooper B J et al 1991 Proceedings of the XIth International Congress on Neuropathology, Kyoto. Neuropathology Supplement 4.

Cork L C 1991 Hereditary canine spinal muscular atrophy: an animal model of motor neuron disease. Canadian Journal of Neurological Sciences 18 (suppl): 432

Cork L C, Price D L, Griffin J W, Sack G H Jr 1990 Hereditary canine spinal muscular atrophy: canine motor neuron disease. Canadian Journal of Veterinary Research 54: 77

Coulton G R, Cutin N A, Morgan J E, Partridge T A 1988a

The mdx mouse skeletal muscle myopathy: II. Contractile properties. Neuropathology and Applied Neurobiology 14: 299

Coulton G R, Morgan J E, Partridge T A, Sloper J C 1988b The mdx mouse skeletal muscle myopathy: I. A histological, morphometric and biochemical investigation. Neuropathology and Applied Neurobiology 14: 53

Cox G A, Cole N M, Matsumura K et al 1993 Overexpression of dystrophin in transgenic mdx mice eliminates dystrophic symptoms without toxicity. Nature 364: 725

Cox J H 1986 An episodic weakness in four horses associated with intermittent serum hyperkalemia and the similarity of the disease to hyperkalemic periodic paralysis in man. Proceedings of the American Association of Equine Practitioners 92: 299

Cribb P H 1988 Malignant hyperthermia in the dog: laboratory investigations. In: Williams C H (ed) Experimental malignant hyperthermia. Springer-Verlag, New York, p 118

Crockett J L, Edgerton V R 1974 Enhancement of muscle protein and tetanic tension after intramuscular spinal homogenate injections in: IIIrd International Congress on Muscle Diseases. International Congress Series No 334, Abstract 22, Exerpta Medica, Amsterdam

Cullen M J, Jaros E 1988 Ultrastructure of the skeletal muscle in the X chromosome-linked dystrophic (mdx) mouse. Comparison with Duchenne muscular dystrophy. Acta Neuropathologica 77: 69

Cummings J F, de Lahunta A, George C et al 1990 Equine motor neuron disease; a preliminary report. Cornell Veterinarian 80: 357

Cummings J F, de Lahunta A, Mohammed H O et al 1991 Equine motor neuron disease: a new neurologic disorder. Equine Practice 13: 15

Cummings J F, de Lahunta A, Summers B A et al 1993 Eosinophilic cytoplasmic inclusions in sporadic equine motor neuron disease: an electron microscopic study. Acta Neuropathologica 85: 291

Cummings J F, George C, de Lahunta A, Valentine B A, Bookbinder P F 1989 Focal spinal muscular atrophy in two German Shepherd pups. Acta Neuropathologica 79: 113

Currie S, Saunders M, Knowles M, Brown A E 1971 Immunological aspects of polymyositis. The in vitro activity of lymphocytes on incubation with muscle antigen with muscle cultures. Quarterly Journal of Medicine 40: 63

Dalldorf G 1950 The Coxsackie viruses. Bulletin of the New York Academy of Medicine 26: 329

Dangain J, Vrbova G 1984 Muscle development in mdx mutant mice. Muscle and Nerve 7: 700

Danko I, Chapman V, Wolff J A 1992 The frequency of revertants in mdx mouse genetic models for Duchenne muscular dystrophy. Pediatric Research 32: 128

Darke P G G, McCullagh K G, Geldart P H 1975 Myasthenia gravis, thymoma and myositis in a dog. Veterinary Record 97: 392

Dau P C, Yano C S, Ettinger S J 1979 Antibody to acetlycholine receptor in canine and human myasthenia gravis: differential cross-reactivity with human and rabbit receptor. Neurology 29: 1065

Davies W, Harbitz I, Fries R, Stranzinger G, Hauge J G 1988 Porcine malignant hyperthermia carrier detection and chromosomal assignment using a linked probe. Animal Genetics 19: 203

Dawkins R L 1965 Experimental myositis associated with

hypersensitivity to muscle. Journal of Pathology and Bacteriology 90: 619

Dawson J R 1970 Myasthenia gravis in a cat. Veterinary Record 86: 562

de Lahunta A 1983 Veterinary neuroanatomy and clinical neurology, 2nd edn. W B Saunders, Philadelphia

De Jong R H, Heavner J E, Amory D W 1974 Malignant hyperpyrexia in the cat. Anesthesiology 41: 608

De Reuck J, De Coster W, Van der Eecken H 1977 The target phenomenon in rat muscle following tenotomy and neurotomy. Acta Neuropathologica 37: 49

Denny-Brown D 1951 The influence of tension and innervation on the regeneration of skeletal muscle. Journal of Neuropathology and Experimental Neurology 10: 94

Di Marco P N, Howell J McC, Dorling P R 1984 Bovine glycogenosis type II. Biochemical and morphological characteristics of skeletal muscle in culture. Neuropathology and Applied Neurobiology 10: 379

Di Marco P N, Howell J M, Dorling P R 1985 Bovine generalised glycogenosis type II. Uptake of lysosomal alpha-glucosidase by cultured skeletal muscle and reversal of glycogen accumulation. FEBS Letters 190: 301

DiMario J, Buffinger N, Yamada S, Strohman R C 1989 Fibroblast growth factor in the extracellular matrix of dystrophic (mdx) mouse muscle. Science 244: 688

DiMario J X, Uzman A, Strohman R C 1991 Fibre regeneration is not persistent in dystrophic (mdx) mouse skeletal muscle. Developmental Biology 148: 314

Divers T J, Mohammed H O, Cummings J F et al 1992 Equine motor neuron disease: a new cause of weakness, trembling, and weight loss. Compendium of Continuing Education for the Practicing Veterinarian 14: 1222

Doizé F, Roux I, Martineau-Doizé B, DeRoth L 1990 Prediction of the halothane (Hal) genotypes by means of linked marker loci (Phi, Po2, Pgd) in Quebec Landrace pigs. Canadian Journal of Veterinary Research 54: 397

Douglas W B 1974 Myographic and electroneurographic responses of leg muscles and cross-innervated sciatic nerves in normal and dystrophic mice (129B6F₁ hybrid) united in parabiosis. In: IIIrd International Congress on Muscle Diseases. International Congress Series No 334 Abstract 19. Excerpta Medica, Amsterdam

Duchen L W 1978 Motor neuron diseases in man and animals. Investigative and Cell Pathology 1: 249

Duncan I D, Griffiths I R 1977 Muscle disease in the chow [letter]. Veterinary Record 100: 476

Dunckley M G, Love D R, Davies K E, Walsh F S, Morris G E, Dickson G 1992 Retroviral-mediated transfer of a dystrophin minigene into mdx mouse myoblasts in vitro. FEBS Letters 296: 128

Dunn J F, Radda G K 1991 Total ion content of skeletal and cardiac muscle in the mdx mouse dystrophy: Ca^{2+} is elevated at all ages. Journal of the Neurological Sciences 103: 226

Dupont-Versteegden E E, McCarter R J 1992 Differential expression of muscular dystrophy in diaphragm versus hindlimb muscles of mdx mice. Muscle and Nerve 15: 1105

Eccles J C 1941 Disuse atrophy of skeletal muscle. Medical Journal of Australia 2: 160

Eccles J C 1944 Investigations on muscle atrophies arising from disuse and tenotomy. Journal of Physiology 103: 252–266

Edström L, Kugelberg E 1968 Histochemical composition distribution of fibres and fatigability of single motor units. Journal of Neurology, Neurosurgery and Psychiatry 31: 424

Edwards J R, Richards R B 1979 Bovine generalized glycogenosis type II. A clinicopathological study. British Veterinary Journal 135: 338

El-Hamidi M, Leipold H W, Vestweber J G E, Saperstein G 1989 Spinal muscular atrophy in Brown Swiss calves. Zentralblatt fur Veterinarmedizin. Reihe A 153: 161

Elder G C B 1992 Beneficial effects of training on developing dystrophic muscle. Muscle and Nerve 15: 672

Engel A G 1979 Myasthenia gravis. In: Vinken P J, Bruyn G W (eds) Handbook of clinical neurology, vol 41. Diseases of muscle part II. North Holland, Amsterdam, ch 4, pp 92–145

Engel W K 1973 Duchenne muscular dystrophy. A histologically based ischaemia hypothesis and comparison with experimental ischaemic myopathy. In: Pearson C M, Mostofi F K (eds). The striated muscle. Williams and Wilkins, Baltimore, p 453

Engel W K, Brooke M H, Nelson P G 1966. Histochemical studies of denervated or tenotomized cat muscle: illustrating difficulties in relating experimental animal conditions to human neuromuscular diseases. Annals of the New York Academy of Sciences 138: 160

England S B, Nicholson L V B, Johnson M A et al 1990 Very mild muscular dystrophy associated with the deletion of 46% of dystrophin. Nature 343: 180

Entrikin R K, Abresch R T, Sharman R B, Larson D B, Levine N A 1987 Contractile and EMG studies of murine myotonia (*mto*) and muscular dystrophy (*dy/dy*). Muscle and Nerve 10: 293

Ervasti J M, Campbell K P 1991 Membrane organization of the dystrophin–glycoprotein complex. Cell 66: 1121

Esiri M M, MacLennan I C M 1975 Some imunological studies of an experimental allergic myositis in rats. In: Bradley W G, Gardner-Medwin D, Walton J N (eds) Recent advances in myology. Excerpta Medica, Amsterdam, p 380

Farrow B R H, Malik R 1981 Hereditary myotonia in the Chow Chow. Journal of Small Animal Practice 22: 451

Fenichel G M, Martin J T 1974 An experimental myopathy in rats produced with imidazole. In: IIIrd International Congress on Muscle Diseases, International Congress Series No 334, Abstract 331. Excerpta Medica, Amsterdam

Ferguson A B, Vaughan L, Ward L 1957 A study of disuse atrophy of skeletal muscle in the rabbit. Journal of Bone and Joint Surgery 39A: 583

Field E J 1960 Virus infections. In: Bourne G H (ed) The structure and function of muscle. Academic Press, New York ch 3, p 85.

Fischbeck K H, Bonilla E, Schotland D L 1984 Distribution of freeze-fracture particle sizes in Duchenne muscle plasma membrane. Neurology 34: 534

Flagstad A 1982 A new hereditary neuromuscular disease in the dog breed 'Gammel Dansk Honsehund'. Genetic investigations. Hereditas 96: 211

Flagstad A, Trojaborg W, Gammeltoft S 1989 Congenital myasthenic syndrome in the dog breed *Gammel Dansk Honsehund*: clinical, electrophysiological, pharmacological and immunological comparison with acquired myasthenia gravis. Acta Veterinaria Scandinavica 30: 89

Fong P, Turner P R, Denetclaw W F, Steinhardt R A 1990 Increased activity of calcium leak channels in myotubes of Duchenne human and mdx mouse origin. Science 250: 673

Francis M J O, Curry O B, Smith R 1974 Vitamin D and muscle: a defect of calcium uptake by sarcoplasmic reticulum in vitamin D deficient rabbits. In: IIIrd International Congress on Muscle Diseases, International Congress Series No 334, Abstract 324. Excerpta Medica, Amsterdam

Franco A Jr, Lansman J B 1990 Calcium entry through stretch-inactivated ion channels in mdx myotubes. Nature 344: 670

Frankel K A, Rosser R J 1976 The pathology of the heart in progressive muscular dystrophy: epimyocardial fibrosis. Human Pathology 7: 375

Fraser D C, Palmer A C, Senior J E, Parkes J D, Yealland M F 1970 Myasthenia gravis in the dog. Journal of Neurology, Neurosurgery and Psychiatry 33: 431

Füchtbauer E-M, Reininghaus J, Jockusch H 1988 Developmental control of the excitability of muscle: transplantation experiments on a myotonic mouse mutant. Proceedings of the National Academy of Sciences USA 85: 3880

Fujii J, Otsu K, Zorzato F et al 1991 Identification of a mutation in porcine ryanodine receptor associated with malignant hyperthermia. Science 253: 448

Fujita T, Nonaka I, Sugita H 1991 Japanese quail and human acid maltase deficiency: a comparative study. Brain and Development 13: 247

Fyfe J C, Giger U, van Winkle T J et al 1992 Glycogen storage disease type IV: inherited deficiency of branching enzyme activity in cats. Pediatric Research 32: 719

Gallant E M 1980 Histochemical observations on muscle from normal and malignant hyperthermia-susceptible swine. American Journal of Veternary Research 41: 1069

Gallant E M, Mickelson J R, Roggow B D, Donaldson S K, Louis C F, Rempel W E 1989 Halothane-sensitivity gene and muscle contractile properties in malignant hyperthermia. American Journal of Physiology 257: C781

Garlepp M, Farrow B, Kay P, Dawkins R L 1979 Antibodies to the acetylcholine receptor in myasthenic dogs. Immunology 37: 807

Garlepp M J, Kay P H, Farrow B R and Dawkins R L 1984 Autoimmunity in spontaneous myasthenia gravis in dogs. Clinical Immunology and Immunopathology 31: 301

Gaschen F P, Hoffman E P, Gorospe J R M et al 1992 Dystrophin deficiency causes lethal muscle hypertrophy in cats. Journal of the Neurological Sciences 110: 149

Gauthier G F, Schaeffer S F 1975 Ultrastructural evidence of early subsarcolemmal protein synthesis in denervated skeletal muscle fibres. In Bradley W G, Gardner-Medwin D, Walton J N (eds) Recent advances in myology. Excerpta Medica, Amsterdam, pp 27–32

Goyer R A, Yin M W 1967 Taurine and creatine excretion after X-irradiation and plasmocid-induced muscle necrosis in the rat. Radiation Research 30: 301

Graham D I, Bonilla E, Gonatas N K, Schotland D L 1976 Core formation in the muscle of rats intoxicated with triethyltin sulfate. Journal of Neuropathology and Experimental Neurology 35: 1

Griffiths I R, Duncan I D 1973 Myotonia in the dog: a report of four cases. Veterinary Record 93: 184

Grounds M D, McGeachie J K 1992 Skeletal muscle regeneration after crush injury in dystrophic mdx mice: an autoradiographic study. Muscle and Nerve 15: 580

Gutmann E, Guttmann L 1942 Effect of electrotherapy on denervated muscles in rabbits. Lancet i: 169

Gutmann E, Hanzlikova V 1975 Factors affecting success of transplantation of skeletal muscle in the rat. In: Bradley W G, Gardner-Medwin D, Walton J N (eds) Recent advances in myology. Excerpta Medica, Amsterdam, p 57

Hadlow W J 1962 Diseases of skeletal muscle. In: Innes J R M, Saunders L Z (eds) Comparative neuropathology. Academic, New York, pp 147–232

Hahn C, Mayhew I G, Shepherd M 1993 Equine motor neuron disease. Veterinary Record 132: 172

Hall G A, Howell J McC, Lewis D G 1972 Thymoma with myasthenia gravis in a dog. Journal of Pathology 108: 178

Harbitz I, Chowdhary B, Thomsen P D et al 1990 Assignment of the porcine calcium release channel gene, a candidate for the malignant hyperthermia locus, to the 6p11–q21 segment of chromosome 6. Genomics 8: 243

Harris A S and Mrak R E 1985 Myotonia congenita. In: Mrak R E (ed) Muscle membranes in diseases of muscle. CRC, Boca Raton, p 81

Hartman K S, Standish S M 1974 Muscle regeneration in the dystrophic Syrian hamster tongue. Effects of a moderately severe crushing injury. Archives of Pathology 98: 126

Harvey J W, Calderwood Mays M B, Gropp K E, Denaro F J 1990 Polysaccharide storage myopathy in canine phosphofructokinase deficiency (type VII glycogen storage disease). Veterinary Pathology 27: 1

Hasty P, Bradley A, Morris J H et al 1993 Muscle deficiency and neonatal death in mice with a targeted mutation in the myogenin gene. Nature 364: 501

Haws C M, Lansman J B 1991 Developmental regulation of mechanosensitive calcium channels in skeletal muscle from normal and mdx mice. Proceedings of the Royal Society of London. Series B: Biological Sciences 245: 173

Head S I, Williams D A, Stephenson D G 1992 Abnormalities in structure and function of limb skeletal muscle fibres of dystrophic mdx mice. Proceedings of the Royal Society of London. Series B: Biological Sciences 248: 163

Heffron J J, Mitchell G, Dreyer J H 1982 Muscle fibre type, fibre diameter and pH1 values of M. longissimus dorsi of normal, malignant hyperthermia- and PSE-susceptible pigs. British Veterinary Journal 138: 45

Heller A H, Eicher E M, Hallet M, Sidman R L 1982 Myotonia, a new inherited muscle disease in mice. Journal of Neuroscience 2: 924

Higuchi I, Nonaka I, Usuki F, Ishiura S, Sugita H 1987 Acid maltase deficiency in the Japanese quail; early morphologic event in skeletal muscle. Acta Neuropathologica 73: 32

Hildebrand S V 1988 Horses and ponies as animal models for malignant hyperthermia. In: Williams C H (ed) Experimental malignant hyperthermia. Springer-Verlag, New York, p 100

Hoffman E P, Brown R H Jr, Kunkel L M 1987 Dystrophin: the protein product of the Duchenne muscular dystrophy locus. Cell 51: 919

Hoffman E P, Morgan J E, Watkins S C, Partridge T A 1990 Somatic reversion/suppression of the mouse mdx phenotype in vivo. Journal of the Neurological Sciences 99: 9

Holmes D, Dickson J A, Pennington R J 1974 Peptide hydrolases in muscle from tumour-bearing rats. In: IIIrd International Congress on Muscle Diseases, International Congress Series No 334, Abstract 326. Excerpta Medica, Amsterdam

Homburger F 1979 Myopathy of hamster dystrophy: history and morphologic aspects. Annals of the New York Academy of Sciences 317: 2

Homburger F, Nixon C W, Eppenberger M, Baker J R 1966 Hereditary myopathy in the Syrian hamster: studies on pathogenesis. Annals of the New York Academy of Sciences 138: 14

Homburger F, Bajusz E 1970 New models of human disease in Syrian hamsters. Journal of the American Medical Association 212: 604

Howell J M, Dorling P R, Shelton J N, Taylor E G, Palmer D G, Di Marco P N 1991 Natural bone marrow transplantation in cattle with Pompe's disease. Neuromuscular Disorders 1: 449

Howell J McC, Dorling P R, Cook R D, Robinson W F, Bradley S, Gawthorne J M 1981 Infantile and late onset form of generalised glycogenosis type II in cattle. Journal of Pathology 134: 266

Howell J McC, Buxton P H 1975 α-Tocopherol responsive muscular dystrophy in guinea pigs. Neuropathology and Applied Neurobiology 1: 49

Howells K F, Goldspink G 1974 The effect of exercise on the progress of the myopathy in dystrophic hamster muscle fibres. Journal of Anatomy 117: 385

Hunter S 1980 The heart in muscular dystrophy. British Medical Bulletin 36: 133

Hutter O F, Burton F L, Bovell D L 1991 Mechanical properties of normal and mdx mouse sarcolemma: bearing on function of dystrophin. Journal of Muscle Research and Cell Motility 12: 585

Iaizzo P A, Klein W, Lehmann-Horn F 1988 Fura-2 detected myoplasmic calcium and its correlation with contracture force in skeletal muscle from normal and malignant hyperthermia susceptible pigs. Pflugers Archiv. European Journal of Physiology 411: 648

Inada S, Simpson C F, Haruta K et al 1978 A clinical study on hereditary progressive neurogenic muscular atrophy in Pointer dogs. Japanese Journal of Veterinary Science 40: 539

Indrieri R J, Creighton S R, Lambert E H, Lennon V A 1983 Myasthenia gravis in two cats. Journal of the American Veterinary Medical Association 182: 57

Ishay J, Lass Y, Sandbank U 1975 A lesion of muscle transverse tubular system by oriental hornet (Vespa orientalis) venom; electron microscopic and histological study. Toxicon 13: 57

Iwata Y, Nakamura H, Fujiwara K, Shigekawa M 1993 Altered membrane-dystrophin association in the cardiomyopathic hamster heart muscle. Biochemical and Biophysical Research Communications 190: 589

Jamison J M, Baird J D, Smith-Maxie L L, Hulland T J 1987 A congenital form of myotonia with dystrophic changes in a quarterhorse. Equine Veterinary Journal 19: 353

Jasmin G, Gareau R 1961 Histopathological study of muscle lesions produced by paraphenylenediamine in rats. British Journal of Experimental Pathology 42: 592

Jasmin G, Eu H Y 1979 Cardiomyopathy of hamster dystrophy. Annals of the New York Academy of Sciences 317: 46

Jenkins W L, Van Dyk E, McDonald C B 1976 Myasthenia gravis in a fox terrier litter. Journal of the South African Veterinary Medical Association 47: 59

Jezyk P F 1982 Hyperkalemic periodic paralysis in a dog. Journal of the American Animal Hospital Association 18: 977

Jockusch H, Friedrich G, Zippel M 1990 Serum parvalbumin, an indicator of muscle disease in murine dystrophy and myotonia. Muscle and Nerve 13: 551

Jockusch H, Reininghaus J, Stuhlfauth I, Zippel M 1988 Reduction of myosin-light-chain phosphorylation and of parvalbumin content in myotonic mouse muscle and its reversal by tocainide. European Journal of Biochemistry 171: 101

Johnson R P, Watson A D, Smith J, Cooper B J 1975 Myasthenia in Springer Spaniel littermates. Journal of Small Animal Practice 16: 641

Johnston D M, Drachman D B 1974 Neurotrophic regulation of dynamic properties of skeletal muscle: effects of botulinum toxin and denervation. In: IIIrd International Congress on Muscle Diseases, International Congress Series No 334, Abstract 21. Excerpta Medica, Amsterdam

Jones B R, Anderson L J, Barnes G R, Johnstone A C, Juby W D 1977 Myotonia in related Chow Chow dogs. New Zealand Veterinary Journal 25: 217

Jones E W, Kerr D D, Nelson T E 1973 Malignant hyperthermia — observations in Poland China pigs. In: Gordon R A, Britt B A, Kalow W (eds) International Symposium on Malignant Hyperthermia. Charles C Thomas, Springfield, p 198

Joseph R J, Carrillo J M, Lennon V A 1988 Myasthenia gravis in the cat. Journal of Veterinary Internal Medicine 2: 75

Kakulas B A 1966 Destruction of differentiated muscle cultures by sensitized lymphoid cells. Journal of Pathology and Bacteriology 91: 495

Kakulas B A 1970 The pathogenesis of human muscle disease. In: Walton J N, Canal N, Scarlato G (eds) Muscle diseases. Excerpta Medica, Amsterdam, p 337

Kakulas B A 1973 Observations on the aetiology of polymyositis. In: Pearson C M, Mostofi F K (eds) The striated muscle. Williams and Wilkins, Baltimore, p 485

Kakulas B A 1975 Experimental muscle diseases. In: Jasmin G, Cantin M (eds) Methods and achievements in experimental pathology, vol 7. Karger, Basel, p 109

Kakulas B A 1982 Toxic and drug-induced myopathies. In: Walton J N, Mastaglia F L (eds) Skeletal muscle pathology. Churchill Livingstone, Edinburgh, ch 13, p 46

Kakulas B A 1988 Animal models of polymyositis/dermatomyositis. In: Dalakas M (ed) Polymyositis and dermatomyositis Butterworths, Boston, pp 133–154

Kakulas B A, Adams R D 1966 Principles of myopathology as illustrated in the nutritional myopathy of the Rottnest quokka (Setonix brachyurus). Annals of the New York Academy of Sciences 138: 90

Kakulas B A, Adams R D 1985 Diseases of muscle. Pathological foundations of clinical myology. Harper and Row, Philadelphia

Kallos P, Pagel W 1937 Experimentelle Untersuchunge uber Asthma bronchiale. Acta Medica Scandinavica 91: 292

Kark R A P, Edgerton V R, Whiteman N 1975 Decreased oxidation by muscle after denervation but not disuse atrophy. In: Bradley W G, Gardner-Medwin D, Walton J N (eds). Recent advances in myology. Excerpta Medica, Amsterdam, p 3

Karpati G, Carpenter S, Eisen A A 1972 Experimental core-like lesions and nemaline rods: a correlative morphological and physiological study. Archives of Neurology 27: 237

Karpati G, Carpenter S, Melmed C, Eisen A A 1974 Experimental ischemic myopathy. Journal of the Neurological Sciences 23: 129

Karpati G, Carpenter S, Prescott S 1982 Prevention of skeletal muscle fibre necrosis in hamster dystrophy. Muscle and Nerve 5: 369

Karpati G, Carpenter S, Prescott S 1988 Small-caliber skeletal muscle fibres do not suffer necrosis in mdx mouse dystrophy. Muscle and Nerve 11: 795

Karpati G, Pouliot Y, Zubrzycka-Gaarn E et al 1989 Dystrophin is expressed in mdx skeletal muscle fibres after

normal myoblast implantation. American Journal of Pathology 135: 27

Karpati G, Zubrzycka-Gaarn E E, Carpenter S, Bulman D E, Ray P N, Worton R G 1990 Age-related conversion of dystrophin-negative to -positive fibre segments of skeletal but not cardiac muscle fibre in heterozygote mdx mice. Journal of Neuropathology and Experimental Neurology 49: 96

Kennedy S, Rice D A, Davidson W B 1987 Experimental myopathy in vitamin E- and selenium-depleted calves with and without added dietary polyunsaturated fatty acids as a model for nutritional degenerative myopathy in ruminant cattle. Research in Veterinary Science 43: 384

Khan M Y 1974 Radiation induced changes in skeletal muscle: an electron microscopic study. Journal of Neuropathology and Experimental Neurology 33: 42

Kirmayer A, Klide A M, Purvance J E 1984 Malignant hyperthermia in a dog: case report and review of the syndrome. Journal of the American Veterinary Medical Association 185: 978

Koenig M, Monaco A P, Kunkel L M 1988 The complete sequence of dystrophin predicts a rod-shaped cytoskeletal protein. Cell 53: 219

Költgen D, Brinkmeier H, Jockusch H 1991 Myotonia and neuromuscular transmission in the mouse. Muscle and Nerve 14: 775

Kornegay J N, Gorgacz E J, Dawe D L, Bowen J M, White N A, DeBuyssscher E V 1980 Polymyositis in dogs. Journal of the American Veterinary Medical Association 176: 431

Kornegay J N, Tuler S M, Miller D M, Levesque D C 1988 Muscular dystrophy in a litter of golden retriever dogs. Muscle and Nerve 11: 1056

Krum S H, Cardinet G H, Anderson B C, Holliday T A 1977 Polymyositis and polyarthritis associated with systemic lupus erythematosis in a dog. Journal of the American Veterinary Medical Association 170: 61

Kugelberg E, Edström L, Abbruzzese M 1970 Mapping of motor units in experimentally reinnervated rat muscle. Interpretation of histochemical and atrophic fibre pattern in neurogenic lesions. Journal of Neurology, Neurosurgery and Psychiatry 33: 319

Leary S L, Anderson L C, Manning P J, Bache R J, Zweber B A 1983 Recurrent malignant hyperthermia in a Greyhound. Journal of the American Veterinary Medical Association 182: 521

Leestma J E 1980 Animal model of human disease. Motor neuron disease in the Wobbler mouse (wr/wr) mouse. American Journal of Pathology 821

Lipicky R J and Bryant S H 1966 Sodium, potassium, and chloride fluxes in intercostal muscle from normal goats and goats with hereditary myotonia. Journal of General Physiology 50: 89

London W T, Sever J L, Madden D L et al 1983 Experimental transmission of simian acquired immunodeficiency syndrome (SAIDS) and kaposi-like skin lesions. Lancet ii: 869

López J R, Allen P D, Alamo L, Jones D, Sreter F A 1988 Myoplasmic free [Ca^{2+}] during a malignant hyperthermia episode in swine. Muscle and Nerve 11: 82

Lorenz M D, de Lahunta A, Alstrom D H 1972 Neostigmine-responsive weakness in the dog, similar to myasthenia gravis. Journal of the American Veterinary Medical Association 161: 795

Lundsgaard E 1930 Üntersuchungen uber Muskelkontraktion ohne Milchsäurebildung, Biochem Zeitschrift 217: 162

MacLennan D H, Phillips M S 1992 Malignant hyperthermia. Science 256: 789

MacLennan P A, McArdle A, Edwards R H T 1991 Effects of calcium on protein turnover of incubated muscles from mdx mice. American Journal of Physiology 260: E594

MacLennan P A, Edwards R H T 1990 Protein turnover is elevated in muscle of mdx mice in vivo. Biochemical Journal 268: 795

Manda P, Kakulas B 1986 The effect of the myotoxic agent iodoacetate on dystrophic mice 129 Journal of the Neurological Sciences 75: 23

Manghani D, Partridge T, Sloper J C, Smith P 1975 Role of myofibrillar antigens in the pathogenesis of experimental myositis with particular reference to lymphocyte sensitization, the transfer of the disease by lymphocytes, and the preferential attachment of lymphocytes from animals with experimental myositis to cultured muscle cells. In: Bradley W G, Gardner-Medwin D, Walton J N (eds) Recent advances in myology. Excerpta Medica, Amsterdam, p 387

Manolov S 1974 Regeneration of rat neuromuscular junctions. In: IIIrd International Congress on Muscle Diseases Series No 334. Abstract 183. Excerpta Medica, Amsterdam

Margreth A, Salviati G, Carraro U 1974 Biochemical characteristics of skeletal muscles in relation to the pattern and rate of activity. In: IIIrd International Congress on Muscle Diseases. International Congress Series No 334 Abstract 10. Excerpta Medica, Amsterdam

Martin A F, Bryant S H, Mandel F 1984 Isomyosin distribution in skeletal muscles of normal and myotonic goats. Muscle and Nerve 7: 152

Marvasti M A, Williams C H 1988 Malignant hyperthermia and the sarcoplasmic reticulum: a review. In: Williams C H (ed) Experimental malignant hyperthermia. Springer-Verlag, New York, p 57

Mascres C, Jasmin G 1975 Changes in the muscle fibre induced in the rat by p-phenylenediamine. Pathology and Biology 23: 193

Mason K V 1976 A case of myasthenia gravis in a cat. Journal of Small Animal Practice 17: 467

Mastaglia F L, Dawkins R L, Papadimitriou J M 1974 A morphological study of muscle grafts in mice. In: IIIrd International Congress on Muscle Diseases, International Congress Series No 334, Abstract 275. Excerpta Medica, Amsterdam

Matsui T, Kuroda S, Mizutani M, Kiuchi Y, Suzuki K, Ono T 1983 Generalized glycogen storage disease in Japanese quail (Coturnix coturnix japonica). Veterinary Pathology 20: 312

Matsumura K, Ervasti J M, Ohlendieck K, Kahl S D, Campbell K P 1992a Association of dystrophin-related protein with dystrophin-associated proteins in mdx mouse muscle. Nature 360: 588

Matsumura K, Tomé F M S, Collin H et al 1992b Deficiency of the 50K dystrophin-associated glycoprotein in severe childhood autosomal recessive muscular dystrophy. Nature 359: 320

Matsumura K, Lee C C, Caskey C T, Campbell K P 1993 Restoration of dystrophin-associated proteins in skeletal muscle of mdx mice transgenic for dystrophin gene. FEBS Letters 320: 276

Mauro A, Shafiq S A, Milhorat A T 1970 Regeneration of striated muscle and myogenesis. International Congress Series No 218. Excerpta Medica, Amsterdam

McArdle A, Edwards R H T, Jackson M J 1991 Effects of contractile activity on muscle damage in the dystrophin-deficient mdx mouse. Clinical Science 80: 367

McMurray C H, Rice D A, Kennedy S 1983 Experimental models for nutritional myopathy. Ciba Foundation Symposium 101: 201

Mehrke G, Brinkmeier H, Jockusch H 1988 The myotonic mouse mutant ADR: electrophysiology of the muscle fibre. Muscle and Nerve 11: 440

Melmed C, Karpati G, Carpenter S 1975 Experimental mitochondrial myopathy produced by in vivo uncoupling of oxidative phosphorylation. Journal of Neurological Sciences 26: 305

Mendell J R 1979 Experimental myopathies: a review of experimental models and their relationship to human neuromuscular diseases. In: Vinken P J, Bruyn G W (eds) Handbook of clinical neurology, vol 30, Part 1. North Holland, Amsterdam, p 133

Mendell J R, Higgins R, Sahenk Z, Cosmos E 1979 Relevance of genetic animal models of muscular dystrophy to human muscular dystrophies. Annals of the New York Academy of Sciences 317: 409

Menke A, Jockusch H 1991 Decreased osmotic stability of dystrophin-less muscle cells from the mdx mouse. Nature 349: 69

Mickelson J R, Gallant E M, Rempel W E et al 1989 Effects of the halothane-sensitivity gene on sarcoplasmic reticulum function. American Journal of Physiology 257: C787

Mickelson J R, Litterer L A, Jacobson B A, Louis C F 1990 Stimulation and inhibition of [^{3}H]ryanodine binding to sarcoplasmic reticulum from malignant hyperthermia susceptible pigs. Archives of Biochemistry and Biophysics 278: 251

Mickelson J R, Ross J A, Reed B K, Louis C F 1986 Enhanced Ca^{2+}-induced calcium release by isolated sarcoplasmic reticulum vesicles from malignant hyperthermia susceptible pig muscle. Biochimica et Biophysica Acta 862: 318

Miller L M, Lennon V A, Lambert E H et al 1983 Congenital myasthenia gravis in 13 smooth fox terriers. Journal of the American Veterinary Medical Association 182: 694

Miranda A F, Gamboa E T, Armstrong C L, Hsu K C 1978 Susceptibility of human skeletal muscle culture to influenza virus infection, Part 2. Ultrastructural cytopathology. Journal of the Neurological Sciences 36: 63

Mitsumoto H and Bradley W G 1982 Murine motor neuron disease (The Wobbler mouse). Degeneration and regeneration of the lower motor neuron. Brain 105: 811

Miyata Y 1983 A new mouse mutant with motor neuron disease. Developmental Brain Research 10: 139

Moise N S, Valentine B A, Brown C A et al 1990 Duchenne cardiomyopathy in a canine model: electrocardiographic and echocardiographic studies. Journal of the American College of Cardiology 17: 812

Montgomery D L, Gilmore W C, Litke L L 1989 Motor neuron disease with neurofilamentous accumulations in Hampshire pigs. Journal of Veterinary Diagnostic Investigation 1: 260

Morgan J E, Coulton G R, Partridge T A 1989 Mdx muscle grafts retain the mdx phenotype in normal hosts. Muscle and Nerve 12: 401

Morgan J E, Hoffman E P, Partridge T A 1990 Normal myogenic cells from newborn mice restore normal histology to degenerating muscles of the mdx mouse. Journal of Cell Biology 111: 2437

Morita H 1926 An experimental study on the pathology of the blackleg. Journal of the Japanese Society of Veterinary Science 5: 1

Morpurgo B 1897 Über activatäts: Hypertrophie de Wilkürliechen Muskeln. Virchow's Archiv für pathologische Anatomie and Physiologie und fur Kliniche Medizin 150: 522

Mumenthaler M, Paakkari I 1974 The needle myopathy. An experimental study. In: IIIrd International Congress on Muscle Diseases, International Congress Series No 334, Abstract 341. Excerpta Medica, Amsterdam

Nabeshima Y, Hanaoka K, Hayasaka M et al 1993 Myogenin gene disruption results in perinatal lethality because of severe muscle defect. Nature 364: 532

Nageotte J 1937 Sur la contraction extreme des muscles squelettiques chez les vertebrés. Zeitschrift für Zellforschung und Mikroskopische Anatomie 26: 603

Naylor J M, Robinson J A, Bertone J 1992 Familial incidence of hyperkalemic periodic paralysis in quarter horses. Journal of the American Veterinary Medical Association 200: 340

Nelson T E 1991 Malignant hyperthermia in dogs. Journal of the American Veterinary Medical Association 198: 989

Nicholson L V B, Davison K, Johnson M A et al 1989 Dystrophin in skeletal muscle. II. Immunoreactivity in patients with Xp21 muscular dystrophy. Journal of the Neurological Sciences 94: 137

Nielsen J S, Andresen E, Basse A, Christensen L G, Lykke T and Nielsen U S 1990 Inheritance of bovine spinal muscular atrophy. Acta Veterinaria Scandinavica 31: 253

O'Brien P J 1986 Porcine malignant hyperthermia susceptibility: hypersensitive calcium release mechanism of skeletal muscle sarcoplasmic reticulum. Canadian Journal of Veterinary Research 50: 318

O'Brien P J 1987 Etiopathogenetic defect of malignant hyperthermia: hypersensitive calcium-release channel of skeletal muscle sarcoplasmic reticulum. Veterinary Research Communications 11: 527

O'Brien P J, Cribb P H, White R J, Olfert E D, Steiss J 1983 Canine malignant hyperthermia: diagnosis of susceptibility in a breeding colony. Canadian Veterinary Journal 24: 172

Oda K, Lambert E H, Lennon V A, Palmer A C 1984a Congenital canine myasthenia gravis: I. Deficient junctional acetylcholine receptors. Muscle and Nerve 7: 705

Oda K, Lennon V A, Lambert E H, Palmer A C 1984b Congenital canine myasthenia gravis: II. Acetylcholine receptor metabolism. Muscle and Nerve 7: 717

Ohlendieck K, Ervasti J M, Snook J B, Campbell K P 1991 Dystrophin-glycoprotein complex is highly enriched in isolated skeletal muscle sarcolemma. Journal of Cell Biology 112: 135

Ohlendieck K, Campbell K P 1991 Dystrophin-associated proteins are greatly reduced in skeletal muscle from mdx mice. Journal of Cell Biology 115: 1685

Ohta T, Endo M, Nakano T, Morohoshi Y, Wanikawa K, Ohga A 1989 Ca-induced Ca release in malignant hyperthermia-susceptible pig skeletal muscle. American Journal of Physiology 256: C358

O'Sullivan B M, Healey P J, Fraser I R, Nieper R E, Whittle R J, Sewell C A 1981 Generalised glycogenosis in Brahman cattle. Australian Veterinary Journal 57: 227

Otsu K, Khanna V K, Archibald A L, MacLennan D H 1991 Cosegregation of porcine malignant hyperthermia and a probable causal mutation in the skeletal muscle ryanodine receptor gene in backcross families. Genomics 11: 744

Palmer A C 1980 Myasthenia gravis. Veterinary Clinics of North America. Small Animal Practice 10: 213

Palmer A C, Lennon V A, Beadle C, Goodyear J V 1980 Autoimmune form of myasthenia gravis in a juvenile Yorkshire Terrier × Jack Russell Terrier hybrid contrasted with congenital (non-autoimmune) myasthenia gravis of the Jack Russell. Journal of Small Animal Practice 21: 359

Palmer A C, Barker J 1974 Myasthenia in the dog. Veterinary Record 95: 452

Palmer E G, Topel D G, Christian L L 1978 Light and electron microscopy of skeletal muscle from malignant hyperthermia susceptible pigs. In: Aldrete J A, Britt B A (eds) Malignant hyperthermia. Grune and Stratton, New York, p 103

Palmer E G, Topel D G, Christian L L 1977 Microscopic observations of muscle from swine susceptible to malignant hyperthermia. Journal of Animal Science 45: 1032

Paola J P, Podell M, Shelton G D 1993 Muscular dystrophy in a Miniature Schnauzer. Progress in Veterinary Neurology (in press)

Papanicolaou G N, Falk E A 1938 General muscular hypertrophy induced by androgenic hormone. Science 87: 238

Partridge T A, Sloper J C 1977 A host contribution to the regeneration of muscle grafts. Journal of the Neurological Sciences 33: 425

Partridge T A, Morgan J E, Coulton G R, Hoffman E P, Kunkel L M 1989 Conversion of mdx myofibres from dystrophin-negative to -positive by injection of normal myoblasts. Nature 337: 176

Pearson C M 1956 Development of arthritis, periarthritis and periosteitis in rats given adjuvants. Proceedings of the Society for Experimental Biology and Medicine 91: 95

Peluchetti D, Mora M, Protti A, Cornelio F 1985 Freeze-fracture analysis of the muscle fibre plasma membrane in Duchenne dystrophy. Neurology 35: 928

Penn A S 1977 Myasthenia gravis, dermatomyositis, and polymyositis: immunopathological diseases. In: Griggs R C, Moxley R T (eds). Advances in neurology, vol 1. Raven, New York, p 41

Perloff J K, de Leon A C, O'Doherty D 1966 The cardiomyopathy of progressive muscular dystrophy. Circulation 33: 625

Peter J B 1973 Skeletal muscle: diversity and mutability of its histochemical, electron microscopic, biochemical and physiologic properties. In Pearson C M, Mostofi F K (eds) The striated muscle. Williams and Wilkins, Baltimore, p 1

Pflugfelder C M, Cardinet G H, Lutz H, Holliday T A, Hansen R J 1981 Acquired canine myasthenia gravis: immunocytochemical localization of immune complexes at neuromuscular junctions. Muscle and Nerve 4: 289

Pickar J G, Spier S J, Snyder J R, Carlsen R C 1991 Altered ionic permeability in skeletal muscle from horses with hyperkalemic periodic paralysis. American Journal of Physiology 260: C926

Pluskal M G, Pennington R J, Johnson M A, Harris J B 1974 Some effects of tiger snake toxin upon skeletal muscle. In: IIIrd International Congress Series No 334, Abstract 327. Excerpta Medica, Amsterdam

Presthus J, Nordstoga K 1989 Probable X-linked myopathy in a Samoyed litter. Proceedings of the European Society for Veterinary Neurology 52

Quinlan J G, Johnson S R, McKee M K, Lyden S P 1992

Twitch and tetanus in mdx mouse muscle. Muscle and Nerve 15: 837

Rafiquzzaman M, Svenkerud R, Strande A, Hauge J G 1976 Glycogenosis in the dog. Acta Veterinaria Scandinavica 17: 196

Ragot T, Vincent N, Chafey P et al 1993 Efficient adenovirus-mediated transfer of a human minidystrophin gene to skeletal muscle of mdx mice. Nature 361: 647

Rand J S, O'Brien P J 1987 Exercise-induced malignant hyperthermia in an English Springer Spaniel. Journal of the American Veterinary Medical Association 190: 1013

Reininghaus J, Füchtbauer E-M, Bertram K, Jockusch H 1988 The myotonic mouse mutant ADR: Physiological and histochemical properties of muscle. Muscle and Nerve 11: 433

Reznik M 1973 Current concepts of skeletal muscle regeneration. In: Pearson C M, Mostofi F K (eds). The striated muscle. Williams and Wilkins, Baltimore, pp 185–225

Rice D A, Blanchflower W J, McMurray C H 1981 Reproduction of nutritional degenerative myopathy in the post ruminant calf. Veterinary Record 109: 161

Richter A, Gerdes C, Löscher W 1992 Atypical reactions to halothane in a subgroup of homozygous malignant hyperthermia (MH)-susceptible pigs: indication of a heterogenous genetic basis for the porcine syndrome. Deutsche Tierarztliche Wochenschrift 99: 401

Roberds S L, Ervasti J M, Anderson R D et al 1993 Disruption of the dystrophin–glycoprotein complex in the cardiomyopathic hamster. Journal of Biological Chemistry 268: 11496

Robinson J A, Naylor J M, Crichlow E C 1990 Use of electromyography for the diagnosis of equine hyperkalemic periodic paresis. Canadian Journal of Veterinary Research 54: 495

Robinson W F, Howell J M, Dorling P R 1983 Cardiomyopathy in generalised glycogenosis type II in cattle. Cardiovascular Research 17: 238

Rosen D R, Siddique T, Patterson D et al 1993 Mutations in Cu/Zn superoxide dismutase gene are associated with familial amyotrophic lateral sclerosis. Nature 362: 59

Rosman N P, Shapiro M B, Haddow J E 1978 Muscle weakness caused by an iodine-deficient diet: investigation of a nutritional myopathy. Journal of Neuropathology and Experimental Neurology 37: 192

Rubin E, Katz A M, Lieber C S, Stein E P, Puszkin S 1976 Muscle damage produced by chronic alcohol consumption. American Journal of Pathology 83: 499

Rudnicki M A, Braun T, Hinuma S, Jaenisch R 1992 Inactivation of MyoD in mice leads to up-regulation of the myogenic HLH gene Myf-5 and results in apparently normal muscle development. Cell 71: 383

Rudnicki M A, Schnegelsberg P N J, Stead R H et al 1993 MyoD or Myf-5 is required for the formation of skeletal muscle. Cell 75: 1351

Rudolph J A, Spier S J, Byrns G, Rojas C V, Bernoco D, Hoffman E P 1992b Periodic paralysis in Quarter horses: a sodium channel mutation disseminated by selective breeding. Nature Genetics 2: 144

Rudolph J A, Spier S J, Byrne G, Hoffman E P 1992a Linkage of hyperkalaemic periodic paralysis in quarter horses to the horse adult skeletal muscle sodium channel gene. Animal Genetics 23: 241

Rustigan R, Pappenheimer M 1949 Myositis in mice following intramuscular injection of viruses of the mouse encephalomyelitis group and of certain other neurotrophic viruses. Journal of Experimental Medicine 89: 69

Ruth G R, Van Vleet J F 1974 Experimentally induced selenium-vitamin E deficiency in growing swine: selective destruction of type I skeletal muscle fibres. American Journal of Veterinary Research 35: 237

Ryder-Cook A S, Sicinski P, Thomas K et al 1988 Localization of the mdx mutation within the mouse dystrophin gene. Embo Journal 7: 3017

Sacco P, Jones D A, Dick J R T, Vrbová G 1992 Contractile properties and susceptibility to exercise-induced damage of normal and mdx tibialis anterior muscle. Clinical Science 82: 227

Sahgal V, Subramani V, Hughes R, Shah A, Singh H 1979 On the pathogenesis of mitochondrial myopathies. An experimental study. Acta Neuropathologica 46: 177

Sandefeldt E, Cummings J F, de Lahunta A, Bjorck G, Krook L 1973 Hereditary neuronal abiotrophy in the Swedish Lapland dog. Cornell Veterinarian 63: 3

Sarnat H B, Portnoy J M, Chi D Y K 1977 Effects of denervation and tenotomy on the gastrocnemius muscle in the frog: a histological and histochemical study. Anatomical Record 187: 335

Sato T, Sakuragawa N, Tsubaki T 1974 Arbovirus myositis: initiation and multiplication of sindbis virus in mouse skeletal muscles. In: IIIrd International Congress on Muscle Diseases, International Congress Series No 334, Abstract 291. Excerpta Medica, Amsterdam

Schiller H H, Esslen E, Weihe W H, Haldermann G, Teelmann K 1974 Investigations on experimental malignant hyperthermia (MH) in pigs. In: IIIrd International Congress on Muscle Diseases, International Congress Series No 334, Abstract 391. Excerpta Medica, Amsterdam

Schimmelpfeng J, Jockusch H, Heimann P 1987 Increased density of satellite cells in the absence of fibre degeneration in muscle of myotonic mice. Cell and Tissue Research 249: 351

Schmalbruch H, Jensen H-J S, Bjaerg M, Kamieniecka Z and Kurland L 1991 A new mouse mutant with progressive motor neuronopathy. Journal of Neuropathology and Experimental Neurology 50: 192

Schotland D L, Bonilla E, Wakayama Y 1981 Freeze fracture studies of muscle plasma membrane in human muscular dystrophy. Acta Neuropathologica 54: 189

Scott-Moncrieff J C, Cook J R Jr, Lantz G C 1990 Acquired myasthenia gravis in a cat with thymoma. Journal of the American Veterinary Medical Association 196: 1291

Sewry C A, Wilson L A, Dux L, Dubowitz V, Cooper B J 1992 Experimental regeneration in canine muscular dystrophy—1. Immunocytochemical evaluation of dystrophin and beta-spectrin expression. Neuromuscular Disorders 2: 331

Sharp N J H, Kornegay J N, Van Camp S D et al 1992 An error in dystrophin mRNA processing in golden retriever muscular dystrophy, an animal homologue of Duchenne muscular dystrophy. Genomics 13: 115

Shell L G, Jortner B S, Leib M S 1987 Familial motor neuron disease in Rottweiler dogs: neuropathologic studies. Veterinary Pathology 24: 135

Shelton G D, Cardinet G H, III and Lindstrom J M 1988 Canine and human myasthenia gravis autoantibodies recognize similar regions on the acetylcholine receptor. Neurology 38: 1417

Shelton G D, Willard M D, Cardinet G H, Lindstrom J 1990 Acquired myasthenia gravis. Selective involvement of esophageal, pharyngeal, and facial muscles. Journal of Veterinary Internal Medicine 4: 281

Shibuya S, Wakayama Y 1988 Freeze-fracture studies of myofibre plasma membrane in X chromosome-linked muscular dystrophy (mdx) mice. Acta Neuropathologica 76: 179

Shibuya S, Wakayama Y 1991 Changes in muscle plasma membranes in young mice with X chromosome-linked muscular dystrophy: a freeze-fracture study. Neuropathology and Applied Neurobiology 17: 335

Shields R P, Vandevelde M 1978 Spontaneous lower motor neuron disease in rabbits (Oryctolagus cuniculus). Acta Neuropathologica 44: 85

Shires P K, Nafe L A, Hulse D A 1983 Myotonia in a Staffordshire terrier. Journal of the American Veterinary Medical Association 183: 229

Shomer N H, Louis C F, Fill M, Litterer L A, Mickelson J R 1993 Reconstitution of abnormalities in the malignant hyperthermia-susceptible pig ryanodine receptor. American Journal of Physiology 264: C125

Shores A, Redding R W, Braund K G, Simpson S T 1986 Myotonia congenita in a Chow Chow pup. Journal of the American Veterinary Medical Association 188: 532

Short C E, Matthews N S 1988 The role of the horse in studies relative to malignant hyperthermia. In: Williams C H (ed) Experimental malignant hyperthermia. Springer-Verlag, New York, p 90

Short C E, Paddleford R R 1973 Malignant hyperthermia in the dog. Anesthesiology 39: 462

Sicinski P, Geng Y, Ryder-Cook A S, Barnard E A, Darlison M G, Barnard P J 1989 The molecular basis of muscular dystrophy in the mdx mouse: a point mutation. Science 244: 1578

Smith C and Bampton P R 1977 Inheritance of reaction to halothane anaesthesia in pigs. Genetical Research 29: 287

Smith G T, Beeuwkes, R, Tomkiewicz Z M, Tadaaki A, Town B 1965 Pathological changes in skin and skeletal muscle following alternation current and capacitor discharge. American Journal of Pathology 47: 1

Smithies O 1993 Animal models of human genetic diseases. Trends in Genetics 9: 112

Sola O M, Christensen D L, Martin A W 1973 Hypertrophy and hyperplasia of adult chicken anterior latissimus dorsi muscles following stretch with and without denervation. Experimental Neurology 41: 76

Sola O M, Dillard D H, Ivey T D, Haneda K, Itoh T, Thomas R 1985 Autotransplantation of skeletal muscle into myocardium. Circulation 71: 341

Spier S J, Carlson G P, Holliday T A, Cardinet G H, III, Pickar J G 1990 Hyperkalemic periodic paralysis in horses. Journal of the American Veterinary Medical Association 197: 1009

Stedman H H, Sweeney H L, Shrager J B et al 1991 The mdx mouse diaphragm reproduces the degenerative changes of Duchenne muscular dystrophy. Nature 352: 536

Steinmeyer K, Klocke R, Ortland C et al 1991 Inactivation of muscle chloride channel by transposon insertion in myotonic mice. Nature 354: 304

Steinmeyer K, Ortland C, Jentsch T J 1991 Primary structure and functional expression of a developmentally regulated skeletal muscle chloride channel. Nature 354: 301

Steiss J E, Naylor J M 1986 Episodic muscle tremors in a Quarter horse: resemblance to hyperkalemic periodic paralysis. Canadian Veterinary Journal 27: 332

Stuhlfauth I, Reininghaus J, Jockusch H, Heizmann C W 1984 Calcium-binding protein, parvalbumin, is reduced in mutant mammalian muscle with abnormal contractile properties. Proceedings of the National Academy of Sciences USA 81: 4814

Sugita H, Arahata K, Ishiguro T et al 1988 Negative immunostaining of Duchenne muscular dystrophy (DMD) and mdx muscle surface membrane with antibody against synthetic peptide fragment predicted from DMD cDNA. Proceedings of the Japan Academy. Series B: Physical and Biological Sciences 64: 37

Sutrave P, Kelly A M, Hughes S H 1990 *ski* can cause selective growth of skeletal muscle in transgenic mice. Genes and Development 4: 1462

Swift L L, Atkinson J B, Lequire V S 1979 The composition and calcium transport activity of the sarcoplasmic reticulum from goats with and without heritable myotonia. Laboratory Investigation 40: 384

Tanabe Y, Esaki K, Nomura T 1986 Skeletal muscle pathology in X chromosome-linked muscular dystrophy (*mdx*) mouse. Acta Neuropathologica 69: 91

Tanaka H, Hayashi K, Ozawa E 1991 Positive immunostaining with dystrophin antibodies in mdx skeletal muscle. Proceedings of the Japan Academy. Series B: Physical and Biological Sciences 67: 148

Tanaka H, Ikeya K, Ozawa E 1990 Difference in the expression pattern of dystrophin on the surface membrane between the skeletal and cardiac muscles of mdx carrier mice. Histochemistry 93: 447

Tannenberg J 1939 Pathological changes in the heart, skeletal musculature and liver in rabbits treated with insulin in shock dosage. American Journal of Pathology 15: 25

Teitz T, Chang J C, Kitamura M, Yen T S, Kan Y W 1993 Rhabdomyosarcoma arising in transgenic mice harboring the beta-globin locus control region fused with simian virus 40 large T antigen gene. Proceedings of the National Academy of Sciences USA 90: 2910

Torres L F B, Duchen L W 1987 The mutant mdx: inherited myopathy in the mouse. Morphological studies of nerves, muscles and end-plates. Brain 110: 269

Trojaborg W, Flagstad A 1982 A hereditary neuromuscular disorder in dogs. Muscle and Nerve 5: S30

Turner P R, Fong P, Denetclaw W F, Steinhardt R A 1991 Increased calcium influx in dystrophic muscle. Journal of Cell Biology 115: 1701

Turner P R, Westwood T, Regan C M, Steinhardt R A 1988 Increased protein degradation results from elevated free calcium levels found in muscle from mdx mice. Nature 335: 735

Usuki F, Ishiura S, Sugita H 1986 Developmental study of α-glucosidases in Japanese quails with acid maltase deficiency. Muscle and Nerve 9: 537

Valentine B A, Blue J T, Cooper B J 1989 The effect of exercise on canine dystrophic muscle. Annals of Neurology 26: 588

Valentine B A, Chandler S K, Cummings J F, Cooper B J 1990a In vitro characteristics of normal and dystrophic skeletal muscle from dogs. American Journal of Veterinary Research 52: 104

Valentine B A, Cooper B J, de Lahunta A, O'Quinn R, Blue J T 1988 Canine X-linked muscular dystrophy. An animal model of Duchenne muscular dystrophy: clinical studies. Journal of the Neurological Sciences 88: 69

Valentine B A, Cooper B J, Cummings J F, de Lahunta A 1990b Canine X-linked muscular dystrophy: morphologic lesions. Journal of the Neurological Sciences 97: 1

Valentine B A, Cooper B J, Cummings J F, de Lahunta A 1986 Progressive muscular dystrophy in a golden retriever dog: light microscope and ultrastructural features at 4 and 8 months. Acta Neuropathologica 71: 301

Valentine B A, Cummings J F, Cooper B J 1989 Development of Duchenne-type cardiomyopathy: morphologic studies in a canine model. American Journal of Pathology 135: 671

Valentine B A, Kornegay J N, Cooper B J 1989 Clinical electromyographic studies of canine X-linked muscular dystrophy. American Journal of Veterinary Research 50: 2145 (abstract)

Valentine B A, Cooper B J 1991 Canine X-linked muscular dystrophy: selective involvement of muscles in neonatal dogs. Neuromuscular Disorders 1: 31

Venable J H 1973 International Symposium on Malignant Hyperthermia. Charles C Thomas, Springfield

Volkmann R 1893 Ueber die Regeneration des quergestreiften Muskelgewebes beim Menschen und Säugethier. Beiträge zue pathologischen Anatomie und zur allgemeinen Pathologie 12: 233

Vora S, Giger U, Turchen S, Harvey J W 1985 Characterization of the enzymatic lesion in inherited phosphofructokinase deficiency in the dog: an animal analogue of human glycogen storage disease type VII. Proceedings of the National Academy of Sciences USA 82: 8109

Vos J H, Van der Linde-Sipman J S, Goedegebuure S A 1986 Dystrophy-like myopathy in the cat. Journal of Comparative Pathology 96: 435

Wakayama Y, Okayasu H, Shibuya S, Kumagai T 1984 Duchenne dystrophy: reduced density of orthogonal array subunit particles in muscle plasma membrane. Neurology 34: 1313

Wakayama Y, Shibuya S 1990 Observations on the muscle plasma membrane-associated cytoskeletons of mdx mice by quick-freeze, deep-etch, rotary-shadow replica method. Acta Neuropathologica 80: 618

Wakeford S, Watt D J, Partridge T A 1991 X-irradiation improves mdx mouse muscle as a model of myofiber loss in DMD. Muscle and Nerve 14: 42

Wallace M E, Palmer A C 1984 Recessive mode of inheritance in myasthenia gravis in the Jack Russell terrier. Veterinary Record 114: 350

Walton J N, Adams R D 1958 Polymyositis. Livingstone, Edinburgh

Walvoort H C 1985 Glycogen storage disease type II in the Lapland dog. Veterinary Quarterly 7: 187

Walvoort H C, Koster J E, Reuser A J J 1985 Heterozygote detection in a family of Lapland dogs with a recessively inherited metabolic disease: canine glycogen storage disease type II. Research in Veterinary Science 38: 174

Walvoort H C, Slee R G, Koster J F 1982 Canine glycogen storage disease type II. A biochemical study of an acid alpha-glucosidase-deficient Lapland dog. Biochimica et Biophysica Acta 715: 63

Ward P, Goldspink G 1974 Response of different fibre types to changes in activity pattern and to protein malnutrition. In: IIIrd International Congress on Muscle Diseases, International Congress Series No 334, Abstract 16. Excerpta Medica, Amsterdam

Warren S 1943 Effects of radiation on normal tissues. XIV. Effects on striated muscle. Archives of Pathology 35: 347

Watkins S C, Hoffman E P, Slayter H S, Kunkel L M 1989 Dystrophin distribution in heterozygote mdx mice. Muscle and Nerve 12: 861

Watkins W J, Watts D C 1984 Biological features of the new A2G-adr mouse mutant with abnormal muscle function. Laboratory Animal 18: 1

Watson A G 1973 Structure of the canine oesophagus. New Zealand Veterinary Journal 21: 195

Webb J N 1970 Experimental immune myositis in guinea pigs. Journal of the Reticuloendothelial Society 7: 305

Wecker L, Dettbarn W D 1977 Effects of denervation on the production of an experimental myopathy. Experimental Neurology 57: 94

Weller B, Karpati G, Carpenter S 1990 Dystrophin-deficient mdx muscle fibers are preferentially vulnerable to necrosis induced by experimental lengthening contractions. Journal of the Neurological Sciences 100: 9

Weller B, Karpati G, Lehnert S, Carpenter S, Ajdukovic B, Holland P 1991b Inhibition of myosatellite cell proliferation by gamma irradiation does not prevent the age-related increase of the number of dystrophin-positive fibers in soleus muscles of mdx female heterozygote mice. American Journal of Pathology 138: 1497

Weller B, Karpati G, Lehnert S, Carpenter S 1991a Major alteration of the pathological phenotype in gamma irradiated mdx soleus muscles. Journal of Neuropathology and Experimental Neurology 50: 419

Wells D J, Wells K E, Walsh F S et al 1992 Human dystrophin expression corrects the myopathic phenotype in transgenic mdx mice. Human Molecular Genetics 1: 35

Wentink G H, Hartman W, Koeman J P 1974a Three cases of myotonia in a family of chows. Tijdschrift voor Diergeneeskunde 99: 729

Wentink G H, Meijer A E F H, Van der Linde-Sipman J S, Hendriks H J 1974b Myopathy in an Irish Terrier with a metabolic defect of the isolated mitochondria. Zentralblatt fur Veterinarmedizin. Reihe A 21: 62

Wentink G H, Van der Linde-Sipman J S, Meijer A E F H et al 1972 Myopathy with a possible X-linked inheritance in a litter of Irish Terriers. Veterinary Pathology 9: 328

Wilkes M K, McKerrell R E, Patterson R C, Palmer A C 1987 Ultrastructure of motor endplates in canine congenital myasthenia gravis. Journal of Comparative Pathology 97: 247

Williams C H, Shanklin M D, Hedrick H B et al 1978 The fulminant hyperthermia-stress syndrome: genetic aspects, hemodynamic and metabolic measurements in susceptible and normal pigs. In: Aldrete J A, Britt B A (eds) Malignant hyperthermia. Grune and Stratton, New York, p 113

Wilson L A, Dux L, Cooper B J, Dubowitz V, Sewry C A 1993 Experimental regeneration in canine muscular dystrophy; 2. Expression of myosin heavy chain isoforms. Neuromuscular Disorders 2: 331

Witkowski J A 1986a Tissue culture studies of muscle disorders: Part I. Techniques, cell growth, morphology, cell surface. Muscle and Nerve 9: 191

Witkowski J A 1986b Tissue culture studies of muscle disorders: Part 2. Biochemical studies, nerve-muscle culture, metabolic myopathies, and animal models. Muscle and Nerve 9: 283

Zacharias J M, Anderson J E 1991 Muscle regeneration after imposed injury is better in younger than older mdx dystrophic mice. Journal of the Neurological Sciences 104: 190

Zacks S I, Shields D R, Steinberg S A 1966 A myasthenic syndrome in the dog: a case report with electron microscopic observations on motor end plates and comparisons with the fine structure of end plates in myasthenia gravis. Annals of the New York Academy of Sciences 135: 79

Zubrzycka-Gaarn E E, Bulman D E, Karpati G et al 1988 The Duchenne muscular dystrophy gene product is localized in sarcolemma of human skeletal muscle. Nature 33: 466

Clinical problems in neuromuscular disease

13. Clinical examination, differential diagnosis and classification

J. Walton   L. P. Rowland

INTRODUCTION

In these days of medical high technology, the diagnosis of neuromuscular diseases may ultimately rely on DNA probes, Western blots, electromyography (EMG), nerve conduction studies, antibody titres, enzyme assays or immunocytochemistry. Nevertheless, an old adage still holds true: '90% of a neurological diagnosis depends upon the medical history'.

There is still much to be learned from the clinical examination (Haerer 1992). Clinicians who have no idea of the clinical differential diagnosis will not know which diagnostic tests are appropriate and will not know how to interpret test results that do not seem to fit in with the clinical evidence.

Hence, in this chapter we shall discuss the central role of symptoms (what the patient tells the doctor) and signs (what the doctor finds on examination) in the diagnosis of neuromuscular disorders.

The neuromuscular disorders are those conditions in which the patient's symptoms result from abnormalities in the motor unit which comprises: the lower motor neurones (including the motor nuclei of the cranial nerves, the anterior horn cells of the spinal cord, the spinal motor roots, the motor fibres of the peripheral nerves); the neuromuscular junction; and the voluntary muscles themselves. Lesions or pathological processes in the spinal cord, spinal roots or peripheral nerves often involve sensory as well as motor pathways, thus causing pain, paraesthesiae and sensory loss which may vary in character and distribution, depending upon the nature and site of the lesion or process concerned. Some such symptoms and their accompanying signs are considered in Chapters 25 and 27. This chapter concentrates upon the clinical manifestations of motor dysfunction resulting from disease of the neuromuscular apparatus.

SYMPTOMS AND SIGNS IN NEUROMUSCULAR DISEASE

Although the neuromuscular disorders are many, the symptoms which they produce are few, pain and weakness being the most frequent; limpness, wasting, twitching in muscles, myotonia, palpable tenderness, local or diffuse swelling of nerves or muscles and contractures are the only others of importance. Often a definite diagnosis can and should be reached only after biochemical, electrophysiological and histological investigation. However, this in no way diminishes the importance of the clinical history and examination, which will usually restrict the differential diagnosis to a few conditions and will also be invaluable in indicating the best site for electromyography and muscle biopsy. These all-important investigations can be inconclusive or even misleading if the muscle chosen is in too advanced or too early a stage of the disease.

In the following catalogue of the clinical features of neuromuscular disease, symptoms and signs are often necessarily discussed together but, as far as possible, points arising from the history are mentioned before the findings on examination. Details of methods of eliciting physical signs are generally omitted but useful accounts of these are given in Haerer (1992), Bickerstaff (1980), Asbury & Gilliatt (1984), Ross Russell & Wiles (1985) and 'Aids to the examination of the peripheral nervous system' (Medical Research Council 1986). Valuable information on the examination of children will be found in Paine & Oppé (1966), Gordon (1976), Dubowitz (1978), Gamstorp (1984) and Pact et al (1984).

Family history

The familial occurrence of a disorder is of obvious diagnostic help. Sometimes, however, the course of the disease may differ greatly in different family members; this can be particularly striking in infan-

tile and juvenile spinal muscular atrophy and in the glycogen-storage disease of muscle due to acid maltase deficiency, where slowly progressive proximal weakness in one sib may bear little resemblance to the severe and rapidly fatal disease in another. Better-understood examples include the homozygous and heterozygous forms of distal muscular dystrophy (Barohn et al 1991), inter-sib variation in the peroneal muscular atrophy syndrome and the subclinical myopathy of female carriers of the Duchenne dystrophy gene.

On the whole it is among the X-linked and autosomal dominant conditions that the family history is most helpful; the early diagnosis of Duchenne, facioscapulohumeral and myotonic muscular dystrophy or of the periodic paralyses is much easier if others in the family have been affected. In obscure myopathies parental consanguinity may, on the other hand, direct attention to the possibility of an autosomal recessive disorder. The patient's statement that there is 'no family history of muscle disease' should not be accepted without a detailed pedigree enquiry. Especially in myotonic dystrophy, facioscapulohumeral dystrophy, peroneal muscular atrophy and its variants and in the congenital myopathies it is a common experience to find previously unrecognised cases when the whole family is carefully examined. In many autosomal dominant diseases presymptomatic individuals can be identified by the application of DNA probes.

There is another consideration emphasising the importance of the family history, because the application of molecular genetics has altered our views about the relationship between genotype and phenotype. For instance, mutations at Xp21 that affect clinical expression are ordinarily expressed in boys or men as either Duchenne or Becker muscular dystrophy. However, similar mutations are found in women who are manifesting carriers of the gene. Also, identical mutations may be found in other X-linked clinical syndromes, including cramps and myoglobinuria, quadriceps myopathy or distal myopathy.

Different clinical syndromes are also associated with the same mutation of mitochondrial DNA, which may be recognised by a pattern of transmission compatible with maternal inheritance.

Therefore it is imperative to take a detailed

family history in each new case of neuromuscular disease. If a first- or second-degree relative has a neurological disorder, even if it seems quite different from that observed in the propositus, the two conditions may be expressions of the same genetic disorder.

Muscle pain at rest

Painful muscular contraction is the basis of many common symptoms, including tension headache, low back pain and 'fibrositis'. Fear, often irrational and unconscious (such as that associated with depression and anxiety), and minor trauma may each be responsible. Among the most mystifying problems are those associated with diffuse and persistent myalgia. In the USA, this symptom is often attributed to a chronic form of Lyme disease, but it is never relieved by any kind of antibiotic therapy. The symptom is often accompanied by oppressive fatigue — the so-called 'chronic (postviral) fatigue syndrome'. Clinicians must be aware that no known muscle disease is manifest by pain alone. Whole-body pain is not due to a myopathy; it is almost always psychogenic. The chronic postviral fatigue syndrome, formerly called benign myalgic encephalomyelitis, for example, is sometimes associated with depression and responds to antidepressive medication; other patients show features of chronic hypochondriasis. Painful, focal and persistent muscle spasm is also a common accompaniment of joint disease. Furthermore, pain is often referred to muscle from other sites. These banal but important conditions are usually easily recognised if considered.

Cramp is a transient, involuntary and painful localised muscular contraction. Common cramps are relieved by stretching or massage. These cramps are most often brought on by plantarflexing the feet in bed (contraction of the gastrocnemius), but other muscles may also be affected. Sodium-depletion, uraemia and pregnancy also increase the likelihood of cramps (Rowland 1985). The EMG recorded from affected muscles shows high frequency discharges during the cramp. Writer's cramp and other occupational cramps are now regarded by many as forms of action dystonia, for several reasons. First, the involuntary twisting motion seen in some cases resembles that observed in other kinds of dystonia. Some patients have relatives with torticollis or other dystonias, and the abnormal motor activity arises in the central nervous system. However, the spasms appear selectively in people who carry out highly skilled and highly repetitive motions — scribes, musicians, telegraphers. In one study 14% of all telegraphers in Sydney were affected; it seems unlikely that so many people in a particular occupation could be suffering a genetic disorder so that some authorities prefer the term 'overuse syndrome'. Others, noting that some individuals with writer's cramp can perform precise and intricate movements, other than those involved in writing, with the affected hand, still believe, in accord with the traditional view, that psychogenic mechanisms also play a part at least in some cases. Nevertheless, the spasms differ from ordinary cramps because they are brought on by specific and focal actions; they do not affect a single muscle; and they are relieved only by ceasing the provocative activity and by the lapse of time, not by any physical manoeuvre or by psychoactive drugs.

In spinal cord lesions, especially multiple sclerosis, *flexor spasms* due to spasticity may be painful. In *compression of spinal roots or nerves* resulting, say, from intervertebral disc disease or peripheral nerve entrapment, pain often radiates along the cutaneous dermatome innervated by the sensory component of the spinal or peripheral nerve concerned, but sometimes dull aching pain is felt in the muscles innervated by its motor component. Nerve trunks may become tender or painful on palpation or stretching when one or more component roots is so affected, or at or near sites of entrapment. Tapping over a nerve at such a site can give not only pain, but also paraesthesiae radiating down its cutaneous sensory distribution (Tinel's sign).

Neuralgic amyotrophy begins with severe aching pain in the shoulder or arm followed after a few days by wasting and weakness that usually involves the serratus anterior, trapezius, deltoid, biceps or spinati. Often there is a preceding febrile illness. The pain generally clears up after a few weeks and the weakness after a few months but both may persist for several months and weakness is very occasionally permanent. In both *poliomyelitis* and the *Guillain–Barré syndrome* the onset of weakness may be preceded by pain, and in poliomyelitis there is often visible fasciculation at this stage. Other painful *polyneuropathies* are those associated with alcoholism, porphyria, arsenic poisoning and polyarteritis nodosa. In yet others, including those due to deficiency of vitamin B_1 or B_{12}, the muscles are tender. In diabetic amyotrophy, usually due to a mononeuropathy of the femoral nerve, less often of the lumbar plexus, there is pain in and atrophy of the quadriceps or rarely of other muscles. Myalgia is common in systemic viral infections and varies in severity from the pain commonly experienced in influenza, to the more severe pain of benign myalgic encephalomyelitis and the very severe diaphragmatic pain of *Coxsackie B myalgia* (*Bornholm disease*). *Polymyalgia rheumatica* affects elderly people who may be severely incapacitated by muscular pains in the arms and legs without weakness or sensory change; the ESR is always raised and the condition responds well to steroid therapy. Thus if weakness is present, the diagnosis is more likely to be one of polymyositis. By contrast, pain is unusual in polymyositis but some myalgia and tenderness of muscles can occur in acute and severe cases.

Pain on exertion

This is usually attributable to muscle ischaemia, illustrated by the familiar experiment of exercising the forearm muscles with a cuff at above arterial pressure around the arm or by 'intermittent claudication' resulting from atherosclerotic occlusion of the iliac or femoro-popliteal arteries. Occasionally the weakness and paraesthesiae in the leg and foot during walking, which result from intermittent ischaemia or 'claudication' of the spinal cord or cauda equina, may cause confusion and are usually due to lumbar canal stenosis. In *McArdle's disease* (myophosphorylase deficiency), and related disorders of muscle glycolytic metabolism including phosphofructokinase deficiency, the earliest symptom is usually an aching sensation in the calves during walking, becoming more painful if the patient perseveres; other muscles become similarly painful, often with temporary contracture, if vigorously exercised. However, many patients with this symptom are investigated enthusiasti-

cally with disappointingly negative results, and the cause of benign exertional cramps in otherwise apparently healthy people is poorly understood. Undoubtedly some patients who complain bitterly of diffuse muscular pain brought on or accentuated by exercise are tense, introspective and obsessional and some respond to treatment with antidepressive or tranquillising remedies. Some are 'fading athletes' who can no longer prevail in competitive sports. Unable to admit the limitations of advancing age (after the age of 30), these people may find the self-image of a muscle disease less threatening. Nevertheless there are some individuals presumed to have an as yet unidentified metabolic disorder of muscle in whom exertional muscle pain may be dramatically relieved by calcium antagonist drugs such as verapamil (Walton 1981, Lane et al 1986). Some such patients may prove to have Ca^{2+} ATPase deficiency (Taylor et al 1988). Other causes of exertional muscle pain, often associated with myoglobinuria, include glycogen storage diseases, carnitine palmitoyl transferase deficiency and mitochondrial myopathies. Sometimes cramp on exertion is a feature of muscular dystrophy, early motor neurone disease or even early spasticity but it is rarely, if ever, a presenting symptom in the absence of other signs of these disorders.

Weakness as a symptom

The disability to which muscle weakness gives rise depends not only on the muscles involved but upon the patient's way of life. Few people use any of their muscles to full capacity and sometimes quite profound weakness goes unnoticed by apparently intelligent people. It is not, therefore, surprising that difficulty in walking is a common presentation of muscle disease, as this is a form of exertion that few escape. Difficulty in running, in climbing stairs or on to bus platforms and in getting out of low chairs are the usual early symptoms of proximal lower limb weakness; often shoulder-girdle weakness is equally severe but asymptomatic. Those whose occupation involves lifting weights or the arrangement of complex hairstyles may, however, notice upper-limb weakness first. Quadriceps weakness sometimes causes sudden falls because of the resulting instability of the knee, and muscle weakness may not even be considered if the idea of 'drop attacks' enters the examiner's mind. Distal weakness leads to tripping over carpets, kerbs and stairs and to weakness of the hands often first described as clumsiness. Patients who complain of difficulty in walking *down* stairs often turn out to have spasticity of the legs or cerebellar ataxia.

Symptoms due to weakness of cranial muscles are limited to only a few conditions. Ptosis and ophthalmoparesis often go together; if the condition is unilateral or notably asymmetrical, myasthenia is more likely. Progressive external ophthalmoplegia syndromes are more likely to be symmetrical and progress more slowly without diurnal fluctuation or remission. Dysarthria and dysphagia are common in myasthenia but may also be prominent in motor neurone disease, pseudobulbar palsy, oculopharyngeal muscular dystrophy or myotonic dystrophy.

The mode of onset and progression of the weakness are very important in neuromuscular disease. A rapid onset after a minor febrile illness may suggest poliomyelitis (within a few days) or the Guillain–Barré syndrome (after 1–4 weeks). It is less well known that the clinical features of spinal musculature atrophy, either Werdnig–Hoffmann disease or its benign variant, may first become apparent after such an illness and may then show further less rapid progression. Benign spinal muscular atrophy is also notable for its tendency to undergo static periods, lasting sometimes for many years, between phases of deterioration. Many of the hereditary myopathies progress steadily at rates that vary widely from one condition to another but tend to be fairly uniform among cases of each disease. The inflammatory myopathies, however, and especially polymyositis, have a wide spectrum of progression from a fulminating course of a few days to an indolent one spanning several decades. The periodic paralyses cause recurrent episodes of weakness which usually give little diagnostic difficulty, especially when there is a family history. In sporadic cases, thyrotoxicosis and hyperaldosteronism must be excluded. Diurnal variation, fluctuation from day to day, and longer periods of remission and exacerbation are characteristic of myasthenia gravis, a pattern that is unlike that noted in any other neuromuscular disease. However, remissions and relapses are also seen in some chronic peripheral neuropathies.

Weakness — the patient in action

The first stage of the examination in a suspected neuromuscular disorder is to watch the patient in action — the posture and gait especially. The facial appearance can be critical in giving the first clue to the diagnosis; myotonic dystrophy is the supreme example of this among muscle disorders because of the many features which are immediately evident — baldness, apathy, wasting of temporal and sternomastoid muscles, masseter weakness, ptosis, drooping of the cheeks and lower lip, and sometimes cataract. In facioscapulohumeral dystrophy only the everted position of the eyelids and lips and the lack of facial lines may be apparent at first. Here the facial weakness must be demonstrated by movement. Lip weakness in myasthenia often produces a characteristic facial appearance (the so-called 'transverse smile') and weakness of the masticators may force the patient to support the jaw with one hand, an almost diagnostic combination. Weakness of neck muscles may make it difficult to hold the head erect (the 'floppy head syndrome'). This can be seen in myasthenia, motor neurone disease, polymyositis or rarely for reasons unknown. In facioscapulohumeral dystrophy the shoulders have a strikingly sloping posture and a characteristic sign is the remarkable elevation of the scapula which occurs when the arm is abducted. *Winging of the scapulae at rest* is seen in facioscapulohumeral dystrophy, in serratus palsies and in limb-girdle muscular dystrophy but it must generally be brought out by putting serratus anterior into action in the many other conditions in which it occurs. *Kyphoscoliosis* is seen early in Friedreich's ataxia and neurofibromatosis. In the muscular dystrophies and in the spinal muscular atrophies it may, if unchecked, become severe, but not until muscular weakness is obvious; thus it is important in management but not in the diagnosis of these conditions. However, contractures of the calf muscles and of the hip flexors can contribute significantly to the lordotic tip-toe position which patients with muscular dystrophy often adopt at a stage when the diagnosis is still in doubt. The posture and appearance of the hands and feet are characteristic and usually easy to recognise in various nerve palsies, tetany, peroneal muscular atrophy and the other hereditary neuropathies, motor neurone disease and syringomyelia. In Emery–Dreifuss muscular dystrophy, a singular appearance is created by contractures and limitation of motion of the neck, elbows, fingers, knees and ankles.

The *gait* can be invaluable in convincing the examiner that weakness is present, and in indicating its approximate distribution. Not too much more should be expected of it and it is a mistake to suggest that any abnormal gait is 'pathognomonic' of a specific neuromuscular disorder. In general the 'steppage' gait of pure peripheral muscle weakness (e.g. in peroneal muscular atrophy) is noticeably more fluent and confident than the combination of foot-drop with sensory ataxia seen in the sensory or mixed neuropathies and in tabes. In the spastic foot-drop of pyramidal tract disease the foot is dragged rather than lifted. Mild weakness of dorsiflexion is easily detected if patients are asked to walk on their heels, and calf weakness when they walk on their toes. The waddling lordotic gait of proximal lower-limb weakness is even less specific. It is seen most typically in the childhood muscular dystrophies when it is often associated with a tip-toe stance. In juvenile spinal muscular atrophy or polymyositis a similar gait is common; in the former the waddle may be even more extreme but the lordosis is often less. The gait in disorders of the hip joint, such as the epiphyseal dysplasias, can be deceptively similar and in young children who cannot co-operate in muscle testing, investigations may be pursued to a late stage before a radiograph reveals the true diagnosis. In early and doubtful cases of proximal weakness it is invaluable to watch the patient running and trying to hurry up stairs. Attempts to run may resemble a 'racing walk' and the hands may push on the knees or pull on the banister when climbing stairs. These signs are usually the earliest detectable in Duchenne dystrophy.

Gowers' sign, illustrated in Chapter 14 (Fig. 14.1), is also valuable but, in the very early stages of pelvic girdle weakness, patients may be able to stand up fairly easily with only perhaps a brief push with a hand on one knee. Weakness of the quadriceps muscle is best shown during attempts to climb stairs or to stand up from a low stool without using the arms. Much can be learned by asking a patient to sit up from the lying position; weakness of the anterior neck muscles causes the head to lag instead of being the first part to be lifted from the couch, weakness of either hip flexion or of abdominal muscles can make the manoeuvre impossible, and localised weakness of upper or lower abdominal muscles will cause the umbilicus to shift from the mid position. Early paraspinal weakness can be tested when the patient is prone by asking him to lift the head and shoulders backwards from the couch.

It is also important to consider methods of assessing clinically respiratory insufficiency secondary to involvement of the muscles of the thoracic cage and diaphragm. Such weakness may develop rapidly, e.g. in acute polymyositis or in the acute polyneuropathies such as the Guillain–Barré syndrome. It sometimes develops, as a rule much more insidiously, in the muscular dystrophies or spinal muscular atrophies and in motor neurone disease, but much less often in the metabolic myopathies, and may then cause alveolar hypoventilation and CO_2 retention which can be easily overlooked. Breathlessness (as a symptom), tachypnoea, shallow breathing and use of the accessory muscles of respiration (as signs), if overt, imply actual or impending respiratory insufficiency, which can be confirmed by respiratory function tests; but, in the first instance, asking the patient to count aloud as quickly as possible without taking a breath is a simple and useful bedside test — inability to count beyond about 15 implies potentially grave insufficiency, possibly requiring assisted respiration. Diaphragmatic movement can be crudely assessed by observing movement of the abdominal wall during deep inspiration and expiration, intercostal efficiency by observing the movements of the chest wall. Indrawing of the lower ribs at the diaphragmatic attachment during inspiration as a result of intercostal weakness is an important (and common) sign in Werdnig–Hoffmann disease; unilateral or bilateral diaphragmatic paralysis develops in some cases of limb-girdle muscular dystrophy, chronic spinal muscular atrophy and motor neurone disease.

For comparative studies and particularly in treatment trials it is useful to record, not only the strength of individual muscles, but also the patient's overall disability. Several different rating systems have been used in therapeutic trials for different neuromuscular diseases. The following scheme modified from Vignos & Archibald (1960) has endured for decades and is suitable for cases of muscular dystrophy but can be adapted for other purposes if, for example, information about early loss of function in the arms or bulbar muscles is important.

Grade 0 Preclinical. All activities normal.
Grade 1 Walks normally. Unable to run freely.
Grade 2 Detectable defect in posture or gait. Climbs stairs without using the banister.
Grade 3 Climbs stairs only with the banister.
Grade 4 Walks without assistance. Unable to climb stairs.
Grade 5 Walks without assistance. Unable to rise from a chair.
Grade 6 Walks only with calipers or other aids.
Grade 7 Unable to walk. Sits erect in a chair. Able to roll a wheelchair and eat and drink normally.
Grade 8 Sits unsupported in chair. Unable to roll wheelchair or unable to drink from a glass unassisted.
Grade 9 Unable to sit erect without support or unable to eat or drink without assistance.
Grade 10 Confined to bed. Requires help for all activities.

In the early stages further quantitative information can be gained by timing the patient walking over measured distances, climbing standard stairs, standing up from the supine position or from a low chair, or from low stools of graded height. In children especially these functional muscle tests are more valid than measurements of strength of individual muscles.

Weakness — detailed muscle testing

The examiner of a patient with muscular weakness must determine whether weakness is genuine or spurious, its degree, distribution and symmetry and whether it changes after exercise. The last point is dealt with in the section on fatiguability.

The question of the reality of the weakness is put first, not through cynicism, but because it poses a common problem. Ill patients can develop severe weakness which is easily missed unless careful muscle testing is performed. Compression neuropathies following general anaesthesia, and drug-induced neuropathies developing in the course of illnesses such as tuberculosis or renal failure are obvious examples, but perhaps most notable is the myopathy associated with osteomalacia in renal failure or malabsorption, which is very commonly ignored. In addition, weakness in myasthenia gravis or thyrotoxic myopathy has been attributed to psychogenic factors. The obverse problem of spurious malingering or psychogenic weakness masquerading as neuromuscular disease is more easily dealt with because the situation invites careful neurological examination. Sometimes a youthful, well-developed and athletic examiner finds weakness in manual muscle testing when an older and feebler clinician examines the same patient and finds no weakness. The goal is to determine whether the patient can exert force deemed normal against resistance. It is not a wrestling match to determine whether the examiner is stronger than the patient. Different muscles normally exert different forces — for instance, the quadriceps muscles are infinitely stronger than the interossei. If the patient has no symptoms suggesting weakness in the muscle being tested, there may still be true weakness, but the examiner should think twice before declaring that it is present. Spasticity and extrapyramidal rigidity or akinesia may give an initial impression of weakness. Pain due to joint disease is a common pitfall in muscle testing and is especially liable to cause confusion at the hips and knees. The position is often made more complex by the genuine weakness and wasting which may develop, e.g. in the quadriceps in rheumatoid disease or osteoarthritis of the knee, or in the small muscles of an arthritic hand. The diagnosis of hysterical weakness or malingering depends chiefly on the discovery of inconsistencies when the clinical signs are considered as a whole, but much can be learned in the course of manual muscle testing. There is often a momentary initial contraction of reasonable strength, followed by a sudden 'give' in the resistance, not found in true weakness, except in the presence of pain. Another version is seen in the familiar 'misdirection of effort' when patients feign weakness. Instead of exerting full force in the muscle being tested, there is little apparent contraction with a great deal of facial grimacing and contraction of other muscles. Sometimes there is also a coarse tremor because the antagonist is contracted in addition to the muscle being tested. In testing the quadriceps, an unobtrusive hand on the hamstrings on the same side may give valuable information. The patient's behaviour during the examination is often indicative of a psychogenic cause for the alleged physical symptoms.

Much can be learned about the extent and severity of muscle weakness by watching the patient in action, walking, hopping, jumping, climbing stairs, getting up from the floor or from a chair, sitting up from a couch, trying to lift his arms above his head or writing his name. A great deal of time can be saved by these tests and, indeed, some muscles such as those of the abdomen and trunk cannot be satisfactorily tested in any other way. In examining young children this may be the only possible approach. However, detailed information is best acquired by manual testing of each muscle or group in turn. The

proper methods for these tests are briefly summarised in Table 13.1 and are more fully described and illustrated in several texts including Bickerstaff (1980), the Medical Research Council memorandum (1986) and Pact et al (1984). A few of the more important tests are illustrated in Figures 13.1–13.5. The precise positioning of the limb and of the examiner's resistance are very important but, with practice, the methods are reliable. Usually isometric resistance is applied to the fully contracted muscle until it gives way (the 'break' test) but in some circumstances it is useful to test a muscle's strength throughout its full range of movement. It is best to palpate the contracting muscle at the same time. The results are usually expressed on the scale used in the Medical Research Council memorandum (1986):

Grade 0 No contraction.
Grade 1 Flicker or trace of contraction.
Grade 2 Active movement with gravity eliminated.
Grade 3 Active movement against gravity.
Grade 4 Active movement against gravity and resistance.
Grade 5 Normal power.

Grades 4–, 4 and 4+ may be used to indicate movement against slight, moderate and strong resistance respectively. For accurate comparative

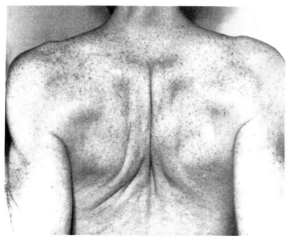
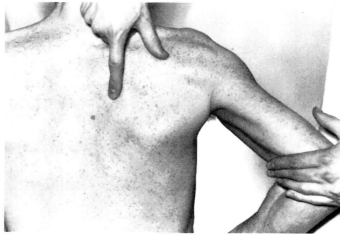

a

Fig. 13.1 a The horizontal fibres of trapezius adduct the scapulae when the shoulders are braced backwards (normal subject). **b** The rhomboids may be felt when the elbow is pushed backwards against resistance. The overlying trapezius is relaxed (normal subject).

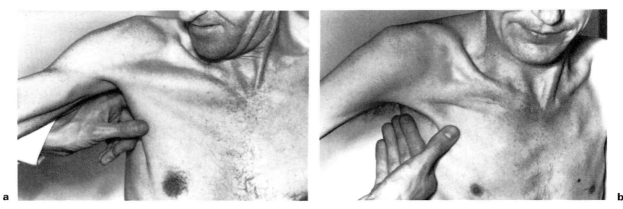

Fig. 13.2   The arm is being adducted and depressed against resistance, the sternocostal fibres of pectoralis major are clearly seen and felt. **a** Normal subject. **b** Becker type of muscular dystrophy.

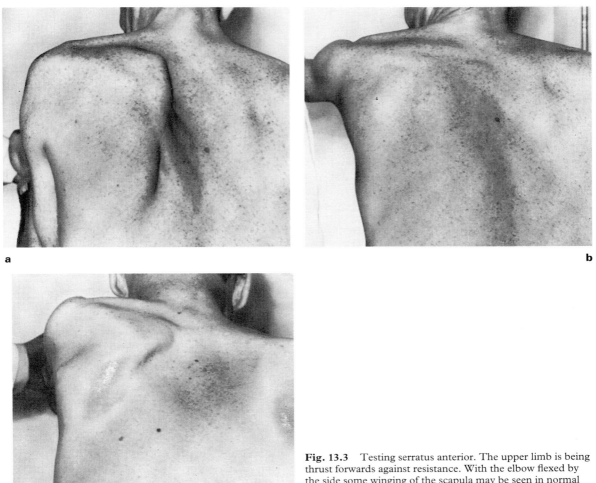

Fig. 13.3   Testing serratus anterior. The upper limb is being thrust forwards against resistance. With the elbow flexed by the side some winging of the scapula may be seen in normal subjects (**a**); but with the arm outstretched there is a clear difference between the normal (**b**) and abnormal (**c**) (Becker dystrophy).

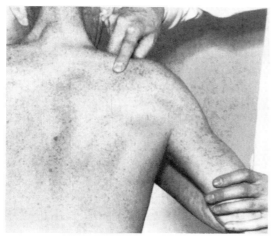
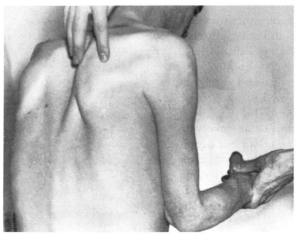

a   b

Fig. 13.4 **a** Supraspinatus acts as the principal abductor with the elbow close to the trunk. Its contraction can easily be felt (normal subject). **b** Infraspinatus is tested during external rotation of the arm against resistance. The wasting of the muscle can be seen and felt (Becker dystrophy).

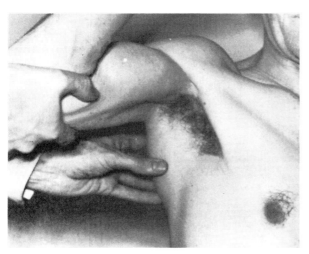
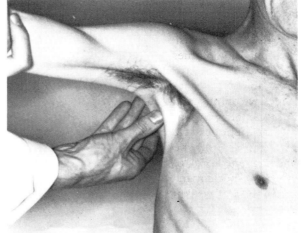

a   b

Fig. 13.5 Latissimus dorsi. The elbow of the externally rotated arm is being pushed downwards against resistance, the difference between the normal bulky muscle (**a**) and the wasted remnant in Becker muscular dystrophy (**b**) is clear.

work there is no substitute for measurement, but here the difficulties of using standard methods and of eliminating gravity and friction are multiplied and skill and experience are required to assess whether the patient is exerting his full strength. Non-extensive strain gauges have theoretical advantages but, in practice, a spring balance held by the examiner is often as good an instrument as any because the 'feel' of the patient's effort can be assessed at the same time. The Hammersmith myometer gives reasonably accurate and reproducible measurements of

muscle power in clinical practice (Edwards & McDonnell 1974, Dubowitz 1978).

Broadly speaking, the interpretation of any muscle weakness which is found is often an exercise in applied anatomy when the lesion is in the lower motor neurone and a matter of pattern recognition in the myopathies. The diagnosis of upper motor neurone lesions requires a combination of these approaches and is beyond the scope of this chapter. Localised weakness in a single limb is usually neurogenic although the effects of muscle trauma such as severe ischaemia or tendon rupture sometimes cause confusion. Details of the root and nerve supply of the principal muscles are given in Table 13.1. When localised weakness seems to fit into no anatomical pattern, poliomyelitis and early motor neurone disease or localised spinal muscular atrophy should be considered. It is difficult to discuss briefly the patterns of muscular involvement in the various myopathies. Nor is it proper to consider the diagnostic value of these patterns without reference to other important points such as the duration and mode of progression of the disease, the presence of other symptoms, the presence or absence of wasting or reflex change, and so on. However, the information given in Table 13.2 may be helpful as an approximate guide and further details are given in the section on differential diagnosis in Chapter 14. It is of special importance to decide whether proximal muscle weakness involves all the shoulder girdle or pelvic muscles to about the same degree (e.g. as in polymyositis or thyrotoxic and other metabolic myopathies) or certain muscles selectively. A selective, symmetrical pattern of involvement in a chronic progressive myopathy is suggestive of muscular dystrophy, although spinal muscular atrophy and other disorders may imitate this. The exact distribution of this selective involvement may be of great help in distinguishing one form of muscular dystrophy from another, especially in the early stages. An atypical distribution of weakness and wasting in a case of apparent muscular dystrophy should arouse immediate suspicions about the diagnosis and will underline the need for full investigation, including muscle biopsy.

Indeed, if a syndrome of proximal limb weakness develops in a patient of any age, without other distinguishing characteristics or family history of a similar disorder, EMG and muscle biopsy are needed to determine whether the condition is neurogenic or myogenic, or whether there are any specific and diagnostic histological features.

Fatiguability

Myasthenia gravis is often defined as a state of abnormal fatiguability. Physiologically, an abnormal decremental response in the evoked muscle potential produced by stimulation of its motor nerve is the diagnostic hallmark electromyographically. However, the symptoms of myasthenia are those of weakness — ptosis, diplopia, dysarthria, dysphagia or weakness of the limbs or neck. For example, patients never start a set of tennis at full strength and suddenly wilt after the first game or set. By contrast, patients who do complain of fatigue usually have a psychological disorder, psychasthenia, not myasthenia. However, during physical examination weakness which is variable in degree and is made worse by repeated contraction is typical of myasthenia. Ptosis may be exaggerated by sustained upgaze for 30 seconds, or relieved by a brief nap (Odel et al 1991). Exaggeration of limb weakness by exercise must be distinguished from simple fatigue due to slight fixed muscular weakness and from stiffness or pain induced by exercise. Clinical demonstration of myasthenia is usually possible if the strength of an affected muscle is compared with its contralateral equivalent before and after repeated contraction. The reverse phenomenon, weakness which improves during the first few contractions following rest, may occur in the myasthenic–myopathic or Eaton– Lambert syndrome. The clinical features of these conditions are described in Chapter 20.

Although typical cases are easily recognised, patients do not always notice the effect of exercise. It is, therefore, wise to try the effect of intravenous edrophonium in every case of obscure muscular weakness; this should be an early investigation whenever muscular weakness is not associated with conspicuous wasting, especially if the tendon reflexes are preserved. Retention of the tendon reflexes is typical of myasthenia gravis, while in the Eaton–Lambert syndrome they are lost early. Another point of distinction between these disorders is the tendency for the lower limbs to be affected first in the myasthenic–myopathic syndrome, while myasthenia gravis rarely presents in this way. Indeed there are almost always ocular or oropharyngeal symptoms and signs in myasthenia. In the Lambert–Eaton syndrome, there may occasionally be ptosis and dysphagia, but these symptoms are likely to be mild and ophthalmoparesis is exceptional. Furthermore, autonomic dysfunction (dry mouth, etc.) is common in the Lambert–Eaton syndrome, not in myasthenia gravis.

Table 13.1 The nerve and root supply of the principal muscles with methods of testing their actions. Modified from Gray's Anatomy (1967) and MRC memorandum (1986). Where any single root supplying a particular muscle is more important than the others it is printed in bold type

Nerve	Muscle	Roots	Action tested
Accessory nerve	Trapezius	Spinal root	Elevation of shoulders. Adduction of scapulae
	Sternocleidomastoid	Spinal root	Tilting of head to same side with rotation to opposite side
Brachial plexus	Pectoralis major		
	Clavicular part	**C5**, C6	Adduction of elevated arm
	Sternocostal part	C6, **C7**, **C8**	Adduction and forward depression of arm
	Serratus anterior	C5, C6, C7	Fixation of the scapula during forward thrusting of the arm
	Rhomboids	C4, C5	Elevation and fixation of scapulae
	Supraspinatus	**C5**, C6	Initiation of abduction of arm
	Infraspinatus	**C5**, C6	External rotation of arm
	Latissimus dorsi	C6, **C7**, C8	Adduction of horizontal, externally rotated arm. Coughing
Axillary nerve	Deltoid	**C5**, C6	Lateral and forward elevation of arm to horizontal
Musculocutaneous nerve	Biceps Brachialis	**C5**, C6	Flexion of the supinated forearm
Radial nerve	Triceps	C6, **C7**, C8	Extension of forearm
	Brachioradialis	C5, **C6**	Flexion of semi-prone forearm
	Extensor carpi radialis longus	**C6**	Extension of wrist to radial side
Posterior interosseus nerve	Supinator	C6, C7	Supination of extended forearm
	Extensor digitorum	**C7**, C8	Extension of proximal phalanges
	Extensor carpi ulnaris	**C7**, C8	Extension of wrist to ulnar side
	Extensor indicis	**C7**, C8	Extension of proximal phalanx of index finger
	Abductor pollicis longus	**C7**, C8	Abduction of first metacarpal in plane at right angle to palm
	Extensor pollicis longus	**C7**, C8	Extension at first interphalangeal joint
	Extensor pollicis brevis	**C7**, C8	Extension at first metacarpophalangeal joint
Median nerve	Pronator teres	C6, C7	Pronation of extended forearm
	Flexor carpi radialis	C6, C7	Flexion of wrist to radial side
	Flexor digitorum superficialis	C7, **C8**, T1	Flexion of middle phalanges
	Abductor pollicis brevis (ulnar nerve rarely)	C8, **T1**	Abduction of first metacarpal in plane at right angle to palm
	Flexor pollicis brevis (more often ulnar nerve)	C8, **T1**	Flexion of proximal phalanx of thumb
	Opponens pollicis (rarely ulnar nerve)	C8, **T1**	Opposition of thumb against fifth finger
	1st and 2nd lumbricals	C8, **T1**	Extension of middle phalanges while proximal phalanges are fixed in extension
Anterior interosseous nerve	Flexor digitorum profundus (lateral part)	**C8**, T1	Flexion of terminal phalanges of index and middle fingers
	Flexor pollicis longus	**C8**, T1	Flexion of distal phalanx of the thumb
Ulnar nerve	Flexor carpi ulnaris	C7, **C8**, T1	Observe tendon during testing abductor digiti minimi
	Flexor digitorum profundus (medial part)	C7, **C8**	Flexion of distal phalanges of ring and little fingers
	Hypothenar muscles	C8, **T1**	Abduction and opposition of little finger
	3rd and 4th lumbricals	C8, **T1**	Extension of middle phalanges while proximal phalanges are fixed in extension
	Adductor pollicis	C8, **T1**	Adduction of thumb against palmar surface of index finger
	Flexor pollicis brevis (sometimes median nerve)	**C8**, T1	Flexion of proximal phalanx of the thumb
	Interossei	C8, **T1**	Abduction and adduction of the fingers

Table 13.1   *Cont'd*

Nerve	Muscle	Roots	Action tested
Femoral nerve	Iliopsoas (and lumbar nerves)	**L1, L2**, L3	Hip flexion from semi-flexed position
	Sartorius	L2, L3	Hip flexion from externally rotated position
	Quadriceps (rectus femoris and the lateral and medial vasti)	**L2, L3, L4**	Extension at the knee
Obturator nerve	Adductor longus magnus* brevis	**L2, L3**, L4	Adduction of the thigh
Superior gluteal nerve	Gluteus medius	**L4, L5**, S1	Abduction of the thigh. Internal rotation of the thigh
	Tensor fasciae latae	L4, L5	
Inferior gluteal nerve	Gluteus maximus	**L5, S1**, S2	Extension of the thigh
Sciatic nerve	Biceps femoris	L5, **S1**, S2	
	Semitendinosus	L5, **S1**, S2	Flexion at the knee
	Semimembranosus	L5, **S1**, S2	
Peroneal nerve (deep)	Anterior tibial	**L4**, L5	Dorsiflexion of the foot
	Extensor digitorum longus	**L5**, S1	Dorsiflexion of the toes
	Extensor hallucis longus	**L5**, S1	Dorsiflexion of great toe
	Extensor digitorum brevis	L5, S1	Dorsiflexion of the toes
Peroneal nerve (superfic.)	Peroneus longus Peroneus brevis	L5, S1	Eversion of the foot
Tibial nerve	Gastrocnemius	**S1**, S2	Plantar-flexion of the foot
	Soleus	S1, **S2**	
	Tibialis posterior	L4, **L5**	Inversion of plantar-flexed foot
	Flexor digitorum longus	L5, **S1, S2**	Flexion of toes (distal phalanges)
	Flexor hallucis longus	L5, **S1, S2**	Flexion of great toe (distal phalanx)
	Flexor digitorum brevis	S1, S2	Flexion of toes (middle phalanges)
	Flexor hallucis brevis	S1, S2	Flexion of great toe (proximal phalanx)
Pudendal nerve	Perineal muscles	S2, S3, S4	Tension of anal sphincter

*Adductor magnus is partly supplied by the sciatic nerve.

Wasting (atrophy)

Atrophy brings patients to the doctor much less often than weakness but may do so in motor neurone disease or syringomyelia, when the small muscles of the hand are affected, and occasionally in other disorders. As a physical sign of muscle disease, however, wasting is second in importance only to weakness. It is particularly valuable to compare the degrees of wasting and weakness in affected muscles; this is illustrated in Table 13.2.

In most patients wasting can be recognised by systematic inspection of the muscles but in some women and in the obese it is difficult to assess. When asymmetry is suspected, limb girth must be measured at points equidistant from well-defined bony landmarks on the two sides. Palpation of the muscles during contraction is often helpful and computed tomography can be very useful (O'Doherty et al 1977). Sometimes confusion is

caused by congenital absence of muscles (most often of pectoralis major, Fig. 13.6). Atrophy may involve only part of a muscle. This is often seen in limb-girdle dystrophy or spinal muscular atrophy, in which localised dimples are seen when muscles are contracted against resistance; in the late stages the uppermost third of the deltoid muscle is often wasted and fibrotic while the lower two-thirds are soft and much bulkier, even hypertrophic. A similar combination of wasting and hypertrophy is sometimes found in quadriceps, usually with atrophy of medial, and partial hypertrophy of lateral, vasti. Another important cause of focal atrophy of part of a muscle is infarction. Focal wasting may be simulated by the appearances after rupture of a tendon (e.g. long head of biceps brachii) or of the perimysial sheath (giving a muscle hernia).

The significance of patterns of muscle involvement is discussed in the section on weakness. In most lower motor neurone disorders and in many

Table 13.2   An outline of some of the common patterns of muscular weakness and atrophy in various disorders

Weakness	Generalised	Mainly distal	Mainly proximal	Symmetrical — highly selective	Asymmetrical
With little or no wasting	Polymyositis Myasthenia gravis Myasthenic-myopathic syndrome Periodic paralyses Hypothyroidism Addison's disease Steroid myopathy	UMN lesions	Polymyositis Myasthenia gravis Myasthenic-myopathic syndrome Myopathy with osteomalacia Periodic paralyses Steroid myopathy Hypothyroidism Upper motor neurone lesions	Periodic paralyses	Periodic (paralyses) Peripheral neuropathy UMN lesion
With wasting	Werdnig–Hoffmann disease Benign congenital myopathies MND (Polymyositis)	Most peripheral neuropathies Peroneal muscular atrophy MND Distal myopathy Myotonic dystrophy* Ocular myopathy (UMN lesions)	Muscular dystrophy† Spinal muscular atrophy Thyrotoxic myopathy Glycogen-storage diseases Lipid storage myopathies Myasthenic-myopathic syndrome Motor neuropathy MND Polymyositis	Muscular dystrophy† Spinal muscular atrophy Thyrotoxic myopathy MND Motor neuropathy Ocular myopathy Glycogen-storage disease (Poliomyelitis)	MND Poliomyelitis Peripheral neuropathy Spinal muscular atrophy (Limb-girdle muscular dystrophy)

MND = motor neurone disease. UMN = upper motor neurone.
Unusual presentations are given in brackets. Causes of purely localised weakness have been excluded.
* In myotonic dystrophy the weakness is semi-distal, i.e. involves the forearm and the leg but not small hand muscles at first.
† 'Muscular dystrophy' refers to the X-linked, limb-girdle and facioscapulohumeral types.

myopathies, muscle wasting and weakness go hand in hand. In motor neurone disease there tends to be proportionately more atrophy and in muscular dystrophy proportionately more weakness, but these points are subtle and often not of much help. However Table 13.2 lists myopathies in which quite severe weakness may be associated with very little wasting; because several of these are treatable, this finding should be recognised as being of great significance. The most important of such conditions are myasthenia gravis, polymyositis, periodic paralysis and the myopathy of osteomalacia; careful investigation to exclude these four conditions (and other metabolic myopathies) is necessary in any case of muscle weakness in which wasting is not prominent. Such investigations should include an edrophonium test, measurement of evoked muscle action potentials during and after repetitive nerve stimulation, electromyography (including single fibre studies with measurement of 'jitter' and 'blocking'), estimation of the serum creatine kinase activity,

calcium, phosphorus, alkaline phosphatase and potassium, assay of circulating antibodies against the acetylcholine receptor (AChR) and muscle biopsy. When the weakness is recent, atrophy may not have had time to develop. Following complete traumatic denervation, clinical atrophy becomes evident after about 2 weeks and is maximal after about 12 weeks. Another potential pitfall is the wasting which may develop after many years in myasthenia gravis, polymyositis, periodic paralysis and in McArdle's disease and other metabolic myopathies.

The reverse situation, muscular wasting with little or no weakness, is common in many systemic diseases such as tuberculosis, malnutrition, carcinomatosis or simple atrophy due to ageing. In fact, muscular atrophy in the elderly, especially in certain lower limb muscles, such as soleus, is associated with histological appearances indistinguishable from those of denervation and seems to be due to a progressive loss of anterior horn cells in the spinal cord consequent upon ageing proces-

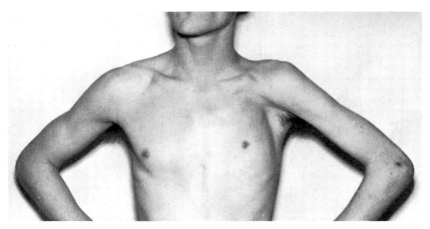

Fig. 13.6 Congenital absence of the left pectoralis major. The patient had developed a secondary brachial plexus lesion and the wasting of the left deltoid can be seen.

ses (Jennekens et al 1971). Some cases of thyrotoxic myopathy are masked by the generalised weight loss which occurs in this condition and similarly the myasthenic–myopathic syndrome of Eaton and Lambert sometimes goes unrecognised in the general malaise and weight loss of carcinomatosis. After weight loss of 20 pounds (12 kg) or more, it may be difficult or impossible to discern focal wasting in the hands.

Muscular hypertrophy and pseudohypertrophy

It is doubtful whether a general increase in muscle bulk is ever a primary pathological phenomenon. Of all the muscle diseases it is seen most strikingly in myotonia congenita, where the muscle hypertrophy may resemble that of a professional weightlifter. The strength of the muscles in this condition is consistent with their bulk, and work hypertrophy induced by the myotonia seems to be responsible. It may even be that the bulky muscles seen in the 'pseudohypertrophic' forms of muscular dystrophy initially pass through a similar phase. Certainly the enlarged muscles seen in early Duchenne dystrophy are relatively strong (e.g. the calves, deltoids and lateral vastus) and contain a high proportion of hypertrophied fibres. Later in the disease replacement by fat and connective tissue sometimes maintains bulk despite

muscle fibre loss. This is the stage of pseudohypertrophy. Failure to distinguish between these two stages is perhaps responsible for contradictory descriptions of the consistency of these muscles as 'rubbery' and 'inelastic' or 'firm' and 'doughy'. In fact they are generally firm while strong and soft when weak but, apart from establishing this fact, palpation of muscle is not of much help in the diagnosis of the muscular dystrophies. Only inspection of the muscles or measurement can make it clear whether they are abnormally bulky or not.

Enlargement of muscles is fairly common in limb-girdle muscular dystrophy and very common in the Becker type as well as in the Duchenne. It is also a fairly common clinical feature in manifesting carriers of the Duchenne gene. It is also seen in the myopathy of hypothyroidism and occasionally in polymyositis or cysticercosis, and localised tender swellings in muscle may be a consequence of infarction (in various vasculitides), of pyogenic infection (in tropical myositis) or of localised nodular myositis (Ch. 16). However, it is not pathognomonic of myopathy as it also occurs in spinal muscular atrophy. There now seems to be general agreement that so-called hypertrophia musculorum vera is not a specific disease entity but a syndrome of diffuse muscular hypertrophy of multiple aetiology. In de Lange's syndrome of athetosis and mental defect (1934), muscle hypertrophy may be the result of continuous muscle spasm.

Spontaneous movements

Two closely similar forms of spontaneous movement may signify neuromuscular disease or dysfunction, viz fasciculation and myokymia. Both are painless contractions of small groups of muscle fibres which cause visible movement of the overlying skin but not usually of neighbouring joints. These points distinguish them not only from the contraction of single fibres (fibrillation) — which is detectable only by electromyography or by examination of the exposed muscle which 'is involved in a confusion of very small twitches', 'without either apparent rhythm or obvious centre of activity' (Denny-Brown & Pennybacker 1938) — but also from tremor, myoclonus, chorea and other more overt movements unrelated to muscular disease. Both fasciculation and myokymia may be felt by the patient.

Fasciculations are brief twitches of groups or bundles of fibres which often involve the same group repetitively over short periods but may be totally irregular. They are best seen where the muscle is superficial, in the hands and especially the tongue and can often be induced by percussing or pinching the muscle. They occur in active degenerative disorders of the anterior horn cell but may be induced in normal individuals by anticholinesterase drugs. Fasciculation is a valuable clue to diagnosis in motor neurone disease and in spinal muscular atrophy and should be sought particularly in the tongue, which should lie relaxed on the floor of the mouth. Absence of fasciculation, however, does not by any means exclude anterior horn cell disease. Spontaneous benign fasciculation is not uncommon in normal subjects, especially in the calf or small hand muscles. It cannot be distinguished with certainty from the pathological type, but fasciculation that is seen *only* after movement or strong contraction, and is not associated with muscle weakness, is usually benign. Both benign fasciculation and the fasciculation of motor neurone diseases are often associated with frequent cramps. The EMG shows similar spontaneous activity in both conditions, although the spontaneous discharges in the benign disorder more often take the form of 'doublets' or 'triplets' than in anterior horn cell disease (Fetell et al 1982, Fleet & Watson 1986)

and there are no signs of denervation in the benign condition; otherwise, it might be difficult to rule out motor neurone disease. Rarely, fasciculation occurs in inflammatory or compressive nerve root lesions, but here its character is different, for it usually involves large fasciculi and tends to occur repetitively in the same fasciculus during minimal contraction but not during complete relaxation. It corresponds to the 'giant units' recorded in the electromyogram.

Myokymia has two definitions, one clinical and the other electromyographic. Clinically, it is used to describe continuous and vigorous twitching of muscle, including slower contraction of small bands or strips of muscle that give an undulating or rippling appearance to the overlying skin.

Electromyographically, the term is used to describe a combination of spontaneous discharges that take the form of singlets, doublets, triplets and multiplets that culminate in bursts or trains of electrical activity. Sometimes the clinical disorder and the EMG pattern go together, as seen in some cases of thyrotoxicosis or tetany due to hypocalcaemia, but more often in cases of Isaacs' syndrome, as described below. However, the EMG pattern of myokymia is often seen without any clinical manifestations, and clinical myokymia may be seen without the EMG pattern.

The manifestations of Isaacs' syndrome have been reported under numerous titles, including 'continuous motor fibre activity' (Isaacs 1961) and 'neuromyotonia' (Mertens & Zschocke 1965). However, the motor fibre activity may not be completely continuous, and there may be no impairment of muscle relaxation, so that neither of these 'specific' names suffices. This is a good example of the justifiable use of an eponym.

Clinical characteristics include abnormal postures of the limbs, especially persistent carpopedal spasm, as well as delayed relaxation (pseudomyotonia); hyperhidrosis; cramps; and myokymia (Gamstorp & Wohlfart 1959, Gardner-Medwin & Walton 1969, Albers et al 1981). The EMG pattern of myokymia is almost always present. In less than 25% of cases there is overt clinical evidence of a sensorimotor peripheral neuropathy (Rowland 1985), but the condition is often ascribed to a peripheral neuropathy because there may be slowing of nerve conduction (Wallis et al

1970) and because the condition is abolished by curare but not by peripheral nerve block, suggesting that the activity arises in distal nerve terminals. Most cases are sporadic and of unknown cause, but some have been familial (Welch et al 1972, Ashizawa et al 1983, Auger et al 1984) and some seem to be precipitated by alcohol (Williamson & Brooke 1972) or exposure to herbicides containing dichlorphenoxyacetate (Wallis et al 1970). Sometimes there is a thymoma, with or without other evidence of myasthenia gravis. The condition responds well to treatment with carbamazepine or phenytoin (Zisfein et al 1983).

The manifestations of Isaacs' syndrome closely resemble those of tetany, but the syndrome is chronic and calcium metabolism is normal. In cases of presumed Isaacs' syndrome with laryngeal stridor (Jackson et al 1979), hyperventilation alkalosis with tetany should be excluded. Unusual forms of the disorder overlap with myoclonus (Leigh et al 1980) and the stiff-man syndrome (Valli et al 1983, Zisfein et al 1983, Auger et al 1984).

Another variety of episodic myokymia, involving one side of the face (facial myokymia) may occur in multiple sclerosis or as an isolated phenomenon (Matthews 1966). The recurrent twitches of the eyelid or of particular parts of muscles, which are commonly experienced by normal people and are often called myokymia, are probably more closely related to benign fasciculations; they have no pathological significance but are often induced by fatigue.

Facial clonic spasm or hemifacial spasm is a recurrent twitch of part, or sometimes the whole, of the musculature supplied by the facial nerve on one side. Rarely it is bilateral. The movement is stereotyped in form but irregular in timing and the former point distinguishes it from chorea and facial dyskinesia. Facial tic or habit spasm is often similar, but less rapidly repeated. Tetany, tetanus and blepharospasm due to ocular irritation, to facial spasticity or to Meige's (Brueghel's) syndrome of blepharospasm-oromandibular-facial dystonia should be considered in differential diagnosis. Hemifacial spasm is an intractable condition usually seen after the fifth decade. It has been attributed to an irritative lesion of the facial nerve in its canal but is more often due to compression of the intracranial trunk of the nerve by an aberrant artery (see Walton 1985). Sometimes it is seen in geniculate herpes or Paget's disease of the skull.

Movement induced by contraction or stimulation

Myotonia is defined by both clinical and EMG criteria. If the latter are absent, the condition may be called 'pseudomyotonia' although this imprecise term has been used to identify the slow contraction and relaxation seen in hypothyroidism and the repetitive electrical high frequency discharges seen in the EMG in some metabolic myopathies. Clinically true myotonia is defined by abnormally slow relaxation after a contraction. The contraction may be induced by either voluntary movement, percussion of the muscle or electrical stimulation. The EMG correlate is a waxing and waning pattern of repetitive discharge. Denny-Brown & Nevin (1941) found that it persisted after nerve block or curarisation, implying that the abnormal activity arises in muscle itself. Molecular genetic studies have indicated that, in hyperkalaemic periodic paralysis and paramyotonia, the myotonia arises from abnormalities of the sodium channel in muscle. In some animal forms of myotonia, and perhaps in myotonia congenita, the condition seems to be due to an abnormality of chloride conductance (Adrian & Marshall 1976). In myotonic muscular dystrophy, the pathophysiological basis is unclear but may be abnormal phosphorylation of a membrane ion channel.

The diseases associated with myotonia and their differentiation are discussed in Chapter 15. In infants with myotonia the face and eyelids may fail to relax for several seconds after a sneeze or cry, the cry itself may sound strangled and the limbs may seem stiff. Later in life, patients complain of stiffness of the limbs, difficulty in walking or inability to relax the grip. Generally myotonia improves after repeated contraction and is worsened by cold. These effects are so striking in paramyotonia that it may be necessary to ask the patient to chill the hands in cold water before any abnormality can be demonstrated. Grip myotonia is shown by failure of relaxation lasting usually for 5–10 seconds after a tight contraction but occasionally for as long as a minute. Often the fingers and thumb remain flexed at the metacarpophalangeal joints while the other joints are extended. Percussion myotonia in the thenar eminence results not only in a dimple but in slow tonic opposition of the thumb and gradual relaxation lasting altogether 2–10 s. A small tendon hammer may be used to percuss the tongue against a spatula (tongue depressor) placed over the lower teeth when a persistent dimple is again seen. There is little difficulty in recognising myotonia once the possibility of its presence has occurred to the examiner. However, percussion myotonia may be confused with *myoidema*, an electrically silent ridge (not a depression) induced by percussion of atrophic muscles in such wasting conditions as tuberculosis and malabsorption (Denny-Brown & Pennybacker 1938, Salick & Pearson 1967). Contraction myotonia can really be mistaken only for the very similar but electrically distinct phenomenon which may be associated with myokymia (Gamstorp & Wohlfart 1959) and with the pseudomyotonia of hypothyroidism (Hoffmann's syndrome) (see Ch. 15). As mentioned above, in these conditions the delayed relaxation is called pseudomyotonia because the characteristic EMG pattern of myotonia is not present. Leyburn & Walton (1959) described a method of quantitative assessment of myotonia for use in trials of treatment.

Tetany may be associated with hypocalcaemia, with alkalosis and possibly with hypomagnesaemia. It is heralded by tingling in the extremities or lips and, in the latent phase, spasms may be induced by nerve percussion (Chvostek's sign) or ischaemia (Trousseau's sign). Later, stridor and dyspnoea may occur and intermittent muscle cramp and spasm develop. Although these spasms can occur spontaneously they are increased by mechanical stimulation or contraction of the muscle as the excitability of both nerve and muscle is increased. They affect chiefly the hands, which adopt the 'main d'accoucheur' position, and the feet. More generalised involvement with opisthotonos may develop in severe cases and may be accompanied by colic and fits. Only in this advanced stage is tetany painful. Although clinical myokymia is not seen in tetany, the clinical spasm may be preceded by visible twitches. The EMG pattern of tetany, however, resembles that of myokymia, with singlets, doublets and multiplets building up to a burst of motor unit potentials that accompany the clinical spasm.

In *tetanus* the hyperexcitability of the nerves and muscles resembles that of tetany. In addition, however, there is usually an underlying state of continuous muscle spasm which results in the well-known features of trismus, neck retraction and the risus sardonicus. This predilection for the face and neck contrasts with the carpopedal spasm of early tetany although the muscles involved early in tetanus may also depend on the site of the infection. Indeed the spasm may remain localised in some cases, usually in partly immunised subjects. In the later stages the spasm usually becomes widespread and any movement or external stimulus induces paroxysmal and painful exacerbations. The bite of the American Black Widow spider (*Lactrodectus mactans*) may result in a similar condition of painful muscle spasm. The *stiff-man syndrome* is a poorly understood disorder that is difficult to define (McEvoy 1991). It is regarded as another syndrome due to abnormal motor unit activity but differs from Isaacs' syndrome in several characteristics. The muscle activity primarily affects the trunk and is manifest by abnormal rigidity and a stiff back, with superimposed painful spasms. The limbs are less affected and the defining features of Isaacs' syndrome are not seen; there is no carpal spasm, myokymia, pseudomyotonia or hyperhidrosis. Also there is no characteristic EMG pattern. It is thought to be an autoimmune disorder, at least in some cases. It is discussed further in Chapter 27.

Physiological contracture (as distinct from physical contracture due to permanent and irreversible shortening) is electrically silent shortening of a muscle induced by exertion. It is seen in McArdle's disease, phosphofructokinase deficiency and in other related forms of glycogen-storage disease of muscle (Lehoczky et al 1965, Satoyoshi & Kowa 1967, and see Ch. 17). Perkoff et al (1966) showed that a similar reversible metabolic disorder with contracture can occur in chronic alcoholism after heavy drinking bouts. The exercised muscle develops aching or cramping pain and then becomes stiff and weak. Continued gentle exercise allows some patients to enter a 'second wind' stage with lessening of the pain as they continue. More often the pain forces them to halt and if the muscle is then examined it is found to be shortened, tense and tender. Only electromyography can distinguish this from true cramp in doubtful cases. The contracture lasts from a few minutes to several hours, depending on its severity. Very severe pain which passes off rapidly is not due to McArdle's disease. The final diagnosis depends on biochemical demonstration of the enzyme abnormality.

Muscle tone

In *infants* hypotonia is an early and important indication of muscle disease. The problem of diagnosis of the 'floppy infant' is dealt with in Chapter 20 and all that needs to be said here is that the cause may lie in the brain (especially the parietal lobes and cerebellum), the anterior horns or posterior columns of the spinal cord, the motor or sensory nerves, the myoneural junctions or the muscle fibres and possibly sometimes in the muscle spindles or ligaments. Hypotonia can also result from malnutrition, malabsorption and metabolic disorders. Part of the diagnostic problem may lie in the failure to define the precise meaning of tone and hypotonia. André-Thomas et al (1960) described methods for testing several different aspects of muscle tone, each of which may be disturbed independently. Thus the *consistency* of a muscle may be tested by wobbling it laterally with a finger, by shaking the limbs and by palpation, its '*extensibilité*' by slow movement of joints through their full range and its '*passivité*' by, for example, measuring the amplitude of the flapping movement when the proximal part of a limb is shaken. The *recoil* of a muscle suddenly released from a fully stretched position is another manifestation of tone. The different functions of tonic and phasic reflexes account for some of the apparent inconsistencies when tone is tested in different ways but, in general, the pathological significance of the various manifestations is not properly understood. In muscle disease consistency and '*passivité*' are more often abnormal than '*extensibilité*'. Other useful signs of hypotonia are the hanging posture of the head and limbs when a baby is lifted supine with the hand under the child's back and the tendency to slip through the hands when the infant is lifted with hands under the axillae. It is important to recall that tone normally decreases from birth until the second to sixth month and gradually increases again in later childhood.

In *children* beyond the 'floppy infant' stage, hypotonia is a valuable sign before full cooperation in muscle strength tests is possible. An important example is the looseness of the shoulders in early Duchenne dystrophy.

In *adults* most myopathies and disorders of the lower motor neurone produce a moderate reduction in muscle tone. Because of the much more definitive information given by assessing muscle wasting and power, tone is rarely of much importance in diagnosis, except when apparently out of keeping with other signs. Thus, in cases of combined pyramidal tract and lower motor neurone involvement, as in some hereditary ataxias and motor neurone disease, spasticity in weak, wasted, areflexic muscles may be the only indication of the upper motor neurone lesion.

Palpation of nerves and muscles

As mentioned above, peripheral nerves may become tender to palpation at sites of entrapment (as with the ulnar nerve behind the medial epicondyle of the humerus) or when their component roots are compressed or irritated (as with the sciatic nerve in sciatica due to lumbar intervertebral disc prolapse). Localised swelling or hypertrophy of peripheral nerves can occur in leprosy or neurofibromatosis, more generalised enlargement, even involving the greater auricular nerve, in cases of hypertrophic neuropathy (as in some cases of peroneal muscular atrophy and related disorders, or in recurrent demyelinating peripheral neuropathy).

The importance of palpation in assessing muscle tone, wasting, hypertrophy or weakness has already been stressed. In addition, local areas of tenderness may be discovered, an event which often provides more satisfaction for the anxious patient than for the thoughtful physician, as the cause of such local tenderness is only rarely found.

Nevertheless in some fairly well-defined syndromes such as 'tennis elbow', attributable to a localised tendonitis at the lateral epicondyle of the humerus or in the region of the neck of the radius resulting from repetitive movement, useful treatment may result. Palpable masses in muscle are generally either areas of local spasm, post-traumatic haematomata or, less commonly, infarcts (in polyarteritis nodosa) or areas of localised nodular myositis. Differentiation between these can be difficult in acute cases. Sometimes the bony swellings of myositis ossificans can be felt and, rarely, a local mass turns out to be a tumour, either primary in muscle (rhabdomyosarcoma), or expanding from deeper structures such as an osteogenic sarcoma. Herniation of muscle fibres through a ruptured perimysial sheath (a muscle hernia) may feel deceptively like a tumour.

Reflex change

Markedly different patterns of reflex change may be found in otherwise similar disorders. In peripheral neuropathy, even without obvious sensory loss, the tendon reflexes are usually abolished early and are often absent in muscles which seem otherwise unaffected. In the muscular dystrophies, loss of reflexes tends to follow closely the degree of weakness and they are absent in any markedly weak muscle. In motor neurone disease, however, substantial wasting and weakness may be found in muscles with brisk reflexes, presumably because of the survival of some motor units with intact peripheral nerve conduction in the presence of corticospinal tract involvement. Polymyositis, myasthenia gravis and the myopathy of osteomalacia or hyperparathyroidism are other disorders in which the reflexes tend to be preserved in weak muscles. They are valuable in distinguishing between myasthenia gravis (in which they are preserved) and the Lambert–Eaton myasthenic syndrome (in which they are abolished early). It is well known that in hypothyroidism, with or without myopathy, the rates of contraction and relaxation in the reflex response are characteristically slow and, less often, excessively rapid responses are found in thyrotoxicosis.

The plantar responses are, of course, generally flexor in neuromuscular disorders. Generally speaking, the discovery of extensor plantar responses in cases of proximal muscle weakness should arouse suspicions of motor neurone disease or of those rare instances of spinal muscular atrophy in which there is evidence of pyramidal tract dysfunction (Gardner-Medwin et al 1967).

Contracture

Contracture is a state of shortening of a muscle not caused by active contraction. It may be acute and spontaneously reversible, as in McArdle's disease, but far more often it is the result of the rearrangement of collagen fibrils within the muscle over a longer period. At this stage it is fully reversible by repeated stretching. Later, actual fibrosis may make it increasingly difficult to treat. Contracture often follows failure of a muscle to grow in length or progressive shortening when its action is not opposed by a sufficiently powerful antagonist or one which is becoming steadily weaker. Palpation of the muscle during attempts at passive movement at the affected joint will rapidly distinguish contracture from joint ankylosis in one case and active contraction in another although, occasionally, examination under general anaesthesia may be necessary when both are present. When the relevant muscles are inaccessible, e.g. at the hip joint or in the 'frozen shoulder' syndrome, these distinctions may be difficult and, indeed, in the latter condition, muscles may pass through all three stages of spasm, contracture and atrophy due to ankylosis. Demonstration of contractures is usually easy, but they may be missed at the shoulder if the scapula is not fixed, and at the hips if the lumbar lordosis is not first eliminated by flexing the opposite hip so that the thigh touches the abdomen.

Contractures develop in many chronic muscle diseases, whether neurogenic or myopathic, and are especially prominent in the syndrome of arthrogryposis multiplex congenita, in muscular dystrophy of the Duchenne type, and in poliomyelitis and the spinal muscular atrophies. In muscular dystrophy they are an important source of early difficulty in walking (see Ch. 14). In acute polymyositis they occasionally develop rapidly within a few weeks, even in muscles with surprisingly little weakness. In progressive myosclerosis (another syndrome of multiple aetiology), contracture may be the major cause of disability; here, no weakness may be detectable, but the muscles have a woody or fibrotic consistency.

Muscles supplied by the cranial nerves

The examination of the *external ocular muscles* is a complex art which is described by Cogan (1978), Glaser (1990) and Leigh & Zee (1991). Only a few points of special relevance to muscle disease are mentioned here. Pareses that do not conform to the pattern of single or multiple nerve palsies suggest a local muscular disorder, but this may be caused by expanding orbital lesions as well as by inflammatory, metabolic or degenerative myopathies. Thus, in polymyositis the ocular muscles are occasionally involved, as they are in the rare orbital myositis and the closely related condition of orbital pseudotumour, which is often unilateral but sometimes bilateral, giving proptosis as well as impaired ocular movement. In the ocular, oculopharyngeal and myotonic muscular dystrophies, ptosis invariably occurs before ocular pareses, and diplopia is only rarely an early symptom. Later, ocular myopathy may progress to complete external ophthalmoplegia. An isolated superior rectus palsy is often the earliest feature of ophthalmic Graves' disease. If proptosis is not obvious in such cases it should be sought using an exophthalmometer; in most cases, conjunctival oedema is also present. Myasthenia gravis is a great imitator of ocular palsies and should be considered wherever diagnosis is uncertain. Maintaining upward gaze for a full minute will usually induce some ptosis in such cases as mentioned earlier but, even if it does not, an edrophonium test should always be tried. Electronystagmographic recording of optokinetic nystagmus or tonometry performed before and after edrophonium has proved helpful in diagnosis but measurement of serum AChR antibodies is more reliable. In children, bilateral facial weakness apparently associated with bilateral sixth nerve palsies suggests Möbius' syndrome, which can be a purely myopathic disorder (sometimes being one manifestation of myotubular myopathy) in some cases,

although it is certainly the result of nuclear agenesis in others. Another imitator of abducens palsy is Duane's syndrome, in which impaired abduction of the affected eye is associated with ptosis and enophthalmos during adduction. It is due to fibrosis of the external rectus muscle and may be bilateral. This anomaly is sometimes dominantly inherited.

The *muscles of mastication* may be affected late in the course of many disorders but are often involved early in myasthenia gravis, in which the hand supporting the lower jaw is a useful clue to diagnosis, in tetanus (trismus) and in myotonic dystrophy, in which wasting of the temporal and masseter muscles and a drooping jaw contribute to the typical facial appearance. The rare branchial myopathy can give bilateral masseter hypertrophy. Trismus may also be of emotional origin or can occur transiently in patients receiving phenothiazines.

The *facial muscles* are commonly involved in myopathies and rather uncommonly in motor neurone disease. A brisk jaw jerk will usually distinguish the latter. Bilateral lower motor neurone weakness, for example, in the Guillain–Barré syndrome, sarcoidosis, acute leukaemia in childhood, poliomyelitis and pontine lesions may sometimes be confirmed by loss of taste, but may closely resemble myopathic weakness. A useful distinguishing point is inability to close the eyes in facial nerve lesions; this is less often seen in myopathy except in advanced facioscapulohumeral dystrophy. In young children, gross facial myopathy is usually due to Möbius' syndrome or myotonic dystrophy. In facioscapulohumeral dystrophy the involvement may be severe or slight and is best shown by asking the patient to shut his eyes tightly, or to hold air in his mouth under pressure. In the middle and late stages of Duchenne dystrophy, facial weakness is rarely absent, though usually slight. Failure to retract the corners of the mouth and to blow out the cheeks are the most useful signs.

Dysarthria and dysphagia are both common in myasthenia gravis and polymyositis. In the myotonic and oculopharyngeal muscular dystrophies dysphagia alone is more frequent. Bulbar involvement in poliomyelitis, motor neurone disease and acute polyneuritis is also well known.

The *sternomastoid* muscles are severely wasted and weak in dystrophia myotonica and often in such neurogenic disorders as motor neurone disease, poliomyelitis and craniovertebral anomalies involving the accessory nerve. Of the other myopathies, myasthenia gravis and polymyositis are two in which weakness of neck flexion or extension may be particularly prominent. Selective trapezius weakness may occur in the limb-girdle type of muscular dystrophy and in accessory nerve lesions.

The *tongue* is important in diagnosis because of the ease with which it shows fasciculation, especially in motor neurone disease and other spinal muscular atrophies, as discussed above. Few myopathies affect the tongue. In dystrophia myotonica, lingual dysarthria is more often a sign of myotonia than of weakness. In Duchenne dystrophy the speech is often indistinct and sometimes the tongue is enlarged. Tongue hypertrophy is also a rare manifestation of late-onset glycogen-storage disease due to acid maltase deficiency. A curiously selective form of atrophy of the tongue is rarely seen in myasthenia gravis.

Important non-muscular symptoms and signs

In polymyositis and dermatomyositis these are particularly important and Raynaud's phenomenon, dysphagia, arthralgia and, above all, skin changes may help in diagnosis. The rash in dermatomyositis may involve the face, trunk or limbs, but in difficult cases the eyelids and nail beds should be examined with particular care. In other obscure myopathies uveitis, erythema nodosum, or dyspnoea with pulmonary infiltration may suggest sarcoidosis; anaemia, proteinuria, rashes, arthropathy, pleurisy or splenomegaly, the collagen diseases; tight shiny skin over the face or fingers, systemic sclerosis; and diarrhoea or steatorrhoea, uraemia, bony tenderness or radiological abnormalities in the bones, osteomalacia or hyperparathyroidism. In all these cases the myopathy may be the presenting feature before the more usual symptoms are obvious. Rarely, this also occurs in thyrotoxic myopathy in which, however, thyroid function tests will be abnormal. The same is true of the myopathy of hypothyroidism (Wilson & Walton 1959) but not in Cushing's syndrome, Addison's disease and acromegaly or hypopituitarism, the myopathy usually amounts to no more than an incidental part of the disease. Severe fatiguability with increased skin pigmentation after bilateral adrenalectomy for Cushing's disease should arouse suspicion of very high levels of circulating ACTH (Nelson's syndrome) (Prineas et al 1968). Myoglobinuria is associated not only with 'idiopathic' paroxysmal rhabdomyolysis but sometimes also with severe necrotising myopathy in polymyositis, acute alcoholism and other intoxications, and after exercise in the anterior tibial syndrome, McArdle's disease or carnitine palmitoyl transferase deficiency (see Chs 17 and 18). The inherited myopathies may be associated with other congenital abnormalities; these are especially prominent in the myotonic and ocular dystrophies (see Ch. 14), in nemaline myopathy (a high-arched palate, long face, protruding jaw and dental malocclusion), in a-β-lipoproteinaemia (steatorrhoea, retinal degeneration, ataxia and acanthocytosis), in ataxia telangiectasia (ataxia, conjunctival telangiectasia and recurrent infections); and in Types II and III glycogen-storage disease in which hepatic involvement and (in Type II) cardiac, cerebral and spinal cord involvement occur.

APPENDIX

World Federation of Neurology Research Group on Neuromuscular Diseases: Classification of Neuromuscular Disorders*

The following classification of neuromuscular disorders has been updated from the original document prepared by J. N. Walton and D. Gardner-Medwin in 1968 for the Research Group on Neuromuscular Diseases of the World Federation of Neurology. In 1988, the classification was revised by Walton, with L. P. Rowland and J. G. McLeod (1988 Journal of the Neurological Sciences 86: 333–360), and we added the catalogue numbers for heritable conditions listed by McKusick in 1986. To accommodate the increasing number of identified diseases, McKusick (1992 Mendelian inheritance in man, 10th edn. Johns Hopkins University Press, Baltimore, MD) had to expand the catalogue

---

*Reproduced here from the Journal of Neurological Sciences by permission.

numbering system and we have followed that precedent. We have also included, where possible, the appropriate three-, four- or five-digit (one letter plus two to four numbers) classification for some of the principal conditions included in the Neurological Adaptation of the 10th International Classification of Disease (ICD-10 NA) (WHO 1994). The 1992 McKusick number is given in parentheses whenever possible. If there is no number, the condition has not yet been listed by McKusick (or the authors did not find the condition in the catalogue). In this system, the first number of the six-digit designation indicates the presumed mode of inheritance; numbers beginning with 1 are autosomal dominant; 2, autosomal recessive; 3, X-linked. Some diseases of the mitochondrial genome were previously given autosomal catalogue numbers but are here grouped together in Appendix A.

Another group of diseases that appears in different modes of inheritance is designated Charcot–Marie–Tooth disease or hereditary sensorimotor neuropathy. These disorders are also denoted by clinical syndrome and pattern of inheritance in the classification; they are grouped in Appendix B.

Another major change since 1988 has been the advent of molecular genetics; we have therefore indicated the chromosome map position for many conditions as well as the affected gene product for some. References are given for some conditions that are not considered elsewhere in the volume or to provide a citation that might otherwise seem obscure.

In keeping with tradition, we use the term amyotrophy, not in the literal sense of 'muscular atrophy' but as the equivalent of 'neurogenic atrophy' as opposed to myopathy or primary disease of muscle.

This is a classification of neuromuscular disorders; but we have also included, for the sake of completeness, peripheral nerve diseases that cause solely sensory manifestations. Questionable entities of doubtful nosology are preceded by a question mark, or are otherwise indicated.

There is likely to be difference of opinion about many aspects of this classification, and we have tried to anticipate differences of view, but some arbitrary choices were necessary. Nowhere is this more evident than in the classification of spinal muscular atrophies, which can be divided according to at least three different sets of criteria: pattern of inheritance; distribution of weakness; or age of onset. With the rapid advance of molecular genetics, we have opted for a genetic classification of the spinal muscular atrophies and other motor disorders. However, disorders of neuromuscular transmission are still separated by clinical or physiological features; genetic differences are indicated, where relevant.

CLASSIFICATION OF NEUROMUSCULAR DISEASES

Index:

I. SPINAL MUSCULAR ATROPHIES AND OTHER DISORDERS OF THE MOTOR NEURONES (G12)

A. Heritable

A-1. Autosomal recessive; biochemical abnormality unknown

1. Spinal muscular atrophy (SMA) type 1. Infantile spinal muscular atrophy, proximal (Werdnig–Hoffmann) (253300). Types 1, 2, and 3 all map to 5q12.2–q13.3 (Gilliam et al 1990 Nature 345: 322; Daniels et al 1992 Genomics 12: 335) but some families do not show this linkage (G12.0)

2. Spinal muscular atrophy type 2. Infantile spinal muscular atrophy, arrested; spinal muscular atrophy, intermediate type, chronic infantile form (253550); presumably allelic to type 1 (G12.100)

3. Spinal muscular atrophy type 3. Proximal spinal muscular atrophy, juvenile (Kugelberg–Welander) (253400), presumably allelic to type 1. Clinically similar disorder may also be autosomal dominant (158600) (G12.101)

4. Spinal muscular atrophy type 4, proximal, of adults (271150), may be indistinguishable from dominant (158590, 182970) and X-linked (313200) forms (G12.102)

5. Spinal muscular atrophy, distal (spinal form of Charcot–Marie–Tooth disease), (271120), autosomal recessive (Meadows, Marsden 1969 Neurology 19: 53; 7. Harding, Thomas 1980 Journal of the Neurological Sciences 45: 337); see also autosomal dominant form (I.A.1.17) as well as III.A.1 and Appendix B (G12.111)

6. Spinal muscular atrophy with microcephaly and mental retardation (271110) (Spiro et al 1967 Developmental Medicine and Child Neurology 9: 594)

7. Spinal muscular atrophy with mental retardation (271109) (Staal et al 1975 Journal of Neurology 25: 57)

8. Spinal muscular atrophy, Ryukyuan type (271200) (Kondo et al 1970 Journal of the Neurological Sciences 11: 359) (G12.117)

9. Spinal muscular atrophy, scapuloperoneal (271220) (Emery 1971 Journal of Medical Genetics 8: 481) (G12.112)

10. Spinal muscular atrophy, type 1, with congenital bone fractures (271225) (Borochowitz et al 1991 Journal of Medical Genetics 28: 345)

11. Arthrogryposis multiplex congenita, neurogenic type (208100) (Drachman, Banker 1961 Archives of Neurology 5: 77; Krugliak et al 1978 Journal of the Neurological Sciences 37: 179; Hageman et al 1984 Brain and Development 6: 273) (Q74.3)

12. Arthrogryposis, distal, with mental retardation and characteristic facies. (208081) (Chitayat et al 1990 American Journal of Medical Genetics 37: 65) (Q74.3)

13. Arthrogryposis, lethal, with whistling face and CNS calcifications (208110 and 208155) (Illum et al 1988 Neuropaediatrics 19: 186)

14. Arthrogryposis multiplex congenita with pulmonary hypoplasia (Pena–Shokier syndrome type 1) (208150) fetal akinesia deformation sequence (FADS) (Moerman et al 1983 Journal of Pediatrics 103: 238; Davis et al 1988 American Journal of Medical Genetics 29: 77)

15. Multiple contracture syndrome, Finnish Type (253310); same as Pena–Shokier syndrome type 1, except fatal in neonatal period, with paucity of motor neurones (Herva et al 1985 American Journal of Medical Genetics 20:

431); may be same as arthrogryposis with pulmonary hypoplasia (208150)

16. Arthrogryposis-like disorder (Kuskokwim disease) (208200), a disorder of Eskimo people, classification uncertain

17. Charcot–Marie–Tooth disease, progressive ataxia, and tremor (214380), consistent with 'neuronal form of Charcot–Marie–Tooth disease' or hereditary motor and sensory neuropathy type II (118210), see III.A.I.b (Bouchard et al 1984 Clinical Genetics 25: 163; Harding, Thomas 1980 Brain 103: 255) (G60.01)

18. Charcot–Marie–Tooth disease (CMT4) (214400); probably same as 17

19. Charcot–Marie–Tooth disease and deafness (214370)

20. Bulbar palsy, progressive, of childhood (Fazio–Londe disease) (211500) (Gomez et al 1962 Archives of Neurology 6: 317; Albers et al 1983 Archives of Neurology 40: 351) (G12.110)

21. Bulbar palsy, progressive, with deafness (pontobulbar palsy with deafness; Brown–Vialetto–van Laere syndrome) (211530) (Hawkins et al 1990 Journal of Medical Genetics 27: 176; Abarbanel et al 1991 Canadian Journal of Neurological Sciences 18: 349)

22. Bulbar palsy, with deafness and retinitis pigmentosa (Alberca et al 1980 Archives of Neurology 37: 214)

23. Bulbar palsy with olivopontocerebellar atrophy (Lapresle, Annabi 1979 Journal of Neuropathology 38: 401)

24. Spinal muscular atrophy with amyotrophic lateral sclerosis, spinocerebellar ataxia and deafness (Geminginani et al 1986 Journal of the Neurological Sciences 3: 125)

25. Spinal muscular atrophy with optic atrophy and deafness (Rosenberg, Chutorian 1967 Neurology 17: 827; Iwashita et al 1970 Achives of Neurology 22: 357; Chalmers, Mitchell 1987 Journal of Neurology, Neurosurgery and Psychiatry 50: 238)

26. Spinal muscular atrophy with deafness (Rosenberg et al 1982 European Neurology 21: 84)

27. Spinal muscular atrophy with ophthalmoplegia (Matsunaga et al 1973 Journal of Neurology, Neurosurgery and Psychiatry 36: 104; Dubrovsky et al 1981 Archives of Neurology 38: 594)

28. Spinal muscular atrophy with retinitis pigmentosa (Pearn et al 1978 Brain 101: 591; Furukawa et al 1968 Neurology 28: 942)

29. Spinal muscular atrophy with retinitis pigmentosa and hereditary spastic paraplegia (Kjellin syndrome) (Kjellin 1959 Archives of Neurology 1: 133; Harding 1984 The hereditary ataxias)

30. Troyer syndrome (spastic paraparesis, childhood onset, with distal muscle wasting) (CMT-5) (275900) (Cross, McKusick 1967 Archives of Neurology 16: 473; Neuhauser et al 1976 Clinical Genetics 9: 315); similar to autosomal recessive, the Silver syndrome (182700). In some there is evidence of demyelination; others seem to be of the neuronal type (Gremignani et al 1992 Acta Neuropathologica 83: 196). Some are associated with poikiloderma or other skin conditions (Antinolo et al 1992 Clinical Genetics 41: 281)

31. Spinal muscular atrophy, mental retardation, seizures, and orofacial dysplasia (Landau et al 1976 Neurology 26: 869)

32. Spinal muscular atrophy, restricted forms, e.g. one hand (Sobue et al 1978 Annals of Neurology 3: 429; Harding et al 1983 Journal of the Neurological Sciences 59: 69);

both hands (Serratrice 1984 Revue Neurologique 140: 368); quadriceps (Furukawa et al 1977 Annals of Neurology 2: 328; Serratrice 1985 Journal of Neurology 232: 150). May be dominant (183020). (See also I.G.I. and I.A.3–3) (G12.26)

33. Spinal muscular atrophy with recessive spinocerebellar degeneration of Friedreich's ataxia (229300) (Singh, Shaw 1964 British Journal of Clinical Practice 18: 91; Boudouresques et al 1971 Revue Neurologique 125: 25). Linked to 9q13–21 (Shaw et al 1990 Cytogenetics and Cell Genetics 53: 221)

34. Spinal muscular atrophy with spastic paraplegia, mental retardation and ichthyosis (Sjögren–Larsson syndrome) (270200) (Sjögren, Larsson 1957 Acta Psychiatrica Neurologica Scandinavica 32 suppl: 113; McNamara et al 1975 Archives of Neurology 32: 699). Fatty aldehyde dehydrogenase deficiency (Rizzo et al 1991 Journal of Clinical Investigation 88: 1643). (See also V.A.2.j for congenital myopathy with Sjögren–Larsson syndrome)

35. Neuronal intranuclear hyaline inclusion disease (Sung et al 1980 Journal of Neuropathology 39: 107); single sporadic case, manifest by amyotrophy, dementia, choreoathetosis, seizures, sphincter disorder

36. Spinal muscular atrophy or axonal neuropathy in xeroderma pigmentosum (192060) (Thrush et al 1974 Journal of the Neurological Sciences 22: 91); spinal cord may be normal at autopsy (Roytta, Antinen 1986 Acta Neurologica Scandinavica 73: 191). May be linked to chromosome 13 (Q82.1)

37. Spinal muscular atrophy in infantile neuroaxonal dystrophy (INAD, Seitelberger disease) (256600) (Huttenlocher, Gilles 1967 Neurology 17: 1174; Ule 1972 Acta Neuropathologica 21: 332)

38. Spinal muscular atrophy in Hallevorden–Spatz disease (neuroaxonal dystrophy, late infantile) (234200) (Bots, Staal 1973, Neurology 23: 35) (G23.0)

39. Spinal muscular atrophy in dominant amyotrophic choreo-acanthocytosis (100500); inheritance is sometimes autosomal recessive (200150) or dominant (Serra et al 1986 Acta Neurologica Scandinavica 73: 481), and X-linked choreo-acanthocytosis is seen with the McLeod syndrome (314850) (G25.53)

A-2. Autosomal recessive, biochemical abnormality known (G12.8)

1. Spinal muscular atrophy with hexosaminidase deficiency (272800)

2. Spinal muscular atrophy with lysosomal enzyme deficiencies (Goto et al 1983 Journal of Neurology 229: 45)

3. Spinal muscular atrophy with phenylketonuria (261600) (Meier et al 1975 Developmental Medicine and Child Neurology 17: 265)

4. Spinal muscular atrophy with hydroxyisovaleric aciduria (Eldjarn et al 1970 Lancet ii: 54)

5. Spinal muscular atrophy in amyotrophic lateral sclerosis with ceroid lipofuscinosis (204200, 204300, 256730) (Iseki et al 1987 Acta Neuropathologica 72: 62; Ashwai et al 1984 Annals of Neurology 16: 184). May be linked to chromosome 1p (E75.4)

A-3. Autosomal dominant, biochemical abnormality unknown

1. Muscular atrophy, ataxia, retinitis pigmentosa, and diabetes mellitus (158500) (Furukawa et al 1968 Neurology 18: 942)

2. Muscular atrophy, juvenile spinal (Kugelberg–Welander) (158600) proximal type usually autosomal recessive, but

dominant forms reported by Tsukagoshi et al (1966 Archives of Neurology 14: 378) and Pearn (1978 Journal of the Neurological Sciences 38: 263). Variants include monomelic form which is usually sporadic (also see I.G.1. and I.A.1.30) (Sobue et al 1978 Annals of Neurology 3: 429) and SMA of facioscapulohumeral distribution (Fenichel et al 1967 Archives of Neurology 17: 257; Furukawa, Toyokura 1976 Journal of Medical Genetics 13: 285); problems of classification discussed by Hausmanowa-Petrusewicz et al 1985 Journal of Medical Genetics 22: 350) and Zerres & Grimm 1983 (Human Genetics 65: 74) (G12.101)

3. Spinal muscular atrophy, segmental (183020) is usually sporadic but may be dominant or recessive, sometimes included in I-A-1 30 (G12.26)

4. Muscular atrophy, progressive, malignant (158650), fatal within 1 year, but not clearly different from autosomal dominant amyotrophic lateral sclerosis (158700) (Zatz et al 1971 Journal de Génetique Humaine 19: 337; Manta et al 1983 Journal of Neurology 230: 141)

5. Muscular atrophy, progressive, with amyotrophic lateral sclerosis (158700); also not clearly different from ALS (105400; I.A-3.6) or 'peroneal muscular atrophy with pyramidal features' (Harding, Thomas 1984 Journal of Neurology, Neurosurgery and Psychiatry 47: 168)

6. Amyotrophic dystonic paraplegia (105300) (Gilman, Horenstein 1964 Brain 87: 51)

7. Amyotrophic lateral sclerosis (105400, 158700), includes typical forms (Mulder et al 1986 Neurology 36: 511), as well as those with degeneration of posterior columns and other tracts in spinal cord (Engel, Klatzo 1959 Brain 82: 203), and forms associated with dementia, parkinsonism or tics (Hudson 1981 Brain 104: 217; Spitz et al 1985 Neurology 35: 366). (G12.2) Inheritance of Madras type uncertain, with predilection for bulbar palsy and hearing loss (Arjundas 1977 Neurology, India 25: 1). The major form of autosomal dominant ALS is linked to 21q22.1–q22.2 (Siddique et al 1991 New England Journal of Medicine 324: 1381). It is uncertain whether ALS with dementia (105550) is different (G12.25)

8. Amyotrophic lateral sclerosis–parkinsonism–dementia complex of Guam (105500), probably not heritable (Garruto et al 1985 Neurology 35: 193; Spencer et al 1987 Science 237: 517), but the cycad nut is probably not responsible (Duncan et al 1988 Lancet 2 631) (G12.240)

9. Spinal muscular atrophy with olivopontocerebellar atrophy type IV (OPCA IV; Schutt–Haymaker type OPCA) (164600) (Landis et al 1974 Archives of Neurology 31: 295) (G11.22)

10. Amyotrophic lateral sclerosis with dementia (105550) said to differ from other forms by Pinsky et al (1975 Clinical Genetics 7: 186)

11. Spinal muscular atrophy, distal, with vocal cord paralysis (158580) (Young, Harper 1980 Journal of Neurology, Neurosurgery and Psychiatry 43: 413; Serratrice et al 1984 Revue Neurologique 140: 657)

12. Spinal muscular atrophy with bulbar palsy (Dobkin, Verity 1976 Neurology 26: 754)

13. Arthrogryposis multiplex congenita, distal, type 1 (108120); uncertain whether this is neurogenic or myopathic (Hall et al 1982 American Journal of Medical Genetics 11: 185; McCormack et al 1980 American Journal of Medical Genetics 6: 163; Fleury, Hageman 1985 Journal of Neurology, Neurosurgery and Psychiatry

48: 1037). Type 2 (108130) has additional congenital anomalies (Hall et al 1986 American Journal of Medical Genetics 24: 255), including craniofacial abnormalities (108140) (Q74.3)

14. Arthrogryposis with oculomotor limitation and electroretinal abnormalities (oculomelic amyoplasia) (108145) (Lai et al 1991 Journal of Medical Genetics 28: 701)

15. Charcot–Marie–Tooth disease, neuronal type (CMT2) (118210), not allelic to CMT1 forms on chromosome 1 or 17 (Hentani et al 1992 Genomics 12: 155). May be related to muscular atrophy, distal type. (CMT syndromes are discussed in III.A.1 and are listed in Appendix B) (G60.01)

16. Scapuloperoneal atrophy with cardiopathy (probably Emery–Dreifuss muscular dystrophy, autosomal dominant type) (181350; also 158700); neurogenic status uncertain (Chakrabati et al 1981 Journal of Neurology, Neurosurgery and Psychiatry 44: 1146; Miller et al 1985 Neurology 35: 1230; Orstavik et al 1990 Clinical Genetics 38: 447) (G71.01)

17. Scapuloperoneal amyotrophy (Kaeser's syndrome) scapuloperoneal syndrome, neurogenic type) (181400) (G12.112)

18. Spastic paraplegia with amyotrophy of hands (Silver's disease) (182700) described by Silver (1966 Annals of Human Genetics 30: 69) and by Van Gent et al (1985 Journal of Neurology, Neurosurgery and Psychiatry 48: 266). May be related to amyotrophic dystonic paraplegia (105300). Similar to autosomal recessive Troyer syndrome (I.A.1, 30)

19. Spinal muscular atrophy, distal (182960); autosomal dominant form similar to recessive form (271120) (Harding, Thomas 1980 Journal of the Neurological Sciences 45: 337); may also be sporadic and confined to the hands (O'Sullivan, McLeod 1978 Journal of Neurology, Neurosurgery and Psychiatry 41: 653) (G12.111)

20. Spinal muscular atrophy, facioscapulohumeral type (182970) (Fenichel et al 1967 Archives of Neurology 17: 257). Linkage is uncertain (Siddique et al 1989 Journal of Medical Genetics 26: 847) (G12.113)

21. Spinal muscular atrophy, proximal, adult type (Finkel late-onset type SMA included) (182980) (Richieri-Costa et al 1981 American Journal of Human Genetics 9: 119). Clinically not different from recessive and X-linked forms

22. Spinocerebellar ataxia with rigidity and peripheral neuropathy (183050) described by Ziegler et al (1972 Archives of Neurology 27: 52), includes fasciculations and parkinsonism as well as signs of peripheral neuropathy (G12.102)

23. Spinal muscular atrophy with myoclonus (Jankovic, Rivera 1979 Annals of Neurology 6: 227)

24. Spinal muscular atrophy with Joseph's disease (109150) (Also, Azorean neurological disease, Machado–Joseph disease, spinopontine atrophy, nigrospinodentatal degeneration) (Rosenberg, Fowler 1981 Neurology 31: 1124; Eto et al 1990 Neurology 40: 968) (G12.80)

25. Scapuloperoneal atrophy with cardiopathy and inflammatory myopathy (Jennekens et al 1975 Brain 98: 709); neurogenic status not certain (G12.112)

26. Amyotrophic lateral sclerosis with Pick's disease of brain (dementia with lobar atrophy and neuronal cytoplasmic inclusions) (172700) (De Morsier 1967 Revue Neurologique 116: 373)

27. Amyotrophic lateral sclerosis with autosomal dominant familial parkinsonism (168600) (Brait et al 1973 Neurology 23: 990)
28. Spinal muscular atrophy with Huntington disease (143100) (Fotopoulos 1966 Psychiatrie, Neurologie und Medizinische Med Psychologie (Leipzig) 18: 129; Serratrice et al 1984 Nouvelle Presse 13: 1274) (G10)
29. Amyotrophic lateral sclerosis with luyso-pallidal-nigral atrophy (Gray et al 1985 Acta Neuropathologica 66: 78) (G12.80)
30. Spinal muscular atrophy with pallidonigral degeneration (Serratrice et al 1983 Neurology 33: 306) (G12.80)
31. Spinal muscular atrophy, infantile, with multiple congenital bone fracture (Borochowitz et al 1991 Medical Genetics 28: 345)

A-4. X-linked recessive, biochemical disorder unknown
1. Spinal and bulbar muscular atrophy (Kennedy's disease); bulbospinal muscular atrophy; X-linked muscular atrophy, benign, with hypertrophy of calves (313200). Kennedy disease localized to Xq13.21 within the gene for the androgen receptor (LaSpada et al 1991 Nature 352: 77); androgen receptor-binding may be abnormal (Warner et al 1992 Neurology 42: 2181). Juvenile form with calf enlargement may be different condition (Bouwsma, van Wijngaarden 1980 Journal of the Neurological Sciences 44: 275; Sakashita et al 1992 Journal of the Neurological Sciences 113: 118) (G12.118)
2. Spinal muscular atrophy, juvenile, proximal, similar to Kugelberg–Welander syndrome but X-linked (Tsukagoshi et al 1970 Neurology 20: 1188) possibly same as Kennedy's syndrome
3. Scapuloperoneal muscular atrophy with cardiopathy, X-linked (Mawatari et al 1973 Archives of Neurology 28: 55); probably Emery–Dreifuss muscular dystrophy (Rowland et al 1979 Annals of Neurology 5: 111) (G71.01)
4. Charcot–Marie–Tooth peroneal muscular atrophy and Friedreich's ataxia, combined (302900); uncertain whether anterior horn cell disease or peripheral neuropathy, based on single report (van Bogaert 1939–41 Encéphale 34: 312)
5. Spinal muscular atrophy, X-linked, facioscapulohumeral distribution (Skre et al 1978 Acta Neurologica Scandinavica 58: 249) (G12.113)
6. Arthrogryposis multiplex congenita with renal and hepatic abnormality (301820); includes rarefaction of anterior horns, reported in only two families (Nezelof et al 1979 Journal of Pediatrics 94: 258; DiRocco et al 1990 American Journal of Medical Genetics 37: 237) (Q74.3)
7. Arthrogryposis multiplex congenita, distal (301830), X-linked; includes one type with anterior horn cell disease; others attributed to non-progressive intrauterine myopathy or connective tissue disease (Hall 1982 Clinical Genetics 21: 81; Hennekam et al 1991 European Journal of Paediatrics 150: 656) (Q74.3)

A-5. X-linked dominant, lethal in males
1. Infantile spinal muscular atrophy in incontinentia pigmenti (Bloch–Sulzberger syndrome) (308300) (Larsen et al 1987 Neurology 37: 446)

B. Congenital and developmental abnormalities
1. Mobius syndrome (agenesis of cranial nerve nuclei) (157900). May appear in autosomal dominant or X-linked patterns but recurrence low when signs restricted to facial paralysis and ophthalmoplegia, especially with limb anomalies (MacDermott et al 1991 Journal of Medical Genetics 28: 18). May occur with peripheral neuropathy and hypogonadism (Abid et al 1978 Journal of the Neurological Sciences 35: 309); or with absence of pectoral muscle (Q81.05)
2. Congenital absence of muscles (e.g. pectorals, abdominals), might better be classed with disorders of muscle, but it is not known whether total motor units (including anterior horn cells) are absent
3. Amyotrophy with developmental anomalies of the spinal cord or nerve roots: hydromyelia, syringomyelia, or syringobulbia (often with Chiari malformation); spinal dysraphism; meningomyelocele; aplasia of spinal cord (amyelia)
4. Spinal muscular atrophy with pontocerebellar hypoplasia (Goutieres et al 1977 Journal of Neurology, Neurosurgery and Psychiatry 40: 370)
5. Arthrogryposis multiplex congenita of non-neural, non-myopathic origin, sporadic, presumably not heritable and presumably intrauterine or developmental disorder of joints, accounts for most cases (Q74.3)

C. Disorders of motor neurones attributed to physical causes
1. Trauma: direct injury of spinal cord (birth injury; spinal fracture); traumatic haematomyelia (S14, S24, S34)
2. Amyotrophy due to destruction or compression or compressive ischaemia of anterior horn cells: intramedullary or extramedullary spinal cord tumours; infectious mass lesions (tuberculoma, gumma, parasitic cysts); spontaneous hydromyelia
3. Amyotrophy due to ischaemia of anterior horns:
   (a) clamping aorta for abdominal vascular surgery
   (b) occlusion or stenosis of anterior spinal artery
   (c) progressive vascular myelopathy (Jellinger, Neumayer 1962 Acta Neurologica Psychiatrica Belgica 62: 944)
4. Amyotrophy after electrical injury, mechanism uncertain (Farrell, Starr 1968 Neurology 18: 60; Holbrook et al 1970 British Medical Journal 4: 659)
5. Amyotrophy after radiotherapy (Lagueny et al 1985 Revue Neurologique 141: 222; Bradley et al 1991 Advances in Neurology 56: 341)

D. Disorders of motor neurones attributed to toxins, chemicals or heavy metal (G62.0)
1. Tetanus toxin (A35)
2. Strychnine
3. Botulinum toxin (adult and infantile forms) (Clay et al 1977 Archives of Neurology 34: 226; Arnon 1980 Annual Review of Medicine 31: 541) (G70.1)
4. Lead (Campbell et al 1970 Journal of Neurology, Neurosurgery and Psychiatry 33: 877; Boothby et al 1974 Archives of Neurology 31: 18)
5. Mercury (Kantarjian 1961 Neurology 11: 639)
6. Organophosphates (TOCP, ginger jake paralysis)
7. Saxitoxin and related marine toxins (G70.1)
8. Dapsone motor neuropathy (not clear whether this is an axonal peripheral neuropathy or motor neurone disorder) (Homeida et al 1980 British Medical Journal 281: 1180)
9. Phenytoin motor neuropathy (Direkze, Fernando 1977 European Neurology 15: 131)

E. Disorders of motor neurones attributed to viral infection

E-1. Acute disorders
1. Paralytic acute anterior poliomyelitis:

(*a*) due to poliomyelitis virus
(*b*) due to other enteroviruses (such as Coxsackie virus) (A80)
2. Amyotrophy in Russian spring-summer encephalitis (A83)
3. Herpes zoster (Thomas, Howard 1972 Neurology 22: 459) (B02)
4. Amyotrophy with acute haemorrhagic conjunctivitis (1972 Lancet 2 970; Kono et al 1974 Journal of Infectious Diseases 129: 590)
5. Amyotrophy with asthma (Beede et al 1980 Johns Hopkins Medical Journal 147: 186), probably same as acute quadriplegic myopathy (Hirano et al 1992 Neurology 42: 2082)
6. Amyotrophy in acute transverse myelitis, cause undetermined

E-2. Subacute or chronic disorders
1. Amyotrophy in Creutzfeldt–Jakob disease (Allen et al 1971 Brain 94: 715) (A81.0, G12.80)
2. Amyotrophy or amyotrophic lateral sclerosis due to human immunodeficiency virus (Hoffman et al 1985 New England Journal of Medicine 313: 324; Horoupian et al 1984 Annals of Neurology 15: 502) (B22)
3. Amyotrophy in HTLV-I infection (A88.8)
4. Persistent infection by poliovirus in agammaglobulinaemia
5. Late post-poliomyelitis muscular atrophy (post-polio syndrome) (Dalakas et al 1984 Reviews of Infections Diseases 6 (suppl 2): S562; Cashman et al 1987 New England Journal of Medicine 317: 7) (B91.0)

F. Disorders of motor neurone with immunological abnormality
1. Motor neurone diseases with monoclonal paraproteinaemia (including Waldenström macroglobulinaemia, multiple myeloma, chronic lymphatic leukaemia) (Shy et al 1986 Neurology 36: 1429) (D89.0)
2. Amyotrophy with Hodgkin's disease (Rowland, Schneck 1963 Journal of Chronic Diseases 16: 777; Walton 1968 Journal of the Neurological Sciences 6: 435; Younger et al 1991 Annals of Neurology 29: 78) (C81)
3. Carcinomatous motor neurone disease (Brain et al 1965 Brain 88: 479); not currently regarded as specific syndrome, but amyotrophy may be seen in paraneoplastic encephalomyelopathy, or may improve after removal of tumour (Evans et al 1990 Neurology 40: 960)

G. Disorders of motor neurone of undetermined aetiology
1. Motor neurone diseases of adults (sporadic): amyotrophic lateral sclerosis, progressive spinal muscular atrophy, progressive bulbar palsy, or mixed forms. Includes sporadic cases with atypical features; e.g. ophthalmoplegia (Harvey et al 1979 Archives of Neurology 36: 615); nystagmus (Kushner et al 1984 Annals of Neurology 16: 71); sporadic multisystem disorders with amyotrophy, cerebellar disorder and ophthalmoplegia (Hayashi et al 1986 Acta Neuropathologica 70: 82); monomelic and other restricted forms (Serratrice 1983 Cardiomyology 2: 255; Hirayama et al 1987 Journal of Neurology, Neurosurgery and Psychiatry 50: 285); or dementia (Caselli et al 1993 Annals of Neurology 33: 200) (G12.2)
2. Juvenile motor neurone disease (sporadic): spinal muscular atrophy or amyotrophic lateral sclerosis (Ben Hamida et al 1990 Brain 113: 347)
3. Amyotrophy in Shy–Drager syndrome (progressive multisystem degeneration, progressive autonomic failure of central origin) with orthostatic hypotension, sphincter disorders, parkinsonism or cerebellar disorder (G12.80)

4. Amyotrophy in sporadic Pick's disease (Minauf, Jellinger 1969 Archiv fur Psychiatre und Nervenkrankheiten 212: 279)
5. Chronic neurogenic atrophy of the quadriceps (sporadic) (Furukawa et al 1977 Annals of Neurology 2: 528; Serratrice et al 1985 Journal of Neurology 232: 150)
6. Amyotrophy in polyglucosan body disease (263620) (Cafferty et al 1991 Muscle and Nerve 14: 102), sometimes with deficiency of branching enzyme. See also III.A.3.m

H. Disorders of motor neurone in metabolic disorders
1. Tetany (hypocalcaemia; hypomagnesaemia; alkalosis)
2. Amyotrophy in hypoglycaemic hyperinsulinism (Harrison 1976 Journal of Neurology, Neurosurgery and Psychiatry 39: 465) (E16.1)
3. Amyotrophy, fasciculation and upper motor neurone signs (syndrome resembling amyotrophic lateral sclerosis) in hyperthyroidism (Mottier et al 1981 Presse Méd 10: 1655; Fisher et al 1985 American Journal of Medicine 78: 1041)
4. Amyotrophy in hyperparathyroidism (Patten, Pages 1984 (E05)Annals of Neurology 15: 453) (E21)

I. Disorders of motor neurone manifest by hyperactivity
(Note: There is debate about the pathogenesis of several syndromes of hyperactivity; many believe that only peripheral nerves are involved but others implicate the perikaryon, alone or in addition to peripheral nerve disorder; discussed in Revue Neurologique (1985; 4: 261). Some may be forms of dystonia or may originate in upper motor neurones)
1. Ordinary muscle cramps
2. Benign fasciculation-cramp syndrome (syndrome of Foley and Denny-Brown) (G64.1)
3. Occupational cramps and writers' cramp (focal action-induced dystonia) (G24.85)
4. Isaacs' syndrome (neuromyotonia; Isaacs–Mertens syndrome) manifest by myokymia, impaired muscle relaxation (pseudomyotonia) and abnormal postures of the limbs (resembling carpal and pedal spasm). Most cases are sporadic but some are heritable (McGuire et al 1984 Archives of Neurology 41: 195) (121020); a few cases are paraneoplastic (Walsh 1976 Journal of Neurology, Neurosurgery and Psychiatry 39: 1976) and may be seen with thymoma (Sintra et al 1991 Lancet 338: 75; Detre et al 1991 Annals of Neurology (29: 218). The syndrome has also been linked to gold therapy for rheumatoid arthritis, or to radiotherapy (see I.1.10) (G64.0)
5. Tetanus (A35)
6. Strychnine intoxication
7. Stiff man syndrome (Moersch–Woltman syndrome), often associated with insulin-dependent diabetes mellitus and with antibodies to glutamate decarboxylase. If corticospinal signs are present should be regarded as a cervical myelopathy or encephalomyelopathy (see no. 9 below) (G25.8)
8. Satoyoshi syndrome (Satoyoshi and Yamada 1967 Archives of Neurology 16: 254)
9. Myelopathy with rigidity, spasm, or continuous motor unit activity (Howell et al 1979 Journal of Neurology, Neurosurgery and Psychiatry 42: 773; Whiteley et al 1976 Brain 99: 220). Should be distinguished from Moersch–Woltman syndrome
10. Myokymia–hyperhidrosis–impaired muscle relaxation (Gamstorp, Wohlfart 1959 Acta Psychiatrica

Scandinavica 34: 181); probably the same as the Isaacs' syndrome, but myokymia may be seen as an isolated phenomenon after gold-salt therapy for rheumatoid arthritis or with thymoma (Garciamerino et al 1991 Annals of Neurology 29: 215) (G64.3)

11. Black widow spider bite
12. Tetany
13. Spinal myoclonus
14. Facial myokymia (G64.4)
15. Hemifacial spasm (see also III C-1 3 a) (G51.3)
16. ? 'Painful legs and moving toes' (Spillane et al 1971 Brain 94: 54)
17. ? Ekbom's syndrome ('restless legs') (Harriman et al 1970 Brain 93: 393)

II. DISORDERS OF MOTOR NERVE ROOTS

A. Congenital (Q05)
1. Associated with meningomyelocele and other anomalies
2. Arthrogryposis multiplex congenita (radicular type) (Pena et al 1968 Neurology 18: 926) (Q75.3)

B. Acquired disorders

B-1. Physical
1. Laceration, contusion, distraction or avulsion of roots (G55)
2. Compression of roots by:
   (a) vertebral osteoarthritis (spondylosis) (G55.2)
   (b) prolapsed intervertebral disc (G55.1)
   (c) Paget's disease (G55.8)
   (d) tumour in the spinal canal or intervertebral foramina
   (e) vertebral collapse

B-2. Ischaemia

B-3. Radiation

B-4. Toxic agents (injected local anaesthetics, phenol, etc.)

B-5. Infective
1. Radiculopathy in meningitis
2. Syphilis (A52.1)
3. Granulomatous arachnoiditis of other causes (including spinal tuberculosis and sarcoidosis)
4. Bilharziasis (B65)

B-6. Post-infective, allergic or immunologically mediated
1. Acute inflammatory (post-infective) polyradiculoneuropathy (Guillain–Barré syndrome). (See also E) (G61.0)
2. Polyradiculoneuropathy after inoculation
3. Serum neuropathy (G61.1)
4. Neuralgic amyotrophy (brachial plexus neuropathy), attributed to plexus rather than nerve roots (Arts et al 1983 Journal of the Neurological Sciences 62: 261) (G54.5)
5. Radiculopathy of Lyme disease (Borreliosis). (See also D1-2) (A69.2)
6. Radiculopathy in AIDS (Cornblath et al 1987 Annals of Neurology 21: 32). (See also D1.1 and D1.2) (B23.8)

B-7 Neoplastic
1. Neurofibroma (M954)
2. Meningioma (M953)
3. Metastases
4. Reticulosis (M967)

B-8. Vascular malformations

III. DISORDERS OF PERIPHERAL NERVE

A. Heritable
1. Hereditary motor and sensory neuropathy (see also Appendix B). The hereditary motor and sensory neuropathies (HMSN) have been classified by Dyck into several different types (see Dyck et al (ed) 1993 Peripheral neuropathy, 3rd edn. Saunders, Philadelphia, pp 1094–1136). Types I and II are commonly known as peroneal muscular atrophy or Charcot–Marie–Tooth disease (Harding, Thomas 1980 Brain 103: 255). Type I (slow nerve conduction form) is usually autosomal dominant (118200); some linked to Duffy blood group at 1q21.1–q23.3 (CMT1B); most are linked to 17p12–p11.2 (CMT1A) (118220). Similar disorders may be autosomal recessive or X-linked dominant (302800). Sometimes associated with deafness (118300 or 214370), ataxia and tremor (214380), Friedreich's ataxia (302900), or ptosis and parkinsonism (118301). A neuronal type has been reported in Guadalajara (118230) (G60.0)
   (a) HMSN I (hypertrophic type); Roussy–Levy syndrome (180800) is a variant, identical to CMT1 except for prominent tremor (G60.00)
   (b) HMSN II neuronal type may be autosomal dominant (118210) or recessive (271120). HMSN II with onset in early childhood (Durries et al 1981 Journal of the Neurological Sciences 51: 181) (G60.01)
   (c) HMSN III (Dejerine–Sottas hypertrophic neuropathy) (145900). May show autosomal recessive inheritance (Ouvrier et al 1987 Brain 110: 121). Cases of congenital hypomyelination neuropathy (Guzetta et al 1982 Brain 105: 395; Kennedy et al 1977 Archives of Neurology 34: 337) are probably variants (G60.02)
   (d) HMSN IV (Refsum's syndrome) (also see III A.3)
   (e) HMSN V (with ataxic paraparesis)
   (f) HMSN VI (with optic atrophy)
   (g) HMSN VII (with retinitis pigmentosa)
   (h) HMSN, X-linked (CMTX) (302801, 302802), apparently X-linked dominant, localised to Xq13 (Hahn et al 1990 Brain 113: 1511); an X-linked recessive form linked to Xp22 and Xq26 (Ionasescu et al 1991 American Journal of Human Genetics 48: 1075; Ionasescu et al 1992 Muscle and Nerve 15: 368). In the Cowchock variety (310490), deafness is an associated feature
   (i) familial Charcot–Marie–Tooth neuropathy with familial trigeminal neuropathy (Coffey et al 1991 Surgical Neurology 49)
   (j) familial multiple symmetric lipomatosis with peripheral neuropathy (Chalk et al 1990 Neurology 27: 1246)
   (k) hereditary motor and sensory neuropathy with calf muscle enlargement (Sakashita et al 1992 Journal of the Neurological Sciences 113: 118)
   (l) hereditary motor and sensory neuropathy with deafness and mental retardation (Mancardi et al 1992 Journal of the Neurological Sciences 110: 121)
2. Hereditary sensory and autonomic neuropathies (HSAN) (G60.8)
   (a) Autosomal dominant hereditary sensory and autonomic neuropathy (HSAN-1) (162400) (Denny-Brown 1951 Journal of Neurology, Neurosurgery and Psychiatry 14: 237; Danon, Carpenter 1985 Neurology 35: 1226). May be associated with ulcerating acropathy because of sensory loss. Rarely,

associated with upper motor neurone signs (162380) (G60.80)

(b) Hereditary sensory and autonomic neuropathy (HSAN-2) (201300), autosomal recessive, with osteolysis (G60.81)

(c) Riley–Day syndrome (familial dysautonomia); hereditary sensory and autonomic neuropathy III (HSAN-3) (223900) (Aguayo et al 1971 Archives of Neurology 24: 105) (G60.82)

(d) neuropathy, congenital sensory, with anhidrosis (familial dysautonomia, type II; congenital insensitivity to pain with anhidrosis of Swanson, hereditary sensory and autonomic neuropathy IV) (HSAN-4) (256800) (Swanson 1963 Archives of Neurology 8: 299) (G60.83)

(e) autosomal recessive sensory neuropathy (256860) (Ohta et al 1973 Archives of Neurology 29: 23)

(f) X-linked recessive sensory neuropathy (256750) (Jestico et al 1985 Journal of Neurology, Neurosurgery and Psychiatry 48: 1259)

(g) congenital sensory neuropathy with selective loss of small myelinated fibres (201300) (HSAN type V) (Low et al 1978 Annals of Neurology 3: 179; Donaghy et al 1987 Brain 110: 563), accounts for some cases of congenital indifference to pain (G60.84)

(h) hereditary dysautonomia with motor neuropathy (252320) (Lisker et al 1981 American Journal of Medical Genetics 9: 255)

(i) congenital indifference to pain (147430; 243000), may be autosomal recessive or dominant

3. Hereditary neuropathies associated with specific biochemical abnormalities.

(a) familial amyloidotic polyneuropathy, autosomal dominant; multiple forms (176300) are attributed to allelic mutations in the gene for transthyretin (formerly 'pre-albumin') which maps to 18 cen-q12.3. Type I, the Portuguese type (176300.0001) was the first described (Andrade 1952 Brain (75: 408). There are now 17 variants of the same gene, some resulting in different clinical syndromes (Saraiva 1991 Neuromuscular Disorders 1: 3) (E85.1, G63.3)

(b) porphyria, autosomal dominant. Usually acute intermittent porphyria (176000) or porphobilinogen deaminase deficiency, which maps to 11q24.1–q24.2. There are now 12 different allelic mutations of the gene, with some clinical variation but including acute polyneuropathy. The Chester type (176010) seems to map to a different locus on chromosome 11. Porphyria variegata, the South African type (176200), also includes polyneuropathy but differs clinically because rash is also common and the affected enzyme differs (protoporphyrinogen oxidase). Hereditary coproporphyria (121300) may include attacks of abdominal pain but polyneuropathy is not characteristic (E80, G63.3)

(c) a-alpha-lipoproteinaemia (Tangier disease) (205400), autosomal recessive (Pollock et al 1983 Brain 106: 911) (E78.60, G63.3)

(d) a-beta-lipoproteinaemia (200100) (Bassen–Kornzweig syndrome), autosomal recessive. Neuropathy probably due to vitamin E deficiency caused by malabsorption (E78.62, G63.3)

(e) metachromatic leukodystrophy (sulphatide lipidosis) (arylsulphatase deficiency) (250100) is autosomal

recessive, mapping distal to 22q13. There are at least nine allelic mutants, including late infantile, juvenile, adult onset, and other variants (E75.23, G63.3)

(f) globoid cell leukodystrophy (Krabbe's disease) (245200), autosomal recessive deficiency of beta-galactosidase, which maps to 14q21–q31. The infantile form is most common but there are late-onset forms (E75.21, G63.3)

(g) Niemann–Pick disease (257200); sphingomyelin lipidosis, autosomal recessive deficiency of sphingomyelinase, maps to 11p15.4–15.1 (Da Veiga Pereira et al 1991 Genomics 9: 229; Landnea, Said 1984 Acta Neuropathologica 63: 66) (E75.26, G63.3)

(h) adrenoleukodystrophy (300100), includes adrenomyeloneuropathy, may combine features of both spastic paraplegia and sensorimotor polyneuropathy (Griffin et al 1977 Neurology 12: 1107; O'Neill et al 1984 Neurology 34: 798). The X-linked recessive defect affects the perioxosomal oxidation of very long chain fatty acids. The deficient enzyme is peroxisomal lignoceroyl-CoA ligase, which maps to Xq28 (Feil et al 1991 American Journal of Human Genetics 49: 1361) (E71.33, G63.3)

(i) Fabry's disease (alpha-galactoside A deficiency; glycosphingolipid lipidosis) (301500) (Bischoff et al 1968 Kliniscke Wochenschrift 46: 666), X-linked recessive. The six known mutations at Xq22-qter include early- and late-onset forms (E75.22, G63.3)

(j) Refsum's syndrome (phytanic acid storage disease, phytanic acid oxidase deficiency) (266500). Symptoms usually appear in adolescence or later, but there is also an infantile form (266510). (HMSN type IV) (G60.1)

(k) glycogen storage diseases with peripheral neuropathy or motor neurone disorder (E74.0, G63.3):

(i) Type II (Pompe's disease) (232300) alpha-1,4-glucosidase deficiency (17q21.2-q23); see also myopathies (Smith et al 1967 Neurology 17: 537) (E74.01)

(ii) Type III (Forbes–Cori disease) debrancher deficiency (232400) (Ugawa et al 1986 Annals of Neurology 19: 294); see also myopathies (E74.02)

(l) primary hyperoxaluria (259900) (Hall et al 1976 Journal of the Neurological Sciences 29: 343) (E74.81)

(m) sensorimotor neuropathy in polyglucosan body disease (263620) (Cafferty et al 1991 Muscle and Nerve 14: 102); brancher enzyme activity is diminished in some patients (Lossos et al 1991 Annals of Neurology 30: 655; Bruno et al 1993 Annals of Neurology 33: 88) (E74.03)

4. Miscellaneous hereditary neuropathies

(a) hereditary liability to pressure palsies. Includes 'tomaculous neuropathies' (162500) (Madrid, Bradley 1975 Journal of the Neurological Sciences 25: 415; Gabreels-Festen et al 1992 Neuropaediatrics 23: 138; autosomal dominant. May be same as 'neuritis with brachial predilection' (162100) or 'hereditary neuralgic amyotrophy' (Thomas, Ormerod 1993 Journal of Neurology, Neurosurgery and Psychiatry 56: 107) Maps to 17p11.2p12 (allelic to CMT-1A) (G60.87)

(b) giant axonal neuropathy (256850), autosomal recessive (Tandon et al 1987 Journal of the Neurological Sciences 87: 205) (G60.85)

(c) ataxia-telangiectasia (208900) (Dunn 1973

Developmental Medicine and Child Neurology 15: 324) maps to 11q22–q23 (G11.30)

(*d*) Cockayne's syndrome (216400) (Moosa, Dubowitz 1970 Archives of Disease in Childhood 45: 474; Smits et al 1982 Neuropediatrics 13: 161) (G87.1)

(*e*) mitochondrial myopathies (251900) (Yiannikas, McLeod 1986 Annals of Neurology 20: 249), may include sensorimotor neuropathy. Mitochondrial encephalomyopathy with lactic acidosis and stroke (MELAS) (251910) and myoclonus epilepsy with ragged red fibres (MERRF) (254775) are listed with autosomal recessive diseases but inheritance is maternal; in both, point mutations have been found in mtDNA. 'Mitochondrial myopathy with lactic acidosis' (251950) is probably an incomplete form of MELAS. Some mitochondrial myopathies are difficult to classify (251945; 252010; 252011) (G71.3). The Kearns–Sayre syndrome is listed with autosomal dominant diseases (165100, 110900) but the responsible molecular lesion is a deletion of mtDNA and familial incidence is exceptional (H49.80)

(*f*) neurofibromatosis (162200) (von Recklinghausen's disease), autosomal dominant, has been mapped to 17q11.2 and at least four allelic mutations have been recognised. In addition to the characteristic neurofibromas, peripheral neuropathy may be seen (Thomas et al 1990 Muscle and Nerve 13: 93) (M9540/1)

(*g*) hereditary hypertrophic neuropathy with paraproteinaemia (162600) (Gibberd, Gavrilescu 1966 Neurology 16: 130)

(*h*) hereditary polyneuropathy with oligophrenia, premature menopause and acromicria (Lundberg 1971 European Neurology 5: 84)

(*i*) neuropathy in the neuroectodermal syndrome with dominant inheritance (Flynn, Aird 1965 Journal of the Neurological Sciences 2: 161)

(*j*) subacute necrotizing encephalomyelopathy (Leigh's disease) (308930) (Goebel et al 1986 Muscle and Nerve 20: 70) (G31.81)

(*k*) peripheral neuropathy associated with xeroderma pigmentosum (278700) (Mimaki et al 1986 Annals of Neurology 20: 70). XP maps to 9q (Q82.1)

(*l*) Marinesco–Sjögren syndrome (248800) may include myopathy or evidence of denervation (Serratrice et al 1973 Revue de Neurologique 128: 432) (G11.16)

(*m*) hereditary parkinsonism and neuropathy (Byrne et al 1982 Journal of Neurology, Neurosurgery and Psychiatry 45: 372)

(*n*) neuropathy in spinocerebellar and cerebellar degenerations

   (*i*) Friedreich's ataxia (Dyck, Lambert 1968 Archives of Neurology 18: 619; McLeod 1971 Journal of the Neurological Sciences 12: 333)

   (*ii*) Other spinocerebellar degenerations (McLeod, Evans 1981 Muscle and Nerve 4: 51)

(o) neuropathy in McLeod's syndrome (Witt et al 1992 Journal of Neurology 239: 302)

(p) neuropathy with multiple symmetric lipomatosis (Chalk et al 1990 Neurology 40: 1246)

B. Congenital

1. Congenital neuropathy with arthrogryposis multiplex congenita (Hooshmand et al 1971 Archives of Neurology 24: 561) (Q07.9)

2. Congenital neuropathy with absence of myelin in the peripheral (Palix, Coignet 1978 Pediatrie 33: 201) and central nervous systems (Schroder, Bohl 1978 In: Canal (ed) Peripheral neuropathies. Elsevier, Amsterdam, pp 49–62)

3. Disorder of axonal development, necrotizing myopathy, cardiomyopathy and cataracts (Lyon et al 1990 Annals of Neurology 27: 193)

C. Traumatic neuropathies

C-1. Physical

1. Laceration, contusion, compression, or distraction of nerves or plexuses

2. Birth trauma to brachial plexus (G54.0):
   (*a*) Erb's paralysis (P14.0)
   (*b*) Klumpke's paralysis (P14.1)

3. Compression neuropathies:
   (*a*) Of cranial nerves:
      (*i*) facial nerve compression in the facial canal (Bell's palsy) (G51.0)
      (*ii*) clonic facial spasm (hemifacial spasm) (G51.3)
      (*iii*) recurrent familial facial palsy (Melkersson syndrome) (G51.2)
   (*b*) Of the upper extremity:
      (*i*) cervical rib or cervical band syndrome (G54.01)
      (*ii*) median nerve in the forearm (pronator syndrome) (G56.12)
      (*iii*) median nerve under the supracondylar process or Struther ligament (G56.11)
      (*iv*) median nerve in the forearm (anterior interosseous syndrome) (G56.13)
      (*v*) median nerve at the wrist (carpal tunnel syndrome) (G56.0)
      (*vi*) ulnar nerve at the elbow (cubital tunnel syndrome) (G56.22)
      (*vii*) ulnar nerve at the elbow (the medial epicondyle) (G56.21)
      (*viii*) ulnar nerve at the wrist or its deep branch in the palm (G56.23, G56.24)
      (*ix*) radial nerve in the spiral groove (G56.31)
      (*x*) radial nerve in the forearm (G56.38)
      (*xi*) posterior interosseous nerve in the forearm (G56.32)
      (*xii*) suprascapular nerve at the shoulder (G58.84)
      (*xiii*) long thoracic nerve at the shoulder (G58.86)
      (*xiv*) axilliary nerve at the shoulder (G58.85)
      (*xv*) musculocutaneous nerve in the upper arm (G56.80)
   (*c*) Of the lower extremity:
      (*i*) sciatic nerve at the pelvic exit (G57.0)
      (*ii*) obturator nerve in the obturator canal (G57.82)
      (*iii*) ilioinguinal nerve at the groin (G57.81)
      (*iv*) genitofemoral nerve (G57.80)
      (*v*) femoral nerve in upper thigh (G57.21)
      (*vi*) lateral cutaneous nerve of the thigh (meralgia paraesthetica) (G57.1)
      (*vii*) common peroneal nerve (G57.3)
      (*viii*) deep peroneal nerve, including compression terminally under the cruciate ligament on the dorsum of the foot (G57.31)
      (*ix*) tibial nerve (G57.4)
      (*x*) posterior tibial nerve in the tarsal tunnel (G57.5)
      (*xi*) medial plantar nerve (G57.61)
      (*xii*) digital nerve (Morton neuroma) (G57.62)

(*d*) Of the trunk:
 (*i*) intercostal neuropathy (G58.0)
 (*ii*) of dorsal branches of thoracic and lumbar spinal nerves (notalgia paresthetica)
(*e*) Multiple entrapments in mucopolysaccharidosis (Karpati et al 1974 Archives of Neurology 31: 418) (E76)
4. Electric shock (Farrell, Starr 1968 Neurology 18: 601) (T75.4)
5. Cold injury ('trench foot', 'immersion foot') (T33)
6. Burns (T20)
7. Vibration injury (vibrating tools) (T75.2)
8. Radiation injury (Stoll, Andrews 1966 British Medical Journal 1: 834) (G62.80)
9. Ischaemic neuropathy★
 (*a*) vasculitis (G63.5)
  (*i*)   polyarteritis nodosa (G63.5, M30.0)
  (*ii*) neuropathy in systemic lupus erythematosus (G63.5, M32)
  (*iii*) Churg–Strauss syndrome (allergic granulomatosis) (G63.5, M30.1)
  (*iv*) diabetes mellitus (some cases) (G63.5, E10.4)
  (*v*)   giant cell (Warrell et al 1968 Lancet i: 1010) (G63.5, M31.5)
  (*vi*) cryoglobinaemia (D891)
  (*vii*) hypersensitivity angiitis (G63.5, M31.0)
  (*viii*) neuropathy in rheumatoid arthritis (Pallis, Scott 1965 British Medical Journal 1: 1141; Dyck et al 1972 Proceedings of the Mayo Clinic 47: 462) (G63.5, M05)
  (*ix*) neuropathy in sarcoidosis — sometimes associated angiitis (Nemni et al, 1981 Neurology 31: 3) (D86.8)
  (*x*)   Wegener's granulomatosis (G63.5, M31.3)
  (*xi*) neuropathy in Lyme disease (Camponovo, Meier 1986 Journal of Neurology 233: 69) (G63.0, A69.2)
 (*b*) arteriosclerotic occlusive disease
 (*c*) thromboangiitis obliterans (Buerger's disease)
 (*d*) embolic infarction of nerve trunks
 (*e*) haemorrhage into nerve trunks
 (*f*) occlusion of large arteries by compression, e.g. tourniquet, trauma
 (*g*) Volkmann's ischaemic contracture (T79.6)
 (*h*) anterior tibial compartment syndrome (see also V.B.-1.3 and 4) (T79.6)

C-2. Toxic
1. Drugs (G62.0, 740–Y59):
amiodarone — carbamazepine — chloroquine — cisplatin — clioquinol (subacute myelo-opticoneuropathy) — cytotoxic agents (especially nitrogen mustard and vincristine) — dapsone — diphenylhydantoin (phenytoin) — disulfiram — emetine — ethionamide — glutethimide — hydralazine — indomethacin — isoniazid — lithium carbonate — methaqualone — metronidazole — misonidazole — nitrofurantoin — perhexiline — phenytoin — pyridoxine — sodium cyanate — stilbamidine — streptomycin — taxol — sulphanilamide — thalidomide — trichloroethylene — vinca alkaloids
2. Inorganic substances (G62.2, 2 × 49):
heavy metals: antimony — arsenic — bismuth — copper —

gold — lead — mercury (Pink disease, Minimata disease) — thallium
3. Organic substances (× 45, × 46, × 47):
acrylamide — alcohol — aniline — bush tea — carbon disulphide — carbon monoxide★ — carbon tetrachloride — dinitrobenzol — dinitrophenol — ethylene oxide — hexachlorophene — n-hexane — methyl butyl ketone — pentachlorophenol and DDT — polychlorinated biphenyl (in cooking oil) (Chia, Chu 1985 Journal of Neurology, Neurosurgery and Psychiatry 48: 894) — tetrachlorethane — trichlorethylene — other organic chlorine derivatives — triorthocresyl-phosphate (G62.1, 62.2)
4. Toxins derived from bacteria (G63):
 (*a*) botulism (A05.1)
 (*b*) diphtheria (A36.8)
 (*c*) tetanus (A35)
5. Toxins derived from other organisms: saxitoxin; cigatuera (Allsop et al 1986 Revue de Neurologique 1986 142: 590) (G70.1)
6. Buckthorn neuropathy (Mitchell et al 1978 Neuropathology and Experimental Neurology 4: 85)
7. Nitrous oxide abuse (× 47)

C-3. Of uncertain aetiology
1. Neuropathy and amyotrophy in:
 (*a*) tropical spastic paraparesis (HTLV-1 infection)
 (*b*) Southern Indian paraplegia
 (*c*) neuropathy in tropical ataxia (Nigeria) (Williams, Osuntokum 1969 Archives of Neurology 21: 475) (G62.8)
2. Neuropathy in the Spanish toxic oil syndrome (Cruz Martinez et al 1984 Muscle and Nerve 7: 12)

D. Infections

D-1. Infective
1. Direct infection of nerves:
 (*a*) leprosy (A30)
 (*b*) herpes simplex (B00)
 (*c*) herpes zoster (B02)
 (*d*) human immunodeficiency virus (HIV) infection; role of direct infection uncertain in prominent sensory neuropathy of late AIDS (Said 1991, Current Opinions in Neurology and Neurosurgery 4: 689). Cytomegalovirus may directly invade and cause peripheral neuropathy in AIDS (Griffin et al 1990 Current Opinions in Neurology and Neurosurgery 1990 3: 697) (B20)
 (*e*) infection with HTLV-1
 (*f*) trypanosomiasis (B56)
 (*g*) nosematosis
2. Neuropathies occurring in other infections:
 (*a*) gonorrhoea (A54)
 (*b*) malaria (B50–53)
 (*c*) meningitis
 (*d*) mumps (B26)
 (*e*) paratyphoid (A01)
 (*f*) puerperal sepsis
 (*g*) septicaemia
 (*h*) smallpox
 (*i*) tuberculosis (A17)
 (*j*) typhoid (A01)

★Peripheral nerve lesions occurring in these disorders are believed to be ischaemic but other pathological processes may well be involved.

★It is possible that neuropathies arising in patients suffering from carbon monoxide poisoning are toxic, but many are probably pressure palsies arising in the unconscious patient.

(*k*) typhus (A75)
(*l*) leptospirosis (A27)
(*m*) subacute bacterial endocarditis
(*n*) AIDS (see III. D-1.1.d) (B23.8)
(*o*) Legionnaire's disease
(*p*) brucellosis (A23)
(*q*) Lyme disease (borelia) (A69.2)

E. Guillain–Barré syndrome and related disorders (probably immunologically mediated)
1. Acute inflammatory neuropathy (acute postinfective polyradiculoneuropathy, Guillain–Barré syndrome) (G61.0)
    (*a*) following identifiable infections, e.g. chicken pox — mumps — measles — rubella — campylobacter jejuni — hepatitis A and B — infectious mononucleosis — influenza — upper respiratory tract infections — AIDS — mycoplasma — cytomegalovirus — bacterial infections
    (*b*) following trauma, surgery
    (*c*) following injection of sera and vaccines
    (*d*) associated with lymphoma and other malignancies
    (*e*) no known preceding events
2. Miller–Fisher syndrome of ophthalmoplegia, ataxia and areflexia (probably a variant of the Guillain–Barré syndrome)
    Other variants: pure motor and sensory forms; polyneuritis cranialis; pure dysautonomia (G61.03)
3. Acute motor axonal neuropathy (Chinese paralysis syndrome) McKhann et al 1993 Annals of Neurology 33: 333)
    Chronic inflammatory demyelinating polyradiculoneuropathy (CIDP; relapsing or recurrent polyneuropathy) (G61.80)
    (*a*) with CNS demyelination (Thomas et al 1987 Brain 110: 53)

F. Neuropathy associated with paraproteinaemia and dysproteinaemia
1. Multiple myeloma (G90.00)
2. Macroglobulinaemia (Waldenström) (D89.00)
3. Cryoglobulinaemia (D89.1)
4. Benign monoclonal gammopathy — IgA, IgG, IgM, sometimes with antibodies to myelin-associated glycoprotein (MAG) (D47.2)
5. Amyloidosis (E85.1)

G. Neuropathy in malignant disease (G63.1, G13.0)
1. Carcinomatous neuropathy, sensorimotor forms; subacute sensory neuropathy with Anti-Hu antibodies (Dalman et al 1991 Medicine 71: 59)
2. Neuropathy in reticulosis — lymphoma, leukaemia, myeloproliferative disorders (see III G 3)

H. Neuropathy associated with connective tissue disorders (see V. C-2.3) (G63.5)
1. Systemic lupus erythematosus (M32)
2. Polyarteritis nodosa (M30)
3. Churg–Strauss syndrome (allergic granulomatosis) (M30.1)
4. Rheumatoid arthritis (M05)
5. Systemic sclerosis (M34.9)
6. Thrombotic thrombocytopenic purpura (thrombotic microangiopathy) (M31.6)
7. Giant cell arteritis (M31.7)

8. Mixed connective tissue disease (M35.1)
9. Sjögren's (sicca) syndrome (M35.0)
10. Non-systemic vasculitic neuropathy (Dyck et al 1987 Brain 110: 843) (M31.9)

I. Metabolic neuropathy (G63.3)
1. Nutritional (G63.4)
    (*a*) (*i*) cyanocobalamin deficiency (D51.9)
        (*ii*) folic acid deficiency (E53.8)
        (*iii*) vitamin E deficiency (E56)
    (*b*) of uncertain aetiology (probably B_1, B_2 and B_6 vitamin deficiency) (E53.8):
        (*i*) in chronic alcoholism
        (*ii*) beri-beri
        (*iii*) burning feet syndrome
        (*iv*) famine oedema and kwashiorkor
        (*v*) in hyperemesis gravidarum
        (*vi*) in pregnancy
2. Neuropathies associated with endocrine disorders (G63.3)
    (*a*) diabetes mellitus (E10.4):
        (*i*) polyneuropathy (G63.2)
        (*ii*) mononeuropathy (including diabetic amyotrophy) (G59.0)
        (*iii*) thoracic radiculopathy (Kikta et al 1982 Annals of Neurology 11: 80)
        (*iv*) autonomic neuropathy (G99.0)
    (*b*) Thyroid disorders:
        (*i*) hyperthyroidism (Feibel, Campa 1976 Journal of Neurology 39: 491) (E05)
        (*ii*) primary hypothyroidism (Dyck, Lambert 1970 Journal of Neuropathology and Experimental Neurology 29: 631) (E03.9)
        (*iii*) hypothyroidism secondary to thyrotropin deficiency (Grabow, Chou 1968 Archives of Neurology 19: 284) (E23.03)
    (*c*) Neuropathy or amyotrophy in organic hyperinsulinism (Mulder et al 1956 Neurology 6: 627) (E16.1)
    (*d*) In acromegaly (Stewart 1966 Archives of Neurology 14: 107) (E22.0)
3. Neuropathy in blood dyscrasias (G63.8)
    (*a*) polycythaemia vera (D45)
    (*b*) myelofibrosis
    (*c*) leukaemia — acute and chronic (G91–95)
    (*d*) bleeding disorders — haemorrhage into nerves (D69.9)
    (*e*) sickle cell disease (D57)
4. Neuropathy in renal failure.
    (*a*) uraemic polyneuropathy (Asbury et al 1963 Archives of Neurology 8: 413) (G63.80, N18.8)
    (*b*) mononeuritis multiplex following dialysis (Meyrier et al 1972 British Medical Journal 2: 252) (G59)
    (*c*) carpal tunnel syndrome due to amyloid deposition (G56.0, E85.1)
5. Neuropathy in acute and chronic liver disease, including primary biliary cirrhosis (Dayan, Williams 1967 Lancet ii: 133; Thomas, Walker 1965 Brain 88: 1079) (G63.81)
6. Neuropathy with giant axons and cardiomyopathy associated with desmin-type intermediate filaments in skeletal muscle (Sabatelli et al 1992 Journal of the Neurological Sciences 109: 1–10)

J. Neuropathy associated with other systemic or non-hereditary degenerative diseases (G63)
1. Sarcoidosis (D86)
2. Chronic obstructive pulmonary disease (Appenzeller et al 1968 American Journal of Medicine 44: 873) (J43)

3. Total lipodystrophy (Tuck, McLeod 1983 Australian and New Zealand Medical Journal 13: 65)
4. Acrodermatitis chronica atrophicans (Hopf 1975 Journal of Neurology, Neurosurgery and Psychiatry 38: 452)
5. Neuropathy associated with critical illness (Zochodne et al 1986 Brain 110: 819) (G63.83)
6. Neuropathy associated with ataxia and retinitis pigmentosa (Tuck, McLeod 1983 Journal of Neurology, Neurosurgery and Psychiatry 46: 206) (G11.15)

K. *Chronic neuropathy with no known cause or association*
1. Chronic sensorimotor neuropathy of undetermined cause (Dyck et al 1981 Annals of Neurology 10: 222; McLeod et al 1984 Journal of Neurology, Neurosurgery and Psychiatry 47: 530) (G62.9)
2. Chronic idiopathic ataxic neuropathy (Dalakas 1986 Annals of Neurology 19: 545)

L. *Tumours of nerves* (D36.1)
1. Arising from supporting structures, axons, or both
   (*a*) plexiform neuroma
   (*b*) traumatic neuroma
2. Arising from supporting structures. (D36.1)
   (*a*) schwannoma (neurinoma, neurofibroma), including acoustic neuroma
   (*b*) fibroma
   (*c*) neurogenic sarcoma
   (*d*) haemangioma
   (*e*) lipoma
   (*f*) neuroepithelioma

IV. DISORDERS OF NEUROMUSCULAR TRANSMISSION

A. *Heritable* (G70.24)
1. Hereditary myasthenia gravis
   (*a*) Congenital (254210) (non-immune) and juvenile (autoimmune) (254200) (Bundey 1972 Journal of Neurology, Neurosurgery and Psychiatry 35: 41; Honeybourne et al 1982 Journal of Neurology, Neurosurgery and Psychiatry 45: 854; Provenzano et al 1988 Journal of Neurology, Neurosurgery and Psychiatry 51: 1228
   (*b*) Myasthenia with myopathy (254300; 159400) (McQuillen 1966 Brain 89: 121)
2. Pseudocholinesterase deficiency (suxamethonium paralysis) (177400) (G70.9)

B. *Congenital or developmental myasthenia (254210)* (G70.2)
For all types, see Engel 1986 In Engel, Banker (eds) Myology, pp 1955–1990; also Matthes et al 1991 Developmental Medicine and Child Neurology 33: 924
1. Putative defect in ACh synthesis or packaging
2. Congenital end-plate acetylcholinesterase deficiency
3. Slow-channel syndrome
4. Congenital end-plate AChR deficiency
5. Decrease of MEPP amplitude without AChR deficiency
6. Abnormality of synaptic vesicles (Morea et al 1987 Neurology 37: 206)

C. *Toxic* (G70.1)
1. Botulism (A05.1)
2. Tick paralysis

3. Puffer-fish paralysis (tetrodotoxin)
4. Magnesium intoxication
5. Kanamycin and other antibiotics (McQuillen et al 1968 Archives of Neurology 18: 402)
6. Penicillamine-induced myasthenia (Garlepp et al 1983 British Medical Journal 1: 338); also anticonvulsants, quinidine

D. *Autoimmune*
1. Myasthenia gravis (G70.0)
   (*a*) transient neonatal myasthenia (Namba et al 1970 Pediatrics 45: 488) (P94.0)
   (*b*) ocular myasthenia with peripheral neuropathy and spastic paraparesis (Brust et al 1974 Neurology 24: 755)
   (*c*) generalised myasthenia:
      (i) severe, especially in young women, correlated with HLA-8 antigen
      (ii) in older patients, often with thymoma and with HL-A2 or A3 antigen
   (*d*) myasthenia with thyrotoxicosis
   (*e*) myasthenia with hypothyroidism (Takamori et al 1972 Archives of Neurology 26: 326)
   (*f*) myasthenia with other autoimmune diseases
   (*g*) myasthenia combined with Lambert–Eaton syndrome (Newsom-Davis et al 1991 Journal of Neurology, Neurosurgery and Psychiatry 44: 542)
   (*h*) myasthenia with the Satoyoshi syndrome (muscle cramps, alopecia and diarrhoea — Satoh et al 1983 Neurology 33: 1209)

E. *Lambert–Eaton syndrome (facilitating disorder of neuromuscular transmission)*
1. With malignant disease (G73.1)
2. Without malignant disease (G70.80)

F. *Cholinergic paralysis* (G70.1)
1. Poisoning with anticholinesterase compounds (e.g. nerve gases)
2. Depolarising drugs
3. Black Widow spider venom

V. DISORDERS OF MUSCLE

A. *Heritable myopathies* (G71.0)
1. The muscular dystrophies
   (*a*) X-linked types:
      (i) X-linked recessive (severe) (Duchenne) (Xp21) (310200) (G71.07)
      (ii) myopathy in manifesting Duchenne carriers (Xp21) (310200)
      (iii) X-linked Duchenne dystrophy (Xp 21) due to chromosomal translocation in females or to Turner's syndrome (Boyd, Buckle 1986 Clinical Genetics 29: 108)
      (iv) X-linked recessive (mild) (Becker) (Xp 21) (310200) is an allelic variant of Duchenne. Atypical forms include X-linked recurrent myoglobinuria, cramps, quadriceps syndrome, distal myopathy (G71.00)
      (v) X-linked recessive myopathy (Xp21) with glycerol kinase deficiency (Guggenheim et al 1980 Annals of Neurology 7: 441)
      (vi) X-linked myopathy (Xp21) with McLeod's

syndrome (314850) (lack of Kell red blood cell antigen and acanthocytes) (Swash et al 1983 Brain 106: 717) or chorea (Cross et al 1985 Archives of Neurology 42: 753)

(*vii*) X-linked recessive with contractures and cardiomyopathy (Emery–Dreifuss) (310300) (Rowland et al 1979 Annals of Neurology 5: 111; Petty et al 1986 Journal of Neurology 233; 108), maps to Xq28. See also (c ii) below and 'rigid spine syndrome' for different myopathies that have similar features (van Munster et al 1986 Journal of Neurology, Neurosurgery and Psychiatry 49: 1292; Bertini et al 1986 Journal of Neurology 233: 248) (G71.01)

(*viii*) X-linked centronuclear myopathy (310400) (Askanas et al 1979 Archives of Neurology 36: 604), may link to Xp28 (Thomas et al 1990 Journal of Medical Genetics 27: 284). Note also autosomal dominant (160150) and recessive (255200) forms (G71.23)

(*ix*) X-linked dominant lethal myopathy in hemizygous boys (309950) (Henson et al 1967, Archives of Neurology 17: 238)

(*x*) muscular dystrophy, cardiac type (309930)

(*xi*) muscular dystrophy, pectorodorsal (310095), not proven to differ from Becker dystrophy

(*xii*) X-linked myotubular myopathy lethal in neonates (Silver et al 1986 Human Pathology 7: 1167); may be same as viii above (centronuclear) (G71.23)

(*xiii*) X-linked scapuloperoneal muscular dystrophy with lethal cardiomyopathy (Bergen et al 1986 Journal of Neurology, Neurosurgery and Psychiatry 49: 143) (G71.06)

(*xiv*) X-linked myopathy with excessive autophagy (MEAX) (310440) (Kalimo et al 1988 Annals of Neurology 23: 258) (G71.083)

(*b*) facioscapulohumeral (Landouzy and Dejerine) (G71.02);

(*i*) autosomal dominant involving face, scapulohumeral and anterior tibial muscles (158900), maps to 4q35-qtr

(*ii*) severe infantile form (Baily et al 1986 Acta Neurologica Scandinavica 74: 51)

(*iii*) childhood form with Möbius syndrome (Hanson, Rowland 1971 Archives of Neurology 24: 31) (Q87.05)

(*iv*) with sensorineural deafness alone (Voit et al 1980 European Journal of Pediatrics 145: 280) or with Coats' disease of the retina (Taylor et al 1982 Annals of Neurology 12: 395; Korf et al 1985 Annals of Neurology 17: 513) or tortuosity of retinal vessels (Gieron et al 1985 American Journal of Medical Genetics 22: 143)

(*v*) facioscapulohumeral phenotype with ragged red fibres, sometimes with cardiomyopathy (Rowland et al 1991 Revue Neurologique 147: 467; Supetz et al 1991 American Journal of Human Genetics 48: 502)

(*c*) scapuloperoneal muscular dystrophy (G71.06):

(*i*) autosomal dominant (181430) (Thomas et al 1975 Journal of Neurology, Neursurgery and Psychiatry 38: 1008); not proven to differ from facioscapulohumeral muscular dystrophy; note possible neurogenic type (181400)

(*ii*) X-linked (Thomas et al 1972 Journal of Neurology, Neursurgery and Psychiatry 35: 208) may be Emery–Dreifuss type (310300), especially when there is also heart-block (181350)

(*iii*) with inflammatory changes and cardiopathy (Jennekens et al 1975 Brain 98: 709)

(*d*) limb-girdle muscular dystrophy (G71.03):

(*i*) autosomal recessive or sporadic (Erb, Leyden and Mobius) (253600)

(*ii*) myopathy limited to quadriceps (310450) (Swash, Heathfield 1983 Journal of Neurology, Neurosurgery and Psychiatry 46: 355); may sometimes be variant of Becker dystrophy (G71.86)

(*iii*) autosomal dominant limb-girdle dystrophy of late onset (159000) (Coster et al 1974 European Neurology 12: 159; Bethlem and van Wijngaarden, 1976 Brain 99: 91; Chutkow et al 1986 Annals of Neurology 20: 240) maps to 5q31.1–q31.3; (Speer et al 1992 American Journal of Human Genetics 50: 1215)

(*iv*) autosomal recessive limb-girdle dystrophy of childhood, also called 'severe childhood autosomal recessive muscular dystrophy' (SCARMD) resembling Duchenne (253600), but more benign and affecting both sexes (especially frequent in Tunisia and other parts of the Middle East) (253700) (Ben Hamida et al 1983 Muscle and Nerve 6: 469), maps to chromosome 13 (Ben Othname et al 1992 Nature Genetics 2: 315). Dystrophin content is normal but there seems to be lack of a dystrophin-associated glycoprotein (Matsumara et al 1992 Nature 359: 320) (G71.080)

(*e*) distal muscular dystrophy (G71.081):

(*i*) autosomal dominant distal myopathy (Welander) (160500); inclusions may resemble those of inclusion body myositis (Borg et al 1991 Acta Neuropathologica 82: 102)

(*ii*) autosomal dominant variety with infantile onset (160300) (Bautista et al 1978 Journal of the Neurological Sciences 37: 149)

(*iii*) autosomal recessive variety (254130) (Scoppetta et al 1984 Muscle and Nerve 7: 478; Barohn et al 1991 Neurology 41: 1365) with rimmed vacuole formation and lamellar (myeloid) bodies (Nonaka et al 1985 Annals of Neurology 17: 51; Mizusawa et al 1987 Journal of Neurology 234: 129) (G71.803)

(*iv*) hereditary distal myopathy with sarcoplasmic bodies and intermediate skeleton filaments (Edstrom et al 1980 Journal of the Neurological Sciences 47: 171); may be the same as Welander type

(*v*) autosomal recessive distal myopathy, with high creatine kinase (Miyoshi et al 1986 Brain 109: 31)

(*f*) autosomal dominant dystrophy with humeropelvic distribution and cardiomyopathy (Fenichel et al 1982 Neurology 32: 1399)

(*g*) autosomal dominant Emery–Dreifuss dystrophy (Galassi et al 1985 Journal of the Neurological Sciences 7: 125; Gilchrist, Leshener 1986 Archives of Neurology 43: 734) (G71.01)

(*h*) benign muscular dystrophy with contractures but no cardiopathy (Bailey et al 1986 Acta Neurologica

Scandinavica 73: 439); may be same as Emery–Dreifuss

(*i*) myositis ossificans (fibrodysplasia ossificans progressiva (135100); autosomal dominant (Pitt, Hamilton 1984 Journal of the Royal Society of Medicine 77: 68; Connor 1982 Journal of Bone and Joint Surgery 64: 76) (M61.1)

(*j*) ocular myopathies (progressive external ophthalmoplegia)★ (G71.04)

(*k*) (*i*) when restricted to ocular myopathy (without CNS abnormalities or cardiopathy), with or without ragged red fibres, syndrome may be apparently congenital or commence later in childhood, adolescence or in adult years. Findings may be restricted to eyes or include neck and limbs; inheritance pattern may seem autosomal dominant (165 000), recessive (258450; 258 470), X-linked (311 000), or maternal. Sporadic cases may show deletions of mitochondrial DNA (mtDNA), which are not found in familial cases. Among those without deletions, some show one of the point mutations of MELAS. The combination of ophthalmoplegia with deafness (165 490) suggests mitochondrial disorder but in the family recorded there was male-to-male transmission (Treft et al 1984 Ophthalmology 91: 908)

(*ii*) with pigmentary retinal degeneration (dominant or sporadic). Ophthalmoplegia is probably an incomplete Kearns–Sayre syndrome, but classification might depend on molecular analysis of mtDNA

(*iii*) with retinal degeneration, short stature, heart block, ataxia and high CSF protein content (165100) (Kearns–Sayre syndrome; Berenberg et al 1977 Annals of Neurology 1: 37). Most of these patients show a deletion of mtDNA; a few Kearns–Sayre patients have been found with the point mutations of MELAS. Almost all are simplex cases, with no others in the family. Survivors of the Pearson marrow-pancreas syndrome (260560) also show deletions of mtDNA and seem especially likely to develop the Kearns–Sayre syndrome (H49.80)

(*iv*) with curare sensitivity (257600)

(*v*) oculopharyngeal muscular dystrophy (Little, Perl 1982 Journal of the Neurological Sciences 53: 145) usually autosomal dominant (164300), sometimes recessive (257950) (G71.05)

(*vi*) oculopharyngeal myopathy with distal myopathy and cardiomoyopathy (Goto et al 1977 Journal of Neurology, Neurosurgery and Psychiatry 40: 600) and other varieties of oculopharyngo-distal myopathy

(*vii*) familial multicore disease (see below) with ophthalmoplegia (255320) (Swash, Schwartz 1981 Journal of the Neurological Sciences 52: 1) (G71.22)

(*viii*) progressive ophthalmoplegia with mental retardation (165150)

(*ix*) congenital ophthalmoplegia in the Goldenhar–Gorlin syndrome (257700) (oculo-auriculo-vertebral) (Aleksic et al 1976 Neurology 26: 638)

(*x*) ophthalmoplegia and myopia (311000), X-linked recessive

(*xi*) neonatal ophthalmoplegia with microfibres (Hanson et al 1977 Neurology 27: 974)

(*xii*) nemaline myopathy (161800; 256030) with ophthalmoplegia and mitochondrial abnormalities (Fukunaga et al 1980 Journal of the Neurological Sciences 46: 169) (G71.24)

(*xiii*) nemaline myopathy with cardiomyopathy (Meier et al 1984 Archives of Neurology 44: 443) (G71.24)

(*xiv*) familial paralysis of horizontal gaze and scoliosis (258460) (Sharpe et al 1975 Neurology 25: 1035)

(*xv*) late-onset 'oculogastrointestinal muscular dystrophy' (Ionasescu et al 1984 American Journal of Medical Genetics 18: 781); same as 'myoneural-gastro-intestinal encephalomyopathy' (MNGIE) (277320), 'polyneuropathy, ophthalmoplegia, leukoencephalopathy, and intestinal pseudo-obstruction' (POLIP)' (263080) 'familial visceral myopathy with ophthalmoplegia' and 'mitochondrial encephalomyopathy with polyneuropathy, ophthalmoplegia, and pseudo-obstruction' (MEPOP). Intestinal pseudo-obstruction due to neuronal disease (243180) is similar. The condition is maternally inherited

(*xvi*) familial static ophthalmoplegia (165000) (Lees 1960 Journal of Neurology, Neurosurgery and Psychiatry 23: 46)

2. Congenital myopathies of unknown aetiology:

(*a*) congenital muscular dystrophy (254100) (including some cases of arthrogryposis multiplex congenita (253900), with infantile cataract (254000) (see k. below), or a 'scleroatonic form' (254090), also with joint contractures. In one form there is also cardiomyopathy with desmin accumulation (253850) (Prelle et al 1992 Neuromuscular Disorders 2: 169) (G71.085)

(*b*) congenital muscular dystrophy with severe mental retardation (253800) (Fukuyama's disease) (Fukuyama et al 1981 Brain and Development 3: 1); described best in Japan but seen throughout the world (Topalogen et al 1991 Journal of Neurology, Neurosurgery and Psychiatry 54: 226). Sometimes associated with abnormality of dystrophin (Beggs et al 1992 Proceedings of the National Academy of Sciences USA 89: 623) (Prelle et al 1992 Journal of Neurology 239: 76) (G71.084)

(*c*) benign congenital myopathy without specific features (Turner 1940 Brain 63: 163; Schmalbruch et al 1987 Journal of Neurology 234: 146) (G71.9)

(*d*) benign congenital or infantile hypotonia (Walton)★ (G72.86)

(*e*) central core disease (117000) maps to same site as malignant hyperthermia, 19q12–q13.2, and patients are especially susceptible to hyperthermic attacks induced by anaesthesia and neuromuscular blocking agents (G71.20)

(*f*) nemaline or rod-body myopathy (161800, 256030), maps to 1q21–q23 (G71.24)

★ The primary myopathic nature of some of these cases is unproven.

★This is not a single entity and many of the cases are probably not myopathic in origin.

(g) myotubular or centronuclear myopathy (255200) (Spiro et al 1966 Archives of Neurology 14: 1; Elder et al 1983 Journal of the Neurological Sciences 60: 79) (G71.23)

   (i) X-linked centronuclear or myotubular myopathy (310400) (van Wijngaarden et al 1969 Neurology 19: 901), maps to Xq28

   (ii) autosomal dominant centronuclear or myotubular (160150) (McLeod et al 1972 Journal of the Neurological Sciences 15: 375)

   (iii) centronuclear with type 1 fibre atrophy (Bethlem et al 1970 Archives of Neurology 23: 70)

(h) familial myosclerosis (myodysplasia fibrosa multiplex) (255600) (G71.806)

(i) myopathy in Marfan's syndrome (Goebel et al 1973 Neurology 23: 1257): centronuclear myopathy with type 1 fibre hypotrophy and 'fingerprint' inclusions with Marfan's syndrome (Jadro-Santel et al 1980 Journal of the Neurological Sciences 45: 43) (Q87.4)

(j) familial congenital myopathy with cataract, gonadal dysgenesis and oligophrenia (Marinesco–Sjögren syndrome) (255170) (Bassoe 1956 Journal of Clinical Endocrinology 16: 1614; Superneau et al 1987 European Neurology 26: 8)

(k) lethal congenital muscular dystrophy with cataracts and minor brain anomaly may be related to Walker–Warburg syndrome (236670) (Wargowski et al 1991 American Journal of Human Genetics 39: 19)

(l) myopathies with characteristic histochemical abnormalities (G71.28):

   (i) type 1 fibre hypotrophy (WK Engel et al 1968 Archives of Neurology 18: 435; Bender, Bender 1977 Neurology 27: 206)

   (ii) congenital fibre type disproportion (255310) (Curless, Nelson 1977 Annals of Neurology 2: 455; Sulaiman et al 1983 Journal of Neurology, Neurosurgery and Psychiatry 46: 175; Argov et al 1984 Archives of Neurology 41: 53; Glick et al 1984 Annals of Neurology 16: 405) (G71.21)

   (iii) congenital myopathy with uniform fibre type (type I) (Oh, Danon 1983 Archives of Neurology 40: 147)

   (iv) congenital fibre type disproportion in Krabbe's disease (245200) (Dehkharghani et al 1981 Archives of Neurology 38: 585) (E75.211)

   (v) reducing body myopathy (Brooke, Neville 1971 Neurology 21: 412; Oh et al 1983 Muscle and Nerve 6: 278) (G71.281)

   (vi) congenital neuromuscular disease with trilaminar muscle fibres (Ringel et al 1978 Neurology 28: 282)

   (vii) congenital myopathy with multifocal degeneration of muscle fibre (AG Engel et al 1971 Proceedings of the Mayo Clinic 46: 666)

(m) the rigid spine syndrome (probably of multiple aetiology but some are myopathic) (Poewe et al 1985 Journal of Neurology, Neurosurgery and Psychiatry 48: 887) (M62.82)

(n) myopathy with features of both centronuclear myopathy and multicores (Lee, Yip 1981 Journal of the Neurological Sciences 50: 227; Fitzsimons, McLeod 1982 Journal of the Neurological Sciences 57: 395)

(o) myopathies with cytoplasmic inclusions (147420) (G71.800):

   (i) (Nakashima et al 1970 Archives of Neurology 22: 270; Patel et al 1983 Journal of the Neurological

Sciences 60: 281; Winter et al 1986 Quarterly Journal of Medicine 61: 1171)

   (ii) with 'fingerprint' inclusions (AG Engel et al 1972 Proceedings of the Mayo Clinic 47: 377) (G71.26)

(p) multicore disease (255320) (Engel, Groover 1971 Neurology 21: 413; Vanneste, Stam 1982 Journal of Neurology, Neurosurgery and Psychiatry 45: 360) (G71.22)

(q) sarcotubular myopathy (Jerusalem et al 1973 Neurology 23: 897) (G71.280)

(r) myopathy with tubular aggregates (Morgan-Hughes et al 1970 Brain 93: 873; Pieroson-Bormioli et al 1985 Muscle and Nerve 8: 291 — see also V.D.-2) (G71.25)

(s) familial neuromuscular disease with type I fibre hypoplasia, tubular aggregates, cardiomyopathy and myasthenic features (Dobkin, Verity 1978 Neurology 28: 1135)

(t) congenital myopathy with type II fibre hypoplasia (Brooke, Engel 1969 Neurology 19: 591)

(u) myopathy with crystalline intranuclear inclusions (Jenis et al 1969 Archives of Neurology 20: 281)

(v) autosomal dominant 'spheroid body' myopathy (Goebel et al 1978 Muscle and Nerve 1: 14)

(w) hypertrophic branchial myopathy (Mancall et al 1974 Neurology 24: 1166) (G71.83)

(x) monomelic hypertrophic myopathy (Celesia et al 1967 Archives of Neurology 17: 69) (G71.82)

(y) cytoplasmic body neuromyopathy with respiratory failure and weight loss (Jerusalem et al 1979 Journal of the Neurological Sciences 41: 1), may be same as V.A-2.o (147420) and V.D-2.12 (G71.800)

(z) zebra body myopathy (Lake, Wilson 1975 Journal of the Neurological Sciences 24: 437) (G71.802)

(a') myopathy with absence of muscle glycogen and neutral lipid in the neuroleptic malignant syndrome

(b') congenital myopathy with oculo-facial abnormalities (Marden–Walker syndrome) (248700) (Linder et al 1991 American Journal of Medical Genetics 39: 377)

(c') myopathy with cylindrical spirals (Tartuto et al 1991 Neuromuscular Disorders 1: 433)

(d') congenital inflammatory myopathy (Shevell et al 1990 Neurology 40: 1111)

(e') familial myopathy with storage of phosphorylated desmin (Rapport et al 1988 FEBS Letters 231: 421; Halbig et al 1991 Revue Neurologique 147: 300)

3. Myotonic disorders (G71.1)

(a) dystrophia myotonica (myotonic muscular atrophy, myotonia atrophica) (160900): maps to 19q13.3 (G71.12)

   (i) adult form (G71.122)

   (ii) infantile form (congenital myotonic dystrophy) (G71.120)

(b) myotonia congenita (autosomal dominant form, Thomsen's disease) (160800) maps to 7q35 (muscle chloride channel); one variant is responsive to acetazolamide (170500) and is related to sodium channel (G71.130)

(c) myotonia congenita, autosomal recessive (Becker's disease) (255700), also maps to 7q35 (muscle chloride channel) (G71.131)

(d) myotonia, dwarfism, diffuse bone disease, with eye and face abnormality (chondrodystrophic myotonia, Schwartz–Jampel syndrome) (255800); possibly related to sodium channel defect (Lehmam-Horn et al 1990 Muscle and Nerve 13: 526) (G71.10)

(e) paramyotonia congenita (Eulenburg) (168300); allelic with hyperkalemic periodic paralysis at 17q13.1–q13.3 (G71.15)

(f) paramyotonia without paralysis on exposure to cold (de Jong) (168350); probably variant of cold-induced myotonia

(g) familial granulovacuolar lobular myopathy with electrical myotonia (254950) (Juguilon et al 1982 Journal of the Neurological Sciences 56: 133); one form with cylindrical spirals (160990) (G71.805)

(h) myotonia with painful cramps (Sanders et al 1976 Archives of Neurology 33: 580)

B. Trauma to muscle by external agents

B-1. Physical

1. Crush syndrome (T04)
2. Ischaemic infarction or atrophy (G72.82)
   (a) in peripheral vascular disease (Engel, Hawley 1977 Journal of Neurology 215: 161) (M62.2)
   (b) in polyarteritis nodosa and other vasculitides (M30)
   (c) in diabetes mellitus (Banker, Chester 1973 Neurology 23: 667)
3. Volkmann's contracture (T79.6)
4. Anterior tibial syndrome (T79.6)
5. Posterior compartment (tibial) syndrome (British Medical Journal 1975 3: 193) (T79.6)
6. Lateral (peroneal) compartment syndrome (T79.6)
7. Triceps surae compartment syndrome (T79.6)
8. Extensor compartment syndrome of the forearm (T79.6)
9. Rectus abdominis compartment syndrome (T79.6)
10. Congenital or idiopathic torticollis (Sarnat, Morrissy 1981 Muscle and Nerve 4: 374) (M62.4)

B-2. Toxic (G72.2)

1. Haff disease (B70.0)
2. Snake-bite by *Enhydrina schistosa* (Malayan sea snake)
3. Saxitoxin poisoning (G70.1)
4. Myoglobinuria caused by hornet venom (Shilkin et al 1972 British Medical Journal 1: 156)
5. Quail myopathy (Ouzonellis 1970 Journal of the American Medical Association 211: 1186)

B-3. Drugs (G72.2)

1. Steroid myopathy
2. Chloroquine myopathy
3. ? Bretylium tosylate myopathy (Campbell, Montuschi 1960 Lancet ii: 789)
4. Emetine
5. Vincristine
6. Diazacholesterol (myotonia)
7. Clofibrate
8. Carbenoxolone (Mohamed et al 1966 British Medical Journal 1: 1581)
9. Amphotericin B (K + depletion)
10. Anodiaquine
11. Colchicine
12. Meperidine (Aberfeld et al 1968 Archives of Neurology 19: 384)
13. Pethidine (Mastaglia et al 1971 British Medical Journal 4: 532)
14. Pentazocine (Steiner et al 1973 Archives of Neurology 28: 408)
15. Polymyxin E (Vanhaeverbeck et al 1974 Journal of Neurology, Neurosurgery and Psychiatry 37: 1343)
16. Triorthocresylphosphate (Prineas 1969 Archives of Neurology 21: 150)
17. Imidazole (Martin et al 1977 Neurology 27: 484)
18. Epsilon-aminocaproic acid (EACA) (Lane et al 1979 Postgraduate Medical Journal 55: 282; Kennard et al 1980 Muscle and Nerve 3: 202)
19. Cimetidine (Feest, Read 1980 British Medical Journal 281: 1284)
20. Ipecac (Rosenberg, Ringel 1986 Western Journal of Medicine 145: 386)
21. Enfluorane anaesthesia (Caccia et al 1978 Journal of Neurological Sciences 39: 61)
22. Iron overload during haemodialysis (Bregman et al 1980 Lancet ii: 876)
23. Gasoline sniffing-myopathy with myoglobinuria (Kovanen et al 1983 Neurology 33: 629)
24. Ziduvodine myopathy (Arnaudo et al 1991 Lancet 337: 508)
25. Steroid therapy with neuromuscular blocking agent, acute quadriplegic myopathy (Danon, Carpenter 1991 Muscle and Nerve 14: 1131)

C. Inflammatory

C-1. Infections of muscle (M60.0)

1. Viral myositis (see Mastaglia, Ojeda 1985 Annals of Neurology 17: 215)
   (a) benign acute myositis due to:
      (i) influenza A and B
      (ii) parainfluenza
      (iii) adenovirus 2
   (b) acute myopathy with myoglobinuria (G72.80):
      (i) influenza A and B
      (ii) Coxsackie B5
      (iii) Echo 9
      (iv) adenovirus 21
      (v) herpes simplex
      (vi) Epstein–Barr
   (c) epidemic pleurodynia due to Coxsackie B5 (also B1, 3 and 4)
   (d) postviral fatigue syndrome or benign postinfectious myositis (Schwartz et al 1978 British Medical Journal 2: 1256); role of virus or autoimmunity fiercely debated (G93.3)
2. Bacterial
   (a) gas gangrene (*Clostridium welchii*)
   (b) tetanus (*Clostridium tetani*) (A35)
   (c) staphylococci and other pyogenic agents (septic myositis) (B95.6)
   (d) leprous myositis (A30)
   (e) tropical myositis (usually pyogenic) (B95.6)
3. Fungal myositis (e.g. disseminated candidiasis) (B37)
4. Protozoal myositis
   (a) toxoplasmosis (Rowland, Greer 1961 Neurology 11: 367; Behan et al 1983 Acta Neuropathologica 61: 246) (B58)
   (b) sarcocystis (B60)
   (c) *Trypanosomiasis cruzi* (Chagas disease) (B57.2)
   (d) amoebiasis (B60)
5. Cestode myositis
   (a) cysticercosis (B69.8)
   (b) coenurosis (multicepts tapeworm) (B83)

(c) hydatidosis (echinococcosis) (B67)
(d) sparganosis (B83)
6. Nematode myositis
    (a) trichinosis (B75)
    (b) toxocariasis (B83)
    (c) cutaneous larva migrans (ancylostma)

C-2. Other inflammatory disorders of muscle
1. Dermatomyositis (M33)
2. Polymyositis (Group I of Walton and Adams) (possibly an organ-specific autoimmune disease) (M33.2)
    (a) acute polymyositis with myoglobinuria
    (b) subacute polymyositis
    (c) chronic polymyositis (including chronic myositis fibrosa)
3. Polymyositis with autoimmune disease.
    (a) polymyositis in systemic lupus erythematosus (M32)
    (b) polymyositis in rheumatic fever
    (c) polymyositis in rheumatoid arthritis (M05.3)
    (d) polymyositis in systemic sclerosis (M34)
    (e) scleroderma (morphoea) with myopathy
    (f) muscle infarction or polymyositis in polyarteritis nodosa or giant cell arteritis (M30)
    (g) myopathy in Sjögren disease (Ringel et al 1982 Archives of Neurology 39: 157; Kaplan et al 1990 Muscle and Nerve 13: 570) (M35)
    (h) myopathy in Werner's disease (nature of muscle atrophy uncertain — Epstein et al 1966 Medicine (Baltimore) 45: 177)
    (i) localised nodular myositis (M60.80)
    (j) myositis of chronic graft versus host disease (Reyes et al 1983 Neurology 33: 1222)
    (k) benign acute childhood myositis (Antony et al 1979 Neurology 29: 1068)
    (l) acne fulminans with inflammatory myopathy (Noseworthy et al 1980 Annals of Neurology 8: 67)
    (m) necrotising myopathy with pipestem capillaries (Emslie-Smith, Engel 1991 Neurology 41: 936)
4. Polymyositis or dermatomyositis (Group IV of Walton and Adams) with malignant disease (M33.11)
5. Polymyositis with associated virus particles (Chou 1967 Science 158: 1453; Carpenter et al 1970 Neurology 20: 889), now regarded as inclusion body myositis
6. Acute fulminant myoglobinuric polymyositis with picornavirus-like particles (Fukuyama et al 1977 Journal of Neurology, Neurosurgery and Psychiatry 40: 775) (G72.80)
7. Eosinophilic polymyositis (Layzer et al 1977 Annals of Neurology 1: 65) (M33.23)
8. Cyclic eosinophilic myositis and hyperimmunoglobulin E (Symmans et al 1986 Annals of Internal Medicine 104: 26)
9. Inclusion body myositis (Carpenter et al 1978 Neurology 28: 8; Julien et al 1982 Journal of the Neurological Sciences 55: 15; Ringel et al 1987 Archives of Neurology 44: 1154). May sometimes be familial (Massa et al 1991 Archives of Neurology 48: 519) (M33.26)
10. Orbital myositis (ocular myositis; pseudotumour of orbit)
11. Polymyositis in AIDS (Snider et al 1983 Annals of Neurology 14: 403) (B23.8)
12. Polymyositis or dermatomyositis due to penicillamine (Carroll et al 1987 Journal of Rheumatology 14: 5) (G72.2)

C-3. Inflammatory disorders of muscle of unknown aetiology
1. Sarcoidosis with myopathy (M63.3)

2. Granulomatous polymyositis (Lynch, Bansal 1973 Journal of the Neurological Sciences 18: 1) and giant cell myositis (Namba et al 1974 Archives of Neurology 31: 27) (M60.80)
3. Polymyalgia rheumatica (M35.3)
4. Localised myositis ossificans (M61.0)
5. Fibrositis and nodular fasciitis; myositis proliferans or pseudotumour (Kern 1960 Archives of Pathology 69: 209; Enzinger, Dulcey 1967 Cancer 20: 2213) (M60.80)
6. ? Myopathy in relapsing panniculitis (Weber–Christian syndrome) (M35.6)
7. Myositis with necrotizing fasciitis (Carruthers et al 1975 British Medical Journal 3: 355) (M35.4)
8. ? Myopathy in psoriasis (Mormum et al 1970 Dermatologia 140: 214)
9. Myopathy in Reye's syndrome (Hanson, Urizar 1977 Annals of Neurology 1: 431) (G93.7)

D. Metabolic myopathies

D-1. Muscle disorders associated with endocrine disease (G73.5)
1. Thyrotoxicosis (G73.53)
    (a) myopathy
    (b) myasthenia gravis (G7.0)
    (c) periodic paralysis, hyperkalaemic (G72.33)
    (d) exophthalmic ophthalmoplegia (infiltrative ophthalmopathy or ophthalmic Graves' disease) (G73.54)
2. Myxoedema (G73.55)
    (a) girdle myopathy
    (b) Debré–Semelaigne syndrome in congenital hypothyroidism (Debré, Semelaigne 1935 American Journal of Diseases of Children 50: 1351) (G73.55)
    (c) Hoffmann syndrome (adults) (Hoffmann, 1897 Deutsche Zeitschrift fur Nervenheilkund 9: 278) (G73.55)
    (d) pseudomyotonia
    (e) ? neuromyopathy following ^{131}I therapy
3. Hypopituitarism with myopathy (G73.58)
4. Acromegaly with muscle hypertrophy or myopathy (Mastaglia et al 1970 Lancet ii: 907) (G73.56)
5. Cushing disease myopathy (and iatrogenic corticosteroid myopathy) (G73.52)
6. ACTH myopathy in Nelson's syndrome (Prineas et al 1968 Quarterly Journal of Medicine 37: 63)
7. Addison's disease with myopathy (G73.57)
8. Primary aldosteronism (with hypokalaemic periodic paralysis) (G72.34)
9. Hyperparathyroidism with myopathy (Cholod et al 1970 American Journal of Medicine 48: 700) (G73.50)
10. Hypoparathyroidism with myopathy (Shane et al 1980 Neurology 30: 192) (G73.51)
11. Myopathy in other forms of metabolic bone disease (G73.58)
    (a) osteomalacia due to:
        (i) idiopathic steatorrhoea
        (ii) malabsorption after partial gastrectomy
        (iii) renal acidosis
        (iv) hypophosphataemia (Schott, Wills 1975 Journal of Neurology, Neurosurgery and Psychiatry 38: 297)
        (v) anticonvulsants (Marsden et al 1973 British Medical Journal 4: 526)
12. Myopathy with calcitonin-secreting medullary carcinoma of the thyroid (Cunliffe et al 1970 American Journal of Medicine 48: 120)

D-2. Heritable myopathies, biochemical abnormality known (G73.6)

1. Glycogen storage disease involving muscle:
   (*a*) glycogenosis type I due to glucose-6-phosphatase deficiency (von Gierke's disease) (232200) (hypotonia but no myopathy) (E74.00)
   (*b*) glycogenosis type II (Pompe's disease) due to amylo-1,4-glucosidase deficiency (232300), maps to 17q23
       (*i*) infantile form
       (*ii*) adult or late-onset variety (Loonen et al 1981 Neurology 31: 1209) (E74.01)
   (*c*) glycogenosis type III (Cori–Forbes disease) due to lack of debrancher enzyme (amylo-1,6-glucosidase) (232400) (DiMauro et al 1979 Annals of Neurology 5: 422) (E74.02)
   (*d*) glycogenosis type IV (Andersen's disease) due to lack of brancher enzyme (1,4-glucan: 1,4-glucan-6-glycosyl transferase) (232500) (Ferguson et al 1983 Journal of the Neurological Sciences 60: 337); adult polyglucosan body myopathy may be related (III.A.3.m.) (E74.03)
   (*e*) Glycogenosis type V (McArdle's disease) due to phosphorylase deficiency (232600), maps to 11q13 (G74.04)
       (*i*) usual form, with onset in childhood or adolescence
       (*ii*) infantile form (DiMauro, Hartlage 1978 Neurology 28: 1124; Cornelio et al 1983 Neurology 33: 1383)
       (*iii*) late-onset myophosphorylase deficiency (Kost, Verity 1980 Muscle and Nerve 3: 195)
   (*f*) glycogenosis type VII (Tarui's disease) due to phosphofructokinase deficiency (G74.06):
       (*i*) typical form, lack of M-subunit (232800) 1cen-q32. (Tarui et al 1965 Biochemical and Biophysical Research Communications 19: 571)
       (*ii*) haemolysis without myopathy, lack of L-subunit (Etiemble et al 1980 Human Genetics 55: 383)
       (*iii*) infantile myopathy (Danon et al 1981 Neurology 31: 1302)
   (*g*) phosphoglycerate kinase deficiency (311800), Xq13 (Bresolin et al 1984 Muscle and Nerve 7: 542) (G74.08)
   (*h*) phosphoglycerate mutase deficiency (261670) (DiMauro et al 1982 Neurology 32: 584) (G74.08)
   (*i*) lactate dehydrogenase deficiency (150000) (Kanno et al 1980 Clinica Chimica Acta 108: 267) (G74.08)
   (*j*) lysosomal glycogen storage disease without acid maltase deficiency (23233) (Danon et al 1981 Neurology 31: 51; Riggs et al 1983 Neurology 33: 873) (G74.08)
   (*k*) mixed enzyme deficiencies (e.g. phosphofructokinase and phosphorylase b kinase — Danon et al 1981 Neurology 31: 1303) (G74.08)
2. Other inherited disorders of carbohydrate metabolism (E74.1):
   (*a*) muscle fructose-1, 6-diphosphatase deficiency (229700) with atypical central core disease (Kar et al 1980 Journal of the Neurological Sciences 48: 243)
   (*b*) myopathy due to glycolytic abnormality involving phosphohexoisomerase (172400) (Satoyoshi, Kowa 1967 Archives of Neurology 17: 248)
3. Myoadenylate deaminase deficiency (with cramps and exertional myalgia) (254740) (DiMauro et al 1980 Journal of the Neurological Sciences 47: 191; Kelemen et al 1982 Neurology 32: 857) (E79.84)
4. Familial periodic paralysis and related syndromes (G72.3):

   (*a*) hypokalaemic periodic paralysis (170400) (G72.30)
   (*b*) hyperkalaemic periodic paralysis (adynamia episodica hereditaria) (170500), sometimes with cardiac arrhythmia (Lisak et al 1972 Neurology (1972) 22: 810; Gould et al 1985 Neurology 35: 208); maps to 17q13.1–q13.3, allelic with paramyotonia congenita; mutations in gene for sodium channel alpha subunit. Autosomal dominant myotonia (160800) may be another variation (G72.31)
   (*c*) normokalaemic periodic paralysis (170600) (variant of b) (Poskanzer, Kerr 1961 American Journal of Medicine 31: 328) (G72.32)
   (*d*) myotonic periodic paralysis (paramyotonia congenita) (168300), allelic with hyperkalaemic periodic paralysis (G71.15)
   (*e*) thyrotoxic periodic paralysis (170600) (G72.33)
5. Mitochondrial and lipid storage myopathies (modified from Morgan-Hughes 1986 In: AG Engel and Banker (eds), Myology, pp. 1709–1743 (G71.3)
   (*a*) Lipid storage myopathies of uncertain origin (255100) (G73.6)
       (*i*) Chanarin–Miranda syndrome: triglyceride lipid storage myopathy and congenital ichthyosis (275630) (Chanarin et al 1975 British Medical Journal 1: 203; Miranda et al 1979 Muscle and Nerve 2: 1)
       (*ii*) congenital myopathies with lipid storage (Jerusalem, Spiess 1975 Journal of the Neurological Sciences 24: 273)
       (*iii*) associated with recognized disease (glycogenosis type I, hyper B-lipoproteinaemia, pyruvate decarboxylase deficiency, arthrogryposis)
       (*iv*) autosomal recessive lipid storage myopathy with electrical myotonia, lipid in leucocytes and defect in long-chain fatty acid utilization (Snyder et al 1982 Neurology 32: 1106)
       (*v*) autosomal dominant lipid storage neuromyopathy with systemic abnormality of fat metabolism (Askanas et al 1985 Neurology 35: 66)
       (*vi*) idiopathic lipid storage myopathies with glycogen storage, and structurally abnormal mitochondria (255100)
       (*vii*) lipid storage myopathy with acyl co-A dehydrogenase, short chain (SCAD) deficiency (201470), (Turnbull et al 1984 New England Journal of Medicine 311: 1232) also long chain (LCAD) (Rocchicciou et al 1990 Pediatric Research 28: 657); and medium chain (MCAD) (Stanley C A, Wale D E, Coates P M et al 1983 17: 877–84), or multiple acyl-coA dehydrogenase deficiency (glutaric acidemia type II with myopathy) (DiDonato et al 1989 Annals of Neurology 25: 479)
   (*b*) alpha-glycerophosphate dehydrogenase deficiency (possible) (DiMauro et al 1973 Archives of Neurology 29: 170)
   (*c*) short chain 3-hydroxyacl-coA dehydrogenase deficiency (SCHAD) with encephalopathy, cardiopathy and myoglobinuria (Tein et al 1991 Annals of Neurology 30: 415)
   (*d*) deficiencies involving the carnitine, acyl-carnitine carrier system:
       (*i*) muscle carnitine deficiency (Engel, Angelini 1973 Science 173: 899) (212160) (E71.34)
       (*ii*) systemic carnitine deficiency (Karpati et al 1975

Neurology 25: 16) — with cardiomyopathy (Walker et al 1982 Journal of Pediatrics 101: 700). Systemic carnitine deficiency may be due to a defect in renal reabsorption of carnitine (212140) or lack of medium chain acyl co-A dehydrogenase (201450), or impaired carnitine transport across the plasma membrane (Treem et al 1988 New England Journal of Medicine 319: 1321; Tein et al 1990 Pediatric Research 28: 247) (E71.35)

   (*iii*) partial muscle carnitine deficiencies or defect in carnitine uptake (Stanley et al 1991 Annals of Neurology 30: 709)

   (*iv*) carnitine palmitoyl transferase (CPT) deficiency (255110, 255120) (DiMauro, Melis-DiMauro 1973 Science 182: 929) including heterogeneous forms (DiDonato et al 1981 Journal of the Neurological Sciences 50: 207); CPT II deficiency with normal CPT I (Scholte et al 1979 Journal of the Neurological Sciences 40: 39; Trevisan et al 1984 Neurology 34: 353); CPT deficiency with myoglobinuria and respiratory failure (Bertorini et al 1980 Neurology 30: 263) and with cold-induced myoglobinuria (Brownell et al 1979 Canadian Journal of Medical Science 6: 367). The gene for liver CPT maps to 1q12–1pter (Finocchiaro et al 1991 Proceedings of the National Academy of Sciences USA 88: 661) (E71.32)

   (*v*) combined carnitine and CPT deficiencies

(*d*) defects of mitochondrial substrate utilization (E74.4, G71.38):

   (*i*) pyruvate decarboxylase deficiency (208800) (E74.40)

   (*ii*) dihydrolipoyl transacetylase deficiency (245348)

   (*iii*) dihydrolipoyl dehydrogenase deficiency (246900)

   (*iv*) pyruvate dehydrogenase phosphatase deficiency (E74.400)

   (*v*) pyruvate carboxylase deficiency

   (*vi*) carnitine acetyltransferase deficiency (E71.31)

Note: Many disorders in this group cause myopathy but the clinical picture is often dominated by progressive encephalopathy, hypotonia, lactic acidosis and respiratory insufficiency.

(*e*) defects of the respiratory chain (G71.30):

   (*i*) defects of NADH oxidation

   (*ii*) cytochrome b deficiency

   (*iii*) cytochrome c oxidase (aa$_3$) deficiency

   (*iv*) combined cytochrome deficiencies (aa$_3$ + b)

   (*v*) encephalomyopathy with decreased succinate-cytochrome c reductase deficiency (Riggs et al 1984 Neurology 34: 48)

(*f*) defects of energy conservation and transduction (G71.33):

   (*i*) hypermetabolic mitochondrial myopathy (Luft's disease)

   (*ii*) other mitochrondrial myopathies with 'loose coupling'

   (*iii*) mitochondrial ATPase deficiency

   (*iv*) myopathy due to a malate-aspartate shuttle defect (Hayes et al 1987 Journal of the Neurological Sciences 82: 27)

   (*v*) mixed respiratory chain defects

Note: The mitochondrial myopathies in e and f are associated with diverse clinical syndromes that include ophthalmoplegia, severe hypotonia, cramps and myoglobinuria, exercise-induced myalgia and limb weakness, occurring at different stages of life. Specific syndromes of uncertain biochemical abnormality include the Kearns–Sayre syndrome and progressive external ophthalmoplegia, which are associated with deletions of mitochondrial DNA. Other syndromes are associated with point mutations of mtDNA, including MELAS, the acronym for 'mitochondrial encephalomyopathy, lactic acidosis and strokes' (Pavlakis et al 1984 Annals of Neurology 16: 481); Fukuhara's syndrome, which comprises myoclonus epilepsy and ragged red fibres (MERRF), and a syndrome of neuropathy, ataxia, and retinitis pigmentosa (NARP). The disorders have been reviewed by Moraes et al 1991 In: Appel (ed) Current neurology, vol 11, St Louis, Mosby Year Book, pp 83–119. See Appendix A.

  6. Malignant hyperthermia, induced by halothane, suxamethonium, ketamine, psychotropic agents and many other anaesthetic agents and drugs (180901, 145600), ryanodine receptor (19q2–q13.2) (Lane, Mastaglia 1978 Lancet ii: 562). Central core disease (117100) maps to the same locus and patients with that congenital myopathy are especially liable to attacks of malignant hyperthermia (Y48, T88.3, G71.84)

  7. Progressive muscle spasm, alopecia, diarrhoea and malabsorption (Satoyoshi's disease) (Satoyoshi 1978 Neurology 28: 458) (G73.6)

  8. Myopathy in lysine-cystinuria (diaminopentanuria) (222350) (Clara, Lowenthal 1966 Journal of the Neurological Sciences 3: 433) (G73.6)

  9. Myopathy in xanthinuria (278300) (Chalmers et al 1969 Quarterly Journal of Medicine 38: 493) (G73.6)

10. Myopathy in Lafora disease (254780) (Coleman et al 1974 Archives of Neurology 31: 396) (G73.7)

11. Myopathy with tubular aggregates, often associated with myalgia (Brumback et al 1981 Journal of Neurology, Neurosurgery and Psychiatry 44: 250; Rohkamm et al 1988 Neurology 33: 331; Niakan et al 1985 Journal of Neurology, Neurosurgery and Psychiatry 48: 882) (G71.25)

12. Cytoplasmic body myopathy (147420) (Kinoshita et al 1975 Archives of Neurology 32: 417; Patel et al 1983 Journal of the Neurological Sciences 60: 281) (G71.800)

13. Benign reducing body myopathy (Oh et al 1983 Muscle and Nerve 6: 278) (G71.281)

D-3. Other metabolic myopathies

1. Alcoholic myopathy (G27.1)

   (*a*) acute, with myoglobinuria

   (*b*) subacute or chronic proximal (Hudgson 1984 British Medical Journal 1: 585)

   (*c*) hypokalaemic (Rubinstein, Wainapel 1977 Archives of Neurology 34: 553)

2. Nutritional myopathy (G73.7, G73.70)

   (*a*) protein deficiency; malnutrition due to anorexia nervosa or malabsorption

   (*b*) human myopathy due to vitamin E deficiency (Neville et al 1983 Neurology 33: 483)

   (*c*) chronic myopathy with hypocalcaemia and hypophosphataemia

3. Myopathy in chronic renal failure (Floyd et al 1974 Quarterly Journal of Medicine 43: 509).

4. Acute polymyopathy during total parenteral nutrition (Stewart, Hensley 1981 British Medical Journal 2: 1578)

5. Potassium depletion myopathy (Comi et al 1985 Muscle and Nerve 8: 17)
6. Carnitine deficiency induced during haemodialysis (Battistella et al 1978 Lancet i: 939)
7. Riboflavin-responsive lipid myopathy with carnitine deficiency (Carroll et al 1981 Neurology 31: 1557)
8. Myoglobinuria (rhabdomyolysis) other than that due to glycogen storage disease, mitochondrial or lipid storage myopathies and CPT deficiency (see Rowland 1984 Canadian Journal of Neurological Science 11: 1) (G72.80)
   (a) exertion (including military training, running, skiing, anterior tibial syndrome, status epilepticus, electric shock, myoclonus, severe dystonia) (T04)
   (b) crush or ischaemic injury to muscle (see above) (T04)
   (c) metabolic depression or distortion including CO or drug intoxication, diabetic ketoacidosis, hyperosmolar states, renal tubular acidosis, hyper- and hyponatraemia, hypokalaemia and hypophosphataemia)
   (d) due to drugs and toxins (see above) (including the ingestion of quail — Bateman 1977 US Office of Naval Research) (G72.0)
   (e) abnormalities of body temperature (including hypothermia due to cold or hypothyroidism, or fever due to toxins, vaccines, heat stroke, malignant hyperpyrexia or the malignant neuroleptic syndrome)
   (f) infections (including viral, bacterial and mycoplasma infections and the toxic shock syndrome)
   (g) autoimmune muscle disease (polymyositis and dermatomyositis) (M33)
   (h) idiopathic recurrent myoglobinuria, sometimes leading to myopathy with persistent weakness (Korein et al 1959 Neurology 9: 767; Favara et al 1967 American Journal of Medicine 42: 196; Bermils et al 1983 Neurology 33: 1613) (G72.81)
9. Chronic myopathy due to drugs (chloroquine, emetine, steroids, penicillin, vincristine, colchicine; repeated intramuscular injections of meperidine or pentazocine) (G72.0)

E. *Myopathy associated with malignant disease (G73.2)*
1. Carcinomatous myopathy (other than polymyositis)
2. Lambert–Eaton syndrome (G73.1)
3. Carcinomatous embolic myopathy (Heffner 1971 Neurology 21: 841)
4. Proximal myopathy due to discrete carcinomatous metastases in muscle (Doshi, Fowler 1983 Journal of Neurology, Neurosurgery and Psychiatry 46: 358)
5. Myopathy in the carcinoid syndrome (Swash et al 1975 Archives of Neurology 32: 572) (G73.7)

F. *Myopathy associated with myasthenia gravis (G70.0)*

G. *Myopathy in thalassaemia (Logothetis et al 1972 Neurology 22: 294) (G73.7)*

H. *Other disorders of muscle of unknown or uncertain aetiology*
1. Acute muscle necrosis
   (a) of unknown cause
   (b) in chronic alcoholism (G72.1)
   (c) in carcinoma (Urich, Wilkinson 1970 Journal of Neurology, Neurosurgery and Psychiatry 33: 398)
2. Amyloid myopathy (E85)
   (a) primary familial
   (b) primary sporadic (sometimes causes pseudohypertrophy of muscle) (Ringel, Claman 1982 Archives of Neurology 39: 413)
   (c) in myelomatosis
   (d) with angiopathy (Bruni et al 1977 Canadian Journal of Neurological Sciences 2: 77)
3. Disuse atrophy (G73.70)
4. Muscle cachexia (in wasting diseases and in the elderly) (G73.70)
5. Muscle wasting in contralateral cerebral lesions (particularly of parietal lobe)
6. Granular nuclear inclusion body disease affecting skeletal muscle and the nervous system (Schroder et al 1985 Muscle and Nerve 8: 52)

I. *Tumours of muscle*
1. Rhabdomyoma (D21)
2. Rhabdomyoscarcoma (C49)
   (a) Adult pleomorphic type
   (b) Embryonal botryoid type
   (c) Embryonal alveolar type
3. Desmoid fibroma
4. Alveolar sarcoma
5. Angioma (D18)
6. Other connective tissue tumours occasionally occurring in muscle

IV. DISORDERS OF SUPRASPINAL TONAL REGULATION WHICH MAY MIMIC NEUROMUSCULAR DISORDERS

A. *Muscular hypertrophy, extrapyramidal disorders and mental deficiency* (de Lange 1934 American Journal of Diseases of Children 48: 243)
B. *Prader–Willli syndrome (176270) (Q87.15)*
C. *Hypotonia in mental defect*
D. *Hypotonia in metabolic disorders*
E. *Hypotonia in cerebral palsy (atonic diplegia)*
F. *Hypotonia in cerebral diplegia and other cerebellar ataxias*
G. *Hypotonia in rheumatic chorea*
H. *Hypotonia in acrodynia (Pink's disease)*
I. *Hypotonia in the cerebrohepatorenal syndrome (Bowen et al 1964 Johns Hopkins Medical Journal 114: 402)*

APPENDIX A: Diseases of mitochondrial DNA

McKusick no. WHO (ICD-IONA)	Name of syndrome	Abbreviation	Mutation
165100	Kearns–Sayre (G71.3)	KSS	Deletion
165000	Progressive external ophthalmoplegia (G71.05)	PEO	Deletion
308900	Leber hereditary optic atrophy (H47.21)	LHON	Mutation
254775	Myoclonus epilepsy, ragged red fibres	MERRF	Mutation

APPENDIX A: *Cont'd*

McKusick no. WHO (ICD-IONA)	Name of syndrome	Abbreviation	Mutation
251910	Mitochondrial encephalopathy, lactic acidosis, stroke	MELAS	Mutation
NL	*Mitochondrial neuromyopathy, gastrointestinal encephalomyopathy	MNGIE	Not known
	*Mitochondrial encephalomyopathy, peripheral neuropathy, ophthalmoplegia, pseudo-obtruction	MEPOP	Not known
NL	Neuropathy, ataxia, retinitis pigmentosa	NARP	Mutation
NL	Diabetes, ataxia, deafness	DAD	Mutation
NL	Cytochrome oxidase deficiency (71.30)		Mutation
266150	Leigh's syndrome (G31.81)		
NL	Benign infantile myopathy		
NL	Fatal infantile myopathy		
NL	Depletion of mtDNA		Not known

NL, not listed; *both names refer to same syndrome; some show multiple deletions.

APPENDIX B: Charcot–Marie–Tooth Diseases (CMT); hereditary motor and sensory neuropathies (HMSN)

WFN and WHO (ICD 10 NA) no.	McKusick no.	Dyck no.	Abbreviations	Name	Map position
G 60.00; III.A.1	118200	1	CMT1, HMSN-1	Charcot–Marie–Tooth (with slow conduction) autosomal dominant	
	118220		CMT 1A		17p12-p11.2
			CMT 1B		1q21.1–q23.3
G 60.01; I.A.1.18		2	CMT, HMSN-2	Neuronal form	
	118210		CMT 2A	Autosomal dominant	
	271120		CMT 2B	Autosomal recessive	
G 60.02	145900	3	CMT-3, HMSN-3	Hypertrophic, infantile (Dejerine–Sottas)	17p12–p11.2 or 1q21–q23.3
G 60.06; I.A.1.5	214400	4	CMT-4, HMSN-4	Dyck lists the multisystem Refsum syndrome as CMT-4; McKusick lists an autosomal recessive form of CMT as CMT-4.	
G 60.03; I.A.1.30	182700	5	CMT-5, HMSN-5	Spastic paraplegia with amyotrophy.	
	275900			Autosomal dominant (Silver's syndrome). Autosomal recessive (Troyer's syndrome).	
G 60.04		6	CMT-6, HMSN-6	CMT with optic atrophy	
G 60.05		7	CMT-7, HMSN-7	CMT with retinitis pigmentosa	
	310490		CMT-X1 HMSN-X1	X-linked dominant	Xq13
	302801		CMT-X2 HMSN-X2	X-linked recessive CMT	Xp22.2, Xq26
	302800				
			'Others'	All others are listed as forms of spinal muscular atrophy or are denoted by associated features such as deafness, skin changes, ptosis, or tremor	

REFERENCES

Adrian R H, Marshall M W 1976 Action potentials reconstructed in normal and myotonic muscle fibres. Journal of Physiology 258: 125

Albers J W, Allen A A, Bastron J A, Daube J R 1981 Limb myokymia. Muscle and Nerve 4: 494

André-Thomas A, Chesni Y, Dargassies S S-A 1960 The neurological examination of the infant. National Spastics Society, London

Asbury A K, Gilliatt R W 1984 Peripheral nerve disorders — a practical approach. Butterworth, London

Ashizawa T, Butler I J, Harati Y, Roongta S M 1983 A dominantly inherited syndrome with continuous motor neuron discharges. Annals of Neurology 13: 285

Auger R G, Daube J R, Gomez M R, Lambert E H 1984 Hereditary form of sustained muscle activity of peripheral nerve origin causing generalised myokymia and muscle stiffness. Annals of Neurology 15: 13

Barohn R J, Miller R G, Griggs R C 1991 Autosomal recessive distal dystrophy. Neurology 41: 1365

Bickerstaff E R 1980 Neurological examination in clinical practice, 4th edn. Blackwell, Oxford

Cogan D G 1978 Neurology of the ocular muscles, 3rd edn. Thomas, Springfield, Illinois

de Lange C 1934 Congenital hypertrophy of muscles, extrapyramidal motor disturbances and mental deficiency. American Journal of Diseases of Childhood 48: 243

Denny-Brown D, Pennybacker J B 1938 Fibrillation and fasciculation in voluntary muscle. Brain 61: 311

Denny-Brown D, Nevin S 1941 The phenomenon of myotonia. Brain 64: 1

Dubowitz V 1978 Muscle disorders in childhood. Saunders, London

Edwards R H T, McDonnell M 1974 Hand-held dynamometer for evaluating voluntary muscle function. Lancet ii: 757

Fetell M R, Smallberg G, Lewis L D, Lovelace R E, Hays A P, Rowland L P 1982 A benign motor neuron disorder: delayed cramps and fasciculation after poliomyelitis or myelitis. Annals of Neurology 11: 532

Fleet W S, Watson R T 1986 From benign fasciculation and cramps to motor neuron disease. Neurology 36: 997

Gamstorp I 1984 Pediatric neurology, 2nd edn. Appleton-Century-Crofts, New York

Gamstorp I, Wohlfart G 1959 A syndrome characterised by myokymia, myotonia, muscular wasting and increased perspiration. Acta Psychiatrica Scandinavica 34: 181

Gardner-Medwin D, Hudgson P, Walton J N 1967 Benign spinal muscular atrophy arising in childhood and adolescence. Journal of the Neurological Sciences 5: 121

Gardner-Medwin D, Walton J N 1969 Myokymia with impaired muscular relaxation. Lancet i: 127

Glaser J 1990 Neuro-ophthalmology, 2nd edn. Lippincott, Philadelphia

Gordon N S 1976 Paediatric neurology for the clinician. Spastics International Medical Publications, Heinemann, London

Gray's Anatomy 1967 34th edn. Davies D V, Coupland R E (eds) Longmans, London

Haerer A F 1992 DeJong's The neurologic examination, 5th edn. Lippincott, Philadelphia

Isaacs H 1961 A syndrome of continuous muscle fibre activity. Journal of Neurology, Neurosurgery and Psychiatry 24: 319

Jackson D L, Satya-Murti S, Davis L, Drachman D B 1979 Isaacs syndrome with laryngeal involvement: an unusual presentation of myokymia. Neurology (Minneapolis) 29: 1612

Jennekens F G I, Tomlinson B E, Walton J N 1971 Histochemical aspects of five limb muscles in old age: an autopsy study. Journal of the Neurological Sciences 14: 259

Lane R J M, Turnbull D M, Welch J, Walton J N 1986 A double-blind, placebo-controlled, crossover study of verapamil in exertional muscle pain.

Lehoczky T, Halasy M, Simon G, Harmos G 1965 Glycogenic myopathy: a case of skeletal muscle-glycogenosis in twins. Journal of the Neurological Sciences 2: 366

Leigh P N, Rothwell J C, Traub M, Marsden C D 1980 A patient with reflex myoclonus and muscle rigidity: 'jerking stiff-man syndrome'. Journal of Neurology, Neurosurgery and Psychiatry 43: 1125

Leigh R J, Zee D S 1991 The neurology of eye movements, 2nd edn. F A Davis, Philadelphia

Leyburn P, Walton J N 1959 The treatment of myotonia: a controlled trial. Brain 82: 81

McEvoy K M 1991 Stiff-man syndrome. Seminars in Neurology 11: 197

Matthews W B 1966 Facial myokymia. Journal of Neurology, Neurosurgery and Psychiatry 29: 35

Medical Research Council 1986 Aids to the examination of the peripheral nervous system, Memorandum no 45, 3rd edn. Baillière Tindall, Eastbourne

Mertens H-G, Zschocke S 1965 Neuromyotonie. Klinische Wochenschrift 43: 917

Odel J G, Winterkorn J M S, Behrens M M 1991 The sleep test for myasthenia gravis. A safe alternative to Tensilon. Journal of Clinical Neuro-ophthalmology 11: 288

O'Doherty D S, Schellinger D, Raptopoulos V 1977 Computed tomographic patterns of pseudohypertrophic muscular dystrophy: preliminary results. Journal of Computer Assisted Tomography 1: 482

Pact V, Sirotkin-Roses M, Beatus J 1984 The muscle testing handbook. Little Brown, Boston, Toronto

Paine R S, Oppé T E 1966 Neurological examination of children. National Spastics Society and Heinemann, London

Perkoff G T, Hardy P, Velez-Garcia E 1966 Reversible acute muscular syndrome in chronic alcoholism. New England Journal of Medicine 274: 1277

Prineas J, Hall R, Barwick D D, Watson A J 1968 Myopathy associated with pigmentation following adrenalectomy for Cushing's syndrome. Quarterly Journal of Medicine 37: 63

Ross Russell R W, Wiles C M 1985 Neurology. Integrated Clinical Science Series. Heinemann, London

Rowland L P 1985 Muscle cramps, spasms, and stiffness. Revue Neurologique (Paris) 141: 261

Salick A I, Pearson C M 1967 Electrical silence of myoidema. Neurology (Minneapolis) 17: 899

Satoyoshi E, Kowa H 1967 A myopathy due to glycolytic abnormality. Archives of Neurology 17: 248

Taylor D J, Brosnan M J, Arnold D L et al 1988 Ca^{2+}-ATPase deficiency in a patient with an exertional muscle pain syndrome. Journal of Neurology, Neurosurgery and Psychiatry 51: 1425

Valli G, Barbieri S, Cappa S, Pellegrini G, Scarlato G 1983 Syndromes of abnormal muscular activity: overlap between continuous muscle fibre activity and the stiff man syndrome. Journal of Neurology, Neurosurgery and Psychiatry 46: 241

Vignos P J, Archibald K C 1960 Maintenance of ambulation in childhood muscular dystrophy. Journal of Chronic Diseases 12: 273

Wallis W E, Poznak A V, Plum F 1970 Generalized muscular stiffness, fasciculation, and myokymia of peripheral nerve origin. Archives of Neurology 22: 430

Walton J N 1981 Diffuse exercise-induced muscle pain of undetermined cause relieved by verapamil. Lancet i: 993

Walton J N 1985 Brain's diseases of the nervous system, 9th edn. Oxford University Press, Oxford, p 116

Welch L K, Appenzeller O, Bicknell J M 1972 Peripheral neuropathy with myokymia, sustained muscular contraction, and continuous motor unit activity. Neurology (Minneapolis) 22: 161

Williamson E, Brooke M H 1972 Myokymia and the motor unit: a histochemical study. Archives of Neurology 26: 11

Wilson J, Walton J N 1959 Some muscular manifestations of hypothyroidism. Journal of Neurology, Neurosurgery and Psychiatry 22: 320

World Federation of Neurology: Research Group on Neuromuscular Diseases 1968 Classification of the neuromuscular disorders. Journal of the Neurological Sciences 6: 165

Zisfein J, Sivak M, Aron A M, Bender A N 1983 Isaacs' syndrome with muscle hypertrophy reversed by phenytoin therapy. Archives of Neurology 40: 241

14. The muscular dystrophies

D. Gardner-Medwin   J. Walton

INTRODUCTION

Definition

The term 'muscular dystrophy', introduced by Erb (1891), is used for a group of progressive, genetically determined, primary, degenerative myopathies (Walton 1961). Each of the known types has a more or less specific clinical pattern in terms of its rate of progression, its pattern of selective muscle involvement and its mode of inheritance. Recent discoveries, discussed below, of the location of the mutant genes and the specific structural-protein deficiencies in some types of muscular dystrophy, starting with the discovery of dystrophin deficiency in Duchenne muscular dystrophy in 1987, have presaged a change in both the definition of the muscular dystrophies as a whole and their classification. But no new definition or classification is possible yet, and for clinical purposes the 1961 definition is comprehensive. Definitions of the individual types are given below.

History

In 1836 Conte & Gioja described two brothers with progressive muscular weakness who were severely disabled by the age of 8 and 10 years and profoundly so by the time of their death at about 17–18 years. There was widespread muscle atrophy but the deltoids and gastrocnemius muscles were three times the ordinary volume. They had cardiac enlargement. These are regarded as the earliest cases of what is now called Duchenne muscular dystrophy. Meryon (1852) gave a clear account of the disease in young boys and demonstrated that it was due to 'granular degeneration' of the muscles without changes in the anterior horns of the spinal cord or in the motor roots. Later, Duchenne (1868) gave a vivid description of this disorder, now given his name, and Gowers' (1879) was the first comprehensive account in English and is still one of the finest. Both Duchenne and Gowers emphasised the 'pseudohypertrophic' enlargement of certain muscles. Meryon (1864; case 87) reported the first pedigree which indicated what we now recognise as X-linked inheritance and Bateson (1909) used this disorder to illustrate the relevant Mendelian principles. In 1979 Lindenbaum et al located the gene at the Xp21 region of the X-chromosome, in 1987 Kunkel's team at Harvard cloned it, and within a few months the structure of the gene product, named dystrophin, had been identified (Koenig et al 1987, 1988). Earlier Becker & Keiner (1955) had proposed that the benign form of X-linked pseudohypertrophic muscular dystrophy, of which examples had been reported by many authors including Meryon (1852; p 81), should be firmly distinguished from the Duchenne type. However, cases of intermediate severity were distinguished (Rideau 1978) and Kingston et al (1983) showed that the Becker and Duchenne types were allelic. When abnormalities of dystrophin were discovered in Becker cases there was again a tendency to think in terms of a spectrum of severity until Bushby et al (1993, 1994) identified a distinctive gene deletion in typical Becker cases which should perhaps be regarded as definitive. Confusion reigns over the names of these disorders. 'Xp21 dystrophies' and 'dystrophinopathies' offend both the eye and the ear. We suggest that 'Meryon muscular dystrophy' for the group as a whole, and 'Meryon–Duchenne' and 'Meryon–Becker' muscular dystrophy for its appropriate components, would pleasantly honour the first man to describe both types and would recognise the hereditary pattern and the significance of the pathology.

The classical description of the facioscapulo-humeral form was by Landouzy & Dejerine (1884) but much earlier cases were recorded and photographed by Duchenne (1855, 1862); indeed a clearly identifiable case, with a detailed account of the surface anatomy, is to be found in a lay publication of 1825, and is effectively the earliest definite case of muscular dystrophy to have been published (Hone 1825). Bell (1943) emphasised the autosomal dominant mode of inheritance. Between 1988 and 1991 international collaboration of a number of research teams resulted in the location of the gene at 4q35-qtr (Wijmenga et al 1991, Upadhyaya et al 1991).

Leyden (1876) and Möbius (1879) described a familial form of degeneration affecting the muscles of the pelvic girdle. In 1884 Erb described a juvenile or scapulohumeral form of the disorder, and stressed that this disease was due to a primary degeneration of the muscles which he later (1891) named muscular dystrophy. Stevenson (1953), in a survey of muscular dystrophy in Northern Ireland, divided his cases into pseudohypertrophic and facioscapulohumeral types and other 'autosomal limb-girdle muscular dystrophies'. Walton & Nattrass (1954) used Stevenson's term to define a limb-girdle type of muscular dystrophy, autosomal recessive in inheritance, comprising the types of Leyden, Möbius and Erb. In time it became apparent that within this category were concealed a number of importantly different disorders, including manifesting female carriers of the Duchenne gene, sporadic cases of Becker dystrophy and a number of subtly different autosomal recessive and autosomal dominant disorders. Only within the last few years has it been possible to define some of these more precisely, as will be discussed below, but it is now clear that the term 'limb-girdle muscular dystrophy' should be abandoned, or at most used broadly, in the stevensonian sense, as a provisional label until a detailed diagnosis is reached. Such a preliminary categorisation should never be used as a basis for genetic counselling. Very recently, as will be discussed below, abnormalities of proteins related to dystrophin have been found to be concerned in the pathology of some autosomal recessive muscular dystrophies, and in some types, gene localisation has been achieved.

Howard (1908) and Batten (1909) suggested that some cases of amyotonia congenita (Oppenheim 1900) were the result of a simple atrophic variety of congenital muscular dystrophy. In 1930 Ullrich reported a distinct 'atonic-sclerotic' type of congenital muscular dystrophy and later another variant associated with cerebral anomalies was reported from Japan by Fukuyama et al (1960). This last type, though congenital in onset and autosomal recessive in inheritance, is severely progressive and has a number of Duchenne-like clinical features, so the recent discovery of a defect in a sarcolemmal 'dystrophin-associated protein' in Fukuyama muscular dystrophy (Matsumura et al 1993) as well as in the, also Duchenne-like, North African type of autosomal recessive childhood muscular dystrophy (Matsumura et al 1992) begins to suggest that a family of related muscular dystrophies exists, with different modes of inheritance, but with a similar underlying molecular pathology.

Welander (1951) gave a full account of a distal muscular dystrophy occurring in Sweden and later two other forms of distal muscular dystrophy were distinguished. A scapuloperoneal distribution of muscular weakness is seen in certain cases of spinal muscular atrophy, of which it seems to form a distinct subtype. In some kindreds a similar disorder of myopathic origin constitutes, in effect, another form of muscular dystrophy (Seitz 1957). It is now apparent that both X-linked and autosomal dominant varieties of scapuloperoneal myopathy exist, the former first characterised by Emery & Dreifuss (1966).

'Muscular dystrophy' in the external ocular muscles was reported by Hutchinson (1879) and by Fuchs (1890). Victor et al (1962) delineated oculopharyngeal muscular dystrophy, separating it from the other ocular myopathies. The discovery in recent years that mitochondrial disorders are responsible for most, if not all, cases of ocular myopathy and many with an oculopharyngeal presentation has made their inclusion with the muscular dystrophies debatable.

Classification

Classification consists in listing those disorders which conform to the operational definition of muscular dystrophy and which seem to be separate entities on genetic, clinical and pathological grounds.

In listing the muscular dystrophies it is customary to include the 'congenital muscular dystrophies', although they infringe the definition since they are by no means always progressive.

Conversely some of the genetically determined 'congenital myopathies', such as nemaline myopathy, are often slowly progressive, thus falling within our definition, yet because of their different and characteristic histology they have never been called muscular dystrophies. Furthermore the concept of primary degenerative disorders in general is being eroded by the discovery of underlying specific metabolic disorders in many conditions. As we mentioned above, the conditions once called the ocular and oculopharyngeal types of muscular dystrophy are now recognised to be mitochondrial disorders and are named, classified and alloted to a different chapter accordingly. Myotonic dystrophy differs in so many respects from the 'pure' muscular dystrophies described here that it too is discussed separately (in Ch. 15). In the list that follows some of the less well-established clinical types are qualified with question marks. Wherever possible each disorder is given the catalogue number used in McKusick's 'Mendelian inheritance in man' (1992) and some category numbers in the International Classification of Disease (ICD-10 NA) will be found in the appendix to Chapter 13.

The muscular dystrophies

(a) X-linked muscular dystrophies
     Meryon   ('dystrophinopathies')   (MIM 310200)
          Duchenne
          Becker
          Intermediate cases
          Manifesting female carriers
     Emery–Dreifuss (MIM 310300)
     Ji (MIM 310095)
     ? Hereditary myopathy limited to females (MIM 309950)
(b) Autosomal recessive muscular dystrophies
     Autosomal recessive in childhood (North African type) (part of MIM 253700). Defect — ? a dystrophin-associated protein
     ?Autosomal recessive in childhood (Western type)(part of MIM 253700)
     Hutterite type (MIM 254110)
     Indiana Amish/Reunion type (part of MIM 253600) gene location 15q
     ?Late onset proximal (lower limbs) (part of

MIM 253600)
Scapulohumeral (part of MIM 253600)
Distal (MIM 254130)
Congenital (Western type) (includes MIM 253900)
Ullrich (MIM 254090)
Eichsfeld (MIM 253850)
Fukuyama (MIM 253800). Defect — ? a dystrophin-associated protein
Walker–Warburg syndrome (MIM 236670 & 253280)

(c) Autosomal dominant muscular dystrophies
Facioscapulohumeral (MIM 158900)
Benign scapuloperoneal (MIM 181430)
Severe scapuloperoneal with cardiomyopathy (MIM 181350)
Gilchrist (late onset proximal, with dysarthria) (part of MIM 159000) — gene location 5q31
? Other late-onset proximal types (part of MIM 159000)
Benign with finger flexion contractures (Bethlem) (MIM 158810)
? Barnes type (MIM 158800)
? Hastings type (with intracellular capillaries) (MIM 159050)
? Quadriceps myopathy (MIM 310450)
Distal (adult-onset) (MIM 160500)
Distal (juvenile) (MIM 160300)
(Ocular) (MIM 165100)
(Oculopharyngeal) (MIM 164300)
(Myotonic) (MIM 160900)

General principles of diagnosis

An unqualified diagnosis of 'muscular dystrophy' is never justifiable. Every case must be allotted firmly to one of the categories listed above; any which seem not to be typical of any specific type should be regarded with great suspicion and should be thoroughly investigated, a point of great importance because several of the other (non-dystrophic) myopathic disorders are treatable.

The differential diagnosis of muscular dystrophy from other disorders is considered in detail in Chapter 13. Special consideration should be given to distinguishing the spinal muscular atrophies, the pseudo-myopathic forms of genetic myasthenia, polymyositis, the congenital myopathies, mitochondrial, lipid-storage and glycogen-storage myopathies and endocrine myopathies, especially those associated with hypothyroidism, hyperthyroidism and metabolic bone disease.

In the early stages of a muscular dystrophy, or in any doubtful case, a firm diagnosis should be made only after investigation, including estimation of serum creatine kinase (CK) activity and muscle biopsy. The discovery of a gene deletion may be diagnostic of one of the Meryon group of dystrophies but, without a muscle biopsy, may give little or no indication of the prognosis; a full deletion screen is also, at present, not a test that can be reported quickly enough to satisfy the need for urgent diagnosis once muscular dystrophy is suspected, especially in negative cases. The search for a specific deletion in secondary cases is of course a quick and effective means of diagnosis, prenatally or later. In cases in which the serum CK activity is very high, electromyography (EMG) has no diagnostic value, but otherwise it may be helpful in differentiating the less aggressive muscular dystrophies from certain other myopathies or from neurogenic or myasthenic disorders.

Nevertheless, the clinical diagnosis of advanced cases of the well-established types is rarely difficult, especially in the Duchenne and facioscapulohumeral types. It is based upon a clear history of the onset and progression of the symptoms, the pattern of inheritance and a detailed examination of the muscles, which will reveal the pattern of selective muscular wasting and weakness that is characteristic of each type of muscular dystrophy.

In the Duchenne and Becker types, the assay of dystrophin in muscle biopsy material and the discovery of a specific gene deletion in blood leucocyte DNA, provide two complementary techniques for specific diagnosis. The differentiation of the many other varieties of muscular dystrophy should be made, ideally, on clinical, pathological and genetic grounds. Unfortunately this is not always possible; many cases have no family history at all and, furthermore, the different genetic varieties of the disease cannot always be distinguished clinically. The problem is most acute in cases of the various autosomal recessive types and also in their differentiation from some manifesting carriers of the Duchenne gene, in which abnormalities of dystrophin may be subtle.

It is obvious that the differentiation of the X-linked disorders from the similar autosomal recessive types is of great importance for genetic counselling. For example, the daughters of a man with Becker dystrophy are all obligate carriers and may transmit the disease to their sons, whereas the daughters of a man with an autosomal recessive muscular dystrophy carry a very small risk of having affected children. The first stage of the differential diagnosis of many of the other muscular dystrophies, even in their early stages, is based on the age of onset, the rate of progression and the pattern of selective muscle involvement. The technique of CT scanning of muscle is potentially a valuable aid to the analysis of selective muscle involvement and may prove helpful in subtle problems of differential diagnosis in the future (Bulcke et al 1981, Jones et al 1983, Stern et al 1984). Ultrasound imaging, though non-invasive, is much less revealing (Heckmatt et al 1982). Further points in differential diagnosis are discussed in relation to the individual types of muscular dystrophy.

General principles of management

1. The first stage of management is diagnosis. Precision in diagnosis is important, not only to exclude treatable disorders but to provide an accurate basis for prognosis and genetic counselling. Furthermore, diagnosis in any disabled patient involves not only identification of the nature of the disease, but also assessment of the nature and degree of the disability, so that appropriate remedial therapy and services can be provided.

2. Telling the patient, or the parents, the diagnosis and prognosis is a vital stage in management, which will often determine their whole subsequent attitude and approach to the disease. It must be done with sensitivity by a physician who knows the patient personally and has a sound understanding of the disease and its implications. We believe that, in general, adult patients or the parents of affected children should be given a full and accurate account in order to allow them to make constructive plans for the future. It is valuable to balance the bad news with an offer of a programme of management and of continuing practical help and support. Most patients also find some comfort in knowing about the extensive worldwide research into the pathogenesis and potential treatment of the muscular dystrophies.

3. Genetic advice must be offered at the earliest opportunity, not only to the immediate family but, in the X-linked and dominant disorders, to other relatives at risk of having affected children.

4. Useful mobility should be maintained as a major priority. Exercise promotes physical fitness and muscle strength, and we believe that regular exercise should become a lifelong habit for all patients. Obesity should be avoided. Contractures can be at least partly controlled by regular gentle but prolonged stretching. Surgery should be undertaken only with great circumspection, should be as simple and brief as possible and must, above all, be done only in conjunction with well-organised programmes for rapid post-operative mobilisation (see Ch. 23). In general, surgical procedures should be done only when they are likely to provide an important functional benefit which can be obtained in no other way. Anaesthesia should be undertaken only with special precautions to avoid respiratory or cardiac complications. Regular breathing exercises and, where appropriate, postural drainage help to delay the onset of respiratory failure.

5. A bewildering variety of practical aids and equipment for the disabled has become available in recent years. Many are invaluable, but careful assessment and trial may be necessary to solve specific problems for individual patients. Wheelchairs and lifting equipment, in particular, must be selected with professional skill. Occasional but regular consultation with an occupational therapist, sometimes linked with visits to one of the many 'Disabled Living Centres' now established in Britain and other countries, may greatly reduce the handicapping effects of the disease. It is of the greatest psychological importance that patients and their families should know in advance of such solutions to problems, so that they may live expecting to remain reasonably independent and successful. Professional help should also be provided in planning for ideal access and convenience in the home, school or place of work.

6. Innumerable practical and emotional problems, large and small, occur during the lives of severely handicapped people, and these commonly affect other members of the family. It is an important part of the management to make sure that an appropriate professional person is available on a continuing basis to suggest solutions and to provide support. A medical social worker or other paramedical health-worker who is trebly qualified, with knowledge of the services available, with counselling skills and with experience of the disease, can often fill this role and may be able to foresee and prevent many difficulties. He or she can also advise on the many grants and special services available for these patients. We have found that psychiatric help is very rarely needed when emotional support and practical help are provided in this way. In Britain the Muscular Dystrophy Group has set up a network of such 'Family Care Officers' whose work has proved to be one of the most important advances of the last two decades in the management of muscular dystrophy.

7. Employment, marriage and child-bearing are feasible, and often very successful, in patients with muscular dystrophy in whom the onset is in adolescence or later. Employment and marriage are very rare in young men with the Duchenne type, although sheltered employment is possible for a short period in some cases. It is an important responsibility of the doctor at the time of diagnosis of the late-onset muscular dystrophies to advise about the aspects of the prognosis affecting employment, so that appropriate training and careers may be planned in advance.

Additional points in the management of specific types of muscular dystrophy are discussed in subsequent sections of this chapter and the principles of management of neuromuscular disease are described in detail in Chapter 22.

THE TYPES OF MUSCULAR DYSTROPHY

The Meryon group of muscular dystrophies

This comprises the Duchenne and Becker types of muscular dystrophy, and some rarer variants, all of them caused by mutations of a very large gene located on the short arm of the X-chromosome at Xp21, and characterised by defects in the product of that gene, which has been called dystrophin. The Duchenne and Becker types are of about equal prevalence in the population and form distinct entities in the clearly bimodal distribution of severity. Cases of greater severity than Duchenne, or milder involvement than Becker dystrophy are rare and 'intermediate' cases are rather uncommon. There is a small but important group of affected females, almost all of them heterozygous for the gene, who manifest signs of the disease for reasons to be discussed below.

The genetic defect. The gene for Duchenne dystrophy was found to be located at the Xp21 site on the short arm of the X-chromosome when translocations resulting from breaks at that site were found in a small number of affected females (Verellen et al 1977, Lindenbaum et al 1979). This led in due course to the discovery of the first of several cloned DNA sequences closely linked to the Duchenne gene (Murray et al 1982). A number of associated disorders, found in a boy with Duchenne muscular dystrophy — chronic granulomatous disease (cytochrome b-245 deficiency), a form of retinitis pigmentosa, congenital adrenal hypoplasia, glycerol kinase deficiency and the McLeod red cell phenotype (Francke et al 1985) — led to the discovery of a rather large Xp21 deletion. It was largely as a result of hybridisation experiments, using DNA material from this patient, that the gene was cloned (Koenig et al 1987). Confirmation of the genetic defect followed, with the demonstration that the gene product, dystrophin, is absent (or virtually so) from skeletal muscle in Duchenne muscular dystrophy and abnormal in structure in Becker muscular dystrophy. The subject is fully discussed in Chapters 2 and 3.

Pathogenesis. This is still not fully understood. The absence or impairment of dystrophin function appears to result in an abnormal relationship between the muscle fibre membrane and the contractile proteins within, possibly as simple as wrinkling of the former during muscle contraction. Whether because of such repeated membrane trauma or for more complex reasons, defects appear to develop in the sarcolemmal membrane which allow a substance or substances, as yet unknown but possibly calcium, to enter the muscle fibre too freely, and there to activate neutral proteases which, in turn, maintain an excessive degree of muscle catabolism and lead to muscle fibre necrosis (Mokri & Engel 1975, Rowland 1976, Ebashi & Sugita 1978, Wakayama et al 1983, see also Chs 8 and 9).

Severe X-linked (Duchenne) muscular dystrophy

Definition

An X-linked, severe, progressive muscular dystrophy defined by the absence or severe deficiency, in the voluntary muscles, of the protein dystrophin.

This, the commonest muscular dystrophy, is X-linked recessive in inheritance and thus, in its typical form, affects only males. Very rarely, females are affected, apparently because of abnormalities of X-chromosome structure or function, including Turner's syndrome, translocations involving part of one X-chromosome at the Xp21 site, or anomalies of X-chromosome inactivation. It is characterised by: (a) onset of symptoms usually before the fourth year, rarely as late as the seventh; (b) symmetrical and at first selective involvement of the muscles of the pelvic and pectoral girdles; (c) hypertrophy of the calves and certain other muscles at some stage of the disease in almost every case; (d) relentlessly progressive weakness in every case, leading to inability to walk before the age of about 12 years and later to contractures and thoracic deformity; (e) invariable cardiac involvement; (f) frequent, but not invariable, intellectual impairment; (g) death by the second or third decade caused by respiratory or, less frequently, cardiac failure, often associated with inanition and respiratory infection; (h) very high activity of certain muscle enzymes, notably creatine kinase (CK) in serum in the early stages of the disease; (i) certain characteristic histological features in muscle; and (j) the occurrence of Xp21 gene deletions in about 65% of cases.

Incidence. The most reliable estimates of the incidence of Duchenne muscular dystrophy range from 18 to 30 per 100 000 liveborn males, and of its prevalence in the population as a whole from 1.9 to 4.8 per 100 000. One-third of cases are new

mutants, one-third have a previous family history and one-third are born to unwitting and often mutant carriers. The mutation rate is about 7–10 $\times 10^{-5}$ per gene per generation (Moser et al 1964, Gardner-Medwin 1970, 1982, Brooks & Emery 1977, Danieli et al 1977, Davie & Emery 1978, Cowan et al 1980, Monckton et al 1982, Nigro et al 1983, Williams et al 1983, Moser 1984, Scheuerbrandt et al 1986, Gardner-Medwin & Sharples 1989; for a comprehensive review see Emery 1991). Experience in the North of England, where systematic carrier counselling has been in place since the early 1960s, shows a fall in prevalence — 4.1/100 000 population in 1968, 3.6 in 1979, 2.4 in 1988 — and in birth incidence in males — 31.2/100 000 in 1952–61, 22.4 in 1962–71, 17.8 in 1972–81 (Gardner-Medwin & Sharples 1989, Bushby et al 1991b).

Occurrence in girls. In the UK, about half of all young girls with a severe progressive muscular dystrophy have the autosomal recessive form (see p. 569). The remainder have a form of Meryon muscular dystrophy. Five different explanations for such cases have been recorded or proposed:

1. Theoretically a girl homozygous for the Duchenne gene might result from the union of a female carrier with an affected man or one in whom a gonadal mutation of the gene had occurred, but this has never been reported.

2. Cases of true Duchenne dystrophy in girls with Turner's syndrome (X0 karyotype) have been reported, but are very rare (Walton 1956a, Ferrier et al 1965, Jalbert et al 1966, Chelly et al 1986). In Chelly's case the sole X-chromosome had an Xp21 deletion.

3. In 1977 a girl with Duchenne muscular dystrophy and a reciprocal translocation of parts of the long arms of chromosomes X and 21 was described by Verellen et al (1977). Subsequently a number of similar cases were reported, and Lindenbaum was the first to realise the significance of the fact that the breakpoints were all at the same site on the X-chromosome, namely Xp21 (Lindenbaum et al 1979 and many others reviewed by Verellen-Dumoulin et al 1984 and Boyd et al 1986). These cases are uncommon; we have still not encountered an example among 14 female cases of severe Duchenne-like muscular

dystrophy seen in Newcastle. Their degree of severity varies over the whole range of the Duchenne and intermediate parts of the spectrum. They appear to manifest the disease, not because they are all carriers of the mutant gene on their other X-chromosome, but because the translocation prevents the random inactivation of the abnormal X-chromosome and thus only the normal X is inactivated in all the relevant cells.

4. A few remarkable pairs of identical twin girls have now been reported, in which one twin has progressive muscular dystrophy while the other is entirely unaffected (Gomez et al 1977, Burn et al 1986, Richards et al 1990, Lupski et al 1991). The dystrophy in such cases appears to be typical of the Duchenne type. No chromosome deletions have been found, but in Lupski's cases both twins had a duplication of part of the gene. Burn has suggested, and has provided some supporting evidence, that in such cases early random inactivation of the normal X-chromosome in some cells and of the other X, containing the mutant Duchenne gene, in other cells might contribute to the *causation* of the twinning process in the early blastocyst stage. The resultant twins, both actually heterozygous for the Duchenne gene, might as a result have quite different phenotypes, one normal and the other typical of Duchenne muscular dystrophy. If this explanation is correct, one might expect early fetal loss of one such twin to result occasionally in apparently isolated heterozygotes of each type (totally non-manifesting carriers, and fully affected girls with a normal karyotype).

5. Since the discovery of dystrophin, it has become possible to diagnose affected females without a chromosome anomaly or discordant twinning. Such cases are usually in the Duchenne or intermediate range of severity, have the same distribution of affected muscles as affected boys, similar cardiac involvement and, as a rule, no other affected members of the family and no detected deletion of the gene. Their intelligence may also be similarly affected, but in one of our cases and that of Maytal et al (1991) intelligence was entirely normal. No adequate search for point mutations or study of X-inactivation patterns has been reported in such affected girls; their pathogenesis remains enigmatic. It is conceivable that all are survivors of cryptic twinning.

More mildly affected 'manifesting heterozygotes' are more frequently seen and may inadvertently be diagnosed as cases of 'limb-girdle dystrophy' (see p 564).

Symptoms. The earliest symptom is usually clumsiness in walking, with a tendency to fall. In many cases, attempts to walk are delayed and awkward from the beginning. About half are still unable to walk at the age of 18 months. General developmental delay, especially involving speech, is not uncommon and may divert the clinician's attention from the neuromuscular problem. In other cases, progress may be apparently normal until the third year and very occasionally parents do not report anything abnormal until the sixth or seventh year. Then the child's walking begins to lack briskness and freedom of movement; often this is erroneously attributed to 'laziness' or flat feet, or some other comparatively trivial complaint. It is common to find that parents who have had a dystrophic child can detect the earliest signs of the disease in a second son, at a time when no abnormal signs can be identified by an experienced clinician. Inability to run, to hop and especially to jump over a small object with both feet together are often useful early guides. Soon the boy has increasing difficulty in climbing stairs and in rising from the floor (Fig. 14.1). The method of rolling from supine to prone and then climbing up the legs to reach a standing position is characteristic (Gowers 1879). He walks with a waddle and protrudes his abdomen, later rising on to his toes with feet wide apart and shoulders and chin drawn back. A detailed study of the pathomechanics of the typical gait was made by Sutherland et al (1981). Weakness of the upper limbs is often not reported until up to 5 years after the onset, but it can be found on examination long before this.

Atypical symptoms. Occasionally hypotonia in the newborn period, and early motor delay may be sufficient to cause temporary confusion with congenital muscular dystrophy. Breningstall et al (1988) reported a case of muscle induration and exceptionally high serum CK activity in an affected neonate. Recurrent myoglobinuria (Meyer-Betz 1910) is a rare feature.

Course. At the age of 4 or 5 years the boy's growth may outstrip the progress of the disease, giving a false impression of improvement, other-

given by Allsop & Ziter (1981), Scott et al (1982) and Brooke et al (1983).

A rapid increase in weakness may follow bed rest for minor illness, fractures or surgery, but the childhood exanthems rarely affect the condition if the child is kept active. Surgical procedures designed to lengthen Achilles tendons are particularly dangerous in this respect. Archibald & Vignos (1959) stressed the importance of early contractures of the hip flexors in accentuating postural difficulties and leading to early confinement to a wheelchair. Contractures of the hip abductors may also become prominent at this time, as the gait becomes broad-based. Regular physiotherapy is capable of preventing these contractures in most cases at this stage. Once the wheelchair stage is reached, contractures at the hips and elsewhere develop rapidly, especially in the hamstrings and biceps, and weakness of spinal muscles almost invariably leads to increasing scoliosis. Eventually the deformity may make even a wheelchair existence impossible and the patient is confined to bed, able to speak, swallow and breathe, but otherwise retaining feeble power only in the movements of the face, in the grip and in plantar-flexion of the feet and toes. Only a quarter of cases survive beyond the age of 21 years and survival beyond 25 years is rare (Gardner-Medwin 1982, Johnston et al 1985). Death usually results from chest infection with respiratory and sometimes cardiac failure.

Relatively mild cases of Duchenne muscular dystrophy are occasionally seen and have been called 'outliers' by some authors (Rideau 1978, Bonsett & Thomson 1987). Typically they remain able to walk until 13–16 years and some of them survive to between 25 and 30 years. This group has been brought into prominence by dystrophin studies, as it is often among such 'intermediate' cases (i.e. those lying between Duchenne and Becker in severity) that small but significant amounts of dystrophin may be demonstrated in muscle, though the correlation is not yet reliable. A few puzzling instances are recorded in which great variation in severity occurs within a family (Furukawa & Peter 1977, Gardner-Medwin 1982) but in general the course of the disease is fairly uniform.

In one striking exception, a very atypical benign early course of the disease was recorded in one of

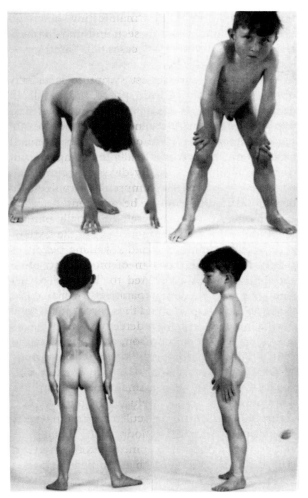

Fig. 14.1   The Duchenne type of muscular dystrophy: note the hypertrophy of the calves and the characteristic method of rising from the floor (Walton 1962).

wise deterioration is continuous and most patients become unable to walk between the ages of 7 and 12 years. The mean age is about 9.5 years (Gardner-Medwin 1982). Despite the apparently intermittent rapid progression of the disease as critical milestones of disability are reached (such as inability to rise from the floor, to climb stairs or to walk), Ziter et al (1977) showed that the decline in measured muscle strength is continuous and linear. In the 1980s efforts to improve the standards of therapeutic trials resulted in a number of studies of the rate of natural progression of the disease. Particularly useful data are

10 affected males in a family. The mildly affected boy also had growth hormone deficiency, a fact of possible pathogenetic importance. He was able to walk until the age of 18 years (Zatz & Betti 1986) but his life was not prolonged (M. Zatz, personal communication).

Physical examination. Weakness and wasting usually begins in the iliopsoas, quadriceps and gluteus muscles and soon spread to involve the anterior tibial group. In the upper limbs, the costal origin of pectoralis major, the latissimus dorsi, the biceps, triceps and brachioradialis muscles are the first involved. Scapular winging occurs, but is not prominent in the early stages. Hypotonia when the child is lifted at the shoulders is a useful early sign. Later, power is better retained in the wrist flexors than extensors, in the hamstrings than in quadriceps, in the invertors of the foot than in the evertors and in neck extension than in flexion. The calf muscles may remain remarkably strong for several years. Slight facial weakness, especially of movements of the mouth, is usual in the later stages. Progressive deterioration of respiratory function occurs and is discussed in a later paragraph.

Muscular hypertrophy, later followed by the pseudohypertrophic phase of fatty replacement of muscle, is commonly seen in the calves (Fig. 14.1), the lateral vasti of quadriceps, the infraspinati and muscles of mastication, less often in the deltoids, wrist extensors, anterior tibial and peroneal muscles and occasionally in other muscles. Denervation of muscle (as in poliomyelitis) may abolish it, and it usually disappears spontaneously as the disease progresses. It is rare for cases of otherwise typical Duchenne muscular dystrophy to show no muscular enlargement at any stage of the disease. Macroglossia is not uncommon.

The tendon reflexes are diminished in the upper limbs early in the disease and the knee jerks also disappear soon. The ankle jerks, however, remain brisk until a comparatively late stage. Contractures generally develop first in the calf muscles and hip flexors and abductors and give rise to progressive plantar-flexion and inversion of the feet, and to hip contractures with compensatory lumbar lordosis; they are seen later in the hamstrings, biceps brachii and flexors of the wrists and fingers. This distribution of contractures at first reflects the weakness of antagonist muscles and later the

customary sitting and sleeping postures, and almost certainly has no more interesting explanation.

Some of the children become generally wasted as the disease progresses, but many become very obese, presumably because of a combination of excessive intake and immobility. Catabolic activity is so low in boys with severe paralysis that calorie requirements in the range of one-quarter to one-sixth of the normal are commonplace, but not easy for families to accept. The obesity is not endocrine in origin. Sexual development is usually normal, but puberty may be delayed. A degree of growth failure in early childhood is almost universal (Eiholzer et al 1988) but in our experience is not continued into adolescence. Constipation is common, as in many other chronic neuromuscular disorders, but there is no impairment of small intestinal function (Korman et al 1991) though colonic motility is, not unnaturally, slow (Gottrand et al 1991). Acute gastric dilatation is an occasional complication (Barohn et al 1988). These gastrointestinal complications may be the result of dystrophin deficiency in smooth muscle but this generally causes significant symptoms.

Intellectual changes. Intellectual retardation is common (Allen & Rodgin 1960, Worden & Vignos 1962). Indeed, it occurred in Duchenne's earliest case and led him to believe at first that the disorder was of cerebral origin. About one-fifth of cases have an intelligence quotient (IQ) below 70 and a significant minority are below 50; about a tenth are above 100. Mean IQ levels in different series vary between about 70 and 85 (Dubowitz 1965, Zellweger & Hanson 1967a, Cohen et al 1968, Prosser et al 1969, Kozicka et al 1971, Marsh & Munsat 1974, Kohno 1978, Leibowitz & Dubowitz 1981, Anderson et al 1988, Billard et al 1992). However, the most thorough population surveys (Cohen et al 1968, Kohno 1978) gave the highest figures for mean IQ. The mean in Emery's (1987) composite survey was 82. Verbal ability is usually most severely affected. Karagan et al (1980) attempted to analyse this verbal deficit in seven selected boys and concluded that verbal expression and memory for patterns, numbers and verbal labels were more severely impaired than some other verbal skills. In addition to the intellectual deficit, Leibowitz & Dubowitz (1981) identified behaviour problems in more than one-third of their cases. There is no evidence of progressive intellectual deterioration however (Marsh & Munsat 1974, Smith et al 1989a) and, except in the series described by Rosman (1970), the severity of the muscular and intellectual involvement are not correlated. The intelligence levels of affected siblings are often similar (Bertolini & Zatz 1986), but no abnormality has been found in non-manifesting carriers, and the sons of known carriers are no more severely affected than are sporadic cases (Prosser et al 1969). Kozicka et al (1971) found that the electro-encephalogram (EEG) was abnormal more often in retarded cases, but the study by Barwick et al (1965) revealed no consistent EEG abnormalities. Rosman & Kakulas (1966) found cerebral-neuronal hetero-topias at autopsy in three retarded boys with Duchenne dystrophy, but not in four patients with normal intelligence. Their cases were somewhat atypical, however, and Dubowitz & Crome (1969) found no significant abnormality in the brain in 21 autopsied patients, in five of whom the IQ had been below 60. The mean head circumference in Duchenne boys is increased but does not correlate with intellectual function (Appleton et al 1991).

Dystrophin is present in the brain. The neuronal protein is encoded from the Xp21 gene, as in muscle, but using a different promoter (Nudel et al 1989, Chelly et al 1990). Deletion of that promoter does not cause exceptional intellectual disability (den Dunnen et al 1991), nor is the presence, size or position of a deletion correlated with IQ (Bushby et al 1993b), with the apparent puzzling exception that deletions at the 5' end of the gene tend to leave intelligence unaffected. In particular, the suggestion by Rapaport et al (1991) that deletion of exon 52 was associated with low IQ has not been confirmed.

Skeletal changes. The pattern of skeletal deformity occurring in patients with the Duchenne type muscular dystrophy was reviewed by Walton & Warrick (1954). The changes, which are secondary to disuse, include narrowing of the shafts and rarefaction of the ends of the long bones (Fig. 14.2), impaired development of flat bones and coxa valga. At a later stage there is almost invariably severe spinal curvature, widespread

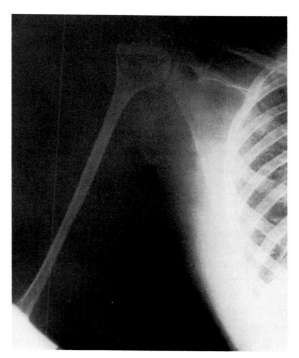

Fig. 14.2 Atrophy of the humerus in an advanced case of Duchenne muscular dystrophy (Walton 1962).

decalcification and eventually gross distortion and disorganisation of the skeletal system. These changes render the affected bones liable to fracture as a result of minimal trauma, and a child may fracture a femur on falling from a wheelchair. A few patients develop a long thoracolumbar lordosis instead of the more usual kyphoscoliosis (Wilkins & Gibson 1976).

Cardiac involvement. This is probably invariable in Duchenne muscular dystrophy, although it may not be detectable in the early stages (Zatuchni et al 1951, Walton & Nattrass 1954, Manning & Cropp 1958, Perloff et al 1966, Slucka 1968, O'Orsognna et al 1988). Persistent tachycardia is common and sudden death from myocardial failure may occur (Berenbaum & Horowitz 1956) but chronic cardiac failure is rare. Of particular importance is the characteristic electrocardiogram (ECG) which shows tall R waves in the right precordial leads and deep Q waves in the limb leads and the left precordial leads (Fig. 14.3). Schott et al (1955), Skyring &

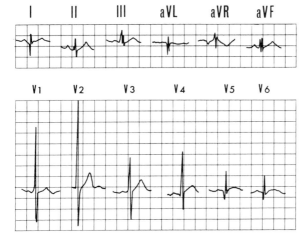

Fig. 14.3 Typical ECG recorded from a boy of 14 with Duchenne muscular dystrophy. There are narrow but deep Q waves in leads I, aVL, V_5 and V_6, and RSR_1 pattern in aVR and dominant R waves in V_1 and V_2.

McKusick (1961), Perloff et al (1966) and Emery (1972) have claimed that this ECG pattern is of diagnostic value in distinguishing between the juvenile forms of muscular dystrophy. Perloff et al (1967) have shown that the pathological basis for this distinctive ECG in two cases was interstitial and replacement fibrosis of the basal part of the left ventricular free wall. Echocardiography has recently indicated relatively good preservation of myocardial function in Duchenne dystrophy, despite the ECG changes. There is, however, some reduction in the rate of diastolic relaxation (Kovick et al 1975, Ahmad et al 1978), impairment of left ventricular contraction and relaxation and, in boys with thoracic distortion, an abnormally high incidence of mitral valve prolapse (Danilowicz et al 1980, Goldberg et al 1980, Reeves et al 1980, Hunsaker et al 1982). Hunsaker et al (1982) documented a decline in function over 10 years.

Hunter (1980) points out that the impairment of physical fitness which results from enforced immobility may contribute to the abnormalities that are found. Despite its usual association with thoracic distortion, mitral valve prolapse seems to result from involvement of the papillary muscle by the cardiomyopathy (Sanyal et al 1980).

A variety of disturbances of rhythm, including labile tachycardia, may be demonstrated by careful investigation (Sanyal & Johnson 1982) but they are relatively uncommon as clinical problems. Disease of the nodal arteries may account for some of these (James 1962, Perloff et al 1967).

Respiratory muscle involvement. The respiratory muscles are always affected in Duchenne dystrophy and when scoliosis and thoracic distortion occur they further diminish the efficiency of respiration. Respiratory failure compounded by infection is the major cause of death.

The vital capacity begins to fall below normal as early as the seventh year, by the age of 14 it is on average only 50% of normal and at 21 only 20% (Rideau 1978, Rideau et al 1981). The expiratory reserve volume component of the vital capacity is affected earlier than the inspiratory component. The tidal volume is relatively preserved but the maximum ventilatory capacity is progressively impaired. The maximum expiratory and inspiratory pressures that can be exerted begin to decline at about the same stage (Inkley et al 1974). The loss of expiratory force is particularly important because it makes attempts to cough ineffective and contributes further to the risk of acquiring and succumbing to infections.

Rideau et al (1981) and Rideau & Delaubier (1987) were able to correlate the age at which the vital capacity reached its plateau with the duration of ultimate survival. Kurz et al (1983) studied the relationship of thoracic spinal curvature to vital capacity and concluded that in addition to the effect of age on the latter, each additional 10° of curvature diminished the vital capacity by 4%.

Only in the last stages of the disease is quiet respiration affected. Because the accessory muscles of respiration are themselves extremely weak, their visible use, often a slight heaving movement of the shoulders, is a very significant bad prognostic sign. The tidal volume, though not reduced, cannot be increased to meet demands and so the respiratory rate increases instead. The central respiratory responses to oxygen and carbon dioxide are normal (Begin et al 1980). Carbon dioxide retention is also a late feature, usually apparent as morning drowsiness but occasionally causing headache and even papilloedema in extreme cases (Burke et al 1971). Fear of falling asleep is a common and disturbing feature for the patient and the whole family as the respiratory reserve fails.

Diagnosis. A definitive diagnosis is based either on finding a deletion in the Xp21 gene or on the absence, or severe deficiency, of dystrophin in muscle biopsy material.

The typical distribution of muscular weakness, wasting and hypertrophy, the characteristic gait, best seen when the child attempts to run or to climb stairs, and the inability to jump or hop provide the basis for the first suspicion of the diagnosis, easily confirmed by the characteristic very high levels of serum CK activity.

Between the ages of 1 and 5 years, serum CK activity in Duchenne muscular dystrophy is 100–300 times the upper limit of the normal range and other muscle enzymes (aldolase, SGOT, pyruvate kinase, lactic dehydrogenase and others) are also grossly elevated. The only other comparable gradually progressive myopathies which may give such high serum enzyme levels are the Becker and automosal recessive types of childhood muscular dystrophy (q.q.v.). The diagnosis may be made at birth (Heyck et al 1966). In the neonatal period the normal range of serum CK activity is higher than in older infants (Gilboa & Swanson 1976) but in a large-scale screening survey the activities in newborn cases of Duchenne muscular dystrophy were at least 2.5 times the highest normal figures and 20–50 times the normal mean (Dellamonica 1978). After birth the serum CK levels rise over the first year or so and then fall gradually from the age of 2–3 years so that, in very advanced cases, they are only one to five times the normal upper limit.

In a first affected case in a family, by the time the serum CK activity has been checked the parents will usually have been concerned about their son for some time and will now be very anxious. It is therefore vital that a definitive diagnosis is reached without further delay. Many laboratory workers have suggested that this should be based on the screening of blood leuco-cyte DNA for a deletion, thus avoiding the need for muscle biopsy. This is acceptable only where facilities exist to complete this laborious process within a matter of days. Even then the 35% of Duchenne cases which have no deletion will require a muscle biopsy. It is our practice to per-form a muscle biopsy in all suspected new cases, thus making it possible to tell the parents the diagnosis without equivocation within 48 hours, based on muscle histology and dystrophin immunocytochemistry.

The muscle biopsy in the first few weeks of life may show only a small excess of endomysial connective tissue and the presence of many large hyaline muscle fibres (see Ch. 7). As the activity of the disease reaches its peak, the muscle fascicles become 'fossilised' by a mesh of perimysial and endomysial connective tissue, the scattered hyaline fibres remain prominent, and active muscle necrosis, phagocytosis and regeneration are conspi-cuous. Gradually the muscle fibres, which are rounded, often showing splitting and central nuclei, and which vary greatly in size, are replaced by increasing quantities of fat. In the late stages of the disease so little muscle may be left in the mass of fat and fibrous tissue that the biopsy is no longer diagnostic, and even the absence of dys-trophin in damaged fibres may be of uncertain significance.

Immunocytochemical staining (see Ch. 8) reveals the absence of dystrophin in most fibres. Some patients have scattered isolated positive fibres, and a very few have small groups of positive fibres or alternatively very faint widespread posi-tive staining. Overall, in the Meryon group of dys-trophies, the amount of residual dystrophin (best measured by immunoblotting) correlates with the severity of the disease, but the presence of small amounts of the protein cannot be relied upon for prognosis in individual cases (Nicholson et al 1993). The analysis of deletions is even less reliable for prognosis within the Duchenne range of severity.

In practice the confirmation of the diagnosis of Duchenne muscular dystrophy is easy. The difficulty lies in early clinical recognition of the disease. The mean age at diagnosis is about 4.7–5.8 years (Gardner-Medwin et al 1978, Crisp et al 1982, Smith et al 1989a). This delay (of 2–4 years from the onset of symptoms) may result in the conception of further preventable cases in the family. The development of a micro-method of CK analysis which can be performed on a dried blood spot (Zellweger & Antonik 1975) has enabled large-scale neonatal screening projects to be set up in several parts of the world (Zellweger & Antonik 1975, Beckmann & Scheuerbrandt 1976, Dellamonica 1978, Dellamonica et al 1978, Drummond 1979, Scheuerbrandt et al 1986, Greenberg et al 1988, Jacobs et al 1989, Bradley et al 1993). Altogether more than 300 000 newborn males have been screened and the incidence of Duchenne muscular dystrophy among them has been about 1 in 3900 males (1 in 3700 of the 176 000 males screened by Scheuerbrandt et al in 1986). At best, neonatal screening can theoretically prevent 12–15% of cases and its effect upon the parents' relationship with their newborn son is unpredictable and potentially psychologically hazardous. The alternative strategy of screening boys with psychomotor developmental delay at the age of about 18 months was put forward as likely to be less effective but still valuable and with probably less harmful emotional consequences (Gardner-Medwin et al 1978, Gardner-Medwin 1979a, Crisp et al 1982, Smith et al 1989a). When put to the test this idea was found to be logistically difficult and not fully effective (Smith et al 1989b, 1990). A trial of neonatal screening by the same team, with immaculate arrangements for counselling, provides early promise of success (Bradley et al 1993), but nowhere in the world has such a project yet provided sufficient evidence of cost-effectiveness to attract government funding for a national scheme for neonatal screening.

Prenatal diagnosis of Duchenne muscular dystrophy, first achieved by the use of linkage markers by Bakker et al (1985), is now reliable in those families where a chorion villus sample can be screened for a known deletion and is discussed in Chapter 26. It is important to recognise that this, and all other techniques of prenatal diagnosis, are essentially methods for permitting couples at risk to have normal children instead of remaining childless. They contribute little to *prevention* of the disease.

Prevention and carrier tracing. About one-third of cases of Duchenne muscular dystrophy in a population not subjected to genetic counselling are theoretically preventable. The contribution which early diagnosis can make to prevention has already been discussed. Considerably more cases could be prevented by the active tracing, and counselling, of potential female carriers. The clini-cian who makes the diagnosis of Duchenne muscular dystrophy thereby acquires the responsibility of making genetic advice available to his patient's female relatives.

Carrier *detection* (whether by serum CK testing, linkage studies, deletion detection or other methods), unlike the active tracing and warning of the potential carriers in affected families, is not concerned with prevention of the disease but with making it safe for women at risk to have a normal family. The principles and techniques of carrier detection are discussed in Chapter 26.

Management. No treatment is at present known which has any definite influence upon muscular dystrophy. The drugs which have been tried in the past, the use of therapeutic trials and the prospects for future gene therapy are discussed in Chapter 22. All that need be said here is that, in the opinion of the authors, the use of cortico-steroids, in any context other than a clinical trial, cannot be justified while the long-term balance of harmful effects against possible benefits remains uncertain.

The absence of specific treatment for muscular dystrophy makes it all the more important to prevent its physical, emotional, social and educational complications and to provide active support for the family throughout the course of the disease. The clinician's first responsibility is to provide an unequivocal diagnosis and enough information and constructive suggestions to enable the family to formulate practical plans for the future. These must be given in relaxed sessions after the initial shock has passed (Firth 1983). Females potentially at risk of being carriers should be actively traced and offered genetic advice at this time. In the early stages, the most useful activities for the parents to encourage are regular physical exercise, appropriate eating habits to prevent obesity, and social activities, sporting and cultural interests, hobbies and education to provide a basis for interests in the later stages of the disease.

Vignos & Watkins (1966) showed that organised programmes of maximum resistance exercise may increase muscular strength in the adult forms of muscular dystrophy. Such programmes are more difficult in childhood and there is still no really satisfactory published trial of the effect of active exercise in Duchenne muscular dystrophy but it is the common experience that Duchenne boys benefit from exercise and, conversely, that rest is detrimental. Bed rest for minor illness or trauma should be avoided whenever possible and regular walking, swimming and games, a little more than the boy really wants to do, should be encouraged. Older boys can do more formal and deliberate exercises and, in the late stages, these should be continued with emphasis on the upper limbs and on breathing exercises. Wheelchair sports provide both exercise and a boost for morale.

Unlike the muscular weakness, contractures are to some extent preventable and reversible. Toe-walking is usually an adaptive response to weakness of the quadriceps (Khodadadeh et al 1986) and should not be interfered with, either by surgery or by the use of walking splints. By contrast equinus *contractures*, once established, generally progress and they can be effectively prevented in the early stages by the use of below-knee night splints (ankle–foot orthoses) to maintain a slight degree of dorsiflexion during sleep. Hip flexion and abduction contractures may significantly alter the stance and interfere with walking at a stage when the muscular weakness alone is not severe enough to prevent ambulation; passive stretching of the hip flexors and iliotibial bands may therefore be an important part of management. Prone lying to prevent hip flexion contracture is useful. Vignos et al (1963) recommended passive stretching for at least 5 seconds repeated 10 times, twice a day. Others suggest more prolonged continuous stretching (Kottke et al 1966) but, in the face of relatively weak antagonist muscles, no intermittent regime of stretching will be entirely successful. Splinting at night, though successful at the ankle, is not feasible at other joints.

The dangers of anaesthesia and the increased weakness which follows immobility demand that minor surgery must be undertaken only if immediate postoperative mobilisation is prepared for in advance. However, surgical management of equinus deformity can be successful in the hands of surgeons with special experience of the postoperative management in muscular dystrophy (Williams et al 1984).

Rideau et al (1986) recommended pre-emptive surgery, at about the age of 6 years, to prevent contractures of the hip flexors and abductors, and claimed that this gave an immediate and continued improvement in gait. A controlled trial (Manzur et al 1992) failed to confirm this, somewhat to the relief of those who regard this period as the best of a Duchenne boy's life and one which should not be intruded upon by unnecessary medical or surgical activity.

Spencer & Vignos (1962) and Vignos et al (1963) pioneered the active management of the combined weakness and contractures in Duchenne muscular dystrophy, recommending a combination of subcutaneous tenotomy (with brief anaesthesia) and subsequent vigorous physiotherapy and bracing in calipers (now often called knee–ankle–foot orthoses). They enabled some of their patients to walk 2 or more years longer than usual. Siegel et al (1968), Roy & Gibson (1970), Miller & Dunn (1982) and Heckmatt et al (1985) recommended similar measures. Later Vignos and his colleagues developed stricter criteria for the application of this technique based on the residual strength and bulk of muscle, the rate of loss of muscle, vital capacity and motivation of the patient (Vignos et al 1983). With time it has become apparent that the surgical component of this process, once regarded as central, is simply a means of reversing established contractures and that a previous programme of physiotherapy, much of it done by the parents, including hip stretching and the use of ankle night-splints, usually makes it possible to mobilise the boy in calipers without the need for surgery. If tenotomies are to be performed, rapid mobilisation and the maintenance of the corrected position with light alloy calipers are essential. Our own experience is that it is both feasible and often very worthwhile to prolong ambulation in this way, but one must set against the advantages of this, the sense of relief which patients often feel on accepting a wheelchair existence after a period of exhaustingly difficult walking with frequent falls, and also the time taken up by physiotherapy and the application of complex braces, often at the expense of schooling, and often for the sake of less useful mobility than is possible in a wheelchair (Gardner-Medwin 1977, 1979b). None the less all families should have the chance to discuss bracing before the need for it arises. When the boy and his parents are both enthusiastic it can be very successful in preserving a useful range of activities and in maintaining morale. There is increasing evidence that it also delays the onset of kyphoscoliosis (Rodillo et al 1988). As walking in calipers gradually becomes impossible (after a period of a few months to as much as 3 years in some cases), periods of standing in the calipers, or with the use of a light 'standing frame' can maintain the upright position for a little longer and can be used for work or play at a high table.

When a wheelchair is required it should at first be hand-propelled to provide exercise, but should be replaced with an electrically propelled chair as soon as it no longer provides independent mobility. It is essential not only to select the right chair for the individual's needs, but to adapt the house and, if necessary, the school, to provide full access for the wheelchair. We often recommend subcutaneous Achilles tenotomy in the early wheelchair stage with subsequent use of below-knee cosmetic splints to prevent the unsightly equinovarus contractures which otherwise occur, simply to allow these boys to wear normal footwear. However, if cosmetic splints are worn consistently from the moment that the ability to walk is lost the need for tenotomy can often be avoided, especially if splints are also worn at night. Contractures at the hips, knees, elbows and wrists occur in the late stages in almost all cases, but these require surgical management only in rare instances where they are persistently painful. At this stage stretching of the muscles of the lower limbs should attempt no more than to maintain a comfortable range of movement. Attempts to *improve* contractures by stretching are painful, doomed to failure and an unwarranted waste of the boy's precious living time. Elbow and wrist contractures can be limited to some extent by regular stretching; prolonged and regular splinting of the upper limbs, by day or at night, is too disabling to be justified.

Progressive scoliosis usually begins soon after patients become unable to walk (Robin & Brief 1971) and the prevention of scoliosis is one practical reason for the artificial maintenance of ambulation in appropriate cases. Once it has become established and fixed it is very difficult to correct or even control and it may go on to cause severe thoracic distortion, respiratory impairment, and a major threat to life.

Attempts at early prevention of scoliosis are usually concentrated on achieving a good posture in the wheelchair. Proper support of the feet and a firm comfortable seat position can encourage a symmetrical upright posture. But Rideau (1978) has suggested that the position in sleep may also be relevant. Discouragement of a single habitual sleeping posture may possibly prevent asymmetrical hip flexion and hip abduction contracures, but the origin of these can often be traced back to asymmetry of stance before the wheelchair stage. Once a curvature appears, some form of spinal support is urgently required, but the *prophylactic* use of spinal orthoses is more controversial (Vignos et al 1963, Young et al 1984). Often they are not well accepted by the boys; the more effectively they support the spine the more they limit activity, so there is some risk that they may actually hasten loss of strength in the muscles of the trunk while also impairing the quality of life. Moulded wheelchair inserts, designed to lock the intervertebral facet joints, and thus to prevent rotation of the spine by inducing an artificial lumbar lordosis, were an important innovation (Wilkins & Gibson 1976) but they depend for their effect on limiting freedom of movement. Low-set, lumbar/thoracic lightweight cosmetic orthoses can induce a lordosis, while allowing more movement and not restricting respiration, and undoubtedly they can help to limit the development of scoliosis, but a cycle of incomplete control of curvature, discomfort, disuse and further curvature is easily set up and failure is frequent (Seeger et al 1984).

Robin & Brief (1971), Robin (1977) and Gibson et al (1978) introduced spinal fusion with insertion of a Harrington rod as an alternative to bracing when scoliosis was uncontrolled. Increasing experience with the methods of anaesthesia and postoperative care required and the proper assessment of respiratory function allowed important advances in the management of scoliosis to be made using this technique (Milne & Rosales 1982, Swank et al 1982, Weimann et al 1983). The introduction of the Luque type of segmental instrumentation and various later modifications (such as the Galveston and Cotrel–Dubousset methods) allowed more rapid postoperative mobilisation and widened the potential scope of surgery (Siegel 1982, Taddonio 1982, Rideau et al 1984, Sussman 1984, 1985, Miller et al 1992, Shapiro et al 1992). It has even been suggested that spinal orthoses should no longer be used because they serve only to delay the development of spinal curvature until respiratory function has deteriorated too far for surgery to be possible (Rideau et al 1984, Sussman 1984). This presupposes the availability of a skilled surgical team which can operate without delay at the critical moment. It may also leave boys who, for any reason, become unsuitable for surgery with an irreversible curvature. It is widely agreed that orthoses rarely control scolioses which start early and quickly reach a Cobb angle of more than 25 degrees, that surgery is often unsuccessful if the curve is greater than 50 degrees and that the hazards of operation become unacceptable if the vital capacity is less than about 35–40% of the predicted normal value. Policies in many units are currently in a state of flux; our own at present is to withhold spinal orthoses (except in cases where surgery seems inappropriate, or likely to be refused), but as soon as the patient is unable to walk, to examine the spine every 3 months and to offer spinal fusion if the curve exceeds 20 degrees at a stage when the vital capacity is still sufficient for safe anaesthesia. In deciding the 'correct' policy it is important to consider not only the effect upon the curvature itself but on the comfort and functional ability of the boys; some, for example, have found the use of their arms restricted after the operation. Most cautious surgeons claim no benefit from the operation in terms of life expectancy.

Many aids such as hoists, bath aids and specially adapted clothing are available; these and adaptations to homes and schools can be provided, after their effectiveness and acceptability for each family have been assessed. An occupational therapist may play a leading part in management when these measures are required. The practical help, advice and emotional support of a social worker are also important. The long, inexorable deterioration of the disease is punctuated by crises occurring, for example, at the time of diagnosis, of inability to walk, of changing or leaving school and of illness. Fears of fatal illness, of another child being affected, or pregnancies either in the mother or in her carrier daughters, may be added to the frequent misguided sense of marital guilt on the part of carriers and to the prolonged maintenance of family facades to avoid sharing knowledge, fears and often myths about the disorder. Social isolation is common. Boys may become over-protected, frightened, petulant, resentful, aggressive and lonely. Reactive depression is far commoner in parents than in boys. A survey of parents' attitudes to their predicaments was reported by Firth et al (1983). Many of these problems can be prevented or alleviated by a medical social worker or Family Care Officer, familiar with both the disease and the family.

The combined physical and intellectual handicap presents formidable educational problems. Psychological assessment of aptitudes as well as limitations can assist in planning both education and hobbies. Many boys with poor verbal skills show special competence in design and modelling. The social isolation of home education should be avoided whenever possible and education should dovetail with the limited opportunities that are likely to be available when the boy leaves school.

Complications include obesity in the wheelchair stage; this is easier to prevent than to treat. The calorie requirements of some immobile boys are very low and expert dietary advice may be required to maintain a balanced diet. In a valuable study, Edwards et al (1984) showed that strict dieting for weight reduction has no deleterious effect on muscle bulk or function in Duchenne boys. Fractures, especially of the lower end of the femur, often occur in the more adventurous wheelchair users. The atrophic bones mend remarkably well and only very limited splinting is needed, especially in the lower limbs. No attempt should be made to correct contractures at the same time. Boys who fracture a femur while still ambulant can often be mobilised in a cast and thus avoid the very grave risk of being unable to walk after a prolonged period of standard immobilisation (Hsu & Garcia-Ariz 1981). Dependent oedema and bedsores are surprisingly rare complications in Duchenne dystrophy.

Anaesthesia may be hazardous (Cobham & Davis 1964, Boba 1970, Genever 1971, Yamashita et al 1976) and should be administered by an experienced anaethestist in hospital, even for minor dental and other procedures. With care, general anaesthesia for muscle biopsy or incidental surgery in young patients with Duchenne muscular dystrophy is usually uneventful. However there are now several case reports of cardiac arrest or rhabdomyolysis induced by anaesthesia (Genever 1971, Watters et al 1977, Miller et al 1978, Seay et al 1978, Bolthauser et al 1980, Lintner et al 1982) and in very occasional cases the full syndrome of malignant hyperpyrexia occurs, confirmed by in vitro tests of muscle sensitivity to halothane or caffeine (Oka et al 1982, Brownell et al 1983, Kelfer et al 1983, Rosenberg & Heiman-Patterson 1983). It is probably wise to avoid using halothane or suxamethonium whenever possible in cases of known or suspected Duchenne muscular dystrophy; certainly dantrolene should be available for immediate use. However, it would be wrong to deny Duchenne patients surgical treatment on the basis of the small number of cases reported as experiencing this complication and in fact, in many of the recorded cases, the muscular dystrophy was recognised only after the anaesthetic problem had occurred.

Respiratory insufficiency often gives rise to no symptoms until sudden decompensation occurs during respiratory infections or other sudden stresses. Death may then occur very suddenly in acute respiratory failure, occasionally with terminal heart failure. Cardiac arrhythmias, although often postulated as a cause of sudden death, are rarely observed and delaying respiratory failure seems to be the only useful approach to prophylaxis. Regular breathing exercises and the prevention of scoliosis are important and all parents should be taught to use postural drainage during respiratory infections, together with appropriate antibiotic therapy. Artificial ventilation during such infections may be appropriate (and effective) in some circumstances.

Chronic respiratory failure may, however, give rise to a number of less specific symptoms including anorexia, weight-loss, apathy, depression and a combination of late-night insomnia, restless fearful sleep and morning headache, somnolence and inertia, sometimes with frank morning cyanosis.

Overnight oximetry recordings will generally reveal baseline levels of 85–90% capillary oxygen saturation, with periods of more severe hypoxia (often below 70%) in deep sleep. Such hypoxia has been shown to accelerate the muscle weakness. It is now clear, from several studies, that the use at home of nocturnal positive-pressure ventilation, using a tightly fitting face mask, will relieve many or all of these symptoms and may improve the quality of life to a degree not enjoyed for several months before its introduction (Rideau et al 1983, Ellis et al 1987, Kerby et al 1987, Miller et al 1988, 1990, Segall 1988, Heckmatt et al 1990). Some of the problems for the family are discussed by Miller et al (1990). Departments of anaesthesia and intensive care in a number of regional centres in Britain provide such a service to neuromuscular patients including, relatively recently, Duchenne patients. This technique is not required or accepted by all cases, but when it is, it may provide benefits for periods of between a few weeks and 3 years in our experience.

Sudden fluctuations in serum potassium, perhaps related to the limited total body (muscle) potassium pool, may cause difficulties in the management of acute illness or in postoperative care.

Useful reviews of the management of Duchenne muscular dystrophy include those of Siegel (1977, 1978), Robin & Falewski de Leon (1977), Dubowitz (1978), Bossingham et al (1979), Emery (1987) and Brooke et al (1989).

Benign X-linked (Becker) muscular dystrophy

Definition. A form of muscular dystrophy, with the onset of symptoms typically in the second decade and with retention of the ability to walk beyond the age of 16 years and typically beyond the age of 30 years, characterised by 'in-frame' deletions (or duplications) of the Xp21 gene, and by the presence in skeletal muscle of dystrophin which is typically of abnormally small or large molecular weight and of normal or only moderately reduced abundance.

It has been customary in recent years to use the ability to walk unaided beyond the age of 16 years as the point of clinical separation from Duchenne muscular dystrophy; indeed before the acceptance of the existence of Duchenne outliers, the conventional cut-off age was 12 years. Bushby et al (1993, 1994) have accumulated evidence for the existence of a specific 'typical Becker' syndrome, based on the rate of progression of the disability and confirmed by the discovery in these same cases of a characteristic 'in-frame' gene deletion restricted to the region of the gene from exon 45 to 59 and, in almost all cases, starting at exon 45. Of 54 cases in this clinically typical group in whom deletion studies were available, 49 had deletions extending from exon 45 to 47, 48, 49 or 54, one a deletion of exons 48–59 and four had no deletion. Of the 11 atypical, more severely disabled, cases none showed the same exon 45- deletion but in contrast they had a variety of other deletions or duplications of the gene, or no deletion. It would be possible to make a case, therefore, for the strict definition of Becker muscular dystrophy to include only such typical cases (to be described in more detail below) and to classify the Meryon group of dystrophies as follows:

Duchenne — various deletions in 65%

Intermediate (Duchenne-outlier) and severe-Becker types — various deletions etc. in 65%

Typical Becker — with a 3-, 4- or 5-exon deletion, starting at exon 45, in 90%

Even milder cases — various, and often large, rod-domain deletions

Background. The existence of a distinct benign X-linked recessive form of muscular dystrophy was first recognised by Becker & Keiner (1955) who described a family and quoted earlier reports of similar pedigrees. Subsequent reports by Becker (1957, 1962), Moser et al (1964), Mabry et al (1965), Rotthauwe & Kowalewski (1965), Markand et al (1969), Emery & Skinner (1976), Ringel et al (1977), Bradley et al (1978) and others made it clear that the benign cases are distinct in the sense that they are part of a bimodal spectrum of severity. Families are occasionally found in which cases of the Becker and Duchenne types seem to coexist (Furukawa & Peter 1977), but these have been thought to reflect the extremes of variation in severity of the two disorders. Genetic linkage data at first suggested that the Duchenne and Becker genes occupied widely separated loci on the X-chromosome (Philip et al 1956, Skinner et al 1974, Zatz et al 1974), but these studies were statistically inconclusive and Kingston et al (1983, 1984) provided firm evidence, based on linkage to cloned DNA sequences, that the Becker and Duchenne genes are both located at Xp21.

Incidence. Since the discovery of dystrophin, earlier suggestions about the prevalence of Becker muscular dystrophy (see the last edition of this book and Emery 1991) have been shown to be serious underestimates. Figures quoted for incidence then varied between 1.7 and 5.5/100 000 male live births (Emery 1991). Bushby et al (1991b) attempted the complete ascertainment of Becker patients in the Northern Region of England, confirming the diagnosis by DNA and dystrophin studies, and showed that the incidence was in fact 5.83/100 000 male live births in 1940–65 (Duchenne incidence 28.8/100 000 for a comparable early date) and the population prevalence in 1988 was 2.38/100 000 (Duchenne 2.48/100 000). In this study the criterion for separating 'mild Duchenne' from 'severe Becker' muscular dystrophy was ability to walk beyond the age of 16 years. Since the population prevalences of Duchenne and Becker dystrophies are nearly equal, it seems likely that all the available birth incidence figures for Becker cases are still underestimates. Bushby & Gardner-Medwin (1993) found the reproductive fitness of typical and severe cases of Becker muscular dystrophy to be respectively 80% and 6% of normal, giving an overall figure of 0.61×10^{-5} for the mutation rate for Becker muscular dystrophy (6.63×10^{-5} for the Meryon muscular dystrophies as a whole). Passos-Bueno & Zatz (1991) also found a very low fitness (12%) in a group of severe Becker cases; Emery & Skinner's (1976) figure for a more typical group was 67%.

Four cases were identified in three neonatal screening programmes (Drummond 1979, Planchu et al 1980, Scheuerbrandt et al 1986) but in an overlapping screening period the French group found two or three possible Becker cases (Guibaud et al 1981) so the identified incidence among 242 000 males was 1.67–2.9 per 100 000. The serum CK activity in the Becker cases at birth was significantly lower than in the Duchenne cases and neonatal screening cannot yet be regarded as reliable in this condition.

Onset and course of the disease. Symptoms may begin as early as 1 and as late as 45 years of age, but in the great majority the onset is between the ages of 5 and 15 years. The first active complaint is usually between the ages of 5 and 20 years (50% by 10 years, almost 90% by 20 years, 98% by 35 years). Walking may be delayed in infancy (mean age 15 months, range 10–36 months) and the mean age of recollected peak performance is 12 years — range 3–25 years– (Bushby & Gardner-Medwin 1993). Toe-walking is a common early feature and is often disregarded for many years. In the early stages muscle cramp, usually occurring in the calves after exercise, occurs in 80% (more frequently than in any other type of muscular dystrophy except myotonic dystrophy). Occasionally this later becomes so severe that decompressive fasciotomy has been suggested (Henry & Neville 1984). The first symptoms otherwise are usually difficulty in running or in hurrying up stairs and, later, in doing heavy work with the arms. Few patients are able to run after the second decade.

The mean ages and ranges for the 'milestones' of the disease are similar in many series: onset 11 years (range 1–45); first upper limb symptoms about 30 years (12–50+); inability to walk 30–40 years (range 12–78); death 42–47 years (range 23–89) (Shaw & Dreifuss 1969, Emery & Skinner 1976, Bradley et al 1978, Bushby & Gardner-Medwin 1993). In the experience of Becker (1964) the age at onset extended from 5 to 30 years and only 10 per cent became unable to walk before the age of 40 years. This accords with the 'typical' (in-frame exon 45-deletion) group in our series in which the mean onset was 12 years, and of 53 cases only four had become unable to walk (at a mean age of 58 years) whereas in the severe group the mean onset was 7.7 years and eight of the ten cases had become unable to walk (at a mean age of 25.6 years).

There is no evidence that the course in Becker dystrophy is intermittently progressive or that the disease arrests at any stage, although progression may be almost imperceptibly slow for long periods.

Physical signs and complications. The selective muscle involvement is virtually identical to that in Duchenne muscular dystrophy. Symptoms are noticed in the lower limbs 5–20 years before the upper limbs, but examination will usually reveal the typically affected shoulder muscles in any patient with symptoms. There is selective bilateral and symmetrical wasting and weakness of the costal origin of pectoralis major, latissimus dorsi, brachioradialis, hip flexors and extensors and medial vastus of quadriceps. Later the supinator, biceps, triceps, serratus anterior and neck flexors become weak, and the adductors and abductors of the thigh and anterior tibial muscles are involved. Deltoids, the flexors and extensors of the wrists and fingers, small hand muscles, hamstrings and calf muscles are relatively preserved. Computed tomography scans are a valuable new means of analysing the selective muscle involvement (de Visser & Verbeeten 1985b). The face is virtually completely spared, even in the late stages. The tendon reflexes are impaired and later absent in affected muscles. Hypertrophy of the calves is a prominent and almost constant feature, and the deltoids, extensor muscles in the forearm, lateral vasti of the quadriceps and anterior tibial muscles are commonly hypertrophic at some stage of the disease. The calf enlargement affects both the gastrocnemii and soleus muscles and may precede all other symptoms by several years. The lordotic standing posture and waddling gait are very similar to those seen in Duchenne muscular dystrophy. Contractures are not a feature in typical Becker dystrophy until the patient is confined to a wheelchair, but pes cavus is reported in between 15% (Bradley et al 1978) and 70% (Ringel et al 1977) of cases. Scoliosis, although emphasised by Ringel et al, is usually not severe and thoracic distortion is very uncommon. Respiratory failure seems to be rare (Rideau et al 1981).

Early cardiac involvement is not a feature in typical Becker dystrophy. In the late stages patients may have significant ECG abnormalities including, in different individuals, bundle-branch block, Q waves, increased R/S ratios and T-wave changes. A few develop clinical cardiac failure and this is sometimes the cause of death (Mabry et al 1965, Markand et al 1969, Emery & Skinner 1976, Bradley et al 1978). Severe cases more often have abnormal ECGs (Bushby & Gardner-

Medwin 1993). Myocardial involvement seems to be more prominent in a few families (Wadia et al 1976, Katiyer et al 1977, Casazzo et al 1988, Donofrio et al 1989) and occasionally progressive cardiomyopathy may require cardiac transplantation (reviewed by Quinlivan & Dubowitz 1992). McKusick includes X-linked dilated cardiomyopathy as allelic with Duchenne and Becker muscular dystrophy, on the basis of tight genetic linkage and abnormal cardiac dystrophin, though skeletal muscle dystrophin is normal (McKusick 1992). Clearly, more work on cardiac dystrophin needs to be done in Becker families.

Although most patients with Becker muscular dystrophy are of normal intelligence, and some are of superior intelligence, there does seem to be a significant minority with mental retardation (Zellweger & Hanson 1967b, Emery & Skinner 1976, Ringel et al 1977, Bradley et al 1978, Karagan & Sorensen 1981). The last-named authors found the mean full scale IQ (WAIS or WISC) in 16 cases to be 94, verbal 90, performance 99. As in patients in Duchenne dystrophy, this retardation appears to be non-progressive and, in our experience, may rarely be the presenting problem with later recognition of muscle weakness. Patients with very delayed early motor development usually have a learning disability. Overall the academic achievements and employment records of Becker patients are disappointing.

Hallen (1970) reported a high incidence of hypogonadism in 'pelvic-girdle' types of muscular dystrophy including the Becker type. We have not encountered this or any other systemic manifestation of this disease, and the reproductive fitness recorded above is not consistent with hypogonadism.

A boy of 6 years with Becker muscular dystrophy and a history of cramps on exercise and episodic, apparently non-exertional, myoglobinuria, died under general anaesthesia with acute rhabdomyolysis, but without hyperthermia (Bush & Dubowitz 1991) as may occasionally happen in Duchenne muscular dystrophy.

Very mild and atypical forms. A widely quoted family in which two generations suffered from muscle cramps and had calf hypertrophy, but no detected muscle weakness, was reported by Gospe et al (1989). They had a large deletion of the rod-domain portion of the gene. Since the three oldest patients were aged 32, 26 and 22 years it is not clear that they fall outwith the range of onset for Becker cases. Another relatively mild case with a large deletion (of 46% of the gene) was reported by England et al (1990). A patient with exertional cramps (and probable myoglobinuria) was found to have a small deletion of the promoter region of the gene (Bushby et al 1991a). Some cases of 'myopathy limited to the quadriceps' turn out to have Becker muscular dystrophy (Sunohara et al 1990).

Diagnosis. The Becker type of muscular dystrophy is generally distinguishable from other muscular dystrophies on clinical grounds, and deletion and dystrophin studies are definitive. The patients reported as cases of X-linked spinal muscular atrophy (SMA) with large calves and high serum CK activity (Pearn & Hudgson 1978) have subsequently been proven to have Becker muscular dystrophy. De Visser & Verbeeten (1985b) showed quite different CT scan appearances of muscle in Becker dystrophy and typical SMA.

The serum CK activity is extremely high in the preclinical and early stages of the disease and falls steeply with age (Rotthauwe & Kowalewski 1965, Emery & Skinner 1976, Bradley et al 1978). In the first 10 years of life the serum CK levels are comparable with those seen in Duchenne cases at the same age (25–200 times normal). After the age of 20 the serum CK levels are lower, 1–10 times normal in the Emery & Skinner (1976) series and usually 2–60 times normal in a Newcastle series (Bradley et al 1978). It seems likely, but is not yet certain, that the disease can be ruled out by a normal serum CK activity in the preclinical age group.

The EMG usually demonstrates a pattern of short-duration low-amplitude polyphasic potentials with some fibrillation potentials and positive waves (Zellweger & Hanson 1967b, Markand et al 1969, Bradley et al 1978). Bradley et al reported that the findings in some cases suggested neurogenic atrophy, but giant motor units and grossly reduced interference patterns are not seen in Becker muscular dystrophy, As in Duchenne muscular dystrophy, high-frequency and myotonic discharges are occasionally seen.

The histological findings in Becker muscular dystrophy have been reviewed by Dubowitz & Brooke (1973), Ringel et al (1977) and Bradley et al (1978). Random variation in fibre size (both atrophy and hypertrophy), fibre splitting, central nuclei and fibrosis are the major features. Active necrosis and regeneration are more prominent in young patients. Bradley et al (1978) discuss the difficulty of differentiating the findings from those of neurogenic atrophy in some cases. The dystrophin immunoblotting and immunocytochemical findings are characteristic (see Ch. 26).

Carrier detection and prevention. All the daughters of affected males are definite carriers of the gene. Carrier detection using serum CK activity is less satisfactory in Becker muscular dystrophy than in the Duchenne type, but the very high incidence of deletions has transformed the situation in recent years. The subject is discussed in Chapter 26.

Manifesting female carriers of X-linked muscular dystrophies

The occasional occurrence of severe Duchenne dystrophy in girls and the problems of identifying non-manifesting potential carriers at risk are discussed elsewhere. Here we are concerned with the fact that female carriers of the Duchenne and Becker genes may have an overt myopathy sufficient to lead to a diagnosis of 'limb-girdle muscular dystrophy' (Fig. 14.4).

Gowers (1879), in his study of Duchenne muscular dystrophy, described one family with evident X-linked inheritance in which a female was severely affected. Moser & Emery (1974) reviewed more than 20 manifesting carriers reported in the previous 40 years adding 22 personal cases and others have been studied since then (Bulcke et al 1981, Yoshioka 1981, Olson & Fenichel 1982, de Visser & Verbeeten 1985a, Hoffman et al 1992). The equivalent situation in Becker dystrophy carriers was reported by Aguilar et al (1978). Overt myopathy appears to be one end of the spectrum of the degree of lyonisation of the X-linked genes and, not surprisingly, the severity of manifestation varies considerably from barely detectable weakness, or isolated calf hypertrophy, to progressive disabling weakness. The special

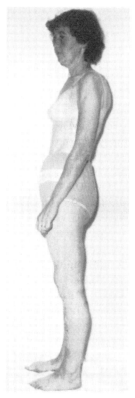

Fig. 14.4 A manifesting carrier of the Duchenne gene, aged 35 with a 3-year history of progressive proximal muscle weakness, diagnosed as 'limb-girdle muscular dystrophy', serum CK activity 11 x normal. Three years later her son, aged five, was found to have Duchenne muscular dystrophy.

case of discordant manifestation in identical twin girls is discussed on page 550. Moser & Emery (1974) showed that the manifesting carrier state often occurs in several members of a family.

The age at the onset of symptoms in manifesting carriers varies from early childhood to the fourth decade and the course is often progressive. We know of three personal cases in which the ability to walk was lost in the fifth or sixth decade. Moser & Emery (1974) reported progression in 12 of 22 cases. All but four had calf muscle hypertrophy and one of these had presented in childhood, 50 years earlier, with swollen calves; she became unable to walk at the age of 53. The weakness and calf hypertrophy are sometimes asymmetrical (Hoffman et al, 1992). The literature is disappointingly silent on the subject of the precise distribution of muscle wasting and weakness but such information as there is suggests that this is the same as in Duchenne cases.

Manifesting carriers usually have very high serum CK activities, except in the late stage of the disorder. The ECG is sometimes abnormal with tall R waves in the right precordial leads, but more often the changes are mild and within the normal range (Emery 1969, Moser & Emery 1974).

Muscle biopsy in manifesting carriers often shows isolated hyaline or necrotic fibres or small foci of necrosis and is sometimes severely dystrophic (Dubowitz 1963, Emery 1965, Pearce et al 1966, Yoshioka 1981, de Visser & Verbeeten 1985a). The use of CT to identify selective muscle involvement in these patients (Bulcke et al 1981, de Visser & Verbeeten 1985a) may prove valuable in the differential diagnosis from other proximal muscular dystrophies.

Moser & Emery (1974) revealingly estimated the prevalence of manifesting carriers in the female population to be 22.4×10^{-6} and pointed out that this was comparable to the incidence of 'limb-girdle dystrophy', and that many females presenting with limb-girdle weakness could be accounted for in this way.

The Duchenne carrier state is the likeliest diagnosis when a female with a normal karyotype presents with progressive proximal myopathy in 'Duchenne' distribution, calf hypertrophy, a very high serum CK activity and randomly scattered necrotic fibres in the muscle biopsy. Additional evidence in favour would be similar symptoms or a raised serum CK level in her mother or other females in the maternal line, asymmetry of the calf hypertrophy or an ECG showing tall R waves over the right precordium. Screening for DNA deletions throughout the Xp21 gene is difficult in females. Even the interpretation of immunocytochemical dystrophin staining of muscle biopsies may be difficult if there is advanced dystrophic change but this, together with the quantitation of dystrophin by immunoblotting, using several different antibodies, is the most reliable diagnostic technique (Hoffman et al 1992). Such patients should be offered appropriate genetic counselling.

Emery–Dreifuss muscular dystrophy

Definition. An X-linked disorder (gene loca-tion Xq28) of which the cardinal features are early muscle contractures of the elbow flexors, the ankle plantiflexors and the paraspinal, especially posterior cervical, muscles; slowly progressive weakness in humeroperoneal distribution; and cardiomyopathy, especially cardiac conduction defects.

A family of eight affected males in three generations with clear evidence of X-linked inheritance was recorded on three occasions by Dreifuss & Hogan (1961), Emery & Dreifuss (1966) and McKusick (1971). The disorder was quite distinct from Becker dystrophy. The symptoms began at 4–5 years and weakness progressed slowly. It was described as affecting only the proximal muscles in the upper and lower limbs but it now appears that the distal muscles of the lower limbs were also affected in the earliest stages (Emery A E H, personal communication). Muscle hypertrophy was absent except in one case. Contractures of the biceps and calf muscles were a striking and early feature. Every patient over the age of 25 had cardiac involvement, either atrial fibrillation or atrio-ventricular block. The serum CK levels were between six and seven times normal in the second decade and fell subsequently. Some female carriers had raised serum CK levels.

Meanwhile cases of a progressive scapuloperoneal syndrome of myopathic origin and with X-linked inheritance were described by Rotthauwe et al (1972), Thomas et al (1972), Waters et al (1975), Hassan et al (1979), Hopkins et al (1981), Dickey et al (1984) and Dubowitz (1985). Rowland et al (1979) described a case, defined the cardinal features and coined the term 'Emery–Dreifuss muscular dystrophy' to include the many cases of X-linked scapulohumeroperoneal myopathy in the literature.

Clinical features. The symptoms begin in early childhood or adolescence, occasionally later, and progress over four to six decades, unless cardiac complications supervene. In young children clinical features are disappointingly non-specific but inability to flex the spine and neck in picking objects up from the floor and very early elbow contractures may sometimes be detected by the age of 2–3 years. Toe-walking usually starts later, from about 10 years. The stride is awkward and restricted before much weakness is apparent.

But gradually wasting and weakness develop in the humeroperoneal distribution, spreading to include scapular winging and proximal lower-limb muscles, with or without mild facial weakness. Muscle hypertrophy is absent. Profound weakness is a rare and late feature, fewer than 10% of cases become confined to a wheelchair. Contractures at the elbows and of the posterior neck, paraspinal and calf muscles are always prominent and in some cases there is pes cavus. Many require (and benefit from) Achilles tenotomies, a potential anaesthetic hazard if the diagnosis has not been made.

Atrio-ventricular conduction defects associated with cardiomyopathy are the most dangerous feature of the disease. Death from heart block is frequent from the twenties onwards, though many cases survive without serious cardiac complications into their 40s, 50s or 60s. Some cases develop a dilating cardiomyopathy. Cardiac pacemakers may be life-saving. The main responsibility in caring for patients with this type of muscular dystrophy is to monitor cardiac function from adolescence onwards, to identify heart block early and to provide a pacemaker at the right moment. In some families the symptoms of heart block were the dominant problem, causing a major threat to life in the third or fourth decade, and evidence of the skeletal myopathy was relatively trivial (Waters et al 1975, Hassan et al 1979, Voit et al 1988); this contrasts with the opposite situation in the original kindred of Emery & Dreifuss (1966). The evolution of the cardiac dysfunction has been reported by Yoshioka et al (1989) and Bialer et al (1991).

The serum CK activity is raised 2- to 20-fold in the first 25–35 years of life but is normal in older cases. Female carriers have normal serum CK levels (see Voit et al 1988 for some exceptions), but may have ECG evidence of premature atrial beats and chronic bradycardia and cardiomegaly, and may even require a pacemaker (Dickey et al 1984, Bialer et al 1991). The EMG suggests myopathy. Occasional necrosis and phagocytosis, central nuclei, type I fibre atrophy, type II predominance and proliferation of connective tissue are the main features of muscle biopsies; but in young children only scattered fibre atrophy and type II fibre predominance may be seen; and in advanced cases there may be full-scale dystrophic changes.

In the family described by Thomas et al (1972) the disorder was closely linked with deutan colour blindness and, since 1985, increasingly precise gene localisation has been achieved, currently to the distal part of Xq28 (Yates et al 1993).

Scapuloperoneal syndromes are much more frequently neurogenic than myopathic in origin (Kaeser 1965, Emery et al 1968; see also Chapter 24). But those cases of the typical Emery–Dreifuss syndrome with (doubtfully) 'neurogenic' features on biopsy (Mawatari & Katayama 1973, Waters et al 1975) are now generally regarded as having the same disorder.

Autosomal dominant scapuloperoneal myopathy may be neurogenic in origin, or may reflect abortive or incompletely expressed examples of facioscapulohumeral muscular dystrophy (Ricker & Mertens 1968, Kazakov et al 1976), but in addition autosomal dominant scapuloperoneal muscular dystrophy and an autosomal dominant form of Emery–Dreifuss-like muscular dystrophy are discussed later in this chapter. Female cases of apparently typical Emery–Dreifuss syndrome cannot at present be firmly classified. They might have the autosomal dominant variety, but by analogy with the Meryon group of muscular dystrophies the occurrence of fully manifesting carriers of the X-linked disorder remains a possibility. The sporadic cases and some of the published small kindreds (Takamoto et al 1984, Miller et al 1985, Merchut et al 1990, Orstavik et al 1990) are compatible with either explanation, and genetic counselling must take this into account.

Useful reviews are those of Rowland et al (1979), Merlini et al (1986), Voit et al (1988), Emery (1989) and Specht (1992).

Ji type of muscular dystrophy

A single large kindred described by Ji et al (1990) appears to represent a new X-linked muscular dystrophy. The shoulder-girdle and paraspinal muscles are mainly involved. Onset is at about 10 years. Neither contractures nor muscle hypertrophy are early features and cardiac function is normal at least until the mid 30s (Ji's oldest case was aged 37 years). The serum CK activity is high.

Hereditary myopathy limited to females

Two reports suggest that X-linked dominant inheritance may occur in a form of muscular dystrophy. The lack of investigation of the muscle disorder in the large pedigree reported by Hertrich (1957) precludes accurate diagnosis. Henson et al (1967) recorded eight cases, all female, in two generations. They had a high incidence of miscarriages. Symptoms of a proximal myopathy began in the first or second decade and progressed to severe disability by the age of 30. They had a waddling gait, lumbar lordosis and weakness of the truncal and proximal muscles of the limbs, especially glutei and hamstrings. The deltoids and medial gastrocnemii were wasted. The facial muscles were spared. Serum CK levels were 9–15 times normal in adults but were normal in two affected children. Muscle biopsy showed a necrotising myopathy.

This may be a separate form of X-linked muscular dystrophy, lethal in affected males before birth.

MUSCULAR DYSTROPHIES WITH AUTOSOMAL RECESSIVE INHERITANCE

These may broadly be divided, according to the age at onset, into congenital, childhood and adult forms. The latter two, together with the proximal muscular dystrophies of autosomal dominant inheritance, are not always easy to separate on clinical grounds, especially in sporadic cases, and have tended in the past to be called 'limb-girdle muscular dystrophy'. In abandoning this term as a definitive diagnosis and in attempting to list and describe the several entities which it disguises, we recognise that research in this long-neglected group of muscular dystrophies is still in an early and transitional stage, that some of the entities we list are tentative and that before the next edition of this book this situation will have changed. Nevertheless, for the patients involved a precise diagnosis is important for prognosis and genetic counselling and by attempting a provisional nosology we hope to help the clinician to give appropriate, if often cautious, advice. It will be seen that the customary description of a specific selective pattern of muscle involvement for each type of muscular dystrophy, so well known and helpful in many of the traditional categories, is not always possible in autosomal recessive types. This may simply be because they have not yet been well described. But it is also possible that we have tended to extrapolate from experience of the Meryon group of dystrophies and the facioscapulohumeral, Emery–Dreifuss and other muscular dystrophies in which consistent patterns occur, to make a false assumption that this must therefore be true of *all* the muscular dystrophies. If so it has been a potent hindrance to progress, and enlightenment may come only from the laboratory, in the form of gene localisation and coding or the discovery of underlying protein defects — a process that has just begun. We must expect and explore the possibility that types which seem clinically very different, perhaps even some of the congenital and adult-onset types, may turn out to be genetically and biochemically related, but at present there is no evidence of this.

Autosomal recessive childhood muscular dystrophy (North African type)

Definition. A progressive muscular dystrophy, fairly closely resembling the Duchenne type in pattern and severity but autosomal recessive in inheritance, which is relatively common in North Africa from Tunisia to Sudan and also in Arabia. There is provisional evidence of a specific defect in a 'dystrophin-associated glycoprotein' with a molecular weight of 50 kDa.

Clinical features. The condition was first described in a number of studies from North Africa (Ben Hamida & Marrakchi 1980, Ben Hamida et al 1983, Salih et al 1983) which characterised a severe autosomal recessive muscular dystrophy seen in large consanguineous kindreds there. Many features were closely similar to those of Duchenne muscular dystrophy, including steadily progressive weakness in a broadly similar distribution, hypertrophy of the calf muscles, in Ben Hamida's cases a very high serum CK activity in the early stages (50–200× the normal limit), and a destructive, necrotising muscle biopsy picture.

Dystrophin is normal (Ben Jelloun-Dellagi et al 1990). In Salih's cases the serum CK levels were only up to $15\times$ normal. The age at the onset varied greatly, even within each family, from 3 to 12 years, and at inability to walk from 10 to 30 years (usually 15–20 years in Ben Hamida's cases and 11–14 years in Salih's). Death, recorded only in Salih's cases, usually occurred at between 15 and 20 years. ECGs were often abnormal (Salih et al 1983) but showed ST depression and T-wave changes and not the deep Q waves seen in Duchenne cases. Impaired respiratory function appeared to be a major cause of death (Salih et al 1984).

In a personal case from Qatar the clinical, CK and biopsy features were indistinguishable from those in Duchenne MD with the striking exception that the hamstring muscles were weaker than the quadriceps. Dystrophin assay on immunoblotting was normal, but immunocytochemical staining showed very little dystrophin associated with the muscle fibre membrane, suggesting faulty attachment of the protein to the membrane. Matsumara et al (1992) found a defective 50 kDa 'dystrophin-associated glycoprotein' in this disorder, a membrane glycoprotein which is concerned with the anchoring of dystrophin to the sarcolemma. This would explain the resemblance to Duchenne muscular dystrophy.

This disorder has not yet been convincingly identified in other ethnic groups. Its relation to cases of autosomal recessive childhood muscular dystrophy as seen elsewhere is not yet known.

Autosomal recessive childhood muscular dystrophy (Hutterite type)

Definition. A mildly progressive autosomal recessive muscular dystrophy with its onset in the first decade, mild facial weakness and predominant involvement of the lower limbs, reported in the Hutterite populations of Manitoba and Saskatchewan.

Clinical features. Symptoms begin at 1–9 years and progress slowly to give difficulty in rising from a chair in the 30s. The pelvic-girdle muscles and quadriceps are the first and most affected; in the arms the trapezius and deltoids are more affected than the pectoral muscles, so that the

shoulders protrude forwards; there is mild facial weakness. Distal weakness is restricted to the brachioradialis and peroneal muscles. The heart and intellect are unaffected. Serum CK level levels are 1–10 times normal and there are apparently non-specific mild myopathic features in the muscle biopsy (Shokeir & Kobrinsky 1976, Shokeir & Rozdilsky 1985). The gene has not been localised.

Indiana Amish and Reunion type of muscular dystrophy

Definition. A progressive, proximal muscular dystrophy, without facial or cardiac involvement, with the onset of symptoms before the age of 20 years, of which the gene maps to chromosome 15.

Background. Fardeau studied a population of related kindreds with a form of 'limb-girdle' muscular dystrophy on the island of Reunion. They could be traced back to an immigrant common ancestor in the mid-seventeenth century. Linkage studies localised the gene to chromosome 15 (Beckmann et al 1991). Use of the same probes confirmed genetic linkage also in the form of muscular dystrophy described 30 years earlier, in an Indiana Amish isolate, by Jackson & Carey (1961) and Jackson & Strehler (1968). Linkage was proved in two 'limb-girdle' pedigrees in Brazil, but excluded in six others (Passos-Bueno et al 1993; see contributions by C E Jackson and others in Clarke 1992).

Clinical features. The onset of symptoms in the Amish cases was at 5–15 years and in Reunion before 20 years, usually 8–15 years. The proximal upper and lower limb muscles were equally and symmetrically involved, together with the anterior and posterior neck muscles. The face was spared, even in the oldest patients, and muscle hypertrophy was uncommon and never a prominent feature.

In Reunion loss of ability to walk was at about 30 years: in Indiana this was much more variable (12–44 years, with few walking beyond 25 years). Five Indiana patients had died, at 15, 24, 41, 48 and 67 years.

Nothing has been published on selective muscle involvement, but Fardeau (personal communication, 1992) provided the following data. *Most affected:* latissimus dorsi, rhomboids, rectus abdominis, gluteus maximus, hip adductors; *next most:* inferior trapezius, deltoid, biceps, gluteus medius, psoas, quadriceps; *moderately:* triceps, serratus anterior, paraspinals, biceps cruri; *less affected:* forearm muscles, triceps surae, tibialis anterior; *least affected or normal:* face and bulbar muscles, small hand muscles, tibialis posterior.

The heart was generally not involved, but several of the cases described by Jackson & Carey (1961) had QRS changes resembling the typical Duchenne pattern.

Serum CK activity in cases below the age of 30 was 8–60 times normal, one to three times normal in older cases (Jackson & Strehler 1968). Muscle biopsies were dystrophic, but no details are available.

Other or undifferentiated childhood muscular dystrophies with autosomal recessive inheritance

The delineation of the above three categories of autosomal recessive, predominantly proximal muscular dystrophy, with an onset in childhood, leaves much uncertainty about the existence of any others.

Gull (1862) gave a very early account of two sisters with 'granular and fatty degeneration' of the muscles. But interest in the probable existence of autosomal recessive inheritance in the childhood muscular dystrophy began in the 1950s (Stevenson 1953, Lamy & de Grouchy 1954) and for many years depended upon the occasional occurrence of muscular dystrophy in girls and on a few families in which consanguinity of the parents made autosomal recessive inheritance likely. As knowledge advanced, earlier studies of female cases of muscular dystrophy were successively discarded because they did not exclude cases of spinal muscular atrophy or of Duchenne females with chromosome translocations. Now, in the dystrophin era, it is apparent that only rather sophisticated studies of dystrophin status are sufficient to distinguish the isolated manifesting carrier of the Duchenne gene from the isolated female case of autosomal recessive muscular dystrophy. Information based on large kindreds remains reliable; hence the basis for delineating all

three of the varieties described above. But undoubtedly the majority of both male and female cases of autosomal recessive dystrophy in most communities are sporadic or at most affect a few sibs in scattered families.

A kindred which may be confidently accepted as an example of autosomal recessive childhood dystrophy, but which has not been assigned to a particular category, was that of Kloepfer & Talley (1958, Pedigree 1). Hazama et al (1979) reported six girls including two sisters who were severely mentally retarded, a feature unique to them. Moser et al (1966), in their review of 'limb-girdle dystrophy' in Switzerland, included 14 cases without facial involvement in whom the lower limb muscles were first affected. In nine, the symptoms began between 3 and 9 years of age and in the rest at 15–27 years. It is interesting that the cases of Jackson & Carey (1961) and Shokeir & Kobrinsky (1976), described in previous sections, were of Swiss descent. The latter cases had some involvement of facial muscles, and Moser et al (1966) also distinguished a separate autosomal recessive group of seven cases, with onset between the ages of 3 and 17 years, in which the facial muscles were affected. Possibly these cases had the 'Hutterite type' of muscular dystrophy. The pure lower limb-girdle group of Moser et al (1966) showed no calf enlargement and their serum CK activities were normal or raised up to 10-fold. The experience of Becker (1964) was different. In south Germany he found that autosomal recessive pelvifemoral dystrophy closely resembled his benign X-linked cases, often showing calf hypertrophy. His recessive cases showed high rates of parental consanguinity and tended to come from small country villages.

Gardner-Medwin & Johnston (1984), in a study of girls with severe muscular dystrophy, flawed by the possible inclusion of some manifesting carriers of the Meryon gene, found six points which appeared to help in the distinction from Duchenne muscular dystrophy. Of these, four remain of some value: (1) brisk toe-walking as a prominent early feature (aged 1–5 years) before the onset of *difficulty* in walking; (2) normal ECG; (3) normal intelligence; (4) relatively less severe destruction of muscle in biopsies performed before the age of 10 years, preservation of the histochemical fibre types and a focal pattern of pathology, typically with foci of tens to hundreds of necrotic, atrophic or regenerating fibres seen against a background of relatively preserved fibres. In a more recent review of eight females in which dystrophin studies showed that four were Meryon carriers and four had normal dystrophin, the latter group provided broad confirmation of the criteria. They should, however, be regarded as suggestive rather than definitive, and as such they may be useful in directing attention to boys who should be investigated with special attention to the possibility of autosomal recessive muscular dystrophy. A similar pattern of biopsy may be seen in early Becker cases, and in the North African form (Ben Hamida et al 1983) but has been recorded by others in sporadic European cases (Kakulas et al 1975, Dubowitz 1978, Figs 2–40).

In summary, therefore, it seems that at least until the North African, Hutterite and Indiana/Reunion types of muscular dystrophy can be specifically identified in individual cases, it will often remain necessary simply to distinguish autosomal recessive from X-linked childhood muscular dystrophy. The former is similar to the Duchenne type but rather more benign. Variation in severity occurs even within families. The birth incidence, based on small numbers, is about 0.3 per 100 000 live births and the prevalence about 0.2 per 100 000 (Gardner–Medwin 1992). The onset may be in the second year or as late as the fourteenth, but is most usual in the second half of the first decade. Early lively toe-walking is a common characteristic. Progression is comparatively slow and patients usually become unable to walk in their early 20s, sometimes as early as 12 years or as late as the fifth decade, and many survive to the fifth decade or later. The weakness is chiefly proximal and has not been differentiated clearly in its distribution from that of Duchenne dystrophy. Muscle hypertrophy is present in some affected families. Intelligence is normal. ECGs are normal. The serum CK activity may be only moderately raised (up to 10 times the normal limit) but in many cases is in the Duchenne range. A strikingly multifocal pattern of necrosis may be a distinctive feature of the pathology.

Dubowitz (1978) described some cases of a 'limb-girdle myopathy' associated with cramps and myoglobinuria, in which glycogen- and lipid-storage diseases had been ruled out. Their significance is not clear.

The principles of management of autosomal recessive childhood muscular dystrophy are the same as for the Duchenne type, taking into account the better prognosis.

Autosomal recessive muscular dystrophy of proximal lower limb distribution and late onset

It is very doubtful if any entity of this type remains after elimination of the four categories discussed above. The review of proximal muscular dystrophies in Switzerland (Moser et al 1966) included five cases affecting the lower limbs with an onset after the age of 15 years. Dubowitz & Brooke (1973) mention reviewing 18 cases of 'limb-girdle dystrophy' and illustrate three of them with a relatively late onset varying from 14 to 33 years. In a second edition (Dubowitz 1985) only one of the three remains. In this case and the four sporadic cases reported by Bethlem et al (1973), of whom two had a suspiciously early onset, lobulated and whorled fibres were prominent but not specific features. The myopathy was relatively slowly progressive. Serum CK levels varied from 86 to 850 iu/l. Two patients had electrophysiological and histological features of denervation as well as of myopathy, a dilemma very commonly posed by cases of the 'limb-girdle syndrome'. Bethlem et al (1973) described similar pathology in two additional sibs with a probably dominant mode of inheritance and it is difficult to know whether rare sporadic cases of this type might be new mutant dominants or are truly examples of a rare autosomal recessive disorder. Similar uncertainties were encountered in the study of Bradley (1979), who found a 2 : 1 male predominance (suggesting contamination of the series by X-linked disorders) and only 33% of cases with no features of a denervating component to the pathology. Panegyres et al (1990) reviewed 33 Western Australian cases, without performing dystrophin studies, with results reminiscent of those of Moser et al (1966); there were eight sporadic, six probably autosomal recessive and four autosomal dominant cases with proximal limb involvement, four early-onset cases with facial involvement, three cases with both proximal and distal involvement, five with mixed neurogenic and myopathic features and three with biopsy evidence of mitochondrial myopathy. Yates & Emery (1985), again at the end of the predystrophin era, commented on the apparent decline in the frequency of 'limb-girdle muscular dystrophy' over the previous 30 years, concluded that it was largely due to attrition as other entities were withdrawn from this category, and found that the maximum prevalance of such cases in the Lothian Region of Scotland was 0.7 per 100 000 and the 'proven' (pre-dystrophin) prevalence was 0.3 per 100 000. Passos-Bueno et al (1993) showed that in most of their large kindreds with 'limb-girdle muscular dystrophy' there was *no* linkage to the 'Reunion gene' on chromosome 15. No other good population study of adult-onset autosomal recessive muscular dystrophies has been reported since dystrophin assay has made it possible to rule out cryptic cases of Becker muscular dystrophy and manifesting carriers of the Meryon gene.

Scapulohumeral muscular dystrophy (Erb 1884)

This is a decidedly uncommon muscular dystrophy which first becomes apparent in early adult life and predominantly affects the upper limb girdle (Fig. 14.5). Becker (1964) did not include any such cases in his comprehensive review of myopathies in Baden. The weakness is at first most prominent in the biceps, triceps, trapezius, rhomboid and serratus anterior muscles, and scapular winging is a major feature. The deltoid is relatively preserved. The proximal muscles of the lower limbs are affected later, especially the hip flexors and quadriceps, with relative preservation of the hamstrings and muscles below the knees. The facial, forearm and hand muscles are also strikingly preserved until the later stages. The condition is usually very slowly but continuously progressive. Ten or even 20 years may elapse before the weakness spreads from the upper to the lower limbs. Moser et al (1966) reported 15 cases of this type from Switzerland where it appears to be relatively common. The sexes were equally affected. The age at onset in their cases varied

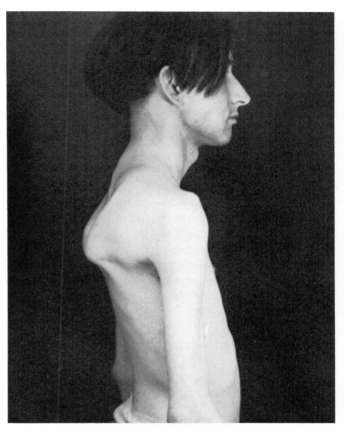

Fig. 14.5 Scapulohumeral muscular dystrophy: note the atrophy of upper limb muscles and the winged scapulae.

from 9 to 31 years but was usually 14–23 years. Hypertrophy of muscles was absent except in one doubtful case, and appears to be rare in this disorder. The serum CK activity was 22 times the normal in the youngest case (aged 14) and normal or only slightly raised (one to five times normal) in cases over 20 years of age. Our experience of a few cases is similar.

Contractures often develop in relation to joints in which the active range of movement is limited, but are not an early feature. The heart is not involved and intelligence is normal.

The differential diagnosis of this clinical syndrome includes the Emery–Dreifuss and facioscapulohumeral types of muscular dystrophy and, above all, spinal muscular atrophy. Any patient showing intermittent progression or asymmetry of muscle weakness is particularly likely to have one of the latter two disorders. Thyrotoxic myopathy (see Ch. 17) may present rather similar features. Diagnosis depends on the clinical and biochemical findings, on the EMG which shows myopathic changes without specific features, and on muscle biopsy to exclude features of the congenital myopathies or denervation. The myopathic features in biopsies of these cases are not well characterised but appear to be relatively indolent. One of the few cases reported under this title with modern published pathological findings seems to be an atypical example with dominant inheritance (Dubowitz 1978, p. 50).

One of the major disabilities in these patients is in raising the arms. The deltoids may be quite strong, but scapular fixation is very poor. Fixing the scapulae by bracing is not easy and contractures at the shoulder joint may limit the benefit of attempting this. Surgical fixation in carefully selected cases may be valuable (Copeland & Howard 1978), but the contractures must be overcome first.

Autosomal recessive distal muscular dystrophy

An autosomal dominant form of distal muscular dystrophy had been recognised for many years (see p. 580). Recently some cases have been described with probable autosomal recessive inheritance and a rather rapidly progressive course from the onset in the second or third decade to the stage of being unable to walk within about 10 years (Markesbery et al 1977, Miller et al 1979, de Visser 1983, Nonaka et al 1985, Miyoshi et al 1986). Nonaka et al and Miyoshi et al reviewed some earlier reports, mainly from the Japanese literature, and reported a total of 22 additional cases. One of the cases of Miyoshi et al was examined at autopsy. Nonaka et al contrasted the dystrophic pathology with that seen in a very similar clinical disorder in which muscle biopsy shows rimmed vacuoles in the muscle fibres and the serum CK activity is only slightly raised (Nonaka et al 1981a). Another less severe autosomal recessive distal myopathy, with filamentous inclusions in muscle fibres, was reported by Matsubara & Tanabe (1982) and Isaacs et al (1988, case 1).

The earliest feature is usually atrophy of the calf muscles and of the small muscles of the hands. The patients find it more difficult to stand on their toes than on their heels. Proximal muscles are more mildly affected. Serum CK activities are 40–100 times normal in the early stages and the muscle biopsy shows evidence of active fibre necrosis and regeneration. The muscle pathology was reviewed by Markesbery et al (1977).

Although most cases have been sporadic, Miyoshi et al (1986) provided strong evidence favouring autosomal recessive inheritance in their cases.

The congenital muscular dystrophies

The congenital muscular dystrophies can be defined as genetically determined necrotising myopathies with muscle weakness evident from the time of birth. With the exception of the Fukuyama type they tend to be relatively non-progressive. There appear to be several different types, in addition to congenital myotonic dystrophy which is discussed in Chapter 15, but much remains to be learned about the nosology of these disorders and some similar cases may even represent non-genetic disorders acquired in utero. The term was first used by Howard (1908) and several cases were recorded over the following 50 years which are now difficult to classify. Since the 1950s numerous *congenital myopathies* with more or less specific histological features have been defined (see Ch. 21), and a somewhat clearer picture of the dystrophies has emerged, though the usual type seen in Western countries is still rather loosely defined.

Three distinctive congenital muscular dystrophies, the hypotonic-sclerotic type of Ullrich and the Fukuyama type, both most commonly seen in Japan, and the type seen in the Eichsfeld isolate in Germany are treated separately.

Related disorders. The large kindred with autosomal recessive inheritance described by Lebenthal et al (1970) is atypical in having invariable congenital arthrogryposis and a high incidence of associated congenital heart disease, though not cardiomyopathy.

Early concepts of congenital muscular dystrophy were also confused by the inclusion of milder and more severe cases which are now thought to be distinct. Thus the benign congenital myopathy classically described by Batten (1903, 1909), Turner (1940) and Turner & Lees (1962) differs from the muscular dystrophies in its non-progressive course and in the absence of dystrophic histological features.

A few cases of a 'rapidly-progressive type of congenital muscular dystrophy' have been reported (de Lange 1937, Lewis & Besant 1962, Short 1963, Wharton 1965). Of these only Wharton's two cases survived beyond the age of 6 months. The clinical features in these cases varied considerably and the pathological evidence was in general inconclusive. The cases of Short (1963) bear a close resemblance to the X-linked type of centronuclear myopathy (see Ch. 21). Further evidence is needed before the existence of a distinct rapidly progressive form of congenital muscular dystrophy can be accepted.

Very uncommonly cases of Duchenne dystrophy are hypotonic at birth, resembling congenital muscular dystrophy, but in such cases dystrophin assay in the muscle biopsy is diagnostic.

Congenital muscular dystrophy in Western countries

Banker et al (1957), Greenfield et al (1958), O'Brien (1962), Pearson & Fowler (1963) and Zellweger et al (1967) described cases with congenital hypotonia and severe but relatively non-progressive muscular weakness, in which the muscle histology was typical of muscular dystrophy. In several children there was associated arthrogryposis multiplex. These cases formed the basis of our current concepts of the usual form of congenital muscular dystrophy seen in Europe and the USA.

In a series of cases from Finland, described by Donner et al (1975), the symptoms progressed slightly in the first few years of life and thereafter remained static. A similar clinical picture was found in the cases reported by Vasella et al (1967), Lazaro et al (1979) and McMenamin et al (1982b). Serratrice et al (1980) reviewed 92 cases from the literature.

The essential features of this disorder are severe hypotonia present from birth, associated with static or very slowly progressive muscular wasting and weakness. Fetal movements are often im-paired. Contractures at birth are common but not invariable, and they often develop later. Some children have difficulty in sucking and breathing in the neonatal period. There is often moderate facial weakness and Donner et al (1975) emphasised severe head lag. The serum CK activity is usually very high in the early stages, but not invariably so. Donner et al (1975) reported figures up to 30 times normal in the first 3 years, falling to one to five times normal by the age of 5 years. In late childhood the serum CK activity is often normal or only a little raised. The diagnosis can be made with confidence only by examination of the muscle histology. The 'dystrophic' appearances are often severe to a degree that seems out of proportion to the clinical disability, although in some mild cases there are simply non-specific myopathic changes without specific features. Afifi et al (1969) and Fidzianska et al (1982) emphasised the excessive collagen proliferation and paucity of muscle fibre regeneration.

Sibs are often affected, and there is increased parental consanguinity (Topaloglu et al 1991).

Most children with congenital muscular dystrophy learn to walk at between 18 months and 8 years, though strenuous efforts to overcome contractures and the use of supporting calipers may be needed (Jones et al 1979). Walking ability is often lost after a few years. Progressive contractures usually affect the flexor muscles in the upper and lower limbs and the paraspinal muscles, especially of the neck. The mortality in early childhood is high despite the non-progressive course of the weakness. Nocturnal hypoventilation may develop in the second decade and responds to face-mask nocturnal ventilation as described in the section above on Duchenne muscular dystrophy.

Intelligence is usually normal. However most cases are found to have a disorder of cerebral myelination on CT and MRI scans. This has been described in the presence of normal intelligence (Nogen 1980, Echenne et al 1986, Topaloglu et al 1991, Pihko et al 1992) or mild non-progressive mental retardation and epilepsy (Echenne et al 1984, 1986, Trevisan et al 1991) or epilepsy and rapidly progressive dementia in the second decade (Egger et al 1983). Among Egger's cases were two affected siblings. Delayed myelination giving a similar CT scan appearance is a frequent feature of Fukuyama muscular dystrophy (q.v.) in which it is non-progressive and usually temporary (Ishikawa 1982, Peters et al 1984). Cerebral atrophy, with normal myelination, may also be seen in cases of congenital muscular dystrophy with normal intelligence or with dementia, and sibs may be discordant in this respect (Pihko et al 1992).

Hypotonic-sclerotic muscular dystrophy (Ullrich). Ullrich described this form of congenital muscular dystrophy in 1930, and descriptions appeared only in the German literature until 1977 since when there have been a few reports in English, mostly originating from Japan (Furukawa & Toyokura 1977, Nihei et al 1979, Nonaka et al 1981b). These authors described 10 cases, and Nihei et al (1979) reviewed 15 cases from the literature.

The features are non-progressive congenital myopathy with slender muscles, contractures of the proximal muscles but hypotonic, hyperextensible distal muscles, relative sparing of the facial muscles, prominence of the calcaneus, high arched palate, hyperhidrosis and normal intelligence. Some cases have preserved tendon reflexes. Secondary scoliosis and torticollis are frequent. Nonaka *et al* (1981b) suggest that some cases may be slowly progressive. The serum CK level is normal or nearly so, EMG studies have shown non-specific myopathic features and muscle biopsies show variation in fibre size, poor histochemical fibre differentiation, often with type I predominance, fatty and connective tissue replacement and relatively little evidence of muscle fibre degeneration.

Siblings of both sexes may be affected and there is an increased rate of consanguinity, suggesting autosomal recessive inheritance (De Paillette et al 1989).

Eichsfeld type of congenital muscular dystrophy. Five cases, four of them related in a manner suggesting autosomal recessive inheritance, were described by Goebel et al (1980). They had congenital weakness, possibly slightly progressive, with progressive scoliosis. In three cases, progressive right ventricular cardiac dilatation, of which the pathology was not established, developed after the age of 9 years and was fatal in

two of them. The muscle pathology was compatible with a congenital dystrophy; the serum CK activities were normal or slightly raised.

Fidzianska et al (1983) described characteristic inclusion bodies in the muscle fibres in this disorder, which stain with desmin-antibodies. McKusick (1992) proposed the name 'Eichsfeld type' for this form of muscular dystrophy.

Fukuyama muscular dystrophy

Definition. A congenital, but severely progressive, muscular dystrophy, inherited as an autosomal recessive trait, with a high gene frequency only in Japan, and associated with cerebral malformation and dysmyelination. Preliminary evidence suggests a causative defect in a dystrophin-associated glycoprotein.

Clinical features. This distinctive type of congenital muscular dystrophy, first described by Fukuyama et al (1960), is now one of the most clearly documented muscular dystrophies (Kamoshita et al 1976, Fukuyama et al 1981). In Japan it is approximately half as frequent as Duchenne dystrophy. Elsewhere only a few reports have appeared (Krijgsman et al 1980, McMenamin et al 1982a, Goebel et al 1983, Peters et al 1984); indeed the very severe cerebral involvement and early mortality in the cases of Krijgsman and Goebel may indicate that they represent yet another separate category of congenital muscular dystrophy, comparable in some respects with the Walker–Warburg group but without eye involvement. Matsumura et al (1993) found a deficiency in 12 cases of the dystrophin-associated proteins in the sarcolemma, particularly the 43 kDa glycoprotein component of the complex. If confirmed, this suggests that the gene for Fukuyama muscular dystrophy, which has not yet been located, may well code for this specific glycoprotein. The closely allied glycoprotein defect in the North African form of autosomal recessive childhood muscular dystrophy (q.v.) is not associated with abnormalities of the brain.

The principal features are progressive muscular dystrophy of early onset, severe mental retardation and epilepsy. The onset is before 8 months but only a few cases have impairment of fetal movements. Congenital arthrogryposis is not a feature. The peak of motor development is at 2–5 years, after which slow deterioration occurs. Many patients learn to crawl but very few to walk. The muscle weakness is generalised with progressive contractures. The facial muscles are affected. Calf hypertrophy is frequent. Mental retardation is severe, the IQ being 30–50 in most cases. About half have some intelligible speech. Mild microcephaly is frequent. Febrile and non-febrile convulsions occur in more than half of all cases, usually with focal paroxysmal discharges in the EEG (Segawa et al 1979). CT brain scans commonly show low-density white matter (Yoshioka et al 1980, Fukuyama et al 1981) in addition to slight cerebral atrophy. Optic atrophy and other eye anomalies are not conspicuous but may be less rare than was suggested in early reports (Yoshioka et al 1990). This reopens the debate over the nosological relationship to the Walker–Warburg syndrome (q.v.), which is now likely to be settled by studies of the dystrophin-associated proteins.

The serum CK activities are comparable to those in Duchenne dystrophy, being 10–50 times the normal limit between 6 months and 6 years, later falling towards the normal range. Muscle biopsy (Fukuyama et al 1981, Nonaka et al 1982) reveals extensive connective tissue infiltration, destruction of the fascicular architecture, a lesser degree of fatty infiltration, muscle fibre atrophy without hypertrophy and type I fibre predominance. Necrosis, phagocytosis and regeneration are less severe than in Duchenne dystrophy but otherwise the appearances are similar.

Mild myocardial abnormalities may be found at autopsy but ECGs during life have been normal.

The cerebral pathology has been described in 24 cases by Fukuyama et al (1981) and in more detail in five cases by Takada et al (1984). Multifocal cerebral and cerebellar cortical dysplasia, micropolygyria, aberrant fascicles of myelinated nerve fibres and a degree of myelin pallor and gliosis in white matter were the main features. The neuropathology suggests a lesion dating from, at the latest, the fifth month of gestation, which has been confirmed in an affected 23-week fetus (Takada & Nakamura 1990).

A detailed genetic study provides strong evidence of autosomal recessive inheritance (Fukuyama & Osawa 1984).

There is little information in the available literature on the management of these cases or on survival. Of the 24 autopsied cases reviewed by Fukuyama et al (1981), four were under 2 years, four aged 2–9 years, 11 aged 10–19 years, four aged 20–22 years and one was unknown.

The Walker–Warburg syndrome and muscle–eye–brain disease

The Walker-Warburg syndrome is an autosomal recessive disorder comprising congenital muscular dystrophy, type II lissencephaly, cerebellar malformation and retinal malformation. Hydrocephalus, encephalocoele, cataracts, glaucoma, retinal detachment and microphthalmos are other common features (Dobyns et al 1989). Variation in fibre size, fibre splitting and endomysial fibrosis are seen in muscle biopsies. The high serum CK activity in early infancy (20–30 times normal) may be picked up in screening programmes for Duchenne muscular dystrophy (Greenberg et al 1992). Congenital 'dystrophic' myopathy, high serum CK activity and cataracts are seen also in the Marinesco–Sjögren syndrome (Tachi et al 1991).

A very similar, and possibly identical, type of congenital muscular dystrophy, associated with severe mental retardation, mild hydrocephalus, congenital glaucoma, cataracts, other eye anomalies and renal anomalies, occurs in Finland (Santavuori et al 1977, 1990, Raitta et al 1978) and has been named muscle–eye–brain disease. The serum CK activity is very high in early childhood but in cases that survive into adult life it falls to normal. Towfighi et al (1984) described seven rather similar cases from the USA, mostly surviving for less than a year, with detailed neuropathological findings, and these cases were given yet a different name, 'cerebro-ocular dysplasia/muscular dystrophy syndrome'. Similar rapidly fatal cases were described by Dobyns et al (1989) and Leyten et al (1989, 1991, 1992).

Dobyns et al (1989) suggested that all three disorders are the same, but Santavuori et al (1990) and Leyten et al (1992) disagree. Fukuyama muscular dystrophy, despite some features in common, seems to be distinct since the eyes are generally not conspicuously abnormal and the neuropathology is different (Leyten et al 1991).

MUSCULAR DYSTROPHIES WITH AUTOSOMAL DOMINANT INHERITANCE

Facioscapulohumeral (FSH) muscular dystrophy

Definition. A form of muscular dystrophy, autosomal dominant in inheritance, with muscular weakness of widely variable severity and age at onset, particularly affecting the facial muscles (eye and mouth closure), the serratus anterior, the humeral muscles (biceps and triceps) and the anterior tibial muscles in the early stages. The gene is located at 4q35 (Wijmenga et al 1991).

The onset may be at any age from childhood until adult life; abortive or mildly affected cases are frequently seen in the same families as more severe cases; after initial involvement of the face and shoulder-girdle muscles, weakness spreads to the distal and later the proximal muscles of the lower limbs; asymmetry of muscle involvement is very frequent; muscular hypertrophy is very rare; contractures and skeletal deformity are infrequent. Although cases occur in which the disease progresses unusually rapidly, most patients survive and remain active to a normal age. Diagnostic criteria have been recommended by Padberg et al (1991).

Atypical features and some similar disorders. This type of muscular dystrophy is one of the more clearly defined forms but some cases may cause confusion. Apparently isolated or recessive cases of facioscapulohumeral muscular dystrophy may occur (Moser et al 1966); their nature remains obscure. Cases with minimal facial involvement must be distinguished from examples of the 'scapuloperoneal syndrome' (q.v. pp. 565 & 579). Cases of spinal muscular atrophy, formerly reported to closely resemble facioscapulohumeral muscular dystrophy, even showing dominant inheritance (Fenichel et al 1967), are now thought to be the result of mistaken histological identity. As in the Becker and Emery–Dreifuss types, the discovery of both 'myopathic' and 'neurogenic' histological findings on muscle biopsy has caused

confusion; current opinion regards such 'neurogenic' changes with suspicion and favours a unitary myopathic facioscapulohumeral disease. Many other disorders with facial weakness which have caused confusion in the past are now recognised as both clinically and pathologically distinct, including the mitochondrial myopathies (Hudgson et al 1972) and atypical polymyositis (Rothstein et al 1971). However a further diagnostic difficulty was first reported by Munsat & Piper (1971) who found inflammatory changes resembling polymyositis in muscle in the early stages of the disease in two families; this is now a recognised feature of the pathology of the disease. Kazakov et al (1974), in a study of 200 cases, divided facioscapulohumeral muscular dystrophy into two groups; in most cases the lower-limb involvement primarily affected the anterior tibial and peroneal muscles while, in a few, the proximal pelvic girdle muscles were more severely affected. The groups in that study appeared to be genetically distinct, but there has been no subsequent confirmation of this finding.

One of the most striking features of this variety, described by Tyler & Wintrobe (1950) and Walton (1955, 1956a), is the occurrence of partly affected or abortive cases. Many of these patients are unaware that they are suffering from the disease in a mild form and it is therefore very important that, in any study of inheritance, all available family members should be examined. In these abortive cases the disease may remain confined to one or two muscle groups indefinitely, although very slow progression of the disease probably continues in all cases.

Cases in which facial weakness is present at birth or in early infancy present special problems (Hanson & Rowland 1971, Brooke 1977, Carroll & Brooke 1979, Bailey et al 1986). Not only may the symptoms be severe, but many patients have been reported as having bilateral progressive sensorineural deafness (Carroll & Brooke 1979, Taylor et al 1982, Wulff et al 1982, Meyerson et al 1984, Korf et al 1985). The deafness is cochlear in origin (Gieron et al 1985). Brouwer et al (1991) showed that subclinical hearing loss is very common in facioscapulohumeral muscular dystrophy, and thus is likely to be an integral feature rather than an occasional complication.

Some but not all of these cases (Taylor et al 1982, Wulff et al 1982) also have Coats' disease of the retina, an association previously noted in four sibs with FSH dystrophy and deafness who were also mentally retarded (Small 1968). Some of these cases have been sporadic but in others FSH dystrophy, both with and without deafness, was seen in affected parents in whom the onset was not in infancy. Coats' disease has sometimes involved affected sibs but not their dystrophic parents. Fitzsimons et al (1987) illuminated this problem by performing retinal fluorescein angiography on 75 cases of facioscapulohumeral muscular dystrophy, of which only three had visible lesions on ophthalmoscopy; 56 had subclinical peripheral retinal vascular disease (telangiectasis, micro-aneurysms, leakage, occlusion). It seems clear that overt Coats' disease is merely a manifestation of a retinopathy which, like the deafness, is an integral, though not invariable, feature of facioscapulohumeral muscular dystrophy. The association between the myopathy, the deafness and the retinal vasculopathy has not been elucidated.

Incidence. Quoted frequencies vary widely, perhaps because of genuine geographical variation. The birth incidence lies between 0.4 and 5.0 per 100 000 and may be about 1.5–3.0 per 100 000 (Becker 1964, Emery 1991). Estimates of the population *prevalence* lie between 0.2 and 4.3 per 100 000 and it may be about 1.5–2.5 per 100 000 overall in Europe and North America (see Emery 1991, Lunt & Harper 1991).

Symptoms. The first symptoms of this form of muscular dystrophy usually appear in the second decade, or less often in the first, while occasionally the onset is apparently delayed until much later in life. Lunt et al (1989) found that diagnostic *physical signs* could be found in 50% by the age of 14 and in 95% by the age of 20 years. Rarely, facial weakness is present at birth or in early infancy. As in scapulohumeral muscular dystrophy the weakness usually begins in the shoulder girdle muscle 50, serratus anterior, rhomboids, triceps and biceps. The pelvic and thigh muscles are affected much later as the disease progresses, but early involvement of the anterior tibial and peroneal muscles is typical. Many patients are aware of the progressive change in their facial appearance and

realise that they are unable to close their eyes properly and that they cannot whistle. When weakness is advanced they cannot pronounce labials and speech becomes characteristically indistinct. Scoliosis may occur, but much more often an extensive and severe lumbar lordosis develops, evident both on standing and sitting. The consequent pelvic tilt, combined with foot-drop and, in some cases, hyperextension of the knees, gives a characteristic gait disturbance, different from that seen in the other muscular dystrophies. The eye movements and bulbar muscles are unaffected.

When sensorineural deafness is present it is usually found at the age of 4–6 years because of speech delay. It has not been documented at birth, and in one case was absent at 2 years and present at 6 years (Korf et al 1985). Coats' disease has developed at various ages between 6 months and 13 years.

Course of the disease. This form of muscular dystrophy is very benign in many cases, and there are many patients who have had the disease since adolescence and who remain active, although with increasing disability, in late life. Only about a fifth of cases over the age of 40 years are unable to walk (Lunt & Harper 1991). Even within the same family there may, however, be considerable variation in severity between individuals. There are some in whom the rate of progression is rapid, and walking becomes impossible in middle life, or even in the second or third decade, but this is unusual and in many there are long periods, often of several years, when there is no apparent progression. Rarely there is sudden loss of power and subsequent atrophy in a muscle or group of adjacent muscles, and this appears to occur after exercise, and often in the dominant upper limb. Lunt and Harper found asymmetry of weakness in 65% of 113 cases, but worse involvement on the dominant side did not reach statistical significance.

The life expectancy in most patients with this form of disease is normal, but in the more rapidly progressive cases, death from respiratory infection can occur in middle life. Rarely the infantile form is severe enough to be fatal in childhood (McGarry et al 1983) or adolescence (Bailey et al 1986).

Physical examination. Muscular hypertrophy is rare in this form, but occasionally occurs in the calves and deltoid muscles. The facial appearance is characteristic; the face is unlined and wrinkles are often missing from the forehead and around the eyes. There is a typical pouting appearance of the lips and a transverse smile. Affected individuals usually cannot close their eyes tightly or bury their eyelashes on command, while few can retain air under pressure within the mouth. Occasionally, the facial weakness is so slight as to be difficult to elicit.

The pattern of muscular involvement in the upper and lower limbs is similar to that described above in scapulohumeral dystrophy, but elevation of the scapulae on attempted abduction of the arms (Fig. 14.6) is rather characteristic of the facioscapulohumeral disorder. The neck flexors, serrati, pectorals, biceps, triceps and extensors of the wrists are selectively involved, with relative sparing of the deltoids and wrist flexors. Abduction of the arms is severely limited by the scapular winging, though the deltoids usually remain quite strong. Some asymmetry of the muscular weakness and wasting is seen in a proportion of cases. Early involvement of the anterior tibial muscles is common, a point of distinction from scapulohumeral dystrophy. Selective lower abdominal muscle weakness commonly gives a positive Beevor's sign (Awerbuch et al 1990). Muscular contractures and skeletal distortion occur late, if at all; cardiac involvement is rare and the range of intelligence is normal.

Diagnosis. Myotonic dystrophy, myotubular, nemaline and mitochondrial myopathies, Möbius syndrome and myasthenia gravis may all present with various combinations of facial and limb muscle weakness. None of these conform to the precise pattern of muscle involvement seen in facioscapulohumeral muscular dystrophy but, once myasthenia and myotonia have been excluded, muscle biopsy is usually essential to make an accurate diagnosis. The serum CK activity is often normal or only slightly raised (up to five times normal, rarely more). The muscle biopsy often shows only minimal myopathic changes. Fibre hypertrophy, scattered very atrophic fibres and occasional 'moth-eaten' fibres are seen (Dubowitz 1985). Lin & Nonaka (1991) emphasise the diagnostic importance of small angular type IIC fibres. Only a minority of preclinical cases have raised serum CK activity (Lunt & Harper, 1991). But in most families the use of linked genetic markers (Lunt & Harper 1991, Upadhyaya et al 1991) is a reliable method of preclinical and (if required) prenatal diagnosis. In few, if

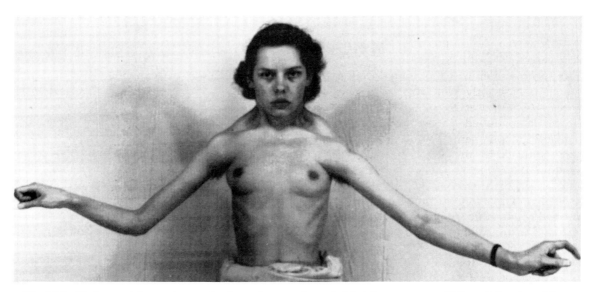

Fig. 14.6 Facioscapulohumeral muscular dystrophy: note the typical facial appearance and bilateral elevation of the scapulae (Walton 1962).

any, patients aged over 25 years are there no signs at all of the disease, but very careful examination may be required to detect signs in slightly affected individuals, even in their 50s and 60s.

Management. The inflammatory changes frequently seen in muscle biopsies are often unassociated with symptoms and then require no treatment, but significant muscular aching does occur quite often in this disease and sometimes responds to a short course of steroids. There is no indication for prolonged steroid therapy nor is any other effective treatment known. A few patients require operations for scapular fixation or spinal fusion (Copeland & Howard 1978) but for most, regular active muscle exercise is the only physical treatment necessary.

Early diagnosis of deafness or retinal disease is important. Early treatment of the latter may prevent or delay the complication of retinal detachment.

Benign autosomal dominant scapuloperoneal myopathy

Cases of sporadic or dominantly inherited scapuloperoneal myopathy have been described by Ricker & Mertens (1968), Thomas et al (1975) and others. They differ from the X-linked cases in having a later onset, in the second to the fifth decade, often with initial foot-drop. The progression is very slow and most patients continue to walk thoughout their lives. The serum CK activity is usually only slightly raised but occasionally is very high (Thomas et al 1975). The condition must be distinguished from the more frequent neurogenic scapuloperoneal syndrome, which may be difficult in the presence of secondary myopathic change in the latter (Feigenbaum & Munsat 1970). Indeed proof, from examination of the spinal cord at autopsy, of the existence of an autosomal myopathic form has not yet been reported. The possibility that some recorded cases have 'incomplete' or abortive forms of facioscapulohumeral muscular dystrophy is suggested by the large kindred reported by Kazakov et al (1976) in which facial weakness was a late and mild feature in many cases.

Severe autosomal dominant scapuloperoneal myopathy and cardiomyopathy: Hauptmann–Thannhauser muscular dystrophy

Cases, probably of this disorder, were reported by Hauptmann & Thannhauser (1941). It resembles Emery–Dreifuss muscular dystrophy (except in its mode of inheritance) but merits a separate eponym.

Chakrabarti & Pearce (1981) reported three siblings and their father with a scapuloperoneal myopathy and a pattern of early contractures and later severe heart block. The onset of muscle symptoms occurred in the first 2 years of life. Similar families, some with male-to-male transmission (which excludes X-linkage), were described by Fenichel et al (1982), Miller et al (1985), Witt et al (1988) and Orstavik et al (1990). The paraspinal and posterior cervical contractures, and the need for a cardiac pacemaker in some cases, closely resembled the features of the Emery–Dreifuss form of muscular dystrophy, from which no clear criteria for distinction of the sporadic case have yet been described. The problem this poses in diagnosing sporadic affected females is discussed on page 566.

Proximal muscular dystrophy of late onset and dominant inheritance

Large pedigrees of individuals affected by a proximal muscular dystrophy with autosomal dominant inheritance have been described by Schneiderman et al (1969), Bacon & Smith (1971), de Coster et al (1974), Chutkow et al (1986), Gilchrist et al (1988), Serratrice & Pellonier (1988) and Marconi et al (1991). The onset of symptoms was between the late teens and the fourth decade (sometimes even later) and weakness progressed very slowly, walking being maintained until after the seventh decade in some cases. Proximal lower limb weakness predominated, but affected the quadriceps particularly in the cases of Bacon & Smith (1971) and relatively mildly in those of Schneiderman and Marconi. In Gilchrist's cases plantar-flexion contractures and absent ankle jerks were an early feature and facial weakness and dysarthria occurred in a few. The myopathic changes on muscle biopsy were in some cases non-specific but deteriorated with increasing age (Bacon & Smith 1971), but in the cases of Schneiderman, Chutkow, Gilchrist and Marconi rimmed vacuolar change was a feature and in Marconi's case there was floccular change in sections stained with NADH-TR. Serum enzyme activities were normal or increased to two to three times normal (up to nine times in Gilchrist's cases). Early diagnosis for genetic counselling appears to depend wholly on careful clinical examination, though in Gilchrist's family the serum CK activity was increased in the clinical and preclinical stages.

In the kindred described by Schneiderman et al (1969) there was genetic linkage with the Pelger–Huet anomaly of polymorphonuclear leucocyte nuclei; the gene for this has not yet been located. In that of Gilchrist et al (1988) linkage with markers at 5q31.3–5q33.5 has been established (Speer et al 1991). This raises acutely the question of the genetic identity or otherwise of the kindreds collected under this heading. Once this has been settled by further linkage studies a clearer definition of the one or more entities involved should emerge.

Other autosomal dominant forms

The 'Barnes type of muscular dystrophy' (Barnes 1932), a dominantly inherited condition of late onset with initial striking muscle hypertrophy, has recently been shown to be of neurogenic origin (D Riddoch, 1974, personal communication).

A type of muscular dystrophy with dominant inheritance, childhood onset, calf hypertrophy and a curious histological picture with capillary proliferation *within* muscle fibres was described by Hastings et al (1980) in a single family.

Quadriceps myopathy

'Myopathy confined to the quadriceps' (Bramwell 1992) should be discussed here. The muscle weakness, of adult onset (20–25 years), rarely remains confined to the quadriceps if cases are re-examined after many years (Turner & Heathfield 1961, Walton 1965b). van Wijngaarden et al (1968) described two brothers with widespread myopathic changes in the EMG although the clinical involvement was limited to the quadriceps. The cases of Espir & Matthews (1973) suggested dominant inheritance. All other cases have been sporadic. Recent reviews suggest that the condition is heterogeneous, some cases having neurogenic atrophy with secondary myopathic change (Boddie & Stewart-Wynne 1974, and possibly the cases of Espir & Matthews 1973), and others a very indolent limb-girdle myopathy (Swash & Heathfield 1983). Some may be sporadic cases of the dominant, late-onset limb-girdle dystrophy of Bacon & Smith (1971) described above and four male cases reported by Sunohara et al (1990) were all shown to have dystrophin deficiency, leading to a revised diagnosis of a forme fruste of Becker muscular dystrophy. The serum CK activity may be raised by up to 10-fold.

Benign myopathy with finger flexion contractures and dominant inheritance

Bethlem & van Wijngaarden (1976) reported three large kindreds with a very slowly progressive myopathy affecting mainly the proximal limb muscles but with torticollis, toe-walking and equinovarus contractures in some cases. A striking feature was flexion contracture of the fingers (not the thumbs) and weakness of finger extension. The onset was at about the age of 5 years and life expectancy was not affected. The serum CK activity was normal. Muscle biopsy showed variation of fibre size, increased fat tissue and, in half the cases, lobulated type I fibres on NADH-TR staining.

A few similar cases have been described (Mohire et al 1988, Somer et al 1991). The benign congenital myopathy of Turner & Lees (1962) differs in presenting with marked congenital hypotonia.

Distal myopathies with dominant inheritance

Distal myopathy was first described by Gowers in 1902; however, many observers now feel that the patient he described may have been suffering from myotonic dystrophy. In 1907 Spiller pointed out the distinction from 'Charcot–Marie–Tooth disease' or hereditary sensorimotor neuropathies (HSMN) with which confusion may still arise because secondary changes suggestive of myopathy may be seen in muscle biopsy specimens (Greenfield et al 1957, Tyrer & Sutherland 1961).

Initial involvement of peripheral limb muscles serves to distinguish these conditions from the scapulohumeral and scapuloperoneal muscular dystrophies, which they otherwise resemble; in the early stages the appearances in the limbs are similar to those of HSMN type 1 but in the latter condition there is usually impairment of vibration sense in the extremities, and impaired nerve conduction. Some cases of mitochondrial myopathy with distal muscle weakness may resemble the juvenile form (Salmon et al 1971, Lapresle et al 1972) and electron-microscopy of muscle may be required to distinguish them (Bautista et al 1978). The difficulty in distinguishing distal myopathy from distal chronic spinal mucular atrophy should not be underestimated (Sumner et al 1971).

Adult form. Welander (1951, 1957) has had a wide experience of the distal form of muscular dystrophy in Sweden, which is inherited as a dominant character, begins usually between the ages of 40 and 60 years and very rarely before 30 years, and affects both sexes, although it is commoner in men than in women. Weakness usually begins in the small muscles of the hands and slowly spreads proximally; in the legs the anterior tibial muscles and the calves are affected first. The condition is comparatively benign, but proximal weakness occurs in a few more severe cases which are probably homozygous for the dominant gene (Welander 1957). Borg et al (1991), recalling that Welander ascribed some mild distal sensory loss found in his cases to ageing, showed that in the early stage of the disease distal stiffness of the fingers is accompanied by impairment of temperature sensation but not of vibration sense. But motor and sensory nerve conduction was normal.

Welander's experience of over 250 cases was unique. In Great Britain and in the USA this form of the disease is rare; in Newcastle upon Tyne most of the few cases we have observed appeared to be sporadic and have probably had the newly described autosomal recessive form (see p. 572). In these patients the rate of progress of the disease was somewhat more rapid than in the Swedish cases, and most of them were severely disabled within 10–15 years of the onset, but the pattern of muscular involvement was similar to that described by Welander. The serum CK activity is as high as 20–100 times normal in sporadic cases but is normal or only slightly raised in cases where the onset is much later. Tomlinson et al (1974) described a non-Scandinavian dominantly inherited case with autopsy findings and Markesbery et al (1977) described the muscle pathology in one such patient.

We conclude that the firmly established Swedish form of dominantly inherited distal myopathy in which the onset is in adult life is occasionally found in non-Swedish patients. But the majority of cases seen elsewhere are probably of the autosomal or recessive juvenile forms.

Another relatively severe distal myopathy with dominant inheritance, described by Edstrom et al (1980), differs clinically in the greater involvement of flexor than extensor muscles in the upper limbs and in being complicated by cardiomyopathy, and histologically in the occurrence of sarcoplasmic bodies, intermediate-sized filaments and leptomeric fibrils in the muscle fibres.

Juvenile form. Biemond (1955) described a juvenile form of distal 'myopathy' which was subsequently found to be neurogenic in origin. Others (Ciani & Gherardi 1963, Magee & de Jong 1965, van der Does de Willebois et al 1968, Bautista et al 1978) have described similar families where the disease seemed more clearly myopathic, although some doubts remain. Like the late form, these early-onset cases are dominant in inheritance. Symptoms begin by the age of 2 years and progress slowly with eventual arrest. The serum CK activity is up to 20 times normal in some early cases but is normal in later life. van der Does de Willebois et al (1968) published histochemical studies in which atrophy of the type I muscle fibres appeared to be a prominent feature.

Ocular myopathy or progressive external ophthalmoplegia

Involvement of the external ocular muscles is

extremely unusual in any of the preceding types of muscular dystrophy, but may occur in myotonic dystrophy. Patients who developed ptosis followed by progressive limitation of ocular movements without significant diplopia were described by Hutchinson (1879) and Fuchs (1890) and were reviewed by Kiloh & Nevin (1951). Fuchs (1890), Sandifer (1946) and Kiloh & Nevin (1951) obtained eyelid muscle during corrective operations and interpreted the histology as showing myopathy. As a result such cases were regarded as having an ocular form of muscular dystrophy. Ross (1963, 1964) found that some such patients are peculiarly sensitive to curare but did not improve on anticholinesterase drugs.

Following the delineation of the Kearns–Sayre syndrome (Kearnes & Sayre 1958) and the discovery of widespread mitochondrial pathology in these cases (Olson et al 1972, Schneck et al 1973) and in uncomplicated progressive external ophthalmoplegia, the term 'ocular muscular dystrophy' fell into disuse as it now seems likely that all such cases are due to mitochondrial disease. Much is now known about these mitochondrial myopathies, and they are discussed elsewhere (see Ch. 18).

Oculopharyngeal muscular dystrophy

Victor et al (1962) separated cases of ocular myopathy with dysphagia as a group to which they gave the name oculopharyngeal myopathy. Bray et al (1965) supported this subdivision and defined the other distinguishing features, of which the most valuable was the age of onset (mean 23 years for the ocular cases and 40 years for the oculopharyngeal). Many of the reported cases have been of French-Canadian stock (Taylor 1915, Hayes et al 1963, Peterman et al 1964, Barbeau 1966, Murphy & Drachman 1968) but occasional cases, often sporadic, have occurred elsewhere. The inheritance in familial cases is dominant. Rebeiz et al (1969), Little & Perl (1982) and several other authors confirmed the primary myopathic nature of cases at autopsy but in the case studied by Schmitt & Krause (1981) there was also evidence of a peripheral neuropathy, possibly incidental. In this type of muscular dystrophy, as in ocular myopathy, muscle biopsy may reveal evidence of a mitochondrial myopathy (Morgan-Hughes & Mair 1973, Julien et al 1974), but more frequently the myopathic findings are less specific including moth-eaten and whorled fibres, rimmed vacuoles and occasional atypical ragged-red fibres. A transient inflammatory response is sometimes seen (Bosch et al 1979).

Typically the disorder starts with ptosis in the fourth to sixth decade and dysphagia a decade or so later. Both progress slowly. The external ophthalmoplegia is evident on examination by the age of about 40–50 but rarely causes symptoms. Mild weakness of the face, neck muscles and proximal limb muscles is commonly seen.

This disorder bears some resemblance to myotonic dystrophy, not only in some of the clinical and genetic features, but in the probable involvement of smooth muscle (Lewis 1966) and reports of gonadal atrophy (Lundberg 1962) and abnormalities of immunoglobulins (Russe et al 1967) in some families.

A closely similar syndrome with autosomal recessive inheritance and an earlier onset has been described by Fried et al (1975). A sporadic case with comparable physical signs progressing since early childhood (Lacomis et al 1991) is unclassifiable at present.

REFERENCES

Afifi A K, Zellweger H, McCormick W F, Mergner W 1969 Congenital muscular dystrophy: light and electron microscopic observations. Journal of Neurology, Neurosurgery and Psychiatry 32: 273

Aguilar L, Lisker R, Ramos G G 1978 Unusual inheritance of Becker type muscular dystrophy. Journal of Medical Genetics 15: 116

Ahmad M, Sanderson J E, Dubowitz V, Hallidie-Smith K A 1978 Echocardiography assessment of left ventricular function in Duchenne's muscular dystrophy. British Heart Journal 40: 734

Allen J E, Rodgin D W 1960 Mental retardation in association with progressive muscular dystrophy. American Journal of Diseases of Childhood 100: 208

Allsop K G, Ziter F A 1981 Loss of strength and functional decline in Duchenne's dystrophy. Archives of Neurolology 38: 406

Anderson S W, Routh D K, Ionasescu V V 1988 Serial position memory of boys with Duchenne muscular dystrophy. Developmental Medicine and Child Neurology 30: 328

Appleton R E, Bushby K M D, Gardner-Medwin D, Welch J,

Kelly P 1991 Macrocephaly and intellectual performance in Duchenne muscular dystrophy. Developmental Medicine and Child Neurology 33: 875

Archibald K C, Vignos P J 1959 A study of contractures in muscular dystrophy. Archives of Physical Medicine 40: 150

Awerbuch G I, Nigro M A, Wishnow R 1990 Beevor's sign and facioscapulohumeral dystrophy. Archives of Neurology 47: 1208

Bacon P A, Smith B 1971 Familial muscular dystrophy of late onset. Journal of Neurology, Neurosurgery and Psychiatry 34: 93

Bailey R O, Marzulo D C, Hans M B 1986 Infantile facioscapulohumeral muscular dystrophy: new observations. Acta Neurologica Scandinavica 74: 51

Bakker E, Goor N, Wrogemann L et al 1985 Prenatal diagnosis and carrier detection of Duchenne muscular dystrophy with closely linked RFLPs. Lancet i: 655

Banker B Q, Victor M, Adams R D 1957 Arthrogryposis multiplex due to congenital muscular dystrophy. Brain 80: 319

Barbeau A 1966 The syndrome of hereditary late onset ptosis and dysphagia in French Canada. In: Kuhn E (ed) Progressive Muskeldystrophie, Myotonie, Myasthenie. Springer, New York.

Barnes S 1932 Report of a myopathic family with hypertrophic, pseudohypertrophic, atrophic and terminal (distal in the upper extremities) stages. Brain 55: 1

Barohn R J, Levine E J, Olson J O, Mendell J R 1988 Gastric hypomotility in Duchenne's muscular dystrophy. New England Journal of Medicine 319: 15

Barwick D D, Osselton J W, Walton J N 1965 Electroencephalographic studies in hereditary myopathy. Journal of Neurology, Neurosurgery and Psychiatry 28: 109

Bateson W 1909 Mendel's principles of heredity. Cambridge University Press, Cambridge, pp 222–232

Batten F E 1903 Three cases of myopathy, infantile type. Brain 26: 147

Batten F E 1909 The myopathies or muscular dystrophies; critical review. Quarterly Journal of Medicine 3: 313

Bautista J, Rafel E, Castilla J M, Alberca R 1978 Hereditary distal myopathy with onset in early infancy. Journal of the Neurological Sciences 37: 149

Becker P E 1957 Neue Ergebnisse der Genetik der Muskeldystrophien. Acta Geneticae medicae et gemellologiae (Roma) 7: 303

Becker P E 1962 Two new families of benign sex-linked recessive muscular dystrophy. Revue Canadienne de Biologie 21: 551

Becker P E 1964 Myopathien. In: Becker P E (ed) Humangenetik: Ein kurzes Handbuch in funf Banden, Band 111/1. George Thieme, Stuttgart, p 411

Becker P E, Keiner F 1955 Eine neue X-chromosomale Muskeldystrophie. Archiv fur Psychiatrie und Nervenkrankheiten 193: 427

Beckmann J S, Richard I, Hillaire D et al, including Fardeau M 1991 A gene for limb-girdle muscular dystrophy maps to chromosome 15 by linkage. Comptes Rendues de l'Academie de Science de Paris 312 ser III: 141

Beckmann R, Scheuerbrandt G 1976 Screening auf erhohte CK-Aktivitaten. Kinderarzt 7: 1267

Begin R, Bureau M-A, Lupien L, Lemieux B 1980 Control of breathing in Duchenne's muscular dystrophy. American Journal of Medicine 69: 227

Bell J 1943 On pseudohypertrophic and allied types of progressive muscular dystrophy. In: Treasury of human inheritance, vol iv, part iv. Cambridge University Press, London

Ben Hamida M, Fardeau M, Attia N 1983 Severe childhood muscular dystrophy affecting both sexes and frequent in Tunisia. Muscle and Nerve 6: 469

Ben Hamida M, Marrakchi D 1980 Dystrophie musculaire progressive de type Duchenne en Tunisie: a propos de 13 familles et 31 cas d'une forme en apparence recessive autosomique. Journal de Génétique Humaine 28: 1

Ben Jelloun-Dellagi S, Chaffey P, Hentati F et al 1990 Presence of normal dystrophin in Tunisian severe childhood autosomal recessive muscular dystrophy. Neurology 40: 1903

Berenbaum A A, Horowitz W 1956 Heart involvement in progressive muscular dystrophy. Report of a case with sudden death. American Heart Journal 51: 622

Bertolini E R, Zatz M 1986 Investigation of genetic heterogeneity in Duchenne muscular dystrophy. American Journal of Medical Genetics 24: 111

Bethlem J, van Wijngaarden G K, de Jong J 1973 The incidence of lobulated fibres in the facioscapulohumeral type of muscular dystrophy and the limb-girdle syndrome. Journal of the Neurological Sciences 18: 351

Bethlem J, van Wijngaarden G K 1976 Benign myopathy, with autosomal dominant inheritance. Brain 99: 91

Bialer M G, McDaniel N L, Kelly T E 1991 Progression of cardiac disease in Emery–Dreifuss muscular dystrophy. Clinical Cardiology 14: 411

Biemond A 1955 Myopathia distalis juvenilis hereditaria. Acta Psychiatrica et Neurologica Scandinavia 30: 25

Billard C, Gillet P, Signoret J L et al 1992 Cognitive functions in Duchenne muscular dystrophy: a reappraisal and comparison with spinal muscular atrophy. Neuromuscular Disorders 2: 371

Boba A 1970 Fatal postanesthetic complications in two muscular dystrophic patients. Journal of Pediatric Surgery 5: 71

Boddie H G, Stewart-Wynne E G 1974 Quadriceps myopathy — entity or syndrome? Archives of Neurology 31: 60

Bolthauser E, Steinmann B, Meyer A, Jerusalem F 1980 Anaesthesia-induced rhabdomyolysis in Duchenne muscular dystrophy. British Journal of Anaesthesia 52: 559

Bonsett C A, Thomson W H S 1987 The Duchenne muscular dystrophy spectrum as clarified by the 'outlier'. Indiana Medicine 80: 742

Borg K, Ahlberg G, Borg J, Edstrom L 1991 Welander's distal myopathy: clinical, neurophysiological and muscle biopsy observations in young and middle aged adults with early symptoms. Journal of Neurology, Neurosurgery and Psychiatry 54: 494

Bosch E P, Gowans J D C, Munsat T 1979 Inflammatory myopathy in oculopharyngeal dystrophy. Muscle and Nerve 2: 73

Bossingham D H, Williams E, Nichols P J R Severe childhood neuromuscular disease: the management of Duchenne muscular dystrophy and spinal muscular atrophy. Muscular Dystrophy Group of Great Britain, London

Boyd Y, Buckle V, Holt S, Munro E, Hunter D, Craig I 1986 Muscular dystrophy in girls with X:autosome translocations. Journal of Medical Genetics 23: 484

Bradley D M, Parsons E P, Clarke A J 1993 Experience with screening newborns for Duchenne muscular dystrophy in Wales. British Medical Journal 306: 357

Bradley W G 1979 The limb-girdle syndromes. In: Vinken P J,

Bruyn G W (eds) Handbook of clinical neurology, vol 40. North Holland, Amsterdam, ch 11

Bradley W G, Jones M Z, Mussini J-M, Fawcett P R W 1978 Becker-type muscular dystrophy. Muscle and Nerve 1: 111

Bramwell E 1922 Observations on myopathy. Proceedings of the Royal Society of Medicine 16: 1

Bray G M, Kaarsoo M, Ross R T 1965 Ocular myopathy with dysphagia. Neurology (Minneapolis) 15: 678

Breningstall G N, Grover W D, Barbera S, Marks H G 1988 Neonatal rhabdomyolysis as a presentation of muscular dystrophy. Neurology 38: 1271

Brooke M H 1977 A clinician's view of neuromuscular disease. Williams and Wilkins, Baltimore

Brooke M H, Fenichel G M, Griggs R C et al and the CIDD Group 1983 Clinical investigation in Duchenne dystrophy: 2. Determination of the 'power' of therapeutic trials based on the natural history. Muscle and Nerve 6: 91

Brooke M H, Fenichel G M, Griggs R C et al 1989 Duchenne muscular dystrophy — patterns of clinical progression and the effects of supportive therapy. Neurology 39: 475

Brooks A P, Emery A E H 1977 The incidence of Duchenne muscular dystrophy in the south east of Scotland. Clincal Genetics 11: 290

Brouwer O F, Padberg G W, Ruys C J M, Brand R, de Laat J A P M, Grote J J 1991 Hearing loss in facioscapulohumeral muscular dystrophy. Neurology 41: 1878

Brownell A K W, Paasuke R T, Elash A et al 1983 Malignant hyperthermia in Duchenne muscular dystrophy. Anesthesiology 58: 180

Bulcke J A, Crolla D, Termote J-L, Baert A, Palmers Y, van den Bergh R 1981 Computed tomography of muscle. Muscle and Nerve 4: 67

Burke S S, Grove N M, Houser C R, Johnson D M 1971 Respiratory aspects of pseudohypertrophic muscular dystrophy. American Journal of Diseases of Childhood 121: 230

Burn J, Povey S, Boyd Y et al 1986 Duchenne muscular dystrophy in one of monozygotic twin girls. Journal of Medical Genetics 23: 494

Bush A, Dubowitz V 1991 Fatal rhabdomyolysis complicating general anaesthesia in a child with Becker muscular dystrophy. Neuromuscular Disorders 1: 201

Bushby K M D, Cleghorn N J, Curtis A et al 1991a Identification of a mutation in the promoter region of the dystrophin gene in a patient with atypical Becker muscular dystrophy. Human Genetics 88: 195

Bushby K M D, Thambyayah M, Gardner-Medwin D 1991b Prevalence and incidence of Becker muscular dystrophy. Lancet 337: 1022

Bushby K M D, Gardner-Medwin D 1993 The clinical, genetic and dystrophin characteristics of Becker muscular dystrophy I: Natural history. Journal of Neurology 240: 98

Bushby K M D, Gardner-Medwin D, Nicholson L V B et al 1993 Idem II: correlation of phenotype with genetic and protein abnormalities. Journal of Neurology 240: 105

Bushby K, Appleton R, Nicholson L, Welch J, Kelly P, Gardner-Medwin D 1994 Deletion status and intellectual impairment in Duchenne muscular dystrophy. (in preparation)

Carroll J E, Brooke M H 1979 Infantile facioscapulohumeral dystrophy. In: Serratrice G, Roux H (eds) Peroneal atrophies and related disorders. Masson, New York

Casazzo F, Bambilla S G, Salvato A, Moraidi L, Gonda E,

Bonacina E 1988 Cardiac transplantation in Becker muscular dystrophy. Journal of Neurology 235: 496

Chakrabarti A, Pearce J M S 1981 Scapuloperoneal syndrome with cardiomyopathy: report of a family with autosomal dominant inheritance and unusual features. Journal of Neurology, Neurosurgery and Psychiatry 44: 1146

Chelly J, Marlhens F, le Marec B et al 1986 De novo DNA microdeletion in a girl with Turner syndrome and Duchenne muscular dystrophy. Human Genetics 74: 193

Chelly J, Hamard G, Koulakoff A, Kaplan J-C, Khan A, Berwald-Netter Y 1990 Dystrophin gene transcribed from different promoters in neuronal and glial cells. Nature 334: 64

Chutkow J G, Heffner R R, Kramer A A, Edwards J A 1986 Adult-onset autosomal dominant limb-girdle muscular dystrophy. Annals of Neurology 20: 240

Ciani N, Gherardi F 1963 Due casi di myopathia distalis juvenilis hereditaria. Rivista di Neurologia 33: 731

Clarke A 1992 Report of ENMC workshop on the limb-girdle muscular dystrophies. Journal of Medical Genetics 29: 753

Cobham I G, Davis H S 1964 Anesthesia for muscular dystrophy patients. Anesthesia and Analgesia — Current Researches 43: 22

Cohen H J, Molnar G E, Taft L T 1968 The genetic relationship of progressive muscular dystrophy (Duchenne type) and mental retardation. Developmental Medicine and Child Neurology 10: 754

Conte G, Gioja L 1836 Scrofula del sistema muscolare. Annali Clinici dell'ospedale degl'incurabili Napoli. (Reprinted 1986 in Cardiomyology 5: 3–4, 14–28)

Copeland S A, Howard R C 1978 Thoracoscapular fusion for facioscapulohumeral dystrophy. Journal of Bone and Joint Surgery 60B: 547

Cowan J, Macdessi J, Stark A, Morgan G 1980 Incidence of Duchenne muscular dystrophy in New South Wales and the Australian Capital Territory. Journal of Medical Genetics 17: 245

Crisp D E, Ziter F A, Bray P F 1982 Diagnostic delay in Duchenne's mucular dystrophy. Journal of the American Medical Association 247: 478

Danieli G A, Mostacciuolo M L, Bonfante A, Angelini C 1977 Duchenne muscular dystrophy: a population study. Human Genetics 35: 225

Danilowicz D, Rutkowski M, Myung D, Schively D 1980 Echocardiography in Duchenne muscular dystrophy. Muscle and Nerve 3: 298

Davie A M, Emery A E H 1978 Estimation of proportion of mutants among cases of Duchenne muscular dystrophy. Journal of Medical Genetics 15: 339

de Coster W, der Reuck J, Thiery E 1974 A late autosomal dominant form of limb-girdle muscular dystrophy: a clinical, genetic and morphological study. European Neurology 12: 159

de Lange C 1937 Studien uber angeborene Lahmugen bzw. angeborene Hypotonie. Acta Paediatrica 20 (suppl III): 33

de Paillette L, Aicardi J, Goutieres F, 1989 Ullrich's congenital atonic-sclerotic muscular dystrophy. Journal of Neurology 236: 108

de Visser M 1983 Computed tomographic findings of the skeletal musculature in sporadic distal myopathy with early adult onset. Journal of Neurological Sciences 59: 331

de Visser M, Verbeeten B 1985a Computed tomographic findings in manifesting carriers of Duchenne muscular dystrophy. Clinical Genetics 27: 269

de Visser M, Verbeeten B 1985b Computed tomography of the skeletal musculature in Becker-type muscular dystrophy and benign infantile spinal muscular atrophy. Muscle and Nerve 8: 435

Dellamonica C 1978 Etude de la réaction couplée, créatine-kinase/luciferase. Application au depistage systematique neonatal de la myopathie de Duchenne de Boulogne. Thesis for the Université Claude Bernard, Lyon

Dellamonica C, Robert J M, Cotte J, Collombel C, Dorche C 1978 Systematic neonatal screening for Duchenne muscular dystrophy. Lancet ii: 1100 (letter)

den Dunnen J T, Casula L, Makover A, Bakker B, Yaffe D, Nudel U, van Ommen G-J B 1991 Mapping of dystrophin brain promoter: a deletion of this region is compatible with normal intellect. Neuromuscular Disorders 1: 327

Dickey R P, Ziter F A, Smith R A 1984 Emery–Dreifuss muscular dystrophy. Journal of Pediatrics 104: 555

Dobyns W B, Pagon R A, Armstrong D, Curry C J R, Greenburg F, Grix A et al 1989 Diagnostic criteria for Walker–Warburg syndrome. American Journal of Medical Genetics 32: 195

Donner M, Rapola J, Somer H 1975 Congenital muscular dystrophy: a clinicopathological and follow-up study of 15 patients. Neuropadiatrie 6: 239

Donofrio D, Challa V, Hackshaw B, Mills S, Cordwell R 1989 Cardiac transplantation in a patient with Becker muscular dystrophy and cardiomyopathy. Archives of Neurology 46: 705

Dreifuss F E, Hogan G R 1961 Survival in X-chromosomal muscular dystrophy. Neurology (Minneapolis) 11: 734

Drummond L M 1979 Creatine phosphokinase levels in the newborn and their use in screening for Duchenne muscular dystrophy. Archives of Disease in Childhood 54: 362

Dubowitz V 1963 Myopathic changes in muscular dystrophy carrier. Journal of Neurology, Neurosurgery and Psychiatry 26: 322

Dubowitz V 1965 Intellectual impairment in muscular dystrophy. Archives of Disease in Childhood 40: 296

Dubowitz V 1978 Muscle disorders in childhood. Saunders, London

Dubowitz V 1985 Muscle biopsy: a practical approach, 2nd edn. Baillière Tindall, London

Dubowitz V, Crome L 1969 The central nervous system in Duchenne muscular dystrophy. Brain 92: 805

Dubowitz V, Brooke M H 1973 Muscle biopsy: a modern approach. Saunders, London

Duchenne G B 1855 De l'électrisation localisée et de son application à la physiologie, à la pathologie et la thérapeutique. Baillière, Paris

Duchenne G B 1862 Album de photographies pathologiques: complémentaire du livre intitulé D'Electrisation Localisée. Baillière, Paris

Duchenne G B 1868 Recherches sur la paralysie musculaire pseudohypertrophique ou paralysie myosclerosique. Archives générales de médécine 11: 5, 178, 305, 421, 552

Ebashi S, Sugita H 1978 The role of calcium in physiological and pathological processes of skeletal muscle. In: Abstracts of the IVth International Congress on Neuromuscular Diseases, Montreal

Echenne B, Pages M, Marty-Double C 1984 Congenital muscular dystrophy with cerebral white matter spongiosis. Brain and Development 6: 491

Echenne B, Arthuis M, Billard C, Campos-Costello J et al 1986 Congenital muscular dystrophy and cerebral CT scan anomalies. Journal of the Neurological Sciences 75: 7

Edstrom L, Thornell L-E, Eriksson A 1980 A new type of hereditary distal myopathy with characteristic sarcoplasmic bodies and intermediate (skeletin) filaments. Journal of the Neurological Sciences 47: 171

Edwards R H T, Round J M, Jackson M J, Griffiths R D, Lilburn M F 1984 Weight reduction in boys with muscular dystrophy. Developmental Medicine and Child Neurology 26: 384

Egger J, Kendall B E, Erdohazi M, Lake B D, Wilson J, Brett E M 1983 Involvement of the central nervous system in congenital muscular dystrophies. Developmental Medicine and Child Neurology 25: 32

Eiholzer U, Bolthauser E, Frey D, Molinari L, Zachmann M 1988 Short stature: a common feature in Duchenne muscular dystrophy. European Journal of Pediatrics 147: 602

Ellis E R, Bye P T B, Bruderer J W, Sullivan C E 1987 Treatment of respiratory failure during sleep in patients with neuromuscular disease: positive-pressure ventilation through a nose mask. American Review of Respiratory Disease 135: 148

Emery A E H 1965 Muscle histology in carriers of Duchenne muscular dystrophy. Journal of Medical Genetics 2: 1

Emery A E H 1969 Abnormalities of the electrocardiogram in female carriers of Duchenne muscular dystrophy. British Medical Journal 2: 418

Emery A E H 1972 Abnormalities of the electrocardiogram in hereditary myopathies. Journal of Medical Genetics 9: 8

Emery A E H 1987 Duchenne muscular dystrophy. Oxford University Press, Oxford

Emery A E H 1989 Emery–Dreifuss muscular dystrophy and other related disorders. British Medical Bulletin 45: 772

Emery A E H 1991 Population frequencies of inherited neuromuscular disorders — a world survey. Neuromuscular Disorders 1: 19

Emery A E H, Dreifuss F E 1966 Unusual type of benign X-linked muscular dystrophy. Journal of Neurology, Neurosurgery and Psychiatry 29: 338

Emery A E H, Skinner R 1976 Clinical studies in benign (Becker type) X-linked muscular dystrophy. Clinical Genetics 10: 189

Emery E S, Fenichel G M, Eng G 1968 A spinal muscular atrophy with scapuloperoneal distribution. Archives of Neurology 18: 129

England S B, Nicholson L V B, Johnson M A et al 1990 Very mild muscular dystrophy associated with the deletion of 46% of dystrophin. Nature 342: 180

Erb W H 1884 Uber die 'juvenile form' der progressiven Muskelatrophie ihre beziehungen zur sogennanten Pseudohypertrophie der Muskeln. Deutsches Archiv fur klinische Medizin 34: 467

Erb W H 1891 Dystrophia muscularis progressiva: Klinische und pathologischanatomische Studien. Deutsche Zeitschrift für Nervenheilkunde 1: 13

Espir M L E, Matthews W B 1973 Hereditary quadriceps myopathy. Journal of Neurology, Neurosurgery and Psychiatry 36: 1041

Feigenbaum J A, Munsat T L 1970 A neuromuscular syndrome of scapuloperoneal distribution. Bulletin of the Los Angeles Neurological Societies 35: 47

Fenichel G M, Emery E S, Hunt P 1967 Neurogenic atrophy simulating facioscapulohumeral dystrophy: a dominant form. Archives of Neurology 17: 257

Fenichel G M, Sul Y C, Kilroy A W, Blouin R 1982 An

autosomal dominant dystrophy with humeropelvic distribution and cardiomyopathy. Neurology 32: 1399

Ferrier P, Bamatter F, Klein D 1965 Muscular dystrophy (Duchenne) in a girl with Turner's syndrome. Journal of Medical Genetics 2: 38

Fidzianska A, Goebel H H, Lenard H G, Heckmann C 1982 Congenital muscular dystrophy (CMD) — a collagen formative disease? Journal of the Neurological Sciences 55: 79

Fidzianska A, Goebel H H, Osborn M, Lenard H G, Osse G, Langenbeck U 1983 Mallory body-like inclusions in hereditary congenital neuromuscular disease. Muscle and Nerve 6: 195

Firth M A 1983 Diagnosis of Duchenne muscular dystrophy: experiences of parents of sufferers. British Medical Journal 286: 700

Firth M A, Gardner-Medwin D, Hosking G, Wilkinson E 1983 Interviews with parents of boys suffering from Duchenne muscular dystrophy. Developmental Medicine and Child Neurology 25: 466

Fitzsimons R B, Gurwin E B, Bird A C 1987 Retinal vascular abnormalities in facioscapulohumeral muscular dystrophy. Brain 110: 631

Francke U, Ochs H D, de Martinville B et al 1985 Minor Xp21 chromosome deletion in a male associated with expression of Duchenne muscular dystrophy, chronic granulomatous disease, retinitis pigmentosa and McLeod syndrome. American Journal of Human Genetics 37: 250

Fried K, Arlozorov A, Spira R 1975 Autosomal recessive oculopharyngeal muscular dystrophy. Journal of Medical Genetics, 12: 416

Fuchs E 1890 Ueber isolieren doppelseitige Ptosia. Archiv für Ophthalmologie 36: 234

Fukuyama Y, Kawazura M, Haruna H 1960 A peculiar form of congenital progressive muscular dystrophy: report of fifteen cases. Paediatria Universitatis, Tokyo 4: 5

Fukuyama Y, Osawa M 1984 A genetic study of the Fukuyama type congenital muscular dystrophy. Brain and Development 6: 373

Fukuyama Y, Osawa M, Suzuki H 1981 Congenital progressive muscular dystrophy of the Fukuyama type: clinical, genetic and pathological considerations. Brain and Development 3: 1

Furukawa T, Peter J B 1977 X-linked muscular dystrophy. Annals of Neurology 2: 414

Furukawa T, Toyokura Y 1977 Congenital hypotonic-sclerotic muscular dystrophy. Journal of Medical Genetics 14: 426

Gardner-Medwin D 1970 Mutation rate in Duchenne type of muscular dystrophy. Journal of Medical Genetics 7: 334

Gardner-Medwin D 1977 Objectives in the management of Duchenne muscular dystrophy. Israeli Journal of Medical Sciences 13: 229

Gardner-Medwin D 1979a Controversies about Duchenne muscular dystrophy. (1) Neonatal screening. Developmental Medicine and Child Neurology 21: 390

Gardner-Medwin D 1979b Controversies about Duchenne muscular dystrophy. (2) Bracing for ambulation. Developmental Medicine and Child Neurology 21: 659

Gardner-Medwin D 1982 The natural history of Duchenne muscular dystrophy. In: Wise G B, Blaw M E, Procopis P G (eds) Topics in child neurology, vol 2. SP Medical & Scientific Books, New York

Gardner-Medwin D 1992 Caring for our genes. D O Butler Memorial Lecture. University of Queensland, Brisbane

Gardner-Medwin D, Bundey S, Green S 1978 Early diagnosis of Duchenne muscular dystrophy. Lancet i: 1102 (letter)

Gardner-Medwin D, Johnston H M 1984 Severe muscular dystrophy in girls. Journal of the Neurological Sciences 64: 79

Gardner-Medwin D, Sharples P 1989 Some studies of the Duchenne and autosomal recessive types of muscular dystrophy. Brain and Development 11: 91

Genever E E 1971 Suxamethonium-induced cardiac arrest in unsuspected pseudohypertrophic muscular dystrophy. British Journal of Anaesthesia 43: 984

Gibson D A, Koreska J, Robertson D, Kahn A, Albisser A M 1978 The management of spinal deformity in Duchenne's muscular dystrophy. Orthopedic Clinics of North America 9: 437

Gieron M A, Korthals J K, Kousseff B G 1985 Facioscapulohumeral dystrophy with cochlear hearing loss and tortuosity of retinal vessels. American Journal of Medical Genetics 22: 143

Gilboa N, Swanson J R 1976 Serum creatine phosphokinase in normal newborns. Archives of Disease in Childhood 51: 283

Gilchrist J M, Pericak-Vance M, Silverman L, Roses A D 1988 Clinical and genetic investigation in autosomal dominant limb-girdle muscular dystrophy. Neurology 38: 5

Goebel H H, Lenard H-G, Lagenbeck U, Mehl B 1980 A form of congenital muscular dystrophy. Brain and Development 2: 387

Goebel H H, Fidzianska S, Lenard H-G, Osse G, Hori A 1983 A morphological study of non-Japanese congenital muscular dystrophy associated with cerebral lesions. Brain and Development 5: 292

Goldberg S J, Feldman L, Reinecke C, Stern L Z, Sahn D J, Allen H D 1980 Echocardiographic determination of contraction and relaxation measurements of the left ventricular wall in normal subjects and muscular dystrophy. Circulation 62: 1061

Gomez M R, Engel A G, Dewald G, Peterson H A 1977 Failure of inactivation of Duchenne dystrophy X-chromosome in one of female identical twins. Neurology (Minneapolis) 27: 537

Gospe S M, Lazaro R P, Lava N S, Grootscholten P M, Scott M O, Fischbeck K H 1989 Familial X-linked myalgia and cramps. Neurology 39: 1277

Gottrand F, Guillonneau I, Carpentier A 1991 Segmental colonic transit time in Duchenne muscular dystrophy. Archives of Disease in Childhood 66: 1262

Gowers W R 1879 Pseudohypertrophic muscular paralysis. Churchill, London

Gowers W R 1902 A lecture on myopathy and a distal form. British Medical Journal 2: 89

Greenberg C R, Jacobs H K, Nylen T E et al 1992 Congenital hydrocephalus secondary to Walker–Warburg syndrome identified on the Manitoba neonatal screening programme for Duchenne muscular dystrophy. Journal of Medical Genetics 29: 583

Greenberg C R, Rohringer M, Jacobs H K et al 1988 Gene studies in newborn males with Duchenne muscular dystrophy detected by neonatal screening. Lancet ii: 425

Greenfield J G, Cornman T, Shy G M 1958 The prognostic value of the muscle biopsy in the 'floppy infant'. Brain 81: 461

Greenfield J G, Shy, G M, Alvord E C, Berg L 1957 An atlas of muscle pathology in neuromuscular diseases. Livingstone, Edinburgh

Guibaud P, Carrier H N, Planchu H, Lauras B, Jolivet M J, Robert J M 1981 Manifestations musculaires précoces, cliniques et histopathologiques, chez 14 garçons presentant dans la premiere année une activité sérique elevée de creatine-phosphokinase. Journale de Génétique Humaine 29: 71

Gull W W 1862 Case of progressive atrophy of the muscles of the hands. Guy's Hospital Reports 8: 244

Hallen O 1970 Zur Frage der Kombination endokriner Symptome und Syndrome mit der Dystrophia musculorum progressiva. Deutsche Zeitschrift für Nervenheilkunde 197: 101

Hanson P A, Rowland L P 1971 Möbius syndrome and facioscapulohumeral muscular dystrophy. Archives of Neurology 24: 31

Hassan Z ul, Fastabend C P, Mohanty P K, Isaacs E R 1979 Atrioventricular block and supraventricular arrythmias with X-linked muscular dystrophy. Circulation 60: 1365

Hastings B A, Groothuis D R, Vick N A 1980 Dominantly inherited pseudohypertrophic muscular dystrophy with internalized capillaries. Archives of Neurology 37: 709

Hauptmann A, Thannhauser S J 1941 Muscular shortening and dystrophy: a heredofamilial disease. Archives of Neurology and Psychiatry 46: 654

Hayes R, London W, Seidman J, Embree L 1963 Oculopharyngeal muscular dystrophy. New England Journal of Medicine 268: 163

Hazama R, Tsujihata M, Mori M, Mori K 1979 Muscular dystrophy in six young girls. Neurology 29: 1486–1491

Heckmatt J Z, Leeman S, Dubowitz V 1982 Ultrasound imaging in the diagnosis of muscle disease. Journal of Pediatrics 101: 656

Heckmatt J Z, Dubowitz V, Hyde S A, Florence J, Gabain A C, Thompson N 1985 Prolongation of walking in Duchenne muscular dystrophy with lightweight orthoses: review of 57 cases. Developmental Medicine and Child Neurology 27: 149

Heckmatt J Z, Loh L, Dubowitz V 1990 Night-time nasal ventilation in neuromuscular diseases. Lancet 335: 579

Henry A N and Neville B G R 1984 Gastrocnemius fasciotomy in Becker muscular dysltrophy. Lancet i: 1350 (letter)

Henson T E, Muller J, De Myer W E 1967 Hereditary myopathy limited to females. Archives of Neurology 17: 238

Hertrich O 1957 Kasuistiche Mitteilung uber eine Sippe mit dominant vererblicher, wahrscheinlich weiblich geschlechtsbebundener progressiver Muskeldystrophe des Schultergurteltyps. Nervenarzt 28: 325

Heyck H, Laudahn G, Carsten P M 1966 Enzymaktivitatsbestimmungen bei Dystrophia musculorum progressiva. IV Mitteilung. Klinische Wochenschrift 44: 695

Hoffman E P, Arahata K, Minetti C, Bonilla E, Rowland L P 1992 Dystrophinopathy in isolated cases of myopathy in females. Neurology 42: 967

Hone W 1825 The every-day book ...., vol I. London, Hunt and Clarke, pp 1017–1034

Hopkins L C, Jackson J A, Elsas L J 1981 Emery–Dreifuss humeroperoneal muscular dystrophy: an X-linked myopathy with unusual contractures and bradycardia. Annals of Neurology 10: 230

Howard R 1908 A case of congenital defect of the muscular system (dystrophia muscularis congenita) and its association with congenital talipes equinovarus. Proceedings of the Royal Society of Medicine (Pathological Section) 1: 157

Hsu J D, Garcia-Ariz M 1981 Fracture of the femur in the Duchenne muscular dystrophy patient. Journal of Pediatric Orthopedics 1: 203

Hudgson P, Bradley W G, Jenkison M 1972 Familial 'mitochondrial' myopathy: a myopathy associated with disordered oxidative metabolism in muscle fibres. Part 1. Clinical, electrophysiological and pathological findings. Journal of the Neurological Sciences 16: 343

Hunsaker R H, Fulkerson P K, Barry F J, Lewis R P, Leier C V, Unverferth D V 1982 Cardiac function in Duchenne's muscular dystrophy: results of 10-year follow-up study and non-invasive tests. American Journal of Medicine 73: 235

Hunter S 1980 The heart in muscular dystrophy. British Medical Bulletin 36: 133

Hutchinson 1879 An ophthalmoplegia externa or symmetrical immobility (partial) of the eye with ptosis. Transactions of the Medico-Chirurgical Society of Edinburgh 62: 307

Inkley S R, Oldenburg F C, Vignos P J 1974 Pulmonary function in Duchenne muscular dystrophy related to stage of disease. American Journal of Medicine 56: 297

Isaacs H, Badenhorst M E, Whistler T 1988 Autosomal recessive distal myopathy. Journal of Clinical Pathology 41: 188

Ishikawa A 1982 Fukuyama-type congenital muscular dystrophy. Archives of Neurology 39: 671

Jackson C E, Carey J H 1961 Progressive muscular dystrophy: autosomal recessive type. Pediatrics 28: 77

Jackson C E, Strehler D A 1968 Limb girdle muscular dystrophy: clinical manifestations and detection of preclinical disease. Pediatrics 41: 495

Jacobs H K, Wrogemann K, Greenberg C R, Seshia S S, Cameron A I 1989 Neonatal screening for Duchenne muscular dystrophy — the Canadian experience. In: Schmidt B J et al (eds) Current trends in infant screening. Amsterdam, Elsevier, pp 361

Jalbert P, Mouriquand C, Beaudoing A, Jaillard M 1966 Myopathie progressive de type Duchenne et mosaique XO/XXX: Considerations sur la génèse de la fibre musculaire striée. Annales Génetiques 9: 104

James T N 1962 Observations on the cardiovascular involvement, including the cardiac conduction system, in progressive muscular dystrophy. American Heart Journal 63: 48

Ji X-W, Tan J, Chen X-Y, Yi S-X, Liang H 1990 New type of X-linked progressive muscular dystrophy involving shoulder girdle and back. American Journal of Medical Genetics 37: 209

Johnston E W, Reynolds T, Stauch D 1985 Duchenne muscular dystrophy: a case with prolonged survival. Archives of Physical Medicine and Rehabilitation 66: 462

Jones D A, Round J M, Edwards R H T, Grindwood S R, Tofts P S 1983 Size and composition of the calf and quadriceps muscles in Duchenne muscular dystrophy: a tomographic and histochemical study. Journal of the Neurological Sciences 60: 307

Jones R, Khan R, Hughes S, Dubowitz V 1979 Congenital muscular dystrophy: the importance of early diagnosis and orthopaedic management in the long term prognosis. Journal of Bone and Joint Surgery 61B: 13

Julien J, Vital C, Vallat J M, le Blanc M 1974 Oculopharyngeal muscular dystrophy: a case with abnormal mitochondria and 'fingerprint' inclusions. Journal of the Neurological Sciences 21: 165

Kaeser H E 1965 Scapuloperoneal muscular atrophy. Brain 88: 407

Kakulas B A, Cullity P E, Maguire P 1975 Muscular dystrophy in young girls. Proceedings of the Australian Association of Neurologists 12: 75

Kamoshita S, Konishi Y, Segawa M, Fukuyama Y 1976 Congenital muscular dystrophy as a disease of the central nervous system. Archives of Neurology 33: 513

Karagan N J, Richman L C, Sorensen J P 1980 Analysis of verbal disability in Duchenne muscular dystrophy. Journal of Nervous and Mental Diseases 168: 419

Karagan N J, Sorensen J P 1981 Intellectual functioning in non-Duchenne muscular dystrophy. Neurology (NY) 31: 448

Katiyer B C, Somani P N, Miscra S, Chaterji A M 1977 Congestive cardiomyopathy in a family of Becker's X-linked muscular dystrophy. Postgraduate Medical Journal 53: 12

Kazakov V M, Bogorodinsky D K, Skorometz A A 1976 The myogenic scapuloperoneal syndrome. Muscular dystrophy in the K kindred: clinical study and genetics. Clinical Genetics 10: 41

Kazakov V M, Bogorodinsky D K, Znoyko Z V, Skorometz A A 1974 The facio-scapulo-limb (or the facioscapulohumeral) type of muscular dystrophy: clinical and genetic study of 200 cases. European Neurology 11: 236

Kearns T P, Sayre G P 1958 Retinitis pigmentosa, external ophthalmoplegia and complete heart block. Archives of Ophthalmology 60: 280

Kelfer H M, Singer W D, Reynolds R N 1983 Malignant hyperthermia in a child with muscular dystrophy. Pediatrics 71: 118

Kerby G R, Mayer L S, Pingleton S K 1987 Nocturnal positive pressure ventilation via nasal mask. American Review of Respiratory Disease 135: 738

Khodadadeh S, McClelland M R, Patrick J H, Edwards R H T, Evans G A 1986 Knee movements in Duchenne muscular dystrophy. Lancet 2: 544

Kiloh L G & Nevin S 1951 Progressive dystrophy of external ocular muscles (ocular myopathy). Brain 74: 115

Kingston H M, Sarfarazi M, Thomas N S T, Harper P S 1984 Localisation of the Becker muscular dystrophy gene on the short arm of the X chromosome by linkage to cloned DNA sequences. Human Genetics 67: 6

Kingston H M, Thomas N S T, Pearson P L, Sarfarazi M, Harper P S 1983 Genetic linkage between Becker muscular dystrophy and a polymorphic DNA sequence on the short arm of the X-chromosome. Journal of Medical Genetics 20: 255

Kloepfer H W, Talley C 1958 Autosomal recessive inheritance of Duchenne type muscular dystrophy. Annals of Human Genetics 22: 138

Koenig M, Hoffman E P, Bertelson C J, Monaco A P, Feener C, Kunkel L M 1987 Complete cloning of the Duchenne muscular dystrophy (DMD) cDNA and preliminary genomic organisation of the DMD gene in normal and affected individuals. Cell 50: 509

Koenig M, Monaco A P, Kunkel L M 1988 The complete sequence of dystrophin predicts a rod-shaped cytoskeletal protein. Cell 53: 219

Kohno K 1978 Mental retardation in Duchenne muscular dystrophy. In: Abstracts of the IVth International Congress on Neuromuscular Diseases, Montreal

Korf B R, Bresnan M J, Schapiro F, Sotrel A, Abrams I F 1985 Facioscapulohumeral dystrophy presenting in infancy with facial diplegia and sensorineural deafness. Annals of Neurology 17: 513

Korman S H, Bar-Oz B, Granot E, Meyer E 1991 Oro-caecal transit time in Duchenne muscular dystrophy. Archives of Disease in Childhood 66: 143

Kottke F J, Pauley D L, Ptak R A 1966 The rationale for prolonged stretching for correction of shortening of connective tissue. Archives of Physical Medicine 47: 345

Kovick R B, Fogelman A M, Abbasi A S, Peter J P, Pearce M L 1975 Echocardiographic evaluation of posterior left ventricular wall motion in muscular dystrophy. Circulation 52: 447

Kozicka A, Prot J, Wasilewski R 1971 Mental retardation in patients with Duchenne progressive muscular dystrophy. Journal of the Neurological Sciences 14: 209

Krijgsman J B, Barth P G, Stam F C, Slooff J L, Jaspar H H J 1980 Congenital muscular dystrophy and cerebral dysgenesis in a Dutch family. Neuropadiatrie 11: 108

Kurz L T, Mubarak S J, Schultz P, Park S M, Leach J 1983 Correlation of scoliosis and pulmonary function in Duchenne muscular dystrophy. Journal of Pediatric Orthopedics 3: 347

Lacomis D, Kupsky W J, Kuban K K, Specht L A 1991 Childhood onset oculopharyngeal muscular dystrophy. Pediatric Neurology 7: 382

Lamy M, de Grouchy J 1954 L'hérédité de la myopathie (formes basses). Journale Génétique Humaine 3: 219

Landouzy L, Dejerine J 1884 De la myopathie atrophique progressive (myopathie héréditaire), débutant, dans l'enfance, par la face, sans alteration due système nerveux. Comptes rendus hebdomadaires des seances de l'Academie des Sciences 98: 53

Lapresle J M, Fardeau M, Godet-Guillain J 1972 Myopathie distale congénitale avec hypertrophie des mollets — presence d'anomalies mitochondriales à la biopsie musculaire. Journal of the Neurological Sciences 17: 87

Lazaro R P, Fenichel G M, Kilroy A W 1979 Congenital muscular dystrophy: case reports and reappraisal. Muscle and Nerve 2: 349

Lebenthal E, Shochet S B, Adam A et al 1970 Arthrogryposis multiplex congenita: twenty-three cases in an Arab kindred. Pediatrics 46: 891

Leibowitz D, Dubowitz V 1981 Intellect and behaviour in Duchenne muscular dystrophy. Developmental Medicine and Child Neurology 23: 557

Lewis A J, Besant D F 1962 Muscular dystrophy in infancy: report of 2 cases in siblings with diaphragmatic weakness. Journal of Pediatrics 60: 376

Lewis I 1966 Late-onset muscular dystrophy: oculopharyngoesophageal variety. Canadian Medical Association Journal 95: 146

Leyden E 1876 Klinik der Ruckenmarks-Krankheiten, vol 2. Hirchwald, Berlin, p 531

Leyten Q H, Gabreels F J M, Renier W O, ter Laak H J, Sengers R C A, Mullaart R A 1989 Congenital muscular dystrophy. Journal of Pediatrics 115: 214

Leyten Q H, Renkawek K, Renier W O et al 1991 Neuropathological findings in muscle–eye–brain disease (MEB-D). Acta Neuropathologica 83: 55

Leyten Q H, Gabreels F J M, Renier W O, Renkawek K, ter Laak H J, Mullaart R A 1992 Congenital muscular dystrophy with eye and brain malformations in six Dutch patients. Neuropediatrics 23: 316

Lin M-Y, Nonaka I 1991 Facioscapulohumeral muscular dystrophy: muscle fiber type analysis with particular reference to small angular fibers. Brain and Development 13: 331

Lindenbaum R H, Clark G, Patel C, Moncrieff M, Hughes J T 1979 Muscular dystrophy in an X;1 translocation female suggests that Duchenne locus is on X chromosome short arm. Journal of Medical Genetics 16: 389

Lintner S P K, Thomas P R, Withington P S, Hall M G 1982 Suxamethonium associated hypertonicity and cardiac arrest in unsuspected pseudohypertrophic muscular dystrophy. British Journal of Anaesthesia 54: 1331

Little B W, Perl D P 1982 Oculopharyngeal muscular dystrophy: an autopsied case from the French-Canadian kindred. Journal of the Neurological Sciences 53: 145

Lundberg P O 1962 Ocular myopathy with hypogonadism. Acta Neurologica Scandinavica 38: 142

Lunt P W, Compston D A S, Harper P S 1989 Estimation of age dependent penetrance in facioscapulohumeral muscular dystrophy by minimising ascertainment bias. Journal of Medical Genetics 26: 755

Lunt P W, Harper P S 1991 Genetic counselling in facioscapulohumeral muscular dystrophy. Journal of Medical Genetics 28: 655

Lupski J R, Garcia C A, Zoghbi H Y, Hoffman E P, Fenwick R G 1991 Discordance of muscular dystrophy in monozygotic female twins: evidence supporting asymmetric splitting of the inner cell mass in a manifesting carrier of Duchenne dystrophy. American Journal of Medical Genetics 40: 354

Mabry C C, Roeckel I E, Munich R L, Robertson D 1965 X-linked pseudohypertrophic muscular dystrophy with a late onset and slow progression. New England Journal of Medicine 273: 1062

Magee K R, de Jong R N 1965 Hereditary distal myopathy with onset in infancy. Archives of Neurology 13: 387

Manning G W, Cropp G J 1958 The electrocardiogram in progressive muscular dystrophy. British Heart Journal 20: 410

Manzur A Y, Hyde S A, Rodillo E, Heckmatt J Z, Bentley G, Dubowitz V 1992 A randomised controlled trial of early surgery in Duchenne muscular dystrophy. Neuromuscular Disorders 2: 379

Marconi G, Pizzi A, Arimondi C G, Vannelli B 1991 Limb girdle muscular dystrophy with autosomal dominant inheritance. Acta Neurologica Scandinavica 83: 234

Markand D N, North R R, D'Agostino A N, Daly D D 1969 Benign sex-linked muscular dystrophy. Clinical and pathological features. Neurology (Minneapolis) 19: 612

Markesbery W R, Griggs R C, Herr B 1977 Distal myopathy: electron microscopic and histochemical studies. Neurology (Minneapolis) 27: 727

Markesbery W R, Griggs R C, Leach R P, Lapham L W 1974 Late onset hereditary distal myopathy. Neurology (Minneapolis) 23: 127

Marsh G G, Munsat T L 1974 Evidence for early impairment of verbal intelligence in Duchenne muscular dystrophy. Archives of Disease in Childhood 49: 118

Matsubara S, Tanabe H 1982 Hereditary distal myopathy with filamentous inclusions. Acta Neurologica Scandinavica 65: 363

Matsumura K, Tomé F M S, Collin H et al 1992 Deficiency of the 50 K dystrophin-associated glycoprotein in severe childhood autosomal recessive muscular dystrophy. Nature 359: 320

Matsumura K, Nonaka I, Campbell K P 1993 Abnormal expression of dystrophin-associated proteins in Fukuyama-type congenital muscular dystrophy. Lancet 341: 521

Mawatari S, Katayama K 1973 Scapulohumeral muscular atrophy with cardiomyopathy: an X-linked recessive trait. Archives of Neurology 28: 55

Maytal J, Shanske A L, Fox J E, Lipper S, Eviatar L 1991 Duchenne muscular dystrophy in a girl identified by dystrophin deficiency. Neuropediatrics 22: 163

McGarry J, Garg B, Silbert S 1983 Death in childhood due to facio-scapulo-humeral dystrophy. Acta Neurologica Scandinavica 68: 61

McKusick V A 1971 X-linked muscular dystrophy, benign form with contractures. Birth Defects VII 2: 113

McKusick V A 1992 Mendelian inheritance in man, 10th edn. Johns Hopkins University Press, Baltimore

McMenamin J B, Becker L E, Murphy E G 1982a Fukuyama-type congenital muscular dystrophy. Journal of Pediatrics 101: 580

McMenamin J B, Becker L E, Murphy E G 1982b Congenital muscular dystrophy: a clinicopathologic report of 24 cases. Journal of Pediatrics 100: 692

Merchut M P, Zdonczyk D, Gujrati M 1990 Cardiac transplantation in female Emery–Dreifuss muscular dystrophy. Journal of Neurology 237: 316

Merlini L, Granata C, Dominici P, Bonfiglioli S 1986 Emery–Dreifuss muscular dystrophy: report of five cases in a family and review of the literature. Muscle and Nerve 9: 481

Meryon E 1852 On granular and fatty degeneration of the voluntary muscles. Medico-Chirurgical Transactions (London) 35: 73

Meryon E 1864 Practical and pathological researches on the various forms of paralysis. Churchill, London

Meyer-Betz F 1910 Beobachtungen an einem eigenartigen mit Muskellahmungen verbundenen Fall von Hamoglobinurie. Deutsches Archiv fur klinische Medizin 101: 85

Meyerson M D, Lewis E, Ill K 1984 Facioscapulohumeral muscular dystrophy and accompanying hearing loss. Archives of Otolaryngology 110: 261

Miller E D, Sanders D B, Rowlingson J C, Berry F A, Sussman M D, Epstein R M 1978 Anesthesia-induced rhabdomyolysis in a patient with Duchenne's muscular dystrophy. Anesthesiology 48: 146

Miller F, Moseley C F, Koreska J 1992 Spinal fusion in Duchenne muscular dystrophy. Developmental Medicine and Child Neurology 34: 775

Miller G, Dunn N 1982 An outline of the management and prognosis of Duchenne muscular dystrophy in Western Australia. Australian Paediatric Journal 18: 277

Miller J R, Cobert A P, Schock N C 1988 Ventilator use in progressive neuromuscular disease: impact on patients and their families. Developmental Medicine and Child Neurology 30: 280

Miller J R, Colbert A P, Osberg J S 1990 Ventilator dependency: decision making, daily functioning and quality of life for patients with Duchenne muscular dystrophy. Developmental Medicine and Child Neurology 32: 1078

Miller R G, Blank N K, Layzer R B 1979 Sporadic distal myopathy with early adult onset. Annals of Neurology 5: 220

Miller R G, Layzer R B, Mellenthin M A, Golabi M, Francoz R A, Mall J C 1985 Emery–Dreifuss muscular dystrophy with autosomal dominant transmission. Neurology 35: 1230

Milne B, Rosales J K 1982 Anaesthetic considerations in patients with muscular dystrophy undergoing spinal fusion and Harrington rod insertion. Canadian Anaesthetic Society Journal 29: 250

Miyoshi K, Kawai H, Iwasa M, Kusaka K, Nishino H 1986 Autosomal recessive distal muscular dystrophy as a new type of progressive muscular dystrophy: seventeen cases in eight families including an autopsied case. Brain 109: 31

Möbius P J 1879 Ueber die hereditaren nervenkrankheiten. Sammlung klinischer Vortage 171: 1505

Mohire M D, Tandan R, Fries T J, Little B W, Pendlebury W W, Bradley W G 1988 Early onset benign autosomal dominant limb-girdle myopathy with contractures (Bethlem myopathy). Neurology 38: 573

Mokri B, Engel A G 1975 Duchenne dystrophy: electron microscopic findings pointing to a basic or early abnormality in the plasma membrane of the muscle fibre. Neurology (Minneapolis) 25: 1111

Monckton G, Hoskin V, Warren S 1982 Prevalence and incidence of muscular dystrophy in Alberta, Canada. Clinical Genetics 21: 19

Morgan-Hughes J A, Mair W G P 1973 Atypical muscle mitochondria in oculoskeletal myopathy. Brain 96: 215

Morton N E, Chung C S 1959 Formal genetics of muscular dystrophy. American Journal of Human Genetics 11: 360

Moser H 1984 Duchenne muscular dystrophy: pathogenetic aspects and genetic prevention. Human Genetics 66: 17

Moser H, Emery A E H 1974 The manifesting carrier in Duchenne muscular dystrophy. Clinical Genetics 5: 271

Moser von H, Weismann U, Richterich R, Rossi E 1964 Progressive Muskeldystrophie. VI Haufigkeit, Klinik und Genetik der Duchenne form. Schweizerische Medizinische Wochenschrift 94: 1610

Moser von H, Weismann U, Richterich R, Rossi E 1966 Progressive Muskeldystrophie. VIII Haufigkeit, Klinik und Genetik der Typen I und III. Schweizerische Medizinische Wochenschrifft 96: 169

Munsat T L, Piper D 1971 Genetically determined inflammatory myopathy with facioscapulohumeral distribution. Neurology (Minneapolis) 21: 440

Murphy S F, Drachman D B 1968 The oculopharyngeal syndrome. Journal of the American Medical Association 203: 1003

Murray J M, Davies K E, Harper P S, Meredith L, Mueller C R, Williamson R 1982 Linkage relationship of a cloned DNA sequence on the short arm of the X chromosome to Duchenne muscular dystrophy. Nature 300: 69

Nicholson L V B, Johnson M A, Bushby K M D et al 1993 Integrated study of 100 patients with Xp 21 linked muscular dystrophy using clinical, genetic, immunochemical and histopathological data. Part 2 Correlations within individual patients. Journal of Medical Genetics 30: 737

Nigro G, Comi L I, Limongelli F M et al 1983 Prospective study of X-linked progressive muscular dystrophy in Campania. Muscle and Nerve 6: 253

Nihei K, Kamoshita S, Atsumi T 1979 A case of Ullrich's disease. Brain and Development 1: 61

Nogen A G 1980 Congenital muscle disease and abnormal findings on computerised tomography. Developmental Medicine and Child Neurology 22: 658

Nonaka I, Sugita H, Takada K, Kumagai K 1982 Muscle histochemistry in congenital muscular dystrophy with central nervous system involvement. Muscle and Nerve 5: 102

Nonaka I, Sunohara N, Ishiura S, Satayoshi E 1981a Familial distal myopathy with rimmed vacuole and lamellar (myeloid) body formation. Journal of the Neurological Sciences 51: 141

Nonaka I, Une Y, Ishihara T, Miyoshino S, Nakashima T, Sugita H 1981b A clinical and histological study of Ullrich's disease (congenital atonic-sclerotic muscular dystrophy). Neuropediatrics 12: 197

Nonaka I, Sunohara N, Satayoshi E, Terasawa K, Yonemoto K 1985 Autosomal recessive distal muscular dystrophy: a comparative study with distal myopathy with rimmed vacuole formation. Annals of Neurology 17: 51

Nudel U, Zuk D, Einat P et al 1989 Duchenne muscular dystrophy gene product is not identical in muscle and brain. Nature 337: 76

O'Brien M D 1962 An infantile muscular dystrophy: report of a case with autopsy findings. Guy's Hospital Reports 111: 98

Oka S, Igarashi Y, Takagi A et al 1982 Malignant hyperpyrexia and Duchenne muscular dystrophy: a case report. Canadian Anaesthetists Society Journal 29: 627

Olson B J, Fenichel G M 1982 Progressive muscle disease in a young woman with family history of Duchenne's muscular dystrophy. Archives of Neurology 39: 378

Olson W, Engel W K, Walsh G O, Einaugler R 1972 Oculocraniosomatic neuromuscular disease with 'ragged-red' fibres: histochemical and ultrastructural changes in limb muscles of a group of patients with idiopathic progressive external ophthalmoplegia. Archives of Neurology 26: 193

O'Orsognna L, O'Shea J P, Miller G 1988 Cardiomyopathy of Duchenne muscular dystrophy. Pediatric Cardiology 9: 205

Oppenheim H 1900 Ueber allgemeine und localisierte atonie der muskulatur (myatonie) im fruhen kindesalter. Monatsschrift für Psychiatrie und Neurologie 8: 232

Orstavik K H, Kloster R, Lippestad C, Rode L, Hovig T, Fuglseth K N 1990 Emery–Dreifuss syndrome in three generations of females, including identical twins. Clinical Genetics 38: 447

Padberg G W, Lunt P W, Koch M, Fardeau M 1991 Diagnostic criteria for facioscapulohumeral muscular dystrophy. Neuromuscular Disorders 1: 231

Panegyres P K, Mastaglia F L, Kakulas B A 1990 Limb girdle syndromes: clinical, morphological and electrophysiological studies. Journal of the Neurological Sciences 95: 201

Passos-Bueno M R, Zatz M 1991 Reproductive fitness and frequency of new mutations in Becker muscular dystrophy. Journal of Medical Genetics 28: 286

Passos-Bueno M R, Richard I, Vainzof M et al 1993 Evidence of genetic heterogeneity in the autosomal recessive adult forms of limb-girdle muscular dystrophy following linkage analysis with 15q probes in Brazilian families. Journal of Medical Genetics 30: 385

Pearce G W, Pearce J M S, Walton J N 1966 The Duchenne type muscular dystrophy: histopathological studies of the carrier state. Brain 89: 109

Pearn J H, Hudgson P 1978 A new syndrome — spinal muscular atrophy with adolescent onset and hypertrophied calves, simulating Becker dystrophy. Lancet i: 1059

Pearson C M, Fowler W G 1963 Hereditary non-progressive muscular dystrophy: inducing arthrogryposis syndrome. Brain 86: 75

Perloff J K, de Leon A C, O'Doherty D 1966 The

cardiomyopathy of progressive muscular dystrophy. Circulation 33: 625

Perloff J K, Roberts W C, de Leon A C, O'Doherty D 1967 The distinctive electrocardiogram of Duchenne's progressive muscular dystrophy. American Journal of Medicine 42: 179

Peterman A F, Lillington G A, Jamplis R W 1964 Progressive muscular dystrophy with ptosis and dysphagia. Archives of Neurology 10: 38

Peters A C B, Bots G T A M, Roos R A C, van Gelderen H H 1984 Fukuyama type congenital muscular dystrophy: two Dutch siblings. Brain & Development 6: 406

Philip U, Walton J N, Smith C A B 1956 Colour-blindness and the Duchenne-type muscular dystrophy. Annals of Human Genetics 21: 155

Pihko H, Louhimo T, Valanne L, Donner M 1992 CNS in congenital muscular dystrophy without mental retardation. Neuropediatrics 23: 116

Planchu H, Dellamonica C, Cotte J, Robert J M 1980 Duchenne muscular dystrophy: systematic neonatal screening and earlier detection of carriers. Journal de Génétique Humaine 28: 65

Prosser E J, Murphy E J, Thompson M W 1969 Intelligence and the gene for Duchenne muscular dystrophy. Archives of Disease in Childhood 44: 221

Quinlivan R M, Dubowitz V 1992 Cardiac transplantation in Becker muscular dystrophy. Neuromuscular Disorders 2: 165 (review)

Raitta C, Santavuori P, Lamminen M, Leisti J 1978 Ophthalmological findings in a new syndrome with muscle, eye and brain involvement. Acta Ophthalmologica 56: 465

Rapaport D, Passos-Bueno M R, Brandao L 1991 Apparent association of mental retardation and specific patterns of deletions screened with probes cf56a and cf23a in DMD. American Journal of Medical Genetics 39: 437

Rebeiz J J, Caulfield J B, Adams R D 1969 Oculopharyngeal dystrophy — a presenescent myopathy: a clinico-pathologic study. In: Progress in neuro-ophthalmology (Excerpta Medica International Congress Series No 176). Excerpta Medica, Amsterdam, p 12

Reeves W C, Griggs R, Nanda N C, Thompson K, Gramiak R 1980 Echocardiographic evaluation of cardiac abnormalities in Duchenne's dystrophy and myotonic muscular dystrophy. Archives of Neurology 37: 273

Richards C S, Watkins S C, Hoffman E P et al 1990 Skewed X inactivation in a female MZ twin results in Duchenne muscular dystrophy. American Journal of Human Genetics 46: 672

Ricker K, Mertens H-G 1968 The differential diagnosis of the myogenic (facio)-scapulo-peroneal syndrome. European Neurology 1: 275

Rideau Y 1978 Outlines of muscular dystrophy. SREREM, Poitiers, France

Rideau Y, Jankowski L W, Grellet J 1981 Respiratory function in the muscular dystrophies. Muscle and Nerve 4: 155

Rideau Y, Gatin G, Bach J, Gines G 1983 Prolongation of life in Duchenne's muscular dystrophy. Acta Neurologica (Napoli) 5 (38): 118

Rideau Y, Glorion B, Delaubier A, Tarle O, Bach J 1984 The treatment of scoliosis in Duchenne muscular dystrophy. Muscle and Nerve 7: 281

Rideau Y, Delaubier A 1987 Neuromuscular respiratory deficit: setting back mortality. Seminars in Orthopaedics 2: 203

Rideau Y, Duport G, Delaubier A 1986 Premieres remissions reproductibles dans l'évolution de la dystrophie musculaire de Duchenne. Bulletin de l'Academie Nationale de Médécine 170: 605

Ringel S P, Carroll J E, Schold C 1977 The spectrum of mild X-linked recessive muscular dystrophy. Archives of Neurology 34: 408

Robin G C 1977 Scoliosis in Duchenne muscular dystrophy. Israel Journal of the Medical Sciences 13: 203

Robin G C, Brief L P 1971 Scoliosis in childhood muscular dystrophy. Journal of Bone and Joint Surgery 53A: 466

Robin G C, Falewski de Leon G (eds) 1977 Symposium on Muscular Dystrophy. Israeli Journal of Medical Sciences 13: 85

Rodillo E, Fernandez-Bermejo E, Heckmatt J, Dubowitz V 1988 Prevention of rapidly progressive scoliosis in Duchenne muscular dystrophy by prolongation of walking with orthoses. Journal of Child Neurology 3: 269

Rosenberg H, Heiman-Patterson T 1983 Duchenne's muscular dystrophy and malignant hyperthermia: another warning. Anesthesiology 59: 362

Rosman N P 1970 The cerebral defect and myopathy in Duchenne muscular dystrophy: a comparative clinico-pathological study. Neurology (Minneapolis) 20: 329

Rosman N P, Kakulas B A 1966 Mental deficiency associated with muscular dystrophy. A neuropathological study. Brain 89: 769

Ross R T 1963 Ocular myopathy sensitive to curare. Brain 86: 67

Ross R T 1964 The effect of decamethonium on curare sensitive ocular myopathy. Neurology (Minneapolis) 14: 684

Rothstein T L, Carlson C B, Sumi S M 1971 Polymyositis with facioscapulohumeral distribution. Archives of Neurology 25: 313

Rotthauwe H-W, Kowalewski S 1965 Klinische und biochemische Untersuchungen bei Myopathien. III. Mitteilung. Recessive X-chromosomale Muskeldystrophie mit relativ gutartigem Verlauf. Klinische Wochenschrift 43: 158

Rotthauwe H-W, Mortier W, Beyer H 1972 Neuer Typ einer recessive X-chromosomal vererten Muskeldystrophie: Scapulo-humero-distale Muskeldystrophie mit fruhzeitigen Kontrakturen and Herzrhythmusstorungen. Humangenetik 16: 181

Rowland L P 1976 Pathogenesis of muscular dystrophies. Archives of Neurology 33: 315

Rowland L P, Fetell M, Olarte M, Hays A, Singh N, Wanat F E 1979 Emery–Dreifuss muscular dystrophy. Annals of Neurology 5: 111

Roy L, Gibson D A 1970 Pseudohypertrophic muscular dystrophy and its surgical management: review of 30 patients. Canadian Journal of Surgery 13: 13

Russe H, Busey H, Barbeau A 1967 Immunoglobulin changes in oculopharyngeal muscular dystrophy. Proceedings of the 2nd International Congress of Neurogenetics, Montreal

Salih M A M, Omer M I A, Bayoumi R A, Karrar O, Johnson M 1983 Severe autosomal recessive muscular dystrophy in an extended Sudanese kindred. Developmental Medicine and Child Neurology 25: 43

Salih M A M, Ekmejian A, Omer M I A 1984 Respiratory insufficiency in a severe autosomal recessive form of muscular dystrophy. Annals of Tropical Paediatrics 4: 45

Salmon M A, Esiri M M, Ruderman N B 1971 Myopathic

disorder associated with mitochondrial abnormalities, hyperglycaemia and hyperketonaemia. Lancet ii: 290

Sandifer P H 1946 Chronic progressive ophthalmoplegia of myopathic origin. Journal of Neurology, Neurosurgery and Psychiatry 9: 81

Santavuori P, Leisti J, Kruus S 1977 Muscle, eye and brain disease: a new syndrome. Neuropadiatrie 8 (Suppl): 550

Santavuori P, Pihko H, Sainio K et al 1990 Muscle-eye-brain disease and Walker–Warburg syndrome. American Journal of Medical Genetics 36: 371

Sanyal S K, Johnson W W, Dische M R, Pitner S E, Beard C 1980 Dystrophic degeneration of papillary muscle and ventricular myocardium: basis for mitral valve prolapse in Duchenne's muscular dystrophy. Circulation 62: 430

Sanyal S K, Johnson W W 1982 Cardiac conduction abnormalities in children with Duchenne's muscular dystrophy. Circulation 66: 853

Scheuerbrandt G, Lundin A, Lovgren T, Mortier W 1986 Screening for Duchenne muscular dystrophy: an improved screening test for creatine kinase and its application in an infant screening program. Muscle and Nerve 9: 11

Schmitt H P, Krause K-H 1981 An autopsy study of a familial oculopharyngeal muscular dystrophy with distal spread and neurogenic involvement. Muscle and Nerve 4: 296

Schneck L, Adachi M, Briet P, Wolintz A, Volk B W 1973 Ophthalmoplegia plus with morphological and chemical studies of cerebellar and muscle tissue. Journal of the Neurological Sciences 19: 37

Schneiderman L J, Sampson W I, Schoene W C, Haydon G B 1969 Genetic studies of a family with two unusual autosomal dominant conditions: muscular dystrophy and Pelger–Huet anomaly. American Journal of Medicine 46: 380

Schott J, Jacobi M, Wald M A 1955 Electrocardiographic patterns in the differential diagnosis of progressive muscular dystrophy. American Journal of Medical Science 229: 517

Scott O M, Hyde S A, Goddard C, Dubowitz V 1982 Quantitation of muscle function in children: a prospective study in Duchenne muscular dystrophy. Muscle and Nerve 5: 291

Seay A R, Ziter F A, Thompson J A 1978 Cardiac arrest during induction of anesthesia in Duchenne muscular dystrophy. Journal of Pediatrics 93: 88

Seeger B R, Sutherland A D'A, Clark M S 1984 Orthotic management of scoliosis in Duchenne muscular dystrophy. Archives of Physical Medicine and Rehabilitation 65: 83

Segall D 1988 Noninvasive nasal mask-assisted ventilation in respiratory failure of Duchenne muscular dystrophy. Chest 93: 1298

Segawa M, Nomura Y, Hachimori K, Shinoyama N, Hosaka A, Mizuno Y 1979 Fukuyama type congenital muscular dystrophy as a natural model of childhood epilepsy. Brain and Development 2: 113

Seitz D 1957 Zur nosologischen Stellung des sogenannten scapulo-peronealen Syndroms. Deutsche Zeitschrift für Nervenheilkunde 175: 547

Serratrice G, Cros D, Pellissier J-F, Gastaut J-L, Pouget J 1980 Dystrophie musculaire congénitale. Revue Neurologique (Paris) 136: 445

Serratrice G, Pellionier J F 1988 Deux familles de myopathies bénignes prédominant sur les cintures d'hérédité autosomique dominante. Revue Neurologique 144: 43

Shapiro F, Sethna N, Colan S, Wohl M E, Specht L 1992 Spinal fusion in Duchenne muscular dystrophy. Muscle and Nerve 15: 604

Shaw R F, Dreifuss F E 1969 Mild and severe forms of X-linked muscular dystrophy. Archives of Neurology 20: 451

Shokeir M H K, Kobrinsky N L 1976 Autosomal recessive muscular dystrophy in Manitoba Hutterites. Clinical Genetics 9: 197

Shokeir M H K, Rozdilsky B 1985 Muscular dystrophy in Saskatchewan Hutterites. American Journal of Medical Genetics. 22: 487

Short J K 1963 Congenital muscular dystrophy: a case report with autopsy findings. Neurology (Minneapolis) 13: 526

Siegel I M 1977 The clinical management of muscle disease. Heinemann, London

Siegel I M 1978 The management of muscular dystrophy: a clinical review. Muscle and Nerve 1: 453

Siegel I M 1982 Spinal stabilization in Duchenne muscular dystrophy: rationale and method. Muscle and Nerve 54: 417

Siegel I M, Miller J E, Ray R D 1968 Subcutaneous lower limb tenotomy in the treatment of pseudohypertrophic muscular dystrophy. Journal of Bone and Joint Surgery 50A: 1437

Skinner R, Smith C, Emery A E H 1974 Linkage between the loci for benign (Becker type) X-borne muscular dystrophy and deutan colour blindness. Journal of Medical Genetics 11: 317

Skyring A, McKusick V A 1961 Clinical, genetic and electrocardiographic studies in childhood muscular dystrophy. American Journal of Medical Science 242: 534

Slucka C 1968 The electrocardiogram in Duchenne progressive muscular dystrophy. Circulation 38: 933

Small R G 1968 Coat's disease and muscular dystrophy. Transactions of the American Academy of Ophthalmology and Otolaryngology 72: 225

Smith R A, Sibert J R, Wallace S J, Harper P S 1989a Early diagnosis and secondary prevention of Duchenne muscular dystrophy. Archives of Disease in Childhood 64: 787

Smith R A, Rogers M, Bradley D M, Sibert J R, Harper P S 1989b Screening for Duchenne muscular dystrophy. Archives of Disease in Childhood 64: 1017

Smith R A, Williams D K, Sibert J R, Harper P S 1990 Attitudes of mothers to neonatal screening for Duchenne muscular dystrophy. British Medical Journal 300: 1112

Somer H, Lautumaa V, Paljarvi L et al 1991 Benign muscular dystrophy with autosomal dominant inheritance. Neuromuscular Disorders 1: 267

Specht L A 1992 In: Case records of the Massachusetts General Hospital: case 34-1992. New England Journal of Medicine 327: 548

Speer M C, Yamaoka L H, Gilchrist J M, Gaskell P C, Stajich J M, Weber J L 1991 Linkage of an autosomal dominant form of limb-girdle muscular dystrophy to chromosome 5q. American Journal of Human Genetics 49 (Suppl): 17

Spencer G E, Vignos P J 1962 Bracing for ambulation in childhood progressive muscular dystrophy. Journal of Bone and Joint Surgery 44A: 234

Spiller W G 1907 Myopathy of the distal type and its relation to the neural form of muscular atrophy (Charcot–Marie–Tooth type). Journal of Nervous and Mental Disease 34: 14

Stern L M, Caudrey D J, Perrett L V, Boldt D W 1984 Progression of muscular dystrophy assessed by computed tomography. Developmental Medicine and Child Neurology 26: 569

Stevenson A C 1953 Muscular dystrophy in Northern

Ireland. Annals of Eugenics 18: 50

Sumner D, Crawfurd M d'A, Harriman D G F 1971 Distal muscular dystrophy in an English family. Brain 94: 51

Sunohara N, Arahata K, Hoffman E P et al 1990 Quadriceps myopathy: forme fruste of Becker muscular dystrophy. Annals of Neurology 28: 634

Sussman M D 1984 Advantage of early spinal stabilization and fusion in patients with Duchenne muscular dystrophy. Journal of Pediatric Orthopedics 4: 532

Sussman M D 1985 Treatment of scoliosis in Duchenne muscular dystrophy. Developmental Medicine and Child Neurology 27: 522

Sutherland D H, Olshen R, Cooper L et al 1981 Pathomechanics of gait in Duchenne muscular dystrophy. Developmental Medicine and Child Neurology 23: 3

Swank S M, Brown J C, Perry R E 1982 Spinal fusion in Duchenne's muscular dystrophy. Spine 7: 484

Swash M, Heathfield K W G 1983 Quadriceps myopathy: a variant of the limb-girdle syndrome. Journal of Neurology, Neurosurgery and Psychiatry 46: 355

Tachi N, Nagata N, Wakai S, Chiba S 1991 Congenital muscular dystrophy in Marinesco-Sjögren syndrome. Pediatric Neurology 7: 296

Taddonio R F 1982 Segmental spinal instrumentation in the management of neuromuscular spinal deformity. Spine 7: 305

Takada K, Nakamura H, Tanaka J 1984 Cortical dysplasia in congenital muscular dystrophy with central nervous system involvement (Fukuyama type). Journal of Neuropathology and Experimental Neurology 43: 395

Takada K, Nakamura H 1990 Cerebellar micropolygyria in Fukuyama congenital muscular dystrophy: observations in fetal and pediatric cases. Brain and Development 12: 774

Takamoto K, Hirose K, Uono M, Nonaka I 1984 A genetic variant of Emery–Dreifuss disease. Archives of Neurology 41: 1292

Taylor E W 1915 Progressive vagus-glossopharyngeal paralysis with ptosis. A contribution to the group of family diseases. Journal of Nervous and Mental Disease 42: 129

Taylor D A, Carroll J E, Smith M E, Johnson M O, Johnston G P, Brooke M H 1982 Facioscapulohumeral dystrophy associated with hearing loss and Coats syndrome. Annals of Neurology 12: 395

Thomas P K, Calne D B, Elliott C F 1972 X-linked scapuloperoneal syndrome. Journal of Neurology, Neurosurgery and Psychiatry 35: 208

Thomas P K, Schott G D, Morgan-Hughes J A 1975 Adult onset scapuloperoneal myopathy. Journal of Neurology, Neurosurgery and Psychiatry 38: 1008

Tomlinson B E, Walton J N, Irving D 1974 Spinal cord limb motor neurones in muscular dystrophy. Journal of the Neurological Sciences 22: 305

Topaloglu H, Yalaz K, Renda Y et al 1991 Occidental type cerebromuscular dystrophy: a report of eleven cases. Journal of Neurology, Neurosurgery and Psychiatry 54: 226

Towfighi J, Sassani J W, Suzuki K, Ladda R L 1984 Cerebro-ocular dysplasia-muscular dystrophy (COD-MD) syndrome. Acta Neuropathologica (Berlin) 65: 110

Trevisan C P, Carollo C, Segalla P, Angelini C, Drigo P, Giordano R 1991 Congenital muscular dystrophy: brain alterations in an unselected series of western patients. Journal of Neurology, Neurosurgery and Psychiatry

54: 330

Turner J W A 1940 The relationship between amyotonia congenita and congenital myopathy. Brain 63: 163

Turner J W A, Heathfield K W G 1961 Quadriceps myopathy occurring in middle age. Journal of Neurology, Neurosurgery and Psychiatry 24: 18

Turner J W A, Lees F 1962 Congenital myopathy — a fifty year follow up. Brain 85: 733

Tyler F H, Wintrobe M M 1950 Studies in disorders of muscle. 1. The problem of progressive muscular dystrophy. Annals of Internal Medicine 32: 72

Tyrer J H, Sutherland J M 1961 The primary spino-cerebellar atrophies and their associated defects, with a study of the foot deformity. Brain 84: 289

Ullrich O 1930 Kongenitale, atonisch-sklerotische Muskeldystrophie. Monatsschrift Kinderheilkunde 47: 502

Upadhyaya M, Lunt P W, Sarfarazi M et al 1991 A closely linked DNA marker for facioscapulohumeral disease on chromosome 4q. Journal of Medical Genetics 28: 665

van der Does de Willebois A E M, Bethlem J, Meijer A E F H, Simons A J R 1968 Distal myopathy with onset in early infancy. Neurology (Minneapolis) 18: 383

van Wijngaarden G K, Hagen C J, Bethlem J, Meijer A E F H 1968 Myopathy of the quadriceps muscles. Journal of the Neurological Sciences 7: 201

Vasella F, Mumenthaler M, Rossi E, Moser H, Weismann U 1967 Die kongenitale Muskeldystrophie. Deutsch Z. Nervenheilk. 190: 349

Verellen C, Freund M, De Meyer R, Laterre C, Scholberg B, Frederic J 1977 Progressive muscular dystrophy of the Duchenne type in a young girl associated with an aberration of chromosome X. In: Littlefield J W (ed) 5th International Congress of Birth Defects, Montreal. Excerpta Medica, Amsterdam, p 42

Verellen-Dumoulin C, Freund M, De Meyer R et al 1984 Expression of an X-linked muscular dystrophy in a female due to translocation involving Xp21 and non-random inactivation of the normal X-chromosome. Human Genetics 67: 115

Victor M, Hayes R, Adams R D 1962 Oculopharyngeal muscular dystrophy. A familial disease of late life characterised by dysphagia and progressive ptosis of the eyelids. New England Journal of Medicine 267: 1267

Vignos P J, Spencer G E, Archibald K C 1963 Management of progressive muscular dystrophy of childhood. Journal of the American Medical Association 184: 89

Vignos P J, Wagner M B, Kaplan J S, Spencer G E 1983 Predicting the success of reambulation in patients with Duchenne muscular dystrophy. Journal of Bone and Joint Surgery 65A: 719

Vignos P J, Watkins M P 1966 The effect of exercise in muscular dystrophy. Journal of the American Medical Association 197: 843

Voit T, Krogmann O, Lenard H G et al 1988 Emery–Dreifuss muscular dystrophy: disease spectrum and differential diagnosis. Neuropediatrics 19: 62

Wadia R S, Wadgaonkar S U, Amin R B, Sardesai H V 1976 An unusual family of benign 'X' linked muscular dystrophy with cardiac involvement. Journal of Medical Genetics 13: 352

Wakayama Y, Bonilla E, Schotland D L 1983 Plasma membrane abnormalities in infants with Duchenne muscular dystrophy. Neurology (Cleveland) 33: 1368

Walton J N 1955 On the inheritance of muscular dystrophy.

Annals of Human Genetics 20: 1

Walton J N 1956a The inheritance of muscular dystrophy: further observations. Annals of Human Genetics 21: 40

Walton J N 1956b Two cases of myopathy limited to the quadriceps. Journal of Neurology, Neurosurgery and Psychiatry 19: 160

Walton J N 1961 Muscular dystrophy and its relation to the other myopathies. Research Publications of the Association of Nervous and Mental Diseases 38: 378

Walton J N, Nattrass F J 1954 On the classification, natural history and treatment of the myopathies. Brain 77: 169

Walton J N, Warrick C K 1954 Osseous changes in myopathy. British Journal of Radiology 27: 1

Waters D D, Nutter D O, Hopkins L C, Dorney E R 1975 Cardiac features of an unusual X-linked humeroperoneal neuromuscular disease. New England Journal of Medicine 293: 1017

Watters G, Karpati G, Kaplan B 1977 Post-anesthetic augmentation of muscle damage as a presenting sign in three patients with Duchenne muscular dystrophy. Canadian Journal of Neurological Sciences 4: 228

Weimann R L, Gibson D A, Moseley C F, Jones D C 1983 Surgical stabilization of the spine in Duchenne muscular dystrophy. Spine 8: 776

Welander L 1951 Myopathia distalis tarda hereditaria. Acta Medica Scandinavica 264: Supplementum 1

Welander L 1957 Homozygous appearance of distal myopathy. Acta Geneticae Medicae et Gemellologiae 7: 321

Wharton B A 1965 An unusual variety of muscular dystrophy. Lancet i: 603

Wijmenga C, Frants R R, Brouwer O F, Moerer P, Weber J L, Padberg G W 1990 Location of facioscapulohumeral muscular dystrophy gene on chromosome 4. Lancet 336: 651

Wijmenga C, Padberg G W, Moerer P et al 1991 Mapping of facioscapulohumeral gene to chromosome 4q35-qter by multipoint linkage analysis and in situ hybridization. Genomics 9: 570

Wilkins K E, Gibson D A 1976 The patterns of spinal deformity in Duchenne muscular dystrophy. Journal of Bone and Joint Surgery 58A: 24

Williams E A, Read L, Ellis A, Morris P, Galasko C S B 1984 The management of equinus deformity in Duchenne muscular dystrophy. Journal of Bone and Joint Surgery 66B: 546

Williams W R, Thompson M W, Morton N E 1983 Complex segregation analysis and computer-assisted genetic risk assessment for Duchenne muscular dystrophy. American Journal of Medical Genetics 14: 315

Witt T N, Garner C G, Pongratz D, Baur X 1988 Autosomal dominant Emery–Dreifuss syndrome: evidence of a neurogenic variant of the disease. European Archives of Psychiatric and Neurological Science 237: 230

Worden D K, Vignos P J 1962 Intellectual function in childhood progressive muscular dystrophy. Pediatrics 29: 968

Wulff J D, Lin J T, Kepes J J 1982 Inflammatory facioscapulohumeral muscular dystrophy and Coats syndrome. Annals of Neurology 12: 398

Yamashita M, Matsuki A, Oyama T 1976 General anaesthesia for a patient with progressive muscular dystrophy. Anaesthetist 25: 76

Yates J R W, Emery A E H 1985 A population study of adult onset limb-girdle muscular dystrophy. Journal of Medical Genetics 22: 250

Yates J R W, Warner J P, Smith J A et al 1993 Emery–Dreifuss muscular dystrophy: linkage to markers in distal Xq28. Journal of Medical Genetics 30: 108

Yoshioka M 1981 Clinically manifesting carriers in Duchenne muscular dystrophy. Clinical Genetics 20: 6

Yoshioka M, Okuno T, Honda Y, Nakano Y 1980 Central nervous system involvement in progressive muscular dystrophy. Archives of Disease in Childhood 55: 589

Yoshioka M, Saida K, Itagaki Y, Kamiya T 1989 Follow up study of cardiac involvement in Emery–Dreifuss muscular dystrophy. Archives of Disease in Childhood 64: 713

Yoshioka M, Kuroki S, Kondo T 1990 Ocular manifestations in Fukuyama type congenital muscular dystrophy. Brain and Development 12: 423

Young A, Johnson D, O'Gorman E, McMillan T, Chase A P 1984 A new spinal brace for use in Duchenne muscular dystrophy. Developmental Medicine and Child Neurology 26: 808

Zatuchni J, Aegerter E E, Molthan L, Schuman C R 1951 The heart in progressive muscular dystrophy. Circulation 3: 846

Zatz M, Betti R T B 1986 Benign Duchenne muscular dystrophy in a patient with growth hormone deficiency: a five years follow-up. American Journal of Medical Genetics 24: 567

Zatz M, Itskan S B, Sanger R, Frota-Pessoa O, Saldanha P H 1974 New linkage data for the X-linked types of muscular dystrophy and G6PD variants, colour blindness and Xg blood groups. Journal of Medical Genetics 11: 321

Zatz M, Vianna-Morgante A M, Campos P, Diament A J 1981 Translocation (X-, 6) in a female with Duchenne muscular dystrophy: implications for the localization of the DMD locus. Journal of Medical Genetics 18: 442

Zellweger H, Antonik A 1975 Newborn screening for Duchenne muscular dystrophy. Pediatrics 55: 30

Zellweger H, Hanson J W 1967a Psychometric studies in muscular dystrophy type IIIa (Duchenne). Developmental Medicine and Child Neurology 9: 576

Zellweger H, Hanson J W 1967b Slowly progressive X-linked recessive muscular dystrophy (type IIIb). Archives of Internal Medicine 120: 525

Zellweger H, Afifi A, McCormick W F, Mergner W 1967 Severe congenital muscular dystrophy. American Journal of Diseases of Childhood 114: 591

Ziter F A, Allsop K G, Tyler F H 1977 Assessment of muscle strength in Duchenne muscular dystrophy. Neurology 27: 981

15. The myotonic disorders

P. S. Harper

INTRODUCTION

The myotonic disorders form a group of characteristic and clinically distinct genetic conditions, whose unifying feature is the occurrence of myotonia. The group (Table 15.1) contains a number of rare non-progressive conditions, together with a single disorder, myotonic dystrophy, which is progressive in nature, and whose frequency exceeds that of all the other myotonic disorders together, being the commonest muscular dystrophy of adult life. Until very recently our understanding of this group has been extremely limited, not only in terms of the pathogenesis of myotonia itself, but regarding the biochemical and molecular basis of the individual conditions. During the past two years this situation has been entirely transformed and specific molecular defects have been discovered for all the major myotonias. Defects have been found in the adult muscle sodium ion channel in paramyotonia and

Table 15.1 The myotonic disorders

Disorder	Primary defect
Myotonic dystrophy	Unstable mutation in myotonin protein kinase gene

Myotonia congenita
  Dominant (Thomsen)
  Recessive (Becker)
	Mutations in skeletal muscle chloride channel

Paramyotonia congenita	Mutations in adult muscle sodium ion channel
Myotonic periodic paralysis (adynamia)	
Chondrodystrophic myotonia (Schwartz–Jampel)	Unknown

Acquired myotonia
  Pharmacological agents (various)
  Associated with malignancy	

myotonic periodic paralysis; myotonia congenita has been shown to result from abnormalities in the skeletal muscle chloride channel. In each case independent evidence from physiological studies had predicted that these specific defects were likely.

In the case of myotonic dystrophy, no clear primary abnormality was predicted from studies of its biochemistry and physiology, and the identification of the primary defect had to await isolation of the gene by positional cloning approaches. This has now been achieved, showing the disorder to result from a mutation in an unstable DNA sequence, the gene itself coding for previously unknown protein kinase.

These very recent developments are already leading to a major reassessment of the classification and pathogenesis of the myotonic disorders, and have initiated new areas of research which are likely to provide new possibilities for therapy as well as for diagnosis and prediction. Much of what is written here is thus likely to be overtaken by work still in progress, and this chapter should be read taking this into consideration.

MYOTONIA

Before describing the individual myotonic disorders, it is necessary to clarify what is meant by the term myotonia. At a clinical level it appears as delayed relaxation of a muscle or group of muscles seen after voluntary contraction, or following a stimulus such as percussion. Symptomatically this state is usually perceived as 'stiffness', although an element of weakness may be noted. The muscle group involved will largely determine the nature of the complaint; stiffness of grip is the most frequent, while involvement of the tongue and pharynx may produce speech disturbances.

As a physical sign, myotonia may be observed in response to a specific action (e.g. delay in relaxation after a firm grip) or in response to direct percussion of a muscle (e.g. the thenar eminence); it is important to note that the percussion should be firm and that the muscle itself, not a tendon, must be percussed.

At the electrophysiological level, described fully elsewhere in this volume (see Chs 11 and 29), the characteristic feature of myotonia is the occurrence of repetitive action potentials after a stimulus, often in sequences of diminishing amplitude and sometimes of diminishing frequency which, when reproduced on a loudspeaker, give the so-called 'dive-bomber' effect. These potentials are absent when the muscle is at complete rest, in contrast to states of increased presynaptic activity; they are unaffected by curarisation, again demonstrating that myotonia is intrinsic to the muscle fibre.

Myotonia has several further general features that help to distinguish it from other states of impaired relaxation. The first of these is 'warm-up', a term that refers to the diminution of myotonia seen with continued exercise of the muscle group over a period of 2–30 min (Cooper et al 1988). This feature is often well recognised by patients, who use it to overcome disability produced by initial myotonia. In occasional patients with myotonia, and notably in the disorder paramyotonia, a paradoxical response is seen, with myotonia aggravated by exercise.

Most patients with myotonia of any type find their symptoms aggravated by cold, even though electrophysiological studies mostly show no change or even improvement (Ricker et al 1977, Cooper et al 1988). Again, paramyotonia shows a specific relationship to cold. A final aspect of myotonia often not fully appreciated is the weakness that may accompany the delayed relaxation; this can be assessed quantitatively (Rüdel & Lehmann-Horn 1985) after the element of stiffness has been blocked by specific drugs and it may exist in the absence of any dystrophic changes in the muscles.

From the above outline it can be seen that the diagnosis of myotonia requires a specific electrophysiological state to be present as well as specific clinical features. A number of other causes of muscle stiffness or impaired relaxation exist, which need careful distinction from true myotonia because their aetiology is entirely different. Familial cramping syndromes are generally painful, while the associated contractures are electrically silent, as are those due to such metabolic causes as McArdle's disease. Brady's disease, due to a deficiency of muscle relaxing factor (see Ch. 17), gives impaired relaxation often called 'silent myotonia' but the electromyogram readily excludes the myotonia. The reflex relaxation delay of hypothyroidism is distinguishable by absence of direct percussion myotonia, although occasional hypothyroid patients may also show true myotonia. Presynaptic disorders characteristically show persistent electrical activity when the muscle is resting, while the repetitive potentials sometimes seen in polymyositis and motor neurone disease are not associated with clinical features of myotonia.

MYOTONIC DYSTROPHY (DYSTROPHIA MYOTONICA; STEINERT'S DISEASE)

This is by far the commonest of the myotonic disorders with a prevalence of about 5 per 100 000 over much of Europe and North America (see Harper 1989). In some isolated populations, notably Northern Quebec, exceptionally high frequencies are seen, up to 1 in 400 individuals being affected (Mathieu et al 1990). The disorder appears to be of comparable frequency in the Japanese and Indian populations (Takeshita et al 1981), but to be very uncommon in Africans (Ashizawa & Epstein 1991, Jenkins 1992). This high frequency of myotonic dystrophy, at least 10 times that of myotonia congenita in most countries, makes it the most likely diagnosis whenever myotonia is encountered, even though the features may not appear typical. It is a disorder that frequently presents to clinicians other than

the neurologist and the uncomplaining attitude of some patients makes it important to have myotonic dystrophy in mind in a wide variety of clinical situations. For a detailed account of this much studied condition readers are referred to the monograph of Harper (1989).

Clinical features

Myotonic dystrophy is one of the most variable of all genetic disorders, a fact long recognised by clinicians, but for which an underlying explanation has only recently been obtained, as discussed later.

Figure 15.1 shows the relative frequency of the various presenting symptoms. Table 15.2 lists the distribution of major muscle atrophy and weakness, which are often characteristic when sought, but which may not always be complained of, or even mentioned by the patient. Myotonia is usually not as severe as in the non-progressive myotonias such as myotonia congenita. It is often accepted as a nuisance rather than being regarded as a symptom of illness; patients presenting in adult life may give a clear history of myotonia extending back for decades, even into childhood. The hands are most affected, although examination will usually show percussion myotonia elsewhere, in particular in the tongue. Generalised severe myotonia affecting gait, speech and eyelids is uncommon but may occur. Such patients can

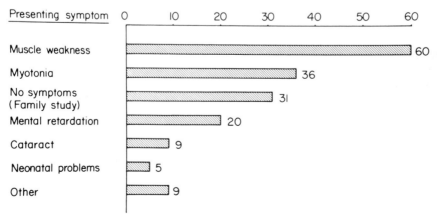

Fig. 15.1 Frequency of presenting symptoms in 170 patients with myotonic dystrophy (from Harper 1979).

Table 15.2   Myotonic dystrophy — distribution of muscle involvement

Usual
  Ptosis
  Facial muscles
  Sternomastoids
  Foot dorsiflexors
  Distal forearm muscles
Frequent
  Small hand muscles
  Palate and pharynx
  Quadriceps
  Diaphragm and intercostals
  Tongue

be extremely difficult to distinguish from those with myotonia congenita, but observation over a prolonged period, or study of relatives, usually clarifies matters. Specific molecular analysis is also now available to help in this situation.

Muscle weakness is the commonest symptom causing referral to the neurologist, but is extre-mely variable in both extent and in rate of progres-sion. The complaint is often of general weakness and fatigue, but the distribution of weakness on examination is more specific. Both upper and lower limbs show predominantly distal weakness, in contrast to the proximal involvement seen in most other muscular dystrophies, while the anterior neck muscles, notably sternomastoids, show a selective involvement that may be extreme. Facial weakness is often marked (Fig. 15.2) and ptosis may be visible as a longstanding feature in photographs. Facial and jaw weakness together may produce dysarthria.

Onset and progression of muscle symptoms are highly variable, even if the congenital form of the disorder, considered below, is omitted. The typical 'adult' form of the disorder may develop at any age from late childhood onwards; usually progression is very slow, with marked loss of function recorded over decades rather than years;

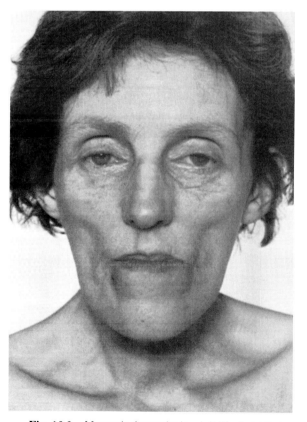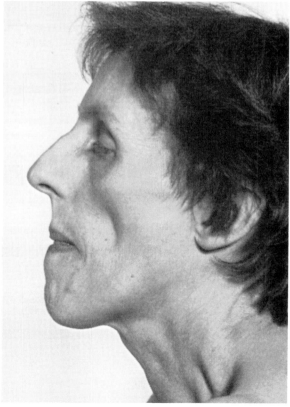

Fig. 15.2   Myotonic dystrophy in adult life: facial features, showing wasting of facial, jaw and sternomastoid muscles.

occasional patients, however, show rapid deterioration and may become wheelchair bound. Since remissions are not a feature of myotonic dystrophy, the best guide to prognosis is the course over the preceding 5–10 years.

Patients with advanced disease may show additional neuromuscular problems. Diaphragmatic involvement may lead to frequent chest infections, to hypoventilation (Coccagna et al 1975, Carroll et al 1977, Begin et al 1980) and to aspiration of food or gastric contents. Foot-drop may be conspicious and can be helped by toe-springs or light splints. Neck weakness may become extreme and be associated with neck pain and headache, due to cervical osteoarthritis in some cases. Myotonia may diminish rather than increase in such severe cases.

Smooth and cardiac muscle involvement

Table 15.3 lists some of the problems that may result from this. Oesophageal function is frequently abnormal, as seen by barium studies and by manometry (Bosma & Brodie 1969, Goldberg & Sheft 1972, Eckardt et al 1986), but dysphagia is not a prominent symptom. Colonic problems are seen principally in childhood cases (Lenard et al 1977), where constipation, 'spastic-colon' symptoms and even faecal soiling can be severe and refractory to treatment. The importance of anal sphincter involvement in children is discussed later. Uterine involvement can lead to maternal complications at delivery (Shore 1975, Sarnat et al 1976), and should be anticipated in any patient who is pregnant or likely to become so.

Cardiac problems have been recognised for many years since the early studies of Evans (1944) and Church (1967). Conduction defects vary from asymptomatic first degree heart block to complex A–V dissociation, while tachyarrhythmias, of which atrial flutter is the commonest, may result in a cardiac referral at a time when the neuromuscular features are unrecognised (Cannon 1962, Holt & Lambert 1964, Olofsson et al 1988). Most instances of sudden death in myotonic dystrophy are likely to occur in patients with at least some evidence of conduction problems, there being no increase in atheroma-

Table 15.3 Smooth muscle involvement in myotonic dystrophy

Pharynx and oesophagus	Delayed relaxation, dysphagia, aspiration
Gallblader	Delayed emptying, frequent calculi
Colon	'Spastic colon' symptoms, megacolon
Anal sphincter	Abnormal dilatation (especially childhood)
Uterus	Incoordinate contraction in labour
Ciliary body	Low intraocular pressure

tous heart disease (Orndahl et al 1964). The neurologist has a special responsibility to ensure that all patients have regular cardiac evaluation including electrocardiography (ECG), since this aspect of the disorder is both more lethal and more treatable than are the neuromuscular features. The use of 24-hour ambulatory ECG recording may be valuable by detecting potentially dangerous ventricular arrhythmias (Forsberg et al 1988). By contrast, mitral valve prolapse, originally thought to represent a significant problem (Winters et al 1977), has since been shown not to be associated with clinical complications in myotonic dystrophy (Morris et al 1982).

The dangers associated with anaesthesia and surgery may appropriately be mentioned. There appears to be a real sensitivity to anaesthetics and muscle relaxants in the sense that conventional doses produce prolonged apnoea and drowsiness (Aldridge 1985, Moore & Moore 1987). Abdominal surgery, such as cholecystectomy and hysterectomy, is more hazardous than procedures such as cataract extraction and orthopaedic measures. It should particularly be noted that it is not only patients with severe muscle disease who are at risk, but those with minimal symptoms, who may not mention their disorder to the surgeon or anaesthetist. Again, the neurologist has a special responsibility to patients and colleagues to ensure that the hazards are both recognised by the patient and noted prominently in the medical record. The legal consequences may be considerable (Brahams 1989).

Other clinical features (Table 15.4)

The most striking feature of many (but by no means all) myotonic dystrophy patients is a marked degree of apathy and inertia, resulting in many fewer symptoms than would seem reasonable for a given degree of weakness and myotonia, but also in a much less adequate level of function. This aspect is most commonly commented on by spouses and other relatives, and may be the deciding factor in determining whether a patient can continue to work. Somnolence can be prominent, even in those with little involvement of respiratory muscles. All these features, along with the occurrence of mental retardation in the congenital form, indicate a degree of central nervous system involvement in the disorder, though the objective radiological and neuropathological changes are not striking (Rosman & Kakulas 1966). Thorough neuropsychiatric studies have been carried out (Woodward et al 1982, Bird et al 1983, Brumback & Wilson 1984). Involvement of peripheral nerve is insignificant at a clinical level, but has been documented pathologically (Panayiotopoulos & Scarpalezos 1976); most of the changes involve the terminal arborisations (Coers & Woolf 1959) and may be secondary to the myotonia; the same is probably true of the changes seen in muscle spindles (Swash 1972, Swash & Fox 1975).

Cataract has been recognised to be an integral part of myotonic dystrophy since the earliest descriptions (Greenfield 1911, Fleischer 1918) and the disorder should be considered in any case of cataract in early adult life. In the older patients cataract may be the only symptomatic clinical problem, with only minimal myotonia to indicate the diagnosis. Such patients commonly remain undiagnosed until more typical myotonic dystrophy is recognised in another relative, and their prognosis for retaining normal muscle function is excellent. The results of cataract surgery are good, but some patients have an associated retinopathy that must be considered if visual acuity remains poor (Burian & Burns 1967). In its early stages the cataract of myotonic dystrophy is characteristic, with multi-coloured, refractile opacities visible in the anterior and posterior subcapsular regions when examined with a slit lamp (Junge 1966). The presence of such opacities is a valuable confirmatory sign in the doubtful case, as well as a useful predictive test in those at risk (Bundey et al 1970, Polgar et al 1972, Harper 1973). It has, however, proved not to be infallible, with recent studies showing that some individuals, predicted to be gene carriers on account of minor lens changes, show no evidence of the myotonic dystrophy mutation on molecular analysis (Brunner et al 1991, Ashizawa et al 1992, Reardon et al 1992a,b).

Endocrine abnormalities are frequent, but do not usually cause serious symptoms. Testicular atrophy is seen in most postpubertal males (Marshall 1959); the atrophy affects the tubular structure more than the interstitial cells (Harper et al 1972a), and does not cause loss of secondary sexual function. Fertility is moderately reduced in both sexes, but there is a high fetal wastage in females (O'Brien & Harper 1984). Alterations in the pituitary fossa and occasional pituitary tumours may result from persistently increased gonadotrophin secretion (Banna et al 1973, Mahler & Parizel 1982), but most patients show a consistent hyperinsulinism and insulin resistance, even at an early stage of their illness (Huff et al 1967, Barbosa et al 1974, Walsh et al 1970, Moxley et al 1984), a finding that has led to suggestions of a defect in insulin metabolism as a primary cause of the disease (see below).

Clinical investigations

Most cases of myotonic dystrophy can be diagnosed without the need for complex investigations; Table 15.5 shows those that are generally most helpful.

The author makes no apology for placing DNA analysis at the top of the list of diagnostic investi-

Table 15.4   Myotonic dystrophy — extramuscular features

CNS	Lethargy, somnolence, mental retardation (children)
Peripheral nerve	Abnormalities in terminal arborisation (usually insignificant clinically)
Ophthalmic	Cataract, retinopathy, blepharitis
Endocrine	Testicular atrophy, complications of pregnancy and labour, diabetes, early balding

gations, now that a specific test for the mutation is available. Although work in progress still has to resolve the optimal techniques and the precise interpretation of the findings, there is no doubt that molecular analysis will rapidly become the benchmark against which other forms of investigation will be gauged (Brunner et al 1992, Reardon et al 1992b).

Electromyography should always be performed where there is doubt as to the diagnosis or where clinical myotonia is equivocal (Streib & Sun 1983). Most patients will show typical myotonic discharges and increased insertion activity, together with a reduced size of the action potential and polyphasic potentials, indicating an active dystrophic process. Absence of the latter may favour the diagnosis of a non-progressive myotonia, but does not prove it. Nerve conduction velocities are normal. Muscle biopsy should be done whenever the diagnosis is not entirely certain. The changes, discussed more fully in Chapters 7 and 8 are often characteristic (Casanova & Jerusalem 1979, Harper 1986), with increased central nuclei in chains, ringed fibres, sarcoplasmic masses and a type I fibre atrophy and predominance, while on electron microscopy Z-band and I-line degeneration with abnormally shaped mitochondria are the most conspicuous features (Aleu & Afifi 1964, Schotland 1970). However, none of the changes can be regarded as absolutely specific, whether in adults or congenital cases, a conclusion recently reinforced by cases where molecular analysis has not confirmed the diagnosis (MacMillan et al 1993). It should be remembered that frozen muscle may itself be a useful source of DNA for analysis in a deceased patient (MacMillan et al 1993).

Ophthalmic assessment for lens opacities has already been mentioned; this has relevance for management as well as for diagnosis. Among the other investigations mainly relevant to management, blood glucose and glucose tolerance tests should be done to exclude incipient diabetes. The ECG will detect most conduction defects; fuller cardiac assessment is needed only if this is abnormal or if episodes of arrhythmia have occurred. Other investigations needed will depend on the presence of specific problems. Finally, a careful family study and documented pedigree should be regarded as an essential investigation: most apparently isolated cases prove not to be so on closer investigation, and it is the undiagnosed family members who may be most at risk, either of unexpected complications, or of having a severely affected child.

Congenital myotonic dystrophy (Vanier 1960, Dodge et al 1966, Dyken & Harper 1973, Harper 1975a,b)

Although the onset of typical myotonic dystrophy can frequently be traced back to childhood, the congenital form of the disorder is a clinically (and probably aetiologically) distinctive form that until recently has been considerably underdiagnosed; even now it is not fully recognised by many adult neurologists and general paediatricians, though with modern techniques of neonatal intensive care and ventilation it is becoming recognised as one of the major neuromuscular causes of respiratory failure.

Some of the prominent features are listed in Table 15.6 and it will be noticed that many of

Table 15.5 Investigations in myotonic dystrophy

Diagnostic
  DNA analysis
  Electromyography
  Muscle biopsy
  Ophthalmological assessment
Management
  Electrocardiogram (conduction defects)
  Ophthalmological assessment (cataract, retinopathy)
  Glucose tolerance test (diabetes)

Table 15.6 Congenital myotonic dystrophy — principal clinical features

Intrauterine
  Hydramnios
  Poor fetal movement
Neonatal
  Hypotonia (no significant myotonia)
  Respiratory failure
  Feeding problems
  Talipes (sometimes more general contractures)
  Disproportionate face and jaw weakness
  Thin ribs, elevated diaphragm on X-ray
Later
  Facial diplegia
  Jaw weakness
  Mental retardation

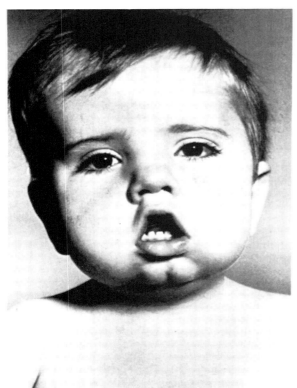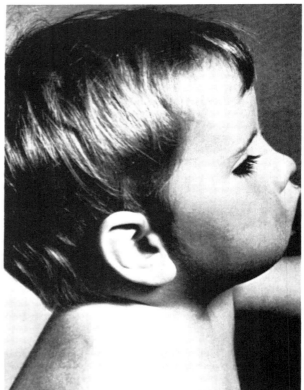

a

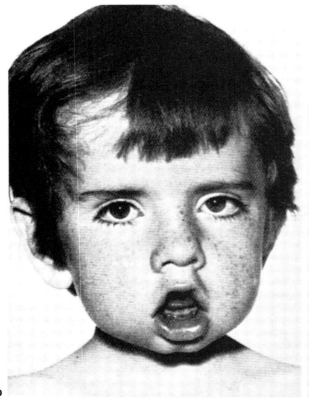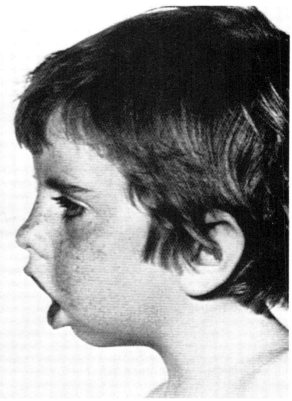

b

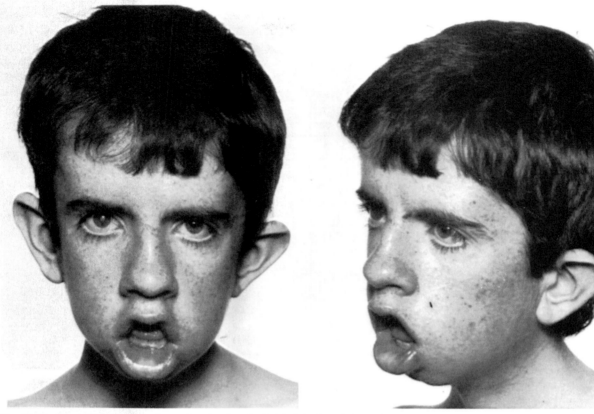

Fig. 15.3 Congenital myotonic dystrophy, showing the facial diplegia and the evolution of the facial appearance in the same patient. **a** Age 2 years; **b** age 6 years; **c** age 15 years.

these are quite unlike those normally seen in myotonic dystrophy of later life; conversely, myotonia is not seen as a clinical feature. Most of the symptoms can be traced back into intrauterine life: indeed, in a pregnancy at risk the disorder can often be predicted by the poor fetal movements and polyhydramnios. The hypotonia and immobility of the affected newborn infant may be profound; the lungs are hypoplastic (Silver et al 1984). Inadequate ventilation previously resulted in death for many without a specific diagnosis, but most now survive following resuscitation to allow recognition that a generalised neuromuscular disorder is present (Rutherford et al 1989).

Unless a family history of myotonic dystrophy has been recognised, it may be difficult to distinguish congenital myotonic dystrophy from other congenital myopathies or allied disorders. Helpful

features include a disproportionate weakness of face and jaw (Fig. 15.3), the occurrence of a greatly raised and hypoplastic diaphragm on chest X-ray and at autopsy (Bossen et al 1974), and thin ribs on X-ray resulting from hypoplastic intercostal muscles. Talipes is frequent, but more general congenital contractures sometimes occur. In most cases confirmation is obtained by the recognition of features of myotonic dystrophy in the mother, which are often mild and relatively symptomless. Careful electromyography may show a few myotonic potentials (Swift et al 1975), but this becomes conspicuous only after infancy. Muscle biopsy is helpful, not only in allowing other specific causes to be recognised, but also in showing unusual features of immature fibres (Sarnat & Silbert 1976, Silver et al 1984) with central nuclei, abundant satellite cells and, on histochemical examination, peripheral regions showing deficiency of oxidative enzymes (Karpati et al 1973, Farkas et al 1974).

The outlook for severely affected congenital cases is poor with regard to both physical and mental function, and mental retardation is present in almost all survivors, even when anoxia has not been a major problem (Harper 1975a). A recent longitudinal study (Reardon et al 1993) has shown that very few patients are able to live an independent adult life. Thus the undertaking of major measures of resuscitation in an infant recognised as being affected in the newborn period deserves careful consideration and discussion with the parents. Death is unusual once neonatal complications are overcome and once an active course is embarked on it is not easy to abandon. The duration of any assisted ventilation that is required gives some guide to likely survival (Rutherford et al 1989).

The factors producing congenital myotonic dystrophy have been the subject of much speculation. The immediate cause is clearly a widespread and severe hypoplasia of muscle; the histology suggests that this results from impairment of growth rather than from degeneration (Sarnat & Silbert 1976). The almost exclusively maternal transmission of truly congenital cases suggests a maternal factor impeding muscle maturation (Harper & Dyken 1972), but it has not been identified; a single experimental study suggesting an effect of maternal serum on rat muscle remains unconfirmed (Farkas-Bargeton et al 1988). Suggestions of an abnormality in bile salts (Tanaka et al 1982) in mothers of affected infants or of hyperinsulinism as a causative factor (Silver et al 1985) have not been confirmed (Soderhall et al 1982), nor has any clear immunological defect, such as that involved in congenital myasthenia gravis, been found. The fact that congenitally affected infants commonly improve in childhood, but later develop more typical 'adult' features, suggests that they possess the gene for the disorder as well as being exposed to the proposed maternal effect; this is confirmed by the finding that approximately half the sibs are unaffected (Harper 1975b), follow-up after a 10-year interval confirming that almost all such sibs are indeed free from the disorder (O'Brien et al 1983).

The recent molecular developments discussed below have explained some, but not all, of the problems related to the basis of congenital myotonic dystrophy. Patients with this form show on average the largest expansions of the mutation, but there is a broad overlap with the range seen in the adult onset form, and no clear molecular difference between the offspring of affected males and females that can explain the exclusively maternal transmission of congenital myotonic dystrophy. The original hypothesis of a transmissible intrauterine factor remains a possibility, but the full situation is not likely to be explained until we have greater understanding of the pathogenesis of the disorder.

Genetic aspects

Myotonic dystrophy has been recognised as following mendelian autosomal dominant inheritance for many years. As far back as 1918 Fleischer showed that most cases were familial, while systematic studies such as that of Bell (1948) confirmed the pattern, with close to 50% of offspring of affected parents of either sex inheriting the disorder. Even at this early stage, however, unusual aspects were noted, many of which have remained unexplained until the recent identification of the molecular basis of the condition. Some of these are summarised in Table 15.7.

Extreme variability of phenotype was the first puzzling finding, with the range of manifestation varying from minimal neuromuscular involvement at one extreme, to profound and fatal neonatal weakness at the other. The range of systems involved was recognised as showing equal variability, as noted earlier in this chapter. The occurrence of this variation within a single kindred was against genetic heterogeneity being the explanation as suggested by Bundey & Carter (1972) and

Table 15.7 Genetic aspects of myotonic dystrophy

Autosomal dominant inheritance
Extreme clinical phenotypic variability, even within a family
Anticipation — earlier onset and greater severity in successive
　　　　　　generations
No new mutations documented
Congenital cases exclusively maternally transmitted

Bundey (1982), a view confirmed when the study of linked markers by numerous groups failed to show more than a single genetic locus.

Related to the observed variability was the concept of *anticipation*, denoting the occurrence of onset of disease at an earlier age or a more severe degree in successive generations. Fleischer (1918) was the first to propose this, after noting that many of his families could be linked through individuals having cataract but no neuromuscular symptoms. His suggestion that there was a progressive deterioration from generation to generation initially found widespread agreement from the clinical observations of others (Henke & Seeger 1927, Bell 1948), but as the understanding of genetic mechanisms increased, it became more difficult to reconcile mendelian inheritance with a changing genetic structure. Penrose (1948) suggested that anticipation could be explained by a combination of inherent variability with observational bias, and that it did not require any unusual biological mechanism, a view widely accepted until very recently. It was only when pedigree studies (Höweler 1986, Höweler et al 1989) showed that anticipation persisted when the biases were removed, that it became clear that a highly unusual genetic mechanism was indeed operating in myotonic dystrophy; the precise nature of this has now been identified as an unstable DNA sequence, as described later.

A third unusual genetic finding in most studies was an almost complete lack of new mutations. Most dominantly inherited disorders show a proportion of new mutations that is directly related to the degree to which the condition impairs fertility, so that a paradox has existed as to why myotonic dystrophy had not died out without new mutations to replace the genes being lost from the population. The very variability of the condition made it difficult to be certain whether any single case was due to a new mutation or not, but the situation again remained unresolved until a molecular explanation was available.

A puzzling observation already noted was the finding that the severe congenital form of the disease was transmitted exclusively by affected mothers (Harper & Dyken 1972), while affecting only 50% of their offspring and not being confined to particular kindreds. This could not be ade-

quately explained by simple mendelian inheritance.

These unusual features not only provided theoretical difficulties in understanding the inheritance of myotonic dystrophy; they also gave (and still give) practical problems relating to genetic counselling and prenatal diagnosis, and for the prognosis of those with early or minimal signs of the disease. Families understandably wished to know the answer to questions such as the likelihood of an apparently healthy person at risk developing the disorder in later life, or the chance of an affected pregnancy resulting in a severely handicapped child. Our inability to provide accurate answers has limited considerably the extent to which we have been able to help families. That these limitations are now disappearing is due to the painstaking and ultimately successful application of molecular genetic techniques to the isolation of the myotonic dystrophy gene, the results of which will now be described.

The molecular genetics of myotonic dystrophy

Work done over the past two years by a number of groups, including that of the author and his colleagues, now enables us to understand the molecular basis of the disorder to an extent that would have seemed inconceivable only recently. However, this satisfying result rests on the solid, if less spectacular foundations of almost a decade of work whose aim was first to map and subsequently to isolate the gene. This *positional cloning* or *reverse genetics* approach was made possible by the discovery of a wealth of inherited variation in DNA, resulting in markers that could map the position of a gene on its chromosome even though, as in the case of myotonic dystrophy, little or nothing might be known about the nature of its primary defect in biochemical or physiological terms (Collins 1992). In the event, the isolation of the myotonic dystrophy gene was entirely achieved by this process, in contrast to the genes for the non-progressive myotonias, whose nature was accurately predicted by previous biochemical and physiological studies.

The mapping of the myotonic dystrophy gene

long antedates the techniques of molecular genetics. One of the earliest studies of blood group markers (Mohr 1954) suggested a hint of linkage between the Lewis blood group and myotonic dystrophy, which was confirmed by more extensive studies (Renwick et al 1971, Harper et al 1972b) that showed linkage between myotonic dystrophy, the secretor locus and the Lutheran blood group system. This group of linked genes was extended to include the complement (C3) locus (Whitehead et al 1982), a finding which allowed a chromosomal assignment for the group when C3 was located on chromosome 19.

With a specific chromosome to focus on, the new DNA techniques could be applied to generating and studying a series of sequences on chromosome 19, an approach which gave the first closely linked marker for myotonic dystrophy, the apolipoprotein C2 gene (Shaw et al 1985). The use of a wide range of techniques for the physical and genetic analysis of the myotonic dystrophy region of chromosome 19 (for review see Wieringa et al 1988, Shaw & Harper 1989) meant that by 1991 there was a detailed map available, with the myotonic dystrophy gene accurately pinned down to a region that included only a small number of genes.

The finding of the myotonic dystrophy gene itself, coming after a prolonged and intensive search, was naturally the cause of much excitement, but it could not have been anticipated how important it would be in general terms, as a result of the unusual nature of the underlying mutation.

The first clue to this came from the findings of two groups (Buxton et al 1992, Harley et al 1992a) of an unusual and variable change in DNA sequence pattern, specific to myotonic dystrophy (Fig. 15.4); this change was detected by two DNA probes, one a cDNA, the other a genomic sequence. Exchange of materials by the two groups showed that they were detecting the same change, and confirmation by a third group (Aslanidis et al 1992) left no doubt that a specific molecular defect for myotonic dystrophy had been detected.

Further study of myotonic dystrophy families showed a remarkable finding which explained at a stroke many of the genetic problems of the disorder

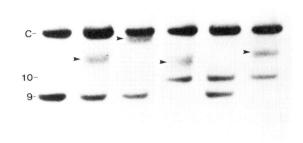

Fig. 15.4 Molecular analysis of the myotonic dystrophy mutation, showing the variable unstable sequence (arrowed) in affected individuals. Lanes 1 and 5 are unaffected individuals, showing the normal polymorphism with 9 and 10 kb fragments from the normal allele. C is a constant band (from Harley et al 1992a).

described above. Not only did the variable sequence differ between affected individuals, but a step-wise increase in fragment size was seen in successive generations (Fig. 15.5), a finding corresponding to and closely correlating with the clinical observation of anticipation, for which an underlying biological mechanism had for so long been sought without success. The interpretation of these observations was made easier by the fact that, 6 months previously (Oberlé et al 1991, Verkerk et al 1991), a similar phenomenon had been encountered as the basis for fragile X mental retardation, in which anticipation is also seen, a finding which had led to the suggestion that a comparable unstable

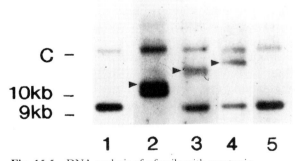

Fig. 15.5 DNA analysis of a family with myotonic dystrophy, demonstrating the molecular basis of anticipation. Lanes 1 and 5 are unaffected individuals. Lanes 2, 3 and 4 are from the minimally affected grandfather, moderately affected mother and congenitally affected child respectively, showing the corresponding small, moderate and large DNA expansions in the gene in successive generations (from Harley et al 1992b).

DNA sequence might be found in myotonic dystrophy (Sutherland et al 1991).

The identification of a specific unstable DNA sequence in myotonic dystrophy led rapidly to two parallel avenues of research, both still in progress: first, the correlation of the molecular abnormality with the known clinical and genetic properties of the disease, and secondly the identification of the nature of the unstable sequence and of the gene in which it is placed. Conclusions from both fields of work, not all yet published, are given here, but should be regarded as provisional (Table 15.8).

The initial observations of the unstable sequence showed that the change was detected by a DNA fragment which showed polymorphism in the normal population, with a 9 kb and 10 kb fragment seen with approximately equal frequency. In myotonic dystrophy patients expansion of the 10 kb fragment was seen (Harley et al 1992a), never the 9 kb fragment, this expansion varying from an additional 0.1 kb to over 6 kb (Harley et al 1992b). Those patients with minimal neuromuscular disease in later life invariably showed a small expansion (Harley et al 1992b, Reardon et al 1992b; see Fig. 15.6), while those with congenital onset showed the largest expansions (Harley et al 1992b, Tsilfidis et al 1992). It can be seen that while there is a degree of overlap between the individual groups, the minimal and severe groups are distinct, a finding that has been confirmed by subsequent studies and which is of considerable importance for genetic counselling and prenatal diagnosis. It has already been mentioned that expansion of the unstable sequence parallels the clinical phenomenon of anticipation; this expansion is seen in the offspring of both male and female patients, so that it cannot alone explain the exclusively maternal transmission of congenital myotonic dystrophy.

Study of the expanded sequence in families has thrown important light on the question of new

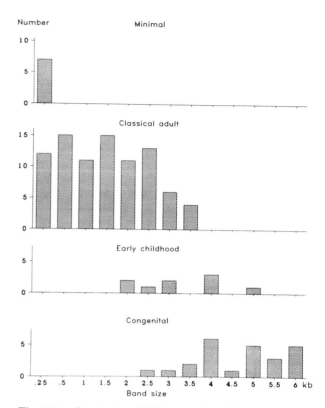

Fig. 15.6 Correlation of DNA expansion with phenotype in myotonic dystrophy. Note that while overlap exists between the different clinical categories, there is a clear distinction between the severe congenital and the minimally affected groups (from Harley et al 1992b).

mutations mentioned earlier. Analysis of a series of families in which neither parent showed any identifiable neuromuscular abnormality has shown that in all cases one parent shows a minimal expansion (Reardon et al 1992b). Thus those rare cases which might have represented new mutations have proved not to be so, a finding of practical consequence for genetic counselling. Current evidence suggests that almost all cases of myotonic dystrophy world-wide may have been derived from a single ancestral mutation of very great antiquity (Harley et al 1992a,b).

Isolation and characterisation of the myotonic dystrophy gene followed rapidly on the initial detection of the unstable sequence (Brook et al 1992, Fu et al 1992, Mahedevan et al 1992) (Table 15.9). The unstable region itself was shown to be a triplet repeat of three bases (CTG),

Table 15.8 The molecular basis of myotonic dystrophy

Gene located on chromosome 19q
Unstable mutation in specific CTG DNA repeat sequence
Progressive expansion of repeat in successive generations
Unique origin of mutation
Mutation located in non-coding region of a protein kinase family gene

Table 15.9 The myotonic dystrophy gene and its protein

Gene relatively small (2400 base pairs cDNA)
15 exons
Unstable mutation located in 3′ untranslated region
Strong cross-species conservation
Protein structure predicts protein kinase activity and transmembrane domain

located within a gene whose sequence showed strong conservation between species and with strongest expression seen in cardiac and skeletal muscle (Brook et al 1992). The cDNA is around 2400 base pairs (bp), with a genomic length of around 30 000 bp and containing 15 exons (Shaw et al 1993). The cDNA sequence predicts a corresponding protein with homology to members of the protein kinase family, but not identical to any known protein. This unique protein, termed myotonin or myotonin protein kinase, has several domains in addition to that with protein kinase activity. Current studies to produce monoclonal antibodies and to analyse the protein in detail should soon produce a wealth of information on it comparable to that now available for dystrophin in relation to Duchenne muscular dystrophy.

Several findings, albeit still at a preliminary stage, suggest that the relationship between myotonin and myotonic dystrophy may be very different from that between dystrophin and Duchenne dystrophy. The unstable mutation lies in the 3′ untranslated sequence of the gene, suggesting that it does not cause an alteration in the primary structure of protein in myotonic dystrophy patients, but rather a secondary disturbance related to the degree of expansion of the mutation. The wealth of variety of mutational defects in Duchenne and Becker dystrophy (Hoffman et al 1988) also contrasts with the universality of the apparently single, but graded myotonic dystrophy mutation. Some of the variability and wide systemic expression seen in myotonic dystrophy could result from the occurrence of alternative splicing and the existence of multiple isoforms of the protein, suggested by Jansen et al (1992). A final point to be considered is whether all the clinical features of myotonic dystrophy can be attributed to dysfunction of the kinase gene, or whether the expansion might affect the function of neighbouring genes, at least one of which is located extremely close to the site of the unstable mutation, and whose properties have been documented in the mouse by Jansen et al (1992) and in the human by Shaw et al (1993). All of this rapidly progressing work will need to be kept under review before we can reach definitive conclusions.

Molecular diagnosis and prediction

The great variety of severity and form of expression in myotonic dystrophy has for many years posed practical problems for neurologists and clinical geneticists in the areas of presymptomatic detection and genetic counselling. Careful clinical assessment has rightly been considered the cornerstone for this (Harper 1973) and remains so now that molecular approaches are possible. Electromyography for myotonic potentials and slit-lamp examination for multi-coloured lens opacities, have also been known to detect some gene carriers with no clinical abnormalities (Bundey et al 1970, Polgar et al 1972), but there has been no objective yardstick against which to assess their value until now.

The new techniques are already proving their practical value in both prediction and diagnosis. Linked DNA markers have been used extensively over the past 5 years (Meredith et al 1988, Norman et al 1989, Reardon et al 1992a), but the value of direct analysis for the unstable mutation has already been demonstrated in prenatal diagnosis (Smeets et al 1991, Myring et al 1992), as well as in neurological practice (MacMillan et al 1993). The recognition of clinically normal carriers of the minimal mutation and its confirmation in those with cataract or equivocal myotonia as the only finding have provided certainty in several previously doubtful situations; equally a number of such individuals thought likely to be minimally affected on clinical grounds have been shown not to have the mutation, an indication that minor neurophysiological and particularly ophthalmological abnormalities may be less specific than was previously thought (MacMillan et al 1993, Reardon et al 1993). The age independence of the mutation analysis also allows a firm prediction to be made in young adults wishing to know their genetic status before embarking on a family. Caution must be expressed in this regard over the testing of children, apart from those with symptoms suspected as being due to the disorder. As with other late-onset genetic diseases, testing for genetic reasons should generally be postponed until adult life, so that the individual at risk can make an informed choice for themselves (Harper & Clarke 1990).

Prenatal diagnosis represents a particular problem in a disorder like myotonic dystrophy, where severity can range from minimal to catastrophic. Linked DNA markers have given considerable experience with this (Norman et al 1989, Reardon et al 1992a) but the inability of such markers to give any indication as to likely severity has been an important limitation for many families. The relationship between DNA expansion and phenotype mentioned earlier, even though approximate, gives a valuable resolution of this difficulty, while the individual specificity of the test and the occurrence of one mutation in virtually all cases so far studied allows it to be applied in those numerous families where family structure makes the use of linked markers difficult or impossible. All couples who wish for prenatal diagnosis can now be offered it, and it is important that they are alerted to the possibility in advance, so that they can make informed and unpressurised decisions, and have first trimester chorion villus sampling if they opt for prenatal diagnosis. It is wise, however, to remain cautious in relating the size of DNA expansion to prognosis, and to establish whenever possible that the mutation is indeed present in some member of the family concerned.

Management

A number of drugs can help to relieve myotonia, but none can alter the natural history of myotonic dystrophy or significantly alter its associated symptoms. Among the anti-myotonic drugs phenytoin is the best first choice in myotonic dystrophy, except for women considering pregnancy, in whom its teratogenic potential must be considered. A relatively low dose, such as 100 mg three times daily, is usually satisfactory. Other useful drugs include procainamide and quinine, but both have effects on cardiac conduction and should be avoided in those patients with clinical or ECG evidence of conduction disorder. Most physicians find out that only a few of their patients, usually those with minimal weakness, continue to take drug therapy for their myotonia; in view of the chronicity of the disorder and potential for iatrogenic drug effects they may be wiser than we think.

Until a drug of real value is found, clinicians should concentrate on educating their patients, and those other doctors whom they may encounter, about the disease, its potential implications, and the importance of avoiding complications from cardiac arrhythmias, anaesthesia and surgery — in other words, how to live with a disorder that is normally relatively benign, and how to keep out of trouble. Such advice may seem obvious, but it is surprising how often it is not given, or not followed, even when the patient has been assessed in a specialist unit. Most clear indications for surgery, such as cataract extraction, or in children, correction of talipes, can be undertaken with care, but the patient should beware of minor surgery for trivial reasons or laparotomy for non-specific abdominal problems. A special card that can be carried, warning of the hazards, is available from the UK lay support group.

On the more active side, benefit can result from simple measures such as provision of head supports in the car or on a chair, with a cervical collar if headache of cervical origin is a problem. A thorough home assessment by a skilled occupational therapist will soon pinpoint which problems are actually hampering the patient's optimal function; a wheelchair commonly helps outdoor mobility, even though few patients become wheelchair-bound. Dietary advice can help those patients with dysphagia or with recurrent chest infection from aspiration. For the present these relatively simple measures, accompanied by the encouragement and support that all families with a chronically disabling disorder need, are the best we can offer, and are much better than the lack of long-term interest that they so often receive. In the near future it is to be hoped that the molecular advances described above will lead to specific therapy, either by modification of the myotonin protein kinase activity or in other ways.

THE NON-PROGRESSIVE MYOTONIAS

This group of rare disorders, even when taken as a whole, is much less common than myotonic dystrophy; in large families, recognition of the specific type is usually straightforward, but isolated cases can be difficult to categorize. The precise relationship between the different types has until recently been uncertain, but identification of their molecular basis has now largely clarified the situation.

Myotonia congenita, dominant type (Thomsen's disease)

This was the first of the myotonic disorders to be documented, the occurrence in his own family being recorded by Dr Julius Thomsen in 1876. Although it is extremely rare, its benign nature and dominant inheritance have resulted in a number of large kindreds being recognised, allowing a clear separation of the condition to be made from myotonic dystrophy, although some early cases of the latter without affected relatives can be difficult to distinguish. Myotonia is the principal feature; in contrast to myotonic dystrophy it is actively complained of and widespread, usually aggravated by cold and reduced by exercise. Eyelid myotonia with lid-lag is prominent; speech may be affected by tongue and jaw stiffness; on examination, myotonia is readily elicited by percussion of most muscle groups. Symptomatically, myotonia is often most severe when movement is initiated rapidly from rest. Some patients show a generalised myotonic reaction to a sudden shock, with widespread rigidity resulting in falling, an occurrence that can be mistakenly attributed to a central nervous system cause.

Onset is commonly in mid-childhood; there is essentially a static course after puberty, although most patients adapt to their symptoms. Men are usually more severely affected than women. No significant or progressive weakness or wasting occurs: indeed, muscle hypertrophy is common, although less marked than in the recessive form discussed below. Lifespan is normal and there are no associated cardiac and extramuscular problems. Histological changes in muscle are usually minimal (Fisher et al 1975), although absence of Group IIB fibres on staining for the myosin ATPase reaction has been noted (Crews et al 1976). Since the molecular basis of dominant and recessive types has been found to be the same, this, along with other experimental studies, will be described for the two together, which may in future be considered as chloride channel disorders.

Myotonia congenita, recessive type

This disorder was recognised as distinct from Thomsen's disease only after the extensive studies by Becker in Germany (1971, 1977), and was first reported in the English literature only 20 years ago (Harper & Johnston 1972). It is probably twice as common as the dominant form, but its recessive mode of inheritance means that it is seen usually only in sibs or as isolated cases. Consanguinity of the healthy parents is frequent. Myotonia is more severe than in Thomsen's disease and may be disabling; some degree of progressive weakness may occur, while muscle hypertrophy can be striking. On muscle biopsy, degenerative changes can be found which might in isolation suggest early myotonic dystrophy, but the clinical features are usually too distinctive for confusion to occur. Myotonia in an infant is very likely to be due to one of the forms of myotonia congenita, not to congenital myotonic dystrophy.

The physiological and molecular basis of myotonia congenita

Experimental studies on the physiology of myotonia have shown that human myotonia congenita is comparable to the animal models provided by the myotonic goat and mouse. Considerable evidence has been produced for these being due to a primary defect in chloride ion conductance, likely to involve the skeletal muscle chloride ion channel. The original experimental work dates from the recognition that the myotonic goat might provide a useful animal model for human myotonia congenita (Kolb 1938). Physiological studies on isolated muscle fibres (Bryant 1969, 1982, Adrian & Bryant 1974) showed a high membrane resistance with normal resting potential; replacement of chloride in the medium by an inert substance such as sulphate produced a very similar situation in normal goat muscle, reproducing the electrophysiological features of myotonia. The conclusion of this and other extensive studies was that the primary abnormality was a defect of chloride conductance in the muscle membrane.

Reproducing this work in human myotonic disorders was not easy, requiring in vivo experiments with intercostal muscle, but in human myotonia congenita, the results were largely comparable to findings in the goat (Lipicky and Bryant 1971, Lipicky 1977, Gruener 1977). By contrast the results in myotonic dystrophy differed considerably and were much less consistent (McComas & Mrozek 1968, Lipicky & Bryant 1973).

Subsequent work has given greater specificity to these conclusions (see Chapter 11) and has been reinforced by studies on another animal model, the myotonic mouse. This defect follows autosomal recessive inheritance whereas the goat disorder is probably dominant, but physiologically it is similar. A combination of gene mapping and direct molecular analyses allowed the mouse gene to be mapped and the mouse skeletal muscle channel to be isolated and its gene cloned (Steinmeyer et al 1991). Specific mutations confirmed that this gene was indeed altered in the myotonic mouse (Steinmeyer et al 1991). The next step was to use the model DNA sequence (in the rat) to isolate the corresponding human gene (Koch et al 1992) and to study this in human myotonia congenita families.

The results of this showed that in both dominant and recessive myotonia congenita there was complete linkage with this gene on human chromosome 7 (the dominant form had already been excluded from other possible regions, such as the myotonic dystrophy region of chromosome 19) (Koch et al 1989). The evidence was strengthened even further by the finding that specific mutations in the chloride ion channel gene could be detected in both the dominant and recessive forms of myotonia congenita (Koch et al 1992) confirming that, despite their different mode of inheritance, they are essentially forms of the same

fundamental condition, and that both are the results of molecular defects of the skeletal muscle chloride channel.

Therapy and management

Therapy for myotonia congenita in both its forms is more effective and more appreciated by the patient than in myotonic dystrophy, where few patients persist with it (Griggs 1977). The agents discussed for myotonic dystrophy are those also suitable for myotonia congenita, including phenytoin, except when there is a possibility of pregnancy. Mexiletine, a drug in wide use for treatment of ventricular arrhythmias, is also effective, but whether it is wise to use this long-term in an essentially benign condition is questionable. Regular ECGs should be taken if it is used. As with myotonic dystrophy, the wider management issues are often more important than specific drug therapy. Establishing the diagnosis of myotonia congenita as not being myotonic dystrophy is in itself an important point in view of the differences in prognosis, complications and genetics. Family analysis of the specific molecular defect will increasingly be important in determining whether an isolated case belongs to the dominant or recessive variety. Anaesthetic management is important; although there is no clear evidence that patients are susceptible to the severe contractures and other effects of malignant hyperpyrexia, the possibility of aggravating the myotonia must be considered in relation to induction of anaesthesia.

Most patients with myotonia congenita will to a large extent adjust their lifestyle, including employment, to avoid major problems with their disorder; the possibility of falls from sudden generalised myotonia should be recognised. Whether cold is an adverse factor is debatable; all objective studies have shown that this actually improves myotonia in this condition, in contrast to paramyotonia. Thus the main help that the physician is likely to be able to give to most patients is an understanding attitude and to help them to know as much as possible about their own complaint. The majority will probably neither need nor wish for drug treatment unless their symptoms are particularly severe or are temporarily exacerbated.

Paramyotonia congenita

The distinguishing feature of this rare condition, first described by Eulenburg in 1886 and reviewed in detail by Lehmann-Horn et al (1993), is the occurrence of prolonged, cold-induced contracture of muscle, which may last for several minutes and may be followed by flaccid weakness in the affected area lasting for hours. More typical myotonic stiffness is also seen, but again differs from that in myotonia congenita in being exacerbated rather than relieved by exercise — 'paradoxical myotonia'. Electromyography shows typical myotonic potentials but the prolonged cold-induced reaction is electrically silent. Electrical recording with the forearm immersed in cold water shows both weakness and delayed relaxation with progressive cooling; this provides a useful diagnostic test which will distinguish paramyotonia from myotonia congenita (Ricker et al 1990). The course of paramyotonia is static with an onset commonly in infancy, and there are no extramuscular features. Muscle biopsy shows variation in fibre diameter, lack of histochemical differentiation into type I and II fibres and some increase in central nuclei, but the extent of the changes seen has varied according to different reports (Thrush et al 1972).

The molecular basis of paramyotonia is discussed below along with that of myotonic periodic paralysis, with which it has been shown to be allelic. The two disorders can be considered as allied disorders of the sodium ion channel, in the same way as the forms of myotonia congenita are chloride channel defects. The detection of specific mutations based on DNA analysis is likely to become an integral part of the investigation of these patients and their family members.

Therapy. Mexiletine may be useful in severe cases especially when cold exposure is unavoidable, but in general the cautions expressed above in relation to myotonia congenita apply equally to paramyotonia. The drug tocainide, particularly effective in relation to cold-induced symptoms (Ricker et al 1980), has been abandoned owing to bone marrow toxicity.

The myotonia of paramyotonia responds to phenytoin or procainamide, but these drugs do not block the cold-induced response significantly. Efficient central heating and avoidance of outdoor occupations in cold climates are as helpful as drug treatment.

Myotonic periodic paralysis (adynamia episodica; Gamstorp's disease)

Myotonia in this dominantly inherited disorder (Gamstorp 1956, Danowski et al 1975, Lehmann-Horn et al 1993) is generally mild and often recorded only on electromyography. The feature that distinguishes it from other myotonic disorders is the occurrence of episodic flaccid weakness in attacks lasting up to several days, usually generalised and sometimes severe, but always sparing the respiratory, bulbar and ocular muscles. The weakness is not cold-induced or localised as in paramyotonia, nor are the episodes sudden as in the generalised myotonic reaction of myotonia congenita. Electrolyte changes are absent or inconsistent, distinguishing the otherwise similar hypokalaemic periodic paralysis, in which myotonia is not found. The disorder is essentially non-progressive, but patients with severe, repeated attacks may show some permanent weakness. The principal change seen on muscle biopsy is dilatation of the sarcoplasmic reticulum.

The most effective therapeutic agent is acetazolamide (Griggs 1977), which diminishes both the severity and the duration of the episodes of weakness, and is more effective than chlorothiazide and other diuretics.

Paramyotonia, myotonic periodic paralysis and the sodium ion channel

Recent molecular studies have made it clear that both of these disorders share a common primary defect, being due to mutations in the adult skeletal muscle sodium ion channel, located on chromosome 17. The initial evidence for this came from the finding of linkage of a large Canadian family with myotonic periodic paralysis to markers on chromosome 17 (Fontaine et al 1990), which was followed by confirmation in other kindreds and demonstration of complete linkage with a polymorphism in the cloned sodium ion channel gene itself (Koch et al 1991). The finding of mutations in this gene in affected individuals (Ptacek et al 1991) has shown that it is indeed directly responsible for the disorder.

Linkage studies on families with paramyotonia had already excluded this from the myotonic dystrophy region of chromosome 19, and analysis of chromosome 17 markers has shown an identical location to that of myotonic periodic paralysis (Koch et al 1991), with a specific mutation showing that the sodium ion channel is responsible for paramyotonia also. This work provides an excellent example of the power of the candidate gene approach (when a convincing candidate is available); it also shows that molecular analysis may result in the unification of disorders previously considered distinct, as well as in the splitting of apparently single conditions that has occurred more frequently.

Chondrodystrophic myotonia (Schwartz–Jampel syndrome)

This unusual disorder, which is recessively inherited, is characterised by the onset in infancy of severe muscle stiffness, giving blepharospasm, painful generalised muscle spasms and feeding difficulty (Schwartz & Jampel 1962, Fitch et al 1971). With increasing age the facial appearance becomes pinched and the voice weak, while muscle hypertrophy may occur. The skeletal features consist of delayed bone growth, particularly involving vertebrae, together with joint contractures; the X-ray appearances of the spine are similar to those seen in Morquio's syndrome.

Electromyography shows both characteristic myotonia and also continuous electrical activity of presynaptic origin (Fowler et al 1974). The latter persists during anaesthesia and may be related to the diffuse distribution of acetylcholinesterase over the muscle fibres, which is seen on histochemical investigation (Fowler et al 1974). There are few other histological changes in muscle. Treatment with benzodiazepines and related drugs is more effective than with anti-myotonic agents.

As yet there is no clear evidence relating to defects in either the sodium or chloride ion channels in this disorder; it seems unlikely that a simple defect in either will be able to explain the clinical or electrophysiological features.

RECENT MOLECULAR ADVANCES

When this chapter was re-written, the myotonic dystrophy gene and mutation had only just been identified and both the clinical and scientific significance of the findings were at an extremely early stage of evaluation. During the subsequent year the field has advanced rapidly, and it is important to draw attention briefly to some of the main advances of recent months.

From the viewpoint of the clinician, the most significant fact is that the unstable CTG repeat sequence has proved to be the underlying mutational basis for virtually all cases of myotonic dystrophy (Shaw & Harper 1992). Those few not showing this abnormality have mostly proved on reassessment to have been misdiagnosed, though a small residue of cases remains unexplained. The practical importance of this is that a single specific molecular test now exists that can confirm or exclude the diagnosis of myotonic dystrophy with a high degree of confidence, as well as providing prediction within a family. Already, studies of molecular diagnosis in neurological and ophthalmic situations have been reported (MacMillan et al 1992, Reardon et al 1993), as have studies of prenatal diagnosis (Myring et al 1992) and of the detection of gene carriers (Brunner et al 1992).

While the previously mentioned correlation between the length of the CTG repeat and the age at onset have been confirmed (Hunter et al 1992, Harley et al 1993, Lavedan et al 1993), it is clear also that there is considerable clinical variation for any value of repeat, so that caution is needed in inferring prognosis from the molecular defect, whether in prenatal or presymptomatic diagnosis. However the group of minimally affected gene carriers do show a correspondingly small DNA expansion that is clearly different from the values seen in more severely affected individuals (Reardon et al 1992). Likewise, congenital cases show the largest expansions, though they overlap considerably with those of later onset (Harley et al 1992, Tsilfidis et al 1992, Lavedan et al 1993).

The variation in repeat size between generations is proving to be of considerable interest. The longstanding debate over the validity of anticipation (Harper et al 1992) has clearly been resolved by the demonstration of progressive expansion of the repeat, but it should be noted that such expansion is not inevitable, and that contraction or even disappearance of the molecular defect may occur, especially in male transmission (Abeliovich et al 1993, Brunner et al 1993). This difference between the sexes may contribute to the molecular basis of congenital myotonic dystrophy (Harley et al 1993, Lavedan et al 1993, Mulley et al 1993), since it appears to be among these offspring of affected women that progressive large expansions are seen.

Population studies have shown considerable geographical variation in the distribution of repeat size in normal individuals (Davies et al 1992), but a single original mutation still seems likely since all patients share a common genetic haplotype (Harley et al 1991, 1992). Rather than postulating that a large number of minimally affected patients exist (e.g. with cataract), it seems probable that there is a pool of entirely normal individuals whose repeat number is in the high normal range (Imbert et al 1993), which over many generations may progressively expand to reach a level (around 50 repeats) at which clinical features first appear.

Compared with these advances, studies of the myotonic dystrophy protein and its relationship to the pathogenesis of the disease remain at a preliminary stage. The genomic structure of the gene has been determined (Mahadevan et al 1993, Shaw et al 1993); it consists of 15 exons in a total length of 13 kb of genomic DNA. In addition to the N-terminal kinase domain, the sequence predicts the protein to have an intermediate filamentous and C-terminal hydrophobic domain. However, whether myotonic dystrophy results from a primary decrease of gene action or some other type of disturbance remains unclear; one study (Fu et al 1993) suggests reduction in levels of mRNA in muscle of affected individuals, while a second (Sabourin et al 1993) has shown an increase. There is evidence that different isoforms may exist in muscle and brain (Jansen et al 1992), possibly as the result of alternative splicing. A number of synthetic antibodies have been developed to detect various parts of the protein, whose molecular weight is around 55 000 daltons (Brewster et al 1993, Fu et al 1993), but no clear data yet exist on the subcellular distribution or other properties of the protein apart from those predicted from the original cDNA sequence.

REFERENCES

Abeliovich D, Lerer I, Pashut-Lavon I, Schueli E, Rass-Rothschild A, Frydman M 1993 Negative expansion of the myotonic dystrophy unstable sequence. American Journal of Human Genetics 52: 1175

Adrian R H, Bryant S H 1974 On the repetitive discharge in myotonic muscle fibres. Journal of Physiology 240: 505

Aldridge L M 1985 Anaesthetic problems in myotonic dystrophy. British Journal of Anaesthesiology 57: 1119

Aleu F P, Afifi A K 1964 Ultrastructure of muscle in myotonic dystrophy. Preliminary observations. American Journal of Pathology 45: 221

Ashizawa T, Epstein H F 1991 Ethnic distribution of myotonic dystrophy gene. Lancet 338: 642

Ashizawa T, Hejtmancik J F, Liu J, Perryman M B, Epstein H F, Koch D D 1992 Diagnostic value of ophthalmologic findings in myotonic dystrophy: comparison with risks calculated by haplotype analysis of closely linked restriction fragment length polymorphisms. American Journal of Medical Genetics 42: 55

Aslanidis C, Jensen G, Amemiya C et al 1992 Cloning of the essential myotonic dystrophy region and mapping of the putative defect. Nature 255: 548

Banna M, Bradley W G, Pearce G W 1973 Massive pituitary adenoma in a patient with dystrophia myotonica. Journal of the Neurological Sciences 20: 1

Barbosa J, Nuttall F Q, Kennedy W, Geotz F 1974 Plasma insulin in patients with myotonic dystrophy and their relatives. Medicine 53: 307

Becker P S 1970 Paramyotonia congenita (Eulenberg). Thieme, Stuttgart

Becker P E 1971 Genetic approaches to the nosology of muscle disease. Myotonias and similar disorders. In: Birth Defects Original Article Series 7: 52

Becker P E 1977 Myotonia congenita and syndromes associated with myotonia. Thieme, Stuttgart

Begin R, Bereau M A, Lupier L, Lemieux B 1980 Control and modulation of respiration in Steinert's myotonic dystrophy. American Review of Respiratory Disease 121: 281

Bell J 1948 Dystrophia myotonica and allied diseases, in Penrose L S (ed) Treasury of human inheritance 4, Part V. Cambridge, Cambridge University Press

Bird T D, Follett C, Griep E 1983 Cognitive and personality function in myotonic muscular dystrophy. Journal of Neurology, Neurosurgery and Psychiatry 46: 971

Bosma J F, Brodie D R 1969 Cineradiographic demonstration

of pharyngeal area myotonia in myotonic dystrophy patients. Radiology 92: 104

Bossen E H, Sehlburne J D, Verkauf B S 1974 Respiratory muscle involement in infantile myotonic dystrophy. Archives of Pathology 97: 250

Brahams D 1989 Postoperative monitoring in patients with muscular dystrophy. Lancet ii: 1053

Brewster B S, Strong P N, Jeal S 1993 Identification of a protein product of the myotonic dystrophy gene using peptide specific antibodies. Biochemical and Biophysical Research Communications 194: 1256

Brook J D, McCurrach M E, Harley H G et al 1992 Molecular basis of myotonic dystrophy: expansion of a trinucleotide (CTG) repeat at the 3' end of a transcript encoding a protein kinase family member. Cell 68: 799

Brumback R A, Wilson H 1984 Cognitive and personality function in myotonic dystrophy. Journal of Neurology, Neurosurgery and Psychiatry 47: 888

Brunner H G, Smeets H J M, Nillesen et al 1991 Myotonic dystrophy. Brain 114: 2303

Brunner H G, Nillesen W, van Oost B A 1992 Presymptomatic diagnosis of myotonic dystrophy. Journal of Medical Genetics 29: 780

Brunner H G, Jansen G, Neilesen W 1993 Reverse mutation in myotonic dystrophy. New England Journal of Medicine 238: 476

Bryant S H 1969 Cable properties of external intercostal muscle fibres from myotonic and non-myotonic goats. Journal of Physiology (London) 204: 539

Bryant S H 1977 The physiological basis of myotonia. In: Rowland L P (ed) Pathogenesis of human muscular dystrophies. Excerpta Medica, Amsterdam, p 715

Bryant S H 1982 Physical basis of myotonia. In: Schotland D L (ed) Disorders of the motor unit. Wiley, New York, p 381

Bundey S 1982 Clinical evidence for heterogeneity in myotonic dystrophy. Journal of Medical Genetics 19: 341

Bundey S, Carter C O, Soothill J F 1970 Early recognition of heterozygotes for the gene for dystrophia myotonica. Journal of Neurology, Neurosurgery and Psychiatry 33: 279

Bundey S, Carter C O 1972 Genetic heterogeneity for dystrophia myotonica. Journal of Medical Genetics 9: 311

Burian H M, Burns C A 1967 Ocular changes in myotonic dystrophy. American Journal of Ophthalmology 63: 22

Buxton J, Shelbourne P, Davies J et al 1992 Detection of an unstable fragment of DNA specific to individuals with myotonic dystrophy. Nature 335: 547

Cannon P I 1962 The heart and lungs in myotonic dystrophy. American Journal of Medicine 32: 765

Carroll J E, Zwillich C W, Weil J V 1977 Ventilatory response in myotonic dystrophy. Neurology 27: 1125

Casanova G, Jerusalem F 1979 Myopathology of myotonic dystrophy. A morphometric study. Acta Neuropathologica (Berlin) 45: 231

Church S C 1967 The heart in myotonica atrophica. Archives of Internal Medicine 119: 176

Coccagna G, Mantouant M, Parch C, Miron F, Lugares E 1975 Alveolar hypoventilation and hypersomnia in myotonic dystrophy. Journal of Neurology, Neurosurgery and Psychiatry 38: 977

Coers C, Woolf A L 1959 The innervation of muscle. Oxford Collins FS 1992 Positional cloning — let's not call it reverse any more. Nature Genetics 1: 3

Cooper R G, Stokes M J, Edwards R H T 1988 Physiological characterisation of the 'warm up' effect of activity in

patients with myotonic dystrophy. Journal of Neurology, Neurosurgery and Psychiatry 51: 1134

Crews J, Kaiser K K, Brooke M H 1976 Muscle pathology of myotonia congenita. Journal of the Neurological Sciences 28: 449

Danowski T S, Fisher E R, Vidalon C 1975 Clinical and ultrastructural observations in a kindred with normal hyperkalaemic periodic paralysis. Journal of Medical Genetics 12: 20

Davies J, Yamagata H, Shelbourne P 1992 Comparison of the myotonic dystrophy associated CTG repeat in European and Japanese populations. Journal of Medical Genetics 29: 766

Dodge P R, Gamstorp I, Byers R K, Russell P 1966 Myotonic dystrophy in infancy and childhood. Paediatrics 35: 3

Dyken P R, Harper P S 1973 Congenital dystrophia myotonica. Neurology (Minneapolis) 23: 465

Eckardt V F, Nix W, Kraus W, Bohl J 1986 Esophageal motor function in patients with muscular dystrophy. Gastroenterology 90: 628

Eulenburg A 1886 Uber sine familiare, durch 6 generationen verfolgbare form congenitaler paramyotonie. Neurol Centralbl 5: 265

Evans W 1944 The heart in myotonia atrophica. British Heart Journal 4: 41

Farkas E, Tomé F M S, Fardeau M, Arsenio-Nunes M L, Dreyfuss P, Doebler M F 1974 Histochemical and ultrastructural study of muscle biopsy in three cases of dystrophica myotonica in the newborn child. Journal of the Neurological Sciences 21: 273

Farkas-Bargeton E, Barbet J P, Dancea S, Wehrle R, Checouri A, Dulac O 1988 Immaturity of muscle fibres in the congenital form of myotonic dystrophy: its consequences and its origin. Journal of the Neurological Sciences 83: 145

Fisher E R, Danowski T S, Ahmad U et al 1975 Electron microscopical study of a family with myotonia congenita. Archives of Neurology 99: 607

Fitch N, Karpati G, Pinsky L 1971 Congenital blepharophimosis, joint contractures and muscular hypotonia. Neurology (Minneapolis) 21: 1214

Fleischer B 1918 Uber myotonischer dystrophie mit katarakt. Albrecht von Graefe's Archives of Ophthalmology 96: 91

Fontaine B, Khurana T S, Hoffman E P et al 1990 Hyperkalemic periodic paralysis and the adult sodium channel alpha-subunit gene. Science 250: 1000

Forsberg H, Oloffson B-O, Andersson S, Henriksson A, Bjerle P 1988 24 hour electrocardiographic study in myotonic dystrophy. Cardiology 75: 241

Fowler W M, Layzer R B, Taylor et al 1974 The Schwartz–Jampel syndrome. Its clinical, physiological and histological expression. Journal of the Neurological Sciences 22: 127

Fu Y-H, Pizzuti A M, Fenwick R G et al 1992a An unstable triplet repeat in a gene related to myotonic muscular dystrophy. Science 255: 1256

Fu Y-H, Mahadevan M, Amemiya C et al 1992b Characterisation of the myotonic dystrophy region predicts multiple protein isoform-encoding mRNAs. Nature Genetics 1: 261

Gamstorp 1956 Adynamia episodica hereditaria. Acta Pediatrica (Uppsala) 45 (Suppl 108): 1

Goldberg J I, Sheft D J 1972 Oesophageal and colon changes in myotonic dystrophica. Gastroenterology 63: 134

Greenfield J 1911 Notes on a family with myotonia atrophica and early cataract with report of an additional case of myotonia atrophica. Rev Neurol Psychiatr 9: 169

Griggs R C 1977 The myotonic disorders and the periodic paralyses. In: Griggs R C, Moxley R T (eds) Advances in neurology, vol 17. Raven, New York, p 143

Gruener R 1977 In vitro membrane excitability of diseases of human muscle In: Rowland L P (ed) Pathogenesis of human muscular dystrophy. Excerpta Medica, Amsterdam, p 242

Harley H G, Brook J D, Rundle S A et al 1992a Expansion of an unstable DNA region and phenotypic variation in myotonic dystrophy. Nature 355: 545

Harley H G, Rundle S A, Reardon W et al 1992b Unstable DNA sequence in myotonic dystrophy. Lancet 339: 1125

Harley H G, Rundle S A, MacMillan J et al 1993 Size of the unstable CTG repeat sequence in relation to phenotype and parental transmission in myotonic dystrophy. American Journal of Human Genetics 52: 1164

Harper P S 1973 Presymptomatic detection and genetic counselling in myotonic dystrophy. Clinical Genetics 4: 134

Harper P S 1975a Congenital myotonic dystrophy in Britain. I. Clinical aspects. Archives of Disease in Childhood 50: 505

Harper P S 1975b Congenital myotonic dystrophy in Britain. II. Genetic basis. Archives of Disease in Childhood 50: 514

Harper P S 1986 Myotonic disorders. In: Angel A G, Banker B Q (eds) Myology. New York: McGraw-Hill, p 1267

Harper P S 1989 Myotonic dystrophy, 2nd edn. W B Saunders, Philadelphia

Harper P S, Clarke A 1990 Should we test children for 'adult' genetic diseases? Lancet 335: 1205

Harper P S, Dyken P R 1972 Early onset dystrophia myotonica — evidence supporting a maternal environmental factor. Lancet 2: 53

Harper P S, Johnston D M 1972 Recessively inherited myotonia congenita. Journal of Medical Genetics 9: 213

Harper P S, Penney R, Foley T Jr, Migeon C J, Blizzard R M 1972a Gonadal function in males with myotonic dystrophy. Journal of Clinical Endocrinology and Metabolism 35: 852

Harper P S, Rivas M L, Bias W B M, Hutchinson J R, Dyken P R, McKusick V A 1972b Genetic linkage confirmed between the loci for myotonic dystrophy. ABH secretion and Lutheran blood group. American Journal of Human Genetics 24: 310

Harper P S, Harley H G, Reardon W, Shaw D J 1992 Anticipation in myotonic dystrophy: new light on an old problem. American Journal of Human Genetics 51: 10

Haynes J, Thrush D C 1972 Paramyotonia congenita: an electrophysiological study. Brain 95: 553

Henke K, Seeger S 1927 Ueber die Verebung der myotonischen Dystrophie. Z Konstitutional 13: 371

Hoffman E P, Fischbeck H K, Brown M D et al 1988 Characterisation of dystrophin in muscle-biopsy specimens from patients with Duchenne or Becker muscular dystrophy. New England Journal of Medicine 318: 1363

Holt J M, Lambert E H 1964 Heart disease as the presenting feature in myotonia atrophica. British Heart Journal 26: 433

Höweler C J 1986 A clinical and genetic study in myotonic dystrophy. Thesis, University of Rotterdam

Höweler C J, Busch H F M, Geraedts J P M, Niermeijer M F,

Staal A 1989 Anticipation in myotonic dystrophy: fact or fiction. Brain 112: 779

Huff R A, Horton E S, Lebovitz H E 1967 Abnormal insulin secretion in myotonic dystrophy. New England Journal of Medicine 277: 837

Hunter A, Tsilfidis C, Mettler G et al 1992 The correlation of age at onset with CTG trinucleotide repeat amplification in myotonic dystrophy. Journal of Medical Genetics 29: 774

Imbert G, Kretz C, Johnson K, Mandel J-L 1993 Origin of the expansion mutation in myotonic dystrophy. Nature Genetics 4: 72

Jansen G, Mahadevan M, Amemiya C et al 1992 Characterisation of the myotonic dystrophy region predicts multiple protein isoform-encoding mRNAs. Nature Genetics 1: 261

Jenkins T. 1992 Personal communication

Junge J 1966 Ocular changes in dystrophia myotonica, paramyotonia and myotonia congenita. Documenta Ophthalmologica 21: 1

Karpati G, Carpenter S, Watters G V, Eisen A E, Andermann F 1973 Infantile myotonic dystrophy. Histochemical and electron microscopic features in skeletal muscle. Neurology 23: 1066

Koch M, Harley H G, Sarfarazi M et al 1989 Myotonia congenita (Thomsen's disease) excluded from the region of the myotonic dystrophy locus on chromosome 19. Human Genetics 82: 163

Koch M C, Ricker K, Otto M et al 1992 Linkage data suggesting allelic heterogeneity for paramyotonia congenita and hyperkalemic periodic paralysis on chromosome 17. Human Genetics 88: 71

Kolb L C 1938 Congenital myotonia in goats. Bulletin of Johns Hopkins Hospital 63: 221

Lavedan C, Hofmann-Radvanyi H, Shelbourne P et al 1993a Myotonic dystrophy: size and sex dependent dynamics of CTG meiotic instability and somatic mosaicism. American Journal of Human Genetics 52: 875

Lavedan C, Hofmann-Radvanyi H, Rabes J P, Roume J, Junien C 1993b Different sex-dependent constraints in CTG length variation as explanation for congenital myotonic dystrophy. Lancet 341: 237

Lenard H G, Goebel H H, Weigel W 1977 Smooth muscle involvement in congenital myotonic dystrophy. Neuropediatrie 8: 42

Lipicky R J 1977 Studies in human myotonic dystrophy. In: Rowland L P (ed) Pathogenesis of human muscular dystrophy. Excerpta Medica, Amsterdam, p 729

Lipicky R J, Bryant S H 1971 Ion content, potassium flux and cable properties of myotonic, human, external intercostal muscle. Transactions of the American Neurological Association 96: 34

Lipicky R J, Bryant S H 1973 A biophysical study of the human myotonias: In: Desmedt J E (ed) New developments in electromyography and clinical neurophysiology. Karger, Basel, p 451

MacMillan H, Myring J, Harley H G, Reardon W, Harper P R, Shaw D J 1992 Molecular analysis for the myotonic dystrophy mutation in neuromuscular disorders. Neuromuscular Disorders 2: 405

Mahadevan M, Tsilfidis C, Sabourin L et al 1992 Myotonic dystrophy mutation: an unstable CTG repeat in the 3' untranslated region of the gene. Science 255: 1253

Mahadevan M et al 1993 Structure and genomic sequence of the myotonic dystrophy (DM kinase) gene. Human Molecular Genetics 2: 299

Mahler C, Parizel G 1982 Hypothalamic pituitary function in myotonic dystrophy. Journal of Neurology 226: 233

Marshall J 1959 Observations on endocrine function in dystrophia myotonica. Brain 82: 221

Mathieu J, De Braekeleer M, Prevost C (1990) Genealogical reconstruction of myotonic dystrophy in the Saguenay-Lac-Saint Jean area. Neurology 40: 839

Meredith A L, Huson S M, Lunt P W et al 1988 Application of a closely linked polymorphism of restriction fragment length to counselling and prenatal testing in families with myotonic dystrophy. British Medical Journal 293: 1353

McComas A J, Mrozek K 1968 The electrical properties of muscle fibre membranes in dystrophia myotonica and myotonia congenita. Journal of Neurology, Neurosurgery and Psychiatry 31: 441

Mohr J 1954 A study of linkage in man. Munksgaard, Copenhagen

Moore J K, Moore A P 1987 Postoperative complications of dystrophia myotonica. Anaesthesia 42: 529

Morris L K, Cuetter A C, Gunderson C H 1982 Myotonic dystrophy, mitral valve prolapse, and cerebral embolism. Stroke 13: 93

Moxley R T, Corbett A J, Minaker M L, Rowe J W 1984 Whole body insulin resistance in myotonic dystrophy. Annals of Neurology 15: 157

Mulley J C, Staples A, Donneally A et al 1993 Explanation for exclusive maternal origin for congenital form of myotonic dystrophy. Lancet 341: 236

Myring J, Meredith A L, Harley H G et al 1992 Specific molecular prenatal diagnosis for the CTG mutation in myotonic dystrophy. Journal of Medical Genetics 29: 785

Norman A M, Floyd J L, Meredith A L, Harper P S 1989 Pre-symptomatic detection and prenatal diagnosis for myotonic dystrophy by means of linked DNA markers. Journal of Medical Genetics 26: 750

Oberlé I, Rousseau P, Heitz D et al 1991 Instability of a 550 base pair DNA segment and abnormal methylation in fragile X syndrome. Science 252: 1097

O'Brien T, Newcombe R G, Harper P S 1983 Outlook for a clinically normal child in a sibship with congenital myotonic dystrophy. Journal of Pediatrics 103: 762

O'Brien T, Harper P S 1984 Reproductive problems and neonatal loss in women with myotonic dystrophy. British Journal of Obstetrics and Gynaecology 4: 170

Olofsson B-O, Forsberg H, Andersson S, Bjerle P, Henriksson A, Wedin I 1988 Electrocardiographic findings in myotonic dystrophy. British Heart Journal 59: 47

Orndahl G, Thulesius O, Enestrom S, Dehlin O 1964 The heart in myotonic disease. Acta Medica Scandinavica 176: 479

Panayiotopoulos C P, Scarpalezos S 1976 Dystrophica myotonica. Peripheral nerve involvement and pathogenetic implications. Journal of the Neurological Sciences 27: 1

Penrose L S 1948 The problem of anticipation in pedigrees of dystrophia myotonica. Annals of Eugenics (Lond) 14: 125

Polgar J G, Bradley W G, Upton A R M et al 1972 The early detection of dystrophia myotonica. Brain 95: 761

Ptacek L J, George A L, Griggs R C et al 1991 Identification of a mutation in the gene causing hyperkalemic periodic paralysis. Cell 67: 1021

Reardon W, Floyd J L, Myring J, Lazarou L P, Meredith A L, Harper P S 1992a Five years experience of predictive testing for myotonic dystrophy using linked DNA markers. American Journal of Medical Genetics 43: 1006

Reardon W, Harley H G, Brook J D et al 1992b Minimal expression of myotonic dystrophy: a clinical and molecular analysis. Journal of Medical Genetics 29: 770

Reardon W, Newcombe R, Fenton I, Sibert J, Harper P S 1993 The natural history of congenital myotonic dystrophy; mortality and long term clinical aspects. Archives of Disease in Childhood 68: 177

Renwick J H, Bundey S E, Ferguson-Smith M A, Izatt M M 1971 Confirmation of the linkage of the loci for myotonic dystrophy and the ABH secretor. Journal of Medical Genetics 8: 407

Ricker K, Haass A, Rudel R, Bohlen R, Mertens H 1980 Successful treatment of paramyotonia congenita (Eulenberg): muscle stiffness and weakness prevented by tocainide. Journal of Neurology, Neurosurgery and Psychiatry 42: 818

Ricker K, Hertel G, Langscheid K, Stodieck G (1977) Myotonia not aggravated by cooling. Force and relaxation of the adductor pollicis in normal subjects and in myotonia as compared to paramyotonia. Journal of Neurology 216: 9

Rosman N P, Kakulas B A 1966 Mental deficiency associated with muscular dystrophy. A neuropathological study. Brain 89: 769

Rüdel R, Lehmann-Horn F 1985 Membrane changes in cells from myotonia patients. Physiological Reviews 65: 310

Rutherford M A, Heckmatt J Z, Dubowitz V 1989 Congenital myotonic dystrophy: respiratory function at birth determines survival. Archives of Disease in Childhood 64: 191

Sabourin L A, Mahadevan M S, Narang M, Lee D S C, Surh L C, Korneluk R G 1993 Effect of the myotonic dystrophy (DM) mutation on mRNA levels of the DM gene. Nature Genetics 4: 233

Sanders D B 1976 Myotonia congenita with painful muscle contractions. Archives of Neurology 33: 580

Sarnat H B, Silbert S W 1976 Maturational arrest of fetal muscle in neonatal myotonic dystrophy. Archives of Neurology 33: 466

Sarnat H B, O'Connor T, Byrne P A 1976 Clinical effects of myotonic dystrophy on pregnancy and the neonate. Archives of Neurology 33: 459

Schotland D L 1970 An electron-microscopic investigation of myotonic dystrophy. Journal of Neuropathology and Experimental Neurology 29: 241

Schwartz O, Jampel R S 1962 Congenital blepharophimosis associated with a unique generalised myopathy. Archives of Ophthalmology 68: 52

Shaw J, Meredith A L, Sarfarazi M et al 1985 The apolipoprotein CII gene: subchromosomal localisation and linkage to the myotonic dystrophy locus. Human Genetics 70: 271

Shaw D J, Harper P S 1989 Myotonic dystrophy: developments in molecular genetics. British Medical Bulletin 45: 745

Shaw D J, Harper P S 1992 Workshop report: myotonic dystrophy — advances in molecular genetics. Neuromuscular Disorders 2: 241

Shaw D J, McCurrach M, Rundle S A et al 1993 Genomic organisation and transcriptional units at the myotonic dystrophy locus. Genomics 18: 673

Shore R N 1975 Myotonic dystrophy: hazards of pregnancy and infancy. Developmental Medicine and Child Neurology 17: 356

Silver M M, Vilos G A, Silver M D, Shaheed W S, Turner K L 1984 Morphologic and morphometric analyses of muscle in the neonatal myotonic dystrophy syndrome. Human Pathology 15: 1171

Silver M M, Hudson A J, Vilos D, Banerjee D 1985 Hyperinsulinemia in myotonic dystrophy. Medical Hypotheses 16: 207

Smeets H J M, Nelen M R, Los F et al 1991 Myotonic dystrophy: prenatal diagnosis using direct mutation analysis. Lancet 340: 73

Soderhall S, Gustafsson J, Bjorkheim I 1982 Deoxycholic acid in myotonic dystrophy. Lancet i: 1068

Streib E W, Sun S F 1983 Distribution of electrical myotonia in myotonic muscular dystrophy. Annals of Neurology 14: 80

Steinmeyer K, Klocke R, Ortland C et al 1991 Inactivation of muscle chloride channel by transposon insertion in myotonic mice. Nature 354: 304

Sutherland G R, Haan E A, Kremer E et al 1991 Hereditary unstable DNA: a new explanation for some old genetic questions? Lancet 338: 289

Swash M 1972 The morphology and innervation of the muscle spindle in dystrophia myotonica. Brain 95: 357

Swash M, Fox K P 1975 Abnormal intrafusal muscle fibres in myotonic dystrophy: a study using serial sections. Journal of Neurology, Neurosurgery and Psychiatry 38: 91

Swift T R, Igancino O J, Dyken P R 1975 Neonatal dystrophia myotonica: electrophysiological studies. American Journal of Diseases of Children 129: 734

Takeshita K, Tanaka K, Nakashima T, Kasagi S 1981 Survey of patients with early-onset myotonic dystrophy in the San-In district, Japan. Japanese Journal of Human Genetics 26: 295

Tanaka K, Takeshita K, Takita M 1982 Abnormalities of bile acids in serum and bile from patients with myotonic muscular dystrophy. Clinical Science 62: 627–642

Thomsen J 1876 Tonische krampfe in willkurlich beweglichen muskeln in folge von erebter psychischer disposition (ataxia muscularis). Archiv fur Psychiatr und Nervenkrank-eiten 6: 702

Thrush D C, Morris C J, Salmon M V 1972 Paramyotonia congenita: a clinical, histochemical and pathological study. Brain 95: 537

Tsilfidis C, MacKenzie A E, Mellter G, Barcelo J, Korneluk R G 1992 Correlation between CTG trinucleotide repeat length and frequency of severe congenital myotonic dystrophy. Nature Genetics 1: 192

Vanier T M 1960 Dystrophia myotonica in childhood. British Medical Journal 2: 1284

Verkerk A J M H, Pieretti M, Sutcliffe J S et al 1991 Identification of a gene (FMR-1) containing a CGG repeat coincident with a break-point cluster region of exhibiting length variation in fragile X syndrome. Cell 65: 905

Vogt A 1921 Die cataract bei myotonische dystrophie. Schweizerische Medizinische Wochenschrift 29: 669

Walsh J C, Turtle J R, Miller S, McLeod J G 1970 Abnormalities of insulin secretion in dystrophia myotonica. Brain 93: 731

Weatherall D J 1992 The new genetics and clinical practice. Oxford, Oxford University Press

Whitehead A S, Solomon E, Chambers S, Bodmer W F, Povey S, Fey G 1982 Assignment of the structural gene for the third component of human complement to chromosome 19. Proceedings of the National Academy of Sciences USA 79: 5021

Wieringa B, Brunner H, Hulsebos T, Schonk D, Ropers H H 1988 Genetic and physical demarcation of the locus for dystrophia myotonica. In: DiDenato et al (eds) Advances in neurology, vol 48, Molecular genetics of neurological and neuromuscular diseases. Raven, New York

Winters S J, Schreiner B, Griggs R C, Rowley P, Nanda N C 1977 Familial mitral valve prolapse and myotonic dystrophy. Annals of Internal Medicine 85: 19

Woodward J B, Heaton R K, Simon D B, Ringel S P 1982 Neuropsychological findings in myotonic dystrophy. Journal of Clinical Neuropsychology 4: 335

16. The inflammatory myopathies

G. Karpati   G. S. Currie

DEFINITION AND CLASSIFICATION

Inflammatory myopathies include acute, subacute or chronic acquired diseases of skeletal muscles of diverse aetiology and pathogenesis. Skeletal muscles contain genuine inflammatory cell infiltrates, although on a single biopsy these may not always be evident. Inflammatory myopathies constitute the largest single group of acquired skeletal muscle diseases. This fact and the treatability of many forms account for the great practical importance of these diseases.

Reliable classification of most inflammatory myopathies based on precise aetiology and pathogenesis is not possible (Dalakas 1988c). However, a practical classification is presented in Table 16.1. The most commonly occurring forms belong to the idiopathic category [(polymyositis (PM), dermatomyositis (DM) and inclusion body myositis (IBM)]. Therefore a major focus of attention in this chapter is directed to these entities which have been the subject of several recent reviews (Whitaker 1982, Mastaglia & Ojeda 1985, Banker & Engel 1986, Dalakas 1988a, Karpati & Carpenter 1988, Engel & Emslie-Smith 1989, Plotz et al 1989, Dalakas 1990a, 1991, Robinson 1991, Rosenberg 1991, Walton 1991, Mastaglia & Walton 1992). Several entities whose names would imply an inflammatory process are discussed in Chapter 27, such as myositis ossificans, eosinophilic fasciitis, polymyalgia rheumatica, etc.

METHODS OF INVESTIGATION

Although the diagnosis of inflammatory myopathies may be suspected on the basis of history and clinical examination, definite diagnosis always

Table 16.1   Classification of human inflammatory myopathies

1. Idiopathic
   Dermatomyositis
   Polymyositis
   Inclusion body myositis
2. Associated with collagen vascular diseases ('overlap syndromes')
   Systemic lupus erythematosus
   Scleroderma
   Rheumatoid arthritis
   Mixed connective tissue disease
   Sjögren's syndrome
3. Microbial
   Viral (influenza A,B, adenoviruses, Coxackie B5, Epstein–Barr virus, HIV, HTLV 1).
   Parasitic (*Trichinella*, toxoplasma, cysticercus)
   Bacterial
   Fungal
4. Specific childhood forms
   Dermatomyositis
   Acute benign myalgic type
   Congenital polymyositis
   Infantile polymyositis with abnormal myonuclei
5. Miscellaneous
   Granulomatous
   Associated with non-specific vasculitis
   Eosinophilic syndromes
   Localised forms (forearm, quadriceps, scapular)
   Drug-induced (systemic or local)
   Graft-versus-host disease
   Inflammatory myopathy with lead pipe capillaries
   Inflammatory myopathy plus mitochondrial myopathy

requires confirmation by laboratory tests. In adults, differentiation may be necessary from various forms of dystrophies and metabolic myopathies, or even from certain forms of denervating diseases. In children, in addition, differentiation may be necessary from congenital myopathies.

Muscle-derived serum enzymes

The most informative and widely used serum enzyme is creatine kinase (CK), which is presumed to be derived from necrotic or otherwise damaged muscle fibres (Banker & Engel 1986). In many but not all types of active inflammatory myopathy the activity of this enzyme is elevated (Oddis & Medsger 1988). The bulk of the increased serum activity of the enzyme is of the MM isoform but some increase of the MB isoform may be present and this is probably related to damage to regenerating fibres. In active polymyositis serum CK activity is invariably elevated to about 5–20-fold above normal, while in some cases of active dermatomyositis serum CK activity may remain normal or is only slightly elevated. The highest serum CK activity occurs in cases of acute rhabdomyolysis that may accompany some forms of acute viral myositis or dermatomyositis associated with extensive muscle infarcts. In inclusion body myositis, CK elevation may be absent or only modest in up to one-half of the cases (Lotz et al 1989). While serum CK levels tend to reflect the activity of disease, they should only be used in conjunction with the overall clinical picture for therapeutic guidance (Oddis & Medsger 1988). Serum CK activity is particularly helpful in distinguishing continually active inflammatory disease from myopathy induced by therapeutic steroid administration in which serum CK activity remains normal. Along with CK, the activity of other enzymes, such as glutamic oxaloacetic transaminase or aldolase, is usually elevated proportionately; this should not be misinterpreted as necessarily being indicative of coexisting liver disease.

Immunological blood tests

Elevation of the erythrocyte sedimentation rate is too inconsistent to be diagnostically useful.

Numerous autoantibodies have been described in patients with DM or PM (Targoff 1989, 1990, Miller et al 1990, Love et al 1991). These may be categorised as either directed to nuclear or cytoplasmic antigens. Antibodies to nuclear antigens include anti-U1 ribonucleoprotein, anti-Ro/SS-A, anti-Sm, anti-La/SS-B and anti-PM-Scl. Some of the ribonucleoproteins which these antibodies recognise are involved in mRNA splicing. Most autoantibodies to nuclear antigens in DM or PM are directed to aminoacyl transfer RNA synthetases which catalyse the linkage of a specific amino acid to its matching tRNA. These autoantibodies include anti-Jo-1 (histidyl transfer RNA), anti-PL-7 (threonyl transfer RNA), anti-PL-12 (alanyl transfer RNA) and anti-OJ (isoleucyl transfer RNA). The anti-KJ antibody is inhibitory to mRNA translation.

The role of these antibodies in the pathogenesis of DM or PM is obscure. The practical usefulness of these antibodies is limited. Most of them are present in fewer than 10% of cases of PM or DM but a higher incidence may occur in the overlap syndromes or in connective tissue diseases. In scleroderma, the presence of anti-PM-Sci antibody suggests a high incidence (40%) of a coexistent myopathy (Mimori 1987). Anti-Jo-1 antibody occurs in 10–30% of DM or PM cases and is associated with a high incidence (50%) of interstitial lung disease (Hochberg et al 1984). The presence of anti-Jo-1 antibodies also correlates with DR3 and/or DRW6 HLA haplotypes.

Electromyography

In active PM, DM or IBM motor unit potentials tend to be of abnormally short duration, small amplitude and polyphasic and show enhanced recruitment (Kimura 1989). Increased spontaneous activity including excessive insertional discharges, single fibre activity indistinguishable from fibrillation and positive sharp waves are common and complex repetitive discharges may also occur. Nerve conduction studies are normal. In IBM, mixed myopathic and neuropathic motor unit action potentials may coexist.

Electromyography can thus be helpful in suggesting an inflammatory myopathy but it is not sufficient to supplant pathological examination of muscle.

Microscopic examination of muscle

For a definite diagnosis of an inflammatory myopathy microscopic examination of a muscle biopsy is indispensable (Carpenter & Karpati 1981, 1984, 1992, Engel & Banker 1986, Mastaglia & Walton 1992). For maximum information three major prerequisites are essential:

1. Proper choice of muscle. As a rule of thumb, a clinically moderate weak muscle offers the best chance for a positive biopsy. Imaging techniques such as computerised tomography or magnetic resonance imaging are rarely required to select an involved region of a muscle. Simultaneous biopsies from more than one site are to be discouraged, although a repeat biopsy from a different site occasionally becomes necessary. Open biopsy done by an expert is strongly recommended in pre-ference to needle biopsy, since open biopsy offers a larger sample and it is far better suited for ultrastructural study.

2. The biopsy specimens should be used for the preparation of cryostat sections, semithin plastic-embedded sections and ultrathin sections for ultrastructural scrutiny. Each of these preparations should be stained by appropriate techniques. Cryostat sections are to be used not only for routine histological and histochemical stains and reactions, but also for special immunocytochemistry for the display of various lymphocytic subsets and the major histocompatibility complex products, as well as immunoglobulins and complements. Semithin plastic-embedded sections offer the most reliable opportunity for the determination of capillary density of muscle which is essential information in the differential diagnosis of DM from PM and IBM (Carpenter 1988). Electron-microscopic examination is required for the detection of tubuloreticular inclusions in endothelial cells of blood vessels in DM or for the identification of the tubular filamentous inclusions in IBM (Carpenter 1988).

3. Interpretation of the biopsy requires special expertise in myopathology to avoid the several pitfalls that can lead to erroneous diagnosis (vide infra).

The principal pathological features in the muscle biopsy may be divided into three major categories:

1. Changes affecting muscle fibres
2. Alterations in blood vessels
3. The inflammatory cell profile, as well as immunopathological features

A constellation of these abnormalities is usually characteristic of DM, PM or IBM and certain other forms of inflammatory myopathy. Table 16.2 summarises these changes in adult DM, as well as PM and IBM.

A number of comments must be made about these changes. Several of these abnormalities are pathognomonic even in isolation. Muscle infarcts, perifascicular atrophy, A-band or focal myofibrillar loss (Carpenter 1988), capillary necrosis (De Visser et al 1989, Emslie-Smith & Engel 1990), membrane attack deposition in vessel walls

Table 16.2 Pathological features in idiopathic inflammatory myopathies

	Dermatomyositis	Polymyositis	Inclusion body myositis
Muscle fibres			
Necrosis of muscle fibres			
Scattered	±	+	+
Infarcts	+	–	–
Sluggish phagocytosis	+	–	–
Regeneration	±	+	+
Atrophy			
Grouped	–	–	–
Scattered	+	+	+
Perifascicular	+	–	–
Hypertrophy	–	–	+
Z-disc streaming	+	+	+
Zonal myofibrillar loss	+	–	–
A band loss	+	–	–
Intrinsic lysosomal activation with exocytosis	–	+	–
Rimmed vacuoles and eosinophilic masses	–	–	+
Nuclear abnormalities (15 nm filaments)	–	–	+
Ragged red fibres	–	–	+
Amyloid staining of inclusions	–	–	+
Ubiquitin-positive inclusions	–	–	+
Blood vessels			
Increased capillarity	–	–	+
Capillary necrosis ± loss	+	± (secondary)	–
Undulating tubules and other endothelial abnormalities	+	–	–
Arterial necrosis or thrombosis	+	–	–
Immunoglobulin deposition	+	–	–
Complement 9 deposition ('membrane attack complex')	+	–	–
Inflammatory and immunopathology			
Lymphocytes			
Endomysial (T helper/inducer)	+	+	+
Septal (B + T helper/inducer)	+	+	–
Partial invasion (T cytotoxic + macrophages)	–	+	+
Plasma cells	–	+	–
Expression of sarcolemmal class 1 major histocompatibility complex protein products	+	+	+
Other			
Marked regional variability of pathology in clinically affected muscles	+	–	–
Interstitial fibrosis	+ (severe cases)	–	+ (focal)

+, Present; –, absent. Since microscopic scrutiny should be directed to muscle fibres, blood vessels and inflammatory cells, changes in these domains are shown separately. Certain highly characteristic pathological changes are marked + and the presence of at least two of these changes in a given biopsy would provide a practically pathognomonic diagnosis for a given entity.

(Kissel et al 1986, 1991b), arterial thrombosis or undulating tubules in endothelial cells are each characteristic for DM. Partial invasion of non-necrotic muscle fibres by cytotoxic lymphocytes and macrophages is typical for PM or IBM but does not occur in DM (Arahata & Engel 1984, 1986, 1988, Engel & Arahata 1984, 1986). The presence of 15–18 nm tubular filamentous masses in nuclei or cytoplasm of muscle fibres is essential for the diagnosis of IBM but its demonstration may require extensive ultrastructural scrutiny (Carpenter 1988, Lotz et al 1989). However, it has become clear that these filamentous masses are not disease-specific for sporadic IBM nor are rimmed vacuoles (Massa et al 1991). The presence of multinucleated giant cells among elongated inflammatory ('epithelioid') cells, macrophages or lymphocytes is characteristic of granulomatous myopathy. The presence of encysted trichinella larvae in muscle fibres in the midst of a florid inflammatory reaction with abundant polymorphonuclear leucocytes is typical for trichinella myositis.

Uniform expression of class 1 major histocompatibility complex (MHC) products at the surface of all muscle fibres is characteristic of PM, whereas in DM this phenomenon may be evident only in the perifascicular or other random regions and in IBM it occurs mainly in fibres that show partial invasion by CD8+ lymphocytes and macrophages (Karpati et al 1988, Emslie-Smith et al 1989). MHC class 1 expression does not occur in limb-girdle dystrophy or denervating diseases or metabolic myopathies (except in regenerating fibres), which makes MHC immunostaining a very helpful diagnostic tool.

The most common cause of a clinical misdiagnosis of inflammatory myopathies is an erroneous pathological interpretation of the biopsy (Karpati & Carpenter 1988).

A relatively common erroneous practice is to lump PM and DM together as the 'DM-PM complex'. Another source of confusion is the failure to distinguish IBM from PM. In the vast majority of the cases, clear distinctions between these entities can be made reliably which is important for investigative, therapeutic and prognostic reasons.

The pitfalls that could lead to erroneous interpretation of the muscle biopsy include the following: failure to assess or appreciate blood vessel pathology may occur because of lack of awareness of its importance or lack of appropriate preparations or stains to assess it. The failure to find IBM filaments is usually related to inadequate electron-microscopy samples and insufficient search. The failure to distinguish between muscle fibre necrosis and partial invasion of muscle fibres by cytotoxic lymphocytes and macrophages is usually related to the lack of awareness of this phenomenon. In dermatomyositis, the pathological involvement may be spotty and a given biopsy may not contain convincing pathological changes. In other instances, even if the biopsy contains changes typical of DM, the lack of inflammatory cell infiltrates in the biopsy could lead to the conclusion of 'non-specific abnormalities'. In

some diseases other than inflammatory myopathies (i.e. Duchenne muscular dystrophy, myasthenia gravis) endomysial infiltration by lymphocytes may occur (Kissel et al 1991a, Maselli et al 1991).

In addition to muscle biopsy, skin biopsy may be indicated in DM, preferably from a clinically involved area but pathological alteration is often present in clinically uninvolved skin. The changes include a thinning of the epithelial cell layer with attenuation or absence of rete pegs, perivascular mononuclear inflammatory cell infiltrates and oedema of the superficial dermis.

CLINICAL FORMS OF INFLAMMATORY MYOPATHIES

Adult dermatomyositis

This is probably the most common form of inflammatory myopathy (Banker & Engel 1986, Karpati & Carpenter 1988, Dalakas 1991). Its overall incidence has been estimated to be two to five cases per million per year (Medsger et al 1979). It occurs twice as often in females than in males. Onset of symptoms is over a wide age range (20–80 years) with a peak occurrence at 40–70 years. Evolution is usually subacute and patients tend to seek medical advice within weeks, or at most a few months after the onset of symptoms. Less frequently, the disease runs a stormy course with rapidly developing quadriparesis and respiratory insufficiency. In hyperacute cases rhabdomyolysis with myoglobinuria can occur.

The natural history of the disease is rarely observed nowadays because of early treatment. However, the disease tends to be remitting or fluctuating in intensity and eventually after several years it usually 'burns itself out'. Late relapses after some years of latency may, however, occur.

Cardinal manifestations include muscle weakness in the limb-girdle and limb muscles mainly in proximal distribution. Neck flexors, trunk and respiratory muscles may become weak. Dysphagia is relatively frequent. Muscle discomfort can take several forms, the most common being exercise-induced pain associated with reduced endurance. In more acute cases, muscles are tender to palpation and/or stretching. Aching in the resting muscles is infrequent.

Skin involvement is present in approximately 90% of cases but in racially pigmented skin it may be masked. Skin manifestations usually precede other symptoms or signs and may be present in the absence of overt muscle weakness. In its typical form there is a violaceous rash of the upper and lower eyelids (Fig. 16.1) and an erythematous rash of the face and upper chest and a scaly purple discolouration of the skin over the knuckles, elbows and knees (Fig. 16.2). Dilated capillaries at the base of the nailbed are characteristic but examination with a magnifying glass may be necessary for visualisation.

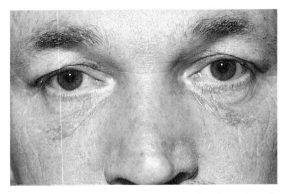

Fig. 16.1 Typical periorbital violaceous discolouration of a patient with dermatomyositis.

Other frequent extramuscular manifestations include arthralgias of both large and small joints, Raynaud's phenomenon and interstitial pulmonary fibrosis (Tazelaar et al 1990). The latter is prone to occur in patients who have anti-Jo-1 serum antibodies (Bernstein et al 1984). Pulmonary fibrosis can be demonstrated by chest X-ray or CT scan or gallium scan. The condition may be asymptomatic or can present with dyspnoea, non-productive cough and even hypoxaemia; it is notoriously resistant to treatment and may lead to death.

Less appreciated extramuscular manifestations include disturbance of oropharyngeal, oesophageal and gastrointestinal motility, cardiac dysfunction manifesting as tachyarrhythmias or impaired ventricular contractility (Haupt & Hutchins 1982). Calcinosis of the subcutaneous connective tissue or intestinal perforation due to vasculitis rarely occur in adult PM but may occur in childhood PM.

There is an association of adult DM and carcinoma that exceeds the rate of chance coincidence (Callen 1988, Lakhanpal et al 1989, Richardson & Callen 1989). PM, IBM or childhood DM show no significant association with carcinoma. In our experience, the incidence is about 20%, mainly in patients over 50 years. Thus, in this age group, a search for latent malignancy is necessary. Lung, breast, colon, prostate, ovary and kidney are the commonest sites. It is unclear whether effective

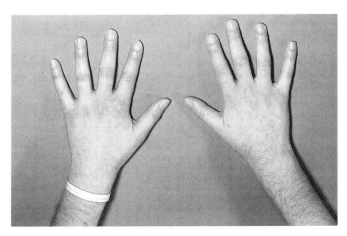

Fig. 16.2 Reddish purple discolouration of the skin over the knuckles in dermatomyositis.

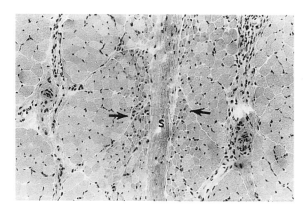

Fig. 16.3 Marked atrophy of muscle fibres (arrows) in the perifascicular zones of each side of an interfascicular connective tissue septum (S). Muscle fibres in the more interior portions of the fascicles (lateral to the arrows) are of normal size. Adult dermatomyositis (haematoxylin & eosin, × 91).

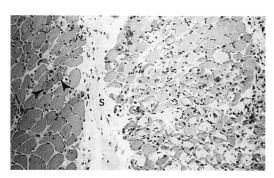

Fig. 16.5 To the right of an interfascicular septum (S) there is severe destruction of muscle fibres, amounting to an infarct. The cell debris in the necrotic fibres is very pale-staining with a great paucity of phagocytes even though on the periphery of such fibres regenerating myoblasts are quite prominent. The fascicle on the left contains no necrotic fibres, but two fibres (arrowheads) show Z-disc streaming. Adult dermatomyositis (haematoxylin and eosin, × 140).

treatment of the carcinoma is beneficial for DM (Basset-Seguin et al 1990). There appear to be no particular clinical or laboratory features that would predict the presence of a latent malignancy, therefore it is not justified to create a separate category of DM associated with malignancy.

The diagnosis of DM can be highly suspected on the basis of the clinical picture alone, but it must be confirmed by determination of serum CK activity, electromyography and characteristic muscle biopsy findings as described in Table 16.2 and illustrated in Figs 16.3–16.13.

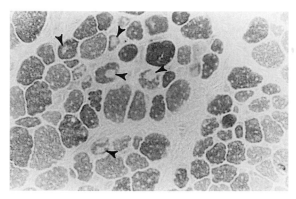

Fig. 16.6 Focal punched-out areas (examples marked by arrowheads) is caused by loss of myofibrils. Adult dermatomyositis (myosin ATP-ase, pH 9.4 perincubation, × 228).

Polymyositis

Polymyositis usually occurs with equal frequency in men and women with its onset peaking at 30–60 years of age (Chiedozi 1979). PM is much more insidious in onset than DM and the course is slowly progressive. Because of the slow evolution, patients may not seek medical advice up to 1–2 years after the onset of symptoms. The chronic course often poses a differential diagnostic dilemma between PM and non-inflammatory chronic neuromuscular diseases. Unlike the situation in DM, appreciable spontaneous fluctuations or remission do not seem to occur. Extramuscular manifestations are less frequent

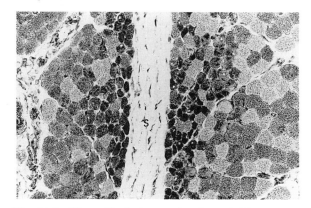

Fig. 16.4 The perifascicular atrophy of muscle fibres on each side of a septum(S) of interfascicular connective tissue: this is very conspicuous because of a marked excess of diformazan in these fibres, obscuring the normal intermyofibrillar staining pattern. Adult dermatomyositis (NADH–tetrazolium reductase, × 130).

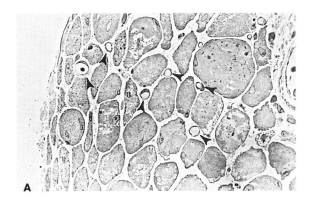

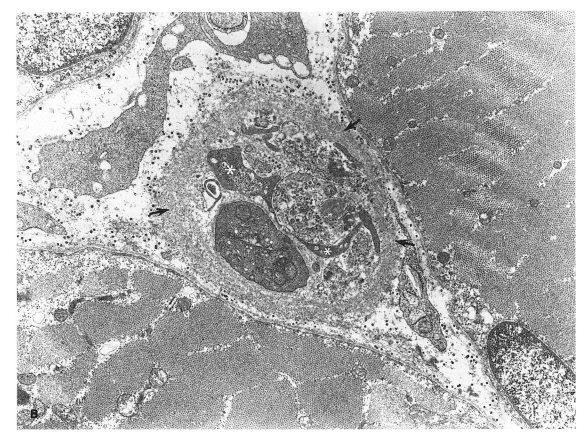

Fig. 16.7   A This plastic-embedded section shows an abnormal paucity of endomysial capillaries particularly in the perifascular region (left). Many of the remaining capillaries (arrowheads) are conspicuously dilated. Several muscle fibres show multifocal punched-out areas of myofibrillar loss. Adult determatomyositis (× 228) (courtesy of Dr S. Carpenter 1982, Muscle and Nerve, John Wiley & Sons, Inc.).
B This electron-micrograph shows a necrotic endomysial capillary in the centre. The lumen is filled with macrophage processes (asterisks) phagocytosing necrotic endothelial cell debris. The basal lamina (arrows) is markedly thickened. Childhood determatomyositis (× 14 000) (courtesy of Dr S. Carpenter 1982, Muscle and Nerve, John Wiley & Sons, Inc.).

and less prominent than in DM. Arthralgia and Raynaud's phenomenon occur much less frequently than in DM. Muscle pain and tenderness do not occur.

The cardinal manifestations consisit of wasting and weakness of limb-girdle and proximal limb muscles. Trunk muscle weakness occurs in the later stages. Respiratory and trunk muscle weakness, as well as craniobulbar involvement, including dysphagia, are rare. The natural history of PM shows a tendency for spontaneous subsidence after years of activity. If untreated,

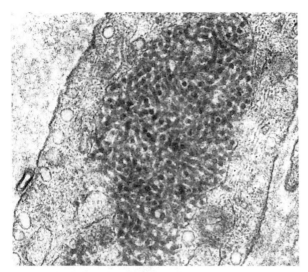

Fig. 16.8 This electron-micrograph shows tubuloreticular inclusions (undulating tubules) in the endoplasmic reticulum of endothelial cells of endomysial capillaries in adult dermatomyositis. Similar structures may be present in disseminated lupus erythematosus, without inflammatory myopathy (× 18 000) (courtesy of Dr S. Carpenter).

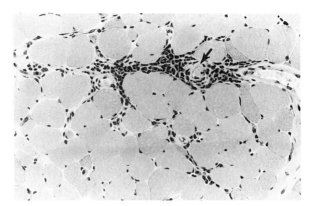

Fig. 16.10 A mononuclear inflammatory infiltrate is present, mainly in a connective tissue septum, in which there are medium-sized blood vessels. The lumen of a blood vessel is obliterated (arrow) presumably by a thrombus, but no major muscle fibre damage is apparent. Adult dermatomyositis (haematoxylin & eosin, × 228).

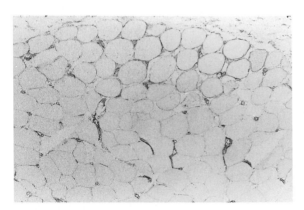

Fig. 16.9 Muscle fibres in the perifascicular region (top) show sarcolemmal expression of class 1 major histocompatibility complex determinants (MHC). Fibres in the interior of the fascicle (bottom) show no such expression as is normally the case. Endomysial blood vessels show strong MHC expression as occurs normally. However, the capillary density is clearly reduced to below normal level. Immunoperoxidase, using a monoclonal antibody to the constant region of class 1 MHC and a biotin-streptavidine peroxidase display system (× 228).

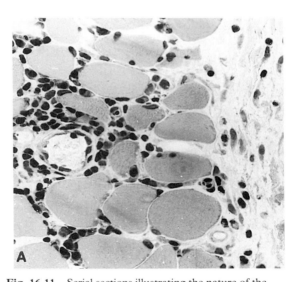

Fig. 16.11 Serial sections illustrating the nature of the mononuclear inflammatory cell infiltrates. **A** Haematoxylin and eosin. **B** CD4+ antigen-bearing lymphocytes constitute the majority of the cells. **C** CD8+ antigen-bearing lymphocytes are scanty. **B** and **C** are immunoperoxidase preparations with monoclonal antibodies specific for CD4 and CD8 antigens respectively. Adult dermatomyositis (× 298).

substantial residual muscle weakness may supervene.

The diagnosis of active PM is confirmed by the demonstration of consistently elevated serum CK values, characteristic EMG findings and a typical constellation of muscle biopsy abnormalities, as described in Table 16.2 and illustrated in Figures 16.14–16.17.

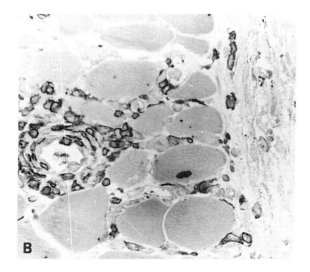

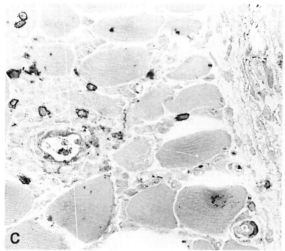

Fig. 16.11   *Contd*

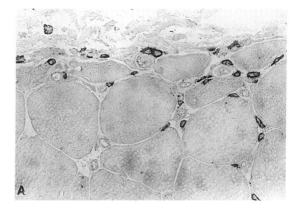

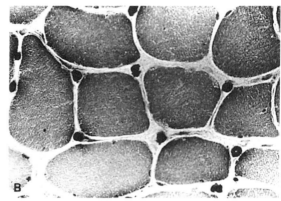

Fig. 16.12   **A** Scattered CD8+ lymphocytes are present in the perifascicular region. Adult dermatomyositis (immunoperoxidase, × 364). **B** Every endomysial capillary shows strong immunoperoxidase staining for complement 9 implying deposition of membrane attack complex. Adult dermatomyositis (× 364).

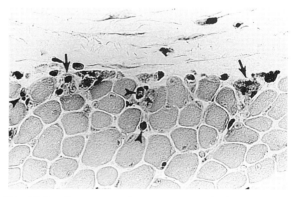

Fig. 16.13   Large macrophages are present in the perifascicular zone. Some of these are phagocytosing necrotic fibres (arrows), others are probably phagocytosing necrotic endothelial cells of capillaries (arrowheads); still others are loose in the connective tissue. Adult dermatomyositis (acid phosphatase, × 228).

Inclusion body myositis

As will be discussed below, there is increasing doubt as to whether IBM truly represents a primary inflammatory myopathy. However, for traditional reasons, IBM is still included as the third major form of idiopathic inflammatory myopathy (Carpenter et al 1978, Eisen et al 1983, Lotz et al 1989).

The male to female incidence of IBM is 3 : 1. In the majority of cases its onset is in the fifth or sixth decade, although in rare instances typical IBM presents as early as the second decade.

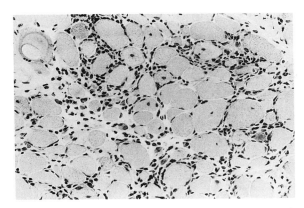

Fig. 16.14 Extensive mononuclear inflammatory reaction is present in the endomysial space. Adult polymyositis (haematoxylin & eosin, × 130).

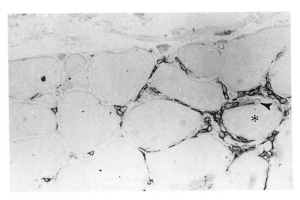

Fig. 16.16 A non-necrotic muscle fibre (asterisk) is partially invaded by CD4+ cells. Some invading cells at the leading edge are CD4– (arrowhead); these are probably macrophages. Adult polymyositis (immunoperoxidase, × 228).

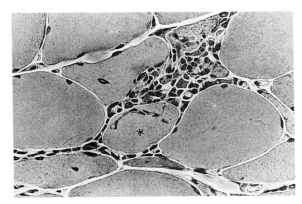

Fig. 16.15 A non-necrotic fibre (asterisk) is invaded by mononuclear inflammatory cell ('partial invasion'). Adult polymyositis (haematoxylin & eosin, × 338).

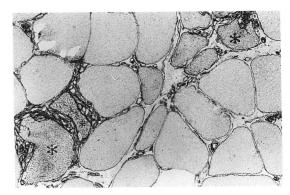

Fig. 16.17 Strong sarcolemmal expression of class 1 major histocompatibility complex determinants is present in all muscle fibres. This is by far the strongest in the three partially invaded fibres (asterisks). The surface of the inflammatory cells and blood vessels are also positive. Adult polymyositis (immunoperoxidase, × 228).

The key manifestation of IBM is limb muscle weakness which, in at least 50% of the cases, is as prominent or even more conspicuous in distal than proximal muscles. Because of this feature, initially IBM is sometimes confused with a denervating disease such as peroneal muscular atrophy. Craniobulbar weakness is exceedingly rare, although dysphagia has been reported due to cricopharyngeus muscle weakness (Verma et al 1991). Respiratory muscle involvement has not been reported.

The evolution of muscle weakness is exceedingly slow and may take up to 5 years before patients seek medical advice. Progression, however, is relentless and about 20 years after onset independent ambulation is usually lost.

Extramuscular manifestations do not occur, except for the fact that an association of IBM with Sjögren's syndrome (Chad et al 1982, Guttman et al 1985) and sarcoidosis (Danon et al 1986) has been observed. A few IBM patients have shown a co-existent chronic axonal peripheral neuropathy (Eisen et al 1983).

Serum CK activity is normal in up to 30% of the cases. The EMG shows a mixed neuropathic and myopathic motor unit potential profile in 30–40% of the cases (Joy et al 1990). The light-microscopic muscle biopsy findings are highly

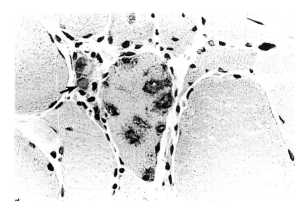

Fig. 16.18 The muscle fibre in the centre contains several rimmed vacuoles. Another fibre to the left has a large intranuclear inclusion (arrow). Inclusion body myositis (haematoxylin & eosin, × 338).

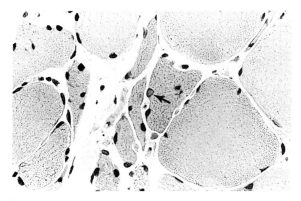

Fig. 16.19 An intranuclear inclusion is present in a muscle fibre (arrow). There is a group of atrophic, somewhat angular fibres in the centre. In the right lower portion of the picture there is a hypertrophied fibre, which is a frequent feature in IBM. Inclusion body myositis (haematoxylin & eosin, × 228).

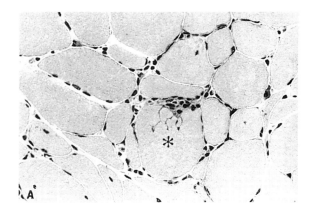

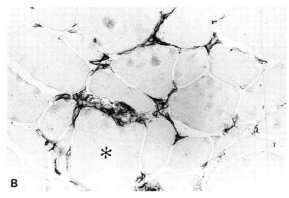

Fig. 16.20 Serial sections showing a partially invaded non-necrotic muscle fibre (asterisk). **A** Haematoxylin & eosin. **B** The invading cells are CD4+ lymphocytes. Inclusion body myositis (immunoperoxidase, × 228).

suggestive of IBM (Table 16.2, Figs 16.18–16.26) but absolute confirmation is dependent on the demonstration of the typical IBM filaments by electron-microscopy. More recent findings indicate that the filamentous masses contain an amyloid-type material (Mendell et al 1991) that reacts with a specific antibody to the Alzheimer's type of beta-amyloid (Askanas et al 1992) but not to the amyloid precursor protein. Some of the IBM filamentous masses also show immuno-staining for ubiquitin (Askanas et al 1991, Albrecht & Bilbao 1992).

Several atypical and rare muscle diseases show a pathological picture indistinguishable from that of IBM. These include an autosomal recessive myopathy with extensive leucoencephalopathy (Cole et al 1988), an autosomal dominant myopathy with a facioscapulohumeral distribution (McKee et al 1992) and an autosomal dominant myopathy with conspicuous quadriceps sparing and a relatively high prevalence among Iranian-Kurdish Jews (Massa et al 1991).

Inflammatory myopathies in collagen vascular diseases

Neuromuscular impairment may occur in any of the collagen-vascular diseases due a variety of causes, such as muscle ischaemia, cachexia, periph-eral nerve involvement, musculoskeletal defor-mities, the therapeutic steroid effect, etc. True inflammatory myopathy is another possible but

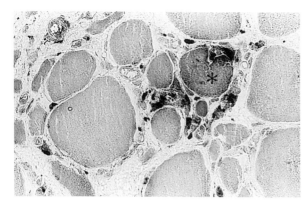

Fig. 16.21 Some of the invading cells of a non-necrotic muscle fibre (asterisk) are macrophages. Inclusion body myositis (acid phosphatase, × 228).

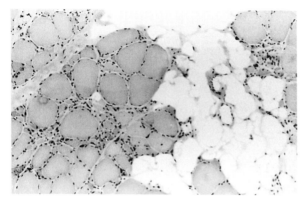

Fig. 16.22 A large area of lost muscle fibres is replaced by adipose tissue. Inclusion body myositis (haematoxylin & eosin, × 130).

relatively infrequent cause (Rosenberg et al 1988). In a large series of patients with systemic sclerosis, a DM-like picture was found in about 12% of the patients, particularly in those having anti-PM-Sci antibodies (Mimori 1987). In systemic lupus the true incidence of clinically evident inflammatory myopathy (Figs 16.27, 16.28) in the form of DM has been estimated at 5–8% (Foote et al 1982). In Sjögren's syndrome both a DM and PM picture have been observed in three out of four patients but the overall incidence is probably much lower (Ringel et al 1982). In rheumatoid arthritis and periarteritis nodosa, clinically evident inflammatory muscle disease is very rare, although muscle biopsies may show focal interstitial or perivascular mononuclear inflammatory cell infiltrates

or necrotic arteritis (Fig. 16.29) respectively, without major muscle fibre damage.

In practical terms, if a patient with any of the above collagenoses as defined by rigorous diagnostic criteria shows undue muscle weakness that cannot otherwise be explained, and particularly if serum CK activity is significantly elevated and if there is an EMG abnormality consistent with an inflammatory myopathy, a muscle biopsy from a carefully selected site is justified.

It appears that either DM or PM in these overlap syndromes show the same pathological features as the ones found in idiopathic DM and PM.

Viral myositis

Numerous viruses have been implicated in the aetiology of inflammatory myopathy (Rosenberg et al 1989), but only two viruses (influenza and Coxsackie) have significant myotropism and, thus, proven cases of acute viral myositis are relatively rare (Ruff & Secrist 1982). The myalgia that often occurs during *influenza infection* does not necessarily imply an inflammatory process, since myalgia can be produced non-specifically by intravenous injection of leucocyte pyrogen. Genuine acute myositis caused by influenza A or B virus has been described in both adults and children. In adults, it is often characterised by variably severe muscle weakness, myalgia and muscle swelling, elevated serum CK activity and frequent rhabdomyolysis with myoglobinuria and a fatal outcome in about 25% of cases (Gamboa et al 1979). Cardiopulmonary complications are common and usually account for the fatalities. Positive viral cultures from muscle, even in severe cases, are difficult to obtain, although muscle biopsy may show intra- and extra-cellular influenza virions and filamentous intranuclear inclusions. In addition, large numbers of necrotic and regenerating fibres are usually present in the acute phase, as well as scattered interstitial or perivascular mononuclear inflammatory infiltrates.

It is not known what predisposes a small minority of patients with generalised influenza infection to developing a significant acute skeletal muscle syndrome. In patients who survive an acute influenza myositis, residual muscle weakness usually does not persist.

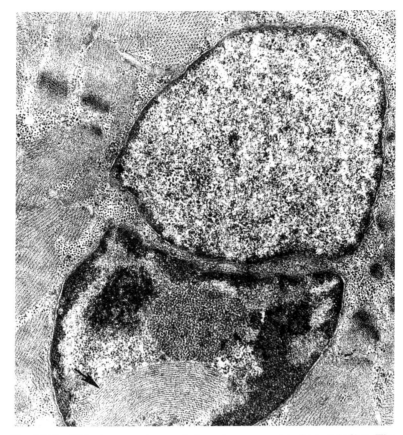

Fig. 16.23 This electron-micrograph shows two myonuclei of a muscle fibre. The one below contains a mass of 18 mm tubular filaments (arrow). Inclusion body myositis ($\times$ 70 000) (courtesy of Dr S. Carpenter).

Coxsackie A virus. This causes mainly an acute myalgic syndrome localised to the thoracic and abdominal muscles. Less often, it causes an acute diffuse myalgic myositis with rhabdomyolysis and myoglobinuria.

Very few cases of acute diffuse myositis caused by human adenovirus 21 and Echo virus 9 have been documented (Wright et al 1979).

The most important viral myopathies are those related to human retroviruses (Dalakas & Illa 1991).

Acquired immunodeficiency syndrome (AIDS). In patients with AIDS several types of skeletal muscle disease have been observed (Dalakas & Pezeshkpour 1988). These include a necrotising myopathy with A-band loss plus nemaline rods and/or cytoplasmic bodies, PM-like

inflammatory myopathy, giant cell myositis and focal myositis. Toxoplasma and sarcosporidia myositis may develop as a result of opportunistic infection. Furthermore, a peculiar myopathy can supervene from therapeutic zidovudine administration in HIV (Human immunodeficiency virus) seropositive patients even without clinical AIDS.

The most important of the AIDS-related muscle diseases is the PM-like inflammatory myopathy (HIV-PM) which is clinically and pathologically very similar to idiopathic PM (Illa et al 1991). It usually occurs in the well-established stage of AIDS but its precise incidence is not known. In a postmortem study, seven out of 14 patients had histological evidence of an inflammatory myopathy. The histological features of

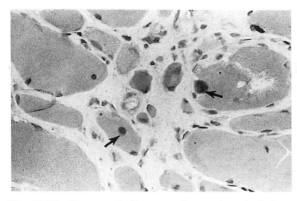

Fig. 16.24   Two muscle fibres contain prominent inclusions (arrows) with staining characteristics of amyloid. The inclusion on the right is possibly being exocytosed. Inclusion body myostitis (crystal violet, × 228).

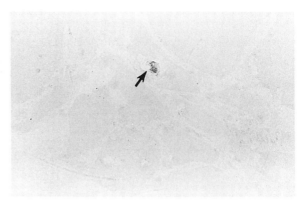

Fig. 16.26   Some nuclear contents (arrow) show immunostaining with an antibody to ubiquitin. Inclusion body myositis (immunoperoxidase, × 228).

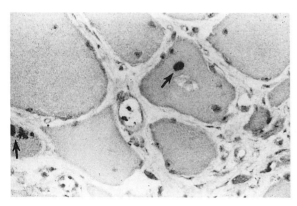

Fig. 16.25   Two muscle fibres contain prominent inclusion bodies (arrows) that show strong immunoreactivity to an antibody against the beta-amyloid of Alzheimer plaques. All nuclei show faint non-specific staining. Inclusion body myositis (immunoperoxidase, × 338).

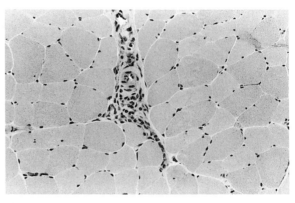

Fig. 16.27   Mononuclear inflammatory infiltrates in an intermyofibrillar septum in a case of disseminated lupus erythematosus (haemotoxylin & eosin, × 228).

HIV-PM are indistinguishable from those of idiopathic PM, including strong sarcolemmal expression of class 1 MHC in all muscle fibres and partial invasion of non-necrotic muscle fibres by CD8+ (cytotoxic) lymphocytes and macrophages. Retroviral antigens could not be demonstrated by in situ hybridization in muscle fibres but they are present in interstitial cells. This implies that retroviruses do not gain entry into muscle fibres but are capable of setting up an inflammatory response from without, that results in muscle fibre damage or destruction. The fact that some antibodies to human ribonucleoproteins cross-react with specific retroviral peptides led to the autosensitisation hypothesis (Rucheton et al 1985).

In HIV-PM, toxoplasmosis must be excluded by serological tests and careful examination of muscle samples for toxoplasma organisms.

Zidovudine-induced myopathy. HIV-PM must be differentiated from zidovudine-induced myopathy (Dalakas et al 1990, Mhiri et al 1991) and the two may actually coexist. In pure zidovudine myopathy, there is prominent myalgia and fatiguability but not much muscle weakness,

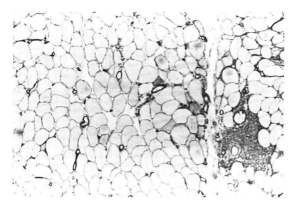

Fig. 16.28 Strong sarcolemmal expression of class 1 MHC determinants is present in all muscle fibres. There is a paucity of endomysial capillaries. In the right lower corner there is a perivascular inflammatory infiltrate. Lupus erythematosus (haematoxylin & eosin, × 130).

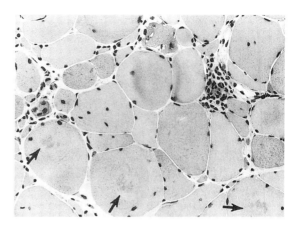

Fig. 16.30 Inflammatory mononuclear cell infiltrate is present in the endomysial space. Targets (arrows) in three muscle fibres indicate a coexisting denervating process. HTLV-1 seropositive spastic paraparesis plus polymyositis (haematoxylin & eosin, × 245).

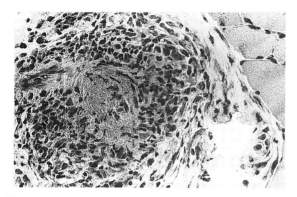

Fig. 16.29 Necrosis and massive inflammatory cell infiltration of an arterial wall in an interfascicular septum. The lumen is occluded by a thrombus. Periarteritis nodosa (haematoxylin & eosin, × 338).

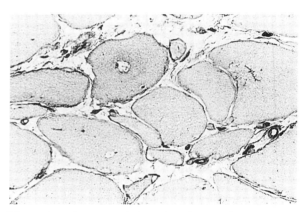

Fig. 16.31 Sarcolemmal class 1 MHC expression is present in all muscle fibres, some of which have denervation characteristics. HTLV-1 seropositive spastic paraparesis plus polymyositis (immunoperoxidase, × 228).

normal or slightly elevated serum CK activity and ragged red fibres in the muscle biopsy. Zidovudine is an inhibitor of γ-DNA polymerase and as a result, the mitochondrial DNA content of muscle fibres is reduced. Thus, zidovudine myopathy is an iatrogenic mitochondrial muscle disease. Zidovudine myopathy is fully reversible upon cessation of administration of the drug.

A PM-like myopathy also occurs in patients who are seropositive for the type 1 *human T cell lymphotrophic virus (HTLV-1)* (Goudreau et al 1988, Morgan et al 1989). These patients may or may not have coexisting spastic paraparesis.

Muscle biopsy shows changes similar to those seen in idiopathic PM (Fig. 16.30) but coexisting denervation related to the spinal cord disease may be present in patients with spastic paraparesis (Figs 16.30, 16.31). Suspicion of an inflammatory myopathy in HTLV-1 disease is raised by a discovery of significantly elevated serum CK activity. In HTLV-1-PM, initial studies suggested the presence of viral components in muscle fibres by in situ hybridization, but later studies disproved this, showing viral-related molecules only in interstitial spaces (Wiley et al 1989, Ishii et al 1991).

Parasitic myositis

Trichinella spiralis. The liberated larvae of the nematode *Trichinella spiralis*, usually derived from ingested poorly cooked pork (containing encysted larvae), have a potent capacity for invading skeletal muscle fibres and initiating a florid inflammatory reaction. The clinical picture is one of an acute diffuse myalgic myositis, often with periorbital oedema. An erythematous skin eruption may occur and because of this, plus periorbital oedema, the task of differentiation of trichinella myositis from acute idiopathic DM may be difficult. The serum CK activity is usually markedly elevated. Muscle biopsy shows a massive interstitial infiltration with lymphocytes, neutrophilic and eosinophilic polymorphonuclear leucocytes, as well as plasma cells. There is partial invasion of muscle fibres by cytotoxic lymphocytes. Extensive muscle fibre necrosis and regeneration are present. Larvae are hard to identify in muscles unless they are encysted; this usually occurs to some extent by the time a muscle biopsy is undertaken in acute trichinella myositis. Encysted larvae are present outside muscle fibres, surrounded by so-called nurse cells in the more acute phase. Encysted larvae may persist indefinitely in muscle but are then asymptomatic. Trichinella myositis is usually a self-limiting disease and residual weakness is rare even in untreated cases.

Toxoplasma gondii. Infection of muscle with the protozoan *Toxoplasma gondii* has rarely been documented in the literature. However, this may change with the increasing incidence of AIDS.

Chronic infection of the muscle by toxoplasma organisms results in a PM-like picture. In fact, according to a once popular hypothesis, idiopathic PM may be due to an occult toxoplasma infection. Muscle biopsy in true toxoplasma myositis shows features of PM. Specific diagnosis requires the demonstration of pseudocysts in muscle fibres. Their identity can be confirmed by immunocytochemistry using specific antibodies. Pseudocysts may persist in muscle after the symptoms subside.

Bacterial and fungal myositis. This is exceedingly rare, since skeletal muscle fibres tend to be resistant to bacterial invasion and suppuration. Even after contaminated muscle biopsies, infection usually involves mainly the skin and subcutaneous tissue but spares the muscle.

Suppurative myositis. In the tropics a curious form of disseminated *suppurative myositis* has been reported with massive polymorphonuclear leucocytic and lymphocytic infiltration of muscles, as well as muscle fibre necrosis, sometimes so massive as to cause myoglobinuria (Muscat et al 1986). Although *Staphylococcus aureus* is usually cultured from the infected tissue, it is not clear whether the infection is a primary or secondary process. The predilection of this myositis for the tropics is unexplained (Shepherd 1983). A necrotising, haemorrhagic myositis (gas gangrene) can develop as a result of infection by the anaerobic bacterium *Clostridium perfringens*, which gains entry to the muscle through open wounds (Wells et al 1985). The muscle damage is due to the clostridial exotoxin that contains collagenase, hyaluronidase and phospholipase.

Lepromatous leprosy. In this condition infiltration of the interstitial space of muscle by clusters of mycobacterium containing macrophages can occur but clinical symptoms of myositis are lacking.

SPECIFIC CHILDHOOD FORMS

Benign acute childhood myositis (BACM)

This syndrome is also called 'myalgia cruris epidemica', since the cardinal manifestations include acute pain and swelling of the muscles in the calves and anterior tibial compartment, and the disease runs a self-limiting course of a few days to up to 2 weeks (Antony et al 1979). Cases tend to cluster, which would be consistent with an infectious aetiology. Influenza A and B virus have been found in patients with BACM (Ruff & Secrist 1982). Muscle biopsy may be normal or it may show intense lymphocytic infiltration and oedema.

Childhood dermatomyositis

This is the most common form of acquired muscle disease in childhood (Carpenter et al 1976, Banker & Engel 1986). Onset of symptoms could occur as early as 2 years. The peak incidence is

10–14 years. The female-to-male ratio of occurrence is about 3 : 2. In approximately 25% of the cases, the onset is preceded by an acute viral-like disease.

The course of the disease is usually subacute but acute cases are not too infrequent. Symptoms include weakness of the shoulder- and hip-girdle muscles, as well as proximal limb muscles. Muscles are often tender to touch and may be swollen. Muscle pain and arthralgia are exaggerated by exercise. The skin rash is similar to that described in adult DM. Raynaud's phenomenon does not occur and carcinoma is not associated with childhood DM.

Extramuscular manifestations are nowadays rare and include ischaemic necrosis of the intestinal wall with perforation, and subcutaneous calcinosis. The latter could cause skin ulceration and limb deformities. Interstitial pulmonary fibrosis is very rare. Childhood DM is self-limiting after a course of 2–4 years but if it is left untreated severe residual muscle wasting and weakness may remain.

The serum CK activity is elevated and the EMG shows a characteristic pattern which is similar to that of adult DM.

The light- and electron-microscopic histological features on muscle biopsy are very similar to those of adult DM (Table 16.3), but perifascicular atrophy and muscle infarcts are more common in childhood DM. The vascular changes include capillary necrosis, reduced capillary density of muscle, endothelial cell abnormalities and thrombosis of medium-sized arteries and veins. These are important features for diagnosis and their demonstration requires the examination of plastic-embedded semithin and ultrathin sections.

Polymyositis in children

Chronic inflammatory myopathy of the adult PM type is exceedingly rare in children (Thompson 1982). Two peculiar types of chronic inflammatory myopathy deserve comment. Although these entities are rare they are still important because they are potentially treatable and require differentiation from congenital dystrophy and other congenital myopathies.

Infantile polymyositis with sick myonuclei (Karpati & Carpenter 1988). Onset is during the

Table 16.3   Salient muscle biopsy features of childhood dermatomyositis

Muscle fibres
Necrosis of muscle fibres
  Scattered
  Perifascicular
  Infarcts
Sluggish phagocytosis
Regeneration
Atrophy of muscle fibres
  Perifascicular
  Scattered
Z-disc streaming
Focal myofibrillar loss
A-band loss
Mitochondrial maldistribution
Class 1 major histocompatibility complex product expression
  (perifascicular or focal)
Lipid globule excess in muscle fibres

Blood vessels
Capillary necrosis → loss (perifascicular or focal)
Undulating tubules
Arterial endothelial swelling
Arterial thrombosis
Membrane attack complex deposition in vessel walls

Inflammation
Lymphocytic infiltration
Septal (helper/inducer T)
Endomysial perivascular (helper/inducer T)
Plasma cells

first year. Early signs include an inability to stand, falling, weak arm elevation and poor head control due to weakness of neck muscles. The atrophy of arm muscles with relatively normal bulk of forearm musculature confers a 'Popeye' type of arm contour (Fig. 16.32). Craniobulbar deficits are lacking and there are no extramuscular manifestations. Tendon reflexes are usually lost early.

The EMG findings are similar to those described for adult idiopathic PM. Serum CK activity is increased 3–10-fold. Muscle biopsy abnormalities include interstitial infiltrates of lymphocytes (Fig. 16.33) but without partial invasion of muscle fibres of the type described in PM, marked smallness of most muscle fibres, scattered muscle fibre necrosis and regeneration. Failed regeneration, however, is common and as a result numerous scattered foci of muscle fibre loss and fibrosis are common features (Fig. 16.34). Sarcolemmal class 1 MHC expression in muscle fibres is present, which tends to confirm the inflammatory nature of this disease.

A distinctive feature of the pathology consists of

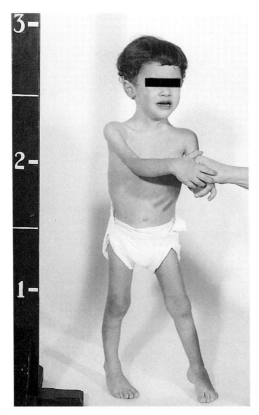

Fig. 16.32 A 4-year-old boy with the syndrome of polymyositis and 'sick' myonuclei. The wasted arm and the more normal forearm give a 'Popeye' configuration to the upper extremities.

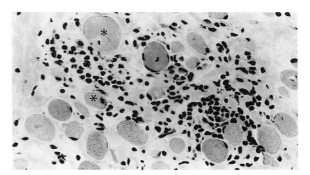

Fig. 16.33 Profuse endomysial inflammatory cell infiltration in the biceps muscle of the patient shown in Figure 16.32. There is marked endomysial fibrosis. Two fibres (asterisks) show partial invasion by inflammatory cells (CD4+ lymphocytes, data not shown).

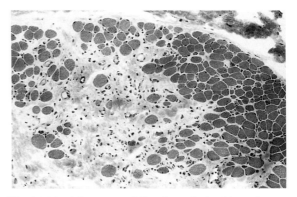

Fig. 16.34 A large area of fibrosis marks focal loss of muscle fibres. Infantile polymyositis (haematoxylin & eosin, × 228).

prominent myonuclear abnormalities (Figs 16.35, 16.36) including abnormally large size, irregular or even bizarre shapes with cytoplasmic invaginations and various inclusions. Inclusions may take the form of 4 nm filaments resembling actin filaments, hexagonal arrays of 22 nm filaments and microtubules. Excess heterochromatin is present in many nuclei.

This disease appears to be self-limiting but even with corticosteroid therapy (which is somewhat helpful) major permanent muscle wasting and weakness remain.

Congenital inflammatory myopathy (Roddy et al 1986, Shevell et al 1990). In this disease fetal movements are reduced and muscular hypotonia is noted at birth. Motor milestones are considerably delayed. Muscle weakness involves the neck, limb, face and respiratory territories. Contractures are common in the limbs. Stretch reflexes are depressed or absent. Most cases show microcephaly and mental subnormality. The muscle biopsy reveals necrosis and regeneration, extensive muscle fibre loss and fibrosis, focal interstitial lymphocytic infiltration and sarcolemmal class 1 HMC expression in large groups of non-regenerating muscle fibres. Dystrophin immunostaining of muscle fibres is normal.

This syndrome must be differentiated from Fukayama's disease (Olney & Miller 1983), as well as the Walker–Warburg syndrome and congenital dystrophy.

Steroid-responsiveness of this disease is variable but never dramatic and CNS features are not affected.

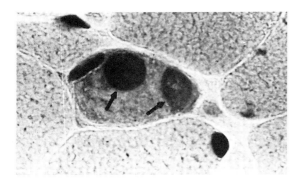

Fig. 16.35   Two massively enlarged myonuclei are marked by arrows in a muscle fibre which shows some streaming of Z discs. There is also a normal myonucleus. Infantile polymyositis (haematoxylin & eosin, × 338).

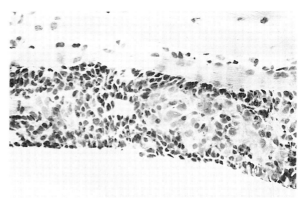

Fig. 16.37   A granulomatous reaction with pleomorphic cell infiltration is present in between muscle fibres. Granulomatous myopathy (haematoxylin & eosin, × 245).

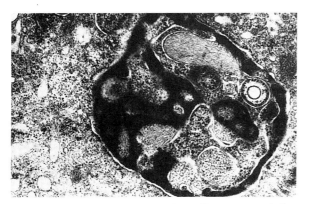

Fig. 16.36   Electron-microscopy shows filamentous, tubular, granular and membranous inclusions in a myonucleus. Infantile polymyositis (× 65 000). (courtesy of Dr S. Carpenter).

Miscellaneous forms of inflammatory myopathies

Granulomatous myopathy (Carpenter & Karpati 1984, Mastaglia & Walton 1992). While many patients with systemic sarcoidosis have asymptomatic microscopic granulomata in muscle that can be helpful in the diagnosis, a clinically manifest myopathy is rare. These patients present with an insidious limb-girdle syndrome and muscle biopsy shows non-caseating granulomas (Fig. 16.37) with giant cells. Muscle fibre damage is usually limited. In some patients, intranuclear filaments can be seen in myonuclei that are indistinguishable from those observed in IBM. In a special group of patients, usually postmenopausal

women, a similar clinical and pathological picture in muscle is present without evidence of systemic sarcoidosis. In some of these patients myasthenia gravis may also develop. The relationship of this granulomatous myopathy to sarcoidosis is unclear.

A granulomatous myopathy may rarely develop in Crohn's disease (Ménard et al 1976) and in association with thymoma.

Myopathy in hypersensitivity vasculitis. Vasculitis in muscle may be present in the many forms of inflammatory myopathy including DM and the collagenoses. In addition, there are patients who present with a non-specific vasculitis which either involves skeletal muscles alone or other tissues as well. In many instances, the aetiological factor remains obscure. In these cases the pathology consists of mononuclear infiltration of vessel walls and their vicinity without necrosis or thrombosis of the vessels themselves. The clinical picture is variable but severe muscle weakness rarely develops.

Eosinophilic syndromes. Three types of inflammatory disease are associated with either prominent presence of eosinophilic polymorphonuclear leucocytes in muscle (or fascia) or systemic eosinophilia or both.

In *eosinophilic polymyositis* (Layzer et al 1977) muscle involvement is part of a systemic hypereosinophilic syndrome. A marked systemic eosinophilia is present. Myocardium is often involved in the inflammatory process. Proximal limb muscles show stiffness, pain and variable weakness.

Serum CK activity is moderately elevated. The pathological picture is similar to that of idiopathic PM, except that there is a conspicuous presence of eosinophilic polymorphonuclear leucocytes in the inflammatory infiltrates.

In *eosinophilic fasciitis* the inflammatory reaction is restricted to the fascia and is best shown by a biopsy of the fascia lata (Simon et al 1982).

The *eosinophilia-myalgia syndrome* is caused by prolonged oral intake of large doses of an L-tryptophan preparation as a therapeutic agent mainly for insomnia (Hertzman et al 1990). There is marked systemic eosinophilia with generalised myalgia and moderate muscle weakness (Martin et al 1990). Another important feature is thickening of the skin mimicking scleroderma. In severe cases, myocarditis and other visceral involvements can supervene. The lymphocytic inflammatory infiltrates (CD8[+] cytotoxic cells) also include either abundant or few eosinophilic polymorphonuclear leucocytes, mainly in the perimysial region, but less often also in the interstitial space of muscle (Emslie-Smith et al 1991). Muscle fibre necrosis is rare and serum CK activity does not rise significantly. Coexisting peripheral neuropathy may cause denervation atrophy. In some cases, the muscle biopsy shows no abnormality, despite clinical symptoms.

The pathogenic factor appears to be a contamination of L-tryptophan with an acetaldehyde ditryptophan derivative which seems to induce an autosensitisation. The disease usually subsides after cessation of exposure but resolution may be slow. Corticosteroid therapy may help to accelerate recovery.

Localised forms. Inflammatory myopathy, usually of the polymyositis type, may be restricted to one muscle or to one group of muscles (Heffner et al 1977, Bharucha & Morgan-Hughes 1981). These localised forms of inflammatory myopathy may involve forearm muscles, quadriceps, sternomastoids, or shoulder-girdle muscles. The latter is probably the best known variety, since it mimics facioscapulohumeral dystrophy (Munsat et al 1972). It may be sporadic or familial (autosomal dominant). The response to corticosteroid therapy is poor.

Another form of localised muscle inflammation can occur in any large muscle presenting as a muscle mass. Necrosis and regeneration of muscle fibres and focal inflammatory infiltrates are present. The aetiology of this peculiar muscle reaction is unknown. It has to be differentiated from neoplasms or abscesses.

Inflammatory myopathy with 'pipe-stem' capillaries (Emslie-Smith & Engel 1991). In three patients a peculiar form of necrotising and to a lesser extent inflammatory myopathy with a microangiopathy was described. The hallmark of the pathology is so-called 'pipe-stem' capillaries which stand out by their thickened wall. Membrane-attack complex was demonstrated in the walls of some of these vessels. The capillarisation of the muscle is usually reduced. While there are similarities between this vascular pathology and that occurring in dermatomyositis, the two entities are different. It should be noted that capillaries with thickened walls, presumably due to a widening of the basal lamina, can occur in a variety of diseases including diabetes and unspecified myopathies and neuropathies.

Drug-induced inflammatory myopathy. Repeated intramuscular injection of pentazocine in habitual users of the analgesic drug produces a necrotic-inflammatory myopathy with massive increase of endomysial and perimysial connective tissue, resulting in joint contractures. A peculiar effect of this process is the inability of the arms to be fully lowered next to the trunk ('arm levitation phenomenon'). It is not known what chemical feature of pentazocine is responsible for this peculiar pathological reaction in muscle.

Systemic use of D-penicillamine (Doyle et al 1983), procainamide and phenytoin may cause vasculitis involving skeletal muscles. Reduced muscle strength, however, is usually mild. D-penicillamine, in fact, causes more often a myasthenia-like picture than vasculitis.

Graft-versus-host reaction. In the graft-versus-host reaction interstitial infiltration of muscle with lymphocytes may occur but clinical muscle weakness is mild or not discernible.

Combined inflammatory and mitochondrial myopathy (Carpenter et al 1992). In three middle-aged patients with a chronic limb-girdle syndrome and markedly elevated serum CK activity, typical muscle pathological features of polymyositis and mitochondrial myopathy were

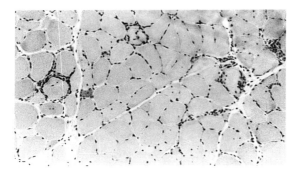

Fig. 16.38 Multiple interstitial mononuclear inflammatory cell infiltrates with partial invasion of muscle fibres. Polymyositis plus mitochondrial myopathy (haematoxylin & eosin × 228).

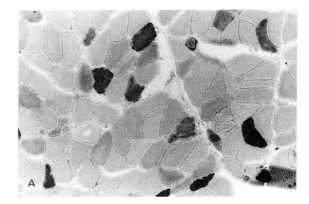

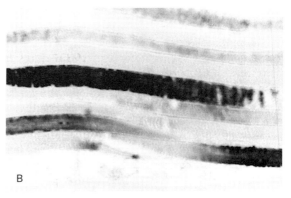

Fig. 16.39 A, B Numerous ragged-red fibre equivalents show abnormally dark staining with succinic dehydrogenase. On the longitudinal view, the involvement is segmental. Same patient as in Figure 16.38 (× 195).

present (Figs 16.38, 16.39). The response to corticosteroids was poor.

AETIOLOGY AND PATHOGENESIS

The aetiology of the inflammatory myopathies is only known in the microbial and toxic varieties. In all other forms, including the common idiopathic types, the primary aetiological factor(s) is still obscure. Attention has recently been focused on picorna viruses as possible triggers of an autoimmune process, since an animal picorna virus coat protein (VP1) shares some amino acid sequence homology with the Jo-1 antigen and myosin light and heavy chains (Walker & Jeffrey 1988). However, evidence for the presence of picorna viruses in PM or DM is highly controversial (Rosenberg et al 1989).

The fact that human retroviruses can also elicit a PM-like reaction in AIDS, apparently by triggering an autoimmune process against some components of muscle fibres, raises the possibility that a hitherto unidentified retrovirus might trigger a destructive autoimmune process in DM or PM (Rucheton et al 1985).

The suggestion that the inclusions in IBM are composed of mumps virus has been disproved (Nishino et al 1989).

More is known about the pathogenesis of DM and PM as well as related disorders. In these diseases, muscle fibres are damaged by immune-mediated processes either directly or indirectly through primary involvement of blood vessels

(Cronin et al 1988, Karpati & Carpenter 1988, Targoff 1989, Engel et al 1990, Griggs & Karpati 1991, Miller 1991). Furthermore, both mechanisms may be operative in parallel.

In DM the primary target of the immunological attack is all types of blood vessels, resulting in either loss of capillaries or occlusion of larger blood vessels. The former causes chronic sublethal ischaemic damage to muscle fibres, particularly those in the perifascicular zones where normally capillarisation is less than inside the fascicles (Emslie-Smith & Engel 1990). Vascular occlusion causes frank infarcts. Thus, in DM muscle fibre damage or death is largely indirect and related to chronic sublethal or acute lethal ischaemia. The evidence suggests that the vascular damage is mediated largely by humoral mechanisms (Griggs & Karpati 1991). The majority of the inflammatory cells are CD4+ helper T lymphocytes, as well as B lymphocytes and plasma cells (Arahata & Engel 1984). Furthermore, there is a lytic membrane attack complex deposition on vessel walls implying a C5b-9 complement activation by antibodies with affinity to vessel walls (Kissel et al 1991b). The significance in this process of the numerous autoantibodies that are found inconsistently in the various forms of inflammatory myopathy is completely unknown and they probably represent a parallel phenomenon. Partial invasion of muscle fibres by CD8+ cells is absent in DM, although class 1 MHC expression at the surface of muscle fibres may be present in focal regions.

In PM (and to some extent IBM) the immuno-effector mechanism that damages muscle fibres is mainly cellular (Engel & Arahata 1986). This is evidenced by the presence of partial invasion of non-necrotic muscle fibres by CD8[+] (CD4[−]) lymphocytes and macrophages (Arahata & Engel 1986). Most of these lymphocytes are bearing α/β T-cell receptors (TCR) but in one patient the CD8[+] cells were demonstrated to bear γ/δ TCR (Hohlfeld et al 1991). Whether a particular cytotoxic lymphocytic subset with a particular TCR profile is characteristic of the various forms of inflammatory myopathies is unknown but is being actively investigated.

The autoinvasive cytotoxic T-cells traverse the basal lamina and often severely indent or even bisect muscle fibres and compromise their function. Additional and probably more severe damage is imparted to muscle fibres by deleterious lymphokines derived from the cytotoxic lympho-cytes, that could eventually lead to necrosis of muscle fibres. The role of perforin may be impor-tant in that respect. The strong expression of sarcolemmal class 1 MHC in practically all muscle fibres in PM is indicative of the fact that the cytotoxic effect of the autoinvasive CD8+ lympho-cytes is class 1 MHC restricted (Karpati et al 1988). The stimulus that triggers class 1 MHC expression is not known, although interferon-γ is capable of such action in vitro. Class 2 MHC expression on the surface of muscle fibres has not been observed by us in any form of muscle disease. The antigens to which the CD8+ cells have become sensitised is unknown. CD8+ cells extracted from muscle of patients with PM or IBM showed a cyto-toxic effect upon autologous myotubes in vitro (Hohlfeld & Engel 1991). This model might be useful in defining the antigen(s) to which cyto-toxic lymphocytes are sensitised in PM or IBM.

While IBM has some features indicating that an autoimmune cytotoxic damage to muscle fibres mediated by CD8+ lymphocytes is present (Engel & Arahata 1984), it is by no means clear whether this is a primary or secondary event. There are several features that raise the possibility that IBM is not a primary inflammatory myopathy and that the inflammatory features are secondary. In up to 50–70% of the cases no major inflammatory cell response is present, class 1 MHC expression is patchy and inconsistent and immunosuppression has no beneficial effect. Furthermore, recent evidence that the inclusions contain a β-amyloid-like material and the ubiquitination of the inclu-sions raises the question of a primary degenerative disorder that creates β-amyloid as a by-product. There may be a parallel mechanism to β-amyloid formation in the brain in Alzheimer's disease and that of muscle in IBM.

It appears that the most important pathological event in IBM is myonuclear destruction and possibly mitochondrial damage. The progressive depletion of myonuclei leads to atrophy and eventually loss of muscle fibres.

THERAPY

The focus of attention here is on the idiopathic inflammatory myopathies. The main aim of therapy in DM or PM is to prevent major muscle damage and irreversible residual weakness by the time the disease spontaneously subsides and also to provide the patient with improved muscular function and freedom from discomfort during the active stage of the disease. There is no consensus regarding the precise treatment regimes for the different types of inflammatory myopathies and it appears that each major neuromuscular group follows a particular therapeutic plan (Rowland et al 1977, Karpati & Carpenter 1988, Dalakas 1989, 1991, Walton 1991).

Adult dermatomyositis

Specific (drug, etc.) and non-specific (diet, exercise) measures should be considered. The mainstay of treatment is glucocorticoids (Dalakas 1988b) and immunosuppressants. The dosage and combination of the drugs and the duration of treatment depend mainly on the severity of the case.

Many types of treatment regimens have been advocated by different groups. At the Montreal Neurological Hospital the following principles have been adopted. Patients are started on azathioprine 2–3 mg/kg/day orally and on oral prednisone that does not exceed a total daily dose of 30 mg/day. If there is an actual or suspected presence of malignancy, azathioprine is not administered. If the severity of the disease requires additional corticosteroids, we provide that in the form of intermittent intravenous large dose solumedrol up to 1 g once or twice per week. This mode of administration is somewhat inconvenient and more costly than the oral one, but it is largely free of the prohibitive side-effects of high-dose oral corticosteroids. Several factors can potentiate the deleterious side-effects of high-dose oral corticosteroids (Dalakas 1990b), including poor protein nutrition, old age and disuse. These factors are often present, particularly in DM. Thus, it is not an uncommon occurrence to find that in a severe case of DM, particularly in a malnourished and elderly person who is no longer able to walk, large oral doses of prednisone are capable of controlling the pathological process of DM; however, the patient may end up worse off than before the treatment due to a devastating steroid-induced myopathy.

Azathioprine administration should continue for at least 2 years but the dosage is usually lowered in the second year. Careful follow-up of liver function and of haematological profiles is mandatory at frequent intervals. In about 5–10% of the patients azathioprine induces an increase of serum activity of liver enzymes which compels withdrawal. The prednisone dose is lowered after 3 months of treatment but is not stopped for at least 1 year or longer. In fact, most patients require some steroid administration for 2–3 years or even longer. If one uses only low-dose oral steroids, alternate-day dosage does not seem to make a great deal of difference. The guidance for adjustment of corticosteroids and immunosuppressive therapy is primarily dictated by the clinical picture, as well as serum CK activity.

If the patient cannot tolerate azathioprine, alternate immunosuppression in the form of cyclosporin A or cyclophosphamide or methotrexate can be used but none of them are superior in therapeutic effect to azathioprine and most have more side-effects and are more cumbersome to administer.

If after tapering or cessation of treatment there is a relapse, one has to start the therapeutic regimen all over again at a dosage range that will be determined by the severity of the relapse.

In relatively rare cases, resistant to the above treatment regimen, or in those who cannot tolerate it, other treatment modalities may be tried. These include large-dose intravenous immunoglobulins (Jan et al 1990) and plasma exchange (Dau 1981, Miller et al 1992). The latter, however, has not been helpful in a moderately large cohort of patients and experience with large-dose intermittent intravenous immunoglobulins is only anecdotal. In extreme situations X-irradiation of the lymphatic system has been found useful (Engel et al 1981, Dalakas & Engel 1988, Kelley et al 1988).

Non-specific measures are equally important in management. A high protein diet, muscle-building exercises and correction of anaemia are essential elements through which damaged muscle can be helped to repair itself and optimal regeneration can be expected. In DM the skin can be treated by topical corticosteroids. In addition, avoidance of direct sunlight is essential.

Polymyositis

The principles and practice of management are quite similar to those in DM. The risk of steroid side-effects, however, appears to be less serious than in DM and, therefore, somewhat larger doses of oral steroids may be possible.

Childhood dermatomyositis

The mainstay of treatment is prednisone in 2 mg/kg/day dosage but tapering should be done as soon as possible, since growth retardation in children is a serious problem. In severe or resistant cases, prednisone should be supplemented with oral or intravenous methotrexate (oral dose = 15 mg/week).

Inclusion body myositis

In this disease administration of prednisone produces no significant or long-term benefit. In fact, in many patients prednisone tends to cause pronounced rapid deterioration. The occasional patient, particularly if the inflammatory element in the muscle is pronounced, may respond with some improvement and stabilisation to steroid administration. Azathioprine and other immunosuppressants are not of proven benefit. In fact no effective treatment can be provided at the present time for patients suffering from IBM, except palliative measures in the form of footdrop braces, tendon transfers in advanced cases and physiotherapy.

Miscellaneous

In some of the microbial inflammatory myopathies specific treatment is available. In trichinella myositis thiabendazole is effective. Active toxoplasmosis responds to a combination of pyrimethamine and sulphadiazine. Folate supplementation is required with the use of these drugs.

The treatment of inflammatory myopathies in the overlap syndromes or granulomatous diseases should include intensive management of the systemic disorder plus the regimen outlined for DM or PM.

In HIV-PM azathiaprine is not used, but the mainstay of treatment is with prednisone and zidovudine.

REFERENCES

Albrecht S, Bilbao J M 1992 Ubiquitin expression in inclusion body myositis. Modern Pathology (in press)

Antony J H, Procopis P G, Ouvrier R A 1979 Benign acute childhood myositis. Neurology 29: 1068

Arahata K, Engel A G 1984 Monoclonal antibody analysis of mononuclear cells in myopathies. I: Quantitation of subsets according to diagnosis and sites of accumulation and demonstration and counts of muscle fibers invaded by T cells. Annals of Neurology 16: 193

Arahata K, Engel A G 1986 Monoclonal antibody analysis of mononuclear cells in myopathies. III Immunoelectron microscopy aspects of cell-mediated muscle fiber injury. Annals of Neurology 19: 112

Arahata K, Engel A G 1988 Monoclonal antibody analysis of mononuclear cells in myopathies. IV: cell-mediated cytoxicity and muscle fiber necrosis. Annals of Neurology 22: 168

Askanas V, Serarogul P, Engel W K, Alvarez R B 1991 Immunolocalization of ubiquitin in muscle biopsies of patients with inclusion body myositis and oculopharyngeal muscular dystrophy. Neuroscience Letters 130: 73

Askanas V, Engel W K, Alvarez R B 1992 Beta-amyloid protein immunoreactivity in muscle of patients with inclusion body myositis. Lancet 339: 560

Banker B Q, Engel A G 1986 The polymyositis and dermatomyositis syndromes. In: Engel A G, Banker B Q (eds) Myology. McGraw-Hill, New York, p 1385

Basset-Seguin N, Roujeau J C, Gherardi R, Guillaume J C, Revuz J, Touraine R 1990 Prognosis factors and predictive signs of malignancy in adult dermatomyositis. Archives of Dermatology 126: 633

Bernstein R M, Morgan S H, Chapman J et al 1984 Anti-Jo-1 antibody: a marker for myositis with interstitial lung disease. British Medical Journal 289: 151

Bharucha N E, Morgan-Hughes J A 1981 Chronic focal polymyositis in the adult. Journal of Neurology, Neurosurgery and Psychiatry 44: 419

Callen J P 1988 Malignancy in polymyositis/dermatomyositis. Clinical Determatology 2: 55

Carpenter S 1988 Resin histology and electron microscopy in inflammatory myopathies. In: Dalakas M C (ed) Polymyositis and dermatomyositis. Butterworths, Boston, pp 195–215

Carpenter S, Karpati G, Rothman S, Watters G 1976 The childhood type of dermatomyositis. Neurology 26: 92

Carpenter S, Karpati G, Heller I, Eisen A 1978 Inclusion body myositis: a distinct variety of idiopathic inflammatory myopathy. Neurology 28: 8

Carpenter S, Karpati G 1981 The major inflammatory myopathies of unknown cause. Pathology Annuals 16: 205

Carpenter S, Karpati G 1984 Pathology of skeletal muscle. Churchill Livingstone, New York

Carpenter S, Karpati G 1992 The pathological diagnosis of specific inflammatory myopathies. Brain Pathology 2: 13

Carpenter S, Karpati G, Johnston W, Shoubridge E, Gavel M 1992 Coexistence of polymyositis (PM) with mitochondrial myopathy (MM). Neurology 42: (Suppl 3) 388 (abstract)

Chad D, Good P, Adelman L, Bradley W G, Mills J 1982 Inclusion body myositis associated with Sjögren's syndrome. Archives of Neurology 39: 186

Chiedozi, I C 1979 Polymyositis. Review of 205 cases in 112 patients. American Journal of Surgery 137: 255

Cole A J, Kuzniecky R, Karpati G, Carpenter S, Andermann E, Andermann F 1988 Familial myopathy with changes resembling inclusion body myositis and periventricular leucoencephalopathy. Brain 111: 1025

Cronin M E, Plots P H, Miller F W 1988 Abnormalities of the immune system in the idiopathic inflammatory myopathies. In Vivo 2: 25

Dalakas, M C (ed) 1988a Polymyositis and dermatomyositis. Butterworths, Boston

Dalakas M C 1988b Treatment of polymyositis and dermatomyositis with corticosteroids: a first therapeutic approach. In: Dalakas M C (ed) Polymyositis and dermatomyositis. Butterworths, Boston, p 235

Dalakas M C 1988c A classification of polymyositis and dermatomyositis. In: Dalakas M C (ed) Polymyositis and dermatomyositis. Butterworths, Boston, p 1

Dalakas M C 1989 Treatment of polymyositis and dermatomyositis. Current Opinion in Rheumatology 1: 443

Dalakas M C 1990a Inflammatory myopathies. Current Opinion in Neurology and Neurosurgery 3: 689

Dalakas M C 1990b Pharmacologic concerns of corticosteroids in the treatment of patients with immune-related neuromuscular diseases. Neurologic Clinics 8: 93

Dalakas M 1991 Polymyositis, dermatomyositis and inclusion-body myositis. New England Journal of Medicine 325: 1487

Dalakas M C, Engel W K 1988 Total body irradiation in the treatment of intractable polymyositis/dermatomyositis. In: Dalakas M C (ed) Polymyositis and dermatomyositis. Boston, Butterworths, pp 281–291

Dalakas M C, Pezeshkpour G H 1988 Neuromuscular diseases associated with human immunodeficiency virus infection. Annals of Neurology 23(S): 38

Dalakas M C, Illa I, Pezeshkpour G H, Laukaitis J P, Cohen B, Griffin J L 1990 Mitochondrial myopathy caused by long-term zidovudine therapy. New England Journal of Medicine 322: 1098

Dalakas M, Illa I 1991 HIV-associated myopathies. In: Pizzo A, Wilfelt C M (eds) Pediatric AIDS. Baltimore, Williams & Wilkins, p 420

Danon M J, Perurena O H, Ronan S, Manaligod J R 1986 Inclusion body myositis associated with systematic sarcoidosis. Canadian Journal of Neurological Science 13: 334

Dau P C 1981 Plasmapharesis in idiopathic inflammatory myopathies. Archives of Neurology 38: 544

De Visser M, Emslie-Smith A M, Engel A G 1989 Early ultrastructural alterations in adult dermatomyositis: capillary abnormalities precede other structural changes in muscle. Journal of Neurological Science 94: 181

Doyle D R, McCurley T L, Sergent J S 1983 Fatal polymyositis in D-penicillamine-treated rheumatoid arthritis. Annals of Internal Medicine 98: 327

Eisen A, Berry K, Gibson G 1983 Inclusion body myositis (IBM): myopathy or neuropathy? Neurology 33: 109

Emslie-Smith A M, Arahata K, Engel A G 1989 Major histocompatibity complex class 1 antigen expression, immunolocalization of interferon subtypes and T-cell-mediated cytotoxicity in myopathies. Human Pathology 20: 224

Emslie-Smith A M, Engel A G 1990 Microvascular changes in early and advanced dermatomyositis: a quantitative study. Annals of Neurology 27: 343

Emslie-Smith A M, Engel A G 1991 Necrotizing myopathy with pipestem capillaries, microvascular deposition of the complement membrane attack complex (MAC) and minimal cellular infiltrations. Neurology 41: 936

Emslie-Smith A M, Engel A G, Duffy J, Bowles C A 1991 Eosinophylia-myalgia syndrome I. Immunocytochemical evidence for a T-cell mediated immune effector response. Annals of Neurology 29: 524

Engel A G, Arahata K 1984 Monoclonal antibody analysis of mononuclear cells in myopathies. II Phenotypes of autoinvasive cells in polymyositis and inclusion body myositis. Annals of Neurology 16: 209

Engel A G, Arahata K 1986 Mononuclear cells in myopathies: quantitation of functionally distinct subsets, recognition of antigen-specific cell-mediated cytotoxicity in some diseases, and implications for the pathogenesis of the different inflammatory myopathies. Human Pathology 17: 704

Engel A G, Banker B Q 1986 Myology. New York, McGraw-Hill, p 1385

Engel A G, Emslie-Smith A M 1989 Inflammatory myopathies. Current Opinion in Neurology and Neurosurgery 2: 695

Engel A G, Arahata K, Emslie-Smith A 1990 Immune effector mechanisms in inflammatory myopathies. Research Publications — Association for Research in Nervous and Mental Disorders 68: 141

Engel W K, Lichter A S, Galdi A P 1981 Polymyositis: remarkable response to total body irradiation. Lancet i: 658 (letter)

Foote R A, Kimbrough S M, Stevens J C 1982 Lupus myositis. Muscle and Nerve 5: 65

Gamboa E T, Eastwood A B, Hays A P, Maxwell J, Penn A S 1979 Isolation of influenza virus from muscle in myoglobinuric polymyositis. Neurology 29: 1323

Goudreau G, Karpati G, Carpenter S 1988 Inflammatory myopathy in association with chronic myelopathy in HTLV I seropositive patients. Neurology 38(suppl 1): 206

Griggs C R, Karpati G 1991 The pathogenesis of dermatomyositis. Archives of Neurology 48: 21

Guttman L, Govindan S, Riggs J E, Schochet S S 1985 Inclusion body myositis and Sjögren's syndrome. Archives of Neurology 42: 1021

Haupt H M, Hutchins G M 1982 The heart and cardiac conduction system in polymyositis-dermatomyositis: a clinicopathologic study of 16 autopsied patients. American Journal of Cardiology 50: 998

Heffner R R, Armbrustmacher V W, Earle K M 1977 Focal myositis. Cancer 40: 301

Hertzman P A, Blevins W L, Mayer J, Greenfield B, Ting M, Gleich G J 1990 Association of the eosinophilia-myalgia syndrome with the ingestion of tryptophan. New England Journal of Medicine 322: 869

Hochberg M C, Feldman D, Stevens M B, Arnett F C, Reichlin M 1984 Antibody to Jo-1 in polymyositis/dermatomyositis: association with interstitial pulmonary disease. Journal of Rheumatology 11: 663

Hohlfeld R, Engel A G 1991 Coculture with autologous myotubes of cytoxic T cells isolated from muscle in inflammatory myopathies. Annals of Neurology 29: 498

Hohlfeld R, Engel A G, Li K, Harper M C 1991 Polymyositis mediated by T lymphocytes that express the γ/δ receptor. New England Journal of Medicine 324: 877

Illa I, Nath A, Dalakas M 1991 Immunocytochemical and virological characteristics of HIV associated inflammatory myopathies: similarities with seronegative polymyositis. Annals of Neurology 29: 474

Ishii K, Yamato K, Iwahara Y et al 1991 Isolates of HTLV-1 from muscle of a patient with polymyositis. American Journal of Medicine 90: 267

Jan S, Beretta S, Maggio M, Alobbati L, Pellegrini G 1990 High-dose intravenous human immunoglobulin in treatment-resistant polymyositis. Neurology 40(S): 120

Joy J L, Oh S J, Baysal A I 1990 Electrophysiological spectrum of inclusion body myositis. Muscle and Nerve 13: 949

Karpati G, Carpenter S 1988 Idiopathic inflammatory myopathies. Current Opinion in Neurology and Neurosurgery 1: 804

Karpati G, Pouliot Y, Carpenter S 1988 Expression of immunoreactive major histocompatibility complex products in human skeletal muscles. Annals of Neurology 23: 64

Kelley J J, Macdoc-Jones H, Andelman L S, Andres P L, Munsat T L 1988 Response to total body irradiation in dermatomyositis. Muscle and Nerve 11: 120

Kimura J 1989 Electrodiagnosis in diseases of nerve and

muscle: Principles and practice, 2nd edn. F A Davis, Philadelphia, p 547

Kissel J T, Mendell J R, Rammohan K W 1986 Microvascular deposition of complement membrane attack complex in dermatomyositis. New England Journal of Medicine 314: 329

Kissel J T, Burrow K L, Rammohan K W, Mendell J R, CIDD Group 1991a Mononuclear cell analysis of muscle biopsies in prednisone-treated and untreated Duchenne muscular dystrophy. Neurology 41: 667

Kissel J T, Halterman R K, Rammohan K W, Mendell J R 1991b The relationship of complement-mediated microvasculopathy to the histologic features and clinical duration of disease in dermatomyositis. Archives of Neurology 48: 26

Lakhanpal S, Bunch T W, Ilstrup D M, Melton L J 3rd 1989 Polymyositis-dermatomyositis and malignant lesions: does an association exist? Mayo Clinic Proceedings 61: 645

Lampert L, Illa I, Dalakas M 1990 In situ hybridization in muscle biopsies from patients with HIV-associated polymyositis (HIV-PM) using labelled HIV-RNA probes. Neurology 40 (suppl 1): 121 (abstract)

Layzer R B, Shearn M A, Satya-Murti S 1977 Eosinophilic polymyositis. Annals of Neurology 1: 65

Lotz B P, Engel A G, Nishino H, Stevens J C, Litcy W J 1989 Inclusion body myositis. Brain 112: 727

Love L A, Leff R L, Fraser D D et al 1991 A new approach to the classification of idiopathic inflammatory myopathy: myositis-specific autoantibodies define useful homogeneous patient groups. Medicine (Baltimore) 70: 360

McKee D, Karpati S, Johnston 1992 Familial inclusion body myositis (IBM) mimics facioscapulohumeral dystrophy (FSHD). Neurology 42 (suppl 3): 302 (abstract)

Martin R W, Duffy J, Engel A G et al 1990 The clinical spectrum of the eosinophilia-myalgia syndrome associated with L-tryptophan ingestion. Annals of Internal Medicine 113: 124

Maselli R A, Richman D P, Wollmann R L 1991 Inflammation at the neuromuscular junction in myasthenia gravis. Neurology 41: 1497

Massa R, Weller B, Karpati G, Shoubridge E, Carpenter S 1991 Familial inclusion body myositis among Kurdish-Iranian Jews. Archives of Neurology 48: 519

Mastaglia F L, Ojeda V J 1985 Inflammatory myopathies. Annals of Neurology 17: 215, 317

Mastaglia F L and Walton J N 1992 Inflammatory myopathies. In: Mastaglia F L, Walton Lord J (eds) Skeletal muscle pathology, 2nd edn, Churchill Livingstone, Edinburgh, p 360

Medsger T A, Dawson W N, Masi A T 1979 The epidemiology of polymyositis. American Journal of Medicine 48: 715

Ménard D B, Haddad H, Blain J G, Beaudry R, Devroede G, Masse S 1976 Granulomatous myositis and myopathy associated with Crohn's disease. New England Journal of Medicine 295: 818

Mendell J R, Shahenk Z, Gales T, Paul L 1991 Amyloid filaments in inclusion body myositis. Archives of Neurology 48: 1229

Mhiri C, Baudrimont M, Bonne G et al 1991 Zidovudine myopathy: a distinctive disorder associated with mitochondrial dysfunction. Annals of Neurology 29: 606

Miller F W 1991 Humoral immunity and immunogenetics in the idiopathic inflammatory myopathies. Current Opinion in Rheumatology 3: 902

Miller F W, Twitty S A, Biswas T, Plotz P H 1990 Origin and regulation of a disease-specific autoantibody response. Journal of Clinical Investigation 85: 468

Miller F, Leitman S, Cronin M E et al 1992 Controlled trial of plasma exchange and leukapheresis in dermatomyositis. New England Journal of Medicine 326: 1380

Mimori R 1987 Scleroderma-polymyositis overlap syndrome: clinical and seriologic aspects. International Journal of Dermatology 26: 419

Morgan O StC, Rodgers-Johnson P, Mora C, Char G 1989 HTLV-1 and polymyositis in Jamaica. Lancet ii: 1184

Munsat T L, Piper D, Cancilla P, Mednick J 1972 Inflammatory myopathy with facioscapulohumeral distribution. Neurology 22: 335

Muscat I, Anthony P P, Cruikshank J G 1986 Non-tropical pyomyositis. Journal of Clinical Pathology 39: 1116

Nishino H, Engel A G, Rima B K 1989 Inclusion body myositis: the mumps virus hypothesis. Annals of Neurology 25: 260

Oddis C V, Medsger T A 1988 Relationship between serum creatine kinase level and corticosteroid therapy in polymyositis/dermatomyositis. Journal of Rheumatology 15: 807

Olney R K, Miller R G 1983 Inflammatory infiltration in Fukuyama type congenital muscular dystrophy. Muscle and Nerve 6: 75

Plots P H, Dalakas M, Leff R L, Love L A, Miller F W, Cronin M E 1989 Current concepts in the ideopathic inflammatory myopathies: polymyositis, dermatomyositis and related disorders. Annals of Internal Medicine 111: 143

Richardson J B, Callen J P 1989 Dermatomyositis and malignancy. Medical Clinics of North America 73: 1211

Ringel S P, Forstot J Z, Tan E M, Wehling C, Griggs R C, Butcher D 1982 Sjögren's syndrome and polymyositis or dermatomyositis. Archives of Neurology 39: 157

Robinson L R 1991 Polymyositis. Muscle and Nerve 14: 310

Roddy S M, Ashwal S, Peckham N, Mortensen S 1986 Infantile myositis: a case diagnosed in the neonatal period. Pediatric Neurology 2: 241

Rosenberg N L 1991 Polymyositis and dermatomyositis — myalgia and inclusion body myositis. Current Opinion in Neurology and Neurosurgery 4: 693

Rosenberg N L, Carry M R, Ringel S P 1988 Association of inflammatory myopathies with other connective tissue disorders and malignancies. In: Dalakas M C (ed) Polymyositis and dermatomyositis. Boston, Butterworths, p 37

Rosenberg N L, Rotbart H A, Abzug M J, Ringel S P, Levin M J 1989 Evidence for a novel picornavirus in human dermatomyositis. Annals of Neurology 26: 204

Rowland L P, Clark C, Olarte M 1977 Therapy for dermatomyositis and polymyositis. Advances in Neurology 17: 63

Rucheton M, Graafland H, Fanton H, Ursule J, Ferrier P, Larsen C J 1985 Presence of circulating antibodies against gag-gene MuLV proteins in patients with autoimmune connective tissue disorders. Virology 144: 468

Ruff R L, Secrist D 1982 Viral studies in benign acute childhood myositis. Archives of Neurology 39: 261

Shepherd J J 1983 Tropical myositis: is it an entity and what is its cause? Lancet ii: 1240

Shevell M, Rosenblatt B, Silver K, Carpenter S, Karpati G 1990 Congenital inflammatory myopathy. Neurology 40: 1111

Simon, D B, Ringel S F, Sufit R I 1982 Clinical spectrum of fascial inflammation. Muscle and Nerve 5: 525

Targoff I N 1989 Immunologic aspects of myositis. Current Opinion in Rheumatology 1: 432

Targoff I N 1990 Immune mechanisms of myositis. Current Opinion in Rheumatology 2: 882

Tazelaar H D, Viggiano R W, Pickersgill J, Colby T V 1990 Interstitital lung disease in polymyositis and determatomyositis: clinical features and prognosis as correlated with histologic findings. American Review of Respiratory Diseases 141: 727

Thompson C E 1982 Infantile myositis. Developmental Medicine and Child Neurology 24: 307

Verma A, Bradley W G, Adesina A M, Sofferman R, Pendlebury W W 1991 Inclusion body myositis with cricopharyngeus muscle involvement and severe dysphagia. Muscle and Nerve 14: 470

Walker E J, Jeffrey P D 1988 Sequence homology between encephalomyocarditis virus protein VPI and histidyl-tRNA synthesase supports of hypothesis of molecular mimicry in polymyositis. Medical Hypotheses 25: 21

Walton J 1991 The idiopathic inflammatory myopathies and their treatment. Journal of Neurology, Neurosurgery and Psychiatry 54: 285

Wells A D, Fletcher M S, Teare E L, Walters H L, Yates-Bell A J 1985 Clostridial myositis of the psoas complicating nephrostomy. British Journal of Surgery 72: 582

Whitaker J N 1982 Inflammatory myopathy: a review of etiologic and pathogenetic factors. Muscle and Nerve 5: 573

Wiley C A, Nerenberg M, Cros D, Soto-Anguilar M C 1989 HTLV-1 polymyositis in a patient also infected with the human immunodeficiency virus. New England Journal of Medicine 320: 992

Wright J, Conconnai G, Hodges G R 1979 Adenovirus type 21 infection: concurrence with pneumonia, rhabdomyolysis and myoglobinuria in an adult. Journal of the American Medical Association 242: 2120

17. Metabolic and endocrine myopathies

R. T. Moxley III

The periodic paralyses
    Primary hypokalaemic periodic paralysis — Thyrotoxic periodic paralysis (TPP) — Hypokalaemic periodic paralysis secondary to urinary or gastrointestinal potassium wastage — Pharmacotherapy-related hypokalaemia — Hypokalaemia related to athletic training and profuse sweating — Barium-induced periodic paralysis — Primary hyperkalaemic periodic paralysis — Paramyotonia congenita — Secondary hyperkalaemic periodic paralysis — Normokalaemic sodium-responsive familial periodic paralysis — Periodic paralysis with cardiac arrhythmia — Histopathological alterations in periodic paralysis — Pathophysiological mechanisms in the periodic paralyses — Treatment of periodic paralyses

The glycogen storage diseases
    Glucose-6-phosphatase deficiency — Acid maltase deficiency — Debranching enzyme deficiency — Branching enzyme deficiency — Myophosphorylase deficiency — Phosphorylase b kinase deficiency — Muscle phosphofructokinase deficiency — Defects in the distal glycolytic pathway — Phosphoglycerate kinase deficiency — Phosphoglycerate mutase deficiency — Lactate dehydrogenase deficiency — Other glycogenoses

Malignant hyperthermia

Muscle AMP deaminase deficiency

Nutritional and toxic myopathies
    Nutritional deficiencies — Myopathy in chronic alcoholism — Other drug-induced myopathies

Diseases associated with myoglobinuria

Endocrine disorders of muscle
    Muscle disorders associated with hyperthyroidism — Muscular disorders in hypothyroidism — Muscle disorders associated with hyperparathyroidism and with osteomalacia — Myopathy associated with hypoparathyroidism — Diseases of the pituitary and suprarenal glands

THE PERIODIC PARALYSES

The recent discovery of the primary structure of the adult human skeletal muscle voltage-dependent sodium channel has led to the discovery of specific gene lesions in different portions of the channel structure that are associated primarily with the potassium-sensitive periodic paralyses (Table 17.1). The gene lesion responsible for the hereditary form of hypokalaemic periodic paralysis appear to involve the DHP-sensitive skeletal muscle calcium channel. Clinical and laboratory investigations are in progress to determine the relationship between the phenotype and the genotype in families having different forms of muscle disease with known gene defects affecting the skeletal muscle sodium channel. Similar investigations are likely to occur in families with hypokalaemic paralysis.

For the present it is convenient to classify the periodic paralyses as primary or secondary and, according to associated changes in the serum K^+ level, as hypokalaemic, normokalaemic or hyperkalaemic. The different types of periodic paralysis share several common features. Paralytic attacks may last from less than 1 hour to several days. Weakness can be localised or generalised. The deep tendon reflexes are diminished or lost in the course of the attacks. The muscle fibres become unresponsive to either direct or indirect electrical stimulation during attacks. The generalised attacks usually begin in proximal muscles and then spread to distal ones. Respiratory and cranial muscles tend to be spared but eventually may also be paralysed. Rest after exercise tends to provoke weakness of the muscles that had been exercised, but continued mild exercise may abort attacks.

Table 17.1   Clinical classification of various forms of periodic paralysis

Features	Hypokalaemic periodic paralysis	Thyrotoxic hypokalaemic periodic paralysis	Hyperkalaemic periodic paralysis — without myotonia	Hyperkalaemic periodic paralysis — with myotonia	Hyperkalaemic periodic paralysis with cardiac arrhythmia	Paramyotonia congenita	Paramyotonia congenita with hyperkalaemic periodic paralysis
Inheritance	Dominant or sporadic	Sporadic (occasional dominant)	Dominant	Dominant	Dominant	Dominant	Dominant
Gene defect	Skeletal muscle calcium channel	Unknown	Skeletal muscle sodium channel	Skeletal muscle sodium channel	Unknown	Skeletal muscle sodium channel	Skeletal muscle sodium channel
Age of onset	1st to 3rd decades	3rd decade (males 20:1)	1st decade	1st decade	1st and 2nd decades	1st decade	1st decade
Myopathy	Moderately common late; vacuoles frequent seen on biopsy	Infrequent	Infrequent	Infrequent	Yes; short stature; dysmorphic features; ventricular bigeminy	Rare	Rare
Myotonia							
Mechanical	No (occasional lid-lag)	No (occasional lid-lag)	No	Yes (especially paradoxical eyelid myotonia)	No	Yes (especially paradoxical eyelid myotonia)	Yes (especially paradoxical eyelid myotonia)
Electrical	No	No	No	Yes	No (rarely the tongue)	Yes	Yes
Potassium-sensitive	No	No	Yes	Yes	Yes (weakens skeletal muscle but occasionally normalises cardiac arrhythmia)	No	Yes
TTX depolarisation block	No, but increased gNa and reduced excitability	Not reported	Yes	Yes	Not known	Yes	Not known
Provocative factors	High carbohydrate meals, rest after exercise, cold, emotional excitement	High carbohydrate meals, rest after exercise, acetazolamide	Rest after exercise, oral potassium	Rest after exercise, cold, oral potassium	Rest after exercise, cold, menses, oral potassium	Cold exposure followed by exercise	Rest after exercise, cold exposure followed by exercise, oral potassium
Palliative factors	Acetazolamide, dichlorophenamide, potassium, spironolactone	Propranolol, restoration of euthyroid state, oral potassium, spironolactone	Mild exercise, glucose, acetazolamide, dichlorophenamide	Mild exercise, glucose, thiazides, acetazolamide, dichlorophenamide	Mild exercise, glucose, high sodium intake, acetazolamide, dichlorophenamide, imipramine	Mexilitene, tocainide, glucose, mild exercise	Mild exercise, thiazides, mexilitine, tocainide

Exposure to cold may provoke weakness in the primary forms of the disease. Complete recovery usually occurs after initial attacks. Permanent weakness and irreversible pathological changes in muscle can develop after repeated attacks.

Primary hypokalaemic periodic paralysis

The disease is transmitted by an autosomal dominant gene on chromosome one that appears to involve the DHP-sensitive skeletal muscle calcium channel (Fontaine et al 1994). The attacks typically begin in the first or second decade and about 60% of the patients are affected before the age of 16 years. Initially the attacks tend to be infrequent, but eventually may recur daily. Diurnal fluctuations in strength may then appear, so that the patient shows the greatest weakness during the night or in the early morning hours and gradually gains strength as the day passes (Allott & McArdle 1938, Engel et al 1965). In major attacks the serum potassium level decreases, but not always to below normal, and there is urinary retention of sodium, potassium, chloride and water (Biemond & Daniels 1934, Aitken et al 1937, Allott & McArdle 1938, Ferrebee et al 1938). Oliguria or anuria develop during such attacks and the patients tend to be constipated. Sinus bradycardia and electrocardiographic (ECG) signs of hypokalaemia (U waves in leads II, V-2, V-3 and V-4, progressive flattening of T waves and depression of the ST segment) appear when the serum potassium falls below normal (Van Buchem 1957, Weisler 1961). In the fourth and fifth decades the attacks become less frequent and may cease altogether. However, repeated attacks may leave the patient with permanent residual weakness (Bekeny 1961, Pearson 1964, Engel et al 1965, Howes et al 1966, Odor et al 1967). The metabolic defect in this form of the disease can be exacerbated or provoked by a high dietary intake of sodium or carbohydrate and by emotional excitement (Aitken et al 1937, Ferrebee et al 1938, Talbott 1941, McArdle 1956, Rowley & Kliman 1960, Shy et al 1961, Engel et al 1965).

The diagnosis is supported by a positive family history and a low serum potassium during major attacks. Depressed serum potassium levels between attacks suggest secondary rather than pri-

Table 17.2 Hand exercise testing for periodic paralysis

Hand exercise with ulnar nerve stimulation (McManis et al 1986)

1. Surface electrodes record the amplitude of the compound muscle action potential (CMAP) from hypothenar muscles given supramaximal stimuli (20–30% over maximal) delivered to the ulnar nerve at the wrist every 30–60 seconds for a period of 2–5 minutes until a stable baseline amplitude is recorded
2. Next the patient contracts his hypothenar muscles isometrically for 2–5 minutes with brief (3–4 second) rest periods every 15 seconds
3. The amplitude of the CMAP is recorded after each minute of exercise (with the muscle relaxed) and then every 1–2 minutes after exercise for a period of 30 minutes or until no further decrease in amplitude occurs
4. Percentage changes in amplitude are calculated as noted:

$$\text{Increase} = \frac{\text{Greatest amplitude after exercise} - \text{amplitude before exercise}}{\text{Amplitude before exercise}}$$

$$\text{Decrease} = \frac{\text{Greatest amplitude after exercise} - \text{smallest amplitude after exercise}}{\text{Greatest amplitude after exercise}}$$

Comment: A decrease of 40% in the amplitude of CMAP after 2–5 minutes of exercise is abnormal and occurs in primary and secondary periodic paralysis and in paramyotonia congenita. However, not all patients have a positive test and some patients are not consistently abnormal on repeated testing. Positive findings in this test help to confirm the clinical suspicion of periodic paralysis (McManis et al 1986 Muscle & Nerve 9: 704–710). This test can be repeated to show improvement in muscle response to a given treatment regimen

mary hypokalaemic periodic paralysis. Tables 17.2 and 17.3 provide an outline of exercise testing (local hand exercise and bicycle ergometry), and Table 17.4 describes hypokalaemia challenge testing. If these tests fail to induce an attack in adults, 30 minutes of bicycle exercise and salt loading (2 g sodium chloride in aqueous solution given orally every hour for a total of 4 doses) may prove effective. Depression of the serum potassium level during the induced attack and a favourable response to 2.5–7.5 g of potassium chloride given orally must be demonstrated. Negative results do not exclude the diagnosis. Glucose and insulin must never be given to patients who are already hypokalaemic and potassium must not be given unless the patient has adequate renal and adrenal reserve. Table 17.4 mentions two specialised provocative tests, the euglycaemic insulin infusion and intra-arterial epinephrine tests, which may be particularly useful

Table 17.3   Bicycle testing for periodic paralysis

Bicycle ergometry testing — 30 minute test (Kantola & Tarssanen, 1992)

1. Patient is tested in early afternoon or late morning. Breakfast is allowed but no strenuous exercise before the test. Each patient lies supine for 15–30 minutes before exercise while baseline ECG monitoring is started. An indwelling intravenous catheter is placed for the collection of free-flowing blood samples. Duplicate samples for potassium are collected at 10 and 5 minutes before the exercise test; at 3, 6, 10, 20 and 30 minutes during the test; and at 3 and 10 minutes after the test
2. Exercise is performed on a bicycle ergometer with the patient seated. The exercise load for men is 100 watts and for women 80 watts. Pedal speed in maintained at 60 r.p.m. No training on the ergometer is allowed. The ECG is monitored throughout all stages of test.
3. After completion of the exercise each patient rests supine for 10 minutes.

Comment: This test is helpful in identifying some patients with hypokalaemic periodic paralysis. The degree of rise in plasma potassium above baseline was significantly low in 11 patients with hypokalaemic periodic paralysis, 0.3 ± 0.1 mmol/l compared to 23 age matched normal controls, 0.8 ± 0.2 mmol/l (Kantola & Tarssanen, 1992). Nine asymptomatic family members out of 105 asymptomatic family members tested had a positive test. Four of these asymptomatic positive testers had muscle biopsies and all showed vacuolar changes despite the absence of definite attacks of weakness. It is noted by Katola and Tarssanen (Neurology 1992; 42: 2158–2161) that patients with hyperkalaemic periodic paralysis and paramyotonia congenita have not yet been systematically tested. Various drugs interfere with this test including beta-agonists, beta-blockers, diuretics, and digitalis

but should be performed by those quite familiar with the techniques. The euglycaemic insulin infusion protocol permits the simultaneous infusion of a fixed dose of insulin in combination with a variable rate of glucose infusion which maintains euglycaemia (Moxley et al 1984). During the controlled insulin infusion serum potassium normally falls over 30–60 minutes and reaches a stable nadir. With very high, supraphysiological doses of insulin the decline in plasma potassium does not fall below 3.0 mmol/l in normal individuals (Minaker & Rowe 1982). Euglycaemic insulin infusion at low physiological and, if necessary, at high physiological rates of insulin infusion has proven to be an easily performed, safe means by which a decline in serum potassium can be induced

and rapidly corrected if an attack of weakness ensues (Minaker et al 1988). The intra-arterial epinephrine test is particularly useful (Engel et al 1965). This local infusion permits a regional decline in serum potassium in blood bathing the forearm and intrinsic hand muscles without producing a significant decline in whole body arterial potassium. This approach produces a focal attack of weakness. Epinephrine (2 µg/min) is infused into the brachial artery for 5 minutes and the amplitude of the evoked compound muscle action potential is recorded from perfused small hand muscles at intervals before, during and for 30 minutes after the infusion. The test, which is positive when the amplitude of the evoked compound potential decreases by more than 30% within 10 minutes after the infusion, is essentially specific for primary hypokalaemic periodic paralysis.

Thyrotoxic periodic paralysis (TPP)

This type resembles the primary hypokalaemic form with regard to changes in serum and urinary electrolytes during attacks and in its response to glucose, insulin and potassium. Carbohydrate ingestion is often a precipitating factor, typically a late night meal (Gastel & Ehrlichman 1978, Conway et al 1974). TPP is six times more common in males than in females. Approximately 75% of the cases occur in orientals; 85% of the patients first exhibit the attacks between the ages of 20 and 39 years, 95% of cases are sporadic and, in all, the attacks cease when the euthyroid state is restored (Engel 1961b). A predisposing genetic factor in Chinese patients is suggested by an increased association with certain HLA haplotypes (Yeo et al 1978, Liu et al 1991). Natural or induced recurrence of the hypermetabolic state causes recurrence of the paralytic attacks (Dunlap & Kepler 1931, Robertson 1954, Okihiro & Nordyke 1966).

Hypokalaemic periodic paralysis secondary to urinary or gastrointestinal potassium wastage

Hypokalaemia, defined as a reduction in plasma potassium concentration to less than 3.5 mmol/l, may be due to a redistribution of potassium away

Table 17.4 Hypokalaemia-provocative testing in patients suspected of having periodic paralysis (adapted from Griggs)

Initial testing:
- Following an overnight fast — *oral glucose load* 1.5 g/kg (maximum of 100 g) over 3 minutes

Monitoring (*with patient at rest*)	1. Obtain free flowing arterialized blood every 30 minutes — baseline to up to 3 hours — for K, Na, Cl, CO_2, glucose, then every 60 minutes to 5 hours postglucose ingestion
	2. Assess strength at 30 minute intervals in four to six muscles based on history of weakness during attacks
	3. Check electrocardiogram every 30 minutes or use continuous monitor if available

Comment The nadir in serum potassium after oral glucose usually coincides with or follows by 30 minutes the peak rise in serum glucose. Potassium levels in normals after oral glucose loading typically do not fall below 3.5 mmol/l. If weakness occurs, treat as indicated below. Challenge testing is best performed in hospital. (See comment below)

If no weakness or adverse effects and if no medical contraindications, follow initial testing with intravenous glucose load and insulin
- Following an overnight fast — infuse intravenously a glucose load of 3 g/kg (maximum of 200 g) in water (2 g/5ml) at a continuous rate over 1 hour. Give a bolus of intravenous insulin (0.1 unit/kg) 30 minutes after initiation of the glucose infusion, and again after 60 minutes

Monitoring (with patient at rest)	1. Obtain free-flowing arterialized blood every 30 minutes from baseline to 3 hours for K, Na, Cl, CO_2, glucose. Obtain additional blood for electrolytes at onset of weakness and every 10–15 minutes thereafter for serum K until the level returns to baseline
	2. Measure strength in muscles used in initial testing every 15 minutes for the initial 2 hours, then at 30 minute intervals for the next hour if no weakness has developed
	3. Check electrocardiogram every 15 minutes or use a continuous monitor if available

Comment: If an attack of weakness occurs, terminate the glucose infusion and maintain the intravenous line with normal saline. Give oral doses of KCl, 30–60 mmol in a sugar-free solution. Repeat oral doses of KCl until serum potassium has returned to baseline and is stable. If vomiting occurs, give intravenous KCl 35 mmol/l in 5% mannitol. Intravenous KCl is not necessary in most attacks. Avoid giving KCl with infusions containing glucose. The nadir for serum potassium usually occurs between 90 and 120 minutes after initiation of the intravenous glucose infusion. Hypoglycaemia can occur 45–60 minutes after completion of the intravenous glucose infusion. Intravenous loading tests require constant physician presence and should not be performed in patients with significant renal, cardiac, or hepatic disease or in diabetes. Intravenous infusion testing should be carried out when the patient is hospitalised

Table 17.4 *Contd*

Specialised provocative hormone infusion tests include:
- Euglycaemic insulin infusion over 2 hours started initially at an insulin dose of 20 mU/m^2/min
- Intrabranchial arterial infusion of epinephrine.

Comment: Both of these specialised tests should be performed in laboratories familiar with the procedures. These tests have the advantage of producing a more reproducible, controlled, fall in circulating potassium for either the whole body (e.g. euglycaemic insulin infusion) or for the forearm tissues (e.g. intrabrachial arterial infusion of epinephrine)

from the plasma into the intracellular compartments or it may be a part of potassium depletion, or it may result from a combination of these conditions (Norgaard & Kjeldsen 1991). Potassium depletion, defined as a reduction in skeletal muscle potassium concentration to less than 75 mmol/g wet weight, may be due to a reduction in the cellular potassium content without a concomitant reduction in cellular volume or mass (Norgaard & Kjeldsen 1991). Hypokalaemia and potassium depletion, individually or in combination, may be caused by a diuretic and other medical treatments, certain diseases, or an insufficient intake of potassium. A low serum potassium, ranging from 3.5 to 3.0 mmol/l, may be associated with whole body potassium depletion. The relationship between serum potassium and skeletal muscle potassium content is close but not exact. One important limitation in the use of serum potassium to give a reliable index of true mild hypokalaemia is related to inaccuracies in the measurement of serum potassium. Potassium may be unintentionally released from intracellular compartments during the collection of venous blood samples, released from platelets as the blood coagulates prior to centrifugation of the sample, or due to mild haemolysis. These factors alone may elevate serum potassium by 0.5 mmol/l or more. True potassium deficiency and mild hypokalaemia may also be masked in the presence of acidosis, renal failure or tissue destruction that is associated with the liberation of potassium. Poor and elderly patients are at special risk for developing hypokalaemia and potassium deficiency, not only because of an increased frequency of medical problems and the use of medications that may produce a potassium wasting, but also because most potassium-rich foods are expensive. Hypokalaemia in the range of 3.5–3.0 mmol/l typically produces fatigue, minimal weakness, myalgia and diminished tendon reflexes. Generalised weakness and frank paralysis do not occur until the serum potassium falls below 3.0 mmol/l. The diagnosis of potassium depletion can be assessed from needle biopsy measurements of muscle potassium (Norgaard & Kjeldsen 1991). The relationship of attacks to excessive ingestion of carbohydrate or sodium has not been clearly established. The diagnosis of excessive urinary potassium loss may be made if, with an average daily intake of sodium or potassium, the daily urinary potassium excretion exceeds 20 mmol on several consecutive days while the serum potassium remains less than 3.0 mmol/l at different times of the day (Mahler & Stanbury 1956, Brooks et al 1957). The normal daily faecal potassium excretion is usually small (10 mmol) (Danowski & Greenman 1953). Because the serum potassium is already decreased, provocative tests that may lower it further are contraindicated.

Mild hypokalaemia and chronic potassium deficiency lead to several potentially serious physiological problems. Ammonia excretion into the urine increases as a result of potassium deficiency (Baertl et al 1963) and eventually leads to the release of amino acids from skeletal muscle to provide glutamine for renal ammonia synthesis. This produces a negative nitrogen balance and loss of muscle ensues. Potassium deficiency further contributes to the loss of muscle tissue by reducing the release of insulin from beta cells (Conn 1965). Skeletal muscle blood flow is reduced by potassium deficiency during exercise since evidence shows that local release of potassium assists in mediating dilatation of arterioles (Knochel 1982). Normal concentrations of intracellular potassium are necessary to maintain glycogen synthesis (Knochel 1982). Studies in animals and man have shown that decreased potassium limits the normal increase in muscle synthesis of glycogen that follows physical conditioning. Diuretic therapy has been shown to depress muscle glycogen levels (Bergstrom & Hultman 1966). Detailed studies to establish precisely the role of potassium deficiency on skeletal muscle glycogen metabolism are needed. However, potassium deficiency may compromise the mobilisation of fuels for muscle contraction, especially during severe exhausting exercise, and may predispose those individuals to rhabdomyolysis. Severe potassium deficiency also compromises smooth muscle function and leads to a dynamic ileus and impairs the normal responses to pressors, such as catecholamines or angiotensin (Knochel 1984). The most serious complication of potassium deficiency is cardiac arrhythmia, especially in patients receiving concomitant digitalis therapy.

Various conditions to be considered in the differential diagnosis of secondary hypokalaemic periodic paralysis are listed in Table 17.5. In addition to periodic or non-periodic weakness, the non-specific effects of chronic potassium depletion may also be present. These include hyposthenuria, polydypsia and vasopressin-resistant polyuria (Conn 1955, Dustan et al 1956, Milne et al 1957, Manitius et al 1960). Chronic pyelonephritis and secondary hypertension leading to secondary aldosteronism and further potassium depletion may develop. Latent or manifest tetany can occur in several types of potassium depletion (Engel et al 1949, Conn 1955). Growth retardation and proportional dwarfism occur in patients whose potassium has been depleted since infancy (Van Buchem et al 1956, Bryan et al 1966).

Pharmacotherapy-related hypokalaemia

Significant hypokalaemia can occur in patients receiving treatment with beta-adrenergic agonists or theophylline (Norgaard & Kjeldsen 1991, Knochel 1987). The hypokalaemia resulting from epinephrine and norepinephrine as well as beta-adrenergic agonists is mediated by stimulation of the beta 2-receptor (Brown et al 1983). Beta 2-receptor agonists have been used for the treatment of patients with asthma and women with premature labour and have been shown to cause hypokalaemia, and terbutaline administration produces a significant fall in plasma potassium in the treatment of patients with respiratory problems. Recently terbutaline treatment has been shown to produce an increase in glucose and serum

Table 17.5 Differential diagnosis of secondary hypokalaemic periodic paralysis

---

Thyrotoxic periodic paralysis
Paralysis secondary to urinary potassium wastage
Hypertension, alkaline urine, metabolic alkalosis
  Primary hyperaldosteronism (Conn 1955)
  Liquorice intoxication (Salassa et al 1962, Achar et al 1989)
  Excessive thiazide therapy for hypertension (Cohen 1959, Knochel 1984)
  Excessive mineralocorticoid therapy for Addison's disease
Normotension, alkaline urine, metabolic alkalosis
  Hyperplasia of juxtaglomerular apparatus with hyperaldosteronism (Bryan et al 1966)
Alkaline urine, metabolic acidosis
  Primary renal tubular acidosis (Owen & Verner 1960)
  Fanconi's syndrome (Milne et al 1952)
Acid urine, metabolic acidosis
  Chronic ammonium chloride ingestion (Goulon et al 1962)
  Recovery phase of diabetic coma (Nabarro et al 1952)
  Bilateral ureterocolostomy (Sataline & Simonelli 1961)
  Recovery phase of acute renal tubular necrosis (Bull et al 1950)
Antibiotic therapy
  Amphotericin B, gentamicin, carbenicillin and ticarcillin (Knochel 1987)
Paralysis secondary to gastrointestinal potassium wastage
  Non-tropical sprue
  Laxative abuse (Schwartz & Relman 1953)
  Pancreatic gastrin-secreting adenoma with severe diarrhoea (Verner & Morrison 1958)
  Villous adenoma of the rectum (Keyloun & Grace 1967)
  Severe or chronic diarrhoea (Keye 1952)
  Draining gastrointestinal fistula
  Prolonged gastrointestinal intubation or vomiting
  Clay ingestion (Severance et al 1988)
  'Spitting' -making weight for wrestlers (Knochel 1987)
Pharmacotherapy
  Beta-adrenergic agonists
  Insulin
Athletic training and profuse sweating
Barium-induced periodic paralysis
  Insecticides and rat poison (Johnson & van Tassell 1991)

---

insulin concentrations along with the fall in serum potassium (Schnack et al 1989), and pretreatment with oral potassium failed to prevent these changes. Combination treatment with bronchodilators such as theophylline and a beta-adrenergic agonist, such as epinephrine (Whyte et al 1988) or albuterol (Lipworth et al 1989), has caused significant lowering of plasma potassium. Hypokalaemia related to beta-adrenergic agonist therapy may be responsible for some cases of unexpected death in asthmatic patients (Wong et al 1990). Hypokalaemia may be aggravated by stress-induced catecholamine responses and by

treatment with corticosteroids as well as with diuretics. Meticulous monitoring of plasma potassium is particularly important during intensive bronchodilator therapy of acute exacerbations of asthma, especially in patients already at risk for hypokalaemia and potassium depletion. Both epinephrine and norepinephrine at physiological concentrations stimulate potassium uptake by the sodium–potassium pump in skeletal muscle through activation of the beta-adrenergic receptors and cyclic AMP.

Insulin also stimulates the activation of the sodium–potassium pump and produces a fall in plasma potassium. Insulin-requiring patients with diabetes mellitus commonly have significant hypokalaemia. This can result from the combined effects of insulin and epinephrine on the sodium–potassium pump in skeletal muscle. A fall in blood glucose caused by insulin-induced hypoglycaemia may activate increased release of epinephrine and exacerbate a fall in plasma potassium which may already be low due to increased renal loss (Clausen & Everts 1989).

Hypokalaemia related to athletic training and profuse sweating

Super-trained athletes may demonstrate hypokalaemia due to a redistribution of potassium to the cellular compartment. The mechanism underlying this finding is unknown, but it is found that athletic training hyperpolarises skeletal muscle cells (Knochel 1987, Knochel et al 1985). Highly trained long-distance runners may have serum potassium levels as low as 2.8 mmol/l. In normal untrained individuals this would represent a moderately severe potassium deficiency. However, athletes have elevated intracellular potassium levels indicating that the hypokalaemia observed in highly trained long-distance runners does not reflect potassium deficiency (Knochel 1987). In contrast to highly trained athletes, normal individuals undergoing severe exhausting exercise may be at risk of developing hypokalaemia and in some individuals rhabdomyolysis develops (Knochel & Schlein 1972, Knochel 1982). Normally potassium is maintained in the range of 3.5–5.0 mmol/l in serum and approximately 160 mmol/l in cells.

All but approximately 2% of the 3500 mmol of total body potassium is contained within cells (Norgaard & Kjeldsen 1991). Because skeletal muscle represents the major reservoir of intracellular potassium, potassium depletion in skeletal muscle can alter the normal rise and fall of local extracellular potassium that is necessary to ensure a normal response to whole body exercise. During exercise the potassium concentration in the interstitial space of normal human skeletal muscle may reach 15 mmol/l (Vyskocil et al 1983), and the plasma potassium concentration can increase by 3–4 mmol/l within the first 10 minutes of exercise (Medbo & Sejersted 1990). Within the first minutes of rest after vigorous physical activity, the plasma potassium concentration may fall 0.5 mmol/l below the usual baseline concentration (Brown 1985). In conditions that produce potassium depletion the normal release of potassium from muscle during exercise is reduced. This in turn decreases normal vasodilatation and leads to muscle fatigue and muscle cell death. The hypokalaemia following exercise has been suspected to be a cause of sudden death in some individuals, especially those with pre-existing hypokalaemia (Nordrehaug and von der Lippe 1983, Brady et al 1989).

Physical exertion for long periods in extreme heat also produces hypokalaemia which primarily results from marked salt and water depletion in association with a significant overproduction of aldosterone (Knochel 1987). Athletes and heavy labourers generally have a high sodium intake. This facilitates renal sodium–potassium exchange and large quantities of potassium may be lost in the urine. This process may continue for several days despite the development of hypokalaemia and in turn can lead to severe potassium deficiency.

Hypokalaemia can occasionally occur in competitive wrestlers due to the practice of 'spitting'. In an attempt to make the proper weight to enter their weight class wrestlers expectorate all of their saliva. Typically they will chew wax flavoured with lemon drops. This may produce large volumes of saliva that exceed 4 litres over 24 hours (Knochel 1987). Potassium concentration averages 20 mmol/l in saliva and this can cause significant hypokalaemia.

Barium-induced periodic paralysis

Barium is a heavy divalent alkaline earth metal that occurs in its natural form as a barite ($BaFO_4$) and witherite ($BaCO_3$) and all water- or acid-soluble barium salts are poisonous (Johnson & Van Tassel 1991). Toxic barium salts are present in many industrial products as carbonates, hydroxides, fluorides, acetates, fluorides, chlorates and sulphides. Insecticides and rat poison are common toxins containing barium salts. The accidental ingestion of absorbable barium salts, such as barium carbonate, induces a haemorrhagic gastroenteritis, hypertension, cardiac arrhythmias, muscle twitching, convulsions, hypokalaemia and muscle paralysis. Barium blocks muscle potassium channels and thereby reduces potassium efflux from muscle; potassium uptake by muscle, mediated by the sodium–potassium pump, continues and hypokalaemia results (Lewi & Bar-Khayim 1964, Gallant 1983).

Primary hyperkalaemic periodic paralysis

The primary hyperkalaemic periodic paralyses represent a group of at least three separate disorders (hyperkalaemic periodic paralysis without myotonia; hyperkalaemic periodic paralysis with myotonia; hyperkalaemic periodic paralysis occurring with paramyotonia congenita). Table 17.1 outlines the major clinical and diagnostic features for these three forms of periodic paralysis as well as important management issues. These diseases are transmitted by an autosomal dominant gene with high penetrance in both sexes (Helweg-Larsen et al 1955, Gamstorp 1956, McArdle 1962, Layzer et al 1967a, Rüdel & Ricker 1985, Ricker et al 1986a, Streib 1987b, Ricker et al 1989, deSilva et al 1990). Rare sporadic cases have been reported (Dyken & Timmons 1963, Riggs et al 1981). Attacks usually begin in childhood and may be brief or last several days (Layzer et al 1967a, Rüdel & Ricker 1985). On average the attacks are shorter in duration and more frequent than those observed in hypokalaemic periodic paralysis. At the onset of the attack patients may develop myalgia. Patients having the form of hyperkalaemic periodic paralysis with myotonia frequently develop muscle stiffness and paradoxical myotonia of the eyelids during attacks of weakness. Similar symptoms occur in those patients having hyperkalaemic periodic paralysis in association with paramyotonia congenita (Rüdel & Ricker 1985). Most families with hyperkalaemic periodic paralysis manifest signs of myotonia, such as a sensation of tension in the back muscles at the onset of an attack, spontaneous runs of action potentials in the electromyogram (EMG), and lid-lag and occasionally eyelid myotonia. The smaller number of families having hyperkalaemic periodic paralysis without myotonia lack these myotonic signs. In the absence of an attack, clinical signs of myotonia, such as muscle stiffness, typically do not occur.

Electromyographic myotonia can be seen frequently. Prominent muscle stiffness typically occurs in those patients having hyperkalaemic periodic paralysis in association with paramyotonia congenita. The specific clinical difference which distinguishies this latter group of patients with periodic paralysis from those families having hyperkalaemic periodic paralysis with myotonia is the differential response of muscular activity. The stiffness and weakness which develops during rest after strenuous work in patients with hyperkalaemic periodic paralysis with myotonia can usually be worked off at the beginning of an attack. In contrast, the stiffness and weakness which occur in patients with paramyotonia congenita alone or in patients with hyperkalaemic periodic paralysis in association with paramyotonia congenita develops only during exercise in a cold environment and usually the weakness and stiffness are mild. Forceful contractions after cooling are required to produce marked paralysis of the muscle (Rüdel & Ricker 1985, Ricker et al 1986b, Ricker et al 1989). Myalgias (McArdle 1962), release of enzymes from muscle into serum and creatinuria (Mertens et al 1964, Hudson et al 1967) can occur during or after paralysis and a permanent myopathy may develop after repeated attacks (French & Kilpatrick 1957, Gruner & Porte 1959, Bekeny 1961, Hudson 1963, McArdle 1963, Pearson 1964, MacDonald et al 1968, Faugere et al 1981). During attacks the serum potassium increases (Gamstorp 1956, French & Kilpatrick 1957, Eagan & Klein 1959, Van der Meulen et al 1961, McArdle 1962, Samaha 1965,

Hudson et al 1967, Layzer et al 1967a, Ricker et al 1989) but may not exceed the normal range, and precordial T waves in the electrocardiogram (ECG) increase in amplitude (French & Kilpatrick 1957, Eagan & Klein 1959). Potassium, water and possibly sodium diuresis occurs during major attacks and the patient may complain of urinary urgency (Gamstorp 1956, Eagan & Klein 1959, Klein et al 1960, Carson & Pearson 1964, Mertens et al 1964). Hypocalcaemia was found during the paralysed state in three patients but their urinary calcium excretion was not studied (Dyken & Timmons 1963, Layzer et al 1967a). The metabolic defect is worsened by exposure to cold, fasting, pregnancy or by potassium administration (Gamstorp 1956, Drager et al 1958, McArdle 1962, Van't Hoff 1962, Herman & McDowell 1963, Hudson 1963, Layzer et al 1967a, Ricker et al 1986a, Streib 1987b, Ricker et al 1989, 1990).

Myotonic phenomena have been demonstrated in some patients and are especially prone to be present in levator palpebrae superioris and other external ocular muscles and in facial, lingual, thenar and finger extensor muscles (French & Kilpatrick 1957, Drager et al 1958, McArdle 1962, Van't Hoff 1962, Hudson 1963, Carson & Pearson 1964, Layzer et al 1967a, Rüdel & Ricker 1985, Ricker et al 1990). However, no myotonia was found in some patients who had all the other typical features of primary hyperkalaemic periodic paralysis (Gamstorp 1956, 1963, Rüdel & Ricker 1985). One report noted abnormal electrical irritability of muscle fibres (Buchthal et al 1958); however, more recent studies have shown an absence of muscle fibre irritability in intercostal muscle biopsies from patients with the nonmyotonic form of hyperkalaemic periodic paralysis (Lehmann-Horn et al 1983). A positive Chvostek sign is frequently observed in attacks (Gamstorp 1956).

The diagnosis of the various forms of primary hyperkalaemic periodic paralysis can be made by searching for the characteristic clinical features outlined in Table 17.1 and performing the provocative testing listed on Tables 17.4 and 17.6. All patients suspected of having some form of primary hyperkalaemic periodic paralysis require a forearm cooling and exercise test

Table 17.6 Hyperkalaemia provocative testing in patients suspected of having some form of potassium-sensitive periodic paralysis (adapted from Griggs)

Initial oral potassium load
• Following an overnight fast give 0.05 g/kg KCl in sugar-free solution over 3 minutes. (If test is negative, repeat testing on another day with a dose of 0.10–0.15 g/kg KCl)

Monitoring   1. Obtain free-flowing arterialised blood every 15 minutes for the initial 2 hours for measurement of K, Na, Cl, CO_2, glucose. Then obtain blood at 30 minute intervals for the next 2 hours if no signs of weakness have occurred. If weakness develops, obtain serum K at 10–15 minute intervals. Intravenous glucose can be given if there is a severe elevation of potassium (>6.5 mmol/l) or prolonged elevation (> 1 hour). As an alternative to intravenous glucose, administration of 100 g of oral glucose can be given. If serum potassium is 7.0 mmol/l or higher, 10–20 units of regular insulin should be administered. Hyperkalaemia usually resolves over 30–90 minutes and the weakness disappears gradually over a few hours
2. Check strength in four to six muscles every 15 minutes for the first 2 hours, then every 30 minutes for the next 2 hours
3. Check electrocardiogram at 15 minute intervals or use a continuous monitor if available

Comment: Often the higher dose of oral KCl, 0.10–0.15 g/kg, is necessary to provoke an attack of weakness. If this fails and suspicion remains high for potassium-sensitive periodic paralysis, use exercise with potassium loading. Oral potassium loading requires constant physician presence, and should not be performed in patients with significant renal, cardiac or hepatic disease or in diabetes. Measures for emergency treatment for hyperkalaemia should be available. Testing should be carried out with the patient hospitalised

Exercise-oral potassium challenge
• Following an overnight fast — have patient perform moderately high level bicycle exercise for 30 minutes (work for men 100 watts; women 80 watts; maintain pedal rate at 60 r.p.m.) then while the patient remains at rest give the high dose of oral KCl, 0.10–0.15 g/kg

Monitoring: Follow the exact protocol noted above
(with the   for oral
patient at rest) potassium loading

Comment: In normal individuals there is a transient rise in serum potassium during exercise with a return to baseline after approximately 30–45 minutes. In patients with hyperkalaemic periodic paralysis there is also an initial transient rise and fall in serum potassium after exercise. However, in these patients the potassium rises again from baseline within 30–90 minutes and climbs to values typically higher than the peak serum potassium observed during exercise

Table 17.7   Forearm cooling and exercise

Isometric forearm exercise before and after cooling (Ricker et al 1990)

This procedure allows for quantitation of changes in strength and in myotonia with exercise after 30 minutes of forearm cooling. This test is especially useful in identifying patients with paramyotonia congenita
1. The forearm and hand of the patient are placed in a trough in a supinated position with the fingers flexed so that the distal phalanges can grip a force transducer attached to the base of the trough
2. The forearm and hand are then secured in such a way to allow contraction of the flexor profundus muscle under isometric conditions
3. Wire electrodes are placed in the flexor profundus muscle 10 mm apart to record electromyographic activity
4. The protocol for exercise is carried out before the trough is filled with cold water, and then again after the forearm is cooled for 30 minutes in water kept at 14–15°C
5. The exercise protocol consists of 60 seconds of maximum isometric contraction interrupted by two 10 second rest periods, first after 20 seconds of exercise and again after 40 seconds of exercise

Comment: In paramyotonia congenita the force of contraction after exercise cooling falls to less than 20% of the force before cooling. A few hours or more are required to recover strength fully after rewarming. Patients with some forms of hyperkalaemic periodic paralysis show a similar decline in strength with exercise after cooling. However, they recover their strength within 45–60 minutes and do not show the prominent spontaneous activity in the EMG that occurs in patients with paramyotonia congenita as the muscle is cooled

(Table 17.7) since some families will have associated paramyotonia congenita. Occasionally the symptoms in patients with hyperkalaemic periodic paralysis will be difficult to distinguish from those of primary hypokalaemic periodic paralysis, and in this instance provocative testing to produce hypokalaemia will also be needed. The hand exercise test and bicycle exercise test (Tables 17.2 and 17.3) are best standardised for identification of patients with primary hypokalaemic periodic paralysis; however, it may be helpful to perform these tests in patients suspected of having primary hyperkalaemic periodic paralysis. These tests can be performed in an outpatient setting and do not require the prolonged time commitment which detailed monitoring of the oral potassium-loading and other provocative tests require.

Paramyotonia congenita

Myotonic hyperkalaemic periodic paralysis and paramyotonia congenita share several common features. The hallmarks of paramyotonia congenita, as described by Eulenburg (1886) and by Rich (1894), were:

1. Dominant inheritance with high penetrance
2. Myotonia provoked especially by exposure to cold
3. Predilection of the myotonia for facial, lingual, neck and hand muscles
4. Attacks of weakness upon exposure to cold and also after exercise.

Subsequently, some patients with features of paramyotonia congenita were also found to fulfill the diagnostic criteria of primary hyperkalaemic periodic paralysis, suggesting that the two disorders were, in fact, a single nosological entity (French & Kilpatrick 1957, Drager et al 1958, Van der Meulen et al 1961).

However, as mentioned above, even in a careful EMG search no myotonia could be found in some cases of hyperkalaemic periodic paralysis. Further, in patients diagnosed as having paramyotonia congenita, potassium loading did not provoke paralytic attacks (Marshall 1952, Gamstorp 1963, Garcin et al 1966, Riggs et al 1977, Griggs et al 1978, Haass et al 1979). Accentuation rather than improvement of the myotonia on repeated muscle contraction ('myotonia paradoxa') has also been cited as a distinguishing feature of paramyotonia (Magee 1963, Garcin et al 1966, Haass et al 1979, Haass et al 1981, Lehmann-Horn et al 1985, Ricker et al 1986b, Moxley et al 1989, Ricker et al 1990). Finally, recent studies, discussed below, provide evidence that specific alterations in the structure of the alpha subunit of the adult skeletal muscle sodium channel are associated with hyperkalaemic periodic paralysis with and without myotonia, with paramyotonia congenita, and with paramyotonia congenita associated with hyperkalaemic periodic paralysis.

Secondary hyperkalaemic periodic paralysis

This is associated with renal or adrenal insufficiency and may occur when the serum potassium exceeds 7 mmol/l. Males tend to be affected more often than females. Rest after exercise provokes weakness as it does in other types of periodic paralysis (Bull et al 1953, Marks & Feit 1953, Richardson & Sibley 1953, Pollen & Williams 1960, Faw & Ewer 1962, Bell et al 1965, Daughaday & Rendleman 1967). Paresthesiae in the distal extremities tend to occur when the serum potassium level exceeds 7.5 mmol/l. ECG abnormalities (T-wave elevation, disappearance of P waves and, eventually, a sinusoidal tracing) evolve as the serum potassium rises from 7 mmol/l to 9.5 mmol/l (Keith et al 1942, Finch et al 1946, Pollen & Williams 1960). The diagnosis is suggested by the very high serum potassium during the attack, persistent hyperkalaemia between attacks and by the associated primary disorder.

Normokalaemic, sodium-responsive familial periodic paralysis

Poskanzer & Kerr (1961) described patients with periodic paralysis that improved following administration of large doses of sodium. The disease is an autosomal dominant condition with high penetrance in both sexes. Paralytic attacks began in the first decade of life and were exacerbated or provoked by rest after exercise, exposure to cold, excess of alcohol, and by potassium loading. Under the conditions of evaluation no consistent changes of serum electrolytes occurred during attacks, but there was an increased sodium excretion and potassium retention. A family described by Meyers et al (1972) suffered from a similar illness but attacks were not provoked by large doses of potassium. These reports of normokalaemic periodic paralysis are difficult to classify and may represent variants of true hyperkalaemic periodic paralysis in which the monitoring of serial changes in serum potassium was not sufficient to detect typical changes. Further studies of these families, including gene analysis as indicated below, will be necessary to determine if this is a true nosological entity.

Periodic paralysis with cardiac arrhythmia

Periodic paralysis associated with extrasystoles

and tachycardia that is often bidirectional has been described in several patients. The disorder is inherited as a dominant trait. The cardiac symptoms are provoked or worsened by hypokalaemia or digitalis, are refractory to disopyramide phosphate, propranolol or phenytoin, but may respond to imipramine. Syncopal attacks and sudden death can occur in the course of the disease. Dysmorphic features, such as short stature, clinodactyly and microcephaly, occur in some cases (Klein et al 1963, Andersen et al 1971, Levitt et al 1972, Stubbs 1972, Yoshimura et al 1983, Gould et al 1985, Fukada et al 1988). The disorder was associated with myotonia in some families (Gould et al 1985), with hyperkalaemia, and after potassium challenge (Yoshimura et al 1983), with hypokalaemia in two patients (Levitt et al 1972, Stubbs 1976), and with normokalaemia in others (Klein et al 1963).

Histopathological alterations in periodic paralysis

The histopathological hallmark of the syndrome is a vacuolar myopathy (Goldflam 1895). This can be seen in either primary or secondary periodic paralysis, but more often in the former than in the latter. The vacuolation is more consistently associated with the permanent myopathy which develops after repeated attacks than with the acute paralysis (Klein et al 1960, McArdle 1963, Samaha 1965, Resnick & Engel 1967, Engel 1977). The vacuoles are typically centrally situated in the muscle fibres and usually one vacuole, but at times several, appear in a fibre in a single plane of sectioning. Some vacuoles are limited by a delicate membrane, some are loculated, and some contain finely granular material staining positively for glycogen.

Numerous ultrastructural studies in the primary and thyrotoxic periodic paralyses can be summarised as follows. Dilatation and proliferation of sarcoplasmic reticulum (SR) components and abundant networks of transverse tubular (T) system origin have been observed in the muscle fibres (Shy et al 1961, Howes et al 1966, Engel 1966a, Gruner 1966, Odor et al 1967, MacDonald et al 1968, Schutta & Armitage 1969, Bergman et al 1970). The larger and light-microscopically visible vacuoles were thought to arise by coalescence of dilated SR components (Shy et al 1961, Odor et al 1967), from fusion of T-system networks (Biczyskowa et al 1969), or to be the endresult of focal fibre destruction (MacDonald et al 1968, Schutta & Armitage 1969). In view of these divergent results, Engel (1970a) re-examined the morphological sequence of fibre vacuolation in the primary hypokalaemic disorder. The steps identified were:

1. Evolving vacuole
2. Intermediate-stage vacuole
3. Mature vacuole
4. Remodelling.

Abnormal fibre regions arise containing myriad dilated and at times mineralised SR vesicles, masses of bizarre tubules or osmiophilic lamellae of T-system origin, or varied cytoplasmic degradation products (evolving vacuole). The T system proliferates and acts as a membrane source for trapping components of the evolving vacuole. These components are degraded by an autophagic mechanism and a membrane-bound space is formed containing remnants of the trapped organelles which are now embedded in an amorphous matrix (intermediate-stage vacuole). When all trapped components have undergone lysis, the entire vacuole is filled with matrix (mature vacuole). The intermediate-stage and mature vacuoles communicate with the extracellular space via T tubules and T networks and there is prompt ingress of peroxidase-labelled extracellular fluid into the matrix compartment. Because these vacuoles are the prevalent ones, most of the vacuolar volume is filled with extracellular fluid. Intermediate-stage and mature vacuoles are remodelled by invaginations of the vacuolar membrane by glycogen-containing sarcoplasm. When the invaginated membrane ruptures, extracellular fluid enters the myofilament space causing fibre injury. Non-vacuolated fibre regions contain numerous focal dilatations of T tubules, T networks and dilated SR vesicles. Subsequent studies also showed that the ultrastructural changes in the different types of periodic paralysis are virtually identical, that electrical inexcitability of a muscle fibre can occur without associated ultrastructural change, and that the morphological changes are reactive, representing delayed consequences of the physiological abnormality (Engel 1977).

Pathophysiological mechanisms in the periodic paralyses

The pathophysiology that underlies primary hypokalaemic periodic paralysis relates to a basic defect in the muscle fibre which causes a reduced excitability and an increased sodium conductance that is not prevented by the application of the sodium channel blocker tetrodotoxin. How this relates to the inherited defect in the skeletal muscle channel requires further study (Fontaine et al 1994).

No specific inherited alteration in the adult skeletal muscle sodium channel has been identified to account for the abnormal regulation of sodium conductance in patients with primary hypokalaemic periodic paralysis. The reduced excitability and increased sodium conductance observed in muscle fibres is aggravated by a reduction in the extracellular potassium concentration. Alterations in the regulation of ion fluxes occur in patients with hypokalaemic periodic paralysis. Movement of potassium into forearm muscle has been observed during a spontaneous attack of weakness (Zierler & Andres 1957) and others have observed decreased urinary potassium excretion and decreased serum potassium levels in these patients (Aitken et al 1937, Ferrebee et al 1938, Shy et al 1961, Engel et al 1965). There is some indirect evidence that patients with hypokalaemic periodic paralysis may have an increased sensitivity of their skeletal muscle insulin receptor (Hofmann et al 1983, Minaker et al 1988) and the normal action of insulin to produce a net uptake of potassium may lead to the attack of weakness. Further investigations of the actions of insulin and other hypokalaemia-producing hormones is necessary to clarify their potential role in the pathophysiology of attacks in primary hypokalaemic periodic paralysis.

In thyrotoxic periodic paralysis the fluid and electrolyte shifts are similar to those noted in the primary hypokalaemic form. In periodic paralysis caused by renal or gastrointestinal potassium wastage the hypokalaemia and body potassium depletion are more marked and episodic paralysis appears when the exchangeable body potassium has fallen to approximately one-half normal levels (Staffurth 1964). The paroxysmal nature of the attacks is unexplained and it is not known whether the ionic shifts during the attacks are the same as in the primary hypokalaemic form. The paroxysmal nature of the attacks may relate to fluctuations in catecholamine levels and associated regulation of sodium potassium ATPase function (Oh et al 1990). Treatment with beta-blockers prevents weakness despite low serum potassium (Conway et al 1974).

In the primary hyperkalaemic periodic paralyses with and without myotonia the movements of potassium are opposite to those which occur in the primary hypokalaemic type: the hyperkalaemia is associated with enhanced urinary excretion of potassium (Gamstorp 1956, Klein et al 1960, Creutzfeldt 1961, Carson & Pearson 1964). Careful studies have demonstrated a decreased serum sodium level and urinary sodium excretion, and a decreased or unaltered serum chloride level (Streeten et al 1971, Clausen et al 1980). These findings are consistent with the egress of potassium and the entry of sodium and possibly of chloride into muscle cells during attacks. Fluid and electrolyte shifts have not been investigated during paroxysmal attacks of secondary hyperkalaemic periodic paralysis.

Abnormalities of carbohydrate metabolism, such as a block in hexose phosphate utilisation (McArdle 1956) or in glycogen synthesis (Shy et al 1961), were postulated to account for the adverse effects of carbohydrate loading in primary hypokalaemic periodic paralysis. Biochemical studies by Engel et al (1967) did not confirm these hypotheses. From a different viewpoint, the opposite effects of carbohydrate loading in the primary hypokalaemic and hyperkalaemic syndromes could be related to ionic movements associated with cellular glucose uptake and utilisation because potassium movements follow the carbohydrate cycle from muscle to liver and back. Such movements could provoke or correct a defect which is not one of carbohydrate metabolism, but which resides in the electrical and biophysical properties of the muscle fibre surface membrane.

The pathophysiological mechanisms associated with the attacks of weakness in hyperkalaemic periodic paralysis with and without myotonia as well as the attacks of weakness in patients with paramyotonia congenita alone or in patients with paramyotonia congenita associated with hyperkalaemic periodic paralysis, all relate to mutations in the adult skeletal muscle sodium channel (Tables 17.1, 17.8, Fig. 17.1). The characterisation of the skeletal muscle sodium channel (Catterall 1986, Catterall 1988, Stuhmer et al 1989, Trimmer et al 1989, Auld et al 1990, George et al 1990, Kallen et al 1990, Ebers et al 1991, George et al 1991, 1992) has led to genetic studies which have localised gene defects to specific portions of the sodium channel gene in the long arm of chromosome 17, 17q23.1–25.3 (Fontaine et al 1990, Ebers et al 1991, Koch et al 1991, Ptacek et al 1991, Rojas et al 1991, Ptacek et al 1992a, b, McClatchey et al 1992a, b, Ptacek et al 1993). A key development in understanding the pathophysiology of hyperkalaemic periodic paralysis and paramyotonia congenita was the recognition that attacks in both diseases are associated with an abnormally increased sodium conductance and by depolarisation block and

paralysis if the muscle fibres are sufficiently depolarised (Lehmann-Horn et al 1983, Ricker et al 1986a, Lehmann-Horn et al 1987, Ricker et al 1989). Although tetrodotoxin (TTX), a blocker of the adult skeletal muscle sodium channel, can reverse the excessive depolarisation associated with failure of contraction of muscle fibres in hyperkalaemic periodic paralysis, it is ineffective in restoring membrane excitability to fibres in paramyotonia congenita that are previously depolarised. The electrophysiological defect in hyperkalaemic periodic paralysis and paramyotonia congenita differs. This difference is apparent in the response of forearm muscle to cooling and exercise. In hyperkalaemic periodic paralysis cooling of forearm muscle followed by forceful contractions leads to significant weakness (Ricker et al 1989), but muscle fibres do not display the marked depolarisation observed in muscle of patients with paramyotonia congenita (Ricker et al 1986b, Lehmann-Horn et al 1987, Ricker et al 1989). Treatment with tocainide did not reduce the weakness provoked by cooling and exercise in hyperkalaemic periodic paralysis, in contrast to its beneficial effect on forearm muscle strength in paramyotonia congenita (Ricker et al 1986a,

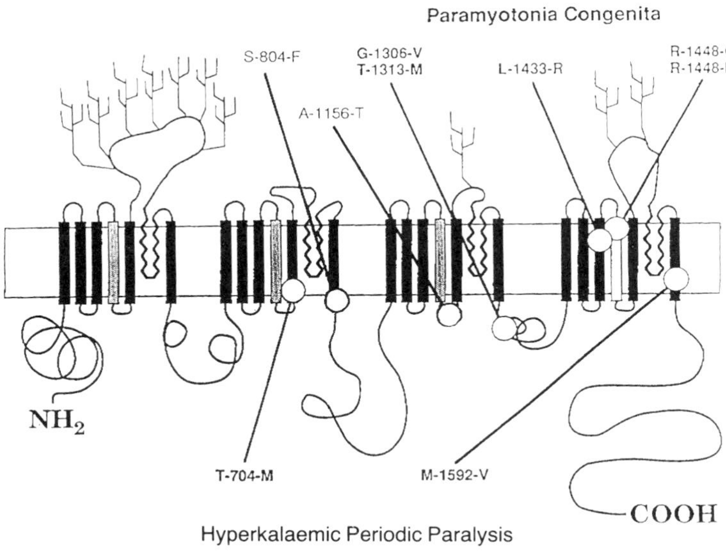

Fig. 17.1 A model of the voltage-dependent skeletal sodium channel, consisting of four homologous domains, each contining six trans-membrane segments, showing the locations of point mutations listed in Table 17.8 (modified from a figure kindly provided by Dr Louis Ptacek).

Table 17.8 Kindreds and mutations in the skeletal muscle sodium channel identified with hyperkalaemic periodic paralysis (HYPP) and with paramyotonia congenita (PC)

Kindred number	Diagnosis	Mutation	Location*	Potassium-sensitive	Cold-sensitive	Reference
No. 1590	HYPP	T704M (thr ⟶ met)	D2/S5			Ptacek et al 1991
No. 1767	HYPP	T704M (thr⟶met)	D2/S5			Ptacek et al 1991
No. 1782	HYPP	T704M (thr⟶met)	D2/S5			Ptacek et al 1991
Pedigree A	HYPP	M1592V (met⟶val)	D4/S6			Rojas et al 1991
Pedigree B	HYPP	M1592V (met⟶val)	D4/S6			Rojas et al 1991
No. 1891	HYPP	M1592V (met⟶val)	D4/S6	Yes	No	Ptacek et al 1993
No. 1894	HYPP	M1592V (met⟶val)	D4/S6	Yes	No	Ptacek et al 1993
Germany	PC	V1589M (val⟶met)	D4/S6			Heine et al 1993
Belgian	PC	G1306V (gly⟶val)	ID3-4			McClatchey et al 1992
Germany	PC	G1306V (gly⟶val)	ID3-4			Lerche et al 1993
North America 1	PC	G1306V (gly⟶val)	ID3-4			McClatchey et al 1992
North America 2	PC	T1313M (thr⟶met)	ID3-4			McClatchey et al 1992
Pedigree 4	PC	T1313M (thr⟶met)	ID3-4			McClatchey et al 1992
No. 1637	PC	R1448C (arg⟶cys)	D4/S4			Ptacek et al 1992
No. 1800	PC	R1448H (arg⟶his)	D4/S4			Ptacek et al 1992
No. 1984	PC	R1448H (arg⟶his)	D4/S4			Ptacek et al 1992
No. 1997	PC	L1448H (leu⟶arg)	D4/S3	No	Yes	Ptacek et al 1993
No. 2034	PC	R1448H (arg⟶his)	D4/S4	No	Yes	Ptacek et al 1993
No. 1995	PC	T1313M (thr⟶met)	ID3-4		Yes	Ptacek et al 1993
No. 2035	PC	T1313M (thr⟶met)	ID3-4	No	Yes	Ptacek et al 1993

*The letter, D, refers to the domain of the alpha subunit of the human skeletal muscle sodium channel that has the alteration caused by the gene mutation. There are four internally repeated domains. The letter, S, refers to one of six putative membrane spanning segments associated with each of the four domains of the sodium channel. The letters, ID, refer to the cytoplasmic loop that connects domains 3 and 4. The specific amino acids involved in each mutation are included adjacent to the mutation.

Moxley et al 1989). The alteration in the muscle fibre that accounts for the release of potassium which occurs during attacks of weakness in hyperkalaemic periodic paralysis (McArdle 1962), is separate from that observed in patients with paramyotonia congenita. Following cooling of forearm muscle and exercise in normals, there is a mild decrease in strength associated with a release of potassium from muscle tissue (Moxley et al 1989), while in patients with paramyotonia congenita or patients with paramyotonia congenita associated with hyperkalaemic periodic paralysis there is a marked uptake of potassium by muscle (Moxley et al 1989). After treatment with tocainide the weakness provoked by forearm cooling and exercise is significantly less in patients with paramyotonia congenita or paramyotonia congenita associated with hyperkalaemic periodic paralysis and the degree of potassium uptake by muscle is less (Moxley et al 1989). These observations indicate normal operation of the sodium–potassium ATPase in paramyotonia congenita during muscle fibre depolarisation caused by cold, and indicate a separate mechanism for the rise in

potassium observed in attacks of hyperkalaemic weakness. Patients with hyperkalaemic periodic paralysis have a strong diurnal sensitivity to attacks of weakness, with attacks occurring primarily in the morning (Ricker et al 1989); however, at present there is no clear explanation for the physiological release of potassium from muscle in this condition. Circulating factors, such as glucocorticoids and beta-adrenergic hormones, may influence the ease with which hyperkalaemic attacks can be provoked. Whether exercise produces a sufficient release of beta-adrenergic hormones to lower extracellular potassium and prevent initiation of muscle fibre depolarisation in hyperkalaemic periodic paralysis is unclear. Salbutamol and metaproteronol, both beta-adrenergic drugs, are capable of increasing muscle force during an attack (Benheim et al 1985, Ricker et al 1989) and the beneficial effect observed with salbutamol was not related to a definite reduction in the high level of serum potassium (Ricker et al 1989).

In paramyotonia congenita, exercise following exposure to cold provokes muscle stiffness and occasionally prolonged paralysis of muscle. The stiffness in part relates to the passive characteristics of muscle (Haass et al 1979) and is poorly understood. The prolonged period of recovery from cold-associated paralysis in paramyotonia is not associated with a fall in high energy metabolites or with a change in intracellular pH (Lehmann-Horn et al 1985). Future studies of the phenomena of muscle stiffness as well as the regulation of serum potassium may help shed light on the pathophysiology of symptoms for both paramyotonia congenita and hyperkalaemic periodic paralysis.

Molecular genetic studies of mutations in the sodium channel have raised interesting hypotheses about the correlation between the symptoms in patients with hyperkalaemic periodic paralysis and paramyotonia congenita and specific functions for different portions of the channel (Ebers et al 1991, Ptacek et al 1991, Rojas et al 1991, McClatchey et al 1992a, b, Ptacek et al 1992a, b, 1993). At present hyperkalaemic periodic paralysis is associated with two different mutations (Fig. 17.1, Table 17.8). There is a suggestion that there may be a greater degree of fixed inter-attack weakness in patients with the D2/S5 mutation (Ptacek et al 1993), but further observations are needed to substantiate this impression. Six distinct mutations are known for paramyotonia congenita (see Table 17.8), and they can be classified into two general groups:

1. Those in the S3–S4 segments in domain 4 near the extracellular surface of the membrane
2. Those in the cytoplasmic loop between domains 3 and 4 (Fig. 17.1, Table 17.8).

Patients with paramyotonia congenita and associated hyperkalaemic periodic paralysis have been found to have a mutation in the cytoplasmic loop between domains 3 and 4 (Ptacek et al 1993). Future studies to correlate phenotype and genotype are necessary. Ultimately, it may be possible to correlate whether specific clinical problems relate directly to defects in those portions of the sodium channel felt to be responsible for voltage gating, inactivation and channel stability (See Chapter 11).

The pathophysiology responsible for hyperkalaemic periodic paralysis associated with cardiac arrhythmia is unclear. Clinically patients have an improvement in their rhythm disturbance with an elevation in serum potassium, but at the same time develop worsening of their skeletal muscle weakness. In association with the bidirectional ventricular tachycardia that typically occurs in these patients, there are some who have intermittent-prolongation of the QT interval (Tawil et al 1994 personal communication). The alterations responsible for prolongation of the QT interval in the long-QT syndrome have suggested that a primary effect could be a delayed outward rectifier potassium channel current (Moss 1992). Genetic linkage of the long QT syndrome and cardiac arrhythmia to the Harvey ras-1 gene has been found and may suggest that the signal transduction from G proteins associated with ion channels could underly the cardiac arrhythmia (Keating et al 1991, Moss 1992). Further investigations are necessary to identify the possible relationship between the prolonged QT syndrome and the patients with hyperkalaemic periodic paralysis with cardiac arrhythmia.

Treatment of periodic paralyses

Primary hypokalaemic periodic paralysis. Acute attacks are treated with 2.0–10.0 g of potassium chloride, given by mouth as an unsweetened 10–25% solution. This dose may be repeated, if necessary, after 3–4 hours (Talbott 1941, McArdle 1963). Intravenous administration of potassium salts is seldom, if ever, required. Utmost care must be exercised in giving potassium intravenously in order to avoid life-threatening hyperkalaemia, and intravenous fluids must contain no glucose or sodium. The patient's strength and serum potassium must be frequently monitored during treatment of major attacks.

Preventive therapy of the primary hypokalaemic variety consists of a relatively low sodium (2.3 g per day) and low carbohydrate (60–80 g per day) diet, avoidance of exposure to cold and overexertion, and supplemental doses of potassium chloride, 2.5–7.5 g, as a 10% aqueous solution taken two to four times daily. The dosage must be adjusted according to attack frequency and severity. Because severely affected patients awaken paralysed, a dose may have to be taken at 02.00 hours (2 a.m.). The serum potassium should not exceed 6 mmol/l during therapy. Acetazolamide (Diamox®) is also highly effective in preventing attacks. Up to 2 g per day of the drug can be used instead of the other preventive measures. The drug probably acts by inducing a mild metabolic acidosis, which prevents an intracellular shift of potassium (Griggs et al 1970, Riggs & Griggs 1979). Treatment with dichlorophenamide (Daranide®) is also effective and may be more useful in preventing the development of permanent muscle weakness (Dalakas & Engel 1983). Doses up to 200 mg per day of dichlorophenamide have proven helpful. Both dichlorophenamide and acetazolamide are carbonic anhydrase inhibitors and their beneficial actions may relate to their direct effects on carbonic anhydrase III which is the major isoform of the enzyme in skeletal muscle (Heath et al 1983, Tashian et al 1990). It is also important to monitor carefully patients with hypokalaemic periodic paralysis during surgery to avoid serious complications (Melnick et al 1983).

Thyrotoxic periodic paralysis. Treatment consists of antithyroid therapy. Until the patient becomes euthyroid, preventive measures and the treatment of the acute attacks are the same as in the primary hypokalaemic form. Acetazolamide is not only ineffective, but may precipitate or worsen symptoms in this form of hypokalaemic periodic paralysis (Shulkin et al 1989) and should be avoided. Propranolol (40 mg q.i.d.) may prevent attacks (Conway et al 1974, Yeung & Tse 1974).

Other forms of secondary hypokalaemic periodic paralysis. Therapy is directed at the primary disorder and potassium is replaced to compensate for both the static deficits and the dynamic losses. Additional treatment is directed against the metabolic acidosis or alkalosis and other associated electrolyte abnormalities that may be present.

Primary sodium-responsive normokalaemic periodic paralysis. In the family studied by Poskanzer & Kerr (1961), therapy with large doses of sodium chloride, or with 0.1 mg 9-α-fluorohydrocortisone and 250 mg acetazolamide per day, was effective in preventing attacks.

Primary hyperkalaemic periodic paralysis. Acute attacks in established cases can be treated with 2 g/kg glucose by mouth and 15–20 units of crystalline insulin subcutaneously, but severe attacks may fail to respond to these measures (Gamstorp 1956, Saglid 1959). Calcium gluconate, 0.5–2 g administered intravenously, has been reported to terminate attacks in some cases (Gamstorp 1959, Van der Meulen et al 1961, Van't Hoff 1962), but not others (McArdle 1962). The inhalation of beta-adrenergic agents, such as metaproterenol every 15 minutes for three doses, has also aborted acute attacks (Benheim et al 1985). Preventive therapy consists of frequent meals of high carbohydrate content, avoidance of fasting or of exposure to cold and overexertion, and use of diuretic-promoting kaliuresis, such as acetazolamide or chlorothiazide. The lowest dose of diuretic required to prevent attacks should be used and the amount given should not lower the serum potassium level below 3.7 mmol/l or the serum sodium below 135 mmol/l (McArdle 1962, Carson & Pearson 1964, Samaha 1965). Daily treatment with small doses of salbuterol has also prevented attacks (Clausen et al 1980, Benheim et al 1985).

Tocainide, an antiarrhythmic drug, can prevent weakness and myotonia induced by cold in paramyotonia congenita and in the myotonic form of hyperkalaemic periodic paralysis. The drug does not prevent hyperkalaemic attacks of weakness in the myotonic form of hyperkalaemic periodic paralysis (Ricker et al 1983, Streit et al 1987a). *The Lancet* (1: 1243–1244; 1987) has advised against the use of tocainide because of arrhythmias. Mexilitine, a related lidocaine derivative antiarrhythmic, has proven an effective alternative in situations in which tocainide is felt to be a significant risk (Kwiecinski & Ryniewicz 1990, Moxley 1990).

Secondary hyperkalaemic periodic paralysis. Therapy is again aimed at the primary disorder and should include restriction of dietary potassium intake until the primary cause can be corrected. Intravenous insulin and glucose therapy can temporarily decrease the serum potassium level. In patients with renal failure, severe hyperkalaemia is an indication for haemodialysis.

THE GLYCOGEN STORAGE DISEASES

Cori (1957) assigned numbers to the glycogen storage diseases in the sequence in which they were discovered. However, those glycogenoses discovered after 1957 were not numbered consistently and recently discovered diseases have been named after the enzyme that is deficient. Skeletal muscle is directly involved in glycogenoses caused by deficiency of acid maltase (type II) (glucan 1,4-d-glucosidase; EC 3.2.1.3), debranching enzyme (type III)(α-dextrin endo-1,6-d-glucosidase; EC 3.2.1.41), branching enzyme (type IV)(1,4-α-glucan branching enzyme, EC 2.4.1.18), myophosphorylase (type V) (EC 2.4.1.1), phosphorylase B kinase deficiency, 6-phosphofructokinase (type VII) (EC 2.7.1.11), phosphoglycerate kinase (EC 2.7.2.3), phosphoglycerate mutase (EC 5.4.2.1) and lactate dehydrogenase (EC 1.1.1.28), and is indirectly involved in glucose-6-phosphatase (EC 3.1.3.9) deficiency (type I). All glycogenoses are autosomal recessive disorders except phosphoglycerate kinase deficiency, which is an X-linked recessive. Considerable phenotype heterogeneity has been observed in each recognised glycogenosis. There are also other glycogen or polysaccharide storage syndromes of muscle for which no enzymatic basis has been uncovered to date.

There are nine identified enzyme defects that affect skeletal muscle alone or in conjunction with brain and peripheral nerve. The genes for seven of these nine enzymes (or their subunits) are noted in Table 17.9. Seven of the defects involve cytoplasmic enzymes which act at different levels in glycogen breakdown and glycolysis; another, branching enzyme deficiency, involves the glycogen synthesis pathway, and the remaining enzyme, acid maltase, involves the intralysosomal glycogen degradation pathway. Muscle weakness may occur in isolation or in association with other systemic complaints in different types of glycogen storage disease. If the inherited enzyme defect exists in a single molecular form that is identical for all tissues, it will cause generalised disease, such as occurs in the infantile form of acid maltase deficiency. Most of the enzymes involved in glycogen metabolism and glycolysis exist in multiple isoforms and are developmentally regulated to appear in fetal or adult form in specific tissues (DiMauro & Servidei 1993). The expression of a fetal isozyme in regenerating muscle may obscure the diagnosis of a disease in which the cell is unable to produce the adult form of the enzyme, as by obtaining a muscle biopsy shortly after an episode of myoglobinuria in a patient with McArdle's disease (Mitsumoto 1979). It may be that the variable severity and varying degrees of organ system involvement in specific disorders of glycogen metabolism and glycolysis relate to the protective effects of uninvolved isoforms of a par-

Table 17.9   Chromosomal assignments of human genes encoding enzymes of glycogen metabolism and glysolysis (adapted from DiMauro & Servidei, 1993)

Enzyme	Subunit of enzyme	Chromosome	References
Acid maltase	—	17(q23 ⟶q25)	D'Ancona et al 1979, Solomon et al 1979, Wail et al 1979, Nickel et al 1982, Martiniuk et al 1985
Phosphorylase	M	11q13	Lebo et al 1990
	L	14	Newgard et al 1986
	B	10, 20	Newgard et al 1988
Phosphorylase b kinase	alpha	Xq12 ⟶q13	Francke et al 1989
	beta	16q12 ⟶q13	Francke et al 1989
	gamma	7, 11	Chamberlain et al 1987 (mouse)
Phosphofructokinase	M	1(cen ⟶q32)	Vora et al 1982
	P	10(p)	Vora et al 1983
	L	21(q22.3)	Van Keuren et al 1986
Phosphoglycerate kinase	A	X(q13)	Meerakhan et al 1971
Phosphoglycerate mutase	M	7	Edwards et al 1989
	B	10	Sakoda et al 1988
Lactate dehydrogenase	M	11	Boone et al 1972
	H	12	Chen et al 1973

* The genes for two other enzyme deficiencies causing muscle symptoms, brancher and debrancher, have not yet been isolated.

ticular enzyme or low residual concentrations of the enzyme in specific target tissues. However, as others have pointed out (DiMauro & Servidei 1993), this leaves many interesting questions to be answered. For example in childhood onset and adult onset forms of acid maltase deficiency, muscle is selectively affected although the enzyme defect is generalised. Debrancher enzyme is felt to exist as a single polypeptide, suggesting it should produce generalised illness, but some patients have sparing of skeletal muscle and heart. It may be that in certain of the disorders of glycogen metabolism there are different amounts of residual enzyme activity in different tissues or different vulnerability of individual tissues to the same amount of residual enzyme activity. If these suggestions are accurate it will be necessary to establish the threshold activity for each enzyme and for each tissue below which glycogen starts accumulating and clinical manifestations appear. These questions and others will need to be addressed in the future.

At present disorders of glycogen metabolism cause two main clinical syndromes: one that involves progressive weakness of the limb and trunk musculature, sparing extraocular and facial muscles, and the other a syndrome of exercise intolerance, muscle cramps and intermittent muscle necrosis and myoglobinuria. In the section that follows the specific enzyme deficiencies are reviewed.

Glucose-6-phosphatase deficiency

The enzyme normally occurs in liver, kidney and small intestine but not in muscle. Deficiency of the enzyme causes no glycogen excess in muscle but profound hypotonia can occur in affected infants. The metabolic fault prevents the release from liver of glucose derived from glycogenolysis or gluconeogenesis. The consequences are severe fasting hypoglycaemia, lactic acidosis and excessive mobilisation of fat from adipose tissue. Chronic lactic acidosis causes osteoporosis and interferes with the renal excretion of uric acid, resulting in hyperuricaemia and secondary gout. Fat mobilisation leads to marked hyperlipidaemia, fatty infiltration of liver and xanthoma formation. A haemorrhagic tendency occurs in many patients.

All manifestations of the disease tend to improve with age (Moses & Gutman 1972, Huijing 1975, Howell 1978).

Acid maltase deficiency

Acid maltase, a lysosomal enzyme, hydrolyses both 1,4- and 1,6-α-glycosidic linkages. It is optimally active between pH 4 and 5 and is capable of degrading glycogen completely. The biosynthesis of acid maltase resembles that of other lysosomal enzymes: a high-molecular-weight precursor synthesised by ribosomes enters the endoplasmic reticulum where it acquires a high-mannose carbohydrate; it then moves to the Golgi apparatus where it becomes phosphorylated, glycosylated and fitted with a special mannose-6-phosphate recognition marker that allows the enzyme to bind to membrane receptors. From the Golgi apparatus the enzyme is exported to lysosomes where it is further modified by proteolysis and stabilised to prevent autolysis (Callahan & Lowden 1981, Barranger & Brader 1984). The synthesis of acid maltase follows the above scheme. An enzyme of molecular weight 110 000 daltons, that already carries the mannose-6-phosphate marker, can be detected in human urine (Oude Elferink et al 1984). In cultured fibroblasts the precursor enzyme is processed through a number of intermediates to become a glycoprotein of molecular weight 76 000 daltons (Hasilik & Neufeld 1980). Although acid maltase deficiency (AMD) was the first lysosomal disorder to be identified (Hers 1963), the precise metabolic role of the enzyme is still enigmatic. Massive amounts of glycogen, and at times acid mucopolysaccharides, accumulate in cells lacking the enzyme and attest to its biological significance, yet severe deficiency of the enzyme can exist in some cells and tissues without glycogen excess or functional impairment. The disease originally described by Pompe (1932) was a generalised glycogenosis invariably fatal in infancy (Sant'Agnese 1959). Subsequently, milder forms of AMD, presenting as myopathy, have been observed in children (Hers & van Hoff 1968, Smith et al 1966, Iancu et al 1988) and adults (Engel & Dale 1968, Hudgson et al 1968, Engel 1970b, Trend et al 1985). All three forms of the disease are transmitted by autosomal recessive inheritance (Williams 1966, Nitowski & Grunfeld 1967, Engel & Gomez 1970) and, with few exceptions (Busch et al 1979, Koster et al 1978, Loonen et al 1981, Hoefsloot et al 1990, Danon et al 1986), the disease breeds true in each family. Not uncommonly adults will present with respiratory insufficiency as their primary myopathic manifestation (Rosenow & Engel 1978, Martin et al 1983, Trend et al 1985, Margolis & Hill 1986), and in a few families adults have presented with intracranial aneurysms felt to be due to glycogen deposition in smooth muscle (Makos et al 1985, Matsuoka et al 1988, Kretzschmar et al 1990).

Infantile AMD presents within the first few months of life with generalised and rapidly progressive weakness and hypotonia, and enlargement of the heart, tongue and liver. Respiratory and feeding difficulties are common and death is usually due to cardiorespiratory failure before the age of 2 years. The ECG typically shows a short P–R interval, high QRS voltage and left ventricular hypertrophy (Sant'Agnese 1959, Caddell & Whitemore 1962, Engel et al 1973). Massive amounts of glycogen accumulate in skeletal muscle, heart and liver. Microscopic examination also shows widespread glycogen deposition in smooth muscle, endothelial and renal tubular cells and in both neural and glial elements of the central nervous system. Most cells of the brain and spinal cord are affected but cerebellar cortical nerve cells are spared. Motor neurones in the brain stem and spinal cord are most severely involved (Mancall et al 1965, Hogan et al 1969). Glycogen also accumulates in Schwann cells in peripheral nerves (Gambetti et al 1971). In addition to glycogen, acid mucopolysaccharides also accumulate in skeletal muscle (Martin et al 1973, Engel et al 1973) and have been noted in muscle, liver, heart leucocytes and cultured fibroblasts (Nitowski & Grunfeld 1967, Danzis et al 1969, Brown et al 1970) but not in kidney (Steinitz & Rutenberg 1967). However, the renal enzyme differs from lysosomal acid maltase (Steinitz & Rutenberg 1967, Salafsky & Nadler 1971, Koster et al 1976, De Burlet & Sudaka 1977, Mehler & DiMauro 1977, Reuser et al 1987). This renal isozyme is present in granulocytes where it may mask the diagnosis of AMD

(DiMauro & Servidei 1993). Diagnostic assays for AMD need to be performed in lymphocytes rather than preparations containing mixed leucocytes (Shanske & DiMauro 1981). A sensitive fluorometric assay, using an artificial substrate, reveals that there is no residual enzyme activity in affected tissues in infantile AMD (Mehler & DiMauro 1977). Catalytically inactive enzyme protein could not be detected by immunological techniques in some patients (De Barsy et al 1972, Reuser et al 1978), but such a protein was abundantly present in at least one infant (Beratis et al 1978). This indicates that even infantile AMD, which seems to be clinically homogeneous, is genetically heterogeneous.

The childhood type of AMD presents clinically in infancy or early childhood as a myopathy. Motor milestones are delayed and weakness is usually greater in proximal than distal limb muscles. Respiratory muscles tend to be selectively severely affected (Martin et al 1983, Rosenow & Engel 1978, Trend et al 1985, Margolis & Hill 1986). Calf enlargement can also occur resulting in a clinical picture which simulates muscular dystrophy (Hers & van Hoff 1968, Swaiman et al 1968, Engel et al 1973). The disease progresses relatively slowly and death usually occurs from respiratory failure after repeated bouts of pneumonia. Few patients survive beyond the second decade. Liver, heart or tongue enlargement occur relatively infrequently. Glycogen excess in muscle is less marked and more variable than in infantile AMD. Autopsy studies reveal little if any increase of glycogen in heart, liver, skin and nervous system (Smith et al 1966, 1967, Engel et al 1973, Martin et al 1976b). The enzyme is deficient in muscle, heart and liver (Hers & van Hoff 1968, Angelini 1972, Mehler & DiMauro 1977, DiMauro & Servidei 1993), cultured fibroblasts (Koster et al 1972) and inconsistently in leucocytes (Brown & Zellweger 1966). Residual acid maltase activity is detected in muscle, liver and heart (Angelini & Engel 1972, Mehler & DiMauro 1977, DiMauro & Servidei 1993).

The adult form of AMD presents after the age of 20 years. The symptoms can be those of a slowly progressive myopathy which clinically mimics polymyositis or limb-girdle dystrophy

(Engel & Dale 1968, Hudgson et al 1968, Engel 1970b, Carrier et al 1975, Gullotta et al 1976, Martin et al 1976a, Karpati et al 1977, DiMauro et al 1978c, Bertagnolio et al 1978, DiMauro & Servidei 1993). However, one-third of the cases present with respiratory failure which may overshadow other manifestations (Rosenow & Engel 1978). Respiratory muscle involvement eventually occurs in all and respiratory failure is the usual cause of death. Heart and liver enlargement does not occur and cardiac manifestations, if present, are those of cor pulmonale secondary to the respiratory failure. Glycogen accumulates in clinically affected muscles but seldom exceeds 5%. In some muscles with histological abnormalities the muscle glycogen content is surprisingly normal. No glycogen excess is found in tissues other than muscle. Acid mucopolysaccharides, which accumulate in muscle in infants and chidren with AMD, are sparse or absent from muscle in affected adults. Deficiency of the enzyme has been found in muscle (Engel & Dale 1968, Hudgson et al 1968), liver (Engel 1970b, Engel et al 1973), heart and central nervous system (DiMauro et al 1978c) as well as in cultured fibroblasts (Angelini et al 1972) and cultured muscle cells (Askanas et al 1976). A lower than normal leucocyte acid maltase level and a depressed acid/neutral maltase ratio were found by Angelini & Engel (1972) and by Koster et al (1974), but not by Bertagnolio et al (1978). Residual acid maltase activity is detectable in muscle and other tissues (Engel et al 1973, Mehler & DiMauro 1977, DiMauro & Servidei 1993).

Serum enzymes of muscle origin, creatine kinase (EC 2.7.3.2) and aspartate aminotransferase (EC 2.6.1.1) are increased in all three types of AMD, but the increases are usually less than 10-fold over the normal upper limit. Electromyographic findings indicate a myopathy in all three types. The abnormalities are more widespread in infants than in older patients. In children and adults, some muscles show no electrical abnormalities whereas others have motor unit potentials of abnormally short duration as well as some of normal duration. Abnormal insertional activity and myotonic discharges (without clinically detectable myotonia) occur in all patients. Other forms of abnormal activity (fibrillation potentials, positive waves and bizarre repetitive discharges) also occur at rest. In adults, the myotonic discharges are less widely distributed and less intense and appear especially in the paraspinal muscles (Engel et al 1973).

The common light-microscopic feature in all cases of AMD is a vacuolar myopathy (Engel 1986, DiMauro & Servidei 1993). In infants, virtually all muscle fibres contain large vacuoles. In children, vacuolation tends to be less marked and some fibres or muscles are spared. In adults, almost all fibres in severely affected muscles show vacuoles. In less severely affected muscles the vacuolation involves 25–75% of the fibres, whereas clinically unaffected muscles show few, if any, such fibres. The vacuoles have a high glycogen content and are strongly reactive for acid phosphatase. Abnormal increases of acid phosphatase activity also occur in fibres with no vacuoles detectable light-microscopically.

Ultrastructural studies show that glycogen accumulates in muscle fibres in four types of space:

1. Dispersed in the sarcoplasm, displacing, replacing or compressing normal organelles
2. In sac-like structures, limited by continuous or discontinuous single or double membranes
3. In ordinary autophagic vacuoles, containing glycogen and miscellaneous cytoplasmic degradation products.
4. In spaces representing transitions between the above.

The limiting membranes are generated by proliferating T-system networks and by the Golgi system. Acid hydrolases are delivered to the vacuoles by vesicles arising from T-system networks (Engel 1970b, Engel et al 1973). Because many vacuoles are membrane-bound and contain acid hydrolases and cytoplasmic degradation products, they represent secondary lysosomes.

Diagnostic clues in AMD consist of organomegaly in infants and children; the firm consistency of the weak muscles; the selectively severe involvement of respiratory muscles, and also of the hip adductor muscles, in some of the adults; the abnormal electrical irritability, including myotonic discharges without clinical myotonia, in the EMG; and a vacuolar myopathy with high glycogen content and acid phosphatase activity of the vacuoles. However, none of the clinical and morphological findings are specific, and confirmatory enzyme studies are essential for diagnosis. Acid maltase can be readily assayed in muscle, cultured fibroblasts and urine (Salafsky & Nadler 1973, Mehler & DiMauro 1976). Prenatal diagnosis is possible by enzyme assays on cultivated amniotic fluid cells obtained during the 14th and 18th weeks of pregnancy (Galjaard et al 1973).

The marked clinical variability of AMD between infants, children and adults is unexplained. Biochemical differences exist between and within the different clinical types of AMD (DiMauro & Servidei 1993). Total absence of enzyme activity, with or without the presence of an inactive enzyme protein, occurs in infantile AMD. However, similar biochemical phenotypes also occur in some childhood and adult cases. In some adults, enzyme activity and enzyme protein are proportionately reduced (De Barsy et al 1972, Beratis et al 1983, Ninomiya et al 1984, Miranda et al 1985). Thus, the different clinical types cannot be readily explained by the remaining residual enzyme activity. Studies of cultured fibroblasts from patients with different types of AMD have revealed five different biochemical defects:

1. No synthesis of the enzyme precursor
2. Reduced synthesis of an enzyme precursor which then matures normally
3. Normal synthesis of an enzyme precursor, most of which is degraded before it is processed by the Golgi apparatus
4. A defect in the phosphorylation of the enzyme precursor
5. A defect in the proteolytic processing of the glycosylated and phosphorylated enzyme (Reuser & Kroos 1982, Steckel et al 1982, Reuser et al 1985).

However, no consistent correlation has been demonstrated between the biochemical and clinical phenotypes. Finally, there is no explanation for the fact that, in childhood or adult AMD, glycogen content in muscle can vary from normal to

moderately high from patient to patient, in different muscles of the same patient, and even in different regions of the same muscle.

Apart from symptomatic management of cardiac and respiratory insufficiency, there is no satisfactory treatment for AMD. Lysosome-labilising agents, such as vitamin A, progesterone or hyperbaric oxygen, have failed to improve symptoms in patients as have the administration of glycogenolytic agents such as epinephrine (DiMauro & Servidei 1993). Enzyme replacement using α-glucosidase prepared from bacteria (Lauer et al 1968) or human placenta (DeBarsy et al 1973) produced no benefit, and even when the enzyme was packaged within liposomes (Tyrrell et al 1976) or bound to albumin (Pozanansky & Bhardwaj 1981) or to low density lipoproteins (Williams & Murray 1980) no improvement occurred. Some promise for improvement has been observed in more recent pilot studies of enzyme replacement using a precursor of acid maltase (van der Ploeg et al 1988, 1991). Intravenous administration of the precursor into mice showed that the enzyme was taken up by muscle and heart but not by brain. This approach may be helpful but limits its application, especially in cases of childhood- and adult-onset AMD when the blood–brain barrier would be impermeable to the precursor.

Patients, especially in childhood and adult life, may need permanent or intermittent mechanically assisted ventilation using options, such as a rocking bed, positive pressure nasal ventilation, the 'sipping' technique, negative-pressure ventilation, or positive-pressure ventilation via a tracheostomy (Martin et al 1983, Rosenow & Engel 1978, Trend et al 1985, Margolis & Hill 1986).

Corticosteroid and thyroid hormone therapy have proven ineffective. Prednisone has been tried in patients who were initially suspected of having polymyositis and has been ineffective (DiMauro & Servidei 1993). Since muscle acid maltase is decreased in hypothyroid myopathy (Engel & Gomez 1970), thyroid hormone administration has been given to euthyroid patients with acid maltase deficiency (Isaacs et al 1986, Braun et al 1982) without clinical benefit.

Dietary intervention has produced mixed results. Low carbohydrate diet with or without epinephrine, and a ketogenic diet have been ineffective (DiMauro & Servidei 1993). However, a high protein diet (1500 calories/day, 50% carbo-hydrate, 20% fat, and 25–30% protein) caused significant improvement in growth, strength, muscle bulk and exercise tolerance in a 5-year-old male (Slonim et al 1983). Subsequent studies of this high protein diet in several patients showed improvement (Margolis & Hill 1986, Isaacs et al 1986, Umpleby et al 1987). However, another study of five adults with AMD showed no improvement on a high protein diet despite evidence of correction of protein catabolism (Umpleby et al 1989). Clearly effective treatment for AMD is not yet available.

Debranching enzyme deficiency

Debranching enzyme is bifunctional: it hydrolyses glycogen branch points (amylo-1,6-glucosidase activity) and transfers those three glucose residues adjacent to the branch points which resist cleavage by phosphorylase (oligo-1,4$\to$1,4-glycan trans-ferase; EC 2.4.1.18) activity (Brown & Illingworth 1962). The two activities are located at separate catalytic sites on the same molecule (Gillard & Nelson 1977). Deficiency of the enzyme leads to the accumulation of glycogen with abnormally short outer chains which resembles limit dextrin (Illingworth & Cori 1952, Illingworth et al 1956). The enzyme is normally present in all tissues and can be assayed in leucocytes, erythrocytes, cultured fibroblasts, muscle, liver and heart (Huijing 1964, van Hoof 1967, Justice et al 1970). The disease is transmitted by autosomal recessive inheritance but is genetically heterogeneous. This is evidenced by the existence of subgroups of the disease according to whether the enzyme deficiency involves some or all tissues, the reactivity of the enzyme towards different substrates and the clinical patterns of the disease.

Van Hoof & Hers (1967) determined debranch-ing enzyme activity with four different substrates in tissues of 45 patients. In 34 cases, debranching enzyme activity was very low in muscle, liver and erythrocytes with each method of assay. The glycogen content of the same tissues was high and the outer chains of glycogen were abnormally short. In the remaining 11 cases, enzyme activity was normal or only moderately reduced in one or more tissues with at least one method of assay, and in most cases the muscle glycogen content was normal. In another series investigated by Brown & Brown (1968), seven of 34 patients had normal glycogen content and enzyme activity in muscle. In other cases enzyme activity was absent from liver and muscle but was preserved in leuco-cytes or erythrocytes (Brandt & De Luca 1966, Williams & Field 1968, Deckelbaum et al 1972). More recently investigators have suggested a simpler classification of glycogenosis type III into three subgroups (Chen et al 1987, Ding et al 1990).

Two major clinical patterns of the disease have been recognised. In the more common form, the metabolic disturbance secondary to the hepatic enzyme deficiency dominates the clinical picture. Hepatomegaly, growth retardation and fasting hypoglycaemia, present since infancy, are the usual findings. In some cases there is also cardiomegaly (Moses & Gutman 1972, Huijing 1975, Howell 1978, Moses et al 1989). The hypo-glycaemia causes increased mobilisation and utili-sation of fat, hyperlipidaemia and a tendency to develop ketosis (Fernandes & Pikaar 1969, 1972). Because the outer chains of glycogen can still con-tribute to blood glucose homeostasis and glucose derived from gluconeogenesis or glycogenolysis can freely leave the liver, the metabolic distur-bance is less profound than in type I glycogenesis. The hepatomegaly and fasting hypoglycaemia diminish or disappear after puberty (Brown & Brown 1968, Cohn et al 1975, Howell 1978). Despite glycogen storage in muscle, the myo-pathic features are seldom disabling (Leving et al 1967).

In a smaller group of patients there is a clinically significant myopathy (Oliner et al 1961, Sidbury 1965, Ozand et al 1967, Badurska et al 1970, Brunberg et al 1971, Murase et al 1973, DiMauro et al 1978b, DiMauro et al 1979, Pellissier et al 1979, Rossignol et al 1979, Slonim et al 1982, Brown 1986, Moses et al 1986, 1989, DiMauro & Servidei 1993). In these patients there may be a history of protuberant abdomen in childhood, decreasing in adolescence, and muscle fatigue or aching on heavy exertion since an early age. Progressive muscle weakness begins in childhood or, more commonly, in adult life and may involve both proximal and distal muscles. Selectively severe involvement of distal forearm muscles occurs in some patients. Persistent hepatomegaly is found in most cases. The ECG revealed biventricular hypertrophy in all of five cases studied by DiMauro et al (1978b) and in two of these there was also congestive heart failure. However, in another report only one of 20 patients had clinically significant cardiac insufficiency while 17 of the 20 had laboratory evidence of cardiac enlargement (Moses et al 1989). Serum enzymes of muscle origin are increased from twice to more than 10 times the upper limit of normal. The EMG shows changes consistent with myopathy. Increased insertional activity, myotonic discharges and fibrillation potentials can also occur (Brunberg et al 1971, DiMauro et al 1978b). The muscle glycogen concentration varies between 3% and 6% and the iodine absorption spectrum of glycogen resembles that of limit dextrin. Histopathological studies show a vacuolar myopathy. The abnormal spaces are filled with glycogen which displaces and replaces normal organelles but is not membrane-bound (Neustein 1969, Brunberg et al 1971, Murase et al 1973). Glycogen excess was also found in erythrocytes in the five cases studied by DiMauro et al (1978c). Glycogen accumulation has also been demonstrated in skin biopsy specimens (Sancho et al 1990), cultured muscle fibres (Miranda et al 1981), intramuscular nerves (Powell et al 1985), in Schwann cells and axons of sural nerve biopsy specimens (Moses et al 1986, Ugawa et al 1986), and in the brain of a patient (Hug & Schubert 1966).

The diagnostic clues in this myopathy consist of a history of hepatic enlargement, and possibly of hypoglycaemic episodes, during childhood; persistent mild hepatomegaly; cardiomyopathy in some patients; easy fatigability on heavy exertion; a diminished or absent glycaemic response to adrenaline or glucagon; an impaired or absent rise of lactic acid in venous blood flowing from muscles after ischaemic exercise (Brunberg et al 1971, DiMauro et al 1978b); abnormal electrical irritability of the muscle fibres in the EMG; and a vacuolar myopathy. Myopathic symptoms in debrancher deficiency typically start in the third or fourth decade (70%) at a time when hepatomegaly may be less prominent or detectable (DiMauro et al 1984, DiMauro & Servidei 1993). Wasting of distal leg muscles and intrinsic hand muscles is common, and can lead to the erroneous diagnosis of motor neurone disease or peripheral neuropathy. Although peripheral neuropathy probably contributes to the distal weakness in these adult patients, sensory findings are rare (Moses et al 1986). Confirmatory biochemical studies include glycogen assay and structural analysis and biochemical determination of debranching enzyme activity by more than one method of assay (van Hoof & Hers 1967, DiMauro et al 1978c, DiMauro & Servidei 1993).

There is no effective treatment of the myopathy. Therapy in younger patients consists of prevention of hypoglycaemia by frequent meals of high protein content. Nocturnal gastric infusions of glucose and uncooked corn starches have been used (Fernandes & Huijing 1968). After the age of 1 year, a diet with 45% of the calories from carbohydrate, 20% from fat and the rest from protein is beneficial (Fernandes & Pikaar 1969). Six months of high protein nocturnal intragastric therapy showed remarkable benefit in a 7-year-old boy (Slonim et al 1982), but 6 months of high protein diet in an adult with myopathy and distal muscle wasting failed to produce improvement (Cornelio et al 1984). Vigorous exercise, which can provoke arrhythmias in patients with cardiomyopathy, should be avoided.

Branching enzyme deficiency

The enzyme introduces branch points into glycogen through its α-1,4-glucan: α-1,4-glucan 6-glycosyl-transferase activity. Deficiency of the enzyme was predicted by Illingworth & Cori (1952) on the basis of structural analysis of glycogen isolated from the liver of an affected boy. This glycogen had abnormally long inner and outer chains and fewer than normal branch points, resembling amylopectin. Andersen (1956) described the clinical aspects of this case and the predicted enzyme deficiency was confirmed by Brown & Brown (1966). As the defect is in the synthetic pathway, glycogen storage would not be expected, but in some cases the liver glycogen content is abnormally high. This is probably due to the poor solubility of the abnormal polysaccharide in the cytosol, which may also explain the hepatocellular injury characteristic of the disease. The abnormal glycogen still contains branch points and is heterogeneous in composition (Reed et al 1968, Mercier & Whelan 1973). Thus, there must be an alternative mechanism for introducing branch points into glycogen: an additional enzyme not detected by the usual assay for branching enzyme (Brown & Brown 1966), or debranching enzyme acting in reverse (Huijing et al 1970).

The disease is transmitted by autosomal recessive inheritance (Legum & Nitowsky 1969, Howell et al 1971). Abnormal glycogen deposits occur in liver, spleen and lymph nodes and, occasionally, in muscle, kidney, adrenals and the central nervous system (Howell et al 1971, Schochet et al 1970). Deficiency of the enzyme has been observed in liver, leucocytes and cultured fibroblasts (Brown & Brown 1966, Fernandes & Huijing 1968, Howell et al 1971), and a deficiency of the enzyme was found in muscle, liver, heart and brain in a female who died of cardiomyopathy with a typical childhood phenotype (Servidei et al 1987b). In contrast, adults with branching enzyme deficiency have decreased activity in leucocytes, peripheral nerve, but normal activity in skeletal muscle (Cafferty et al 1991, Lossos et al 1991). Another report describing adult type brancher deficiency suggests genetic heterogeneity in that branching enzyme activity was normal in leucocytes and nerve biopsy tissue (DiMauro & Servidei 1993).

The typical early onset form of branching enzyme deficiency presents during the first year of life with progressive enlargement of liver and spleen and failure to thrive. The abnormal polysaccharide in liver induces nodular cirrhosis, hepatoparenchymal insufficiency and portal hypertension. Carbohydrate tolerance remains normal. Muscle weakness and atrophy appear in some patients (Sidbury et al 1962, Hollerman et al 1966, Levin et al 1968, Reed et al 1968, Zellweger et al 1972), but not in others (Brown & Brown 1966). Death occurs in infancy or early childhood due to hepatic or cardiac failure.

The abnormal polysaccharide stains positively with periodic acid-Schiff (PAS), alcian blue and colloidal iron, gives a brown-blue colour with iodine and resists diastase digestion. It consists of finely filamentous and granular material which intermingles with normal glycogen particles in affected tissues. The presence of normal glycogen particles again suggests that an alternative mechanism for glycogen synthesis is still operative. Deposits in the central nervous system, conspicuous in astroglial cells, resemble Lafora bodies. Different muscles are affected to different extents, but the tongue appears to be particularly severely affected (Schochet et al 1970).

The diagnosis of this enzyme deficiency is suggested by progressive hepatosplenomegaly and failure to thrive in infancy, muscle weakness (if present), and PAS-positive, diastase-fast deposits in affected tissues. Enzyme assays and structural analysis of glycogen are confirmatory. Antenatal diagnosis is possible by enzyme assays on fibroblasts cultured from amniotic fluid cells (Howell et al 1971, Brown & Brown 1989). Diagnosis in the adult-onset form of the disease typically shows mild abnormalities in liver function, cardiomegaly on chest X-ray, left ventricular dilatation on echocardiography, an axonal sensory motor neuropathy on electrodiagnostic studies, and a neurogenic bladder on cystometrogram (DiMauro & Servidei 1993). In these adult-onset cases of branching enzyme deficiency, sural nerve biopsy and leucocyte analysis confirm the diagnosis (Cafferty et al 1991, DiMauro & Servidei 1993).

Therapy with fungal α-glucosidase was attempted in two cases (Fernandes & Huijing 1968). Although the liver glycogen content was reduced, the course of the disease was not altered. Long-term steroid administration, high protein, low carbohydrate diet, and glucagon therapy have proven ineffective (DiMauro & Servidei 1993). In two children with the unusual finding of fasting hypoglycaemia, nutritional treatment to insure normoglycaemia improved their hepatic function and survival (Greene et al 1988). Liver transplantation has been beneficial in 10 children (Selby et al 1991). However, this procedure does not protect patients from developing the disease in other organs. Two years after liver transplantation a child with brancher deficiency died of intractable cardiomyopathy (Sokal et al 1992).

Myophosphorylase deficiency

McArdle in 1951 described the clinical features of the disease and attributed them to a deficiency of muscle phosphorylase. This prediction was confirmed by Schmidt & Mahler (1959) and by Mommaerts et al (1959).

Phosphorylase catalyses the cleavage of $1,4-\alpha$-glucosidic linkages, releasing glucose 1-phosphate from non-reducing ends of exposed glycogen chains. Its action comes to a halt when the chain length is reduced to four glucose residues which are then removed by the debranching enzyme complex. In resting muscle, phosphorylase is mostly in an inactive b form which phosphorylase b kinase converts to an active form. Activation of the kinase, and hence of phosphorylase, is mediated by cyclic AMP via activation of adenyl cyclase by adrenaline (in muscle and liver) or glucagon (in liver). Electrical stimulation or exercise activates phosphorylase, probably through calcium release from the sarcoplasmic reticulum. Phosphorylase a is reconverted to phosphorylase b by a specific phosphatase which, in turn, is inhibited by cyclic AMP (for reviews see Huijing 1975, Howell 1978, Servidei et al 1988b, Lewis & Haller 1991).

Different tissues contain different phosphorylase isoenzymes, and different structural genes code for the isoenzymes present in skeletal muscle, liver and smooth muscle. Cardiac muscle contains isoenzymes found in smooth and skeletal muscles as well as hybrid isoenzymes (Yunis et al 1962, Davis et al 1967, Miranda et al 1979). Deficiency of muscle phosphorylase occurs independently of other isoenzymes and only skeletal muscle is affected clinically. The syndrome, however, is genetically heterogeneous. This is evinced by subgroups of the disease defined according to mode of inheritance, clinical patterns, and the presence or absence of catalytically active enzyme protein in muscle (DiMauro & Servidei 1993).

In most instances the disease is transmitted by autosomal recessive inheritance, but there is an unexplained preponderance of males (Huijing 1975). Possibly, some females remain undiagnosed, being less likely to engage in the type of exercise which provokes symptoms. Autosomal dominant transmission of phosphorylase

deficiency was reported in one family (Chui & Munsat 1976).

Symptoms may date from early childhood, but more typically the capacity for exercise is unimpaired until the second half of the second decade. In contrast to this common pattern, a fatal infantile case, with death due to respiratory insufficiency at the age of 13 weeks, has been reported (DiMauro & Hartlage 1978, Miranda et al 1979, Milstein et al 1989). 'Late-onset' cases have been described in a brother and sister who did not develop symptoms until their fiftieth year (Engel et al 1963), in a 73-year-old man with cardiac alterations and weakness (Servidei et al 1988b), and in a patient who presented with muscle weakness at the age of 74 years (Hewitt & Gardner-Thorpe 1978).

Catalytically inactive enzyme protein is present in some cases but not in others (DiMauro & Servidei 1993). The inactive protein has been detected by immunological tests (Dreyfus & Alexandre 1971) or by SDS–polyacrylamide electrophoresis (Feit & Brooke 1976, Koster et al 1979). In one case, the electrophoretic method detected inactive enzyme protein when the immunological method did not (Koster et al 1979). Most patients lack immunologically reactive enzyme protein in muscle. It was absent in 41 of 48 cases in one report (Servidei et al 1988b) and in 10 of 11 patients in another report (McConchie et al 1991). Normal mature skeletal muscle has just one isozyme of skeletal muscle type. Cardiac muscle and brain show three isozymes with the brain-type isozyme contributing 58% to the total activity in cardiac muscle and 64% to the activity in brain (DiMauro & Servidei 1993). It is possible that the lack of cardiomyopathy in most patients with McArdle's disease relates to the contribution of the brain isoenzyme (DiMauro & Servidei 1993).

The typical symptoms consist of muscular pain, weakness and stiffness during slight to moderate exertion. Pain on exercise, which is the most prominent feature, can occur in any muscle, even those of the jaw. Rest rapidly relieves the symptoms after moderate exercise, but the more severe or protracted the exercise, the longer symptoms persist (McArdle 1951). The pain may disappear with continued exercise if stiffness has not developed. This 'second wind' is related to increased muscle blood flow, and the augmented utilisation by muscle of plasma free fatty acids (Pernow et al 1967, Haller et al 1985, Braakhekke et al 1986, Mineo et al 1990, Lewis et al 1991) and amino acids (Wahren et al 1973, Slonim & Goans 1985) as energy sources. A frequent and characteristic symptom is inability to extend the fingers fully after sustained gripping movements against resistance; full recovery may take many minutes. After severe exercise, muscle pain, weakness and swelling may persist for several days. Myoglobinuria after exercise occurs at least once in the course of the disease in one-half to two-thirds of cases (Dawson et al 1968, Fattah et al 1979). Muscle weakness and atrophy are detected in about one-third and are usually mild. Muscles of the pectoral girdle are more likely to be affected than those of the pelvic girdle, and calf muscle bulk may be larger than normal. Moderate exercise provokes the typical muscle symptoms as well as tachycardia, dyspnoea, exhaustion and rarely nausea and vomiting. Ischaemic exercise of forearm muscles results in rapid fatigue and shortening of forearm flexors which may persist for some minutes after return of the circulation. It is not a true cramp but a physiological contracture during which affected muscles remain electrically silent (McArdle 1951, Rowland et al 1966). To perform the test, a blood-pressure cuff is placed on the upper arm and is maximally inflated to occlude arterial blood flow. Exercise is by squeezing a rubber bulb against a fixed resistance at a rate of one per second. Normal subjects can readily do this for a minute. In occasional patients, weakness develops during the test, preventing them from exercising to the point of developing a contracture. Because the muscles cannot degrade glycogen to lactic acid during the exercise, there is no rise in lactate in venous blood taken from forearm muscles after release of the circulation (McArdle 1951). Normal subjects exhibit a threefold to five-fold increase of lactate within 5 minutes of the end of exercise and the lactate level returns to baseline in about 30 minutes. Normal subjects also show a rise in venous alanine following ischaemic forearm exercise. In contrast, patients with McArdle's disease show a net uptake of alanine (Wahren et al 1973).

The mechanism of the electrically silent muscle contractures is not understood. One possible explanation would be a deficiency of ATP required for the operation of the sarcoplasmic reticulum (SR) calcium pump. However, Rowland et al (1965) could not demonstrate a decrease of ATP in muscle during a contracture induced by ischaemic exercise. On the other hand, Gruener et al (1968) found that microapplications of a calcium-containing solution to skinned muscle fibres elicited prolonged contractures, and Brody et al (1970) noted that isolated SR vesicles accumulated calcium normally in the presence of ATP. The latter two studies are consistent with the view that the SR calcium pump fails when ATP becomes unavailable. However, ^{31}P-nuclear magnetic resonance studies show normal levels of ATP but a reduced concentration of phosphocreatine in fatigued myophosphorylase-deficient muscle (Ross et al 1981). Increasing evidence suggests that premature fatigue in McArdle's disease may be due to impaired excitation–contraction coupling mediated by an excessive accumulation of ADP as opposed to deficiency in muscle ATP (Lewis & Haller 1991). Excessive accumulation of ATP may mediate contracture by various mechanisms. These include:

1. An addition of ADP disassociation from actomyosin resulting in increased percentage time that cross-bridges spend in a force-generating state
2. Direct interaction of ADP with thin filaments increasing their calcium sensitivity
3. Alteration of sarcoplasmic reticulum function resulting in increased calcium concentration in the myoplasm (DiMauro & Servidei 1993).

The serum levels of muscle enzymes are usually raised at rest. Following exercise, these levels increase markedly within a few hours (Hammett et al 1966). EMG studies may show alterations in motor unit potentials indicative of a myopathy and there is electrical silence of muscle fibres during contracture. Repetitive stimulation of motor nerves at 18 Hz was reported to produce an abnormal decrement of the amplitude of the evoked compound muscle action potential (Dyken et al 1967) but this finding has not been confirmed.

Muscle glycogen is usually raised, often to between 2% and 5%, but very occasionally it is normal. Glycogen accumulates subsarcolemmally in blebs and between myofibrils, especially adjacent to I bands (Schotland et al 1965). Small pockets of glycogen may also become invaginated into mitochondria (Gruener et al 1968). Lack of phosphorylase can be demonstrated histochemically in cryostat sections of fresh-frozen muscle. Characteristically, enzyme activity is absent from muscle fibres but is preserved in the smooth muscle cells of blood vessels. The histochemical demonstration of phosphorylase in muscle depends on the presence of glycogen primer, and the enzyme cannot be demonstrated even in normal muscle depleted of glycogen as, e.g., after prolonged storage of a muscle specimen at room temperature, or after death. Biochemical assay of the enzyme is independent of the muscle glycogen content. Although mature skeletal muscle fibres of affected patients lack phosphorylase, regenerating fibres and muscle cells cultured in vitro do show enzyme activity (Roelofs et al 1971). This has been attributed to the synthesis of a fetal isozyme by immature muscle cells (Sato et al 1977, DiMauro et al 1978a). Synthesis of the fetal isozyme is repressed by the time of birth.

The diagnosis of myophosphorylase deficiency is suggested by weakness, pain and contractures of muscle on exertion, a history of myoglobinuria, failure to form lactic acid on ischaemic exercise and by histochemical studies of the muscle biopsy specimen. Biochemical assay of the enzyme is required to confirm the diagnosis.

The ingestion of glucose or fructose increases exercise tolerance, but their long-term use has proved disappointing. They are awkward to take, predispose to obesity, and fructose may cause colicky pain. Injections of glucagon have proven impractical and inconsistent in attempting to maintain high blood glucose during exercise. Another potentially rational approach to treatment is to imitate the metabolic changes associated with the 'second wind' phenomenon by administering free fatty acids. An infusion of emulsified fat, administration of nor-epinephrine or heparin, and fasting have all increased exercise tolerance in patients with McArdle's disease, but practical measures, such as consumption of a high-fat, low-carbohydrate diet proved ineffective (DiMauro & Servidei 1993). Because branch-chain amino acids can serve as an alternative fuel, one patient was treated with a high protein diet and improvement was observed (Slonim & Goans 1985). However, others have found no improvement in energy metabolism-based magnetic resonance spectroscopy or formal exercise testing (Argov et al 1987b, Jensen et al 1990). All patients should be advised to keep within the limits of exertion causing significant pain and, as far as possible, to precede vigorous exertion by a period of more gentle activity.

Phosphorylase b kinase deficiency

Phosphorylase b kinase is a multimeric enzyme composed of four different subunits, alpha, beta, gamma and delta with molecular weights of 145 000, 28 000, 45 000 and 18 000. The enzyme composition is $(\alpha\,\beta\,\gamma\,\delta)^4$, for a molecular weight of 1.28×10^6 (van der Berg & Berger 1990). The gamma subunit is catalytic, and the activity of the enzyme is regulated by the degree of phosphorylation of the alpha and beta subunits. Calcium sensitivity is conferred by the delta subunit, which is calmodulin. Two isoforms of the alpha subunit have been described, alpha and alpha prime, alpha prime being present in heart and type I muscle fibres (DiMauro & Servidei 1993). Two principal mechanisms lead to activation of phosphorylase b kinase in muscle:

1. A cascade of reactions starting with activation by epinephrine of adenylate cyclase via G proteins, followed by cyclic AMP-mediated activation of protein kinase, which activates phosphorylase b kinase through phosphorylation of the alpha and beta subunits.
2. Direct activation through binding of calcium (release from the sarcoplasmic reticulum during contraction) to the delta subunit (DiMauro & Servidei 1993).

There are four different clinical syndromes associated with deficiency of phosphorylase b kinase. One presents in infancy or childhood manifesting as liver disease associated with hepatomegaly, growth retardation, delayed motor development and fasting hypolygcaemia (DiMauro & Servidei 1993). Inheritance is X-linked recessive but autosomal recessive transmission has also been reported (van der Berg & Berger 1990). Another form of the disease has autosomal recessive transmission and affects liver and muscle with hepatomegaly that usually resolves with age, and a non-progressive myopathy (van den Berg & Berger 1990). A third form of phosphorylase b kinase deficiency is primarily myopathic and has been described in hypotonic young children (Ohtani et al 1982, Iwamasa et al 1983), in later childhood with exercise intolerance and myalgias (Abarbanel et al 1986), and in adult life presenting with exercise intolerance, or pigmenturia following vigorous exercise (Abarbanel et al 1986, Servidei et al 1987a, Carrier et al 1990, Clemens et al 1990). Inheritance is autosomal recessive. The fourth form of phosphorylase b kinase deficiency presents with autosomal recessive inheritance and has primarily cardiomyopathic symptoms. The cardiac dysfunction led to death in infancy in two unrelated patients (Mizuta et al 1984, Servidei et al 1988a).

In patients with myopathy serum creatine kinase activity is elevated to a variable degree. The venous lactate response to forearm ischaemic exercise has been reported as normal in two of six patients, impaired but not flat in three, and flat in only one patient, who also developed a contracture (Abarbanel et al 1986). Electromyographic study showed non-specific myopathic changes.

Light microscopy of muscle biopsy specimens shows subsarcolemmal accumulations of glycogen predominantly in type II b fibres (DiMauro & Servidei 1993). By electron-microscopy the vacuoles correspond to pools of free, normal-appearing glycogen particles. No glycogen storage is present in satellite cells, fibroblasts, endothelial cells, pericytes, smooth muscle of intramuscular blood vessels, or in axons or Schwann cells of intramuscular nerves (Clemens et al 1990). Histochemical staining for phosphorylase is normal.

No effective therapy has been described in patients with myopathy due to a deficiency of phosphorylase b kinase. One patient received prednisone 30 mg/day for 3 months without improvement (Clemens et al 1990). New approaches to therapy are necessary. There are similarities in the clinical and biochemical features of both phosphorylase b kinase deficiency and phosphorylase deficiency. It may be helpful to attempt a high protein diet in phosphorylase b kinase-deficient patients.

Muscle phosphofructokinase deficiency

Phosphofructokinase (PFK) is a tetrameric enzyme under the control of three structural genes located on chromosomes 1, 10 and 21 which encode muscle-type (M), liver-type (L), and fibroblast- or platelet-type (P) subunits respectively. The three genes are differentially expressed in various tissues, resulting in tissue-specific isozyme patterns. The various homotetrameric and heterotetrameric enzymes can be distinguished by subunit-specific monoclonal antibodies and ion-exchange chromatography (reviewed by Vora 1983, Vora et al 1987). Muscle and liver contain homotetramers M_4 and L_4 respectively, whereas erythrocytes contain five enzymes made up of M and L subunits in various combinations (Vora et al 1983a, Vora et al 1987). Cultured muscle fibres express all three subunits and contain multiple homotetrameric and heterotetrameric isozymes (Davidson et al 1983).

Muscle PFK deficiency was first described by Tarui et al (1965); a second case was investigated by Layzer et al (1967b). More than 20 cases of the disease have been described (Rowland et al 1986, Mineo et al 1987, Vora et al 1987, Danon et al 1988, Haller & Lewis 1991).

The enzyme catalyses the conversion of fructose-6-phosphate to fructose-1,6-diphosphate. The reaction requires ATP and is irreversible. Absence of the enzyme completely inhibits the Embden–Meyerhof pathway and blocks glucose utilisation. Glucose-1-phosphate and glucose-6-phosphate levels are increased, and fructose-1,6-diphosphate is markedly reduced in muscle (Tarui et al 1965). There is an associated partial enzyme deficiency in erythrocytes which lack the M isoenzyme (Tarui et al 1965, Layzer et al 1967b, Tarui et al 1969, Danon et al 1988, Vora et al 1987).

The clinical picture can be similar to that seen with myophosphorylase deficiency and the ischaemic exercise test is positive. In addition, there is a mild haemolytic disease, secondary to the partial erythrocyte enzyme defect (Tarui et al 1969). Hyperuricaemia and gout occur in a proportion of the patients. This may be related to the accelerated erythropoiesis, or to the stimulation of nucleotide metabolism by another mechanism. Exercise results in an abnormal rise of inosine, hypoxanthine, uric acid and ammonia in venous blood flowing from exercised muscle (Kono et al 1986, Mineo et al 1987). Autosomal recessive inheritance operates in some families (Tarui et al 1965, Layzer et al 1967b, Dupond et al 1977) but, in the family reported by Serratrice et al (1969), the trait was probably autosomal dominant. In the latter family, the propositus was also atypical in that he had hepatomegaly and suffered from progressive muscle weakness.

Other 'atypical' cases of PFK deficiency have also been observed, attesting to the heterogeneity of the syndrome. In two sibs (Guibaud et al 1978) and in an isolated case (Danon et al 1981a) of PFK deficiency, muscle weakness and joint contractures were present from birth. Two of the three patients died in infancy or early childhood. Further evidence of clinical heterogeneity is emphasised by the existence of two groups of patients, one with haemolytic anaemia without myopathy, and the other with fixed weakness of early or late onset. One report described a 37-year-old male with hepatomegaly who since age 15 had slowly progressive weakness and wasting typical of the scapuloperoneal syndrome (Serratrice et al 1969). Another report describes a 60-year-old woman who tired easily since childhood but was normal until age 55 at which time she developed proximal weakness (Hays et al 1981). Another patient was 75 years old with a history of tiring easily as a youngster but did not seek medical evaluation until the age of 65 at which time proximal weakness was a major complaint (Danon et al 1988).

Some patients have partial erythrocyte PFK deficiency and a haemolytic syndrome but no muscle symptoms and produce lactate normally on ischaemic exercise. This syndrome has been attributed to an unstable or deficient L subunit or to kinetically abnormal M or L subunits (Vora 1983, Vora et al 1983a, Rowland et al 1986, Vora et al 1987, Danon et al 1988).

The subsarcolemmal glycogen deposits in muscle resemble those seen in myophosphorylase deficiency. Structurally abnormal glycogen, resembling amylopectin that accumulates in branching enzyme deficiency, has also been observed in some muscle fibres in a few patients (Agamanolis et al 1980, Hays et al 1981). Absence of phosphofructokinase can be demonstrated histochemically (Bonilla & Schotland 1970) but the diagnosis is best established by biochemical assay of the enzyme in muscle. Cultured muscle cells express the M, L and P subunits of PFK in multiple tetrameric combinations. However, the M subunit is catalytically inactive in muscle cells cultured from patients with PFK deficiency (Davidson et al 1983). This suggests a structural mutation involving the catalytic site of the M subunit. The clinical laboratory results are similar in myophosphorylase deficiency and phosphofructokinase deficiency. In patients with PFK deficiency serum creatine kinase is variably but consistently increased, there is a moderate reticulocytosis and increased bilirubin due to the haemolytic trait, and the serum uric acid is increased in most patients. Electromyographic findings are variable occasionally, showing myopathic features. Contractures induced by ischaemic exercise are electrically silent as they are in phosphorylase deficiency. The magnetic resonance spectroscopic findings differ from those seen in myophosphorylase deficiency because in PFK deficiency, as with other defects of distal glycolysis, glycolytic intermediates accumulate as phosphorylated mono-esters. These are seen as a discrete peak on magnetic resonance spectroscopy (Argov & Bank 1991). The peak of phosphorylated mono-esters is not present at rest but occurs during mild exercise and is proportional to the severity of the block in glycolysis (Argov & Bank 1991). During recovery, these phosphorylated mono-esters are dephosphorylated with the liberation of inorganic phosphate. This explains why there is a slower return to normal of the inorganic phosphate peak after exercise in patients with PFK deficiency compared to those with phosphorylase deficiency (Argov & Bank 1991).

Treatment for the metabolic derangements in PFK deficiency are similar to those described for phosphorylase deficiency, with one important additional problem, that glucose is not an alternative substrate for patients with PFK deficiency. Theoretically a high protein diet may prove useful as it has in some patients with phosphorylase deficiency. This has not been reported at present as a treatment in PFK deficiency.

Defects in the distal glycolytic pathway

Deficiencies of phosphoglycerate kinase (PGK), phosphoglycerate mutase (PGAM), and lactate dehydrogenase (LDH) have been recognised to date. The three disorders share certain common features (reviewed by DiMauro & Servidei 1993):

1. As in myophosphorylase and PFK deficiencies, severe exercise is poorly tolerated and provokes attacks of myoglobinuria.
2. There is mild or no glycogen accumulation in the muscle fibres.
3. The ischaemic exercise test is either positive, or there may be a modest (less than two-fold) rise of lactate in venous blood flowing from the ischaemically exercised muscles.
4. Residual enzyme activity can be detected in the muscle fibres.

Phosphoglycerate kinase deficiency

This is the only glycogenosis transmitted by X-linked recessive inheritance. PGK is a monomer; tissue-specific PGK isozymes are lacking, and the enzyme defect is expressed in cultured cells. Mutations involving PGK are asymptomatic, or result in severe haemolytic anaemia associated with neurological deficits (reviewed by DiMauro & Servidei 1993), or produce a myopathy with the features described above (Rosa et al 1982, DiMauro et al 1983). Mutant PGKs differ in their kinetic and physical properties. The mutant enzyme studied by DiMauro et al (1983) had reduced substrate affinity, altered electrophoretic mobility, and an abnormal pH profile. Muscle contained reduced amounts of the immunologically recognisable but abnormal enzyme protein (Bresolin et al 1984). The mutant enzyme observed by Rosa et al (1982) had increased affinity for ATP, increased heat lability and abnor-

mal electrophoretic mobility. As PGK has no tissue-specific isozymes, the fact that a given mutation affects either erythrocytes, or muscle fibres, or neither, remains unexplained. Four patients had myopathic symptoms (Rosa et al 1982, DiMauro et al 1983, Tonin et al 1989, Sugie et al 1989). Three had myopathic symptoms alone, a 13-year-old boy (DiMauro et al 1983), a 31-year-old man (Rosa et al 1982) and a 37-year-old man (Tonin et al 1989). All had intolerance to exercise, cramps and myoglobinuria. One, a 37-year-old man, died suddenly in his sleep. A fourth patient, an 11-year-old boy, had recurrent myoglobinuria but also haemolytic anaemia and mental retardation (Sugie et al 1989). Serum CK activity was variably elevated in all patients, ischaemic forearm exercise showed no rise of venous lactate in two patients (an 18-year-old boy and a 37-year-old man) and an inadequate rise in another (a 31-year-old man). Studies of magnetic resonance spectroscopy revealed findings similar to those seen in PFK deficiency with a marked rise in phosphorylated mono-esters after exercise (Duboc et al 1987).

No specific treatment is known. The therapeutic issues would be similar to those in PFK deficiency.

Phosphoglycerate mutase deficiency

This is an autosomal recessive disorder. PGAM is a dimeric enzyme composed of muscle (M) and brain (B) subunits giving rise to MM, MB and BB isozymes (reviewed by DiMauro & Servidei 1993). The expression of the various isozymes in different tissues is developmentally regulated. In mature muscle, the MM isozyme predominates. Deficiency of PGAM has been reported in four patients, two men and two women (DiMauro et al 1981, DiMauro et al 1982, Bresolin et al 1983, Kissel et al 1985, Vita et al 1990), and all patients had intolerance to intense exercise with myalgia, cramps and recurrent myoglobinuria. Forearm ischaemic exercise was associated with low but not absent elevations in venous lactate (1.5–2 fold increases of resting values)(DiMauro & Servidei 1993). Muscle biopsy is usually normal but may show diffuse (DiMauro et al 1982) or patchy (Bresolin et al 1983) glycogen accumulation.

PGAM deficiency is transmitted as an autosomal recessive trait. All patients reported were sporadic cases, but partial PGAM deficiency was documented in one set of parents (Bresolin et al 1983). Magnetic resonance spectroscopy in one patient showed findings virtually identical to those in a patient with PGK deficiency (Argov et al 1987a). No specific approaches to treatment have been reported.

Lactate dehydrogenase deficiency

This is also an autosomal recessive disorder. LDH is a tetrameric enzyme composed of various combinations of muscle (M) and heart (H) subunits. As in the case of PGAM, the expression of the various isozymes in different tissues is developmentally regulated. The M_4 form predominates in mature muscle. LDH deficiency has been reported in three patients. Two young men displayed intolerance to intense exercise and had recurrent myoglobinuria (Kanno et al 1980, Bryan et al 1990) and an asymptomatic young woman was detected through blood screening (Maekawa et al 1984). In all three patients forearm ischaemic exercise showed an inadequate rise of venous lactate; a deficiency of LDH was demonstrated in muscle as well as serum erythrocytes and leucocytes. Biochemical studies have confirmed autosomal recessive inheritance (Kanno et al 1980).

Other glycogenoses

Other glycogenoses have been reported, some affecting muscle, in which only a single patient or a single family have been described, or in which the enzymatic disorder has been insufficiently defined. An example was the disorder described by Satoyoshi & Kowa (1967) in two brothers. Both, when 35 years old, developed muscle pain, stiffness and weakness occurring a few hours after moderately heavy exercise. Blood lactate failed to rise after ischaemic exercise except following fructose ingestion. Biopsy studies showed an apparent block at the level of phosphohexose-isomerase (glucose-6-phosphate isomerase; EC 5.3.1.9), thought to be due to inhibition of the enzyme, associated with a decreased activity of phosphofructokinase. Exercise tolerance improved considerably following fructose, but not glucose, ingestion.

Another example was the 8-year-old boy with pains on exercise, described by Strugalska-Cynowska (1967); he had a very delayed rise in blood lactate following ischaemic exercise. This was attributed, on histochemical grounds, to a disturbance in the activity of phosphorylase-b-kinase (EC 2.7.1.38) which converts phosphorylase from the inactive to the active form.

Another glycogenesis was noted in the 4-year-old boy described by Thomson et al (1963) with a mild myopathy and marked contracture of his calves, having only a slight rise in blood lactate after ischaemic exercise. His muscles were loaded with glycogen of normal structure. It was thought that there was a partial deficiency of phosphoglucomutase and possibly of other glycolytic enzymes.

Holmes et al (1960) studied a female patient who presented at the age of 21 with symptoms of a myopathy and died at the age of 31 years. Cardiac and skeletal muscle contained basophilic, PAS-positive, diastase-fast polysaccharide deposits. Similar material was found in hepatocytes and in the lumen of the convoluted tubules. Enzyme assays and structural analysis of the polysaccharide were not performed. A similar disorder was reported by Karpati et al (1969) in a male patient who died of cardiac failure at the age of 19 years. Post-mortem examination was restricted to muscle and liver. The abnormal polysaccharide had a filamentous fine structure and was especially abundant in type II muscle fibres.

A cardioskeletal lysosomal glycogenosis without acid maltase deficiency has been observed in children and young adults (Danon et al 1981b, Riggs et al 1983b). Mental retardation and abnormal liver functions are variable associated features. The cardiomyopathy distinguishes the disorder clinically from adult AMD. An infantile variant of this syndrome may also exist (Atkin et al 1984). All patients described to date were male. The mode of inheritance is still uncertain.

MALIGNANT HYPERTHERMIA

Since its recognition (Denborough & Lovell

1960), this syndrome has aroused great interest among anaesthetists. Recent reports have emphasised the importance of standardization of diagnosis using the muscle contracture response to halothane and caffeine (The European Malignant Hyperpyrexia Group 1984, Ording 1988, Larach for the North American Malignant Hyperthermia Group 1989, Larach et al 1992). In most cases susceptibility to the disorder is thought to be transmitted via an autosomal dominant gene with variable penetrance (MacLennan & Phillips 1992). Recent genetic studies in swine susceptible to malignant hyperthermia (Mickelson et al 1989, Ervasti et al 1991, Fletcher et al 1991, Fujii et al 1991) and in humans (MacLennan et al 1990, McCarthy et al 1990, Healy et al 1991, Kausch et al 1991, Levitt et al 1991, MacKenzie et al 1991, Deufel et al 1992, Fagerlund et al 1992, Otsu et al 1992) have shown that susceptibility to malignant hyperthermia both in swine and humans relates to abnormalities in the calcium-release channel of the skeletal muscle sarcoplasmic reticulum (the ryanodine receptor). In swine all cases of malignant hyperthermia in all breeds point to a single founder mutation (MacLennan & Phillips 1992). The gene for the ryanodine receptor in humans localises to chromosome 19 (MacLennan et al 1990). Unlike bovine MHS the human disorder appears to have different forms in view of the recently described genetic heterogeneity (Deufel et al 1992, Fagerlund et al 1992). Prior to the demonstration that the ryanodine receptor and associated gene lesions are responsible for malignant hyperthermia, the muscle contracture test following exposure to halothane and caffeine was the only means of confirming the diagnosis. It is now apparent that the muscle contracture test is not specific for malignant hyperthermia and Table 17.10 lists a newly proposed classification for malignant hyperthermia susceptibility and identifies other groups of disorders that may have alterations on the muscle contracture test. The rationale for developing this classification is based on the different pathogenetic mechanisms that can lead to the positive muscle contracture response. This indicates that there can be different substances that trigger muscle contraction, different drugs to reverse that type of contracture and possibly different animal models in which to study

Table 17.10 Classification of malignant hyperthermia susceptibility (MHS) (adapted from scheme presented by Dr Frank Lehmann-Horn at the International Workshop on Malignant Hyperthermia in Hershey, Pennsylvania)

Definition	MHS = positive test in a family without clinical myopathy	
Rationale for classification	— Different pathomechanisms exist in MHS — Contracture test not specific	
Myopathies	Group 1	Triad channelopathies = MHS
	Group 2	Other channelopathies (sodium, chloride)
	Group 3	Enzymopathies (eg CPT deficiency, etc.)
	Group 4	Cytoskeletonopathies (Duchenne–Becker dystrophy, etc.)
	Groups 2–4	Calcium dysregulation syndrome or non-MHS calcium dysregulation syndromes

these disorders. In a study of 44 patients with myotonia, 10 patients had equivocal findings and four positive responses to the muscle contracture test (Lehmann-Horn & Iaizzo 1990). These investigators point out that the positive and equivocal test results may be accounted for solely by electrical after-activity in the patients with pure myotonia and by increased resting myoplasmic calcium in those patients with myotonic dystrophy. The results emphasise that the in vitro contracture test lacks specificity. Takagi et al (1989) reported an abnormally enhanced caffeine contracture test response in 11 out of 13 patients with Duchenne dystrophy. They compared the response in the Duchenne dystrophy patients to those with documented episodes of malignant hyperthermia and concluded that different mechanisms were involved to produce the positive test. Another report described the presence of susceptibility to malignant hyperthermia in a patient, a 6-year-old boy, with McArdle's disease (Isaacs et al 1989). There is also an association between susceptibility to malignant hyperthermia and central core disease, and it has been suggested that the two disorders may result from allelic gene alterations (Kausch et al 1991).

As noted above, the most commonly used and most sensitive laboratory test for predicting malignant hyperthermia susceptibility is the caffeine halothane contracture test (Ording 1988, Larach for the North American Malignant Hyperthermia Group 1989, Larach et al 1992). The report by Ording (1988) reviews in detail the wide variety of tests that have been considered as predictors of susceptibility to malignant hyperthermia. These tests have included serum tests (creatine kinase, cholinesterase), erythrocyte tests (osmotic fragility, chemiluminescence), platelet tests (platelet aggregation, platelet nucleotide depletion), white cell tests (human leucocyte antigen type, calcium concentration in lymphocytes), electrophysiological tests (motor unit counting, tourniquet tests, relaxation rates of twitch response, recruitment pattern after halothane and suxamethonium), biochemical muscle tests (ATP depletion, glycolytic metabolites, myophosphorylase ratio, adenylate kinase deficiency, adenylate cyclase activity in cyclic AMP, adenylate deaminase deficiency, low weight molecular proteins, calcium uptake by sarcoplasmic reticulum, intracellular ionised calcium concentration, heat production), nuclear magnetic resonance (NMR) scanning (muscle histology), and contracture tests (caffeine, halothane). Ording (1988) concludes his review by indicating that of all the tests suggested for the diagnosis of susceptibility to malignant hyperthermia only the invasive, cumbersome, halothane and caffeine contracture tests have been proven reliable. Unfortunately, even with this type of testing, control data of good quality are scarce. The results of more recent investigations that have sought to find better alternative diagnostic procedures to identify patients susceptible to malignant hyperthermia have supported the conclusion of Ording. Investigations of NMR spectroscopy (Olgin et al 1988, Webster et al 1990, Olgin et al 1991), electron paramagnetic resonance spectroscopic measurements in erythrocytes (Cooper et al 1992), measurements of twitch properties in ankle dorsiflexor muscles (Quinlan et al 1989), and multiple pulse stimulation during intravenous infusion of dantrolene (Quinlan et al 1990) all proved less accurate when

compared to the muscle contracture test with caffeine and halothane. There is an ongoing effort to improve the reliability and sensitivity of performing muscle contracture testing (Melton et al 1989, Fletcher et al 1991, Iaizzo et al 1991, MacKenzie et al 1991, Heytens et al 1992, Larach et al 1992). To help establish the specificity and sensitivity of the proposed guidelines of the North American Malignant Hyperthermia Group (Larach and the North American Malignant Hyperthermia Group 1989), muscle contracture testing was performed in tissue obtained from 176 subjects not felt to be at risk for malignant hyperthermia (there was no abnormal response to triggering anaesthetic agents, no evidence of myopathy, no family history of malignant hyperthermia susceptibility). The investigators analysed the responses of 1022 muscle fascicles to the following: separate administration of 3% halothane or incremental caffeine concentrations, or the joint administration of 1% halothane and incremental concentrations. The results of these studies led the authors to conclude that there were sources of error in the test related to the number of muscle fascicles that were tested and the different concentrations of halothane and caffeine given; however, the major source of variation in the results occurred between the laboratories in the different centres. The authors have concluded that their data demonstrate that the proposed diagnostic guidelines need to be modified to improve the specificity estimates for malignant hyperthermia susceptibility before adopting a specific test methodology as the definitive diagnostic procedure. However, contracture testing will remain the gold standard for diagnosis in patients who have not experienced an acute crisis of malignant hyperthermia.

The malignant hyperthermia reaction is triggered by potent inhalation anaesthetics (halothane, ether, cyclopropane, methoxyflurane, enflurane) or succinylcholine. Premonitory signs include tachycardia, tachypnoea, dysrhythmias, skin mottling, cyanosis, rising body temperature, muscle rigidity, sweating and unstable blood pressure. Failure to obtain muscle relaxation with adequate doses of succinylcholine can also be an early warning sign. The fully developed syndrome is associated with a rapid rise of body temperature (up to 1°C every 5 minutes); rapidly evolving metabolic acidosis with lactic acidaemia; often, also, respiratory acidosis due to carbon dioxide overproduction; muscle rigidity in 75% of the cases; hyperkalaemia; variable alterations of the serum calcium; very high serum CK activity; myoglobinaemia and myoglobinuria. Despite wide awareness of the syndrome and symptomatic therapy, the mortality rate remains high.

Treatment of the acute syndrome consists of termination of anaesthesia, body cooling, intravenous hydration, sodium bicarbonate administration to combat metabolic acidosis, mechanical hyperventilation to decrease the respiratory acidosis, and mannitol or frusemide, as needed, to maintain urine flow. More specific treatment consists of dantrolene, given intravenously, 1–2 mg/kg, which may be repeated each 5–10 minutes, up to 10 mg/kg (Faust et al 1979, Gronert 1980, Amiel & Nivoche 1989, Cornet et al 1989, Meier-Hellmann et al 1990, Akasaka et al 1991). Vecuronium and doxapram are agents that can be safely administered to patients with susceptibility to malignant hyperthermia (Ording & Fonsmark 1988) and a new dantrolene-like drug, Azumolene, may prove useful as another effective medication to prevent and to treat malignant hyperthermia (Dershwitz & Sreter 1990, Foster et al 1991). There are recent reviews of the approach to nursing care following crisis in malignant hyperthermia (Ashby 1990, Newberry 1990, Sinkovich & Mitch-Reisgnalo 1991, Wlody 1991) and of the diagnosis and management of susceptibility to malignant hyperthermia in pregnancy (Sorosky et al 1989).

Screening of relatives of affected patients for susceptibility to malignant hyperthermia is important. Seventy percent of the cases at risk have increased serum CK activities (Britt et al 1976). Without this finding, in vitro testing of muscle strips for an abnormal contracture response to halothane, caffeine or a combination of both agents can be done.

MUSCLE AMP DEAMINASE DEFICIENCY

AMP deaminase (EC 3.5.4.6) converts AMP to IMP with liberation of ammonia. The biological role of the enzyme is not understood; possibly it participates in regulation of ATP levels in muscle. In 1978, Fishbein et al found deficiency of the muscle enzyme in five young men with complaints, often since childhood, of muscle weakness or cramping after exercise. Three patients had mild increases in serum CK and two had abnormal EMGs. Muscle histology was normal except for mild type I fibre atrophy in one case. Erythrocyte enzyme activity was normal. Ammonia levels failed to rise but lactate values rose normally in venous blood flowing from ischaemically exercised muscles. Muscle AMP deaminase deficiency had also been reported in a single case of primary hypokalaemic periodic paralysis (Engel et al 1964). Fishbein (1985, 1986) now distinguishes between inherited and acquired forms of AMP deaminase deficiency. The primary deficiency is transmitted by autosomal recessive inheritance and may or may not manifest clinically in adult life with muscle cramping and exercise intolerance. The prognosis is benign. The secondary type, in which residual enzyme activity is higher (1–10%) than in the primary type, can occur in a variety of neurogenic and myopathic disorders. In view of the marked clinical heterogeneity, the significance of muscle AMP deaminase deficiency remains uncertain.

NUTRITIONAL AND TOXIC MYOPATHIES

Nutritional deficiencies

Although malnutrition is common in many parts of the world, its effects on skeletal muscle have not been thoroughly investigated. Negative nitrogen balance and lack of essential nutrients can be expected to cause muscle weakness and wasting, but their relative significance is not clearly understood.

Vitamin E deficiency has been shown to cause a disorder associated with progressive gait and limb ataxia, sensorimotor neuropathy, extraocular muscle paresis, and a myopathy in which giant abnormal lysosomes accumulate in muscle. The cause is a malabsorption syndrome, as in chronic cholestasis or with cystic fibrosis of the pancreas (Blanc et al 1958, Tomasi 1979, Burck et al 1981, Neville et al 1983, Werlin et al 1983). The patient with giant lysosomes in muscle, peripheral neuropathy and hyperparathyroidism studied by Gomez et al (1972) was also subsequently shown to have vitamin E deficiency (M. R. Gomez & A. G. Engel, unpublished observations). Malabsorption of vitamin E also occurs in abetalipoproteinaemia and treatment with high doses of vitamin E arrests the neuropathy and myopathy in this disease (Hegele & Angel 1985).

The muscle weakness in nutritional osteomalacia has been attributed partly to disuse and partly to malnutrition (Dastur et al 1975). The myopathy of osteomalacia is discussed together with the myopathy of hyperparathyroidism.

Deficiencies of various electrolytes can produce myopathy and the deficiency of potassium is reviewed in the section on secondary causes of hypokalaemia as well as in the subsequent portion of this chapter on endocrine-related myopathies. Phosphate depletion as an associated provocative factor of myopathy and rhabdomyolysis is important to consider (Knochel 1984, Knochel 1987). Phosphate repletion along with repletion of potassium stores is important in hypokalaemia associated with chronic alcoholism or renal disease producing both kaliuresis and loss of phosphate. Chronic magnesium deficiency can produce myopathic changes. A 3-year-old child with a magnesium-losing nephropathy developed cardiomyopathy with convulsions (Riggs et al 1992). Muscle magnesium content was markedly decreased. Chronic oral and intermittent intravenous magnesium supplementation were not effective in controlling the muscle symptoms.

Myopathy in chronic alcoholism

Alcohol may have a direct toxic effect on muscle, or its effects can be mediated by malnutrition and fluid and electrolyte disturbances (Preedy & Peters 1990, Chen et al 1991, Conde-Martel et al 1992). Song & Rubin (1972) found that ingestion of ethanol (42% of calories) without malnutrition induced increased serum CK activity and nonspecific ultrastructural changes in muscle in human volunteers. In ethanol-fed rats, mitochondria show reduced ability to oxidise various substrates, energy production with NAD-dependent substrates, calcium uptake, activity of several enzymes and cytochrome content. These effects may be mediated by acetaldehyde rather than ethanol (Cederbaum & Rubin 1975).

Two types of clinically distinct myopathy, acute and subacute, have been described in chronic alcoholics. The acute type (Hed et al 1962) occurs after a bout of acute drinking. In these patients, muscle swelling and tenderness are associated with weakness and myoglobinuria. Hyperkalaemia and renal insufficiency develop in the more severely affected. A painless variety of acute alcoholic myopathy associated with severe hypokalaemia, marked serum CK elevation, vacuolar myopathy and focal fibre necrosis has also been described (Rubenstein & Wainapel 1977). The hypokalaemia may be secondary to the combined effects of sweating, vomiting, diarrhoea or renal potassium wastage. The hypokalaemia may be followed by hyperkalaemia as rhabdomyolysis, myoglobinuria and secondary renal failure develop. Histochemical studies in acute alcoholic myopathy reveal focal decreases in oxidative enzyme activity in type I muscle fibres and in necrotic fibres. Ultrastructural changes occur in mitochondria, but some of these changes are secondary to fibre necrosis (Martinez et al 1973). Other causes of severe hypokalaemia can also produce a necrotising myopathy (Knochel 1982, Knochel 1984, Victor 1986, Knochel 1987). The subacute alcoholic myopathy described by Ekbom et al (1964) is associated with symmetrical proximal weakness with little loss of muscle bulk, EMG changes and increased serum levels of muscle enzymes. In some alcoholics, serum enzyme and EMG abnormalities occur without muscle weakness. However, Faris & Reyes (1971) suggest that the subclinical group is neuropathic rather than myopathic. Alternatively, a chronic, mild neuropathy can exist in alcoholics who also develop a myopathy. The subacute syndrome is reversible within a few months of alcohol withdrawal.

Perkoff et al (1966) drew attention to impaired production of lactate by ischaemically exercised muscle in chronic alcoholics within 48 hours after intoxication. Muscle phosphorylase activity was reduced or low normal in six of seven biopsies. Muscle symptoms, when present, resembled those of phosphorylase deficiency. Other reports have also emphasised alterations in energy metabolism in patients abusing alcohol with myopathy. One report showed a selective reduction in the area of type II muscle fibres with a relative preservation of type I fibre diameter in patients having low plasma alpha-tocopherol and selenium levels (Preedy & Peters 1990). The authors suggest that alterations in energy metabolism and protein synthesis are related to the decreased levels of tocopherol and selenium and have proposed a rat model to study this derangement. Another report investigating 28 cases of chronic alcoholism with myopathic problems has found total or partial myophosphorylase deficiency in 33% (Chen et al 1991). The authors note that many patients also had angular atrophic fibres and fibre-type grouping suggesting co-existing chronic denervation. At present there is still an incomplete understanding of the myopathy that accompanies chronic alcoholism and a lack of a true animal model of this disorder. For an extensive review of acute and chronic alcoholic myopathy the reader is referred to Victor (1986).

Other drug-induced myopathies (see Ch. 28)

Chloroquine myopathy. This quinoline derivative, introduced as an antimalarial drug but useful in the treatment of amoebiasis and certain collagen-vascular diseases, causes undesirable side-effects involving the macula, cornea, skeletal muscle and peripheral nerves. The first cases of myopathy were described by Whisnant et al (1963). Most patients who became weak during chloroquine treatment received 500 mg of the drug per day for a year or longer. Pathologically, it is a vacuolar myopathy mainly affecting type I fibres (Garcin et al 1964, MacDonald & Engel 1970, Hughes et al 1971). The vacuoles contain cytoplasmic degradation products and are autophagic in character. In an experimental study, MacDonald & Engel (1970) found that the initial ultrastructural change was a proliferation of the internal membrane system (both T system and SR) and the encirclement of small cytoplasmic areas. Larger vacuoles arose by fusion of smaller ones. The entrapped membranous organelles were degraded by myeloid structures. The limiting membranes of the vacuoles were derived from tubules and labyrinthine networks of T-system

origin, and the degraded vacuolar contents reacted strongly for acid phosphatase. Exocytosis of vacuolar contents and frequent fibre splitting occurred after other pathological changes were well established. Chloroquine myopathy is a prototype for those muscle disorders in which an autophagic mechanism becomes excited. The myopathy presents with proximal weakness after months or years of use at doses as low as 200 mg/day. There is a mild elevation in serum creatine kinase activity and often electromyographic changes of myopathy. Hydroxychloroquine also produces a neuromyopathy similar to that caused by chloroquine but is milder (Estes et al 1987). Both chloroquine and hydroxychloroquine increase lysosomal cathepsins in experimental models and the use of a lysosomal cysteine proteinase inhibitor can abolish the myopathy in this model (Sugita et al 1987, Tågerud et al 1986). Discontinuation of treatment usually leads to improvement in the human myopathy.

Emetine myopathy. Emetine, an ipecac alkaloid used in the treatment of amoebiasis, inhibits protein synthesis in many cell types (Grollman 1968). Side-effects include cardiotoxicity and muscle weakness (Klatskin & Friedman 1948). In experimental animals the drug induces focal decreases in muscle mitochondria, associated with focal myofibrillar degeneration in type I fibres (Duane & Engel 1970). The lesions in type I fibres resemble those observed in multicore disease (Engel et al 1971). More advanced pathological changes induced by emetine include muscle fibre necrosis (Bradley et al 1976). A reversible myopathy has been observed in patients with major eating disorders who abuse ipecac to induce vomiting (Mateer et al 1985, Palmer & Guay 1985, Pope et al 1986) and in chronic alcoholics receiving emetine (about 500 mg over 11–14 days) for aversion therapy (Sugie et al 1984). The pathological findings resembled those described in experimental animals.

Lovastatin myopathy. Lovastatin (Mevacor) is an inhibitor of cholesterol synthesis used in treating hypercholesterolaemia. It may occasionally produce mild elevations in serum CK activity (Thompson et al 1986) and can in some cases, especially in combination with gemfibrozil, another cholesterol-lowering drug, cause severe myonecrosis and myoglobinuria (East et al 1988, Pierce et al 1990, Manoukian et al 1990, Spach et al 1991, Suki 1991, Wallace & Mueller 1992). The risk of myopathy occurring from lovastatin treatment (less than 1%) is increased to 5% in patients who take concomitant gemfibrozil and to 30% in patients taking lovastatin and cyclosporin (Kuncl & Wiggins 1988). The exact mechanism by which gemfibrozil interacts with lovastatin to cause myalgias and muscle weakness is unknown. However, a recent case report indicates that gemfibrozil in the absence of lovastatin can cause myopathy (Magarian et al 1991). Myopathic symptoms usually resolve completely following discontinuation of these cholesterol-lowering drugs.

Clofibrate myopathy. Clofibrate and related drugs are branched chain fatty acid esters used to treat hyperlipidaemia, and all can cause a necrotizing myopathy in humans (Kuncl & Wiggins 1988). Clofibrate has effects on fatty acid and branch chain amino acid oxidation and on carnitine palmityl-transferase activity. Which of these different actions or other unknown effects cause the myopathy is unclear. Patients with renal insufficiency are more predisposed to clofibrate myopathy (Bridgman et al 1972, Pierides et al 1975, Rimon et al 1984, Rush et al 1986). The myopathy often presents as a painful weakness within 2–3 months of starting the drug and is associated with an elevation in serum CK activity and occasionally myoglobinuria (Rush et al 1986). Cautious monitoring of serum CK, muscle strength and renal function is necessary to anticipate potential problems when this family of medications is used.

Epsilon-aminocaproic acid. Epsilon-aminocaproic acid (Amicar; EACA), is used to improve haemostasis in life-threatening fibrinolytic bleeding. The drug acts to inhibit the activator which converts plasminogen to plasmin. In skeletal muscle the drug inhibits the lyososomal enzyme cathepsin D without affecting other proteases (Kuncl & Wiggins 1988). Whether this action or some other mechanism is responsible for the muscle injury that occurs occasionally with this drug is unknown. Case reports describe necrotising myopathy with rhabdomyolysis and renal failure (Brodkin 1980, Brown et al 1982, Galassi

et al 1983, Morris et al 1983, Vanneste & van Wijngaarden 1982). Epsilon-aminocaproic acid is sometimes used to prevent subarachnoid haemorrhage prior to aneurysm surgery and is often given in a dose of 36 g/day. This treatment is often over a few weeks or more. Necrotising myopathy due to this drug can occur at doses as low as 10 g/day for a duration as brief as 14 days (Kuncl & Wiggins 1988). Patients should be monitored closely for signs of muscle pain and weakness, especially when treatment has exceeded 2 weeks.

Amiodarone neuromyopathy. Amiodarone produces neuromyopathy that may appear within weeks or several months after initiation of treatment. It produces phosholipid-containing myeloid inclusions in peripheral nerve and skeletal muscle (Kuncl & Wiggins 1988). These alterations may persist in muscle and nerve for as long as 2 years after discontinuing the drug (Alderson et al 1987). Patients are usually more symptomatic from their neuropathy caused by this drug than from the mild vacuolar myopathy that it causes or the additional hypothyroid myopathy that can be induced with treatment (Alderson et al 1987, Mason 1987).

Colchicine myopathy and neuropathy. Colchicine myoneuropathy has occurrred in patients receiving this drug for gout (Kuncl et al 1987, Kuncl & Wiggins 1988, Kuncl et al 1988). Typically patients are men over 50 with secondary gout who receive colchicine in doses of 0.5–0.6 mg twice daily. Proximal weakness develops over 1–6 months, serum CK is elevated (up to 50-fold in symptomatic cases, 1–3-fold in subclinical cases). Electromyographic investigation shows myopathic changes with increased spontaneous activity (Kuncl et al 1987). The major risk factor for this drug-induced myoneuropathy is renal insufficiency (Kuncl & Wiggins 1988). Recent reports have described colchicine-induced myopathy in a renal transplant patient (Johnsson et al 1992), and in a 24-year-old patient receiving colchicine for treatment of familial Mediterranean fever which was complicated by renal amyloidosis (Himmelmann & Schroder 1992). Muscle biopsy reveals membranous and vacuolar inclusions which on electron-microscopy are autophagic vacuoles (Kuncl & Wiggins 1988). Based upon the findings on muscle biopsy some investigators have hypothesised that colchicine myopathy is caused by disruption of microtubules (Kuncl & Wiggins 1988).

Selected toxic myopathies and associated conditions. Several drugs lead to toxic myopathy associated with neuropathy. These are: amiodarone, chloroquine, clofibrate, colchicine, doxorubicin, ethanol, hydroxychoroquine, organophosphates, perhexiline, vincristine (Kuncl & Wiggins 1988). Some of these same drugs have a separate association with cardiomyopathy. These are: chloroquine, clofibrate, colchicine, doxorubicin, emetine, ethanol, hydroxychoroquine, metronidazole. These possible associated conditions with toxic myopathy need to be monitored frequently during the course of clinical treatment with these drugs.

Risk factors known to provoke certain drug-induced myopathies. Chronic renal insufficiency increases the likelihood of toxic myopathy resulting from clofibrate (and related compounds) and colchicine (Kuncl & Wiggins 1988). The nephrotic syndrome also increases the likelihood of clofibrate myopathy. Fasting enhances the toxic effects of ethanol abuse and hypokalaemia, while bulimia and anorexia increase the possibility of myopathy related to emetine. The concomitant use of cyclosporine with lovastatin, primarily in renal transplant patients, increases the likelihood of toxic myopathy due to lovastatin (Kuncl & Wiggins 1988).

L-tryptophan myopathy: eosinophilia-myalgia syndrome. Since 1989 a syndrome typified by generalised, disabling myalgias (without any other recognised cause) and peripheral blood eosinophilia (eosinophil count greater than 1.0×10^9/l) has occurred in some individuals taking varying amounts of L-tryptophan. A wide spectrum of symptoms has been described in different patients which include eosinophilia and myalgia alone, or in association with eosinophilic fasciitis, pneumonitis, myocarditis, peripheral neuropathy, respiratory failure, encephalopathy, sclerodermatous skin changes and alopecia, and venous thromboses (Catton et al 1990, Estrada et al 1990, Hertzman et al 1990, Glickstein et al 1990, Gresh et al 1990, Kaufman et al 1990, Martin et al 1990, Strongwater et al

1990, Hollander & Adelman 1991, Ivey et al 1991). While some patients had relatively mild symptoms that resolved without treatment, others have had profound weakness and respiratory failure (Catton et al 1991, Hollander & Adelman 1991, Ivey et al 1991). Treatment with high-dose corticosteroids has led to improvement in many patients with the eosinophilia-myalgia syndrome (Glickstein et al 1990, Gresh et al 1990, Hertzman et al 1990, Catton et al 1991, Hollander & Adelman 1991, Ivey et al 1991, Martin et al 1991). Patients may have taken L-tryptophan for as little as 3 weeks to $2\frac{1}{2}$ years and in doses of 1.2–2.4 g/day (Hertzman et al 1990) before developing symptoms. Muscle biopsy typically reveals a mononuclear infiltrate with a variable mixture of eosinophils, and similar findings are observed in biopsies of skin, fascia and some viscera (Martin et al 1990). Immunofluorescence staining showed a major basic protein deposited outside the eosinophils in affected tissues and suggested that toxic granule proteins are released as a part of the pathomechanism (Martin et al 1990). Testing sera for autoantibodies has shown an antibody which recognises epitopes in a nuclear lamin fraction (Varga et al 1992). The positive antinuclear antibody (ANA) test suggests that an autoimmune response may mediate the symptoms in the eosinophilia-myalgia syndrome. Present evidence suggests that the ingestion of L-tryptophan may produce the eosinophilia-myalgia syndrome by an associated contamination involved in the preparation of this product (Roufs 1992) and this contaminant may be a chemical constituent such as a toxic oil compound (Belongia et al 1990, Adachi et al 1991, Kaufman & Seidman 1991, Kilbourne et al 1991). At present the presumed contaminant has not been definitively identified and the final pathomechanism for the production of the eosinophilia-myalgia is not known. However, the results suggest that many people exposed to the agent responsible for the syndrome may develop illness, and that the dose of the presumed contaminated L-tryptophan is the single most important predictor of the severity of the eosinophilia-myalgia syndrome (Kamb et al 1992). The broad spectrum of signs and symptoms observed in patients using L-tryptophan emphasises the difficulty in developing a strict definition to identify all affected cases. At present the use of L-tryptophan supplements is to be discouraged.

Zidovudine (AZT) myopathy. Both infection with human immunodeficiency virus HIV-1 and zidovudine (AZT) cause myopathy (Dalakas et al 1990). Patients typically present with myalgia and proximal muscle weakness and an elevation in serum CK activity (Chalmers et al 1991). Most patients with HIV-1 receiving treatment with zidovudine have inflammatory abnormalities on muscle biopsy that are also observed in patients with muscle weakness related to HIV-1 in the absence of zidovudine treatment (Dalakas et al 1990). However, patients with zidovudine-related myopathy have characteristic findings on muscle biopsy including ragged red fibres indicating abnormal mitochondria with paracrystalline inclusions (Dalakas et al 1990, Arnaudo et al 1991, Mhiri et al 1991, Pezeshkpour et al 1991). The mitochondrial abnormalities are unique to the HIV patients treated with zidovudine. Zidovudine is a DNA chain terminator that inhibits the mitochondrial gamma-DNA polymerase and is toxic to muscle mitochondria. Cessation of zidovudine therapy leads to prompt disappearance of myalgia and gradual recovery of muscle strength and a return of CK to the normal range (Chalmers et al 1991).

Muscle relaxant-steroid treatment induced myopathy. Recently a small number of patients receiving a combination of muscle relaxants and high-dose steroids for treatment of status asthmaticus have developed a generalised flaccid quadriplegia with areflexia following treatment (Danon & Carpenter 1991, Sitwell et al 1991, Kupfer et al 1992). A 20-year-old female with status asthmaticus was initially treated with bronchodilators, antibiotics and high-dose corticosteroids and given vecuronium for 10 days while receiving mechanical ventilation. After discontinuation of her ventilator therapy she was found to have a flaccid quadriplegia with areflexia and a four-fold elevation in serum creatine kinase activity (Danon & Carpenter 1991). Muscle biopsy revealed loss of thick myofilaments with relative preservation of thin filaments and Z discs. Muscle strength returned to normal after 2 months. The pathological changes observed on the muscle biopsy resembled those in experimentally treated rats receiving high doses of corticosteroids following denervation. The combination of continuous vecuronium (a putative form of denervation) combined with steroid treatment may in some way account for the prolonged weakness. A similar case has been reported after long-term infusion of vecuronium (Kupfer et al 1992) and after a combination of high-dose intravenous methylprednisolone and pancuronium therapy (Sitwell et al 1991). Patients receiving this form of treatment for status asthmaticus or for other related problems need careful monitoring after discontinuation of ventilation. Whether some other type of muscle relaxant drug or a lower dose of corticosteroids might ameliorate this disorder is unknown. The mechanism requires further investigation.

DISEASES ASSOCIATED WITH MYOGLOBINURIA

Myoglobin is a 17 000 dalton protein with a prosthetic heme group, located in red skeletal muscle fibres and cardiac muscle; it binds one molecule of oxygen, and has a concentration in muscle about 1 mg/g (Kagen & Christian 1966, Odeh 1991). Myoglobin appears in urine at serum concentrations ranging from 300 ng/ml to 2 µm/ml (Odeh 1991). Oliguric renal failure has developed in patients with straw-coloured urine. Normal individuals have a serum myoglobin ranging from 3 to 80 ng/mol and urine concentrations ranging from trace to 12 ng/ml (Penn 1986, Odeh 1991). The appearance of myoglobin in the urine is both an indication of severe and acute muscle injury, and a warning that renal damage may result. Any injury to muscle fibres which abnormally increases the permeability or disrupts the integrity of the surface membrane entails leakage of myoglobin into the plasma. The renal threshold for myoblobin is relatively low (Koskelo et al 1967) but massive and relatively synchronous injury to muscle (rhabdomyolysis) is required before brown discolouration of urine, caused by myoglobin plus metmyoglobin, is observed. The urinary pigment reacts positively with benzidine. If there is no haemoglobinaemia and no haematuria, the test strongly suggests myoglobin-uria. However, microhaematuria can also develop with myoglobinuria. Positive identification of myoglobin requires specific chemical, spectrophotometric or immunological tests. The last are the most sensitive and the immunoprecipitation assay is both quantitative and simple (Markowitz & Wobig 1977).

Acute attacks of myoglobinuria are characterised by the onset, over a few hours, of muscle weakness, swelling and pain. In addition to myoglobin, phosphate, potassium, creatine, creatinine and muscle enzymes are released into the circulation. The haem pigment in the glomerular filtrate and myoglobin casts in renal tubules may cause proteinuria, haematuria and renal tubular necrosis. Renal failure is more likely if the attack is complicated by hypovolaemia, hypotension or metabolic acidosis. With increasing renal insufficiency, hyperphosphataemia with secondary hypocalcaemia and tetany, life-threatening hyperkalaemia may develop (Hed 1955, Bowden et al 1956, Pearson et al 1957, Savage et al 1971, Rowland & Penn 1972, Penn 1986). Death can result from renal or respiratory failure. If the patient survives, the myoglobinuria and proteinuria tend to disappear by the third to fifth day after the onset of the attack; marked hyperenzymaemia, present initially, subsides more gradually; muscle strength returns relatively slowly after major attacks. EMG abnormalities (fibrillation potentials, increased insertional activity and motor unit potential alterations) may persist for several months after severe attacks (Haase & Engel 1960).

The syndrome has many known causes but in many cases the aetiology remains elusive. The immediate biochemical mechanism which disrupts the plasma membrane remains to be determined; however, the major life-threatening complications of myoglobinuria are primarily related to renal damage due to acute tubular necrosis. Tubular damage may result from hypovolaemia, circulating toxins (such as tumour necrosis factor alpha) and oxygen free radical formation which damages tubular membranes (Odeh 1991). For descriptive purposes, it is convenient to classify the syndrome as metabolic, postinfectious, toxic, ischaemic and/or traumatic, secondary to inflammatory or other myopathies, and idiopathic.

Metabolic. The common denominator is impaired substrate utilisation for energy metabolism, or a critical substrate deficiency in the face of excessive demands for energy. Certain diseases in this group were considered earlier in this chapter, specifically those dealing with glycogen metabolism and glycolysis, while other disorders including mitochrondial disease and the metabolism of fatty acids are covered in Chapter 18. Phosphorylase, phosphofructokinase, phosphoglycerate kinase, phosphoglycerate mutase, and lactate dehydrogenase deficiencies block anaerobic glycolysis, and carnitine palmityltransferase deficiency impairs oxidation of long-chain fatty acids. Rare instances of muscle carnitine deficiency and conditions in which there is an impairment in utilisation of fatty acids may also contribute to myoglobinuria (see Ch. 18).

Critical substrate deficiency in the face of excessive demands for energy probably accounts for the myoglobinuria which occurs in malignant hyperthermia, after unusually severe exercise in untrained but otherwise healthy individuals, performing weight lifting (Doriguzzi et al 1988, Aranyi & Rado 1992), after severe whole body exercise (Demos et al 1974, Nilne 1988, Hurley 1989), or in conga drummers (Furie & Penn 1974, Hurley 1989).

Myoglobinuria also occurs with marked muscle rigidity and hyperthermia in the malignant neuroleptic syndrome (Guzé & Baxter 1985) and in some patients with parkinsonism when drug therapy is abruptly withdrawn (Friedman et al 1985).

Postinfectious. Myoglobinuria has been reported after infections with influenza A, herpes simplex, Epstein–Barr and Coxsackie viruses (Simon et al 1970, DiBona & Morens 1977, Schlesinger et al 1978). Virus-like structures have been demonstrated by electron-microscopy in affected muscle by Gamboa et al (1979). The latter workers were also able to isolate influenza B virus from muscle of a patient who had a fatal attack. The muscle biopsy in this individual showed inflammatory changes as well as perifascicular atrophy. The precise mechanism by which viral infections cause rhabdomyolysis is not understood. Myoglobinuria can also occur with bacterial infections accompanied by high fever and sepsis and with muscle gangrene caused by clostridial infection (Penn 1986).

Toxic. Myoglobinuria complicating chronic alcoholism is not uncommon and has been discussed previously. Almost any other extreme metabolic insults may produce it. These include carbon monoxide poisoning, extreme hypoglycaemia, severe hypokalaemia, hypernatraemia or water intoxication, diabetic acidosis, barbiturate, narcotic and amphetamine intoxication and uraemic hyperparathyroidism (reviewed by Penn 1986, Kuncl & Wiggins 1988, Tein et al 1990). In Haff's disease the eating of fish contaminated by an unidentified toxin induced an epidemic of myoglobinuria along the Baltic coast (Berlin 1948). In Malayan waters, fisherman bitten by the sea snake *Enhydrina schistosa* develop myalgias, flaccid paralysis, trismus and myoglobinuria (Reid 1961).

Ischaemic and traumatic. Prolonged massive ischaemia of muscle from whatever cause results in necrosis of muscle fibres and can induce myoglobinuria and renal failure (Bywaters et al 1941, Bywaters & Stead 1945). Localized ischaemic necrosis of muscle and occasionally myoglobinuria may occur in severe forms of the anterior tibial syndrome.

Traumatic rhabdomyolysis (crush syndrome) results in disintegration of muscle tissue and the influx of myoglobin, potassium and phosphorus into the circulation. The hypovolaemic shock and hyperkalaemia which occur are often followed by acute renal failure in the absence of treatment (Odeh 1991). The conversion of xanthine dehydrogenase to xanthine oxidase during ischaemia occurs within 10 seconds in the gut, within 8 minutes in cardiac muscle, and within the liver, spleen, kidney and lung within 30 minutes (Odeh 1991). This conversion does not occur during ischaemia of skeletal muscle, but develops following muscle protein breakdown associated with reperfusion of skeletal muscle after prolonged ischaemia (Odeh 1991). The production of xanthine oxidase, the activation of leucocytes, the production of prostaglandin synthetase and catecholamine autooxidation all produce oxygen free radicles which lead to damage of tubular membranes. Other circulating toxins (such as tumour necrosis factor) are also released following tissue damage. In association with these changes, there is an influx of calcium into muscle fibres during reperfusion. The influx of calcium activates phospholipase A-2 which in turn stimulates production of leukotrines and prostaglandins (Odeh 1991). Collectively these changes lead to renal tubular damage and to subsequent renal failure. Treatment including vigorous hydration, alkalinisation of the urine, intravenous mannitol and allopurinol may help to prevent the need for dialysis treatment (Odeh 1991).

Secondary to other myopathies. Myoglobinuria has been described in dermatomyositis (Kessler et al 1972), and in fulminant polymyositis (Sloan et al 1978, Gamboa et al 1979). In some patients, the myoglobinuria could have been related to a concurrent or underlying viral infection (Gamboa et al 1979). Recurrent myoglobinuria was observed by Dr A. G. Engel in one patient with classic systemic lupus erythematosus. Finally, anaesthesia-induced myoglobinuria without rigidity or hyperthermia was reported in a patient with Duchenne dystrophy (Miller et al 1978).

Idiopathic. It is likely that at least some cases initially classified as idiopathic will eventually be shown to have a metabolic or postinfectious aetiology.

ENDOCRINE DISORDERS OF MUSCLE

Muscle disorders associated with hyperthyroidism

Some of these disorders are a direct consequence of the endocrinopathy: others occur more often with thyroid dysfunction than predicted by chance and may or may not be affected by the altered endocrine state. Thyrotoxic myopathy, thyrotoxic hypokalaemic periodic paralysis, myasthenia gravis and exophthalmic ophthalmoplegia are the currently recognised neuromuscular diseases associated with hyperthyroidism. (For a more detailed review of endocrine myopathies, including myopathies associated with hyperthyroidism, the reader may wish to consult the detailed review by Kaminski & Ruff 1994.)

Thyrotoxic myopathy. Both acute and chronic forms have been described but it is doubtful that the rare acute type exists as a distinct entity. More probably, it represents cases of acute myasthenia gravis associated with severe thyrotoxicosis (Millikan & Haines 1953, Engel 1961a, Kaminski & Ruff 1994).

Muscle weakness occurs in about 80% of untreated cases of hyperthyroidism (Ramsey 1965). Men are affected more often than women and the average duration of muscle symptoms before diagnosis is about 6 months. Proximal muscle weakness is present in about two-thirds, and both proximal and distal muscle weakness in another one-fifth of the cases. The thyrotoxicosis is relatively mild and of long duration, or present for only a few weeks before the onset of weakness. The weakness is often out of proportion to the visible muscle atrophy, although severe atrophy can occur. Shortness of breath can occur in patients, and even respiratory insufficiency (Mier et al 1989, McElvaney et al 1990). Oesophageal motility impairment and bulbar muscle weakness may also occur (Sweatman & Chambers 1985). The deep tendon reflexes are usually normal or hyperactive with almost 25% of the patients having shortened relaxation times (Lambert et al 1951), and only seldom are the tendon reflexes decreased or absent. The serum CK activity is not increased as a rule (in contrast to myxoedema in which it is usually increased, but weakness is uncommon) (Ramsey 1965, 1968, Fleisher et al 1965). EMG abnormalities are found in about 90% of patients with hyperthyroidism (Havard et al 1963, Ramsey 1965). These abnormalities consist of a decrease in the mean duration of motor unit potentials and an increase in the incidence of polyphasic potentials. Spontaneous electrical activity (fibrillation potentials, fasciculation, or repetitive discharges) is absent as a rule. After correction of the hyperthyroidism, the EMG reverts to normal.

Light-microscopic studies of muscle may show no abnormality or varying degrees of fatty infiltration and fibre atrophy. Ultrastructural studies have revealed mitochondrial hypertrophy; focal loss of mitochondria from muscle fibres; focal myofibrillar degeneration beginning at the Z disc; focal dilatations of the transverse tubular system; sub-sarcolemmal glycogen deposits; and papillary projections of the surface of the muscle fibres, probably resulting from fibre atrophy (Engel 1966b, 1972). The duration of hyperthyroidism not only correlates with greater muscle weakness and wasting, but with a greater likelihood of abnormalities on muscle biopsy (Satoyoshi et al 1963b). Approximately 85% of the patients with thyrotoxicosis of more than 1 year's duration showed abnormalities on muscle biopsy. Other studies have shown a lower proportion of type I fibres, a higher capillary density, a lower glycogen content, and a higher hexokinase activity in quadriceps femoris muscle in patients with hyperthyroid myopathy in muscle tissue obtained at the time of diagnosis and compared to findings in a repeat biopsy obtained after 10 months of treatment (Celsing et al 1986). None of the ultrastructural changes are specific for thyrotoxic myopathy.

The precise mechanism responsible for the muscle weakness in thyrotoxic myopathy remains unclear. A detailed discussion of different contributing metabolic and electrophysiological changes is available in an excellent review by Kaminski & Ruff (1994). The muscle weakness probably results from several different combined effects rather than from the single action of an elevation in thyroxine. Excessive levels of thyroid hormone (T_4 and T_3) increase mitochondrial respiration (Satoyoshi et al 1963b, Schwartz & Oppenheimer 1978, Janssen et al 1981), but there is no evidence that thyrotoxicosis uncouples oxidative phosphorylation in human skeletal muscle (Ernster et al 1959, Stocker et al 1968). Abnormal elevations of thyroid hormone accelerate protein degradation (Yates et al 1981, Morrison et al 1988), increase lipid oxidation (Lithell et al 1985, Asayama & Kato 1990), and enhance beta-adrenergic sensitivity (Kaminski & Ruff 1994). Unlike thyrotoxic animal models patients with thyrotoxic myopathy do not have a reduction in protein degradation in response to treatment with beta-adrenergic drugs (Hasselgren et al 1984). The fatigability that patients frequently display may relate to a combination of glycogen depletion and impaired glucose uptake that occurs (Celsing et al 1986). Thyrotoxic patients are resistant to insulin (Celsing et al 1986) and have an impaired regulation of glycogen stores (Kabadi & Eisenstein 1980) which probably contributes both to glucose intolerance and muscle wasting.

Electrophysiological alterations occur in skeletal muscle. There is a shortening of contraction time (Wiles et al 1979) which may result from the combined effects of an accelerated rate of action of myosin ATPase, a preferential expression of fast-type myosin, and an enhanced calcium uptake by the sarcoplasmic reticulum (Kaminski & Ruff 1994). There is a reduction in the surface membrane excitability of skeletal muscle (Gruener et al 1975, McArdle et al 1977) and this probably results from depolarisation-induced sodium channel inactivation (Ruff et al 1988). Studies in skeletal muscle (Kjeldsen et al 1984, Norgaard & Kjeldsen 1991), in isolated human lymphocytes (Oh et al 1990), and in cultured muscle cells (Bannett et al 1984) demonstrate that excessive levels of thyroid hormone increase the activity of the sodium–potassium ATPase and lead to alterations in intracellular electrolyte distribution. In addition toxic levels of thyroid hormone may indirectly reduce the expression of the sodium channel (Brodie & Sampson 1989) and impair action potential propagation into the muscle fibres (Dulhunty et al 1986). Cell injury may be mediated by an increase in intracellular calcium, other electrolyte disturbances, activation of intracellular proteases, and reduction of oxygen-free radicals (Kaminski & Ruff 1994).

No specific treatment is available for thyrotoxic myopathy other than the re-establishment of the euthyroid state. Muscle weakness, including weakness of respiratory muscles, may be significantly improved with beta-adrenergic blocking drugs (Wang 1986). Studies in thyrotoxic rats have suggested that glucocorticoids block the peripheral conversion of T_4 to T_3 and because of this effect may be useful in the initial treatment of thyrotoxicosis (Heyma & Larkins 1982).

Thyroid dysfunction and myasthenia gravis. The incidence of thyroid disorders is much greater in patients with myasthenia gravis than could occur by chance: 5.7% of myasthenic patients are hyperthyroid, 5.3% hypothyroid and 2.1% have non-toxic goitre (Engel 1961a). Approximately 0.35% of patients with hyperthyroidism have myasthenia gravis, a prevalence

30 times higher than that of myasthenia gravis in the general population (Kaminski & Ruff 1989). Thyrotoxicosis usually precedes or develops simultaneously with myasthenia gravis. Infrequently thyrotoxicosis will develop after the diagnosis of myasthenia gravis is established (Swanson et al 1981, Ruff & Weissman 1988). Thyroid disease (hyperthyroidism and hypothyroidism) worsens the course of myasthenia gravis (Engel 1961a). About 8–17% of euthyroid and 40% of thyrotoxic patients have circulating antibodies directed against thyroid cell antigens (Osserman et al 1967, Kaminski & Ruff 1994). The association between myasthenia gravis and Graves' disease probably reflects their autoimmune origins (Engel 1984, Kaminski et al 1990).

Myasthenia gravis seldom occurs with spontaneous myxoedema but 19% of myasthenic patients, compared with less than 1% of the general population, have evidence of thyroiditis at autopsy (Becker et al 1964).

Exophthalmic ophthalmoplegia (Graves' ophthalmopathy). Exophthalmos occurs with both hyperthyroidism due to Graves' disease and as a separate autoimmune disease known as Graves' ophthalmopathy (Feldon 1990). For a more detailed discussion of this problem, the reader may want to consult the excellent review by Kaminski & Ruff (1994). In hyperthyroidism due to Graves' disease exophthalmos is typically painful, and diplopia is the most frequent symptom, related to enlargement of the orbital contents (Kaminski & Ruff 1994). Elevation and abduction are the eye movements most affected and the symptoms are usually bilateral. Swelling of the orbital contents increases intraorbital pressure and compression of the vascular supply to the optic nerve may lead to loss of vision (Hallin 1988, Kaminski & Ruff 1994). Computerized tomographic imaging of the orbits and magnetic resonance imaging are useful in distinguishing thyroid ophthalmopathy from orbital myositis (Rothfus & Curtin 1984, Hosten et al 1989). Ultrasound studies have demonstrated subclinical ophthalmopathy in as many as 90% of patients, while clinical evidence indicates an incidence of only 5% (Werner et al 1974). Eighty per cent of patients with prominent exophthalmos are hyperthyroid, 10% have Hashimoto's disease or primary hypothyroidism, and 10% have no demonstrable thyroid disease (Wall & Kuroki 1985).

The pathogenesis of the eye findings and the thyroid disease is complex. The inflammatory oedema that develops in the contents of the orbit is likely to result from autoimmune processes. In Graves' disease, thyroid-stimulating antibodies appear to initiate immune-mediated destruction of the thyroid and produce thyrotoxicosis (Wall et al 1991). These antibodies may cross-react with orbital membranes and lead to the ophthalmopathy that occurs in some patients. A second form of ophthalmopathy, Graves' ophthalmopathy, is considered to be a separate autoimmune disorder (Feldon 1990) and is probably mediated by antibodies which react specifically with extraocular muscles (Ahman et al 1987, Hiromatsu et al 1988). Cytotoxic lymphocytes and alterations in lymphatic drainage may be additional factors in producing the ophthalmopathy (Kaminski & Ruff 1994).

Treatment of the ophthalmopathy includes topical adrenergic-blocking agents. Guanethidine eyedrops (5%) have been used for prolonged periods without systemic side-effects. Prevention of exposure keratitis caused by severe lid retraction includes protection of the eye during the day with glasses and ophthalmic ointment and taping the eyelids closed at night. If adrenergic-blocking agents are not sufficient to prevent lid retraction, surgery may be necessary. Oedema of the eyelids and conjunctiva often responds to local injections of glucocorticoids (Bouzas 1980). Systemic treatment with glucocorticoids or azathioprine is not successful (Kaminski & Ruff 1994). Thyroid hormone replacement in hypothyroid patients may help control ophthalmopathy. However, in refractory cases, orbital decompression surgery may be necessary (Small and Meiring 1981, Mouritis et al 1990).

Muscle disorders in hypothyroidism

The main manifestations of the various types of muscle disorder described in hypothyroidism are weakness, cramps, aching or painful muscles, sluggish movements and reflexes, myoidema (i.e. ridging of muscle on percussion) and in some an increase in muscle bulk. The reflex changes are seen in most cases, myoidema and myalgia are less common and weakness occurs in but a few. The serum CK activity is typically elevated even if there are no other clinical symptoms of muscle involvement (Fleisher et al 1965, Giampietro et al 1984, Khaleeli & Edwards 1984, Frank et al 1989). Electrical recording of the slow contraction and relaxation of the tendon reflex (Lambert et al 1951, Khaleeli & Edwards 1984) and of the myoidema (Salick & Pearson 1967, Salick et al 1968, Mizusawa et al 1984) would suggest that it is the contractile mechanism of the muscle that is predominantly involved.

It seems possible that many enzyme systems are affected in hypothyroid myopathy and the degree of involvement of each system may influence the pattern of clinical involvement. An impairment in energy metabolism may lead to the muscle weakness, cramps, and slowed movement. Hypothyroidism reduces muscle oxygen consumption, decreases mitochondrial oxidation capacity, decreases glucose uptake, impairs muscle glycogenolysis, and reduces muscle acid maltase activity (McDaniel et al 1977, Schwartz & Oppenheimer 1978, Argov et al 1988, Ho 1989). Hypothyroidism alters the normal pattern of protein expression during development and decreases protein turnover (Mahdavi et al 1987, Russell 1988, Morrison et al 1988, Moussavi et al 1988, D'Albis et al 1990). Both protein synthesis and degradation are reduced, but the net effect is one of protein catabolism. There is a decrease in adrenergic activity in hypothyroidism. There is a decrease in beta-adrenergic receptors on muscle cells (Sharma & Banerjee 1978), decreased beta-adrenergic glycogenolysis (Chu et al 1985), and a decreased activity of sodium–potassium ATPase (Kjeldsen et al 1984, Norgaard & Kjeldsen 1991). Fluid and electrolyte balance is also impaired with a decreased resorption of sodium in the distal tubules (Ruff & Weissman 1988). Hypothyroidism also produces a significant hypercholesterolaemia (Schwartz & Oppenheimer 1978), reduced cholesterol esterase activity (Demartino & Goldberg 1981), and diminished muscle uptake of triglyceride (Kaciuba-Uscilko et al 1980). Taken together, the above derangements in metabolism may restrict the repair and replacement of myo-fibrillar proteins, slow the contraction and relaxation of muscle, diminish cardiac output and produce a significant decrease in exercise tolerance (Kaminski & Ruff 1994).

Muscle hypertrophy, with weakness and slowness of movement, constitute the syndrome of Debré–Semelaigne (Debré & Semelaigne 1935) which occurs predominantly in cretinous children; when accompanied by painful spasms it is given the name of Hoffmann's syndrome and is then seen in myxoedematous adults. However, the two conditions tend to merge into each other and may even occur, although at different times, in the same patients (Wilson & Walton 1959, Norris & Panner 1966). Slow relaxation and myoidema are prominent features of Hoffmann's syndrome; superficially, therefore, it resembles myotonia congenita or the very rare cases of true myotonia associated with myxoedema, either iatrogenic or resulting from disease. In the two patients reported by Jarcho & Tyler (1958) the myxoedema probably exacerbated a pre-existing mild myotonia, because symptomless myotonia was demonstrated in some relatives. The occasional association of a girdle myopathy causing mild proximal weakness and atrophy has been described by Åström et al (1961). Morphological studies reveal non-specific alterations in hypothyroid myopathy. These include fibre enlargement, increased central nuclei, glycogen and mitochondrial aggregates, dilated SR and proliferating T-system profiles, and focal myofibrillar degeneration (Norris & Panner, 1966, Afifi et al 1974, Emser & Schimrigk 1977, Mukherjee et al 1984, Ho 1989, Evans et al 1990, Riggs 1990). The specific explanation for the muscle enlargement that occurs in hypothyroidism remains unclear and is not accounted for by the microscopic studies (Kaminski & Ruff 1994).

Typically patients with long-standing hypothyroidism have slowly progressive proximal muscle weakness often associated with compression neuropathies that rapidly recover with treatment and restoration of the euthyroid state. Occasionally hypothyroidism may present with rhabdomyolysis (Riggs 1990) or respiratory muscle weakness (Martinez et al 1989). Treatment must be tailored to the specific abnormality. There is no evidence that dietary manipulation or exercise improves muscle function in hypothyroid conditions (Kaminski & Ruff 1994).

Muscle disorders associated with hyperparathyroidism and with osteomalacia

Parathormone and biologically active forms of vitamin D are important regulators of calcium metabolism and of the serum calcium level. Parathormone mobilises calcium from bone, increases the reabsorption of calcium and excretion of phosphate by the kidney, and stimulates the renal conversion of 25-hydroxycholecalciferol to 1,25-dihydroxycholecalciferol, a highly potent form of vitamin D. Parathormone increases cyclic AMP in skeletal muscle (Ritz et al 1980) and stimulates protein breakdown in skeletal muscle (Garber 1983). The mechanism by which parathormone may produce muscle weakness is unknown, but a recent hypothesis was given in the detailed review of this subject by Kaminski & Ruff (1994). Excessive amounts of parathormone may lead to an elevation in cytoplasmic calcium which in turn produces both an activation of a neutral cell protease and a reduction in the calcium sensitivity of the contractile system. These changes may impair the bioenergetics of skeletal muscle. Parathormone also acts to inhibit the reabsorption of phosphate by the kidney as noted above, but the associated hypophosphataemia is typically not sufficient to impair muscle function (Knochel 1977a). Biologically active vitamin D promotes intestinal calcium absorption and facilitates mineralisation of osteoid and of newly formed enchondral bone (Haussler & McCain 1977, Habener & Potts 1978). Studies in vitamin D-deficient animals also suggest that vitamin D has a direct effect on muscle in augmenting SR and mitochondrial calcium uptake, protein synthesis, ATP stress and force generation (Curry et al 1974, Birge & Haddad 1975, Rodman & Baker 1978, Pleasure et al 1979, Ritz et al 1980).

Cholecalciferol is derived from dietary consumption or produced within the body from pro vitamin D following exposure of the skin to ultraviolet radiation. Formation of the active form of vitamin D requires an initial hydroxylation of cholecalciferol in the liver to form 25-hydroxy-cholecalciferol and a second hydroxylation in the kidney to form 1,25-dihydroxycholecalciferol. Renal disease and hypoparathyroidism inhibit this second hydroxylation. Skeletal muscle from uraemic subjects shows changes comparable to those in vitamin D-deficient animals (Henderson et al 1974), and patients with muscle weakness associated with chronic renal failure often show improved muscle strength following administration of 1,25-dihydroxycholecalciferol (Henderson et al 1974), emphasising the clinical importance of the impairment in vitamin D metabolism in producing muscle weakness in uraemia.

Muscle weakness can occur in primary and secondary hyperparathyroidism and in osteomalacia. Further, conditions that lead to osteomalacia, such as vitamin D deficiency, renal tubular acidosis or chronic renal failure, are also typically associated with secondary hyperparathyroidism. Vicale in 1949 observed a distinctive syndrome in two cases of primary hyperparathyroidism and in one case of renal tubular acidosis. It was characterised by symmetrical weakness and fatigability involving especially the proximal muscles, pain on muscular effort, slow, waddling gait, muscle atrophy, creatinuria, weight loss, hyperactive deep tendon reflexes, guarding against passive movement of limbs and tenderness of bone. The EMG showed no fibrillations or fasciculations. Subsequent reports confirmed the existence of the syndrome in both primary hyperparathyroidism and in osteomalacia (Murphy et al 1960, Bischoff & Esslen 1965, Prineas et al 1965, Smith & Stern 1967, Frame et al 1968, Cholod et al 1970, Floyd et al 1974, Schott & Wills 1975, Skaria et al 1975, Irani 1976, Mallette et al 1975, Rutz et al 1980). The serum alkaline phosphatase level is usually raised; the serum calcium is typically increased in primary hyperparathyroidism but is low or normal in osteomalacia; the serum phosphate tends to be low, except in the presence of chronic renal failure. (A more detailed description of the myopathic disorders associated with both primary and secondary hyperparathyroidism is provided in the excellent review by Kaminski & Ruff 1994.)

Muscle biopsy studies have revealed simple atrophy (Bischoff & Esslen 1965), minimal vacuolar change (Cholod et al 1970), type II fibre atrophy and changes that may indicate mild denervation atrophy (Patten et al 1974, Mallette et al 1975, Ljunghall et al 1984). The latter authors speculate that the muscle damage in both primary and secondary hyperparathyroidism may be neuropathic.

A clearly myopathic and highly malignant syndrome may occur in uraemic hyperparathyroidism. Here, metastatic calcification of vessels causes ischaemia of tissues. This results in gangrenous skin lesions arising on ulcerating areas of livedo reticularis, a necrotising myopathy with increased serum CK activity, myoglobinuria, and visceral infarcts (Richardson et al 1969, Goodhue et al 1972).

Therapy of the various syndromes is directed at removal of the primary cause. Patients with primary hyperparathyroidism improve with removal of the adenoma. Muscle weakness in osteomalacia improves with vitamin D replacement. Patients with chronic renal failure often improve after partial removal of an overfunctioning parathyroid gland and concomitant treatment with 1,25-dihydroxycholecalciferol or 1-α-hydroxycholecalciferol (Henderson et al 1974, Davie et al 1976). Renal trasplantation can also improve the myopathy (Boland 1986).

Myopathy associated with hypoparathyroidism

This endocrine disorder is not definitely known to be associated with a myopathy. Increased serum CK activity, but normal muscle histology, has been observed in a few cases by Hower & Struck (1972), Shane et al (1980), and by Yamaguchi et al (1987), who noted that the conditions resolved partially with calcium and vitamin D treatment, correcting the hypocalcaemia, hypomagnesaemia and hyperphosphataemia. A similar syndrome associated with an elevation in serum CK activity, with minimal weakness and muscle discomfort, has been reported in patients with pseudohypoparathyroidism whose muscle biopsies revealed diminished glycogen phosphorylase activity (Piechowaik et al 1981). Cape (1969) found histochemical deficiency of phosphorylase a, but not of phosphorylase b, in a case of pseudohypoparathyroidism.

Treatment of hypoparathyroidism is directed to correcting the decreased concentrations of calcium and magnesium associated with the tetany of skeletal muscle and the prominence of a Chvostek sign (spasm provoked by tapping facial muscles) and Trousseau sign (carpopedal spasm following occlusion of venous drainage from the arm). Tetany, Chvostek sign, and carpopedal spasm are aggravated by hyperventilation and other causes of alkalosis. The preferred treatment is intravenous infusion of 15–20 mg of calcium per kg of body weight over several hours. Patients having seizures should receive a slow intravenous bolus of calcium gluconate while monitoring pulse and blood pressure. Intravenous administration of magnesium sulphate, 1 g, is helpful if hypomagnesaemia is present. If renal insufficiency is present, a lower dose of magnesium should be given. Long-term treatment of hypocalcaemia includes dietary supplements of 2–5 g of elemental calcium daily and vitamin D_2 (50 000 to 100 000 units daily). The doses of vitamin D and calcium need to be adjusted to achieve a blood calcium of 8.5–9 mg/100 ml (2.0–2.25 mmol/l). If this treatment is unsuccessful, 1,25-dihydroxycholecalciferol or 1-hydroxycholecalciferol may be tried to circumvent a presumed impairment in the activation of vitamin D. Magnesium supplements are necessary if hypomagnesaemia is present.

Disease of the pituitary and suprarenal glands

Acromegaly and hypopituitarism. Acromegaly in its earlier stages can cause increased muscle bulk and strength, especially if its onset precedes cessation of growth. Later it results in generalised muscle weakness and wasting. Mastaglia et al (1970) noted mild weakness in six of 11 acromegalics with raised serum CK activity in five. The EMG showed a decrease in the mean duration of motor unit potentials. Muscle biopsy studies revealed segmental fibre degeneration, foci of small round cell infiltration, thickening of capillary basement membranes, variable hypertrophy and atrophy involving either type I or type II fibres, lipofuscin accumulation, large nuclei with prominent nucleoli and prominent Golgi systems (Mastaglia et al 1970, Mastaglia 1973). Pickett

et al (1975) found clinical and EMG evidence of myopathy in nine of 17 acromegalics. More recent studies (Khaleeli et al 1984) noted proximal muscle weakness and decreased exercise tolerance in approximately 50% of patients with acromegaly. The muscle weakness was insidious in onset, gradually progressive, and associated with only minimal muscle wasting; there may be a slight elevation in serum CK activity. A carpal tunnel syndrome was a frequent associated finding (Pickett et al 1975, Jamal et al 1987). Pickett et al (1975) found no abnormalities in muscle biopsies in three patients and no patient had increased serum CK activity. The weakness improved slowly after surgical therapy for the acromegaly.

Multiple factors are likely to account for the myopathy in acromegaly. A detailed overview is presented in a review by Kaminski & Ruff (1994). There is a decrease in the force generated by skeletal muscle despite a larger than normal fibre diameter (Bigland & Young 1954). Acromegaly leads to insulin resistance and impairs carbohydrate and protein metabolism (Kaminski & Ruff 1994). The impairment in carbohydrate metabolism and the narrowing of capillaries in muscle (Pickett et al 1975) may account in part for the decreased exercise tolerance in acromegaly. The myopathy usually resolves after restoration of normal circulating levels of growth hormone. Surgical removal of the underlying pituitary adenoma is the preferred treatment. Bromocriptine is useful as an adjunct to surgical or radiation therapy of these tumours (Tindall & Barrow 1986).

Severe weakness and fatigability without a significant loss of muscle mass occurs with pituitary failure in adults. These symptoms are due to the loss of hormones from the thyroid and adrenal cortex and a loss of their synergistic actions with growth hormone (Kaminski & Ruff 1994). Stroke or masses producing thrombosis of the pituitary circulation, pituitary or hypothalamic tumours, head injury, meningitis, and granulomatous disease can cause adult pan-hypopituitarism. Idiopathic hypopituitarism in children gives rise to dwarfism and poor muscle development. Growth hormone release leads to the production of insulin-like growth factor 1 which plays a major role in the development of muscle (Froesch et al 1985). In normal muscle development, there is a coordinated interaction between insulin, glucocorticoids and insulin-like growth factor 1 (Ball & Sanwal 1980, Ewton & Florini 1981, Schoenle et al 1992, Froesch et al 1985, DeVol et al 1990). For a discussion of the physiology of growth hormone, insulin-like growth factor 1 and their interaction with other hormones, the reader may wish to read reviews by Froesch et al (1985) and Kaminski & Ruff (1994). Children with hypopituitarism require appropriate circulating levels of human growth hormone for normal muscle development. Thyroid hormone (T_3) and growth hormone synergise to control normal protein synthesis, and thyroid hormone simultaneously helps to modulate the rate of muscle protein breakdown (Kaminski & Ruff 1994). These hormones act as powerful homeostatic regulators of muscle mass along with other critical factors including muscular exercise, the circulating levels of insulin and cortisone.

Cushing's syndrome and steroid myopathy. Muscle weakness develops in 50–80% of patients suffering from Cushing's syndrome (Plotz et al 1952, Müller & Kugelberg 1959, Golding et al 1961, Pleasure et al 1970) and can also occur as a complication of glucocorticoid hormone treatment (Perkoff et al 1959, Williams 1959, Golding et al 1961, Byers et al 1962, Coomes 1965, Askari et al 1976, Urbanic & George 1981, Khaleeli et al 1983, Rebuffe-Scrive et al 1988, Kaminski & Ruff 1994). Fluorinated steroids (dexamethasone, triamcinolone) appear to be more pathogenic for muscle than non-fluorinated ones (prednisone, cortisone), but the latter also cause myopathy in sufficiently high dosages (Askari et al 1976, Bunch et al 1980, Rothstein et al 1983, Shee 1990, Kaminski & Ruff 1994). The lowest dosage which can induce myopathy is not know for any steroid, and considerable individual variation must exist. This variation may in large part be due to variations in the level of free concentrations of the specific corticosteroid in the plasma related to the amount of binding proteins produced by the liver. Over 90% of corticosteroid is usually bound to circulating proteins and the amount of binding proteins is diminished by hepatic or renal disease and in older individuals (Frey & Frey 1990). Certain medications, such as ketaconazole and birth control pills, influence the level of free corticosteroid (Frey & Frey 1990). However, for a given dose of prednisone, women are more susceptible to developing steroid myopathy than men (Bunch et al 1980).

The onset of steroid myopathy is usually insidious, but occasionally it can be sudden and accompanied by diffuse myalgia (Askari et al 1976). Muscles of the pelvic girdle are affected earlier and more severely than those of the pectoral girdle. Proximal muscles are typically weaker than distal, but relatively severe weakness of anterior tibial muscles can occur. Patients who have received corticosteroids for less than 4 weeks rarely develop severe steroid myopathy (Askari et al 1976). Normal muscle bulk was found in Cushing's syndrome by Müller & Kugelberg (1959) but muscle atrophy can occur in steroid myopathy (Engel 1966b). Studies in animals indicate that the primary alteration responsible for the weakness and wasting of muscle in steroid myopathy is an increase in protein breakdown (Mayer & Rosen 1977, Clark & Vignos 1979, Elia et al 1981, Tomas et al 1984, Shoji 1989), despite other evidence suggesting that a decrease in the rate of muscle protein synthesis contributes to the muscle wasting (Pacy & Halliday 1989, Shoji 1989). EMG studies have not shown a consistent alteration (reviewed by Askari et al 1976) but typically there is no spontaneous electrical activity and no abnormality in morphology of motor unit potentials in patients with no associated myopathy or neuropathy. The serum CK activity is not increased but creatinuria is constant (Askari et al 1976). The muscle biopsy in Cushing's syndrome shows type II fibre atrophy (Pleasure et al 1970). Many light-microscopic abnormalities have been described in human steroid myopathy (reviewed by Askari et al 1976), but earlier reports, based on paraffin sections, included descriptions of artefacts. While focal increases and decreases in oxidative enzyme activity and focal myofibrillar degeneration can occur in human steroid myopathy, the predominant abnormality, as in Cushing's disease, is atrophy of type II fibres (Engel 1966b, Afifi et al 1968). Experimental steroid myopathy in animals has emphasised this prominent feature (Gardiner et al 1978, Gardiner & Edgerton 1979,

Clark & Vignos 1979, Robinson & Clamann 1988, Ferguson et al 1990).

The diagnosis of steroid myopathy poses no problem when the drug is given for diseases which cause no muscle weakness, such as asthma or psoriasis. However, in polymyositis and in other collagen-vascular diseases treated by steroids, weakness may result from the primary disease as well as the treatment. In such cases, the following favour the diagnosis of steroid myopathy: a temporal relationship between the exacerbation of the weakness and the appearance of other manifestations of hypercorticism; increased weakness within a few weeks of the time when steroid dosage was raised; absence of spontaneous electrical activity in the EMG; normal serum CK activity but significant creatinuria; and type II fibre atrophy but no inflammation in the muscle biopsy. In practice, the differential diagnosis is difficult because none of the criteria are entirely reliable: high doses of steroids are often started when the primary disease itself becomes more severe, and weakness due to the primary disease and due to steroids can coexist.

The pathogenesis of steroid myopathy is not fully understood. An excellent discussion of possible mechanisms is presented in the review by Kaminski & Ruff (1994). An acceleration of protein degradation and the development of type II muscle fibre atrophy were mentioned above. Steroid treatment also increases the fatigability of fast twitch muscles (Gardiner et al 1978, Botterman et al 1983, Robinson & Clamann 1988). While skeletal muscle does contain a high concentration of glucocorticoid receptors (Almon & Dubois 1990), the degree of muscle fibre atrophy does not correlate in a direct fashion, since type I soleus muscle has a higher density of receptors than do type II fibres (Shoji & Pennington 1977). Glucocorticoid treatment also produces an insulin-resistant state which may antagonise the normal anabolic actions of insulin which include a slowing of the rate of muscle breakdown and a stimulation of amino acid uptake in protein synthesis (Block & Buse 1990, Smith et al 1990). Muscle atrophy associated with glucocorticoid treatment is exacerbated by disuse (Almon & Dubois 1990), denervation (Rouleau et al 1987, Massa et al 1992), and by sepsis which

leads to the release of cytokines (Fischer & Hasselgern 1991) and tumour necrosis factor (Hall-Angeras et al 1990) which stimulate protein breakdown. Steroid myopathy also results in an abnormal accumulation of glycogen in muscle (Bullock et al 1972, Tan & Bonen 1985), and changes in the structure (Engel 1966b, Bullock et al 1972) and function (Koski et al 1974, Almon & Dubois 1990) of mitochondria. Treatment with glucocorticoids can cause a transient decrease in muscle potassium content (Klein et al 1962) but as steroid myopathy develops, muscle potassium content (Ruff et al 1982b), serum potassium (Askari et al 1976) and total body potassium (Bauer et al 1960) are normal. Dietary supplements of potassium do not prevent steroid myopathy (Askari et al 1976). Glucocorticoid therapy also causes hypophosphataemia due to an increased renal clearance of phosphate and occasionally severe phosphate depletion results in muscle necrosis. However, phosphate depletion does not appear to have an important role in steroid myopathy since there is only a slight depletion caused by chronic steroid therapy. The histological appearance of muscle is unlike the marked muscle fibre necrosis seen in phosphate depletion, and there is no elevation of muscle-associated enzymes (Knochel 1977a). A study in mice has suggested that glucocorticoid treatment may decrease the excitability of skeletal muscle sarcolemma (Gruener & Stern 1972a,b), and these investigators found that glucocorticoid-treated mice experienced an improvement in their clinical weakness when treated with phenytoin. Subsequent investigations have failed to demonstrate a decrease in membrane excitability associated with glucocorticoid therapy (Ruff et al 1982a, Robinson & Clamann 1988, Grossie & Albuquerque 1978). Additional studies have shown that in single fibres glucocorticoid treatment does not affect excitation–contraction coupling (Laszewski & Ruff 1985, Ruff et al 1982b). Steroid myopathy is not associated with alterations in motor nerve conduction (Askari et al 1976, Afifi et al 1977, Sakai et al 1978) or in neuromuscular transmission (Grossie & Albuquerque 1978, Ribera & Nastuk 1988). As stated above, it appears that the major change in steroid myopathy is related to an increased muscle protein catabolism. Despite significant muscle atrophy the force-generating capacity of muscle is relatively spared with glucocorticoid treatment. This may represent a potentiation of excitation–contraction coupling with glucocorticoid treatment (Kaminski & Ruff 1994). Further studies are necessary to clarify the specific factors responsible for the myopathy. It may be that glucocorticoids deplete muscle of a protein not essential for contraction but necessary for maintaining adequate muscle fibre diameter and bioenergetics (Kaminski & Ruff 1994).

Therapy of steroid myopathy requires withdrawal, if possible, of the offending hormone, or use of the minimum effective dose of a non-fluorinated preparation for control of the primary disease. Muscle strength usually returns to normal within 1–4 months of cessation of steroid therapy (Askari et al 1976). Avoidance of starvation and bouts of sepsis during steroid treatment will lessen the likelihood of steroid myopathy. Inactivity worsens steroid myopathy (Strausz & Janikovsky 1960, Jaspers & Tischler 1986) and increased muscle activity may have a beneficial effect (Falduto et al 1990, Hickson et al 1990). For this reason physical therapy may be a beneficial adjunct in reversing steroid myopathy. The potential benefit of androgen therapy in preventing glucocorticoid-induced myopathy remains to be established (Kaminski & Ruff 1994) and studies of other anabolic agents, such as growth hormone and insulin-like growth factor 1, as treatments to prevent steroid myopathy, remain to be explored.

Primary hyperaldosteronism. The muscular weakness occurring in this condition was discussed earlier in the chapter.

Myopathy and pigmentation after adrenalectomy for Cushing's syndrome. Prineas et al (1968) reported a series of patients who developed diffuse pigmentation and severe myopathy accompanied by lipid excess in muscle fibres after adrenalectomy for Cushing's syndrome. The pathogenesis remains obscure.

Addison's disease. Generalised weakness is a characteristic feature of Addison's disease. It is closely related to plasma and muscle water and electrolyte changes and possibly to the associated hypotension. When these are adequately treated, the weakness rapidly disappears. Joint contractures, especially of the knees, have been observed in Addison's disease. They may be caused by a disorder of tendon and fascia rather than by a primary disease of muscle (Thorn 1949, Ebinger et al 1986).

ACKNOWLEDGEMENTS

The author expresses appreciation to Dr Salvatore DiMauro, Dr Louis Ptacek, Dr Andrew Engel, Dr Frank Lehmann-Horn, Dr Henry Kaminski and Dr Kenneth Ricker for their help in preparing and identifying the most appropriate material to include in this chapter, some of which is based upon the chapter by Dr Andrew Engel in previous editions of this book. Thanks go to the Muscular Dystrophy Association of America, The Saunders Foundation, Wayne C. Gorell Jr. Research Fund, and to NIH for additional support provided by NINDS Grant 5RO1 AR 38894, NIH GLRC 5MO1-RR00044. Special thanks go to Jean Ellinwood and to Barbara Hayes for their exceptional efforts in organising and typing this chapter.

REFERENCES

Abarbanel J M, Bashan N, Potashnik R et al 1986 Adult muscle phosphorylase b kinase deficiency. Neurology 36: 560

Adachi J, Yamamoto K, Ogawa Y et al 1991 Endogenous formation of 1-methyl-1,2,3,4-tetrahydro-beta-carboline-carboxylic acid in man as the possible causative substance of eosinophilia-myalgia syndrome associated with ingestion of L-tryptophane. Archives of Toxicology 65: 505

Afifi A K, Bergman R A, Harvey J C 1968 Steroid myopathy. Clinical, histologic and cytologic observations. Johns Hopkins Medical Journal 123: 158

Afifi A, Najjar S, Mire-Salman J et al 1974 The myopathology of the Kocher–Debré–Semelaigne syndrome. Journal of the Neurological Science 22: 445

Afifi A, Al-Gailany A, Salman J et al 1977 Nerve and muscle in steroid-induced weakness in the rabbit. Archives of Physical Medicine and Rehabilitation 58: 143

Agamanolis D P, Askari A D, DiMauro S et al 1980 Muscle phosphofructokinase deficiency: two cases with unusual polysaccharide accumulation and immunologically active enzyme protein. Muscle and Nerve 3: 456

Ahman A, Baker J, Weetman A et al 1987 Antibodies to porcine eye muscle in patients with Graves' ophthalmopathy: Identification of serum immunoglobins directed against unique determinants by immunoblotting and enzyme-linked immunosorbent assay. Journal of Clinical Endocrinology and Metabolism 64: 454

Aitken R S, Allott E N, Castleden L I M, Walker M 1937 Observations on a case of familial periodic paralysis. Clinical Science and Molecular Medicine 3: 47

Akasaka T, Ogura Y, Anbe J et al 1991 Correction of tetralogy of Fallot accompanied by malignant hyperthermia. Journal of Cardiovascular Surgery 32: 581

Alderson K, Griffin J W, Cornblath D R et al 1987 Neuromuscular complications of amiodarone therapy. Neurology 37 (suppl): 355

Allott E N, McArdle B 1938 Further observations on familial periodic paralysis. Clinical Science and Molecular Medicine 3: 229

Almon R R, Dubois D C 1990 Fiber-type discrimination in disuse and glucocorticoid-induced atrophy. Medicine & Science in Sports & Exercise 22: 304

Amiel I, Nivoche Y 1989 Treatment of malignant hyperthermia crisis during anesthesia. Annales Françaises d'Anesthesie et de Reanimation 8: 427

Andersen D H 1956 Familial cirrhosis of the liver with storage of abnormal glycogen. Laboratory Investigation 5: 11

Andersen E D, Krasilnikoff P A, Overvad H 1971 Intermittent muscular weakness, extrasystoles, and multiple developmental anomalies. Acta Paediatrica Scandinavica 60: 559

Angelini C, Engel A G, Titus J L 1972 Adult acid maltase deficiency. Abnormalities in fibroblasts cultured from patients. New England Journal of Medicine 287: 948

Angelini C, Engel A G 1972 Comparative study of acid maltase deficiency. Archives of Neurology 26: 344

Aranyi J, Rado J 1992 Rhabdomyolysis in a medical student induced by body-building exercise (rhabdomyolysis following acute muscular exertion). Orvosi Hetilap 2: 133 (31).

Argov Z, Bank W J 1991 Phosphorus magnetic resonance spectroscopy (^{31}P MRS) in neuromuscular disorders. Annals of Neurology 30: 90

Argov Z, Bank W J, Boden B et al 1987a Phosphorus magnetic resonance spectroscopy of partially blocked muscle glycolysis. Neurology 44: 614

Argov Z, Bank W J, Maris J et al 1987b Muscle energy metabolism in McArdle's syndrome by in vivo phosphorus magnetic resonance spectroscopy. Neurology 37: 1720

Argov Z, Renshaw P, Boden B et al 1988 Effects of thyroid hormones on skeletal muscle bioenergetics. In vivo phosphorus-31 magnetic resonance spectroscopy study of humans and rats. Journal of Clinical Investigation 81: 1695

Arnaudo E, Dalakas M, Shanske S, Moraes C T et al 1991 Depletion of muscle mitochondrial DNA in AIDS patients with zidovudine-induced myopathy. Lancet 337: 508

Asayama K, Kato K 1990 Oxidative muscular injury and its relevance to hyperthyroidism. Free Radical Biology and Medicine 8: 293

Ashby D 1990 Malignant hyperthermia: a potential crisis in the postanesthesia care unit. Journal of Post Anesthesia Nursing 5: 279

Askanas V, Engel W K, DiMauro S, Brooks D R, Mehler M 1976 Adult onset acid maltase deficiency. Morphological and biochemical abnormalities reproduced in cultured muscle. New England Journal of Medicine 294: 573

Askari A, Vignos P, Moskowitz R 1976 Steroid myopathy in connective tissue disease. American Journal of Medicine 61: 485

Åström K E, Kugelberg E, Muller R 1961 Hypothyroid myopathy. Archives of Neurology 5: 472

Atkin J, Snow J W, Zellweger H, Rhead W J 1984 Fatal infantile cardiac glycogenosis without acid maltase deficiency presenting as congenital hydrops. European Journal of Pediatrics 142: 150

Auld V J, Goldin A L, Krafte D S et al 1990 A neutral amino acid change in segment IIS4 dramatically alters the gating properties of the voltage-dependent sodium channel. Proceedings of the National Academy of Science USA 87: 323

Badurska G, Fidzianska A, Kwiatkowska Z 1970 Muscular glycogenosis type III in a 15-year-old boy. Neuropathology Policy 8: 265

Baertl J M, Sancetta S M, Gabuzda J 1963 Relation of acute potassium depletion to renal ammonium metabolism in patients with cirrhosis. Journal of Clinical Investigation 42: 696

Ball E, Sanwal B 1980 A synergistic effect of glucocorticoids and insulin on the differentiation of myoblasts. Journal of Cell Physiology 102: 27

Bannett R, Sampson S, Shainberg A 1984 Influence of thyroid hormone on some electrophysiological properties of developing rat skeletal muscle cells in culture. Brain Research 294: 75

Barranger J A, Brader R O (eds) 1984 Molecular basis of lysosomal storage disorders. Academic Press, New York

Bauer F, Dubois E, Teleer N 1960 Total exchangeable potassium in SLE with reference to triamcinolone myopathy. Proceedings of the Society of Experimental Biology and Medicine 105: 671

Becker K, Titus J, McConahey W, Wollner L 1964 Morphologic evidence of thyroiditis in myasthenia gravis. Journal of the American Medical Association 187: 994

Bekeny G 1961 Über irreversible Muskelveränderungen, bei der paroxysmalen Lähmung auf grund bioptischer Muskeluntersuchungen. Deutsche Zeitschrift für Nervenheilkunde 1982: 119

Bell H, Hayes W L, Vosburgh J 1965 Hyperkalaemic paralysis due to adrenal insufficiency. Archives of Internal Medicine 115: 418

Belongia E A, Hedberg C W, Gleich G J et al 1990 An investigation of the cause of the eosinophilia-myalgia syndrome associated with tryptophan use. New England Journal of Medicine 323: 357

Benheim P E, Dostarczyk R, Berg B O 1985 β-Adrenergic treatment of hyperkalaemic periodic paralysis. Neurology 35: 746

Beratis N G, Labadie G U, Hirschhorn K 1978 Characterization of the molecular defect in infantile and adult acid α-glycosidase deficiency in fibroblasts. Journal of Clinical Investigation 62: 1264

Beratis N G, LaBadie G U, Hirschhorn K 1983 Genetic heterogeneity in acid alpha-glucosidase deficiency. American Journal of Human Genetics 35: 21

Bergman R A, Afifi A K, Dunkle L M, Johns R J 1970 Muscle pathology in hypokalaemic periodic paralysis with hyperthyroidism. Bulletin of the Johns Hopkins Hospital 126: 100

Bergstrom J, Hultman E 1966 The effect of thiazides, chlorthalidone and furosemide on muscle electrolytes and muscle glycogen in normal subjects. Acta Medica Scandinavica 180: 363

Berlin R 1984 Haff disease in Sweden. Acta Medica Scandinavica 129: 560

Bertagnolio S, DiDonato S, Peluchetti D, Rimoldi M, Storchi G, Cornelio F 1978 Acid maltase deficiency in adults. Clinical, morphological and biochemical study of three patients. European Neurology 17: 193

Biczyskowa W, Fidzianska A, Jedrzejowska H 1969 Light and electron microscopic study of the muscles in hypokalaemic periodic paralysis. Acta Neuropathologica 12: 329

Biemond A, Daniels A P 1934 Familial periodic paralysis and its transition into spinal muscular atrophy. Brain 57: 91

Bigland B, Young F 1954 Influence of growth hormone on the protein composition of rat muscle. Journal of Endocrinology 10: 179

Birge S, Haddad J 1975 25-Hydroxycholecalciferol stimulation of muscle metabolism. Journal of Clinical Investigation 56: 1100

Bischoff A, Esslen E 1965 Myopathy with primary hyperparathyroidism. Neurology (Minneapolis) 15: 64

Blanc W A, Reid J D, Andersen D H 1958 Avitaminosis E in cystic fibrosis of the pancreas. A morphologic study of gastrointestinal and striated muscle. Pediatrics 22: 494

Block K, Buse M 1990 Glucocorticoid regulation of muscle branched-chain amino acid metabolism. Medical Science Sports Exercise 22: 316

Boland R 1986 Role of vitamin D in skeletal muscle function. Endocrine Review 7: 434

Bonilla E, Schotland D L 1970 Histochemical diagnosis of muscle phosphofructokinase deficiency. Archives of Neurology 22: 8

Botterman B, Eldred E, Edgerton V 1981 Spindle discharges in glucocorticoid-induced muscle atrophy. Experimental Neurology 72: 25

Bouzas A 1980 Endocrine ophthalmopathy. Transactions in Ophthalmology 100: 511

Bowden D H, Fraser D, Jackson S H, Walter N F 1956 Acute recurrent rhabdomyolysis (paroxysmal myohaemoglobinuria). Medicine (Baltimore) 35: 335

Braakhekke J P, deBruin M I, Stegeman D F et al 1986 The second wind phenomenon in McArdle's disease. Brain 198: 1087

Bradley W G, Fewings J D, Harris J B, Johnson M A 1976 Emetine myopathy in the rat. British Journal of Pharmacology 57: 29

Brady H R, Kinirons M, Lynch T et al 1989 Heart rate and metabolic response to competitive squash in veteran players: identification of risk factors for sudden cardiac death. European Heart Journal 10: 1029

Brandt I K, De Luca V A 1966 Type III glycogenosis: a family with unusual tissue distribution of the enzyme lesion. American Journal of Medicine 40: 779

Braun N, Marino W, Jacobs T et al 1982 Therapeutic trial of thyroid hormone in patients with acid maltase deficient myopathy: a preliminary report. 5th International Congress on Neuromuscular Diseases, Abstract 38.6

Bresolin N, Ro Y-I, Reyes M, Miranda A F, Di Mauro S 1983 Muscle phosphoglycerate mutase (PGAM) deficiency: a second case. Neurology 33: 1049

Bresolin N, Miranda A F, Chang H W, Shanske S, Di Mauro S 1984 Phosphoglycerate kinase deficiency myopathy: biochemical and immunological studies of the mutant enzyme. Muscle and Nerve 7: 542

Bridgman J F, Rosen S M, Thorp J M 1972 Complications during clofibrate treatment of nephrotic-syndrome hyperlipoproteinemia. Lancet ii: 506

Britt B A, Endrenyi L, Peters P L 1976 Screening of malignant hyperthermia susceptible families by creatine phosphokinase measurement and other clinical investigations. Canadian Anaesthetists' Society Journal 23: 263

Brodie C, Sampson S 1989 Characterization of thyroid hormone effects on Na channel synthesis in cultured skeletal myotubes: role of Ca^{2+}. Endocrinology 125: 842

Brodkin H M 1980 Myoglobinuria following epsilon-aminocaproic acid (EACA) therapy. Journal of Neurosurgery 53: 690

Brody I A, Gerber C J, Sidbury J B 1970 Relaxing factor in McArdle's disease. Calcium uptake by sarcoplasmic reticulum. Neurology (Minneapolis) 20: 555

Brooks R V, McSwiney R R, Prunty T F G, Wood F J Y 1957 Potassium deficiency of renal and adrenal origin. American Journal of Medicine 23: 391

Brown B I 1986 Debranching and branching enzyme deficiencies. In: Engel A G, Banker B Q, eds. Myology. McGraw Hill, New York, p 1653

Brown B I, Brown D H 1966 Lack of an α-1, 4-glucan: α-1,4-glucan 6-glycosyl transferase in a case of type IV glycogenosis. Proceedings of the National Academy of Sciences USA 56: 725

Brown B I, Zellweger H 1966 α-1, 4-Glucosidase activity in leukocytes from the family of two brothers who lack this enzyme in muscle. Biochemical Journal 101: 16c

Brown B I, Brown D H 1968 Glycogen storage diseases: Types I, III, IV, V, VII and unclassified glycogenosis. In: Dickens F, Randle P J, Whelan W J (eds) Carbohydrate metabolism and its disorders, vol 2. Academic Press, New York, p 123

Brown B I, Brown D H 1989 Branching enzyme activity of cultured amniocytes and chorionic villi: prenatal testing for type IV glycogen storage disease. American Journal of Human Genetics 44: 378

Brown B I, Brown D H, Jeffrey P L 1970 Simultaneous absence of α-1, 6-glucosidase activities (pH 4) in tissues of children with type II glycogen storeage disease. Biochemical Journal 9: 1423

Brown D H, Illingworth B 1962 The properties of an oligo-1, $4 \rightarrow 1$, 4 glucantransferase from animal tissue. Proceedings of the National Academy of Sciences USA 48: 1783

Brown J A, Wollmann R L, Mullan S 1982 Myopathy induced by epsilon-aminocaproic acid. Case report. Journal of Neurosurgery 57: 130

Brown M J 1985 Hypokalaemia from beta₂-receptor stimulation by circulating epinephrine. American Journal of Cardiology 56: 3D

Brown M J, Brown D C, Murphy M B 1983 Hypokalaemia from beta₂-receptor stimulation by circulating epinephrine. New England Journal of Medicine 309: 1414

Brunberg J A, McCormick W F, Schochet S S 1971 Type III glycogenosis. An adult with diffuse weakness and muscle wasting. Archives of Neurology 25: 171

Bryan G T, MacCardle R C, Bartter F C 1966 Hyperaldosteronism, hyperplasia of the juxtaglomerular complex, normal blood pressure, and dwarfism. Pediatrics 37: 43

Bryan W, Lewis S F, Bertocci L et al 1990 Muscle lactate dehydrogenase deficiency: a disorder of anaerobic glycogenolysis associated with exertional myoglobinuria. Neurology 40 (suppl 1): 203

Buchthal F, Engback L, Gamstorp I 1958 Paresis and hyperexcitability in adynamia episodica hereditaria. Neurology (Minneapolis) 8: 347

Bull G M, Carter A B, Lowe K G 1953 Hyperpotassaemic paralysis. Lancet ii: 60

Bullock G, Carter E, Elliot P et al 1972 Relative changes in the function of muscle ribosomes and mitochondria during early phase of steroid-induced catabolism. Biochemical Journal 127: 881

Bunch T, Worthington J, Combs J, Ilstrup D, Engel A 1980 Azathioprine with prednisone for polymyositis: a controlled, clinical trial. Annals of Internal Medicine 92: 365

Burck U, Goebel H H, Kuhlendahl H D, Meier C, Goebel K M 1981 Neuromyopathy and vitamin E deficiency in man. Neuropediatrics 12: 267

Busch H F M, Koster J F, Van Weerden T W 1979 Infantile and adult-onset acid maltase deficiency occurring in the same family. Neurology (Minneapolis) 29: 415

Byers R K, Bergman A B, Joseph M C 1962 Steroid myopathy: report of five cases occurring during treatment of rheumatic fever. Pediatrics 29: 26

Bywaters E G L, Stead J K 1945 Thrombosis of the femoral artery with myoglobinuria and low serum potassium concentration. Clinical Science 5: 195

Bywaters E G L, Delory G E, Rimington C, Smiles J 1941 Myohaemoglobin in the urine of the air raid casualties with crushing injury. Biochemical Journal 35: 1164

Caddell J, Whitemore R 1962 Observations on generalised glycogenosis with emphasis on electrocardiographic changes. Pediatrics 29: 743

Cafferty M S, Lovelace R E, Hays A P et al 1991 Polyglucosan body disease. Muscle and Nerve 14: 102

Callahan J W, Lowden J A (eds) 1981 Lysosomes and lysosomal storage diseases. Raven, New York

Cape C 1969 Phosphorylase A deficiency in pseudohypoparathyroidism. Neurology (Minneapolis) 19: 167

Carrier H, Lebel M, Mathieu M, Pialat J, Oevic M 1975 Late familial pseudo-myopathic muscular glycogenosis with α-1, 4-glucosidase deficiency. Pathologica Europea (Bruxelles) 10: 51

Carrier H, Maire I, Vial C et al 1990 Myopathic evolution of an exertional muscle pain syndrome with phosphorylase b kinase deficiency. Acta Neuropathology 81: 84

Carson M J, Pearson C M 1964 Familial hyperkalaemic periodic paralysis with myotonic features. Journal of Pediatrics 64: 853

Catterall W A 1986 Molecular properties of voltage-sensitive sodium channels. Annual Review of Biochemistry 55: 953

Catterall W A 1988 Structure and function of voltage-sensitive ion channels. Science 242: 50

Catton C K, Elmer J C, Whitehouse A C et al 1991 Pulmonary involvement in the eosinophilia-myalgia syndrome. Chest 99: 327

Cederbaum A I, Rubin E 1975 Molecular injury to mitochondria produced by ethanol and acetaldehyde. Federation Proceedings 34: 2045

Celsing F, Blomstrand E, Melichna J et al 1986 Effect of hyperthyroidism on fibre-type composition, fibre area, glycogen content and enzyme activity in human skeletal muscle. Clinical Physiology 6: 171

Chalmers A C, Greco C M, Miller R G 1991 Prognosis in AZT myopathy. Neurology 41: 1181

Chen S S, Pena M J, Chen T J 1991 Study of myopathy in chronic alcoholics with neurological complications. Kaoo-Hsiung I Hsueh Ko Hsueh Tsa Chih 7: 296

Chen Y-T, He J-K, Ding J-H et al 1987 Glycogen debranching enzyme: purification, antibody characterization, and immunoblot analyses of type III glycogen storage disease. American Journal of Human Genetics 41: 1002

Cholod E, Haust M, Hudson A, Lewis F 1970 Myopathy in primary familial hyperparathyroidism. Clinical and morphological studies. American Journal of Medicine 48: 700

Chu D, Shikama H, Khatra B et al 1985 Effects of altered thyroid status on beta-adrenergic actions on skeletal muscle glycogen metabolism. Journal of Biology and Chemistry 260: 9994

Chui L A, Munsat T L 1976 Dominant inheritance of McArdle syndrome. Archives of Neurology 33: 636

Clark A, Vignos P 1979 Experimental corticosteroid myopathy: effect on myofibrillar ATPase activity and protein degradation. Muscle and Nerve 2: 265

Clausen T, Everts M E 1989 Regulation of the Na,K-pump in skeletal muscle. Kidney International 35: 1

Clausen T, Wang P, Orskov H, Kristensen O 1980 Hyperkalemic periodic paralysis: relationship between changes in plasma water, electrolytes, insulin and catecholamines during the attacks. Scandinavian Journal of Clinical and Laboratory Investigation 40: 211

Clemens P R, Yamamoto M, Engel A G 1990 Adult phosphorylase b kinase deficiency. Annals of Neurology 28: 529

Cohn J, Wang P, Hauge M, Henningsen K, Jensen B, Sveigaard A 1975 Amylo-1, 6-glucosidase deficiency (glycogenosis type III) in the Faroe Islands. Human Heredity 25: 115

Conde-Martel A, Gonzalez-Reimers E, Santolaria-Fernandez F et al 1992 Pathogenesis of alcoholic myopathy: roles of ethanol and malnutrition. Drug and Alcohol Dependence 30: 101

Conn J W 1955 Presidential address I. Painting background. II. Primary aldosteronism. Journal of Laboratory and Clinical Medicine 45: 3

Conn J W 1965 Hypertension, the potassium ion and impaired carbohydrate tolerance. New England Journal of Medicine 273: 1135

Conway M J, Seibel J A, Eaton R P 1974 Thyrotoxicosis and periodic paralysis: Improvement with beta blockade. Annals of Internal Medicine 81: 332

Coomes E N 1965 Corticosteroid myopathy. Annals of Rheumatic Diseases 24: 465

Cooper P, Kudynska J, Buckmaster H A 1992 An EPR investigation of spin-labelled erythrocytes as a diagnostic technique for malignant hyperthermia. Biochimica et Biophysica Acta 9: 1139

Cori G T 1957 Biochemical aspects of glycogen deposition diseases. Modern Problems in Paediatrics 3: 344

Cornelio F, Bresolin N, Singer P A et al 1984 The clinical varieties of neuromuscular disease in debrancher deficiency. Archives of Neurology 41: 1027

Cornet C, Moeller R, Laxenaire M C 1989 Clinical features of malignant hyperthermia crisis. Annales Françaises d'Anesthesie et de Reanimation 8: 435

Creutzfeldt O D 1961 Die episodiche Adynamie (Adynamia episodica hereditaria Gamstorp) eine familiäre hyperkalämische Lähmung. Forschritte der Neurologie, Psychiatrie und Irhe Gerenzgebiete 29: 529

Curry O B, Basten J F, Francis M J O et al 1974 Calcium uptake by sarcoplasmic reticulum of muscle from vitamin D-deficient rabbits. Nature 249: 83

Dalakas M C, Engel W K 1983 Treatment of 'permanent' muscle weakness in familial hypokalemic periodic paralysis. Muscle and Nerve 6: 182

Dalakas M C, Illa I, Pezeshkpour G H et al 1990 Mitochondrial myopathy caused by long-term zidovudine therapy. New England Journal of Medicine 322: 1098

D'Albis A, Chanoine C, Janmot C, Mira J, Couteaux R 1990 Muscle-specific response to thyroid hormone of myosin isoform transitions during rat postnatal development. European Journal of Biochemistry 193: 155

Danon M J, Carpenter S 1991 Myopathy with thick filament (myosin) loss following prolonged paralysis with vecuronium during steroid treatment. Muscle and Nerve 14: 1131

Danon M J, Carpenter S, Manaligod J R, Schliselfeld L H 1981a Fatal infantile glycogen storage disease: Deficiency of phosphofructokinase and phosphorylase b kinase. Neurology 31: 1303

Danon M J, Oh S J, DiMauro S et al 1981b Lysosomal glycogen storage with normal acid maltase. Neurology 31: 51

Danon M J, DiMauro S, Shanske S et al 1986 Juvenile onset acid maltase deficiency with unusual familial features. Neurology 36: 818

Danon M J, Servidei S, DiMauro S et al 1988 Late-onset muscle phosphofructokinase deficiency. Neurology 38: 956

Danowksi T S, Greenman L 1953 Changes in fecal and serum constituents during ingestion of cation and anion exchange. Annals of the New York Academy of Sciences 57: 273

Danzis J, Hutzler J, Lynfield J et al 1969 Absence of acid maltase in glycogenosis type II (Pompe's disease) in tissue culture. American Journal of Diseases of Children 117: 108

Dastur D K, Gagrat B M, Wadia N H, Desai M M, Bharucha E P 1975 Nature of muscular change in osteomalacia: light and electronmicroscope observations. Journal of Pathology 117: 221

Daughaday W H, Rendleman D 1967 Severe symptomatic hyperkalemia in an adrenalectomized woman due to enhanced mineralocorticoid requirement. Annals of Internal Medicine 66: 1197

Davidson M, Miranda A F, Bender A N, Di Mauro S, Vora S 1983 Muscle phosphofructokinase deficiency. Biochemical and immunological studies of phosphofructokinase isozymes in muscle culture. Journal of Clinical Investigation 72: 545

Davie M W J, Chalmers T M, Hunter J O et al 1976 1-Alpha-hydroxycholecalciferol in chronic renal failure: studies of the effect of oral doses. Annals of Internal Medicine 84: 281

Davis C H, Schliselfeld L H, Wolf D P, Leavitt C A, Krebs E G 1967 Interrelationships among glycogen phosphorylase isoenzymes. Journal of Biological Chemistry 242: 4824

Dawson D M, Spong F Z, Harrington J F 1968 McArdle's disease: lack of muscle phosphorylase. Annals of Internal Medicine 69: 229

De Barsy T, Jacquemin P, Devos P, Hers H G 1972 Rodent and human acid α-glucosidase: Purification, assay and inhibition by antibodies. Investigations in type II glycogenosis. European Journal of Biochemistry 31: 156

De Barsy T, Jacquemin P, Van Hoof F, Hers H G 1973 Enzyme replacement in Pompe's disease: an attempt with purified human α-glucosidase. Birth Defects 9: 184

De Burlet G, Sudaka P 1977 Properties catalitiques de l'α-glucosidase neutre du rein humain. Biochimie 59: 7

Debré F, Semelaigne G 1935 Syndrome of diffuse muscular hypertrophy in infants causing athletic appearance; its connection with congenital myxedema. American Journal of Diseases of Children 50: 1351

Deckelbaum R J, Russell A, Shapira E, Cohen T, Agam G, Gutman G 1972 Type III glyocogenosis: atypical enzyme activities in blood cells in two siblings. Journal of Pediatrics 81: 955

Demartino G, Goldberg A 1981 A possible explanation of myxedema and hypercholesterolemia in hypothyroidism: control of lysosomal hyaluronidase and cholesterol esterase by thyroid hormones. Enzyme 26: 1

Demos M A, Gitin E L, Kagen L J 1974 Exercise myoglobinemia and acute exertional rhabdomyolysis. Archives of Internal Medicine 134: 669

Denborough M A, Lovell R R H 1960 Anaesthetic deaths in a family. Lancet ii: 45

Dershwitz M, Sreter F A 1990 Azumolene reverses episodes of malignant hyperthermia in susceptible swine. Anesthesia and Analgesia 70: 253

deSilva S M, Kuncl R W, Griffin J W, Cornblath D R, Chavoustie S 1990 Paramyotonia congenita or hyperkalemic periodic paralysis? Clinical and electrophysiological features of each entity in one family. Muscle and Nerve 13: 21

Deufel T, Golla A, Illes A et al 1992 Evidence for genetic heterogeneity of malignant hyperthermia susceptibility. American Journal of Human Genetics 50: 1151

DeVol D, Rotwein P, Sadow J, Novakofski J, Bechtel P 1990 Activation of insulin-like growth factor gene expression during work-induced skeletal muscle growth. American Journal of Physiology 259: E89

DiBona F J, Morens D M 1977 Rhabdomyolysis associated with influenza A. Report of a case with unusual fluid and electrolyte abnormalities. Journal of Pediatrics 91: 943

DiMauro S, Hartlage P L 1978 Fatal infantile form of muscle phosphorylase deficiency. Annals of Neurology 28: 1124

DiMauro S, Servidei S 1993 Disorders of carbohydrate metabolism: Glycogen storage diseases. In: Rosenberg R, Pruisner S B, Di Mauro S et al (eds) The molecular and genetic basis of neurological disease Butterworth Heinemann, Boston p. 93

DiMauro S, Arnold S, Miranda A, Rowland L P 1978a McArdle disease: the mystery of reappearing phosphorylase activity in muscle culture — a fetal isozyme. Annals of Neurology 3: 60

Di Mauro S, Hartwig G B, Hays A et al 1978b Debrancher enzyme deficiency: neuromuscular disorder in 5 adults. Annals of Neurology 5: 422

DiMauro S, Stern L Z, Mehler M, Nagle R B, Payne, C 1978c Adult-onset acid maltase deficiency: a postmortem study. Muscle and Nerve 1: 27

DiMauro S, Hartwig G B, Hays A P et al 1979 Debrancher deficiency: neuromuscular disorder in five adults. Annals of Neurology 5: 422

DiMauro S, Miranda A F, Khan S et al 1981 Human muscle phosphoglycerate mutase deficiency: a new cause of recurrent myoglobinuria. Science 212: 1277

Di Mauro S, Miranda A F, Olarte M, Friedman R, Hays A P 1982 Muscle phosphoglycerate mutase deficiency. Neurology 32: 548

DiMauro S, Dalakas M, Miranda A F 1983 Phosphoglycerate kinase (PGK) deficiency: new cause of recurrent myoglobinuria. Annals of Neurology 13: 11

DiMauro S, Bresolin N, Hays A P 1984 Disorders of glycogen metabolism. In: Roses A D (ed) Critical reviews in clinical neurobiology. CRC Press, Boca Raton, FL, p 83

Ding J-H, DeBarsy Th, Brown B L et al 1990 Immunoblot analyses of glycogen debranching enzyme in different subtypes of glycogen storage disease type III. Journal of Pediatrics 116: 95

Doriguzzi C, Palmucci L, Mongini T et al 1988 Body building and myoglobinuria: report of three cases. British Medical Journal – Clinical Research 296: 826

Drager G A, Hammill J F, Shy G M 1958 Paramyotonia congenita. Archives of Neurology 80: 1

Dreyfus J C, Alexandre Y 1971 Immunological studies on glycogen storage disease type III and V. Demonstration of the presence of an immunoreactive protein in one case of muscle phosphorylase deficiency. Biochemical and Biophysical Research Communications 44: 1364

Duane D D, Engel A G 1970 Emetine myopathy. Neurology (Minneapolis) 20: 733

Duboc D, Jehenson P, Dinh S T et al 1987 Phosphorous NMR spectroscopy study of muscular enzyme deficiencies involving glycogenolysis and glycolysis. Neurology 37: 663

Dulhunty A, Gage P, Lamb G 1986 Differential effects of thyroid hormone on T-tubules and terminal cisternae in rat muscles: an electrophysiological and morphometric analysis. Journal of Muscle Research and Cell Motility 7: 225

Dunlap H F, Kepler E J 1931 Occurrence of periodic paralysis in the course of exophthalmic goiter. Proceedings of the Staff Meetings of the Mayo Clinic 6: 272

Dupond J L, Robert M, Carbillet J P, Leconte Des, Floris R 1977 Glycogénose musculaire et anémie hémolytique par déficit enzymatique chez aux germains. La Nouvelle Presse Médicale 6: 2665

Dustan H P, Corcoran A C, Page I H 1956 Renal function in primary aldosteronism. Journal of Clinical Investigation 35: 1357

Dyken M L, Timmons G D 1963 Hyperkalemic periodic paralysis with hypocalcemic episode. Archives of Neurology 9: 508

Dyken M L, Smith D M, Peake R L 1967 An electromyographic diagnostic screening test in McArdle's disease and a case report. Neurology (Minneapolis) 17: 45

Eagan T J, Klein R 1959 Hyperkalemic familial periodic paralysis. Pediatrics 24: 761

East C, Alivizatos P A, Grundy S M et al 1988 Rhabdomyolysis in patients receiving lovastatin after cardiac transplantation. New England Journal of Medicine 318: 47

Ebers G C, George A L, Barchi R L et al 1991 Paramyotonia congenita and hyperkalemic periodic paralysis are linked to the adult muscle sodium channel gene. Annals of Neurology 30: 810

Ebinger G, Roland S, Brugland M, Samers G 1986 Flexion contracture: a forgotten symptom in Addison's disease and hypopituitarism. Lancet ii: 858

Ekbom K, Hed R, Kirstein L, Åström K E 1964 Muscular affections in chronic alcoholism. Archives of Neurology 10: 449

Elia M, Carter A, Bacon S, Winearls C, Smith R 1981 Clinical usefulness of urinary 3-methylhistidine excretion in indicating muscle protein breakdown. British Medical Journal (Clinical Research) 282: 351

Emser W, Schimrigk K 1977 Myxedema myopathy: a case report. European Neurology 16: 286

Engel A G 1961a Thyroid function and myasthenia gravis. Archives of Neurology 4: 663

Engel A G 1961b Thyroid function and periodic paralysis. American Journal of Medicine 30: 327

Engel A G 1966a Electron microscopic observations in primary hypokalemic and thyrotoxic periodic paralysis. Mayo Clinic Proceedings 41: 797

Engel A G 1966b Electron microscopic observations in thyrotoxic and corticosteroid-induced myopathies. Mayo Clinic Proceedings 41: 785

Engel A G 1970a Evolution and comment on vacuoles in primary hypokalemic periodic paralysis. Mayo Clinic Proceedings 45: 774

Engel A G 1970b Acid maltase deficiency in adults: studies in four cases of a syndrome which may mimic muscular dystrophy or other myopathies. Brain 93: 599

Engel A G 1972 Neuromuscular manifestations of Graves' disease. Mayo Clinic Proceedings 47: 919

Engel A G 1977 Hypokalemic and hyperkalemic periodic paralysis. In: Goldensohn E S, Appel S H (eds) Scientific approach to clinical neurology. Lea and Febiger, Philadelphia, p 1742

Engel A 1984 Myasthenia gravis and myasthenic syndrome. Annals of Neurology 16: 519

Engel A G 1986 Acid maltase deficiency. In: Engel A G, Banker B Q (eds) Myology, vol 2. McGraw-Hill, New York, p 1629

Engel A G, Dale A J D 1968 Autophagic glycogenesis of late onset with mitochondrial abnormalities: light and electron microscopic observations. Mayo Clinic Proceedings 43: 233

Engel A G, Gomez M R 1970 Acid maltase levels in human heterozygous acid maltase deficiency and in non-weak and neuromuscular disease controls. Journal of Neurology, Neurosurgery and Psychiatry 33: 801

Engel A G, Potter C S, Rosevear J W 1964 Nucleotides and adenosine monophosphate deaminase activity of muscle in primary hypokalemic periodic paralysis. Nature 292: 670

Engel A G, Lambert E H, Rosevear J W, Tauxe W N 1965 Clinical and electromyographic studies in a patient with primary hypokalemic periodic paralysis. American Journal of Medicine 38: 626

Engel A G, Potter C S, Rosevear J W 1967 Studies on carbohydrate metabolism and mitochondrial respiratory activities in primary hypokalemic periodic paralysis. Neurology (Minneapolis) 17: 329

Engel A G, Gomez M R, Groover R V 1971 Multicore disease. A recently recognized congenital myopathy with multifocal degeneration of muscle fibers. Mayo Clinic Proceedings 46: 666

Engel A G, Gomez M R, Seybold M E, Lambert E H 1973 The spectrum and diagnosis of acid maltase deficiency. Neurology (Minneapolis) 23: 95

Engel F L, Martin S P, Taylor H 1949 On the relation of potassium to the neurological manifestations of hypocalcemic tetany. Bulletin of the Johns Hopkins Hospital 84: 285

Engel W K, Eyerman E L, Williams H E 1963 Late-onset type of skeletal muscle phosphorylase deficiency. New England Journal of Medicine 268: 135

Ernster L, Ikkos D, Luft R 1959 Enzymatic activities of human skeletal muscle mitochondria: a tool in clinical metabolic research. Nature 184: 1851

Ervasti J M, Strand M A, Hanson T P 1991 Ryanodine receptor in different malignant hyperthermia-susceptible porcine muscles. American Journal of Physiology 260: C58

Estes M L, Ewing-Wilson D, Chou S M et al 1987 Chloroquine neuromyotoxicity: clinical and pathologic perspective. American Journal of Medicine 82: 447

Estrada C A, Harrington D W, Glasberg M R 1990 Eosinophilic myositis an expression of L-tryptophan toxicity? Journal of Rheumatology 17: 1554

Eulenburg A 1986 Über eine familiäre, durch 6

Generationen verfolgbere form kongenitaler Paromyotonie. Nerologisches Zentralblatt 5: 508

European Malignant Hyperpyrexia Group 1984 A protocol for the investigation of malignant hyperpyrexia (MH) susceptibility. British Journal of Anaesthesia 56: 1267

Evans R, Watanabe I, Singer P 1990 Central changes in hypothyroid myopathy: a case report. Muscle and Nerve 13: 952

Ewton D, Florini J 1981 Effects of the somatomedins and insulin on myoblast differentiation in vivo. Developmental Biology 86: 31

Fagerlund T, Islander G, Ranklev E et al 1992 Genetic recombination between malignant hyperthermia and calcium release channel in skeletal muscle. Clinical Genetics 41: 270

Falduto M T, Czerwinski S M, Hickson R C 1990 Glucocorticoid-induced muscle atrophy prevention by exercise in fast-twitch fibers. Journal of Applied Physiology 69: 1058

Faris A A, Reyes M G 1971 Reappraisal of alcoholic myopathy. Clinical and biopsy study on chronic alcoholics without muscle weakness or wasting. Journal of Neurology, Neurosurgery and Psychiatry 34: 86

Fattah S M, Rubulis A, Faloon W W 1979 McArdle's disease: metabolic studies in a patient and review of the syndrome. American Journal of Medicine 48: 693

Faugere M C, Pellisier J F, Toga M 1981 Subsequent morphological changes in periodic paralysis: a study of seven cases. Acta Neuropathology (Berlin) Suppl VII: 301

Faust D K, Gergis S D, Sokoll M D 1979 Management of suspected hyperpyrexia in an infant. Anesthesia and Analgesia 58: 33

Faw M L, Ewer R W 1962 Intermittent paralysis and chronic adrenal insufficiency. Annals of Internal Medicine 57: 461

Feit H, Brooke M H 1976 Myophosphorylase deficiency: two different molecular forms of etiology. Neurology (Minneapolis) 26: 963

Feldon S 1990 Graves' ophthalmopathy. Is it really thyroid disease? Archives of Internal Medicine 150: 948

Ferguson G, Irvin C, Cherniack R 1990 Effect of corticosteroids on respiratory muscle histopathology. American Review of Respiratory Disease 142: 1047

Fernades J, Huijing F 1968 Branching enzyme deficiency glycogenosis: studies in therapy. Archives of Diseases in Childhood 43: 347

Fernades J, Pikaar N A 1969 Hyperlipidemia in children with liver glycogen disease. American Journal of Clinical Nutrition 22: 617

Fernades J, Pikaar N A 1972 Ketosis in hepatic glycogenosis. Archives of Diseases of Childhood 47: 41

Ferrebee J W, Atchley D W, Loeb R F 1938 A study of the electrolyte physiology in a case of familial periodic paralysis. Journal of Clinical Investigation 17: 504

Finch C A, Sawyer C G, Flynn J M 1946 Clinical syndrome of potassium intoxication. American Journal of Medicine 1: 337

Fischer J, Hasselgren P 1991 Cytokines and glucocorticoids in the regulation of the 'hepato-skeletal muscle axis' in sepsis. American Journal of Surgery 161: 266

Fishbein W N 1985 Myoadenylate deaminase deficiency: inherited and acquired forms. Biochemical Medicine 33: 158

Fishbein W N 1986 Myoadenylate deaminase deficiency. In: Engel A G, Banker B Q (eds) Myology. McGraw-Hill, New York, p 1745

Fishbein W N, Armbrustmacher V W, Griffin J L 1978 Myoadenylate deaminase deficiency: a new disease of muscle. Science 200: 545

Fleisher G A, McConahey W M, Pankow M 1965 Serum creatine kinase, lactic dehydrogenase and glutamic-oxaloacetic transaminase in thyroid diseases and pregnancy. Mayo Clinic Proceedings 40: 300

Fletcher F E, Conti P A, Rosenberg H 1991 Comparison of North American and European malignant hyperthermia group halothane contracture testing protocols in swine. Acta Anaesthesiologica Scandinavica 35: 483

Fontaine B, Vale-Santos J, Jurkar-Rott K et al 1994 Mapping of the hypokalemic periodic paralysis locus to chromosome 1g 31–32 in three European families. Nature Genetics 6: 267

Fontaine B, Khurana T S, Hoffman E P et al 1990 Hyperkalemic periodic paralysis and the adult sodium channel alpha-subunit gene. Science 250: 1000

Foster P S, Hopkinson K C, Payne N et al 1991 The effect of azumolene on hypercontractility and sarcoplasmic reticulum Ca(2+)-dependent ATPase activity of malignant hyperpyrexia-susceptible porcine skeletal muscle. Clinical and Experimental Pharmacology and Physiology 18: 489

Frame B, Heinze E, Block M, Manson G 1968 Myopathy in primary hyperparathyroidism. Annals of Internal Medicine 68: 1022

Frank B, Schonle P, Klingehlofer J 1989 Autoimmune thyroiditis and myopathy; reversibility of myopathic alterations under thyroxine therapy. Clinical Neurology Neurosurgery 91: 251

French E G, Kilpatrick R 1957 A variety of paramyotonia congenita. Journal of Neurology, Neurosurgery and Psychiatry 20: 40

Frey B M, Frey F J 1990 Clinical pharmacokinetics of prednisone and prednisolone. Clinical Pharmacokinetics 19: 126

Friedman J H, Feinberg S F, Feldman R G 1985 A neuroleptic malignant syndrome due to levodopa therapy withdrawal. Journal of the American Medical Association 254: 2792

Froesch E, Schmid C, Schwander J, Zapf J 1985 Actions of insulin-like growth factors. Annual Review of Physiology 47: 443

Fujii J, Otsu K, Zorzato F 1991 Identification of a mutation in porcine ryanodine receptor associated with malignant hyperthermia. Science 253: 448

Fukada K, Ogawa S, Yolozuka H et al 1988 Long-standing bidirectional tachycardia in a patient with hypokalemic periodic paralysis. Journal of Electrocardiology 21: 71

Furie B, Penn A S 1974 Pigmenturia from conga drumming. Annals of Internal Medicine 80: 727

Galassi G, Gibertoni M, Corradini L et al 1983 Why may epsilon-aminocaproic acid (EACA) induce myopathy in man? Report of a case and literature review. Italian Journal of Neurological Science 4: 489

Galjaard H, Menkes M, De Josselin de Jong J E, Niermeijer M F 1973 A method for rapid prenatal diagnosis of glycogenosis II (Pompe's disease). Clinica Chimica Acta 49: 361

Gallant E M 1983 Barium-treated mammalian skeletal muscle: similarities to hypokalemic periodic paralysis. Journal of Physiology (London) 335: 577

Gambetti P L, Di Mauro S, Baker L 1971 Nervous system in Pompe's disease. Journal of Neuropathology and Experimental Neurology 30: 412

Gamboa E T, Eastwood A B, Hays A P, Maxwell J, Penn A S

1979 Isolation of influenza virus from muscle in myoglobinuric polymyositis. Neurology (Minneapolis) 29: 1323

Gamstorp I 1956 Adynamia episodica hereditaria. Acta Paediatrica Scandinavica 45: 1

Gamstorp I 1963 Adynamia episodica hereditaria and myotonia. Acta Neurologica Scandinavica 39: 41

Garber A 1983 Effects of parathyroid hormone on skeletal muscle protein and amino acid metabolism in the rat. Journal of Clinical Investigation 71: 1806

Garcin R, Rondot P, Fardeau M 1964 Sur les accidents neuromusculaires et en particulier sur une myopathie vacuolare observés au cours d'un traitement prolongé par la chloroquine. Amélioration rapid apres arrêt du médicament. Revue Neurologique 111: 117

Garcin R, Legrain M, Rondot P, Fardeau M 1966 Étude clinique et métabolique d'une observation de paramyotonie congénitale d'Eulenberg. Documents ultrastructuraux concenant la biopsie musculaire. Revue Neurologique 115: 295

Gardiner P, Edgerton V 1979 Contractile responses of rat fast-twitch and slow-twitch muscles to glucocorticoid treatment. Muscle and Nerve 2: 274

Gardiner P, Botterman B, Eldred E, Simpson S, Edgerton V 1978 Metabolic and contractile changes in fast and slow muscle of the cat after glucocorticoid-induced atrophy. Experimental Neurology 62: 241

Gastel B, Ehrlichman R J 1978 Hypokalemic periodic paralysis. Johns Hopkins Medical Journal 143: 148

George A L, Kallen R G, Barchi R L 1990 Isolation of a human skeletal muscle Na$^+$ channel cDNA clone. Biophysics Journal 57: 108a

George A L, Ledbetter D H, Kallen R G, Barchi R L 1991 Assignment of a human skeletal muscle sodium channel-subunit gene (SCN4A) to 17q-1-25-3. Genomics 9: 555

George A L Jr, Komisarof J, Kallen R G, Barchi R L 1992 Primary structure of the adult human skeletal muscle voltage-dependent sodium channel. Annals of Neurology 31: 131

Giampietro O, Clerico A, Buzzigoli G et al 1984 Detection of hypothyroid myopathy by measurement of various serum muscle markers — myoglobin, creatine kinase, lactate dehydrogenase and their isoenzymes. Correlations with thyroid hormone levels (free and total) and clinical usefulness. Hormone Research 19: 232

Gillard B K, Nelson T E 1977 Amylo-1, 6-glucosidase/4-α-glucano-transferase: use of reversible substrate model inhibitors to the binding and active sites of rabbit muscle debranching enzyme. Biochemistry 16: 3978

Glickstein S L, Gertner E, Smith S A et al 1990 Eosinophilia-myalgia syndrome associated with L-tryptophan use. Journal of Rheumatology 17: 1534

Goldflam S 1895 Weitere Mittheilung über die paroxysmale, familiäre Lähmung. Deutsche Zeitschrift für Nervenheilkundle 7: 1

Golding D N, Murray S M, Pearce G W et al 1961 Corticosteroid myopathy. Annals of Physical Medicine 6: 171

Gomez M R, Engel A G, Dyck P J 1972 Progressive ataxia, retinal degeneration, neuromyopathy, and mental subnormality in a patient with true hypoparathyroidism, dwarfism, malabsorption and cholelithiasis. Neurology (Minneapolis) 22: 849

Goodhue W, Davis J, Porro R 1972 Ischemic myopathy in uremic hyperparathyroidism. Journal of the American Medical Association 221: 911

Gould R J, Steeg C N, Eastwood A B, Penn A S, Rowland L P, DeVivo D 1985 Potentially fatal cardiac dysrrythmia and hyperkalemic periodic paralysis. Neurology 35: 1208

Greene H L, Ghishan F K, Brown B L et al 1988 Type IV glycogenosis: improvement in two patients treated by maintenance of normal blood glucose levels. Journal of Pediatrics 112: 55

Gresh J P, Vasey F B, Espinoza L R et al 1990 Eosinophilia-myalgia syndrome in association with L-tryptophan ingestion. Journal of Rheumatology 17: 1557

Griggs R C, Engel W K, Resnick J S 1970 Acetazolamide treatment of hypokalemic periodic paralysis. Annals of Internal Medicine 73: 39

Griggs R C, Moxley R T, Riggs J E et al 1978 Effects of acetazolamide on myotonia. Annals of Neurology 3: 531

Grollman A P 1968 Inhibitors of protein biosynthesis. V. Effects of emetine on protein and nucleic acid biosynthesis in HeLa cells. Journal of Biological Chemistry 243: 4089

Gronert G A 1980 Malignant hyperthermia. Anesthesiology 53: 395

Grossie H, Albuquerque E 1978 Extensor muscle response to triamcinolone. Experimental Neurology 58: 435

Gruener R G, Stern L Z 1972a Diphenylhydantoin reverses membrane effects in steroid myopathy. Nature New Biology 235: 41

Gruener R G, Stern L 1972b Diphenylhydantoin reverses membrane effects in steroid myopathy. Nature 235: 54

Gruener R, McArdle B, Ryman B E, Weller R O 1968 Contracture of phosphorylase deficient muscle. Journal of Neurology, Neurosurgery and Psychiatry 31: 268

Gruener R G, Stern L Z, Payne C, Hannapel L 1975 Hyperthyroid myopathy. Intracellular electrophysiological measurements in biopsied human intercostal muscle. Journal of the Neurological Sciences 24: 339

Gruner J E 1966 Anomalies due réticulum sarcoplasmique et prolifération de tubules dans le muscle d'une paralysie périodique familiale. Comptes Rendus des Seances de la Société de Biologie et de ses Filiales 160: 193

Gruner J E, Porte A 1959 Les lesions musculaires de la paralysie periodique familiale. Revue Neurologie 100: 501

Guibaud R, Carrier H, Mathieu M et al 1978 Observation familiale de dystrophie musculaire congenitale par deficit en phosphofructokinase. Archives Françaises Pediatrics 35: 1105

Gullotta F, Stefan H, Mattern H 1976 Pseudodystrophoische Muskelglykogenose In Erwachsenenalter (Saure-Maltase-Mangle-Syndrome). Journal of Neurology 213: 199

Guzé B H, Baxter L R 1985 Neuroleptic malignant syndrome. New England Journal of Medicine 313: 163

Haase G R, Engel A G 1960 Paroxysmal recurrent rhabdomyolysis. Archives of Neurology 2: 410

Haass A, Ricker K, Hertel G, Heene R 1979 Influence of temperature on isometric contraction and passive muscular tension in paramyotonia congenita (Eulenburg). Journal of Neurology 221: 151

Haass A, Ricker R, Rüdel R, Lehmann-Horn F, Böhlen R, Dengler R, Mertens H G 1981 Clinical study of paramyotonia congenita with and without myotonia in a warm environment. Muscle and Nerve 4: 388

Habener J F, Potts J T 1978 Parathyroid physiology and primary hyperparathyroidism. In: Avioli L V, Krane S M (eds) Metabolic bone disease, vol 2. Academic, New York, p 1

Hall-Angeras M, Angeras U, Zamir O, Hasselgren P 1990 Interaction between corticosterone and tumor necrosis factor stimulated protein breakdown in rat skeletal muscle, similar to sepsis. Surgery 108: 460

Haller R G, Lewis S F 1991 Glucose-induced exertional fatigue in muscle phosphofructokinase deficiency. New England Journal of Medicine 324: 364

Haller R G, Lewis S F, Cook J D et al 1985 Myophosphorylase deficiency impairs muscle oxidative metabolism. Annals of Neurology 17: 196

Hallin E, Sverker, Feldon S 1988 Graves'ophthalmopathy: correlation of clinical signs with measures derived from computed tomography. British Journal of Ophthalmology 72: 678

Hammett J F, Bale P, Basser L S, Neale F C 1966 McArdle's disease: three cases in an Australian family. Proceedings of the Australian Association of Neurologists 4: 21

Hasilik A, Neufeld E F 1980 Biosynthesis of lysosomal enzymes in fibroblasts: phosphorylation of mannose residues. Journal of Biological Chemistry 255: 4946

Hasselgren P, Adlerberth A, Angeras U 1984 Protein metabolism in skeletal muscle tissue from hyperthyroid patients after preoperative treatment with antithyroid drug or selective beta-blocking agent. Results from a prospective, randomized study. Journal of Clinical Endocrinology and Metabolism 59: 835

Haussler M R, McCain T A 1977 Basic and clinical concepts related to vitamin D metabolism and action. New England Journal of Medicine 297: 974

Havard C, Cambell E, Ross H, Spence A 1963 Electromyographic and histological findings in the muscles of patients with thyrotoxicosis. Quarterly Journal of Medicine 32:

Hays A, Hallett M, Delf J et al 1981 Muscle phosphofructokinase deficiency: abnormal polysaccharide in a case of late-onset myopathy. Neurology 31: 1077

Healy S J, Heffron J J, Lehane M et al 1991 Diagnosis of susceptibility to malignant hyperthermia with flanking DNA markers. British Medical Journal 16: 1225

Heath R, Schwartz M S, Brown I R F, Carter N D 1983 Carbonic anhydrase III in neuromuscular disorders. Journal of Neurological Sciences 59: 383

Hed R 1955 Myoglobinuria in man, with special reference to familial form. Acta Medica Scandinavica 151 (suppl 303): 1

Hed R, Lundmark C, Fahlgren H, Orell S 1962 Acute muscular syndrome in chronic alcoholism. Acta Medica Scandinavica 171: 585

Hegele A R, Angel A 1985 Arrest of neuropathy and myopathy in a-betalipoproteinemia with high-dose vitamin E therapy. Canadian Medical Association Journal 132: 41

Helweg-Larsen H F, Hauge M, Sagild U 1955 Hereditary transient muscular paralysis in Denmark. Acta Geneticae Medicae et Gemellologiace (Rome) 5: 263

Henderson R, Ledingham J, Oliver D et al 1974 Effects of 1,25-dihydroxycholecalciferol on calcium absorption, muscle weakness, and bone disease in chronic renal failure. Lancet i: 279

Herman R G, McDowell M K 1963 Hyperkalemic paralysis (adynamia episodica hereditaria). American Journal of Medicine 35: 749

Hers H G 1963 α-Glucosidase deficiency in generalized glycogen storage disease (Pompe's disease) Biochemical Journal 86: 11

Hers H G, Van Hoff F 1968 Glycogen storage diseases: type II and type VI glycogenosis. In: Dickens F, Randle P J, Whelan W J (eds) Carbohydrate metabolism and its disorders, vol 2. Academic Press, New York, p 151

Hertzman P A, Blevins W L, Mayer J et al 1990 Association of the eosinophilia-myalgia syndrome with the infestion of tryptophan. New England Journal of Medicine 322: 869

Hewitt R H, Gardner-Thorpe C 1978 McArdle's disease — what limit to the age of onset? South African Medical Journal 53: 60

Heyma P, Larkins R 1982 Glucocorticoids decrease the conversion of thyroxine into 3,5,3,triiodothyronine by isolated rat renal tubules. Clinical Science 62: 215

Heytens L, Martin J J, Bossaert L L 1992 In vitro diagnosis of malignant hyperthermia: influence of electrical stimulation on the contracture response to caffeine. British Journal of Anaesthesia 69: 87

Hickson R, Czerwinski S, Falduto M, Young A 1990 Glucocorticoid antagonism by exercise and adrenergic-anabolic steroids. Medical Scientific Exercise 22: 331

Himmelmann F, Schroder J M 1992 Colchicine myopathy in a case of familial Mediterranean fever: immunohistochemical and ultrastructural study of accumulated tubulin-immunoreactive material. Acta Neuropathologica 83: 440

Hiromatsu Y, Fukazawa H, Guinard F et al 1988 A thyroid cytotoxic antibody that cross-reacts with an eye muscle cell surface antigen may be the cause of thyroid-associated ophthalmopathy. Journal of Clinical Endocrinology and Metabolism 67: 565

Ho K 1989 Basophilic bodies of skeletal muscle in hypothyroidism: enzyme histochemical and ultrastructural studies. Human Pathology 20: 1119

Hoefsloot L H, van der Ploeg A T, Kroos M A et al 1990 Adult and infantile glycogenosis type II in one family, explained by allelic diversity. American Journal of Human Genetics 46: 45

Hofmann W W, Adornato B T, Reich H 1983 The relationship of insulin receptors to hypokalemic periodic paralysis. Muscle and Nerve 6: 48

Hogan G R, Gutmann L, Schmidt R, Gilbert E 1969 Pompe's disease. Neurology (Minneapolis) 19: 894

Hollander D, Adelman L S 1991 Eosinophilia-myalgia syndrome associated with ingestion of L-tryptophane: muscle biopsy findings in 4 patients. Neurology 41: 319

Hollerman L W J, Van Der Haar J A, De Vaan G A M 1966 Type IV glycogenosis. Laboratory Investigation 15: 357

Holmes J M, Houghton C R, Woolf A L 1960 A myopathy presenting in adult life with features suggestive of glycogen storage disease. Journal of Neurology, Neurosurgery and Psychiatry 23: 302

Hosten N, Sander B, Cordes M et al 1989 Graves ophthalmopathy: MR imaging of the orbits. Radiology 172: 759

Howell R R 1978 The glycogen storage diseases. In: Stanbury J B, Wyngaarden J B, Frederickson D S (eds) The metabolic basis of inherited disease, 4th edn. McGraw-Hill, New York, p 137

Howell R R, Kaback M M, Brown B I 1971 Type IV glycogen storage disease: Branching enzyme deficiency in skin fibroblasts and possible heterozygote detection. Journal of Pediatrics 78: 638

Hower J, Struck H 1972 CPK activity in hypoparathyroidism (Letter to the editor). New England Journal of Medicine 287: 1096

Howes E L, Price H M, Blumberg J M 1966 Hypokalemic periodic paralysis. Neurology (Minneapolis) 16: 242

Hudgson P, Gardner-Medwin D, Worsfold M, Pennington R J T, Walton J N 1968 Adult myopathy from glycogen storage disease due to acid maltase deficiency. Brain 91: 435

Hudson A J 1963 Progressive neurological disorder and myotonia congenita associated with paramyotonia. Brain 86: 811

Hudson A J, Strickland K P, Wilensky A J 1967 Serum enzyme studies in familial hyperkalemic periodic paralysis. Clinical Chimica Acta 17: 331

Hug G, Schubert W K 1966 Glycogenosis associated with degenerative disease of the brain: Biochemical and electron microscopy findings (abstr). Clinical Research 14: 441

Hughes J T, Esiri M, Oxbury J M, Whitty C W M 1971 Chloroquine myopathy. Quarterly Journal of Medicine 40: 85

Huijing F 1964 Amylo-1, 6-glucosidase activity in normal leukocytes and in leukocytes of patients with glycogen storage disease. Clinica Chimica Acta 9: 269

Huijing F 1975 Glycogen metabolism and glycogen storage diseases. Physiological Reviews 55: 609

Huijing F, Lee E Y C, Carter J H, Whelan W J 1970 Branching action of amylo-1, 6-glucosidase/oligo 1, 4→1, 4-glucantransferase. FEBS Letters 7: 251

Hurley J K 1989 Severe rhabdomyolysis in well conditioned athletes. Military Medicine 154: 244

Iaizzo P A, Wedel D J, Gallagher W J 1991 In vitro contracture testing for determination of susceptibility to malignant hyperthermia: a methodologic update: Mayo Clinic Proceedings 66: 998

Iancu T C, Lerner A, Shiloh H et al 1988 Juvenile acid maltase deficiency presenting as paravertebral pseudotumor. European Journal of Pediatrics 147: 372

Illingworth B, Cori G T 1952 Structure of glycogen and amylopectins: III. Normal and abnormal human glycogen. Journal of Biological Chemistry 199: 653

Illingworth B, Cori G T, Cori C F 1956 Amylo-l, 6-glucosidase in muscle tissue in generalized glycogen storage disease. Journal of Biological Chemistry 213: 123

Irani P 1976 Electromyography in nutritional osteomalacic myopathy. Journal of Neurology, Neurosurgery and Psychiatry 39: 585

Isaacs H, Savage N, Badenhorst M et al 1986 Acid maltase deficiency: a case study and review of the pathophysiological changes and proposed therapeutic measures. Journal of Neurology, Neurosurgery and Psychiatry 49: 1011

Isaacs H, Badenhorst M E, Du Sautoy C 1989 Myophosphorylase B deficiency and malignant hyperthermia. Muscle and Nerve 12: 203

Ivey M, Eichenhorn M S, Glasberg M R et al 1991 Hypercapnic respiratory failure due to L-tryptophan-induced eosinophilic polymyositis. Chest 99: 756

Iwamasa T, Fukuda S, Tokumitsu S et al 1983 Myopathy due to glycogen storage disease. Experimental Molecular Pathology 38: 405

Jamal G, Kerr D, McLellan A, Weir A, Davies D 1987 Generalised peripheral nerve dysfunction in acromegaly: a study by conventional and novel neurophysiological techniques. Journal of Neurology, Neurosurgery and Psychiatry 50: 886

Janssen J, Delange-Berkout I, Van Hardeveld C, Kassenaar A 1981 The disappearance of L-thyroxine and triiodothyronine from plasma and red and white skeletal muscle after administration of one subcutaneous dose of L-thyroxine to hyperthyroid and euthyroid rats. Acta Endocrinologica 97: 226

Jarcho L W, Tyler F H 1958 Myxedema, pseudomyotonia and myotonia congenita. Archives of Internal Medicine 102: 357

Jaspers S, Tischler M 1986 Role of glucocorticoids in the response of rat leg muscles to reduced activity. Muscle and Nerve 9: 554

Jensen K E, Jakobsen J, Thomsen C et al 1990 Improved energy kinetics following high protein diet in McArdle's syndrome. A ^{31}P magnetic resonance spectroscopy study. Acta Neurologica Scandinavica 81: 499

Johnson C H, Van Tassell V J 1991 Acute barium poisoning with respiratory failure and rhabdomyolysis. Annals of Emergency Medicine 126: 1138

Johnsson J, Gelpi J R, Light J A et al 1992 Colchicine-induced myoneuropathy in a renal transplant patient. Transplantation 53: 1369

Justice P, Ryan C, Hsia D Y, Kromptik E 1970 Amylo-1, 6-glucosidase in human fibroblasts: studies in type III glycogen-storage disease. Biochemical and Biophysical Research Communications 39: 301

Kabadi U, Eisenstein A 1980 Glucose intolerance in hyperthyroidism: role of glucagon. Journal of Clinical Endocrinology 50: 392

Kaciuba-Uscilko H, Dudley G, Terjung R 1980 Influence of thyroid status on skeletal muscle LPL activity. American Journal of Physiology 238: E518

Kagen L J, Christian C L 1966 Immunologic measurements of myoglobin in human and fetal skeletal muscle. American Journal of Physiology 211: 656

Kallen R G, Sheng Z H, Yang J et al 1990 Primary structure and expression of a sodium channel characteristic of denervated and immature rat skeletal muscle. Neuron 4: 233

Kamb M L, Murphy J J, Jones J L et al 1992 Eosinophilia-myalgia syndrome in L-tryptophan-exposed patients. Journal of American Medical Association 267: 77

Kaminski H, Ruff R 1989 Neurologic complications of endocrine diseases. Neurology Clinic 7: 489

Kaminski H F, Ruff R L 1994 Endocrine myopathies. In: Engel A G, Banker B Q (eds) Myology. McGraw-Hill, New York (in press)

Kaminski H, Maas E, Spiegel P, Ruff R 1990 Why are eye muscles frequently involved by myasthenia gravis? Neurology 40: 1663

Kanno T, Sudo K, Takeuchi I et al 1980 Hereditary deficiency of lactate dehydrogenase M subunit. Clinica Chimica Acta 108: 267

Karpati G, Carpenter S, Wolfe L S, Sherwin A 1969 A peculiar polysaccharide accumulation in muscle in a case of cardioskeletal myopathy. Neurology (Minneapolis) 19: 553

Karpati G, Carpenter S, Eisen A, Abue M, Di Mauro S 1977 The adult form of acid maltase (α-1, 4-glucosidase) deficiency. Annals of Neurology 1: 276

Kaufman L D, Siedman R J 1991 L-Tryptophan-associated eosinophilia-myalgia syndrome: perspective of a new illness. Rheumatic Diseases Clinics of North America 17: 427

Kaufman L D, Siedman R J, Phillips M E et al 1990 Cutaneous manifestations of the L-tryptophan-associated eosinophilia-myalgia syndrome: a spectrum of sclerodermatous skin disease. Journal of the American Academy of Dermatology 23: 1063

Kausch K, Lehmann-Horn F, Janka M, Wieringa B, Grimm T, Müller 1991 Evidence for linkage of the central core disease locus to the proximal long arm of human chromosome 19. Genomics 10: 765

Keating M, Atkinson D, Dunn C, Timothy K, Vincent G, Leppert M 1991 Linkage of a cardiac arrhythmia, the long QT syndrome, and the Harvey ras 1 gene. Science 252: 704

Keith N M, Osterberg A E, Burchell H B 1942 Some effects of potassium salts in man. Annals of Internal Medicine 16: 879

Kessler E, Weinberger I, Rosenfeld J B 1972 Myoglobinuric acute renal failure in a case of dermatomyositis. Israel Journal of Medical Science 8: 978

Khaleeli A, Edwards R 1984 Effect of treatment on skeletal dysfunction in hypothyroidism. Clinical Science 66: 63

Khaleeli A, Betteridge D, Edwards R et al 1983 Effect of treatment of Cushing's syndrome on skeletal muscle structure and function. Clinical Endocrinology 19: 547

Khaleeli A, Levy R, Edwards R et al 1984 The neuromuscular features of acromegaly: a clinical and pathological study. Journal of Neurology, Neurosurgery and Psychiatry 47: 1009

Kilbourne E M, Posada de la Paz M, Abaitua Borda I et al 1991 Toxic oil syndrome: a current clinical and epidemiologic summary, including comparisons with the eosinophilia-myalgia syndrome. Journal of the American College of Cardiology 18: 711

Kissel J T, Beam W, Bresolin N, Gibbons G, Di Mauro S, Mendell J R 1985 The physiologic assessment of a newly described metabolic myopathy, phosphoglycerate mutase deficiency, through incremental exercise testing. Neurology 35: 828

Kjeldsen K, Norgaard A, Gotzsche C O, Thomassen A 1984 Effect of thyroid on number of Na–K pumps in human skeletal muscle. Lancet 8393: 8

Klatskin G, Friedman H 1948 Emetine toxicity in man: studies on the nature of early toxic manifestations, their relationship to the dose level, and their significance in determining safe dosage. Annals of Internal Medicine 28: 892

Klein R, Egan T, Usher P 1960 Changes in sodium, potassium and water in hyperkalemic familial periodic paralysis. Metabolism 9: 1005

Klein R, Ganelin R, Zelkowitz P, Hays P, Richards C 1962 Effects of quinidine, ouabain, and corticosteroids on muscle sodium, potassium, and water content. Proceedings of the Society of Experimental Biology and Medicine 110: 280

Klein R, Ganelin R, Marks J F, Usher P, Richards C 1963 Periodic paralysis with cardiac arrhythmia. Journal of Pediatrics 62: 371

Knochel J 1977a The pathophysiology and clinical characteristics of severe hypophosphatemia. Archives of Internal Medicine 137: 203

Knochel J P 1977b Role of glucoregulatory hormones in potassium homeostasis. Kidney International 11: 443

Knochel J P 1982 Neuromuscular manifestations of electrolyte disorders. American Journal of Medicine 72: 521

Knochel J P 1984 Hypokalemia. Advances in Internal Medicine 30: 317

Knochel J P 1987 Etiologies and management of potassium deficiency. Hospital Practice 1: 153

Knochel J P, Schlein E M 1972 On the mechanism of rhabdomyolysis in potassium depletion. Journal of Clinical Investigation 51: 1750

Knochel J P et al 1985 Muscle cell electrical hyperpolarization and reduced exercise hyperkalemia in physically conditioned dogs. Journal of Clinical Investigation 75: 740

Koch M C, Ricker K, Otto M 1991 Linkage data suggesting allelic heterogeneity for paramyotonia congenita and hyperkalemic periodic paralysis on chromosome 17. Human Genetics 88: 71

Kono N, Mineo I, Shimizu T et al 1986 Increased plasma uric acid after exercise in muscle phosphofructokinase deficiency. Neurology 36: 106

Koskelo P, Kekki M, Wager O 1967 Kinetic behaviour of ^{131}I-labelled myoglobin in human beings. Clinica Chimica Acta 17: 339

Koski C, Rifenberick D, Max S 1974 Oxidative metabolism of skeletal muscle in steroid atrophy. Archives of Neurology 31: 407

Koster J F, Slee R G, Hulsmann W C, Neimeijer M F 1972 The electrophoretic pattern and activities of acid and neutral maltase of cultivated fibroblast and amniotic fluid cells from controls and patients with the variant of glycogen storage disease type II (Pompe's disease). Clinica Chimica Acta 40: 294

Koster J F, Slee R G, Hulsmann W C 1974 The use of the leukocytes as an aid in the diagnosis of glycogen storage disease type II (Pompe's disease). Clinica Chimica Acta 51: 319

Koster J F, Slee R G, Van Der Klei-Van Moorsel J M, Rietra P J G M, Lucas C J 1976 Physicochemical and immunologic properties of acid α-glucosidase from various human tissues in relation to glycogenosis type II (Pompe's disease). Clinica Chimica Acta 68: 49

Koster J F, Busch H F M, Slee R G et al 1978 Glycogenosis type II: the infantile and late-onset acid maltase deficiency observed in one family. Clinica Chimica Acta 87: 451

Koster J F, Slee R G, Jennekens F G I, Wintzen A R, Van Berkel T J C 1979 McArdle's disease: a study of the molecular basis of two different etiologies of myophosphorylase deficiency. Clinica Chimica Acta 94: 229

Kretzschmar H A, Wagner H, Hubner G et al 1990 Aneurysm and vacuolar degeneration of cerebral arteries in late-onset acid maltase deficiency. Journal of Neurological Science 98: 169

Kuncl R W, Wiggins W W 1988 Toxic myopathies. Neurologic Clinics 6: 593

Kuncl R W, Duncan G, Watson D et al 1987 Colchicine myopathy and neuropathy. New England Journal of Medicine 316: 1562

Kuncl R W, Cornblath D R, Avila O, Duncan G 1989 Electrodiagnosis of human colchicine myoneuropathy. Muscle Nerve 12: 360

Kupfer Y, Namba T, Kaldawi E, Tessler S 1992 Prolonged weakness after long-term infusion of vecuronium bromide. Annals of Internal Medicine 117: 484

Kwiecinski H, Ryniewicz B 1990 A comparative study of disopyramide, diphenylhydantion, mexiletine and tocainide in the treatment of myotonia. Journal of Neurological Sciences 98: 113

Lambert E, Underdahl L, Beckett S, Mederos L 1951 A study of the ankle jerk in myxedema. Journal of Clinical Endocrinology and Metabolism 11: 1186

Larach M G for the North American Malignant Hyperthermia Group 1989 Standardization of the caffeine halothane muscle contracture test. Anesthesia and Analgesia 69: 511

Larach M G, Landis J R, Bunn J S et al 1992 Prediction of malignant hyperthermia susceptibility in low-risk subjects. An epidemiologic investigation of caffeine halothane contracture responses. The North American Malignant Hyperthermia Registry. Anesthesiology 76: 16

Laszewski B, Ruff R 1985 The effects of glucocorticoid treatment on excitation-contraction coupling. American Journal of Physiology 248: E363

Lauer R M, Mascarinas T, Racela A S et al 1968 Administration of a mixture of fungal glucosidases to a patient with type II glycogenosis (Pompe's disease). Pediatrics 42: 672

Layzer R G, Lovelace R E, Rowland L P 1967a Hyperkalemic periodic paralysis. Archives of Neurology 16: 455

Layzer R G, Rowland L P, Ranney H M 1967b Muscle phosphofructokinase deficiency. Archives of Neurology 17: 512

Legum C P, Nitowsky H M 1969 Studies on leukocyte brancher enzyme activity in a family with type IV glycogenosis. Journal of Pediatrics 74: 84

Lehmann-Horn F, Iaizzo P A 1990 Are myotonias and periodic paralyses associated with susceptibility to malignant hyperthermia? British Journal of Anaesthesia 65: 692

Lehmann-Horn F, Rüdel R, Ricker K, Lorkoniv H, Dengler R, Hopf H C 1983 Two cases of adynamia episodica hereditaria: in vitro investigation of muscle cell membrane and contraction parameters. Muscle and Nerve 6: 113

Lehmann-Horn F, Höpfel D, Rüdel R, Ricker R, Küther G 1985 In vivo P-NMR spectroscopy: muscle energy exchange in paramyotonic patients. Muscle and Nerve 8: 606

Lehmann-Horn F, Rüdel R, Ricker K 1987 Membrane defects in paramyotonia congenita. Muscle and Nerve 10: 633

Levin B, Burgess E A, Mortimer P E 1968 Glycogen-storage disease type IV, amylopectinosis. Archives of Diseases in Childhood 43: 548

Levin S, Moses S W, Chayoth R, Jagoda N, Steinitz K 1967 Glycogen storage disease in Israel. Israel Journal of Medical Sciences 3: 397

Levitt L P, Rose L I, Dawson D M 1972 Hypokalemic periodic paralysis with arrhythmia. New England Journal of Medicine 286: 253

Levitt R C, Norui N, Jedlicka A E et al 1991 Evidence for genetic heterogeneity in malignant hyperthermia susceptibility. Genomics 11: 543

Lewi Z, Bar-Khayim Y 1964 Food poisoning from barium carbonate. Lancet ii: 342

Lewis S F, Haller R G 1991 Fatigue in skeletal muscle disorders. In: Atlan G, Beliveau L, Bouissou P (eds) Muscle fatigue: biochemical and physiological aspects. Masson, Paris, p 119

Lewis S F, Vora S, Haller R G 1991 Abnormal oxidative fructokinase deficiency. Journal of Applied Physiology 70: 391

Lipworth B J, McDevitt D G, Struthers A D 1989 Prior treatment with diuretic augments the hypokalemic effects of fenoterol, salbutamol, and terbutaline in asthma. Lancet 336: 1396

Lithell H, Vessby B, Selinus I, Daahlberg P 1985 High muscle lipoprotein lipase activity in thyrotoxic patients. Acta Endocrinology (Copenhagen) 109: 227

Liu W H, Liu C D, Zhang J Y 1991 Association of HLA antigens with thyrotoxic periodic paralysis. Chung-Hua Nei Ko Tsa Chih 30: 395

Ljunghall S, Akerstrom G, Johansson G, Olsson Y, Stalberg E 1984 Neuromuscular involvement in primary hyperparathyroidism. Journal of Neurology 231: 263

Loonen M C B, Busch H F M, Koster J F et al 1981 A family with different clinical forms of acid maltase deficiency (glycogenosis type II): biochemical and genetic studies. Neurology 31: 1209

Lossos A, Barash V, Soffer D et al 1991 Hereditary branching enzyme dysfunction in adult polyglucosan body disease. Annals of Neurology 30: 665

McArdle B 1951 Myopathy due to a defect in muscle glycogen breakdown. Clinical Science 10: 13

McArdle B 1956 Familial periodic paralysis. British Medical Bulletin 12: 226

McArdle B 1962 Adynamia episodica hereditaria and its treatment. Brain 85: 121

McArdle B 1963 Metabolic myopathies. American Journal of Medicine 35: 661

McArdle J, Garnes R, Sellin L 1977 Membrane electrical properties of fast- and slow-twitch muscles from rats with experimental hyperthyroidism. Experimental Neurology 56: 168

McCarthy T V, Healy J M, Heffron J J et al 1990 Localization of the malignant hyperthermia susceptibility locus to human chromosome 19q12–13.2. Nature 343: 562

McClatchey A I, Trofatter J, McKenna-Yasek D et al 1992a Dinucleotide repeat polymorphisms at the SCH4A locus suggest allelic heterogeneity of hyperkalemic periodic paralysis and paramyotonia congenita. American Journal of Human Genetics 50: 896

McClatchey A I, Van den Bergh P, Pericak-Vance M A et al 1992b Temperature-sensitive mutations in the III–IV cytoplasmic loop region of the skeletal muscle sodium channel gene in paramyotonia congenita. Cell 68: 769

McClatchey A I, McKenna-Yasek D, Cros D et al 1992c Novel mutations in families with unusual and variable disorders of the skeletal muscle sodium channel. Nature Genetics 2: 148

McConchie S M, Coakley J, Edwards R H T et al 1991 Molecular heterogeneity in McArdle's disease. Biochimica et Biophysica Acta 1096: 26

McDaniel H, Pitman C, Oh S, DiMauro S 1977 Carbohydrate metabolism in hypothyroid myopathy. Metabolism 26: 867

MacDonald R D, Engel A G 1970 Experimental chloroquine myopathy. Journal of Neuropathology and Experimental Neurology 29: 479

MacDonald R D, Rewcastle N B, Humphrey J G 1968 The myopathy of hyperkalemic periodic paralysis. Archives of Neurology 19: 274

McElvaney G, Wilcox P, Fairbarn M, Hilliam C, Wilkins G 1990 Respiratory muscle weakness and dyspnea in thyrotoxic patients. American Review of Respiratory Disease 141: 1221

MacKenzie A E, Allen G, Lahey D et al 1991 A comparison of the caffeine halothane muscle contracture test with the molecular genetic diagnosis of malignant hyperthermia. Anesthesiology 75: 4

MacLennan D H, Phillips M S 1992 Malignant hyperthermia. Science 256: 789

MacLennan D H, Duff C, Zorzato F et al 1990 Ryanodine receptor gene is a candidate for predisposition to malignant hyperthermia. Nature 343: 559

Maekawa M, Kanda S, Sudo K et al 1984 Estimation of the gene frequency of lactate dehydrogenase subunit deficiencies. American Journal of Human Genetics 36: 1204

Magarian G J, Lucas L M, Colley C 1991 Gemfibrozil-induced myopathy. Archives of Internal Medicine 151: 1873

Magee K R 1963 A study of paramyotonia congenita. Archives of Neurology 8: 461

Mahdavi V, Izumo S, Nadal-Ginard B 1987 Developmental and hormonal regulation of sarcomeric myosin heavy chain gene family. Circulatory Research 60: 804

Mahler R F, Stanbury S W 1956 Potassium-losing renal disease. Quarterly Journal of Medicine 25: 21

Makos M M, McComb R D, Adickes E D et al 1985 Acid maltase deficiency and basilar artery aneurysms: a report of a sibship. Neurology 35 (suppl 1): 193

Mallette L, Pattern B, Engel W 1975 Neuromuscular disease in secondary hyperparathyroidism. Annals of Internal Medicine 82: 474

Mancall E L, Aponte G E, Berry R G 1965 Pompe's disease (diffuse glycogenosis) with neuronal storage. Journal of Neuropathology and Experimental Neurology 24: 85

Manitius A, Levitin H, Beck D, Epstein F H 1960 On the mechanism of impairment of renal concentrating ability in potassium deficiency. Journal of Clinical Investigation 39: 684

Manoukian A A, Bhagavan N V, Hayashi T et al 1990 Rhabdomyolysis secondary to lovastatin therapy. Clinical Chemistry 36: 2145

Margolis M L, Hill A R 1986 Acid maltase deficiency in an adult. American Review of Respiratory Disease 134: 328

Markowitz H, Wobig G H 1977 Quantitative method for estimating myoglobin in urine. Clinical Chemistry 23: 1689

Marks L J, Feit E 1953 Flaccid quadriplegia, hyperkalemia and Addison's disease. Archives of Internal Medicine 91: 56

Marshall J 1952 Observations on a case of myotonia paradoxa. Journal of Neurology, Neurosurgery and Psychiatry 15: 206

Martin J J, De Barsy T, Van Hoof F, Palladini G 1973 Pompe's disease: an inborn lysosomal disorder with storage of glycogen. A study of brain and striated muscle. Acta Neuropathologica (Berlin) 23: 229

Martin J J, De Barsy T, Den Tandt W R 1976a Acid maltase deficiency in non-identical adult twins. A morphological and biochemical study. Journal of Neurology 213: 105

Martin J J, De Barsy T, De Schrijver R, LeRoy J G, Palladini G 1976b Acid maltase deficiency (type II glycogenosis). Morphological and biochemical studies of a childhood type. Journal of the Neurological Sciences 30: 155

Martin R J, Sufit R L, Ringel S T et al 1983 Respiratory improvement by muscle training in adult-onset acid maltase deficiency. Muscle and Nerve 6: 201

Martin R W, Duffy J, Engel A G et al 1990 The clinical spectrum of the eosinophilia-myalgia syndrome associated with L-tryptophan infestion. Clinical features in 20 patients and aspects of pathophysiology. Annals of Internal Medicine 113: 124

Martinez A J, Hooshmand H, Faris A A 1973 Acute alcoholic myopathy. Enzyme histochemistry and electron microscopic findings. Journal of the Neurological Sciences 20: 245

Martinez F, Bermudez-Gomez M, Celli B 1989 Hypothyroidism. A reversible cause of diaphragmatic dysfunction. Chest 96: 1059

Mason J W 1987 Amiodarone. New England Journal of Medicine 316: 455

Massa R, Carpenter S, Holland P et al 1992 Loss and renewal of thick myofilaments in glucocorticoid-treated rat soleus after denervation and reinnervation. Muscle and Nerve 15: 1290

Mastaglia F 1973 Pathological changes in skeletal muscle in acromegaly. Acta Neuropathologica (Berlin) 24: 273

Mastaglia F L, Barwick D D, Hall R 1970 Myopathy in acromegaly. Lancet ii: 907

Mateer J E, Farrell B J, Chou S S, Gutmann L 1985 Reversible ipecac myopathy. Archives of Neurology 42: 188

Matsuoka Y, Senda Y, Hirayama M et al 1988 Late-onset acid maltase deficiency associated with intracranial aneurysm. Journal of Neurology 235: 371

Mayer M, Rosen F 1977 Interaction of glucocorticoid and androgens with skeletal muscle. Metabolism 26: 937

Medbo J I, Sejersted O M 1990 Plasma potassium change with high intensity exercise. Journal of Physiology (London) 421: 105

Mehler M, Di Mauro S 1976 Late-onset acid maltase deficiency. Detection of patients and heterozygotes by urinary enzyme assay. Archives of Neurology 33: 692

Mehler M, Di Mauro S 1977 Residual acid maltase activity in late-onset acid maltase deficiency. Neurology (Minneapolis) 27: 178

Meier-Hellmann A, Romer M, Hannemann L et al 1990 Early recognition of malignant hyperthermia using capnometry. Anaesthesist 39: 41

Melnick B, Chang J L, Larson C E, Bedger R C 1983 Hypokalemic familial periodic paralysis. Clinical Reports 58: 263

Melton A T, Martucci R W, Kien N D et al 1989 Malignant hyperthermia in humans — standardization of contracture testing protocol. Anesthesia and Analgesia 69: 437

Mercier C, Whelan W J 1973 Further characterization of glycogen from type IV glycogen-storage disease. European Journal of Biochemistry 40: 22

Mertens H G, Schimrigk K, Volkwein U, Voigt K D 1964 Elekrolyt- und Aldosteronestoffwechsel bei der Adynamia episodica hereditaria, der hyperkaliämschen Form der periodischen Lähmung. Klinische Wochenschrift 42: 65

Meyers K R, Gilden D H, Rinaldi C F, Hansen J L 1972 Periodic muscle weakness, normokalemia and tubular aggregates. Neurology (Minneapolis) 22: 269

Mhiri C, Baudrimont M, Bonne B et al 1991 Zidovudine myopathy: a distinctive disorder associated with mitochondrial dysfunction. Annals of Neurology 29: 606

Mickelson J R, Gallant E M, Rempel W E et al 1989 Effects of the halothane-sensitivity gene on sarcoplasmic reticulum function. American Journal of Physiology 257: C787

Mier A, Brophy C, Wass J, Besser G, Green M 1989 Reversible respiratory muscle weakness in hyperthyroidism. American Review of Respiratory Disease 139: 529

Miller E D, Sanders D B, Rowlinson J C, Berry F A, Sussman M D, Epstein R M 1978 Anesthesia-induced rhabdomyolysis in a patient with Duchenne's muscular dystrophy. Anesthesiology 48: 146

Millikan C H, Haines S F 1953 The thyroid gland in relation to neuromuscular disease. Archives of Internal Medicine 92: 5

Milne M D, Muchrcke R C, Heard B E 1957 Potassium deficiency and the kidney. British Medical Bulletin 13: 15

Milstein J M, Herron T M, Haas J E 1989 Fatal infantile phosphorylase deficiency. Journal of Child Neurology 4: 186

Minaker K L, Rowe J W 1982 Potassium homeostasis during hyperinsulinemia: effective insulin level, beta-blockade and age. American Journal of Physiology 242: 373

Minaker K L, Meneilly G S, Flier J S, Rowe J W 1988 Insulin-mediated hypokalemia and paralysis in familial hypokalemic periodic paralysis. American Journal of Medicine 84: 1001

Mineo I, Kono N, Hara N et al 1987 Myogenic hyperuricemia. New England Journal of Medicine 317: 75

Mineo I, Kono N, Yamada Y et al 1990 Glucose infusion abolishes the excessive ATP and degradation in working muscles of a patient with McArdle's disease. Muscle and Nerve 13: 681

Miranda A F, Nette G, Hartlage P et al 1979 Phosphorylase isoenzymes in normal and myophosphorylase deficient human heart. Neurology 29: 1538

Miranda A F, DiMauro S, Antler A et al 1981 Glycogen debrancher deficiency is reproduced in muscle culture. Annals of Neurology 9: 283

Miranda A F, Shanske S, Hays A P, Di Mauro S 1985 Immunocytochemical analysis of normal and acid maltase-deficiency muscle cultures. Archives of Neurology 42: 371

Mitsumoto H 1979 McArdle disease: phosphorylase activity in regenerating muscle fibers. Neurology 29: 258

Mizusawa H, Takagi A, Nonaka T et al 1984 Muscular abnormalities in experimental hypothyroidism of rats with special reference to mounding phenomenon. Experimental Neurology 85: 480

Mizuta K, Kashimoto E, Tsutou A et al 1984 A new type of glycogen storage disease caused by deficiency of cardiac phosphorylase kinase. Biochemical and Biophysical Research Communications 119: 582

Mommaerts W F H M, Illingworth B, Pearson C M, Guillory R J, Seraydarian K 1959 A functional disorder of muscle associated with the absence of phosphorylase. Proceedings of the National Academy of Sciences USA 45: 791

Morris C D W, Jacobs P, Berman P A et al 1983 Epsilon-aminocaproic acid-induced myopathy: a case report. South African Medical Journal 64: 363

Morrison W, Gibson J, Jung R, Rennie M 1988 Skeletal muscle and whole body protein turnover in thyroid disease. European Journal of Clinical Investigations 18: 62

Moses S W, Gutman A 1972 Inborn error of glycogen metabolism. Advances in Pediatrics 19: 95

Moses S W, Gadoth N, Bashan N et al 1986 Neuromuscular involvement in glycogen storage disease type III. Acta Paediatrica Scandinavica 5: 289

Moses S W, Wanderman K L, Myroz A et al 1989 Cardiac involvement in glycogen storage disease type III. European Journal of Pediatrics 148: 764

Moss A J 1992 Molecular genetics and ventricular arrhythmias. New England Journal of Medicine. 327: 885

Mouritis M, Koorneef L, Van Mourik-Noordenbos A et al 1990 Extraocular muscle surgery for Graves ophthalmopathy: does prior treatment influence surgical outcome. British Journal of Ophthalmology 1990: 481

Moussavi R, Meisami E, Timiras P 1988 Early responses of skeletal muscle in recovery from hypothyroidism. Mechanisms of Ageing and Development 45: 285

Moxley R T 1990 New therapies for the non-dystrophic hereditary myotonias and paramyotonias. Journal of the Neurological Sciences 98: 111

Moxley R T, Corbett A J, Minaker K L et al 1984 Whole body insulin resistance in myotonic dystrophy. Annals of Neurology 15: 57

Moxley R T, Ricker K, Kingston W J, Bohlen R 1989 Potassium uptake in muscle during paramyotonic weakness. Neurology 39: 952

Mukherjee J A, Moitra S, Bhattacharyya A, Sengupta P 1984 Kocher-Debre-semelaigne syndrome. Journal of Indian Medical Association 82: 21

Muller R, Kugelberg E 1959 Myopathy in Cushing's syndrome. Journal of Neurology, Neurosurgery and Psychiatry 22: 314

Murase T, Ikeda H, Muro T, Nakao K, Sugita H 1973 Myopathy associated with type III glycogenosis. Journal of the Neurological Sciences 20: 287

Murphy T, Retline W, Burbank M 1960 Hyperparathyroidism: report of a case in which parathyroid adenoma presented primarily with profound muscular weakness. Mayo Clinical Proceedings 35: 629

Neustein H B 1969 Fine structure of skeletal muscle in type III glycogenosis. Archives of Pathology (Chicago) 88: 130

Neville H E, Ringel S R, Guggenheim M A, Wehling C A, Starcevich J M 1983 Ultrastructural and histochemical abnormalities of skeletal muscle in patients with chronic vitamin E deficiency. Neurology 33: 483

Newberry J E 1990 Malignant hyperthermia in the postanesthesia care unit: a review of current etiology, diagnosis, and treatment. Journal of Post Anesthesia Nursing 5: 25

Nilne C J 1988 Rhabdomyolysis, myoglobinuria and exercise. Sports Medicine 6: 93

Ninomiya N, Matsuda I, Matsuoka T, Iwamasa T, Nonaka I 1984 Demonstration of acid alpha-glucosidase in different types of Pompe disease by use of an immunochemical method. Journal of the Neurological Sciences 66: 129

Nitowski H M, Grunfeld A 1967 Lysosomal α-glucosidase activity in type II glycogenosis: activity in leukocytes and cell cultures in relation to genotype. Journal of Laboratory and Clinical Medicine 69: 742

Nordrehaug J E, von der Lippe G 1983 Hypokalaemia and ventricular fibrillation in acute myocardial infarction. British Heart Journal 50: 525

Norgaard A, Kjeldsen K 1991 Interrelation of hypokalaemia and potassium depletion and its implications: a re-evaluation based on studies of the skeletal muscle sodium-potassium-pump. Clinical Science 81: 449

Norris F, Panner B 1966 Hypothyroid myopathy. Archives of Neurology 14: 574

Odeh M 1991 Role of reperfusion-induced injury in the pathogenesis of crush syndrome. New England Journal of Medicine 324: 1417

Odor D L, Patel A N, Pearce L A 1967 Familial hypokalemic periodic paralysis with permanent myopathy. Journal of Neuropathology and Experimental Neurology 26: 98

Oh, V M, Taylor E A, Yeo S H, Lee K O 1990 Cation transport across lymphocyte plasma membranes in euthyroid and thyrotoxic men with and without hypokalaemic periodic paralysis. Clinical Science 78: 199

Ohtani Y, Matsuda I, Iwamasa T et al 1982 Infantile glycogen storage myopathy in a girl with phosphorylase kinase deficiency. Neurology 32: 833

Okihiro M M, Nordyke R A 1966 Hypokalemic periodic paralysis. Journal of the American Medical Association 198: 949

Olgin J, Argov Z, Rosenberg H et al 1988 Non-invasive evaluation of malignant hyperthermia susceptibility with phosphorus nuclear magnetic resonance spectroscopy. Anesthesiology 68: 507

Olgin J, Rosenberg H, Allen G et al 1991 A blinded comparison of noninvasive, in vivo phosphorus nuclear magnetic resonance spectroscopy and the in vitro halothane/caffeine contracture test in the evaluation of malignant hyperthermia susceptibility. Anesthesia and Analgesia 72: 36

Oliner L, Schulman M, Larner J 1961 Myopathy associated with glycogen deposition from generalized lack of amylo-1, 6-glucosidase. Clinical Research 9: 243

Ording H 1988 Diagnosis of susceptibility to malignant hyperthermia in man. British Journal of Anaesthesia 60: 287

Ording H, Fonsmark L 1988 Use of vecuronium and doxapram in patients susceptible to malignant hyperthermia. British Journal of Anaesthesia 60: 445

Osserman K E, Tsairis P, Weiner L B 1967 Myasthenia gravis and thyroid disease: clinical and immunological correlation. Mount Sinai Journal of Medicine (New York) 34: 469

Otsu K, Phillips M S, Khanna V K et al 1992 Refinement of diagnostic assays for a probable causal mutation for porcine and human malignant hyperthermia. Genomics 13: 835

Oude Elferink R P J, Brouwer-Kelder E M, Surya I 1984 Isolation and characterization of a precursor form of lysosomal alpha-glucosidase from human urine. European Journal of Biochemistry 139: 489

Ozand P, Tikatli M, Amiri S 1967 Biochemical investigation of an unusual case of glycogenosis. Journal of Pediatrics 71: 225

Pacy P J, Halliday D 1989 Muscle protein synthesis in steroid-induced proximal myopathy: a case report. Muscle and Nerve 12: 378

Palmer E P, Guay A T 1985 Reversible myopathy secondary to abuse of ipecac in patients with major eating disorders. New England Journal of Medicine 313: 1457

Patton B, Bilezikian J, Mallette L, Prince A, Engel W, Auerbach G 1974 Neuromuscular disease in primary hyperparathyroidism. Annals of Internal Medicine 80: 182

Pearson C M 1964 The periodic paralyses: differential features and pathological observations in permanent myopathic weakness. Brain 87: 341

Pearson C M, Beck W S, Blahd W H 1957 Idiopathic paroxysmal myoglobinuria. Archives of Internal Medicine (Chicago) 99: 376

Pellissier J F, DeBarsy Th, Faugere M C et al 1979 Type III glycogenosis with multicore structures. Muscle and Nerve 2: 124

Penn A S 1986 Myoglobinuria. In: Engel A G, Banker B Q (eds) Myology. McGraw-Hill, New York, p 1785

Perkoff G T, Silber R, Tyler F H, Cartwright G E, Wintrobe M M 1959 Studies on disorders of muscle XII. Myopathy due to the administration of therapeutic amounts of 17-hydroxycorticosteroids. American Journal of Medicine 26: 891

Perkoff G T, Hardy P, Velez-Garcia E 1966 Reversible acute muscular syndrome in chronic alcoholism. New England Journal of Medicine 274: 1277

Pernow B B, Havel R J, Jennings D B 1967 The second-wind phenomenon in McArdle's syndrome. Acta Medica Scandinavica 472 (suppl): 294

Pezeshkpour G, Illa I, Dalakas M C 1991 Ultrastructural characteristics and DNA immunocytochemistry in human immunodeficiency virus and zidovudine-associated myopathies. Human Pathology 22: 1281

Pickett J, Layzer R, Levin S et al 1975 Neuromuscular complications of acromegaly. Neurology 25: 638

Piechowiak H, Grobner W, Kremer H et al 1981 Pseudohypoparathyroidism and hypocalcemia. Klinische Wochenschrift 59: 1195

Pierce L R, Wysowski D K, Gross T P 1990 Myopathy and rhabdomyolysis associated with lovastatin-gemfibrozil combination therapy. Journal of the American Medical Association 264: 71

Pierides A M, Alvarez-Ude F, Kerr D N S et al 1975 Clofibrate-induced muscle damage in patients with renal failure. Lancet ii: 1279

Pleasure D E, Walsh G O, Engel W K 1970 Atrophy of skeletal muscle in patients with Cushing's syndrome. Archives of Neurology 22: 118

Pleasure D, Wyszynski B, Sumner D et al 1979 Skeletal muscle calcium metabolism and contractile force in vitamin D-deficient chick. Journal of Clinical Investigation 64: 1157

Plotz C M, Knowlton A I, Ragan C 1952 The natural history of Cushing's syndrome. American Journal of Medicine 13: 597

Pollen R H, Williams R H 1960 Hyperkalemic neuromyopathy in Addison's disease. New England Journal of Medicine 262: 273

Pompe J C 1932 Over idiopatsche hypertrophic van het hart. Nederlands Tijdschrift voor Geneeskunde 76: 304

Pope H G Jr, Hudson J I, Nixon R A, Herridge P L 1986 The epidemiology of ipecac abuse. New England Journal of Medicine 314: 245

Poskanzer D C, Kerr D N S 1961 A third type of periodic paralysis with normokalemia and favourable response to sodium chloride. American Journal of Medicine 31: 328

Powell H C, Haas R, Hall C H et al 1985 Peripheral nerve in type III glycogenosis: selective involvement of unmyelinated fiber Schwann cells. Muscle and Nerve 8: 667

Poznansky M J, Bhardwaj D 1981 Antibody-mediated targeting of alpha-1, 4-glucosidase-albumin polymers to rat hepatocytes. Biochemical Journal 196: 89

Preedy V R, Peters J J 1990 Alcohol and skeletal muscle disease. Alcohol and Alcoholism 25: 177

Prineas J W, Mason A S, Henson R A 1965 Myopathy in metabolic bone disease. British Medical Journal 1: 1034

Prineas J W, Hall R, Barwick D D et al 1968 Myopathy associated with pigmentation following adrenalectomy for Cushing's syndrome. Quarterly Journal of Medicine 37: 63

Ptacek L J, George A L, Griggs R C et al 1991 Identification of a mutation in the gene causing hyperkalemic periodic paralysis. Cell 67: 1021

Ptacek L J, Tawil R, Griggs R C, Storvick D, Leppert M 1992a Linkage of atypical myotonia congenita to a sodium channel locus. Neurology 42: 431

Ptacek L J, George A L Jr., Barchi R L et al 1992b Mutations in an S4 segment of the adult skeletal muscle sodium channel cause paramyotonia congenita. Neuron 8: 891

Ptacek L J, Gouw L, Kwiecinski H et al 1993 Sodium channel mutations in paramyotonia congenita and hyperkalemic periodic paralysis. Annals of Neurology 33: 300

Quinlan J G, Iaizzo P A, Lambert E H et al 1989 Ankle dorsiflexor twitch properties in malignant hyperthermia. Muscle and Nerve 12: 119

Quinlan J G, Wedel D J, Iaizzo P A 1990 Multiple-pulse stimulation and dantrolene in malignant hyperthermia. Muscle and Nerve 13: 904

Ramsey I D 1965 Electromyography in thyrotoxicosis. Quarterly Journal of Medicine 34: 255

Ramsey I D 1968 Thyrotoxic muscle disease. Postgraduate Medical Journal 44: 385

Rebuff'e-Scrive M, Krotkiewski M, Elfverson J, Bjorntorp P 1988 Muscle adipose tissue morphology and metabolism in Cushing's syndrome. Journal of Clinical Endocrinology and Metabolism 67: 1122

Reed G B, Dixon J F P, Neustein H B, Donnell G N, Landing B H 1968 Type IV glycogenosis: patient with absence of a branching enzyme α-1, 4-glucan 6-glucosyl transferase. Laboratory Investigation 19: 546

Reid H A 1961 Myoglobinuria in sea-snake-bite poisoning. British Medical Journal 1: 1284

Resnick J S, Engel W K 1967 Myotonic lid lag in hyperkalaemic periodic paralysis. Journal of Neurology, Neurosurgery and Psychiatry 30: 478

Reuser A J J, Kroos M 1982 Adult forms of glycogenosis type II: a defect in an early stage of alpha-glucosidase relatization. FEBS Letters 146: 361

Reuser A J J, Koster J F, Hoogeveen A, Galjaard H 1978 Biochemical, immunochemical and cell genetic studies in glycogenosis type II. American Journal of Human Genetics 30: 132

Reuser A J J, Kroos M, Oude Elferink R P J, Tager J M 1985 Defects in synthesis, phosphorylation, and maturation of acid alpha-glucosidase in glycogenosis type II. Journal of Biological Chemistry 260: 8336

Reuser A J J, Kroos M, Willemsen R et al 1987 Clinical diversity in glycogenosis type II. Journal of Clinical Investigation 79: 1689

Ribera A, Nastuk W 1988 Effects of chronic prednisolone treatment on post-junctional membrane responses to agonist. Muscle and Nerve 11: 265

Rich E C 1894 A unique form of motor paralysis due to cold. Medical News 65: 210

Richardson G O, Sibley J C 1953 Flaccid quadriplegia associated with hyperpotassemia. Canadian Medical Association Journal 69: 504

Richardson J, Herron G, Reitz R, Layzer R 1969 Ischemic ulcerations of the skin and necrosis of muscle in azotemic hyperparathyroidism. Annals of Internal Medicine 71: 129

Ricker K, Böhlen R, Rohkamm R 1983 Different effectiveness of tocainide and hydrochlorothiazide in paramyotonia congenita with hyperkalemic episodic paralysis. Neurology 33: 1615

Ricker K, Rohkamm R, Bohlen R 1986a Adynamia episodica and paralysis periodica paramyotonia. Neurology 36: 682

Ricker K, Rüdel R, Lehmann-Horn F, Küther G 1986b Muscle stiffness and electrical activity in paramyotonia congenita. Muscle and Nerve 9: 299

Ricker K, Camacho L M, Grafe P, Lehmann-Horn F, Rudel R 1989 Adynamia episodic hereditaria: What causes the weakness? Muscle and Nerve 12: 883

Ricker K, Lehmann-Horn F, Moxley R T 1990 Myotonia fluctuans. Archives of Neurology 47: 268

Riggs J 1990 Acute exertional rhabdomyolysis in hypothyroidism: the result of a reversible defect in glycogenolysis? Military Medicine 155: 171

Riggs J E, Griggs R C 1979 Diagnosis and treatment of the periodic paralyses. In: Klawans H L (ed) Clinical neuropharmacology, vol 4. Raven, New York, p 123

Riggs J E, Griggs R C, Moxley R T 1977 Acetazolamide-induced weakness in paramyotonia congenita. Annals of Internal Medicine 86: 169

Riggs J E, Moxley R T, Griggs R C, Horner F A 1981 Hyperkalemic periodic paralysis: an apparent sporadic case. Neurology 31: 1157

Riggs J E, Schochet S S, Gutman L et al 1983 Lysosomal glycogen storage disease without acid maltase deficiency. Neurology 33: 873

Riggs J F, Klingberg W G, Flink E B et al 1992 Cardioskeletal mitochondrial myopathy associated with chronic magnesium deficiency. Neurology 42: 128

Rimon D, Ludatscher R, Cohen L 1984 Clofibrate-induced muscular syndrome. Case report with ultrastructural findings and review of the literature. Journal of Medical Science 20: 1082

Ritz E, Boland R, Kreusser W 1980 Effects of vitamin D and parathormone on muscle: potential role in uremic myopathy. American Journal of Clinical Nutrition 33: 1522

Robertson E G 1954 Thyrotoxic periodic paralysis. Australian and New Zealand Journal of Medicine 3: 182

Robinson A, Clamann H 1988 Effects of glucocorticoids on motor units in cat hindlimb muscles. Muscle and Nerve 11: 703

Rodman J, Baker T 1978 Changes in the kinetics of muscle contraction in vitamin D depleted rats. Kidney International 13: 189

Roelofs R I, Engel W K, Chauvin P 1971 Demonstration of myophosphorylase activity in muscle grown in tissue culture from patients with muscle phosphorylase deficiency (McArdle's disease). Journal of Histochemistry and Cytochemistry 19: 715

Rojas C V, Wang J, Schwartz L S et al 1991 A met-to-val mutation in the skeletal muscle Na^+ channel α-subunit in hyperkalemic periodic paralysis. Nature 354: 387

Rosa R, George C, Fardeau M, Calvin M C, Rapin M, Rosa J 1982 A new case of phosphoglycerate kinase deficiency: PGK Creteil associated with rhabdomyolysis and lacking hemolytic anemia. Blood 60: 84

Rosenow E C, Engel A G 1978 Acid maltase deficiency in adults presenting as respiratory failure. American Journal of Medicine 64: 485

Ross B D, Radda G K, Gadian D G, Rocker G, Esiri M, Falconer-Smith J 1981 Examination of a case of suspected McArdle's syndrome by ^{31}P nuclear magnetic resonance. New England Journal of Medicine 304: 1338

Rossignol A M, Meyer M, Rossignol B et al 1979 La myocardiopathie de la glycogenose type III. Archives de France Pediatrics 36: 303

Rothfus W, Curtin H 1984 Extraocular muscle enlargement: a CT review. Radiology 151: 677

Rothstein J, Delitto A, Sinacore D, Rose S 1983 Muscle function in rheumatic disease patients treated with corticosteroids. Muscle and Nerve 6: 128

Roufs J B 1992 Review of L-tryptophan and eosinophilia-myalgia syndrome. Journal of the American Diabetic Association 92: 844

Rouleau G, Karpati G, Stirling C, Soza M, Prescott S, Holland P 1987 Glucocorticoid excess induces preferential depletion of myosin in denervated skeletal muscle fibers. Muscle and Nerve 10: 428

Rowland L P, Penn A S 1972 Myoglobinuria. Medical Clinics of North America 56: 1233

Rowland L P, Araki S, Carmel P 1965 Contracture in McArdle's disease. Archives of Neurology 13: 541

Rowland L P, Lovelace R E, Schotland D L, Araki S, Carmel P 1966 The clinical diagnosis of McArdle's disease. Identification of another family with deficiency of muscle phosphorylase. Neurology (Minneapolis) 16: 93

Rowland L P, Di Mauro S, Layzer R B 1986 Phosphofructokinase deficiency. In: Engel A G, Banker B Q (eds) Myology. McGraw-Hill, New York, p 1603

Rowley P T, Kliman B 1960 The effect of sodium loading and depletion on muscular strength and aldosterone excretion in familial periodic paralysis. American Journal of Medicine 28: 376

Rubenstein A E, Wainapel S F 1977 Acute hypokalemic

myopathy in alcoholism. A clinical entity. Archives of Neurology 34: 553

Rüdel R, Ricker K 1985 The primary periodic paralyses. Trends in Neurosciences 8: 467

Ruff R, Weissman J 1988 Endocrine myopathies. Neurological Clinics 6: 575

Ruff R, Martyn D, Gordon A 1982a Glucocorticoid-induced atrophy is not due to impaired excitability in rat muscle. American Journal of Physiology 243: E512

Ruff R, Stühmer W, Almers W 1982b Effect of glucocorticoid treatment on the excitability of rat skeletal muscle. Pflugers Archives 395: 132

Ruff R, Simoncini L, Stühmer W 1988 Slow sodium channel inactivation in mammalian muscle: a possible role in regulating excitability. Muscle and Nerve 11: 502

Rush P, Baron M, Kapusta M 1986 Clofibrate myopathy: a case report and a review of the literature. Seminar Arthritis and Rheumatism 15: 226

Russell S 1988 Thyroid hormone induces a nerve-independent precocious expression of fast myosin heavy chain mRNA in rat hindlimb skeletal muscle. Journal of Biology and Chemistry 263: 6370

Saglid U 1959 Hereditary transient paralysis. Ejnar Munkgaard, Copenhagen

Sakai Y, Kobayashi K, Twata N 1978 Effects of an anabolic steroid and vitamin D complex upon myopathy induced by corticosteroids. European Journal of Pharmacology 52: 353

Salafsky I S, Nadler H L 1971 Alpha-1, 4-glucosidase activity in Pompe's disease. Journal of Pediatrics 79: 794

Salafsky I S, Nadler H L 1973 Deficiency of acid alpha-glucosidase in the urine of patients with Pompe's disease. Journal of Pediatrics 82: 294

Salick A I, Pearson C M 1967 Electrical silence of myoedema. Neurology (Minneapolis) 17: 899

Salick A, Colachis S J, Pearson C 1968 Myxedema myopathy: clinical electrodiagnostic and pathologic findings in an advanced case. Archives of Physical and Medical Rehabilitation 49: 230

Samaha F J 1965 Hyperkalemic periodic paralysis. Archives of Neurology 12: 145

Sancho S, Navarro C, Fernandez J M et al 1990 Skin biopsy findings in glycogenosis III: clinical, biochemical, and electrophysiological correlations. Annals of Neurology 27: 480

Sant'Agnese P A 1959 Diseases of glycogen storage with special reference to the cardiac type of generalized glycogenosis. Annals of the New York Academy of Sciences 72: 439

Sato K, Imai F, Hatayama I, Roelofs R I 1977 Characterization of glycogen phosphorylase isoenzymes present in cultured skeletal muscle from patients with McArdle's disease. Biochemical and Biophysical Research Communications 78: 663

Satoyoshi E, Kowa H 1967 A myopathy due to glycolytic abnormality. Archives of Neurology 71: 248

Satoyoshi E, Murakami K, Koine H, Kinoshita M, Nishiyama Y 1963a Periodic paralysis in hyperthyroidism. Neurology 13: 746

Satoyoshi E, Murakami K, Kowa H et al 1963b Myopathy in thyrotoxicosis: with special emphasis on an effect of potassium ingestion on serum and urinary creatine. Neurology 13: 645

Savage D C L, Forbes M, Pearce G W 1971 Idiopathic rhabdomyolysis. Archives of Disease in Childhood 46: 594

Schlesinger J J, Gandara D, Bensch K G 1978 Myoglobinuria associated with herpes-group viral infection. Archives of Internal Medicine 138: 422

Schmidt R, Mahler R 1959 Chronic progressive myopathy with myoglobinuria: demonstration of a glycogenolytic defect in the muscle. Journal of Clinical Investigation 38: 2044

Schnack C, Podolsky A, Watzke H et al 1989 Effects of somatostatin and oral potassium administration on terbutaline-induced hypokalemia. American Review of Respiratory Diseases 139: 176

Schochet S S Jr, McCormick W F, Zellweger H 1970 Type IV glycogenosis (amylopectinosis). Archives of Pathology 90: 354

Schoenle E, Zapf J, Humbel R, Froesch E 1982 Insulin-like growth factor I stimulates growth in hypophysectomized rats. Nature 296: 252

Schotland D L, Spiro D, Rowland L P, Carmel P 1965 Ultrastructural studies of muscle in McArdle's disease. Journal of Neuropathology and Experimental Neurology 24: 629

Schott G, Wills M 1975 Myopathy and hypophosphotaemic osteomalacia presenting in adult life. Journal of Neurology, Neurosurgery and Psychiatry 38: 297

Schutta H S, Armitage J L 1969 Thyrotoxic hypokalemic periodic paralysis. Journal of Neuropathology and Experimental Neurology 28: 321

Schwartz H, Oppenheimer J 1978 Physiologic and biochemical actions of thyroid hormone. Pharmacological Therapy (B)3: 349

Selby R, Starzl T E, Yunis E et al 1991 Liver transplantation for type IV glycogen storage disease. New England Journal of Medicine 324: 39

Serratrice G, Monges A, Roux H, Aquaron R, Gambarelli D 1969 Myopathic form of phosphofructokinase deficit. Revue Neurologique 120: 271

Servidei S, Metlay L A, Booth C A et al 1987a Clinical and biochemical heterogeneity of phosphorylase b kinase deficiency. Neurology 37(suppl 1): 139

Servidei S, Riepe R E, Langston C et al 1987b Severe cardiopathy in branching enzyme deficiency. Journal of Pediatrics 111: 51

Servidei S, Metlay L A, Chodosh J et al 1988a Fatal infantile cardiopathy caused by phosphorylase b kinase deficiency. Journal of Pediatrics 113: 82

Servidei S, Shanske S, Zeviani M et al 1988b McArdle disease: biochemical and molecular genetic studies. Annals of Neurology 24: 774

Shane E, McClane K A, Olarte M R et al 1980 Hypoparathyroidism and elevated muscle enzymes. Neurology 30: 192

Shanske S, DiMauro S 1981 Late-onset acid maltase deficiency: biochemical studies of leukocytes. Journal of Neurological Science 50: 57

Sharma V, Banerjee S 1978 Beta-adrenergic receptors in rat skeletal muscle. Effects of thyroidectomy. Biochimica et Biophysica Acta 539: 538

Shee C D 1990 Risk factors for hydrocortisone myopathy in acute severe asthma. Respiratory Medicine 84: 229

Shoji S 1989 Myofibrillar protein catabolism in rat steroid myopathy measured by 3-methylhistidine excretion in the urine. Journal of the Neurological Sciences 93: 333

Shoji S, Pennington R 1977 Binding of dexamethasone and cortisol to cytosol receptors in rat extensor digitorum longus and soleus muscles. Experimental Neurology 57: 342

Shulkin D, Olson B R, Levey G S 1989 Thyrotoxic periodic paralysis in a Latin-American taking acetazolamide. American Journal of the Medical Sciences 297: 337

Shy G M, Wanko T, Rowley P T, Engel A G 1961 Studies in familial periodic paralysis. Experimental Neurology 3: 53

Sidbury J B 1965 The genetics of the glycogen storage diseases. Progress in Medical Genetics 4: 32

Sidbury J B Jr, Mason J, Burns W B Jr, Ruebner B H 1962 Type IV glycogenosis: report of a case proven by characterization of glycogen and studies at necropsy. Bulletin of the John Hopkins Hospital 57: 157

Simon N M, Rovner R N, Berlin B S 1970 Acute myoglobinuria with type A2 (Hong Kong) influenza. Journal of the American Medical Association 212: 1704

Sinkovich D D, Mitch-Resignalo A E 1991 Malignant hyperthermia. Orthopaedic Nursing 10: 39

Sitwell L D, Weinshenker B G, Monpetit V, Reid D 1991 Complete ophthalmoplegia as a complication of acute corticosteroid- and pancuronium-associated myopathy. Neurology 41: 921

Skaria J, Katiyar B, Srivastave T, Dube D 1975 Myopathy and neuropathy associated with osteomalacia. Acta Neurologica Scandinavica 51: 37

Sloan M F, Franks A J, Exley K A, Davison A M 1978 Acute renal failure due to polymyositis. British Medical Journal 1: 1457

Slonim A E, Goans P J 1985 Myopathy in McArdle's syndrome: improvement with a high-protein diet. New England Journal of Medicine 312: 355

Slonim A E, Weisberg C, Benke P et al 1982 Reversal of debrancher deficiency myopathy by the use of high-protein nutrition. Annals of Neurology 11: 420

Slonim A E, Coleman R A, McElligot M A et al 1983 Improvement of muscle function in acid maltase deficiency by high-protein therapy. Neurology 33: 34

Small R, Meiring N 1981 A combined orbital and antral approach to surgical decompression of the orbit. Ophthalmology 99: 542

Smith H L, Amick L D, Sidbury J B Jr 1966 Type II glycogenosis: Report of a case with four-year survival and absence of acid maltase associated with an abnormal glycogen. American Journal of Diseases of Children 111: 475

Smith J, Zellweger H, Afifi A K 1967 Muscular form of glycogenosis, type II (Pompe): report of a case with unusual features. Neurology (Minneapolis) 17: 537

Smith O, Wong C, Gelfand R 1990 Influence of glucocorticoids on skeletal muscle proteolysis in normal and diabetic-adrenalectomized eviscerated rats. Metabolism 39: 641

Smith R, Stern G 1967 Myopathy, osteomalacia and hyperparathyroidism. Brain 90: 593

Sokal E M, Van Hoof F, Alberti D et al 1992 Progressive cardiac failure following successful orthotopic liver transplantation for type IV glycogenosis. European Journal of Pediatrics 151: 200

Song S K, Rubin E 1972 Ethanol produces muscle damage in human volunteers. Science 175: 327

Sorosky J I, Ingardia C J, Botti J J 1989 Diagnosis and management of susceptibility to malignant hyperthermia in pregnancy. American Journal of Perinatology 6: 46

Spach D H, Bauwens J E, Clark C D, Burke W G 1991 Rhabdomyolysis associated with lovastatin and erythromycin use. Western Journal of Medicine 154: 213

Staffurth J S 1964 The total exchangeable potassium in patients with hypokalemia. Postgraduate Medical Journal 40: 4

Steckel F, Gieselmann V, Waheed A 1982 Biosynthesis of acid alpha-glucosidase in late-onset forms of glycogenosis type II (Pompe's disease). FEBS Letters 150: 69

Steinitz K, Rutenberg A 1967 Tissue α-glucosidase activity and glycogen content in patients with generalized glycogenosis. Israel Journal of Medical Sciences 3: 411

Stocker W, Samaha F, DeGroot L 1968 Coupled oxidative phosphorylation in muscle of thyrotoxic patients. American Journal of Medicine 44: 900

Strausz I, Janikovsky B 1960 Corticosteroid myopathy. Orvosi Hetilap 101: 946

Streeten D H P, Dalakos T G, Fellerman H 1971 Studies on hyperkalemic periodic paralysis: evidence of changes in plasma Na and Cl and induction of paralysis by adrenal glucocorticosteriods. Journal of Clinical Investigation 40: 152

Streib E W 1987a Paramyotonia congenita: successful treatment with tocainide. Clinical and electrophysiologic findings in seven patients. Muscle and Nerve 10: 155

Streib E W 1987b AAEE minimonograph 27: Differential diagnosis of myotonic syndromes. Muscle and Nerve 10: 603

Strongwater S L, Woda B A, Yood R A et al 1990 Eosinophilia-myalgia syndrome associated with L-tryptophan ingestion. Analysis of four patients and implications for differential diagnosis and pathogenesis. Archives of Internal Medicine 150: 2178

Strugalska-Cynowska M 1967 Disturbances in the activity of phosphorylase b-kinase in a case of McArdle myopathy. Folia Histochemica et Cytochemica 5: 151

Stubbs W A 1976 Bidirectional ventricular tachycardia in familial hypokalaemic periodic paralysis. Proceedings of the Royal Society of Medicine 69: 223

Stuhmer W, Conti F, Suzki H et al 1989 Structural parts involved in activation and inactivation of the sodium channel. Nature 339: 597

Sugie H, Russin R, Verity M A 1984 Emetine myopathy: two case reports with pathobiochemical analysis. Muscle and Nerve 7: 54

Sugie H, Sugie Y, Nishida M et al 1989 Recurrent myoglobinuria in a child with mental retardation: phosphoglycerate kinase deficiency. Journal of Child Neurology 4: 95

Sugita H, Higuchi I, Sano M, Ishiura S 1987 Trial of a cysteine proteinase inhibitor, EST, in experimental chloroquine myopathy in rats. Muscle and Nerve 10: 516

Suki W N 1991 Myopathic effects of lovastatin (editorial). Western Journal of Medicine 154: 223

Swaiman K F, Kennedy W R, Sauls H S 1968 Late infantile acid maltase deficiency. Archives of Neurology 18: 642

Swanson J, Kelly J, McConahey W 1981 Neurologic aspects of thyroid dysfunction. Mayo Clinic Proceedings 56: 504

Sweatman M, Chambers L 1985 Disordered oesophageal motility in thyrotoxic myopathy. Postgraduate Medical Journal 61: 619

Tägerud S, Jirmanova I, Libelius R 1986 Biochemical and ultrastructural effects of chloroquine on horseradish peroxidase uptake and lysosomal enzyme activities in innervated and denervated mouse skeletal muscle. Journal of the Neurological Sciences 75: 159

Takagi A, Kojima S, Arki M 1989 Clinical implication of enhanced caffeine contracture in malignant hyperthermia (MH) and Duchenne muscular dystrophy (DMD). Rinsho Shinkeigaku — Clinical Neurology 29: 301

Talbott J H 1941 Periodic paralysis. Medicine (Baltimore) 20: 85

Tan M, Bonen A 1985 The in vitro effect of corticosterone on insulin binding and glucose metabolism in mouse skeletal muscles. Canadian Journal of Physiology and Pharmacology 63: 1133

Tarui S, Okuno G, Ikura Y, Tanaka T, Suda M, Nishikawa M 1965 Phosphofructokinase deficiency in skeletal muscle. A new type of glycogenosis. Biochemical and Biophysical Research Communications 19: 517

Tarui S, Kono N, Nasu T, Nishikawa M 1969 Enzymatic basis for coexistence of myopathy and hemolytic disease in inherited muscle phosphofructokinase deficiency. Biochemical and Biophysical Research Communications 34: 77

Tashian R E, Venta P J, Nicewander P H, Hewett-Emmet D 1990 Evolution, structure, and expression of the carbonic anhydrase multi-gene family. In: Isozymes: structure, function and use in biology & medicine. Wiley-Liss, p 159

Tawil R, Ptacek L J, Pavalakis S G et al 1994 Andersen's syndrome: potassium-sensitive periodic paralysis, ventricular ectopy, and dysmorphic features. Annals of Neurology 35: 326

Tein I, Di Mauro S, DeVivo D C 1990 Recurrent childhood myoglobinuria. Advances in Pediatrics 37: 77

Thompson G R, Ford J, Jenkinson M, Trayner I 1986 Efficacy of mevinolin as adjuvant therapy for refractory familial hypercholesterolaemia. Quarterly Journal of Medicine 232: 803

Thomson W H S, MacLaurin J C, Prineas J W 1963 Skeletal muscle glycogenosis: an investigation of two dissimilar cases. Journal of Neurology, Neurosurgery and Psychiatry 26: 60

Thorn G W 1949 The diagnosis and treatment of adrenalin insufficiency. Thomas, Springfield, Illinois, p 44

Tindall G, Barrow D 1986 Disorders of the pituitary. C V Mosby, St Louis

Tomas F, Murray A, Jones L 1984 Interactive effects of insulin and corticosterone on myofibrillar protein turnover in rats as determined by N tau-methylhistidine excretion. Biochemical Journal 220: 469

Tomasi L G 1979 Reversibility of human myopathy caused by vitamin E deficiency. Neurology (Minneapolis) 29: 1183

Tonin P, Shanske S, Brownell A K et al 1989 Phosphoglycerate kinase (PGK) deficiency: a third case with recurrent myoglobinuria. Neurology 39 (suppl 1): 359

Trend P St J, Wiles C M, Spencer G T et al 1985 Acid maltase deficiency in adults. Brain 108: 845

Trimmer J S, Cooperman S S, Tamiko S A et al 1989 Primary structure and functional expression of a mammalian skeletal muscle sodium channel. Neuron 3: 33

Tyrrell D A, Ryman B E E, Keeton B R et al 1976 Use of liposome in treating type II glycogenosis. British Medical Journal 2: 88

Ugawa Y, Inoue K, Takemura T et al 1986 Accumulation of glycogen in sural nerve axons in adult-onset type III glycogenosis. Annals of Neurology 19: 294

Umpleby A M, Wiles C M, Trend P St J et al 1987 Protein turnover in acid maltase deficiency before and after treatment with a high protein diet. Journal of Neurology, Neurosurgery and Psychiatry 50: 587

Umpleby A M, Trend P St J, Chubb D et al 1989 The effect of a high protein diet on leucine and alanine turnover in acid maltase deficiency. Journal of Neurology, Neurosurgery and Psychiatry 52: 954

Urbanic R, George J 1981 Cushing's disease — 18 years experience. Medicine 60: 14

Van Buchem F S P 1957 The electrocardiogram and potassium metabolism. American Journal of Medicine 23: 376

Van Buchem F S P, Doorenbos H, Elings H S 1956 Conn's syndrome, caused by adrenocortical hyperplasia. Acta Endocrinologica 23: 313

van der Berg I E T, Berger R 1990 Phosphorylase b kinase deficiency in man: a review. Journal of Inherited Metabolic Disease 13: 442

Van der Meulen J P, Gilbert G J, Kane C A 1961 Familial hyperkalemic paralysis with myotonia. New England Journal of Medicine 264: 1

van der Ploeg A T, Bolhuis P A, Wolterman R A et al 1988 Prospect for enzyme therapy in glycogenosis type II variants: a study on cultured muscle cells. Journal of Neurology 235: 392

van der Ploeg A T, Kroos M A, Willemsen R et al 1991 Intravenous administration of phosphorylated acid alpha-glucosidase leads to uptake of enzyme in heart and skeletal muscle of mice. Journal of Clinical Investigation 87: 513

Van Hoof F 1967 Amylo-l, 6-glucosidase activity and glycogen content of the erythrocytes of normal subjects, patients with glycogen-storage disease and heterozygotes. European Journal of Biochemistry 2: 271

Van Hoof F, Hers H G 1967 The subgroups of type III glycogenosis. European Journal of Biochemistry 2: 271

Vanneste J A L, van Wijngaarden G K 1982 Epsilon-aminocaproic acid myopathy. Report of a case and literature review. European Neurology 21: 242

Van't Hoff W 1962 Familial myotonic periodic paralysis. Quarterly Journal of Medicine 31: 385

Varga J, Maul G G, Jimenez S A 1992 Autoantibodies to nuclear lamin C in the eosinophilia-myalgia syndrome associated with L-tryptophan ingestion. Arthritis and Rheumatism 35: 106

Vicale C T 1949 The diagnostic features of a muscular syndrome resulting from hyperparathyroidism, osteomalacia owing to renal tubular acidosis and perhaps to related disorders of calcium metabolism. Transactions of the American Neurological Association 74: 143

Victor M 1986 Toxic and nutritional myopathies. In: Engel A G, Banker B Q (eds) Myology. McGraw-Hill, New York, p 1807

Vita G, Toscano A, Bresolin N et al 1990 Muscle phosphoglycerate mutase (PGAM) deficiency in the first caucasian patient. Neurology 40 (suppl 1): 297

Vora S 1983 Isozymes of human phosphofructokinase. Biochemical and genetic aspects. In: Ratazzi J G, Scandalios J G, Whitt G S (eds) Isozymes: current topics in biological and medical resarch, vol II. Alan Liss, New York, p 3

Vora S, Davidson M, Seaman C et al 1983a Heterogeneity of the molecular lesions in inherited phosphofructokinase deficiency. Journal of Clinical Investigation 72: 1995

Vora S, Miranda A F, Hernandez E et al 1983b Regional assignment of the human gene for platelet-type phosphofructokinase (PFKP) to chromosome 10p: novel use of polyspecific rodent antisera to localize human enzyme genes. Human Genetics 63: 374

Vora S, DiMauro S, Spear D, Harker D, Danon M J 1987 Characterization of the enzyme defect in late-onset muscle phosphofructokinase deficiency. Journal of Clinical Investigations 80: 1479

Vyskocil F, Hnik P, Rehfeldt H, Vejsada R, Ujec E 1983 The measurement of K^+_c concentration changes in human muscle during volitional contractions. Pflügers Archives 399: 235

Wahren J, Felig P, Havel R J, Jorfeldt L, Pernow B, Saltin B 1973 Amino acid metabolism in McArdle's syndrome. New England Journal of Medicine 288: 774

Wall J, Kuroki T 1985 Immunological factors in thyroid disease. Medical Clinics of North America 69: 913

Wall J, Salvi M, Bernard N et al 1991 Thyroid-associated ophthalmopathy — a model for the association of organ-specific autoimmune disorders. Immunology Today 12: 150

Wallace C S, Mueller B A 1992 Lovastatin-induced rhabdomyolysis in the absence of concomitant drugs. Annals of Pharmacotherapy 26: 190

Wang Y 1986 Lung function and respiratory muscle strength after propanolol in thyrotoxicosis. Australia/New Zealand Journal of Medicine 16: 496

Webster D W, Thompson R T, Gravelle D R et al 1990 Metabolic response to exercise in malignant hyperthermia-sensitive patients measured by ^{31}P magnetic resonance spectroscopy. Magnetic Resonance in Medicine 15: 81

Weisler M J 1961 The electrocardiogram in periodic paralysis. Chest 4: 217

Werlin S L, Harb J M, Swick H, Bank E 1983 Neuromuscular dysfunction and ultrastructural pathology in children with chronic cholestasis and vitamin E deficiency. Annals of Neurology 13: 291

Werner S, Coleman D, Frazen L 1974 Ultrasonographic evidence of a consistent orbital involvement in Graves' disease. New England Journal of Medicine 290: 1447

Whisnant J P, Espinosa E R, Kierland R R, Lambert E H 1963 Chloroquine neuromyopathy. Proceedings of the Staff Meetings of the Mayo Clinic 38: 501

Whyte K F, Reid C, Addis G J, Whitesmith R, Reid J L 1988 Salbutamol induced hypokalaemia: the effect of theophylline alone and in combination with adrenaline. British Journal of Clinical Pharmacology 25: 571

Wiles C, Young A, Jones D, Edwards R 1979 Muscular relaxation in rate, fibre-type composition and energy turnover in hyper- and hypothyroid patients. Clinical Science 57: 375

Williams C, Field J B 1968 Studies in glycogen-storage disease: limit dextrinosis, a genetic study. Journal of Pediatrics 72: 214

Williams H E 1966 α-Glucosidase activity in human leukocytes. Biochimica et Biophysica Acta 124: 34

Williams J C, Murray A K 1980 Enzyme replacement in Pompe's disease with an alpha-glucosidase-low-density lipoprotein complex. Birth Defects 16: 415

Williams R S 1959 Triamcinolone myopathy. Lancet i: 698

Wilson J, Walton J 1959 Some muscular manifestations of hypothyroidism. Journal of Neurology, Neurosurgery and Psychiatry 22: 320

Wlody G S 1991 Malignant hyperthermia. Critical Care Nursing Clinics of North America 3: 129

Wong C S, Pavord I D, Williams J, Britton J R, Tattersfield A E 1990 Bronchodilator, cardiovascular, and hypokalaemic effects of fenoterol, salbutamol, and terbutaline in asthma. Lancet 336: 1396

Yamaguchi H, Okamoto K, Shooji M, Morimatsu M, Hirai S 1987 Muscle histology of hypocalcemic myopathy in hypoparathyroidism. Journal of Neurology, Neurosurgery and Psychiatry 50: 8177

Yates R O, Connor H, Woods H F 1981 Muscle breakdown in thyrotoxicosis assessed by urinary 3-methylhistidine excretion. Annals of Nutrition and Metabolism 25: 262

Yeo P P B, Chan S H, Lui K F, Wee G B, Lim P, Cheah J S 1978 HLA and thyrotoxic periodic paralysis. British Medical Journal 2: 930

Yeung R T T, Tse T F 1974 Thyrotoxic periodic paralysis. Effect of propranolol. American Journal of Medicine 57: 584

Yoshimura T, Kaneuji M, Okuno T et al 1983 Periodic paralysis with cardiac arrhythmia. European Journal of Pediatrics 140: 338

Yunis A A, Fischer E H, Krebs E G 1962 Comparative studies on glycogen phosphorylase. Journal of Biological Chemistry 237: 2809

Zellweger H, Mueller S, Ionnasescu V, Schochet S S, McCormick W F 1972 Glycogenosis IV: a new cause of infantile hypotonia. Journal of Pediatrics 80: 842

Zierler K L, Andres R 1957 Movement of potassium into skeletal muscle during spontaneous attacks in family periodic paralysis. Journal of Clinical Investigation 28: 376

18. Mitochondrial and lipid storage disorders of muscle

L. A. Bindoff   Sandra Jackson   D. M. Turnbull

HISTORICAL PERSPECTIVE

Disorders of mitochondrial function, including the pathways of ATP production and fat metabolism, are capable of producing a wide range of diseases in which muscle involvement is often the primary or predominant clinical feature. Historically, the first clear link between mitochondrial dysfunction and disease was made by Luft and colleagues (1962). Subsequent studies concentrated on morphological abnormalities in muscle and led to the appreciation that disease was linked both to abnormalities of structure and distribution of mitochondria (Shy et al 1966). By the application of vital stains (Olsen et al 1972), abnormal collections of mitochondria could be identified using light-microscopy. The hallmark of respiratory chain disease was thus established and, although not pathognomonic or indeed constant, such studies often provide the first substantial clue to the presence of mitochondrial disease. To a certain extent a similar situation exists with the so-called lipid storage myopathies—appreciation that a metabolic disturbance may be the underlying cause coming from morphological studies. Progress in both areas means that, in a significant number of cases, it is now possible to identify not only morphological abnormalities but also to define the precise biochemical and molecular defect responsible.

Since this is primarily a book on muscle and its disorders we will concentrate on how disorders of mitochondrial function manifest in this tissue and will divide this chapter into two major sections dealing with: (a) disorders due to abnormalities of the respiratory chain; and (b) lipid storage myopathies due to defects of mitochondrial fatty acid oxidation. Both types of mitochon-drial disorder are often systemic and may present with disease outside the neuromuscular system. These disorders will also be described with appro-priate reference to the presence or absence of muscle involvement.

BACKGROUND BIOCHEMISTRY

All cells require energy to maintain function and integrity. Cellular energy, in the form of ATP, is generated predominantly by oxidative metabolism occurring within mitochondria. The energy required to drive ATP production is provided by the breakdown of metabolic fuels, principally glucose, free fatty acids, ketone bodies and amino acids. The balance of metabolism, that is which fuels are consumed to generate ATP, depends on the tissue and prevailing state, i.e. the degree of physical activity and whether the individual is fed or fasted. Following a meal, glucose and fatty acids are the major fuels, whereas during fasting, oxidation of fatty acids predominates. Exercise also influences substrate usage. During short-duration, high-intensity, exercise, glucose, either released from glycogen stores or delivered direct from the blood stream, is metabolised via glyco-lysis to generate ATP. Lactate generated by this process is converted back to glucose in the liver once exercise stops (the basis of the oxygen debt). During prolonged, submaximal, exercise fatty acids are the major source of energy. Under aerobic conditions, both glucose and fatty acid oxidation generate acetyl-CoA which can be further metabolised via the tricarboxylic acid cycle (TCA) to yield carbon dioxide and water. This yields a greater amount of energy than glycolysis alone.

Apart from glycolysis, the major pathways of substrate oxidation and ATP production occur within mitochondria. The conversion of pyruvate to acetyl-CoA, the majority of fatty acid oxida-tion, the TCA cycle and the respiratory chain all take place either within the mitochondrial matrix or inner mitochondrial membrane. These processes are closely linked and an abnormality in one pathway will often cause dysfunction in others.

DEFECTS OF THE MITOCHONDRIAL RESPIRATORY CHAIN

Biochemistry

The mitochondrial respiratory chain is composed of a series of multisubunit complexes situated within the inner mitochondrial membrane. It has two major functions: reoxidation of reduced cofactors (NADH and reduced flavoproteins) generated by substrate oxidation; and the synthe-sis of ATP (Fig. 18.1). Linkage of substrate oxida-tion with the phosphorylation of ADP to ATP is termed oxidative phosphorylation (for review see Sherratt & Turnbull 1990). Table 18.1 describes the components of the respiratory chain and pro-vides a brief explanation of their function. Figure 18.2 is a diagrammatic representation of these components and illustrates important features of their role in respiratory chain activity.

The reoxidation of NADH and reduced flavo-proteins is achieved by the transfer of electrons from reduced cofactor to respiratory chain com-plexes. Electrons from NADH are transferred to ubiquinone from complex I whilst electrons from other flavoproteins are passed either directly to ubiquinone (from glycerol-3-phosphate dehydro-genase), to ubiquinone via complex II (through succinate dehydrogenase) or via electron transfer flavoprotein (ETF) and ETF: ubiquinone oxido-reductase (from several dehydrogenases including the fatty acyl-CoA, isovaleryl and sarcosine dehy-drogenases). The respiratory chain complexes act as a series of graded, redox couples. Electrons are passed from complex I and complex II to complex III via the mobile electron-carrier ubiquinone. From complex III, electrons are transferred to complex IV via cytochrome c. Complex IV donates electrons directly to mole-cular oxygen. Sufficient energy is generated at three steps (at complexes I, III and IV) to drive the extrusion of protons (H^+) across the inner mitochondrial membrane and out of the mito-chondria. Because of the insulating properties of the inner mitochondrial membrane, these protons cannot return to the matrix side of the inner membrane. This creates an electrochemical or proton gradient across the inner membrane which is subsequently discharged by complex V (ATP synthase); the energy this releases is

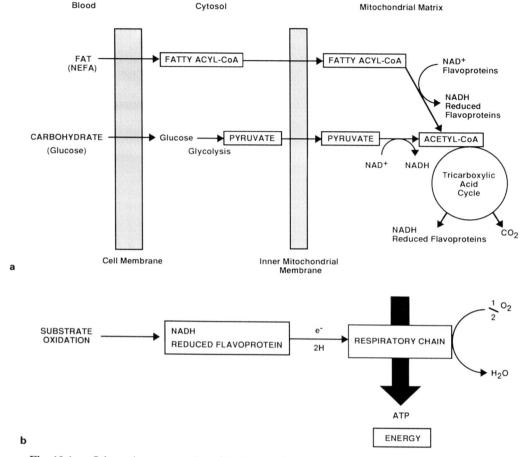

Fig. 18.1 **a** Schematic representation of the important elements involved in substrate oxidation. Metabolic fuels, predominantly carbohydrates and fats, are delivered either from the blood stream or mobilised from cellular stores. Skeletal muscle contains both fat and glycogen stores. Fatty acids (NEFA, non-esterified fatty acids) are activated to their acyl-CoA esters in the outer mitochondrial membrane/intramembranous space and transported into the mitochondrial matrix. Once inside the mitochondrion, fatty acyl-CoA esters are broken down by the process of β-oxidation. This process generates large amounts of reduced cofactors — NADH and reduced flavoproteins. Glucose is metabolised to pyruvate in the cytosol by the process of glycolysis. Pyruvate enters the mitochondria where it is converted to acetyl-CoA. Acetyl-CoA, also the end-product of β-oxidation, is broken down by the citric acid cycle with production of reduced cofactors together with carbon dioxide (CO_2). So that metabolism may proceed, and in order to generate cellular energy in the form of adenosine triphosphate (ATP), the reduced cofactors are reoxidised by the respiratory chain.
b The link between substrate oxidation and energy production — the respiratory chain. This diagram shows that ATP production is linked to substrate oxidation by the respiratory chain. The process is dependent upon the reduction of molecular oxygen and is, therefore, termed oxidative metabolism.

used to drive ATP synthesis (Senior 1988) (Fig. 18.2b).

Genetics

Two genomes control the production of respiratory chain proteins; the majority are encoded by chromosomal DNA whilst a small number are produced from an extrachromosomal genome found within mitochondria. Mitochondrial DNA (mtDNA) is a small (16.5 kb), circular genome that encodes 13 proteins, 22 transfer (tRNA) and two ribosomal RNA (rRNA) (Anderson et al 1981) (Fig. 18.3). All of the 13 polypeptides

Table 18.1 Components of pathways of oxidative phosphorylation

Component	Function	Number of subunits/molecular weight	Comments
Complex I (NADH–ubiquinone oxidoreductase)	Reoxidises NADH to NAD$^+$. Electrons are passed to ubiquinone within the inner membrane. Proton pump, i.e. H$^+$ are pumped out of the matrix linked to the transfer of electrons within the complex (Weiss et al 1991)	>30	Complex I spans the inner mitochondrial membrane and contains a flavin prosthetic group (FMN) and several iron-sulphur centres necessary for electron transport within the complex. Seven of the >30 subunits are encoded by mtDNA
Ubiquinone (UQ)	Mobile electron carrier that diffuses through lipid bilayer. Reduction of UQ→UQH$_2$ is effected either by complexes I or II	830 daltons	Ubiquinone, otherwise known as coenzyme Q$_{10}$ is a benzoquinone with an isoprenoid side-chain containing 10 isoprenoid units. It is likely that different molecules of UQ exist, both linked to complexes and as free molecules
Complex II (succinate–ubiquinone oxidoreductase)	Oxidises succinate to fumarate and transfers electrons to UQ (Ackrell et al 1992)	4	Complex II is transmembraneous but not a proton pump. It contains covalently bound flavin (FAD), three iron-sulphur centres involved in electron transport and also contains a b-type cytochrome. Succinate dehydrogenase forms part of this complex and, therefore, complex II has a role in two major metabolic pathways—the TCA cycle and respiratory chain
Complex III (ubiquinol–cytochrome c oxidoreductase)	Reoxidises ubiquinol, i.e. UQH$_2$→UQ, donating electron to cytochrome c. Proton pump (Weiss 1987)	11	Also known as the bc$_1$ complex, there are two cytochromes in this complex, b and c$_1$. The cytochrome b apoprotein, encoded by mtDNA, coordinates two b-type haems. Complex III contains a single iron-sulphur protein — the Rieske protein
Cytochrome c	Accepts single electrons from complex III and donates to complex IV. Predominantly found in the intermembrane space it can interact with other electron donors	13 kDa	
Complex IV (cytochrome c oxidase)	Reoxidation of reduced cytochrome c passing electrons to molecular oxygen with the consequent formation of water. Proton pump (Capaldi 1990)	13	Final step in electron transport catalysing the transfer of electrons from cytochrome c to oxygen. It contains two a-type cytochromes and at least two copper atoms which are involved in electron transport. The three largest subunits are encoded by mtDNA
Complex V (ATP synthetase)	Uses electrochemical gradient to drive reaction: ADP + P$_i$ →ATP	approx. 14	The extrusion of protons (H$^+$) across the inner membrane creates an electrochemical gradient with the matrix negative with respect to the external environment. ATP synthetase discharges this gradient and the movement of protons through this complex and back into the matrix drives ATP synthesis
Cardiolipin	Phospholipid involved in insulating properties of inner membrane		

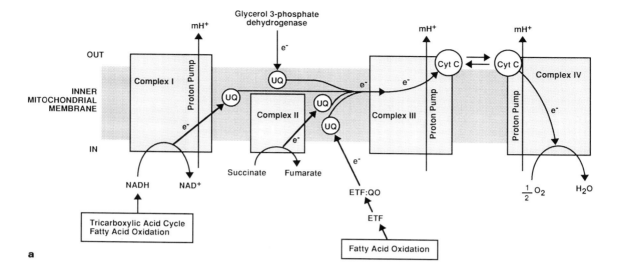

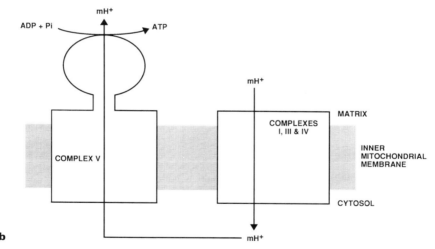

Fig. 18.2 Details of the reoxidation of cofactors and production of ATP by the respiratory chain. **a** Electron transport. NADH produced either from the TCA cycle or fatty acid oxidation is reoxidised by complex I of the respiratory chain. This involves the transfer of electrons from NADH through complex I to the mobile electron acceptor, ubiquinone. Energy released by this process is sufficient for this complex to pump protons (mH+) out of the mitochondrial matrix; thus, complex I both pumps protons and transfers electrons. Complex II is involved in the oxidation of succinate to fumarate. Succinate dehydrogenase is an integral part of this complex and electrons are transferred from succinate to ubiquinone (UQ). Ubiquinone also accepts electrons from the flavoprotein dehydrogenase involved in fatty acid oxidation (ETF dehydrogenase) and from glycerol-3 phosphate dehydrogenase in the intramembranous space. The reduction of ubiquinone generates ubiquinol which is reoxidised by complex III. Electrons are transferred from ubiquinol to the cytochrome b component of this complex. Complex III is also a proton pump similar to complex I. From complex III electrons are passed to another mobile electron carrier, cytochrome c, which donates electrons to complex IV (cytochrome c oxidase). From this terminal electron transporting complex electrons are passed to molecular oxygen which then combines with two H+ to form water. Cytochrome c oxidase is also a proton pump. **b** The production of ATP. By pumping protons out of the mitochondrial matrix, the respiratory chain generates an electrochemical gradient or proton gradient across the inner mitochondrial membrane. This gradient is discharged through complex V (mitochondrial ATP synthetase) which uses the energy involved to drive ATP synthesis. Thus, it can be seen that substrate oxidation which generates the electrochemical gradient through the respiratory chain is linked to the phosphorylation of ADP to ATP, hence the term *oxidative phosphorylation*.

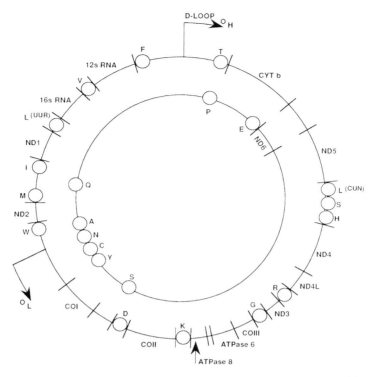

Fig. 18.3 Schematic representation of mitochondrial DNA. Mitochondrial DNA only encodes 13 proteins, all subunits of the respiratory chain. There are seven subunits of complex I (ND1-6), one of complex III (cytochrome b, cyt b), three of complex IV (CO I-III) and two of complex V (ATPase 6 and 8). In addition, there are two ribosomal RNA (16s and 12s) and 22tRNA (represented as circles with the amino acid single letter code as identification). MtDNA can be separated into two strands, heavy (H) and light (L), on the basis of buoyant density. The D-loop is the only non-coding sequence and this contains the promoters for transcription of both H- and L-strands plus the origin of replication of the H-strand. The transcription of both strands produces a large polycistronic message which is then cleaved into the individual mRNA, tRNA and rRNA. Replication of mtDNA begins with the H-strand and L-strand replication only occurring when the start site (O_L) is exposed by H-strand synthesis.

encoded by this genome are components of the respiratory chain and are synthesised inside the mitochondrion using the tRNA and rRNA found on mtDNA. mtDNA shows great economy of organisation with only a small section, the D-loop, lacking assignable coding frames. Even this is functionally active, however, since it contains promoters for transcription and replication of mtDNA.

mtDNA has several unique properties relevant to its association with disorders of the respiratory chain:

1. It is predominantly, if not exclusively, inherited from the mother. At fertilisation, few if any mitochondria from sperm appear to survive. Thus, the fertilised egg contains only maternal mitochondria and only maternal mtDNA.

2. Mitochondria usually contain more than one copy of mtDNA. In skeletal muscle the number may be as high as 10–100 copies. This means that in muscle, there may be many thousands of copies per cell.

The nuclear-encoded proteins destined for both the respiratory chain and all other intramitochondrial pathways (including fatty acid oxidation) are synthesised on cytosolic ribosomes. These proteins are transported into mitochondria by specific mechanisms often involving the presence of an N-terminal leader sequence which targets the protein to mitochondria and is then subsequently cleaved (Hartl & Neupert 1990). Currently, no disease has been shown to be due to this multistep process but this is likely to change.

It is apparent that the inheritance of respiratory chain disorders will be complicated by the presence of two genomes. Diseases due to mtDNA defects should be maternally inherited and this is indeed true in some, but not all cases. Many appear sporadic. Nevertheless, when taken as a group, analysis of those in which a family history exists show a preponderance of mother to child transmission (Harding et al 1988).

Investigation of respiratory chain defects

Due to the complexity of this pathway, difficulties still surround the identification and classification of respiratory chain disease. In the following section, the clinical, biochemical and genetic abnormalities associated with respiratory chain disease will be described. Methods of investigation will be discussed in general terms with appropriate references for those interested in greater detail. Clearly, the information from the history and examination may suggest the possibility of respiratory chain disease and will indicate its extent (i.e. which tissues might be involved).

Clinical. The search for an elevated venous lactate and an elevated lactate : pyruvate ratio are perhaps the commonest screening investigations used. The increase in lactate may be modest (2–3 mM) or extreme (we have found concentrations of 28 mM). In some individuals, basal levels may be normal so that some form of provocation (e.g. fasting, carbohydrate load or exercise) is necessary. Occasionally, in patients with predominantly CNS symptoms, abnormal elevation of lactate is maximal or even confined to the cerebrospinal fluid (CSF); in these patients it is valuable to measure both venous and CSF lactate after fasting. Spurious elevations of venous lactate concentration are common and may be due to venous stasis and/or an upset and struggling child. Venous blood should, therefore, be taken without stasis or, failing this, and of particular importance in children, arterial samples may be necessary.

Computerised tomographic (CT) scanning and magnetic resonance imaging (MRI) are both useful for detecting disease within the central nervous system (CNS). In some cases characteristic lesions are present, e.g. low-density slit-like areas in the basal ganglia seen in Leigh's syndrome (see below). Rather characteristic changes are seen by MRI in those mitochondrial disorders associated with encephalopathy and stroke-like episodes (Matthews et al 1991). However, both techniques will still only define the site of abnormality and not its nature.

Electrophysiological studies including electromyography (EMG) and electroencephalography (EEG) may also be of value. These studies are relatively non-invasive and again help define the extent of the disease, which is clearly important for prognosis. For example, in patients with clinical evidence of myopathy or cardiomyopathy only, an abnormal EEG strongly suggests CNS involvement. The EMG may be entirely normal in respiratory chain disease even when the patient appears clinically to have a myopathy.

Phosphorus magnetic resonance spectroscopy has been used and will add further information, although the changes seen, low phosphocreatine and impaired conversion of ADP to ATP, are fairly non-specific and do not allow differentiation between different biochemical defects or clinical syndromes (Arnold et al 1985). One major advantage of the technique is that, being non-invasive, repeated measurements can be made to follow the effects of treatment. Positron emission tomography (PET) is also informative, since it is possible to show uncoupling of the normal ratio of oxygen consumed per molecule of glucose metabolised. When uncoupling occurs it suggests that anaerobic metabolism is being used to provide energy in cells where normal respiratory chain function is deficient.

In certain centres, whole-body investigation measuring metabolic rate, fuel consumption, energy turnover, etc. has provided a great deal of information concerning the general metabolism in patients with respiratory chain disease. These facilities are not widely available, so most centres screen by assessment of the clinical features, measuring serum lactate concentration and CNS imaging.

Morphological studies. Historically, morphological abnormalities in skeletal muscle mitochondria provided one of the earliest indications that disease may be caused by altered mitochondrial function. Muscle fibre necrosis and atrophy may be seen in patients with respiratory chain disease. More specifically, qualitative and quantitative abnormalities of mitochondria have been found in these patients. Perhaps the most well-known finding is the 'ragged-red fibre' which describes the abnormal accumulation of normal and abnormal mitochondria beneath the muscle cell membrane, giving it a ragged edge. When stained by the Gomori trichrome method, the accumulated mitochondria are stained red (Olsen et al 1972). Such changes are more specifically demonstrated by using enzyme reactions such as succinate dehydrogenase (SDH) (Fig. 18.4).

In addition to changes in mitochondrial number and structure, the use of tissue sections now permits considerable insight into the nature of respiratory chain dysfunction.

1. Direct enzyme measurements. The activity of both SDH and cytochrome c oxidase can be measured in thin sections using a specially adapted spectrophotometer. Since cytochrome c oxidase deficiency is one of the most common of these disorders, this provides a rapid method for diagnosis (Johnson et al 1993).

2. The identification of associated metabolic defects. Abnormal storage of lipid is a common finding in muscle from patients with respiratory chain dysfunction. This is due to a secondary effect on β-oxidation (Watmough et al 1990).

3. Immunocytochemistry. This technique involves the localisation of proteins using specific antisera and is of great importance since it can demonstrate whether low activity correlates with an abnormal amount of protein/complex (Johnson 1991).

4. In situ hybridization. Detection of DNA or RNA using specific probes is possible in tissue sections (Mita et al 1989). It is possible to show: (a) whether lowered activity correlates with lowered transcription of RNA; and (b) whether abnormal mtDNA is uniformly distributed.

Morphological changes in mitochondria are best seen using electron-microscopy. A variety of abnormalities have been described including intramitochondrial inclusions. Paracrystalline inclusions are characteristic but not pathognomonic of respiratory chain disease.

Biochemical studies. Accurate definition of the site and extent of the biochemical defect is essential if we are to understand the pathogenesis of these disorders. A great deal of information is provided by morphological and histochemical analysis, but these techniques cannot assess all components of the respiratory chain. Preparation of mitochondrial fractions from fresh muscle is required for full biochemical characterisation of the defect.

Analysis of respiratory chain function may be divided into three broad categories:

1. Measurement of activity in the whole or segments of the pathway (flux measurement)
2. Measurement of activity in individual complexes
3. Measurement of the steady-state levels of components of individual complexes.

Each is important and provides complementary information. For a full description of the techniques see Birch-Machin et al (1993).

Molecular studies. What understanding we have of the genetic basis of respiratory chain disorders is relatively recent. Much of the work has involved analysis of mitochondrial DNA and we will concentrate on this genome. Nuclear gene defects must occur since autosomal patterns of inheritance are present in some individuals. The genes involved are, however, yet to be identified.

Abnormalities of mtDNA include major rearrangement (deletions and duplications), point mutations and depletion (loss of mtDNA relative to normal levels). The latter is an interesting phenomenon and appears to affect very young children. That mtDNA depletion is due to a nuclear gene defect is suggested by the relative normality of the remaining mtDNA, the tendency for it to affect one or only a few tissues and the similarity between what is found in these patients and the depletion of mtDNA caused by the drug zidovudine (AZT) which affects mitochondrial DNA polymerase (Arnaudo et al 1991).

Two important points require further discussion. First, whether mtDNA abnormalities are causally related to disease, and secondly, the

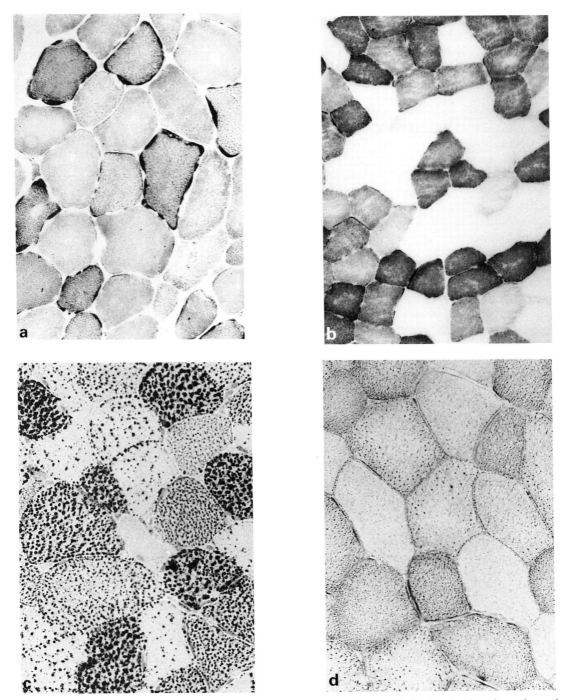

Fig. 18.4 Morphological changes in muscle. **a** Succinate dehydrogenase reaction specifically showing the subsarcolemmal accumulation of mitochondria in muscle from a patient with a defect of the respiratory chain (SDH, × 200). **b** Cytochrome c oxidase reaction showing the presence of cytochrome c oxidase positive and negative fibres in muscle from a patient with a defect of the respiratory chain (CCO, × 120). **c** Marked lipid storage, particularly in type I muscle fibres, in muscle from a patient with acyl-CoA dehydrogenase deficiency (Oil Red O, × 280). **d** Normal or very mildly increased lipid in muscle from a patient with acyl-CoA dehydrogenase deficiency (Sudan Black, × 240).

significance of the occurrence of both normal and abnormal mtDNA in the same individual. That abnormal mtDNA may cause disease was established by some elegant experiments using cultured cells depleted of mitochondrial DNA (rho° cells) (King & Attardi 1989). Fusion of mitochondria and cytoplasm from cells of patients harbouring mtDNA mutations with these rho° cells allows biochemical analysis of mitochondria in a neutral nuclear environment. Such studies showed that the fused cells were respiration deficient, thus confirming that mtDNA from the patient directed the biochemical defect (Chomyn et al 1991). The presence of both normal and abnormal mtDNA in one individual is termed heteroplasmy. The degree of heteroplasmy can vary between different tissues and the percentage of abnormal mtDNA seems to be highest in non-dividing tissues such as muscle and nerve. In the case of mtDNA deletions the amount of abnormal mtDNA increases with time and disease progression (Larsson et al 1990).

Deletions, duplications and mtDNA depletion may be detected by Southern blotting (Fig. 18.5). In addition, deletions can be detected by the polymerase chain reaction (PCR) and, whilst this technique is extremely sensitive, quantitation is difficult. Known point mutations can be detected by PCR amplification followed by sequencing or, if the mutation creates or destroys a restriction endonuclease site, by PCR amplification and restriction digest (Hammans et al 1991).

Classification of respiratory chain defects

Attempts at classifying respiratory chain defects have been based on clinical, biochemical or, more recently, genetic criteria. Difficulties arise with each and in the following section we shall explore some of these problems.

Clinical. Initially, mitochondrial respiratory chain diseases were described in muscle and gave rise to the term *mitochondrial myopathy*. Involvement of other tissues, especially brain, led to the use of terms such as *mitochondrial encephalomyopathy* or *mitochondrial cytopathy*, the latter term highlighting that mitochondrial disease is commonly systemic. In addition to these generic descriptions, a number of acronyms and eponymous titles have arisen. Since these do not necessarily reflect a common biochemical defect their use in classifica-

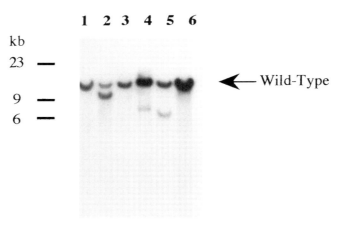

Fig. 18.5   Southern blot of mitochondrial DNA. Genomic DNA was digested with a restriction endonuclease (to cut mitochondrial DNA into a linear strand) and separated according to size on an agarose gel. The DNA was then transferred to a nylon membrane by Southern blotting and the different spacies of mtDNA hybridised with a radioactively labelled probe which can be detected by autoradiography. Mitochondrial DNA from control subjects is shown in lanes 1, 3 and 6 and from patients with the Kearns–Sayre syndrome or chronic progressive external ophthalmoplegia (lanes 2, 4 and 5). The normal mitochondrial genome (wild-type) is shown at 16.5 kb whilst the rearranged mtDNA are shown as the smaller species in the patients. The patients demonstrate heteroplasmy, i.e. the presence of normal and abnormal mtDNA.

tion has been questioned. Progress in genetic definition is helping to clarify the situation but this remains a contentious area.

Biochemical. Definition of respiratory chain diseases by which enzyme(s) is involved presupposes that measurement of these activities is uniform. This is not the case. Previously, we have grouped cases according to which complex or complexes was reported to be affected, but acknowledged that in many instances more than one complex activity was lowered (Bindoff & Turnbull 1990). Certainly, our own observations suggest that the commonest finding is for multiple respiratory chain complexes to be affected in any single patient.

In many instances biochemical evaluation of the respiratory chain is both inadequate and incomplete. This in part reflects the difficulty of this evaluation and the variety of the different techniques used in different laboratories. Because of this, it is not possible to construct a rational classification based on which enzymes are affected.

Genetic. Deletions of mtDNA were discovered in 1988 (Holt et al 1988) and this finding was quickly followed by the identification of duplications and point mutations. The more common mtDNA mutations are shown in Figure 18.6. These genetic abnormalities show greater congruence with clinical subtypes than biochemical findings. Thus, the majority of patients with

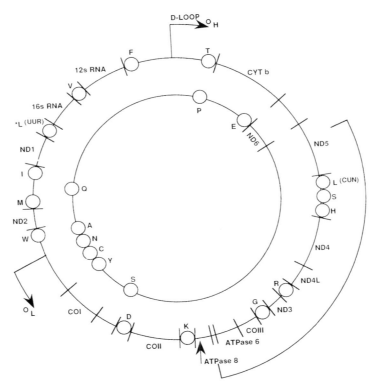

Fig. 18.6 Mutations of mitochondrial DNA. Several of the commoner mtDNA mutations are shown. The 'common' deletion occurs between ND5 and ATPase 6 and at each breakpoint there are 13 base pair repeats (ACCACTCCCTCCA) which may be involved in the mechanism of deletion. The majority of other deletions found in the Kearns–Sayre syndrome or in chronic progressive external ophthalmoplegia are found in the same region. The MELAS syndrome is most commonly associated with a mutation in tRNA$^{Leu(UUR)}$. This tRNA appears to be a 'hot spot' for mutations since several different mutations have been identified. The MERRF mutation occurs in tRNA^{Lys}, whilst Leber's optic neuropathy is most commonly associated with primary mutations in ND4 and ND1.

the syndrome of MELAS (see below) have a particular point mutation in tRNA$^{Leu (UUR)}$. There is, however, undoubted overlap in the clinical features observed and the different genetic defects. In addition, there are still many patients in whom the molecular defect has not been identified, making genetic classification alone inadequate. Until more information provides a clearer understanding of the disorders a combination of all three parameters should be used. In the following section ('Clinical syndromes') the recognised syndromes have been grouped according to the broad categories described earlier. Information concerning the biochemical and genetic findings will be given for each category.

Clinical syndromes

Isolated myopathy. Despite the early concentration on muscle-related disease, isolated myopathy is uncommon. Patients present with non-specific symptoms such as cramp-like pain, burning discomfort in the muscles, weakness and fatigue. These symptoms are usually provoked or worsened by exertion but a clear relationship between pain and exercise is not always present. The distribution of weakness is proximal/axial and may also involve the face, giving a facioscapulohumeral picture (FSH). Neck flexion weakness is almost uniform. These patients do not have ophthalmoplegia, ptosis or retinopathy.

Excluding myopathy occurring in infancy, adults with myopathy can present from their teens into their forties and fifties. Progression too is variable but those affected earlier tend to progress more rapidly. Bulbar weakness can develop and poses major management problems. Death is usually secondary to respiratory muscle weakness and concurrent bulbar muscle weakness may be a contributory factor.

Clinical investigation often shows elevation of serum lactate at rest which increases with exercise. The serum creatine kinase activity is usually normal or only slightly elevated. Electromyography (EMG) usually demonstrates myopathic changes, although it can be normal. EEG, CT and NMR imaging and psychometric testing are normal in these patients, compatible with the absence of CNS symptoms. Morphological examination of muscle usually shows the typical subsarcolemmal mitochondrial accumulation and histochemical analysis will in most cases show cytochrome c oxidase-negative fibres. In addition, atrophy and necrosis may be present as can significant abnormal lipid storage. Biochemical analysis of mitochondrial fractions isolated from muscle biopsy specimens have shown multiple respiratory chain defects and no consistent molecular abnormality has been identified.

Chronic progressive external ophthalmoplegia (CPEO). This is one of the commonest adult presentations of respiratory chain dysfunction. It may occur as an isolated finding or more usually in association with myopathy, pigmentary retinopathy and/or CNS disease, particularly ataxia. Presentation is with ptosis, fatigue or unsteadiness. Interestingly, diplopia is not often troublesome, despite marked ophthalmoplegia, and this probably reflects the very gradual onset of the eye movement disorder.

Lactate levels in blood are often normal or only mildly elevated. CT/MRI may show atrophy confined to the cerebellum, although occasionally it is more generalised. Muscle histochemistry shows subsarcolemmal accumulation of mitochondria and cytochrome c oxidase-deficient fibres. Biochemical analysis of mitochondrial fractions shows that whilst a defect of complex IV is most commonly found, multiple respiratory chain defects are also present. Genetic analysis shows that most patients with CPEO have a deletion of mtDNA (Moraes et al 1989). Deletions vary from approximately 1 kb to over 7 kb and are invariably heteroplasmic (i.e. there is a mixture of wild-type and mutant mtDNA). Many of the deletions occur in the same region of mtDNA, the 'common' deletion. Studies have shown that in many instances, and this is particularly true of the common deletion, the deleted region is flanked by repeated sequences and it has been suggested that recombination between these regions causes the loss of intermediary mtDNA (Schon et al 1989).

Conditions with predominant CNS disease. Many respiratory chain diseases have multisystem involvement with the major clinical manifestation being CNS dysfunction, e.g. encephalopathy, seizures, dementia. Overlap exists and although the following categories are useful, it is not always possible to categorise individual patients.

Kearns–Sayre syndrome (KSS). This disorder, also called the oculocraniosomatic syndrome, is characterised by progressive external ophthalmoplegia, pigmentary retinopathy and heart block but may include a number of other, distinctive features (Table 18.2). It is by definition a disorder with onset of symptoms before the age of 20. What is of interest, however, is the similarity between this syndrome and CPEO which may also manifest deafness, ataxia, etc. Presentation may be with eye problems (diminished vision or ptosis), syncope due to heart block or encephalopathy. Muscle involvement is common but often over-shadowed by CNS disease.

Clinical investigation often demonstrates a range of features; lactate is usually elevated in blood and CSF and muscle histology characteristically shows mitochondrial accumulation and cytochrome c oxidase negative fibres. Since KSS has a major central component, neurogenic changes such as atrophy and fibre loss occasionally occur in biopsy specimens. Peripheral nerve involvement can also occur.

Biochemical studies commonly show multiple defects (complexes I, III and IV), although isolated complex I or complex IV deficiency has also been reported. At the genetic level, almost all cases of KSS have a major rearrangement of mtDNA; in the majority this is a deletion and once again the majority of these cases have the so-called 'common' deletion. In rare cases, duplication of mtDNA has been documented (Poulton et al 1989).

Myoclonus epilepsy with ragged red fibres (MERRF). As the name suggests, myoclonus is a major feature of this disorder. Weakness, ataxia, deafness and dementia are also found (Table 18.2). The finding of morphological abnormalities in skeletal muscle (the ragged-red fibre) gave the initial clue that this disorder may be due to mitochondrial dysfunction and indeed this has been confirmed. Biochemical studies usually show multiple defects suggesting once again that mtDNA is affected. MERRF was one of the first of the mitochondrial disorders to be linked with a point mutation in the mitochondrial genome (Shoffner et al 1990). This mutation affects a tRNA (that for lysine) and is found in most, but not all, cases with

this syndrome. Additional reports are appearing of patients initially diagnosed as having MERRF but who later develop stroke-like episodes (see below, 'MELAS'). As would be expected for a mitochondrial genetic disorder maternal transmission is found in many of the cases.

Mitochondrial myopathy, encephalopathy, lactic acidosis and stroke-like episodes (MELAS). The feature that separates this syndrome is the occurrence of stroke-like episodes. These are so termed because although they mimic stroke clinically their nature is uncertain. Whilst they may be due to vascular insufficiency, an alternative possibility is that they result from metabolic insufficiency within the CNS. Characteristic lesions are seen on CT and MRI; these lesions may resolve rapidly or proceed to an established neurological defect. The onset of symptoms is before the age of 15 years in most patients. Cortical blindness and hemianopia are present in virtually all patients and stroke-like episodes may be preceded by a migraine-like headache together with nausea and vomiting (Ciafaloni et al 1992). Focal and generalised seizures are common, as is dementia (Table 18.2). Myopathy is a part of this condition but is usually overshadowed by the more catastrophic CNS disease. There may be overlap between MELAS and other mitochondrial encephalomyopathies, with some patients having myoclonus, ophthalmoplegia, retinopathy and ptosis.

Lactate levels are often high, especially within the CSF. The MELAS syndrome has been associated with different biochemical findings, although complex I deficiency appears by far the most common. As in the MERRF syndrome, a mutation in mtDNA has been demonstrated but in MELAS the majority of mutations occur within the tRNA for leucine (UUR) (Goto et al 1990). Although the abnormal mitochondrial DNA is maternally inherited, familial cases are relatively uncommon. Clinical expression may be dependent not just on the dose of mutant *versus* wild-type mitochondrial DNA but also on other, as yet unidentified, modifying factors.

Neurogenic weakness, ataxia and retinitis pigmentosa (NARP). This clinical syndrome is inherited in a maternal manner and the predominant clinical features are retinitis pigmentosa, epilepsy, ataxia, neurogenic weakness and peripheral

Table 18.2   Clinical, biochemical and molecular features of defects of mitochondrial genome

Clinical feature	KSS	MERRF	MELAS	Depletion	NARP
Ophthalmoplegia	+	–	–	–	–
Retinal degeneration	+	–	–	–	–
Heart block	+	–	–	–	–
CSF protein >100 mg/dl	+	–	–	–	–
Myoclonus	–	+	–	–	–
Ataxia	+	+	–	–	+
Weakness	+	+	+	+	+
Episodic vomiting	–	–	+	–	–
Headache	–	–	+	–	–
Cerebral blindness	–	–	+	–	–
Hemiparesis, hemianopia	–	–	+	–	–
Seizures	–	+	+	+	+
Dementia	+	+	+	+	+
Short stature	+	+	+	–	–
Sensorineural hearing loss	+	+	+	–	–
Lactic acidosis	+	+	+	+	–
Family history	–	M	M	A	M
Ragged red fibres	+	+	+	+	–
Leigh's phenotype	–	–	–	–	+
mtDNA duplication	+	–	–	–	–
mtDNA deletion	–	–	–	+	–
mtDNA point mutation	–	tRNA^{Lys} (8344)	tRNA$^{LEU(UUR)}$ (3243)	–	ATPase 6^{8993}

KSS, Kearns–Sayre syndrome; MERRF, myoclonus epilepsy with ragged red fibres; MELAS, mitochondrial myopathy, encephalopathy, lactic acidosis and stroke-like episodes; NARP, neurogenic weakness, ataxia and retinitis pigmentosa; M, maternal (mitochondrial) transmission; A, autosomal recessive transmission.

neuropathy (Holt et al 1990) (Table 18.2). In one family a severely affected child had the clinical and pathological features of Leigh's disease (Tatuch et al 1992) (see below). Unlike the syndromes described above there are no morphological changes in skeletal muscle. There is a point mutation in the ATPase 6 gene which does not seem to affect ATP hydrolysis by this enzyme but presumably affects ATP synthesis.

Other conditions.

Luft's disease. Historically, this was the first condition to be linked with abnormal mitochondrial function. Paradoxically, it is extremely rare and only a single case has been added to that described by Luft and colleagues in 1962. Mitochondria in this disorder show poor respiratory control but normal phosphorylation capacity—a state termed 'loose coupling'. It is suggested that the cause of this disorder is an inability of mitochondria to retain calcium ions so that the constant recycling of calcium results in sustained, maximal respiration and hypermetabolism. The two individuals described have presented with euthyroid hypermetabolism.

Ubiquinone deficiency. This encephalomyopathic disorder has been described in only two individuals (sisters) (Ogasahara et al 1989). Both sisters had normal early development but developed abnormal fatigability on exertion and slowly progressive weakness of truncal and proximal limb muscles. Subsequently, both developed CNS symptoms with ataxia, dysarthria and seizures. Laboratory analysis demonstrated that flux through the respiratory chain was slow, whilst activity of the individual complexes, measured with artificial electron acceptors, was normal. This paradox suggested a disorder of ubiquinone rather than of one of the individual complexes. Confirmation is by direct measurement of ubiquinone concentration.

Multiple mtDNA deletions. Whilst this syndrome clearly has a similar phenotype to KSS, the molecular basis is different (Zeviani et al 1989). The patients described had chronic progressive external ophthalmoplegia, proximal myopathy, sensorineural deafness, cataracts and peripheral neuropathy. Muscle histology showed subsarcolemmal accumulation of mitochondria, decreased cytochrome c oxidase activity and some neurogenic changes. Biochemical studies showed multiple respiratory chain defects and molecular studies showed multiple DNA deletions. Most deletions spanned a mtDNA region of several kilobases between the end of the D loop and the region encompassing genes for ATPase 8 and 6, and CO I (Fig. 18.6). The syndrome is inherited in an autosomal dominant manner which implies a mutation in a nuclear encoded gene. The mechanism by which this nuclear gene defect results in multiple deletions is unknown. A similar syndrome has also been reported in two brothers, but the transmission in these cases was probably autosomal recessive.

Leigh's syndrome. Also called subacute necrotising encephalomyelopathy, this syndrome is essentially diagnosed by the neuropathological findings of symmetrical necrotic lesions, glial reaction and vascular proliferation in the mid-brain, pons, basal ganglia, thalamus and optic nerves. It usually presents as a devastating encephalopathy in infancy or childhood, although an adult onset is recorded. The major impact of this disorder is within the CNS but ophthalmoplegia has been reported.

Lactate and pyruvate concentrations are frequently elevated in blood and CSF; CT/MRI scans show very characteristic (but not pathognomonic) low density areas within the basal ganglia or less commonly cerebellum. In those individuals with respiratory chain disease as the underlying defect (probably the majority, through the exact proportion is still uncertain), single complex deficiency involving either complex I or IV appears to be more common than in other respiratory chain syndromes. When complex IV is the cause, diagnosis on muscle biopsy is possible using microspectrophotometric techniques (Johnson et al 1993). The systemic nature of the disease and the occasional autosomal recessive pattern of inheritance has led to the presumption that most cases of Leigh's syndrome are caused by a nuclear gene rather than a mitochondrial gene defect. However, cases with Leigh's syndrome phenotype have been found in patients with a mutation in mtDNA (Tatuch et al 1992).

Other encephalopathies. As stated earlier, it is often difficult to fit individuals into the above categories. We have seen a number of patients presenting with features such as dementia, eye movement disorder (ophthalmoplegia or disorders of conjugate gaze), epilepsy, muscle weakness and peripheral neuropathy. Most of these patients have shown multiple defects of respiratory chain complexes suggesting that mtDNA is once again affected.

Involvement of other tissues in respiratory chain disease. Since this chapter concerns disorders of muscle, we have concentrated on this area. It is important to realise, however, that respiratory chain defects may produce a wide range of diseases and the following section will discuss these briefly.

Optic neuropathy: Leber's hereditary optic neuropathy. This disorder merits special attention since it is: (a) a common cause of blindness affecting mainly young men; (b) clearly maternally inherited and due to a defect of mtDNA. Mutations in several mtDNA genes are now associated with this disorder (Wallace et al 1988, Howell et al 1991) and biochemical studies in muscle (as well as platelets and fibroblasts) have documented abnormal respiratory chain activity.

Gastrointestinal involvement. Although relatively uncommon compared with other manifestations, gastrointestinal disease is recognised and probably under-reported. Anorexia and vomiting may be general indicators of disease whilst abdominal pain is seen in many patients with systemic lactic acidosis. The myo-, neuro-, gastro-intestinal encephalopathy syndrome (MNGIE) has been coined to describe a single case which presented external ophthalmoplegia, muscular atrophy, peripheral neuropathy, malabsorption and a disorder of white matter within the brain. A partial decrease in cytochrome c oxidase activity was reported as the cause (Bardosi et al 1987).

Cardiomyopathy. The cardiac conduction system is affected in KSS/CPEO and these patients often develop complete heart block. This is thought to be a significant cause of mortality, should be actively sought and may require treatment by pacemaker insertion. In other patients, there is involvement of the heart muscle itself leading to heart failure. Nevertheless, the biochemical diagnosis in these patients is still usually made using skeletal muscle mitochondria, suggesting, therefore, that the disease process is more diffuse. Clearly this must be borne in mind when considering treatment for the cardiac failure, as the options may include transplantation.

Renal disease. A proximal renal tubular defect (de Toni–Fanconi–Debré syndrome) has been described in several patients with respiratory chain disease. Most of these had cytochrome c oxidase deficiency diagnosed in skeletal muscle mitochondria. Renal impairment or renal failure has rarely, if ever, been documented alone.

Haematopoetic system. Pearson's syndrome presents at birth or in early infancy with refractory sideroblastic anaemia, thrombocytopenia, neutropenia, metabolic acidosis, pancreatic insufficiency and hepatic dysfunction. Renal dysfunction, diarrhoea, steatorrhoea and ill-defined skin lesions are also reported. Children usually die from liver failure. Deletions of mtDNA have now been identified in a significant proportion of children with this syndrome (Rötig et al 1989). Furthermore, there are recorded cases of children presenting initially with Pearson's syndrome who later develop a disease identical to the Kearns–Sayre syndrome.

Disorders of the respiratory chain presenting in infancy. Whilst any of the above syndromes may present in the very young, several conditions appear confined to infants and it is worthwhile discussing this group in isolation. It is important to remember that due to their lack of motor and intellectual development, especially lack of language, presentation of disease in infancy follows different patterns from that seen in children and adults; for example, muscle weakness will manifest as a floppy infant, systemic disease may cause failure to thrive, whilst acidosis will provoke vomiting which is itself a common feature of disease in infancy.

Fatal infantile lactic acidosis. Profound lactic acidosis presenting from birth to around 3 months of age is highly suggestive of a respiratory chain defect. Hypotonia, vomiting and ventilatory distress are all commonly associated features and death from respiratory failure is the usual outcome, often before the age of 6 months. Apart from the elevated blood lactate, several reports have mentioned generalised amino aciduria (de Toni–Fanconi–Debré syndrome), seizures, ele-

vated calcium, liver dysfunction and hypoglycaemia. Isolated defects of complexes I, III and IV have been described (Moreadith et al 1984, DiMauro et al 1986, Birch-Machin et al 1989).

Benign infantile lactic acidosis. Benign infantile lactic acidosis presents a similar initial picture (DiMauro et al 1983). Failure to thrive, hypotonia and ventilatory difficulties are all features of this condition and lactic acid levels may be as high in this disorder as in the fatal form. Despite this, the condition gradually remits and by 12–18 months these infants are often normal. Biochemical studies have shown that all reported cases have been due to an initial, severe defect of cytochrome c oxidase. This deficiency improves with age and it has been postulated that the defect involves a fetal isoform of a nuclear-encoded subunit of complex IV, the switch to the adult form being associated with the resolution of the disease. Immunohistochemical studies have suggested that it may be possible to differentiate the fatal and benign forms (Tritschler et al 1992).

The syndrome of mtDNA depletion. This recently described syndrome affects neonates and infants (Moraes et al 1991). Weakness, hypotonia and ventilatory difficulty are once again common and renal involvement and seizures may occur (Table 18.2). The family history in some cases is suggestive of an autosomal recessive pattern of inheritance, indicating that the disease may itself be due to a nuclear gene defect. Interestingly, the degree of mtDNA depletion may vary between tissues in the same individual and this has led to clinical presentation outside the neuromuscular system, e.g. with liver disease. Biochemical studies have shown that complexes I, III and IV are affected, with the major deficiency apparently involving cytochrome c oxidase. The condition is fatal in the majority of cases, usually before the age of 12 months.

Treatment

The treatment of patients with respiratory chain defects is difficult and in our experience often unsuccessful. This difficulty is partly due to the nature of the biochemical defect involving as it does the final common pathway of oxidative metabolism. This means that it is impossible to bypass the defect by giving alternative metabolic fuels. In addition, relatively little is understood about the secondary biochemical changes in these conditions.

There have been conflicting results of treatment in patients with apparently similar biochemical abnormalities. Most success has been achieved with substances that act as artificial electron acceptors, vitamin C (ascorbate 4 g per day), vitamin K_3 (menadione up to 80 mg per day) (Argov et al 1986) and ubiquinone (up to 150 mg per day) (Ogasahara et al 1986). Objective increases in muscle strength have been reported with all three treatments. Improvements in muscle energetic processes have been suggested by NMR studies in these patients. No improvement in the ophthalmoplegia or ptosis has been reported.

Other attempts at treating respiratory chain disorders include the use of thiamine, biotin, carnitine, riboflavin and dichloracetate. For many of these treatments there are either single case reports or anecdotal evidence of clinical improvement, but none has been consistently shown to be of therapeutic benefit. The mitochondrial respiratory chain generates free radicals and their production may be increased in the presence of respiratory chain disease. Therefore, the use of free radical scavengers such as vitamin E could, in theory, help prevent further damage but there is little evidence, as yet, to justify their use.

An important aspect of patient care is rehabilitation and supportive care, since at present many of these conditions are progressive and associated with significant disability. Patients with respiratory muscle involvement may need ventilatory support.

Access to genetic counselling is important for patients and their families, especially since many of these disorders are inherited in a maternal manner. Prenatal diagnosis of some of the most severe presentations is now possible in a very few instances either by identifying a biochemical abnormality in cultured cells from a chorionic villus biopsy or amniocentesis, or by genetic analysis of fetal material (Harding et al 1992). In families in which the disease is clearly maternally inherited, ovum donation will prevent the birth of an affected child.

LIPID STORAGE MYOPATHIES AND DEFECTS OF FATTY ACID OXIDATION

Biochemistry and genetics of mitochondrial fatty acid oxidation

The major site for the oxidation of fat is in the mitochondria, although oxidation of long-chain fatty acids also occurs in peroxisomes. The peroxisomal β-oxidation pathway is of minor importance in muscle and disorders of this pathway do not present with primary muscle disease.

Free fatty acids (FFA) are taken up by muscle cells and then transported through the cytosol to the mitochondria. Before they can undergo β-oxidation, fatty acids must first be activated to the corresponding acyl-CoA ester, a reaction catalysed by the acyl-CoA synthetases. Long-chain fatty acids are activated to acyl-CoA esters by long-chain acyl-CoA synthetase on the outer mitochondrial membrane. The acyl-CoA esters thus formed are transported into the matrix in a carnitine-dependent manner in a process which involves the carnitine palmitoyltransferases (CPT I and II) and carnitine-acylcarnitine translocase (Fig. 18.7). Short-chain and medium-chain fatty acids are able to enter the mitochondria directly. They are converted to their acyl-CoA esters by acyl-CoA synthetases present in the matrix. The acyl-CoA esters then undergo β-oxidation, a complicated pathway requiring repeated cycles of four reactions: flavoprotein dehydrogenation, hydration, NAD^+-linked dehydrogenation and thiolysis. The result of one cycle of β-oxidation is chain-shortening of the fatty acid by a two-carbon unit, i.e. acetyl-CoA. β-Oxidation proceeds to completion which results in the complete degradation of long-chain fatty acids into two carbon units. The different enzymes involved are described in detail in Table 18.3.

The control of mitochondrial fatty acid oxidation occurs at several sites, the importance of each site varying depending on the prevailing metabolic environment. Potentially important factors include substrate supply, entry of fatty acids into mitochondria, recycling of cofactors and disposal of acetyl-CoA. Mitochondrial fatty acid oxidation is also regulated by the redox state of the mitochondria. If respiratory chain activity is impaired, both the acyl-CoA dehydrogenase and 3-hydroxy-

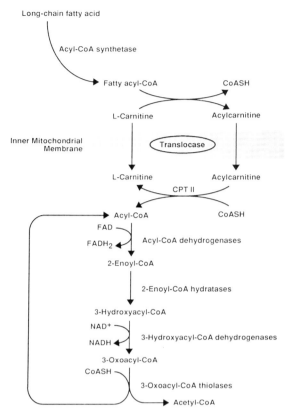

Fig. 18.7   Mitochondrial oxidation of long-chain fatty acids.

acyl-CoA dehydrogenase enzymes will be inhibited. This is presumably the mechanism of the lipid storage myopathy seen in patients with respiratory chain defects.

Unlike the proteins of the respiratory chain, all the enzymes involved in fatty acid oxidation are encoded by nuclear genes. The pattern of inheritance is, therefore, much simpler and in all cases described so far the pattern of inheritance has been autosomal recessive.

Investigation

The investigation of patients with defects of fatty acid oxidation involves a combination of clinical, morphological, biochemical and molecular studies. In many patients it is a combination of all these studies which results in a diagnosis, although the introduction of molecular techniques may simplify the diagnosis in some patients.

Clinical studies. An important component of any investigation is identifying patients who may have a fatty acid oxidation disorder, including an appreciation that whilst the presentation may be of muscle disease, other tissues, e.g. heart, may be involved. Screening procedures to identify involvement of other organs including heart and liver should, therefore, be performed on all patients. Since these defects are inherited errors in metabolism, assessment of other family members is essential.

Morphological studies. In the presence of a fatty acid oxidation defect, free fatty acids in muscle are diverted to triacylglycerol synthesis and this results in a lipid storage myopathy. The lipid storage is usually most severe in the oxidative type I fibres (Fig. 18.4). In patients with recent episodes of rhabdomyolysis due to a fatty acid oxidation defect, evidence of muscle necrosis may be present. Two important reservations must be mentioned, however. First, there may be no or only slight lipid accumulation in a patient with a fatty acid oxidation defect (Fig. 18.4). This is particularly true for patients with carnitine palmitoyltransferase (CPT) deficiency but is also found in other fatty acid oxidation disorders. The lipid accumulation is dependent both on the severity and site of the metabolic defect, and the metabolic state of the patient. Second, lipid storage may be seen in patients with respiratory chain defects due to the secondary effect on fatty acid oxidation.

Biochemical studies.

Concentration of metabolic fuels and intermediary metabolites in blood. Valuable information concerning the presence of abnormal β-oxidation may be obtained by studying the concentrations of metabolic fuels (glucose, ketone bodies, glycerol, free fatty acids) and intermediary metabolites (pyruvate, lactate, alanine) in blood. These patients have an impaired ability to withstand stress or fasting. Since they have impaired energy production from fat they depend upon glycogen stores and circulating carbohydrate. When these stores are depleted, hypoglycaemia will result. Since ketone body production is dependent upon fatty acid oxidation in the liver, hypoglycaemia in these patients is associated with hypoketonaemia. Moreover, since lipolysis is stimulated by a drop in circulating glucose, hypoglycaemia in this situa-

Table 18.3 Mitochondrial fatty acid oxidation

Enzyme	Functions	Comments
Acyl-CoA synthetases	These enzymes catalyse the conversion of fatty acids to acyl-CoA esters (Londesborough & Webster 1974)	There are at least three enzymes; long-chain acyl-CoA synthetase is present on the outer mitochondrial membrane whilst the short-chain and medium-chain specific synthetases are in the mitochondrial matrix
Carnitine palmitoyl transferases (CPT)	The acyl groups are transferred from CoA to carnitine by CPT I which is situated on the outer mitochondrial membrane. The long-chain acyl-CoA is then reformed at the inner surface of the inner membrane by CPT II (Woeltje et al 1990)	CPT I and CPT II are different proteins. CPT I is a major site of regulation of fatty acid oxidation in some tissues, e.g. liver
Carnitine-acylcarnitine translocase	The acylcarnitine esters cross the mitochondrial inner membrane in exchange for carnitine in a reaction catalysed by the carnitine-acylcarnitine translocase (Pande 1975)	The carnitine-acylcarnitine translocase is one of the closely related membrane proteins that shuttle substrates between the cytosol and the intramitochondrial matrix space
Acyl-CoA dehydrogenases	These catalyse the dehydrogenation of acyl-CoA to form the 2-trans-enoyl-CoA which is the first of the four reactions of mitochondrial β-oxidation (Finocchiaro et al 1987)	There were thought to be three acyl-CoA dehydrogenases — short-chain, medium-chain, long-chain — named according to the chain length of their preferred substrate. Recently, a fourth enzyme, very-long-chain acyl-CoA dehydrogenase, has been purified from rat liver (Izai et al 1992)
Electron transfer flavoprotein (ETF) and electron transfer flavoprotein : ubiquinone oxidoreductase (ETF : QO)	The reducing equivalents from the acyl-CoA dehydrogenases are transferred to ETF and then to the iron-sulphur protein ETF : QO. ETF : QO then transfers electrons to the ubiquinone pool (McKean et al 1983, Beckmann & Frerman 1985)	Both ETF and ETF : QO are involved in electron transfer not only from fatty acyl-CoA dehydrogenases but also branched chain acyl-CoA esters from amino acids, glutaryl-CoA and oxidation of intermediates of choline metabolism
2-Enoyl-CoA hydratases	The second reaction of β-oxidation is the hydration of 2-enoyl-CoA esters to form 3-hydroxyacyl-CoA esters and is catalysed by the 2-enoyl-CoA hydratases	A short-chain 2-enoyl-CoA hydratase has been purified but hydration of long-chain enoyl-CoA esters is by the trifunctional protein of β-oxidation (Carpenter et al 1992, Uchida et al 1992).
3-Hydroxyacyl-CoA dehydrogenase	The dehydrogenation of 3-hydroxyacyl-CoA esters to form 3-oxoacyl-CoA esters is catalysed by the 3-hydroxyacyl-CoA dehydrogenases	A short-chain enzyme has been purified. Long-chain 3-hydroxyacyl-CoA dehydrogenase activity is part of the trifunctional protein
3-Oxoacyl-CoA thiolase	These enzymes catalyse the final reaction of β-oxidation, the thiolytic cleavage of 3-oxoacyl-CoA esters, to form acetyl-CoA and an acyl-CoA ester that is shortened by two carbon atoms	The trifunctional enzyme catalyses the thiolysis of long-chain 3-oxoacyl-CoA esters. There appear to be two additional thiolases, a general 3-oxo-acyl-CoA thiolase most active towards medium-chain substrates and an acetoacetyl-CoA-specific thiolase

tion will also be associated with a high concentration of free fatty acids.

The abnormal relationship between metabolic fuels and intermediary metabolites may only occur under conditions of stress. For this reason it is vital that blood samples are obtained when the patient is ill. Furthermore, similar information may be obtained under conditions of 'controlled-stress', e.g. fasting (Bartlett et al 1991), but these studies are potentially dangerous, must only be performed under carefully controlled conditions and are not recommended for patients who give a history of myoglobinuria.

Measurement of carnitine and acylcarnitines. Low blood and tissue carnitine concentration is a common finding in patients with defects of β-oxidation. In primary carnitine deficiency it tends to be profound, often 10% or less of control values. Secondary carnitine deficiency is more common and reflects the mechanism whereby the body copes with abnormal fat metabolism. In the presence of abnormal fatty acid oxidation, acyl-CoA esters which cannot be metabolised accumulate within the mitochondrial matrix. These acyl-CoA esters combine with carnitine (a reaction catalysed by the carnitine acyltransferases) and the carnitine esters are transported out of the mitochondrion. This results in a higher percentage of measured carnitine being present in the acylated form, the excretion of specific acylcarnitines and secondary carnitine deficiency. The presence of specific acylcarnitines in blood and urine can be detected by fast atom bombardment tandem mass spectrometry (Millington et al 1989) and this may be very valuable in the investigation of β-oxidation defects.

Measurement of organic acids and acylglycines in urine. In addition to mitochondrial β-oxidation, fatty acids are also oxidised by omega oxidation in the endoplasmic reticulum and by β-oxidation in peroxisomes. When mitochondrial fatty acid oxidation is impaired, long-chain fatty acids are oxidised by these alternative pathways, generating dicarboxylic acids which are then excreted in the urine. The finding of a marked dicarboxylic aciduria in the absence of significant ketonuria is an important indication of disordered fatty acid oxidation. Diagnosis of defects of mitochondrial β-oxidation on the basis of organic acid findings is difficult, however, since not only may the urinary abnormalities be present intermittently, but the patterns of metabolite excretion may be complex and very variable even within a single disorder (Pollitt 1990). Acyl-CoA esters accumulating in liver mitochondria as a result of abnormal β-oxidation are converted to acylglycines by the action of glycine-N-acylase. The acylglycine formed will depend upon the site of the defect, and determination of the acylglycines in blood and urine may therefore be helpful in the diagnosis of fatty acid oxidation defects (Rinaldo et al 1988).

Measurement of activity of the individual enzymes. Despite advances in the techniques described above, identification of a defect of fatty acid oxidation still requires measurement of enzyme activity. Radiochemical, spectrophotometric and fluorometric assays have been devised to measure all the enzymes involved (Birch-Machin et al 1993), but this remains a difficult process because of the number of enzymes and the lack of commercial availability of some of the substrates.

Molecular studies. Recently, cDNA sequences for several enzymes of mitochondrial fatty acid oxidation have been identified, including CPT II (Finocchiaro et al 1991), the acyl-CoA dehydrogenases (Kelly et al 1987, Naito et al 1989, Indo et al 1991) and electron transfer flavoprotein (ETF) (Finocchiaro et al 1988). This has allowed the molecular characterisation of the deficiency in some patients with fatty acid disorders. Combined with the recent advances in molecular techniques, the identification of the same genetic defect present in many patients can improve the diagnosis and give important information on the incidence of fatty acid oxidation disorders. For example, probably the most common defect of fatty acid oxidation in people of European origin is medium-chain acyl-CoA dehydrogenase (MCAD) deficiency. Approximately 85% of mutant alleles have an A to G transition at position 985 (G985A) of the coding sequence (Fig. 18.8). The prevalence of the G985A mutation in MCAD deficiency has allowed several important observations to be made concerning the incidence of MCAD deficiency and thus of fatty acid oxidation disorders in general. In the UK the carrier frequency is about 1 in 40–68 (Blakemore et al 1991, Matsubara et al 1991) and since MCAD is inherited as an autosomal recessive disorder, the predicted frequency of the disease due to the G985A mutation would be between 1 in 6400 and 1 in 18 500 live births. Since G985A represents only 85% of mutant alleles, the frequency of MCAD deficiency in the population will be higher (Editorial 1991).

Clinical features

Clinical presentation of patients with abnormal fatty acid oxidation falls into two broad categories: those with isolated organ involvement and those with systemic symptoms. Isolated organ involvement most commonly affects skeletal muscle, heart or liver. This commentary will concentrate on the enzyme defects presenting with muscle involvement.

The muscle symptoms in these patients are predominantly of exercise-induced muscle pain and/or muscle weakness. In most patients the muscle pain is associated with prolonged exercise when fatty acids become an essential metabolic fuel. This symptom was thought to be characteristic of CPT deficiency, but recently it has been

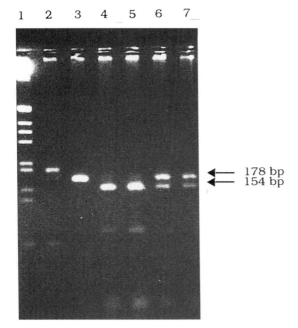

1 2 3 4 5 6 7

←— 178 bp
←— 154 bp

Fig. 18.8 PCR-based test showing the prevalent mutation in medium-chain acyl-CoA dehydrogenase (MCAD) deficiency. Genomic DNA is amplified by PCR; the products are digested with a restriction endonuclease (Ncol) and then separated on the basis of size by agarose gel electrophoresis. All the PCR products contain an Ncol site near one end. Near the other end the PCR primer generates an Ncol site only in alleles with the prevalent mutation (G985A). Lane 1 is a DNA ladder for measuring size. Lane 2 shows the 199 bp PCR product prior to digestion. Lanes 3–7 show PCR products after digestion. In a normal individual (lane 3) the PCR product is cut once, generating a 178 bp fragment. In two siblings with MCAD deficiency (lanes 4 and 5) the PCR product is cut twice leaving a 154 bp fragment. Their parents (lanes 6 and 7) are clearly heterozygous.

shown that other fatty acid oxidation defects may present in an identical manner. In some patients the muscle pain may also be induced by fasting. Defects of fatty acid oxidation may lead to muscle necrosis with rhabdomyolysis and myoglobinuria which may be severe enough to lead to acute renal failure. The muscle weakness in these patients may be severe, especially in young children where it can cause profound hypotonia and difficulty in feeding. In adults it tends to follow a pattern of a proximal myopathy.

Several enzyme defects may present in a similar manner and it is important to use the investigations outlined above to identify the site of the enzyme defect. It is also important to appreciate that the same enzyme defect may present with muscle pain in one patient and profound hypoglycaemia in another. That the variability of clinical presentation may even occur within the same family emphasises the importance of screening other family members once a metabolic defect has been identified.

Carnitine palmitoyltransferase (CPT) deficiency. CPT deficiency was the first defect of fatty acid oxidation to be described (DiMauro & DiMauro 1973). The most common clinical presentation of this deficiency is exercise-induced muscle pain and most patients present between late teenage and 30. The muscle pain is often induced by prolonged exercise, although in some, it is worse following fasting and may be relieved by taking carbohydrates. Myoglobinuria occurs in most patients and may be severe enough to lead to acute renal failure. In approximately 20% of patients mild muscle weakness has been documented. Whilst the majority of affected individuals are male, the pattern of inheritance is autosomal recessive and the biochemical defect involves CPT II. A different presentation of CPT II deficiency has been reported recently with severe disease in infancy (DeMaugre et al 1991, Hug et al 1992). These children all presented in the first few days or months of life with hypoglycaemia, cardiomegaly, hypotonia, renal cysts and fatty infiltration of several organs. The third presentation of CPT deficiency is of recurrent hypoglycaemic episodes in the absence of muscle or other symptoms (DeMaugre et al 1988). The two children described with this presentation have an abnormality of CPT I, and are now symptom-free aged 10 and 11 years.

Primary carnitine deficiency. This condition is due to impaired carnitine transport across the plasma membrane (Treem et al 1988). The majority of patients have presented in childhood (2–7 years) with progressive proximal muscle weakness and hypertrophic cardiomyopathy (Tein et al 1990, Stanley et al 1991). In some, the onset of symptoms is earlier (1–2 years) and in these children hypoglycaemic episodes are common. Primary carnitine deficiency is inherited in an autosomally recessive manner, although one report suggests that a heterozygote may manifest the cardiac symptoms (Garavaglia et al 1991).

Acyl-CoA dehydrogenase deficiency.

Short-chain acyl-CoA dehydrogenase (SCAD) deficiency. SCAD deficiency has been identified in only a few patients and the clinical and laboratory findings are variable. It can present as a severe illness in childhood with poor feeding, hypoglycaemic episodes, vomiting, lethargy, hypotonia and respiratory muscle weakness leading to death in the first few days of life (Amendt et al 1987). Delayed motor development with microcephaly and cognitive impairment were described in another child (Coates et al 1988). These children all had systemic SCAD deficiency. SCAD deficiency limited to skeletal muscle has been described in an adult with slowly progressive muscle weakness (Turnbull et al 1984). It is possible that this patient had a variant of a multiple acyl-CoA dehydrogenation deficiency (see below).

Medium-chain acyl-CoA dehydrogenase (MCAD) deficiency. MCAD deficiency appears to be one of the most common inborn errors of fatty acid oxidation with a proposed incidence of 1 in 6000 to 10 000 in the UK (Editorial 1991). Presentations include acute encephalopathy and hepatomegaly sometimes resembling Reye's syndrome, sudden and unexpected death, near-miss cot death and lipid storage myopathy (Roe & Coates 1989). Symptoms are often precipitated by metabolic stress such as fasting or infection and between episodes patients may be perfectly well. Whilst the majority of cases reported are in young children, patients may present in adult life with muscle pain and rhabdomyolysis.

Long-chain acyl-CoA dehydrogenase (LCAD) deficiency. The majority of patients with LCAD deficiency have presented in the first few months and years of life and the clinical phenotypes may be divided into three groups (Hale et al 1990). The first group is characterised by onset in the first 6 months of life and is associated with a high mortality (Hale et al 1985, Treem et al 1991). Clinical manifestations in this group include severe hypoglycaemic episodes, skeletal muscle weakness, hepatomegaly, cardiomyopathy and sudden infant death. The second group all presented with hypoglycaemic coma associated with fasting. The third group is associated with a later onset (18 months to 20 years), often with an absence of fasting-induced coma, but with a prominence of muscle symptoms including exercise-induced muscle pain and myoglobinuria (Naylor et al 1980). The symptoms in these patients may be very similar to those described for CPT deficiency and the lipid storage in muscle may be mild.

Multiple acyl-CoA dehydrogenase deficiency. A number of patients with low activity of two or more of the acyl-CoA dehydrogenases have been described (Turnbull et al 1988a, DiDonato et al 1989). These patients presented predominantly in their teens or adult life with muscle pain and weakness. Whilst the underlying biochemical abnormality is unknown, these patients often respond to administration of riboflavin with resolution of both their symptoms and the lipid storage myopathy.

Glutaric aciduria Type II.

This condition can be due to a defect of either ETF or ETF: ubiquinone oxidoreductase. Presentation ranges from the severe with multiple congenital abnormalities and death within the first few weeks of life to episodic hypoglycaemia, acidosis and hepatomegaly in children (Loehr et al 1990). Some individuals present later with muscle weakness associated with lipid storage (Dusheicko et al 1979, Turnbull et al 1988b).

Long-chain 3-hydroxyacyl-CoA dehydrogenase/trifunctional enzyme deficiency.

This recently described enzyme has been associated with a similar range of disease to that described above. Symptoms include non-ketotic hypoglycaemia, sudden infant death, cardiomyopathy, hepatomegaly, sensorimotor polyneuropathy and muscle weakness (Jackson et al 1991). Interestingly, patients deficient in one or more components of the enzyme often have elevated lactate levels and in one instance pigmentary retinopathy. Muscle weakness has been described in several children and has been associated with myoglobinuria and respiratory failure (Jackson et al 1992).

Treatment

Fatty acid oxidation defects can often be treated successfully if recognised at an early stage.

Clearly, this is dependent on clinical recognition of the syndromes and an ability to identify a defect. The therapy for these conditions is divided into the following:

1. Diet. In all patients with mitochondrial β-oxidation defects it is vital to provide sufficient calories as carbohydrate and to ensure that prolonged fasting does not occur. This is particularly important for infants and young children who may die suddenly if prolonged fasting occurs. Thus, overnight fasts should be avoided and adequate carbohydrate intake maintained during intercurrent infection. Episodes of hypoglycaemia must be treated immediately with intravenous glucose infusions aimed at completely suppressing lipolysis. A low-fat, high-carbohydrate diet is recommended for most patients, although medium-chain triglycerides are helpful for patients with defects of long-chain specific enzymes. For instance, in a patient with trifunctional enzyme deficiency a diet including medium-chain triglycerides contributed to improvement in muscle

strength and cardiac function (Jackson et al 1991).

2. Carnitine. Administration of L-carnitine (100 mg/kg/day in children) to patients with primary carnitine deficiency results in marked improvement in muscle strength and cardiac function (Stanley et al 1991). Carnitine supplementation also improves the metabolic response to fasting in these children. It has been proposed that carnitine therapy is of benefit in the treatment of other patients with β-oxidation defects by correcting the secondary carnitine deficiency which develops.

3. Riboflavin. Riboflavin is the precursor of FAD, the coenzyme essential as a prosthetic group for ETF, ETF : ubiquinone oxidoreductase and the acyl-CoA dehydrogenases. Some patients with multiple acyl-CoA dehydrogenase deficiency and some with apparent glutaric aciduria Type II have responded to pharmacological doses of riboflavin (100–300 mg per day) (Turnbull et al 1988b, DiDonato et al 1989).

REFERENCES

Ackrell B A C, Johnson M K, Gunsalus R P, Cecchini G 1992 Structure and function of succinate dehydrogenase and fumarate reductase. In: Muller F (ed) Chemistry and biochemistry of flavoproteins, vol 3. CRC Press, Boca Raton, Florida, p 229

Amendt B A, Green C, Sweetman L et al 1987 Short-chain acyl-coenzyme A dehydrogenase deficiency: clinical and biochemical studies in two patients. Journal of Clinical Investigation 79: 1303

Anderson S, Bankier A T, Barrell B G et al 1981 Sequence organisation of the human mitochondrial genome. Nature 290: 457

Argov Z, Bank W J, Maris J et al 1986 Treatment of mitochondrial myopathy due to complex III deficiency with vitamins K₃ and C: a ³¹P-NMR follow-up study. Annals of Neurology 19: 598

Arnaudo E, Dalakis M, Shanske S, Moraes C T, DiMauro S, Schon E A 1991 Depletion of muscle mitochondrial DNA in AIDS patients with zidovudine-induced myopathy. Lancet 337: 508

Arnold D L, Taylor D J, Radda G K 1985 Investigation of human mitochondrial myopathies by phosphorus magnetic spectroscopy. Annals of Neurology 18: 189

Bardosi A, Creutzfeldt W, DiMauro S et al 1987 Myo-, neuro-, gastro-intestinal encephalopathy (MNGIE syndrome) due to partial deficiency of cytochrome c oxidase. Acta Neuropathologica (Berlin) 74: 248

Bartlett K, Aynsley-Green A, Leonard J V, Turnbull D M 1991 Inherited disorders of mitochondrial β-oxidation. In: Schob J, Van Hoof F, Vis H L (eds) Nestle nutrition workshop series, vol 24, inborn errors of metabolism. Vevey/Raven Press, New York, p 19

Beckmann J D, Frerman F E 1985 Electron transfer oxidoreductase from pig liver: purification and molecular, redox and catalytic properties. Biochemistry 24: 3913

Bindoff L A, Turnbull D M 1990 Defects of the respiratory chain. In: Harris J B, Turnbull D M (eds) Metabolic myopathies. Baillière-Tindall, p 583

Birch-Machin M A, Jackson S, Singh Kler R, Turnbull D M 1993 Study of skeletal muscle mitochondrial dysfunction. Methods in Toxicology 2: 51–69

Birch-Machin M A, Shepherd I M, Watmough N J et al 1989 Fatal lactic acidosis in infancy with a defect of complex III of the respiratory chain. Paediatric Research 25: 553

Blakemore A I F, Singleton H, Pollitt R J et al 1991 Frequency of the G985 MCAD mutation in the general population. Lancet 337: 298

Capaldi R A 1990 Structure and assembly of cytochrome c oxidase. Archives of Biochemistry and Biophysics 280: 252

Carpenter K, Pollitt R J, Middleton B 1992 Human liver long-chain 3-hydroxyacyl-coenzyme A dehydrogenase is a multifunctional membrane-bound β-oxidation enzyme of mitochondria. Biochemical and Biophysical Research Communications 183: 443

Chomyn A, Meola G, Bresolin N, Lai S T, Scarlato G, Attardi G 1991 In vitro genetic transfer of protein synthesis and respiration defect to mitochondrial DNA-less cells with myopathy-patient mitochondria. Molecular and Cellular Biology 11: 2236

Ciafaloni E, Ricci E, Shanske S et al 1992 MELAS: clinical features, biochemistry, and molecular genetics. Annals of Neurology 31: 391

Coates P M, Hale D E, Finocchiaro G, Tanaka K, Winter S C 1988 Genetic deficiency of short-chain acyl-coenzyme A dehydrogenase in cultured fibroblasts from a patient with muscle carnitine deficiency and severe skeletal muscle weakness. Journal of Clinical Investigation 81: 171

DeMaugre F, Bonnefont J P, Mitchell G et al 1988 Hepatic and muscular presentations of carnitine palmitoyltransferase deficiency: two distinct entities. Pediatric Research 24: 308

DeMaugre F, Bonnefont J P, Colonna M, Cepanec C, Leroux J-P, Saudubray J-M 1991 Infantile form of carnitine palmitoyltransferase II deficiency with hepatomuscular symptoms and sudden death. Journal of Clinical Investigation 87: 859

DiDonato S, Gellera C, Peluchetti D et al 1989 Normalization of short-chain acyl-coenzyme A dehydrogenase after riboflavin treatment in a girl with multiple acylcoenzyme A dehydrogenase-deficient myopathy. Annals of Neurology 25: 479

DiMauro S, Nicholson J F, Hays A P et al 1983 Benign infantile mitochondrial myopathy due to reversible cytochrome c oxidase deficiency. Annals of Neurology 14: 226

DiMauro S, DiMauro P P 1973 Muscle carnitine palmitoyltransferase deficiency and myoglobinuria. Science 182: 929

DiMauro S, Zeviani M, Servidei S et al 1986 Cytochrome c oxidase deficiency: clinical and biochemical heterogeneity. Annals of the New York Academy of Sciences 488: 19

Dusheiko G, Kew M G, Joffe B I, Lewin J R, Mantagos S, Tanaka K 1979 Recurrent hypoglycaemia associated with glutaric aciduria type II in an adult. New England Journal of Medicine 301: 1405

Editorial 1991 Medium-chain acyl-CoA dehydrogenase deficiency. Lancet i: 544

Finocchiaro G, Ito M, Tanaka K 1987 Purification and properties of short-chain acyl-CoA, medium-chain acyl-CoA and isovaleryl-CoA dehydrogenases from human liver. Journal of Biological Chemistry 262: 9782

Finocchiaro G, Ito M, Ikeda Y, Tanaka K 1988 Molecular cloning and nucleotide sequence of cDNA encoding the α-subunit of human electron transfer flavoprotein. Journal of Biological Chemistry 263: 15773

Finocchiaro G, Taroni F, Rocchi M et al 1991 cDNA cloning, sequence analysis, and chromosomal localisation of human carnitine palmitoyltransferase. Proceedings of the National Academy of Science USA 88: 661

Garavaglia B, Uziel G, Dworzak F, Carrara F, DiDonato S 1991 Primary carnitine deficiency: heterozygote and intrafamilial phenotypic variation. Neurology 41: 1691

Goto Y-I, Nonaka I, Horai S 1990 A mutation in the tRNA$^{Leu(UUR)}$ gene associated with the MELAS subgroup of mitochondrial encephalopathies. Nature 348: 651

Hale D E, Batshaw M L, Coates P M et al 1985 Long-chain acyl coenzyme A dehydrogenase deficiency: an inherited cause of nonketotic hypoglycaemia. Pediatric Research 19: 666

Hale D E, Stanley C A, Coates P M 1990 The long-chain acyl-CoA dehydrogenase deficiency. In: Tanaka K, Coates P M (eds) Fatty acid oxidation: clinical, biochemical and molecular aspects. Alan R Liss, New York, p 303

Hammans S R, Sweeney M G, Brockington M, Morgan-Hughes J A, Harding A E 1991 Mitochondrial encephalopathies: molecular genetic analysis from blood samples. Lancet 337: 1311

Harding A E, Petty R K H, Morgan-Hughes J A 1988 Mitochondrial myopathy: a genetic study of 71 cases. Journal of Medical Genetics 25: 528

Harding A E, Holt I J, Sweeney M G, Brockington M, Davis M B 1992 Prenatal diagnosis of mitochondrial DNA$^{8993T→G}$ disease. American Journal of Human Genetics 50: 629

Hartl F-U, Neupert W 1990 Protein sorting to mitochondria: evolutionary conservations of folding and assembly. Science 247: 930

Holt I J, Harding A E, Morgan-Hughes 1988 Deletions of muscle mitchondrial DNA in patients with mitochondrial myopathies. Nature 331: 717

Holt I J, Harding A E, Petty R K H, Morgan-Hughes J A 1990 A new mitochondrial disease associated with mitochondrial DNA heteroplasmy. American Journal of Human Genetics 46: 428

Howell N, Bindoff L A, McCullough D A et al 1991 Leber's hereditary optic neuropathy: identification of the same ND1 mutation in six pedigrees. American Journal of Human Genetics 49: 939

Hug G, Bove K E, Solikup S 1992 Lethal neonatal multiorgan deficiency of carnitine palmitoyltransferase II. New England Journal of Medicine 325: 1862

Indo Y, Yang-Feng T, Glassberg R, Tanaka K 1991 Molecular cloning and nucleotide sequence of cDNA encoding human long-chain acyl-CoA dehydrogenase and assignment of the location of its gene (ACADL) to chromosome 2. Genomics 11: 609

Izai K, Uchida Y, Orii T, Yamamoto S, Hashimoto T 1992 Novel fatty acid β-oxidation enzymes in rat liver mitochondria. I Purification and properties of very-long-chain acyl-coenzyme A dehydrogenase. Journal of Biological Chemistry 267: 1027

Jackson S, Bartlett K, Land J, Moxon E R, Pollitt R J, Leonard J V, Turnbull D M 1991 Long-chain 3-hydroxyacyl-7-CoA dehydrogenase deficiency. Pediatric Research 29: 406

Jackson S, Singh Kler R, Bartlett K et al 1992 Combined enzyme defect of mitochondrial fatty acid oxidation. Journal of Clinical Investigation 90: 1219

Johnson M A 1991 Cytochemical and immunocytochemical investigation of respiratory chain complexes in individual fibres of human skeletal muscle. In: Gorrod J W, Albano O, Ferrari E, Papa S (eds) Molecular basis of neurological disorders and their treatment. Chapman and Hall, London, p 40

Johnson M A, Bindoff L A, Turnbull D M 1993 Cytochrome c oxidase activity in single muscle fibres: assay techniques and diagnostic applications. Annals of Neurology 33: 28–35

Kelly D P, Kim J-J, Billadello J J, Hainline B E, Chu T W, Strauss A W 1987 Nucleotide sequence of medium-chain acyl-CoA dehydrogenase mRNA and its expression in enzyme-deficient human tissue. Proceedings of the National Academy of Sciences USA 84: 4068

King M P, Attardi G 1989 Human cells lacking mtDNA: repopulation with exogenous mitochondria by complementation. Science 246: 500

Larsson N-G, Holme E, Kristiansson B, Oldfors A, Tulinius M 1990 Progressive increase of the mutated mitochondrial DNA fraction in Kearns–Sayre syndrome. Pediatric Research 28: 13

Loehr J P, Goodman S I, Frerman F E 1990 Glutaric acidemia type II: Heterogeneity of clinical and biochemical phenotypes. Pediatric Research 27: 311

Londesborough J C, Webster J R 1974 Fatty acyl-CoA synthetases. In: Boyer P D (ed) The enzymes. Academic, New York 10: 469

Luft R, Ikkos D, Palmieri G, Ernster L, Afzelius B 1962 A case of severe hypermetabolism of non-thyroid origin with a defect in the maintenance of mitochondrial respiratory control: a correlated clinical, biochemical and morphological study. Journal of Clinical Investigation 41: 1776

McKean M C, Beckmann J D, Frerman F E 1983 Subunit structure of electron transfer flavoprotein. Journal of Biological Chemistry 258: 1866

Matsubara Y, Narisawa K, Tada K et al 1991 Prevalence of K329E mutation in medium-chain acyl-CoA dehydrogenase gene determined from Guthrie cards. Lancet 338: 552

Matthew P M, Tampieri D, Berkovic S F et al 1991 Magnetic resonance imaging shows specific abnormalities in the Melas syndrome. Neurology 41: 1043

Millington D S, Norwood D K, Kodo N, Roe C R, Inoue F 1989 Application of fast atom bombardment with tandem mass spectrometry and liquid chromatography/mass spectrometry to the analysis of acylcarnitines in human urine, blood and tissue. Analytical Biochemistry 180: 331

Mita S, Schmidt B, Schon E A et al 1989 Detection of 'deleted' mitochondrial genomes in cytochrome c oxidase deficient muscle fibres of a patient with Kearns–Sayre syndrome. Proceedings of the National Academy of Science USA 86: 9509

Moraes C T, DiMauro S, Zeviani M et al 1989 Mitochondrial DNA deletions in progressive external ophthalmoplegia and Kearns–Sayre syndrome. New England Journal of Medicine 320: 1293

Moraes C T, Shanske S, Tritschler H-J et al 1991 Mitochondrial DNA depletion with variable tissue specificity: a novel genetic abnormality in mitochondrial diseases. American Journal of Human Genetics 48: 492

Moreadith R W, Batshaw M L, Ohnishi T et al 1984 Deficiency of the iron-sulphur clusters of mitochondrial reduced nicotinamide-adenine dinucleotide-ubiquinone oxidoreductase (complex I) in an infant with congenital lactic acidosis. Journal of Clinical Investigation 74: 685

Naito E, Indo Y, Tanaka K 1989 Molecular cloning and nucleotide sequence of complementary cDNAs encoding human short-chain acyl-Coenzyme A dehydrogenase and the study of the molecular basis of human short-chain acyl-Coenzyme A dehydrogenase deficiency. Journal of Clinical Investigation 83: 1605

Naylor E W, Mosovich L L, Guthrie R, Evans J E, Tieckelmann H 1980 Intermittent non-ketotic dicarboxylic aciduria in two siblings with hypoglycaemia: an apparent defect in β-oxidation of fatty acids. Journal of Inherited Metabolic Disease 3: 19

Ogasahara S, Nihikawa Y, Yoritugi S et al 1986 Treatment of Kearns–Sayre syndrome with coenzyme Q_{10}. Neurology 36: 45

Ogasahara S, Engel A G, Frens D, Mack D 1989 Muscle coenzyme Q deficiency in familial mitochondrial encephalomyopathy. Proceedings of the National Academy of Sciences USA 86: 2379

Olsen W, Engel W K, Walsh G O, Einangler R 1972 Oculocraniosomatic neuromuscular disease with 'ragged-red' fibres. Archives of Neurology 26: 193

Pande S V 1975 A mitochondrial carnitine acyltransferase translocase system. Proceedings of the National Academy of Sciences USA 72: 883

Pollitt R J 1990 Clinical and biochemical presentations in twenty cases of hydroxydicarboxylic aciduria. In: Tanaka K & Coates P M (eds) Fatty acid oxidation: clinical, biochemical and molecular aspects. Alan R Liss, New York, pp 495–502

Poulton J, Deadman M E, Gardiner R M 1989 Duplications of mitochondrial DNA in mitochondrial myopathy. Lancet i: 236

Rinaldo P, O'Shea J J, Coates P M, Hale D E, Stanley C A, Tanaka K 1988 Medium-chain acyl-CoA dehydrogenase deficiency: diagnosis by stable isotope dilution measurement of urinary n-hexanoylglycine and 3-phenylpropionylglycine. New England Journal of Medicine 319: 1308

Roe C R, Coates P M 1989 Acyl-CoA dehydrogenase deficiencies. In: Scriver C R, Beaudet A L, Sly W S, Valle D (eds) The metabolic basis of inherited disease. McGraw Hill, New York, p 889

Rötig A, Colonna M, Bonnefont J P et al 1989 Mitochondrial DNA deletion in Pearson's marrow/pancreas syndrome. Lancet i: 902

Schon E A, Rizzuto R, Moraes C T et al 1989 A direct repeat is a hot spot for large-scale deletion of human mitochondrial DNA. Science 244: 346

Senior A E 1988 ATP synthesis by oxidative phosphorylation. Physiological Review 68: 177

Sherratt H S A, Turnbull D M 1990 Mitochondrial oxidations and ATP synthesis in muscle. In: Harris J B, Turnbull D M (eds) Metabolic myopathies. Baillière-Tindall, London, p 523

Shoffner J M, Lott M T, Lezza A M S et al 1990 Myoclonic epilepsy and ragged-red fibre disease (MERRF) is associated with a mitochondrial DNA tRNA[Lys] mutation. Cell 61: 931

Shy G M, Gonatas N K, Perez M 1966 Two childhood myopathies with abnormal mitochondria. I Megaconial myopathy. II Pleoconial myopathy. Brain 89: 133

Stanley C A, Deleeuw S, Coates P M et al 1991 Chronic cardiomyopathy and weakness or acute coma in children with a defect in carnitine uptake. Annals of Neurology 30: 709

Tatuch Y, Christodoulou J, Feigenbaum A et al 1992 Heteroplasmic mtDNA mutation (T-G) at 8993 can cause Leigh disease when the percentage of abnormal mtDNA is high. American Journal of Human Genetics 50: 842

Tein I, DeVivo D C, Bierman F et al 1990 Impaired fibroblast carnitine upake in primary systemic carnitine deficiency manifested by childhood carnitine responsive cardiomyopathy. Pediatric Research 28: 247

Treem W R, Stanley C A, Finegold D N, Hale D E, Coates P M 1988 Primary carnitine deficiency due to a failure of carnitine transport in kidney, muscle and fibroblasts. New England Journal of Medicine 319: 1331

Treem W R, Stanley C A, Hale D E, Leopold H B, Hyams J S 1991 Hypoglycaemia, hypotonia and cardiomyopathy: the evolving clinical picture of long-chain acyl-CoA dehydrogenase deficiency. Pediatrics 87: 328

Tritschler H J, Bonilla E, Lombes A et al 1992 Differential diagnosis of fatal and benign cytochrome c oxidase-deficient myopathies of infancy: an immunological approach. Neurology 41: 300

Turnbull D M, Bartlett K, Stevens D L, Alberti K G M M et al 1984 Short-chain acyl-CoA dehydrogenase deficiency associated with a lipid-storage myopathy and secondary carnitine deficiency. New England Journal of Medicine 311: 1232

Turnbull D M, Shepherd I M, Ashworth B et al 1988a Lipid storage myopathy associated with low acyl-CoA dehydrogenase activities. Brain 111: 815

Turnbull D M, Bartlett K, Eyre J A et al 1988b Lipid storage myopathy due to glutaric aciduria type II: treatment of a potentially fatal myopathy. Developmental Medicine Child Neurology 30: 667

Uchida Y, Izai K, Orii T, Hashimoto T 1992 Novel fatty acid β-oxidation enzymes in rat liver mitochondria, II. Purification and properties of enoyl-Coenzyme A (CoA) hydratase/3-hydroxyacyl-CoA dehydrogenase/3-ketoacyl-CoA thiolase trifunctional protein. Journal of Biological Chemistry 267: 1034

Wallace D C, Singh G, Lo H M T et al 1988 Mitochondrial DNA mutation associated with Leber's hereditary optic neuropathy. Science 242: 1427

Watmough N J, Bindoff L A, Birch-Machin M A et al 1990 Impaired mitochondrial β-oxidation in a patient with an abnormality of the respiratory chain: studies in skeletal muscle mitochondria. Journal of Clinical Investigation 85: 177

Weiss H 1987 Structure of mitochondrial ubiquinol–cytochrome c reductase (complex III). Current Topics in Bioenergetics 15: 67

Weiss H, Friedrich T, Hofhaus G, Preis D 1991 The respiratory chain NADH dehydrogenase (complex I) of mitochondria. European Journal of Biochemistry 197: 563

Woeltje K F, Esser V, Weis B C et al 1990 Inter-tissue and inter-species characteristics of the mitochondrial carnitine palmitoyltransferase system. Journal of Biological Chemistry 265: 10714

Zeviani M, Gellera C, Antozzi C et al 1989 Maternally inherited myopathy and cardiomyopathy: association with mutation in mitochondrial DNA tRNA Leu(UUR). Lancet 338: 143

19. Involvement of human muscle by parasites

C. A. Pallis   P. D. Lewis

INTRODUCTION

A large body of data concerning parasitic involvement of human muscle is available to workers in tropical medicine and related fields. In this review we have attempted to summarise this information, emphasising features — both clinical and pathological — of relevance to neurological practice.

Muscle lesions (of varying severity and clinical relevance) are encountered in at least four protozoal diseases of man (toxoplasmosis, sarcosporidiosis, African and American trypanosomiasis). The larval stages of the life cycle of at least five cestodes (tapeworms) may develop in human muscle and result in conditions known as cysticercosis, coenurosis, unilocular and alveolar hydatidosis, and sparganosis. Finally the larvae of various nematodes may be found in muscle, causing diseases such as trichinosis and toxocariasis. In the following short accounts of these conditions parasitological and epidemiological data are kept to a minimum, and the clinical accounts emphasise muscle involvement. The parasitic disorders which may affect muscle are summarised in Table 19.1.

PROTOZOAL DISORDERS

Sarcosporidiosis and toxoplasmosis

Protozoal parasites of the class Sporozoasida may be found in the striated muscle of many mammals and birds: amongst the creatures recorded in 1990 as being infected were cougars, ibex, raccoons, a grand electus parrot and a Moluccan cockatoo. Such parasites have also occasionally been reported in man. They are given the generic name *Sarcocystis*. The muscle lesions are known as sar-

Table 19.1 Some clinical and pathological features of parasitic involvement of human muscle*

Parasite	Refs†	Disease	Weakness	Wasting	Pain	Tenderness	Nodules	Local mass	Diffuse enlargement	Cardiac muscle involvement	Systemic illness	Calcification in muscle	Parasites in muscle fibres	Parasites between fibres	Diffuse inflammatory change	Abscesses	Inflammatory cell aggregates without parasites	'Tracks' in muscle	Involvement of central nervous system	Comments
1. Protozoa																				
Toxoplasma gondii	1–5	Toxoplasmosis	o	o	o	o	o	o	o	+	+	o	+	o	+	o	+	o	+	Possible relation to polymyositis
Sarcocystis lindemanni	6–11	Sarcosporidiosis	[±]	[±]	[±]	[±]	o	o	o	+	o	o	+	o	+	o	+	o	+	Sarcocysts. Possible relation to polymyositis
Trypanosoma gambiense	12–16	African trypanosomiasis	+	+	o	o	o	o	o	+	+	o	o	o	+	o	+	o	+	Not known in what proportions terminal weakness and wasting are 'myopathic', 'neuropathic' or 'cachectic'
Trypanosoma cruzi	17–18	American trypanosomiasis (Chagas' disease)	o	o	o	o	o	o	o	+	+	o	+	o	+	o	+	o	+	Leishmanial phase in muscle 'pseudocysts'
2. Cestodes																				
Taenia solium	19–25	Cysticercosis	[±]	o	[±]	[±]	+	o	[++]	+	[±]	+	o	+	[±]	o	±	o	+	Occasional weakness, pain and tenderness (in pseudohypertrophic type only)
Multiceps brauni	26–30	Coenurosis of muscle	o	o	o	o	o	+	o	o	o	o	o	+	[±]	o	[+]	o	o	Cerebral coenurosis is due to a different species (*M. multiceps*)
Echinococcus granulosus	31–37	Unilocular hydatidosis	o	o	[+]	o	o	+	o	+	+	+	+	+	o	o	[+]	o	+	Rupture may cause severe pain and oedema
Echinococcus multilocularis	38–40	Alveolar hydatidosis	o	o	[+]	[+]	o	[+]	o	−	[+]	o	−	+	+	[+]	−	o	+	No capsule. Locally invasive. May metastasise
Spirometra mansonoides, erinacei	41–46	Sparganosis	o	o	+	+	o	+	o	o	o	o	o	+	+	+	+	+	+	Local mass may be mobile
3. Nematodes																				
Trichinella spiralis	47–55	Trichinosis	[++]	o	++	++	o	o	[+]	+	[++]	o	+	o	++	o	+	o	+	Profuse fibrillation (intracellular parasite 'denervates' part of muscle fibre). Calcification, visible microscopically, *not* visible radiologically
Toxocara canis T. cati	56–58	Toxocariasis (visceral larva migrans)	o	o	[±]	o	o	o	o	[+]	+	o	o	+	+	o	+	+	+	Possible relation to 'eosinophilic myositis'

Table 19.1 *Contd*

Parasite	Refs†	Disease	Weakness	Wasting	Pain	Tenderness	Nodules	Local mass	Diffuse enlargement	Cardiac muscle involvement	Systemic illness	Calcification in muscle	Parasites in muscle fibres	Parasites between fibres	Diffuse inflammatory change	Abscesses	Inflammatory cell aggregates without parasites	'Tracks' in muscle	Involvement of central nervous system	Comments
Ascaris lumbricoides A. sui, A. devosi, A. columnaris Neoascaris vitulorum Parascaris equorum Toxascaris leonina T. transfuga	59–60	? Visceral larva migrans	o	o	o	o	o	o	o	o	+	o	o	+	+	o	+	[+]	o	Doubtful involvement of nervous system (? coincidental toxocariasis)

*Decreasing degrees of severity are indicated on a scale ranging from + + to±. Absence of a feature is shown by o. Parentheses indicate that a particular feature has occasionally been reported. The absence of a symbol implies that information was not available to us.

†*References* (key references are italicised).
[1]Faust et al 1975. [2]Frenkel 1973. [3]Kagan et al 1974. [4]Rabinowicz 1971. [5]Samuels & Rietschel 1976. [6]Kean & Breslau 1964. [7]Jeffery 1974. [8]Liu & Roberts 1965. [9]Markus et al 1974. [10]McGill & Goodbody 1957. [11]Pamphlett & O'Donoghue 1990. [12]Goodwin 1970. [13]Janssen et al 1956. [14]Koten & de Raadt 1969. [15]Losos & Idede 1972. [16]Poltera et al 1977. [17]Faust et al 1970. [18]Köberle 1968. [19]Dixon & Lipscomb 1961. [20]Jacob & Mathew 1968. [21]Jolly & Pallis 1971. [22]MacArthur 1950. [23]McGill 1948. [24]Sawhney et al 1976. [25]Slais 1970. [26]Fain 1956. [27]Orihel et al 1970. [28]Raper & Dockeray 1956. [29]Templeton 1968. [30]Wilson et al 1972. [31]Arana-Iñiguez 1978. [32]Blanco et al 1949. [33]Dévé 1936. [34]Dévé 1949. [35]Dew 1951. [36]Lorenzetti 1962. [37]Pearson & Rose 1960. [38]Abuladze 1964. [39]Hunter et al 1976. [40]Schimrigk & Emser 1978. [41]Ali-Khan et al 1973. [42]Cho & Patel 1978. [43]Mueller 1938. [44]Mueller et al 1963. [45]Nakamura et al 1990. [46]Wirth & Farrow 1961. [47]Brashear et al 1971. [48]Davis et al 1976. [49]Despommier et al 1975. [50]Drachman & Tuncbay 1965. [51]Gould 1954. [52]Gould 1970. [53]Gross & Ochoa 1979. [54]Marcus & Miller 1955. [55]Stoll 1947. [56]Beaver et al 1952. [57]Dent et al 1956. [58]Woodruff 1970. [59]Nichols 1956. [60]Sprent 1965.

cocysts. *Sarcocystis* and certain species of *Isospora* are probably different stages in the life cycle of the same parasite.

Carnivorism is important in the transmission of this infection. It is believed that the life cycle involves two vertebrate hosts: a 'prey' (ungulates, rodents, birds, etc.) and a 'predator' (dog, cat, cheetah, etc.). The prey is infected by eating sporocysts passed in the faeces of the predator. Asexual multiplication takes place in the lymphoid cells of the prey. When predator eats prey, sexual reproduction of the parasite takes place in the intestinal submucosa of the predator and free sporocysts are discharged into the lumen of the gut. There is thus a biologically intriguing alternation of generations in two different vertebrate hosts. Man's fate is sometimes to act as an *Isospora*-passing predator, sometimes as a sarco-cyst-ridden prey. The sporocysts most readily available to modern man for ingestion are probably those in his own faeces.

Sarcocysts are cylindrical bodies, usually 400–1000 μm in length and about 100 μm in diameter. They are sometimes much longer and may then be visible to the naked eye as minute white threads. *Sarcocystis lindemanii* (the species found in man) may produce cysts 5 cm long. These cylindrical structures (sometimes referred to as Miescher's tubes) have a hyaline, radially striated limiting membrane, from which septa arise (Fig. 19.1). These divide the tube into compartments containing round, oval or sickle-shaped bodies, 12–16 μm long and 4–10 μm wide, called sporozoites or 'Rainey's corpuscles'. Microscopic calcification may occur (Greve 1985), but this is never radiologically evident. Electron-microscopic

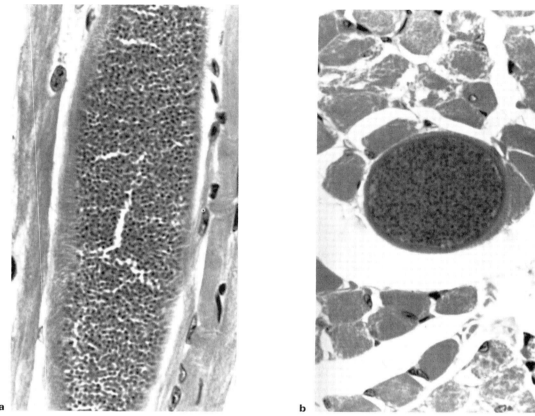

Fig. 19.1   Sarcocysts in muscle. **a** Longitudinal section. Radial striations of the limiting membrane are clearly visible. **b** Transverse section (H & E × 600).

findings have been described by Pamphlett & O'Donoghue (1990).

The only other parasite forming morphologically similar structures in human muscle is *Toxoplasma gondii*. Differentiation is based on the length and diameter of the cysts (smaller in toxoplasmosis), on the thickness and striations of the capsule, on the division of the cyst by septa, and on the size of the sporozoites (more than twice as large in sarcosporidiosis).

Patients have occasionally presented with features conceivably related to the presence of parasites in muscle. Thus Liu & Roberts (1965) described a patient with a chronic, painful, indurated area of the chest wall. This was excised and showed sarcocysts, surrounded by areas of lymphocytic and eosinophilic cellular infiltration, giant cells and interstitial fibrosis. Jeffery (1974) reviewed the

whole subject of human sarcosporidiosis in some detail. His report included the description of a 21-year-old Gurkha soldier presenting with a painful lump in the thigh. Necrotic muscle tissue was evacuated and sarcocysts were found in an area of relatively unaffected muscle taken from the periphery of the lesion.

Rarely sarcosporidiosis is found in association with other disease (see e.g. McGill & Goodbody 1957, Agarwal & Srivastava 1983). However the weight of evidence suggests coincidence rather than a causal relationship; human sarcosporidiosis is generally an asymptomatic disorder.

African trypanosomiasis

African trypanosomiasis is transmitted by the 'bite' of tsetse flies of the genus *Glossina*. These act as biological vectors: part of the life cycle of the parasite takes place in their tissues.

The trypanosomes (*T. rhodesiense* and *T. gambiense*) multiply in the gut of the fly, but do not involve cells. Crithidial forms metamorphose into metacyclic (infective) trypanosomes. It is this form which is 'injected' when man is 'bitten'.

Myositis is a feature of trypanosomal infections in rats (Losos & Idede 1972). Patients with African trypanosomiasis may show gross muscle wasting, but this could be largely 'cachectic' in origin (many patients dying of this disease have concomitant illnesses such as tuberculosis). It is possible, however, that the wasting may sometimes be due to primary changes in muscle (perhaps immunologically induced). Occasionally it may even be neurogenic. Examination of skeletal muscle has seldom been carried out. Lesions of spinal roots have been reported (Janssen et al 1956, Poltera et al 1977). In the otherwise very detailed study by the latter group of workers, systematic investigation of skeletal muscle was undertaken in only one instance, samples being obtained from the upper and lower limbs, the recti abdominis and the diaphragm. The striated muscles showed atrophic fibres, sometimes accompanied by a patchy chronic cellular infiltration. There were eosinophilic degenerative changes of variable severity. The changes were most marked in the diaphragm. The illustrated appearance was not that of neural atrophy. Further studies are needed.

American trypanosomiasis

American trypanosomiasis (caused by *Trypanosoma cruzi*) is transmitted through the infected faeces, deposited on human skin, of several species of reduviid or triatomine bugs which 'bite' and defaecate after feeding. Opossums, armadillos, wood and water rats and raccoons act as natural reservoirs. The spread of the disease to man is related to the adaptation of the vector bugs to living and breeding in and around primitive rural habitations. Man himself then becomes an important reservoir host.

Many infections are clinically silent. Swelling is an early local response to the inoculation of infective material and may characteristically involve one eye and one side of the face. There may be generalised lymphadenopathy, fever and malaise. Trypanosomal forms of the parasite are present in the blood during this stage.

The parasites show a predilection for cells of neuroectodermal or mesenchymal origin (cardiac and skeletal muscle, and lymphoid cells). There may be early myocarditis or meningoencephalitis. In infected cells the organism goes into a leishmanial phase (unlike what happens in African trypanosomiasis). The *Leishmania* multiply by binary fission, distend the cell, and produce a leishmanial pseudocyst. Cyst rupture releases crithidial and further trypanosomal forms which re-enter the circulation causing febrile relapses. Death of intracellular *Leishmania* produces an inflammatory reaction, which may be severe in non-immune individuals.

Skeletal muscle involvement may be florid but is usually asymptomatic. Chronic myocarditis is common. Chronic Chagas' disease is a late complication. It is characterised by megacolon and megaoesophagus, brought about by lesions of the intrinsic autonomic innervation of the gastrointestinal tract. Pathogenetic mechanisms are still poorly understood.

CESTODES

Cysticercosis

Man is the only definitive host of the cestodes *Taenia solium* and *Taenia saginata*. Ripe proglottids are shed in human faeces. The ova released are consumed by an intermediate host. The pig (occasionally sheep, bears, cats, dogs and monkeys) has this role in the *T. solium* cycle. Various bovidae are involved in the life cycle of *T. saginata*.

The embryos, freed in the gut of the intermediate host, burrow through the intestinal mucosa and spread widely via mesenteric venules and lymphatic channels, to skeletal and cardiac muscle, the nervous system and other tissues where, within 2–3 months, they develop into infective bladder worms or cysticerci. The larval forms of *T. solium* and *T. saginata* are known respectively as *Cysticercus cellulosae* and *Cysticercus bovis*. These forms were recognised and named before their relationship to their parent worms was recognised. The pseudo-generic names have no taxonomic significance.

When parasitised undercooked pork or beef is eaten by man, the scolex (head) of the cysticercus evaginates like the finger of a glove and attaches to the gut wall. The human host then develops an adult tapeworm, *not* cysticercosis. The point needs emphasis as it is still widely misunderstood.

Probably the only way in which man can contract *cysticercosis* is by doing what the pig normally does, i.e. by eating *T. solium* ova (his own or someone else's—usually the latter). It should be noted, that, for reasons that are poorly understood, the ingestion by man of the ova of *T. saginata* hardly ever produces cysticercosis.

T. solium taeniasis has virtually disappeared from Europe. The same has happened in many other places. In the Middle East, Muslim Africa, and Indonesia it was always a very rare or non-existent condition because of religious practices which forbid the consumption of pork. Human cysticercosis continues to occur, however, in India, Mongolia, Korea, China, Central and South American and South Africa (Slais 1970).

Muscle involvement. Involvement of the central nervous system in cysticercosis is common and will not be discussed further. Involvement of skeletal muscle has been known since the condition was first recognised. In early accounts it was thought to be rare, but is now known to be common. There was positive evidence of such invasion in 429 of the 450 cases of cysticercosis surveyed by Dixon & Lipscomb (1961). Its morbid anatomy is well described in standard textbooks and articles (MacArthur 1950, Trelles & Trelles 1978 and notably by Slais 1970).

Pseudohypertrophic myopathy. Although it had been described earlier, pseudohypertrophic myopathy in cysticercosis was first drawn to the attention of neurologists by Jacob & Mathew in 1968. In 1971 Jolly & Pallis reviewed seven previously reported cases and described two of their own. Since then, further cases have been reported, and it is now possible to detail the clinical and pathological features of this condition.

All but one of the 16 cases of muscular pseudo-hypertrophy shown by biopsy to be due to cysticercosis have been reported from India. The main features are summarised in Table 19.2. Eleven males and five females have been affected, their ages ranging from 10 to 45 years.

The thighs, calves, glutei and shoulder girdles are, as a rule, massively enlarged, the patients often being described as having developed a 'Herculean' appearance (Fig. 19.2). The nuchal musculature, erector spinae, masseters and forearm muscles may be notably involved. The pseudohypertrophy is invariably bilateral and symmetrical.

The enlarged muscles are usually firm. There may be slight overlying oedema. No individual nodules can usually be felt, probably because the muscles are so tightly packed with cysticerci. The nodules may occasionally be felt on contraction.

In six cases there was no detectable weakness in the enlarged muscles. In seven there was mild to moderate, predominantly proximal weakness and in one case it seemed to be confined to the calf musculature. Two patients were described as very weak. In no case was power increased commensurate with the muscle bulk.

Muscle pain was experienced before the onset of the pseudohypertrophy in several instances, but at the time of presentation was seldom prominent. In most patients the muscular enlargement was entirely painless throughout. Definite muscle tenderness was elicited in two of the 16 cases and in a further two slight tenderness may have been present.

The muscle enlargement had come on insidiously in all cases, over a period varying from a few weeks to 18 months or more. In six cases an initial illness was described, often consisting of fever, pain in the limbs and occasionally urticaria or pruritus. Muscular enlargement was sometimes noted within 2 to 3 weeks of such an illness.

In 14 of the 16 patients, muscular enlargement was found associated with palpable subcutaneous nodules, i.e. clinically obvious cysticercosis. Lingual cysticerci were seen in no fewer than 10 cases and ocular cysticerci in two. Two patients had cardiac failure and a further three had abnormal electrocardiograms. There was evidence of nervous system involvement in 14 instances (usually epilepsy, but occasionally mental change or a focal neurological deficit). Calcification of the parasites in muscle was found only twice and seemed to be early (i.e. confined to the scolices).

Table 19.2 Summary of clinical and laboratory findings in reported cases of pseudohypertrophic myopathy due to cysticercosis

Authors	Year	Cases reported	Sex	Age (years)	Identifiable initial illness	Weakness	Pain	Tenderness	Subcutaneous nodules	Tongue involvement	Eye involvement	Heart involvement	CNS involvement	Calcified muscle cysts	Ova in stool or history of taeniasis	EMG	CPK	Eosinophilia
Priest	1926	1	M	24	+	+	+I	+	+	+	+	+	+	NI	o	o	o	o
McRobert	1944	1	M	25	o	o	o	o	+	o	o	NI	+	o	o	o	o	+
McGill	1947, 1948*	2	M	25 20	+ o	++ I (calves)	++ I	+ o	+ +	+ o	+ o	NI	+ +	? scolices only	o o	o o	o o	+ +
Singh & Jolly	1957	1	F	22	o	o	o	+	+	o	papillitis	NI Abnormal ECG	+ +	? scolices only	+ o	o	o	+ o
Prakash & Kumar	1965	1	M	14	o	o	o	±	+	+	o	Abnormal ECG	+	? scolices only	o	NI	NI	+
Jacob & Mathew	1968	1	M	30	+	±	I	±	+	+	+	o	+	o	+ o	NI	NI	o +
Armbrust-Figueiredo et al	1970	1	F	35	+	±	I	o	o	o	o	Cardiac failure	+	o	o	NI	NI	NI
Jolly & Pallis	1971	2†	M	22	o	o	o	o	o	+	+	Abnormal ECG	+	o	o	o	o	NI
Rao et al	1972	1	M	25	o	o	o	o	+	+	o	o	+ o	o	o	NI o	NI o	+ o
Salgaokar & Watcha	1974	1	M	11	+	±	o	o	+	+	proptosis; swollen disc	o	+	o	o	o	o	+
Vigg & Rai	1975	2	F	45 35	o +	+ ±	++ ±	NI o	+ +	+	o o	o o	+ +	o o	o o	o o	o o	+ +
Sawhney et al	1976	1	F	24	o	+	+	o	+	o	+	Non-specific T-wave changes	+	NI	NI	Abnormal	N	+
Vijayan et al	1977	1	M	17	o	+	o	o	+	+	+	NI	+	o	o	o	o	NI

I, Initial muscle pain; NI, no information.
* Same cases described in two communications.
† Cases 3 and 4.

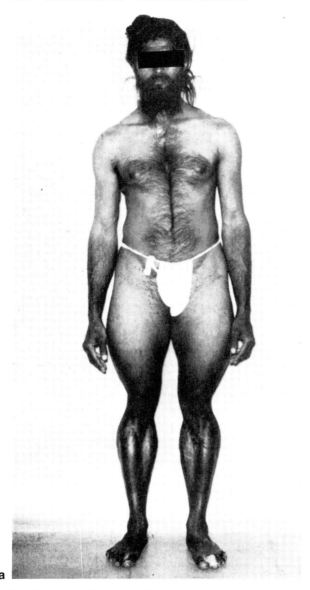
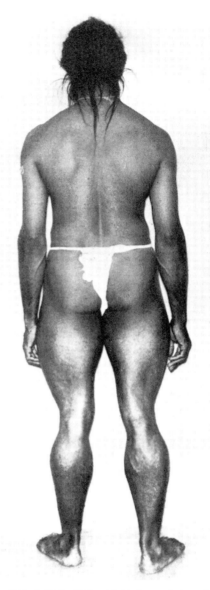

a   b

Fig. 19.2   Pseudohypertrophic myopathy due to cysticercosis (reproduced from Jolly & Pallis 1971 with kind permission of the authors, editor and publisher).

Muscle biopsy usually reveals numerous tense cysts, 1 cm or more in length (Fig. 19.3). The muscle fibres are not hypertrophied. Regions in the immediate vicinity of the cysticerci occasionally show variable cellular infiltration with polymorphs, lymphocytes, plasma cells and/or eosinophils, and degenerative changes with areas of focal fibrosis. Sawhney et al (1976), however, illustrated changes 'not in continuity with the inflammatory reaction seen around the cysts'. These consisted of swollen muscle fibres with loss of cross-striation and central migration of nuclei. Their finding implied, they thought, 'an affection of the muscle fibres per se in the disease process'. They did not report, however, on the appearances in sections of muscle from above and below the affected areas. We believe that as likely an explanation for their observations is the phenomenon

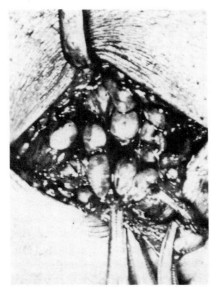

Fig. 19.3 Numerous tense cysticerci, presenting at the biopsy site in gastrocnemius muscle (case of Prakash & Kumar 1965 reproduced with kind permission of the authors, editor and publisher).

reported by Drachman & Tuncbay (1965)—in cases of obvious trichinosis—to account for 'extensive myositis without trichinae'.

Fine needle aspiration biopsy of a muscle lesion may produce a diagnostic yield if the tissue sample includes the cyst wall (Kung et al 1989).

Electromyography was used in such cases by Salgaokar & Watcha (1974), who reported normal findings in the proximal muscle groups of their patient. Sawhney et al (1976) reported motor units 'averaging' 300–800 μV and 4–8 ms in duration, 10–15% of which were polyphasic. They interpreted these findings as indicative of myopathy.

We believe muscle enlargement in cysticercosis to be related to larval death, not the initial dissemination. Cysts found in such cases are invariably very tense and never contain viable parasites. Very little is known of the natural history of the disorder but some evidence suggests that it may be a spontaneously reversible condition.

Treatment. Intestinal taeniasis, if present, should be treated. Drug-induced larval death, and the subsequent appearance of further tense cysts, may for a while aggravate the pseudohypertrophy.

The pyrazino-isoquinoline anthelminthic praziquantel is clinically effective against a wide spectrum of cestode and trematode infections in animals and humans (Andrews et al 1983, Pearson & Guerrant 1983). At low concentrations the drug paralyses adult worms, causing them to loosen their attachment to host tissues. At higher concentrations it produces vesiculation of the tegument of susceptible parasites (including the larval form of *T. solium*) and release of the contents of the parasite with activation of host defence mechanisms and eventual destruction of the worms. Massive cysticercosis of muscle should be treated cautiously, for the abrupt destruction of large numbers of larvae and the associated oedema may have deleterious effects, particularly if the nervous system is also massively involved. The use of biphasic courses of dexamethasone and praziquantel has been described by de Ghetaldi et al (1983). The dose of praziquantel used was 50 mg/kg/day (given in three divided doses) for 14 days. Caution has been expressed over the use of prolonged high-dose praziquantel therapy for human cysticercosis (Sotelo et al 1984).

Coenurosis

The word coenurus refers to the polycephalous larval form of certain taeniid worms of the genus *Multiceps*, the adults of which inhibit the intestine of dogs and other canidae. The term is descriptive and has no taxonomic significance.

On farm or field, herbivorous mammals may swallow the ova passed by dogs infected by *Multiceps multiceps*. The embryos burrow through the intestinal mucosa and disseminate widely. Affected sheep may develop a neurological disorder known as 'staggers'. Other possible intermediate hosts include rabbits, wild rodents, certain monkeys and, occasionally, man, in whom cerebral symptoms may also be prominent. The cycle is completed when dogs gain access to infected sheep tissue.

In parts of tropical Africa where *M. multiceps* seems to be very rare the taeniid *M. brauni* is found in the gut of the domestic dog, fox and jackal, the usual intermediate hosts being wild rodents or porcupines. Cases of human coenurosis reported from such areas all seem to have shown predominant subcutaneous or muscle involvement.

Coenuri are glistening, globular or ovoid unilocular cysts, each containing several scolices which seem to bud from the inner surface of the cyst wall. The cysts vary in size from that of an almond to that of an apricot. They are usually filled with a milky, gelatinous fluid. They contain neither brood capsules nor daughter cysts. They are surrounded by an adventitious capsule derived from the host, composed of dense collagenous fibrous tissue infiltrated with plasma cells, lymphocytes and occasional histiocytes and eosinophils.

A coenurus is one of the causes of a palpable, occasionally slightly tender, 'tumour' in muscle. The 'tumour' is usually solitary and—in muscle—almost invariably unilocular. The vast majority occur on the trunk. The intercostal and anterior abdominal muscles are favourite sites (Templeton 1971). Coenuri may also be found in the neck, in relation to the sternomastoid or trapezius muscles.

The preoperative diagnosis is usually fibroma or lipoma. When the excised 'tumour' is cut across, and the multiple scolices are revealed in the cyst, macroscopic diagnosis should be obvious.

Hydatidosis

The two canid tapeworms (*Echinococcus granulosus* and *Echinococcus multilocularis*) may cause hydatid disease in man. Muscle involvement has been reported with both types of infection.

Ova of *E. granulosus*, discharged in dogs' faeces, are ingested by the intermediate host (usually sheep but occasionally goats, cattle, pigs, wild herbivores or man). After hatching, embryos penetrate the venules of the intestinal wall and settle in the liver. If they can pass the hepatic circulation they lodge in the lungs. A small number may reach other tissues such as muscle or bone. The natural cycle is completed when dogs eat ovine offal. In echinococcosis due to *E. multilocularis*, the natural reservoir is in foxes, although dogs and cats may also harbour the parent tapeworm. The usual intermediate hosts are wild rodents. Man may become infected by consuming fruit and vegetables contaminated by fox excreta.

The classic morphological appearance of hydatid cysts due to *E. granulosus* is well described in standard textbooks. Unlike the large single cysts produced by this tapeworm the larval stage of *E. multilocularis* consists of a honeycomb-like aggregate in innumerable small cysts. There is no proper limiting capsule. The lesion may look like the cut surface of a slice of bread. It may have a necrotic centre, resembling an abscess. It behaves locally like an invasive tumour and true metastases may occur.

In sheep-rearing countries, where hydatidosis is common, hydatid disease of muscle is not rare. Muscle is the third most frequent site (after liver and lung) in which cysts may be found. Over 5% of cases of human hydatid disease show lesions of muscle (Dévé 1949, Dew 1951). Goinard & Salasc (1931) reported a personal series of 33 cases.

The initial lesion probably occurs within an individual muscle fibre (Dévé 1936). Only about one-third of muscle hydatids contain viable scolices. They are most often encountered in the paravertebral gutters and in limb-girdle musculature, particularly the thigh. They are rare distally.

In many parts of the world a hydatid is the commonest benign muscle tumour. Physical examination will reveal a deep, slowly growing, poorly mobile, spherical or lobulated mass, of variable size and firm consistency. The exact shape of the tumour will often be influenced by adjacent bone and limiting fascia. Pain is rare, although patients may complain of a dull ache in the relevant muscle after use. A hydatid 'thrill' can seldom be elicited. The lesion may occasionally calcify. Secondary infection is not uncommon. The condition may then present as an abscess.

Hydatids in muscle cause neither weakness nor tenderness. The finding of myotonia in three out of five members of a family with muscle involvement due to *E. multilocularis* (Schimrigk & Emser 1978) was probably fortuitous. The family probably had myotonia congenita.

Sparganosis

The term sparganosis refers to the extraintestinal infection of vertebrate hosts by the plerocercoid larvae (or spargana) of pseudophyllidean (diphyllobothriid) tapeworms of the genus *Spirometra*. These tapeworms are related to *D. latum* (well known to haematologists and neurologists as an occasional cause of vitamin B_{12} deficiency) but differ in that they cannot complete their life cycle and develop their adult form in man. Two intermediate hosts are needed: the first a copepod crustacean, the second a vertebrate.

The adult worms live in the gut of carnivores. In the Far East '*Spirometra mansoni*' is a common intestinal parasite of dogs and cats. In the USA *Spirometra mansonoides* has been found in bobcats, occasionally in domestic cats and—more rarely—in dogs.

Infected carnivores pass mature proglottids. The ova hatch in ponds or streams, liberating a ciliated coracidium. The coracidia are swallowed by water-fleas of the genus *Cyclops* in whose haemocoele they mature, becoming procercoid larvae. When such larvae are then eaten by frogs, lizards, snakes, birds or small mammals the procercoid larva is liberated in the gut of the vertebrate host, penetrates the intestinal wall and is distributed to the tissues, where it matures to a migrating, plerocercoid larva.

In the USA, natural paratenic (carrier) hosts include mice, rhesus monkeys, water snakes and the pig, raccoon and opossum. In Korea various species of snake have been incriminated. Unlike *Diphyllobothrium*, the plerocercoids are not found in fish. It is only when the paratenic host is consumed by the definitive (carnivore) host that the life cycle is completed and that an adult tapeworm can again develop.

Man can become infected in one of four ways:

1. By the accidental ingestion of procercoid-infected copepods (as in drinking unboiled, unfiltered, infected water). The procercoid will then penetrate the human gut and become a plerocercoid.

2. By eating the infected, uncooked, plerocercoid-containing flesh of frogs, snakes or certain fish, for purposes of nutrition or—more often in parts of South East Asia—as a 'tonic'. The plerocercoid is then transmitted from one paratenic (carrier) host to another. It remains a plerocercoid however, for the adult worm cannot develop in man.

3. Through eating uncooked pork (Becklund 1962, Corkum 1966). Spargana are known to develop in pigs allowed to forage in woodland areas, where they may become infected through the ingestion of snakes, frogs or small mammals infected with plerocercoids—or through drinking water from ponds containing infected copepods.

4. By using the raw flesh of plerocercoid-infected 'split frogs' or snakes as poultices. The practice, long prevalent in Thailand and Vietnam, of dressing ulcers, wounds or infected eyes with such poultices doubtless accounted for many cases of ocular sparganosis.

Clinical features. In ocular sparganosis there is often an intense inflammatory reaction with periorbital oedema. Retrobulbar lesions produce lagophthalmos and the threat of corneal ulceration. The early phases of infection by the gastrointestinal route are usually asymptomatic. In soft tissues the clinical features vary. The usual presentation is as a slightly fluctuant subcutaneous or superficial intramuscular lump, about 5 cm in diameter, often suspected of being a lipoma. Occasionally the lump presents with signs of inflammation. A characteristic if uncommon feature is the tendency of the lumps to move slowly downwards, over several weeks or months—as correctly observed by many patients and repeatedly doubted at first interview by many doctors.

Involved muscles have included the rectus abdominis, thigh muscles, pectoralis major and calf muscles. In many cases, other parts of the body will have been involved, although from the descriptions it is not always clear whether the lesions were entirely subcutaneous or could have extended deeper. In a given lesion there is usually a single, viable larva.

A case in which a live sparganum was extracted from the biceps muscle was reported by Ali-Khan et al (1973). Cho & Patel (1978) report a case in which the parasite, deep in the right thigh, was surrounded by granulomatous tissue showing a striking histological similarity to the nodules of rheumatoid arthritis. The length of the excised parasite may lead to misdiagnosis of guinea-worm (dracunculiasis).

The rare human disease proliferative sparganosis, in which muscles are involved in the course of lethal systemic asexual proliferation of parasites, occurs in the Far East and in the Americas. An account by Nakamura et al (1990) contains data linking the culprit plerocercoid to *Spirometra erinacei*.

NEMATODES

Trichinosis

The larvae of *Trichinella spiralis* may be found in the muscles of many facultative or obligatory carnivores. Natural infection is readily transmitted between species—or by cannibalism within a given species.

Trichinosis, among carnivores, is world-wide, its distribution independent of climate. It is encountered from equatorial to arctic regions. The prevalence of human trichinosis, however, is patchy and deeply influenced by cultural factors.

Human infection takes place through eating parasitised ('measly') pork in the form of raw or undercooked sausage, smoked ham or pickled trotters—or more exotic foods such as boar, bear or walrus meat. (Pigs are infected by eating infected rats, or by being fed uncooked swill containing, inter alia, the offal of other pigs.) Recent outbreaks in Italy and the Auvergne region of France have been ascribed to the ingestion of horseflesh à la tartare (Editorial 1990).

After ingestion of infected meat, viable larvae are released and pass into the duodenum and jejunum where, after moulting, they very rapidly develop into adult worms. The male dies after copulation but the viviparous female (which may reach a size of 4 mm) burrows into the intestinal mucosa and starts producing larvae within a week of ingestion. During the next 2 or 3 weeks each female may produce over a thousand 'second-generation larvae' which enter the systemic circulation (via the lymphatics and the right side of the heart) and seed into many tissues.

In striated muscle the larvae penetrate the sarcolemma and grow, until after 16 days they reach a length of 800–1000 μm and a width of 30 μm. They show no preference for any particular fibre type (Ochoa & Pallis 1980) (Fig. 19.4). Three weeks after penetration they have increased their length tenfold, becoming coiled in the process (Fig. 19.5). An ellipsoidal collagenous capsule about 500 μm long and 250 μm wide is formed by the muscle cell around the coiled-up larvae. It takes about 3 months for this capsule to develop fully. Although widely distributed, the larvae seem to encyst in this manner in striated muscle only. Encysted larvae may remain viable for many years.

Calcification may begin within 6–9 months. Following death of the trichinae some cysts may be completely resorbed. The penetration of a striated muscle fibre by a larva results in the destruction both of the penetrated fibre and of some adjacent ones.

The extraocular muscles, masseters, diaphragm, muscles of the tongue, larynx and neck, intercostals and deltoid are most heavily involved. In some epidemics parasites predominated in diaphragm, calves and forearm muscles. Sites of attachment to tendons are particularly prone to be affected.

Many infections are asymptomatic, with diaphragm counts of less than 10 larvae per gram. Muscular symptoms probably arise when the larval count reaches 100 per gram. One patient (Davis et al 1976) survived a deltoid concentration of 4000 larvae per gram. Fatal cases, according to Gould (1970), may carry up to 100 million larvae to the grave with them. A worm's eye view of the human connection could only be depressing, for this massive parasitisation of man is clearly a demographic dead-end.

Clinical features. The first diagnostically helpful sign is often periorbital oedema. The whole face may be grotesquely bloated. Patients may be misdiagnosed as suffering from angioneurotic oedema or even from renal disease. There may be chemosis, a widespread facial erythema and subconjunctival haemorrhages. Patients may present to ophthalmologists with complaints of conjunctivitis or of pain in one or both eyeballs often related to eye movement. The combination of severe photophobia, fever and headache may lead to misdiagnoses of meningitis. Diagnosis may be very difficult as there may be neck stiffness, probably from myositis of the nuchal musculature. A macular rash, more persistent than that of typhoid, is seen in 10% of cases. Subungual 'splinters' and retinal haemorrhages are not uncommon.

Myalgia is an early and common complaint, although often preceded by periorbital oedema. Involvement of the ocular muscles, masseters and tongue influences the symptomatology. Masticatory difficulties or even trismus may occur. Oedema of the tongue and pharyngeal muscles may cause dysphagia. The calves and forearms are usually painful. Lumbar pains may be excruciating.

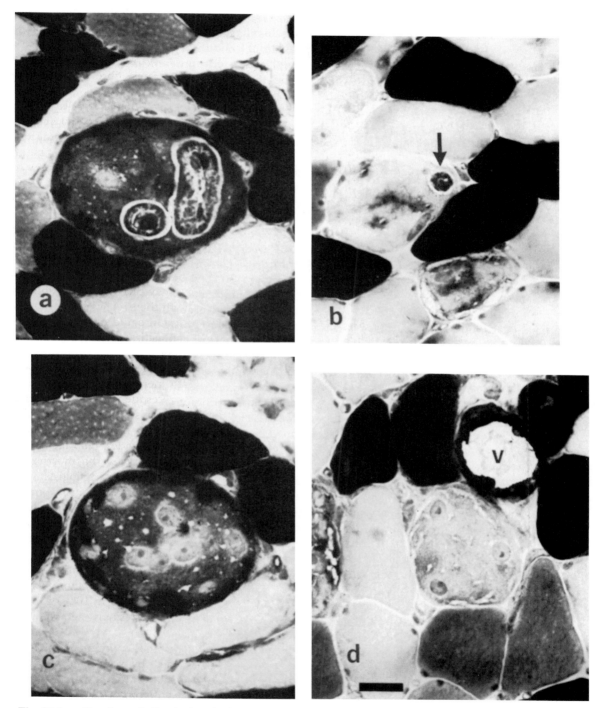

Fig. 19.4   a Type I muscle fibre harbouring larvae of *Trichinella spiralis*. **b** Type II (A?) fibre cut across parasite (arrowed). **c** Distended type I fibre with reactive nuclei, probably cut close to a parasite. **d** Type II (A?) fibre showing similar changes to those in the fibre in **c**. V = blood vessel. ATPase pH 4.6: black = Type I; white = Type IIA; intermediate = Type IIB (scale bar = 25 μm).

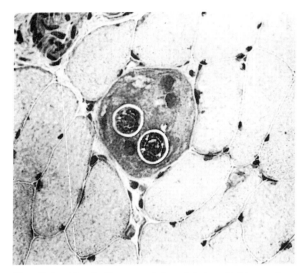

Fig. 19.5   Muscle fibre containing slightly coiled larva of *Trichinella spiralis*, cut across twice.

Myalgia reaches its height during the third week of the illness, seldom extending into the fourth or fifth.

The involved muscles may be patchily tender but the most striking feature is their weakness. In part, this is genuine paresis. But there is also a considerable reluctance to move, as movement tends to produce 'tension pain' in both agonists and antagonists. Occasionally, limb muscles may be grossly swollen. An 'oedematous' patient with puffy face, swollen legs and tender muscles will almost certainly prove to have trichinosis.

The weakness may be extreme, patients rapidly becoming tetraplegic from muscle involvement. There is probably no other disorder of muscle, except periodic paralysis, in which such severe weakness develops in so short a time. The tendon reflexes may be impaired.

Calf pain may result in early reluctance to stand, of a degree that would not be warranted by paresis or general prostration. Patients may attempt to remain ambulant by walking on their toes. When they take to bed, they tend to remain immobile. Early contractures may ensue.

Involvement of the central nervous system is well documented in the more massive infections. Its manifestations are protean and include stupor, frank meningitis, brain-stem involvement and various combinations of upper motor neurone

and radicular signs. These are of variable pathogenesis (haemorrhage, vasculitis, oedema, granulomatous nodules). Larval embolisation into capillaries is encountered but is much less common than vasculitis. The marked response of neurological signs to steroid medication probably relates to these manifestations of hypersensitivity. Confusing symptoms may be encountered. Diplopia is more often than not myopathic. Dyspnoea may be due to asthma, the pain of deep breathing, cardiac failure or ventilatory insufficiency of myopathic type. Misdiagnoses of poliomyelitis, polyneuritis and even myasthenia have been reported.

In severe cases the illness reaches its height in 2 to 4 weeks. Paresis and asthenia may be protracted and convalescence delayed. In various epidemics, 2–10% of recognised cases have proved fatal. Death usually results from non-specific myocarditis, pneumonia or encephalitis.

Electromyography. Marcus & Miller (1955) described a patient with widespread, severe trichinosis who exhibited 'the most profuse fibrillation of denervation the examiner had ever seen'. There was gross weakness and some wasting. Although the authors attributed the fibrillation, wasting and weakness to 'lower motor neurone changes', a more likely mechanism is the one suggested to account for 'profuse spontaneous fibrillation in all muscles sampled' in the case described by Gross & Ochoa (1979). These authors incriminated 'disconnection of fragments of muscle fibres from their end-plate regions due to focal muscle necrosis'. The implications of this mechanism are considerable. They might help in the electromyographic differentiation of those parasitic myopathies in which the parasites lie *within* muscle fibres from those in which the parasites lie *between* them.

Treatment. The antihelminthic thiabendazole (2-(thiazolyl)-benzimidazole) was introduced into the therapy of human trichinosis in 1964. It has a profound effect on larvae already in muscle, damaging or killing many of them. The suggested intake is 50 mg/kg/day, taken in divided doses. Medication should be continued until symptoms subside or incapacitating side-effects appear, but should not be continued for more than a week. Side-effects include anorexia and gastrointestinal upsets, slight dizziness, and occasionally, drowsiness.

Treatment with thiabendazole alone may result in a Herxheimer-like reaction, probably due to massive dissolution of larvae with abrupt release of protein-breakdown products into the circulation. Corticosteroids are therefore usually prescribed concurrently with—or even a little earlier than—thiabendazole. Such a regimen involves the larvicidal effect of one drug, the immunosuppressive effect of the other and the combined anti-inflammatory effects of both.

Toxocariasis

Toxocara canis is a widely distributed ascarid of dogs, in which species its life cycle resembles that of *Ascaris lumbricoides* in man. Its ova are infective to man. *Toxocara cati* (a common feline ascarid) may also cause human toxocariasis.

Human toxocariasis occurs when ova, present in dog or cat faeces, get into the mouths of children, playing in yards or gardens. The ova hatch in the child's jejunum and the liberated larvae enter mesenteric venules or lymphatics. They are then carried to extraintestinal sites, usually the liver but sometimes to the lungs and even beyond: to brain, eye or muscle. The larvae may remain alive and actively motile in such tissues, boring their way in various directions.

Granulomatous lesions caused by larvae may be few or many, depending on the number of ingested eggs, and on the degree of sensitisation of the invaded host. In the liver they appear as subcapsular white nodules or plaques, 5–10 mm in diameter and easily visible to the naked eye. Lesions in human muscle are less numerous but may be detected by the use of a hand lens (Dent et al 1956). Using a pepsin technique these workers recovered a mean of 5 larvae per gram of skeletal muscle in a child with toxocariasis who had died from a post-transfusion hepatitis. They suggested that the recovery of *Toxocara* larvae by this technique might be applied to muscle and liver biopsy specimens, as a diagnostic procedure in suspected cases. As far as we know, muscle biopsy has seldom been used for this purpose.

Florid disease is rare, the most usual presentation being a chronically ill child with an enlarged liver, pneumonitis and sustained eosinophilia. Muscle pain is an occasional feature (Hunter et al 1976). Diagnostic procedures were reviewed by Woodruff (1970). The morphological differentiation of various larvae capable of causing visceral larva migrans was discussed by Nichols (1956).

REFERENCES

Abuladze K I 1964 Alveococci as parasites in man. In: Taeniata of animals and man and diseases caused by them. Iztadel'stvo 'Nauka', Moscow (English version: Israel Program for Scientific translations, 1970, Jerusalem) pp 379–383

Agarwal P K, Srivastava A N 1983 Sarcocystis in man: a report of two cases. Histopathology 7: 783

Ali-Khan Z, Irving R T, Wingnall N, Bowmer E J 1973 Imported sparganosis in Canada. Canadian Medical Association Journal 108: 590

Andrews P, Thomas H, Pohlke R, Seubert J 1983 Praziquantel. Medical Research Review 3: 147

Arana-Iñiguez R 1978 Echinococcus. In: Vinken P J, Bruyn G W (eds) Handbook of clinical neurology, vol 35. North-Holland, Amsterdam, pp 175–208

Armbrust-Figueiredo J, Speciali J G, Lison M P 1970 Forma miopatica da cisticercose. Arquivos de Neuropsiquiatria 28: 385

Beaver P C, Synder C H, Carrera G M, Dent J H, Lafferty J W 1952 Chronic eosinophilia due to visceral larva migrans. Pediatrics 9: 7

Becklund W W 1962 Occurrence of a larval trematode (Diplostomatidae) in a larval cestode (Diphyllobothriidae) from Sus scrofa in Florida. Journal of Parasitology 48: 286

Blanco A E, Mozador J L, Minetti R 1949 Los quistes hidatidicos musculares. Archivos internacionales de la Hidatidosis 9: 221

Brashear R E, Martin R R, Glover J L 1971 Trichinosis and respiratory failure. American Review of Respiratory Disease 104: 245

Cho C, Patel S P 1978 Human sparganosis in Northern United States. New York State Journal of Medicine 78: 1456

Corkum K C 1966 Sparganosis in some vertebrates in Louisiana and observations of a human infection. Journal of Parasitology 55: 444

Davis M J, Cilo M, Plaitakis A, Yahr M D 1976 Trichinosis: a severe myopathic involvement with recovery. Neurology (Minneapolis) 26: 37

De Ghetaldi L D, Norman R M, Douville A W 1983 Cerebral cysticercosis treated biphasically with dexamethasone and praziquantel. Annals of Internal Medicine 99: 170

Dent J H, Nichols R L, Beaver P C, Carrera G M, Staggers R J 1956 Visceral larva migrans with a case report. American Journal of Pathology 32: 777

Despommier D, Aron L, Turgeon L 1975 Trichinella spiralis:

Growth of the intracellular (muscle) larva. Experimental Parasitology 37: 108

Dévé F 1936 Sur le siège initial des kystes hydatiques musculaires. Comptes rendus de la Société de Biologie 123: 764

Dévé F 1949 L'échinococcose primitive. Masson, Paris, p 79

Dew R H 1951 Hydatid disease. In: Lord Horder (ed) British encyclopaedia of medical practice, 2nd edn, vol 4. Butterworth, London, pp 587–614

Dixon H B F, Lipscomb F M 1961 Cysticercosis: an analysis and follow-up of 450 cases. In: Special report series. Medical Research Council, London

Drachman D A, Tuncbay T O 1965 The remote myopathy of trichinosis. Neurology (Minneapolis) 15: 1127

Editorial 1990 Walrus without tears. Lancet 335: 202

Fain A 1956 Coenurus of Taenia brauni Setti parasitic in man and animals from the Belgian Congo and Ruanda-Urundi. Nature 178: 1353

Faust E C, Russell P F, Jung R C 1970 Craig and Faust's clinical parasitology, 8th edn. Lea and Febiger, Philadelphia

Faust E C, Beaver P C, Jung R C 1975 Animal agents and vectors of human disease, 4th edn. Lea and Febiger, Philadelphia, pp 92–96

Frenkel J K 1973 Toxoplasmosis: Parasite life cycle, pathology and immunology of toxoplasmosis. In: Hammond D M, Long P (eds) The Coccidia: Eimeria, Toxoplasma, Isospora and related genera. University Park Press, Baltimore, pp 343–410

Goinard P, Salasc J 1931 Sur les kystes hydatiques des muscles volontaires. Journal de Chirurgie 54: 320

Goodwin L G 1970 The pathology of African trypanosomiasis. Transactions of the Royal Society of Tropical Medicine and Hygiene 64: 797

Gould S E 1954 Eye and orbit in trichinosis. Bulletin of the New York Academy of Medicine 30: 726

Gould S E 1970 Trichinosis in man and animals. Thomas, Springfield, Illinois, pp 147–189

Greve E 1985 Sarcosporidiosis—an overlooked zoonosis. Danish Medical Bulletin 32: 228

Gross B, Ochoa J 1979 Trichinosis: A clinical report and histochemistry of muscle. Muscle and Nerve 2: 394–398

Hunter G W, Swatzwelder J C, Clyde D E 1976 Tropical Medicine, 5th edn. Saunders, Philadelphia

Jacob J C, Mathew N T 1968 Pseudohypertrophic myopathy in cysticercosis. Neurology (Minneapolis) 18: 767

Janssen P, van Bogaert L, Haymaker W 1956 Pathology of the peripheral nervous system in African trypanosomiasis. Study of 7 cases. Journal of Neuropathology and Experimental Neurology 15: 269

Jeffery H C 1974 Sarcosporidiosis in man. Transactions of the Royal Society of Tropical Medicine and Hygiene 68: 17

Jolly S S, Pallis C 1971 Muscular pseudohypertrophy due to cysticercosis. Journal of the Neurological Sciences 12: 155

Kagan L J, Kimball A C, Christian C L 1974 Serologic evidence of toxoplasmosis among patients with polymyositis. American Journal of Medicine 56: 186

Kean B H, Breslau R C 1964 Cardiac sarcosporidiosis. In: Parasites of the human heart. Grune and Stratton, New York, pp 74–83

Köberle F 1968 Chagas' disease and Chagas' syndromes: the pathology of American trypanosomiasis. Advances in Parasitology 6: 63

Koten J W, de Raadt 1969 Myocarditis in Trypanosoma rhodesiense infections. Transactions of the Royal Society of Tropical Medicine and Hygiene 63: 485

Kung I T, Lee D, Hip Cho Yu 1989 Soft tissue cysticercosis. Diagnosis by fine-needle aspiration. American Journal of Clinical Pathology 92: 834

Liu C T, Roberts L M 1965 Sarcosporidiosis in a Bantu woman. American Journal of Clinical Pathology 44: 639

Lorenzetti L 1962 Contributo alla conoscenza dell'echinococcosi primitiva dei muscoli. Gazzetta internazionale di medicine e chirurgia 67: 2775

Losos G J, Idede B O 1972 Review of pathology of diseases in domestic and laboratory animals caused by Trypanosoma congolense, T. vivax, T. brucei, T. rhodesiense and T. gambiense. Veterinary Pathology 9 (suppl): 1–56

MacArthur W P 1950 In: Lord Horder (ed) British encyclopaedia of medical practice, vol 4, 2nd edn. Butterworth, London, p 111

McGill R J 1947 Cysticercosis resembling a myopathy. Indian Journal of Medical Sciences 1: 109

McGill R J 1948 Cysticercosis resembling myopathy. Lancet 2: 728

McGill R J, Goodbody R A 1957 Sarcosporidiosis in man with periarteritis nodosa. British Medical Journal 2: 333

McRobert G R 1944 Somatic taeniasis (solium cysticercosis). Indian Medical Gazette 79: 399

Marcus S, Miller R V 1955 An atypical case of trichinosis with report of electromyographic findings. Annals of Internal Medicine 43: 615

Markus M B, Killick-Kendrick R, Garnham P C 1974 The coccidial nature and life-cycle of Sarcocystis. Journal of Tropical Medicine and Hygiene 77: 248

Mueller J F 1938 Studies on Sparganum mansonoides and Sparganum proliferum. American Journal of Tropical Medicine 18: 303

Mueller J F, Hart E P, Walsh W P 1963 Human sparganosis in the United States. Journal of Parasitology 48: 294

Nakamura T, Hara M, Matsuoka M, Kawabata M, Tsuji M 1990 Human proliferative sparganosis. A new Japanese case. American Journal of Clinical Pathology 94: 224

Nichols R L 1956 The etiology of visceral larva migrans. II. Comparative larval morphology of Ascaris lumbricoides, Necator americanus, Strongyloides stercoralis and Ancylostoma caninum. Journal of Parasitology 42: 363

Ochoa J, Pallis C 1980 Trichinella thrives in both oxidative and glycolytic human muscle fibres. Journal of Neurology, Neurosurgery and Psychiatry 43: 281

Orihel T C, Gonzales F, Beaver P C 1970 Coenurus from neck of Texas woman. American Journal of Tropical Medicine and Hygiene 19: 255

Pamphlett R, O'Donoghue P 1990 Sarcocystis infection of human muscle. Australian and New Zealand Journal of Medicine 20: 705

Pearson C M, Rose A S 1960 The inflammatory disorders of muscle. In: Adams R D, Eaton L M, Shy G M (eds) Neuromuscular disorders (the motor unit and its disorders), vol 38. Williams and Wilkins, Baltimore, p 433

Pearson R D, Guerrant R L 1983 Praziquantel: Major advance in anthelminthic therapy. Annals of Internal Medicine 99: 195

Poltera A A, Owor R, Cox J N 1977 Pathological aspects of human African trypanosomiasis (HAT) in Uganda. A postmortem study of 14 cases. Virchows Archiv A. Pathological Anatomy and Histology 373: 249

Prakash C, Kumar A 1965 Cysticercosis with taeniasis in a vegetarian. Journal of Tropical Medicine and Hygiene 68: 100

Priest R 1926 A case of extensive somatic dissemination of cysticercus cellulosae in man. British Medical Journal 2: 471

Rabinowicz J 1971 A case of acquired toxoplasmosis in the adult. In: Hentsch D (ed) Toxoplasmosis. Huber, Berne, pp 197–219

Rao C M, Sattar S A, Gopal P S, Reddy C C M, Sadasivudu B 1972 Cysticercosis resembling myopathy. Report of a case. Indian Journal of Medical Sciences 26: 841

Raper A B, Dockeray G D 1956 Coenurus cysts in man: five cases form East Africa. Annals of Tropical Medicine and Parasitology 50: 121

Salgaokar S V, Watcha M F 1974 Muscular hypertrophy in cysticercosis: a case report. Journal of Postgraduate Medicine 20: 148

Samuels B S, Rietschel R L 1976 Polymyositis and toxoplasmosis. Journal of the American Medical Association 235: 60

Sawhney B B, Chopra J S, Banerji A K, Wahi P L 1976 Pseudohypertrophic myopathy in cysticercosis. Neurology (Minneapolis) 26: 270

Schimrigk K, Emser W 1978 Parasitic myositis caused by *Echinococcus alveolaris*. European Neurology 17: 1

Singh A, Jolly S S 1957 Cysticercosis: case report. Indian Journal of Medical Sciences 11: 98

Slais J 1970 The morphology and pathogenicity of bladder worms: *Cysticercus cellulosae* and *Cysticercus bovis*. Academia, Prague

Sotelo J, Escobedo, F, Rodriguez-Carbajal, Torres B, Rubio-

Donnadieu F 1984 Therapy of parenchymal brain cysticercosis with praziquantel. New England Journal of Medicine 310: 1001

Sprent J F A 1965 Ascaridoid larva migrans: differentiation of larvae in tissues. Transactions of the Royal Society of Tropical Medicine and Hygiene 59: 365

Stoll N R 1947 This wormy world. Journal of Parasitology 33: 1

Templeton A C 1968 Human coenurus infection. A report of 14 cases from Uganda. Transactions of the Royal Society of Tropical Medicine and Hygiene 62: 251

Templeton A C 1971 Anatomical and geographical location of human coenurus infection. Tropical and Geographical Medicine 23: 105

Trelles J O, Trelles L 1978 In: Vinken P J, Bruyn G W (eds) Handbook of clinical neurology, vol 35. North Holland, Amsterdam, pp 291–320

Vigg B, Rai 1975 Muscular involvement in cysticercosis with pseudohypertrophy of muscles. Journal of the Association of Physicians of India 23: 593

Vijayan G P, Venkataraman S, Suri M L, Seth H M, Hoon R S 1977 Neurological and related manifestations of cysticercosis. Tropical and Geographical Medicine 29: 271

Wilson C V L C, Wayte D M, Addae R O 1972 Human coenurosis: the first reported case from Ghana. Transactions of the Royal Society of Tropical Medicine and Hygiene 66: 611

Wirth W A, Farrow C C 1961 Human sparganosis. Case report and review of the subject. Journal of the American Medical Association 177: 6

Woodruff A W 1970 Toxocariasis. British Medical Journal 3: 663

20. Myasthenia gravis and related syndromes

J. Newsom-Davis

OVERVIEW

The neuromuscular junction seems especially vulnerable to autoimmune attack, perhaps because it lacks the protection that the blood–brain barrier provides for synapses in the central nervous system. It is also the site of rare congenital/hereditary abnormalities.

The autoimmune hypothesis for *myasthenia gravis (MG)*, first formulated by Simpson (1960), has now been validated. Anti-acetylcholine receptor (AChR) antibodies, detectable in 85% of MG patients, lead to AChR loss, and fully account for the physiological findings. Even in those patients apparently 'seronegative' in the radioimmunoassay for anti-AChR antibodies, humoral factors – probably antibodies – appear to underlie the transmission disorder in many.

The advances in MG were followed by the discovery that autoimmunity underlies the *Lambert–Eaton myasthenic syndrome (LEMS)*, the target here being presynaptic voltage-gated calcium channels (VGCCs). This is the commonest and best-characterised of the paraneoplastic neurological syndromes, and was the first in which cross-reactive autoantibodies were directly implicated as the link between the cancer and the nervous system. Anti-VGCC antibodies, initially detected by a bioassay, are present both in those with the associated small cell lung cancer and those without.

Very recent evidence now suggests that *acquired neuromyotonia* (Isaacs' syndrome), a disorder characterised by hyperexcitability of peripheral nerves leading to continuous muscle fibre activity, is also antibody-mediated. The target in this instance may possibly be voltage-gated potassium channels (VGKC) at the nerve terminal.

NEUROMUSCULAR JUNCTION

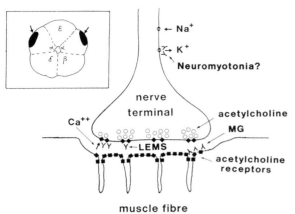

Fig. 20.1   The main events underlying neuromuscular transmission are as follows. Depolarisation of the nerve terminal membrane (dependent on voltage-gated sodium channels) opens voltage-gated calcium channels (VGCC) until repolarisation occurs (dependent on inactivation of the sodium channels and opening of voltage-gated potassium channels (VGKC)). The resulting local Ca^{2+} influx leads to the release by exocytosis of 50 or more packages (quanta) of acetylcholine, each quanta containing about 10 000 molecules. Binding of acetylcholine to its receptor site on the two α-subunits (inset: arrows) of the postsynaptic acetylcholine receptors (AChR) opens the central cation channel. This allows an influx of small cations, mainly Na^+, that generates the end-plate potential and activates postsynaptic voltage-gated sodium channels, thereby triggering the action potential. Propagation of the action potential along the muscle fibre membrane activates muscle contraction. Single quanta are also released spontaneously, generating a miniature end-plate potential. The inset shows the structure of the acetylcholine receptor that comprises five subunits forming a central ion channel. The α-subunit is represented twice, and occurs as two isoforms (Beeson et al 1990). The γ-subunit in fetal (and denervated) muscle is replaced by an ε at junctional acetylcholine receptors. The figure also illustrates the presence of anti-AChR antibodies in myasthenia gravis (MG), anti-VGCC antibodies in the Lambert-Eaton myasthenic syndrome and, in acquired neuromyotonia, the possible presence of anti-VGKC antibodies.

Figure 20.1 outlines the main events accompanying neuromuscular transmission, and indicates the targets for the autoantibodies in MG, LEMS and acquired neuromyotonia.

These aetiological discoveries have led to new — immunological — approaches to diagnosis, and have had an important influence on management. They have also helped to define as a separate group patients with *congenital/hereditary myasthenia*, in whom there is no immunological abnormality but where the defect is due to inherited or congen-ital defects at the nerve–muscle junction. Here, neurophysiological, biological and molecular approaches are beginning to define their several natures.

MYASTHENIA GRAVIS

Clinical subtypes

The clinical expression of MG is heterogeneous, but several distinct groups can be identified (Table 20.1). About 10% of patients have an associated thymoma, the peak age at onset in this group being in the fifth decade. In non-thymoma cases, Compston et al (1980) described an early-onset (<40 years) group, in which females predominate (4 : 1), the thymic medulla shows changes of hyperplasia and anti-AChR antibody titres tend to be high. This group was distinguished from a late-onset group where males predominate and the thymus appears atrophic. Anti-AChR antibody titres in the late-onset group tend to be lower, while those for thymoma are intermediate. Immunogenetic studies (see below) show a difference in HLA and Ig heavy chain gene associations between the old-onset and young-onset non-thymomatous cases.

To these three groups can be added another, those who are 'seronegative' in the standard radio-immunoprecipitation assay using human AChR as antigen. In this group, the thymus is typically atrophic, or may show minor abnormalities of T-cell areas, but lacks the germinal centres seen in the young-onset group (Willcox et al 1991). Restricted ocular symptoms are most common in the sero-negative and late-onset groups.

Racial differences. Although affecting all races, the clinical expression of MG can differ. A comparison of 258 Chinese (Taiwan) with 258 Caucasian (UK) patients showed that the former had a greater proportion of early-onset and ocular cases, lacked the late-onset peak of the latter group and had fewer severe cases (Chiu et al 1987b). Immunogenetic associations also differ (see below).

Penicillamine-induced MG. This has been observed most frequently in rheumatoid arthritis patients, but has also been reported in Wilson's disease (Czlonkowska 1975) and primary biliary

Table 20.1 Clinical heterogeneity in myasthenia gravis: typical features

	'Early onset' (55%)	'Thymoma' (10%)	'Late onset' (20%)	'Seronegative' (15%)
Thymus	Hyperplasia	Thymoma	Atrophy	? ↑ T-cell areas
Sex incidence	F >>M	M = F	M > F	M >F
Anti-AChR	High	Intermediate	Low	Not detectable
Immune response gene associations				
HLA-B8	++	–	–	–
-DR3	+	–	–	–
-B7	–	–	+	–
-DR2	–	–	+/–	–
Ig heavy chain (Sμ: 2.6/2.6 kb)	–	–	++	Not available
Weakness	Generalised	Generalised	Generalised or ocular	Generalised or ocular

cirrhosis (Marcus et al 1984) treated with penicillamine. Serum anti-AChR is detectable, and its characteristics do not differ from those found in recent-onset idiopathic MG (Vincent & Newsom-Davis 1982a). The pathophysiological features are also similar (Kuncl et al 1986). There is an association with HLA-Bw35 and -DR1 (Garlepp et al 1993). Symptoms usually decline over several months following drug withdrawal.

Neonatal MG. This occurs in 10–15% of babies born to MG mothers, and differs from other forms of myasthenia in being a 'passive' rather than an 'active' disorder. It is due to placental transfer of maternal anti-AChR antibodies. It has been observed even in the absence of detectable anti-AChR in the mother, i.e. in a 'seronegative' case, nature's passive transfer experiment indicating the presence of a humoral factor. In the mothers of babies with neonatal MG, no clear difference was found in the characteristics of their anti-AChR antibodies compared with MG mothers who had healthy babies (Tzartos et al 1990). Arthrogryposis is a rare complication (Morel et al 1988, Stoll et al 1991).

Symptoms usually disappear within 3 weeks (Namba et al 1970) and anti-AChR antibodies become undetectable in 1–5 months (Morel et al 1988), although in occasional cases they may persist for a few months (Lefvert & Osterman 1983).

Familial MG. This describes MG occurring within families. It should be distinguished from familial infantile myasthenia which is a form of congenital myasthenia and is non-immunological in origin (see below). MG has been reported in monozygotic twins (Murphy & Murphy 1986). To date, a total of 18 sets of monozygotic twins appear to have been reported, seven of whom were concordant for the presence of MG and/or anti-AChR antibodies. This contrasts with 13 sets of dizygotic twins in whom none were concordant.

Epidemiology

MG can affect all races. The prevalence of MG has been variably estimated at 5–10 per 100 000. A recent survey by Somnier et al (1991) in Denmark gave a point prevalence (in 1988) of 9.6 per 100 000 for women and 5.7 per 100 000 for men. The annual incidence in this population was 4.4 per million. Earlier studies in other populations are reviewed by Kurtzke (1978).

Clinical features

Ocular symptoms (diplopia or ptosis) are the commonest at presentation, as illustrated in Figure 20.2, but any striated muscle group can be involved, including respiratory muscles. The characteristic features of the weakness in MG are its variability within the day or even within the hour, its exacerbation by muscle usage and improvement with rest. Emotional stress and infection will also increase symptoms.

Signs that may be present are those of progressive weakness during sustained effort

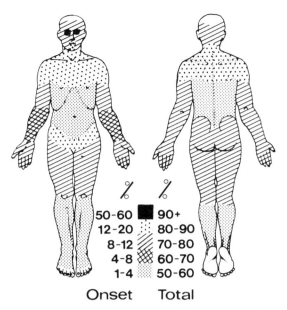

%   %
50-60 ■ 90+
12-20 ░ 80-90
8-12 ▨ 70-80
4-8 ▩ 60-70
1-4 ░ 50-60

Onset   Total

Fig. 20.2 Percentage of cases in which various muscle groups are affected at the onset (left of key) and at some time during the illness (right of key).

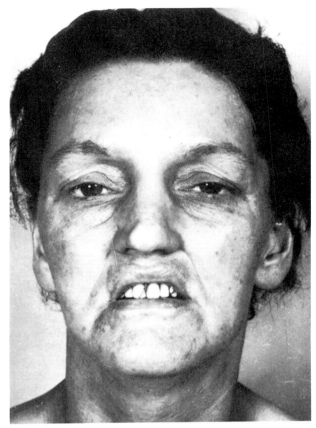

Fig. 20.3 The characteristic myasthenic 'snarl' in myasthenia gravis (from Engel et al 1977a with permission)

(i.e. 'fatiguable' ptosis). There may be variable diplopia, occasionally 'pseudo'-nystagmus, nasal speech, nasal regurgitation, difficulty with swallowing, weakness of jaw closure, and weakness also of neck extension leading to jaw propping and head droop. The smile has a highly characteristic snarling quality (Fig. 20.3). Elevation of the arms, elbow extension, finger abduction and hip flexion are commonly affected, often with sparing of ankle dorsiflexion. Weakness increases with repeated effort. Wasting is a relatively rare occurrence. Tendon reflexes are typically brisk and sphincter control is usually unaffected.

Central nervous system (CNS) features. Levels of anti-AChR in the cerebrospinal fluid (CSF) suggest passive diffusion rather than active synthesis within the CNS (Keesey et al 1977). Mavra et al (1990) found no evidence of CSF oligoclonal bands in 17 of 19 patients, positivity in the two remaining patients being attributed to co-existing non-myasthenic disorders (multiple sclerosis and systemic lupus erythematosus). Whether there are subtle associated cognitive defects is not yet resolved. Tucker et al (1988) found a memory disorder which improved after plasma exchanges, whereas Lewis et al (1989) detected no change in

an auditory vigilance task before and after plasma exchange. Psychiatric disturbances were noted in 38 of 74 patients, especially depressed mood and emotional disorders, but no controls were studied (Magni et al 1988). When appropriate disease controls are evaluated, no differences are observed (Cordess et al 1983).

Cardiac abnormalities. Hofstad et al (1984) found signs of MG-related heart disease in 17 of 108 patients (16%). Interestingly, a control group of spinal muscular atrophy patients showed a similar frequency of heart disease, but the proportion who were symptomatic was smaller (2% versus 10%). Cardiac involvement was commonest in thymoma patients (5 of 10), and focal myocarditis was seen in the three patients examined at autopsy. Arrhythmias were the commonest manifestation, sudden death occurring in five. Mygland et al (1991) detected heart muscle antibodies by

ELISA in 29 of 30 thymoma patients, in none of 30 early-onset cases with thymic hyperplasia, and in seven of 15 late-onset patients with thymic atrophy. The antibodies cross-reacted with skeletal muscle in most cases.

Natural history

The progress of the disease is variable (Oosterhuis 1989). In some, the disorder remains confined to the eye muscles (ocular MG) and if this lasts for 2 years or more, the chance of generalised MG developing is greatly diminished. Earlier observations in patients receiving only anticholinesterase treatment (that does not interfere with the underlying autoimmune process) show that the disease typically reaches maximum severity in most patients within the first 5–7 years. Oosterhuis (1981) found a remission rate of about 1% per year in over 180 patients with generalised MG treated with anticholinesterase medication alone, followed for a mean period of 17 years. The annual remission rate in similarly treated ocular cases was about twice this.

Immunopathogenesis

Immunological associations. One of the earliest clues to the immunological nature of MG was its association with other autoimmune disorders, particularly thyroid disease. In a personal consecutive series of 600 cases, history of hyperthyroidism was present in 3%, rheumatoid arthritis in 2%, SLE in 1%, polymyositis in 0.5%. MG can also be associated with the Lambert–Eaton myasthenic syndrome (Taphoorn et al 1988, Newsom-Davis et al 1991). Similarly, other organ-specific and non-organ-specific autoantibodies are detected at increased frequencies.

Immune response gene associations. Particular immune response genes appear to confer susceptibility to MG, as in many other autoimmune disorders, and analysis of patient populations in terms of their immune response gene associations has provided further evidence to support the clinical evidence for heterogeneity. As shown in Table 20.1, for a Caucasian population, the early-onset patient group shows an increased frequency of the HLA-A1, B8, DR3 haplotype (Compston et al

1980). Interestingly, the association is strongest with HLA B8 (class I) rather than with DR3 (class II). The late-onset cases, by contrast, show an association – rather less strong – with B7 and DR2. This distinction in terms of HLA association is supported by studies of Ig heavy chain polymorphisms. Typing by restriction fragment length polymorphisms using probes for the switch (S) region of the μ constant domain showed a highly significant increase for a particular allele in the late-onset cases that was not observed in the early-onset group (Table 20.1), further underlining the immunogenetic heterogeneity (Demaine et al 1992), and arguing against a single susceptibility gene for MG. No clear immune response gene associations in Caucasian patients have been observed in the thymoma, seronegative or ocular subgroups.

Several studies have shown very different HLA associations in non-Caucasian patients. In Chinese MG patients, the associations were with Bw46 and DRw9 (Chiu et al 1987a). Matsuki et al (1990) found strong associations with DRw9, and also with DRw13 and DQw3 in young-onset Japanese patients.

Pathophysiology. The primary defect in MG is a reduction in the number of functional AChRs at the neuromuscular junction (Fig. 20.1), as shown by the use of α-bungarotoxin (BuTx) that binds with high affinity to the α-subunits of the AChR (Fambrough et al 1973). This reduction results in a decreased amplitude of the end-plate potential that may fail to reach the critical firing threshold for the muscle cell, leading to conduction block, as first shown in biopsied intercostal muscle in MG patients by Elmqvist et al (1964). Miniature end-plate potential (mepp) amplitudes are also reduced.

In established MG cases, the end-plate can show striking morphological abnormalities, characterised by widening of the synaptic cleft and a reduction in the folding of the postsynaptic membrane (Engel 1980).

Anti-acetylcholine receptor (AChR) antibodies. Loss of functional AChRs in MG is due to binding of anti-AChR antibodies (Fig. 20.1). Animals immunised with purified AChR develop experimental autoimmune (EA)MG (Patrick & Lindstrom 1973) which in primates closely resembles the human disease (Tarrab-Hazdai et al

1975). Mice injected with immunoglobulins from MG patients show reduced mepp amplitudes and AChR loss and some became weak (Toyka et al 1977).

AChRs have an active turnover, new receptors being synthesised and assembled in the muscle cell before insertion into the cell membrane. Antibodies can cause AChR loss by: (1) complement-mediated lysis (Engel 1980, Engel & Arahata 1987); (2) cross-linking of adjacent AChRs, leading to an increased rate of internalisation and down-regulation (Drachman et al 1980); (3) blocking of agonist binding to the ACh recognition site (Drachman et al 1982, Burges et al 1990).

Anti-AChR antibodies are of IgG class and are heterogeneous, i.e. they differ in their sites of binding to the AChR. Many of them bind to sites within the main immunogenic region of the α subunit, that includes amino acids 60–75 on the extracellular domain (Tzartos & Lindstrom 1980, Tzartos et al 1991), but some do not (Heidenreich et al 1988). Both κ and λ light chains are represented (Vincent & Newsom-Davis 1982b). The antibodies also differ in their idiotypes. For example, anti-idiotypic polyclonal antisera raised in rabbits against a particular patient's AChR antibodies will inhibit their binding to AChR, but have only a minor inhibition of the binding of another patient's anti-AChR antibodies (Lang et al 1985).

The antibodies are normally assayed using human muscle AChRs either extracted from amputated calf muscle or from human muscle cell lines that express AChR. The use of AChR from other species (e.g. rat, calf) leads to a lower yield of positive results. The AChRs are labelled with [^{125}I]α-BuTx, and [^{125}I]BuTx–AChR complexes are then precipitated with an anti-human Ig polyclonal serum (Vincent & Newsom-Davis 1985).

Anti-AChR antibodies can be detected in the serum in about 85–90% of patients with generalised MG and in about 50–60% of those with ocular myasthenia. They have only very rarely been detected in patients who have no history of MG (Vincent & Newsom-Davis 1985), and their detection is thus, for all practical purposes, diagnostic of the disorder.

The absolute titre of anti-AChR antibody is not an index of disease severity. For example, a patient with severe disease may have a much lower titre than another with mild disease, or one who is even in remission. This may reflect the antibody heterogeneity mentioned above. The titre within an individual, by contrast, relates directly to disease severity. For instance, the decline in anti-AChR following plasma exchange shows an inverse relationship to muscle strength (Newsom-Davis et al 1978), and patients who have entered remission following thymectomy or immunosuppressive drug treatment will generally have lower anti-AChR titres than before treatment began (Oosterhuis et al 1983).

AChR-reactive T cells. Anti-AChR antibody production in MG is believed to be dependent on T helper cells, as it is in experimental autoimmune MG. Hohlfeld et al (1984) pioneered the raising of AChR reactive T-cell lines from MG patients, using *Torpedo* AChR as antigen and showing that responses to the α-subunit appeared to be dominant. *Torpedo* AChR was used since amounts of AChR that can be purified from amputated human calf muscle are insufficient. However, *Torpedo* AChR is not the ideal antigen since it has only about 75% homology with human AChR. An alternative has been to use a recombinant approach for expressing the protein products of the human AChR subunit cDNAs in *E. coli* (Beeson et al 1989). Several T-cell epitopes of the α-subunit have been identified in this way (Newsom-Davis et al 1989), together with their class II restriction, and, in one clone, T-cell receptor gene usage also (Ong et al 1991). The functional role of these T cells – in particular whether they are able to provide cognate help for antibody production – has not yet been determined.

Seronegative MG. In about 15% of patients with generalised MG, and up to 50% of those with restricted ocular MG, anti-AChR antibody cannot be detected in the standard radioimmunoprecipitation assay (Table 20.1). However, there is strong clinical evidence that the nature of their disorder is not substantially different from that of the seropositive cases. The clinical spectrum of the disease is broadly similar in the two groups (Soliven et al 1988), and it seems likely that a humoral factor, probably an antibody, underlies their disorder. The evidence for this is as follows:

1. Neonatal MG has been observed in an infant born to a 'seronegative' mother who nevertheless

had clinical features of severe MG. The infant recovered fully in due course, as typically occurs in other cases of neonatal MG from seropositive mothers.

2. Patients with seronegative MG often show a clear response to a course of plasma exchange that removes circulating factors including antibodies (Mossman et al 1986).

3. Long-term treatment with immunosuppressive drugs, in those with generalised weakness, can induce a sustained remission (Birmanns et al 1991).

4. Plasma or immunoglobulin from seronegative patients transfers a defect of neuromuscular transmission when injected into mice (Mossman et al 1986).

Recent studies suggest that the causative humoral factor in a proportion of these patients co-purifies with IgM, and might thus be an IgM antibody (Yamamoto et al 1991). Its target at the neuromuscular junction has not yet been clearly identified. Some patients have antibodies to defined end-plate determinants (e.g. Vinculin), but their functional role is unknown (Yamamoto et al 1987).

Role of the thymus. Differences in thymic pathology contribute to the evidence for clinical heterogeneity in MG (Table 20.1). In the early-onset group, hyperplasia of the thymic medulla is almost always observed in those who are seropositive for AChR antibodies. These changes are characterised by lymphoid follicles with germinal centres that, together with their surrounding T-cell areas, appear to invade the thymic medulla. In well-advanced cases, there is a breakdown in the laminin layer that would otherwise separate the T-cell areas from the medullary epithelial bands.

Functional studies reveal spontaneous anti-AChR production by thymic cell cultures in about two-thirds of patients in this early-onset group (Newsom-Davis et al 1981, Scadding et al 1981). The rate of antibody production *in vitro* correlates with the serum anti-AChR titre (Newsom-Davis et al 1987), and studies of the fine specificities of the anti-AChR produced in culture show that they closely match those in the patient's serum (Heidenreich et al 1988).

The hyperplastic thymus is enriched for AChR-reactive T-cells (Sommer et al 1990). This observation, together with the spontaneous production of anti-AChR, points to the presence of antigen in the thymus as earlier proposed by Wekerle & Ketelsen (1977). It might thus be relevant that thymic myoid cells both in MG patients and controls have been shown to express AChR *in situ* (Schluep et al 1987), and in MG may perhaps be the target of immune attack (Kirchner et al 1988a).

In the late-onset cases, the thymus is typically atrophic, and anti-AChR production is minimal or undetectable. The thymus is also usually atrophic in seronegative cases, and clearly differs from young-onset seropositive cases by the absence of germinal centres (Willcox et al 1991). However, an increase in thymic 'lymph-node type' T-cell areas distinguished these patients from controls.

Thymomata appear to arise from rare cortical epithelial cells that are positive both for cortical and medullary epithelial cell markers (Willcox et al 1987). They are characterised by the presence of large numbers of lymphocytes, giving them their characteristic lympho-epithelial character, and they are enriched for AChR-reactive T cells (Sommer et al 1990). About 30% of tumours are locally invasive (Monden et al 1984). AChR-like determinants appear to be present in thymoma, as indicated by the binding of a particular anti-AChR monoclonal antibody (Kirchner et al 1988b, Marx et al 1989), but mRNA for the AChR α-subunit was not detected in thymoma (Geuder et al 1989), and ACh-induced currents were not found in their epithelial cells (Siara et al 1991).

Investigations

Detection of serum anti-AChR antibodies at raised titre (>0.5 nmol/l) is essentially specific for MG and, if the test is positive, further diagnostic tests for the presence of MG are not usually required. In seronegative cases, however, additional investigation is needed. The intravenous edrophonium (Tensilon) test is widely used, but is not specific for MG, producing improvement in other myasthenic disorders and sometimes in other neuromuscular diseases. After a 30-second latent period it induces a brief (2–3 minute) period of improvement in myasthenic symptoms and signs. Adverse effects occasionally occur, so resuscitation equipment should be available and a test dose (2 mg in adults) should be given, preferably after a premedicating intravenous dose of atropine (0.6 mg). Some patients will respond to the test dose, removing the need for the full dose (5–8 mg).

Electromyography (EMG) is valuable in demonstrating a defect in neuromuscular transmission, although it cannot always discriminate between MG and other disorders of transmission. The methods are described in greater detail in Chapter 29 but, in brief, decrement exceeding 10% in the compound muscle action potential amplitude at 3 per second stimulation (fifth compared to the first response) is abnormal. A more sensitive method is to use single fibre electromyography (SFEMG) (Stålberg & Trontelj 1979), which detects abnormalities (increased jitter) in the great majority of MG patients (Sanders & Howard 1986). In ocular MG, jitter studies in orbicularis oculi may be particularly helpful (Trontelj et al 1988).

The thymus is currently best imaged by computerised tomography, although this cannot always distinguish thymoma from normal thymus (Brown et al 1983, Janssen et al 1983, Moore 1989). Magnetic resonance imaging may prove to be useful, but is not yet adequately evaluated. Imaging should be undertaken in all patients in whom thymoma is suspected – which in general would mean all seropositive patients since thymoma appears to be exceedingly rare in seronegative MG. Anti-striated muscle antibody is detectable in about 85% of thymoma patients (Gilhus et al 1984), but is also present in a proportion of non-tumour cases. Some of these antibodies recognize titin (Aarli et al 1990).

In seronegative MG, plasma exchange is sometimes useful as an investigative technique. A clear-cut clinical response, coupled with electromyographic monitoring, strengthens the case for long-term immunosuppressive treatment (see below).

Investigations may also be needed to exclude other autoimmune diseases, e.g. thyrotoxicosis or associated polymyositis.

Differential diagnosis

The principal disorders to be considered in the differential diagnosis are those that can also produce fatigable weakness. The majority are dealt with elsewhere in this chapter. The Lambert–Eaton myasthenic syndrome is distinguished by a different pattern of weakness, depressed tendon reflexes, autonomic changes and a reduced compound muscle action potential amplitude that increases by more than 100% following maximum voluntary contraction of the muscle. Congenital/hereditary myasthenia is a heterogeneous group of disorders of which most present within the first 2 years of life. Onset of MG before 2 years is very rare. There may be a family history, or consanguineous parents and anti-AChR antibody is not present. The possibility of botulinum toxin poisoning should be kept in mind in those who may have eaten infected food, or have a wound infection, and in infants in whom the toxin may be produced in the gastrointestinal tract. Autonomic features and ocular symptoms occur early. The chronic fatigue syndrome does not usually present diagnostic difficulties since the typical myasthenic history of fluctuating ocular and limb involvement is lacking, fatigable weakness is not demonstrable clinically and the EMG changes of a neuromuscular transmission defect are absent.

Ocular myasthenia can cause special diagnostic difficulty, and it is necessary to consider ophthalmic Graves' disease, intracranial lesions such as parasellar tumours and aneurysms (Moorthy et al 1989), and also mitochondrial myopathy which when presenting with unilateral ptosis, can closely mimic MG. Such patients may also show an increase in jitter in single fibre EMG studies.

Management

Following the diagnosis of MG, most patients will be prescribed anticholinesterase medication at low dosage (e.g. pyridostigmine 30–60 mg, 4 or 5 times daily). This will often adequately control mild symptoms, but patients who fail to respond will sometimes find the side-effects of higher dosage unacceptable. There is also a risk of cholinergic paralysis as the dose is increased. Chronic treatment at high dosage could theoretically lead to AChR loss, as has been shown in animals (Chang et al 1973, Gwilt and Wray 1986).

A flow diagram provides a useful way of reviewing further management (Fig. 20.4). If a thymoma is detected, thymectomy is indicated because of

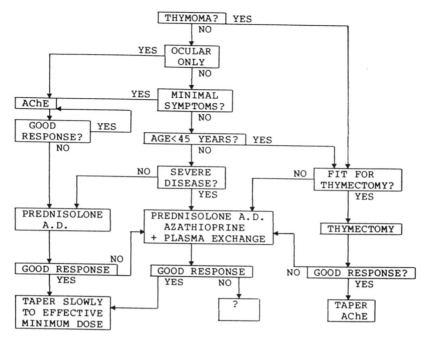

Fig. 20.4 A 'flow diagram' of the management of myasthenia gravis. AChE, anticholinesterase (pyridostigmine, prostigmine); A.D., alternate days; ?, consider alternative therapy. Thymectomy is probably not indicated in those who are seronegative (modified from Newsom-Davis 1992, with permission).

the risk of local invasion, although removal does not usually result in improvement of the myasthenia. Should the patient not be well enough for surgery, plasma exchange, possibly coupled with immuno-suppressive drug treatment, can be undertaken first. Thymectomy may not be indicated in very elderly patients with thymoma, since the tumours may be slow-growing. Patients who retain their tumours can still respond to immunosuppressive drugs. If removal of the tumour is incomplete, or it is inoper-able, local radiotherapy or chemotherapy will be needed (Daugaard et al 1983, Monden et al 1984). Occasional tumours will recede simply with steroid treatment (Tandan et al 1990).

Patients whose symptoms are confined to eye muscles (ocular MG), who usually have low or absent anti-AChR antibodies, are best treated with alternate-day prednisolone if they have not responded adequately to anticholinesterase med-ication. Because of the risk of steroid-induced deterioration, the dose should be given as alter-nate-day medication (Seybold & Drachman 1974), and increased slowly (e.g. by 5 mg weekly)

from a low initial dose, until remission is achieved or an acceptable upper dose is reached. Symptoms typically fluctuate during the initiation of therapy. The dose should then be held constant until the patient has been in remission for about 3 months, before reducing it slowly (e.g. 5 mg per month) and making final adjustments to define the effec-tive minimal dose, which will usually need to be maintained in the long term. The majority of patients will achieve full remission, but in resistant cases extraocular surgery can be considered (Acheson et al 1991). Although thymectomy has been reported to benefit some patients in this group (Schumm et al 1985), this has not been gen-erally accepted as a treatment option in restricted ocular cases. Complete absence of response to cor-ticosteroids in seronegative patients suspected to have ocular MG casts doubt on the diagnosis (see 'Differential diagnosis' above).

Thymectomy, by the trans-sternal route, appears to be indicated in the early-onset group of seropositive cases, although this therapy has never been subjected to a randomised trial. A computerised retrospective study (Buckingham et al 1976), however, showed clear benefits following thymectomy compared with results achieved in patients treated by anticholinesterase medication alone. Similar results are described for thymectomy in childhood MG (Rodriquez et al 1983). Pooled results from several different series indicate an expected remission rate in this group of about 30%, and improvement in a further 40–50%. The effects of thymectomy in the remaining 25% appear neutral.

Evidence that thymectomy is beneficial in the late-onset cases is not compelling and the thymus in these patients is often atrophic. In such patients, and also in those who have failed adequately to respond to thymectomy, prednisolone is the first line of treatment, to which many patients respond (Pascuzzi et al 1984, Sghirlanzoni et al 1984). Prednisolone is best given on alternate days, with 5–10 mg dose increments from a low initial dose up to a maximum of 1–1.5 mg/kg body weight. It may be combined with azathioprine (2.5 mg/kg body weight). In severely weak patients, initiation of treatment should be covered by a 5-day course of plasma exchange, that can be repeated at regular 4–6-week intervals if required. Such patients require to be treated initially in hospital, especially if bulbar or respiratory muscles are involved, because of the risk of steroid-induced exacerbation. Subject to side-effects, dosage should be maintained until remission has been present for 3 months, when the dose can be reduced by 5 mg per month and adjusted to define the effective minimal dose. Prednisolone is faster in its action than azathioprine, but improvement may still take 2–3 months to develop, while the response to azathioprine may take 6–12 months. The latter is valuable as a steroid-sparing drug (Mantegazza et al 1988), but some patients are intolerant (Hohlfeld et al 1988). Its benefits have been clearly shown by reactivation of disease 3–11 months after drug withdrawal (Hohlfeld et al 1985). Patients on azathioprine should have full blood count and liver function tests weekly for the first 8 weeks and 1–3 monthly thereafter.

In patients who fail to respond to the above regimen, the use of other immunosuppressive drugs should be considered, such as cyclosporin A (Tindall et al 1987), cyclophosphamide or methotrexate. Total lymphoid irradiation has also been used. Case reports of the benefits of intravenous immunoglobulin need to be confirmed in a controlled trial.

Plasma exchange is typically followed by symptomatic improvement for 3–5 weeks (Pinching et al 1976). It can be used to prepare patients for thymectomy, to cover deterioration in the post-thymectomy period and during initiation of prednisolone therapy, and to control symptoms during an acute relapse, allowing immunosuppressive drug therapy to be instituted. There appears to be no synergy between immunosuppressive drugs and plasma exchange.

Drugs that can interfere with neuromuscular transmission. Medications that should be used with caution in poorly controlled myasthenic patients include quinine, quinidine, procainamide, aminoglycoside antibiotics, and β-blockers. Neuromuscular blocking agents used in anaesthesia may reveal clinically silent MG.

LAMBERT–EATON MYASTHENIC SYNDROME (LEMS)

Clinical subtypes

LEMS was first recognised as an unusual form of myasthenia occurring in association with lung cancer (Anderson et al 1953). Its distinction from MG was defined electromyographically by Lambert et al (1961) and its presynaptic nature was established in further studies on biopsied intercostal muscle (Lambert & Elmqvist 1971). It later became clear that LEMS could occur not only in association with cancer (C-LEMS), but also in its absence (NC-LEMS) in patients who were non-smokers and where long-term follow-up had clearly excluded an occult tumour. From a survey of 50 consecutive LEMS cases, O'Neill et al (1988) found the association was predominantly with small cell lung cancer (SCLC) and estimated that a patient presenting with LEMS had a 62% risk of underlying SCLC. This risk decreases sharply after 2 years because in most cases the tumour has declared itself by then, but in a recent case of the author's, the interval between the onset of LEMS and the radiological appearance of the tumour was 5 years. This suggests that

LEMS can occur very early in the life of the tumour. The distribution of the age of onset of NC-LEMS is shifted to the left compared with C-LEMS, some patients first developing symptoms in their second decade.

Associations of LEMS with other cancers (e.g. lymphoma) have been reported, but it has proved difficult to show that such an association could not have occurred by chance.

Epidemiology

No epidemiological survey of the prevalence or incidence of LEMS within a general population appears to have been done. Assessment is complicated by the presence of the two distinct subtypes outlined above, survival time in the SCLC group being much shorter, and to the fact that the diagnosis is often overlooked (O'Neill et al 1988). Nevertheless, the prevalence is clearly very much lower than MG, probably at least ten-fold.

The results of a prospective survey of 150 SCLC patients undertaken by Elrington et al (1991), taken together with earlier studies (e.g. Hawley et al 1980), suggest an overall prevalence in this tumour population of about 3%. Extrapolating from the incidence of SCLC in the UK population, one can estimate an incidence in this subgroup of LEMS patients in the UK as 260 per annum, i.e. approximately 4–5 per million, a broadly similar incidence value to that for MG. The incidence of NC-LEMS is clearly very much lower.

Clinical features

The presenting symptom is usually difficulty in walking, described as weakness, heaviness or stiffness of the legs (O'Neill et al 1988). Autonomic symptoms are nearly always present, although not usually volunteered. On being questioned, most patients will acknowledge dryness of the mouth, and some patients will have constipation and, in the case of males, sexual impotence. Upper limb weakness is less evident to the patient. Occasionally the disorder can present acutely with ventilatory failure.

Examination may reveal mild bilateral ptosis, proximal limb weakness with an augmentation of strength over the first few seconds of a maximum effort (that is easy to overlook), and depressed or absent tendon reflexes that often show post-tetanic potentiation after 15 seconds of maximum voluntary contraction. There is no sensory involvement.

No neurological differences were detected between C-LEMS and NC-LEMS patients (O'Neill et al 1988).

Immunopathogenesis

Immunological associations. The incidence of other autoimmune disease is increased in LEMS, as reported by Lennon et al (1982). In the patients reported by O'Neill et al (1988), 26% had associated organ-specific autoimmune disease, equally distributed between C- and NC-LEMS cases, vitiligo and thyroid disease being predominant. As expected, there was an increased incidence of other autoantibodies. LEMS occasionally occurs in association with MG (Newsom-Davis et al 1991).

Immune response gene associations. In NC-LEMS, there is an increased association with HLA-B8 and -DR3 (Willcox et al 1985), that with B8 being significantly the stronger as in young-onset MG cases. There is also an increase in the frequency of the Ig heavy chain marker G1m(2) in all patients, implying as in MG that there is more than one inherited susceptibility factor.

Pathophysiology. The primary defect in LEMS is a reduction in the number of acetylcholine packages (quanta) released by the nerve impulse (Lambert & Elmqvist 1971). This results in a decreased amplitude of the end-plate potential (EPP). As in other conditions in which the quantal content of the EPP (i.e. number of quanta released) is reduced, it increases progressively during the first few impulses in a nerve train, probably because of mobilisation of Ca^{2+} from nerve terminal stores. This underlies the post-tetanic potentiation observed clinically. The amplitude, time-course and frequency of the miniature end-plate potentials in resting muscle is unchanged.

There are no gross pathological changes at the neuromuscular junction. In occasional cases, there may be a striking loss of type I muscle fibres (Squier et al 1991).

Anti-voltage gated calcium channel

(VGCC) antibodies. The defect in quantal release in LEMS appears to be due to an antibody-mediated reduction in the number of functional voltage-gated calcium channels (VGCCs) at motor nerve terminals (Fig. 20.1). LEMS IgG injected into mice leads to a highly significant reduction in the quantal content of the end-plate potential, as occurs in the human disease (Lang et al 1981, 1983). Freeze-fracture electron-microscopy of the end-plate region in healthy individuals reveals parallel double row arrays of active zone particles, each of about 10 nm diameter. These are believed to represent voltage-gated calcium channels. Fukunaga et al (1982) showed that the normal orderly array of active zone particles was disorganised in LEMS muscle, and that the total number of active zones was decreased. They suggested that the active zone particles might therefore be the targets for the pathogenic antibodies described by Lang et al (1981). In a collaborative study, it was then shown that mice injected with LEMS IgG that caused a decrease in quantal content also resulted in the typical disorganisation and paucity of active zones as occurs in the human disease (Fukunaga et al 1983). Further physiological studies indicated an approximately 40% decrease in the number of functional VGCCs at the nerve terminal of injected mice (Lang et al 1987).

The mechanism of VGCC loss does not appear to be complement-dependent (Prior et al 1985). Physiological studies in mice injected with Lambert–Eaton IgG showed a time-course for the decline and recovery of quantal content that closely followed the level of human IgG in the mouse serum and which had a $t_{1/2}$ of about 1.5 days in each case. This finding argued against a direct blocking action of the antibodies. The LEMS IgG was localised at the active zones of injected mice by immuno-electron-microscopy (Fukuoka et al 1987a). A freeze-fracture electron-microscopic study of the earliest changes indicates that they result from cross-linking of adjacent active zone particles by the divalent antibody (Fukuoka et al 1987b), leading to a reduction in their density. This effect was still observed when the divalent antibody fraction ($F(ab')_2$) was applied to organ cultures of mouse diaphragm, but not with the monovalent fraction (Fab') (Nagel et al 1988).

Role of small cell cancer (SCLC). SCLC is believed to be of neuroectodermal origin, raising the possibility that it might express antigenic determinants shared by the nervous system. Roberts et al (1985) demonstrated $^{45}Ca^{2+}$ influx into a human SCLC cell line under depolarising conditions (i.e. high external K^+ concentration), confirming the presence of tumour VGCCs. Influx was significantly reduced in cells exposed to LEMS IgG, whether from cancer or non-cancer cases. Moreover, inhibition of Ca^{2+} influx correlated significantly with disease severity (Lang et al 1989). These findings thus suggested that tumour VGCCs were triggering the anti-VGCC antibody response, cross-reactivity of these antibodies with nerve terminal VGCCs leading to the neurological disorder. Further support for this was provided by the clinical observation that seven of 11 patients surviving for 2 months or more after specific tumour therapy (surgery, radiotherapy or chemotherapy) showed substantial neurological improvement (Fig. 20.5; Chalk et al 1990), one of these patients being in complete remission from both tumour and LEMS 9 years later. Thus tumour VGCCs appear to be driving the autoimmune response in these cases. An immunocytochemical comparison of the tumours in patients with and without LEMS showed a greater infiltration of the SCLC by activated macrophages in the LEMS patients, and also a reduced expression by the tumour cells of the 200 kDa neurofilament antigen and of HLA-class I (Morris et al 1992).

Anti-VGCC antibody assays. There are several subtypes of VGCCs (T-, L-, N-, P-), and the question thus arises as to which of these are targeted by LEMS antibodies. Neurophysiological studies on bovine adrenal chromaffin cells by Kim & Neher (1988), and by Peers et al (1990) on the neuroblastoma cell line NG108, indicated that LEMS IgG can inhibit the action of L-type channels, but not T-type. However, L-type VGCCs do not appear to control ACh release at the motor nerve terminals. Recent evidence suggests that this may be a function of P-type channels (Uchitel et al 1992), but the electrophysiological effects of LEMS IgG on P-type channels has not yet been investigated.

An alternative approach to identifying anti-VGCC antibodies has been to use an immunoprecipitation assay to detect antibodies binding to

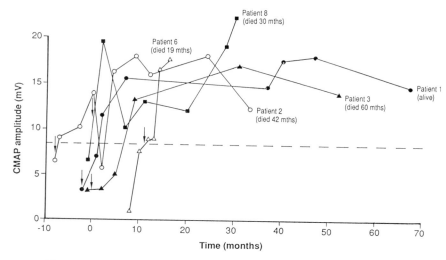

Fig. 20.5 Serial measurements of the amplitude of the compound muscle action potential (CMAP) in patients with C-LEMS who received specific tumour therapy at time zero. Arrows indicate a course of plasma exchange. Dashed line indicates lower limit for CMAP amplitude in a control population (reproduced from Chalk et al 1990 with permission).

labelled VGCCs. The marine fish-eating snail *Conus geographus* secretes a toxin (ω-CgTx) that binds N-type channels, and can be labelled ($[^{125}I]$CgTx). An assay using this toxin detects anti-VGCCs antibodies in a proportion of LEMS patients, as reported by Sher et al (1988), Lennon & Lambert (1989) and Leys et al (1991). The proportion of seropositive patients varies in these different series (91%, 54% and 42% respectively), depending on where the 'normal' cut-off line is placed. In longitudinal studies over several years the anti-$[^{125}I]$ω-CgTx-VGCC antibodies correlated with disease severity (Leys et al 1991). However, a high titre was recently reported in a patient with SCLC and paraneoplastic cerebellar degeneration who did not have LEMS (Clouston et al 1992). These data suggest that anti-N-type VGCC antibodies may not be the only pathogenic antibodies in LEMS. Further evidence that the conotoxin assay may not be detecting all the relevant antibodies comes from the Ca^{2+} flux studies described in the preceding section. Using an SCLC line (MB) derived from a patient with LEMS, Lang et al (1993) found a significant inhibition of flux by IgGs from some patients who were seronegative in the $[^{125}I]$ω-CgTx assay.

Investigations

The diagnosis of LEMS presently depends principally on the EMG findings. These are characterised by a reduced compound muscle potential amplitude, measured for example in a small muscle of the hand, that typically shows an increase greater than 100% following maximum voluntary contraction of the muscle for 15 seconds (Lambert et al 1961). High frequency (40 Hz) nerve stimulation is a less well-tolerated means of observing this effect. There is also an increase in voluntary single fibre EMG jitter (Schwartz & Stålberg 1975) and in stimulated SFEMG (Chaudhry et al 1991). Decrement (at 3 per second stimulation) may also be increased in some patients.

The presence of a raised titre of anti-VGCC antibodies in the $[^{125}I]$ω-conotoxin assay provides further support for the diagnosis (see above).

Investigations for SCLSC need to be undertaken regularly in those especially at risk (i.e. smokers), bearing in mind the long interval that can separate the onset of LEMS from the radiological or other evidence of the cancer.

Differential diagnosis

The commonest alternative diagnosis in the cases reported by O'Neill et al (1988) was MG (in 20%). The disorder can also sometimes be mis-diagnosed as a myopathy. The simple EMG measurement of the compound muscle action po-tential amplitude with supramaximal stimulation of the nerve should prevent the correct diagnosis being overlooked in such cases.

Management

3,4-Diaminopyridine is the drug of choice for the symptomatic treatment of LEMS and is available at special centres. It acts by blocking voltage-gated potassium channels at the nerve terminal, thereby prolonging the depolarising phase of the nerve action potential and allowing a greater influx of calcium to the nerve terminal with each nerve impulse. It is well-tolerated in doses up to 100 mg daily (Lundh et al 1984, McEvoy et al 1989). Excessive dosage can lead to central excitation and seizures. It is preferable to guanidine, as this can have serious side-effects including bone marrow depression.

In SCLC cases, treatment of the tumour will often lead to neurological improvement (Fig. 20.5, Chalk et al 1990). This may be helped by the addi-tion of alternate-day prednisolone therapy.

Where an underlying SCLC is very unlikely (i.e. in non-smokers and young patients), prednisolone combined with azathioprine (2.5 mg/kg body-weight) can be very effective (Newsom-Davis & Murray 1984), leading to complete remission in some cases.

In severe cases, plasma exchange can be a useful way of controlling symptoms, while treatment of the cancer, or immunosuppressive drug therapy, is instituted.

ACQUIRED NEUROMYOTONIA (ISAACS' SYNDROME)

Clinical features

Acquired neuromyotonia is a rare syndrome of spontaneously occurring muscle fibre activity that is of peripheral nerve origin (Isaacs 1961). It pre-sents with stiffness, cramps and weakness of muscle and in most cases there is visible myokymia that has an undulating quality (Denny-Brown & Foley 1948). Muscles may be hypertrophied, especially those of the calf. Sweating may be excessive and in some cases there may be psychological features including hallucinations (Morvan 1890, Halbach et al 1987). In severe cases, movements may be greatly compromised and contractures may occur (Issacs 1961). Some patients have EMG evidence of an associated neuropathy. Transient spontaneous remissions can occur (Isaacs & Heffron 1974).

The characteristic EMG change, first reported by Denny-Brown & Foley (1948), is the occur-rence of spontaneous doublet, triplet or multiplet single unit discharges that have a high intraburst frequency, the frequency of the bursts themselves being irregular (Fig. 20.6). Fasciculation and fibrillation potentials may also be present.

Evidence that the disorder originated in periph-eral nerve was first provided by Isaacs (1961), who showed its abolition by curare and its persistence with proximal peripheral nerve block by local anaesthetic, and suggested its origin in the termi-nal arborisation of motor nerves. In some cases

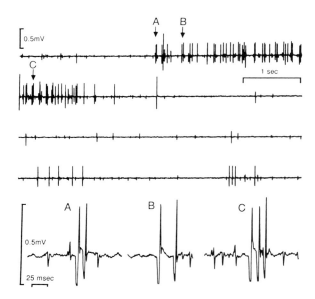

Fig. 20.6 Electromyographic recording with a concentric needle electrode from the muscle of a patient with acquired neuromyotonia. The upper four traces are continuous and show a neuromyotonic discharge lasting about 4 seconds. Within the discharge, single motor units fire as doublets (at A and B, see below), or triplets (at C, see below) (reproduced from Newsom-Davis & Mills 1993 by permission of Oxford University Press).

Table 20.2 Congenital/hereditary myasthenia: Principal disorders

Disorder	Inheritance	Age at onset	Response to AChE	EMG response	
				Single shock	Train
Familial infantile myasthenia	Recessive	Infancy	+	Single	Decrement
Paucity of synaptic vesicles	Recessive	Infancy	+	Single	Decrement
Acetylcholinesterase deficiency	Recessive	Infancy	−	Repetitive	Decrement
Slow channel	Dominant	Infancy to adulthood	−	Repetitive	Decrement
AChR deficiency	Recessive	< 2 years	+	Single	Decrement

the origin may lie more proximally in the nerve or even in the motor neurone itself since in these patients proximal nerve block abolishes the neuromyotonic discharge (for review, see Newsom-Davis & Mills 1993).

Immunopathogenesis

Immunological associations. Despite its rarity, neuromyotonia has been reported in association with thymoma in five cases published in the English literature over the last 20 years, of which two had clinical evidence of MG and two others had raised anti-AChR antibodies without evidence of MG (Newsom-Davis & Mills 1993). Penicillamine treatment has also been reported to induce neuromyotonia (Reeback et al 1979). Three patients reported by Newsom-Davis & Mills (1993) had oligoclonal bands in their cerebrospinal fluid, indicating abnormal IgG synthesis within the central nervous system. Occasional cases have had associated lung cancer (Partanen et al 1980), raising the possibility of an immunologically mediated paraneoplastic basis for the disorder in these patients.

Evidence for an antibody mechanism

Several patients have recently been reported to improve for a few weeks following plasma exchange, pointing to a humoral factor (Sinha et al 1991, Bady et al 1991, Newsom-Davis & Mills 1993). More direct evidence for a causative antibody was the finding that neuromyotonic IgG (or plasma), injected into mice, increased resistance to d-tubocurarine at the nerve terminal in the phrenic nerve diaphragm preparation, compared to mice injected with control human IgG (Sinha et al 1991). This suggested an increase in nerve-evoked acetylcholine release that might result from an antibody-mediated reduction in functional VGKC that normally control peripheral nerve excitability (Fig. 20.1). Subsequent experiments were confirmatory in showing a significant increase in the quantal content of the end-plate potential in mice injected with IgG from neuromyotonia patients without neuropathy (Shillito et al 1993a). Further studies will be needed, however, before it can be concluded that VGKC are the targets for IgG antibodies in some patients with this disorder.

Investigations

Diagnosis is made by the characteristic EMG findings described above. Their origin from peripheral nerve can be confirmed by peripheral nerve block, and by the persistence of the discharges during sleep or general anaesthesia.

Management

Many patients will respond to phenytoin or carbamazepine. It has not yet been shown whether patients failing to respond to this regimen benefit from immunosuppressive drug treatment.

CONGENITAL/HEREDITARY MYASTHENIA

This heterogeneous group of disorders is rare. The disorders are distinguished from MG and LEMS by their non-immunological origins. They are dealt with in further detail in Chapter 21, and have recently been reviewed by Shillito et al (1993b). Table 20.2 provides a classification for the principal disorders in this category and brief clinical features.

REFERENCES

Aarli J A, Stefansson K, Marton L S G, Wollmann R L 1990 Patients with myasthenia gravis and thymoma have in their sera IgG autoantibodies against titin. Clinical and Experimental Immunology 82: 284

Acheson J F, Elston J S, Lee J P, Fells P 1991 Extraocular muscle surgery in myasthenia gravis. British Journal of Ophthalmology 75: 232

Anderson H J, Churchill-Davidson H C, Richardson A T 1953 Bronchial neoplasm with myasthenia. Lancet ii: 1291

Bady B, Chauplannaz G, Vial C, Savet J-F 1991 Autoimmune aetiology for acquired neuromyotonia. Lancet 338: 1330

Beeson D, Brydson M, Wood H, Vincent A, Newsom-Davis J 1989 Human muscle acetylcholine receptor: cloning and expression in *E. coli* of cDNA for the α-subunit. Biochemical Society Transactions 17: 219

Beeson D, Morris A, Vincent A, Newsom-Davis, J 1990 The human muscle nicotinic acetylcholine receptor α-subunit exists as two isoforms: a novel exon. EMBO Journal 9: 2101

Birmanns B, Brenner T, Abramsky O, Steiner I 1991 Seronegative myasthenia gravis: clinical features, response to therapy and synthesis of acetylcholine receptor antibodies *in vitro*. Journal of the Neurological Sciences 102: 184

Brown L R, Muhm J R, Sheedy P F, Unni K K, Bernatz P E, Hermann R C 1983 The value of computed tomography in myasthenia gravis. American Journal of Roentgenology 140: 31

Buckingham J M, Howard F M, Bernatz P E et al 1976 The value of thymectomy in myasthenia gravis: a computer-matched study. Annals of Surgery 184: 453

Burges J, Wray D W, Pizzighella S, Hall Z, Vincent A 1990 A myasthenia gravis plasma immunoglobulin reduces miniature endplate potentials at human endplates in vitro. Muscle and Nerve 13: 407

Chalk C H, Murray N M, Newsom-Davis J, O'Neill J H, Spiro S G 1990 Response of the Lambert–Eaton myasthenic syndrome to treatment of associated small-cell lung carcinoma. Neurology 40: 1552

Chang C C, Chen T F, Chuang S-T 1973 Influence of chronic neostigmine treatment on the number of acetylcholine receptors and the release of acetylcholine from the rat diaphragm. Journal of Physiology 230: 613

Chaudhry V, Watson D F, Bird S J, Cornblath D R 1991 Stimulated single-fiber electromyography in Lambert–Eaton myasthenic syndrome. Muscle and Nerve 14: 1227

Chiu H C, Hsieh R P, Hsieh K H, Hung T P 1987a Association of HLA-DRw9 with myasthenia gravis in Chinese. Journal of Immunogenetics 14: 203

Chiu H C, Vincent A, Newsom-Davis J, Hsieh K H, Hung T 1987b Myasthenia gravis: population differences in disease expression and acetylcholine receptor antibody titers between Chinese and Caucasians. Neurology 37: 1854

Clouston P D, Saper C B, Arbizu T et al 1992 Paraneoplastic cerebellar degeneration. III. Cerebellar degeneration, cancer and the Lambert–Eaton myasthenic syndrome. Neurology 42: 1944

Compston D A S, Vincent A, Newsom-Davis J, Batchelor J R 1980 Clinical, pathological, HLA antigen and immunological evidence for disease heterogeneity in myasthenia gravis. Brain 103: 579

Cordess C, Folstein M F, Drachman D B 1983 Quantitative psychiatric assessment of patients with myasthenia gravis. Journal of Psychiatric Treatment and Evaluation 5: 381

Czlonkowska A 1975 Myasthenia syndrome during penicillamine treatment. British Medical Journal 1: 726

Daugaard G, Hansen H H, Rørth M 1983 Combination chemotherapy for malignant thymoma. Annals of Internal Medicine 99: 189

Demaine A, Willcox N, Janer M, Welsh K, Newsom-Davis J 1992 Immunoglobulin heavy chain gene associations in myasthenia gravis: new evidence for disease heterogeneity. Journal of Neurology 239: 53

Denny-Brown D, Foley J M 1984 Myokymia and the benign fasciculation of muscular cramps. Transactions of the Association of American Physicians 61: 88

Drachman D B, Adams R N, Stanley E F, Pestronk A 1980 Mechanisms of acetylcholine receptor loss in myasthenia gravis. Journal of Neurology, Neurosurgery and Psychiatry 43: 601

Drachman D B, Adams R N, Josifek L F, Self S G 1982 Functional activities of autoantibodies to acetylcholine receptors and the clinical severity of myasthenia gravis. New England Journal of Medicine 307: 769

Elmqvist D, Hofmann W W, Kugelberg J, Quastel D M J 1964 An electrophysiological investigation of neuromuscular transmission in myasthenia gravis. Journal of Physiology 174: 417

Elrington G M, Murray N M G, Spiro S G, Newsom-Davis J 1991 Neurological paraneoplastic syndromes in patients with small cell lung cancer: a prospective survey of 150 patients. Journal of Neurology, Neurosurgery and Psychiatry 54: 764

Engel A G 1980 Morphologic and immunopathologic findings in myasthenia gravis in congenital myasthenic syndromes. Journal of Neurology Neurosurgery and Psychiatry 43: 577

Engel A G, Arahata K 1987 The membrane attack complex of complement at the endplate in myasthenia gravis. Annals of the New York Academy of Sciences 505: 326

Fambrough D M, Drachman D B, Satyamurti S 1973 Neuromuscular junction in myasthenia gravis: decreased acetylcholine receptors. Science 182: 293

Fukunaga H, Engel A G, Osame M, Lambert E H 1982 Paucity and disorganisation of presynaptic membrane active zones in the Lambert–Eaton myasthenic syndrome. Muscle and Nerve 5: 686

Fukunaga H, Engel, A G, Lang B, Newsom-Davis J, Vincent A 1983 Passive transfer of Lambert–Eaton myasthenic syndrome with IgG from man to mouse depletes the presynaptic membrane active zones. Proceedings of the National Academy of Sciences USA 80: 7637

Fukuoka T, Engel A G, Lang B, Newsom-Davis J, Vincent A 1987a Lambert–Eaton myasthenic syndrome: II. Immunoelectron microscopy localization of IgG at the mouse motor end-plate. Annals of Neurology 22: 200

Fukuoka T, Engel A G, Lang B, Newsom-Davis J, Prior C, Wray D W 1987b Lambert–Eaton myasthenic syndrome: I. Early morphological effects of IgG on the presynaptic membrane active zones. Annals of Neurology 22: 193

Garlepp M J, Dawkins R L, Christiansen F T 1983 HLA antigens and acetylcholine receptor antibodies in penicillamine induced myasthenia gravis. British Medical Journal 286: 338

Geuder K I, Schoepfer R, Kirchner Th, Marx A, Müller-Hermelink H K 1989 The gene of the α-subunit of the acetylcholine receptor: molecular organization and transcription in myasthenia-associated thymomas. Thymus 14: 179

Gilhus N E, Aarli J A, Matre R 1984 Myasthenia gravis: difference between thymoma-associated antibodies and cross-striational skeletal muscle antibodies. Neurology 34: 246

Gwilt M, Wray D 1986 The effect of chronic neostigmine treatment on channel properties at the rat skeletal neuromuscular junction. British Journal of Pharmacology 88: 25

Halbach M, Hömberg V, Freund H-J 1987 Neuromuscular, autonomic and central cholinergic hyperactivity associated with thymoma and acetylcholine receptor-binding antibody. Journal of Neurology 234: 433

Hawley R J, Cohen M H, Saini N, Armbrustermacher V W 1980 The carcinomatous neuromyopathy of oat cell lung cancer. Annals of Neurology 7: 65

Heidenreich F, Vincent A, Newsom-Davis J 1988 Differences in fine specificity of anti-acetylcholine receptor antibodies between subgroups of spontaneous myasthenia gravis of recent onset, and of penicillamine induced myasthenia. Autoimmunity 2: 31

Hofstad H, Ohm O-J, Mork S J, Aarli J A 1984 Heart disease in myasthenia gravis. Acta Neurologica Scandinavica 70: 176

Hohlfeld R, Toyka K V, Heininger K, Gross-Wilde H, Kalies I 1984 Autoimmune human T lymphocytes specific for acetylcholine receptor. Nature 310: 244

Hohlfeld R, Toyka K V, Besinger U A, Gerhold B, Heininger K 1985 Myasthenia gravis: reactivation of clinical disease and of autoimmune factors after discontinuation of long-term azathioprine. Annals of Neurology 17: 238

Hohlfeld R, Michels M, Heininger K, Besinger U, Toyka K V 1988 Azathioprine toxicity during long-term immunosuppression of generalized myasthenia gravis. Neurology 38: 258

Isaacs H 1961 A syndrome of continuous muscle-fibre activity. Journal of Neurology, Neurosurgery and Psychiatry 24: 319

Isaacs H, Heffron J J 1974 The syndrome of 'continuous muscle-fibre activity' cured: further studies. Journal of Neurology, Neurosurgery and Psychiatry 37: 1231

Janssen R S, Kaye A D, Lisak R P, Schatz N J, Arger P A, Savino P J 1983 Radiologic evaluation of the mediastinum in myasthenia gravis. Neurology 33: 534

Keesey J, Linstrom J M, Cokely H, Herrmann C 1977 Anti-acetylcholine receptor antibody in neonatal myasthenia gravis. New England Journal of Medicine 296: 55

Kim Y I, Neher E 1988 IgG from patients with Lambert–Eaton syndrome blocks voltage dependent calcium channels. Science 239: 405

Kirchner T, Hoppe F, Schalke B, Muller-Hermelink H K 1988a Microenvironment of thymic myoid cells in myasthenia gravis. Virchows Archiv. B. Cell Pathology 54: 295

Kirchner T, Tzartos S, Hoppe F, Schalke B, Wekerle H, Muller-Hermelink H K 1988b Pathogenesis of myasthenia gravis: acetylcholine receptor-related antigenic determinants in tumour-free thymuses and thymic epithelial tumours. American Journal of Pathology 130: 268

Kuncl R W, Pestronk A, Drachman D B, Rechthand E 1986 The pathophysiology of pencillamine-induced myasthenia gravis. Annals of Neurology 20: 740

Kurtzke J F 1978 Epidemiology of myasthenia gravis. Advances in Neurology 19: 549

Lambert E H, Rooke E D, Eaton L M, Hodgson C H 1961 Myasthenic syndrome occasionally associated with bronchial neoplasm: neurophysiologic studies. In: Viets H R (ed) Myasthenia gravis. Charles Thomas, Springfield, p 362

Lambert E H, Elmqvist D 1971 Quantal components of end-plate potentials in the myasthenic syndrome. Annals of the New York Academy of Sciences 183: 183

Lang B, Newsom-Davis J, Wray D, Vincent A, Murray N M F 1981 Autoimmune aetiology for myasthenic (Eaton–Lambert) syndrome. Lancet ii: 224

Lang B, Newsom-Davis J, Prior C, Wray D 1983 Antibodies to motor nerve terminals: an electrophysiological study of a human myasthenic syndrome transferred to mouse. Journal of Physiology 344: 335

Lang B, Roberts A J, Vincent A, Newsom-Davis J 1985 Anti-acetylcholine receptor idiotypes in myasthenia gravis analysed by rabbit anti-sera. Clinical and Experimental Immunology 60: 637

Lang B, Newsom-Davis J, Peers C, Prior C, Wray D W 1987 The effect of myasthenic syndrome antibody on presynaptic calcium channels in the mouse. Journal of Physiology 390: 257

Lang B, Vincent A, Murray N M, Newsom-Davis J 1989 Lambert–Eaton myasthenic syndrome: immunoglobulin G inhibition of Ca^{2+} flux in tumor cells correlates with disease severity. Annals of Neurology 25: 265

Lang B, Johnston I, Leys K et al 1993 Autoantibody specificities in Lambert–Eaton myasthenic syndrome. Proceedings of VIIIth International Conference on Myasthenia Gravis. Annals of New York Academy of Sciences 681: 382

Lefvert A K, Osterman P O 1983 Newborn infants to myasthenic mothers: a clinical study and an investigation of acetylcholine receptor antibodies in 17 children. Neurology 33: 133

Lennon V A, Lambert E H, Whittingham S, Fairbanks V 1982 Autoimmunity in the Lambert–Eaton myasthenic syndrome. Muscle and Nerve 5: S21

Lennon V A, Lambert E H 1989 Autoantibodies bind solubilised calcium channel-omega-conotoxin complexes from small cell lung carcinoma: a diagnostic aid for Lambert–Eaton myasthenic syndrome. Mayo Clinic Proceedings 64: 1498

Lewis S W, Ron M A, Newsom-Davis J 1989 Absence of central functional cholinergic deficits in myasthenia gravis. Journal of Neurology, Neurosurgery and Psychiatry 52: 258

Leys K, Lang B, Johnston I, Newsom-Davis J 1991 Calcium channel autoantibodies in the Lambert–Eaton myasthenic syndrome. Annals of Neurology 29: 307

Lundh H, Nilsson O, Rosén I 1984 Treatment of Lambert–Eaton syndrome: 3,4-diaminopyridine and pyridostigmine. Neurology 34: 1324

Magni G, Micaglio G F, Lalli R et al 1988 Psychiatric disturbances associated with myasthenia gravis. Acta Psychiatrica Scandinavica 77: 443

Mantegazza R, Antozzi C, Peluchetti D, Sghirlanzoni A, Cornelio F 1988 Azathioprine as a single drug or in combination with steroids in the treatment of myasthenia gravis. Journal of Neurology 235: 449

Marcus S N, Chadwick D, Walker R J 1984 D-Penicillamine-induced myasthenia gravis in primary biliary cirrhosis. Gastroenterology 86: 166

Marx A, Kirchner T, Hoppe F et al 1989 Proteins with epitopes of the acetylcholine receptor in epithelial cell cultures of thymomas in myasthenia gravis. American Journal of Pathology 134: 865

Matsuki K, Juji T, Tokunaga K et al 1990 HLA antigens in Japanese patients with myasthenia gravis. Journal of Clinical Investigation 86: 392

Mavra M, Apostolski S, Nikolic J, Thompson E J 1990 Oligoclonal immunoglobulin G in cerebrospinal fluid of myasthenia gravis patients. Acta Neurologica Scandinavica 81: 250

McEvoy K M, Windebank A J, Daube J R, Low P A 1989 3,4-Diaminopyridine in the treatment of Lambert–Eaton myasthenic syndrome. New England Journal of Medicine 321: 1567

Monden Y, Nakahara K, Nanjo S et al 1984 Invasive thymoma with myasthenia gravis. Cancer 54: 2513

Moore N R 1989 Imaging in myasthenia gravis. Clinical Radiology 40: 115

Moorthy G, Behrens M M, Drachman D B et al 1989 Ocular pseudomyasthenia or ocular myasthenia 'plus': a warning to clinicians. Neurology 39: 1150

Morel E, Eymard B, Vernet-Der Garabedian B, Pannier C, Dulac O, Bach J F 1988 Neonatal myasthenia gravis; a new clinical and immunologic appraisal on 30 cases. Neurology 38: 138

Morris C S, Esiri M N, Marx A, Newsom-Davis J 1992 Immunocytochemical characteristics of small cell lung carcinoma associated with the Lambert–Eaton myasthenic syndrome. American Journal of Pathology 140: 839

Morvan A 1890 De la chorée fibrillaire. Gaz Hebd Med Chir 27: 173

Mossman S, Vincent A, Newsom-Davis J 1986 Myasthenia gravis without acetylcholine receptor antibody: a distinct disease entity. Lancet i: 116

Murphy J, Murphy S F 1986 Myasthenia gravis in identical twins. Neurology 36: 78

Mygland A, Aarli J A, Hofstad H, Gilhus N E 1991 Heart muscle antibodies in myasthenia gravis. Autoimmunity 10: 263

Nagel A, Engel A G, Lang B, Newsom-Davis J, Fukuoka T 1988 Lambert–Eaton myasthenic syndrome IgG depletes presynaptic membrane active zone particles by antigenic modulation. Annals of Neurology 24: 552

Namba T, Brown S B, Grob D 1970 Neonatal myasthenia gravis: report of two cases and review of the literature. Pediatrics 45: 488

Newsom-Davis J, Pinching A J, Vincent A, Wilson S G 1987 Function of circulating antibody to acetylcholine receptor in myasthenia gravis: investigation by plasma exchange. Neurology 28: 266

Newsom-Davis J, Willcox H N A, Calder L 1981 Thymus cells in myasthenia gravis selectively enhance production of anti-acetylcholine receptor antibody by autologous blood lymphocytes. New England Journal of Medicine 305: 1313

Newsom-Davis J, Murray N M 1984 Plasma exchange and immunosuppressive drug treatment in the Lambert–Eaton myasthenic syndrome. Neurology 34: 480

Newsom-Davis J, Willcox N, Schluep M et al 1987 Immunological heterogeneity and cellular mechanisms in myasthenia gravis. Annals of the New York Academy of Sciences 505: 12

Newsom-Davis J, Harcourt G, Sommer N, Beeson D, Willcox N, Rothbard J B 1989 T-cell reactivity in myasthenia gravis. Journal of Autoimmunity 2 (Suppl): 101

Newsom-Davis J, Leys K, Vincent A, Ferguson I, Modi G, Mills K 1991 Immunological evidence for the co-existence of the Lambert–Eaton myasthenic syndrome and myasthenia gravis in two patients. Journal of Neurology, Neurosurgery and Psychiatry 54: 452

Newsom-Davis J 1992 Diseases of the neuromuscular junction. In: Asbury A K, McKhann G M, McDonald W I (eds) Diseases of the nervous system. WB Saunders, Philadelphia, pp 197–212

Newsom-Davis J, Mills K R 1993 Immunological associations of acquired neuromyotonia (Isaac's syndrome): report of 5 cases and literature review. Brain 116: 453

O'Neill J H, Murray N M, Newsom-Davis J 1988 The Lambert–Eaton myasthenic syndrome. A review of 50 cases. Brain 111: 577

Ong B, Willcox N, Wordsworth P et al 1991 Critical role for the Val/Gly[86] HLA-DRβ dimorphism in autoantigen presentation to human T cells. Proceedings of the National Academy of Sciences USA 88: 7343

Oosterhuis H J 1981 Observations of the natural history of myasthenia gravis and the effects of thymectomy. In: Grob D (ed) Myasthenia gravis: pathophysiology and management. Annals of the New York Academy of Sciences 377: 678

Oosterhuis H J G H, Limburg P C, Hummel-Tappel E, The T H 1983 Anti-acetylcholine receptor antibody in myasthenia gravis. II. Clinical and serological follow-up of individual patients. Journal of Neurological Sciences 58: 371

Oosterhuis H J G H 1989 The natural course of myasthenia gravis: a long term follow up study. Journal of Neurology, Neurosurgery and Psychiatry 52: 1121

Partanen V S J, Soininen H, Saksa M, Riekkinen P 1980 Electromyographic and nerve conduction findings in a patient with neuromyotonia, normocalcemic tetany and small-cell lung cancer. Acta Neurologica Scandinavica 61: 216

Pascuzzi R M, Branch Coslett H, Johns T R 1984 Long-term corticosteroid treatment of myasthenia gravis: report of 116 patients. Annals of Neurology 15: 291

Patrick J, Lindstrom J 1973 Autoimmune response to acetylcholine receptor. Science 180: 871

Peers C, Lang B, Newsom-Davis J, Wray D W 1990 Selective action of myasthenic syndrome antibodies on calcium channels in a rodent neuroblastoma × glioma cell line. Journal of Physiology 421: 293

Pinching A J, Peters D K, Newsom-Davis J 1976 Remission of myasthenia gravis following plasma exchange. Lancet ii: 1373

Prior C, Lang B, Wray D, Newsom-Davis J 1985 Action of Lambert–Eaton myasthenic syndrome IgG at mouse motor nerve terminals. Annals of Neurology 17: 587

Reeback J, Benton S, Swash M, Schwartz M S 1979 Penicillamine-induced neuromyotonia. British Medical Journal 1: 1464

Roberts A, Perera S, Lang B, Vincent A, Newsom-Davis J 1985 Paraneoplastic myasthenic syndrome IgG inhibits $^{45}Ca^{2+}$ flux in a human small cell carcinoma line. Nature 317: 737

Rodriguez M, Gomez M R, Howard F M, Taylor W F 1983 Myasthenia gravis in children: long term follow-up. Annals of Neurology 13: 504

Sanders D B, Howard J F 1986 AAEE minimonograph #25: single-fiber electromyography in myasthenia gravis. Muscle and Nerve 9: 809

Scadding G K, Vincent A, Newsom-Davis J, Henry K 1981 Acetylcholine receptor antibody synthesis by thymic lymphocytes: correlation with thymic histology. Neurology 31: 935

Schluep M, Willcox N, Vincent A, Dhoot G K, Newsom-Davis J 1987 Acetylcholine receptors in human thymic myoid cells in situ: an immunohistological study. Annals of Neurology 22: 212

Schumm F, Wiethölter H, Fareh-Moghadam A, Dichgans J 1985 Thymectomy in myasthenia with pure ocular symptoms. Journal of Neurology, Neurosurgery and Psychiatry 48: 332

Schwartz M S, Stålberg E 1975 Myasthenic syndrome studied with single fiber electromyography. Archives of Neurology 32: 815

Seybold M E, Drachman D B 1974 Gradually increasing dose of prednisolone in myasthenia gravis. New England Journal of Medicine 290: 81

Sghirlanzoni A, Peluchetti D, Mangegazza R, Fiacchino F, Cornelio F 1984 Myasthenia gravis: prolonged treatment with steroids. Neurology 34: 170

Sher E, Pandiella A, Clementi F 1988 Ω-conotoxin binding and effects on calcium channel function in human neuroblastoma and rat pheochromocytoma cell lines. FEBS Letters 235: 178

Shillito P, Lang B, Newsom-Davis J, Bady B, Chauplannaz G 1993a Evidence for an autoantibody mediated mechanism in acquired neuromyotonia. Journal of Neurology, Neurosurgery and Psychiatry (abstract, in press)

Shillito P, Vincent A, Newsom-Davis J 1993b Congenital myasthenic syndromes. Neuromuscular Disorders 3: 183

Siara J, Rüdel R, Marx A 1991 Absence of acetylcholine-induced current in epithelial cells from thymus glands and thymomas of myasthenia gravis patients. Neurology 41: 128

Simpson J A 1960 Myasthenia gravis: a new hypothesis. Scottish Medical Journal 5: 419

Sinha S, Newsom-Davis J, Mills K, Byrne N, Lang B, Vincent A 1991 Autoimmune aetiology for acquired neuromyotonia (Isaacs' syndrome). Lancet 338: 75

Soliven B C, Lange D J, Penn A S et al 1988 Seronegative myasthenia gravis. Neurology 38: 514

Sommer N, Willcox N, Harcourt G C, Newsom-Davis J 1990 Myasthenic thymus and thymoma are selectively enriched in acetylcholine receptor-reactive T cells. Annals of Neurology 28: 312

Somnier F E, Keiding N, Paulson O B 1991 Epidemiology of myasthenia gravis in Denmark: a longitudinal and comprehensive population survey. Archives of Neurology 48: 733

Squier M, Chalk C, Hilton-Jones D, Mills K R, Newsom-Davis J 1991 Type 2 fiber predominance in Lambert–Eaton myasthenic syndrome. Muscle and Nerve 14: 625

Stålberg E, Trontelj J V 1979 Single fibre electromyography. Mirvalle Press, Old Woking, Surrey, p 1

Stoll C, Ehret-Mentre M-C, Treisser A, Tranchant C 1991 Prenatal diagnosis of congenital myasthenia with arthrogryposis in a myasthenic mother. Prenatal Diagnosis 11: 17

Tandan R, Taylor R, DiCostanzo D P, Sharma K, Fries T, Roberts J 1990 Metastasizing thymoma and myasthenia gravis. Cancer 65: 1286

Taphoorn M J B, Van Duijn H, Wolters E C H 1988 A neuromuscular transmission disorder: combined myasthenia gravis and Lambert–Eaton syndrome in one

patient. Journal of Neurology, Neurosurgery and Psychiatry 51: 880

Tarrab-Hazdai R, Aharonov A, Silman I, Fuchs S 1975 Experimental autoimmune myasthenia induced in monkeys by purified acetylcholine receptor. Nature 256: 128

Tindall R S A, Rollins J A, Phillips J T, Greenlee R G, Wells L, Belendiuk G 1987 Preliminary results of a double-blind, randomized, placebo-controlled trial of cyclosporin in myasthenia gravis. New England Journal of Medicine 316: 719

Toyka K V, Drachman D B, Griffin D E et al 1977 Myasthenia gravis: study of humoral immune mechanisms by passive transfer to mice. New England Journal of Medicine 296: 125

Trontelj J V, Khuraibet A, Mihelin M 1988 The jitter in stimulated orbicularis oculi muscle: technique and normal values. Journal of Neurology, Neurosurgery and Psychiatry 51: 814

Tucker D M, Roeltgen D P, Wann P D, Wertheimer R I 1988 Memory dysfunction in myasthenia gravis: evidence for central cholinergic effects. Neurology 38: 1173

Tzartos S J, Lindstrom J M 1980 Monoclonal antibodies used to probe acetylcholine receptor structure: localization of the main immunogenic region and detection of similarities between subunits. Proceedings of the National Academy of Sciences USA 77: 755

Tzartos S J, Efthimiadis A, Morel E, Eymard B, Bach J-F 1990 Neonatal myasthenia gravis: antigenic specificities of antibodies in sera from mothers and their infants. Clinical and Experimental Immunology 80: 376

Tzartos S J, Barkas T, Cung M T et al 1991 The main immunogenic region of the acetylcholine receptor: structure and role in myasthenia gravis. Autoimmunity 8: 259

Uchitel O D, Protti D A, Sanchez V, Cherskey B D, Sugimori M, Llinas R 1992 P-type voltage-dependent calcium channel mediates presynaptic calcium influx and transmitter release in mammalian synapses. Proceedings of the National Academy of Sciences USA 89: 3330

Vincent A, Newsom-Davis J 1982a Acetylcholine receptor antibody characteristics in myasthenia gravis. II. Patients with penicillamine-induced myasthenia or idiopathic myasthenia of recent onset. Clinical and Experimental Immunology 49: 266

Vincent A, Newsom-Davis J 1982b Acetylcholine receptor antibody characteristics in myasthenia gravis. I. Patients with generalised myasthenia or disease restricted to ocular muscles. Clinical and Experimental Immunology 49: 257

Vincent A, Newsom-Davis J 1985 Acetylcholine receptor antibody as a diagnostic test for myasthenia gravis: results in 153 validated cases and 2967 diagnostic assays. Journal of Neurology, Neurosurgery and Psychiatry 48: 1246

Wekerle H, Ketelsen U-P 1977 Intrathymic pathogenesis and dual genetic control of myasthenia gravis. Lancet i: 678

Willcox H N, Newsom-Davis J, Calder L R 1984 Cell types required for anti-acetylcholine receptor antibody synthesis by cultured thymocytes and blood lymphocytes in myasthenia gravis. Clinical and Experimental Immunology 58: 97

Willcox N, Demaine A G, Newsom-Davis J, Welsh K I, Robb S A, Spiro S G 1985 Increased frequency of IgG heavy chain marker G1m(2) and of HLA-B8 in Lambert–Eaton myasthenic syndrome with and without associated lung carcinoma. Human Immunology 14: 29

Willcox N, Schluep M, Ritter M A, Schuurman H J, Newsom-Davis J, Christensson B 1987 Myasthenic and nonmyasthenic thymoma. An expansion of a minor cortical epithelial cell subset? American Journal of Pathology 127: 447

Willcox N, Schluep M, Ritter M A, Newsom-Davis J 1991 The thymus in seronegative myasthenia gravis patients. Journal of Neurology 238: 256

Yamamoto T, Sato T, Sugita H 1987 Antifilamin, antivinculin and antitropomyosin antibodies in myasthenia gravis. Neurology 37: 1329

Yamamoto T, Vincent A, Ciulla T A, Lang B, Johnston I, Newsom-Davis J 1991 Seronegative myasthenia gravis: a plasma factor inhibiting agonist-induced acetylcholine receptor function copurifies with IgM. Annals of Neurology 39: 550

21. Neuromuscular disorders in infancy and childhood

D. Gardner-Medwin

INTRODUCTION

This chapter attempts two tasks: to give an account of some disorders, particularly the congenital myopathies and congenital myasthenias, which are not covered elsewhere in this volume and then to describe in broader terms the various clinical presentations of the neuromuscular diseases in childhood. Professor Sir Peter Tizard wrote the corresponding chapter in earlier editions and much of the matter, especially in the section on hypotonia, is his and is gratefully acknowledged.

Children present special problems to the neurologist: they demand special approaches to history-taking and examination; their disorders are superimposed on the shifting ground of continuous development, and they are subject to a very wide variety of disorders, many of them rare, of which a high proportion are unknown in adult life. Most of the serious neuromuscular diseases which affect children are genetically determined and so the need for genetic counselling pervades the strategies of management and may impose a sense of urgency for accurate diagnosis and prognosis even on clinical situations which might otherwise properly be subjected to the test of time.

Normal muscle activity in young infants is evident mainly in their tone and posture, so hypotonia is the dominant presenting feature of most neuromuscular disorders presenting in the first year or so of life. However, hypotonia is also the earliest sign of many systemic illnesses and disorders of the central nervous system, so a discussion of the hypotonic infant must cover a wide field. Other important presenting features of congenital neuromuscular disorders are contractures (arthrogryposis) and dysfunction of certain critical muscles, especially those of sucking, swallowing and respiration, but also those of eye movement and facial expression.

Later in childhood the disorders causing progressive muscle weakness dominate the scene but the intermittent paralyses, muscle pain and stiffness or myoglobinuria may be the principal problems in various disorders. Each of these will be discussed in turn after an initial account of the congenital myopathies.

More detailed accounts of neuromuscular disease in childhood include those of Brooke (1977), Dubowitz (1978, 1980, 1985), Brooke et al (1979), Engel & Banker (1986), Vinken et al (1992) and (for the spinal muscular atrophies) Hausmanowa-Petrusewicz (1978) and Gamstorp & Sarnat (1984). Quantitative data for muscle-power in normal children are given by Hosking et al (1976) and Newman et al (1984). The technique and use of needle muscle biopsy in children will be found in Heckmatt et al (1984) and Dubowitz (1985).

The genetic and developmental disorders of the neuromuscular system in childhood may be listed conveniently (not really classified) as follows:

1. Genetic myopathies with specific biochemical defects
    Glycogen storage diseases
    Lipid storage diseases
    Disorders of fatty acid metabolism
    Cytochrome disorders
    Other disorders of mitochondrial function or structure
2. Genetic myopathies with periodic metabolic manifestations
    Periodic paralyses
    Malignant hyperpyrexia
    Familial paroxysmal rhabdomyolysis
    Other myoglobinurias
3. Genetic myopathies with specific structural changes in fibres
    Central core disease
    Minicore (multicore) myopathy
    Nemaline myopathy
    The centronuclear myopathies etc
4. Genetic myopathies with changes in the histochemical fibre type

5. Genetic myopathies with necrotic degeneration (the muscular dystrophies)
6. Genetic myopathies with non-specific histology
7. Disorders of muscle development
    Amyoplasia
    Local absence of muscles
    Arthrogryposis multiplex congenita
    Congenital fibre-type disproportion
8. Genetic disorders of neuromuscular transmission
9. Genetic disorders with abnormal muscle fibre activity
    Myotonic disorders
    Myokymia
    Muscle rigidity
10. Progressive fibrodysplasia ossificans (myositis ossificans)
    Myosclerosis

Only a few of the categories in this list are discussed below; descriptions of the others can be found in Chapters 15, 17, 18 and 27.

THE CONGENITAL MYOPATHIES

Most of the true myopathies present at birth are genetically determined, and in the rest the cause is usually unknown. On the other hand, many of the genetic disorders customarily described as congenital myopathies may not cause symptoms until later in childhood or even adult life, by which time many acquired myopathies including polymyositis and the endocrine disorders must be considered in the differential diagnosis. It is best, therefore, to consider these myopathies as 'genetic and idiopathic myopathies'.

This chapter concentrates on clinical aspects of the congenital myopathies because their pathological features are described in Chapters 7, 8 and 9.

Genetic myopathies with specific structural changes in fibres

Central core disease. Although it was the first of this group of myopathies to be described (Shy & Magee 1956), central core disease is uncommon. It can be recognised only by histochemical and ultrastructural examination of the muscle.

The cores in the muscle fibres may be single or multiple, central or peripheral but they extend for a considerable distance along the fibre. They are seen almost exclusively in type I fibres and are devoid of mitochondria, myophosphorylase and oxidative enzymes; the myofibril structure in the core may be disrupted or may be intact and the fibres are otherwise normal. Type I fibre predominance is usual and sometimes type II fibres are virtually absent. Morgan-Hughes et al (1973) reported a mother with central core disease whose two clinically affected children had muscle with type I predominance but no cores.

Three or more clinical syndromes of central core disease seem to exist, but cores have also been described after experimental tenotomy and in association with other types of muscle pathology, so their presence should be interpreted with caution if the clinical situation is unusual.

Most cases present with moderate infantile hypotonia and often with delay in walking until three or four years of age. Thereafter there is no deterioration, but hurried walking and climbing stairs remain difficult. Brooke (1977) has pointed out that affected families often recognise and make light of the symptoms and may come under observation only incidentally. The weakness is greater in the legs than in the arms, and muscle wasting is usually slight. The facial muscles are usually, but not always, spared. The tendon reflexes are diminished but present in most cases. A common feature is congenital dislocation of the hips (Armstrong et al 1971) and in some families talipes is prominent either from birth or later in life while others have flat feet. Kyphoscoliosis may occur. Late respiratory failure is a rare feature. Although the onset in this typical form is almost always in infancy, a minority of cases develop weakness in adult life which may then be slowly progressive; infantile and adult forms may occur in the same family (Patterson et al 1979).

The serum creatine kinase (CK) activity is usually normal, but may be increased, occasionally to 6–10 times normal. Electromyographic (EMG) abnormalities are often slight and unhelpful. Cruz Martinez et al (1979) reviewed the EMG findings and reported an increase in the density of muscle fibres belonging to individual motor units, a finding presumably related to the predominance of type I fibres. Isaacs et al (1975) reported a reduction in calcium uptake by the sarcoplasmic reticulum in two cases. Although both Cruz Martinez et al and Isaacs et al interpreted their findings as giving evidence of denervation, more direct and definite evidence of a neurogenic basis for central core disease is lacking, its pathogenesis remains obscure and it is probably best to classify it for the present among the congenital myopathies. Inheritance in this typical form of central core disease is autosomal dominant; the gene has been linked to 19q12-13.2 (Haan et al 1990, Kausch et al 1991).

Dubowitz & Platts (1965) reported an affected brother and sister whose unaffected parents were first cousins, making autosomal recessive inheritance likely. These cases were atypical also in both having focal wasting of the muscles of the right arm from childhood and more generalised weakness in the fourth decade.

The family reported by Bethlem et al (1966) was unique in having only minimal weakness and in having suffered since childhood from severe painless stiffness of the muscles induced by running, climbing stairs or walking on tiptoe, and lasting for several minutes.

In addition, various sporadic and atypical cases have been reported, including one with congenital contractures, who had an unaffected identical twin (Cohen et al 1978) and another with late-onset pes cavus with no clinical abnormality of muscle (Telerman-Toppet et al 1973).

Denborough et al (1973) described a patient with central core disease who had an extensive family history of malignant hyperpyrexia and was herself susceptible. Eng et al (1978) and Frank et al (1980) reviewed the association of these two disorders and concluded that it was rare but not coincidental. An atypically elevated serum CK activity in central core disease appears to indicate a risk of susceptibility to malignant hyperpyrexia. The association is presumably related to the linkage of the gene for both disorders to the same region of chromosome 19.

Minicore (multicore) disease. Most authors have followed Engel et al (1971) and Heffner et al (1976) in calling this condition multicore disease. 'Minicore', proposed by Currie et al (1974) distinguishes the typical appearance of the muscle biopsy more precisely from that of central core disease. The minicores extend for only a few sarcomeres, but have the same histochemical and ultrastructural appearance as central cores. Type I fibre predominance is usual but, unlike central cores, minicores occur in both fibre types.

Ten reported cases were reviewed by Taratuto et al (1978); Dubowitz (1985) recorded seven more and several others have been reported. In the typical form of the disease the clinical features have been rather uniform. There is infantile hypotonia, delay in motor development and continuing but non-progressive muscle weakness tending to be proximal in distribution, modest wasting, often some mild asymmetry of involvement, and impairment, rarely absence, of the tendon reflexes. The face is often affected, neck flexion may be weak and typically the ocular muscles are unaffected. The serum CK activity is normal and the EMG usually indicates a myopathic disorder. In several personal cases proximal weakness was more evident in the upper than lower limbs, and triceps biopsy revealed the diagnosis when earlier quadriceps biopsy findings had been non-specific.

One of the cases of Engel et al (1971) had a family history of neuromuscular symptoms in three generations and Vanneste & Stam (1982) found minicores in muscle biopsies from the asymptomatic mother and sister of their patient; other autosomal dominant pedigrees were recorded and reviewed by Paljarvi et al (1987); otherwise only sibs or sporadic cases have been affected and the inheritance in most cases is therefore probably autosomal recessive. No clear clinical distinction, however, between autosomal recessive and dominant cases has yet emerged.

There have been reports of several atypical cases. A child reported by Gadoth et al (1978) had muscle biopsy findings perhaps more akin to minicore than central core disease. The patient's non-progressive myopathy was punctuated by exacerbations of weakness during, and for some time after, febrile illnesses. Koch et al (1985) described a severely affected infant who also had an atrial septal defect and who died after anaesthesia. Cardiomyopathy has developed some years after initial diagnosis in some cases (de Lumley et al 1976). One personal case required cardiac trans-

plantation at the age of 10 years. A late-onset case with proximal weakness progressing from the age of 33 years was reported by Bonnette et al (1974). Chudley et al (1985) reported two affected sibs who also had severe mental retardation, vertical ophthalmoplegia, facial anomalies, short stature, hypogonadism and hypoplasia of the pituitary fossa. Swash & Schwartz (1981) discussed a possibly separate variant of minicore disease in which there is associated ophthalmoplegia and, in addition to minicores, the muscle biopsy shows focal loss of cross-striations. Curiously McKusick (1992) regards this variant and the Chudley kindred as the only two autosomal recessive forms of minicore myopathy.

Nemaline (rod body) myopathy. This condition was first described by Shy et al (1963) and by Conen et al (1963) and has since become the most frequently reported and most intensively studied of the congenital myopathies. It has been reviewed by Kuitonnen et al (1972), Brooke et al (1979) and Banker (1986a). The pathogenesis is unknown but a deficiency of depeptidyl peptidase 1 has been found in two cases (Stauber et al 1986).

The characteristic tiny rod bodies (they are not really 'nemaline' or thread-like) are derived from the disorganisation of the material from which the Z bands of the sarcomeres are formed. They may reflect a defect in the regulation of the length of actin filaments (Yamaguchi et al 1982) with an associated partial deficiency in α-actinin (Wallgren-Pettersson et al 1990a). They form clusters or irregular palisades and are often seen near active vesicular nuclei. They may be inconspicuous and are best seen in thick sections stained with toluidine blue or trichrome stains, or under phase contrast when they are usually refractile. Their ultrastructure is also characteristic. As in central core disease, type I fibre predominance is usual and, indeed, rods and cores or minicores may occur together (Afifi et al al 1965, Dubowitz 1978 p. 83). Rods are seen in a variety of clinical and experimental myopathies and are, therefore, not in themselves specific; nevertheless, the typical clinical features of the congenital myopathy with which they are usually associated have now been so well defined as to leave no doubt that 'nemaline myopathy' is a specific genetic disorder.

In addition, however, nemaline rods may be seen in adults with a late-onset progressive myopathy (Heffernan et al 1968) and it is still not clear whether such cases should be considered to be distinct or part of a spectrum of disease severity; the latter seems more likely. The pathogenesis is unknown and, although various pieces of evidence have indicated a neurogenic lesion in some cases, notably the post-mortem evidence (discounted by Banker 1986a) of loss of anterior horn cells in a patient with abundant nemaline rods in the muscle fibres (Dahl & Klutzow 1974) and the occurrence of minipolymyoclonus in one case (Colamaria et al 1991), the overall evidence seems still to point to a primary myopathy.

The typical patient is hypotonic in infancy with delayed motor development and with strikingly slender muscles, which are often not as weak as they look. There is usually definite facial weakness (Fig. 21.1a) and often nasal speech due to palatal

weakness. The muscle involvement is indeed universal and the cases of Conen et al (1963) and Hopkins et al (1966) were initially diagnosed as having 'Krabbe's universal muscle hypoplasia' (Krabbe 1958), a term no longer in use. The tendon reflexes are reduced or absent. Various skeletal features including a high-arched palate, dental malocclusion, scoliosis and pes cavus, although by no means confined to nemaline myopathy, are common and combine with the facial weakness and muscle hypoplasia to present a striking clinical picture from which the diagnosis may often be suspected. Most cases are moderately severely disabled throughout childhood. In the neonatal period the disease may be severe and cause early death (Shafiq et al 1967, Eeg-Olofsson et al 1983) and there is some inconclusive evidence that this form of nemaline myopathy is a distinct autosomal recessive entity (Schmalbruch et al 1987) (Fig. 21.1b). The disorder is usually

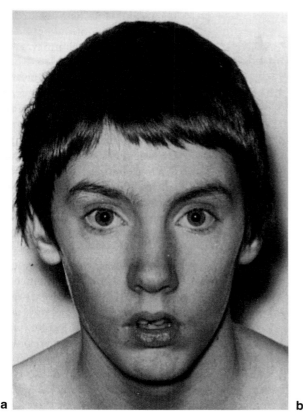
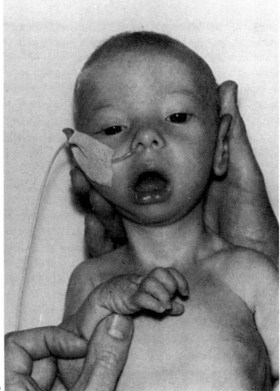

a   b

Fig. 21.1 Nemaline myopathy. **a** Facies, a boy aged 12 years. **b** Severe neonatal form, a boy at 3 weeks old. **c** A girl of 13 years, shortly after she had developed severe nocturnal respiratory failure.

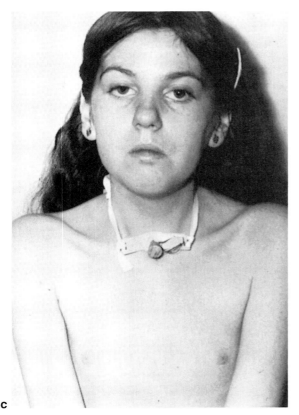

c

Fig. 21.1 c

considered to be non-progressive, but undoubtedly deterioration can occur; e.g. some relatives may be found to have subclinical involvement and it is likely that in some cases they will develop symptoms in adult life (Hopkins et al 1966). Furthermore, progressive respiratory failure is now frequently recognised in the first and second decades (Kuitonnen et al 1972, Dubowitz 1978) and often proves fatal. Serial testing of respiratory function may reveal striking abnormalities months or years before serious respiratory symptoms occur, but excessive fatigue and morning headaches are warning symptoms. One of Dubowitz's cases first presented with acute respiratory failure while hill-walking (Dubowitz 1978). A patient described by us in 1969 (Fulthorpe et al 1969) later developed severe disabling respiratory failure at the age of 13 years (Fig. 21.1c). Regular overnight use of a negative pressure cuirass ventilator at home, together with tracheostomy, controlled this and

she remained fully ambulant for a further 14 years. Loss of central respiratory drive and muscle weakness may both be factors in such cases (Riley et al 1977). Deterioration of nemaline myopathy in the third or fourth decade may also be attributable to cardiomyopathy, either with nemaline rods in the heart muscle (Meier et al 1984) or without (Stoessl et al 1985).

Many families have now been described with affected parents and children, and autosomal dominant inheritance is very likely (Kondo & Yuasa 1980); however, no very extensive pedigrees have been recorded. Subtle weakness or dysmorphic signs, with or without nemaline rods in the muscle biopsy, may be found in ostensibly 'normal' parents. Sporadic cases with normal biopsies in both parents have been reported but in other families rods have been found in *both* asymptomatic parents, suggesting autosomal recessive inheritance (Arts et al 1978, Wallgren-Pettersson et al 1990b). Even X-linked dominant inheritance has been suggested because of an apparent excess of female patients and the predominance of affected mothers (see Brooke et al 1979) but this is improbable because the disorder may apparently be transmitted by a father to his sons (Gonatas et al 1966). This confusing genetic situation makes nemaline myopathy a candidate for the discovery of the occurrence of variable repeat segments of the gene, such as have been found in myotonic dystrophy and Huntington's chorea. The gene locus is at 1q21–23 (Laing et al 1991).

Centronuclear (myotubular) myopathies. One of the histological characteristics of myopathic disorders in general is the tendency for muscle fibre nuclei to drift from their normal subsarcolemmal position towards the centre of the fibre. In the centronuclear myopathies, however, central nuclei dominate a histological picture in which abnormal variation in fibre size and often a tendency to type I fibre predominance are the only other major features. Spiro et al (1966), who first drew attention to this disorder, described a boy aged 12 years with congenital but progressive muscle weakness and ophthalmoplegia. His muscle fibres contained central nuclei, often vesicular with prominent nucleoli, which were surrounded by clear areas devoid of myofibrils and ATPase activity, and sometimes lacking oxidative enzyme activity also, but containing mitochondria. They likened these fibres to the myotubes found in early fetal muscle, postulated that the disorder might represent arrested maturation of muscle fibres and named it 'myotubular myopathy'. Since then many cases have been described and the more non-committal name 'centronuclear myopathy' is now generally preferred because the fibres usually lack the perinuclear clear areas and differ in several other respects from fetal myotubes. In at least some cases the central position of the nuclei is an aquired phenomenon, and the immuno-chemical staining pattern of various cytoskeletal proteins is abnormal (van der Ven et al 1991). Much overlapping clinical, genetic and pathologi-cal variation has emerged; for the present purpose a genetic and clinical classification seems to be appropriate. Banker (1986a) and de Angelis et al (1991) gave useful reviews.

Early infantile ophthalmoplegic myopathy with probable autosomal recessive inheritance. Patients in this category resemble that described by Spiro et al (1966) and include those reported by Sher et al (1967), Bethlem et al (1968), Coleman et al (1968), Campbell et al (1969), Oritz de Zarate & Maruffo (1970) and Bill et al (1979). The condi-tion is apparent in the first year of life because of developmental delay, usually without severe hypo-tonia at first although this may appear later. By the time of diagnosis in the first or second decade there has usually been slight deterioration in gait or some other evidence of gradual progression. Ptosis, strabismus, partial external ophthalmo-plegia (for all directions of gaze), facial weakness (not invariable), generalised muscular weakness and wasting, and tendon areflexia are the usual features. Sternomastoid weakness and foot drop are prominent in some cases. Dysarthria and nasal speech are frequent but dysphagia is uncom-mon. The face may be long and thin and foot deformities and scoliosis may develop. Most patients become unable to walk in the second decade. Intelligence is generally normal but several patients (Banker 1986a says 18%) have had con-vulsions, including the patient described by Spiro et al (1966), whose history was complicated by subdural haematomas; it is not yet certain whether the association with convulsions is coincidental. The serum CK activity is normal or, more often,

raised two- or three-fold and the EMG shows myopathic abnormalities. The genetic position is puzzling: both sexes are affected; most cases are sporadic but affected sibs have been recorded (Sher et al 1967, Bradley et al 1970) and in some families subclinical centronuclear myopathy has been found in the mother (Sher et al 1967, Coleman et al 1968). It is, therefore, not yet possi-ble to distinguish autosomal recessive inheritance with manifestation in the heterozygote from auto-somal dominant inheritance with variable ex-pressivity. Indeed, de Angelis et al (1991) who reviewed the clinical and genetic data from 136 kin-dreds (288 cases) concluded that autosomal reces-sive inheritance was uncommon and difficult to document. Their (slightly discrepant) figures were: autosomal dominant 14 (plus six possible) kin-dreds, X-linked recessive 14 (plus nine possible) kindreds, possible autosomal recessive seven kin-dreds, with 85 isolated cases (32 female, 53 male). It is possible that the brother and sister reported by Hurwitz et al (1969), with hypotonia and oph-thalmoplegia and a family history of amino-aciduria, may have had centronuclear myopathy, as both the clinical and histological features were compatible.

Possibly this category should be defined a little less strictly. In the otherwise typical case described by Kinoshita & Cadman (1968) the symptoms developed at the age of 4 years and there was ptosis but no ophthalmoplegia. Similarly, the patient of Bethlem et al (1970) had no involve-ment of the cranial musculature; the symptoms developed at 5 years and had progressed only slowly at 35 years. A boy with a mild clinical myopathy and with 'hypotrophy' of type I fibres was reported by Inokuchi et al (1975): he had areflexia; the eye movements were not mentioned; sucking had been abnormal in infancy. Ten cases in which the onset was in infancy, the eye move-ments were normal and the biopsy showed type I fibre atrophy with central nuclei were reviewed by Peyronnard et al (1982); these may represent a separate autosomal recessive entity. The noso-logical situation overlaps here with that of the 'fibre-type disproportions'. The affected broth-ers described by Bradley et al (1970) did have ophthalmoplegia but the onset was at eight and 15 years respectively and they deteriorated and died at the age of 34 years. In contrast, the patient of Campbell et al (1969) died at the age of 27 months and in occasional cases there have been life-threatening hypotonia and respiratory difficulties in the neonatal period (Coleman et al 1967, Bender & Bender 1977).

Cases with autosomal dominant inheritance and late onset. The family reported by McLeod et al (1972) is unique in having 16 affected members in five generations. Biopsies were taken from two members. In most, symptoms began in the third decade but in three (including two of the only three children at risk) the disease began in early childhood (in the second year). The myopathy was usually proximal in emphasis but in some cases showed a scapuloperoneal distribution. The eye muscles were spared, although some had slight facial weakness. While the symptoms were slowly progressive, lifespan was normal. The serum CK activity was normal.

There have been other cases with dominant inheritance, mostly with a relatively late onset (Karpati et al 1970, Edstrom et al 1982; see de Angelis et al 1991) and other adult-onset cases have been reported by Vital et al (1970), Harriman & Haleem (1972) and Misra et al (1992). In Misra's cases intrafibrillar perinuclear desmin and vimentin were present in the muscle fibres which resembled, in this respect, fetal myotubes. Involvement of extraocular muscles is uncommon in adult-onset cases.

Severe X-linked centronuclear myopathy. X-linked centronuclear myopathy was first reported in two unrelated Dutch families by van Wijngaarden et al (1969) and Barth et al (1975). The males involved were severely affected, often fatally, with polyhydramnios and impaired fetal movements followed by hypotonia, inability to suck and respiratory insufficiency at birth (Fig. 21.2), but the survivors tended to improve and two aged 26 and 33 years were not severely disabled. In the patients of van Wijngaarden et al (1969) the clinical features, including ophthalmoplegia and facial weakness, as well as the pathology, were remarkably similar to those of the autosomal recessive cases already described. Further severe X-linked cases were described by Bruyland et al (1984) and Heckmatt et al (1985). They showed that female carriers of the gene may have mild clinical signs of a myopathy, or an excess of central nuclei in the muscle biopsy. The gene is located at Xq28 (Thomas et al 1990).

Askanas et al (1979) found persistent ultrastructural abnormalities in cultured muscle cells from two affected infants and a deficiency of adenylate cyclase associated with the muscle fibre membrane. Abnormal expression of the fetal isoform of the heavy chain of myosin has been

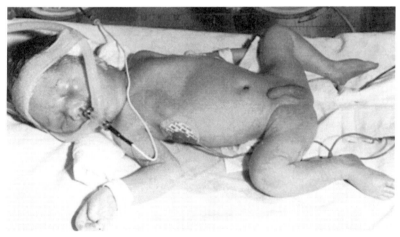

Fig. 21.2   X-linked centronuclear myopathy. A boy born 7 weeks preterm, photographed at 10 days of age. Severe hypotonia and ophthalmoplegia. Needed assisted ventilation for 6 weeks. Died at 5 months old.

reported in muscle in the X-linked but not in the autosomal recessive form (Sawchak et al 1991).

Earlier, Engel et al (1968) had reported a similar severely hypotonic male infant who died aged 18 months. The pathology was reported under the title of 'Type I fibre hypotrophy and central nuclei' which for a time was regarded as a disorder separate from centronuclear myopathy. Then Meyers et al (1974) studied a second affected brother and obtained a family history of recurrent male stillbirths in the mother's generation, suggesting X-linked inheritance. The second child was apnoeic at birth and profoundly hypotonic, and died at seven months. These brothers had no facial weakness, and eye movements were normal. The serum CK activities were normal and the EMGs were inconclusive. These cases are now widely regarded as examples of X-linked centronuclear myopathy. A boy with similar clinical and pathological features in infancy who showed striking improvement by the age of 6 years was reported by Ricoy & Cabello (1985).

Unusual features associated with centronuclear myopathy. The patient of Harriman & Haleem (1972), a woman of 67 years, had marked hypertrophy of the calves. A case with generalised muscle hypertrophy, with muscle weakness since infancy and progressive weakness and hypertrophy since the second decade, was reported by Matsushita et al (1991).

The association of cardiomyopathy with centronuclear myopathy is recorded by Bethlem et al (1969) in a girl of 16 years, and by Verhiest et al (1976) in two brothers. The boys had early sucking difficulties, delayed motor development and generalised myopathy with ptosis, but the eye movements were not mentioned.

Hawkes & Absolon (1975) reported a man of 29 with typical features of the ophthalmoplegic form but, in addition, cataracts and electromyographic myotonia. His father had cataracts and unilateral congenital ptosis. The cataracts were seen only with a slit lamp. A similar case, but without ptosis or ophthalmoplegia, was reported by Vallat et al (1985). Gil-Peralta et al (1978) described two affected sibs with clinical myotonia. This condition seems to be distinct both from the typical centronuclear myopathies and from myotonic dystrophy.

Other congenital myopathies with structural abnormalities in muscle fibres

Finger-print inclusion myopathy. Six cases have been reported by Engel et al (1972), Gordon et al (1974), Fardeau et al (1976) and Curless et al (1978a). They include identical twin brothers (Curless et al) half brothers (Fardeau et al) and isolated female cases, in one of which non-progressive congenital myopathy had been present for 54 years before diagnosis (Gordon et al). Subsarcolemmal inclusions resembling fingerprints were associated with a few small areas of focal loss of myofibrillar structure (not unlike minicores) and, in some cases, type I fibre predominance.

All cases were hypotonic in infancy with delayed motor development (walking at between two years and, in Gordon's patient, 12 years) and with no deterioration. The muscles were slim with retained reflexes and mild to moderate weakness. The cranial musculature was normal. Four of the six cases were mildly mentally retarded. Serum CK levels were normal or slightly raised. One patient was thought to show some beneficial response to neostigmine but had no other evidence of myasthenia (Gordon et al 1974). Finger-print inclusions have also been seen in various other disorders including dermatomyositis, myotonic dystrophy, oculopharyngeal dystrophy and distal myopathy with rimmed vacuoles (see Curless et al 1978a, Banker 1986a), but the features of the six cases mentioned are sufficiently similar to comprise a clinical entity. The genetic situation is obscure.

Reducing body myopathy. A rather heterogeneous group of isolated cases has been described by Brooke & Neville (1972), and by Dubowitz (1985) (see also Dubowitz 1978, Tomé & Fardeau 1975, Dudley et al 1978, Oh et al 1983, Carpenter et al 1985). The common factor is the presence of subsarcolemmal inclusion bodies rich in RNA and sulphydryl groups and capable of reducing nitroblue tetrazolium stain. Their ultrastructure is also diagnostic. Two sibs were reported by Hübner and Pongratz (see Carpenter et al 1985) suggesting a genetic basis. However, in two other cases (Dubowitz 1978, Carpenter et al 1985) there have been high serum antibody titres against Coxsackie virus, the significance of which is not clear.

The patients of Brooke and Neville were hypotonic in infancy. Their weakness progressed and both died, at nine months and two years of age respectively. The older child had facial weakness and contractures and was of normal intelligence. The serum CK activity was normal. Another infant (Dudley et al 1978) died at 2.5 months of age after a different type of illness consisting of respiratory paralysis due to progressive board-like rigidity of the muscles of the neck, chest and abdomen, and finally of the limbs; his parents were a father and daughter.

Dubowitz's patient developed a progressive asymmetrical myopathy at the age of four years and died three years later. In addition to reducing bodies, she had histological evidence of a severe degenerative myopathy. Her Coxsackie B virus antibody titre was high and she was treated as having a possible subacute viral polymyositis, responding temporarily to cyclophosphamide but not to steroids. The patients described by Oh et al (1983) and Carpenter et al (1985) developed a slowly progressive proximal myopathy from the age of about one year; the weakness fluctuated in Oh's patient.

The less severely affected patient of Tomé & Fardeau (1975) had a non-progressive proximal myopathy without facial involvement and with normal serum CK activity. In an adult patient with scapuloperoneal myopathy reported by Sahgal & Sahgal (1977) the ultrastructural findings were atypical. A patient reported by Nomizu et al (1992) first developed weakness at the age of 13 years and by 17 required nocturnal ventilation following surgical treatment of scoliosis. She also had mitral valve prolapse and evidence suggesting abnormal circulating immune complexes. There is currently no clear evidence that reducing body myopathy is genetically determined.

Other congenital myopathies with inclusions. Adams et al (1965) reported a man with lifelong weakness culminating in rapid deterioration for two years. He had a necrotising myopathy and the muscle fibres contained a variety of sarcoplasmic and nuclear inclusions.

Jenis et al (1969) described an infant with severe hypotonia and weakness who died, aged two months, of respiratory failure. There were numerous crystalline inclusions in muscle fibre nuclei and in the cytoplasm.

'*Sarcotubular myopathy*' was reported by Jerusalem et al (1973) in two brothers with consanguineous parents. There was mild non-progressive myopathy dating from early infancy. The muscle fibres contained vacuoles derived from the sarcoplasmic reticulum and the T system.

Subsarcolemmal '*tubular aggregates*' are found in some patients with muscle cramp on exercise (Lazaro et al 1980) and in a wide variety of other neuromuscular disorders, but they have also been seen in a form of very slowly progressive myopathy, beginning in the second decade, in families with autosomal dominant inheritance (Rohkamm et al 1983, Pierobon-Bormioli et al 1985) and in one of the genetically determined myasthenic syndromes (Engel et al 1982 and see pp. 796–800).

Tubular masses and coated vesicles in central inclusions in muscle fibres were the characteristic feature of a case of chronic non-progressive congenital myopathy reported by Carpenter et al (1992).

An X-linked recessive myopathy (with mild signs in a carrier female) has been reported from Finland, in which autophagic vacuoles are the only diagnostic feature of the muscle histology. Slowly progressive muscle weakness began in childhood and apparently affected the shoulder muscles and both proximal and distal muscles in the lower limbs (Kalimo et al 1988). Linkage to the distal long arm of the X-chromosome was suggested (Saviranta et al 1988).

'*Zebra-body*' inclusions were found in the muscle of a boy of 15 years with a relatively benign congenital vacuolar myopathy (Lake & Wilson 1975) and in a second case by Reyes et al (1987). Their specificity is uncertain.

'*Cap disease*'. Fidzianska et al (1981) reported a single case of a boy with a severe non-progressive congenital myopathy with facial and general muscle weakness and wasting, and a scoliosis. In 70% of the muscle fibres a peripheral ring or a segment ('cap') was deficient in ATPase and myosin and on electron microscopy these zones were shown to contain disorganised myofibrils. The authors postulated a defect in myofilament synthesis or myoblast fusion.

Dense '*cytoplasmic bodies*', differing from nemaline rods, have been described in a form of non-progressive congenital proximal myopathy with mildly raised serum CK activity, but also in a variety of other myopathies (Goebel et al 1981, Patel et al 1983, Mizumo et al 1989, Bertini et al 1990).

Typically the disorder causes infantile hypotonia, weakness of the face, bulbar muscles and neck and of proximal limb muscles. Progressive respiratory failure and scoliosis are frequent, especially in cases with a postnatal onset (Patel et al 1983, Mizuno et al 1989). Patients with progressive skeletal muscle weakness with subsequent cardiomyopathy (Pellissier et al 1989) or vice versa (Vajsar et al 1993), 17 in all, have been found to have eosinophilic subsarcolemmal inclusions in muscle fibres, with the electron-microscopic appearance of granular material with intermediate filaments and the staining characteristics of desmin and ubiquitin. The onset varied from early childhood to middle age. A similar case, without cardiomyopathy (aged 5 years), was reported by Paelle et al (1992). Rather similar structures, 'spheroid bodies', were found in the muscle fibres of several members of a family who had an autosomal dominant slowly progressive proximal myopathy with the onset of symptoms varying from early childhood to the fourth decade (Goebel et al 1978).

Yet another 'granular myopathy' in which the granules were in vacuoles and 30% of the muscle fibres also had a lobular appearance was reported in three young adults (two of them sibs). Profound weakness of the muscles spared the posterior neck, hand and quadriceps muscles in two of the cases. All had electrical (but not clinical) myotonia (Juguilon et al 1982).

Other 'structural' congenital myopathies. Ringel et al (1978) reported a remarkable child with severe muscular rigidity at birth and very high serum CK activity (45 times normal) who gradually improved over 10 months. The EMG was electrically silent. Muscle biopsy revealed that the fibres had an unusual trilaminar structure.

Brooke (1977, p. 217) described a lace-like structure of the sarcoplasm of type II fibres on oxidative enzyme staining in two members of a large family of 'toe-walkers'. Electron microscopy gave normal results.

Cancilla et al (1971) reported a brother and sister aged two and five years with infantile hypotonia, delayed motor development and mild weakness without areflexia, whose muscle biopsies showed atrophy of type I fibres and apparent lysis of their myofibrils.

Genetic myopathies with changes in the histochemical fibre types

Details of the techniques of histochemical fibre typing and of the patterns found at various stages of the development of normal muscles in man will be found in Chapter 8.

It has already been made clear that in many of the congenital myopathies, notably central core disease, nemaline myopathy and centronuclear myopathy, an abnormal predominance of type I fibres (those concerned with slow, oxidative, postural activity) is found. Sometimes affected members in families with central core disease may have evidence only of type I fibre predominance on muscle biopsy (Morgan-Hughes et al 1973). It is not unusual, when investigating a hypotonic child, to find no other pathological change and because such cases tend to improve they are ipso facto included in the category 'benign congenital hypotonia'. Indeed, it is not yet clear whether fibre-type predominance is a cause of hypotonia or a result of it. Very similar patterns of fibre-type predominance have been found in muscle biopsies from hypotonic children with primary disorders of the central nervous system (Curless et al 1978b). Occasionally virtually all the fibres are of one type (mostly type I) for many years in children or young adults with symptoms suggesting a congenital myopathy (Oh & Danon 1983). Whether this is an entity or a prolonged transitional phase of some more specific pathology is uncertain.

However, in addition to inequality of the numbers of type I and II fibres there may be inequality in their size. Usually the small fibres are of type II and this pattern may be found in a wide variety of disorders, especially muscle disuse. Children with small type I fibres have been described as having 'congenital fibre-type disproportion'.

Congenital fibre-type disproportion. Brooke (1973) suggested this name for a group of hypotonic children with no significant pathology other than the numerical predominance and small size of their type I fibres. The pattern had emerged from a previous wider analysis of the histochemical patterns found in children's muscle biopsies (Brooke & Engel 1969). Other patients with the same biopsy findings had been found to have cerebellar disease or myotonic dystrophy, but 22 cases seemed to comprise a clinical entity. There was hypotonia, often quite severe, at or soon after birth, which might deteriorate for up to one year but thereafter remained static. Congenital contractures, often with dislocation of the hips, were frequent and high-arched palates, short stature and later kyphoscoliosis were each seen in about half the cases (Fig. 21.3). The tendon reflexes were usually diminished but present, the serum CK activity was normal or slightly

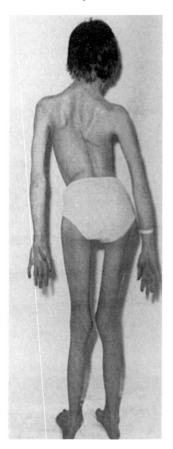

Fig. 21.3 Congenital fibre-type disproportion. A girl of 16 years. Hypotonia since birth; sat at 12 months; walked at 20 months; scoliosis and respiratory insufficiency for 3 years; stature below 3rd centile. Sister affected.

increased and the EMG was normal or mildly 'myopathic'. Walking was delayed beyond 18 months in all but one case and in some beyond three years. Brooke emphasised the relatively good prognosis, but later modified this because most of his cases remained significantly disabled (Brooke et al 1979). One patient turned out to have facioscapulohumeral dystrophy. Mild neuromuscular symptoms were present in first-degree or more distant relatives of several cases.

Other cases, subsequently described by Fardeau et al (1975), Lenard and Goebel (1975), Martin et al (1976), Dubowitz (1978), Sulaiman et al (1983) and many others, have on the whole tended to confirm the existence of this disorder as an entity, although some doubts remain. For instance Martin et al (1976) reported that their patient's mother had been alcoholic during her pregnancy and they also found identical biopsy appearances in two cases of globoid cell leucodystrophy and one of Pompe's glycogenosis. Dubowitz pointed out the importance of making the diagnosis only when the type II muscle fibres were normal or large, in order to avoid confusion with congenital myotonic dystrophy. Lenard & Goebel (1975) reported a child with life-threatening hypotonia and respiratory insufficiency in the neonatal period. The occurrence of an apparently dominant mode of transmission in some families was confirmed by Fardeau et al (1975) and apparently autosomal recessive inheritance is sometimes seen (Jaffe et al 1988). Fibre-type disproportion may be seen in the 'rigid-spine syndrome' (q.v.).

When the clinical and histochemical findings are typical, one is justified in making a provisional diagnosis of congenital fibre-type disproportion, but follow-up assessments for some years are essential. Some cases may be found later to have central hypotonia. Because of the relatively good long-term outlook it is important to prevent and treat spinal deformities enthusiastically to avoid further respiratory insufficiency; the contractures should also be given vigorous attention. Mizuno & Komiya (1990) reviewed the occurrence of late respiratory failure and in their own case suggested 'dysmaturation' of spinal motor neurones innervating type I fibres (based on repeated muscle biopsy). There is little doubt that the next few years will bring a clearer understanding of the nature of this disorder and its pathogenesis. Its status as an entity is fragile and as a primary myopathy even more so.

Other abnormalities of size and number of histochemical fibre types. Given two basic fibre types of which either may predominate, or which may be equal in number, and of which either or both may be small or normal (or rarely large) in size, there is wide scope for variation. One may add the presence or absence of central nuclei in the centronuclear myopathies. In practice many of the possible combinations have been reported, and Farkas-Bargeton et al (1978) and Argov et al (1984) suggested that defective neural control of the functional maturation of the muscle fibres might be responsible.

In congenital myotonic dystrophy there may be relatively small type I fibres, but the type II fibres also are often smaller than normal. Relatively small type II fibres are unusual in the context of congenital myopathy. Brooke & Engle (1969) and Matsuoka et al (1974) described children with this finding who had infantile hypotonia, markedly delayed motor development, normal facial and eye movements, preserved reflexes, a non-progressive course and normal intelligence. One of the patients of Argov et al (1984) with type II fibre hypoplasia had impaired central control of vertical gaze. Dubrovsky et al (1978) reported a different clinical pattern associated with type II fibre hypoplasia in a 6-year-old child with non-progressive distal muscle weakness and atrophy, bilateral external ophthalmoplegia and cataracts. The EMG suggested neurogenic atrophy. A similar histological picture has been reported in the Marshall–Smith syndrome of accelerated growth and mental retardation (Roodhooft et al 1988). A case with uniformly small type IIA fibres and a lifelong slowly progressive proximal myopathy at the age of 12 years was reported by Gallanti et al (1992).

Extremely small fibres of both types in a very hypotonic baby aged 2 weeks reverted to normal at 10 months, together with the hypotonia, but severe congenital ophthalmoplegia and slight facial weakness persisted (Hanson et al 1977).

Congenital myopathies with muscle fibre necrosis

The muscular dystrophies are discussed in detail in Chapter 14. It is only necessary to mention here that both 'congenital muscular dystrophy' and congenital myotonic dystrophy (Ch. 15) differ sharply from the other muscular dystrophies in being virtually non-progressive and, indeed, necrosis is not a feature of the muscle pathology in myotonic dystrophy. Nevertheless, both may cause profound and life-threatening hypotonia and muscular paralysis in the first few days and weeks of life. Infants born before term, as they often are, with myotonic dystrophy are particularly at risk. Both may give rise to congenital contractures which are often widespread in congenital muscular dystrophy, but tend to be restricted to the ankles in myotonic dystrophy. Necrotising myopathy, with a very high serum CK level, is a feature of the Marinesco–Sjögren syndrome in which congenital cataracts, mental retardation and cerebellar ataxia are other cardinal features (Tachi et al 1991).

Thompson (1982) reported three cases of a congenital necrotising myopathy with some inflammatory features and an apparent response to steroids, and suggested that they were suffering from an acquired 'infantile myositis'. Shevell et al (1990) reviewed the seven cases in the literature and presented three more. A high serum CK level and positive staining for immune complexes in muscle were helpful in diagnosis. Several cases had severe associated cerebral and ocular malformations, in one case resembling the Walker–Warburg syndrome (see Ch. 14). The aetiology remains obscure and may be heterogeneous. Steroids have been helpful in several cases, but not in all (Nagai et al 1992).

Genetic myopathies with non-specific changes in fibres: 'minimal change myopathy'

Everyone who investigates children with neuromuscular disorders is familiar with patients who have undoubted muscular weakness without helpful diagnostic features and whose muscle biopsies show equally non-specific changes. When the symptoms date from infancy and the myopathic features include muscle destruction, fatty replacement, fibrosis and marked variation in the fibre size the label is often 'congenital muscular dystrophy' (q.v., Ch. 14). When the changes are milder, the term 'benign congenital myopathy', 'minimal change myopathy' (Dubowitz 1985) or some other non-committal term is applied. Such cases are by no means uncommon but are, naturally, reported in the medical literature only when the author is drawing attention to the problems they pose (Fenichel & Bazelon 1966, Lenard & Goebel 1980) or when they have some unusual feature such as an extensive family history (Turner & Lees 1962) or associated external ophthalmoplegia (Ohtaki et al 1990). Undoubtedly, many of the cases diagnosed in the past would have been classified differently had they undergone full histochemical or ultrastructural investigations; in others, no doubt, ill-luck or ill-judgement in choosing the site for muscle biopsy led to the failure to reach a more definite conclusion. One wonders, for example, whether the case of Ohtaki et al may have had the Swash–Schwartz variant of minicore myopathy, which it clinically resembles, or even centronuclear myopathy.

In the cases reported by Turner & Lees (1962), six of 13 sibs were affected with hypotonia from birth and had been followed up without evidence of progression of the disorder for 50 years. The pathology was confined to one post-mortem examination of a bedridden patient, but served to confirm the primary myopathic nature of the disorder. Flexion deformities of the fingers occurred in the adult affected members and in an unaffected aunt and a daughter.

Bethlem & van Wijngaarden (1976) described three kindreds in which dominant inheritance of a benign myopathy occurred over four and five generations. Some had congenital torticollis; otherwise the symptoms had started at about 5 years of age and had progressed extremely slowly. Proximal muscles were mainly affected, but flexion contractures of the fingers were a prominent feature. The muscle biopsy findings were non-specific, but lobulated fibres, of the type often seen in the late-onset types of muscular dystrophy, were prominent. In this situation the distinc-

tion between a 'benign familial myopathy' and a very mild muscular dystrophy is semantic.

'Myosclerosis'. Sometimes, non-specific myopathic features in the muscle biopsy may be accompanied by an apparently disproportionate amount of fibrous tissue around and within the fascicles of muscle fibres. The muscles may feel hard and have striking contractures and the electromyographer may encounter a grating sensation as he inserts his needle. Such cases raise the question of whether such a condition as 'primary myosclerosis' exists. Cases have been reported by Löwenthal (1954) and by Bradley et al (1973) but considerable doubt remains as to whether they constitute a specific entity. In isolated cases, especially if the pathology is confined to a few muscles, the possibility of fibrosis induced by previous intramuscular drug injection must be considered (see Ch. 28). Chronic spinal muscular atrophy and the congenital muscular dystrophies sometimes give a similar picture.

DISORDERS OF NEUROMUSCULAR TRANSMISSION

Myasthenia

Myasthenia is relatively uncommon in infancy or childhood. Of 447 cases collected by Millichap & Dodge (1960), 16 showed signs of the disease at, or soon after, birth and 35 presented between the ages of one and 16 years. In a series of 217 cases presenting in infancy, childhood or adolescence (Osserman 1958), 34 had symptoms at, or within a few days of birth and eight more within the first 2 years of life. In a Mayo Clinic series of 157 cases whose symptoms began before the age of 17 years, only eight had symptoms before the age of 1 year (Rodriguez et al 1983).

For many years it has been recognised that some cases of infantile myasthenia are genetically determined; Bundey (1972) demonstrated that autosomal recessive inheritance made a major contribution in those cases presenting before the age of 2 years. However, the ability to distinguish autoimmune myasthenia gravis from other myasthenic syndromes by measuring serum antibodies against the acetylcholine receptor (AChR), and the development of in vitro techniques for studying the structure and function of the neuromuscular junction have together led to the recognition of a number of new entities (Engel 1984, 1992) and to a clearer understanding of some of the traditional categories (Fenichel 1978, 1983). Amongst children the incidence of symptomatic myasthenia of autoimmune and genetic aetiology is approximately equal (Gardner-Medwin 1993). The current position may be summarised as follows:

Autoimmune myasthenia gravis
1. Generalised
2. Ocular
3. Transient neonatal
   Genetically determined myasthenia (see p. 796)
   Other disorders of neuromuscular transmission
1. Botulism
   a. Acute intoxication
   b. Infantile form
2. Eaton–Lambert syndrome
3. Other toxic causes

Autoimmune myasthenia in childhood. Children as young as 1–2 years may develop myasthenia gravis, either generalised or restricted to the external ocular muscles. They never have thymomas. The disorder is essentially identical to that seen in other age groups and is fully described in Chapter 20. The patient of Oberklaid & Hopkins (1976) was 6 months old at the onset and died at 10 months. Without AChR antibody titres it is impossible to distinguish in this kind of case between extremely early autoimmune myasthenia and a genetic disorder. Similarly, some early descriptions of a fulminatingly acute form, threatening life within 24 hours of the onset, were not backed up by AChR antibody assays but may well be genuine examples of this disorder (see Fenichel 1978).

Fukuyama et al (1973) discussed the outcome in 51 patients aged between nine months and 11 years at the onset, who had apparently not been subjected to thymectomy; very few had remitted within 12 years, although most had 'improved'. Cavanagh (1980) and Bjerre & Hallberg (1983) pointed out the sketchy nature of the published evidence about the role of thymectomy in children. In the series of Rodriguez et al (1983) the 10-year remission rate was under 20% without and 50% after thymectomy (and was higher when thymectomy was done within a year of the onset).

The usual policy in children with generalised myasthenia and AChR antibodies (as in older people) is to perform a thymectomy as soon as possible, to use steroids if necessary to induce a remission and to rely upon anticholinesterase drugs as sparingly as possible for the control of symptoms. Even infants may very occasionally require plasmapheresis (Snead et al 1987). The position regarding purely (or predominantly) ocular autoimmune myasthenia is difficult. Few regard it as justifying thymectomy, yet it tends to be relatively difficult to control by other means.

Transient neonatal myasthenia gravis. In most cases of myasthenia presenting at birth, the mother is affected and the baby's transient weakness is attributed to the placental transfer of maternal antibodies. Nevertheless, very few babies born to myasthenic mothers (10 out of 71 in Osserman's series; Osserman 1958) have symptoms of the condition, and the severity of their symptoms bears no obvious relation to the severity or duration of the mother's illness or to her AChR antibody titre. Even the baby's titre is not a wholly reliable guide (Morel et al 1988, Engel 1992). There is evidence that such babies also produce endogenous AChR antibodies (Lefvert & Osterman 1983).

Early diagnosis is important because, although the myasthenia is transient, lasting for a few days to a few weeks, it is generalised and may be severe or even fatal unless appropriate treatment is given. Signs may be present at birth, or may be delayed for as long as three days, and they often deteriorate over the first few days. The main features are generalised hypotonia, a weak cry, respiratory insufficiency, intermittent cyanosis especially during feeds, and difficulty and fatigue in sucking and swallowing. In a hypotonic baby, reduced mobility of the face, with constantly open eyes and mouth or (less often) ptosis, should suggest the diagnosis.

An intramuscular test dose of 0.05 mg prostigmine or 0.3 mg pyridostigmine bromide, or a subcutaneous dose of 0.1 ml Tensilon® (edrophonium chloride 1 mg) will confirm the diagnosis. Tube feeding and assisted ventilation may be required. Maintenance therapy, when necessary, consists of 1–5 mg of prostigmine or 4–20 mg of pyridostigmine bromide orally with feeds. The size and frequency of the dose will have to be adjusted according to the degree and duration of relief of symptoms and must be reduced as spontaneous recovery takes place.

In extreme cases of this syndrome maternal myasthenia gravis may paralyse the fetus, leading to congenital arthrogryposis; Carr et al (1991) described a programme of maternal therapy with steroids and plasmapheresis to prevent this from recurring in subsequent children, and gave a useful review.

Genetically determined myasthenias

Research in this field, and hence up-to-date clinical investigation, requires complex techniques available in only a few centres, notably the Mayo Clinic. From this work a logical classification, based on pathophysiology and genetics, is beginning to emerge (see below). But for most clinicians this has two fatal drawbacks — the tests are not available to them (and are anyway too invasive for small children), and two of the most numerous clinical groups ('congenital myasthenia' and the 'limb-girdle myasthenias') have so far eluded precise physiological characterisation and so cannot be classified. For this chapter, therefore, after setting out the gold standard, a more practical clinical arrangement is adopted.

*Genetically determined myasthenias**

With well-characterised presynaptic physiological defect:
    Familial infantile myasthenia (defect in acetylcholine resynthesis or packaging), AR
    Paucity of synaptic vesicles and reduced quantal release
With well-characterised postsynaptic physiological defect:
    End-plate acetylcholinesterase deficiency, AR
    Combined defect in function and numbers of AChRs
        Slow-channel syndrome, AD
        Long-channel open-time, low conductance, epsilon-subunit mutation
        Short-channel open-time
    Defect in function of AChRs
        High-conductance fast-channel syndrome, AR

        Abnormal ACh–AChR interaction
With partially characterised defects:
    With possible resynthesis defect and brisk decremental response to repetitive stimuli (Albers)
    AChR deficiency with paucity of secondary synaptic clefts. AR
    Other AChR defects
        'Congenital myasthenia', AR
        In myopathy with tubular aggregates (Morgan–Hughes)
        'Limb-girdle myasthenia', AR
Clinical entities with defect not yet characterised
    Congenital myasthenia with facial malformation (Goldhammer) AR

*Considerably modified from Engel (1992). AR and AD indicate autosomal recessive and autosomal dominant inheritance respectively; the inheritance in the other syndromes is uncertain, though probably autosomal recessive.

'Congenital myasthenia'. This name is by convention applied to a disorder present from birth (but not always noticed until later) in which ptosis and external ophthalmoplegia are the dominant features; there may also be mild involvement of the facial and skeletal muscles. There is a good response to anticholinesterase drugs and a decremental response can be found on electromyography even in clinically normal limb muscles. The condition usually remains relatively mild over many years but does not improve, and some patients develop progressive skeletal muscle weakness (Ford 1966, see Fenichel 1978, 1983) while in others the condition remains localised for many years (Whiteley et al 1976). AChR antibodies are absent (Vincent & Newsom-Davis 1979, Engel 1992). Thymectomy is contraindicated in this, as in all other non-autoimmune myasthenic disorders. The condition may be genetically heterogeneous, but in any case appears to be autosomal recessive in inheritance.

Vincent et al (1981) studied five patients with myasthenia dating from birth, of whom three had the features of this syndrome. In all these three cases there were findings indicating a defect in the acetylcholine receptors. These patients had a partial response to anticholesterase drugs, possibly enhanced by treatment with 3,4-diaminopyridine (Palace et al 1991). A fourth child (case 3) with more generalised symptoms in infancy and the later development of ophthalmoplegia (by the age of 13 years) had a different postsynaptic defect.

A single patient (their case 2) conforming to this clinical pattern was investigated by Lecky et al (1986) and the findings also suggested a postsynaptic defect, possibly in the structure of the AChR macromolecule.

Recently Slater et al (1994) have demonstrated a specific deficiency of the dystrophin-related protein (DRP or utrophin) at the neuromuscular junction in a patient with the clinical features of 'congenital myasthenia', and a reduction in the number of acetylcholine receptors.

It should be noted that one of the families with the 'slow-channel syndrome' described by Engel et al (1982) presented with ophthalmoparesis and weakness of neck flexion in infancy. Early infantile ophthalmoplegia with facial weakness was also the presenting feature of a child with 'congenital AChR deficiency and short channel-open time' (Engel et al 1990, case 4) but she also had recurrent respiratory insufficiency. There was a decremental response and she responded to pyridostigmine.

Myasthenia with facial malformation. A distinct autosomal recessive disorder affecting 10 Iraqi and Iranian Jewish families (eight of them consanguineous) was reported by Goldhammer et al (1990). Ptosis, facial weakness, and fatigue of speech and less often of swallowing dating from early childhood, were associated with elongation of the face, prognathism and a high-arched palate. There was a decremental response of evoked potentials, and a good response to pyridostigmine. The underlying defect is unknown.

Familial infantile myasthenia. Again by convention this term is used for patients with an autosomal recessive disorder causing generalised and often life-threatening myasthenia in the newborn period (Fenichel 1978, 1983). Ocular muscle involvement is absent or at least not a prominent feature. Respiratory failure, recurrent severe apnoeic attacks during crying, and choking and cyanosis during feeding are the dominant symptoms. There is a useful response to anticholinesterase drugs but ventilation and tracheostomy are sometimes required in the early stages. The myasthenia tends to improve over several weeks and it may be possible to withdraw medication but recurrent acute exacerbations pose a threat throughout infancy and early childhood and many of the reported cases have died unexpectedly. In the family reported by Gieron & Korthals (1985) exacerbations continued in adult life. Affected sibs may show a wide variation in the severity of symptoms; the patient of Robertson et al (1980) required continuous anticholinesterase treatment at the age of 14 years but a brother had had only recurrent respiratory depression in infancy with complete remission. The AChR antibody titres are normal (Robertson et al 1980, Gieron & Korthals 1985). Steroid therapy and thymectomy are valueless. In addition to the generally cited reports, some typical cases have escaped notice because of confusion over nomenclature (e.g. McLean et al 1973).

A typical case of this type studied by Hart et al (1979) was found to have evidence of a presynaptic transmission defect of acetylcholine resynthesis or packaging (see also Engel 1984, Mora et al 1987). A decremental response of the muscle action potential could be obtained only after prolonged nerve stimulation. This is a potent cause of diagnostic delay (Matthes et al 1991).

Other myasthenic syndromes present from birth. A boy with lifelong generalised myasthenia dating from the first week of life and including bulbar and ocular muscle involvement was found by Engel et al (1977) to have a deficiency of acetylcholinesterase in the end-plates. Five further cases were subsequently described (see Engel 1992), all very similar, though only three had ocular weakness. There was no response to anticholinesterase drugs, repetitive stimuli gave a decremental response and single stimuli applied to motor nerves induced repetitive muscle action potentials.

A baby with hypotonia and respiratory failure with absent AChR antibody and a normal routine EMG was found to have a striking decremental response (thus differing from familial infantile myasthenia) and no response to pyridostigmine.

He died at 8 months. A presynaptic defect was suggested (Albers et al 1984).

The only patient described with the 'high conductance: fast closure syndrome' (Engel et al 1990, 1993) was clinically rather similar to familial infantile myasthenia, with neonatal weakness, motor developmental delay and intermittent ptosis with fatigue, and showed no decrement on routine testing. She responded partially to pyridostigmine.

A patient with fatigable ocular, bulbar, cervical and limb weakness since infancy with a decremental response, who responded to pyridostigmine, had a defect of synaptic vesicles (Engel et al 1990, case 1). A briefly described, apparently similar case had 'abnormal ACh–AChR interaction' (Engel et al 1990, Engel 1992), while two others had a deficiency of ACh receptors with a prolonged channel open-time and absence of the epsilon-subunit of the receptors (Engel 1992).

Smit et al (1984, 1988) described two patients born with multiple contractures and severe generalised myasthenic weakness whose fetal movements had been impaired. The eye movements were normal. They had recurrent myasthenic crises but improved with treatment with pyridostigmine. Study of biopsy samples revealed too few secondary synaptic clefts, an altered distribution of the acetylcholine receptors and an increased number of end-plates. Two sibs aged 64 and 58, who had lifelong ptosis and mild weakness, with progression from the fourth decade to give external ophthalmoplegia and paralysis, were found to have an identical end-plate lesion. There was a partial response to pyridostigmine (Wokke et al 1989).

Slowly progressive weakness. For many years patients have been described with 'benign congenital myopathy' who survived into adult life with some elements of fluctuation or fatigability but with a limited response to anticholinesterase drugs (Rowland & Eskanazi 1956, Walton et al 1956).

McQuillen (1966) described a brother and sister who developed a 'limb-girdle' syndrome of proximal and distal weakness in the early teens and who showed a striking response to prostigmine. The ocular and bulbar muscles were not involved. Other similar cases have been described

(Fenichel 1978, 1983, Husain et al 1989), some of them with tubular aggregates in the muscle fibres on biopsy, but the pathogenesis of this condition remains obscure.

However, Morgan-Hughes et al (1981) found tubular aggregates in the muscle biopsy and evidence both of reduced numbers of AChRs and of a reduction in their affinity for ACh in a man of 32 years. This patient presented with a 14-month history of myasthenia resembling the autoimmune disease clinically and electrophysiologically, but with absent AChR antibody and no response to anticholinesterase drugs.

The slow channel syndrome. Engel et al (1982) described and investigated six patients who all had lifelong muscle weakness and who were shown to have identical postsynaptic neuromuscular transmission defects with a prolonged open-time of the acetylcholine-induced ion channel. The inheritance was autosomal dominant. From early infancy they had weakness of the neck and scapular muscles, the finger extensors, usually (but not always) the external ocular muscles and sometimes other muscles including the face. Periodic exacerbations of the weakness occurred but apparently not typical myasthenic fatigue. Their symptoms progressed gradually and as adults they had muscle wasting but in most cases normal reflexes. The overall picture resembled a congenital muscular dystrophy or myopathy more than myasthenia. AChR antibody titres and serum CK activity were normal. The EMG showed a characteristic repetitive firing response after single nerve stimuli, and a decremental response in affected muscles. Muscle biopsies showed variation in fibre size, fibre splitting, some mild fibrosis, type I fibre predominance and grouping (which could be mistaken for neurogenic atrophy) and tubular aggregates and vacuoles. It is likely that patients with this disorder are usually overlooked. Treatment with anticholinesterase drugs, however, has been disappointing. Two further cases were reported by Oosterhuis et al (1987).

Other 'limb-girdle' myasthenias with partially characterised transmission defects. A patient of Lecky et al (1986, case 1) had lifelong muscle weakness without diurnal fluctuation which involved the face and proximal limb muscles more than the distal ones. There was ptosis but the eye movements were not recorded. The tendon reflexes were sluggish. There was no response to edrophonium but some improvement with 3,4-diaminopyridine. The serum AChR antibody titre and CK activity were normal. The patient had delayed puberty and an impaired growth hormone response to insulin. EMG showed a limited decremental response and no repetitive firing but there was increased jitter. Muscle biopsy was normal. In vitro studies suggested a reduced amount of ACh per quantum but did not exclude a postsynaptic defect in ACh sensitivity. In one of the patients (case 1) of Vincent et al (1981) there were similar clinical features and findings and on investigation this patient responded to treatment with 4-aminopyridine. He had full external ocular movements. The response to treatment in such patients, who lack obvious clinical evidence of myasthenia, makes it particularly important to use sophisticated electrophysiological studies to identify them.

Seven patients seen in Newcastle, in a series of 27 cases of childhood myasthenia, displayed a fairly uniform clinical picture more suggestive of a congenital myopathy than myasthenia (Gardner-Medwin 1993). A brother and sister were affected and five were sporadic cases, three male, two female. The onset was at 6–14 months with motor delay in four cases, and between 2 and 7 years with fluctuating abnormality of gait in the others. The gait disturbance fluctuated gradually and for no obvious reason over weeks or months and typical myasthenic fatigability or diurnal fluctuation were uncommon. When weakness increased after exercise it often lasted for many days. The weakness in four cases gradually increased over a decade or more. The eye movements were spared, ptosis and facial weakness were absent or a late and slight feature. Limb-muscle weakness was mainly proximal, with little wasting and generally preserved tendon reflexes. The striking features were the stance and gait and the consistently and enigmatically normal results of repeated investigations. The stance was lordotic with some neck extension and with inward rotation of the hips so the feet were at right angles. When the weakness was more severe the rotated knees were rested against each other. The gait preserved this posture in a sinuous waddle that is virtually diagnostic.

Serum creatine kinase activity and routine EMG were normal. The seven patients were subjected to 14 muscle biopsies, all normal or at most showing variation of fibre size, and type I fibre predominance and an increase in IIc fibres. One had a few tubular aggregates. The diagnosis was based on single-fibre EMG and a decremental response to repetitive stimulation, sometimes with post-tetanic facilitation. Motor point biopsies in four cases showed evidence of a presynaptic defect, not further characterised (Slater C, Walls T J and Fawcett P R W in preparation). One of these cases (Fig. 21.4) was earlier reported as a congenital myopathy (Young & Anderson 1987) with another unrelated case who was shown also to be similarly affected (Walls T J, personal communication). Pyridostigmine may improve the symptoms in very small doses, or not at all, and in

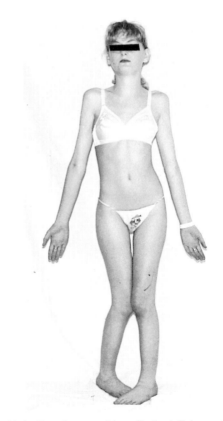

Fig. 21.4 Pseudomyopathic or 'limb-girdle' myasthenia.

one case caused sudden worsening. The combination of this drug with 3,4-diaminopyridine improved one case more than either alone.

Other defects of neuromuscular transmission

Infantile botulism. Two infants, aged two and three months, who became hypotonic over a period of a few days and had difficulty in sucking and swallowing, were found to have evidence of neuromuscular blockade on electromyography and both had *Clostridium botulinum* organisms and toxin in the faeces. Both made a spontaneous recovery (Pickett et al 1976). Other cases have been described, all with a similar history, the great majority of them from the USA (Midura & Arnon 1976, Turner et al 1978, Long et al 1985, Schreiner et al 1991). The pupils are fixed and dilated and other signs of autonomic failure are common. Constipation is an early and constant feature, perhaps related to the production of toxin in the bowel. This disorder is quite distinct from the acute effects of ingestion of *C. botulinum* toxin. It may momentarily be mistaken for myasthenia, or even Werdnig–Hoffmann disease.

The Eaton-Lambert syndrome (see Ch. 20) is exceedingly rare in childhood but has been described in association with leukaemia (Shapira et al 1974) and in children with no detectable tumour (Chelmicka-Schorr et al 1979, Bady et al 1987). A similar electrophysiological situation has been described in a 2-year-old, lasting for 6 weeks following the continuous use of muscle relaxant drugs for a week (Benzing et al 1990).

CLINICAL PROBLEMS IN CHILDREN WITH NEUROMUSCULAR DISORDERS

Hypotonia

'Hypotonia' alone is an inadequate clinical term and its analysis requires assessment of posture, spontaneous movement and reflex responses as well as of the power, extensibility and resistance to rapid passive movements of the muscles.

The differential diagnosis of infantile hypotonia may arise either when a baby is relatively immobile and limp at birth or in the first few days and weeks of life or, more often, because of delay in the development of control of posture at about six months of age and onwards.

The normal infant at birth. Even when a newborn baby is quiet it exhibits marked flexor tone when lying or suspended prone or supine, and it is not possible fully to extend the thighs or legs by passive stretching. Passive movements of the limbs give the impression of hypertonia which should, of course, be equal bilaterally provided that the head is kept in a central position to eliminate the influence of the asymmetrical tonic neck reflex on the limbs. A beat or two of ankle clonus is normal. Even at birth there is some postural control of the head: on being sat up, the newborn baby will balance its head for a brief period in the upright position before it flops forward; an anencephalic baby will keep its head upright.

The development of postural control in the normal infant. It is important to realise that the muscle tone of the normal infant diminishes during the first month of life to be regained later. The newborn baby may take his weight on his legs more firmly than he will do again until the age of 6–9 months.

By about 6 weeks of age a baby can extend its head against gravity to the midline when held prone, by three months it can flex against gravity when held supine. By three months it will raise the shoulders and fully extend the head when lying prone; by 5–6 months a baby lying supine will raise its head in anticipation of being picked up.

By three months a baby lying supine will extend its *arms* towards a proferred object and by five months will reach out and grasp the object with one hand. At 6 months most babies will sit with support and even for brief periods without support, propping themselves up by the arms placed between the abducted thighs; 50% of normal Newcastle infants are sitting unsupported at 6.4 months, 90% at 8.1 months and 97% at 9.3 months; 50% are walking unaided at 12.8 months, 90% at 15.8 months and 97% at 18.4 months (Neligan & Prudham 1969). The percentile figures for Denver infants are a little different, but the Denver Developmental Screening Test is useful and straightforward to apply (Frankenburg & Dodds 1967, Bryant et al 1979).

The hypotonic infant. The sight of a newborn hypotonic infant lying awake and motionless with outstretched limbs is in striking contrast to the appearance of the normal baby. Typically the hips are fully abducted, the knees flexed and the elbows extended. Hypotonia can be confirmed on handling and lifting the infant, when instead of its curling up, the head, trunk and limbs will flop about under the influence of gravity (Fig. 21.5a). Resistance to passive movement of the limbs and head will be decreased, passivité will be increased and so will extensibilité, as evinced by wrapping each arm round the neck (the 'scarf' sign) or by flexing the thighs on the trunk with the legs fully extended at the knees.

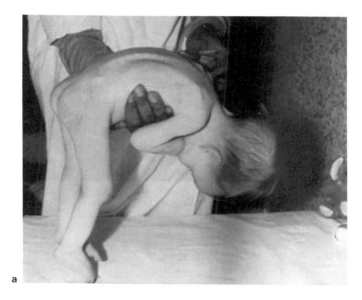

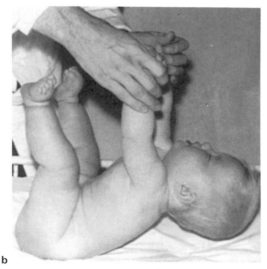

Fig. 21.5   Two infants with severe central hypotonia and no neuromuscular disease. **a** Severe mental retardation; a boy 11 months old. **b** Prader–Willi syndrome; a boy of 9 months. Abnormal 'passivité' contrasts with active contraction against gravity.

Almost all hypotonic infants move less actively than normal babies. Dubowitz (1978, 1980) emphasises the difference between the paralysed floppy baby with neuromuscular disease and the baby with central hypotonia but without significant weakness who can withdraw from a painful stimulus or support the limbs briefly against gravity (Fig. 21.5b). The distinction is important and useful but by no means always easy to see; some disorders of the central nervous system may give rise to severe paralysis.

Asking the mother about the fetal movements may elicit some evidence about the duration of the hypotonia before birth. Contractures at birth imply fetal immobility, and dislocation of the hips is quite frequent when prenatal hypotonia of the muscles of the lower limbs has diminished the normal forces required to form the acetabula properly. Fetal impairment of swallowing is an important cause of polyhydramnios.

Causes of hypotonia. Diminished movement and limpness in the *newborn baby* may be caused by extreme prematurity, by any severe systemic illness, by drugs given to the mother or by lesions of the brain, spinal cord, peripheral nerves, myoneural junction, muscles and ligaments. Severe generalised illness (such as respiratory distress or septicaemia) or cerebral disorders (especially malformation, bleeding, infection or the effects of asphyxia) are by far the commonest causes but, in the absence of obvious illness, and especially when the baby is alert, one must consider the possibility of a number of less common disorders in the differential diagnosis. These include the neuromuscular disorders.

There are also numerous causes for *delay in the development of postural control* and many babies who display retarded motor development give the clinical impression of hypotonia. Attempts to measure muscle tone objectively have been made (Rondot et al 1958) but not applied in a systematic fashion to this problem. It is uncommon for muscular hypotonia and weakness to develop in a previously normal infant so rapidly that they command attention in themselves, or cause actual regression in development. Such an event clearly implies a progressive disorder, whether cerebral, spinal or neuromuscular in origin. Even these more often result in developmental delay before any regression is seen, and so timing the 'onset' of the disease, an important point in differential diagnosis, may be a difficult matter, greatly influenced by the parents' experience, powers of observation and memory (Pearn 1974).

Paine's follow-up study (Paine 1963) put the differential diagnostic problem into perspective. The following were the final diagnoses in 111 'floppy' infants reviewed at from six months to 20 years of age: various forms of cerebral palsy 48; cerebral degenerative disease 3; brain tumour one; mental retardation 28; spinal cord injury 1; spinal muscular atrophy 4; myopathy 4; benign congenital hypotonia 18; and disease outside the nervous system 4. In contrast, no fewer than 67 of Walton's series of 109 cases (Walton 1956) were eventually diagnosed as having spinal muscular atrophy, but here the initial diagnosis in each case was 'amyotonia congenita' whereas Paine's series of children simply presented with delay in postural control.

Some non-neuromuscular causes of hypotonia

Any chronic debilitating illness in early infancy and many conditions adversely affecting growth (malnutrition, malabsorption syndromes, metabolic diseases, congenital heart malformations, congenital defects of the renal tract, chronic pulmonary diseases, etc.) may result in delayed motor control and hypotonia, but can usually be differentiated fairly easily by the history, symptoms and signs. Mental handicap may not be as easily distinguished because the conventional yardsticks of mental development in infancy are so dependent on motor performance; attention must be directed to alertness, awareness, and language development as well as to the specific dysmorphic or other characteristics of the different conditions underlying the mental handicap. It is important not to confuse the absence of facial expression caused by muscle weakness with that of retardation.

It is not uncommon to find delay in postural control and hypotonia, otherwise inexplicable, in infants who have lacked normal care in the early weeks of life (Buda et al 1972). In such cases the cause may be apparent in simple parental neglect, frequent change of foster parent or institutional life, but in other cases the lack of normal mothering is by no means always obvious to the clinician — the mother's anxiety being attributed to the baby's condition, rather than vice versa.

Acute metabolic disease in the newborn. An inborn error of metabolism — particularly an organic acidaemia, aminoacidaemia or hyperammonaemia — should be suspected in a baby who is well at birth but develops profound hypotonia, respiratory failure, poor feeding and drowsiness within the first few days, without evidence of infection or intracranial haemorrhage. Hyperventilation is an important clue to the underlying metabolic acidosis in these disorders. Checking for hypoglycaemia, ketonuria, an unusual odour of the urine and acidosis are important initial stages in their investigation.

These metabolic disorders may, incidentally, present only much later when an acute illness causes a catabolic state and decompensation.

Spinal cord injury, tumours and myelodysplasia. Deformity or injury of the spinal cord at birth may result in the classic picture of the floppy infant, but the arms are often spared. Birth injury to the spinal cord was first accurately described by Crothers (1923). The cord is damaged by stretching or by avulsion of the spinal roots forming the brachial plexus. Most cases follow difficult breech delivery which may be complicated by the rare distal form of brachial plexus palsy (Klumpke) causing paralysis of the small muscles of the hand and the long flexors of the hand and fingers. A minority of spinal cord injuries, namely those complicating difficult vertex delivery, are more usually associated with brachial plexus palsy of the proximal type (Erb) involving mainly the abductors of the upper arm and flexors and supinators of the forearm (Crothers & Putnam 1927).

The initial complete flaccidity and immobility of the lower limbs and trunk in spinal cord injury may result in a mistaken diagnosis of a general neuromuscular disorder, especially if there are also brachial plexus lesions. However, the presence of sphincter and sensory abnormalities will reveal the true diagnosis even if the localised nature of the paralysis is not at first obvious.

There is likely to be retention of urine and a patulous anus for several days and pinching the skin of the lower half of the body, although it may later cause reflex withdrawal, will not result in a cry or grimace. After the first few days, however, normal sphincter action may be regained and sensory loss may be difficult to detect. The CSF may contain blood. The subject is reviewed by Towbin (1969) and Byers (1975).

Spinal tumours in infancy are uncommon and are easily overlooked at first if there is extensive paralysis involving the intercostal or abdominal muscles as well as the limbs. Tumours extending over many segments of the cord, whether intramedullary (glioma or ependymoma) or extramedullary such as a neuroblastoma, are fairly characteristic at this age. They provide the same pitfalls in diagnosis as extensive cord injury.

Myelodysplasia is usually obvious at birth in the form of meningomyelocele. In cases where the deformity is hidden, however, there are nearly always overlying skin defects (hair, haemangioma, lipoma or congenital dermal sinus) and X-rays will reveal the spinal deformity.

Cerebral causes of hypotonia at birth. The higher control of muscle tone in the newborn is not well understood. Anencephalic and grossly hydranencephalic newborn infants may exhibit normal muscle tone, but whereas *absence* of cerebral hemispheres may not be associated with hyper- or hypotonicity, *damage* to or disease of the hemispheres may.

Muscular hypotonia is characteristic of asphyxia at birth, in which apnoea is associated with pallor, bradycardia and unresponsiveness to physical stimuli. 'Cerebral depression' in the first few days of life may follow severe asphyxia at birth or a traumatic labour, or may occur unexpectedly in the presence of prenatally determined disease or deformity of the brain. Temporary cerebral depression may follow administration of sedative drugs to the mother in labour and hypotonia is a particularly striking feature when diazepam is used in cases of pre-eclamptic toxaemia. The appearance of a pallid, motionless, hypotonic baby with open eyes and with increasingly frequent periods of apnoea and cyanosis is characteristic of cerebral depression in the newborn. Automatisms, such as the Moro, rooting, nasopalpebral and sucking reflexes are absent. The mortality is high, especially in the first 48 hours of life, and massive intracranial haemorrhage is a common post-mortem finding. In those who survive, the hypotonia usually gives place after a day or two either to normal muscle tone and movement or to a clinical state suggesting cerebral irritation, signs of which include hypertonia, hyperactivity, easily elicited automatisms and multifocal fits. The hypotonia caused by a cerebral lesion acquired at birth only infrequently persists after the first few days of life and in these cases lack of alertness or responsiveness, and preservation of the tendon reflexes usually help to differentiate the condition from lower motor neurone or muscular disorders.

Hypotonia as a feature of cerebral palsy. Persistent hypotonia following a perinatal cerebral catastrophe is very rare and its pathological basis is uncertain. It is of interest in this context that Woolf (1960) reported the case of one infant with bilateral cerebral softening secondary to birth asphyxia, accompanied by vacuolar degeneration of anterior horn cells. Flaccidity is, however, often seen in the early months in infants who later prove to be cases of spastic diplegia, athetosis, ataxia or mental defect (as Sigmund Freud realised nearly a century ago). Most infants with more persistent central hypotonia will be found to have a chromosomal disorder, the Prader–Willi syndrome, or other disorders of cerebral or cerebellar development associated with mental defect or persistent congenital ataxia respectively (Lesny 1979). There is thus no evidence to support the widespread concept of a permanent hypotonic category of cerebral palsy. Some infants with cerebral disorders originating before or at birth are found to have delayed maturation of muscle fibres — a fetal or neonatal pattern persisting for longer than usual (Fenichel 1967, Curless et al 1978b), and some cases of 'fibre-type disproportion' seem to fall into this category.

Spastic diplegia is the typical type of cerebral palsy seen in preterm infants, although it is not confined to this group. Ingram (1955) found that 40% of his cases went through a hypotonic stage in early infancy. Within a few weeks after birth physical examination shows hypotonia and diminished tendon reflexes, but automatisms such as the Moro reflex and palmar grasp reflexes are too easily elicited and tonic neck reflexes are conspicuous. Transition to a dystonic stage usually takes place within six months. By then early spasticity is indicated by hyperadduction of the thighs and plantar flexion of the feet on upright suspension, and spread of the knee jerk to the adductors of one or both thighs.

Hypotonia is also characteristic of athetosis and choreoathetosis in infancy, but the tendon reflexes tend to be brisk in contrast to the diminished muscle tone, and tonic neck reflexes are usually easily elicited. Polani (1959) studied the natural history of choreoathetosis. About one-third of his patients displayed marked muscular hypotonia from about the second month and this might still be apparent by one year of age. Usually opisthotonic episodes and athetoid tongue-thrusting begin within the first year.

Muscular hypotonia and delay in postural control are often the presenting symptoms of ataxic syndromes of infancy and childhood, whether attributable to prenatal cerebellar hypoplasia, to perinatal events or to degenerative processes. An important minority of these cases results from congenital hypothyroidism. At first, congenital ataxia presents a clinical picture of generalised hypotonia, paucity of spontaneous movement, hyperextensibility of joints, absent automatisms and poor postural control. Intention tremor and incoordination of voluntary movement emerge as the child begins to reach out for objects.

Similarly, degenerative diseases producing ataxia, such as Friedreich's and other hereditary ataxias and ataxia telangiectasia, may present with delay in acquisition of motor control and hypotonia. *Intermittent* ataxia (Blass et al 1971), whether caused by intoxication, benign paroxysmal vertigo, a IVth ventricular tumour, an aminoacidaemia or lactic acidosis, or the syndrome of idiopathic familial intermittent ataxia, may be difficult at first to distinguish from periodic paralysis in very young children.

Mental handicap. Delay in motor development in the first year of life is frequently the presenting symptom of mental retardation and is often accompanied by hypotonia. Later, the child generally proves to have no detectable motor defect while the learning difficulties gradually become apparent. However, there are several conditions, of which Down syndrome and the Prader–Willi syndrome are the best known, in which hypotonia in the early stages is particularly conspicuous.

The Prader–Willi syndrome is an entity characterised by short stature, obesity, mild to moderate mental retardation, cryptorchidism and genital hypoplasia (Prader et al 1956, Laurence 1967, Zellweger & Schneider 1968) and is associated in many cases with a deletion of part of chromosome 15 at 5q11.2–12 (Fear et al 1985, Robinson et al 1991). Most cases have from birth shown marked generalised hypotonia, areflexia, paucity of movement and feeble sucking. Tube feeding is commonly required in the first few weeks of life. After several months the infants become more active and the tendon reflexes are elicitable but moderate hypotonia persists. Excessive appetite and obesity develop in the second or third year. Children with the Prader–Willi syndrome (Fig. 21.6) have recognisably similar faces (Laurence 1967, Dubowitz 1980, Stephenson 1980).

Muscular hypotonia is a feature of *several other*

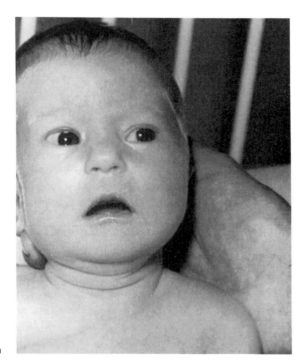

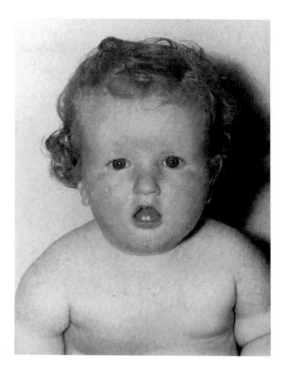

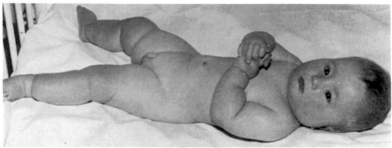

Fig. 21.6 Prader–Willi syndrome. **a** Facies, a girl at 3 weeks old. Severe hypotonia, needed tube-feeding for 10 weeks. At 5 years her stature was below the 3rd centile, her weight near the 97th. **b** Facies, hypotonic posture, hypogenitalism, obesity at 9 months of age. Same patient as 21.5(b). **c** Facies, a boy aged 9 months.

chromosomal defects, but peripheral nerve and muscle have rarely been studied in these conditions. Muscular hypotonia and multiple malformations are prominent in trisomy 13, and in trisomy 18 initial hypotonia is later replaced by hypertonia. Hypotonia is also characteristic of infants with the cri du chat syndrome (partial deletion of the short arm of chromosome 5). Three chromosomal disorders which may present with hypotonia as the dominant clinical problem are ring chromosome 14 (Fig. 21.7), ring chromosome 22 and possibly translocation of the long arm of chromosome 10; but even in these disorders minor dysmorphic features provide a clue to the diagnosis. One-third of cases of XXXXY karyotype have been noted to be hypotonic (Smith 1982).

The association of mental retardation with hypotonia by no means rules out serious neuromuscular disease. Both in Duchenne muscular dystrophy and in congenital myotonic dystrophy, mental retardation may be severe and may divert attention from the muscular weakness. Boys with unexplained delay in walking or in speech development should be tested for Duchenne muscular dystrophy by estimation of the serum CK activity (see Ch. 14). Mental retardation is a major feature of Fukuyama muscular dystrophy (Ch. 14), of Lowe syndrome (X-linked hypotonia, myopathy, cataracts and renal aminoaciduria), of a syndrome of retardation, eye anomalies and progressive myopathy (Santavuori et al 1977) and of another with similar features associated with mucolipidosis type

IV (Zlotogora et al 1983), of Pompe disease, systemic carnitine deficiency and of certain lipid storage and mitochondrial diseases.

Mental retardation is also found with severe hypotonia, although not with overt myopathy, in Zellweger's cerebrohepatorenal syndrome (Fig. 21.8), neonatal adrenoleucodystrophy (Aubourg et al 1986) and the Smith–Lemli–Opitz syndrome (Smith 1982). In the early stages of certain neurodegenerative diseases (especially Tay–Sachs and Niemann–Pick diseases, generalised gangliosidosis and infantile neuroaxonal dystrophy) the motor disturbance is first evident as hypotonia. In the leucodystrophies and in Tay–Sachs disease, hypotonia of the neck and trunk muscles may co-exist with spasticity of the limbs (Fig. 21.9). In the Krabbe and metachromatic types of leucodystrophy the associated peripheral neuropathy also causes areflexia in the presence of spasticity.

Skeletal, tendinous and ligamentous causes of hypotonia. It may be difficult to make a clinical distinction between ligamentous laxity and muscular hypotonia in early infancy. Later in childhood the hyperextensibility of the joints with otherwise relatively normal muscle tone becomes apparent. Certain congenital disorders of connective tissue may be accompanied by delay in postural control and apparent hypotonia due to hyperextensibility of joints.

In Marfan's syndrome and especially in a similar 'marfanoid' syndrome (Walker et al 1969) joint laxity is prominent and in the former some muscular weakness occurs. 'Marfanoid' features

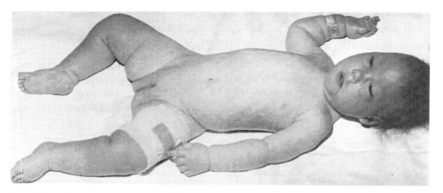

Fig. 21.7 Chromosome anomaly (ring chromosome 14). Hypotonia and weakness were the dominant problems. Mild facial dysmorphism. EMG and needle muscle biopsy normal. Here aged 10 months.

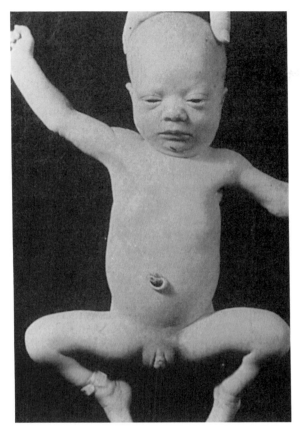

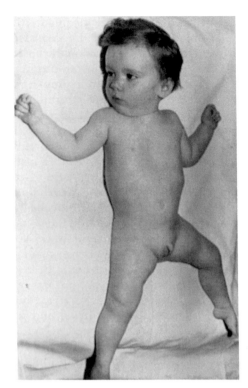

Fig. 21.9   Tay–Sachs disease. Progressive hypotonia, blindness and megalencephaly since 7 months. Here aged 21 months. Note the asymmetrical tonic neck reflex.

Fig. 21.8   Zellweger (cerebrohepatorenal syndrome), profound hypotonia, areflexia and seizures from day 1; liver dysfunction. Here aged 2 weeks.

have often been mentioned in nemaline myopathy but in fact bear little resemblance to true Marfan's disease. Ehlers–Danlos syndrome must also be considered in the differential diagnosis of the limp child. Eight varieties of this are now recognised of which two (types III and VII) present with joint laxity and recurrent dislocations of joints as the main features while, in the other types, elastic skin, bruising and other features are more prominent (Byers et al 1983). Osteogenesis imperfecta has been reported as presenting with delay in walking and hypotonia (Tizard 1949); the mild autosomal dominant form (type 1) is the relevant one of the four types described and ligamentous laxity and deep blue sclera are striking features (Sillence et al 1979).

Benign congenital hypotonia. This much-maligned term arose from the work of Walton (1956, 1957) who obtained follow-up information on 109 infants diagnosed as having 'amyotonia congenita' during the period 1930–54. Oppenheim's concept of 'myatonia', put forward in 1900 for hypotonic children with a favourable prognosis, had become debased and Walton found that, half a century later, the terms 'myatonia' or 'amyotonia congenita' were sometimes used to encompass all of the infantile hypotonias including Werdnig–Hoffmann disease. Seventeen of his 109 cases had hypotonia of unknown cause, but with recovery which was complete in eight and incomplete in nine cases. The term 'benign congenital hypotonia' was 'used as a descriptive title' for these cases whose 'condition appears to have been due to a widespread congenital muscular hypotonia of undetermined aetiology which eventually recovered completely' (Walton 1956). In the same year, central core disease was first described and, in the period of nearly 40 years which has passed since then, many other disorders giving hypotonia with incomplete recovery have been recognised and are now generally classified among the congenital myopathies described earlier in this chapter. The nature of those cases which show complete recovery, and for which Walton now reserves the term 'benign congenital hypotonia', has been less satisfactorily clarified. Brooke & Engel (1969) found that some of them had type I fibre predominance in the muscle biopsy but others have no histological abnormality at all on the evidence of current techniques. No doubt, entities within this group will be identified in the future; meanwhile 'benign congenital hypotonia' remains, at any particular state of the art, a valuable term for those residual cases for whom, after full investigation, no more accurate label exists. It should be reserved for patients: (1) who are hypotonic at or soon after birth, sometimes quite severely; but (2) who retain active limb movements and tendon reflexes; and (3) whose motor development is delayed but shows improvement, over a period of months or years; and (4) whose serum enzyme activities, EMGs and biopsies are essentially normal. However, it is quite reasonably argued that muscle biopsy is not justified in an apparently benign situation when it can lead to no effective treatment, unless genetic counselling will be influenced by the result. Certainly, biopsy should be performed in this situation only when full histochemical and electron-microscopic studies will be done, for otherwise it is certain to be inconclusive.

The paediatrician with an interest in the development of the child's motor functions tends to look at hypotonia in a different light. For instance Lundberg (1979) reviewed 78 children who had delayed development of gross motor functions, such as sitting and walking, but had relatively well-developed manipulative functions and no abnormal neurological signs. She found that only three were diagnosed as having neuromuscular disease. Of 65 children whose walking was delayed beyond 27 months, 72% had been significantly hypotonic in infancy, and 28% had a family history of late walking. Half of them were 'bottom shufflers' and 30% had a family history of bottom-shuffling. A common sign among the late walkers in whom no cause for the delay was found

was the 'sitting on air' posture of flexion of the hips and extension of the knees while being suspended under the arms.

Whether one thinks of such children as having 'benign congenital hypotonia' or 'dissociated motor development', the essential need in management is to provide the child with the stimulation and equipment and the family with the understanding of the situation and the support that they need, to allow him to develop without the loss of opportunities which may, in the long run, prove more handicapping than the neuromuscular problem itself.

The place of neuromuscular investigations in infantile hypotonia. It will be evident that most hypotonic newborn infants are not suffering from neuromuscular disorders. Most will be found to be ill or mentally retarded or in the early stages of cerebral palsy. On the other hand the baby may become asphyxiated or otherwise ill *because* of neuromuscular problems and when there is apparently disproportionate hypotonia or muscle atrophy, or unexplained respiratory failure, neuromuscular disease must be suspected. Recognition of a neuromuscular problem is much easier when the baby is fully alert with no signs of central nervous system dysfunction and no dysmorphic features, and especially when there is a history of diminished fetal movement, or if weakness of the cranial muscles or the presence of congenital contractures draw attention to the muscles. Early resort to muscle biopsy has the dual disadvantage that the passage of time may, within a few weeks, reveal evidence for an alternative cause for the hypotonia and that muscle histology and histochemistry in the newborn are more difficult to interpret than in older children. In many of the congenital myopathies and in Werdnig–Hoffmann disease, very early biopsy may be misleading.

However it is obviously important to diagnose myasthenia as quickly as possible. Disorders of life-threatening severity and those that are clearly progressive must also be diagnosed as soon as possible, not only to rule out treatable conditions, but for the sake of future genetic counselling.

The serum CK activity is rarely very helpful in neonatal myopathies, but it does provide a valuable clue to the diagnosis of congenital muscular dystrophy if it is very high. Similarly, electromyography may be difficult to interpret in the newborn but in difficult cases is sometimes helpful. Nerve conduction studies are valuable in ruling out peripheral neuropathies. Ultrasonic or CT scanning of muscle are non-specific tests which, however, may provide enough evidence for or against a neuromuscular disorder to help in planning a strategy of early management of the problem.

The following strategy of management may be found helpful in suspected neuromuscular disease of the newborn:

1. Rule out myasthenia, transplacental drug intoxication and metabolic acidosis. Consider the Prader–Willi syndrome (facies, genitalia, swallowing) and other chromosome anomalies. Consider congenital myotonic dystrophy (examine the mother).

2. In all uncertain cases check the serum CK level, nerve conduction velocity and if necessary do an ultrasound muscle scan.

3. In life-threatening cases proceed to EMG and muscle biopsy. Be prepared to repeat these later if they give an uncertain result.

4. In less severe cases, after full consultation with the parents, delay further investigation until after a period of follow-up. This may last a few weeks to a few years depending (inversely) on the severity of the residual problem. Repeated clinical examination over a period will usually allow a provisional diagnosis to be made and an appropriate moment for further investigation to be chosen. In cases that improve considerably or remain mild, remember that a biopsy that is 'within normal limits' or 'non-specific' can inspire little confidence if it is performed too early. Above all, muscle biopsy should never be performed unless experienced laboratory services are available for histochemical and electron-microscopic examination.

Arthrogryposis multiplex congenita

The presence of multiple joint contractures at birth is clearly a situation with many causes, and individual appraisal of each patient is essential if one is to avoid overlooking the relatively unusual cases which have a simple genetic basis, an underlying progressive disease or important associated anomalies. The condition in most patients follows a non-progressive course and most are of normal intelligence. Arthrogryposis is seen in about one in 10 000 live births.

To qualify as having arthrogryposis multiplex congenita (AMC) a patient must have joint contractures present at birth in at least two different areas of the body (Fisher et al 1970). The more limited condition of congenital talipes, however, is analogous in having many different causes which include denervation of the lower limbs (as in spina bifida), oligohydramnios (which perhaps acts by restricting movement) and a large group of cases of unknown origin. Similarly, anterior horn cell aplasia confined to the cervical cord, with congenital non-progressive upper limb weakness and contractures has been described (Hageman et al 1993). In a typical case of AMC there is equinovarus deformity of the feet, the hips are abducted and flexed or extended, the knees and elbows incompletely extended, the forearms pronated and the hands flexed with a claw-like apposition of thenar and hypothenar eminences. There may be considerable variation upon this distribution. The muscles acting at the affected joints are typically wasted.

It is currently thought that the condition can result from a number of different pathological processes which cause immobilisation of the limbs during, or shortly after, the embryonic formation of joints (Dodge 1960). In support of this view, Jago (1970) described a typical case of arthrogryposis in an infant born to a mother who had had tetanus at the tenth to twelfth week of pregnancy and was treated with D-tubocurarine for 10 days. Arthrogryposis in the offspring of myasthenic mothers is described earlier in this chapter (Carr et al 1991).

Arthrogryposis, then, may result from immobility imposed on the fetus by external factors, including oligohydramnios, but it also occurs in a number of rare complex syndromes which affect the fetal muscles directly or indirectly: Beckerman & Buchino (1978), Hall et al (1982) and Hall (1983) provided extensive lists of these. The current London Neurogenetics Database (Baraitser & Winter 1991) has 88 entries under

congenital arthrogryposis. However, the most frequent causes, and those most relevant to this
chapter are disorders of nerve and muscle.

Most cases are found to have a neurogenic basis
(Brandt 1947, Drachman & Banker 1963, Besser
& Behar 1967, Banker 1986b). In Banker's series,
largely based on autopsy experience, there were
84 neurogenic and five myopathic cases. Typically
there is asymmetry of the weakness and joint
involvement suggesting patchy loss of anterior
horn cells (although this was not Banker's
(1986b) experience in her neurogenic cases, in
which symmetry was usual), and the spinal cord
lesion appears to be non-progressive in almost all
cases. Although joint contractures may be found at
birth in Werdnig–Hoffmann disease, these are
uncommon and never severe, and the joint deformity is fully correctable by passive stretching.
Clarren & Hall (1983) compared the pathology in
the two conditions and found that in Werdnig–
Hoffmann disease there was a general loss of the
anterior horn cells, whereas in neurogenic arthrogryposis only the alpha motor neurones were lost
and the smaller neurones were present in increased
numbers. It seems clear, therefore, that neurogenic
arthrogryposis is not simply a variant of Werdnig–
Hoffmann disease and indeed the two conditions
appear to be unrelated entities.

Krugliak et al (1978) described an infant with
arthrogryposis in whom post-mortem examination demonstrated apparently total agenesis of the
muscle spindles in addition to loss of the anterior
horn cells.

Another relatively common entity is amyoplasia (Hall et al 1983) in which a rather stereo-
typical pattern of contractures occurs (shoulders
inwardly related, elbows extended, wrists and
fingers flexed, hips and knees flexed and talipes
equinovarus) with appropriately distributed
severe muscle weakness due to aplasia. Biopsy
reveals islands of small muscle fibres in fascicles
surrounded by extensive areas of fat cells and
some connective tissue. The condition is strictly
sporadic, even to the point of discordance in
monozygotic twins, and the cause is unknown.

A primary myopathy with features of 'congenital muscular dystrophy' (q.v. Ch. 14) is much
more rarely the basis of arthrogryposis (Banker
et al 1957, 1986b, Pearson & Fowler 1963).

The former authors suggested that the posture
induced by the contractures was characteristically
different in the myopathic disorders, with flexion
of the hips and knees and adduction of the legs,
as well as kyphoscoliosis, chest deformity and
torticollis. It is unlikely that these criteria are
reliable for clinical diagnosis. The 'dystrophic'
nature of the muscle pathology in myopathic
AMC has been questioned by many authors,
notably by Dastur et al (1972) who studied
the histological and histochemical features of
26 cases of all types. A primary failure of
muscle embryogenesis with secondary fibrosis
and disorganisation of muscle architecture seems
more likely than a degenerative process in these
cases. In the Ullrich type of muscular dystrophy
the proximal muscles of both the upper and
lower limbs show contractures while the distal
joints are hyperextensible (Ch. 14).

Der Kaloustian et al (1972) reported a myopathic form of arthrogryposis in which massive
accumulation of glycogen in muscle fibres was
found on biopsy.

There is no doubt that both the EMG and the
muscle histology may be difficult to interpret in
arthrogryposis, presumably because of the chronicity of the lesion, the associated disuse atrophy
and the problems of 'secondary myopathic change
in denervated muscle'. Nevertheless, investigation will permit most cases to be assigned to a
neurogenic or myopathic category (Bharucha et al
1972, Dastur et al 1972). CT scanning may make
a contribution to this assessment (Abbing et al
1985).

Neurogenic AMC may be associated with
severe malformation of the brain causing severe
retardation, microcephaly and optic atrophy
(Fowler 1959, Frischknecht et al 1960) and sometimes with more subtle cerebral atrophy and mild
educational subnormality (Ek 1958, Bharucha et
al 1972) but most patients, whether of the neurogenic or myopathic type, are intellectually normal
(Wynne-Davies & Lloyd-Roberts 1976). Bargeton
et al (1961) and Peña et al (1968) described cases
of arthrogryposis of autosomal recessive genetic
origin, in which the pathology consisted of a peculiar nodular fibrosis of the anterior spinal roots.
Congenital familial polyneuropathy may also
cause arthrogryposis confined, however, to the

lower limbs (Yuill & Lynch 1974). A similar clinical pattern, due probably to anterior horn cell disease, in an extensive family with dominant inheritance was recorded by Fleury & Hageman (1985).

Autosomal recessive inheritance occurs in myopathic AMC (Lebenthal et al 1970). Dominant inheritance was reported in a father and two daughters with relatively mild myopathic features (Daentl et al 1974). In Banker's series she was able to identify genetic myopathies (congenital muscular dystrophy, central core disease or nemaline myopathy) in all five of her myopathic cases (Banker 1986b).

Although most neurogenic cases are sporadic it is crucial, before giving the parents a low genetic risk, to exclude the likelihood of one of the many genetic forms now described. This is a task for a geneticist skilled in dysmorphology. As a single example, the Pena–Shokeir syndrome type I comprises arthrogryposis, pulmonary hypoplasia and a subtly characteristic facies. Some cases are autosomal recessive in inheritance but even within this syndrome genetic heterogeneity (and some non-genetic phenocopies) seem likely (McKusick 1992). However, in a survey of all the cases of AMC seen in four large centres in Great Britain, Wynne-Davies & Lloyd-Roberts (1976) found none that were familial and concluded that a variety of environmental factors acting in utero were responsible, although these could rarely be identified. Wynne-Davies et al (1981) confirmed these conclusions in a wider study of an epidemic of arthrogryposis which occurred in the 1950s and 1960s in three widely separated parts of the world. They were unable to identify the causative factors involved, but complications early in pregnancy were a frequent concomitant.

Early and vigorous orthopaedic management of the deformities of arthrogryposis is usually successful in correcting them and because the underlying disorder in the great majority of cases is non-progressive the effort is well worth while. The treatment has been reviewed by Friedlander et al (1968) and Lloyd-Roberts & Lettin (1970). A hypermetabolic reaction to anaesthesia is reported in occasional cases (Hopkins et al 1991).

Muscle contractures and spinal deformities later in childhood

Congenital contractures, not usually amounting to arthrogryposis multiplex, occur in several of the congenital myopathies, notably in central core disease, congenital myotonic dystrophy and fibre-type disproportion, and also in nemaline myopathy, some of the congenital polyneuropathies and in some cases of infantile spinal muscular atrophy (SMA). In SMA fixed contractures at birth suggest a degree of chronicity of the lesion that makes it more likely that the case may fall into the slowly progressive or static type II category rather than into the inevitably progressive type I (Werdnig–Hoffmann disease).

Later in childhood contractures develop especially in the most severe neuromuscular diseases including Duchenne muscular dystrophy and SMA; they may contribute substantially to the child's disability. Regular stretching of the shortened muscles by the parents and the school physiotherapist, while by no means completely successful, makes a major contribution and attention to the sitting posture and sometimes the use of night splints may be valuable. Except at the ankles, where stretching techniques are rarely totally effective, tenotomy is not usually needed when a child has been regularly supervised. The use of tenotomy in the late stages of diseases with a poor prognosis must have a clear purpose, such as improving the child's appearance, posture, or handling, because it will rarely achieve any improvement in function. This is in sharp contrast to its value in arthrogryposis and other congenital contractures with relatively good muscle power. Contractures acquired later, either in the feet or elsewhere, following fractures, immobilisation or neglect, may benefit from the same approach.

Localised contractures in otherwise normal muscles are usually the sequel of earlier intramuscular injections of drugs (Norman et al 1970, Hoefnagel et al 1978).

In some cases of polymyositis in childhood, contractures may develop in a matter of a few days or weeks. Recurrent inflammatory lesions in muscle going on to ossification and contractures are characteristic of fibrodysplasia ossificans progressiva (see Ch. 27).

The management of kyphoscoliosis is discussed in relation to Duchenne muscular dystrophy in Chapter 14. The importance of preventive bracing applies a fortiori to disorders with a potentially better prognosis, such as spinal muscular atrophy and fibre-type disproportion, in which, however, increasing thoracic distortion may pose a major threat to life.

A disorder in which contractures play a major part is the *rigid spine syndrome*, so named by Dubowitz (1973, 1978). Further cases have been described by Goebel et al (1977), Seay et al (1977) and Goto et al (1979). The syndrome has been recorded only in males, although Dubowitz (1978) mentions seeing a female patient. The patients described had noted the cervical contractures by the age of six or seven years. Some had been normal until that time, others had had earlier muscle weakness and delay in walking. The condition is usually diagnosed late in the second decade, by which time the affected boy has severe contracture of the posterior cervical and paraspinal muscles and slighter elbow and knee contractures. The muscles are generally very thin but only slightly weak. A patient of Professor Sir John Walton's was able to run upstairs but had difficulty in walking down because of severe neck retraction. Neck flexion, however, is very weak and there is no doubt that there is a generalised mild myopathy. Respiratory failure is the major threat to life and may be alleviated by elective nocturnal ventilation (Morita et al 1990). Muscle biopsy of the rigid muscles reveals excessive endomysial and perimysial fibrosis, and variation in fibre size. Goebel et al (1977) and Seay et al (1977) found fibre-type disproportion in biceps in their cases. There are no reports of familial cases of the typical syndrome at present. However, somewhat similar contractures and muscle weakness are seen in the Emery–Dreifuss type of muscular dystrophy and of the similar autosomal dominant genotype (see Ch. 14). Indeed it is of the greatest importance in any patient suspected of having the 'rigid-spine syndrome' to consider the possibility of Emery–Dreifuss muscular dystrophy and to investigate carefully for cardiac involvement.

Acute muscular weakness

In the countries which provide immunisation against poliomyelitis it has become a rare event to see a child who has developed severe generalised muscular weakness over a period of hours or a few days.

Poliomyelitis must still be considered, especially in travellers from abroad. ECHO and Coxsackie viruses very occasionally cause an almost indistinguishable illness. The multifocal distribution of the weakness, the relation to a preceding febrile illness and the development of a purely motor deficit over a few days sometimes accompanied by pain and by fasciculation are all characteristic. Poliomyelitis has been reported as an uncommon occurrence in newborn babies (Pugh & Dudgeon 1954, Bates 1955). It seems clear, from the onset of the disease within the first few days of life, that the virus can be transmitted via the placenta. In many cases the mother has had the paralytic form of the disease shortly before or after the birth of the infant. In other cases, infection through faecal contamination from the mother in the birth process or postnatal infection may have taken place. The infant may have little fever and no diarrhoea. The extent of the paralysis is variable, but in many cases has been widespread with a fatal outcome. Focal myocarditis has been a common post-mortem finding in addition to the typical central nervous system changes.

Some patients who later are shown to have chronic spinal muscular atrophy develop symptoms for the first time very suddenly over a few days or even hours in an illness which may resemble poliomyelitis. This often occurs, however, during the course of one of the common childhood fevers or may follow immunisation. Recovery, if any occurs, is usually very slight after such an episode. Later in the course of the disease, episodes of deterioration are quite often a feature, again with very limited improvement or none at all, so that the disability in these patients tends to deteriorate in a series of steps rather than taking the more continuous downhill course which is seen in the muscular dystrophies and indeed in many other cases of spinal muscular atrophy. However, Robb et al (1991) described two sisters with spinal muscular atrophy who both had an initial rapidly progressive course leading to severe paralysis within two weeks (at the age of 4 and 10 months respectively) with considerable subsequent improvement.

Other causes of rapidly progressive paralysis which must be considered and which are more fully described in other chapters are acute polyneuritis, the periodic paralyses, myasthenia gravis, acute myositis and acute rhabdomyolysis. Botulism causes bulbar weakness, blurred vision and diplopia followed by generalised flaccid paralysis and areflexia. Poisoning with organophosphorus compounds, curare or an overdose of an anticholinesterase drug may have to be considered in some cases. In young infants, quite acute weakness and hypotonia may occur in Leigh's disease and the organic acidaemias.

Acute post-infectious polyneuritis (Ch. 25) is uncommon before the age of four years and rare before two years. The presenting symptoms and course of the illness are similar in childhood and adult life. It is not uncommon to be able to diagnose the preceding infection serologically and *Campylobacter jejuni* and the Epstein–Barr virus are important among many other causative agents. The disease as it affects children has been reviewed by Peterman et al (1959), Paulson (1970), Eberle et al (1975) and Aicardi (1992). Acute neuropathy in porphyria is extremely rare in childhood.

Acute transient viral myositis (Ch. 16) may cause a rather painful generalised paralysis after a prodromal febrile illness of several days; the serum CK level is 5–50 times normal; recovery occurs in a few days. McKinlay & Mitchell (1976) described eight patients aged between five and nine years.

Acute weakness may result from fluctuations in serum potassium levels (Ch. 17). Any condition causing considerable hypokalaemia is likely to be associated with muscular weakness, hypotonia and areflexia. Cushing's disease and primary aldosteronism are rare in young children, but gastrointestinal and renal losses of potassium may occur in a number of infantile diseases such as chronic diarrhoea and vomiting, congenital alkalosis of gastrointestinal origin, renal tubular acidosis and galactosaemia, and the hypokalaemia produces muscular weakness, hypotonia and depres-

sion of tendon reflexes. The hypokalaemic, hyperkalaemic and normokalaemic forms of periodic paralysis may all be seen in childhood: indeed, the hyperkalaemic form almost always begins in the first decade. In their series of 108 cases, Gamstorp et al (1957) found that 45% had attacks before the age of 5 years and 90% before the age of 10 years. Their youngest patient was 8 months old at the onset. The symptoms last a few minutes at first but become more prolonged in adolescence. The treatment of attacks of hyperkalaemic periodic paralysis with inhaled salbutamol, introduced by Wang & Clausen (1976) has proved useful in children. The hypokalaemic form tends to start later but may do so at as early as three years (Howes et al 1966, Buruma et al 1985). As the attacks continue, a permanent myopathy may develop and this may be seen even in children (Pearson 1964, Dyken et al 1969). The normokalaemic form of periodic paralysis also begins before the age of 10 years (Poskanzer & Kerr 1961) and causes recurrent severe tetraparesis lasting usually for several days or even weeks. A similar clinical pattern of weakness was described by Shy et al (1966) in the 'pleoconial' type of mitochondrial myopathy.

Acute focal muscular weakness of lower motor neurone type may result from birth trauma or other injuries to the brachial plexus, or from poliomyelitis. Acute radiculitis or mononeuritis multiplex are two of the many potential neurological complications of tick-borne *Borrelia* infection (Lyme disease) (Reik et al 1979, Bruhn 1984).

Two other conditions are of special interest in children. Recurrent attacks of neuralgic amyotrophy (brachial neuritis) occur in some families in which the trait is inherited as an autosomal dominant (Geiger et al 1974, Dunn et al 1978, Airaksinen et al 1985). As in the sporadic adult disease, quite severe local pain precedes acute weakness, usually in certain proximal muscles of the upper limb but sometimes in the forearm. There is profound atrophy; recovery takes many months and may be incomplete. Sometimes there is autonomic involvement. Attacks may occur from the first year of life but do so at long intervals, usually of several years. Rarely there is vocal cord paresis. Several authors have noted hypotelorism in affected members of the families. A more indolent lumbosacral plexus neuropathy, with preceding buttock pain and eventual spontaneous recovery was reported in two children in South Africa (Thomson 1993).

Amyotrophy following asthma ('post-asthmatic pseudo-poliomyelitis') was first described by Hopkins (1974) in a series of 10 cases. Three more were reported by Danta (1975) and Ilett et al (1977). Acute paralysis, preceded in most cases by pain, occurred four to ten days after an acute asthmatic attack. The weakness resolved slowly and very incompletely. In several of Hopkins' patients the leg was affected, a situation which is very rare in neuralgic amyotrophy if, indeed, it ever occurs. In Hopkins' series, CSF pleocytosis was the rule, often with a raised protein level, but in one of the patients of Ilett et al (1977) the CSF was normal. Shahar et al (1991) reviewed 22 similar cases aged between 13 months and 11 years, all with permanent, usually monoplegic, paralysis. There seemed to be no consistent relationship to any of the drugs given for the asthma, or to any particular virus infection.

The quite separate acute *myopathy* which may follow status asthmaticus appears to be drug-induced (Waclawik et al 1992).

Fluctuating and intermittent muscular weakness

In addition to the periodic paralyses there are several disorders in which muscular weakness varies from time to time.

Repeated episodes of temporary paralysis occur also in mitochondrial myopathy as Shy et al (1966) pointed out nearly 30 years ago. Recurrent subacute attacks of muscular weakness, especially if they follow physical stress and are associated with nausea or vomiting, should arouse suspicion of a disorder of fatty-acid metabolism or mitochondrial myopathy. The discrete episodes of focal neuropathic paralysis in familial brachial neuritis have been mentioned and families have been reported in which recurrent pressure palsies occur against a background of a permanent subclinical generalised peripheral neuropathy (Madrid & Bradley 1975). The acute attacks may be steroid-responsive (Barisic et al 1990). Chronic relapsing inflammatory polyneuropathy is a sporadic disorder in which recurrent episodes of severe demyelinating motor and sensory neuropathy occur and lead to permanent weakness. It is important to recognise this because of the good response to steroids in most cases. The CSF protein is increased and oligoclonal bands are present. Attacks may start in childhood and the disorder has occurred in early infancy (Pasternak et al 1982). There is an association with certain HLA haplotypes (Thomas 1979).

The fluctuating weakness and fatigability which occur in myasthenia gravis are rarely mimicked by any other disorder. A degree of fluctuation over a longer time-scale is often seen in the myopathy of carnitine deficiency and has been reported in reducing-body myopathy. A striking sense of fatigue which seems out of proportion to the muscular weakness is a feature of some of the mitochondrial myopathies, but it is not possible to induce true loss of power by repeated muscle contraction in these cases. The degree of weakness in the mitochondrial myopathies may also vary from time to time, but not to a great degree. A sense of fatigue without demonstrable weakness or physiological fatigue (Barnes et al 1993) is seen in the 'chronic fatigue syndrome' which is not infrequent in adolescence (Smith et al 1991). Rarely one encounters cases of apparent congenital myopathy in which slow fluctuation in symptoms is a prominent feature and some of these cases are unrecognised examples of genetic disorders of neuromuscular transmission (pp 798–800).

Progressive muscular weakness

The rate at which muscular weakness develops and progresses is of vital importance both in diagnosis and prognosis. Table 21.1 gives an indication of the rate of progression of the most important neuromuscular disorders which may be considered in differential diagnosis at various periods of childhood. This approach has its limitations, however, because the rate of progression may vary from case to case, may change during the course of the illness and in any case may be difficult to gauge in the early stages.

Other valuable clues to diagnosis include the degree of muscle atrophy in relation to the weak-

Table 21.1   Progressive muscular weakness

Apparent rate of progression at time of presentation	Onset			
	First 6 months	First 2 years	2–10 years	Adolescence
Progressive over hours or days	Myasthenia disease Werdnig–Hoffmann disease Spinal tumour Metabolic acidoses Cytochrome oxidase deficiency Carnitine deficiency (Chronic SMA) (Poliomyelitis) (Rhabdomyolysis) (Botulism)	Poliomyelitis Myasthenia gravis Chronic SMA Hyperkalaemic P.P. Rhabdomyolysis (Guillain–Barré) Organicacidaemia Leigh's disease Mitochondrial myopathies	Poliomyelitis Guillain–Barré syndrome Hyperkalaemic P.P. Hypokalaemic P.P. Myasthenia gravis Rhabdomyolysis Acute myositis Mitochondrial myopathies CPT deficiency Other lipid myopathies	Poliomyelitis Guillain–Barré syndrome All 3 periodic paralyses Myasthenia gravis Acute myositis
Weeks or months	Werdnig–Hoffmann disease Pompe's disease Mitochondrial myopathy Nemaline myopathy Centronuclear myopathy Leigh's disease Congenital polyneuropathy Metabolic myopathies	Chronic SMA Dermatomyositis Myasthenia Carnitine disorders Leigh's disease Metabolic myopathies	Dermatomyositis Chronic SMA Kearns–Sayre syndrome Lipid storage myopathies Myasthenia gravis Metabolic myopathies (Refsum's disease)	Myasthenia Polymyositis Lipid storage myopathies Metabolic myopathies (MLD neuropathy) (Dermatomyositis) (Refsum's disease)
Years	Chronic SMA Nemaline myopathy Centronuclear myopathy Rarely FSH MD Mitochondrial myopathy HMSN type III Hypothyroidism Congenital MD	Duchenne MD Autosomal recessive MD Rarely polymyositis Chronic SMA Glycogen storage disease Kearns–Sayre syndrome Lipid storage myopathies Other mitochondrial myopathies Myasthenic myopathies Distal MD & SMA Fukuyama MD Centronuclear myopathy	Duchenne MD Becker MD Emery–Dreifuss MD Autosomal recessive MD Chronic SMA Scapuloperoneal SMA Kearns–Sayre syndrome Glycogen storage disease Lipid storage myopathies Mitochondrial myopathies HMSN I and II (Polymyositis)	Becker MD Emery–Dreifuss MD FSH MD Chronic SMA Glycogen storage disease Lipid storage myopathies HMSN I and II Myotonic MD Desmin myopathy
Static or progressive over decades	Chronic SMA Central core disease Minicore disease Fibre-type disproportion Congenital myotonic MD Duchenne MD Congenital MD Fingerprint myopathy	Duchenne MD Autosomal recessive MD Fingerprint myopathy Central core disease	Duchenne MD Autosomal recessive MD Myotonic MD Becker MD Emery–Dreifuss MD (Central core disease)	Becker MD Myotonic MD FSH MD Manifesting female DMD carriers

ness, the broad pattern of distribution of the weakness (whether proximal, distal or generalised), whether the weakness within this broad pattern is highly selective for particular muscles or not, whether the face and other cranial muscles are involved, the presence or absence of fasciculation, fatigability, reflex changes or symptoms and signs of involvement of other tissues, the degree of abnormality in serum CK activity and in other enzymes, and the findings in the EMG and muscle biopsy. Many of these points are discussed in Chapter 13, and here we confine discussion of the progressive disorders to a few comments upon some of the most important conditions.

Duchenne muscular dystrophy. The diagnosis is easy to confirm (Ch. 14). The problem is to remember to consider it when a child presents with the early symptoms. It is not uncommonly overlooked until after another affected child has been born in the family. The earliest sign in most cases is delay in walking (50% walk only after the age of 18 months). General psychomotor delay is quite frequent and speech may be immature. At first the gait disturbance is easier to recognise when the patient tries to run or to climb stairs. From an early age, boys with this condition are unable to jump with both feet together and they roll on to their faces before standing up from the floor. The full 'Gowers' manoeuvre' of climbing up the legs is not apparent until the age of 4–6 years. A few are hypotonic during the first few months of life. Unexplained developmental delay in any young boy warrants an estimation of his serum CK activity. Although the very high serum CK levels, present from birth, indicate that active destruction of muscle occurs from the beginning, clinical evidence of progression may not be apparent until the age of 4–7 years.

Spinal muscular atrophy (SMA). After Duchenne muscular dystrophy, SMA is by far the commonest neuromuscular disorder in childhood. The nosology of the spinal muscular atrophies is complex. They vary greatly in age at onset, rate of progression and distribution of weakness, and attempts to classify them on these grounds have often proved to be genetically invalid (see Chs 24, 26), while purely genetic classifications lead to a state of apparent clinical confusion. The following list of apparent genetic entities, modified from

Pearn (1980), in no sense comprises a nosological classification because the criteria for inclusion in the categories are so mixed, but it does provide a basis for a brief discussion of the diagnosis and management in childhood. More detail will be found in Chapter 24.

Autosomal recessive
(1) Progressive infantile spinal muscular atrophy ('Acute Werdnig–Hoffmann disease') McK 253300
(2) Chronic childhood SMA (proximal or generalised) including the phenotypes 'Arrested Werdnig–Hoffmann disease', 'Intermediate SMA' 'Kugelberg–Welander syndrome' McK 253550 and 253400
(3) Infantile SMA with initial diaphragmatic paralysis
(4) Infantile SMA with cerebellar hypoplasia
(5) Adult-onset SMA (proximal) McK 271150
(6) Distal SMA (infantile onset) McK 271120
(7) Bulbar SMA (Fazio-Londe disease) McK 211500
(8) SMA in hexosaminidase deficiency McK 272800 and 268800

Autosomal dominant
(9) Autosomal dominant scapuloperoneal SMA McK 181400
(10) Distal SMA (juvenile onset) McK 182960
(11) Distal, with vocal cord paresis McK 158580
(12) ? Facioscapulohumeral SMA (a doubtful entity) McK 182970
(13) Other autosomal dominant SMAs (adult onset) McK 182980, 158580 and 158590

X-linked
(14) X-linked bulbar/distal SMA McK 313200 (adult onset)

Most cases fall into one of the first two categories. Progressive infantile SMA may present at any time in the first five months of life and is best distinguished from the chronic cases, not by the age at onset which may be evident from diminished fetal movement as early as the thirty-fifth week of gestation in both acute and chronic cases, but by its relentlessly progressive course. It is therefore prudent to wait for clear evidence of deterioration before offering a firm prognosis when the clinical picture of severe paralytic hypotonia, areflexia and fasciculation of the tongue makes the diagnosis of infantile SMA obvious. Muscle biopsy appears not to be of help in distinguishing progressive from non-progressive cases. Other conditions which may present a very similar clinical picture are congenital peripheral neuropathy of the type reported by Lyon (1969), described below, and perhaps infantile botulism.

At least two other distinct genetic forms of acute infantile spinal muscular atrophy have been described. In one the infants present with diaphragmatic paralysis within the first few months of life, and may only later develop limb paralysis (Mellins et al 1974, McWilliam et al 1985, Murphy et al 1985, Schapira & Swash 1985). This situation contrasts with the usual relative preservation of the phrenic motor neurones in Werdnig–Hoffmann disease (Kuzuhara & Chou 1981). A comparable variant, in which predominant weakness of the anterior and posterior neck muscles is the presenting feature, was described by Goutières et al (1991), and presentation with vocal cord paresis has been reported (Roulet & Deonna 1992). Infantile spinal muscular atrophy of fetal onset with multiple bone fractures is another proposed entity, but the available evidence is not yet convincing (Borochowitz et al 1991, Garcia-Alix et al 1992). In the other distinct form, neuropathological examination reveals hypoplasia of the cerebellum and ventral pons, and sometimes of the thalamus, as well as anterior horn cell degeneration. Some cases have more widespread degenerative change in grey and white matter. During life, both the motor and sensory nerve conduction velocities are very slow. Such children are usually already severely hypotonic at birth and may be less socially responsive than children with typical Werdnig–Hoffmann disease (Norman 1961, Weinberg & Kirkpatrick 1975, Goutières et al 1977, Steiman et al 1980, de Leon et al 1984). Dubowitz & Davies (1993) ruled out chromosome 5q-linkage in one affected sibship, thus showing that this disorder is genetically distinct from SMA type I.

The discovery of apparent vitamin E deficiency in Werdnig–Hoffmann disease has, unfortunately, not been shown to have any aetiological or therapeutic relevance (Shapira et al 1981).

The term *chronic childhood SMA* embraces cases of Kugelberg–Welander syndrome (type III SMA) and of the intermediate or type II variety (Emery 1971). Although the gene for these chronic forms and for type I SMA has been shown to be identical, and localised at 5q13, they remain clinically distinct in prognosis and management. Chronic SMA covers a wide range of cases in which the onset may be as early as fetal life or as late at least as the end of the first decade, and the severity may vary equally widely. The fact that such variation may occur within a single family confirms that only one genetic entity is involved but undoubtedly the severely affected infant who never learns to sit unsupported and who survives in a helpless condition with major contractures and spinal deformity for anything from a few months to three or more decades presents a very different problem in clinical management from the previously normal 5-year-old who begins to develop a waddling gait. It is also characteristic of chronic SMA that it may progress irregularly, intermittently or not at all, and it is therefore exceptionally difficult to give an accurate prognosis in an individual case, even after a considerable period of observation. A few cases present with the sudden development of weakness over a matter of hours or days, usually in association with an infection or immunisation, and with subsequently a relatively static or chronic course. The Kugelberg–Welander syndrome resembles the muscular dystrophies (and very few other neuromuscular disorders) in causing strikingly selective muscular weakness. It differs in causing no recognisable pattern of selection and in often being asymmetrical. Fasciculation, so helpful in diagnosis when present, may be absent or inconspicuous in as many as 50% of cases. The feet tend to evert rather than adopting the equinovarus position seen in Duchenne muscular dystrophy. The serum CK may be normal or slightly increased. Where it is considerably elevated it should alert the clinician to the possibility of mistaken diagnosis. Many apparent SMAs (e.g. the autosomal dominant facioscapulohumeral, the X-linked scapuloperoneal and the X-linked with large calves) are now regarded as 'pseudo-neurogenic' cases of muscular dystrophy of, respectively, the FSH, Emery–Dreifuss and Becker types. Even the EMG, so valuable in cooperative adult patients, may be confusing or quite often even normal in children if they are unable to maintain a strong volitional contraction of the needled muscle. It is therefore particularly important to select an appropriate and moderately severely affected muscle for biopsy in trying to reach a definitive diagnosis. It is difficult to assess the power of individual muscles in an unco-operative or obese child; careful palpation of the degree of atrophy will often be helpful in diagnosis and in choosing a muscle for biopsy. When the choice is difficult, visualising the muscles by ultrasound or even CT scanning may be helpful.

Investigation of the cause of SMA is almost always disappointing. A few cases of juvenile SMA (with onset at 5–16 years) have been found to have hexosaminidase A deficiency. Some of them, but not all, had additional features such as dysarthria, ataxia, pyramidal signs, mild dementia or episodic psychosis (Johnson et al 1982, Mitsumoto et al 1985, Parnes et al 1985).

A number of restricted non-progressive forms of congenital anterior horn cell disease exist, probably not of genetic origin and probably akin to neurogenic arthrogryposis multiplex (q.v.). Often only the lower limbs are affected, but cases in which amyotrophy is confined to the upper limbs are also described (Darwish et al 1981). Segmental upper limb *progressive* amyotrophy of the type seen in young adults, especially in the Far East, may also occur in children and may be autosomal recessive in inheritance (Sobue et al 1978, Gucuyener et al 1991, Liu & Specht 1993). In Liu's cases the lower limbs were eventually affected.

Rapidly fatal forms of juvenile anterior horn cell disease include the bulbar (Fazio–Londe) type (q.v.) and juvenile motor neurone disease (Nelson & Prensky 1972), both mercifully rare.

The principles of management of spinal muscular atrophy follow in many respects those laid down for Duchenne muscular dystrophy in Chapters 14, 22 and 23. Active orthopaedic measures to deal with contractures and spinal deformity are, however, even more important because of the possibility of prolonged arrest of progression of the disease and because thoracic distortion due to kyphoscoliosis presents one of the major hazards to life by contributing to respiratory insufficiency. Rigid spinal braces applied to very late and advanced cases of spinal curvature may actually make the respiratory function worse (Noble-Jamieson et al 1986). Active spinal bracing as soon as a hypotonic child begins to sit up is therefore usually the best policy, but spinal fusion during adolescence is often necessary. It must be expertly performed after very careful assessment of respiratory function (Aprin et al 1982, Riddick et al 1982). Active and intensive postoperative care, including active exercise of limb muscles, is a vital component of this type of management. The provision of lightweight walking calipers is useful in some cases and is worth trying in very young children (from 2 years of age) if they have strong enough trunk muscles (Granata et al 1987).

Other progressive myopathies. The other important conditions to consider in a progressive muscular disorder in childhood include dermatomyositis or, much less commonly, pure polymyositis (see Ch. 16), glycogen storage disease (especially the juvenile forms of acid maltase deficiency and debrancher enzyme deficiency), lipid storage diseases, mitochondrial myopathy, nemaline myopathy, centronuclear myopathy, the Becker, autosomal recessive and facioscapulohumeral types of muscular dystrophy, myotonic dystrophy and the myopathies associated with renal failure, metabolic bone disease, malabsorption, chronic cholestasis, hypothyroidism, Cushing's syndrome (and steroid therapy), some of the genetically-determined myasthenias and the various peripheral neuropathies. Some of the myopathies may mimic muscular dystrophy, especially dermatomyositis, lipid storage myopathy, acid maltase and debrancher enzyme deficiency and sometimes the myopathy of metabolic bone disease — a point of great importance because several of these disorders are potentially treatable. The myopathy associated with vitamin E deficiency in chronic cholestasis is also treatable with high doses of the vitamin (Guggenheim et al 1982). Vitamin E deficiency is seen also as a consequence of the malabsorption in a-β-lipoproteinaemia, and was reported by Burck et al (1981) in a child with an autosomal recessive neuromyopathy and ataxia. Further discussion of these important disorders of childhood will be found elsewhere in this volume.

Skeletal myopathy and cardiomyopathy.

Cardiomyopathy is a constant feature of Pompe's disease and a frequent one of certain types of lipid storage myopathy, particularly disorders of carnitine metabolism, and mitochondrial myopathy in childhood (see Ch. 18). Other rare metabolic myopathies with cardiac involvement in childhood include β-galactosidase deficiency (Kohlschutter et al 1982) and a polysaccharide storage disease described by Karpati et al (1969). An inherited myopathy (possibly X-linked dominant), in which mental retardation and cardiomyopathy are associated with a skeletal myopathy with autophagic vacuoles, was reviewed by Hart et al (1987). The onset varied from 2 to 19 years in males and the serum CK level was high. Heart block is a frequent component of the Kearns–Sayre syndrome, and may be seen in various other mitochondrial myopathies in childhood. It is a rare feature in children with myotonic dystrophy although the ECG is frequently abnormal (Morgenlander et al 1993). Cardiac involvement is an important feature but usually a late feature in Duchenne, Becker and especially Emery–Dreifuss muscular dystrophy and the Eichsfeld type of congenital muscular dystrophy (q.v. Ch. 14), and has been described as a late feature in nemaline myopathy, minicore disease (see p. 783) and centronuclear myopathy (Verhiest et al 1976). All of these possibilities must be considered when a child presents with combined skeletal and cardiac myopathy. The familial occurrence of cardiomyopathy with necrotising vacuolar skeletal myopathy, cataracts and atrophy of the corpus callosum (due to abnormal axonal development) was described by Lyon et al (1990). Severe hypotonia and cerebral atrophy developed in the first 3 months of life and survival varied from 5 to 16 months. A cardiomyopathy followed by progressive skeletal myopathy is characteristic of the myopathy with subsarcolemmal accumulation of desmin intermediate filament proteins (Vajsar et al 1993). A peripheral neuropathy with giant axons containing abundant neurofilaments, but without the other clinical features of 'giant axonal neuropathy' is found in at least some such cases (Sabatelli et al 1992).

However, it is not unusual to encounter children with this combination of features in whom no satisfactory diagnosis emerges on investigation — or even at post-mortem examination — for such children usually have only moderate skeletal muscle weakness while their cardiomyopathy may progress relentlessly. Only a few such cases appear in the literature (e.g. Fried et al 1979, Dubowitz 1985), (pp 623–633) but the author has seen four cases, all with a fatal outcome. The muscles are strikingly hypotonic, muscle biopsy has revealed type II fibre atrophy or no significant abnormality and the cardiac pathology has been a cardiomyopathy with or without associated endocardial fibroelastosis. A boy aged 18 years (case 11) reported by Shafiq et al (1972), who had cardiomyopathy and mild myopathy with type I fibre atrophy, in retrospect seems to have had the clinical features of Emery–Dreifuss muscular dystrophy. Lenard & Goebel (1980) did muscle biopsies in 10 children with cardiomyopathy but with clinically normal skeletal muscle and found type II fibre atrophy in four of them. The X-linked mitochondrial disorder described by Barth et al (1983) has a similar cardiac presentation, in infancy, but with additional problems due to neutropenia, and subclinical or mild skeletal myopathy.

Myopathy and bone disorders.

A number of genetically determined bone dysplasias may cause a pseudomyopathic waddling gait because of involvement of the hips or spine. In at least one condition, however, progressive diaphyseal dysplasia (Camurato-Engelmann disease), striking muscular atrophy and weakness appears to be an integral feature of the pathology (Sparkes & Graham 1972, Naveh et al 1985) and muscle pain and fatigue are prominent symptoms. X-rays show thickening and hyperostosis of the diaphyses of the long bones; growth is not affected.

In childhood, as in adult life, chronic osteomalacia in nutritional or renal disorders may be associated with a reversible myopathy. Coeliac disease has been described as presenting with a dystrophy-like progressive myopathy (Hardoff et al 1980).

Both bone and muscle may be involved in thalassaemia major. Logothetis et al (1972) found myopathic features in one-fifth of their 138 cases and muscle atrophy in one-third. Those with myopathy tended to be of shorter stature with more bone complications than those without.

Facial, bulbar and external ocular muscle weakness in infancy

Traumatic unilateral *facial weakness* is not uncommon in the newborn and usually disappears in a few days or weeks. Persistent congenital paralysis is much rarer, and may reflect nuclear agenesis.

Bell's palsy occurs in young children and may be associated with acute viral infections or occasionally with arterial hypertension. Recurrent attacks, especially if bilateral, raise the possibility of Melkersson's syndrome or very rarely sarcoidosis (Jasper & Denny 1968). The silent development of facial weakness, first on one side and then on the other, occurs especially in meningeal leukaemia or pontine glioma. Subacute progression of facial and other cranial nerve palsies may occur in the tick-borne infection Lyme disease, which responds to treatment with penicillin.

Bilateral facial weakness in the newborn may result from bilateral nuclear agenesis (Moebius syndrome) when it is usually accompanied by bilateral lateral rectus palsies and sometimes by bulbar paresis and mild amyotrophy of the limbs. A few patients are also mentally handicapped. In the most typical form, primary skeletal defects (syndactyly, short or absent fingers) are often a feature and such cases are almost always sporadic. The association with arthrogryposis is a risk factor for autosomal dominant transmission, as is a chromosome deletion or translocation at 13q12–13 (Ziter et al 1977, Slee et al 1991). Recurrence in sibs is a risk where skeletal defects or rectus palsies are absent, or deafness, more extensive ophthalmoplegia or finger contractures are present. The nosology and genetics are reviewed by MacDermot et al (1991), Kumar (1990) and McKusick (1992). A rare association of Moebius syndrome with the Poland anomaly (unilateral absence of the pectoralis major muscle) has also been established (Parker et al 1981). In an apparently distinct disorder the features of Moebius syndrome are associated with hypogonadotrophic hypogonadism and a late-onset progressive neuropathy (Abid et al 1978, Kawai et al 1990).

Several of the congenital myopathies may produce prominent facial weakness, especially centronuclear myopathy, nemaline myopathy, minicore disease and less often mitochondrial myopathy, carnitine deficiency, central core disease and fibre-type disproportion. Myasthenia gravis must be ruled out. Congenital myotonic dystrophy causes very prominent facial diplegia with a triangular open mouth together with hypotonia and feeding difficulties, and an infantile form of facioscapulohumeral dystrophy exists in which difficulty in closing the mouth to suck or inability to smile or to close the eyes may be a first symptom. In both of these diseases, examination of the parents gives the essential clue to the diagnosis. Infantile SMA (Werdnig–Hoffmann disease) may affect the face, but rarely profoundly. In Fazio–Londe disease (Gomez et al 1962) progressive bulbar paralysis may be accompanied by facial weakness and eventually by paralysis of all the cranial muscles, including those of the eyes. Some cases, but not all, also have signs of limb muscle weakness. In the similar but more slowly progressive Brown–Vialetto–van Laere syndrome there is also sensorineural deafness (Gallai et al 1981, Hawkins et al 1990). Cranial polyneuritis, meningeal lymphoma or leukaemia and pontine glioma must be excluded before either of these rare diseases can justifiably be diagnosed.

Apart from rare congenital or post-infectious lesions, isolated paralyses affecting the *Xth and XIIth cranial nerves* are uncommon. A unilateral XIIth nerve lesion may be seen in the Arnold–Chiari malformation. Bulbar paralysis may occur in meningeal and medullary neoplasm. Bulbar paralysis in the neonate, in association with more generalised hypotonia or paralysis, suggests myasthenia, Werdnig–Hoffmann disease or congenital myotonic dystrophy, but may also occur in nemaline and centronuclear myopathy, the fibre-type disproportion Moebius syndrome and the Prader–Willi syndrome. Later in childhood, bulbar paralysis as an important feature of a generalised muscular problem should bring to mind myasthenia, botulism or the Guillain–Barré syndrome or, if the pace is slower, dermatomyositis, myotonic dystrophy, nemaline myopathy or centronuclear myopathy.

External ocular palsies are not uncommon in the newborn period, and must be distinguished from the Duane syndrome and from more extensive external ophthalmoplegia. The congenital neuromuscular disorders most often associated with external ophthalmoplegia are myasthenia, centronuclear myopathy and the Moebius syndrome; but it may occur in minicore disease. The later development of ophthalmoplegia may be seen in the same disorders but is also a major feature of the Kearns–Sayre syndrome and very occasionally of other variants of mitochondrial myopathy and of Fazio–Londe disease. None of these should be diagnosed until the possibility of a brain stem lesion or of myasthenia gravis has been considered.

Peripheral motor neuropathy

The distinction between a predominantly motor neuropathy in a child and the very similar distal form of SMA and, even rarer, the distal type of muscular dystrophy, can really be made only on the basis of electrophysiological and histological investigations. The distal forms of spinal muscular atrophy seen in children are the autosomal recessive type and the autosomal dominant form with vocal cord paresis (Young & Harper 1980, Pridmore et al 1992). Some cases of mitochondrial myopathy also present with distal weakness and, in the facioscapulohumeral and scapuloperoneal sydromes, the distal lower limb involvement may be sufficiently predominant in the early stages to cause confusion.

No attempt is made here to cover all the peripheral neuropathies of childhood and a systematic account will be found in Chapter 25. Nutritional deficiencies and diphtheria are now rare diseases in developed countries and so is acrodynia (pink disease), since the elimination of mercury from teething powders. Lead poisoning causes an encephalopathy rather than a polyneuropathy in childhood. Certain insecticides and drugs may produce peripheral neuropathy (Watters & Barlow 1967). This problem is mostly encountered during the treatment of children with malignant tumours with cytotoxic drugs, especially vincristine or cisplatin. Abuse of solvents such as hexane may cause a peripheral neuropathy. Otherwise in clinical practice the Guillain–Barré syndrome and Charcot–Marie–Tooth disease (hereditary motor and sensory neuropathy type I–HMSN I) are seen far more frequently than other types. The former has been mentioned above in relation to acute muscular weakness.

HMSN I. 'Peroneal muscular atrophy' often begins in childhood and in some cases as early as the first year of life. The foot deformity usually causes more disability than the weakness itself at first, and responds well to orthopaedic treatment. Weakness of the hands may become a serious problem during the school years. The CSF protein content may be increased though less frequently than in HMSN III (Hagberg & Lyon 1981). Diagnosis is straightforward on the basis of profound slowing of nerve conduction. It is a common experience to find subclinical involvement in one of the parents and it is important to seek this by clinical and, if necessary, neurophysiological examination for genetic counselling purposes. Nerve conduction velocities are abnormal from the first year of life (Feasby et al 1992) but preclinical diagnosis is of little practical use. There are two genotypes mapping to chromosomes 17p11.2 and 1q23–25 respectively.

HMSN II. The axonal form of 'peroneal muscular atrophy' is also seen in childhood but much less frequently. Both sporadic cases (possibly recessive) and, more often, families with dominant inheritance occur. The onset is usually a little later than in HMSN I, but the clinical problems are similar.

HMSN III. Dejerine–Sottas disease is a rare but very disabling demyelinating neuropathy, usually producing symptoms in the first two years of life, rarely later. Hypertrophic nerves (also seen in HMSN I), a high CSF protein, and early ataxia and severe weakness and deformity are the helpful diagnostic features. Scoliosis is common. Inheritance is autosomal recessive though McKusick (1992) demurs. The milder form of 'autosomal recessive form of HMSN I' may be a separate disorder (Vance 1991).

Giant axonal neuropathy. Cases of this rare disorder were first described by Asbury et al (1972) and Carpenter et al (1974). Tandan et al (1987) reviewed 22 reported cases. A progressive peripheral motor and sensory neuropathy of axonal type begins at the age of 2–3 years and progresses to become severe within a few years. Children in these reports were intelligent and like all subsequently reported cases they had abnormal tightly curled hair which is often blond. The stance is memorable with the knees close together, the legs splayed rather widely and the medial arches of the feet very flat. Later case reports have mentioned various additional features including ataxia, learning disorders and sexual precocity, and in some cases the neuropathy has taken a much slower course (Ionasescu et al 1983). In some patients central nervous system dysfunction, particularly of the cerebellum, predominates (Stollhoff et al 1991, Lampl et al 1992). Nerve biopsy shows remarkable segmental enlargement of axons, distended with neurofilaments. Abnormal cytoplasmic filaments may possibly also be found in other intraneural cells including fibroblasts and endothelial cells. Affected sibs have been recorded and consanguinity is a frequent factor (Takebe et al 1981, Tandan et al 1987).

Congenital peripheral neuropathies. Charcot–Marie–Tooth disease (HMSN I) may present at birth in rare instances (Vanasse & Dubowitz 1979, Hagberg & Lyon 1981). One type of congenital peripheral neuropathy resembles Werdnig–Hoffmann disease in presenting with severe hypotonia and areflexia in early infancy, but with profound slowing of nerve conduction, a raised CSF protein level (usually) and, in the peripheral nerve, virtually total absence of myelin sheaths and hypertrophic reduplication of the basement membrane (Lyon 1969, Anderson et al 1973, Kasman & Bernstein 1974, Karch & Urich 1975, Goebel et al 1976, Kennedy et al 1977, and others reviewed by Harati & Butler 1985, Balestrini et al 1991). Both parents of one child had slight slowing of nerve conduction (Kennedy et al 1977). Joosten et al (1974) described two sibs aged 12 and 14 years in whom the symptoms had started in the second or third year of life and had progressed much more in one than the other, but whose nerve pathology was similar to that in the Lyon type. This disorder may be fatal in infancy but most of the cases described have survived at least into their second decade.

A much milder form of congenital peripheral neuropathy was described by Yuill & Lynch (1974) and was inherited as a dominant trait, but there was no information about histology and in only one case were nerve conduction studies performed.

Other genetically determined peripheral neuropathies seen in childhood include Refsum disease, por-phyria, and several others in which the clinical features of the neuropathy are largely sensory rather than motor (including Friedreich's ataxia, Fabry disease, Tangier disease, a-β-lipoproteinaemia and the various disorders classified as hereditary sensory neuropathies). A clinically overt peripheral neuropathy may also occur in some of the progressive degenerative disorders of the central nervous system, particularly in metachromatic leucodystrophy, infantile neuroaxonal dystrophy and the Cockayne syndrome, while a subclinical neuropathy, of no significance to the patient but helpful in diagnosis, may be found by nerve conduction studies in Krabbe (globoid cell) leucodystrophy (Moosa 1971) and in Canavan disease.

In the typical infantile form of metachromatic leucodystrophy, deterioration of gait and speech begin at about the age of 1 year and progress over several months to a state of severe retardation with a spastic tetraparesis, optic atrophy and severe distal muscle wasting. The tendon reflexes are diminished soon after the onset. In some cases the disorder presents later, usually with cerebral symptoms but occasionally with a pure progressive demyelinating peripheral neuropathy (Yudell et al 1967). In all forms of the disease the CSF protein level is raised, metachromatic staining may be seen in the nerve biopsy and the underlying deficiency or abnormality of the enzyme aryl-sulphatase A may be demonstrated in white blood cells.

In infantile neuroaxonal dystrophy, progressive mental retardation and optic atrophy in the first year of life are sometimes associated with severe hypotonia and muscle paralysis resembling that of SMA (Huttenlocher & Gilles 1967). The diagnosis is difficult without a brain biopsy but can be achieved in at least some cases by the biopsy of muscle (Kimura & Sasaki 1988) or peripheral nerve or even by examination of the nerve twigs in skin (Özmen et al 1991) or a conjunctival biopsy (Arsenio-Nunes & Goutières 1978).

In Cockayne dwarfism, progressive growth failure and dementia starting in the first 5 years of life are associated with a characteristic light-sensitive rash, deep-set eyes and a peripheral neuropathy (Ohnishi et al 1987). Other features are intracranial calcification, leucodystrophy and a mild retinal pigmentary degeneration.

Cramps and abnormal muscle contraction

Cramp, although less frequent in childhood than in later life, is no better understood. Limb pains are a common stress symptom in children. Muscle rigidity and weakness in the newborn are an uncommon but long-established manifestation of congenital hypothyroidism (the Debré–Semelaigne syndrome) and acquired hypothyroidism later in childhood may also present with painful muscle cramps after exercise.

Of the overt muscle disorders, patients with the myotonic and, for some reason, the Becker type of muscular dystrophy are chiefly plagued by cramps. Stiffness on exertion, sometimes amounting to cramp, is a feature of the early stages of McArdle disease, phosphofructokinase deficiency, carnitine palmityl transferase deficiency and certain disorders of the cytochrome system. In persistent cases of exertional or postexertional cramp it is therefore appropriate to do an ischaemic lactate test and to measure the serum CK activity after exercise performed during a fast (see Ch. 18). The urine should also be examined for myoglobin. Similar symptoms, starting in childhood, may occur in muscle adenylate deaminase deficiency (Fishbein et al 1978, Kelemen et al 1982, Ashwal & Peckham 1985). The serum CK activity is often increased during attacks of pain. Painless stiffness of the muscles after exertion may also occur in a variant of central core disease (Bethlem et al 1966) and in a myopathy with subsarcolemmal tubular aggregates (Lazaro et al 1980). Brody (1969) described a single case in which muscle contracture induced by exercise appeared to result from a defect in a 'muscle relaxing factor' subsequently identified as calcium ATPase deficiency, possibly autosomal dominant in inheritance (Karpati et al 1986, Danon et al 1988).

Dystonia and tetany must be considered as possible causes of persistent cramping of muscle during activity. Rigidity, equal in degree to that seen in tetanus, has already been mentioned as one of the presentations of reducing-body myopathy (Dudley et al 1978) and of a myopathy with trilaminar fibres (Ringel et al 1978).

The myotonic disorders occurring in childhood are discussed in Chapter 15.

Myokymia with impaired muscular relaxation (also called 'neuromyotonia' and 'continuous muscle fibre activity') is a slowly progressive disorder, which usually begins between the ages of 15 and 25 years but may do so earlier, even in infancy, and gives rise to muscular stiffness and cramps (Isaacs 1961, Gardner-Medwin & Walton 1969). The distal muscles of the feet and hands are mainly affected, but disabling laryngeal spasm occurs in some cases; there may be associated hyperhidrosis. Claw-like deformities of the feet are common and close inspection of the muscles, especially the small hand muscles, reveals irregular undulating contractions which have been likened to a 'bag of worms'. Distal muscle atrophy is usual but secondary muscle hypertrophy may occur if the myokymia is very active. The EMG shows continuous motor unit activity at rest and the activity can be blocked by curare but not by peripheral nerve blockade. Some cases show evidence of a mild peripheral neuropathy; it is not certain whether this is a secondary phenomenon. Almost all cases are sporadic but dominant inheritance has been described (McGuire et al 1984). The condition usually responds to treatment with carbamazepine or, less certainly, phenytoin (also see Ch. 20). Similar activity occurs in chondrodystrophic myotonia (see Ch. 15).

Myoglobinuria

Children, like adults, may develop myoglobinuria as a result of crush injury or intoxication (see Chs 13, 28). Acute rhabdomyolysis after abuse of the drug methylenedioxymethamphetamine ('ecstasy') perhaps merits special mention in this chapter (Henry et al 1992).

Paroxysmal myoglobinuria occurring after exertion is a rare phenomenon in childhood. Tein et al (1990) found only 26 such cases (with the onset of myoglobinuria before the age of 16 years) in a review of the literature from 1910 to 1988 and added 10 of their own. The great majority were boys. McArdle's disease, although causing stiffness on exertion in some cases during the first decade of life (Williams & Hosking 1985), hardly ever causes myoglobinuria at such an early stage. Deficiency of phosphofructokinase or phosphoglycerate mutase or, even more rarely, of one of several other glycolytic enzymes may do so (Tein et al 1990). Carnitine palmityl transferase deficiency not uncommonly first presents with myoglobinuria in childhood, the mean age in Tein's selected review series was 10 years. Fasting combined with exercise is an important precipitant in CPT deficiency. A few cases occur in which these clinical symptoms in childhood are associated with no detectable evidence of glycogen- or lipid-storage myopathy and, no doubt, other comparable metabolic disorders remain to be discovered.

Paroxysmal myoglobinuria occurring without exertion is a much more devastating illness in which large amounts of muscle undergo acute necrosis (rhabdomyolysis). It typically affects children under 5 years of age and may occur as early as the first few months of life. Acute muscle weakness with respiratory and, less often, cardiac failure may be complicated further by renal failure as a result of heavy myoglobinuria, and by high serum levels of calcium and potassium. Serum CK levels may reach 20 000–100 000 units. The mortality is high but children who survive generally make a full recovery. Recurrent attacks may affect several sibs in a family (Bowden et al 1956, Favara et al 1967, Savage et al 1971, Ramesh & Gardner-Medwin 1992). The pathogenesis is unknown and to label such cases as 'toxic' is unhelpful. Some of these cases have CPT deficiency or various acyl CoA dehydrogenase deficiencies (Vici et al 1991, Tein 1993). In others, attacks tend to follow viral infections; Coxsackie virus has been implicated in a few cases, and evidence may be found of a fulminating viral myositis (Fukuyama et al 1977). Cold has been suggested as another precipitant (Raifman et al 1978). Fasting may well be the common factor in the precipitating minor illnesses, and indeed one of my cases was plunged from perfect health into a life-threatening attack by a controlled overnight fast of only 16 hours, with a normal ketotic response. She and another case (both of whom had sibs who died

of the disease) have remained well for several years following advice to avoid fasting for more than 12 hours, and the use of IV glucose infusions to cover vomiting or anorexic illnesses, surgical operations, etc. (Ramesh & Gardner-Medwin 1992). In the face of this evidence it seems prudent initially to assume the danger of fasting in all cases of paroxysmal non-exertional myoglobinuria. However Tein et al (1990) and Tein (1993) reported fasting as only a minor factor in their large series and it seems likely that a number of different metabolic causes for this syndrome may await discovery. Adequate calorie intake, intensive respiratory care and often renal dialysis are vital in the emergency treatment of this dangerous disorder.

Malignant hyperpyrexia, like acute rhabdomyolysis, may cause sufficient myoglobinuria to induce uraemia in those patients who survive the initial emergency.

Rarely, recurrent myoglobinuria may accompany a progressive myopathy comparable to muscular dystrophy. Meyer–Betz (1910) described this situation in a boy of 13 years and Dubowitz (1978, p. 48) illustrates the case of a boy of seven years with cramps and myoglobinuria associated with a chronic 'dystrophic' myopathy.

Malignant hyperpyrexia. The incidence in children is high, one in 15 000 anaesthetics administered. Apart from the usual dominantly inherited syndrome of susceptibility, an association has been suggested with several conditions in childhood including central core disease (q.v.), Duchenne muscular dystrophy (q.v.), myotonia congenita, a family history of the sudden infant death syndrome (Denborough et al 1982) and a syndrome occurring in males of ptosis, low-set ears, hypoplasia of the mandible, thoracic kyphosis, short stature and cryptorchidism (King et al 1972). The associations with all of these except the first and the last are weak and such patients should not be denied anaesthesia; it is prudent, however, to avoid the use of halothane or suxamethonium.

REFERENCES

Abbing P J R, Hageman G, Willemse J 1985 CT-scanning of skeletal muscle in arthrogryposis multiplex congenita. Brain and Development 7: 484

Abid F, Hall R, Hudgson P, Weiser R 1978 Moebius syndrome, peripheral neuropathy and hypogonadotrophic hypogonadism. Journal of the Neurological Sciences 35: 309

Adams R D, Kakulas B A, Samaha F A 1965 A myopathy with cellular inclusions. Transactions of the American Neurological Association 90: 213

Afifi A K, Smith J W, Zellweger H 1965 Congenital non-progressive myopathy: central core disease and nemaline myopathy in one family. Neurology (Minneapolis) 15: 371

Aicardi J 1992 Diseases of the Nervous System in Childhood. Mac Keith Press, London

Airaksinen E M, Iivanainen M, Karli P, Sainio K, Haltia M 1985 Hereditary recurrent brachial plexus neuropathy with dysmorphic features. Acta Neurologica Scandinavica 71: 309

Albers J W, Faulkner J A, Dorovini-Zis K, Barald K F, Must R E, Ball R D 1984 Abnormal neuromuscular transmission in an infantile myasthenic syndrome. Annals of Neurology 16: 28

Anderson R M, Dennett X, Hopkins I J, Shield L K 1973 Hypertrophic interstitial polyneuropathy in infancy: clinical and pathologic features in two cases. Journal of Pediatrics 82: 619

Aprin H, Bowen J R, MacEwen G D, Hall J E 1982 Spine fusion in patients with spinal muscular atrophy. Journal of Bone and Joint Surgery 64A: 1179

Argov Z, Gardner-Medwin D, Johnson M A, Mastaglia F L 1984 Patterns of muscle fiber-type disproportion in hypotonic infants. Archives of Neurology 41: 53

Armstrong R M, Koenigsberger R, Mellinger J, Lovelace R E 1971 Central core disease with congenital hip dislocation: study of two families. Neurology (Minneapolis) 21: 369

Arsenio-Nunes M L, Goutières F 1978 Diagnosis of infantile neuroaxonal dystrophy by conjunctival biopsy. Journal of Neurology, Neurosurgery and Psychiatry 41: 511

Arts W F, Bethlem J, Dingemans K P, Eriksson A W 1978 Investigations on the inheritance of nemaline myopathy. Archives of Neurology 35: 72

Asbury A K, Gale M K, Cox S C, Baringer J R, Berg B O 1972 Giant axonal neuropathy — a unique case with segmental neurofilamentous masses. Acta Neuropathologica (Berlin) 20: 237

Ashwal S, Peckham N 1985 Myoadenylate deaminase deficiency in children. Pediatric Neurology 1: 185

Askanas V, Engel W K, Reddy N B et al 1979 X-linked recessive congenital muscle fiber hypotrophy with central nuclei: abnormalities of growth and adenylate cyclase in muscle tissue cultures. Archives of Neurology 36: 604

Aubourg P, Scotto J, Rocchiccioli F, Feldmann-Pautrat D, Robain O 1986 Neonatal adrenoleukodystrophy. Journal of Neurology, Neurosurgery and Psychiatry 49: 77

Bady B, Chauplannaz G, Carrier H 1987 Congenital Lambert–Eaton myasthenic syndrome. Journal of Neurology, Neurosurgery and Psychiatry 50: 476

Balestrini M R, Cavaletti G, D'Angelo A, Tredici G 1991. Infantile hereditary neuropathy with hypomyelination: report of two siblings with different expressivity. Neuropediatrics 22: 65

Banker B Q 1986a The congenital myopathies. In: Engel A G, Banker B Q (eds) Myology: basic and clinical. McGraw-Hill, New York, ch 51

Banker B Q 1986b Congenital deformities. In: Engel A G, Banker B Q (eds). Myology: basic and clinical. McGraw-Hill, New York, ch 73

Banker B Q, Victor M, Adams R D 1957 Arthrogryposis multiplex due to congenital muscular dystrophy. Brain 80: 319

Bargeton E, Nezelof C, Guran P, Job J-C 1961 Étude anatomique d'un cas d'arthrogrypose multiple congénitale et familiale. Revue Neurologique 104: 479

Baraitser M, Winter R M 1991 The London Neurogenetics Database. Oxford University Press, Oxford

Barisic N, Skarpa D, Jusic A, Jadro-Santel D 1990 Steroid responsive familial neuropathy with liability to pressure palsies. Neuropediatrics 21: 191

Barnes P R J, Taylor D J, Kemp G J, Radda G J 1993. Skeletal muscle bioenergetics in the chronic fatigue syndrome. Journal of Neurology, Neurosurgery and Psychiatry 56: 679

Barth P G, van Wijngaarden G K, Bethlem J 1975 X-linked myotubular myopathy with fatal neonatal asphyxia. Neurology (Minneapolis) 25: 531

Barth P G, Scholte J A, Berden J A et al 1983 An X-linked mitochondrial disease affecting cardiac muscle, skeletal muscle and neutrophil leucocytes. Journal of the Neurological Sciences 62: 327

Bates T 1955 Poliomyelitis in pregnancy, fetus and newborn. American Journal of Diseases of Children 90: 189

Beckerman R C, Buchino J J 1978 Arthrogryposis multiplex congenita as part of an inherited symptom complex: two case reports and a review of the literature. Pediatrics 61: 417

Bender A N, Bender M B 1977 Muscle fiber hypotrophy with intact neuromuscular junctions: a study of a patient with congenital neuromuscular disease and ophthalmoplegia. Neurology (Minneapolis) 27: 206

Benzing G, Iannacco S T, Bove K E, Keebler P J, Shockley L L 1990 Prolonged myasthenic syndrome after one week of muscle relaxants. Pediatric Neurology 6: 190

Bertini E, Ricci E, Boldrini R et al 1990 Involvement of respiratory muscles in cytoplasmic body myopathy — a pathological study. Brain and Development 12: 798

Besser M, Behar A 1967 Arthrogryposis accompanying congenital spinal-type muscular atrophy. Archives of Disease in Childhood 42: 666

Bethlem J, van Gool J, Hulsmann W C, Meijer A E F H 1966 Familial non-progressive myopathy with muscle cramps after exercise. A new disease associated with cores in the muscle fibres. Brain 89: 569

Bethlem J, Meijer A E F H, Schellens J P M, Vroom J J 1968 Centronuclear myopathy. European Neurology 1: 325

Bethlem J, van Wijngaarden G K, Meijer A E F H, Hulsmann W C 1969 Neuromuscular disease with type 1 fiber atrophy, central nuclei, and myotube-like structures. Neurology (Minneapolis) 19: 705

Bethlem J, van Wijngaarden G K, Mumenthaler M, Meijer A E F H 1970 Centronuclear myopathy with Type 1 fiber atrophy and 'myotubes'. Archives of Neurology 23: 70

Bethlem J, van Wijngaarden G K 1976 Benign myopathy, with autosomal dominant inheritance: a report on three pedigrees. Brain 99: 91

Bharucha E P, Pandya S S, Dastur D K 1972 Arthrogryposis multiplex congenita. Journal of Neurology, Neurosurgery and Psychiatry 35: 425

Bill P L A, Cole G, Proctor N S F 1979 Centronuclear myopathy. Journal of Neurology, Neurosurgery and Psychiatry 42: 548

Bjerre I, Hallberg A 1983 Myasthenia gravis: immunological studies in a young child treated with thymectomy and immunosuppressive drugs. Neuropediatrics 14: 106

Blass J P, Kark R A P, Engel W K 1971 Clinical studies of a patient with pyruvate decarboxylase deficiency. Archives of Neurology 25: 449

Bonnette H, Roelofs R, Olson W H 1974 Multicore disease: report of a case with onset in middle age. Neurology (Minneapolis) 24: 1039

Borochowitz Z, Glick B, Blazer S 1991 Infantile spinal muscular atrophy (SMA) and multiple congenital bone fractures in sibs: a lethal new syndrome. Journal of Medical Genetics 28: 345

Bowden D H, Fraser D, Jackson S H, Walker N F 1956 Acute recurrent rhabdomyolysis (paroxysmal myohaemoglobinuria): a report of 3 cases and a review of the literature. Medicine 35: 335

Bradley W G, Price D L, Watanabe C K 1970 Familial centronuclear myopathy. Journal of Neurology, Neurosurgery and Psychiatry 33: 687

Bradley W G, Hudgson P, Gardner-Medwin D, Walton J N 1973 The syndrome of myosclerosis. Journal of Neurology, Neurosurgery and Psychiatry 36: 651

Brandt S 1947 A case of arthrogryposis multiplex congenita. Acta Paediatrica 34: 365

Brody I A 1969 Muscle contracture induced by exercise: a syndrome attributable to decreased relaxing factor. New England Journal of Medicine 281: 187

Brooke M H 1973 Congenital fiber type disproportion. In: Kakulas B A (ed) Clinical studies in myology, part 2. Excerpta Medica, Amsterdam, p 147

Brooke M H 1977 A clinician's view of neuromuscular disease. Williams and Wilkins, Baltimore

Brooke M H, Engel W K 1969 The histographic analysis of human muscle biopsies with regard to fiber types: 4. Children's biopsies. Neurology (Minneapolis) 19: 591

Brooke M H, Neville H E 1972 Reducing body myopathy. Neurology (Minneapolis) 22: 829

Brooke M H, Carroll J E, Ringel S P 1979 Congenital hypotonia revisited. Muscle and Nerve 2: 84

Bruhn F W 1984 Lyme disease. American Journal of Diseases of Children 138: 467

Bruyland M, Liebaers I, Sacre L, Vandeplas Y, De Meirleir L, Martin J J 1984 Neonatal myotubular myopathy with a probable X-linked inheritance; observations on a new family with a review of the literature. Journal of Neurology 231: 220

Bryant G M, Davies K J, Newcombe R G 1979 Standardisation of the Denver developmental screening test for Cardiff children. Developmental Medicine and Child Neurology 21: 353

Buda F B, Rothney W B, Rabe E F 1972 Hypotonia and the maternal–child relationship. American Journal of Diseases of Children 124: 906

Bundey S 1972 A genetic study of infantile and juvenile myasthenia gravis. Journal of Neurology, Neurosurgery and Psychiatry 35: 41

Burck U, Goebel H H, Kuhlendahl H D, Meier C, Goebel K M 1981 Neuromyopathy and vitamin E deficiency in man. Neuropediatrics 12: 267

Buruma O J S, Bots G T A M, Went L N 1985 Familial hypokalemic periodic paralysis: 50-year follow-up of a large family. Archives of Neurology 42: 28

Byers P H, Holbrook K A, Barsh G S 1983 Ehlers–Danlos syndrome. In: Emery A E H, Rimoin D L (eds) Principles and practice of medical genetics. Churchill Livingstone, Edinburgh, ch 58

Byers R K 1975 Spinal-cord injuries during birth. Developmental Medicine and Child Neurology 17: 103

Campbell M J, Rebeiz J J, Walton J N 1969 Myotubular, centronuclear or pericentronuclear myopathy? Journal of the Neurological Sciences 8: 425

Cancilla P A, Kalyanaraman K, Verity M A, Munsat T, Pearson C M 1971 Familial myopathy with probable lysis of myofibrils in type 1 fibers. Neurology (Minneapolis) 21: 579

Carpenter S, Karpati G, Andermann F, Gold R 1974 Giant axonal neuropathy: A clinically and morphologically distinct neurological disease. Archives of Neurology 31: 312

Carpenter S, Karpati G, Holland P 1985 New observations in reducing body myopathy. Neurology 35: 818

Carpenter S, Karpati G, Holland P 1992 A chronic myopathy with coated vesicles and tubular masses. Neuromuscular Disorders 2: 209

Carr S R, Gilchrist J M, Abuelo D N, Clark D 1991 Treatment of antenatal myasthenia gravis. Obstetrics and Gynecology 78: 485

Cavanagh N P C 1980 The role of thymectomy in childhood myasthenia. Developmental Medicine and Child Neurology 22: 668

Chelmicka-Schorr E, Bernstein L P, Zurbrugg E B, Huttenlocher P R 1979 Eaton–Lambert syndrome in a 9-year-old girl. Archives of Neurology 36: 572

Chudley A E, Rozdilsky B, Houston C S, Becker L E, Knoll J H 1985 Multicore disease in sibs with severe mental retardation, short stature, facial anomalies, hypoplasia of the pituitary fossa, and hypogonadotrophic hypogonadism. American Journal of Medical Genetics 20: 145

Clarren S K, Hall J G 1983 Neuropathic findings in the spinal cords of 10 infants with arthrogryposis. Journal of the Neurological Sciences 58: 89

Cohen M E, Duffner P K, Heffner R 1978 Central core disease in one of identical twins. Journal of Neurology, Neurosurgery and Psychiatry 41: 659

Colamaria V, Zanetti R, Simeone M et al 1991 Minipolymyoclonus in congenital nemaline myopathy: a nonspecific clinical marker of neurogenic dysfunction. Brain and Development 13: 358

Coleman R F, Nienhuis A W, Brown W J, Munsat T L, Pearson C M 1967 New myopathy with mitochondrial enzyme hyperactivity. Journal of the American Medical Association 199: 624

Coleman R F, Thompson L R, Nienhuis A W, Munsat T L, Pearson C M 1968 Histochemical investigation of 'myotubular' myopathy. Archives of Pathology 86: 365

Conen P E, Murphy E G, Donohue W L 1963 Light and electron microscopic studies of 'myogranules' in a child with hypotonia and muscle weakness. Canadian Medical Association Journal 89: 983

Crothers B 1923 Injury of the spinal cord in breech extractions as an important cause of foetal death and paraplegia in childhood. American Journal of Medical Science 165: 94

Crothers B, Putnam M C 1927 Obstetrical injuries of the spinal cord. Medicine (Baltimore) 6: 41

Cruz Martinez A, Ferrer M T, López-Terradas J M, Pascual-Castroviejo I, Mingo P 1979 Single fibre electromyography in central core disease. Journal of Neurology, Neurosurgery and Psychiatry 42: 662

Curless R G, Payne C M, Brinner F M 1978a Fingerprint body myopathy: a report of twins. Developmental Medicine and Child Neurology 20: 793

Curless R G, Nelson M B, Brinner F 1978b Histological patterns of muscle in infants with developmental brain abnormalities. Developmental Medicine and Child Neurology 20: 159

Currie S, Noronha M, Harriman D 1974 'Minicore' disease. In: Bradley W G (ed) Abstracts of the IIIrd International Congress on Muscle Diseases. Excerpta Medica, Amsterdam, p 12

Daentl D L, Berg B O, Layzer R B, Epstein C J 1974 A new familial arthrogryposis without weakness. Neurology (Minneapolis) 24: 55

Dahl D S, Klutzow F W 1974 Congenital rod disease: further evidence of innervational abnormalities as the basis for the clinico-pathologic features. Journal of the Neurological Sciences 23: 371

Danon M J, Karpati G, Charuk J, Holland P 1988 Sarcoplasmic reticulum adenosine triphosphatase deficiency with probable autosomal dominant inheritance. Neurology 38: 812

Danta G 1975 Electrophysiological study of amyotrophy associated with acute asthma (asthmatic amyotrophy). Journal of Neurology, Neurosurgery and Psychiatry 38: 1016

Darwish H, Sarnat H, Archer C, Brownell K, Kotagal S 1981 Congenital cervical spinal atrophy. Muscle and Nerve 4: 106

Dastur D K, Razzak Z A, Bharucha E P 1972 Arthrogryposis multiplex congenita: part 2: Muscle pathology and pathogenesis. Journal of Neurology, Neurosurgery and Psychiatry 35: 435

de Angelis M S, Palmucci L, Leone M, Doriguzzi C 1991 Centronuclear myopathy: clinical, morphological and genetic characters. Journal of the Neurological Sciences 103: 2

de Leon G A, Grover W D, D'Cruz D A 1984 Amyotrophic cerebellar hypoplasia: a specific form of infantile spinal atrophy. Acta Neuropathologica (Berlin) 63: 282

Denborough M A, Dennett X, Anderson R M 1973 Central-core disease and malignant hyperpyrexia. British Medical Journal 1: 272

Denborough M A, Galloway G J, Hopkinson K C 1982 Malignant hyperpyrexia and sudden infant death. Lancet 2: 1068

Der Kaloustian V M, Afifi A K, Mire J 1972 The myopathic variety of arthrogryposis multiplex congenita: A disorder with autosomal recessive inheritance. Journal of Pediatrics 81: 76

Dodge P R 1960 Neuromuscular disorders. Research Publications of the Association for Research into Nervous and Mental Disease 38: 497

Drachman D B, Banker B Q 1963 Arthrogryposis multiplex congenita: case due to disease of the anterior horn cells. Archives of Neurology 8: 77

Dubowitz V 1973 Rigid spine syndrome: a muscle syndrome in search of a name. Proceedings of the Royal Society of Medicine 66: 219

Dubowitz V 1978 Muscle disorders in childhood. Saunders, London

Dubowitz V 1980 The floppy infant, 2nd edn. Spastics International Medical Publications, London

Dubowitz V 1985 Muscle biopsy: a practical approach, 2nd edn. Baillière Tindall, London

Dubowitz V, Platts M 1965 Central core disease of muscle with focal wasting. Journal of Neurology, Neurosurgery and Psychiatry 28: 432

Dubowitz V, Davies K 1993 Pontocerebellar hypoplasia with severe infantile SMA does not map to chromosome 5q. Presentation to the Annual Meeting of the British Paediatric Neurology Association, London

Dubrovsky A L, Taratuto A L, Martino R 1978 Type II hypotrophy and ophthalmoplegia: another congenital neuromuscular disease? In: Abstracts of the IVth International Congress of Neuromuscular Diseases (Montreal)

Dudley A W, Dudley M A, Varakis J M, Blackburn W R 1978 Progressive tetany and reducing bodies in a neonate: A new myopathy. In: Abstracts of the IVth International Congress of Neuromuscular Diseases (Montreal)

Dunn H G, Daube J R, Gomez M R 1978 Heredofamilial brachial plexus neuropathy (hereditary neuralgic amyotrophy with brachial predilection) in childhood. Developmental Medicine and Child Neurology 20: 28

Dyken M, Zeman W, Rusche T 1969 Hypokalemic periodic paralysis: children with permanent myopathic weakness. Neurology (Minneapolis) 19: 691

Eberle E, Brinke J, Azen S, White D 1975 Early predictors of incomplete recovery in children with Guillain–Barré polyneuritis. Journal of Pediatrics 86: 356

Edstrom L, Wroblewski R, Mair W G P 1982 Genuine myotubular myopathy. Muscle and Nerve 5: 604

Eeg-Olofsson O, Henriksson K-G, Thornell L-E, Wesstrom G 1983 Early infant death in nemaline (rod) myopathy. Brain and Development 5: 53

Ek J I 1958 Cerebral lesions in arthrogryposis multiplex congenita. Acta Paediatrica Scandinavica 47: 302

Emery A E H 1971 The nosology of the spinal muscular atrophies. Journal of Medical Genetics 8: 481

Eng G D, Epstein B S, Engel W K, McKay D W, McKay R 1978 Malignant hyperthermia and central core disease in a child with dislocating hips: case presentation and review. Archives of Neurology 35: 189

Engel A G 1984 Myasthenia gravis and myasthenic syndromes. Annals of Neurology 16: 519

Engel A G 1992 Myasthenia gravis and myasthenic syndromes. In: Vinken P J, Bruyn G W, Klawans H L (eds) Handbook of clinical neurology, vol 62, ch 14

Engel A G, Gomez M R, Groover R V 1971 Multicore disease: a recently recognised congenital myopathy associated with multifocal degeneration of muscle fibres. Mayo Clinic Proceedings 10: 666

Engel A G, Angelini C, Gomez M R 1972 Fingerprint body myopathy. Mayo Clinic Proceedings 47: 377

Engel A G, Lambert E H, Gomez M R 1977 A new myasthenic syndrome with end-plate acetylcholinesterase deficiency, small nerve terminals, and reduced acetylcholine release. Annals of Neurology 1: 315

Engel A G, Lambert E H, Mulder D M, Torres C F, Sahashi K, Bertorini T E, Whitaker J N 1982 A newly recognised congenital myasthenic syndrome attributed to a prolonged open time of the acetylcholine-induced ion channel. Annals of Neurology 11: 553

Engel A G, Banker B Q 1986 Myology, basic and clinical. McGraw-Hill, New York

Engel A G, Walls T J, Nagel A, Uchitel O 1990 Newly recognised congenital myasthenic syndromes. I. Congenital paucity of synaptic vesicles and reduced quantal release. II. High-conductance fast-channel syndrome. III. Abnormal acetylcholine receptor (AChR) interaction with acetylcholine. IV. AChR deficiency and short channel-open time. In: Aquilonius S M, Gillberg P G (eds) Progress in brain research. vol 84, ch 14, p 125

Engel A G, Uchitel O D, Walls T J, Nagel A, Harper C M, Bodensteiner J 1993 Newly recognised congenital myasthenic syndrome associated with high conductance and fast closure of the acetylcholine receptor channel. Annals of Neurology 34: 38

Engel W K, Gold G N, Karpati G 1968 Type I fiber hypotrophy and central nuclei. Archives of Neurology 18: 435

Fardeau M, Harpey J-P, Caille B, Lafourcade J 1975 Hyptonies neo-natales avec disproportion congénitale des differents types de fibre musculaire, et petitesse relative des fibres de type I: demonstration du caractère familial de cette nouvelle entité. Archives Françaises de Pédiatrie 32: 901

Fardeau M, Tomé F M S, Derambure S 1976 Familial fingerprint body myopathy. Archives of Neurology 33: 724

Farkas-Bargeton E, Aicardi J, Arsenio-Nunes M L, Wehrle R 1978 Delay in the maturation of muscle fibers in infants with congenital hypotonia. Journal of the Neurological Sciences 39: 17

Favara B E, Vawter G F, Wagner R, Kevy S, Porter E G 1967 Familial paroxysmal rhabdomyolysis in children: a myoglobinuric syndrome. American Journal of Medicine 42: 196

Fear C N, Mutton D E, Berry A C, Heckmatt J Z, Dubowitz V 1985 Chromosome 15 in Prader–Willi syndrome. Developmental Medicine and Child Neurology 27: 305

Feasby T E, Hahn A F, Bolton C F, Brown W F, Koopman W J 1992 Detection of hereditary motor sensory neuropathy type 1 in childhood. Journal of Neurology, Neurosurgery and Psychiatry 55: 895

Fenichel G M 1967 Abnormalities of skeletal muscle maturation in brain damaged children: a histochemical study. Developmental Medicine and Child Neurology 9: 419

Fenichel G M 1978 Clinical syndromes of myasthenia in infancy and childhood: a review. Archives of Neurology 35: 97

Fenichel G M 1983 Myasthenia gravis. In: Emery A E H, Rimoin D L (eds) Principles and practice of medical genetics. Churchill Livingstone, Edinburgh, ch 34

Fenichel G M, Bazelon M 1966 Myopathies in search of a name: benign congenital forms. Developmental Medicine and Child Neurology 8: 532

Fidzianska A, Badurska B, Ryniewicz B, Dembek I 1981 'Cap disease': new congenital myopathy. Neurology (New York) 31: 1113

Fishbein W N, Armbrustmacher V W, Griffin J L 1978 Myoadenylate deaminase deficiency: a new disease of muscle. Science 200: 545

Fisher R L, Johnstone W T, Fisher W H, Goldkamp O G 1970 Arthrogryposis multiplex congenita: A clinical investigation. Journal of Pediatrics 76: 255

Fleury P, Hageman G 1985 A dominantly inherited lower motor neuron disorder presenting at birth with associated arthrogryposis. Journal of Neurology, Neurosurgery and Psychiatry 48: 1037

Ford F R 1966 Diseases of the nervous system in infancy, childhood and adolescence, 5th edn. Charles C Thomas, Springfield, Ill

Fowler M 1959 A case of arthrogryposis multiplex congenita with lesions in the nervous system. Archives of Disease in Childhood 34: 505

Frank J P, Harati Y, Butler I J, Nelson T E, Scott C I 1980 Central core disease and malignant hyperthermia syndrome. Annals of Neurology 7: 11

Frankenburg W K, Dodds J B 1967 The Denver developmental screening test. Journal of Pediatrics 71: 181

Fried K, Beer S, Vure E, Algom M, Shapira Y 1979 Autosomal recessive sudden unexpected death in children probably caused by a cardiomyopathy associated with a myopathy. Journal of Medical Genetics 16: 341

Friedlander H L, Westin G W, Wood W L 1968 Arthrogryposis multiplex congenita. A review of 45 cases. Journal of Bone and Joint Surgery 50A: 89

Frischknecht W, Bianchi L, Pilleri G 1960 Familial arthrogryposis multiplex congenita. Neuroarthromyodysplasia congenita. Helvetica Paediatrica Acta 15: 259

Fukuyama Y, Sugiura S, Hirayama Y, Segawa M G 1973 The prognosis of myasthenia gravis in infancy and childhood. In: Kakulas B A (ed) Clinical studies in myology: Part II. Excerpta Medica, Amsterdam, p 552

Fukuyama Y, Ando T, Yokota J 1977 Acute fulminant myoglobinuric polymyositis with picornavirus-like crystals. Journal of Neurology, Neurosurgery and Psychiatry 40: 775

Fulthorpe J J, Gardner-Medwin D, Hudgson P, Walton J N 1969 Nemaline myopathy: a histological and ultrastructural study of skeletal muscle from a case presenting with infantile hypotonia. Neurology (Minneapolis) 19: 735

Gadoth N, Margalit D, Shapira Y 1978 Myopathy with multiple central cores: a case of hypersensitivity to pyrexia. Neuropädiatrie 9: 239

Gallai V, Hockaday J M, Hughes J T, Lane D J, Oppenheimer D R, Rushworth G 1981 Ponto-bulbar palsy with deafness (Brown–Vialetto–Van Laere syndrome): a report on three cases. Journal of the Neurological Sciences 50: 259

Gallanti A, Prelle A, Chianese L et al 1992 Congenital myopathy with type 2A muscle fibre uniformity and smallness. Neuropediatrics 23: 10

Gamstorp I, Hauge M, Helweg-Larsen H F, Mjönes H, Sagild U 1957 Adynamia episodica hereditaria: A disease clinically resembling familial periodic paralysis but characterised by increasing serum potassium during the paralytic attacks. American Journal of Medicine 23: 385

Gamstorp I, Sarnat H B (eds) 1984 Progressive spinal muscular atrophies. Raven, New York

Garcia-Alix A, Rodriguez J I, Quero J 1992 A new form of infantile spinal muscular atrophy. Journal of Medical Genetics 29: 215

Gardner-Medwin D, Walton J N 1969 Myokymia with impaired muscular relaxation. Lancet i: 127

Gardner-Medwin D 1993 Clinical experience with the genetic myasthenias. In: Fejerman N, Chamoles N A (eds) New trends in pediatric neurology. Excerpta Medica, Amsterdam, p 117

Geiger L R, Mancall E L, Penn A S, Tucker S H 1974 Familial neuralgic amyotrophy: report of three families with review of the literature. Brain 97: 97

Gieron M A, Korthals J K 1985 Familial infantile myasthenia gravis: Report of three cases with follow-up until adult life. Archives of Neurology 42: 143

Gil-Peralta A, Rafel E, Bautista J, Alberca R 1978 Myotonia in centronuclear myopathy. Journal of Neurology, Neurosurgery and Psychiatry 41: 1102

Goebel H H, Zeman W, DeMyer W 1976 Peripheral motor and sensory neuropathy of early childhood, simulating Werdnig–Hoffmann disease. Neuropädiatrie 7: 182

Goebel H H, Lenard H G, Görke W, Kunze K 1977 Fibre type disproportion in the rigid spine syndrome. Neuropädiatrie 8: 467

Goebel H H, Muller J, Gillen H W, Merritt A D 1978 Autosomal dominant 'spheroid body myopathy'. Muscle and Nerve 1: 14

Goebel H H, Schloon H, Lenard H G 1981 Congenital myopathy with Cytoplasmic bodies. Neuropediatrics 12: 166

Goldhammer Y, Blatt I, Sadeh M, Goodman R M 1990 Congenital myasthenia associated with facial malformations in Iraqi and Iranian Jews: a new genetic syndrome. Brain 113: 1291

Gomez M R, Clermont V, Bernstein J 1962 Progressive bulbar paralysis in childhood (Fazio–Londe's disease): report of a case with pathologic evidence of nuclear atrophy. Archives of Neurology 6: 317

Gonatas N K, Shy G M, Godfrey E H 1966 Nemaline myopathy: the origin of nemaline structures. New England Journal of Medicine 274: 535

Gordon A S, Rewcastle N B, Humphrey J G, Stewart B M 1974 Chronic benign congenital myopathy: finger print body type. Canadian Journal of Neurological Sciences 1: 106

Goto I, Nagasaka S, Nagara H, Kuroiwa Y 1979 Rigid spine syndrome. Journal of Neurology, Neurosurgery and Psychiatry 42: 276

Goutières F, Aicardi J, Farkas E 1977 Anterior horn cell disease associated with pontocerebellar hypoplasia in infants. Journal of Neurology, Neurosurgery and Psychiatry 40: 370

Goutières F, Bogicevic D, Aicardi J 1991 A predominantly cervical form of spinal muscular atrophy. Journal of Neurology, Neurosurgery and Psychiatry 54: 223

Granata C, Cornelio F, Bonfiglioli S, Mattutini P, Merlini L 1987 Promotion of ambulation of patients with spinal muscular atrophy by early fitting of knee–ankle–foot orthoses. Developmental Medicine and Child Neurology 29: 221

Gucuyener K, Aysun S, Topaloglu H, Inan L, Varli K 1991 Monomelic amyotrophy in siblings. Pediatric Neurology 7: 220

Guggenheim M A, Ringel S P, Silverman A, Grabert B E 1982 Progressive neuro-muscular disease in children with chronic cholestasis and vitamin E deficiency: diagnosis and treatment with alpha tocopherol. Journal of Pediatrics 100: 51

Haan E A, Freemantle C J, McCure J A, Friend K L, Mulley J C 1990 Assignment of the gene for central core disease to chromosome 19. Human Genetics 86: 187

Hagberg B, Lyon G 1981 Pooled European series of hereditary peripheral neuropathies in infancy and childhood. Neuropediatrics 12: 9

Hageman G, Ramaekers V T, Hilhorst B G J, Rozeboom A R 1993 Congenital cervical spinal muscular atrophy: a non-familial, non-progressive condition of the upper limbs. Journal of Neurology, Neurosurgery and Psychiatry 56: 365

Hall J G 1983 Arthrogryposes (congenital contractures) In: Emery A E H, Rimoin D L (eds) Principles and practice of medical genetics. Churchill Livingstone, Edinburgh, ch 55

Hall J G, Reed S D, Greene G 1982 The distal arthrogryposes: delineation of new entities — review and nosologic discussion. American Journal of Medical Genetics 11: 185

Hall J G, Reed S D, Driscoll E P 1983 Amyoplasia: a common, sporadic condition with congenital contractures. American Journal of Medical Genetics 15: 571

Hanson P A, Mastrianni A F, Post L 1977 Neonatal ophthalmoplegia with microfibers: a reversible myopathy? Neurology (Minneapolis) 27: 974

Harati Y, Butler I J 1985 Congenital hypomyelinating neuropathy. Journal of Neurology, Neurosurgery and Psychiatry 48: 1269

Hardoff D, Sharf B, Berger A 1980 Myopathy as a presentation of coeliac disease. Developmental Medicine and Child Neurology 22: 781

Harriman D G F, Haleem M A 1972 Centronuclear myopathy in old age. Journal of Pathology 108: 237

Hart Z, Sahashi K, Lambert E H, Engel A G, Lindstrom J M 1979 A congenital familial myasthenic syndrome caused by a presynaptic defect of transmitter resynthesis or mobilization. Neurology 29: 556

Hart Z H, Servidei S, Peterson P L, Chang C-H, DiMauro S 1987 Cardiomyopathy, mental retardation, and autophagic vacuolar myopathy. Neurology 37: 1065

Hausmanowa-Petrusewicz I 1978 Spinal muscular atrophy: Infantile and juvenile type. National Science Foundation, Washington DC and National Centre for Scientific, Technical and Economic Information, Warsaw, Poland

Hawkes C H, Absolon M J 1975 Myotubular myopathy associated with cataract and electrical myotonia. Journal of Neurology, Neurosurgery and Psychiatry 38: 761

Hawkins S A, Nevin N C, Harding A E 1990 Pontobulbar palsy and neurosensory deafness (Brown–Vialetto–Van Laere syndrome) with possible autosomal dominant inheritance. Journal of Medical Genetics 27: 176

Heckmatt J Z, Moosa A, Hutson C, Maunder-Sewry C A, Dubowitz V 1984 Diagnostic needle muscle biopsy: a practical and reliable alternative to open biopsy. Archives of Disease in Childhood 59: 528

Heckmatt J Z, Sewry C A, Hodes D, Dubowitz V 1985 Congenital centronuclear (myotubular) myopathy: a clinical, pathological and genetic study in eight children. Brain 108: 941

Heffernan L P, Rewcastle N B, Humphrey J G 1968 The spectrum of rod myopathies. Archives of Neurology 18: 529

Heffner R, Cohen M, Duffner P, Daigler G 1976 Multicore disease in twins. Journal of Neurology, Neurosurgery and Psychiatry 39: 602

Henry J A, Jeffreys K J, Dawling S 1992 Toxicity and deaths from 3,4-methylenedioxymethamphetamine ('ecstasy'). Lancet 340: 384

Hoefnagel D, Jalberg E O, Publow D G, Richtsmeier A J 1978 Progressive fibrosis of the deltoid muscles. Journal of Pediatrics 92: 79

Hopkins I J 1974 A new syndrome: poliomyelitis-like illness associated with acute asthma in childhood. Australian Paediatric Journal 10: 273

Hopkins I J, Lindsey J R, Ford F R 1966 Nemaline myopathy. A long-term clinicopathologic study of affected mother and daughter. Brain 89: 299

Hopkins P M, Ellis F R, Halsall P J 1991 Hypermetabolism in arthrogryposis multiplex congenita. Anaesthesia 46: 374

Hosking G P, Bhat U S, Dubowitz V, Edwards R H T 1976 Measurements of muscle strength and performance in children with normal and diseased muscle. Archives of Disease in Childhood 51: 957

Howes E L, Price H M, Pearson C M, Blumberg J M 1966

Hypokalemic periodic paralysis: electronmicroscopic changes in the sarcoplasm. Neurology (Minneapolis) 16: 242

Hurwitz L D, Carson N A J, Allen I V, Chopra J S 1969 Congenital ophthalmoplegia, floppy baby syndrome, myopathy and aminoaciduria. Journal of Neurology, Neurosurgery and Psychiatry 32: 495

Husain F, Ryan N J, Hogan G R 1989 Concurrence of limb girdle muscular dystrophy and myasthenia gravis. Archives of Neurology 46: 101. See also letter to the editor by Rowland L P Archives of Neurology 46: 1047

Huttenlocher P R, Gilles F H 1967 Infantile neuroaxonal dystrophy. Clinical, pathologic and histochemical findings in a family with 3 affected siblings. Neurology (Minneapolis) 17: 1174

Ilett S J, Pugh R J, Smithells R W 1977 Poliomyelitis-like illness after acute asthma. Archives of Disease in Childhood 52: 738

Illingworth R S 1972 The development of the infant and young child, normal and abnormal, 5th edn. E & S Livingstone, Edinburgh

Ingram T T S 1955 The early manifestations and course of diplegia in childhood. Archives of Disease in Childhood 30: 244

Inokuchi T, Umezaki H, Santa T 1975 A case of type I muscle fibre hypotrophy and internal nuclei. Journal of Neurology, Neurosurgery and Psychiatry 138: 475

Ionasescu V, Searby C, Rubenstein P, Sandra A, Cancilla P, Robillard J 1983 Giant axonal neuropathy: normal protein composition of neurofilaments. Journal of Neurology, Neurosurgery and Psychiatry 46: 551

Isaacs H 1961 A syndrome of continuous muscle fibre activity. Journal of Neurology, Neurosurgery and Psychiatry 24: 319

Isaacs H, Heffron J J A, Bandenhorst M 1975 Central core disease: a correlated genetic, histochemical, ultramicroscopic and biochemical study. Journal of Neurology, Neurosurgery and Psychiatry 38: 1177

Jaffe M, Shapira J, Borochowitz Z 1988 Familial congenital fiber type disproportion (CFTD) with an autosomal recessive inheritance. Clinical Genetics 33: 33

Jago R H 1970 Arthrogryposis following treatment of maternal tetanus with muscle relaxants. Archives of Disease in Childhood 45: 277

Jasper P L, Denny F W 1968 Sarcoidosis in children: with special emphasis on the natural history and treatment. Journal of Pediatrics 73: 499

Jenis E H, Lindquist R R, Lister R C 1969 New congenital myopathy with crystalline intranuclear inclusions. Archives of Neurology 20: 281

Jerusalem F, Engel A G, Gomez M R 1973 Sarcotubular myopathy: a newly recognised, benign, congenital muscle disease. Neurology (Mineapolis) 23: 897

Johnson W G, Wigger H J, Karp H R, Glaubiger L M, Rowland L P 1982 Juvenile spinal muscular atrophy: a new hexosaminidase deficiency phenotype. Annals of Neurology 11: 11

Joosten E, Gabreëls F, Gabréels-Festen A, Vrensen G, Korten J, Notermans S 1974 Electron-microscopic heterogeneity of onion-bulb neuropathies of the Déjerine–Sottas type: two patients in one family with the variant described by Lyon (1969). Acta Neuropathologica (Berlin) 27: 105

Juguilon A, Chad D, Bradley W G et al 1982 Familial granuolar vacuolar lobular myopathy with electrical myotonia. Journal of the Neurological Sciences 56: 133

Kalimo H, Savontaus M-L, Lang H et al 1988. X-linked myopathy with excessive autophagy: a new hereditary muscle disease. Annals of Neurology 23: 258

Karch S B, Urich H 1975 Infantile polyneuropathy with defective myelination: an autopsy study. Developmental Medicine and Child Neurology 17: 504

Karpati G, Carpenter S, Wolfe L S, Sherwin A 1969 A peculiar polysaccharide accumulation in muscle in a case of cardioskeletal myopathy. Neurology (Minneapolis) 19: 553

Karpati G, Carpenter S, Nelson R F 1970 Type I muscle fibre atrophy and central nuclei: a rare familial neuromuscular disease. Journal of the Neurological Sciences 10: 489

Karpati G, Charuk J, Carpenter S, Jablecki C, Holland P 1986 Myopathy caused by deficiency of Ca(2+)-adenosine triphosphatase in sarcoplasmic reticulum (Brody's disease). Annals of Neurology 20: 38

Kasman M, Bernstein L 1974 Chronic progressive polyradiculoneuropathy of infancy. Neurology (Minneapolis) 24: 367

Kausch K, Lehmann-Horn F, Janka M, Wieringa B, Grimm T, Muller C 1991. Evidence for linkage of the central core disease locus to the proximal long arm of human chromosome 19. Genomics 10: 765

Kawai M, Momoi T, Fujii T, Nakano S, Itagaki Y, Mikawa H 1990 The syndrome of Moebius sequence, peripheral neuropathy, and hypogonadotrophic hypogonadism. American Journal of Medical Genetics 37: 578

Kelemen J, Rice D R, Bradley W G, Munsat T L, DiMauro S, Hogan E L 1982 Familial myoadenylate deaminase deficiency and exertional myalgia. Neurology (New York) 32: 857

Kennedy W R, Sung J H, Berry J F 1977 A case of congenital hypomyelination neuropathy: clinical, morphological and chemical studies. Archives of Neurology 34: 337

Kimura S, Sasaki Y 1988 Ultrastructural muscle pathology in infantile neuroaxonal dystrophy. Brain and Development 10: 327

King J O, Denborough M A, Zapf P W 1972 Inheritance of malignant hyperthermia. Lancet i: 365

Kinoshita M, Cadman T E 1968 Myotubular myopathy. Archives of Neurology 18: 265

Koch B M, Bertorini T E, Eng G D, Boehm R 1985 Severe multicore disease associated with reaction to anesthesia. Archives of Neurology 42: 1204

Kohlschutter A, Sieg K, Schulte F J, Hayek H W, Goebel H H 1982 Infantile cardiomyopathy and neuromyopathy with β-galactosidase deficiency. European Journal of Pediatrics 139: 75

Kondo K, Yuasa T 1980 Genetics of congenital nemaline myopathy. Muscle and Nerve 3: 308

Krabbe K H 1958 Congenital generalised muscular atrophies. Acta Psychiatrica 33: 94

Krugliak L, Gadoth N, Behar A J 1978 Neuropathic form of arthrogryposis multiplex congenita: report of 3 cases with complete necropsy, including the first reported case of agenesis of muscle spindles. Journal of the Neurological Sciences 37: 179

Kuitonnen P, Rapola J, Noponen A L, Donner M 1972 Nemaline myopathy. Report of 4 cases and review of the literature. Acta Paediatrica Scandinavica 61: 353

Kumar D 1990 Moebius syndrome. Journal of Medical Genetics 27: 122

Kuzuhara S, Chou S M 1981 Preservation of the phrenic motoneurons in Werdnig-Hoffmann disease. Annals of Neurology 9: 506

Lake B D, Wilson J 1975 Zebra body myopathy: Clinical, histochemical and ultrastructural studies. Journal of the Neurological Sciences 24: 437

Laing N, Majda B, Akkari P 1991 Assignment of nemaline myopathy (MIM 161800, NEM 1) to chromosome 1. Cytogenetics and Cell Genetics 58: 1858

Lampl Y, Eshel Y, Ben-David E, Gilad R, Sarova-Pinhas I, Sandbank U 1992 Giant axonal neuropathy with predominant central nervous system manifestations. Developmental Medicine and Child Neurology 34: 164

Laurence B M 1967 Hypotonia, mental retardation, obesity and cryptorchidism associated with dwarfism and diabetes in children. Archives of Disease in Childhood 42: 126

Lazaro R P, Fenichel G M, Kilroy A W, Saito A, Fleischer S 1980 Cramps, muscle pain and tubular aggregates. Archives of Neurology 37: 715

Lebenthal E, Shocket S B, Adam A et al 1970 Arthrogryposis multiplex congenita: Twenty-three cases in an Arab kindred. Pediatrics 46: 891

Lecky B R F, Morgan-Hughes J A, Murray N M F, Landon D N, Wray D, Prior C 1986 Congenital myasthenia: further evidence of disease heterogeneity. Muscle and Nerve 9: 233

Lefvert A K, Osterman P O 1983 Newborn infants to myasthenic mothers: a clinical study and an investigation of acetylcholine receptor antibodies in 17 children. Neurology 33: 133

Lenard H G, Goebel H H 1975 Congenital fibre type disproportion. Neuropädiatrie 6: 220

Lenard H-G, Goebel H-H 1980 Congenital muscular dystrophies and unstructured congenital myopathies. Brain and Development 2: 119

Lesny I 1979 Follow up study of hypotonic forms of cerebral palsy. Brain and Development 1: 87

Liu G T, Specht L A 1993 Progressive juvenile segmental spinal muscular atrophy. Pediatric Neurology 9: 54

Lloyd-Roberts G C, Lettin A W F 1970 Arthrogryposis multiplex congenita. Journal of Bone and Joint Surgery 52B: 494

Logothetis J, Constantoulakis M, Economidou J et al 1972 Thalassemia major (homozygous beta-thalassemia): a survey of 138 cases with emphasis on neurologic and muscular aspects. Neurology (Minneapolis) 22: 294

Long S S, Gajewski J L, Brown L W, Gilligan P H 1985 Clinical, laboratory, and environmental features of infant botulism in southeastern Pennsylvania. Pediatrics 75: 935

Löwenthal A 1954 Un groupe hérédodégénératif nouveau: les myoscléroses hérédofamiliales. Acta Neurologica et Psychiatrica Belgica 54: 155

Lundberg A 1979 Dissociated motor development: Developmental patterns, clinical characteristics, causal factors and outcome, with special reference to late walking children. Neuropädiatrie 10: 161

Lyon G 1969 Ultrastructural study of a nerve biopsy from a case of early infantile chronic neuropathy. Acta Neuropathologica (Berlin) 13: 131

Lyon G, Arita F, Le Galloudec E, Valle L, Misson J-P, Ferriere G 1990 A disorder of axonal development, necrotising myopathy, cardiomyopathy and cataracts: a new familial disease. Annals of Neurology 27: 193

MacDermot K D, Winter R M, Taylor D, Baraitser M 1991 Oculofacialbulbar palsy in mother and son: review of 26 reports of familial transmission within the "Möbius spectrum of defects". Journal of Medical Genetics 28: 18

McGuire S A, Tomasovic J J, Ackerman N 1984 Hereditary continuous muscle fiber activity. Archives of Neurology 41: 395

McKinlay I A, Mitchell I 1976 Transient acute myositis in childhood. Archives of Disease in Childhood 51: 135

McKusick V A 1992 Mendelian inheritance in man, 10th edn Baltimore, Johns Hopkins University Press

McLean W T, McKone R C 1973 Congenital myasthenia gravis in twins. Archives of Neurology 29: 223

McLeod J G, Baker W de C, Lethlean A K, Shorey C D 1972 Centronuclear myopathy with autosomal dominant inheritance. Journal of the Neurological Sciences 15: 375

McQuillen M P 1966 Familial limb-girdle myasthenia. Brain 89: 121

McWilliam R C, Gardner-Medwin D, Doyle D, Stephenson J B P 1985 Diaphragmatic paralysis due to spinal muscular atrophy: an unrecognised cause of respiratory failure in infancy? Archives of Disease in Childhood 60: 145

Madrid R, Bradley W G 1975 The pathology of neuropathies with focal thickening of the myelin sheath (tomaculous neuropathy): studies on the formation of the abnormal myelin sheath. Journal of the Neurological Sciences 25: 415

Martin J J, Clara R, Ceuterick C, Joris C 1976 Is congenital fibre type disproportion a true myopathy? Acta Neurologica Belgica 76: 335

Matsuoka Y, Gubbay S S, Kakulas B A 1974 A new myopathy with type II muscle fibre hypoplasia. Proceedings of the Australian Association of Neurologists 11: 155

Matsushita S, Ikeda S, Hanyu N, Yamamoto K, Yanagisawa N 1991 Muscular pseudohypertrophy in an adult case with centronuclear myopathy. European Neurology 31: 172

Matthes J W A, Kenna A P, Fawcett P R W 1991 Familial infantile myasthenia: a diagnostic problem. Developmental Medicine and Child Neurology 33: 924

Meier C, Voellmy W, Gertsch M, Zimmermann A, Geissbuhler J 1984 Nemaline myopathy appearing in adults as cardiomyopathy: a clinicopathologic study. Archives of Neurology 41: 443

Mellins R B, Hays A P, Gold A P, Berdon W E, Bowdler J D 1974 Respiratory distress as the initial manifestation of Werdnig–Hoffmann disease. Pediatrics 53: 33

Meyer-Betz F 1910 Beobachtungen an einem eigenartigen mit Muskellahmungen verbundenen Fall von Hamoglobinurie. Deutsches Archiv für klinische Medizin 101: 85

Meyers K R, Golomb H M, Hansen J L, McKusick V A 1974 Familial neuromuscular disease with 'myotubes'. Clinical Genetics 5: 327

Midura T F, Arnon S S 1976 Infant botulism: identification of Clostridium botulinum and its toxins in faeces. Lancet ii: 934

Millichap J G, Dodge P R 1960 Diagnosis and treatment of myasthenia gravis in infancy, childhood and adolescence. Neurology (Minneapolis) 10: 1007

Misra A K, Menon N K, Mishra S K 1992 Abnormal distribution of desmin and vimentin in myofibers in adult onset myotubular myopathy. Muscle and Nerve 15: 1246

Mitsumoto H, Sliman R J, Schafer I A et al 1985 Motor neuron disease and adult hexosaminidase A deficiency in two families: evidence for multisystem degeneration. Annals of Neurology 17: 378

Mizuno Y, Komiya K 1990 A serial muscle biopsy study in a case of congenital fiber-type disproportion associated with progressive respiratory failure. Brain and Development 12: 431

Mizuno Y, Nakamura Y, Kamiya K 1989 The spectrum of cytoplasmic body myopathy: report of a congenital severe case. Brain and Development 11: 20

Moosa A 1971 Peripheral neuropathy and ichthyosis in Krabbe's leucodystrophy. Archives of Disease in Childhood 46: 112

Mora M, Lambert E H, Engel A G 1987 Synaptic vesicle abnormality in familial infantile myasthenia. Neurology 37: 206

Morel E, Eymard B, Vernet-der Garabedian B, Pannier C, Dulac O, Bach J F 1988 Neonatal myasthenia gravis: a new clinical and immunologic appraisal on 30 cases. Neurology 38: 138

Morgan-Hughes J A, Brett E M, Lake B D, Tomé F M S 1973 Central core disease or not? Observations on a family with non-progressive myopathy. Brain 96: 527

Morgan-Hughes J A, Lecky B R F, Landon D N, Murray N M F 1981 Alterations in the number and affinity of junctional acetylcholine receptors in a myopathy with tubular aggregates: a newly recognized receptor defect. Brain 104: 279

Morgenlander J C, Nohria V, Saba Z 1993 EKG Abnormalities in pediatric patients with myotonic dystrophy. Pediatric Neurology 9: 124

Morita H, Kondo K, Hoshino K, Maruyama K, Yanagisawa N 1990 Rigid spine syndrome with respiratory failure. Journal of Neurology, Neurosurgery and Psychiatry 53: 782

Murphy N P, Davidson D C, Bouton J 1985 Diaphragmatic paralysis due to spinal muscular atrophy. Archives of Disease in Childhood 60: 495

Nagai T, Hasegawa T, Saito M, Hayashi S, Nonaka I 1992 Infantile polymyositis: a case report. Brain and Development 14: 167

Naveh Y, Ludatshcer C, Alon U, Sharf B 1985 Muscle involvement in progressive diaphyseal dysplasia. Pediatrics 76: 944

Neligan G, Prudham D 1969 Norms for four standard developmental milestones by sex, social class and place in family. Developmental Medicine and Child Neurology 11: 413

Nelson J S, Prensky A L 1972 Sporadic juvenile amyotrophic lateral sclerosis: a clinicopathological study of a case with neuronal cytoplasmic inclusions containing RNA. Archives of Neurology 27: 300

Newman D G, Pearn J, Barnes A, Young C M, Kehoe M, Newman J 1984 Norms for hand grip strength. Archives of Disease in Childhood 59: 453

Noble-Jamieson C M, Heckmatt J Z, Dubowitz V, Silverman M 1986 Effects of posture and spinal bracing on respiratory function in neuromuscular disease. Archives of Disease in Childhood 61: 178

Nomizu S, Person D A, Saito C, Lockett L J 1992 A unique case of reducing body myopathy. Muscle and Nerve 15: 463

Norman M G, Temple A R, Murphy J V 1970 Infantile quadriceps-femoris contracture resulting from intramuscular injections. New England Journal of Medicine 282: 964

Norman R M 1961 Cerebellar hypoplasia in Werdnig–Hoffmann disease. Archives of Disease in Childhood 3: 96

Oberklaid F, Hopkins I J 1976 'Juvenile' myasthenia gravis in early infancy. Archives of Disease in Childhood 51: 719

Oda K, Fukushima N, Shibasaki H, Ohnishi A 1989 Hypoxia-sensitive hyperexcitability of the intramuscular nerve axons in Isaacs' syndrome. Annals of Neurology 25: 140

Oh S J, Danon M J 1983 Nonprogressive congenital neuromuscular disease with uniform type 1 fiber. Archives of Neurology 40: 147

Oh S J, Meyers G J, Wilson E R, Alexander C B 1983 A benign form of reducing body myopathy. Muscle and Nerve 6: 278

Ohnishi A, Mitsudome A, Murai Y 1987 Primary segmental demyelination in the sural nerve in Cockayne's syndrome. Muscle and Nerve 10: 163

Ohtaki E, Yamaguchi Y, Yamashita Y et al 1990 Complete external ophthalmoplegia in a patient with congenital myopathy without specific features (minimal change myopathy). Brain and Development 12: 427

Oosterhuis H J G H, Newsom-Davis J, Wokke J H J et al 1987 The slow channel syndrome. Brain 110: 1061

Ortiz de Zarate J C, Maruffo A 1970 The descending ocular myopathy of early childhood. Myotubular or centronuclear myopathy. European Neurology 3: 1

Osserman K E 1958 Myasthenia gravis. Grune & Stratton, New York

Ozmen M, Caliskan M, Goebel H H, Apak S 1991 Infantile neuroaxonal dystrophy: diagnosis by skin biopsy. Brain and Development 13: 256

Paine R S 1963 The future of the 'floppy infant'. A follow up study of 133 patients. Developmental Medicine and Child Neurology 5: 115

Palace J, Wiles C M, Newsom-Davis J 1991 3,4-Diaminopyridine in the treatment of congenital (hereditary) myasthenia. Journal of Neurology, Neurosurgery and Psychiatry 54: 1069

Päljarvi L, Kalimo H, Lang H, Savontaus M-L, Sonninen V 1987 Minicore myopathy with dominant inheritance. Journal of the Neurological Sciences 77: 11

Parker D L, Mitchell P R, Holmes G L 1981 Poland–Möbius syndrome. Journal of Medical Genetics 18: 317

Parnes S, Karpati G, Carpenter S et al 1985 Hexosaminidase-A deficiency presenting as atypical juvenile-onset spinal muscular atrophy. Archives of Neurology 42: 1176

Pasternak J F, Fulling K, Nelson J, Prensky A L 1982 An infant with chronic, relapsing polyneuropathy responsive to steroids. Developmental Medicine and Child Neurology 24: 504

Patel H, Berry K, MacLeod P, Dunn H G 1983 Cytoplasmic body myopathy: report on a family and review of the literature. Journal of the Neurological Sciences 60: 281

Patterson V H, Hill T R G, Fletcher P J H, Heron J R 1979 Central core disease: clinical and pathological evidence of progression within a family. Brain 102: 581

Paulson G W 1970 The Landry–Guillain–Barré syndrome in childhood. Developmental Medicine and Child Neurology 12: 604

Pearn J H 1974 The use of motor milestones to determine retrospectively the clinical onset of disease. Australian Paediatric Journal 10: 147

Pearn J 1980 Classification of spinal muscular atrophies. Lancet i: 919

Pearson C M 1964 The periodic paralyses. Differential features and pathology in permanent myopathic weakness. Brain 87: 341

Pearson C M, Fowler W G 1963 Hereditary non-progressive muscular dystrophy inducing arthrogryposis syndrome. Brain 86: 75

Pellissier J F, Pouget J, Charpin C, Figarella D 1989 Myopathy associated with desmin type intermediate filaments. An immunoelectron microscopic study. Journal of the Neurological Sciences 89: 49

Peña C E, Miller F, Budzilovich G B, Feigen I 1968 Arthrogryposis multiplex congenita. Neurology (Minneapolis) 18: 926

Peterman A F, Daly D D, Dion F R, Keith H M 1959 Infectious neuronitis (Guillain–Barré syndrome) in children. Neurology (Minneapolis) 9: 533

Peyronnard J-M, Charron L, Ninkovic S 1982 Type I fiber atrophy and internal nuclei: a form of centronuclear myopathy? Archives of Neurology 39: 520

Pickett J, Berg B, Chaplin E, Brunstetter-Shafer M-A 1976 Syndrome of botulism in infancy: clinical and electrophysiologic study. New England Journal of Medicine 295: 770

Pierobon-Bormioli S, Armani M, Ringel S P, Angelini C, Vergani L, Betto R, Salviati G 1985 Familial neuromuscular disease with tubular aggregates. Muscle and Nerve 8: 291

Polani P E 1959 The natural clinical history of choreoathetoid cerebral palsy. Guy's Hospital Reports 108: 32

Poskanzer D C, Kerr D N S 1961 A third type of periodic paralysis, with normokalemia and favourable response to sodium chloride. American Journal of Medicine 31: 328

Prader A, Labhart A, Willi H 1956 Ein Syndrome von Adipositas, Kleinwuchs, Kryptorchismus und Oligophrenie nach myatonieartigem Zustand im Neugeborenalter. Schweizerische medizinische Wochenschrift 86: 1260

Prelle A, Moggio M, Comi G P et al 1992 Congenital myopathy associated with abnormal accumulation of desmin and dystrophin. Neuromuscular Disorders 2: 169

Pridmore C, Baraitser M, Brett E M, Harding A E 1992 Distal spinal muscular atrophy with vocal cord paralysis. Journal of Medical Genetics 29: 197

Pugh R C B, Dudgeon J A 1954 Fatal neonatal poliomyelitis. Archives of Disease in Childhood 29: 381

Raifman M A, Berant M, Lenarsky C 1978 Cold weather and rhabdomyolysis. Journal of Pediatrics 93: 970

Ramesh V, Gardner-Medwin D 1992 Familial paroxysmal rhabdomyolysis: management of two cases of the non-exertional type. Developmental Medicine and Child Neurology 34: 73

Reik L, Steere A C, Bartenhagen N H, Shope R E, Malawista S E 1979 Neurologic abnormalities of Lyme disease. Medicine (Baltimore) 58: 281

Reyes M G, Goldbarg H, Fresco K, Bouffard A 1987 Zebra body myopathy: a second case of ultrastructurally distinct congenital myopathy. Journal of Child Neurology 2: 307

Ricoy J R, Cabello A 1985 Hypotrophy of type 1 fibres with central nuclei: recovery 4 years after diagnosis. Journal of Neurology, Neurosurgery and Psychiatry 48: 167

Riddick M F, Winter R B, Lutter L D 1982 Spinal deformities in patients with spinal muscle atrophy: a review of 36 patients. Spine 7: 476

Riley D J, Santiago T V, Daniele R P, Schall B, Edelman N H 1977 Blunted respiratory drive in congenital myopathy. American Journal of Medicine 63: 459

Ringel S P, Neville H E, Duster M C, Carroll J E 1978 A new congenital neuromuscular disease with trilaminar muscle fibers. Neurology (Minneapolis) 28: 282

Robb S A, McShane M A, Wilson J, Payan J 1991 Acute onset spinal muscular atrophy in siblings. Neuropediatrics 22: 45

Robertson W C, Chun R W M, Kornguth S E 1980 Familial infantile myasthenia. Archives of Neurology 37: 117

Robinson W P, Bottani A, Yagang X et al 1991 Molecular, cytogenetic, and clinical investigations of Prader–Willi syndrome patients. American Journal of Human Genetics 49: 1219

Rodriguez M, Gomez M R, Howard F M, Taylor W F 1983 Myasthenia gravis in children: long-term follow-up. Annals of Neurology 13: 504

Rohkamm R, Boxler K, Ricker K, Jerusalem F 1983 A dominantly inherited myopathy with excessive tubular aggregates. Neurology (Cleveland) 33: 331

Rondot P, Dalloz J-C, Tardieu G 1958 Mesure de la force des réactions musculaires a l'étirement passif aux cours des raideurs pathologiques par lésions cérébrales. Revue Française d'Études Cliniques et Biologiques 3: 585

Roodhooft A M, van Acker K J, van Thienen M N, Martin J J, Ceuterick C 1988 Marshall–Smith syndrome: new aspects. Neuropediatrics 19: 179

Roulet E, Deonna T 1992 Vocal cord paralysis as a presenting sign of acute spinal muscular atrophy (SMA type 1). Archives of Disease in Childhood 67: 352

Rowland L P, Eskenazi A N 1956 Myasthenia gravis with features resembling muscular dystrophy. Neurology (Minneapolis) 6: 667

Sabatelli M, Bertini E, Ricci et al 1992 Peripheral neuropathy with giant axons and cardiomyopathy associated with desmin type intermediate filaments in skeletal muscle. Journal of the Neurological Sciences 109

Sahgal V, Sahgal S 1977 A new congenital myopathy: a morphological cytochemical and histochemical study. Acta Neuropathologica (Berlin) 37: 225

Santavuori P, Leisti J, Kruus S 1977 Muscle, eye and brain disease: a new syndrome. Neuropädiatrie 8 (suppl): 553

Savage D C L, Forbes M, Pearce G W 1971 Idiopathic rhabdomyolysis. Archives of Disease in Childhood 46: 594

Saviranta P, Lindlof M, Lehesjoki A-E et al 1988 Linkage studies in a new X-linked myopathy, suggesting exclusion of the DMD locus and tentative assignment to distal Xq. American Journal of Human Genetics 42: 84

Sawchak J A, Sher J H, Norman M G, Kula R W, Shafiq S A 1991 Centronuclear myopathy heterogeneity: distinction of clinical types by myosin isoform patterns. Neurology 41: 135

Schapira D, Swash M 1985 Neonatal spinal muscular atrophy presenting as respiratory distress: a clinical variant. Muscle and Nerve 8: 661

Schmalbruch H, Kamieniecka Z, Arroe M 1987 Early fatal nemaline myopathy: case report and review. Developmental Medicine and Child Neurology 29: 800

Schreiner M S, Field E, Ruddy R 1991 Infant botulism: a review of 12 years' experience at The Children's Hospital of Philadelphia. Pediatrics 87: 159

Seay A R, Ziter F A, Petajan J H 1977 Rigid spine syndrome: a type I fiber myopathy. Archives of Neurology 34: 119

Shafiq S A, Dubowitz V, Peterson H de C, Milhorat A T 1967 Nemaline myopathy: report of a fatal case, with histochemical and electron miscroscopic studies. Brain 90: 817

Shafiq S A, Sande M A, Carruthers R R, Killip T, Milhorat A T 1972 Skeletal muscle in idiopathic cardiomyopathy. Journal of the Neurological Sciences 15: 303

Shahar E M, Hwang P A, Niesen C E, Murphy E G 1991 Poliomyelitis-like paralysis during recovery from acute bronchial asthma: possible etiology and risk factors. Pediatrics 88: 276

Shapira Y, Cividalli G, Szabo G, Rozin R, Russell A 1974 A myasthenic syndrome in childhood leukemia. Developmental Medicine and Child Neurology 16: 668

Shapira Y, Amit R, Rachmilewitz E 1981 Vitamin E deficiency in Werdnig–Hoffmann disease. Annals of Neurology 10: 266

Shevell M, Rosenblatt B, Silver K, Carpenter S, Karpati G 1990 Congenital inflammatory myopathy. Neurology 40: 1111

Sher J H, Rimalovski A B, Athanassiades T J, Aronson S M 1967 Familial myotubular myopathy: a clinical, pathological, histochemical and ultrastructural study. Journal of Neuropathology and Experimental Neurology 26: 132

Shy G M, Engel W K, Somers J E, Wanko T 1963 Nemaline myopathy: a new congenital myopathy. Brain 86: 793

Shy G M, Gonatas N K, Perez M 1966 Two childhood myopathies with abnormal mitochondria I. Megaconial myopathy. II. Pleoconial myopathy. Brain 89: 133

Shy G M, Magee K R 1956 A new congenital non-progressive myopathy. Brain 79: 610

Sillence D O, Senn A S, Danks D M 1979 Genetic heterogeneity in osteogenesis imperfecta. Journal of Medical Genetics 16: 101

Slater C R, Baxter P, Young C et al 1994 Reduction of dystrophin-related protein (utrophin) at the neuromuscular junction in a case of congenital myasthenia with acetylcholine receptor deficiency. In preparation

Slee J J, Smart R D, Viljoen D L 1991 Deletion of chromosome 13 in Möebius syndrome. Journal of Medical Genetics 28: 413

Smit L M E, Jennekens F G I, Veldman H, Barth P G 1984 Paucity of secondary synaptic clefts in a case of congenital myasthenia with multiple contractures: ultrastructural morphology of a developmental disorder. Journal of Neurology, Neurosurgery and Psychiatry 47: 1091

Smit L M E, Hageman G, Veldman H, Molenaar P C, Oen B S, Jennekens F G I 1988 A myasthenic syndrome with congenital paucity of secondary synaptic clefts: CPSC syndrome. Muscle and Nerve 11: 337

Smith D W, Jones K L 1988 Recognisable patterns of human malformation, 4th edn. Saunders, Philadelphia

Smith M S, Mitchell J, Corey L et al 1991 Chronic fatigue in adolescents. Pediatrics 88: 195

Snead O C, Kohaut E C, Oh S J, Bradley R J 1987 Plasmapheresis for myasthenic crisis in a young child. Journal of Pediatrics 110: 740

Sobue I, Saito N, Iida M, Ando K 1978 Juvenile type of distal and segmental muscular atrophy of upper extremities. Annals of Neurology 3: 429

Sparkes R S, Graham C B 1972 Camurati–Engelmann disease: genetics and clinical manifestations with a review of the literature. Journal of Medical Genetics 9: 73

Spiro A J, Shy G M, Gonatas N K 1966 Myotubular myopathy — persistence of fetal muscle in an adolescent boy. Archives of Neurology 14: 1

Stauber W T, Riggs J E, Schochet S S, Gutmann L,

Crosby T W 1986 Nemaline myopathy; evidence of dipeptidyl peptidase 1 deficiency. Archives of Neurology 43: 39

Steiman G S, Rorke L B, Brown M J 1980 Infantile neuronal degeneration masquerading as Werdnig–Hoffmann disease. Annals of Neurology 8: 317

Stephenson J B P 1980 Prader–Willi syndrome: neonatal presentation and later development. Developmental Medicine and Child Neurology 22: 792

Stoessl A J, Hahn A F, Malott D, Jones D T, Silver M D 1985 Nemaline myopathy with associated cardiomyopathy: report of clinical and detailed autopsy findings. Archives of Neurology 42: 1084

Stollhoff K, Albani M, Goebel H H 1991 Giant axonal neuropathy and leukodystrophy. Pediatric Neurology 7: 69

Sulaiman A R, Swick H M, Kinder D S 1983 Congenital fibre type disproportion with unusual clinico-pathological manifestations. Journal of Neurology, Neurosurgery and Psychiatry 46: 175

Swash M, Schwartz M S 1981 Familial multicore disease with focal loss of cross-striations and ophthalmoplegia. Journal of the Neurological Sciences 52: 1

Tachi N, Nagata N, Wakai S, Chiba S 1991 Congenital muscular dystrophy in Marinesco–Sjögren syndrome. Pediatric Neurology 7: 296

Takebe T, Koide N, Takahashi G 1981 Giant axonal neuropathy: report of two siblings with endocrinological and histological studies. Neuropediatrics 12: 392

Tandan R, Little B W, Emery E S, Good P S, Pendlebury W W, Bradley W G 1987 Childhood giant axonal neuropathy: case report and review of the literature. Journal of the Neurological Sciences 82: 205

Taratuto A L, Sfaello Z M, Rezzonico C, Morales R C 1978 Multicore disease: report of a case with lack of fibre type differentiation. Neuropädiatrie 9: 285

Tein I 1993 Recurrent childhood myoglobinuria. In: Fejerman N, Chamoles N A (eds) New trends in pediatric neurology. Excerpta Medica, Amsterdam, p 185

Tein I, DiMauro S, DeVivo D C 1990 Recurrent childhood myoglobinuria. Advances in Pediatrics 37: 77

Thomas N S T, Williams H, Cole G et al 1990 X linked neonatal centronuclear/myotubular myopathy: evidence for linkage to Xq28 DNA marker loci. Journal of Medical Genetics 27: 284

Telerman-Toppet N, Gerard J M, Coërs C 1973 Central core disease: a study of clinically unaffected muscle. Journal of the Neurological Sciences 19: 207

Thomas P K 1979 Chronic relapsing idiopathic inflammatory polyneuropathy. Neuropädiatrie 10 (suppl): 452

Thompson C E 1982 Infantile myositis. Developmental Medicine and Child Neurology 24: 307

Thomson A J C 1993 Idiopathic lumbosacral plexus neuropathy in two children. Developmental Medicine and Child Neurology 35: 258

Tizard J P M 1949 Osteogenesis imperfecta presenting with delay in walking. Proceedings of the Royal Society of Medicine 42: 80

Tomé R M S, Fardeau M 1975 Congenital myopathy with 'reducing bodies' in muscle fibres. Acta Neuropathologica (Berlin) 31: 207

Touwen B 1976 Neurological development in infancy. Heinemann, London

Towbin A 1969 Latent spinal cord and brain stem injury in newborn infants. Developmental Medicine and Child Neurology 11: 54

Turner H D, Brett E M, Gilbert R J, Ghosh A C, Liebeschuetz H J 1978 Infant botulism in England. Lancet i: 1277

Turner J W A, Lees F 1962 Congenital myopathy — a fifty-year follow up. Brain 85: 733

Vajsar J, Becker L E, Freedom R M, Murphy E G 1993 Familial desminopathy: myopathy with accumulation of desmin-type intermediate filaments. Journal of Neurology, Neurosurgery and Psychiatry 56: 644

Vallat J M, Hugon J, Fressinaud C, Outrequin G, Dumas M, Vallat M 1985 Centronuclear myopathy, cataract and electrical myotonia: a new case. Muscle and Nerve 8: 807

Vanasse M, Dubowitz V 1979 Hereditary motor and sensory neuropathy type I in infancy and childhood: a clinical, electro-diagnostic, genetic and muscle biopsy study. Neuropädiatrie 10 (suppl): 454

Vance J M 1991 Hereditary motor and sensory neuropathies. Journal of Medical Genetics 28: 1 (review)

van der Ven P F M, Jap P H K, Wetzels R H W et al 1991 Postnatal centralization of muscle fibre nuclei in centronuclear myopathy. Neuromuscular Disorders 1: 211

Vanneste J A, Stam F C 1982 Autosomal dominant multicore disease. Journal of Neurology, Neurosurgery and Psychiatry 45: 360

van Wijngaarden G K, Fleury P, Bethlem J, Meijer A E F H 1969 Familial 'myotubular' myopathy. Neurology (Minneapolis) 19: 901

Verhiest W, Brucher J M, Goddeeris P, Lauweryns J, de Geest H 1976 Familial centronuclear myopathy associated with 'cardiomyopathy'. British Heart Journal 38: 504

Vici C D, Burlina A B, Bertini E et al 1991 Progressive neuropathy and recurrent myoglobinuria in a child with long-chain 3-hydroxyacyl-coenzyme A dehydrogenase deficiency. Journal of Pediatrics 118: 744

Vincent A, Newsom-Davis J 1979 Absence of anti-acetylcholine receptor antibodies in congenital myasthenia gravis. Lancet i: 441

Vincent A, Cull-Candy S G, Newsom-Davis J, Trautmann A, Moleaar P C, Polak R L 1981 Congenital myasthenia: end-plate acetylcholine receptors and electrophysiology in five cases. Muscle and Nerve 4: 306

Vinken P J, Bruyn G W, Klawans H L, Rowland L P, DiMauro S (eds) 1992 Myopathies. In: Handbook of clinical neurology, vol 62. Elsevier, Amsterdam

Vital C, Vallat J-M, Martin F, LeBlanc M, Bergouignan M 1970 Étude clinique et ultrastructurale d'un cas de myopathie centronucléaire (myotubular myopathy) de l'adulte. Revue Neurologique 123: 117

Waclawik A J, Sufit R L, Beinlich B R, Schutta H S 1992 Acute myopathy with selective degeneration of myosin filaments following status asthmaticus treated with methylprednisolone and vecuronium. Neuromuscular Disorders 2: 19

Walker B A, Beighton P H, Murdoch J L 1969 The marfanoid hypermobility syndrome. Annals of Internal Medicine 71: 349

Wallgren-Pettersson C, Arjomaa P, Holnberg C 1990a Alpha-actinin and myosin light chains in congenital nemaline myopathy. Pediatric Neurology 6: 171

Wallgren-Pettersson C, Kaariainen H, Rapola J, Salmi T, Jaaskelainen J, Donner M 1990b Genetics of congenital nemaline myopathy: a study of 10 families. Journal of Medical Genetics 27: 480

Walton J N 1956 Amyotonia congenita: a follow-up study. Lancet i: 1023

Walton J N 1957 The limp child. Journal of Neurology, Neurosurgery and Psychiatry 20: 144

Walton J N, Geshwind N, Simpson J A 1956 Benign congenital myopathy with myasthenic features. Journal of Neurology, Neurosurgery and Psychiatry 19: 224

Wang P, Clausen T 1976 Treatment of attacks in hyperkalaemic familial periodic paralysis by inhalation of salbutamol. Lancet i: 221

Watters G V, Barlow C F 1967 Acute and subacute neuropathies. Pediatric Clinics of North America 14: 997

Weinberg A G, Kirkpatrick J B 1975 Cerebellar hypoplasia in Werdnig–Hoffmann disease. Developmental Medicine and Child Neurology 17: 511

Whiteley A M, Schwartz M S, Sachs J A, Swash M 1976 Congenital myasthenia gravis: clinical and HLA studies in two brothers. Journal of Neurology, Neurosurgery and Psychiatry 39: 1145

Williams J, Hosking G 1985 Type V glycogen storage disease. Archives of Disease in Childhood 60: 1184

Wokke J H J, Jennekens F G I, Molenaar P C, van den Oord C J M, Oen B J, Busch H F M 1989 Congenital paucity of synaptic clefts (CPSC) syndrome in 2 adult sibs. Neurology 39: 648

Woolf A L 1960 Muscle biopsy in the diagnosis of the 'floppy baby' (infantile hypotonia). Cerebral Palsy Bulletin 2: 19

Wynne-Davies R, Lloyd-Roberts G C 1976 Arthrogryposis multiplex congenita: search for prenatal factors in 66 sporadic cases. Archives of Disease in Childhood 51: 618

Wynne-Davies R, Williams P F, O'Connor J C B 1981 The 1960s epidemic of arthrogryposis multiplex congenita: a survey from the United Kingdom, Australia and the United States of America. Journal of Bone and Joint Surgery 63B: 76

Yamaguchi M, Robson R M, Stromer M H, Dahl D S, Oda T 1982 Nemaline myopathy rod bodies: structure and composition. Journal of the Neurological Sciences 56: 35

Young I D, Harper P S 1980 Hereditary distal spinal muscular atrophy with vocal cord paralysis. Journal of Neurology, Neurosurgery, and Psychiatry 43: 413

Young J A, Anderson J M 1987 Infantile myopathy with type I fibre specific hypertrophy. Developmental Medicine and Child Neurology 29: 680

Yudell A, Gomez M R, Lambert E H, Dockerty M B 1967 The neuropathy of sulfatide lipidosis (metachromatic leukodystrophy). Neurology (Minneapolis) 17: 103

Yuill G M, Lynch P G 1974 Congenital non-progressive peripheral neuropathy with arthrogryposis multiplex. Journal of Neurology, Neurosurgery and Psychiatry 37: 316

Zellweger H, Schneider H J 1968 Syndrome of hypotonia–hypomentia–hypogonadism–obesity (O) or Prader–Willi syndrome. American Journal of Diseases of Children 115: 588

Ziter F A, Wiser W C, Robinson A 1977 Three-generation pedigree of a Moebius syndrome variant with chromosome translocation. Archives of Neurology 34: 437

Zlotogora J, Ben Ezra D, Livni N, Ashkenazi A, Cohen T 1983 A muscle disorder as presenting symptom in a child with mucolipidosis IV. Neuropediatrics 14: 104

22. Medical and psychological management of neuromuscular disease

R. H. T. Edwards   *Robert C. Griggs*

INTRODUCTION

This chapter deals with practical aspects of the medical treatment and psychological management of patients with neuromuscular disease. Specific treatment is now available for many disorders (Table 22.1) and is considered in appropriate detail in the chapters dealing with each disease. The number of pharmacological agents not yet subjected to rigorous testing is, however, of concern to all clinicians treating patients with neuromuscular disease. With the strong likelihood that the molecular defect will be known in most hereditary neuromuscular diseases within the next decade, there will be new opportunities for treatment and the need to have adequate methods for studying the efficacy of each new strategy. The methods used to study new treatments are also considered in this chapter.

The patient with progressive, disabling weakness for whom there is no specific, pharmacological treatment presents a major challenge to the physician. Patients who require a wheelchair may even be unable to reach physicians' offices. Much can be done to maintain function in such patients despite inexorably progressive weakness. As a rule, only respiratory and cardiac complications are life-threatening. Treatment of these complications is often successful. The consequences of immobility often take an unnecessary toll on life quality in patients and add to the burden imposed upon carers: oedema, obesity, constipation and other gastrointestinal problems, bone loss, and pressure sores are all preventable and most are treatable.

Table 22.1   Specific treatments for neuromuscular diseases

	Modality
Anterior horn cell disorders	
Rabies	Preventive: active and passive immunisation
Poliomyelitis	Preventive: active immunisation
Peripheral nerve disorders	
Guillain-Barré syndrome	Plasma exchange; intravenous immunoglobulin
Chronic inflammatory demyelinating polyneuropathy	Corticosteroids; immunosuppression; plasma exchange; intravenous immunoglobulin
Refsum's disease	Plasma exchange; intravenous immunoglobulin; chlorophyll-free diet
Neuromyotonia	Plasma exchange
Toxic neuropathies	Toxin withdrawal
Neuromuscular junction disorders	
Myasthenia gravis	Anticholinesterases; immunosuppression; thymectomy; plasma exchange; intravenous immunoglobulin
Myasthenic syndrome	3,4-Diaminopyridine; immunosuppression; plasma exchange
Congenital myasthenias	Anticholinesterases; 3,4-diaminopyridine (only some are treatable)
Myopathies	
Duchenne muscular dystrophy	Prednisone (slight-moderate benefit)
Dermatomyositis	Corticosteroids; azathioprine and other immunosuppressants; plasma exchange
Polymyositis, other inflammatory myopathy	Corticosteroids; azathioprine and other immunosuppressants
Endocrine deficiency/excess	Hormone replacement/reduction
Hypokalaemic periodic paralysis	Acetazolamide; dichlorphenamide
Hyperkalaemic periodic paralysis; paramyotonia congenita	Acetazolamide; thiazides
Myotonia	
Autosomal dominant	Phenytoin; quinine; procainamide
Autosomal recessive	Mexiletine; phenytoin
Carnitine deficiency	Corticosteroids; riboflavin; carnitine; propranolol

RESPIRATORY MANAGEMENT

Two important considerations that obtain in following all patients with chronic progressive neuromuscular disease are:

1. Recognition of a second and treatable, coincidental illness
2. Recognizing the presence of atypical manifestations of the underlying neuromuscular disease that might suggest a second diagnosis to the unwary or naive clinician.

In the second instance, inappropriate diagnostic and therapeutic measures may be applied. Both considerations require familiarity with the spectrum of medical illness complicating neuromuscular disease. As an example of coincidental illness that might be overlooked, a patient with severe, wheelchair-bound facioscapulohumeral muscular dystrophy who presents with acute respiratory symptoms, hypoxia and CO_2 retention might

be considered to have end-stage neuromuscular disease. However, since facioscapulohumeral muscular dystrophy seldom causes ventilatory failure (Griggs & Donohoe 1982), it is overwhelmingly likely that a treatable intercurrent illness is present. In this instance, aggressive respiratory support would be indicated. As an example of an unrecognised but well-known manifestation of underlying neuromuscular disease, a child with myotonic dystrophy who presents with colicky abdominal pain and is found to have elevated liver function test results including an abnormal glutamyl transpeptidase (γ-GT) might be suspected of having liver disease. Although a coincidental illness *could* be present, unexplained abdominal pain is a frequent manifestation of childhood myotonic dystrophy (Harper 1989) and the γ-GT and other liver function studies are often elevated in this disease. In practice, one would simply follow the patient with myotonic dystrophy to see if the symptoms and laboratory abnormalities were progressive.

Table 22.2 lists the chronic neuromuscular disorders causing respiratory insufficiency. The availability of techniques for home management of what was once considered 'terminal respiratory failure' and the increasing awareness that ventilator-dependency can be prevented for many years by appropriate treatment, has prompted careful study of the mechanisms leading to ventilatory failure in patients with muscular dystrophy (Smith et al 1991).

Patients with neuromuscular disease characteristically develop a restrictive defect with a reduction in total lung capacity (Newsom-Davis et al 1976, Roussos & Macklem 1982). This fall in lung capacity is the result of a combination of factors: impaired ventilatory musculature leads to chest wall stiffness resulting from a combination of kyphoscoliosis, fibrosis of dystrophic chest muscles, pulmonary microatelectasis, aspiration, and impaired clearing of secretions because of reduced ability to cough (McCool et al 1981, Smith et al 1991). The inability to expand the lungs by a sigh as well as inability to change posture may contribute to restrictive lung disease. The earliest detectable abnormality easily recognised by clinical tests is a reduction in static pressures: maximum expiratory pressure is reduced to a greater extent than maximum inspiratory pressure (Black & Hyatt 1971, Saunders et al 1978, Griggs et al 1981). Other factors contributing to respiratory difficulties include ineffective cough because of impaired glottic function as well as respiratory muscle weakness, impaired central nervous system ventilatory drive, and upper airway obstruction during sleep. Sleep-related respiratory abnormalities have recently been shown to have a major role in ventilatory failure; nocturnal hypoxaemia develops and contributes to cardiac failure (cor pulmonale) and hypercapnia. Nocturnal hypoxaemia first occurs during REM sleep and may be present when other signs of hypoxaemia such as daytime hypoxaemia, carbon dioxide retention and associated symptoms are lacking (Coakley et al 1990). Duchenne muscular dystrophy (Smith et al 1988, 1989a,b, Carroll et al 1991), myotonic dystrophy (Gilmartin et al 1991), as well as other myopathies (Ellis et al 1987) have been shown to have sleep-related hypoxaemia well in advance of other signs of ventilatory failure. Since treatment of this process with nocturnal respiratory support is now practical (Garay et al 1981, Ellis et al 1987, Heckmatt et al 1990) and since studies to detect hypoxaemia can be obtained with no morbidity and can even be done as an outpatient (Carroll et al 1991), patients with neuromuscular disease must be followed prospectively for the possibility of impending ventilatory difficulties.

Acute respiratory failure

Acute respiratory failure is usually precipitated by a readily apparent event such as pneumonitis, bronchitis, atelectasis, aspiration, pneumothorax, congestive heart failure, or some other intercurrent process (Griggs & Donohoe 1985). In follow-

Table 22.2 Chronic respiratory muscle insufficiency with neuromuscular diseases

Anterior horn cell disease	Motor neurone disease (amyotrophic lateral sclerosis)[*] Spinal muscular atrophy (especially Werdnig–Hoffman disease); late progression of poliomyelitis
Peripheral neuropathy	Charcot–Marie–Tooth disease Neuralgic amyotrophy [†] Chronic relapsing polyneuritis[†]
Neuromuscular junction disorders	Myasthenia gravis[*]; Lambert–Eaton syndrome[*]
Myopathy	Muscular dystrophies: Duchenne dystrophy; Becker dystrophy [†]; autosomal recessive childhood dystrophy; myotonic dystrophy[*]; limb-girdle dystrophy; facioscapulohumeral dystrophy[†], scapuloperoneal dystrophy Metabolic disorders: acid maltase deficiency[*]; carnitine deficiency Congenital myopathies: centronuclear myopathy; nemaline myopathy Polymyositis/dermatomyositis[†]

[*] May present with respiratory failure prior to other signs of weakness.
[†] Respiratory muscle insufficiency uncommon.

ing patients with neuromuscular disease, when the forced vital capacity falls below 30% of normal, both the patient and family should be warned of the risk of both acute and chronic ventilatory failure and management options should be discussed. A decision about providing ventilatory assistance is complex and depends upon the availability of carers and of appropriate social and financial support, the tempo of the disease, the life-style, and the wishes of the patient. A number of thoughtful discussions and studies of this problem are now available and all physicians caring for chronic neuromuscular disease must be attuned to this issue (Madorsky et al 1984, Mendell & Vaughn 1984, Goldblatt 1984, Silverstein et al 1991).

Prevention of respiratory complications

In neuromuscular diseases where respiratory muscle involvement is expected (Table 22.2) the forced vital capacity should be obtained at least annually. If respiratory symptoms develop, both the forced vital capacity and static pressure (particularly maximum expiratory pressure) should be obtained. A reduction of forced vital capacity with the preservation of maximum expiratory pressure indicates that respiratory symptoms are not due to the restrictive effect of neuromuscular weakness (Griggs et al 1981, Griggs & Donohoe 1985). A coincidental process is likely to be present. Chronic obstructive lung disease, for example, is present in at least 25% of patients over the age of 50 and is frequently confused with the results of 'end-stage' neuromuscular disease.

If the forced vital capacity is reduced to less than 50% of normal, respiratory exercises should be instituted, and a chest radiograph and electrocardiogram (EGG) should be obtained. All patients should receive a single programme of immunisation against pneumococcal infections (Schwartz 1982) and in patients with a vital capacity of less than 30%, annual immunisation for influenza viral infection should be administered (ACIP 1984). The major exception to the use of respiratory exercises is in disorders characterised by fatigability such as myasthenia gravis where exercise may pose hazards. Although intermittent positive pressure breathing has been recommended in the past as a means of improving lung compliance, there is evidence that it is ineffective in neuromuscular disease patients (McCool et al 1981).

Expectant management of respiratory failure

Patients with amyotrophic lateral sclerosis, Duchenne dystrophy, and the late stages of other neuromuscular diseases need to be told the risk of both acute and chronic ventilatory failure and management options discussed. It is important that a plan of action (or inaction) be charted and discussed carefully. Patients, even boys with Duchenne dystrophy, are well aware of the likelihood that respiratory failure will develop eventually and are reassured by such discussions. Patients often mistakenly anticipate that death is imminent at a time when their respiratory function is adequate or even normal.

Management of acute respiratory failure

Patients who are obtunded or dyspnoeic associated with hypoxia and hypercapnia usually require emergency endotracheal intubation. If hypoxia alone is present and the patient is alert, low flow oxygen (less than 1 l/min) may correct hypoxia without causing hypercapnia. Special equipment is often necessary to provide reliable low flow rates. If oxygen is administered in the acute setting, it is essential to obtain blood gases frequently to exclude the development of hypercapnia. Oxygenation can be monitored by digital oximetry. Patients with respiratory muscle weakness are often intermittently hypercapnic and the administration of oxygen may further depress already decreased ventilatory drive and worsen hypoventilation (Weinberger et al 1989). Specific treatment of ventilatory failure depends on the cause. The commonest event to precipitate ventilatory failure is atelectasis which can be improved by ventilatory support, appropriate suctioning of secretions, hydration, and postural drainage. Pathogens are seldom cultured from bronchial secretions at the time of acute presentation. Antibiotics are indicated if the sputum is purulent or there are other clinical findings to support the presence of infection.

Long-term ventilatory support

Negative pressure ventilation such as the cuirass (Holtackers et al 1982) and plastic 'raincoat' (Griggs & Donohoe 1982) devices are occasionally helpful but are not well tolerated by alert patients with normal sensation. Over the past decade, positive pressure nasal mechanical ventilation during sleep has been applied with success to patients with neuromuscular disease. Duchenne dystrophy (Rideau et al 1981, Heckmatt et al 1990), amyotrophic lateral sclerosis and many other disorders (Ellis et al 1987) are amenable to such treatment. If glottic dysfunction impairs cough, the retention of secretions ultimately poses an insurmountable problem for the use of negative pressure ventilators or positive pressure nasal ventilation and in this situation tracheostomy is necessary. Most end-stage patients with motor neurone disease, Duchenne dystrophy, myotonic dystrophy, and Becker dystrophy in whom assisted respiration is considered appropriate will ultimately require tracheostomy and positive pressure ventilation. Tracheostomy permits normal speech and provides an easy means of clearing tracheal secretions. If tracheostomy is performed, it must be done in hospital and usually requires 1–3 days of intensive care unit hospita-

lisation and subsequently 1–2 weeks of training for patients and carers to help them develop the necessary skills for outpatient management. Atelectasis often develops in the postoperative period and may necessitate longer respiratory care in the hospital. The goal of ventilatory support is to return the patient to an active life-style and to permit both patient and family to maintain activities outside the home. With lightweight, portable, rechargeable ventilators, portable suction equipment, and a wheelchair that accommodates the equipment, patients who require ventilatory support can often continue attending school and even maintain employment. The possibility of providing long-term ventilatory support for patients with neuromuscular disease poses both ethical and economic issues that have been considered in recent reviews (Goldblatt 1984, Goldblatt & Greenlaw 1989, Silverstein et al 1991). An account of one Duchenne dystrophy patient's decision to pursue ventilatory support makes compelling reading (Eberhardt 1988).

CARDIAC COMPLICATIONS

Symptomatic cardiac disease is relatively uncommon in neuromuscular disease (Table 22.3). Histopathological, electrocardiographic and ultrasonographic studies, however, indicate that myocardial involvement is extremely frequent in myopathies (Reeves et al 1980, Nippoldt et al

Table 22.3 Chronic neuromuscular diseases with cardiac disease

Congestive cardiomyopathy	
Muscular dystrophy	Limb-girdle, myotonic, Duchenne, Becker, Emery–Dreifuss[*]
Congenital myopathy	Nemaline
Metabolic myopathy	Acid maltase (infantile disease), carnitine deficiency, X-linked glycogen storage diseases, Type III glycogen storage disease
Inflammatory myopathy	Polymyositis/dermatomyositis
Cor pulmonale	
Muscular dystrophy	Duchenne, Becker, myotonic, limb-girdle
Congenital	Nemaline myopathy
Metabolic	Acid maltase deficiency
Arrhythmias	
Muscular dystrophy	Myotonic[*], limb-girdle, Emery–Dreifuss[*]
Metabolic	Kearns–Sayre syndrome, Andersen's syndrome[*], hyperkalaemic periodic paralysis
Inflammatory	Polymyositis/dermatomyositis
Mitral valve prolapse	
Muscular dystrophy	Myotonic, Duchenne

[*] May present with cardiac disease.

1982). Primary myocardial involvement with a congestive cardiomyopathy occurs in a proportion of patients with Duchenne and Becker muscular dystrophy (Brooke et al 1989). Prospective studies indicate that patients with relatively preserved ambulation are more likely to develop clinical cardiac disease (Brooke et al 1989). Cardiomyopathy is occasionally the presenting manifestation of a neuromuscular disorder (Norris et al 1966, Griggs 1974) (Table 22.3). In such patients, as in all instances of apparent primary myocardial disease in association with neuromuscular disease, the possibility that cardiac failure may be the direct result of respiratory insufficiency and consequent cor pulmonale must be carefully pursued. Oximetry should be performed in all instances. Even patients with normoxaemia during the day may have severe sleep apnoea or hypoventilation with nocturnal hypoxia (see above). Night-time respiratory support that eliminates this hypoxia will correct heart failure.

If cardiac failure is indeed present as a result of myocardial involvement treatment options are limited. Fluid restriction, diuretics such as frusemide and after-load reduction with agents such as the angiotensin-converting enzyme inhibitors may be of benefit. Patients with ejection fractions of <50% should be anticoagulated to prevent emboli. In unusual patients where primary myocardial disease has been the dominant feature of an illness with mild skeletal muscle weakness, cardiac transplantation has been performed with successful return to near-normal activities (Donofrio et al 1989).

Cardiac arrhythmias commonly complicate several neuromuscular diseases. Complete heart block requiring pacemaker implantation is frequent in myotonic dystrophy (Griggs et al 1975, Moorman et al 1985, Editorial 1992), Emery–Dreifuss muscular dystrophy and mitochondrial myopathies. Life-threatening tachyarrhythmias are infrequent in most myopathies but are characteristic of Andersen's syndrome (Andersen et al 1971) (hyperkalemic periodic paralysis with bidirectional tachycardia). Myotonic dystrophy, Duchenne dystrophy, Becker dystrophy and occasional patients with humeroperoneal or scapuloperoneal muscular dystrophy can have atrial or ventricular arrhythmias that require therapy.

PREVENTION OF OEDEMA

Oedema of the feet, ankles, or in the bed-bound patient, the presacral region, is frequent in the severely immobilised patient with neuromuscular disease. The appearance of oedema should prompt clinical evaluation for:

1. Respiratory failure and cor pulmonale
2. Cardiomyopathy, or
3. A coincidental illness such as renal disease, hypoalbuminaemia, or drug-related fluid retention.

In most patients with neuromuscular disease, however, ankle oedema is the combined result of a loss of muscle pumping action and the dependency of the legs. Oedema is a particular hazard in patients with neuromuscular disease because it increases the weight of the extremities, further compromising mobility. Oedema also causes tissue damage leading to skin infection and ulceration.

Prevention and treatment of ankle oedema

Medications that cause or worsen ankle oedema should be avoided: amitriptyline and other tricyclic antidepressants, non-steroidal anti-inflammatory agents, and β-adrenergic blocking agents and calcium channel blocking agents are particularly likely to precipitate or exacerbate ankle oedema. Wheelchair-bound patients should have elevating leg rests to avoid the complete dependency of the lower extremities. Elevation of the foot of the bed at night by placing a cushion between a mattress and the inner springs (not under the legs themselves) is often well tolerated and will lessen oedema in patients who can spend a period of the day in bed. Elastic support stockings may decrease oedema but are often uncomfortable and require frequent reapplication so that both patient and carers are reluctant to use them. Sodium restriction has theoretical benefits but is often unacceptable to patients. Patients often request diuretics; anecdotally, frusemide is effective in eliminating ankle oedema. Diuretic treatment poses the risk of electrolyte imbalance and should be avoided where possible.

GASTROINTESTINAL COMPLICATIONS

All portions of the alimentary system are subject to involvement by one or more neuromuscular diseases (Table 22.4). Although most myopathies have their major impact on skeletal muscle, emerging data on diseases such as Duchenne muscular dystrophy, where it is clear that that dystrophin is deficient in smooth muscle, indicate that major, symptomatic involvement of the gastrointestinal tract is a direct consequence of the disease (Barohn et al 1988). In other instances, gastrointestinal complications may be the result of immobility.

Abnormalities of deglutition

Patients with bulbar weakness may develop nasal regurgitation of liquids when they swallow. Myasthenia gravis, the Kennedy syndrome (bulbar spinal muscular atrophy) and congenital myasthenic disorders are notable examples. Impaired function of pharyngeal muscles results in pooling of secretions in the hypopharynx and usually leads to aspiration. Atelectasis and pulmonary infection may result but are not frequent unless there is coincidental weakness of respiratory and glottic muscles that impairs cough. Patients with abnormalities of swallowing usually recognise their problem and localise the difficulty. Patients with oculopharyngeal muscular dystrophy, inclusion body myositis, dermatomyositis and motor neurone disease (progressive bulbar palsy) are susceptible to cricopharyngeal achalasia and indicate the site of obstruction by pointing to the submental and glottic regions. These disorders affect the striated muscle of the upper one-third of the oesophagus. If the obstruction or motility disturbance is located in the lower portion of the oesophagus (as occurs in scleroderma, the mixed connective tissue syndrome, and uncommonly in dermatomyositis) the patient will point to the substernal region as the site of obstruction or pain.

Occasionally patients with severe swallowing dysfunction have no spontaneous complaints referable to deglutition. Such unrecognised difficulty with swallowing is frequently seen in oculopharyngeal muscular dystrophy and myotonic dystrophy. Patients may present with unexplained cough, unexplained dyspnoea at mealtimes, recurrent pulmonary infection because of aspiration, and remarkably, may even lose weight to the point of inanition while not directly complaining of swallowing difficulties.

Cricopharyngeal achalasia Cricopharyngeal achalasia is important to recognise because it can be corrected surgically by the cricopharyngeal myotomy. If the cricopharyngeus muscle does not contract normally, food remains in the hypopharynx. Cricopharyngeal achalasia is frequent in oculopharyngeal muscular dystrophy and occurs in other syndromes with progressive external ophthalmoplegia. It is also prominent in a subset of

---

Table 22.4   Gastrointestinal manifestations of neuromuscular disease

Abnormalities of deglutition
   Nasal regurgitation: myasthenia gravis; motor neurone disease (progressive bulbar palsy, amyotrophic lateral sclerosis);
      Kennedy syndrome
   Dysphagia:
     Pain — dermatomyositis; polymyositis
     Inability to swallow — dermatomyositis; polymyositis; myotonic dystrophy; motor neurone disease
   Cricopharyngeal achalasia: oculopharyngeal muscular dystrophy; inclusion body myositis; dermatomyositis; polymyositis;
     myotonic dystrophy; motor neurone disease
   Oesophageal hypomotility: dermatomyositis; polymyositis; myotonic dystrophy
Abnormalities of gastrointestinal function
   Gastroparesis or gastric dilatation: Duchenne dystrophy; mitochondrial myopathies
   Intestinal hypomotility: pseudo-obstruction; Duchenne dystrophy; Becker dystrophy; mitochondrial myopathies
   Megacolon: myotonic dystrophy; mitochondrial myopathies
   Constipation: Duchenne dystrophy; Becker dystrophy; myotonic dystrophy; most neuromuscular diseases resulting in loss of
     ambulation
Biliary tract disease; Myotonic dystrophy

patients with polymyositis and inclusion body myositis (Palmer 1976, Kagen et al 1985, Lotz et al 1989, Verma et al 1991). Patients with these diseases should be followed expectantly for the development of swallowing difficulties. Patients with oculopharyngeal muscular dystrophy, in particular, should have studies of swallowing function once their disease has reached the point of marked ptosis and ophthalmoparesis (Weitzner 1969).

Patients with neuromuscular disease and abnormal swallowing function who develop severe weight loss or recurrent aspiration need studies of swallowing function. In motor neurone disease, in particular, cricopharyngeal myotomy may restore swallowing capability at least for a few weeks or months; when dysphagia becomes intolerable, however, an invasive procedure will be needed to provide adequate nutrition. Percutaneous gastrostomy is now the procedure of choice for virtually all patients with the inability to maintain alimentation. The sole exceptions are patients with previous gastric surgery, and the ambulatory patient with selective involvement of muscles of deglutition such as is occasionally seen in dermatomyositis, polymyositis, and inclusion body myositis. Here, an open gastrostomy is necessary in order to position the feeding tube high in the abdomen (avoiding problems of acid reflux).

Gastric and intestinal abnormalities

Duchenne dystrophy patients have impaired gastric motility and may present with severe gastric dilatation and intestinal pseudo-obstruction (Barohn et al 1988). Treatment consists of decompression of the dilated stomach with a nasal gastric tube and *parenteral* fluids. Low-dose metaclopramide 10–20 mg/day has been helpful in preventing this complication in our anecdotal experience. In the MNGIE syndrome (mitochondrial myopathy, peripheral neuropathy, gastrointestinal disease, and encephalopathy) involvement of intestinal muscles results in episodes of pseudo-obstruction caused by visceral neuropathy (Cevera et al 1988, Blake et al 1990). The syndrome occurs with cytochrome oxidase deficiency and may well reflect a mitochondrial disorder of visceral nerves. Dermatomyositis, particularly in childhood, is associated with a vasculitis that can culminate in

intestinal perforation (Banker & Victor 1966). This complication is rarely encountered in adequately treated patients. Patients with polymyositis and inclusion body myositis are not susceptible to this abnormality. Other disorders of gastric and oesophageal function also occur in various myopathies (Swick et al 1981, Horowitz et al 1986, Yoshida et al 1988, Camilleri 1990).

Constipation. Management of constipation represents a major treatment problem in most bed-bound patients with neuromuscular disease. The inconvenience of toileting results in most patients electing to restrict their own fluids severely (often to less than 500 ml a day) and choosing a low-residue, low-fibre diet. Patients can be encouraged to improve constipation by taking larger fluid amounts and eating high residue foods only if there is sufficient attention to making it easy for them to void and defaecate. Medications are usually necessary. Stool softeners and natural or synthetic cellulose moistening agents are preferable to bowel-irritating laxatives. Magnesium-containing preparations such as magnesium sulphate are often necessary on an intermittent basis. Magnesium-containing agents are potentially hazardous in patients with neuromuscular junction diseases or any neuromuscular disorder associated with coincidental renal insufficiency.

Both children and adults always have questions concerning bowel function which they will raise in the setting of a private, supportive consultation. It is our impression that adequate attention to these questions will prevent the severe obstipation which is unfortunately common in end-stage neuromuscular disease. Rectal suppositories, various forms of enema, and manual disimpaction often become necessary if preventive measures are delayed. Lactulose (30 ml 1–3 times a day) and pyridostigmine bromide (15–60 mg) have the potential hazards of producing electrolyte imbalance and parasympathetic toxicity respectively but are occasionally helpful. In following patients with neuromuscular disease it is important to prevent hypokalaemia which will lead to intestinal ileus and may exacerbate weakness. Patients with gastric dilatation, intestinal pseudo-obstruction, or those that require frequent enemas are particularly vulnerable to this problem.

Dietary treatment and prevention of obesity

There is no evidence that any dietary modification improves muscle strength or function in patients with neuromuscular disease. Prevention of obesity in both young and old patients with neuromuscular disease is extremely important and requires careful prospective dietary management and follow-up of weight. Excessive weight is both cosmetically disabling and limiting to mobility. It is difficult, but no less important, to determine the weight of wheelchair-bound and bed-bound adult patients. Patients must be followed in facilities that have wheelchair-weighing and bed-weighing capability. If patients are not losing weight as their disease progresses, they are gaining adipose tissue. As with children, prospective dietary counselling is essential. Once obesity is established, severe dietary restriction is necessary, depriving the patient of one of their few physical pleasures. Severe dietary restriction can, however, reduce obesity without compromising muscle mass (Edwards et al 1984). The normal growth and development charts used by clinical nutritionists and dietitians make no allowance for the progressive loss of muscle that occurs in childhood muscular dystrophy or spinal muscular atrophy. Unless the child appears somewhat cachectic, excess body fat is almost certainly present. An ideal weight centile chart for Duchenne dystrophy is useful in the management of patients (Griffiths & Edwards 1988) (Fig. 22.1).

Only a limited number of studies of metabolic rate have been performed but these confirm that the basal metabolic rate declines in the wasted patient with diseases such as myotonic dystrophy. Muscle mass as assessed by creatinine excretion (Griggs et al 1983) correlates well with the reduction in metabolic rate (Jozefowicz et al 1987). In practice it is more important to follow weight than to assess muscle mass in following patients.

PRESSURE-RELATED (DECUBITUS) ULCERS

Patients with progressive neuromuscular disease cannot 'fidget' and reposition themselves nor-

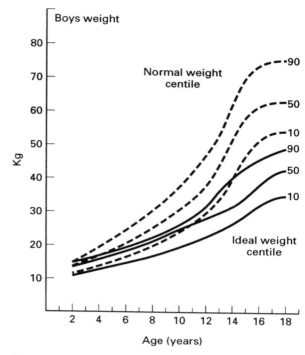

Fig. 22.1 Ideal weight centile chart for boys with Duchenne muscular dystrophy. Assumes a 4% per year decline in muscle bulk (Griffiths & Edwards 1988).

mally. They are also unable to turn themselves at night in contrast to normal subjects where unconscious repositioning occurs 10–20 times per night. Normal subjects awaken only one to three times per night and such movements are largely unconscious. Neuromuscular patients, in contrast, awaken because they are uncomfortable and as a result have severe interruption of sleep. Patients are, however, surprisingly free of decubitus ulcers unless sensory involvement decreases the awareness of pressure. Duchenne dystrophy and motor neurone disease respectively, the commonest childhood and adult neuromuscular diseases resulting in quadriplegia, do not usually develop pressure-related ulcers. The Duchenne patient, in particular, becomes increasingly difficult to manage because of his needs to be repositioned frequently at night — often at 20–30 minute intervals, a trial for the patient and parents.

However, in diseases where sensation is disturbed, pressure necrosis is common and must be prevented by appropriate precautions. Older patients with diseases sparing sensory systems including motor neurone disease and myasthenia gravis commonly have coincidental peripheral nerve, spinal cord or central nervous system disease which decreases the perception of pain or increases pain tolerance.

Alert young patients demand frequent repositioning and carers will be equally insistent on finding aids to decrease the need for repositioning. Older, immobile patients should be provided with the same equipment to prevent pressure necrosis. Electrical alternating pressure mattresses for night-time use are helpful. Waterbeds or equally weight-distributing (but expensive) bead-filled mattresses are helpful in improving sleep quality and decrease the number of repositionings necessary. Wheelchair-bound patients benefit from gel cushions in the chair. Body jackets used to treat scoliosis and calipers (orthoses) must be carefully padded and skin inspected regularly.

Patients with peripheral neuropathy (or their carer) must be taught to inspect areas of pressure. The feet are vulnerable in hereditary neuropathies with decreased distal sensation. Perforating ulcers, osteomyelitis and Charcot joints are frequent. Not uncommonly, the first and presenting symptom of a foot ulcer that penetrates deeply to the bone is that the feet are malodorous. Patients should inspect the soles of their feet with a mirror daily. The inside of shoes must also be inspected and palpated (by someone other than the patient if hand sensation is reduced) for small nails and pebbles.

PSYCHOLOGICAL SUPPORT

The effect of childhood neuromuscular disease on family life

The presence of a patient with Duchenne muscular dystrophy or other childhood neuromuscular disease in a family creates great stress and anxiety in addition to a host of practical problems (Firth 1983, Firth et al 1983). In many Duchenne families there are two or more brothers with the disease because the cause of delayed walking was not diagnosed before the time the second son was conceived. Once diagnosis is confirmed in the index case the second is diagnosed at an earlier

age, although this is scarcely a consolation or help. Mobilisation of family, neighbourhood and social resources usually follows, though some families remain isolated and disadvantaged. The Muscular Dystrophy Group of Great Britain, the Muscular Dystrophy Association (in the USA) and equivalent organisations in other countries provide an important practical source of education and support as well as an opportunity to work towards the goal of rational treatment of the disease and, where possible, its prevention.

Group sessions where patients and families share the experience of dealing with practical problems in everyday life are helpful in coping. They also learn of the benefits of involvement in integrated treatment programmes which combine rational care and trials of putative therapeutic agents. Neuromuscular disease clinics play a valuable role in giving a specialist diagnostic service and genetic counselling. Because of disease rarity the patient's family doctor may be at a disadvantage because he or she may never have had personal experience of managing the disease. Too often in the past families were frustrated by the time taken to secure a specialist opinion and hence a diagnosis. Then when given the bad news the impression is gained that nothing can be done and families are left with the burden of caring while waiting for the premature death of their child. It is necessary to be sensitive in recommending literature for patients which describes the course and complications of the disease. The literature provides information relevant to the problems of patients at varying stages. It is potentially hurtful for the family to learn of disease progression too soon, since the time-course of the disease can vary from one patient to the next and most importantly depends on how vigorously the patient and his family determine to avoid complications. It can be helpful to remind the parents, on being informed of the diagnosis (first in a provisional form, to be confirmed after a period of observation) that their child has not changed at all *that day* as a consequence of the diagnosis.

Presenting the diagnosis

It is wise for a senior specialist in neuromuscular disease to discuss diagnosis with the patient or the family. It should not be delegated to a more junior individual or to the general practitioner. When the diagnosis is muscular dystrophy, the confirmation of the parent's suspicion by a specialist may leave them numbed and frightened with confused emotions of denial, rejection and often the reactions through which the recently bereaved pass. For the parents of a child with muscular dystrophy or other severe childhood neuromuscular disease, as for the bereaved, it is important to work through these emotions by articulating fears, resentments and worries to a sympathetic person who can explain in an honest but positive way what lies ahead while suggesting means by which the family achieve a coping strategy.

It is important to deal with parents' questions fully at the initial discussion of diagnosis but one should not talk at length about other issues. Once the parents hear the diagnosis, they are often unable to assimilate other information. Further discussion of management should be deferred to subsequent visits. It is unhelpful and indeed a dereliction of the medical advisor's duty to present the diagnosis and leave the family unsupported. It is illogical and unkind to change the attitudes of the parents to their child as a result of telling them what may happen at some future date. For the time being the realisation that their child is not as others is the first step towards rational coping with their problem. The next is to ensure that they realise that what may happen in the future and indeed the timescale over which deterioration can occur is going to depend on how the problems of the present are dealt with from day to day. It is therefore in a spirit of determination to face and overcome difficulties as they occur that the family can afford to be optimistic in their endeavours to support research for effective treatment, and in the case of Duchenne dystrophy, for example, it is now reasonable to discuss the prospect that effective gene therapy may become available in the not too distant future. What is understandable but less than satisfactory is the wish for a 'cure' which will put all to right without any effort on the part of the patient or his family to prevent or to correct complications.

Schooling

Considerable anxieties occur over the question of schooling. The aim is to provide the education that the child's intellectual endowment allows him or her to attain while sustaining the necessary care in the form of physiotherapy and orthotics. Important for the child's emotional development is his opportunity to take part in as many experiences as possible with normal children of similar age. Duchenne muscular dystrophy patients often have impaired intellectual capacity with approximately a 20% downward shift in the distribution of intelligence quotient (Dubowitz 1965).

Intellectual impairment is also common in early-onset myotonic dystrophy (Harper 1989). Patients with other childhood neuromuscular diseases are usually of normal intelligence and patients with spinal muscular atrophy often of *above* average IQ (Worden et al 1962). Remarkably, some patients with a decreased IQ and severe disability show talent in drawing or other non-physically demanding activities and most are able to perform activities such as computer studies.

The later years

For the patient with Duchenne muscular dystrophy it is distressing to see his contemporaries deteriorating and eventually dying while he becomes aware of his own progressive weakness and further disability. So far little has been done formally to explore the attitudes of the patient to his impending demise. Our own discussions with individuals who have approached their end with more or less equanimity indicate a progressive weariness with the struggles of life.

In 'So briefly my son' Joan Neville described (Neville 1962) the last illness of her son with Duchenne muscular dystrophy who died of pneumonia 12 days before he would have become 13 years of age. Today in the UK and other countries of Europe or North America there must be very few patients with Duchenne muscular dystrophy who die as young as this. Antibiotics, physiotherapy, nursing care, spinal surgery and respiratory care have increased the life expectancy by 10 or more years. It is unwise and unkind for the doctor to attempt to be too precise in predicting the eventual life expectancy. Rather it is to be hoped that by dealing promptly and appropriately with each problem the illness which could be the last may be averted to some future date.

THERAPEUTIC TRIALS IN NEUROMUSCULAR DISEASE

The prospect for the development of new treatments for chronic, progressive neuromuscular disease is bright. The steps necessary for such discoveries have been carefully reviewed in the past (Brooke et al 1981, 1983, Brooke & CIDD Group 1984, Edwards 1984, Armitage 1985). In general, the first step in developing therapy is to characterise the course of the untreated disease by charting the natural history. Such natural history studies must:

1. Be longitudinal (i.e. following patients for many months or even years depending on the rate of disease progression)
2. Be cross-sectional (i.e. determining the findings of a large group of patients at each age and stage of disease)
3. Be conducted in a homogeneous, defined population of patients with the disease
4. Employ quantitative measures that can be used to derive statistically analysable data. For weakness, forced vital capacity (Griggs 1990), manual muscle testing (Brooke et al 1983, Florence et al 1992), quantitative myometry (Edwards et al 1987, Brussock et al 1992) and timed functional testing (Brooke et al 1983, Moxley 1990) can all be employed. There are other important manifestations of neuromuscular disease that require similar quantitation such as myotonia (Torres et al

1983) and dysphagia (Nathadwarawala et al 1992).

Using natural history data it is then possible to determine:

1. The variability of a quantitative measurement between different tests in the same patient, tests by different examiners, and variation amongst patients
2. The rate of change of the measurement over time
3. The number of patients and extent of treatment response necessary to produce a statistically significant change in the natural history over any specified interval of time (Brooke et al 1983).

The introduction of a therapeutic modality is usually conducted in a small group of patients to establish safety. Even a single patient, carefully studied, can provide important information. If the natural history has been charted, it is possible to perform a relatively small controlled therapeutic trial using historical controls (Mendell et al 1987). The randomised, double-masked controlled trial remains the 'gold standard' for therapeutic trials but can seldom be performed until there is preliminary evidence for safety and efficacy of the proposed treatment. Fortunately, many groups have begun to address the quantitation of the natural history of many of the neuromuscular diseases: Duchenne dystrophy, myotonic dystrophy, facioscapulohumeral dystrophy, amyotrophic lateral sclerosis, periodic paralysis, spinal muscular atrophy and others.

REFERENCES

ACIP 1984 Prevention and control of influenza. MMWR 33: 252, 365
Andersen E D, Krasilnikoff P A, Overvad H 1971 Intermittent muscular weakness, extrasystoles, and multiple developmental anomalies. Acta Paediatrica Scandinavica 60: 559
Armitage P 1985 The search for optimality in clinical trials. International Statistical Review 53: 15
Banker B Q, Victor M 1966 Dermatomyositis (systemic angiopathy) of childhood. Medicine 45: 261
Barohn R J, Levin E J, Olson J O, Mendell J R 1988 Gastric motility in Duchenne's muscular dystrophy. New England Journal of Medicine 319: 15

Black L F, Hyatt R E 1971 Maximal static respiratory pressures in generalized neuromuscular disease. American Review of Respiratory Disease 103: 641
Blake D, Lombes A, Minetti C et al 1990 MNGIE syndrome: report of 2 new patients. Neurology 40: 294
Brooke M H, CIDD Group 1984 Therapeutic trials in Duchenne muscular dystrophy — the scientific difference between 'didn't' and 'doesn't'. Italian Journal of Neurological Sciences 1 (suppl 3 Muscular dystrophy facts and perspectives): 127
Brooke M H, Fenichel G M, Griggs R C, Mendell J R, Moxley R T, Miller J P, and the CIDD Group 1989 Duchenne muscular dystrophy: patterns of clinical

progression and effects of supportive therapy. Neurology 39: 475

Brooke M H, Fenichel G M, Griggs R C et al 1983 Clinical investigation in Duchenne muscular dystrophy: 2 Determination of the 'power' of therapeutic trials based on the natural history. Muscle and Nerve 6: 91

Brooke M H, Griggs R C, Mendell J R, Fenichel G M, Shumate J B, Pellegrino R J 1981 Clinical trial in Duchenne muscular dystrophy. I. The design of the protocol. Muscle and Nerve 4: 186

Brussock C M, Haley S M, Munsat T L, Bernhardt D B 1992 Measurement of isometric force in children with and without Duchenne's muscular dystrophy. Physical Therapy 72: 105

Camilleri M 1990 Subject review: disorders of gastrointestinal motility in neurologic diseases. Mayo Clinic Proceedings 65: 825

Carroll N, Bain R J I, Smith P E M, Saltissi S, Edwards R H T, Calverley P M A 1991 Domiciliary investigation of sleep-related hypoxaemia in Duchenne muscular dystrophy. European Respiratory Journal 4: 434

Cevera R, Bruix J, Bayes A et al 1988 Chronic intestinal pseudoobstruction and ophthalmoplegia in a patient with mitochondrial myopathy. Gut 29: 544

Coakley J H, Edwards R H T, Calverley P M A 1990 Sleep and breathing pattern in myotonic dystrophy: effect of mazindol. Thorax 45: 336

Donofrio P D, Challa V R, Hackshaw B T, Mills S A, Cordell A R 1989 Cardiac transplantation in a patient with muscular dystrophy and cardiomyopathy. Archives of Neurology 46: 705

Dubowitz V 1965 Intellectual impairment in muscular dystrophy. Archives of Disease in Childhood 40: 296

Eberhardt M 1988 Mark's test. Vantage, New York

Editorial 1992 The heart in myotonic dystrophy. Lancet 339: 528

Edwards R H T 1984 Nuclear magnetic resonance and other new techniques for the study of metabolism in human muscular dystrophy. Italian Journal of Neurological Sciences 1 (suppl 3 Muscular dystrophy, facts and perspectives): 75

Edwards R H T, Chapman S J, Newham D J, Jones D A 1987 Practical analysis of variability of muscle function measurements in Duchenne muscular dystrophy. Muscle and Nerve 10: 6

Edwards R H T, Round J M, Jackson M J, Griffiths R D, Lilburn M F 1984 Weight reduction in boys with muscular dystrophy. Developmental Medicine and Child Neurology 26: 375

Ellis E R, Bye P T P, Bruderer J W, Sullivan C E 1987 Treatment of respiratory failure during sleep in patients with neuromuscular disease. American Review of Respiratory Disease 135: 148

Firth M A 1983 Diagnosis of Duchenne muscular dystrophy: experiences of parents of sufferers. British Medical Journal 286: 700

Firth M A, Gardner-Medwin D, Hosking G, Wilkinson E 1983 Interviews with parents of boys suffering from Duchenne muscular dystrophy. Developmental Medicine and Child Neurology 25: 466

Florence J M, Pandya S, King W M et al 1992 Intrarater reliability of manual muscle test (Medical Research Council Scale) grades in Duchenne's muscular dystrophy. Physical Therapy 72: 115

Garay S M, Turino G M, Goldring R M 1981 Sustained

reversal of chronic hypercapnia in patients with alveolar hypoventilation syndromes: long-term maintenance with noninvasive nocturnal mechanical ventilation. American Journal of Medicine 70: 269

Gilmartin J J, Cooper B G, Griffith C J et al 1991 Breathing during sleep in patients with myotonic dystrophy and non-myotonic respiratory muscle weakness. Quarterly Journal of Medicine 78: 21

Goldblatt D 1984 Decisions about life support in amyotrophic lateral sclerosis. Seminars in Neurology 4: 104

Goldblatt D, Greenlaw J 1989 Starting and stopping the ventilator for patients with amyotrophic lateral sclerosis. Neurology Clinics 7: 789

Griffiths R D, Edwards R H T 1988 A new chart for weight control in Duchenne muscular dystrophy. Archives of Disease in Childhood 63: 1256

Griggs R C 1974 Hypertrophy and cardiomyopathy in the neuromuscular diseases. Circulation Research 34, 35 (suppl) 2: 145

Griggs R C 1990 The use of pulmonary function testing as a quantitative measurement for therapeutic trial. Muscle and Nerve (Supplement): S30

Griggs R C, Davis R J, Anderson D C, Dove J T 1975 Cardiac conduction in myotonic dystrophy. American Journal of Medicine 59: 37

Griggs R C, Donohoe K M 1982 The recognition and management of respiratory insufficiency in neuromuscular disease. Journal of Chronic Disease 35: 497

Griggs R C, Donohoe K M 1985 Emergency management of neuromuscular disease. In Henning R J, Jackson D L (eds) Handbook of critical care neurology and neurosurgery. Praeger, New York, p 201

Griggs R C, Donohoe K M, Utell M J, Goldblatt D, Moxley R T III 1981 Evaluation of pulmonary function in neuromuscular disease. Archives of Neurology 38: 9

Griggs R C, Forbes G, Moxley R T, Herr B E 1983 The assessment of muscle mass in progressive neuromuscular disease. Neurology (NY) 33: 158

Harper P S 1989 Myotonic dystrophy, 2nd edn. Saunders, Philadelphia

Heckmatt J Z, Loh L, Dubowitz V 1990 Clinical practice. Night-time nasal ventilation in neuromuscular disease. Lancet 335: 579

Holtackers T R, Loosbrock L M, Gracey D R 1982 The use of the chest cuirass in respiratory failure of neurologic origin. Respiratory Care 27: 271

Horowitz M, McNeil J D, Maddern G J, Collins P J, Shearman D J C 1986 Abnormalities of gastric and esophageal emptying in polymyositis and dermatomyositis. Gastroenterology 90: 434

Jozefowicz R F, Welle S L, Nair K S, Kingston W J, Griggs R C 1987 Basal metabolic rate in myotonic dystrophy: evidence against hypometabolism. Neurology 37: 1021

Kagen L J, Hochman R B, Strong E W 1985 Cricopharyngeal obstruction in inflammatory myopathy (polymyositis/dermatomyositis): report of three cases and review of literature. Arthritis and Rheumatism 28: 630

Lotz B P, Engel A G, Nishino M, Stevens J C 1989 Inclusion body myositis. Brain 112: 727

Madorsky J G B, Radford L M, Newman E M 1984 Psychosocial aspects of death and dying in Duchenne muscular dystrophy. Archives of Physical Medicine and Rehabilitation 65: 79

McCool F D, Mayewski R J, Shayne D S, Hyde R W, Griggs R C, Gibson C J 1981 Short term effects of IPPB on patients with neuromuscular restrictive lung disease. Respiratory Disease 123: 188

Mendell J R, Province M, Moxley R T, Griggs R C et al 1987 Clinical investigation of Duchenne dystrophy. A methodology for therapeutic trials based on natural history controls. Archives of Neurology 44: 808

Mendell J R, Vaughn J 1984 Duchenne muscular dystrophy: Ethical and emotional considerations in long-term management. Seminars of Neurology 4: 98

Moorman J R, Coleman R E, Packer D L et al 1985 Cardiac involvement in myotonic muscular dystrophy. Medicine 64: 371

Moxley R T 1990 Functional testing. Muscle and Nerve 13 (suppl): S26

Nathadwarawala K M, Nicklin J, Wiles C M 1992 A timed test of swallowing capacity for neurological patients. Journal of Neurology, Neurosurgery, and Psychiatry 55: 822

Neville J 1962 So briefly my son. Hutchinson, London, pp 1–80

Newsom-Davis J, Goldman M, Loh L, Casson M 1976 Diaphragm function and alveolar hypoventilation. Quarterly Journal of Medicine 45: 87

Nippoldt T B, Edwards W D, Holmes Jr D R, Reeder G S, Hartzler G O, Smith H C 1982 Right ventricular endomyocardial biopsy: clinicopathologic correlates in 100 consecutive patients. Mayo Clinic Proceedings 57: 407

Norris Jr F H, Moss A J, Yu P N 1966 On the possibility that a type of human muscular dystrophy commences in myocardium. Annals of the New York Academy of Science 138: 342

Palmer E D 1976 Disorders of the cricopharyngeus muscle: a review. Gastroenterology 71: 510

Reeves W, Griggs R, Nanda N C, Thomson K, Gramiak R 1980 Echocardiographic evaluation of cardiac abnormalities in Duchenne's dystrophy and myotonic muscular dystrophy. Archives of Neurology 37: 273

Rideau Y, Jankowski L W, Grellet J 1981 Respiratory function in the muscular dystrophies. Muscle and Nerve 4: 155

Roussos C, Macklem P T 1982 The respiratory muscles. New England Journal of Medicine 307: 786

Saunders N A, Rigg J R A, Pengelly L D, Campbell E J M 1978 Effect of curare on maximum static PV relationships of the respiratory system. Journal of Applied Physiology 44: 589

Schwartz J S 1982 Pneumococcal vaccine: clinical efficacy and effectiveness. Annals of Internal Medicine 96: 208

Silverstein M D, Stocking C B, Antel J P 1991 Amyotrophic lateral sclerosis and life-sustaining therapy: patients' desires for information, participation in decision making, and life-sustaining therapy. Mayo Clinic Proceedings 66: 906

Smith P E M, Calverley P M A, Edwards R H T 1988 Hypoxemia during sleep in Duchenne muscular dystrophy. American Review of Respiratory Disease 137: 884

Smith P E M, Edwards R H T, Calverley P M A 1989a Ventilation and breathing pattern during sleep in Duchenne muscular dystrophy. Chest 96: 1346

Smith P E M, Edwards R H T, Calverley P M A 1989b Protriptyline treatment of sleep hypoxaemia in Duchenne muscular dystrophy. Thorax 44: 1002

Smith P E M, Edwards R H T, Calverley P M A 1991 Mechanisms of sleep-disordered breathing in chronic neuromuscular disease: implications for management. Quarterly Journal of Medicine 296: 961

Swick H M, Werlin S L, Dodds W J, Hogan W J 1981 Pharyngoesophageal motor function in patients with myotonic dystrophy. Annals of Neurology 10: 454

Torres C T, Griggs R C, Moxley R T 1983 Quantitative testing of handgrip strength, myotonia, and fatigue in myotonic dystrophy. Journal of Neurological Sciences 60: 156

Verma A, Bradley W G, Adesina A M, Sofferman R, Pendlebury W W 1991 Inclusion body myositis with cricopharyngeus muscle involvement and severe dysphagia. Muscle and Nerve 14: 470

Weinberger S E, Schwartzstein R M, Weiss J W 1989 Hypercapnia. New England Journal of Medicine 321: 1223

Weitzner S 1969 Changes in the pharyngeal and esophageal musculature in oculopharyngeal muscular dystrophy. American Journal of Digestive Diseases 14: 805

Worden D K, Vignos P J Jr 1962 Intellectual function in childhood progressive muscular dystrophy. Pediatrics 29: 968

Yoshida M M, Krishnamurthy S, Wattchow D A, Furness J B, Schuffler M D 1988 Megacolon in myotonic dystrophy caused by a degenerative neuropathy of the myenteric plexus. Gastroenterology 95: 820

23. The orthopaedic management of neuromuscular disease

C. S. B. Galasko

INTRODUCTION

The orthopaedic management of patients with neuromuscular disorders is aimed at obtaining the maximum quality of life by preventing deformity or treating it when it has occurred. Furthermore, the prevention and treatment of scoliosis is associated with an improved prognosis in some disorders, notably Duchenne muscular dystrophy. However, orthopaedic treatment will not do anything for the underlying neuromuscular disorder.

The vast majority of patients treated are children, although adults (e.g., following a stroke) may also require orthopaedic management. That problem is beyond the scope of this chapter.

Multidisciplinary approach

Ideally, the patient should be treated via a multidisciplinary approach. The members of the team will depend on the disease, e.g. in spina bifida, a team could consist of a paediatric surgeon, neurosurgeon, orthopaedic surgeon, physiotherapist, occupational therapist, orthotist and social worker; in cerebral palsy essential members of the team include a paediatric neurologist or paediatrician, speech therapist, teacher, orthopaedic surgeon, orthotist, occupational therapist, physiotherapist, social worker and, depending on the associated abnormalities, the child may require help with hearing, vision or perceptual difficulties. For the dystrophies, other myopathies and spinal muscular atrophies, essential team members include a paediatric neurologist, orthopaedic surgeon, clinical geneticist, orthotist, occupational therapist and physiotherapist.

Diagnosis

Early diagnosis of the affected child is important: it relieves parental anxiety and allows early counselling, particularly important in hereditary conditions. Methods of diagnosis are beyond the scope of this chapter, but unfortunately, diagnosis is often delayed. Retrospective analysis of patients with Duchenne muscular dystrophy referred to our Muscle Clinic after a diagnosis was made showed an average delay of 2 years (range 0–6 years). Many of these children had been 'treated' for clumsiness, abnormal gait and flat feet for months or years before diagnosis (Read & Galasko 1986). An underlying neuromuscular disorder should be considered in patients presenting with these non-specific complaints.

Assessment

Before embarking upon treatment, these children require a detailed assessment. This includes an assessment of their overall functional capability (Table 23.1), of their muscle power, the range of movement of each joint and measurement of any joint contractures. All deformities must be noted and the ability of the child to co-operate determined. This will depend on the intelligence of the child, his or her physical development, the psychological attitude of the child and family, and the child's age. This assessment is usually carried out by the physiotherapist, and is repeated at regular intervals. As part of our initial assessment we obtain an erect anteroposterior radiograph of the spine, a radiograph of the pelvis and, in patients who can co-operate, lung function tests.

Deformity

The deformities vary in the different diseases (Galasko 1977) and will be discussed separately. Several mechanisms may be involved in their development (Table 23.2).

Provided that the agonists and antagonists acting on a joint are balanced, deformity tends not to occur, irrespective of whether the muscles are hypertrophied, spastic, normal or weak. If there is imbalance between the power of the agonist and antagonist the joint will be pulled in the direction

Table 23.1 Functional assessment in neuromuscular disease

Grade	Functional ability
1	Walks; climbs stairs without assistance
2	Walks; climb stairs with aid of rail
3	Walks; unable to climb stairs; able to get out of chair
4	Walks unassisted; able to get out of chair
5	Walks with assistance of calipers
6	Stands in calipers; unable to walk with assistance or calipers
7	In wheelchair; can roll chair
8	In wheelchair; able to perform bed and chair activities
9	In wheelchair; sits erect with support. Minimal activities
10	In bed; unable to perform activities of daily living

Table 23.2 Mechanisms of development of deformity in neuromuscular disease

Muscle imbalance
Unequal growth of fibrotic muscle and adjacent bone
Gravity plus weak musculature
Pressure, e.g. bed clothes

of the more powerful muscle. This occurs if one muscle is spastic and the other normal, one is normal and the antagonist is weak or both muscles are weak but to different degrees. The redundant capsule and ligaments fibrose on the contracted side of the joint, producing secondary joint contractures. At this stage, rebalancing the muscles will not correct the deformity: a soft-tissue release is also required. In the growing child, if the muscles are attached beyond a growth plate, the bone will tend to be deformed in the direction of the more powerful muscle. Treatment will depend on the stage of deformity but techniques include tendon division (tenotomy), elongation, transfer, soft tissue release, osteotomy and arthrodesis.

Fibrotic muscle grows more slowly than the adjacent bone. This may cause the deformity, and is probably the main cause of recurrence. Before embarking upon surgical correction, the family, and the patient (if old enough), must appreciate that the deformity may recur and that the operation may have to be repeated before growth ceases. Postoperatively, in many circumstances, the patient is provided with night splints in an attempt to prevent recurrence of the deformity,

Table 23.3 Comparison of spinal and hip surgery required in Duchenne muscle dystrophy and cerebral palsy

Disease	Patients (no.)	Patients undergoing spinal fusion (no.)	Dislocated hips (no.)	Hips requiring surgery for subluxation (no.)
Duchenne	169	41	0	0
Cerebral palsy	322	17	59	99

and ideally patients should wear the night splints until growth has ceased.

The aetiology of scoliosis, a common complication of many neuromuscular disorders, is not fully understood. One factor responsible for progressive scoliosis is the effect of gravity on a trunk with weak musculature. The process may start when the patient leans to one side to support his trunk. Gravity may also be partly responsible for the common development of equinovarus deformities in wheelchair-bound patients.

Local pressure on an area with gross muscle weakness may also produce deformity. The pressure of bedclothes may be sufficient to produce an equinus deformity in a flail foot.

The type of deformity varies in the different conditions and depends on which muscle groups are affected as well as the other factors discussed above. Table 23.3 contrasts the incidence of scoliosis treated by spinal fusion, dislocation of the hip and subluxation requiring surgery in patients with Duchenne dystrophy and cerebral palsy followed for 1–5 years.

DUCHENNE MUSCULAR DYSTROPHY

This is the commonest of the neuromuscular disorders considered in this chapter. It is associated with progressive and rapid increase in weakness, most of the boys losing their ability to walk independently between the ages of 8 and 11 years. Most die in their late teens from respiratory infection or cardiomyopathy.

Discussion with the parents of boys attending our Muscle Clinic indicated that there are four main areas of concern where orthopaedic management may help:

1. Delay in diagnosis
2. Loss of independent ambulation
3. Scoliosis
4. Foot deformity.

Delay in diagnosis (see above)

Gardner-Medwin (1979) reported that in the UK the average age at diagnosis was 5.8 years, and in the US the average time which elapsed between initial parental concern and ultimate diagnosis was 3.0 years (range 1.5–5.5 years) (Crisp et al 1982). In our study (Read & Galasko 1986) the average age at diagnosis was 5.2 years (range 1.5–9 years). Although the condition is hereditary, many parents were not aware of their family background until the diagnosis was made in their son (Read & Galasko 1986).

The diagnosis should not be missed if the possibility of muscle dystrophy is considered when a boy is late in walking, is clumsy, has difficulty with climbing stairs or running, has a tendency to fall often or his walking deteriorates.

Mobility

Many parents stated that the morale of their son deteriorated significantly when he lost the ability to walk independently. Provision of orthoses can maintain weight-bearing for several years (Spencer & Vignos 1962, Roy & Gibson 1970, Miller & Dunn 1982, Heckmatt et al 1985). However, the orthoses must be fitted before the boy goes off his feet. It is extremely difficult to mobilise a child with Duchenne dystrophy once he is chairbound, in contrast to many other neuromuscular disorders. The orthoses are usually prescribed when the child is still able to walk on the flat, but cannot climb stairs or get out of a chair. The patient uses them for 20–30 minutes each day, and as he goes off his feet he gradually becomes more dependent upon them.

Several types of orthoses are available, but they all rely on extending the hip, either with an elasticated strap or an ischial seat (Fig. 23.1). The patient leans back, tightening the Y ligament, stabilising the hips.

Frequently, these patients lose their independent ambulation after they have been confined to

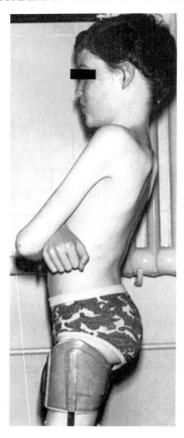

Fig. 23.1 The type of orthosis most frequently used in Duchenne muscular dystrophy. The ischial-bearing moulded thigh piece allows the patient to lean back, extending and stabilising his hips. It also produces a lumbar lordosis.

bed for an intercurrent illness, following an operation or injury. In general terms, they should not be confined to bed. Fractures should be treated by plaster of Paris or lightweight casts and immediate mobilisation. If a child is operated on in the morning, he should be stood with the help of the physiotherapist that afternoon. If surgery is carried out in the afternoon he should be stood the following morning.

Not every child, nor every family, will accept orthoses. They are cumbersome and slow the patient down. Some centres prefer to prescribe a wheelchair to allow the boy to keep up with his peers. Learning to use orthoses requires a lot of effort and, unless the family co-operates, the child will not succeed.

Scoliosis

This is the most important and most serious deformity that can occur in these patients. It is not just a cosmetic deformity, but is associated with significant morbidity. In Duchenne dystrophy, like many other neuromuscular disorders, the scoliosis eventually involves the pelvis and results in an increasing pelvic obliquity. The patient can no longer sit squarely and weight is increasingly taken on one buttock and subsequently the lumbar spine. Sitting becomes uncomfortable and the patient is confined to bed, not because of the underlying neuromuscular disorder, but as a result of the progressive scoliosis. The Cobb angle is used as a measure of the lateral curvature of the spine. It is the angle between a line drawn as an extension of the upper border of the upmost vertebral body involved in the curve and a similar line extending from the lower border of the lowest. Hsu (1983) reported that progression of the curve beyond 40 degrees was associated with diminished sitting tolerance and use of the arms and hands to prop the body up when seated. Furthermore, the scoliosis continues to deteriorate after growth has ceased, probably due to the effect of gravity.

Progressive scoliosis is also associated with diminished lung function. Kurz and colleagues (1983) showed that the vital capacity peaked at approximately the age when standing ceased and then declined rapidly. Age and thoracic scoliosis together were better predictors of the forced vital capacity (FVC) than either one alone. The vital capacity deteriorated approximately 4% for each year of life after the patient became wheelchair bound. For every 10 degrees of thoracic scoliosis there was an additional 4% loss of vital capacity. We found that the yearly decrease in forced vital capacity in patients with scoliosis who refused spinal stabilisation was 8%, whereas it remained static in patients who underwent spinal stabilisation for their scoliosis, during the first 36 months following surgery, and then fell slightly (Galasko et al 1992).

Obesity is another factor which may affect pulmonary function. It is important that the parents and patients alike understand the potential ill-effects. Because of loss of muscle bulk, the ideal

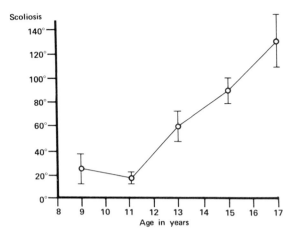

Fig. 23.2   The progression of scoliosis with increasing age in patients with Duchenne muscular dystrophy.

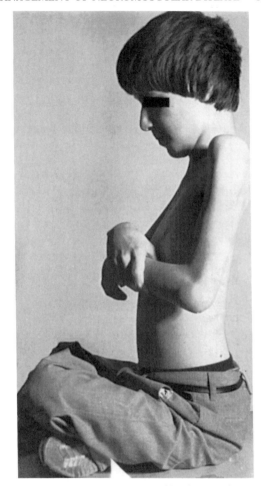

Fig. 23.3   Lordotic posture due to fibrotic extension contracture of the spine in a patient who was no longer ambulant.

weight of these patients is less than the normal for their height and age (Edwards et al 1984).

Prevention. The scoliosis increases with increasing age (Gibson & Wilkins 1975). Under the age of 8 years scoliosis is uncommon. This is thought to be due to the lordotic posture adopted by patients who are still mobile. Once the patient is confined to a wheelchair the curve deteriorates rapidly (Fig. 23.2). Very rarely, patients develop fibrotic extension contractures of the spine, with fixed lordosis and a mild scoliosis (Gibson & Wilkins 1975). Two of our 169 patients have developed such a contracture (Fig. 23.3). Provision of the ischial-bearing knee-ankle-foot orthoses (KAFOs) not only maintains mobility, but also seems to maintain the lordotic posture (Fig. 23.1) and slows the development of scoliosis (Fig. 23.4). At the age of 13 years the mean curve in our chairbound patients was 62 ± 12 degrees, compared with 13 ± 3 degrees in patients who were still mobile in their orthoses.

Standing, even when the patient is no longer mobile, also protects the spine (Miller & Dunn 1982). We now encourage our patients to stand for 2–3 hours per day, even when they are no longer independently mobile in their orthoses. When they are no longer stable in the orthoses we provide them with a swivel walker and when they can no longer use the swivel walker, it is converted to a standing frame (Fig. 23.5).

Several centres have tried to modify the wheelchair to help obtain a lordotic posture, or support the spine. These have all failed to prevent the development of scoliosis or its progression, although in some cases they may have slowed the progression of the curve (Fig. 23.6). As a result, the use of these modified wheelchairs has been largely abandoned in patients with Duchenne muscular dystrophy. However, moulded chairs or the Matrix seating system (Trail & Galasko 1990) are very useful in patients with scoliosis associated with severe cerebral palsy.

The arms of the wheelchair are sometimes removed to allow the child easier access to the

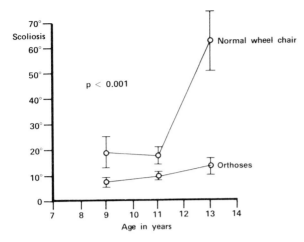

Fig. 23.4   The effect of ischial-bearing KAFOs in preventing scoliosis in patients with Duchenne muscular dystrophy. Patients who wore the orthoses had a significantly smaller curve than those confined to a wheelchair.

wheels. This situation results in further lack of support to the trunk, the patient leaning to one side, and may start the scoliotic process. It is essential that arm rests are fitted to the wheelchair to provide maximum support. These patients need powered chairs with a central control to obviate the necessity of leaning to one side (Fig. 23.7).

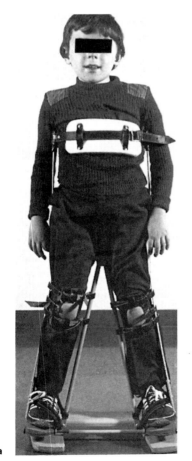

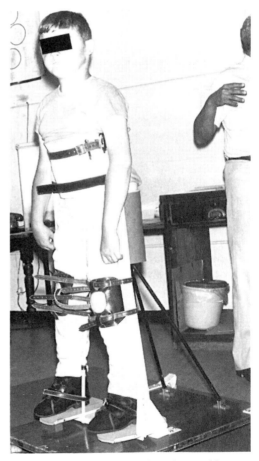

a   b

Fig. 23.5   **a** Use of a swivel walker in a patient with Duchenne muscular dystrophy who is no longer able to stand with calipers. **b** Modified swivel walker for use as a standing frame.

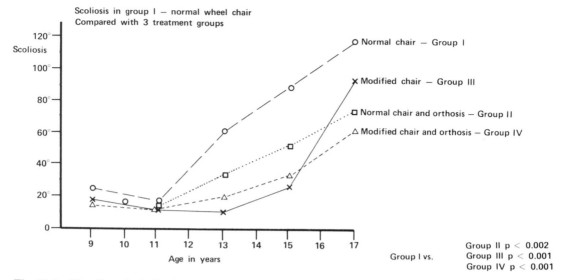

Fig. 23.6   The effect of spinal orthoses and modified wheelchairs on the progression of scoliosis in Duchenne muscular dystrophy. Although there was some slowing of the rate of progression of the scoliosis, these forms of treatment did not prevent the development of a severe deformity.

A variety of spinal orthoses have been tried. They may slow the scoliotic process, but there are inherent difficulties: because the patients are sedentary the orthoses are more difficult to fit and tend to ride up even if carefully moulded; they are often uncomfortable and, if they are too well fitting, may interfere with respiration; many patients will not use them regularly. Our results (Fig. 23.6) show that they slow the progression of the curve but do not prevent it; this may partly be due to lack of patient co-operation.

Hsu (1983) reported that spinal orthoses were capable of slowing the progression of curves of less than 25 degrees, but had little or no effect on more severe curves, and Colbert & Craig (1987) concluded that spinal bracing did not ultimately prevent severe scoliosis. Miller & O'Connor (1985) found that spinal orthoses diminished the already limited lung function in these patients,

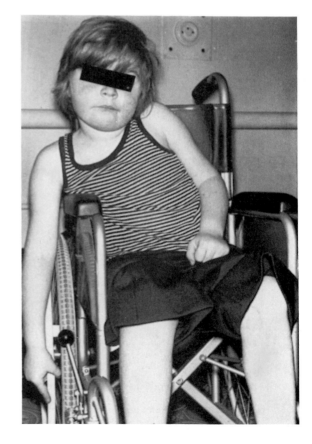

Fig. 23.7   With a manual chair the patient tends to lean to the side to propel the chair. This may start the scoliotic process, and is worsened if the arms of the chair are removed to provide easier access to the wheels. These patients should be provided with powered chairs, with a central control to obviate the necessity of leaning to one side.

and Noble-Jamieson et al (1986) reported that the forced vital capacity fell by an average of 22%.

Treatment. Once a scoliosis has developed, the use of a modified chair or orthosis may slow the progression of the curve, but will not prevent it (Fig. 23.6). Seeger and colleagues (1984) reported that modular seats and custom-moulded seats had no effect on the rate of progression of the curve in patients of 14 years of age and older. Furthermore, once the curve has reached 45–50 degrees it deteriorates rapidly.

The optimum treatment for a progressive curve is surgical stabilisation of the spine. However, in Duchenne dystrophy the patient may no longer be fit for surgery because of rapid and progressive deterioration in lung function by the time he has developed a major curve. Fig. 23.8 shows the radiographs of a patient in whom spinal stabilisation was advised when the curve was 34 degrees and he was fit for surgery: the operation was refused as he had minimal side-effects from the curve. Nine months later the curve had doubled, sitting was becoming awkward because of the associated pelvic obliquity, and surgery was requested; but he was no longer fit, his vital capacity having fallen to 19% of normal. The concept of 'prophylactic' surgery has therefore arisen, i.e. stabilisation of the spine when the patient is still fit for major surgery even though the curve is relatively small. The optimum time to stabilise the spine in a patient with Duchenne dystrophy is soon after he loses his ability to walk independently, when his lung function is adequate for major spinal surgery, before he has developed cor pulmonale or severe cardiomyopathy and when his curve is still mobile and preferably less than 30 degrees. Despite the risks of major surgery in these children it is the author's opinion that such prophylactic surgery is well worth while, in avoiding the problems associated with a late severe scoliosis. Successful spinal stabilisation not only prevents the progressive deteri-

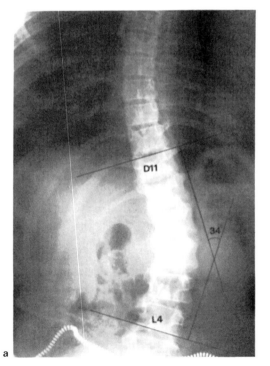
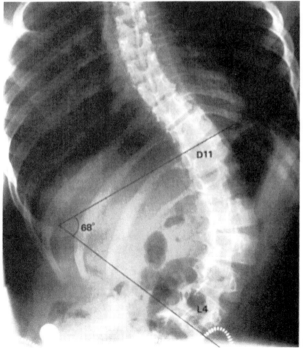

Fig. 23.8   Patient with Duchenne muscular dystrophy. **a.** Surgical stabilisation was advised when his curve measured 34 degrees, and he was fit for surgery. Operation was refused. **b.** Nine months later the curve had progressed to 68 degrees. Surgery was requested by the family, but the patient's pulmonary function had deteriorated to such an extent that he was no longer fit for the operation.

oration of the curve with the associated pelvic obliquity, resultant sitting intolerance, and difficulty with toileting, but is also associated with maintenance of lung function and improved survival (Galasko et al 1992). Figure 23.9 shows the differences in forced vital capacity, peak expiratory flow rate and severity of scoliosis in two groups of patients. The groups were the same in terms of the severity of their Duchenne dystro-

phy, their lung function, and their scoliosis at the start of the study. All patients were offered spinal stabilisation and the results were compared between those who accepted surgery and those who refused surgery. At 5 years 17% of the patients who refused surgery were alive, compared with 67% of those who had undergone spinal stabilisation. No patient was lost to follow-up though some missed one or more 6-monthly assessments.

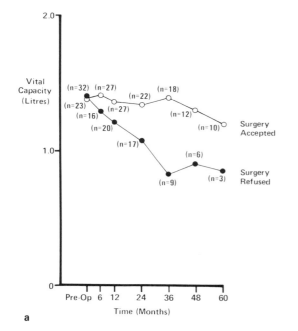

a

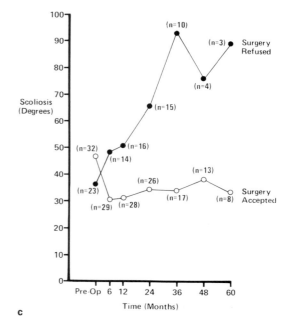

c

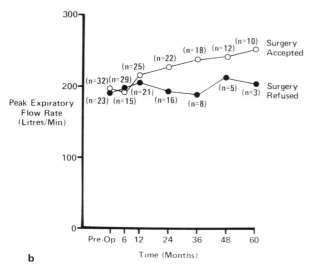

b

Fig. 23.9 The effect of spinal stabilisation in patients with scoliosis secondary to Duchenne muscular dystrophy. **a** Forced vital capacity (FVC). The mean FVC decreased at a rate of 8% per annum in the non-operated group, but remained static for 36 months in the operated group, after which it diminished slightly. The difference between the two curves is significant (P<0.0002). The decreasing numbers of patients (n) are due to patients dying, and to variable follow-up. **b** The mean expiratory flow rate diminished slightly in the first 6 months following spinal surgery, and thereafter increased. It remained the same in the patients who refused surgery. The difference is significant (P<0.02). **c** The severity of scoliosis was measured by the Cobb angle. The mean Cobb angle measured on sitting posteroanterior radiographs was corrected by surgery from a mean of 47 degrees to 30 degrees and thereafter altered little. In the patients who refused surgery, the mean Cobb angle had increased to 93 degrees by 36 months. The difference between the two curves is significant (P<0.001) (reproduced with permission from Galasko et al 1992).

The patients require a 6-monthly erect radiograph of their spine and 6-monthly lung function tests. Rapid deterioration in lung function or progression of the curve suggests earlier stabilisation of the spine. We are also concerned about the cardiac status, and electrocardiograms and echocardiography are required before surgery (Morris & Galasko 1988). Provided that their cardiac status is reasonable, we have operated on patients whose vital capacity was only 23% of the expected normal for their age and arm span, although Swank and colleagues (1982), who reported on 14 boys with Duchenne dystrophy who had undergone spinal fusion with Harrington instrumentation, did not recommend surgery if the vital capacity was less than 40%, if the patient had a non-functional cough, symptoms due to cardiomyopathy, or rapidly progressive deterioration in muscle strength.

These patients must not be placed on a long waiting list, but must be given priority, to obviate the risk of them becoming unfit for the operation while waiting.

The operation is a major one. The spine is stabilised from the 3rd or 4th dorsal vertebra to the sacrum. We now use a square-ended U-shaped rod, each arm being fixed to each vertebra by sublaminar wires. The square end is wired to the sacrum (Fig. 23.10). Other methods of stabilising the spine are available (Figs 23.11, 23.12). The facet joints are excised and the spine grafted. The average operating time is 5–7 hours and the blood loss (average 3–4 litres) is very much greater than in non-neuromuscular scoliosis, because of the length of the stabilisation and fusion, poor muscle contractility and the deliberate non-use of hypotensive anaesthesia in those patients with cardiac conduction defects (p. 865). Although the patients are weak they have normal sphincteric control and sensation. Spinal cord monitoring

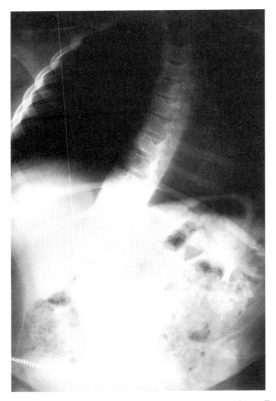

a

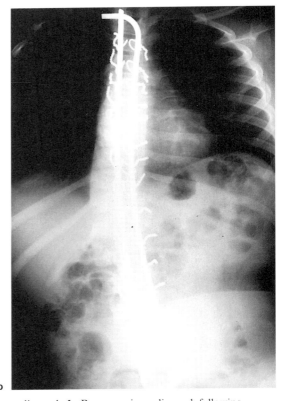

b

Fig. 23.10   Patient with Duchenne muscular dystrophy. **a** Preoperative radiograph. **b.** Postoperative radiograph following correction of the scoliosis using the 'U'-shaped rod.

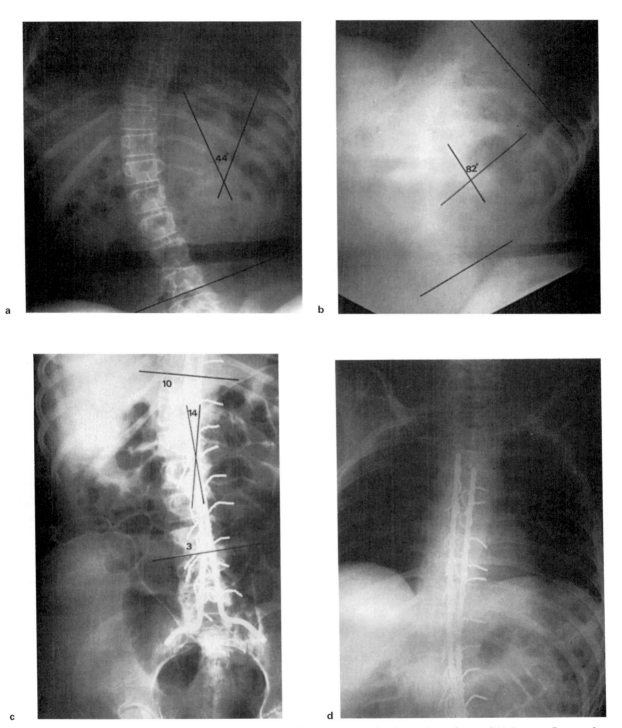

Fig. 23.11   Luque stabilisation of the spine in a patient with Duchenne muscular dystrophy. **a** Curve of 44 degrees. Consent for surgical stabilisation was refused. **b** One year later the curve had deteriorated to 82 degrees. Fortunately, the patient was still fit for surgery. **c** Immediate postoperative radiograph showing the large bowel ileus, the fixation of the Luque rods into the pelvis and the drains. **d** The Luque rods are fixed from L3 or 4 to the pelvis or sacrum.

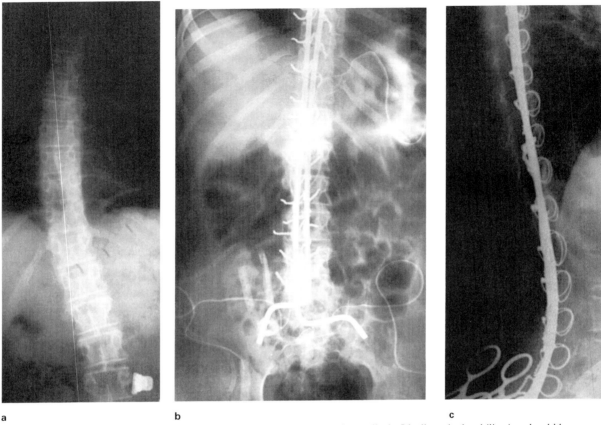

a   b   c

Fig. 23.12 Patient with Duchenne muscular dystrophy. **a** Early progressive scoliosis. Ideally, spinal stabilisation should be carried out at this stage. **b** Immediate postoperative radiograph showing the large bowel ileus and the drains. The fixation extended to D3. **c** Lateral view indicating the lumbar lordosis moulded into the rods.

should be used to minimise the risk of damaging the spinal cord or cauda equina.

The postoperative regimen is critical. The patients require nursing in an intensive care unit for at least 24 hours, and they may require intubation for the first 12–24 hours. Analgesia is provided via an intravenous morphine drip, the drip rate being increased or decreased as required. Virtually all the patients develop a profound ileus and require nasogastric suction and intravenous feeding for 3–4 days.

We have stabilised the spine in 41 patients with Duchenne muscular dystrophy. Radiographs of three of the patients are shown in Figs 23.10–23.12.

Treatment of the gross curve (Fig. 23.13) is unsatisfactory. At this stage the patients are unfit for major surgery. Attempts have been made to pad the chair or provide moulded inserts, but they usually fail and often the patient cannot be sat up without discomfort. Treatment must be aimed at preventing such gross curves and the consequential severe morbidity.

Foot deformity

Mobile patients. The development of an equinus deformity in an independently mobile patient makes walking even more difficult in a child with inherent muscle weakness (Fig. 23.14). Contractures should be avoided or minimised by physiotherapy in the form of gentle ankle stretching exercises and night ankle–foot orthoses (AFOs). The stretching exercises must be care-

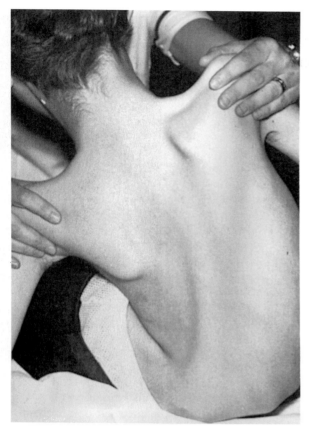

Fig. 23.13 A 16-year-old boy with Duchenne muscular dystrophy. He has progressive scoliosis with a rigid curve. He is unable to sit unsupported. When he sits, his weight is taken on the lumbar spine and his pelvis is almost vertical.

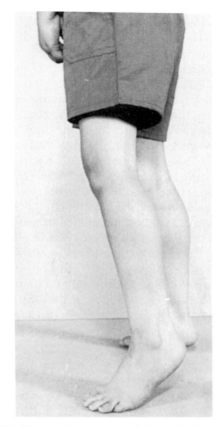

Fig. 23.14 Equinus deformity in an independently mobile patient with Duchenne muscular dystrophy.

fully carried out to avoid reflex contracture of the calf muscles. The parents should be taught the exercises so that they can be carried out daily. Once an equinus or equinovarus deformity has occurred, surgical correction should be considered (Williams et al 1984). The deformity can usually be corrected by simple elongation of the tendo Achilles, but it is essential not to overlengthen the tendon, as this may result in excessive dorsiflexion in the standing position with loss of balance. Some authors combine elongation of the tendo Achilles with a 'prophylactic' transfer of the tendon of tibialis posterior to the dorsum of the foot (Shapiro & Bresnan 1982). However, surgery should not be undertaken unless the equinus deformity has affected the patient's mobility, as there is a risk that the patient may lose his independent mobility following surgery.

Postoperatively the limbs are immobilised in below-knee plaster casts and the patients are mobilised, with the aid of the physiotherapist, within 12–16 hours of surgery. The casts are changed at 2–3 weeks, when the sutures are removed and casts are taken for night splints, which are provided when the plaster casts are finally removed at approximately 6 weeks.

Patients in KAFOs. Equinus or equinovarus deformities should be corrected before a patient is fitted with the orthoses. Following surgery the limbs are immobilised in long-leg casts and the patient is mobilised within 12–16 hours. The casts are usually changed at three weeks and the patients provided with KAFO's at 6 weeks, when the casts are removed.

Chairbound patients. Most of the equinus and equinovarus deformities occur after the patients have gone off their feet (Williams et al 1984, Fig. 23.15). Progressive equinovarus is often associated with pain which may be due to a stress fracture of an osteoporotic bone or simply secondary to the contractures, pressure sores over bony prominences, and inability to fit footwear. Attempts have been made to prevent the development of these deformities by providing adequate foot support with wheelchair footplates, by modifying the footplate, the use of night AFOs and the provision of lightweight moulded day AFOs which fit into the shoes and hold the feet in a neutral or slightly dorsiflexed position (Galasko 1986, 1987a).

If the deformity causes symptoms, surgical correction is indicated. Elongation of the tendo Achilles alone is usually insufficient and elonga-

tion or transfer of the tibialis posterior tendon with tenotomy of the tendons of flexor hallucis and flexor digitorum longus, and a posterior capsulotomy of the ankle joint, may be required (Williams et al 1984). The deformity tends to recur after surgical correction, but at a slower rate than in unoperated patients (Williams et al 1984). Transfer of the tibialis posterior tendon (Miller et al 1982) may prevent the recurrence. Siegel (1980) advised curettage of part of the cancellous bone from the head of the talus and distal calcaneus in equino-cavo-varus.

Postoperatively, the limb is immobilised in a below-knee plaster cast until the wounds have healed, after which day and night AFOs are worn.

Contractures of the hip and knee

Contractures should be avoided or minimised in mobile patients by daily prone lying and stretching exercises. Contracture of the tensor fascia latae may affect the gait and require surgical release. Contractures may have to be corrected before orthoses are fitted; this is rarely required.

Flexion contractures of the hips and knees always develop in wheelchair-bound patients, but seem to be of little significance. Flexion of the hip is not associated with dislocation in Duchenne dystrophy, despite the pelvic obliquity (Fig. 23.16), and contractures of the hips or knees do not produce symptoms unless attempts are made forcibly to correct them. We have not found that surgical correction of these contractures was necessary in any wheelchair-bound patient.

Fractures

In our experience fractures are not a common complication of Duchenne muscular dystrophy although Matejczyk & Rang (1983) recorded an incidence of 18% during the course of the disease. Fractures of the long bones occur from falls out of a wheelchair as well as in ambulatory patients (Siegel 1977, Hsu 1979, Hsu & Garcia-Ariz 1981), the commonest site being the femoral supracondylar region (Matejczyk & Rang 1983). Patients in wheelchairs should have safety belts applied for transport over rough outdoor terrain. When a braced child falls, the orthoses tend to

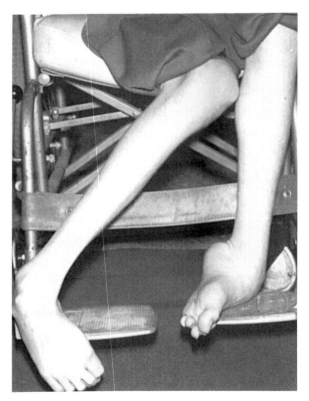

Fig. 23.15 Gross equinovarus deformities in a wheelchair-bound patient with Duchenne muscular dystrophy.

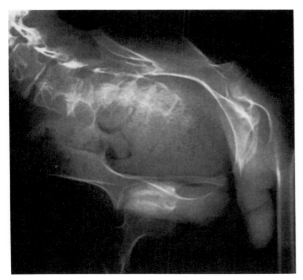

Fig. 23.16   Gross pelvic obliquity in a patient with Duchenne muscular dystrophy. Neither hip is dislocated; however, there is marked varus moulding of the more cranially situated femur. In many other forms of neuromuscular disorders, pelvic obliquity of this degree would have been associated with a dislocation of the more cranially sited hip joint.

protect his lower limbs from direct trauma (Siegel 1977).

The fractures heal rapidly and should be immobilised in the lightest possible cast. In the mobile child, fractures of the lower limbs should be treated in a weight-bearing cast and the patient may require admission to hospital so that intensive physiotherapy, including ambulation, can be supervised on a daily basis.

Anaesthesia

Complications of anaesthesia in children with Duchenne muscular dystrophy include sudden death (Boba 1970, Ellis 1980), anaesthesia-related cardiac arrest (Seay et al 1978), rhabdomyolysis (Miller et al 1978, Boltshauser et al 1980) and malignant hyperthermia (Oka et al 1982, Brownell et al 1983). Hyperpyrexia has also been described in other types of neuromuscular disease (Denborough et al 1973). Suxamethonium, a neural blocking agent sometimes used in general anaesthesia, should be strictly avoided as it may be responsible for hyperkalaemic cardiac arrest and sudden death (Genever 1971).

In the later stage of the disease cardiomyopathy may occur, resulting in a lowering of cardiac reserve. This is not necessarily a contraindication to surgery, two of our patients undergoing foot surgery and three undergoing spinal stabilisation having shown these changes. Conduction defects occur most commonly. Most of our patients with Duchenne dystrophy had a bundle branch block or some other form of conductive cardiac abnormality at the time of spinal stabilisation. Congestive heart failure does not respond to conventional therapy and progresses rapidly (Mattioli & Melhorn 1982).

Table 23.4 shows our experience with cardiac and respiratory problems in patients with neuromuscular disease. One hundred and twenty patients have been operated upon for scoliosis. One patient with minicore disease (a congenital myopathy) had a cardiac arrest; he was successfully resuscitated but died 4 years later from cor pulmonale. One patient with Friedreich's ataxia died 3 weeks postoperatively from cardiac failure. One patient with spinal muscle atrophy required

Table 23.4   Cardiac and pulmonary complications in patients with neuromuscular disease undergoing spinal stabilisation

	Patients (no.)
Duchenne dystrophy	41
Spinal muscle atrophy	17
Cerebral palsy	17
Spina bifida	14
Friedreich's ataxia	6
Congenital myopathies	6
Miscellaneous	19
Total	120

Cardiac and respiratory complications in these 120 patients	
Perioperative deaths	0
Cardiac arrest (resuscitated)	1 (Minicore disease)
Postoperative death	1 (Friedreich's ataxia — cardiac failure 3 weeks postoperatively)
Atrial flutter with 2:1 heart block	1 (Duchenne)
Temporary tracheostomy	1 (Duchenne)
Required serial postoperative bronchoscopies	1 (Spinal muscle atrophy)
Required single postoperative bronchoscopy	1 (Duchenne)
Chest infection	5
Pulmonary atelectasis	5

serial bronchoscopies and suction postoperatively as she was not able to co-operate with the physiotherapists and one patient with Duchenne muscular dystrophy required a bronchoscopy for a postoperative chest infection. One patient with Duchenne muscular dystrophy required a temporary tracheostomy. Five patients developed a chest infection and five patients pulmonary atelectasis. One patient with Duchenne dystrophy developed a 2 : 1 heart block with an atrial flutter.

In two patients (not included in the 120 patients shown in Table 23.4), the operation was abandoned. One patient with Friedreich's ataxia developed severe hypotension during induction of the anaesthetic. She was resuscitated, and the operation was abandoned. One patient with Duchenne muscular dystrophy was unable to breathe when placed prone, even with an endotracheal tube in situ. His operation was also abandoned. One patient with nemaline myopathy died while awaiting surgery; she had nocturnal apnoea and was on nocturnal cuirass ventilation.

OTHER DYSTROPHIES

This section covers a number of conditions which may require orthopaedic management, but perhaps less frequently than Duchenne dystrophy. The orthopaedic problems differ in the different disorders; e.g., congenital dystrophy is associated with a high incidence of scoliosis, hip dislocation which is often present at birth, severe talipes equinovarus and contractures (Jones et al 1979). In the limb girdle dystrophies the main problem is weakness of abduction at the shoulders. The limb-girdle syndrome embraces a number of different disorders, the primary condition often being spinal muscular atrophy. In such cases there is slowly progressive weakness of the proximal upper and lower limb muscles, often less rapid than in the muscle dystrophies and sometimes becoming arrested (Walton 1983).

Patellar subluxation due to weakness of the quadriceps muscles is a recognised complication. It has been described in Becker dystrophy (Khan & MacNicol 1982), although this complication is not common because isolated wasting of a single muscle group is rare in any form of muscle dystrophy.

Scoliosis

The optimum form of treatment is surgical stabilisation using segmental sublaminal wiring. As in Duchenne dystrophy, I prefer to stabilise the spine from D4 to the sacrum. Except for congenital dystrophy the other forms of muscular dystrophy seldom cause a significant scoliosis, presumably because their muscle weakness is mild during the growth period.

Mobility

Where indicated, KAFOs should be used, but they are usually unnecessary.

Foot deformities

Equinus and equinovarus deformities occur commonly in many of these conditions (Galesko 1987b). Contractures should be prevented by physiotherapy, if possible. If the tendo Archilles is tight, regular gentle stretching exercises and night AFOs are indicated. Established equinus deformity usually requires surgical correction, the extent of surgery depending on the severity of the deformity.

Hip and/or knee contractures

If the contractures interfere with gait, surgical release is required. This may include release of the hip flexors, ilio-tibial band and hamstrings.

Dislocation/subluxation of the hip

Dislocation of the hip should be avoided. Progressive subluxation of the hip should be treated by releasing soft tissue contractures, balancing the muscle pull across the hip joint and by femoral and/or pelvic osteotomy. Usually the femoral neck is in valgus and a varus osteotomy is required. If the acetabulum is deficient a pelvic osteotomy will also be required. If the hip has already dislocated, and if the patient is grossly disabled (mentally and physically), or will not be expected to stand or walk (with or without the use of aids) and has no pain, treatment is usually not indicated. If he or she is likely to be able to stand or walk (with or without aids) the hip should be stabilised. The hip muscles must be balanced and the femoral head reduced into the acetabulum. As with subluxing hips, an upper femoral varus osteotomy with or without femoral shortening is usually required and if acetabular development is poor, some form of pelvic osteotomy is needed. If the dislocated hip is painful, surgery is indicated: however, reduction of the hip may not reduce pain, particularly if the femoral head is already deformed.

Loss of shoulder abduction

Many of these patients learn trick manoeuvres, but abduction of the shoulder can be helped by stabilising the scapula to the chest wall. This minimises the winging of the scapula and gives the residual musculature optimum mechanical advan-

tage. However, scapular stabilisation may be of little value if the deltoids are atrophied (Copeland & Howard 1978), and surgery should be postponed until growth is complete.

SPINAL MUSCULAR ATROPHY

Orthopaedic management is usually required in the intermediate variety, but only rarely is it indicated in the mild form (Kugelberg–Welander syndrome), where the children are ambulant and should be encouraged to remain so, or in the severe form (Werdnig–Hoffman disease), when the patient usually dies within the first year of life.

Mobility

Most children with intermediate spinal muscular

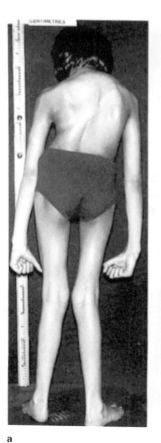 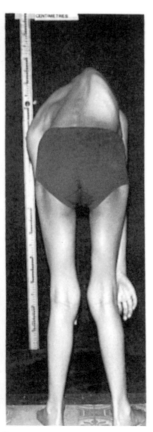 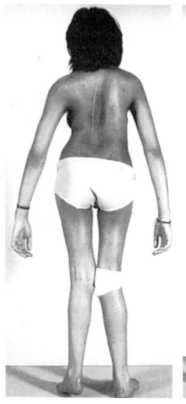 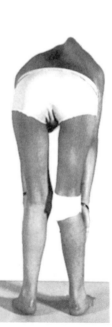

a   b   c   d

Fig. 23.17 Patient with spinal muscle atrophy. **a, b** Rigid thoracic curve of 121 degrees. **c, d** Twelve months postoperatively. The curve has been corrected to 78 degrees. A long posterior fusion was carried out with Harrington instrumentation.

atrophy are unable to walk when first seen. It is not usually possible to provide orthoses until the child is three or four years old and during this period active physiotherapy is encouraged, provided that the child will co-operate. Most children will manage with reciprocating gait orthosis or ischial-bearing KAFOs, although occasionally a rollator is also needed with the younger child. Unlike Duchenne dystrophy patients with spinal muscular atrophy can sometimes be mobilised, even though they have been chairbound for some time.

Scoliosis

As with Duchenne dystrophy, the most important deformity in these children is scoliosis. A curve was already present in nearly half of our patients when first seen at our clinic. It is our policy to obtain an erect (sitting) anteroposterior radiograph of their spine at 6-monthly intervals. Progressive curves, or curves of more than 20 degrees are braced until the patient is old enough for surgical stabilisation. Aprin and colleagues (1982) reported that bracing was ineffective in preventing the progression of scoliosis and recommended a long posterior fusion with Harrington rod instrumentation (Fig. 23.17), but we now prefer segmental spinal stabilisation with sublaminal wiring, as this avoids the necessity for a postoperative plaster of Paris cast or spinal orthosis. However, these patients can tolerate a postoperative jacket and a posterior fusion with Harrington instrumentation or combined posterior and anterior correction and fusion (Riddick et al 1982) is feasible.

The type of bracing depends on the age of the child. In the first 2–3 years of life a plastazote jacket may suffice. In older children a moulded underarm orthosis is usually used, although curves greater than 70 degrees may require periods of immobilisation in a plaster cast. If bracing does not hold the curve, earlier surgery may be required.

Hips

Unlike Duchenne dystrophy, dislocation of the hip does occur in patients with spinal muscular

atrophy, although much less frequently than in spina bifida or cerebral palsy (Galasko 1986). Dislocation is secondary to muscle imbalance and is preceded by progressive subluxation. Serial radiographs will indicate which hips are at risk, and dislocation can usually be prevented by balancing the musculature (which usually requires release of the hip flexors and adductors) and a varus upper femoral osteotomy in hips which are progressively subluxing. A pelvic osteotomy may also be required. Dislocated hips require open reduction, muscle-balancing procedures and often femoral and pelvic osteotomies. If there is an associated scoliosis with pelvic obliquity, this should be corrected first before the hip is reduced.

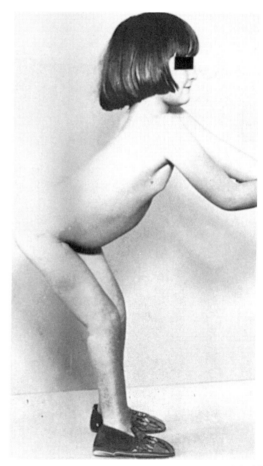

Fig. 23.18 Ninety degree fixed flexion deformity of the hips in a patient with spinal muscle atrophy. Following surgical release of the contractures, she regained her independent mobility.

Flexion contractures may be gross (Fig. 23.18), can interfere with mobility and may require surgical correction. Regular prone lying should be encouraged in an attempt to prevent these deformities.

Knees and feet

The principles of management are similar to those for Duchenne dystrophy. Regular stretching exercises are encouraged and, if the tendo Achilles are tight, night AFOs are provided. Surgical release is required for those deformities which interfere with ambulation, before the fitting of orthoses and for symptomatic deformities.

Shoulders

In some patients weakness of the shoulder girdle muscles may result in winging of the scapula which limits flexion and abduction. Stabilisation of the scapula to the chest wall usually provides a more stable fulcrum, resulting in a better range of abduction and flexion (Fig. 23.19).

CONGENITAL MYOPATHY

This includes several conditions: many are associated with a cardiomyopathy and preoperative cardiac investigations are essential. Anaesthesia carries the risk of malignant hyperpyrexia.

Most of the patients with a congenital myopathy are mobile, their commonest deformity being scoliosis. The principles of treatment are similar to those of spinal muscular atrophy, but the risk with anaesthesia is greater.

NEUROPATHIES AND ATAXIAS

Neuropathies

This group also embraces many conditions. In hypertrophic neuropathy (peroneal muscular atrophy, Charcot–Marie–Tooth syndrome, HMSN type I), pes cavus is often noted in early childhood before the onset of symptoms. Later there is involvement of the hands with difficulty in fine manipulation. In the Dejerine–Sottas syndrome (hypertrophic neuropathy of infancy), the onset is usually in infancy with delay in early milestones

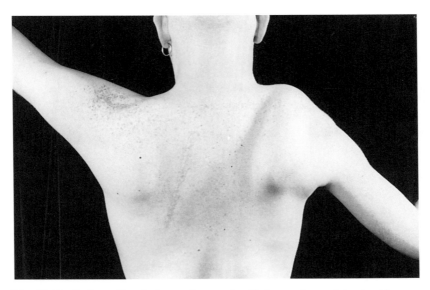

Fig. 23.19 Patient with spinal muscular atrophy. He has weakness of the shoulder girdle muscles resulting in winging of the scapula. This interfered with abduction and flexion. The left scapula has been stabilised by fixation to the chest wall, resulting in improved flexion and abduction of his shoulder. This photograph was taken when he was admitted to hospital for surgery to his right side.

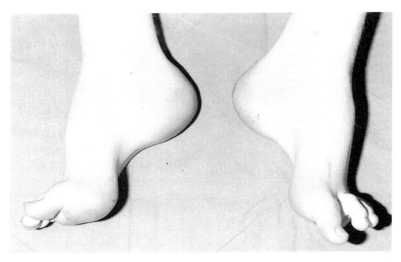

Fig. 23.20 Patient with spinal cerebellar ataxia who has early pes cavus. The deformity is still mobile. He has equinus of the forefoot and a cavo-varus foot. The tightness of the structures in the sole of his feet can be seen, as well as the prominence of the metatarsal heads and the secondary clawing deformities. He was treated by an extensive plantar release, a modified Jones' procedure to the great toe, and a transfer of the extensor digitorum longus tendons to the forefoot.

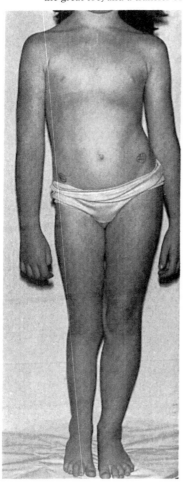

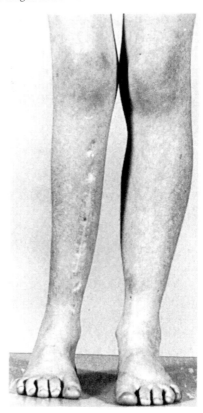

b

Fig. 23.21 Patient with polyneuropathy. **a** Forty-two-millimetre limb-length discrepancy, the shortening being in the lower leg. The anterior superior iliac spines have been marked. **b** Following tibial lengthening her discrepancy has been corrected.

a

and walking may be achieved only by the third or fourth year.

In the neuronal type of peroneal muscular-atrophy (HMSN type 2), there is marked atrophy of muscle and there may be an associated pes cavus. The commonest early symptom is difficulty with walking, but the onset may not be until middle age and the patient may have excelled at sports in his youth.

The commonest orthopaedic problem is foot deformity. This is usually a pes cavus, but equinus and equinovarus deformities also occur. The latter are treated by soft tissue releases, whereas a significant cavus deformity requires wedge tarsectomy or triple arthrodesis. Early cavus deformities, that are still mobile, can often be corrected by a radical plantar release and tendon transfers (Fig. 23.20).

Scoliosis may also occur in these conditions and the management is similar to that of spinal muscular atrophy. Asymmetrical lower limb involvement may result in limb-length inequality (Fig. 23.21) and if this is greater than 3 cm, a limb-lengthening procedure may be required to improve the gait and to avoid the back pain which is often associated with significant limb-length inequality.

Sensory neuropathies may present with trophic ulceration, osteomyelitis or septic arthritis (Fig. 23.22). These lesions also occur with congenital insensitivity to pain (Greider 1983).

It may not be possible to use spinal cord monitoring in patients with sensory neuropathy, because of inability to stimulate a peripheral nerve (Arafa et al 1987).

Friedreich's ataxia

This is commonly associated with scoliosis and pes cavus. The scoliosis frequently requires surgical correction to allow for comfortable sitting (Figs. 23.23, 23.24). Cady & Bobechko (1984) suggested that bracing was of no value and recommended a long posterior spinal fusion as soon as the curve reached 40–50 degrees. In independently mobile patients, locomotion may be dependent on trunk movement and they may lose their mobility following upper thoracic to pelvic stabilisation. If the curve is still localised to the thoracic

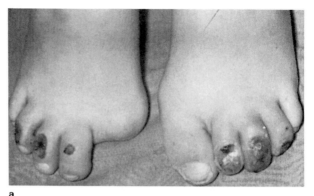

a

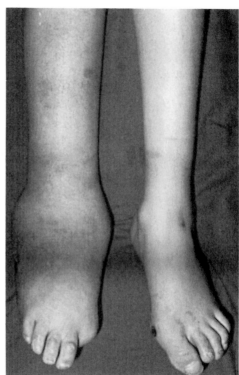

b

Fig. 23.22 Patient with a sensory neuropathy. **a** Trophic ulceration affecting several of his toes. He already has had an amputation of his right great toe. **b** Two years later he developed septic arthritis of his right ankle.

spine, a localised stabilisation should be carried out to preserve trunk mobility and allow for independent walking. If the curve subsequently involves the lumbar spine, a secondary procedure may be required.

The cavus deformity may require treatment if the patient is ambulatory. A flexible deformity can

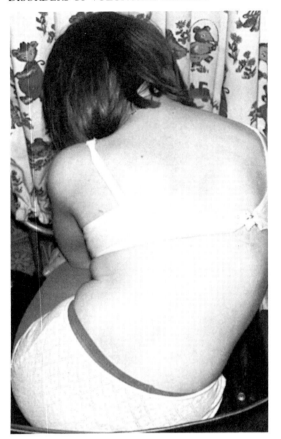
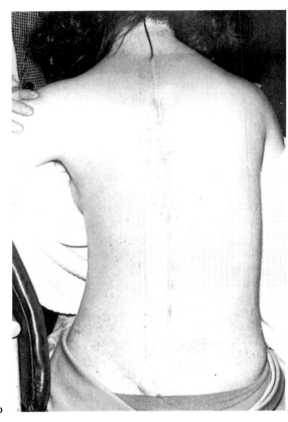

a   b

Fig. 23.23   A 17-year-old wheelchair-bound girl with Friedreich's ataxia. **a** She was unable to sit for more than an hour at a time because of pain under her right buttock. **b** Following spinal fusion using Harrington rod instrumentation. Routine evaluation at 6 months postoperatively revealed a pseudoarthrosis and she required a supplementary bone graft. Following the fusion she was able to sit unsupported without pain.

be corrected by combining a plantar release with tendon transfers and a Dwyer calcaneal osteotomy if required, but a triple arthrodesis is required if the cavus is rigid.

Friedreich's ataxia may be associated with cardiac abnormalities (Table 23.4) and a careful cardiac assessment is required prior to major reconstructive surgery. Taddonio (1982) analysed segmental spinal stabilisation in 17 patients with a variety of neuromuscular disorders. The only death occurred 36 hours postoperatively in one of the two patients with Friedreich's ataxia, who also had a cardiomyopathy. His series included two patients with Duchenne dystrophy, two with spinal muscular atrophy and one with congenital myopathy.

Hereditary telangiectatic ataxia is frequently associated with scoliosis, which may require surgical correction for comfortable sitting.

MISCELLANEOUS CONDITIONS

There are a variety of miscellaneous neurological and neuromuscular conditions which may require orthopaedic management, and which do not fit into any of the above categories. They include conditions such as hereditary spastic paraparesis, where release of tight hip adductors for a scissoring gait, or elongation of the tendo Achilles for an equinus deformity may be beneficial; inflammatory myopathies, which may be associated with an equinus deformity or other contractures; myotonic syndromes where the patient may

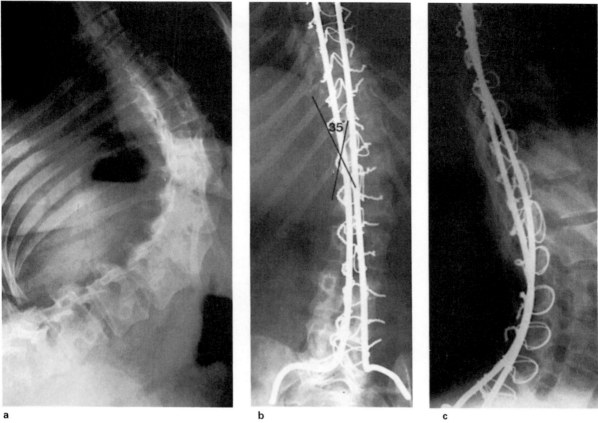

a   b   c

Fig. 23.24 A 32-year-old patient with Friedreich's ataxia. **a** She had a 96 degree curve and associated pelvic obliquity.
b. Following segmental stabilisation from D4 to the pelvis her curve has been corrected to 35 degrees and her pelvis is horizontal.
c. Lateral view showing the lumbar lordosis, which is necessary for comfortable sitting.

present with a scoliosis (Fig. 23.25) or foot deformity: and the rigid spine syndrome. In the latter condition, hyperextension of the cervical spine may be so severe as to create difficulties with deglutition. Release of the posterior spinal muscles is required but the deformity creates major anaesthetic difficulties. Cardiac muscle is frequently affected in dystrophia myotonica and in these patients thiopentone must be avoided. Congenital talipes equinovarus often occurs in this condition.

Arthrogryposis probably includes a number of conditions as yet undefined, where muscle is replaced by fibrous tissue. Multiple deformities may occur, especially talipes equinovarus, fixed flexion deformities of the knee (Fig. 23.26) and hip dislocation. Recurrence of the deformity following

surgery is common, because the fibrotic muscle does not grow as rapidly as the adjacent bone.

SUMMARY

Deformities occur commonly in the dystrophies, myopathies, atrophies, neuropathies and ataxias. The incidence and type of deformity varies between the different conditions.

The most significant deformity is scoliosis. Progressive neuromuscular scoliosis produces increasing respiratory insufficiency and increasing pelvic obliquity with loss of sitting balance. In Duchenne dystrophy it may be possible to control the scoliosis by prolonging standing. Irrespective of the underlying disorder, surgical stabilisation is

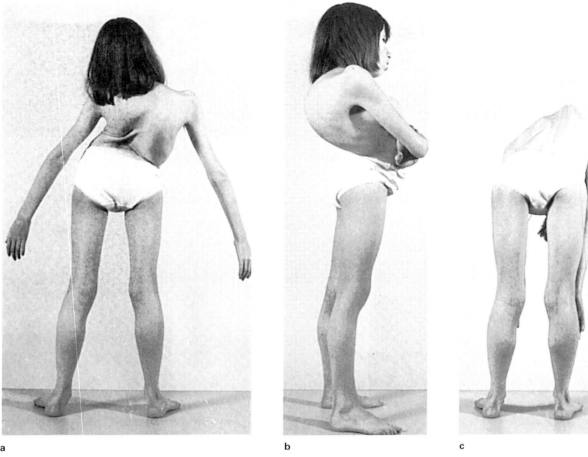

a   b   c

Fig. 23.25   Patient with myotonic dystrophy who had developed a gross scoliosis. Patients should be referred for orthopaedic management before they develop such severe deformities.

indicated for a progressive curve, provided the patient is fit enough for major surgery. At the moment, segmental stabilisation with sublaminal wiring seems to offer considerable advantages as a postoperative plaster jacket or spinal orthosis is avoided. Ideally, the operation should not be carried out under the age of 11 or 12 years; however, if the curve is progressive and cannot be adequately controlled, earlier stabilisation may be necessary.

Contractures can occur in any joint. Contractures of the upper limb rarely require surgical correction in this group of patients. Contractures occur most often in the feet and ankles, the commonest being equinus and equinovarus deformities, although any type of deformity can occur.

Surgical correction is required if the contracture interferes with gait, interferes with the fitting of orthoses or is symptomatic. Equinus or equinovarus deformities can be corrected by soft tissue release whereas a rigid pes cavus deformity usually requires a wedge tarsectomy or a triple arthrodesis.

Contractures of the hips and knees occur less often. They always develop in children confined to a wheelchair, but then rarely produce problems. Regular stretching exercises and prone lying may help prevent these deformities. If contractures do occur, do not respond to physiotherapy and interfere with gait or the fitting of orthoses, surgical correction is indicated.

Winging of the scapula and limb length dis-

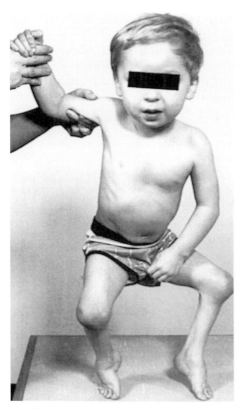
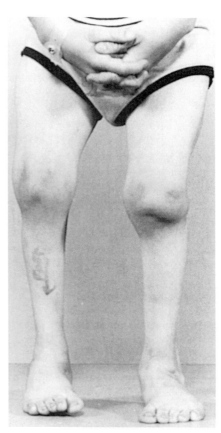

a   b

Fig. 23.26 Patient with arthrogryposis. **a** Gross fixed flexion deformities of the knees. As a result the patient walked on his knees . Note the thickened skin over the front of the knees. **b** Following bilateral femoral osteotomies to correct the deformities.

crepancy are other complications of specific neuromuscular conditions and may require surgery.

It must be emphasised that orthopaedic management is part of the continuing treatment of these patients. Orthopaedic management must be associated with a careful assessment, preoperative physiotherapy programme and detailed postoperative rehabilitation: it forms part of the overall management of the child.

Orthopaedic surgery can do nothing to cure the underlying neurological disorder: it is aimed at preventing and correcting deformity. Major reconstructive surgery in these patients is not undertaken purely for cosmetic reasons, but is used to aid mobility, to alleviate discomfort and to improve the quality of life of these patients.

ACKNOWLEDGEMENTS

I am grateful to my colleagues who have referred patients with neuromuscular diseases from a wide area. I am particularly grateful to my colleagues and the nursing staff at the Royal Manchester Children's Hospital, without whose skill and expertise the procedures described in this chapter could not have been carried out.

I wish to thank the Department of Medical Illustration at Hope Hospital and the Royal Manchester Children's Hospital for the illustrations, Blackwell Scientific Publications and the Journal of Bone and Joint Surgery for permission to reproduce those already published.

REFERENCES

Aprin H, Bowen J R, MacEwen G D, Hall J E 1982 Spine fusion in patients with spinal muscular atrophy. Journal of Bone and Joint Surgery 64-A: 1179

Arafa M, Morris P, Galasko C S B 1987 Spinal cord monitoring during surgery for scoliosis. In: Noble J, Galasko C S B (eds) Recent developments in orthopaedic surgery. Manchester University Press

Boba A 1970 Fatal postanaesthetic complications in two muscular dystrophic patients. Journal of Paediatric Surgery 5: 71

Boltshauser E, Steinmann B, Meyer A, Jerusalem F 1980 Anesthesia induced rhabdomyolysis in Duchenne muscular dystrophy. British Journal of Anaesthesia 52: 559

Brownell A K W, Paasuke R T, Elash A et al 1983 Malignant hyperthermia in Duchenne muscular dystrophy. Anesthesiology 58: 180

Cady R B, Bobechko W P 1984 Incidence, natural history and treatment of scoliosis in Friedreich's ataxia. Journal of Pediatric Orthopaedics 4: 673

Colbert A P, Craig C 1987 Scoliosis in Duchenne muscular dystrophy: prospective study of modified Jewett hyperextension brace. Archives of Physical Medicine Rehabilitation 68: 302

Copeland S A, Howard R C 1978 Thoracoscapular fusion for facioscapulohumeral dystrophy. Journal of Bone and Joint Surgery 60-B: 547

Crisp D E, Ziter F A, Bray P F 1982 Diagnostic delay in Duchenne's muscular dystrophy. Journal of the American Medical Association 347: 478

Denborough M A, Dennett L, Anderson R M 1973 Central core and malignant hyperpyrexia. British Medical Journal 1: 272

Edwards R H, Round J M, Jackson M J, Griffiths R D, Lilburn M F 1984 Weight reduction in boys with muscular dystrophy. Developmental Medicine and Child Neurology 26: 384

Ellis F R 1980 Inherited muscle disease. British Journal of Anaesthesia 52: 153

Galasko C S B 1977 Incidence of orthopaedic problems in children with muscle disease. Israel Journal of Medicine Sciences 13: 165

Galasko C S B 1986 Orthopaedic management of children with neurological disorders. In: Gordon N, McKinlay I (eds) Neurologically handicapped child, treatment and management. Blackwell Scientific Publications, Oxford, p 109

Galasko C S B 1987a The orthopaedic management of the dystrophies, myopathies, atrophies, neuropathies and ataxias. In: Galasko C S B (ed) Neuromuscular problems in orthopaedics. Blackwell Scientific Publications, Oxford, p 83

Galasko C S B 1987b The management of foot deformities in neuromuscular diseases. Seminars in Orthopaedics 2: 183

Galasko C S B, Delaney C, Morris P 1992 Spinal stabilisation in Duchenne muscular dystrophy. Journal of Bone and Joint Surgery 74B: 210

Gardner-Medwin D 1979 Controversies about Duchenne muscular dystrophy: (1) Neonatal screening. Developmental Medicine and Child Neurology 21: 390

Genever E E 1971 Suxamethonium-induced cardiac arrest in unsuspected pseudohypertrophic muscular dystrophy: a case report. British Journal of Anaesthesia 43: 984

Gibson D A, Wilkins K E 1975 The management of spinal

deformities in Duchenne muscular dystrophy. A new concept of spinal bracing. Clinical Orthopaedics and Related Research 108: 41

Greider T D 1983 Orthopaedic aspects of congenital insensitivity to pain. Clinical Orthopaedics and Related Research 172: 117

Heckmatt J Z, Dubowitz V, Hyde S A, Florence J, Gabain A C, Thompson N 1985 Prolongation of walking in Duchenne muscular dystrophy with lightweight orthoses: review of 57 cases. Developmental Medicine and Child Neurology 27: 149

Hsu J D 1979 Extremity fractures in children with neuromuscular diseases. The Johns Hopkins Medical Journal 145: 89

Hsu J D 1983 The natural history of spine curvature progression in the non-ambulatory Duchenne muscular dystrophy patient. Spine 8: 771

Hsu J D, Garcia-Ariz M 1981 Fracture of the femur in the Duchenne muscular dystrophy patient. Journal of Pediatric Orthopaedics 1: 203

Jones R, Khan R, Hughes S, Dubowitz V 1979 Congenital muscular dystrophy. The importance of early diagnosis and orthopaedic management in the long-term prognosis. Journal of Bone and Joint Surgery 61B: 13

Khan R H, MacNicol M F 1982 Bilateral patellar subluxation secondary to Becker muscular dystrophy. Journal of Bone and Joint Surgery 64A: 777

Kurz L T, Mubarak S J, Schultz P, Park S M, Leach J 1983 Correlation of scoliosis and pulmonary function in Duchenne muscular dystrophy. Journal of Pediatric Orthopaedics 3: 347

Matejczyk M B, Rang M 1983 Fractures in children with neuromuscular disorders. In: Houghton G R, Thompson G D (eds) Problematic musculo-skeletal injuries in children. Butterworth, London, p 178

Mattioli L, Melhorn M 1982 Duchenne's muscular dystrophy. The diagnosis and management of cardiac involvement. The Journal of the Kansas Medical Society 83: 115

Miller E D, Sanders D B, Rowlingson J C, Berry F A, Sussman M D, Epstein R M 1978 Anesthesia-induced rhabdomyolysis in a patient with Duchenne's muscular dystrophy. Anesthesiology 48: 146

Miller G, Dunn N 1982 An outline of the management and prognosis of Duchenne muscular dystrophy in Western Australia. Australian Paediatric Journal 18: 277

Miller G M, Hsu J D, Hoffer M M, Rentfro R 1982 Posterior tibial tendon transfer: a review of the literature and analysis of 74 procedures. Journal of Pediatric Orthopaedics 2: 363

Miller G, O'Connor J 1985 Spinal bracing and respiratory function in Duchenne muscular dystrophy. Clinical Pediatrics (Philadelphia) 24: 94

Morris P, Galasko C S B 1988 Anaesthesia for spinal stabilisation in children and adolescents with neuromuscular disease. In: Galasko C S B, Noble J (eds) Current trends in orthopaedic surgery. Manchester University Press, Manchester, p 203

Noble-Jamieson C M, Heckmatt J Z, Dubowitz V, Silverman M 1986 Effects of posture and spinal bracing on respiratory function in neuromuscular disease. Archives of Disease in Childhood 61: 178

Oka S, Igarashi Y, Takagi A et al 1982 Malignant

hyperpyrexia and Duchenne muscular dystrophy. A case report. Canadian Anaesthetists' Society Journal 29: 627

Read L, Galasko C S B 1986 Delay in diagnosing Duchenne muscular dystrophy in orthopaedic clinics. Journal of Bone and Joint Surgery 68B: 481

Riddick M F, Winter R B, Lutter L D 1982 Spinal deformities in patients with spinal muscle atrophy. A review of 36 patients. Spine 7: 476

Roy L, Gibson D A 1970 Pseudohypertrophic muscular dystrophy and its surgical management: review of 30 patients. Canadian Journal of Surgery 13: 13

Seay A R, Ziter F A, Thompson J A 1978 Cardiac arrest during induction of anaesthesia in Duchenne muscular dystrophy. Journal of Paediatrics 93: 88

Seeger B R, Sutherland A D'A, Clark M S 1984 Orthotic management of scoliosis in Duchenne muscular dystrophy. Archives of Physical Medicine and Rehabilitation 65: 83

Shapiro F, Bresnan M J 1982 Current concepts review: orthopaedic management of childhood neuromuscular diseases. Part III: diseases of muscle. Journal of Bone and Joint Surgery 64A: 1102

Siegel I M 1977 Fractures of long bones in Duchenne muscular dystrophy. Journal of Trauma 17: 219

Siegel I M 1980 Maintenance of ambulation in Duchenne muscular dystrophy. The role of the orthopaedic surgeon. Clinical Paediatrics 19: 383

Spencer G E, Vignos P J Jr 1962 Bracing for ambulation in childhood progressive muscular dystrophy. Journal of Bone and Joint Surgery 44A: 234

Swank S M, Brown J C, Perry R E 1982 Spinal fusion in Duchenne's muscular dystrophy. Spine 7: 484

Taddonio R F 1982 Segmental spinal instrumentation in the management of neuromuscular spinal deformity. Spine 7: 305

Trail I A, Galasko C S B 1990 The matrix seating system. Journal of Bone and Joint Surgery 72B: 660–669

Walton J 1983 Changing concepts of neuromuscular diseases. Hospital Update 949

Williams E A, Read L, Ellis A, Galasko C S B, Morris P 1984 The management of equinus deformity in Duchenne muscular dystrophy. Journal of Bone and Joint Surgery 66B: 546

24. Motor neurone diseases

Malcolm J. Campbell   Theodore L. Munsat

INTRODUCTION

This chapter is concerned with human diseases of motor neurones of which the archetype is adult motor neurone disease (more often called amyotrophic lateral sclerosis, or ALS in the USA). Few, if any, of these clinical syndromes are exclusive to the motor systems although in some diseases the non-motor involvement may be mild or subclinical. Furthermore, the motor system within the CNS may be selectively affected, with involvement of the upper or lower motor neurones at cerebral, brain-stem or spinal cord level, or even restricted with sparing of some neuronal group, e.g. the nucleus of Onufrowicz in the sacral cord supplying the external sphincteric muscles, or the oculomotor nuclei in the brainstem which are motor to the external ocular musculature. Many of these conditions are inherited, and recently several of the genes involved have been mapped to specific chromosomes.

Much research has been directed to studying neuronal function and metabolism, especially in relation to the role of various polypeptide neurotransmitters, to try to differentiate specific neuronal cell types. Understanding at the molecular genetic level will undoubtedly be the key to characterising motor neurones and to determining the specific abnormalities related to individual motor neurone diseases. Only then are rational treatments likely to be feasible.

The neuronal cell body or soma undertakes a high level of protein synthesis, largely through ribosomes associated with the endoplasmic reticulum. These proteins, macromolecules, neurotransmitters and enzymes required by the axon and the target tissues are then conveyed by active transport into the nerve fibres to effect normal neuronal function. This involves primarily the conduction of the nerve impulse, neurotransmitter release and transport of neurotrophic factors, as well as maintaining the structure and functional integrity of the axonal membrane. Dyck and co-workers (Dyck et al 1971, Dyck & Lais 1973) showed that neuronal degeneration may give axonal atrophy, maximal distally, with myelin wrinkling, nodal lengthening and internodal demyelination causing slowing of impulse conduction. Attempts at remyelination of Schwann cell proliferation may lead to nerve hypertrophy. If the metabolic failure proceeds, then axonal degeneration spreads proximally (dying-back), leading to loss of the axon. Recovery of metabolic activity leads to restoration of axonal structure and function. Thus the rigid separation of motor neurone disease from peripheral neuropathy is not always possible (Dyck 1982). Wallerian degeneration is associated with a decline of the membrane potential and failure of excitability in the nerve distal to transection. The atrophy and other regressive changes in the target muscle cell after nerve section or block of axoplasmic transport indicate a failure to supply some (unknown) neurotrophic substances. Thus some motor neuronal diseases may be due to a deficiency of neurotrophic substances or a defect of axoplasmic transport. Changes in the electrical activity of neurones and patterns of stimulation of muscle probably also play a part.

Fast axoplasmic transport is dependent on oxidative metabolism involving high-energy ATP provision and calcium ions and takes place at a rate of approximately 400 mm/24 h (reviewed by Ochs 1984). Identified compounds carried down nerve fibres by fast transport include glycoproteins, glycolipids, lipids, cholesterol and acetylcholinesterase (AChE). Many studies have shown retrograde transport of labelled proteins, horseradish peroxidase (HRP), toxins, nerve growth factor (NGF) and viruses at roughly half the antegrade rate. This retrograde transport has been related to chromatolysis of the neurone cell body and an increased neuronal protein synthesis after nerve injury; the signal substance is unknown. It is not known whether there is a single or multiple transport mechanism.

It is postulated that some substances taken up from muscle and other cells by nerve terminals and carried back to the cell body may be required to maintain normal neuronal function. Interference with such processes or the uptake of abnormal substances such as chemicals or toxins, may be responsible for neuropathological changes in the motor unit (Ochs 1984). This might also be an explanation for the apparent loss of motor units in certain muscle diseases such as myotonic dystrophy (Ch. 15). How far axons of peripheral nerves rely on their satellite Schwann cells for metabolic support is not yet known.

The excitability and axoplasmic transport of mammalian nerves fail quickly under conditions of anoxia or ischaemia. Fast axoplasmic transport is related to the integrity of the microtubular system within the axon. Certain drugs, e.g. colchicine or vincristine, which cause a transport block, are associated with the disaggregation or reduction in the number of microtubules and in some cases an accumulation of neurofilamentous material in the axon. Abnormalities of axoplasmic transport have been described in motor neurone disease, both in man (Norris 1979, Bradley et al 1983) and in animal models (Griffin et al 1982).

Retrograde labelling of anterior horn cells (AHC) with HRP in experimental animals has permitted a direct correlation of neuronal size and nerve fibre diameter with nerve conduction velocity and the physiological characteristics of motor units (reviewed by Burke 1982). The largest motor neurones in the lateral part of the ventral grey matter (Rexed layer IX) innervate the Type II fast twitch motor units and the intermediate size cells innervate Type I slower twitch units. The smallest motor neurones of under 35 μm diameter are largely gamma cells innervoting the muscle spindle. Campa & Engel (1970) showed that large AHC neurones of >30 μm diameter had high phosphorylase and low succinic dehydrogenase histochemical activity, implying a mainly anaerobic metabolic pathway, compared with small < 30 μm motor neurones which had a reversed metabolic profile, that is, an aerobic pattern. Burke (1982) concluded that there is no clear histochemical difference between motor neurones that innervate the different types of extrafusal motor units, and there is no clear evidence of any affinity of specific disease processes for certain motor unit types in ALS.

The physiological effect of motor neurone disease may be motor overactivity or under-activity. Overactivity is commonly associated with muscle fasciculation and cramp, or less commonly focal myokymia or painful spasms, as in tetanus. Fasciculations may persist after nerve block or spinal anaesthesia (Forster & Alpers 1944, see Layzer 1982), which suggests that an independent peripheral process can be established; they are also triggered or exacerbated by anticholinesterase drugs. Underactivity of the motor unit commonly leads initially to abnormal fatigability. Strength may be maintained for a time by the compensatory reinnervative activity of residual healthy motor neurones and axons. This leads to increased muscle fibre density within a motor unit but with variability of terminal nerve fibre branch conduction and depolarisation of individual muscle cells within the unit (Stålberg 1982). This conductive defect can be shown electrophysiologically by single-fibre electromyography (SFEMG) as 'jitter' and correlates with neuromuscular fatigue. Progressive neuronal loss leads to weakness and wasting of muscles. Such changes are seen to a degree as a natural consequence of ageing (Campbell et al 1973). Muscle wasting in the elderly, often selectively of type II units, correlates with measured loss of peripheral nerve fibres, ventral nerve roots and anterior horn cells (Tomlinson & Irving 1977, Kawamura et al 1981).

The differential diagnosis of motor neuronal diseases includes distinction from structural diseases of the spinal grey matter, as in intrinsic cord tumours or syringomyelia, compressive lesions of the spinal cord, particularly in the neck region, chronic polyradiculopathies or peripheral neuropathies and inflammatory muscle diseases (polymyositis). Cervical spondylosis may cause particular difficulty because of its frequent occurrence in the elderly, especially men, and because it often co-exists with motor neurone diseases.

The following account concerns those conditions where motor neuronal disease with neurogenic muscular atrophy and weakness are the predominant disorder leading to disability. Other conditions where amyotrophy, i.e. neurogenic muscular atrophy, is a significant secondary feature of more generalised disease are discussed briefly as study of such conditions has provided clues to the metabolic disorders present in the primary diseases. A classification of motor neurone diseases is given in Table 24.1

ADULT MOTOR NEURONE DISEASE (MND)

Adult motor neurone disease (MND) is a progressive degenerative disease of the motor system that encompasses several different clinical syndromes. It includes the features of progressive muscular atrophy (PMA), first described by Aran (1850), progressive bulbar palsy (PBP) (Duchenne 1860, Duchenne & Joffroy 1870) and primary lateral sclerosis (Charcot 1865), a purely upper motor neurone disorder. The descriptive term amyotrophic lateral sclerosis (ALS) coined by Charcot

Table 24.1   Motor neurone diseases

1. Adult motor neurone disease (ALS) includes:
   progressive muscular atrophy
   progressive bulbar palsy
   primary lateral sclerosis
   amyotrophic lateral sclerosis
   a. Sporadic forms
   b. Heredofamilial forms
   c. Western Pacific types

2. Hereditary motor neuropathies
   a. Spinal muscular atrophies (SMA)
   b. Hereditary motor and sensory neuropathies (HMSN) including Charcot–Marie–Tooth disease
   c. Spino-cerebellar ataxias including familial spastic paraplegia with amyotrophy, Friedreich's ataxia

3. Infections
   including poliomyelitis (and post-poliomyelitis muscular atrophy or PPMA), tetanus, rabies, zoster, CJD

4. Metabolic disorders
   including storage diseases, e.g. lipid (adrenomyeloneuropathy) and glycogen (Pompe's disease)
   hexosaminidase A deficiency
   diabetes and hypoglycaemia
   thyrotoxicosis
   hyperparathyroidism

5. Toxicity — heavy metals, organophosphorus compounds

6. Ischaemic myelopathy including radiation injury

7. Trauma including electrical injury

8. Immune disorders
   including plasma cell dyscrasia with paraproteinaemias
   cancers and lymphoma
   anti-ganglioside antibodies

9. Non-familial CNS degenerative disorders with amyotrophy
   including dementias, basal ganglia disease, Shy–Drager syndrome

(1874) combines all these clinical features in single patients with the pathological findings in the disease. Hence motor neurone disease and amyotrophic lateral sclerosis have come to be used by some as synonyms identifying the same disease complex. It is generally agreed that there is a similar clinical picture in the sporadic and the rare hereditary forms and in the Western Pacific form of the disease.

Clinical features

Progressive muscular atrophy syndrome.
Progressive muscular atrophy of skeletal muscles reflects involvement of motor neurones in the anterior horn of the spinal grey matter. The syndrome most commonly presents in one or other upper limb (40%), usually with wasting and weakness of the muscles of one hand. The muscles of the thenar eminence are frequently involved and this prevents opposition and abduction of the thumb. Thus the patient complains of loss of fine finger control and difficulty in fastening buttons, turning keys, picking up small objects and writing. Alternatively, more proximal arm weakness may be associated with difficulty in lifting up heavier objects, especially shopping bags, cooking utensils or during occupations. Leg weakness may present with a limping gait, foot drop or difficulty in ascending steps or stairs. Often the weakness is preceded, over several months, by symptoms of motor unit over-activity. Frequent muscle cramps are accompanied by visible muscle fasciculation. Recurrent muscle cramps in the hand or forearm are almost diagnostic of MND. Progressive atrophy of the interossei and lumbrical muscles of the hand allows the unopposed action of the long extensor and flexor muscles, causing clawing of the fingers. The atrophy and weakness commonly ascend progressively up the arm to the shoulder girdle muscles and then usually involve the contralateral hand and upper limb. The disease may then spread to the cranial musculature, as in bulbar palsy, or to the lower limbs and trunk musculature. The latter may lead to respiratory difficulty, which is discussed later.

The patchy asymmetrical wasting and weakness is associated with progressive weight loss. One hallmark of MND is the preservation or enhancement of tendon reflexes in the presence of signs of overt lower motor neurone disease. This is due to involvement of the upper motor neurones which later becomes more apparent in the fully manifest ALS picture. A pure progressive muscular atrophy picture with loss of tendon reflexes occurs in fewer than 10% of patients and should raise the question of an alternative diagnosis with a more favourable prognosis, e.g. hereditary spinal muscular atrophy or motor polyneuropathy.

Progressive bulbar palsy may be a presenting feature in 25% of patients, especially in elderly females, and often heralds a subacute disease. This causes difficulty with speech and swallowing. Indistinct or blurred speech is often the first symptom but inability to sing, whistle or speak rapidly or simply a change in tone or volume (dysphonia) may be the presenting complaint. Dysarthria arises from loss of speech muscle strength or co-ordination. This is a variable mixture of flaccid (LMN) and spastic (UMN) weakness depending on the chronology of the disease (see Aronson 1980). Whilst speech may remain intelligible for some time, it can be distorted by exhibiting audible prolongations, inappropriate pause times, imprecise articulation of consonants, hypernasality and vocal harshness (Caruso & Burton 1987). These features are distinctive and can be distinguished from other types of dysarthria (Enderby 1988). Dysphonia arises from altered muscle tone of the extra- and intralaryngeal muscles in addition to the weakness of the intercostal and diaphragmatic muscles. The former tends to affect the pitch and tone whereas the latter causes reduction of volume; normal speech is said to require a tidal air volume of 500 ml (Aronson 1980). The dysphonia is accompanied by an increased frequency of respirations during speech and a decreased length of utterances. Spasticity may give glottal constriction and a strained harshness of the voice typical of the disorder. Pooling of secretions and food particles in the hypopharynx adds a tell-tale wet, gurgling component to speech, often with an occasional coughing or choking fit. Flaccidity of the hypopharynx and larynx gives adductor muscle weakness and dysphonia and often difficult, heavy breathing or inspiratory stridor. In addition, palatal weakness allows nasal escape of air with hypernasality and decreased intra-oral pressure, which reduces friction and plosion required for articulating some consonants, leading to blurring of speech. Articulation is dependent on the precise action of many muscles including those of the tongue, lips and cheeks. An early difficulty commonly arises from wasting and immobility of the tongue, especially of the tip (Colmant 1975). Dworkin et al (1980) showed considerable reduction of tongue protrusion force in ALS. Reduction of tongue strength and speed causes distortion of many consonants as the tongue is no longer able to make firm contact with the teeth and hard palate (Aronson 1980). Slowness of tongue movements and hence of speech is evident from the reduced number of syllables per second, from an average of six to a maximum of four (Dworkin et al 1980). With general weakness of the tongue the vowels 'u' and 'o' become progressively difficult to pronounce as these require subtle movements (Böhme 1974). Weakness of the circumoral musculature reduces lip mobility and seal pressure and lowers intra-oral pressure during speech: thus plosive sounds become difficult and then impossible (see Darley et al 1975). In the late stages all speech is lost (anarthria). In addition to the primary speech disorder there may be pathological laughter or crying from corticobulbar (pseudobulbar) involvement.

Difficulty with swallowing (dysphagia) may emanate from weakness of the lips making it difficult to retain material in the mouth or weakness of the tongue which normally controls the propulsion of the bolus in the oral phase and pushes it posteriorly into the oral pharynx. Masticatory muscle weakness causes difficulty in chewing and may even result in subluxation of the jaw, either spontaneously or during involuntary yawning. The soft palate should lift to prevent nasal regurgitation. Simultaneously the larynx should rise to assist with closure of the epiglottis and the pharyngeal constrictor muscles contract to move food down into the oesophagus. In the oesophagus reflex peristaltic waves move the food bolus down to the stomach. In a survey of 31 patients with MND 73% were found to have dysphagia, 42% had difficulty swallowing both food and liquid, 37% more difficulty with solids and 21% more difficulty with liquids (Mayberry &

Atkinson 1986). Bosma & Brodie (1969) have demonstrated several kinds of pharyngeal dysfunction in ALS, especially failure to prevent laryngeal penetration. Such penetration may not occur at the time of swallowing but during respiration afterwards. This is related to pooling of food particles in the hypopharynx, either as a result of flaccidity or due to hypertonicity of the cricopharyngeus muscle from UMN involvement. Oesophageal motility has been studied by cinéradiological techniques and by measurement of intraluminar pressure using catheters connected to pressure transducers. Smith et al (1957) reported that, of 19 ALS patients studied, most had abnormalities of the middle and lower oesophagus with feeble contractions; some of their patients had weak upper and lower oesophageal sphincteric function. Smith et al (1980) reported that the low resting pressure seen in the upper sphincter could be augmented by administration of intravenous edrophonium chloride (Tensilon®) resulting in improved motility; however, they found that lower oesophageal sphincter pressures were generally normal. Dysphagia is often aggravated by troublesome pooling of saliva, often resulting in drooling and a spluttering cough.

In some cases, visible wasting of the tongue with fasciculations may precede any bulbar symptoms. In others, physical signs in the bulbar musculature may not be apparent in the early stages and may lead erroneously to a diagnosis of hysteria. Later, wasting and fasciculation of the tongue, together with weak force and slowness of alternating movements, become obvious. Poor voluntary palatal or pharyngeal movement may be associated with a brisk gag reflex or jaw jerk from supranuclear (UMN) involvement.

Primary lateral sclerosis. This much-debated entity as described by Charcot (1865) is a rare presenting form of MND in fewer than 10% of cases. With the advent of magnetic resonance imaging it has become clear that the vast majority of patients with this syndrome have a demyelinating disorder indistinguishable from late-onset progressive multiple sclerosis (Younger et al 1988). Slowly progressive spasticity and weakness of the limbs, usually the lower extremities, together with pathologically brisk tendon reflexes, are the sole presenting clinical features. Its differentiation from other causes of spastic paraparesis or quadriparesis is usually made by the appearance of visible fasciculations and wasting or by electrophysiological findings of LMN involvement. There have been few clinicopathological correlative studies describing complete preservation of anterior horn cells in such cases, but some have shown intracytoplasmic hyaline inclusions, similar to those described in familial ALS (Fisher 1977, Beal & Richardson 1981).

Amyotrophic lateral sclerosis (ALS). In a large series of MND patients Bonduelle (1975) found that 66% had ALS. This is the combined UMN and LMN disease state that is virtually always present terminally and is the commonest clinical syndrome. It is responsible for the common 'strained-strangled voice' disorder of bulbar involvement. Spasticity is rarely severe in the limbs, despite the very brisk reflexes and the extension plantar (Babinski) responses. The clinical picture is one of steadily progressive weakness of all limb and bulbar muscles, with increasing disability. Recent quantitative studies have shown that deterioration rates are remarkably linear but variable between patients (Munsat et al 1988). Respiratory muscles are also involved, although dyspnoea is usually a late symptom. Very occasionally, alveolar hypoventilation can be a presenting symptom of MND. The diaphragm is the main muscle used in quiet breathing, and intercostal and accessory muscles can compensate for diaphragmatic weakness, but not during exertional breathing. Breathing difficulties may be apparent during speech. Spirometric studies have shown that the forced vital lung capacity (FVC) is the most useful measure of respiratory function in MND and correlates with the progression of the disease. A fall of the FVC by 25% between the upright and supine positions is indicative of diaphragmatic weakness. It declines slowly until the terminal months when it falls below 50% of the predicted normal (Fallat et al 1979). The maximum inspiratory and expiratory pressures (PI max and PE max) are more sensitive tests of respiratory muscle function (Hyatt & Black 1971, Griggs et al 1981), but these are often difficult to record because of poor lip seal. The arterial blood gases are rarely abnormal even when the predicted FVC is less than 50% (Fallat & Norris 1980). Chronic respiratory failure often indicates co-existing lung disease. If it is present, it can only be treated with mechanical ventilatory support. Studies of autonomic nerve function, both of the vagal parasympathetic and sympathetic systems, have shown normal results (Sachs et al 1985). Some patients demonstrate breath-holding attacks in sleep (sleep apnoea) which may be responsible for respiratory arrest.

Respiratory complications are the most frequent terminal event. These include restricted ventilation causing chronic respiratory failure, pharyngeal or laryngeal weakness causing poor airway protection and bronchopulmonary aspiration, impaired cough response and inability to clear airway and sudden vagal arrest from choking or cough stimulation.

Familial forms of adult MND. The familial incidence of MND with pyramidal tract (UMN) signs, i.e. ALS, is 5–10% world-wide with a 1:1 sex distribution ratio and commonly with an autosomal dominant pattern of inheritance (Emery & Holloway 1982). Recent linkage analysis of large pedigrees have demonstrated that in most, but not all families, the ALS gene maps to chromosome 21 (Siddique et al 1991). The various forms of spinal muscular atrophy without UMN signs are dealt with below.

The clinical picture in general is similar to that in sporadic cases except for the earlier age of onset, mean 45.1 compared with 56.2 years for sporadic cases (Emery & Holloway 1982), the more frequent onset of weakness in the legs, especially in juvenile-onset cases, and the higher concurrence with other features of CNS disease, e.g. dementia, extrapyramidal disease (reviewed by Bonduelle 1975). Amyotrophy or motor neurone disturbance as part of multisystem degenerative disease is discussed later. Juvenile MND (ALS) is considered here, as a high proportion of cases are familial. Three separate forms have been identified:

1. An early childhood form, with bulbar features in 80% of cases, has an autosomal recessive pattern of inheritance.
2. A slowly progressive late juvenile form with autosomal dominant inheritance has early involvement of the legs and no bulbar signs (Emery & Holloway 1982).

3. An autosomal recessive form reported from Tunisia with upper and lower motor neurone signs sometimes with a pseudobulbar picture, and very slow progression (Ben Hamida et al 1990).

The clinical course of familial MND varies widely, even among some family pedigrees. Overall there is a shorter duration to death (Engel et al 1959, Campbell 1979), but some familial cases, especially the juvenile forms, are extremely chronic (Horton et al 1976).

Western Pacific forms of adult MND. An abnormally high prevalence of MND was previously found in the indigenous Chamorro population of Guam and other Mariana islands (Reed & Brody 1975, Reed et al 1975), as well as in certain other foci: on the Kii peninsula of Honshu island, Japan (Kondo 1979), in West New Guinea (Gajdusek 1963, 1982) and in Groote Eylandt and the adjacent coastland of Northern Australia (Kiloh et al 1980) (Fig. 24.1). The clinical picture of MND in these high-incidence foci differs from the ubiquitous form in an earlier age of onset, the predominance of spasticity and leg involvement and the longer clinical course. There is also an inter-relationship with another high-incidence disease, the parkinsonism–dementia complex (P–D) which occurs in the Marianas. About 10% of MND patients on Guam show extrapyramidal or intellectual deficit (Kurland & Brody 1975); in the P–D complex about 30% of patients show evident muscle wasting. The epidemiological and pathological features of this disease are discussed later.

Unusual clinical features

Intellectual impairment or mental deficit have been described in a small proportion of typical MND patients, especially among familial cases (Wikstrom et al 1982); systematic investigation of cognitive function in a group of sporadic cases showed mild significant cognitive deficit but no memory impairment or behavioural disturbances (Gallassi et al 1985). The syndromes of ALS with dementia have been reviewed by Salazar et al (1983) in relation to transmissible Creutzfeldt–Jakob disease (CJD). Their review included 231 patients with dementia and early LMN signs: in

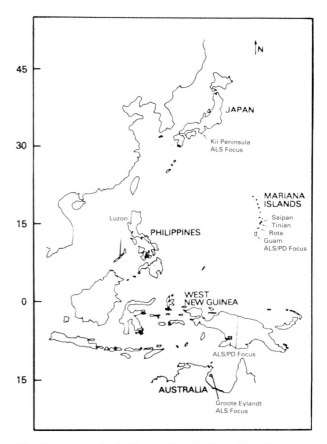

Fig. 24.1 Areas in the Western Pacific affected by a high incidence of adult MND

these cases the clinical course was slower than that in CJD and there was little, if any, spongiform change in the brain at autopsy; only two out of 33 brains transmitted a spongiform change to inoculated primates. This is in contrast to the typical subacute transmissible CJD where LMN involvement occurs late in the course of the disease.

Ocular muscle involvement is seldom observed clinically in MND (Harvey et al 1979), although defective eye movements have been detected by electro-oculography (Leveille et al 1982) and nystagmus has also been observed in a few cases (Kushner et al 1984).

Sensory symptoms of numbness, deadness or tingling in the extremities are often mentioned by patients but routine sensory testing is normal even in those familial cases who are subsequently demonstrated to have spinal sensory tract degeneration. However, careful quantitative sensory testing has revealed a 40% incidence of impaired touch-pressure sensibility (Dyck et al 1975). Automated thermal sensory threshold studies have also shown mild abnormalities (Jamal et al 1985). This would correlate with the minor non-motor and sensory abnormalities which have been found in pathological studies (see Hirano et al 1969). Chronic pain has been described in MND but it is uncertain whether this is a primary disorder or secondary to the problems of immobility and pressure deformities (Drake 1983, Newrick & Hewer 1984). Pressure sores or other skin damage are unusual in MND and probably reflect normal autonomic function. Bladder, bowel and sexual dysfunction are unusual even in the terminal stages. The unaffected autonomic sphincter function correlates with the histological preservation of motor neurones in the nucleus of Onufrowicz area of the sacral spinal cord and of the external anal sphincteric muscle in ALS patients (Mannen et al 1982). Constipation may result from the enforced immobility and low-fibre dietary intake. This may account for the occasional urinary retention. Libido and sexual function can be retained up to the final weeks of the illness (Jokelainen & Palo 1976). Normal cardiovascular responses reflecting vagal nerve function have also been reported (Sachs et al 1985).

Clinical course and prognosis

The usual course of the disease is a relentless spread of wasting and weakness of all skeletal and cranial musculature towards total paralysis, with the exception of the extra-ocular muscles. Diaphragmatic paralysis is usually incomplete for the probable reason that respiratory failure, often complicated by lung infection, is the usual terminal event. A number of patients have an acute arrhythmia or myocardial ischaemia, sometimes stimulated by troublesome coughing or choking. In some patients the course is unusually prolonged or rarely appears to arrest. These patients typically have little if any VMN deficit (Mulder & Howard 1976, Norris et al 1980). Most studies have shown a better prognosis for those patients presenting with LMN disease as progressive muscular atrophy, but care must be taken in dis-tinguishing late-onset forms of hereditary spinal muscular atrophy. A shorter mean survival occurs in cases of bulbar palsy and/or those patients with early-onset bulbar symptoms, with death on average within 18 months. Overall in ALS, Mulder & Howard (1976) reported a 50% survival of less than 3 years, but 20% survived 5 years and 10% survived 10 years from initial symptoms.

Epidemiology

Adult MND has been described world-wide and in Western countries is responsible for approximately 1 in 1000 adult deaths, with a higher rate in men. The crude death rate is 0.5–1.1 per 100 000 population, centring near 0.8 (Kurtzke 1982). The age-adjusted mortality figure in the USA is 0.6–0.7, being 0.8 for men and 0.4 for women (Juergens & Kurland 1980). The age-specific mortality rates appear to increase steadily up to the 65+ age groups, especially in males, to 5–8 for men and 3–5 per 100 000 for women; recent studies suggest that there may not be a subsequent decline (Li et al 1985).

The annual incidence of MND (ALS) varies between 0.4 and 1.8 per 100 000 population, except in certain foci in the Western Pacific area where the incidence and prevalence was previously much higher. Recent studies for Rochester, Minnesota, USA, suggest that the age-specific incidence continues to rise with age up to 75+ like that of any degenerative or ageing disease (Juergens et al 1980), whereas earlier studies showed a peak at 65–70 years with a subsequent decline. There is generally more variation in prevalence rates than reported for incidence, but an overall figure of 4–6 per 100 000 is an average figure (Kurtzke 1982): this would correspond to an average duration of MND of 3–4 years. Between 5% and 10% of cases in most countries are familial, with an equal sex distribution and an autosomal dominant pattern of inheritance (Kurland & Mulder 1955). Recently, the gene has been mapped to chromosome 21 by two groups (Siddique et al 1991). Linkage data suggests that there is some non-allelic heterogeneity, although this remains to be elucidated. Several foci of high incidence of MND (ALS) have been extensively reported in the

Western Pacific area, starting with Guam. Initially, incidence and mortality rates there were 50–100 times greater than average world-wide figures; however, there has been a steady decline from these high rates to less than 5 per 100 000 population on Guam for 1980–82 (Garruto et al 1985). Similar declining rates have been reported for the Kii peninsula in Japan and a focus in West New Guinea. The significance of this rapid decline is discussed later, but it is inconsistent with a primary genetic origin.

Laboratory investigations

There are still no specific biochemical tests for MND but the most helpful findings are revealed by electro-diagnostic tests (Bradley 1987). Routine needle electromyography (EMG) demonstrates scattered spontaneous fibrillation and fasciculation potentials, and enlarged polyphasic volitional units in muscles from two or more extremities, indicative of denervative and reinnervative muscle disease. The spontaneous motor unit discharges, or fasciculation potentials, are frequently polyphasic and discharge at a slower rate (average every 4–5 seconds) than in the benign fasciculation syndrome (Hjorth et al 1973, Trojaborg & Buchthal 1965 and see Ch. 13). The motor unit potentials (MUP) are often prolonged in duration and enlarged in amplitude, indicative of reinnervative activity with increased muscle-fibre density (FD). These changes are more easily seen with macro-EMG studies (Stålberg 1982). The enlarged MUP often has a variable shape or amplitude during consecutive discharges, indicating impaired transmission in new terminal nerve endings. This is best seen as abnormal jitter with single-fibre EMG (SFEMG) studies. An abnormal EMG picture including abnormal jitter in 30% of recordings can be found in clinically normal muscles in MND, or in patients with UMN signs only, but the abnormalities are maximal in the weakest muscles (Stålberg 1982). In slowly progressive disease a high FD (twice to four times the normal level) with high-amplitude macro MUPs (up to 15–20 times normal) and mild to moderate jitter is seen (Swash & Schwartz 1982). With moderately severe weakness the FD and MUP amplitudes are markedly elevated but

the maximal reinnervative response is insufficient to compensate for motor unit loss. With increasing weakness the MUP amplitudes progressively decrease as the motor neurones are unable to maintain the maximal degree of reinnervation (Stålberg & Sanders 1984). A rapid clinical progression is associated with a moderately increased FD, normal or mildly increased macro EMG potentials but with very abnormal jitter and frequent impulse blocking on SFEMG (Swash & Schwartz 1982).

The fastest motor and sensory nerve conduction velocities (NCV) are frequently normal, except in severe denervation where the maximal evoked muscle response is less than 10% of normal (Lambert 1969). However, mild slowing and increased F-wave latencies are frequently found (Stålberg & Sanders 1984); sensory velocities were slightly abnormal in four of 18 patients. This probably reflects secondary demyelinative changes in degenerating axons. Abnormal neuromuscular transmission has been found in a high proportion of MND patients studied by repetitive nerve stimulation and is partly improved by anticholinesterase drug administration (Lambert & Mulder 1957, Mulder et al 1959, Denys & Norris 1979). This corresponds to the abnormal jitter found by SFEMG studies and is thought to relate to inefficient reinnervative sprouting rather than terminal fibre degeneration (Stålberg 1982). Slowing of electrical conduction in the central motor pathways of the brain and spinal cord has been demonstrated recently in MND (Ingram & Swash 1987). The changes were more marked in patients with UMN signs but a relative inexcitability of the motor cortex and spinal cord in other early cases was thought to reflect subclinical UMN cell loss, axonal degeneration and secondary demyelination in the central motor pathways. Similar findings of mild CNS slowing have been reported using the new technique of transcutaneous magnetic stimulation of the brain and spinal nerve roots (Barker et al 1985, Ingram et al 1988).

Routine blood investigations are generally normal apart from a mild to moderate increase in the serum creatine kinase (CK) activity in about 40% of MND patients (Williams & Bruford 1970, Harrington et al 1983). Increased serum CK cardiac isoenzyme (MB) has been described in more than one-half of all ALS patients and has been correlated with muscle-fibre regeneration, as seen histologically on muscle biopsy (Koller & Engel 1984). An abnormal blood glucose in response to a glucose loading test, together with a high circulating pyruvate level, has been repeatedly demonstrated in MND (Steinke & Tyler 1964). This was thought to be due to subnormal pancreatic insulin secretion (Gotoh et al 1972), or insulin resistance but this finding was not confirmed by others (Astin et al 1975). Similarly, earlier claims for an abnormal pancreatic exocrine function (Quick & Greer 1967) have not been substantiated.

Standard cerebrospinal fluid analyses are generally normal in MND, but the presence of a high protein content and oligoclonal immunoglobin bands, raised the possibility of an associated paraproteinaemia in 10% of MND patients (Shy et al 1986, Younger et al 1990). Latov and coworkers (1988) found high titres of antibodies to GM_1 ganglioside in some of these patients but this is not a finding specific to MND. A number of these patients have now been found to have lymphoma (Younger et al 1991).

Increased lead content in the blood and cerebrospinal fluid (CSF) has been reported in MND patients by Conradi and colleagues (see Conradi et al 1982) but has not been found by others (Manton & Cook 1979). A high incidence of radiographic abnormalities of the spine (Campbell et al 1970) has been found also by others and correlated with abnormalities of calcium metabolism in a proportion of MND patients. Abnormal blood calcium levels, usually high rather than low, and elevated concentrations of serum parathormone have been reported in 20% or more of ALS patients (Patten 1982). These changes are thought to represent a secondary hyperparathyroid reaction to hypocalcaemia but no improvement in the neurological state occurred with restoration of the calcium homeostasis. The reason for these changes remains unknown.

Blood group or histocompatibility antigen (HLA) studies have revealed no clear relationship with MND or ALS. Some reports have suggested an over-representation of A3 in ALS patients or an excess of B12 in slow progressive disease (Antel

et al 1982, Kott et al 1979). Other studies have reported an excess of BW35 (Kott et al 1976, Bartfeld et al 1982b). Guamanian ALS patients with HLA-BW35 showed impaired cell-mediated immunity and T-cell mitogen reactivity, and a shorter disease duration, compared with Guamanian patients who lacked this antigen (Hoffman et al 1978). The total T-lymphocyte counts, and T-cell subset analyses and serum and CSF immunoglobulins have been unchanged from normal in most studies (Antel et al 1982, Bartfeld et al 1982a), but others have found decreased T-cell reactivity to non-specific mitogens (Hoffman et al 1977, Behan 1979, Aspin et al 1986). Kott et al (1979) reported increased cell-mediated immunity to pooled polio antigens and this has been confirmed by Bartfeld et al (1982a). Serological studies have not shown raised complement-fixing or neutralising antibodies to polio or other viruses in blood or CSF of MND patients (Kascsak et al 1982, Harter 1982). Virus-related antigens or nucleic acid sequences have not been identified in ALS tissue (See Fallis & Weiner 1982). Circulating immune complexes were reported by Oldstone and colleagues (1976) but were undetected in the CSF by Bartfeld et al (1982a); however, Digby et al (1985) reported that MND sera contain immunoglobulins that bind to spinal cord cells in culture. Studies of cell count and total protein levels in CSF are normal in MND.

Pathology

The gross pathological features described by Charcot (1874) have been little modified since (see review by Hughes 1982). The overall picture in the CNS is of selective neuronal loss with secondary motor tract degeneration in the brain stem and spinal cord maximal caudally. There may be substantial loss of the large pyramidal cells from layer V of the motor cortex plus corticospinal tract degeneration through the posterior limb of the internal capsule, the cerebral peduncles, brain stem and spinal cord. Such pyramidal tract degeneration is found even in cases without clinically detectable UMN involvement (Friedman & Freedman 1950). Neuronal loss and degeneration is seen in the motor nuclei of the brain stem, especially of the Vth, VIIth, Xth and XIIth cranial nerves. Mild changes may be seen in the oculomotor nuclei of the mid-brain. Degenerative changes include cell shrinkage and neuronophagia. In the spinal cord, neuronal changes are confined to the anterior horn neurones, especially at cervical and lumbar level but with selective sparing of motor neurones in the lateral parts of the sacral cord (nucleus of Onufrowicz) (Mannen et al 1982). This selective sparing has also been seen in poliomyelitis (Kojima et al 1989). The depletion of large neurones is associated with gliosis in the ventral grey matter. Chromatolysis and 15 nm neurofilamentous accumulation may be found; some containing ubiquitin resemble heavy bodies (Leigh et al 1988). Spheroidal axonal swellings on the proximal nerve roots were first described by Wohlfart (1959) and were rediscovered by Carpenter (1968). Electron-microscopy reveals that the swellings consist of bundles of 100 nm diameter filaments. Non-motor neurones and myelinated tracts may show minor degenerative changes in sporadic cases of ALS, especially in cases of prolonged survival with ventilatory support (Hayashi & Kato 1989). Familial forms of the disease frequently include degeneration of the posterior myelinated sensory tracts and of the anterior and posterior spinocerebellar tracts, as well as of Clarke's column, despite the absence of clinical sensory involvement (Hirano et al 1969). Ubiquitin inclusions in motor neurones are more common and striking (Mizusawa et al 1989).

Histochemical studies of normal spinal cords show a heavy concentration of acetylcholinesterase (AChE), choline acetyltransferase (ChAT) and muscarinic cholinergic receptors in Rexed layer IX (Villiger & Faull 1985). In ALS, ChAT levels (Gillberg et al 1982) and muscarinic receptors (Whitehouse et al 1983) are markedly reduced. Various other polypeptide neurotransmitters have been studied: glycine levels are normal but glycine receptors are reduced (Hayashi et al 1981, Whitehouse et al 1983). Plaitakis et al (1988), reporting increased levels of the excitatory neurotransmitter amino acid glutamate in the CSF and low levels in the brain and spinal cord in ALS, advocated branched-chain amino acid (BCAA) therapy to stimulate glutamate oxidation to lower levels of the excitotoxin in motor neurones.

Others failed to find the changes (discussed by Young 1990). Thyrotrophin-releasing hormone (TRH) terminals, which are normally restricted to medial layer VII and layer IX (Hokfeld et al 1975, Schoenen et al 1985), are markedly reduced in ALS (Manakar et al 1985). Substance P (SP) studies have given variable results but SP fibres in layer IX of cervical and lumbar ALS cords have been reported as markedly reduced, even when degenerating motor neurones are inconspicuous (Schoenen et al 1985). ChAT activity in ALS peripheral nerves was reduced to 20% of control values and AChE to about 45%, with a greater loss distally (Bradley et al 1983).

Mann & Yates (1974) demonstrated decreased RNA content in the cytoplasm of anterior horn cells of two patients with ALS and postulated that the primary lesion was degeneration of neuronal nuclear DNA with secondary loss of RNA production. These findings have been confirmed by Hartmann & Davidson (1982) in both the cervical and lumbar motor neurones. Ribosomal RNA (rRNA) constitutes 80% of cellular RNA. The 40% reduction in RNA in motor but not in sensory neurones, presumably of rRNA, would deter neuronal protein synthesis.

The anterior nerve roots are thin and pale from depletion of axons and of large myelinated fibres, together with fibrosis. Smaller-diameter myelinated fibres, probably gamma efferents to the muscle spindles, are well preserved (Sobue et at 1981). These ventral root changes are maximal in the cervical and lumbar cord levels and correspond to the selective vulnerability of the large alpha motor neurones in MND (Kawamura et al 1981). Teased-fibre preparations of the ventral roots have demonstrated fibres undergoing axonal degeneration and, to a lesser extent, segmental demyelination (Hanyu et al 1981). The latter abnormality is probably a secondary Schwann-cell change and would correspond to the delayed F-wave nerve conduction seen in electrophysiological studies (Stålberg 1982). Similar degenerative changes have been demonstrated at proximal and distal levels of the phrenic nerve in keeping with a neuronopathy (Bradley et al 1983). Peripheral nerve trunks may appear normal because of the predominant large afferent sensory fibres, although degeneration and demyelination of sensory fibres to a mild extent are well established in MND (Dayan et al 1969, Dyck et al 1975). These sensory nerve changes correlate with reports that neurones in the lumbar dorsal root ganglia are reduced to 46% of control numbers (Kawamura et al 1981). Degeneration and regenerative sprouting of motor nerve endings, together with denervated atrophic motor end-plates, are seen in muscle biopsy specimens (Bjornskov et al 1984, Tsujihata et al 1984). Skeletal muscles show the typical changes of chronic denervation with grouped fibre atrophy, often of the same histochemical type. Inflammatory changes are not present but occasional regenerating fibres may be seen, especially in rapidly progressive clinical cases.

Aetiology

Epidemiological factors. Approximately 90–95% of cases of adult MND (ALS) seen to be sporadic. Familial cases of ALS show a greater degree of non-motor involvement pathologically but the motor neuronal changes are thought to be identical to those found in sporadic cases. The rapid decline in incidence of ALS on Guam and other foci in the Western Pacific area (Garruto et al 1985) is inconsistent with a primary genetic disease; the offspring of index cases have not shown an increased risk of developing ALS (Plato et al 1984). In addition, Chamorros on the neighbouring Mariana islands, Saipan and Tinian, do not have an increased incidence of ALS (Yanagihara et al 1983). Hence the earlier high incidence on Guam and the Kii peninsula of Japan has been suggested as resulting from environmental factors. The absence of any clear blood group or HLA association is also evidence against a genetically determined metabolic defect.

Ageing. Progressive neuronal loss occurs in the ventral horn of the spinal grey matter with normal ageing (Tomlinson & Irving 1977); this correlates with the finding of neurogenic muscular atrophy in skeletal muscles of the elderly (Tomlinson et al 1969) and electrophysiological evidence of progressive loss of motor units after the age of 60 years (Campbell et al 1973). Hence the suggestion has been made that MND is due to an accelerated ageing process (McComas et al

1973b). This suggestion would be more tenable if recent work suggesting an increasing incidence of MND with age were substantiated (Juergens et al 1980) rather than the more common finding of a peak incidence at about 65 years and a decline thereafter. The accelerated ageing could be due to as yet unknown exogenous factors.

Molecular biology. The observation of a low RNA content in MND motor neurones led Mann & Yates (1974) to postulate a primary defect of nuclear DNA with decreased RNA synthesis and subsequent protein synthesis. Such a theory is supported by the observation of a 30% reduction in RNA content and nuclear RNA synthesis in the spinal motor neurones of the wobbler mouse, an animal model of human MND (Murakami et al 1981). Actinomycin D, a specific RNA polymerase inhibitor that inhibits RNA and protein synthesis, and the 5-fluoropyrimidines that disturb biosynthesis of pyrimidine nucleotides, RNA and protein, when injected intrathecally into cats, both lead to neuronal degeneration (Koenig 1969). Thus there are several possible mechanisms for the reduced level of ribosomal RNA in ALS motor neurones, although Bradley & Krasin (1982) have postulated aberrant transcription caused by accumulation of unrepaired DNA damage arising from a deficiency of DNA repair enzymes.

Intoxication. The superficial similarity to PMA of various motor neuropathies attributable to intoxication with heavy metals, notably lead, has resulted in repeated searches for their involvement in MND, but an increased incidence of the disease has not been reported among lead or manganese workers. A higher incidence of exposure to the heavy metals, lead and mercury, participation in athletics and consumption of large quantities of milk, was reported for a group of 25 ALS patients (Felmus et al 1976). Several previous studies have reported failure of treatment with various chelating agents in MND or ALS patients who gave a history of exposure to lead, mercury or arsenic (Currier & Haerer 1968, Engel et al 1969, Campbell et al 1970). The reports by Conradi and colleagues (1982) of increased levels of lead in blood and CSF of ALS patients have not been confirmed by others (Manton & Cook 1979), although a high level of lead in spinal cord tissue from ALS patients has been demonstrated

(Kurlander & Patten 1979). The mode of entry of lead into the nervous system in ALS has not been established. The search for local environmental factors in the high-incidence Western Pacific areas revealed a low calcium and magnesium concentration in garden soil and drinking water and a higher content of heavy or trace metals, e.g. manganese and aluminium (Yase 1972, 1984). Analyses of brain tissue from ALS cases on Guam and Japan showed a high intraneuronal content of calcium and aluminium (Garruto et al 1984) and also a high manganese level in spinal cord tissue (Miyata et al 1983). X-ray analysis has shown metal-related calcification in degenerating areas of the cervical cord in ALS (Yoshida 1977, 1979, quoted by Yanagihara 1982). Selective motor neurone involvement may occur because of the requirement for high levels of calcium ions. Yase (1984) has postulated that chronic nutritional deficiencies of calcium and magnesium may cause secondary hyperparathyroidism leading to increased bone resorption and release of calcium and other cations, as well as increased intestinal absorption of trace metals, thus leading to ectopic calcification and deposition of heavy metals. The deposition of heavy metals including manganese, aluminium and lead in the CNS may be a secondary phenomenon, as a consequence of an altered blood–brain barrier or as a result of neuronal degeneration and reactive gliosis (Mandybur & Cooper 1979). However, Yase (1984) cites experiments with rats maintained on a low calcium and magnesium diet which results in ectopic calcification in kidney, muscle and the CNS, and is associated with increased gliosis and anterior horn cell degeneration in the spinal cord. Such changes are said to occur only in the presence of parathormone. Patients with primary or secondary hyperparathyroidism have been reported to have neuromuscular disorders and signs suggestive of MND (Patten 1982), but treatment of some typical MND patients with abnormal calcium metabolism showed no improvement in neurological function.

An alternative theory for a toxic cause of the earlier high incidence and prevalence of ALS on Guam has been related to the dietary use of the Cycad nut. This was a major source of edible starch for the native Chamorros. It is known to contain certain neurotoxic compounds including cycasin, or methylazoxymethanol, a lathyrogenic factor (Kurland & Molgaard 1982). More recently, Spencer and colleagues (1986) were able to reproduce a lathyrism-like syndrome in macaques by the oral ingestion of the excitatory amino acid L-β methylaminoalanine (BOAA) extracted from the chickling pea. Similarly, these workers have provided experimental evidence that ALS in Guam might be caused by an excitotoxin contained in the Cycad nut (Spencer et al 1987). The decline in ALS on Guam has coincided with a striking reduction in the use of cycad as the Chamorros have changed from a horticultural and fishing subsistence economy to a westernised culture (Garruto et al 1985).

Viruses. A number of viruses selectively infect neurones and in some cases motor neurones, e.g. poliovirus. The production of new viral particles is the result of an ordered sequence of virus–cell interactions within a permissive cell. Susceptible cells may initiate translation of early viral proteins, but fail to form complete viruses, i.e., they are non-permissively infected. Non-permissive infections can lead to cell death, cell transformation or metabolic deficits, even though the infected cell does not contain infectious virus or morphologically discernible viral particles (Johnson 1982a). Polioviruses in man and the neurotrophic leukaemia retrovirus in the mouse (MuLV)(Gardner et al 1973) both cause paralytic disease with acute pathological changes in the spinal motor neurones. Polio infection excites an intense inflammatory response with neuronal degeneration and an acute cytolytic reaction in some cells. In MuLV infection of susceptible species there is a long incubation period resulting in a chronic non-inflammatory infection with neuronal degeneration (Andrews & Gardner 1974). The selective involvement of motor neurones in poliomyelitis and MND has led to many attempts to isolate poliovirus, or to demonstrate virus structures, antigens or raised antibody responses in ALS patients, all with negative results. Molecular genetic studies of the paralytic induction by MuLV have suggested that the retrovirus binds to a specific cellular receptor on motor neurones leading to degeneration (Paquette et al 1989). Certain mouse strains infected with lactate dehydrogenase elevating virus (LDV) show extensive motor neurone destruction; this correlates with increased MuLV expression in susceptible species with increasing age, after X-irradiation and immunosuppression (Contag et al 1989). This may be a model for post-poliomyelitis muscular atrophy (PPMA). There is no evidence for retroviral infection in ALS although occasional patients from populations infected with HTLV-I virus have been seropositive. HTLV-I infection is normally associated with a chronic paralytic myelopathy. These studies were prompted by reports of a higher incidence of previous poliomyelitis infections in MND patients. The situation has been complicated by the frequent description of chronic MND in patients occurring many years after acute paralytic poliomyelitis (Campbell et al 1969, Mulder et al 1972, Dalakas et al 1986). This disease, perhaps better named post-poliomyelitis muscular atrophy (PPMA), becomes symptomatic some 15–54 years after acute poliomyelitis (Munsat 1991). The new weakness and muscular atrophy develop in muscles previously affected and fully or partly recovered, or in clinically unaffected muscles. Occasional fasciculations are seen but bulbar symptoms or UMN signs do not appear during the slow progressive course. Electrodiagnostic tests show the typical appearances of a very chronic denervation disorder with giant MUP, but abnormal jitter and frequent blocking are seen in most muscles (Dalakas et al 1986). This indicates poor function in the terminal nerve fibres and correlates with the old observations of myasthenic-like neuromuscular fatigue in surviving muscles (Hodes 1948). Histological studies of muscle biopsies from PPMA have shown scattered isolated angulated atrophic fibres and no grouped atrophy. This has been interpreted as indicative of degeneration of individual nerve terminals in the hypertrophied motor unit rather than as a result of complete motor unit loss from neuronal death (Dalakas et al 1986). It has been proposed that the motor neurone is unable to maintain the metabolic demands of the extended territory and target cells. Cerebrospinal fluid studies have shown normal protein and IgG levels and no evidence of in situ antibody production to poliovirus. This does not entirely rule out the possibility of chronic or reactivated polio infection, as

animal studies with Theiler's virus or murine poliomyelitis have shown a delayed immune response to the chronic mild inflammatory disease (Lipton & Dal Canto 1976). A case of chronic progressive poliomyelitis secondary to live virus vaccination has been reported in an immunodeficient child (Davis et al 1977). A search for other viruses in MND has produced no substantiated results. Repeated transmission studies of ALS material into primates have been negative (Gibbs & Gajdusek 1982). Similar negative results of attempts to isolate viruses in tissue culture from muscle were reported by Cremer et al (1973). Sera and CSF samples from 10 ALS patients tested negative for anti-HTLV-I antibodies (Annunziata et al 1989).

As mentioned in the section on investigations (pp 887–888), no strong link with an HLA antigen has been reported in MND: thus there is no evidence for a genetically determined immune responsiveness. Circulating immune complexes have been detected in ALS sera; when used to immunise rabbits, the complexes induced an antibody response to enterovirus-infected cells including Coxsackie A9 and B4, and poliovirus type 3 (Bartfeld et al 1989). Reports that MND sera has a toxic effect on spinal cord explants (Wolfgram 1976), contained immunoglobulins binding to cultured spinal neurones (Digby et al 1985), and auto-antibodies directed against muscle-derived nerve growth factor (Gurney et al 1984) have not been reproducible in cultures of human fetal spinal cord (Erkman et al 1989). Serum antibodies to gangliosides have been demonstrated by several groups (Pestronk et al 1989) but the significance of these findings is uncertain. Drachman & Kuncl (1989) have summarised the evidence for an autoimmune process in ALS. The finding of an oncogenic retrovirus causing both lymphoma and chronic motor neuronal disease in mice (Gardner et al 1973) has raised the question of a relationship between lymphoma and MND (Younger et al 1991). The rare reports of MND occurring in association with bronchial carcinoma probably represent a chance association. There is a more direct link between plasma cell dyscrasias and paraproteinaemia and motor neuropathies. Plasma paraproteins of the IgG, IgM and IgA type have all been associated with LMN disease or a demyelinative neuropathy but only rarely with an ALS picture (Latov 1982). Most ALS patients lack IgM monoclonal antibodies and anti-GM1 or anti-GD1 antibodies which have been associated with a lower motor neurone syndrome that is sometimes responsive to imunosuppressive therapy (Latov et al 1988). Patients with this syndrome have a progressive distal weakness and multiple nerve conduction block, and usually have high titres of anti-GM1 antibody (Pestronk et al 1989).

Treatment

Not surprisingly for a condition of unknown cause, many treatments have been tried, based on theories of the aetiology and generally with negative results. Initial anecdotal or uncontrolled studies have not been substantiated in clinical trials. The latter have been reviewed extensively elsewhere (Festoff & Crigger 1980) and this Chapter endeavours to summarize these and more recent reports. Some drugs do have an effect in modifying the symptoms or pathophysiological effects of the disease.

The early reports of ALS-like disorders associated with hypoglycaemia or insulinomas led to studies of glucose metabolism and then of pancreatic or gastrointestinal function. Pancreatic extract and tocopherol (vitamin E) have been tried therapeutically but without benefit (Quick & Greer 1967, Brown & Kater 1969, Dorman et al 1969). Hydroxycobalamin (vitamin B_{12}) injections, either parenterally or intrathecally, were unhelpful (Peiper & Fields 1959). The reports of abnormal calcium metabolism in some ALS patients led to unsuccessful treatment with vitamin D preparations (Patten 1982). The association of ALS with parkinsonism on Guam led to unsuccessful therapeutic trials of levodopa in Guamanians and sporadic cases of ALS (Mendell et al 1971). Similarly, amantadine, an antiviral agent which also enhances dopamine release in the CNS, was unhelpful (Norris 1972a). Bovine brain gangliosides, which promote axonal sprouting, were not beneficial in two more recent trials (Bradley et al 1984, Harrington et al 1984).

The reports of abnormal exposure to lead or other heavy metals in MND patients led to several unsuccessful therapeutic trials with the chelating agents dimercaprol, EDTA and penicillamine (Kantarjian 1961, Campbell et al 1970, Conradi et al 1982). Reports of circulating neurotoxins (Wolfgram 1976) may have been the basis for treatment with modified snake neurotoxins (Sanders & Fellowes 1975) but initial enthusiasm was not borne out in controlled trials (Tyler 1979). Plasma exchange with or without immunosuppression has been ineffective in ALS patients (Silani et al 1980, Kelemen et al 1983).

The possible association of MND with polio or other virus infection has led to many negative studies with antiviral agents (Server & Wolinsky 1982). These have included idoxuridine (Liversedge et al 1970), inosiplex (isoprinosine) (Percy et al 1971), amantadine (Norris 1972a), cytosine arabinoside (Ara-C) and guanidine (Norris et al 1974, Munsat et al 1981). Drugs which modify or improve the host defences against viral infection have also been tried unsuccessfully. These include levamisole (Olarte & Shafer 1985), interferons (Cook et al 1979, Rissanen et al 1980), tilorone (Olson et al 1978) polyinosinic-polycytidylic acid (Poly-ICIC) (Engel et al 1978), which are interferon-inducing drugs, and transfer factor (Olarte et al 1979). The corticosteroids and more powerful immunosuppressive drugs, including intrathecal hydrocortisone (Peiper & Fields 1959) and azathioprine, have also been tried with negative results in ALS. Currently trials with cyclophosphamide and cyclosporin are in progress. Plasmapheresis to remove any possible humoral factors has also given negative results (Olarte et al 1980).

The demonstration of low levels of TRH in spinal grey matter of ALS patients led to therapeutic trials. Further studies with TRH infusions and with RX 77368, a long-acting TRH analogue, have shown a weak, insignificant benefit only (reviewed by Brooke 1989). Recently experimental studies in animal models with neurotrophic factor have reported marked improvement in strength and muscle mass (Sendtner et al 1992); this is now the subject of human clinical studies.

Considerable benefit in relieving spasticity may be obtained from the synthetic GABA-like compound baclofen, but alternative treatment with dantrolene usually causes unacceptable enhancement of weakness and may precipitate respiratory failure. The earlier reports of benefit from an uncontrolled trial of guanidine therapy (Norris 1973) probably related to its action in facilitating the release of acetylcholine at the neuromuscular junction (Otsuka & Endo 1960). Similar symptomatic benefits may be seen in some MND patients, especially with bulbar weakness, with the anticholinesterase drugs neostigmine and pyridostigmine. Unfortunately, the improvement is usually short-lived and may be masked by troublesome side effects of muscle cramps or increased salivation. The latter can be improved with anticholinergic compounds such as atropine or its synthetic analogues.

Management

The good management of a patient with MND requires considerable expertise in interpersonal relationships with the patient and his family, plus the support and help of other professional health care workers. A simple understanding of the nature of their progressive neuromuscular disorder leading to increasing disability must be imparted to the sufferers. This is helped by explaining the sparing of intellectual functioning and the absence of incontinence, together with a knowledge of the variable prognosis. In later stages of the disease, mood-elevating drugs may be necessary for the understandable depression. The need for attendance at special clinics is controversial but it is generally accepted that one medical adviser should undertake the supervision of care and co-ordination of various necessary aids. Contact with volunteer support organisations such as the Motor Neurone Disease Association (MNDA) or the ALS Society may be considered appropriate.

Many drug trials are taking place, as discussed previously, but essentially no effective treatment is available at present. Symptomatic treatment can be tried: for weakness, especially of bulbar musculature, pyridostigmine (Mestinon®) 60–90 mg 4-hourly; for spasticity, baclofen (Lioresal®) 10–30 mg 6-hourly; for hypersalivation, atropine sulphate 0.6–1.2 mg 6-hourly, benzhexol hydrochloride (Artane®) 2–5 mg 6-hourly or hyoscine

skin patches (Scopoderm TTS®); as well as appropriate psychotropic drugs.

The management of bulbar palsy involves treatment of dysphagia, of choking, drooling and of speech difficulty (Campbell & Enderby 1984). Dysphagia may be managed more successfully if positioning, texture of the diet, food supplements and a swallow routine are attended to by a therapist. In the case of more spastic difficulty, relaxation of muscles by sucking an ice cube prior to meals may facilitate swallowing. The drugs pyridostigmine or baclofen may be tried as detailed above. Progressive dysphagia may result in pooling of secretions and food in the hypopharynx, which predisposes to tracheo-bronchial aspiration. Teaching relatives how to use suction devices can be helpful. Benefits may be obtained from cricopharyngeal myotomy, which lowers the resting intrapharyngeal pressure (Mills 1973, Lebo et al 1976). The operative mortality in one series of 25 patients was 20% and this was thought to be due to severe limitation of ventilatory capacity and effective coughing (Loizou et al 1980). This may be overcome by advising myotomy at an earlier stage in the disease when respiratory involvement is limited. Severe drooling, unresponsive to anticholinergic drugs, may be helped by salivary gland irradiation or denervation; division of the chorda tympani nerve by transtympanic surgery can be performed under local anaesthesia and can result in a 95% reduction of salivation (Zalin & Cooney 1974, Mullins et al 1979). Unfortunately, a drier mouth may have negative effects on speech, particularly if the tongue has LMN involvement causing generalised weakness. Occasionally tracheostomy and the use of a cuffed airway is necessary to prevent distressing choking or spluttering on natural secretions or food particles. Various means have been advocated for the treatment of severe dysphagia and maintenance of adequate nutrition, with additional food supplements being the primary course, but later surgical techniques including gastrotomy and cervical oesophagostomy may be considered. We now favour percutaneous gastrostomy tube feeding, although small bore nasogastric tubes can be well tolerated for many months. Adequate nutrition will prevent some weight loss and will optimise strength.

Dyspnoea is a late symptom of ventilatory weakness in MND and usually arises only when the FVC is below 50% of the predicted normal, or where there is co-existing lung disease. Physiotherapy with inspiratory muscle training may improve ventilatory function in neuromuscular disease (Martin et al 1983). Some patients benefit from ventilatory support with or without a tracheostomy. This can be provided with a cuirass, continuous positive airway pressure (CPAP) or nocturnal intermittent CPAP (Howard et al 1989). This is best reserved for those patients who at least have good upper limb function which enables them to continue useful activities. Long-term management with portable mechanical ventilatory support at home is possible, provided that the necessary support of family or others is available. The physical and psychological problems associated with such long-term support have been discussed by Sivak and colleagues (1982), and by Braun (1987).

Physiotherapy for limb weakness is helpful psychologically and allows evaluation of the needs for mechanical aids, such as foot drop splints, wrist supports, cervical collars for neck muscle weakness or suitable wheelchairs with adequate head rests or mobile arm supports. The help of an occupational therapist may prolong independence with dressing by the adaptation of clothing fasteners, or with eating by the provision of suitable large-handled cutlery and cups, or with writing by similar large-handled implements (Cochrane et al 1987).

Speech therapy is useful on several counts. In the early stages of speech difficulty, deliberate slowing of the rate of speech may considerably aid intelligibility. More specific exercises, especially of the tongue, may help to overcome localised weakness for a short period. Modification of speech patterns may help to overcome hypernasality. In some cases a palatal lift incorporated into an upper denture will avoid nasal escape and increase intraoral pressure. Relaxation exercises may help to overcome spasticity but the anti-spasmodic drug baclofen should also be tried, as mentioned above. Marked fatigability of the voice with dysphonia may be eased by pyridostigmine therapy or by a simple amplifier. The availability of a portable suction apparatus may facilitate speech by removing excess secretions and distressing gurgling. Eventually, communication aids are required, ranging from a simple alphabet board to portable electronic communicators, or to more elaborately activated electronic display systems triggered by head or eye movements (Campbell & Enderby 1984). The latter may be incorporated into a comprehensive environmental control system (e.g. POSSUM) which opens doors, or operates controls of telephone, radio or television sets, etc. Attention to appropriate computerised equipment can assist patients to extend their productive life, even to continue working when very severely disabled (e.g. Hawkins 1990).

The management of end-stage MND is concerned with maintaining a quality of life rather than prolonging misery and more suffering (Campbell 1980, Carey 1986). It is of prime importance that the patient and relatives do not feel abandoned at this stage. The development of the hospice service has been a welcome boon for the terminally ill (O'Brien et al 1992). Rational symptomatic treatment, as described above, is insufficient and psychotropic drugs may be required to allay mental anguish. Narcotic medication, including opiates, is safe and effective, and is useful to control anxiety, dyspnoea, pain and insomnia. We commonly use diamorphine 2.5–5 mg orally or subcutaneously 4- to 6-hourly, despite the increased risk of central respiratory depression, sleep apnoea and respiratory arrest.

HEREDITARY SPINAL MUSCULAR ATROPHIES

These are a heterogeneous group of heredofamilial disorders of the motor neurones, predominantly of the spinal cord but occasionally affecting the motor nuclei of the brainstem and without clinical evidence of involvement of sensory or UMN pathways (Harding 1984). The various types can generally be distinguished clinically by the distribution of weakness, the pattern of inheritance and by the age of onset. Family studies show virtually no overlap between the acute generalised, benign proximal, scapuloperoneal and distal forms of the disease, thus suggesting a different genetic cause (Emery 1971, Pearn et al 1978a,c). Some overlap occurs in relation to age of onset and prognosis of the acute and chronic infantile forms (Pearn 1980, 1982).

Infantile spinal muscular atrophy (Werdnig–Hoffmann disease: SMA Type I)

Recently the genes for acute (Type I) and chronic (Types II and III) childhood, autosomal recessive spinal muscular atrophy (SMA) have been mapped to the same locus on chromosome 5q11.2–13.3 (Brzustowicz et al 1990, Gilliam et al 1990), raising the likelihood that these disorders are allelic. The clinical heterogeneity of families mapping to this region has now been established (Munsat et al 1990). Although it is still possible that other loci may produce the same phenotype, this is not yet established and is considered unlikely. Prenatal testing using informative markers and based on linkage analysis is now available for SMA with a high degree of reliability. It is hoped and anticipated that the gene will be cloned in the near future.

The acute infantile form (SMA Type I) was first described by Sevestre (1899). It is characterised by its severe generalised muscle involvement and fatal outcome before 3 years of age (Brandt 1950, Byers & Banker 1961). In at least one-third of cases the disease is manifest, before or at birth, either by decreased fetal movements or by congenital skeletal deformities, usually of the chest, hips or feet. In a large study by Pearn & Wilson (1973a) the onset occurred before 5 months of age, and before 3 months in 95% of cases. Generalised weakness and hypotonia with areflexia was the commonest presenting feature in two-thirds, and feeding difficulties in 40% of cases. Breathing difficulties are usually responsible for the inevitably fatal outcome. Fasciculations may be evident in the wasted tongue but are generally invisible elsewhere. Buchthal & Olsen (1970) failed to find any true fasciculation potentials on EMG in the limbs but did document a unique finding of regularly discharging motor units every 5–15 seconds in relaxed muscles or during sleep. Other EMG features of severe denervation with a central motor neuropathy are commonly found. The mean age at death is 6 to 9 months, depending on the pre- or postnatal onset, and 95% of infants died before 18 months of age.

Pathological studies of the brain and spinal cord show severe loss of motor neurones but some remaining cells are chromatolytic (Byers & Banker 1961, Chou & Fakadej 1971). The anterior motor roots are very atrophic and sensory roots and spinal cord tracts appear normal, although careful studies have found mild abnormalities of the dorsal root ganglia and non-motor pathways (Carpenter et al 1978, Marshall & Duchen 1978). Histological studies of skeletal muscle show severe denervation changes with scattered small groups, or single hypertrophied fibres, usually of Type I and also apparent preservation of muscle spindles.

SMA Type II

The chronic infantile form (SMA Type II), first described by Werdnig (1891, 1894) and by Hoffmann (1893, 1897), is a more slowly progressive generalised disease with a variable prognosis. It appears to have a slightly later onset than SMA Type I and rarely presents before 6 months of age, but 75% are manifest in the first year (Pearn et al 1978b). Less than 25% of infants are ever able to sit unsupported and none learn to crawl or walk (Pearn & Wilson 1973b). Atrophy and fasciculation is seen in the tongue. Spontaneous tremor of the fingers may be evident and correlates with the EMG findings of spontaneous motor unit discharges (Buchthal & Olsen 1970). Tendon reflexes are depressed or absent, especially by 2 years of age. Clinical progression is slow or appears even to arrest, although sudden deterioration may be associated with intercurrent infection (Munsat et al 1969). All children, if untreated, develop scoliosis with further compromise of respiratory ventilation and increased risk of pneumonia. Life expectancy is very variable, ranging up to adult life in some cases.

Chronic proximal spinal muscular atrophy (Kugelberg–Welander disease: SMA Type III)

Kugelberg & Welander (1954, 1956) and Wohlfart et al (1955) described a progressive proximal muscular weakness in young adults, clinically resembling a muscular dystrophy but showing fasciculations and investigational findings of a neuropathic disorder. Kugelberg (1975) later defined the clinical picture as proximal muscular atrophy and weakness especially in the legs, pseudohypertrophy of the calves, absent knee jerks with other tendon reflexes preserved, no pyramidal signs and normal intelligence. Patients are able to walk for more than 10 years after the onset and are capable of normal survival. Fasciculations in limb muscles are seen in at least 50% of cases, but are rarely evident in the tongue; bulbar involvement is rare. The usual presentation is difficulty in walking, especially up steps or stairs, together with a waddling gait. Later there is difficulty in lifting the arms and winging of the scapulae. The posture is hyperlordotic with a protuberant abdomen. Joint contractures and kyphoscoliosis are common later.

Kugelberg & Welander (1956) found EMG evidence of spontaneous fasciculations and chronic denervation changes with giant residual units. Muscle biopsy in five cases showed fibre-type grouping, both of the small atrophic and of the hypertrophied muscle fibres, thus indicating the neuropathic nature of the disease. Wohlfart (1942) had previously described two similar clinical cases, also with evident fasciculations, but on finding 'myopathic' changes in a muscle biopsy he ascribed the disease to a muscular dystrophy. He subsequently reassessed these two cases, together with seven others, and confirmed the findings of Kugelberg & Welander (Wohlfart et al 1955). The secondary myopathic abnormalities often found in muscle sections appear to correlate with the presence of 'myopathic' motor units on EMG studies (Gath et al 1969) and also with the frequent finding of an increased serum CK activity (Mastaglia & Walton 1971). The few autopsy reports have confirmed the spinal motor neuronal loss and have shown no evidence of corticospinal or sensory tract involvement (Gardner-Medwin et al 1967, Kohn 1968).

Juvenile proximal SMA was familial in about two-thirds of cases reviewed by Namba et al (1970). The majority of families have shown an autosomal recessive pattern of inheritance, but both dominant and X-linked recessive forms of the disease have been described (see Emery 1971). Adult onset of typical cases showing a benign course was first described by Finkel (1962) and Wiesendanger (1962) and the clinical symptoms of such patients resemble those in cases of Becker or limb-girdle muscular dystrophy (Pearn et al 1978c). However, the importance of their differentiation lies in distinguishing such cases from adult MND with its wretched prognosis.

Chronic distal spinal muscular atrophy

This group of disorders is very heterogeneous, both clinically and genetically. Sporadic and familial cases have been described with many different ages of onset. Autosomal dominant and recessive patterns of inheritance have been described. Atrophy and weakness usually start in the lower extremities and later spread to involve the hands and lower forearms (Dyck & Lambert 1968b, McLeod & Prineas 1971). However, Meadows & Marsden (1969) described three siblings with onset in the hands in childhood and with spread to the lower legs in later life. Pes cavus is more prominent in the early-onset cases. The condition is relatively benign and severe disability is uncommon. Some of the adult cases may be indistinguishable from early forms of the scapuloperoneal syndrome or the neuronal/axonal form of peroneal muscular atrophy (HMSN type II) (Harding & Thomas 1980). The latter condition is distinguished by the presence of minor sensory abnormalities found either clinically or on electrodiagnostic tests (Dyck & Lambert 1968b), whereas motor and sensory conduction velocities in distal SMA are normal. With genetic definition now becoming more readily available it will be interesting to see whether these forms are allelic variants or due to different genes.

Bulbo-spinal muscular atrophy

This X-linked recessive disorder of late onset, which is clinically different from the proximal forms of spinal muscular atrophy (SMA), was first described by Kennedy et al (1968). The age of onset varies but most cases occur at 20–40 years of age. Proximal weakness usually begins in the lower limbs, then spreads to the shoulder girdle, face and bulbar musculature. Fasciculation is prominent, especially in the face and tongue.

Postural tremor of the outstretched hands occurs frequently (Harding 1984). Dysphagia and dysarthria develop some 10–20 years after the onset of weakness. Gynaecomastia is common and diabetes may also occur. Life expectancy may be normal. Electrodiagnostic tests show evidence of severe denervation. Motor nerve conduction velocity is normal or slightly reduced; some cases have shown absent or reduced sensory potentials (Kennedy et al 1968, Stefanis et al 1975, Harding et al 1982). Sobue et al (1989) in a clinicopathological study of nine cases reported consistent sensory involvement due to a distal axonopathy giving a loss of myelinated fibres in the distal peripheral nerves, and in the rostral fasciculus gracilis of the spinal cord. Unlike ALS, there is no evidence of corticospinal tract degeneration but the motor nerve loss in the brainstem and spinal cord is similar.

The responsible gene and the CAG repeat sequence on the X-chromosome which codes for the androgen receptor was identified on the proximal long arm by Fischbeck and colleagues (Fischbeck et at 1991, La Spada 1991). It has subsequently been shown that the onset of the limb weakness and the severity of the disability correlate with the size of the CAG repeat (Doyu et al 1992).

Scapuloperoneal form

The scapuloperoneal syndrome includes a variety of disorders giving rise to proximal weakness around the shoulders and distal weakness in the lower limbs. Some cases appear to be myopathic (see Kaeser 1975), generally with an onset around the shoulder girdle and with features resembling those of facioscapulohumeral muscular dystrophy except that the face is spared (see below). Kaeser (1964, 1965) reported the findings in 12 members of a family extending through five generations and with an autosomal dominant pattern of inheritance. The onset was in adult life with symmetrical weakness and wasting of the long extensor muscles of the toes and ankles. After many years the muscles around the shoulder girdle became involved, producing winging of the scapulae and difficulty in raising the arms. The weakness of the legs also spread to involve the calves and quadriceps muscles. In two cases, in the fourth and fifth generations, bulbar muscles became involved, resulting in dysphagia, dysphonia and facial weakness; extraocular weakness was present in one case. Tendon reflexes were diminished or absent; sensory examination revealed no abnormal findings. EMG studies in three affected members (Kaeser 1975) revealed abundant fibrillation and fasciculation potentials in some muscles. Severe denervation changes were evident in the legs but a mixed pattern was found in the facial muscles and in muscles around the shoulder girdle. Motor conduction velocities and sensory nerve studies were normal. Muscle biopsies from the lower extremities gave findings which were consistent with chronic denervation but specimens from the deltoid or triceps muscle were thought to be myopathic or pseudomyopathic. An autopsy study of one case showed clear evidence of degeneration of anterior horn cells and bulbar motor nuclei and a neurogenic type of muscle atrophy including muscles of the upper extremity.

Sporadic cases with a similar distribution of muscle involvement have been described in infancy (Feigenbaum & Munsat 1970). Zellweger and McCormick (1968) described a single congenital case with talipes equinovarus and progressive inspiratory stridor due to bilateral vocal cord paralysis. A family of three affected sibs with an onset in childhood and a mildly affected mother has been studied personally in conjunction with Dr B. Berg. The propositus presented with acute bulbar weakness and bilateral vocal cord paralysis requiring tracheostomy. She later developed a scapuloperoneal distribution of muscular atrophy which was evident in two of three brothers and in her mother. The EMG findings in this family, as in the other childhood cases, were those of chronic denervation with normal motor conduction velocities.

Facioscapulohumeral form

Conditions resembling facioscapulohumeral muscular dystrophy in the distribution of muscular atrophy and weakness have been described in a mother and daughter, with onset in adolescence but with pathological evidence of a neuropathy (Fenichel et al 1967). Facial weakness was the first symptom, followed by involvement of the proximal limb muscles. Two other sporadic cases with a similar picture were reported by Furukawa et al 1969). There are also some forms of the scapuloperoneal syndrome which could alternatively be included here (Kaeser 1975).

Progressive juvenile bulbar palsy (Fazio–Londe disease)

There appear to be two forms of this rare disease — the Vialetto–van Laere syndrome and Fazio-Londe disease. The Vialetto–van Laere syndrome is an autosomal recessive disorder usually presenting in the second decade with facial weakness, dysphagia and dysarthria, and associated with sensorineural deafness. The weakness later spreads to affect the limbs and sometimes the trunk, causing respiratory difficulty, sometimes with sleep apnoea (Vialetto 1936, van Laere 1966, Gallai et al 1981). Autopsy reports have described degeneration and atrophy of cranial nuclei VI to XII.

Cases of Fazio–Londe disease do not have deafness and generally begin in early childhood. Fazio (1892) described the disease in a mother and son, and Londe (1894) described a more rapid disease in two brothers. Excessive drooling from facial weakness, repeated respiratory infections and stridor are the usual presenting features. Dysphagia and ocular paresis as well as generalised limb weakness may follow. Death is usually from respiratory failure and/or infection. Autopsied cases have shown degeneration and atrophy of the brainstem nuclei including the oculomotor nerves, and a variable loss of anterior horn cells in the cervical and dorsal spinal cord; the pyramidal tracts were normal (Gomez et al 1962, Alexander et al 1976).

Motor neuropathy with hexosaminidase A deficiency

Neurogenic muscular atrophy may be a common feature of hexosaminidase deficiency disease causing GM2-gangliosidosis. Hexosaminidase A (Hex.A) is a heteropolymer of alpha and beta polypeptides. The gene for the alpha subunit is on chromosone 15 and that for the beta subunit on chromosone 5. Recently it has been demonstrated that the gene for the locus of the beta subunit is close to that for childhood SMA (Kleyn et al 1991). Hexosaminidase B (Hex.B) is a tetramer of beta subunits. Patients with Hex. B deficiency have visceral storage of globoside, and of other sialic acid-derived conjugates in addition to GM2 gangliosides.

Adult onset GM2 gangliosidosis causes a slowly progressive multisystem degeneration and motor neurone disease resembling a spinocerebellar degeneration. Some patients have had psychosis and dementia but others retain normal cognition and viscera (Mitsumoto et al 1986). Membranous cytoplasmic bodies of the type seen in infantile Tay–Sachs disease occur in the rectal ganglion cells. Serum, leucocyte and fibroblast Hex.A activity is markedly reduced in patients and partially reduced in heterozygous relatives. Recently a similar disorder has been reported in a patient with a beta-locus defect giving absent Hex.B and partial Hex.A activity (Cashman et al 1986).

Johnson and colleagues (1982) have described two late-onset phenotypes of Hex.A deficiency in which motor neuropathy was a presenting manifestation. In one family a progressive adolescent-onset spinal muscular atrophy syndrome resembled Kugelberg–Welander disease (SMA type III). There were no UMN findings or macular abnormality (cherry-red spot) and no dementia. Biochemically there was severe deficiency of hexosaminidase A (Hex.A). Rectal ganglion cells were filled with classic membranous cytoplasmic bodies. Presumably the spinal motor neurones were similarly affected. The second type concerns a single case of an ALS-like syndrome commencing in late adolescence with cramps, progressive proximal atrophy and weakness and dysarthria. Generally brisk tendon reflexes were accompanied by extensor plantar responses. The principal biochemical finding was of severe Hex.A deficiency. Rectal neurones were enlarged and contained membranous cytoplasmic bodies.

Focal or monomeltic amyotrophy

In 1959 Hirayama et al described a new clinical entity which they entitled 'juvenile muscular atrophy of unilateral upper extremity' and in 1987 Hirayama and his colleagues reported the first autopsy findings in a single case, noting that some 150 cases had been reported in the interim from Japan and many from other countries including South India (Gourie-Devi & Suresh 1988). The condition occurs predominantly in males aged 15–25 years, is usually sporadic and develops insidiously with muscular weakness and atrophy beginning in the hand and generally limited to the hand and forearm, ceasing to progress after 1 or 2 years. Pathologically they found atrophy of the anterior horns of the spinal cord at C5–T1 with degeneration of large and small nerve cells and some gliosis. The aetiology is unknown.

HEREDITARY MOTOR AND SENSORY NEUROPATHIES (HMSN)

A detailed description of all these conditions is outside the scope of this chapter and is dealt with more fully elsewhere (see Dyck 1984).

The separation of these conditions from hereditary spinal muscular atrophies, especially in the distal forms is somewhat arbitrary. All have selective neuronal degeneration and atrophy but the conditions discussed here are not exclusive for motor neurones, that is both motor and sensory peripheral neurones are affected. The clinical features affect both sides of the body symmetrically and the course is chronic and fairly progressive. These are inherited disorders and hence are assumed to be related to inborn errors of metabolism; but in most cases the nature of this is unknown. The identification of biochemical abnormalities, and sometimes of the enzyme deficiency, has been made in a few cases, e.g. in Refsum's disease, metachromatic leucodystrophy and hexosaminidase A deficiency.

Many of these conditions are included in the peroneal muscular atrophy syndrome (Charcot–Marie–Tooth disease). This is a heterogeneous group, both clinically and genetically. All patients have predominant involvement of peripheral motor neurones, with lesser disease of peripheral sensory and autonomic neurones. The disorders are inherited, are slowly progressive and cause

symmetrical distal muscular atrophy and weakness affecting the feet initially, together with some distal sensory loss (see Dyck 1984). Dejerine & Sottas (1893) described the pathological findings of hypertrophic interstitial neuritis in two siblings with typical features of HMSN. Subsequently it has been shown many times that nerve hypertrophy can be present in many different types of the disease, including the common form, HMSN type I. Dyck & Lambert (1968a) proposed a classification based on motor nerve conduction velocity measurements. In HMSN type I the conduction velocity is markedly slowed due to severe demyelinative and remyelinative changes along the degenerating axons. Type II HMSN was associated with normal or mildly slowed conduction related only to the minimal secondary demyelinative change in peripheral nerves. Subsequently, subgroups based on the clinical picture and pattern of inheritance have been proposed (Dyck 1984).

HMSN type I includes the commonest clinical type inherited as an autosomal dominant trait as described by Charcot & Marie (1886) and concurrently by Tooth (1886). Separate rare autosomal recessive forms include those described by Dejerine & Sottas (1893) and Refsum (1946). The dominantly inherited form may be very variable in its severity and even asymptomatic. The onset is usually apparent in the second to fourth decades, with abnormalities of the feet, usually pes cavus, steppage gait and atrophy and weakness of the small muscles of the feet and peronei. Later cases show atrophy and clawing of the hands and sometimes wasting and weakness of the lower thigh muscles. Tendon reflexes are usually absent or severely diminished. Mild distal sensory loss is commonly found clinically. Severe disability and loss of walking ability are rare; life expectancy is normal. Kinships with identical features to those described above, but including tremor, were described by Roussy & Levy (1926). Pathological features of these diseases are confined to the spinal cord and peripheral nerves. Atrophy and loss of anterior horn cells are present, together with loss of myelinated fibres in the dorsal ascending tracts, especially in the cervical region.

HMSN type II has been called the neuronal form of peroneal muscular atrophy. It is inherited as an autosomal dominant trait but differs from

HMSN type I in having a later onset of symptoms, less severe deformities of the feet and difficulties with balance and walking as well as less involvement of the hands. Fasciculations may be observed but peripheral nerve thickening is not a clinical feature. Some tendon reflexes may be obtained, especially in the arms. The motor and sensory nerve conduction velocities are normal or only mildly slowed. Digital sensory nerve action potentials are unobtainable or diminished, in contradistinction to the findings in the distal type of spinal muscular atrophy (SMA).

AMYOTROPHY IN THE HEREDITARY ATAXIAS

A detailed discussion of these diverse CNS disorders is outside the remit of this book. The classification of these conditions is difficult but has been considered in a recent monograph (Harding 1984). In general peripheral sensory neurones are affected more than lower motor neurones but neurogenic muscular atrophy (amyotrophy) is a feature in a number of these system degenerations (Rosenberg 1982). The purely peripheral diseases which present as hereditary motor neuropathies (SMA) or HMSN have already been discussed. The archetype of the spinal ataxic form is Friedreich's ataxia, although the spastic UMN forms comprise the various types of familial spastic paraplegia, some with prominent LMN involvement. Basal ganglia involvement occurs in the olivo-ponto-cerebellar ataxias and in certain dementias, e.g. Huntington's chorea.

The clinical and pathological features of Friedreich's ataxia as described in a series of papers between 1863 and 1877 by Friedreich, have been reviewed recently by Harding (1984). This is an autosomal recessive disorder, with onset usually by puberty, causing ataxia and dysarthria, associated with foot deformity, absent ankle jerks and extensor plantar responses. There is a progressive pyramidal-type weakness of the legs and sensory loss, usually of proprioception, together with generalised wasting of the lower limbs; distal amyotrophy is common in the hands. Electrodiagnostic studies show normal or slightly reduced motor nerve conduction velocities (MNCV) and

absent median and ulnar sensory action potentials (SAP) (Dyck & Lambert 1968b, McLeod 1971). Pathological studies show a small spinal cord with degeneration of the dorsal, pyramidal and spinocerebellar tract, and also of the dorsal root ganglia. Some loss of AHC is seen, especially in the cervical cord. Mild degenerative changes are seen in the brain and cerebellum. Peripheral nerves show loss of large myelinated fibres to a greater extent distally than proximally, thus providing a pathological correlate for the 'dying-back' concept (Dyck & Lais 1973).

Two other forms of hereditary ataxia associated with peripheral neuropathy and muscle wasting are ataxia telangiectasia and xeroderma pigmentosa. Both are associated with abnormalities of DNA repair and increased risk of malignancies. Ataxia telangiectasia (Louis-Bar 1941) is associated with progressive cerebellar incoordination and choreo-athetosis but normal power until the later stages when general or distal weakness and atrophy occur. Tendon reflexes are depressed early and absent later (Sedgwick & Boder 1960, 1972). The spinal cord shows relatively few pathological changes (compared with Friedreich's ataxia), apart from some posterior column demyelination and mild loss of lumbar AHC and of neurones in the sensory and autonomic ganglia (Aguilar et al 1968).

Xeroderma pigmentosa is a skin condition with abnormal sensitivity to sunlight causing multiple skin cancers. Neurological disorder (de Sanctis–Cacchioni syndrome) occurs in 40% of cases, Mental subnormality, deafness, athetosis and ataxia are associated with areflexia and a variable sensorimotor polyneuropathy. Motor NCV is normal or slightly slowed, SAP are small or absent and muscle biopsy shows denervation atrophy (Thrush et al 1974).

Hereditary spastic paraplegia (HSP) in its pure form was first described by Strumpell (1880). This is inherited as an autosomal dominant trait with a variable age of onset and varying severity of weakness in the lower limbs. Distal amyotrophy, especially of the hands, is commoner in the older age group, who also show mild sensory loss. Normal MNCV and SAP studies have been reported, despite the wasting, distal sensory loss and ankle areflexia (McLeod et al 1977, Harding

1981). This has been explained on the basis of a central axonopathy and is supported by the report of absent or reduced somato-sensory evoked potentials (SSEP) in all of 18 patients, four of whom had sensory loss (Thomas et al 1981). Pathological studies have shown marked degeneration of the posterior sensory columns and pyramidal tracts, especially in the thoracic cord, despite the fact that the dorsal root ganglia and posterior roots appear normal. The AHC have appeared normal even in cases with distal amyotrophy (Van Bogaert 1952), giving further support for the concept of an axonopathy with 'dying-back'.

Some cases of HSP are associated with marked amyotrophy. Certain forms resemble peroneal muscular atrophy (HMSN type II) with pyramidal signs (Dyck & Lambert 1968b, Harding & Thomas 1984). Another autosomal recessive form, resembling ALS, was described by Refsum & Skillicorn (1954), with an early childhood onset of spastic paraparesis spreading to involve the arms and then, in adolescence, developing generalised wasting with fasciculations. The patients also developed bulbar symptoms.

Amyotrophy is often a late manifestation of olivo-ponto-cerebellar degeneration. Landis and colleagues (1974), in reviewing the family described by Schut (1950), found amyotrophy in 78% of cases and 50% with tongue wasting and fasciculations. Bulbar symptoms, especially dysphagia, may occur (see Harding 1984). Loss of AHC and sensory neurones have been described by several authors. Huntington's chorea may be associated with amyotrophy late in the disease. Pathological studies have shown involvement of the spinal cord, including pallor of the pyramidal tracts and some loss of AHC with occasional vacuolated cells (Bruyn et al 1979).

Typical motor neurone disease has been associated with familial parkinsonism (see Emery & Holloway 1982). The two disorders may show considerable variation in expressivity within families (Campbell 1979). Sporadic cases of Parkinson's disease with the late development of ALS have also been described (Bonduelle 1975). Several of these cases have followed encephalitis lethargica (Pallis 1976, Brait et al 1973). Some families, apart from those in the Western Pacific islands, have shown features of MND, parkinsonism and dementia with variable expression (see Tyler 1982).

Amyotrophy in non-familial CNS degenerative disorders

The association of MND with dementia has been reviewed recently by Salazar et al (1983) in relation to transmissible Creutzfeldt–Jakob disease. In a review of more than 2000 cases they found 231 patients with dementia and early LMN signs causing amyotrophy. They showed that, in general, these cases had a much slower disease course and that pathological studies could not detect any spongiform change. In only two cases could the condition be transmitted to primates and these cases had the more typical subacute course, with myoclonus but presenting with amyotrophy (Allen et al 1971). Of the typical transmissible cases, approximately 15% showed fasciculations or amyotrophy late in the disease. Similarly, amyotrophy has been reported late in the course of Alzheimer's or Pick's disease. This may be simply an ageing phenomenon (Tomlinson et al 1969), as similar pathological changes have been found in elderly, non-demented patients (Jennekens et al 1971). The association of typical ALS with Alzheimer's or Pick's disease may be a chance association (reviewed by Brion et al 1980). Similarly, the association of parkinsonism–dementia and ALS in Guam is thought to be an overlap of two separate diseases which are common locally.

The presence of amyotrophy in sporadic cases of parkinsonism was mentioned previously. Other sporadic forms of basal ganglia disease may be associated with neurogenic muscular atrophy including pallido-nigral degeneration (Gray et al 1985), dystonia musculorum deformans (Tyler 1982), Hallervorden–Spatz disease (Seitelberger et al 1963), progressive supranuclear palsy (Steele et al 1964) and the Shy–Drager syndrome (Tyler 1982). Primary orthostatic hypotension (Shy–Drager syndrome) is said to be associated with mild amyotrophy, usually in the legs, in more than 50% of patients. Bulbar features have not been described. Mild changes of AHC degeneration including chromatolysis have been reported and were indicated as the cause of the lax anal sphincter, as well as the distal limb wasting (Shy & Drager 1960).

MISCELLANEOUS DISEASES

Infections

Acute poliomyelitis is the archetype of a necrotising infection of the large motor neurones of the spinal cord, brain stem and cortex. Poliovirus is an enterovirus which may exist as a commensal in the bowel and causes a mild systemic upset only, without neurological features, in most cases. This may be associated with features of an aseptic meningitis. Paralytic disease occurs in fewer than 10% of infected individuals and may show familial clustering, even during severe epidemics (Aycock 1942). This suggests a genetic predisposition to the development of poliomyelitis (Addair & Snyder 1942, Herndon & Jennings 1951). An association between HLA-A3 and poliomyelitis has been reported by Pietsch & Morris (1975) but denied by others (Lasch et al 1979).

After a prodromal illness for one to four days with fever, headache and neck stiffness, muscle stiffness with hyper-reflexia and fasciculations ensue, before the onset of asymmetrical muscle weakness and corresponding tendon reflex loss (Johnson 1982b). Maximum severity is reached within a few days and recovery may start within a week of the onset of paralysis. The brain-stem vital centres are involved in 10–15% of cases, especially the IXth and Xth cranial nuclei. Cardiorespiratory difficulties may develop, including hypertension and arrhythmias, but respiratory paralysis may also occur from peripheral involvement of the diaphragm and intercostal muscles. Fortunately, relatively few affected muscles become permanently paralysed, but it is uncertain whether this implies that affected neurones are capable of recovery from viral infection and replication. The recovery of muscle power may be the result of sparing of individual motor neurones, but certainly electrophysiological studies demonstrate that reinnervative sprouting in surviving motor units occurs to produce greatly enlarged units (McComas et al 1971). Probably suboptimal conduction in these reinnervative terminal nerve fibres accounts for the neuromuscular transmission defects which are demonstrable (Dalakas et al 1986). Pathological studies of acute fatal cases show inflammation and neuronal destruction, mainly in the spinal anterior horns, bulbar motor

nuclei, reticular formation, thalamus and motor cortex (Bodian 1949). Treatment of acute paralytic poliomyelitis is supportive and may require tracheostomy and ventilatory assistance. The mortality appears to vary between 5% and 30%.

The clinical syndrome of paralytic poliomyelitis was caused initially almost exclusively by polioviruses. With the advent of widespread immunisation, other enteroviruses, including Coxsackie and ECHO viruses, have rarely been associated with the syndrome, although 40% of the few cases in the USA are now associated with live vaccine virus infection (Johnson 1982b). Chronic progressive poliomyelitis has been reported secondary to vaccination in an immunodeficient child (Davis et al 1977). The encephalomyelitic picture which very occasionally complicates neoplastic disease, especially lymphomas, may also be attributable to viral infection, although full virological studies have not been undertaken (Walton et al 1968, Castleman 1970).

Herpes zoster or shingles is an acute viral infection of sensory ganglion cells, which produces a painful vesicular rash. Very occasionally, the viral infection spreads to adjacent areas of the spinal cord to produce a segmental myelitis (Thomas & Howard 1972) and sometimes a generalised encephalomyelitis occurs (Gardner-Thorpe et al 1976). Segmental myelitis may be associated with local invasion and destruction of motor neurones, resulting in localised muscular atrophy and weakness. Such motor complications generally involve the lower spinal cord or cauda equina. Recovery from such weakness is possible but is usually incomplete. Cranial motor nerve involvement is also known, but may result from peripheral infection and swelling which is local rather than in the brainstem, e.g. oculomotor paralysis from orbital infection with ophthalmic zoster, or facial nerve paralysis from geniculate ganglion herpes (Ramsay–Hunt syndrome).

Metabolic disorders with amyotrophy

Several workers have suggested an association between motor neurone disease and previous gastrectomy, but this is probably fortuitous (Norris 1975). A progressive muscle-wasting disorder has been described in patients with hypoglycaemic symptoms following partial gastrectomy (Williams 1955) but most cases of hypoglycaemic amyotrophy are associated with insulin-secreting tumours (Silfverskiold 1946, Tom & Richardson 1951, Mulder et al 1956). Such patients commonly experience paraesthesiae, although the sensory loss has been minimal. Surgical removal of the tumour has led to disappearance of the paresthesiae and to stabilisation of the muscle weakness; in some cases electrophysiological evidence of improvement has been shown (Lambert et al 1960). The evidence that this disease is neuronal rather than due to an axonopathy is uncertain.

Diabetic amyotrophy is characterised by asymmetrical proximal wasting and weakness of the legs, often accompanied by severe local pain in the anterior thighs and sometimes in the lumbar region or perineum. Garland & Taverner (1953) pointed to the frequent finding of extensor plantar responses which, together with the appearance of fasciculations, can cause confusion with motor neurone disease. The patients are invariably middle-aged or elderly and the neuromuscular syndrome may be the presenting feature of maturity-onset diabetes. Good metabolic control may be associated with excellent recovery of function (Casey & Harrison 1972). Garland & Taverner (1953) initially attributed the disorder to a myelopathy but later coined the term diabetic amyotrophy (Garland 1955). The condition has been attributed to a local femoral neuropathy because of the prolonged latency of the knee jerk (Gilliatt & Willison 1962) and a prolonged femoral conduction time (Chopra & Hurwitz 1968, Lamontagne & Buchthal 1970), but the frequent involvement of other muscle groups and the absence of sensory loss makes this an incomplete explanation. Pathological involvement of the femoral nerve has been shown in some cases (Raff et al 1968).

Chronic renal failure or uraemia is usually associated with a mixed motor and sensory polyneuropathy. However, the motor involvement may predominate and cause distal weakness of the legs and, to a lesser extent, of the arms, with depressed tendon reflexes. Distal dysaesthesiae are common, though rarely painful, and may be associated with muscle cramps and a 'restless legs' syndrome (Asbury 1984). There have been variable reports of benefit from long-term haemodialysis but rapid recovery has followed successful renal transplantation (Asbury 1984). Electrophysiological studies show mild slowing of motor and sensory conduction (Jebsen et al 1967). Recently, electrophysiological studies have shown that late responses using H-reflex and F-wave studies are abnormally slowed early in the disease course when MNCV is still normal (Knoll & Dierker 1980, Panayiotopoulos & Lagos 1980). Asbury and colleagues (1963), in an autopsy study of four cases, found a striking loss of nerve fibres in the distal parts of the nerves, with little or no involvement of the proximal portions or nerve roots. They also noted striking myelin breakdown. Central chromatolysis was noted in spinal motor neurones. They concluded that the changes are those of axonal degeneration. Demyelinative changes in fresh sural nerve biopsies have been stressed by some workers (Dinn & Crane 1970) but, in an elegant combined electrophysiological and histological study by Dyck and colleagues (1971), the demyelination was shown to be non-random and present in nerve fibres undergoing axonal degeneration.

Chronic hepatic failure is commonly associated with mild muscle wasting and weakness. In many cases, mild abnormalities of peripheral nerve function may be present but a frank neuropathy is unusual unless alcoholism or diabetes is also present (Kardel & Nielson 1974). Pathological studies on sural nerve biopsies have shown a mild, usually asymptomatic, demyelinating neuropathy in patients with liver disease, and this finding was not restricted to alcoholic cases (Dayan & Williams 1967). However, it is still not clear whether or not the demyelination is non-random and secondary to axonal degeneration. Electrophysiological studies have demonstrated a significant incidence of subclinical polyneuropathy, affecting sensory fibres more than motor, including non-alcoholic cases (Seneviratne & Peiris 1970, Morgan et al 1979). The mild slowing of nerve conduction suggests that this is primarily an axonal disorder similar to that seen in uraemia, but further studies are needed.

Muscle wasting in hyperthyroidism is generally thought to be myopathic, but histological studies have shown remarkably little abnormality in most cases. Neither specific myopathic nor denervation changes have been described. McComas et al

(1973a) described electrophysiological findings of a reversible motor neuropathy in thyrotoxicosis, but this awaits independent confirmation. Hypothyroidism commonly causes local entrapment mononeuropathies, especially in the carpal tunnel, but a polyneuropathy is rarely seen and is predominantly sensory with mild motor weakness (Dyck & Lambert 1970).

Muscle weakness may also be a feature of acromegaly or gigantism caused by a growth-hormone secreting pituitary tumour. In some cases this may be rapidly reversed with treatment; no adequate explanation for this phenomenon has been given. The carpal tunnel syndrome is common in acromegaly and a diffuse hypertrophic neuropathy has been described occasionally since the last century (Marie & Marinesco 1891). Histological studies have shown an increase of endoneural and perineural connective tissue with loss of myelinated nerve fibres (Stewart 1966) and Dinn (1970) found evidence of a primary demyelinating disorder. However, nerve conduction is slowed only mildly in addition to a moderate reduction in nerve action potentials, suggesting a mainly axonal degeneration with non-random demyelination (Low et al 1974, Pickett et al 1975).

Hyperlipoproteinaemia has been associated with progressive muscular atrophy, but it is uncertain whether such cases represent an adult-onset form of spinal muscular atrophy with an associated genetic abnormality of lipid metabolism (Quarfordt et al 1970).

Toxic motor neuropathies

Many exogenous toxins have been associated with peripheral neuropathies but few cause a predominantly motor syndrome. The possible association of chronic lead poisoning and motor neurone disease has been discussed earlier. Lead intoxication may affect the central nervous system or the peripheral nerves. Motor involvement predominates, although paraesthesiae and pain are common. Motor weakness is greatest in muscles receiving most use: hence the wristdrop in painters intoxicated by lead paints. In children, CNS involvement predominates, but foot-drop may be evident in association with brisk reflexes and extensor plantar responses (Seto & Freeman 1964). Pathological studies show axonal degeneration and also dose-dependent demyelination (Fullerton 1966).

Several other heavy metal intoxications cause peripheral neuropathy. In arsenic poisoning, sensory involvement is prominent and causes painful dysaesthesiae in addition to distal weakness. In other metal intoxications the initial sensory disturbances may subside and produce a predominantly distal motor weakness, e.g. in gold therapy for rheumatoid arthritis (Katrak et al 1980, Windebank et al 1984). It is not clear whether gold neuropathy is a direct neuronal toxicity or an immunologically mediated demyelinating polyradiculopathy.

The effects of mercury on the nervous system depend on the chemical state of the element. Inorganic mercuric chloride, when discharged into the sea of Minamata Bay, Japan, was converted to organic methylmercury by micro-organisms, and then concentrated in the bodies of fish and shellfish. Organic mercury intoxication affects the central nervous system and produces mental and extrapyramidal disorders (McAlpine & Araki 1958, Kurland et al 1960). Inorganic mercury intoxication, usually due to inhalation of vapour, generally causes a personality change and tremor, but a few cases of predominantly distal motor neuropathy have been described (Ross 1964, Swaiman & Flagler 1971, Windebank et al 1984). The significance of an ALS-like syndrome following chronic mercurialism reported by Kantarjian (1961) is uncertain.

Organophosphorus compounds have been widely used in industry, mainly as pesticides. They are powerful inhibitors of carboxylic esterase enzymes, including cholinesterase. In man, acute intoxication causes inhibition of acetylcholinesterase in the nervous system, resulting in accumulation of acetylcholine at the synapses and a paralytic cholinergic crisis. If respiratory paralysis is treated and the airway is protected from excessive secretions, complete recovery occurs within 10 days (Namba et al 1971). Bidstrup et al (1953) described three cases of a delayed neuropathy after an acute cholinergic illness in workers manufacturing the compound 'Mipafox'. However, the delayed neuropathy in organophosphorus poisoning generally occurs without an antecedent cholinergic illness. Tri-orthocresyl phosphate (TOCP), a weak insecticide and a high-temperature industrial lubricant, has been responsible for the greatest number of cases of neuropathy in man. The largest outbreak of poisoning occurred in 1930–31 in the USA when alcoholic extracts of ginger and rum were adulterated by TOCP and freely used as an alcoholic drink. An estimated 16 000 cases of polyneuropathy (ginger jake paralysis) occurred at that time (Namba et al 1971), and several other major outbreaks have resulted from contaminated cooking oil since then. The neuropathy develops after an interval of 7–21 days, beginning with paraesthesiae swiftly followed by spreading distal weakness (Hopkins 1975). The paralysis progresses rapidly over several days: the affected muscles waste; sensory loss is trivial or absent and paresthesiae disappear early. The tendon reflexes may be lost, but are sometimes increased because of pyramidal tract involvement; spasticity may develop later. Recovery from any neuropathy attributable to organophosphorus poisoning is poor. Pathological studies in man and experimental animals have shown axonal degeneration (present only in the distal ends of the motor nerves) and changes in the spinal cord (Cavanagh 1964).

Ischaemic myelopathy

Acute occlusion of arteries supplying the spinal cord causes an initial paraplegia with sensory loss up to the level which is ischaemic, but in certain cases good sensory recovery has occurred, leaving a residual motor neuropathy (Dodson & Landau 1973). Less acute aortic disease has been associated with selective poliomyelomalacia, particularly of the ventral grey matter of the spinal cord (Herrick & Mills 1971), and a chronic motor neurone syndrome has been described in relation to arteriosclerosis or hypertension (Jellinger & Neumayer 1962, Hughes & Brownell 1966, Jellinger 1967). The latter is a progressive disease with a picture of weakness and wasting, mainly in the lower limbs, and mild but definite sensory impairment. The pathological changes are confined to the territory of the anterior spinal artery. Ischaemic lacunae are present in the spinal grey matter involving the motor neurones, and the lesions may

extend laterally into the territory of the spinothalamic tracts or dorsally into the base of the posterior columns. Atherosclerosis does not appear to occur in the anterior spinal artery or its branches, but mesial thickening of the wall has been found, particularly in hypertensive patients. It seems unlikely that this condition, largely restricted to the lower limbs, could be confused with MND. Its restriction to the territory of the anterior spinal artery probably relates to the architectural deficiency of the blood supply to the anterior two-thirds of the spinal cord, and its vulnerability to ischaemia (Jellinger & Neumayer 1969).

Radiation injury. The occasional chronic myelopathy with progressive muscle wasting and weakness which follows radiation therapy to the spinal region, including the spinal cord, is thought to be largely due to ischaemia. Prominent abnormalities of small and medium-sized arterioles are found in damaged areas. Hyalinisation, fibrinoid necrosis and thrombosis of vessels are seen with local necrosis and astrocytosis (Pennybacker & Russell 1948). Several authors have described a clinical syndrome of muscular atrophy and weakness in the lower limbs, with preserved sensation, which has occurred several months after irradiation (Greenfield & Stark 1948, Sadowsky et al 1976).

Trauma, including electrical injury

Cases of motor neurone disease with a previous history of significant trauma have been reported by many authors, but are thought to be chance associations (see Bonduelle 1975). However, a distinctive syndrome of benign post-traumatic amyotrophy developing several months after major local trauma has been described (Norris 1972b). The wasting was confined to the injured limb and after several months there was complete recovery; this was reminiscent of neuralgic amyotrophy or allergic brachial neuritis. A few cases of apparent post-traumatic MND were subsequently proved to be attributable to cervical arachnoiditis (Puech et al 1947, Kissel 1948).

The neurological effects of electrical trauma were comprehensively reviewed by Panse (1970). Transient sensorimotor paralysis of limbs, persisting for up to 2 weeks, has been described in survivors of severe electrical trauma involving moderate or high energies (voltages of 1000 V or more and current in the range 25 mA–5 A) and also in those struck by lightning. The site of damage has depended on the path taken by the electrical current through the body. Spinal amyotrophy following lightning accidents has been known for more than a century. It is also well known after passage of electricity from limb to limb, or trunk to limb. The muscular atrophy is commonly unilateral and is roughly confined to the neurological distribution of sensory dermatomes related to the point of contact. Hence, weakness and wasting around the shoulder and upper arm may develop after electrical burns to the thumb and index fingers. Not all victims show electrical burns or scars at the site of contact and roughly only one-half have suffered loss of consciousness at the time of injury. Apparently, the weakness may be immediate or delayed by as long as a few months and the atrophy can be progressive for a few months before becoming static or showing regression. Loss of local tendon reflexes is the general rule, but sensory loss is usually slight. Spasticity or other pyramidal signs have been described and indicate more extensive spinal cord damage. There have been a few descriptions of typical clinical cases of MND following electrical trauma, but these are generally regarded as coincidental.

Plasma cell dyscrasias and motor neurone disease

The neuromuscular complications of plasma cell dyscrasias may be in the form of a spinal muscular atrophy, a motor polyneuropathy or as an ALS-like syndrome (Latov 1982). The plasma cell dyscrasia produces a paraproteinaemia in 80% of patients, usually IgG in about 50% and IgA in 20% of cases. The neurological disease may begin in association with an isolated plasmacytoma, but it is usually related to multiple myeloma by the time that the patient is seen. The disease may produce lambda light chains and cause amyloidosis but this is not thought to be the direct cause of the neuropathy in myeloma (McLeod et al 1984). Benign monoclonal gammopathy, where there is a monoclonal paraproteinaemia but no evidence of a malignant B-cell disorder, may be present in 6%

of patients with peripheral neuropathy (Kelly et al 1981) and in an even higher proportion of elderly patients. IgG, IgM and IgA paraproteinaemia have been described.

Clinical sensorimotor neuropathy is present in about 15% of patients with multiple myeloma. Chazot et al (1976) demonstrated binding of paraproteins to the perineurium and endoneurium of peripheral nerves in IgA and IgG myeloma. Motor neurone syndromes (Patten 1984) and an ALS-like syndrome (Krieger & Melmed 1982) have been associated with paraproteinaemia. The association of motor neurone syndromes with paraproteins has been reported with increasing frequency (Parry et al 1986, Shy et al 1986, Rudnicki et al 1987) with suggestive evidence that some of these patients may respond to immunosuppression or plasmapheresis (Rudnicki et al 1987). The added association of lymphoma in both LMN disease and ALS has recently been reported (Younger et al 1991). About 25% of patients with macroglobulinaemia have neurological complications, including neuropathies (Logothetis et al 1960). Sensory symptoms are usually prominent but the distal motor weakness and wasting may be very severe and often associated with fasciculations (Layani et al 1955, Saric et al 1967). Very occasionally the neuropathy may be acute, resembling a Guillain–Barré syndrome (Bing & Neel 1936, Logothetis et al 1960). A spinal muscular atrophy syndrome (Peters & Clatanoff 1968) and a motor neurone syndrome have been described in association with IgM paraproteinaemia (Bauer et al 1977, Rowland et al 1982). Amyloidosis, either primary or secondary to myeloma, usually gives a polyneuropathy without CNS signs (Kyle & Greipp 1985) but UMN signs have been described in a recent case (Abarbanel et al 1986).

Antiglycolipid antibodies and motor neurone disease

Considerable interest has been generated recently in the association of motor neurone disorders and antineural antibodies, particularly antibodies directed against the ganglioside GM1. There is general agreement that anti-GM1 antibodies occur with significant frequency in patients with motor neuropathies, especially those associated with conduction blocks (Pestronk 1991). Recognition of this association is of particular importance, since some of these patients will respond to immunosuppressive therapy, particularly cyclophosphamide (Pestronk et al 1988). The association of anti-ganglioside antibodies with ALS is less certain and although some have reported an association as high as 78% (Pestronk et al 1989) this has not been confirmed by others (Salazar-Grueso et al 1990). Nonetheless, it has become common practice to measure serum anti-ganglioside antibodies in patients with motor neurone disorders, particularly those with mainly LMN forms, and to institute immunosuppressive therapy if elevations are found.

Non-metastatic carcinomatous neuromuscular disease

The various forms of neuromuscular disease occurring in association with lymphoma and cancer are discussed fully in Chapter 27. Reference here is limited to those cases where a direct involvement of motor neurones is apparent. Non-inflammatory degeneration of anterior horn cells and of dorsal ganglion cells has been described in sensorimotor polyneuropathies (Norris et al 1964, Victor 1965, Henson & Urich 1970). However, the direct association of cancer with a pure motor neurone disease state remains controversial and in most cases is coincidental (Norris & Engel 1965, Norris et al 1969, Brownell et al 1970).

Modern electrophysiological techniques have revealed evidence of subclinical neuropathy in up to 50% of cases of malignancy, usually lung cancer (McLeod 1984). These cases correspond to the carcinomatous 'neuromyopathy' of Brain & Henson (1958) and in some cases to the 'mild terminal neuropathy' which complicates known cancer (Croft et al 1967, Croft & Wilkinson 1969, Hawley et al 1980). This disorder presents with symmetrical, mainly proximal, limb weakness and wasting in association with minor sensory symptoms such as paraesthesiae or mild numbness. The examination findings are of depressed tendon reflexes and, frequently, occasional fasciculations or distal sensory loss, especially to vibration. Electromyography reveals a high incidence of chronic denervation changes together with spontaneous discharge of fibrillation and short-duration fasciculation potentials; active 'myopathic' units may also be found, particularly in proximal muscles (Trojaborg et al 1969, Campbell & Paty 1974). Motor conduction velocity is frequently normal but may be mildly slowed, especially in the terminal nerve segments. Sensory conduction is frequently impaired and sensory action potentials may be absent or markedly reduced. It has been suggested that the disorder is a progressive neuronal dysfunction with an involvement of motor to a greater extent than of sensory neurones (Campbell & Paty 1974).

The mechanism by which non-metastatic polyneuropathy and neuronal disease are produced is unknown. The possibility that they are caused by toxic factors released by the tumour has been suggested by many authors (Costa & Holland 1965). Certainly, the incidence of clinical neurological disease is apparently higher in association with undifferentiated cell tumours of the lung, which may produce a wide range of hormone-like compounds (Lebovitz 1965, Ross 1972). The possibility of neuronal damage from viral invasion was discussed earlier and this could be linked with an immune mechanism. Brain & Henson (1958) speculated on a crossed reaction to shared antigenic sites between tumour and nervous tissue proteins. This was supported by the finding of anti-CNS antibodies in the serum of four patients with subacute sensory neuropathy but not in other forms of neuropathy (Wilkinson 1964). The demonstration of circulating lymphocytes sensitised to peripheral nervous tissue was thought, like the serum antibodies, to be a secondary phenomenon to sequestrated or damaged neural proteins (Paty et al 1974).

ACKNOWLEDGEMENTS

We would like to thank Dr Pam Enderby for her critical help on the sections about bulbar palsy and their management.

REFERENCES

Abarbanel J M, Frisher S, Osimani A 1986 Primary amyloidosis with peripheral neuropathy and signs of motor neuron disease. Neurology 36: 1125

Addair J, Snyder L H 1942 Evidence for an autosomal recessive gene for susceptibility to paralytic poliomyelitis. Journal of Heredity 33: 306

Aguilar M J, Kamoshita S, Landing B H, Boder E, Sedgewick R P 1968 Pathological observations in ataxia telangiectasia. Journal of Neuropathology and Experimental Neurology 27: 659

Alexander M P, Emery E S, Koerner F C 1976 Progressive bulbar paresis in childhood. Archives of Neurology 33: 66

Allen I V, Dermott E, Connelly J H, Hurwitz L J 1971 A study of a patient with the amyotrophic form of Creutzfeld-Jakob disease. Brain 94: 715

Andrews J M, Gardner M B 1974 Lower motor neuron degeneration associated with type C RNA virus infection in mice. Neuropathological features. Journal of Neuropathology and Experimental Neurology 33: 285

Annunziata P, Giarrtana M, Ancone A M et al 1989 Anti HTLV-I antibodies in the serum and CSF from amyotrophic lateral sclerosis patients: negative findings. Journal of Neurology 236: 185

Antel J P, Noronha A C C, Oger J J F, Arnason B G W 1982 Immunology of amyotrophic lateral sclerosis. In: Rowland L P (ed) Human motor neuron diseases. Raven, New York, p 395

Aran F 1850 Recherches sur une maladie non encore décrite de système musculaire (atrophie musculaire progressive). Archives Générales de Médecin, Paris 24: 4

Aronson A E 1980 Definition and scope of the communication disorder. In: Mulder D W (ed) The diagnosis and treatment of amyotrophic lateral sclerosis. Houghton Mifflin, Boston, p 225

Asbury A K 1984 Uremic neuropathy. In: Dyck P J, Thomas P K, Lambert E H, Bunge R (eds) Peripheral neuropathy. 2nd edn. Saunders, New York, p 1811

Asbury A K, Victor M, Adams R D 1963 Uremic polyneuropathy. Archives of Neurology 8: 413

Aspin J, Harrison R, Jehanli A, Lunt G, Campbell M J 1986 Stimulation by mitogen and neuronal membranes of lymphocytes from patients with motor neurone disease. Journal of Neuroimmunology. 11: 31

Astin K J, Wilde C E, Davies-Jones G A B 1975 Glucose metabolism and insulin response in the plasma and cerebrospinal fluid in motor neurone disease. Journal of the Neurological Sciences 25: 205

Aycock W L 1942 Familial aggregation in poliomyelitis. American Journal of the Medical Sciences 203: 452

Barker A T, Jalinous R, Freeston I L 1985 Magnetic stimulation of the human brain. Lancet i: 1106

Bartfeld H C, Dham H, Donnenfeld L et al 1982a Immunological profile of amyotrophic lateral sclerosis patients and their cell mediated immune responses to viral and CNS antigens. Clinical and Experimental Immunology 48: 137

Bartfeld H, Pollack M S, Cunningham-Rundles S, Donnenfeld H 1982b HLA frequencies in amyotrophic lateral sclerosis. Archives of Neurology 39: 270

Bartfeld H, Dham C, Donenfield D et al 1989 Entero-viral related antigen in circulating immune complexes of amyotrophic lateral sclerosis patients. Intervirology 30: 202

Bauer M, Bergstrom R, Ritter B, Olsson Y 1977 Macroglobulinemia Waldenstrom and motor neuron syndrome. Acta Neurologica Scandinavica 55: 245

Beal M F, Richardson E P 1981 Primary lateral sclerosis. A case report. Archives of Neurology 38: 630

Behan P O 1979 Cell mediated immunity in motor neurone disease and poliomyelitis. In: Rose F Clifford (ed) Clinical neuroimmunology. Blackwell, London, p 259

Ben Hamida M, Hentati F, Ben Hamida C 1990 Hereditary motor system disease (chronic juvenile amyotrophic lateral sclerosis). Brain 113: 347

Bidstrup P L, Bonnell J A, Beckett A G 1953 Paralysis following poisoning by a new organic phosphorus insecticide (mipafox). Report on two cases. British Medical Journal 1: 1068

Bing J, Neel A V 1936 Two cases of hyperglobulinaemia with affection of the central nervous system on a toxic-infectious basis. Acta Medica Scandinavica 88: 492

Bjornskov E R, Norris F H, Kirby-Mower J 1984 Quantitative axon terminal and end-plate morphology in amyotrophic lateral sclerosis. Archives of Neurology 41: 527

Bodian D 1949 Poliomyelitis: Pathological anatomy. In: Poliomyelitis. Papers and discussion presented at the First International Poliomyelitis Conference. Lippincott, Philadelphia p 62

Böhme G 1974 Stimm-, Sprech-und Hörstörungen. Aetiologie, Diagnostik, Therapie. Fischer Verlag, Stuttgart

Bonduelle M 1975 Amyotrophic lateral sclerosis. In: Vinken P J, Bruyn G W (eds) Handbook of clinical neurology, vol 22. North Holland, Amsterdam p 281

Bosma J F, Brodie D R 1969 Disabilities of the pharynx in amyotrophic lateral sclerosis as demonstrated by cineradiography. Radiology 92: 97

Bradley W G, Krasin F 1982 A new hypothesis of the etiology of amyotrophic lateral sclerosis: the DNA hypothesis. Archives of Neurology 39: 677

Bradley W G, Good P, Rassool C G, Adelman L S 1983 Morphometric and biochemical studies of peripheral nerves in amyotrophic lateral sclerosis. Annals of Neurology 14: 267

Bradley E G, Hedlund W, Cooper C et al 1984 A double-blind controlled trial of bovine brain gangliosides in amyotrophic lateral sclerosis. Neurology (Cleveland) 34: 1079

Bradley W G 1987 Recent views on amyotrophic lateral sclerosis with emphasis on electrophysiologic studies. Muscle and Nerve 10: 490

Brain W R, Henson R A 1958 Neurological syndromes associated with carcinoma. Lancet ii: 971

Brait K, Fahn S, Schwartz G A 1973 Sporadic and familial parkinsonism and motor neuron disease. Neurology 23: 990

Brandt S 1950 Course and symptoms of progressive infantile muscular atrophy. A follow-up study of 112 cases in Denmark. Archives of Neurology and Psychiatry 63: 218

Braun S R 1987 Respiratory system in amyotrophic lateral sclerosis. Neurology Clinics 5: 9

Brion S, Psimzrus A, Chevalier J P et al 1980 Association of Pick's disease and amyotrophic lateral sclerosis. Encéphale 6: 259

Brooke M H 1989 Thyrotrophin-releasing hormone in ALS: are the results of clinical studies inconsistent? Annals of the New York Academy of Sciences 553: 422

Brown J C, Kater R M H 1969 Pancreatic function in patients

with amyotrophic lateral sclerosis. Neurology (Minneapolis) 19: 1985

Brownell D B, Oppenheimer D R, Hughes J T 1970 The central nervous system in motor neurone disease. Journal of Neurology, Neurosurgery and Psychiatry 33: 338

Bruyn G W, Bots G T A M, Dom R 1979 Huntington's chorea: Current neuropathological status. In: Chase T N, Wexler N S, Barbeau A (eds) Huntington's disease. Advances in Neurology 23: 83

Brzustowicz L M, Lehner T, Castilla L G et al 1990 Genetic mapping of childhood-onset spinal muscular atrophy to chromosome 5q11.2–13.3. Nature 344: 540

Buchthal F, Olsen P Z 1970 Electromyography and muscle biopsy in infantile spinal muscle atrophy. Brain 93: 15

Burke R E 1982 Motor units in cat muscles: Anatomical considerations in relation to motor unit types. In: Rowland L P (ed) Human motor neuron diseases. Raven, New York, p 31

Byers R K, Banker B Q 1961 Infantile muscular atrophy. Archives of Neurology 5: 140

Campa J F, Engel W K 1970 Histochemistry of motor neurons and interneurons in the cat lumbar spinal cord. Neurology 20: 559

Campbell A M G, Williams E R, Pearce J 1969 Late motor neuron degeneration following poliomyelitis. Neurology 19: 1101

Campbell A M G, Williams E R, Barltrop D 1970 Motor neurone disease and exposure to lead. Journal of Neurology, Neurosurgery and Psychiatry 33: 872

Campbell M J 1979 Genetic aspects of motor neurone disease. In: Behan P O, Rose F C (eds) Progress in neurological research. Pitman, London, p 135

Campbell M J 1980 Management of patients with motor neurone disease. International Rehabilitation Medicine 2: 111

Campbell M J, McComas A J, Petito F 1973 Physiological changes in ageing muscle. Journal of Neurology, Neurosurgery and Psychiatry 36: 174

Campbell M J, Paty D W 1974 Carcinomatous neuromyopathy; an electrophysiological and immunological study of patients with carcinoma of the lung. I. Electrophysiological studies. Journal of Neurology, Neurosurgery and Psychiatry 37: 131

Campbell M J, Enderby P M 1984 Management of motor neurone disease. Journal of the Neurological Sciences 64: 65

Carey J S 1986 Motor neuron disease — a challenge to medical ethics: discussion paper. Journal of the Royal Society of Medicine 79: 216

Carpenter S 1968 Proximal axonal enlargement in motor neuron disease. Neurology (Minneapolis) 18: 841

Carpenter S, Karpati G, Rothman S, Watters G, Andermann F 1978 Pathological involvement of primary sensory neurons in Werdnig–Hoffmann disease. Acta Neuropathologica 42: 91

Caruso A, Burton E K 1987 Temporal measures of dysarthria associated with amyotrophic lateral sclerosis. Journal of Speech and Hearing Research 30: 80

Casey E B, Harrison M J G 1972 Diabetic amyotrophy: a follow-up study. British Medical Journal 1: 656

Cashman N R, Antel J P, Hancock L W et al 1986 N-acetyl-beta-hexosaminidase beta locus defect and juvenile motor neuron disease: a case study. Annals of Neurology 20: 568

Castleman B (ed) 1970 Case records of the Massachusetts General Hospital (case 42–1970). New England Journal of Medicine 283: 806

Cavanagh J B 1964 Peripheral nerve changes in orthocresyl phosphate poisoning in the cat. Journal of Pathology and Bacteriology 87: 365

Charcot J M 1865 Sclérose de cords lateraux de la moelle spineuse chez une femme hysterique atteinte de contracture peiman de quatre menieres. Bulletin de la Societé Médicale des Hopitaux (Paris) 2 (suppl 2): 24

Charcot J M 1874 De la sclérose latérale amyotrophique. Progrès Médicale (Paris) 2: 325, 341, 453

Charcot J M, Marie P 1886 Sur une forme particulière d'atrophie musculaire progressive, souvent familiale, débutant par les pieds et les jambes et atteignant plus tard les mains. Revue de Médecine (Paris) 6: 97

Chazot G, Berger G, Carrier H et al 1976 Manifestations neurologiques des gammapathies monoclonales. Revue Neurologique 132: 195

Chopra J S, Hurwitz L J 1968 Femoral nerve conduction in diabetes and chronic occlusive vascular disease. Journal of Neurology, Neurosurgery and Psychiatry 31: 28

Chou S M, Fakadej A V 1971 Ultrastructure of chromatolytic motoneurons and anterior spinal roots in a case of Werdnig–Hoffmann disease. Journal of Neuropathology and Experimental Neurology 30: 368

Cochrane G 1987 Increasing reliance on others. In: Cochrane G (ed) The management of motor neurone disease. Churchill Livingstone, London, p 65

Colmant H J 1975 Progressive bulbar palsy in adults. In: Eds. Vinken P J, Bruyn G W (eds) Handbook of clinical neurology, Vol. 22. North Holland, Amsterdam, p 111

Conradi S, Ronnevi L-O, Norris F H 1982 Motor neuron disease and toxic metals. In: Rowland P (ed) Human motor neuron diseases. Raven, New York, p 201

Contag C A, Harty J T, Plagemann P G W 1989 Dual virus etiology of age dependent poliomyelitis of mice. A potential model for human motor neurone disease. Microbial Pathology 6: 391

Cook A W, Pertschuk L P, Gupta K et al 1979 The effect of antiviral agents on jejunal immunopathology in amyotrophic lateral sclerosis. In: Behan P O, Rose F C (eds) Progress in neurological research. Pitman, London, p 62

Costa G, Holland J F 1965 Systemic effect of tumours with special reference to the nervous system. In: Lord Brain, Norris F H (eds) The remote effects of cancer on the nervous system. Grune and Stratton, New York, p 125

Cremer N E, Oshiro L S, Norris F H, Lennette E H 1973 Cultures of tissues from patients with amyotrophic lateral sclerosis. Archives of Neurology 29: 331

Croft P B, Urich H, Wilkinson M 1967 Peripheral neuropathy of sensorimotor type associated with malignant disease. Brain 90: 31

Croft P B, Wilkinson M 1969 The course and prognosis in some types of carcinomatous neuropathy. Brain 92: 1

Currier R D, Haerer A F 1968 Amyotrophic lateral sclerosis and metallic toxins. Archives of Environmental Health 17: 712

Dalakas M C, Elder G, Hallett M et al 1986 A long-term follow-up study of patients with post-poliomyelitis neuromuscular symptoms. New England Journal of Medicine 314: 959

Darley F L, Aronson A E, Brown J R 1975 Motor speech disorders. Saunders, Philadelphia

Davis L E, Bodian D, Price D, Butler I J, Vickers J H 1977

Chronic progressive poliomyelitis secondary to vaccination of an immunodeficient child. New England Journal of Medicine 297: 241

Dayan A D, Williams R 1967 Demyelinating peripheral neuropathy and liver disease. Lancet ii: 133

Dayan A D, Graveson G S, Illis L S, Robinson P K 1969 Schwann cell damage in motor neuron disease. Neurology (Minneapolis) 19: 242

Dejerine J, Sottas J 1893 Sur la névrite interstitelle, hypertrophique et progressive de l'enfance. Comptes Rendus des Séances de la Société de Biologie et de ses filiales (Paris) 45: 63

Denys E H, Norris F H 1979 Amyotrophic lateral sclerosis. Impairment of neuromuscular transmission. Archives of Neurology 36: 202

Digby J, Harrison R, Jehanli A, Lunt G G, Rose F C 1985 Cultured rat spinal cord neurones: interaction with motor neurone disease immunoglobulins. Muscle and Nerve 8: 595

Dinn J J 1970 Schwann cell dysfunction in acromegaly. Journal of Clinical Endocrinology and Metabolism 31: 140

Dinn J J, Crane D L 1970 Schwann cell dysfunction in uraemia. Journal of Neurology, Neurosurgery and Psychiatry 33: 605

Dodson W E, Landau W M 1973 Motor neuron loss due to aortic clamping in repair of coarctation. Neurology (Minneapolis) 23: 539

Dorman J D, Engel W K, Fried D M 1969 Therapeutic trial in amyotrophic lateral sclerosis. Journal of the American Medical Association 209: 257

Doyu M, Sobue G, Mikai E et al 1992 Severity of linked recessive bulbo-spinal neuronopathy correlates with size of the tandem CAG repeat in androgen receptor gene. Annals of Neurology 32: 707

Drachman D B, Kuncl R W 1989 Amyotrophic lateral sclerosis: an unconventional autoimmune disease? Annals of Neurology 26: 269

Drake M E Jr 1983 Chronic pain syndrome in amyotrophic lateral sclerosis. Archives of Neurology 40: 453

Duchenne G 1860 Paralysie musculaire progressive de la langue, du voile du palais et des lèvres. Archives Générales de Médecine 16: 283

Duchenne G, Joffroy A 1870 De l'atrophie aigue et chronique des cellules nerveuses de la moelle et du bulbe rachidien, à propos d'une observation de paralysie glossolabio-laryngée. Archives de Physiologie 3: 499

Dworkin J P, Aronson A E, Mulder D W 1980 Tongue force in normals and in dysarthric patients with amyotrophic lateral sclerosis. Journal of Speech and Hearing Research 23: 828

Dyck P J 1982 Are motor neuropathies and motor neuron diseases separable? In: Rowland L P (ed) Human motor neuron diseases. Raven, New York, p 105

Dyck P J 1984 Inherited neuronal degeneration and atrophy affecting peripheral motor, sensory and autonomic neurons. In: Dyck P J, Thomas P K, Lambert E H, Bunge R (eds) Peripheral neuropathy, 2nd edn. Saunders, Philadelphia, p 1600

Dyck P J, Lais A C 1973 Evidence of segmental demyelination secondary to axonal degeneration in Friedreich's ataxia. In: Kakulas B A (ed) Clinical studies in myology. Excerpta Medica, Amsterdam, p 253

Dyck P J, Lambert E H 1968a Lower motor and primary sensory neuron diseases with peroneal muscular atrophy. I. Hereditary polyneuropathies. Archives of Neurology 18: 603

Dyck P J, Lambert E H 1968b Ibid. II Various neuronal degenerations. Archives of Neurology 18: 619

Dyck P J, Lambert E H 1970 Polyneuropathy associated with hypothyroidism. Journal of Neuropathology and Experimental Neurology 29: 631

Dyck P J, Johnson W J, Lambert E H, O'Brien P C 1971 Segmental demyelination secondary to axonal degeneration in uremic neuropathy. Mayo Clinic Proceedings 46: 400

Dyck P J, Stevens J C, Mulder D W, Espinosa R E 1975 Frequency of nerve fiber degeneration of peripheral motor and sensory neurons in amyotrophic lateral sclerosis. Morphometry of deep and superficial peroneal nerves. Neurology (Minneapolis) 25: 781

Emery A E H 1971 The nosology of the spinal muscular atrophies. Journal of Medical Genetics 8: 481

Emery A E H, Holloway S 1982 Familial motor neuron diseases. In: Rowland L P (ed) Human motor neuron diseases. Raven, New York, p 139

Enderby P 1988 The assessment of dysarthria: a challenge to more than the ears. Clinical Rehabilitation 2: 267

Engel W K, Kurland L T, Klatzo I 1959 An inherited disease similar to amyotrophic lateral sclerosis with a pattern of posterior column involvement. An intermediate form? Brain 82: 203

Engel W K, Hogenhuis L A H, Collis W J, Schalch D S, Barlow M H, Gold E N, Dorman J D 1969 Metabolic studies and therapeutic trials in amyotrophic lateral sclerosis. In: Norris F H, Kurland L T (eds) Motor neuron diseases. Grune and Stratton, New York, p 199

Engel W K, Cuneo R A, Levy H B 1978 Polyinosinicytidylic acid treatment of neuropathy (letter). Lancet i: 503

Erkman I, Touzeau G, Bertrand D et al 1989 Characterization of dissociated monolayer cultures of human spinal cord. Brain Research Bulletin 22: 57

Fallat R J, Jewitt B, Bass M, Kamm B, Norris F H Jr 1979 Spirometry in amyotrophic lateral sclerosis. Archives of Neurology 36: 74

Fallat R J, Norris F H Jr 1980 Respiratory problems. In: Mulder D W (ed) The diagnosis and treatment of amyotrophic lateral sclerosis. Houghton Mifflin, Boston, p 301

Fallis R J, Weiner L P 1982 Further studies in search of a virus in amyotrophic lateral sclerosis. In: Rowland L P (ed) Human motor neuron diseases. Raven, New York, p 363

Fazio M 1892 Erediatrieta della paralise bulbare progressiva. Riforma Medica 8: 327

Feigenbaum J A, Munsat T L 1970 A neuromuscular syndrome of scapuloperoneal distribution. Bulletin of the Los Angeles Neurosurgical Society 35: 47

Felmus M T, Patten J P, Swanke D 1976 Antecedent events in amyotrophic lateral sclerosis. Neurology (Minneapolis) 26: 167

Fenichel G M, Emery E S, Hunt P 1967 Neurogenic atrophy simulating facio-scapulo-humeral dystrophy. A dominant form. Archives of Neurology 17: 257

Festoff B W, Crigger N J 1980 Therapeutic trials in amyotrophic lateral sclerosis; a review. In: Mulder D W (ed) The diagnosis and treatment of amyotrophic lateral sclerosis. Houghton Mifflin, Boston p 337

Finkel N 1962 A forma pseudomiopatica tardia da atrophia muscular progressiva heredo-familial. Archives de Neuropsiquiatria 4: 307

Fischbeck K H, Saunders D, La Spada A 1991 A candidate

gene for X-linked spinal muscular atrophy. Advances in Neurology 56: 209

Fisher C M 1977 Pure spastic paralysis of corticospinal origin. Canadian Journal of Neurological Sciences 4: 252

Forster F M, Alpers B J 1944 Site of origin of fasciculations in voluntary muscle. Archives of Neurology and Psychiatry 51: 264

Friedman A P, Freedman D 1950 Amyotrophic lateral sclerosis. Journal of Nervous and Mental Disease 111: 1

Fullerton P M 1966 Chronic peripheral neuropathy produced by lead poisoning in guinea-pigs. Journal of Neuropathology and Experimental Neurology 25: 214

Furukawa T, Tsukagoshi H, Sugita H, Toyokura Y 1969 Neurogenic muscular atrophy simulating facioscapulohumeral muscular dystrophy. Journal of the Neurological Sciences 9: 389

Gajdusek D C 1963 Motor neuron disease in natives of New Guinea. New England Journal of Medicine 268: 474

Gajdusek D C 1982 Foci of motor neurone disease in high incidence in isolated populations of East Asia and the Western Pacific. In: Rowland L P (ed) Human motor neuron diseases. Raven, New York, p 363

Gallai V, Hockaday J M, Hughes J T, Lane D J, Oppenheimer D R, Rushworth G 1981 Ponto-bulbar palsy with deafness (Brown–Vialetto–van Laere syndrome). A report on 3 cases. Journal of the Neurological Sciences 50: 250

Gallassi R, Montagua P, Ciardulla C, Lorusso S, Mussuto V, Stracciari A 1985 Cognitive impairment in MND. Acta Neurologica Scandinavica 71: 480

Gardner M B, Henderson B E, Officer J E et al 1973 A spontaneous lower motor neuron disease apparently caused by indigenous Type-C RNA virus in wild mice. Journal of the National Cancer Institute 51: 1243

Gardner-Medwin D, Hudgson P, Walton J N 1967 Benign spinal muscular atrophy arising in childhood and adolescence. Journal of the Neurological Sciences 5: 121

Gardner-Thorpe C, Foster J B, Barwick D D 1976 Unusual manifestations of herpes zoster: a clinical and electrophysiological study. Journal of the Neurological Sciences 28: 427

Garland H 1955 Diabetic amyotrophy. British Medical Journal 2: 1287

Garland H, Taverner D 1953 Diabetic myelopathy. British Medical Journal 1: 1405

Garruto R M, Yanagihara R, Gajdusek D C, Arion D M 1984 Concentrations of heavy metals and essential minerals in garden soil and drinking water in the Western Pacific. In: Chen K M, Yase Y (eds) Amyotrophic lateral sclerosis in Asian and Oceania. National Taiwan University, Taipei, p 265

Garruto R M, Yanagihara R, Gajdusek D C 1985 Disappearance of high-incidence amyotrophic lateral sclerosis and parkinsonism-dementia on Guam. Neurology 35: 193

Gath I, Sjaastad O, Loken A C 1969 Myopathic electromyographic changes correlated with histopathology in Wohlfart–Kugelberg–Welander disease. Neurology (Minneapolis) 19: 344

Gibbs C J, Gajdusek D C 1982 An update on long-term in vivo and in vitro studies designed to identify a virus as the cause of amyotrophic lateral sclerosis, parkinsonism-dementia and Parkinson's disease. In: Rowland L P (ed) Human motor neuron diseases. Raven, New York, p 343

Gillberg P G, Aquilonius S M, Eckernas S A 1982 Choline acetyltransferase and substance P-like immunoreactivity in the human spinal cord: changes in amyotrophic lateral sclerosis. Brain Research 250: 394

Gilliam T C, Brzustowicz L M, Castilla L H et al 1990 Genetic homogeneity between acute (SMA I) and chronic (SMA II & III) forms of spinal muscular atrophy. Nature 345: 823

Gilliatt R W, Willison R G 1962 Peripheral nerve conduction in diabetic neuropathy. Journal of Neurology, Neurosurgery and Psychiatry 25: 11

Gomez M R, Clermont V, Bernstein J 1962 Progressive bulbar palsy in children (Fazio–Londe's disease). Archives of Neurology and Psychiatry 6: 317

Gotoh F, Kitamura A, Koto A, Kataoka K, Atsuji H 1972 Abnormal insulin secretion in amyotrophic lateral sclerosis. Journal of the Neurological Sciences 16: 201

Gourie-Devi M, Suresh T G 1988 Madras pattern of motor neurone disease in South India. Journal of Neurology, Neurosurgery and Psychiatry 51: 773

Gray F, Eizenbaum J F, Ghervardi R, Degos J D, Poirier J 1985 Luyso-pallido-nigral atrophy and amyotrophic lateral sclerosis. Acta Neuropathologica 66: 78

Greenfield J G, Stark F M 1948 Post-irradiation neuropathy. American Journal of Roentgenology, Radium Therapy and Nuclear Medicine 60: 617

Greenfield J G, Matthews W B 1954 Post-encephalitic parkinsonism and amyotrophy. Journal of Neurology, Neurosurgery and Psychiatry 17: 50

Griffin J W, Cork L C, Adams R J, Price D L 1982 Axonal transport in hereditary canine spinal muscular atrophy (HCSMA). Journal of Neuropathology and Experimental Neurology 41: 370

Griggs R C, Donohoe K M, Utell M J et al 1981 Evaluation of pulmonary function in neuromuscular disease. Archives of Neurology 38: 9

Gurney M E, Belton A C, Cashman N, Antel J P 1984 Inhibition of terminal axon sprouting by serum from patients with amyotrophic lateral sclerosis. New England Journal of Medicine 311: 933

Hanyu N, Oguchi K, Yangisawa N, Tsukagoshi H 1981 Degeneration and regeneration of ventral root motor fibers in amyotrophic lateral sclerosis. Journal of the Neurological Sciences 55: 99

Harding A E 1981 Hereditary 'pure' spastic paraplegia: a clinical and genetic study of 22 families. Journal of Neurology, Neurosurgery and Psychiatry 44: 871

Harding A E 1984 The hereditary ataxias and related disorders. Churchill Livingstone, Edinburgh

Harding A E, Thomas P K 1980 Hereditary distal spinal muscular atrophy. A report on 34 cases and a review of the literature. Journal of the Neurological Sciences 45: 337

Harding A E, Thomas P K, Baraitser M, Bradbury P G, Morgan-Hughes J A, Ponsford J R 1982 X-linked recessive bulbospinal neuronopathy: a report of ten cases. Journal of Neurology, Neurosurgery and Psychiatry 45: 1012

Harding A E, Bradbury P G, Murray N M F 1983 Chronic asymmetrical spinal muscular atrophy. Journal of the Neurological Sciences 59: 69

Harding A E, Thomas P K 1984 Peroneal muscular atrophy with pyramidal features. Journal of Neurology, Neurosurgery and Psychiatry 47: 168

Harrington H, Hallet M, Tyler H R 1984 Ganglioside therapy for amyotrophic lateral sclerosis: a double-blind controlled trial. Neurology (Cleveland) 34: 1083

Harrington T M, Cohen M D, Batheson J D, Ginsburg W W 1983 Elevation of creatine kinase in amyotrophic lateral sclerosis. Potential confusion with polymyositis. Arthritis and Rheumatism 26: 201

Harter D H 1982 Viruses other than poliovirus in human amyotrophic lateral sclerosis. In: Rowland L P (ed) Human motor neuron diseases. Raven, New York, p 339

Hartmann H A, Davidson T J 1982 Neuronal RNA in motor neuron disease. In: Rowland L P (ed) Human motor neuron diseases. Raven, New York, p 89

Harvey D, Torack R, Rosenbaum H 1979 Amyotrophic lateral sclerosis with ophthalmoplegia: a clinicopathologic study. Archives of Neurology 36: 615

Hawkins S 1990 Motor neurone disease: a brief history of disability. Rehabilitation Network, London, p 7

Hawley R J, Cohen M H, Saini N, Armbrustmacher V M 1980 The carcinomatous neuromyopathy of oat-cell lung cancer. Annals of Neurology 7: 65

Hayashi H, Suga M, Satake M, Tsubaki T 1981 Reduced glycine receptor in the spinal cord in amyotrophic lateral sclerosis. Annals of Neurology 9: 292

Hayashi H, Kato S 1989 Total manifestations of amyotrophic lateral sclerosis (ALS) in the totally locked in state. Journal of the Neurological Sciences 93: 19

Henderson C E, Camu W, Mettling C et al 1993 Neurotrophins promote motor neuron survival and are present in embryonic limb bud. Nature 363: 266

Henson R A, Urich H 1970 Peripheral neuropathy associated with malignant disease. In: Vinken P J, Bruyn G W (eds) Handbook of clinical neurology, vol 8. North Holland, Amsterdam, p 131

Herndon C N, Jennings R G 1951 A twin-family study of susceptibility to poliomyelitis. American Journal of Human Genetics 3: 17

Herrick M K, Mills P E 1971 Infarction of the spinal cord. Archives of Neurology 24: 228

Hirano A, Malamud N, Kurland L T, Zimmerman H W 1969 A review of the pathological findings in amyotrophic lateral sclerosis. In: Norris F H, Kurland L T (eds) Motor neuron diseases. Grune and Stratton, New York, p 51

Hirayama K, Toyokura Y, Tsubaki T 1959 Juvenile muscular atrophy of unilateral upper extremity: a new clinical entity. Psychiatry Neurology Japan 61: 2190

Hirayama K, Tomonaga M, Kitano K, Yamada T, Kojima S, Arai K 1987 Focal cervical poliopathy causing juvenile muscular atrophy of distal upper extremity: a pathological study. Journal of Neurology, Neurosurgery and Psychiatry 50: 285

Hjorth R J, Walsh J C, Willison R G 1973 The distribution and frequency of spontaneous fasciculations in motor neurone disease. Journal of the Neurological Sciences 18: 469

Hodes R 1948 Electromyographic study of defects of neuromuscular transmission in human poliomyelitis. Archives of Neurology and Psychiatry 60: 457

Hoffmann J 1893 Uber chronische spinale Muskelatrophie im Kindesalter, auf familiarer Basis. Deutsche Zeitschrift für Nervenheilkunde 3: 427

Hoffmann J 1897 Weiter Beitrag zur Lehre von der hereditaren progressiven spinalen. Muskelatrophie im Kindesalter. Deutsche Zeitschrift für Nervenheilkunde 10: 292

Hoffmann P M, Robbins D S, Gibbs C J, Gajdusek D C, Garruto R M, Terasaki P I 1977 Histocompatability antigens in amyotrophic lateral sclerosis and parkinsonism-dementia on Guam. Lancet ii: 717

Hoffman P M, Robbins D S, Nolte M T, Gibbs C J, Gajdusek D C 1978 Cellular immunity in Guamanians with amyotrophic lateral sclerosis and parkinsonism-dementia. New England Journal of Medicine 299: 680

Hokfeld T, Fuxe K, Johansson O et al 1975 Distribution of thyrotrophin releasing hormone (TRH) in the central nervous system as revealed with immunohistochemistry. European Journal of Pharmacology 34: 389

Hopkins A 1975 Toxic neuropathy due to industrial agents. In: Dyck P J, Thomas P K, Lambert E H (eds) Peripheral neuropathy. Saunders, New York, p 1207

Horton W A, Eldridge R, Brody J A 1976 Familial motor neuron disease: evidence for at least three different types. Neurology (Minneapolis) 26: 460

Howard R S, Wiles C M, Loh L 1989 Respiratory complications and their management in motor neurone disease. Brain 112: 1155

Hughes J T 1982 Pathology of amyotrophic lateral sclerosis. In: Rowland L P (ed) Human motor neuron diseases. Raven, New York, p 61

Hughes J T, Brownell D B 1966 Spinal cord ischaemia due to arteriosclerosis. Archives of Neurology 15: 189

Hyatt R E, Black L F 1971 Maximal static respiratory pressures in generalised neuromuscular disease. American Review of Respiratory Diseases 103: 641

Ingram D A, Swash M 1988 Central motor conduction is abnormal in motor neurone disease. Journal of Neurology, Neurosurgery and Psychiatry 50: 159

Ingram D A, Thompson A J, Swash M 1987 Abnormalities of central motor conduction in multiple sclerosis revealed by transcutaneous magnetic stimulation of the brain. Journal of Neurology, Neurosurgery and Psychiatry 51: 487

Jamal G A, Hansen S, Weir A I, Ballantyne J P 1985 An improved automated method for the measurement of thermal thresholds in patients with peripheral neuropathy. Journal of Neurology, Neurosurgery and Psychiatry 48: 361

Jebsen R H, Tenckhoff H, Honet J C 1967 Natural history of uremic polyneuropathy and effects of dialysis. New England Journal of Medicine 277: 327

Jellinger K 1967 Arteriosclerosis of the spinal cord and progressive vascular myelopathy. Journal of Neurology, Neurosurgery and Psychiatry 30: 195

Jellinger K, Neumayer E 1962 Myelopathie progressive d'origine vasculaire. Revue Neurologique 106: 666

Jellinger K, Neumayer E 1969 Intermittent claudication of the cord and cauda equina. In: Vinken P J, Bruyn G W (eds) Handbook of clinical neurology, vol 13: North Holland, Amsterdam, p 507

Jennekens F G I, Tomlinson B E, Walton J N 1971 Data on the distribution of fibre types in five human limb muscles. An autopsy study. Journal of the Neurological Sciences 14: 245

Johnson R T 1982a Selective vulnerability of neural cells to viral infection. In: Rowland L P (ed) Human motor neuron diseases. Raven, New York, p 331

Johnson R T 1982b Viral infections of the nervous system. Raven, New York

Johnson W G, Wigger H J, Karp H R et al 1982 Juvenile spinal muscular atrophy; a new hexosaminidase deficiency phenotype. Annals of Neurology 11: 11

Jokelainen M, Palo J 1976 Amyotrophic lateral sclerosis and autonomic nervous system (letter). Lancet i: 1246

Juergens S M, Kurland L T 1980 Epidemiology. In:

Mulder D W (ed) The diagnosis and treatment of amyotrophic lateral sclerosis. Houghton Mifflin, Boston, p 35

Juergens S M, Kurland L T, Okazaki H, Mulder D W 1980 ALS in Rochester, Minnesota, 1925–1977. Neurology (New York) 30: 463

Kaeser H E 1964 Die familiare scapulo-peroneale Muskelatrophie. Deutsche Zeitschrift für Nervenheilkunde 186: 379

Kaeser H E 1965 Scapuloperoneal muscular atrophy. Brain 88: 407

Kaeser H E 1975 Scapulo-peroneal syndrome. In: Vinken P J, Bruyn G W (eds) Handbook of clinical neurology, vol 22. North Holland, Amsterdam, p 57

Kantarjian A D 1961 A syndrome clinically resembling amyotrophic lateral sclerosis following chronic mercurialism. Neurology (Minneapolis) 11: 639

Kardel T, Nielson V K 1974 Hepatic neuropathy, a clinical and electrophysiological study. Acta Neurologica Scandinavica 50: 513

Kascsak R J, Carp R I, Vilcek J T et al 1982 Virological studies in amyotrophic lateral sclerosis. Muscle and Nerve 5: 93

Katrak S M, Pollock M, O'Brien C P et al 1980 Clinical and morphological features of gold neuropathy. Brain 103: 671

Kawamura Y, Dyck P J, Shimono M et al 1981 Morphometric comparison of the vulnerability of peripheral motor and sensory neurons in amyotrophic lateral sclerosis. Journal of Neuropathology and Experimental Neurology 40: 667

Kelemen J, Hedlund W, Orlin J B, Berkman E M, Munsat T L 1983 Plasmapheresis with immunosuppression in amyotrophic lateral sclerosis. Neurology 40: 752

Kelly J J, Kyle R A, Miles J M, O'Brien P C, Dyck P J 1981 The spectrum of peripheral neuropathy in myeloma. Neurology (New York) 31: 24

Kennedy W R, Alter M, Sung J H 1968 Progressive proximal spinal and bulbar muscular atrophy of late onset; a sex-linked recessive trait. Neurology (Minneapolis) 18: 671

Kiloh K G, Lethlean A K, Morgan G, Cawte J E, Harris M 1980 An endemic neurological disorder in tribal Australian aborigines. Journal of Neurology, Neurosurgery and Psychiatry 43: 661

Kissel P 1948 Syndrome de sclérose latérale amyotrophique avec paralysie labio-glosso-laryngée par arachnoidite cervicale post-traumatique. Verification operatoire. Revue Neurologique 80: 771

Kleyn P W, Brzustowicz L M, Wilhelmsen K C et al 1991 Spinal muscular atrophy is not the result of mutations at the beta-hexosaminidase or GM$_2$-activator loci. Neurology 41: 1418

Knoll O, Dierker E 1980: Detection of uremic neuropathy by reflex response latency. Journal of the Neurological Sciences 47: 305

Koenig H 1969 Neurobiologic effects of agents which alter nucleic acid metabolism. In: Norris F H, Kurland L T (eds) Motor neuron diseases: Research on amyotrophic lateral sclerosis and related disorders. Grune & Stratton, New York, p 347

Kohn R 1968 Postmortem findings in a case of Wohlfart–Kugelberg–Welander disease. Confinia Neurologica 30: 253

Kojima H, Furata Y, Fujita M et al 1989 Onuf's motor neurone is resistant to polio virus. Journal of the Neurological Sciences 93: 85

Koller M, Engel W K 1984 Increased serum creatine kinase (CK) MB isozyme and alkaline phosphate positive (AP + ve) regenerative muscle fibers in amyotrophic lateral sclerosis (abst). Neurology (Cleveland) 34: 84

Kondo K 1979 Population dynamics of motor neuron disease. In: Tsubaki T, Toyokura Y (eds) Amyotrophic lateral sclerosis. University Park Press, Baltimore, p 61

Kott E, Livni E, Zamir R, Kuritzky A 1976 Amyotrophic lateral sclerosis: cell-mediated immunity to polio virus and basic myelin protein in patients with high frequency of HLA-BW35. Neurology (Minneapolis) 26: 376

Kott E, Livni E, Zamir R, Kuritzky A 1979 Cell-mediated immunity to polio and HLA antigens in amyotrophic lateral sclerosis. Neurology (Minneapolis) 29: 1040

Krieger C, Melmed K A 1982 A case of amyotrophic lateral sclerosis and paraproteinemia. Neurology (New York) 32: 896

Kugelberg E 1975 Chronic proximal (pseudomyopathic) spinal muscular atrophy. Kulgelberg–Welander syndrome. In: Vinken P J, Bruyn G W (eds) Handbook of clinical neurology, vol 22(11). Elsevier, New York, p 67

Kugelberg E, Welander L 1954 Familial neurogenic (spinal?) muscular atrophy simulating ordinary proximal dystrophy. Acta Psychiatrica Scandinavica 29: 42

Kugelberg E, Welander M 1956 Heredofamilial juvenile muscular atrophy simulating muscular dystrophy. Archives of Neurology and Psychiatry 75: 500

Kurland L T, Mulder D W 1955 Epidemiologic investigations of amyotrophic lateral sclerosis: 2 Familial aggregations indicative of dominant inheritance. Neurology 5: 192–196, 249

Kurland L T, Faro S N, Siedler H 1960 Minamata disease: the outbreak of a neurological disorder in Minamata, Japan, and its relationship to the ingestion of seafood contaminated by mercuric compounds. Neurology (Minneapolis) 1: 370

Kurland L T, Brody J A 1975 Amyotrophic lateral sclerosis Guam type. In: Vinken P J, Bruyn G W (eds) Handbook of clinical neurology, vol 22. Elsevier, New York, p 339

Kurland L T, Molgaard C A 1982 Guamanian ALS: Hereditary or acquired? In: Rowland L P (ed) Human motor neuron diseases. Raven, New York, p 165

Kurlander H M, Patten B M 1979 Metals in spinal cord tissue of patients dying of motor neuron disease. Annals of Neurology 6: 21

Kurtzke J F 1982 Epidemiology of amyotrophic lateral sclerosis. In: Rowland L P (ed) Human motor neuron disease. Raven, New York, p 281

Kushner M J, Parrish M, Burke A et al 1984 Nystagmus in motor neuron disease: clinicopathological study of two cases. Annals of Neurology 16: 71

Kyle R A, Greipp P R 1985 Amyloidosis. Clinical and laboratory features in 229 cases. Mayo Clinic Proceedings 58: 665

Lambert E H 1969 Electromyography in amyotrophic lateral sclerosis. In: Norris F H, Kurland L T (eds) Motor neuron diseases. Grune and Strattton, New York, p 135

Lambert E H, Mulder D W 1957 Electromyographic studies in amyotrophic lateral sclerosis. Proceedings of the Staff Meetings of the Mayo Clinic 32: 441

Lambert E H, Mulder D W, Bastron J A 1960 Regeneration of peripheral nerves and hyperinsulin neuronopathy. Neurology (Minneapolis) 10: 851

Lamontagne A, Buchthal F 1970 Electrophysiological studies

in diabetic neuropathy. Journal of Neurology, Neurosurgery and Psychiatry 33: 442

Landis D M, Rosenberg R N, Landis S C, Schut L, Nyhan W L 1974 Olivopontocerebellar degeneration. Archives of Neurology 31: 295

Lasch E E, Joshua K, Gazit E, El Nasri M, Marcus O, Zamir R 1979 Study of the HLA antigens in Arab children with paralytic poliomyelitis. Israel Journal of Medical Sciences 15: 12

La Spada A R, Wilson E M, Lubahn D B et al 1991 Androgen receptor gene mutations in X linked spinal and bulbar muscular atrophy. Nature 352: 77

Latov N 1982 Plasma cell dyscrasia and motor neuron disease. In: Rowland L P (ed) Human motor neuron diseases. Raven, New York, p 273

Latov N, Hays A P, Donofrio P D 1988 Monoclonal IgM with unique reactivity to gangliosides GM1 and GD1B and to lacto-N-tetraose in two patients with motor neurone disease. Neurology 38: 763

Layani F, Ashkenasy A, Bengui A 1955 Macroglobulinémie avec lesions du squelette. Presse Médicale 63: 44

Layzer R B 1982 Diagnostic implications of clinical fasciculation and cramps. In: Rowland L P (ed) Human motor neuron diseases. Raven, New York, p 23

Lebo C P, U K S, Norris F H Jr 1976 Cricopharyngeal myotomy in amyotrophic lateral sclerosis. Laryngoscope 86: 862

Lebovitz H E 1965 Endocrine-metabolic syndromes associated with neoplasms. In: Brain Lord, Norris F H Jr (eds) Remote effects of cancer on the nervous system. Grune and Stratton, New York, p 104

Leigh P N, Anderton B H, Dodson A et al 1988 Ubiquitin deposits in anterior horn cells in motor neurone disease. Neuroscience Letters 93: 197

Leveille A, Kiernan J, Goodwin J A, Antel J 1982 Eye movements in amyotrophic lateral sclerosis. Archives of Neurology 39: 684

Li T M, Swash M, Alberman E 1985 Morbidity and mortality in motor neurone disease; comparison with multiple sclerosis and Parkinson's disease; age and sex specific rates and cohort analyses. Journal of Neurology, Neurosurgery and Psychiatry 48: 320

Lipton H L, Dal Canto M C 1976 Theiler's virus-induced CNS disease in mice. In: Andrews J M, Johnson R T, Brazier M (eds) Amyotrophic lateral sclerosis. Recent research trends. Academic Press, New York, p 263

Liversedge L A, Swinburn W R, Yuill G M 1970 Idoxuridine and motor neurone disease. British Medical Journal 1: 755

Logothetis J, Silverstein P, Coe J 1960 Neurologic aspects of Waldenstrom's macroglobulinemia. Archives of Neurology 3: 564

Loizou L A, Small M, Dalton G A 1980 Cricopharyngeal myotomy in motor neurone disease. Journal of Neurology, Neurosurgery and Psychiatry 43: 42

Londe P 1894 Paralysie bulbaire progressive infantile et familiale. Revue Médicale 14: 212

Louis-Bar D 1941 Sur un syndrome progressif comprenant des telangiectasies capillaires, cutanées et conjonctivales symmetriques, a disposition naevoide et des troubles cerebelleux. Confinia Neurologica (Basel) 4: 32

Low P A, McLeod J G, Turtle J R, Donnelly P, Wright R G 1974 Peripheral neuropathy in acromegaly. Brain 97: 139

McAlpine D, Araki S 1958 Minamata disease: an unusual neurological disorder caused by contaminated fish. Lancet ii: 629

McComas A J, Sica R E P, Campbell M J, Upton A R M 1971 Functional compensation in partially denervated muscles. Journal of Neurology, Neurosurgery and Psychiatry 34: 453

McComas A J, Sica R E P, McNabb A R, Goldberg W, Upton A R M (1973a) Neuropathy in thyrotoxicosis. New England Journal of Medicine 289: 219

McComas A J, Upton A R M, Sica R E P 1973b Motor neurone disease and aging. Lancet ii: 1474

McLeod J G 1971 An electrophysiological and pathological study of peripheral nerves in Friedreich's ataxia. Journal of the Neurological Sciences 12: 333

McLeod J G 1984 Carcinomatous neuropathy. In: Dyck P J, Thomas P K, Lambert E H, Bunge R (eds) Peripheral neuropathy, 2nd edn. Saunders, New York, p 2180

McLeod J G, Prineas J W 1971 Distal type of chronic spinal muscular atrophy: clinical, electrophysiological and pathological studies. Brain 94: 703

McLeod J G, Morgan J A, Reye C 1977 Electrophysiological studies in familial spastic paraplegia. Journal of Neurology, Neurosurgery and Psychiatry 40: 611

McLeod J G, Walsh J C, Pollard J D 1984 Neuropathies associated with paraproteinemias and dysproteinemias. In: Dyck P J, Thomas P K, Lambert E H, Bunge R (eds) Peripheral neuropathy. 2nd edn. Saunders, New York, p 1847

Manakar S, Shulman L H, Winokur A, Rainbow T C 1985 Autoradiographic localisation of thyrotrophin releasing hormone receptors in amyotrophic lateral sclerosis spinal cord. Neurology 35: 1650

Mandybur T I, Cooper G P 1979 Increased spinal cord lead content in amyotrophic lateral sclerosis — possibly a secondary phenomenon. Medical Hypotheses 5: 1313

Mann D M A, Yates P O 1974 Motor neurone disease: the nature of the pathogenic mechanism. Journal of Neurology, Neurosurgery and Psychiatry 37: 1036

Mannen T, Iwata M, Toyokura Y, Nagashima K 1982 The Onuf's nucleus and the external anal sphincter muscle in amyotrophic lateral sclerosis and Shy–Drager syndrome. Acta Neuropathologica (Berlin) 58: 255

Manton W J, Cook J D 1979 Lead content of cerebrospinal fluid and other tissue in amyotrophic lateral sclerosis (ALS). Neurology (New York) 29: 611

Marie P, Marinesco G 1891 Sur l'anatomie pathologique de l'acromegalie. Archives de Médecine experimental et d'Anatomie Pathologique (Paris) 3: 539

Martin R J, Sufit R L, Ringel S P et al 1983 Respiratory improvement by muscle training in adult-onset acid maltase deficiency. Muscle and Nerve 6: 201

Marshall A, Duchen L W 1978 Sensory system involvement in infantile spinal muscular atrophy. Journal of the Neurological Sciences 26: 349

Mastaglia F L, Walton J N 1971 Histological and histochemical changes in skeletal muscle from cases of chronic juvenile and early adult spinal muscular atrophy (the Kugelberg–Welander syndrome). Journal of the Neurological Sciences 12: 15

Mayberry J F, Atkinson M 1986 Swallowing problems in patients with motor neurone diseases. Journal of Clinical Gastroenterology 8: 233

Meadows J C, Marsden C D 1969 A distal form of chronic spinal muscular atrophy. Neurology (Minneapolis) 19: 53

Mendell J R, Chase T N, Engel W K 1971 Amyotrophic lateral sclerosis. A study of central monamine metabolism and a therapeutic trial of levodopa. Archives of Neurology 25: 320

Mills C P 1973 Dysphagia in pharyngeal paralysis treated by cricopharyngeal sphincterotomy. Lancet i: 455

Mitsumoto H, Sliman R J, Schafer I A et al 1986 Motor neuron disease and adult hexosaminidase A deficiency in two families: evidence for multisystem degeneration. Annals of Neurology 17: 378

Miyata S, Nakamura S, Nagata H, Kameyama M 1983 Increased manganese level in spinal cords of amyotrophic lateral sclerosis determined by radiochemical neutron activation analysis. Journal of the Neurological Sciences 61: 283

Mizusawa H, Matsumoto F, Yen S-H et al 1989 Focal accumulation of phosphorelated neurofilaments within anterior horn cells in familial amyotrophic lateral sclerosis. Acta Neuropathologica 79: 37

Morgan M H, Read A E, Campbell M J 1979 Clinical and electrophysiological studies of peripheral nerve function in patients wth chronic liver disease. Clinical Science 57: 31

Mulder D W, Howard F M 1976 Patient resistance and prognosis in amyotrophic lateral sclerosis. Mayo Clinic Proceedings 51: 537

Mulder D W, Bastron J A, Lambert E H 1956 Hyperinsulin neuropathy. Neurology (Minneapolis) 6: 627

Mulder D W, Lambert E H, Eaton L M 1959 Myasthenic syndrome in patients with amyotrophic lateral sclerosis. Neurology (Minneapolis) 9: 627

Mulder D W, Rosenbaum R A, Layton D D 1972 Late progression of poliomyelitis or forme fruste amyotrophic lateral sclerosis? Mayo Clinic Proceedings 47: 756

Mullins W M, Gross C W, Moore J M 1979 Long-term follow-up of tympanic neurectomy for sialorrhoea. Laryngoscope 89: 1219

Munsat T L (ed) 1991 Post-polio syndrome. Butterworth-Heinemann, Boston

Munsat T L, Woods R, Fowler W, Pearson C M 1969 Neurogenic muscular atrophy of infancy with prolonged survival. Brain 92: 9

Munsat T L, Easterday C S, Levy S, Wolff S M, Hiett R 1981 Amantadine and guanidine are ineffective in ALS. Neurology 31: 1054

Munsat T L, Andres P L, Finison L et al 1988 The natural history of motoneuron loss in ALS. Neurology 38: 409

Munsat T L, Skerry L, Korf B et al 1990 Phenotypic heterogeneity of spinal muscular atrophy mapping to chromosome 5q11.2-13.3 (SMA 5q). Neurology 40: 1831

Murakami T, Mastaglia F L, Mann D M A, Bradley W G 1981 Abnormal RNA metabolism in spinal motor neurons in the wobbler mouse. Muscle and Nerve 4: 407

Namba T, Aberfeld D C, Grob D 1970 Chronic proximal spinal muscular atrophy. Journal of the Neurological Sciences 11: 401

Namba T, Nolte C T, Jackrel J, Grob D 1971 Poisoning due to organophosphate insecticides. Acute and chronic manifestations. American Journal of Medicine 50: 475

Newrick P G, Hewer R L 1984 Motor neuron disease: can we do better? A study of 42 patients. British Medical Journal 289: 539

Norris F H 1972a Amantadine in Jakob-Creutzfeld disease. British Medical Journal 2: 349

Norris F H 1972b Benign post-traumatic amyotrophy. Archives of Neurology 27: 269

Norris F H 1973 Guanidine in amyotrophic lateral sclerosis. New England Journal of Medicine 288: 690

Norris F H 1975 Adult spinal motor neuron disease. In:

Vinken P J, Bruyn G M (eds) Handbook of clinical neurology, vol 22. North Holland, Amsterdam, p 156

Norris F H 1979 Moving axon particles of intercostal nerve terminals in benign and malignant ALS. In: Tsubaki T, Toyokura Y (eds) Amyotrophic lateral sclerosis. University Park Press, Baltimore, p 375

Norris F H, Rudolf J H, Barney M 1964 Carcinomatous neuropathy. Neurology (Minneapolis) 14: 202

Norris F H, Engel W K 1965 Carcinomatous amyotrophic lateral sclerosis. In: Brain W R, Norris F H (eds) The remote effects of cancer on the nervous system. Grune and Stratton, New York, p 24

Norris F H, McMenemey W H, Barnard R O 1969 Anterior horn cell pathology in carcinomatous neuromyopathy compared with other forms of motor neurone disease. In: Norris F H, Kurland L T Motor neurone diseases. Grune and Stratton, New York, p 100

Norris F H, Calanchini P R, Fallat R J, Panchari R P T, Jewett B 1974 The administration of guanidine in amyotrophic lateral sclerosis. Neurology (Minneapolis) 24: 721

Norris F H, Denys E H, U K S 1980 Differential diagnosis of adult motor neuron disease. In: Mulder D W (ed) The diagnosis and treatment of amyotrophic lateral sclerosis. Houghton Mifflin, Boston, p 53

O'Brien T, Kelly M, Saunders C 1992 Motor neurone disease: a hospice perspective. British Medical Journal 304: 471

Ochs S 1984 Basic properties of axoplasm transport. In: Dyck P J, Thomas P K, Lambert E H, Bunge R (eds) Peripheral neuropathy, 2nd edn. Saunders, New York, p 453

Olarte M R, Gersten J C, Zabriskie J, Rowland L P 1979 Transfer factor is ineffective in amyotrophic lateral sclerosis. Annals of Neurology 5: 385

Olarte M R, Schoenfeldt R S, McKiernan G, Rowland L P 1980 Plasmapheresis in amyotrophic lateral sclerosis. Annals of Neurology 8: 644

Olarte M R, Shafer S R 1985 Levamisole is ineffective in the treatment of amyotrophic lateral sclerosis. Neurology 35: 1063

Oldstone M B A, Perrin L H, Wilson C B, Norris F H 1976 Evidence for immune-complex formation in patients with 'ALS'. Lancet ii: 169

Olson W H, Simons J A, Halaas G W 1978 Therapeutic trial of tilorone in ALS. Lack of benefit in a double-blind placebo-controlled study. Neurology (Minneapolis) 28: 1293

Oppenheim R W, Qin-Wei Y, Prevette D, Yan Q 1992 Brain-derived neurotrophic factor rescues developing avian motoneurons from cell death. Nature 360: 755

Otsuka M, Endo M 1960 The effect of guanidine on neuromuscular transmission. Journal of Pharmacology and Experimental Therapeutics 128: 273

Pallis C 1976 In: Rose F C (ed) Motor neurone disease. Pitman, London

Panayiotopoulos C P, Lagos G 1980 Tibial nerve H-reflex and F-wave studies in patients with uremic neuropathy. Muscle and Nerve 3: 423

Panse F 1970 Electrical lesions of the nervous system. In: Vinken P J, Bruyn G W (eds) Handbook of clinical neurology, vol 7. North Holland, Amsterdam, p 344

Paquette Y, Hanna Z, Savard P et al 1989 Retrovirus-induced murine motor neuron disease: mapping the determinant of spongiform degeneration within the envelope gene. Proceedings of the National Academy of Sciences USA 86: 3896

Parhad I M, Clark A W, Barron K D, Staunton S B 1978 Diaphragmatic paralysis in motor neuron disease: report of two cases and a review of the literature. Neurology (New York) 28: 18

Parry G J, Holtz S J, Ben-Zeev D, Drori J B 1986 Gammopathy with proximal motor axonopathy simulating motor neuron disease. Neurology 36: 273

Patten B M 1982 Phosphate and parathyroid disorders associated with the syndrome of amyotrophic lateral sclerosi. In: Rowland L P (ed) Human motor neuron diseases. Raven, New York, p 181

Patten B M 1984 Neuropathy and motor neuron syndromes associated with plasma cell disease. Acta Neurologica Scandinavica 69: 47

Paty D W, Campbell M J, Hughes D 1974 Carcinomatous neuromyopathy; an electrophysiological and immunological study of patients with carcinoma of the lung. II Imunological studies. Journal of Neurology, Neurosurgery and Psychiatry 37: 142

Pearn J 1980 Classification of spinal muscular atrophies. Lancet i: 919

Pearn J 1982 Infantile motor neuron diseases. In: Rowland L P (ed) Human motor neuron diseases. Raven, New York, p 121

Pearn J H, Wilson J 1973a Acute Werdnig-Hoffmann disease. Archives of Disease in Childhood 48: 425

Pearn J H, Wilson J 1973b Chronic generalised spinal muscular atrophy of infancy and childhood. Archives of Disease in Childhood 48: 768

Pearn J H, Bundey S, Carter C O, Wilson J, Gardner-Medwin D, Walton, J N 1978a A genetic study of subacute and chronic spinal muscular atrophy in childhood — a nosological analysis of 124 index patients. Journal of the Neurological Sciences 37: 227

Pearn J, Gardner–Medwin D, Wilson J 1978b A clinical study of chronic childhood spinal muscular atrophy. A review of 141 cases. Journal of the Neurological Sciences 38: 23

Pearn J, Hudgson P, Walton J N 1978c A clinical and genetic study of adult-onset spinal muscuar atrophy. The autosomal recessive form as a discrete disease entity. Brain 101: 591

Peiper S J, Fields W S 1959 Failure of amyotrophic lateral sclerosis to respond to intrathecal steroid and vitamin B 12 therapy. Archives of Neurology 9: 522

Pennybacker J, Russell D S 1948 Necrosis of the brain due to radiation therapy. Journal of Neurology, Neurosurgery, and Psychiatry 11: 183

Percy A K, Davis L E, Johnston D M, Drachman D B 1971 Failure of isoprinosine in amyotrophic lateral sclerosis. New England Journal of Medicine 285: 689

Pestronk A 1991 Motor neuropathies, motor neuron disorders, and antiglycolipid antibodies. Muscle and Nerve 14: 927

Pestronk A, Adams R N, Cornblath D, Kuncl R W 1989 Patterns of serum IgM antibodies to GM1 and GD1a gangliosides in amyotrophic lateral sclerosis. Annals of Neurology 25: 98

Pestronk A, Cornblath D, Ilyeas A A et al 1988 A treatable multifocal motor neuropathy with antibodies to GM1 ganglioside. Annals of Neurology 24: 730

Peters H A, Clatanoff D V 1968 Spinal muscular atrophy secondary to macroglobulinemia. Neurology (Minneapolis) 18: 101

Pickett J B E, Layzer R N, Levin S R, Schneider V, Campbell M J, Sumner A J 1975 Neuromuscular complications of acromegaly. Neurology (Minneapolis) 25: 638

Pietsch M C, Morris P J 1975 An association of HLA 3 and HLA 7 with paralytic poliomyelitis. Tissue Antigens 4: 50

Plaitakis A, Caroscio J T 1987 Abnormal glutamate metabolism in amyotrophic lateral sclerosis. Annals of Neurology 22: 575

Plaitakis A, Mandeli J, Smith J, Yahr M D 1988 Pilot trial of branched-chain amino acids in amyotrophic lateral sclerosis. Lancet ii: 1015

Plato C C, Garruto R M, Fox K M 1984 Familial and epidemiological studies of amyotrophic lateral sclerosis and parkinsonism-dementia of Guam. A twenty-five year prospective patient control study. American Journal of Epidemiology 120: 478

Puech P, Grossiard A, Brun M, Denis J P 1947 Tableau clinique de sclérose latérale amyotrophique. Arachnoidite cervicale en virole à l'intervention. Revue Neurologique 79: 358

Quarfordt S H, Devino D C, Engel W K, Levy R I, Fredrickson D S 1970 Familial adult-onset proximal spinal muscular atrophy. Archives of Neurology 22: 541

Quick D T, Greer M 1967 Pancreatic dysfunction in amyotrophic lateral sclerosis. Neurology (Minneapolis) 17: 112

Raff M C, Sangalang V, Asbury A K 1968 Ischemic mononeuropathy multiplex associated with diabetes mellitus. Archives of Neurology 18: 487

Reed D A, Brody J A 1975 Amyotrophic lateral sclerosis and parkinsonism-dementia on Guam, 1945–1972. I. Descriptive epidemiology. American Journal of Epidemiology 101: 287

Reed D A, Torres J M, Brody J A 1975 Amyotrophic lateral sclerosis and parkinsonism-dementia on Guam, 1945–1972. II Familial and genetic studies. American Journal of Epidemiology 101: 302

Refsum S 1946 Heredopathia atactica polyneuritiformis: a familial syndrome not hitherto described. Acta Psychiatrica Scandinavica (Suppl) 38: 1

Refsum S, Skillicorn S A 1954 Amyotrophic familial spastic paraplegia. Neurology (Minneapolis) 4: 40

Riggs J E, Schochet S S, Gutman L 1984 Benign focal amyotrophy. Variant of chronic spinal muscular atrophy. Archives of Neurology 41: 678

Rissanen A, Palo J, Myllyla G, Cantell K 1980 Interferon therapy for ALS. Annals of Neurology 7: 392

Rosenberg R N 1982 Amyotrophy in multisystem genetic diseases. In: Rowland L P (ed) Human motor neuron diseases. Raven, New York, p 149

Ross A T 1964 Mercuric polyneuropathy with albumino-cytologic dissociation and eosinophilia. Journal of the American Medical Association 188: 830

Ross E J 1972 Endocrine and metabolic manifestations of cancer. British Medical Journal 1: 735

Rothstein J D, Tsai G, Kuncl R W et al 1990 Abnormal excitatory amino acid metabolism in amyotrophic lateral sclerosis. Annals of Neurology 28: 18

Roussy G, Levy G 1926 Sept cas d'une maladie familiale particulière. Revue Neurologique 1: 427

Rowland L P, Defendini R, Sherman W et al 1982 Macroglobulinemia with peripheral neuropathy simulating motor neuron disease. Annals of Neurology 11: 532

Rudnicki S, Chad D A, Drachman D A et al 1987 Motor neuron disease and paraproteinemia. Neurology 37: 335

Sachs C, Conradi S, Kaijsu 1985 Autonomic function in ALS: a study of cardiovascular responses. Acta Neurologica Scandinavica 71: 373

Sadowsky C H, Sachs E, Ochoa J 1976 Post-radiation motor neuron syndrome. Archives of Neurology 33: 786

Salazar-Grueso E, Routbort M J, Martin J et al 1990 Polyclonal IgM anti-GM1 ganglioside antibody in patients with motor neuron disease and variants. Annals of Neurology 27: 558

Salazar A M, Masters C L, Gajdusek D C, Gibbs C J Jr 1983 Syndromes of amyotrophic lateral sclerosis and dementia: relation to transmissible Creutzfeldt–Jakob disease. Annals of Neurology 14: 17

Sanders M, Fellowes J 1975 Use of detoxified snake neurotoxin as a partial treatment for amyotrophic lateral sclerosis. Journal of Cancer and Cytology 15: 26

Saric R, Moreau F, Tignol J 1967 Neuropathie précédant de loin une maladie de Waldenstrom: effet du traitement prolongé par le melphalan. Journal Médicale Bordeaux 114: 1301

Schoenen J, Resnik M, Delwaide P J, Vanderhaeghen J J 1985 Etude immunocytoclinique de la distribution spinale de sub. P, des encéphalines, de cholecystokinene et de serotonine dans las sclérose latérale amyotrophique. Comptes Rendus des Séances de la Sociéte de Biologie et de ses Filiales (Paris) 179: 528

Schut J W 1950 Hereditary ataxia: clinical study through six generations. Archives of Neurology and Psychiatry (Chicago) 63: 535

Sedgwick R P, Boder E 1960 Progressive ataxia in childhood with particular reference to ataxia-telangiectasia. Neurology 10: 705

Sedgwick R P, Boder E 1972 Ataxia-telangiectasia. In: Vinken P J, Bruyn G W (eds) Handbook of clinical neurology, vol 14. North Holland, Amsterdam, p 267

Seitelberger F, Gootz E, Gross H 1963 Beitrag zur spatinfantilen Hallevorden-Spatzchen Krankheit. Acta Neuropathologica (Berlin) 3: 16

Sendtner M, Schmalbruch H, Stockli K A et al 1992 Ciliary neurotrophic factor prevents degeneration of motor neurons in mouse mutant progessive motor neuronopathy. Nature 358: 502

Seneviratne K N, Peiris O A 1970 Peripheral nerve function in chronic liver disease. Journal of Neurology, Neurosurgery and Psychiatry 33: 609

Server A C, Wolinsky J S 1982 Approaches to antiviral therapy. In: Rowland L P (ed) Human motor neuron diseases. Raven, New York, p 519

Seto D S Y, Freeman J M 1964 Lead neuropathy in childhood. American Journal of Diseases of Children 107: 337

Sevestre M 1899 Paralysie flasque des quatre membres et des muscles du tronc (sauf le diaphragme) chez un nouveauné. Bulletin des Sociétés Pédiatriques Paris 1–2: 7

Shy G M, Drager G A 1960 A neurological syndrome associated with orthostatic hypotension. Archives of Neurology 2: 511

Shy M E, Rowland L P, Smith L et al 1986 Motor neuron disease and plasma cell dyscrasia. Neurology 36: 1429

Siddique T, Feglewicz D, Pericak-Vance M A et al 1991 Linkage of a gene causing familial amyotrophic lateral sclerosis to chromosome 21 and evidence for genetic locus heterogeneity. New England Journal of Medicine 324: 1418

Silani V, Scarlato G, Valli G, Marconi M 1980 Plasma exchange ineffective in amyotrophic lateral sclerosis. Archives of Neurology 37: 511

Silfverskiold B P 1946 Polyneuritic hypoglycaemia. Late peripheral paresis after hypoglycemic attacks in two insulinoma patients. Acta Medica Scandinavica 125: 502

Sivak E D, Gipson W T, Hanson M R 1982 Long-term management of respiratory failure in amyotrophic lateral sclerosis. Annals of Neurology 12: 18

Smith A W M, Mulder D W, Code C F 1957 Esophageal motility in amyotrophic lateral sclerosis. Proceedings of the Staff Meetings of the Mayo Clinic 32: 438

Smith R A, Dawson A, Foroozan P 1980 Pharmacology and surgical modalities. In: Mulder D W (ed) The diagnosis and treatment of amyotrophic lateral sclerosis. Houghton Mifflin, Boston, p 241

Sobue G, Matsouka Y, Mukai E et al 1981 Pathology of myelinated fibers in cervical and lumbar ventral spinal roots in amyotrophic lateral sclerosis. Journal of the Neurological Sciences 50: 413

Sobue G, Hashizume Y, Mukai E et al 1989 X-linked bulbo-spinal neuronopathy. A clinico-pathological study. Brain 112: 209

Spencer P S, Ludolph A, Dwineda M P et al 1986 Lathyrism: evidence for role of the neuroexcitatory amino acid, BOAA. Lancet ii: 1066

Spencer P S, Nunn P B, Hugon J et al 1987 Guam amyotrophic lateral sclerosis-parkinsonism-dementia linked to a plant excitant neurotoxin. Science 237: 517

Stålberg E 1982 Electrophysiological studies of reinnervation in ALS. In: Rowland L P (ed) Human motor neuron diseases. Raven, New York, p 47

Stålberg E, Sanders D B 1984 The motor unit in ALS studied with different electrophysiological techniques. In: Rose F C (ed) Progress in motor neurone disease. Pitman, London

Steele J C, Richardson J C, Olszewski J 1964 Progressive supranuclear palsy. Archives of Neurology 10: 333

Stefanis C, Papapetropoulos T, Scarpalezos S, Lygidarkis G, Panayiotopoulous C P 1975 X-linked spinal and bulbar muscular atrophy of late onset. Journal of the Neurological Sciences 24: 493

Steinke J, Tyler R H 1964 The association of amyotrophic lateral sclerosis (motor neuron disease) and carbohydrate intolerance, a clinical study. Metabolism 13: 1376

Stewart B M 1966 The hypertrophic neuropathy of acromegaly: a rare neuropathy associated with acromegaly. Archives of Neurology 14: 107

Stumpell A 1880 Beitrage zur Pathologie des Ruckenmarks. Archiv für Psychiatrie und Nervenkrankheiten 10: 676

Swaiman K F, Flagler D G 1971 Penicillamine therapy of the Guillain–Barré syndrome caused by mercury poisoning. Neurology 21: 456

Swash M, Schwartz M S 1982 A longitudinal study of changes in motor units in motor neurone disease. Journal of the Neurological Sciences 56: 185

Thomas J E, Howard F M 1972 Segmental zoster paresis. A disease profile. Neurology (Minneapolis) 22: 459

Thomas P K, Jefferys J G R, Smith I S, Loulakakis D 1981 Spinal somatosensory evoked potentials in hereditary spastic paraplegia. Journal of Neurology, Neurosurgery and Psychiatry 44: 243

Thrush D C, Holti G, Bradley W G, Campbell M J, Walton J N 1974 Neurological manifestations of xeroderma pigmentosum in two siblings. Journal of the Neurological Sciences 22: 91

Tom M I, Richardson J C 1951 Hypoglycaemia from islet cell tumour of pancreas with amyotrophy and cerebrospinal nerve cell changes. Journal of Neurology, Neurosurgery and Psychiatry 10: 51

Tomlinson B E, Walton J N, Rebeiz J J 1969 The effects of ageing and of cachexia upon skeletal muscle. A histopathological study. Journal of the Neurological Sciences 9: 321

Tomlinson B E, Irving D 1977 The numbers of limb motor neurons in the human lumbosacral cord throughout life. Journal of the Neurological Sciences 34: 213

Tooth H H 1886 The peroneal type of progressive muscular atrophy. H K Lewis, London

Trojaborg W, Buchthal F 1965 Malignant and benign fasciculations. Acta Psychiatrica et Neurologica Scandinavica (Suppl 13) 41: 251

Trojaborg W, Frantzen E, Andersen I 1969 Peripheral neuropathy and myopathy associated with carcinoma of the lung. Brain 92: 71

Tsujihata M, Hazama R, Yoshimura T, Sotcoh A, Moir M, Nagataki S 1984 The motor end-plate fine structure and intrastructural localisation of acetylcholine receptors in amyotrophic lateral sclerosis. Mucle and Nerve 7: 243

Tyler H R 1979 Double-blind study of modified neurotoxin in motor neurone disease. Archives of Neurology 29: 77

Tyler H R 1982 Nonfamilial amyotrophy with dementia or multisystem degeneration and other neurological disorders. In: Rowland L P (ed) Human neuron diseases. Raven, New York, p 173

Van Bogaert L 1952 Etudes sur la paraplégie spasmodique familiale V. Acta Neurologica et Psychiatrica Belgica 52: 795

Van Laere J 1966 Paralysie bulbo-pontine chronique progressive familiale avec surdité. Revue Neurologique 115: 289

Vialetto E 1936 Contributo alla forma ereditaria della paralisi bulbare progressiva. Rivista Spir de Fren. 40: 1

Victor M 1965 The effects of nutritional deficiency on the nervous system. A comparison with the effects of carcinoma. In: Brain Lord, Norris F H (eds) The remote effects of cancer on the nervous system. Grune and Stratton, New York, p 134

Villiger J W, Faull R L 1985 Muscarinic cholinergic receptors in the human spinal cord: differential localization of (3H). Brain Research 14: 196

Walton J N, Tomlinson B E, Pearce G W 1968 Subacute 'poliomyelitis' and Hodgkin's disease. Journal of the Neurological Sciences 6: 435

Werdnig G 1891 Zwei fruhinfantile hereditare Fälle von progressiver Muskelatrophie unter dem bilde der Dystrophie, aber auf neurotischer Grundlag. Archiv Psychiatrie und Nervenkrankheiten 22: 437

Werdnig G 1894 Die fruh-infantile progressive spinale Amyotrophie. Archives of Psychiatry 26: 706

Whitehouse P J, Wamsley J K, Zarbin M A et al 1983 Amyotrophic lateral sclerosis: alterations in neurotransmitter receptors. Annals of Neurology 14: 8

Wiesendanger M 1962 Uber die hereditare, neurogene proximale Amyotrophie (Kugelberg–Welander). Archiv der Julius Klaus-Stiftung für Vererungsforschung 37:147

Wikstrom J, Paetau A, Palo J et al 1982 Classic amyotrophic lateral sclerosis with dementia. Archives of Neurology 39: 681–683

Wilkinson P C 1964 Serological findings in carcinomatous neuropathy. Lancet i: 1301

Williams C J 1955 Amyotrophy due to hypoglycaemia. British Medical Journal 1: 707

Williams E R, Bruford A 1970 Creatine phosphokinase in motor neurone disease. Clinical Chimica Acta 27: 53

Windebank A J, McCall J T, Dyck P J 1984 Metal neuropathy. In: Dyck P J, Thomas P K, Lambert E H, Bunge R (eds) Peripheral neuropathy. 2nd edn. Saunders, New York, p 2133

Wohlfart G 1942 Zwei Fälle von Dystrophia musculorum progressiva mit fibrillaren Zuckungen und atypischen Muskelbefund. Deutsche Zeitschrift für Nerveheilkuncle 153: 189

Wohlfart G 1959 Degenerative and regenerative axonal changes in the ventral horns, brain stem and cerebral cortex in amyotrophic lateral sclerosis. Acta Universitatis Lundensis (New Series 2): 56, 1

Wohlfart G, Fex J, Eliasson S 1955 Hereditary proximal spinal muscle atrophy simulating progressive muscular dystrophy. Acta Psychiatrica et Neurologica 30: 395

Wolfgram F 1976 Blind studies on the effect of amyotrophic lateral sclerosis sera on motor neurons in vitro. In: Andrews J M, Johnson R T, Brazier M (eds) Amyotrophic lateral sclerosis. Recent research trends. Academic Press, New York, p 145

Yan Q, Elliott J, Snider W D 1992 Brain-derived neurotrophic factor rescues spinal motor neurons from axotomy-induced cell death. Nature 360: 753

Yanagihara R 1982 Heavy metals and essential minerals in motor neuron disease. In: Rowland L P (ed) Human motor neuron diseases. Raven, New York, p 233

Yanagihara R T, Garruto R M, Gajdusek D C 1983 Epidemiological surveillance of amyotrophic lateral sclerosis and parkinsonism-dementia in the Commonwealth of the Northern Mariana Islands. Annals of Neurology 13: 79

Yase Y 1972 The pathogenesis of amyotrophic lateral sclerosis. Lancet ii: 292

Yase Y 1984 Environmental contribution to the amyotrophic lateral sclerosis process. In: Serratrice G, Desnuelle C, Pellissier J–F et al (eds) Neuromuscular disease. Raven, New York, p 335

Yoshida S 1977 X-ray microanalytic studies on amyotrophic lateral sclerosis. I Metal distribution compared with neuropathological findings in cervical spinal cord. Rinsho Shinkeigaku 17: 299

Yoshida S 1979 X-ray microanalytic studies on amyotrophic lateral sclerosis. III Relationship of calcification and degeneration found in cervical spinal cord of ALS. Rinso Shinkeigaku 19: 641

Young A B 1990 What's the excitement about excitatory amino acids in amyotrophic lateral sclerosis? Annals of Neurology 28: 9

Younger D S, Chow S, Hays A P et al 1988 Primary lateral sclerosis. A clinical diagnosis re-emerges. Archives of Neurology 45: 1304

Younger D S, Rowland L P, Latov N et al 1990 Motor neurone disease and amyotrophic lateral sclerosis: relation of high CSF protein content to paraproteinemia and clinical syndromes. Neurology 40: 595

Younger D S, Rowland L P, Latov N et al 1991 Lymphoma, motor neuron diseases, and amyotrophic lateral sclerosis. Annals of Neurology 29: 78

Zalin H, Cooney T C 1974 Chorda tympani neurectomy — a new approach to sub-mandibular salivary obstruction. British Journal of Surgery 61: 391

Zellweger H, McCormick W F 1968 Scapuloperoneal dystrophy and scapuloperoneal atrophy. Helvetia Paediatrica Acta 6: 643

25. Peripheral nerve disease

P. K. Thomas

INTRODUCTION

This book deals with disorders of voluntary muscle, and the primary symptom of such disorders is weakness. Weakness may also be caused by disorders of the neuromuscular junction, peripheral nerve, anterior horn cell and central nervous system. Voluntary effort is required for muscle contraction and therefore simulated weakness can be due to malingering or a complaint of weakness can be related to psychiatric disorders. This chapter provides an outline of disorders of the peripheral nerves as they enter into the differential diagnosis of disorders of skeletal muscle.

CLINICAL PATTERNS OF PERIPHERAL NERVE DISEASE

Anatomy

The nervous system is divided into two parts, comprising the brain and spinal cord, in which oligodendroglial cells are responsible for myelination, and the peripheral nervous system, consisting of the cranial nerves (with the exception of the second), the spinal nerve roots and sensory ganglia, the peripheral nerves and the autonomic nerves and their ganglia. The limits of the peripheral nervous system are defined by the association of axons with Schwann cells. This distinction has a rational basis in terms of many of the diseases which separately affect the two parts of the nervous system. Two neuronal systems, however, lie in both the central and the peripheral nervous systems. In the efferent systems, the perikarya and proximal axons of the anterior horn cells (alpha and gamma motor neurones), cranial nerve motor nuclei and preganglionic parasympathetic and sympathetic neurones lie within the central nervous system, whereas their distal axons run in the peripheral nerves. Similarly, the centrally directed axons of the primary sensory neurones run in the central nervous system, while their cell bodies and peripheral axons lie within the peripheral nervous system.

The peripheral nervous system is divided into the somatic motor, the sensory and the autonomic systems. The motor system innervates the skeletal (alpha motor neurones) and fusimotor (gamma motor neurones) muscle fibres. The sensory nerves run from free nerve endings or specialised receptors in the skin, subcutaneous tissue, muscles, joints, ligaments and bones to the spinal cord, predominantly via the posterior roots. The autonomic nervous system provides motor innervation to glands, the smooth muscle of the eyes and viscera, blood vessels, and the sweat glands and arrector pili muscles of the skin. The autonomic nervous system is divided into two separate subdivisions. The preganglionic fibres of the sympathetic nervous system leave the spinal cord from the T1–L2 segments and pass to the sympathetic chain. Postganglionic fibres then join visceral plexuses and peripheral nerves to innervate the distal structures. The preganglionic fibres of the parasympathetic nervous system run in the third, seventh and tenth cranial nerves and in the sacral nerves, to reach the eyes, glands and the viscera, where they synapse on short postganglionic neurones.

The perikarya and axons of neurones of the different components of the peripheral nervous system are of different sizes. The alpha motor neurones tend to be large, and their axons are all myelinated. The sensory axons have a very wide range of diameters from the largest myelinated A-alpha fibres, through the smaller myelinated A-delta fibres, to the unmyelinated C fibres, the latter two categories conveying pain and temperature sensation. The autonomic preganglionic fibres are myelinated, and the postganglionic axons are of small diameter and unmyelinated. The structure of the mammalian body results in some nerve fibres, such as those going to the hands and feet, being extremely long, while others, such as those in most of the cranial nerves, are extremely short (e.g. those to the external ocular muscles).

The anatomical arrangement of the peripheral nervous system is based upon the segmental development of the embryo, with a series of dermatomes, sclerotomes and myotomes, and a bilaterally symmetrical pattern. The distal arrangements of the nerve fibres, however, show a dazzling array of plexiform interchanges both in the upper and lower limb plexuses and in the individual nerve fasciculi themselves.

The structural characteristics of the peripheral nervous system explain many of the features of peripheral nerve disorders. Both the neurone and the Schwann cell are cells under considerable metabolic stress. The axons of many of the neurones of the peripheral nervous system are extremely long for their diameter. Moreover all of the protein of the neurone has to be synthesised by the Nissl substance within the perikaryon. An indication of the geometrical asymmetry of the neurone can be gauged from the following analogy. The perikaryon of a human S1 anterior horn cell is approximately 100 μm in diameter. An axon running from the sacral spinal cord to the extensor digitorum brevis muscle of the foot is about 1 m long, and about 10 μm in diameter. If the neurone were magnified so that the perikaryon became the size of a man's head, it would be 1.3 km high, and the axon 1.2 cm in diameter. The volume of axoplasm in the axon is at least 150 times that of the perikaryon. It is for this reason that the neurones have such abundant Nissl substance, and such a high rate of protein synthesis. The axoplasmic transport of material down the axon is an energy-dependent and very important process. Impairment of either perikaryal synthesis of macromolecules or of their axoplasmic transport may underlie the distal degeneration of axons in many neuropathies. The Schwann cell is under a different form of metabolic stress from the neurone. It is a very thin cell with little cytoplasm and a very large surface area. This would be clear if a Schwann cell from a large myelinated fibre could be unwrapped and laid flat. The Schwann cell covers approximately 1 mm of the axon, and is about 3 mm wide when unwrapped. Only a thin sliver of about 2 μm diameter of Schwann cell cytoplasm is present around the complete periphery of the cell, with lesser amounts of Schwann cell cytoplasm connecting the outer and inner portions of cytoplasm and corresponding to the Schmidt–Lanterman clefts. The remainder of the Schwann cell consists of two apposed layers of

Schwann cell plasmalemma, which comprises the myelin sheath. For the Schwann cell, the surface-to-volume ratio is approximately 75 while that of a lymphocyte is less than one. Thus the Schwann cell has a great deal of immunogenic cell membrane, which it continually maintains metabolically. This explains the vulnerability of the myelin sheath, and the frequency of demyelinating neuropathies.

The peripheral neuropathies can be motor, sensory or autonomic or any combination of these. Single or multiple nerves or nerve roots can be involved. Disorders may affect only large or small fibres, or long or short fibres. Disease processes may lead to the loss of nerve cell bodies as well as their axons (neuronopathies), the distal axons only (axonopathies), or the Schwann cells and the myelin derived from them (demyelinating neuropathies).

Clinical patterns of disorders

There is an extremely wide range of patterns of disorders of the peripheral nerves. The distribution may be distal, proximal, restricted to the cranial nerves or diffuse. The pattern may be symmetrical or asymmetrical. It may involve single nerves (mononeuropathy), multiple single nerves (multiple mononeuropathy), nerve roots (radiculopathy), nerve plexuses (plexopathy) or affect the peripheral nervous system diffusely (polyneuropathy). A polyneuropathy may be distal, proximal or generalised. The involvement may be motor, sensory, autonomic or a combination of any of these. The disorder may develop acutely (over a few days), subacutely (over several weeks) or chronically. Motor or predominantly motor neuropathies, especially those with a symmetrical proximal distribution or, less importantly, a symmetrical distal distribution, must be considered in the differential diagnosis of myopathy.

PATTERNS OF PERIPHERAL NERVE DISEASE WHICH ENTER INTO THE DIFFERENTIAL DIAGNOSIS OF DISORDERS OF SKELETAL MUSCLE
(See Table 25.1)

Distal symmetrical motor polyneuropathy

The longest and often the largest diameter motor nerves are affected in a number of different disorders of peripheral nerves, with consequent distal amyotrophy, muscle weakness and loss of tendon reflexes. The clinical picture can be very similar to that of distal spinal muscular atrophy, progressive muscular atrophy or distal myopathy. Peripheral nerve diseases which can produce this pattern of clinical involvement include hereditary motor and sensory neuropathy (Charcot–Marie–Tooth disease), chronic inflammatory demyelinating polyneuropathy, toxic neuropathy, many of the peripheral nerve disorders associated with metabolic diseases, vitamin deficiencies and neoplasms such as carcinoma, lymphoma and paraproteinaemia. In many such cases no cause can be identified and the disease must be classified as a cryptogenic or idiopathic polyneuropathy. Disorders of the peripheral nerves usually involve some abnormality of sensation; this is helpful diagnostically. Anterior horn cell disorders and less commonly axonopathies are often associated with muscle fasciculation, but fasciculation may also occur in demyelinating neuropathies. Full laboratory investigation is frequently required to separate the possible diseases responsible for the clinical picture of a distal symmetrical motor polyneuropathy.

Proximal symmetrical motor polyneuropathy

In a few disorders of the peripheral nerves, there is a predominantly proximal motor neuropathy, producing proximal muscle weakness and sometimes wasting. Such a pattern is much more commonly produced by muscular dystrophy, polymyositis or dermatomyositis, spinal muscular atrophy or even a disorder of neuromuscular transmission such as myasthenia gravis. The disorders of the peripheral nerves causing such a pattern of involvement include the neuropathy of acute intermittent porphyria, acute inflammatory polyneuropathy (Guillain–Barré syndrome) and chronic inflammatory demyelinating polyneuropathy. Many cases have some degree of sensory involvement, most often distal or diffuse, and rarely proximal, which can be helpful in separating the neuropathies from the other conditions. The distribution of muscle involvement in the muscular dystrophies is usually specific in that it involves some muscles severely

Table 25.1   The main patterns of muscle weakness and their differential diagnosis

Distribution of muscle weakness	Differential diagnosis	
	Peripheral nerve disorders	Muscle, motor neurone, and neuromuscular junction disorders
Distal symmetrical weakness and wasting	Hereditary motor and sensory neuropathy (Charcot–Marie–Tooth disease) Chronic inflammatory demyelinating polyneuropathy Chronic polyneuropathy of many aetiologies or idiopathic	Distal myopathy Distal spinal muscular atrophy Progressive muscular atrophy Myotonic dystrophy Inclusion body myositis
Chronic proximal symmetrical weakness (± wasting)	Chronic inflammatory demyelinating polyneuropathy	Muscular dystrophies Polymyositis Motor neurone disorders (ALS, spinal muscular atrophy) Neuromuscular junction disorders (myasthenia gravis, myasthenic syndrome) Metabolic myopathies
Acute severe diffuse muscle weakness	Guillain–Barré syndrome Porphyric neuropathy Toxic neuropathy Diphtheritic neuropathy	Acute polymyositis or dermatomyositis Rhabdomyolysis Toxic myopathy Periodic paralysis Myasthenia gravis
Cranial muscle weakness	Guillain–Barré syndrome Diphtheritic neuropathy Bell's palsy Sarcoidosis and other structural lesions around base of skull Borreliosis	Ocular myopathy Oculopharyngeal muscular dystrophy Chronic progressive external ophthalmoplegia Myotonic dystrophy Facioscapulohumeral muscular dystrophy Myasthenia gravis Congenital myopathies Motor neurone diseases
Asymmetrical muscle weakness (± wasting)	Vasculitic neuropathy Proximal diabetic plexopathy Other plexopathies Focal inflammatory demyelinating polyneuropathy	Motor neurone diseases (spinal muscular atrophy, progressive muscular atrophy) Muscular dystrophies

and, to a large extent, spares others. The principal idiopathic inflammatory myopathies (polymyositis and dermatomyositis) may be associated with muscle tenderness and a skin rash. Anterior horn cell disorders are often associated with visible fasciculations which can be increased by neostigmine. In myasthenia gravis, the muscle fatiguability may be evident from the history or on examination and wasting is not usually pronounced.

Acute severe diffuse motor polyneuropathies

Acute severe muscle weakness can be produced by a number of disorders of the peripheral nerves including acute inflammatory polyneuropathy (Guillain–Barré syndrome), the neuropathy of acute intermittent and variegate porphyria, diphtheritic neuropathy and sometimes neuropathies related to pharmaceutical and environmental neurotoxins such as thallium and various industrial solvents. The condition can simulate acute inflammatory myopathy, rhabdomyolysis, toxic myopathy, periodic paralysis and myasthenia gravis. The severity of the patient's condition can sometimes make it difficult to recognise minor sensory involvement in such acute neuropathies. The release of creatine kinase into the blood and myoglobin into the urine can help to point to conditions damaging muscles rather than nerves, although a moderate increase in the serum creatine kinase level is not infrequent in denervating disorders. Relapses and remissions and variability can point towards a diagnosis of periodic paralysis, myasthenia gravis, or metabolic myopathy.

Cranial neuropathies

The cranial motor nerves are affected in a number

of local and general conditions. Symmetrical or asymmetrical cranial muscle weakness can occur in the Miller Fisher syndrome, diphtheritic neuropathy, borreliosis and sarcoidosis. The distribution of muscle weakness may suggest a motor neuropathy, but ocular myopathy, facioscapulohumeral muscular dystrophy and myasthenia gravis will often enter into the differential diagnosis. Many of the cranial neuropathies involve both sensory and motor nerves, which can help to clarify the differential diagnosis.

Asymmetrical motor neuropathies and plexopathies

The peripheral nerves can be damaged by various focal phenomena, including nerve compression in anatomical tunnels such as the carpal tunnel, or can be damaged by adjacent tumours or fractures. Focal nerve ischaemia can occur with disorders that affect the vasa nervorum, such as polyarteritis nodosa and other vasculitides, or diabetic vasculopathy. A focal form of chronic inflammatory polyneuropathy can produce multiple asymmetrical mononeuropathies and plexopathies. Generally, the anatomical distribution, the presence of sensory abnormalities and pain help to separate these conditions from the disorders of anterior horn cells and muscles which may present with asymmetrical focal weakness and wasting.

INVESTIGATIONS TO SEPARATE PERIPHERAL NERVE DISORDERS FROM OTHER CAUSES OF MUSCLE WEAKNESS

Clinical examination and laboratory investigations can help to distinguish disorders of the peripheral nerves from other causes of muscle weakness. The presence of significant sensory abnormality, in the absence of any other cause, suggests that the weakness is due to peripheral nerve dysfunction. Needle electromyography (see Ch. 29) is a powerful tool for separating conditions causing denervation of muscle from primary disorders of muscle, although the changes are similar in peripheral neuropathy and in anterior horn cell disorders. Single-fibre EMG and repetitive nerve stimulation studies are particularly helpful in diagnosing disorders of the neuromuscular junction.

Studies of sensory and motor nerve conduction, including the latency of late waves, can often be shown to be abnormal in peripheral neuropathies. If there is severe demyelination, conduction velocity will be markedly reduced and the phenomenon of multifocal block may be observed. Strict electrophysiological criteria must be fulfilled before the presence of conduction block is accepted (see Cornblath et al 1991a). Sensory nerve action potentials may be desynchronised and of reduced amplitude because of temporal dispersion of conduction. Motor neuronopathies and axonopathies cause loss of nerve fibres, with consequent reduction in amplitude of evoked compound muscle action potentials. In mixed neuropathies sensory nerve action potentials will also be reduced in amplitude, or lost. There is, however, a wide range of normal amplitudes for sensory and motor evoked action potentials, and modest loss of axons may not be shown by this technique. The routinely applied clinical electrophysiological studies examine only the largest (fastest-conducting) axons, and disease of small myelinated and unmyelinated axons can go undetected by these methods.

Repetitive nerve-stimulation studies help to demonstrate neuromuscular junction failure, such as occurs in myasthenia gravis, and the changes associated with the Lambert–Eaton syndrome.

Cerebrospinal fluid (CSF) examination may show raised protein concentrations in patients with demyelinating neuropathies, particularly where the nerve roots are involved. Biopsy of a skeletal muscle, studied with histochemistry, can be of diagnostic help in separating myopathy and myositis from chronic denervating conditions including peripheral neuropathy. At times a biopsy of a nerve may be required, but nerve biopsy is usually undertaken to establish the nature of, rather than the presence of, neuropathy. Biopsies are usually taken from the sural, superficial peroneal or terminal radial nerves, which are all sensory. Fascicular biopsies may be taken from mixed motor nerves; this is rarely indicated for clinical diagnosis, and has a significant potential morbidity.

DISEASES OF PERIPHERAL NERVES

A list of many of the causes of peripheral neuropathy is given in Chapter 13. This section provides an outline of the clinical and electrophysiological features of the main disorders of peripheral nerves which have to be considered in the differential diagnosis of skeletal muscle weakness. These conditions may all cause a virtually pure motor neuropathy, although in many patients there will also be some degree of sensory nerve involvement.

Guillain–Barré syndrome

Guillain et al (1916) reported a series of patients with acute polyradiculoneuritis, stressing the albumino-cytological dissociation in the CSF. Many such patients have been described since and much is known about the aetiology of the condition, although the criteria for diagnosis still remain difficult to define. There is considerable variation in the rapidity of onset and in the severity of weakness. For research purposes, diagnostic criteria have been defined that have proved useful (Ad Hoc NINCDS Committee 1978). Emphasis is particularly given to the duration between the onset and peak of the weakness, and generally 4 weeks is the maximum accepted for the diagnosis.

The clinical features of the Guillain–Barré syndrome (GBS) have been reviewed by Hughes (1990) and Ropper et al (1991). Over 50% of patients give a history of some preceding viral infection 2–4 weeks before the onset of the neuropathy. Over one-quarter begin with paraesthesiae in the feet, spreading proximally and then involving the hands. Over one-third have moderately severe pain, particularly in the back and limbs, which may cause diagnostic difficulties. Sensory loss is usually slight and is absent in about one-third of patients, while motor involvement is the most striking feature. In one-half of the patients, weakness is diffuse from the onset, whereas in the remainder it spreads from the lower limbs to involve the upper limbs, the respiratory and then bulbar muscles in the most severe cases. A completely 'locked-in' state may develop. On average the condition progresses for 2–4 weeks and, at its maximum, respiratory support is required in about 10–20% of cases. In terms of a peripheral neuropathy, such a progress is *acute*. Cases with a *subacute* evolution over 4–8 weeks are also encountered. They may constitute a separate category (Hughes et al 1992b).

For the average patient, the paresis is at its maximum for 1–4 weeks, and thereafter there is gradual recovery, although it may take several months and full recovery may not occur. The range of duration of severe disability is wide. About 3–6% of patients have relapses.

The CSF protein concentration is raised in almost all patients at some time during the illness. The maximum rise is seen from the tenth to twentieth day and the level may rise to 20 g/l. The proportion of IgG is raised in most cases. Although Guillain et al (1916) emphasised the albumino-cytological dissociation, about one-quarter of patients have a raised cell count in the CSF, but rarely to more than 40 cells/mm^3. Inflammatory infiltration with lymphocytes and segmental demyelination involve both the roots and peripheral nerves. Involved nerves may show either complete or partial conduction block, or may show a decrease of maximum conduction velocity of up to 50% of normal. Studies undertaken early in the condition may give normal results for motor conduction velocity, but investigation of the late (F and H) waves of the evoked muscle action potential may help to demonstrate proximal nerve and root involvement.

The overall prognosis for recovery is good, considering the poor state of some patients. Most series have a mortality rate of about 10%, mainly in respirator-dependent patients but lower values are recorded in some series (Ropper & Shahani 1984). About 20% of patients followed for more than 3 years have some permanent residual signs and symptoms. Older patients and those more severely paralysed have a worse prognosis, as do those with extensive axonal degeneration. The existence of a separate axonal form (Feasby et al 1986) is still under discussion. Of those on a respirator, 17% remain severely disabled and an additional 10% have residual signs but lead a normal life (Hewer et al 1968).

An interesting variant of the GBS is the Chinese paralytic syndrome (McKhann et al 1991) which affects children in northern China in annual epidemics and gives rise mainly to axonal degeneration.

Autonomic involvement can also occur in the GBS. Orthostatic hypotension is relatively common, but spontaneous episodes of hypotension, hypertension and cardiac dysrrhythmia may also occur. These may result from partial blockade of the afferent and efferent portions of the cardiovascular reflexes. Bladder atony and paralytic ileus may also occur, as may hyponatraemia.

The Miller Fisher syndrome is probably a variant of the GBS. It is characterized by external ocular and other cranial nerve palsies, ataxia and tendon areflexia. It has a good prognosis for recovery (Fisher 1956, Elizan et al 1971).

Aetiology. Uncertainty still exists concerning the exact causation of this condition. Although it is clear that a preceding viral or other infection is often important, many organisms have been implicated and the condition may occur following other precipitants such as surgical operations (Arnason & Asbury 1968) and immunising procedures (Schonberger et al 1981). In recent years, intestinal infection with *Helicobacter jejuni* has emerged as an important precipitant (Kaldor & Speed 1984, Winer et al 1988b) and may be associated with a particular tendency to give rise to axonal degeneration. The histological features in typical cases suggest a cell-mediated disorder and there is evidence of accompanying disturbances of cellular immunity. There is also evidence that humoral factors may be implicated. The immunological mechanisms involved in the GBS are still uncertain but have been reviewed by Hughes (1990) and Ropper et al (1991).

An experimental model that duplicates some features of this condition is available, namely experimental allergic neuritis (EAN) produced by the injection of peripheral nerve antigens together with Freund's adjuvant (Waksman & Adams 1955). This is primarily a T-cell-mediated delayed hypersensitivity reaction (Linington et al 1984), but humoral factors may also be involved. The principal antigen involved is myelin P_2 protein (Kadlubowski et al 1980). Many of the details of the immunological mechanisms still require elucidation, in particular, the factors involved in the natural termination of the disease. An antibody-mediated experimental neuropathy has also been produced in rabbits by hyperimmunisation with galactocerebroside (Saida et al 1979).

Treatment. Early reports of benefit produced by ACTH or corticosteroids have not been confirmed by subsequent controlled trials (Hughes et al 1978, 1992a). The multicentre North American trial of plasma exchange in over 200 patients with severe GBS has demonstrated the efficacy of this form of treatment if given within the first 14 days of the illness (McKhann et al 1985), a conclusion that has been confirmed in other smaller trials. More recently the use of high-dose intravenous human immunoglobulin (HIG) has been studied. A controlled trial comparing this with plasma exchange (Van der Meché et al 1992) reported greater benefit for HIG. However, this is difficult to interpret as the patients treated by plasma exchange fared less well than in the North American multicentre trial. Supportive measures are of considerable importance in the treatment of severely affected patients, including ventilatory assistance, control of autonomic dysfunction and prevention of thromboembolic complications.

Chronic inflammatory demyelinating polyneuropathy has been defined by continued deterioration after 8 weeks (Cornblath et al 1991b). There are indications that patients with a subacute course who deteriorate for periods of between 4 and 8 weeks may respond to corticosteroids (Hughes et al 1992b).

Chronic inflammatory demyelinating polyneuropathy (CIDP)

This has a much more diverse clinical presentation than the acute syndrome. Some cases have a picture resembling acute inflammatory polyneuropathy but the disorder continues to progress for more than 8 weeks. Some have a relapsing–remitting course; others, usually with a later age of onset, have a chronic progressive picture (McCombe et al 1987). The distribution is generally distal or diffuse, but may rarely be proximal. A hypertrophic neuropathy with thickened nerves may develop; nerve biopsies show onion bulbs from chronic repetitive segmental demyelination and remyelination. In all these conditions there may be inflammatory cell infiltration, maximal in the proximal parts of the nerves, together with segmental demyelination and remyelination (Thomas et al 1969, Dyck et al 1975). These syndromes are usually predominantly motor but ataxic sensory forms are encountered rarely. Multifocal variants with relatively pure motor involvement occur. Lewis et al (1982) identified some such cases that showed persistent multifocal conduction block. Similar cases have been reported subsequently (Parry & Clarke 1985, Van den Bergh et al 1989), some of which have been shown to be associated with antiGM1 ganglioside antibodies in the serum (Pestronk et al 1988). Whether the cases associated with such antibodies represent a separate disorder or whether they are a variant of CIDP is not yet established. Strictly focal examples of inflammatory demyelinating polyneuropathy affecting the brachial plexus (Cusimano et al 1988) or limb nerves (Mitsumoto et al 1990) are also recognised. CIDP is accepted as an autoimmune disorder but the precise immunopathogenetic mechanisms are not established.

CIDP may respond to treatment with corticosteroids, as in the original case reported by Austin (1958) and confirmed by a controlled clinical trial (Dyck et al 1982). The benefits of cytotoxic drugs have been reported anecdotally, but this has not been established by a formal trial (Dyck et al 1985). Plasma exchange has also been shown to be effective (Dyck et al 1986). It is likely that high-dosage intravenous human immunoglobulin (HIG) is beneficial in some cases. The variable response to these different treatment modalities may depend upon variation in the underlying disease mechanisms between patients and in variation between batches of pooled HIG.

Diphtheritic neuropathy

Diphtheria was once a scourge in many parts of the world, but immunisation in early childhood and the frequent use of antibiotics have now made it a rare disease in developed countries. It was first described by Trousseau & Lassegue (1851). The responsible organism is *Corynebacterium diphtheriae*, which usually causes an acute pharyngitis characterised by a grey membrane, but which can infect a skin wound. The dangerous complications are delayed and are due to cardiotoxicity and neurotoxicity. In experimental animals, the severity of the disease is proportional to the dose of neurotoxin used. However, the amount of neurotoxin produced by the *Corynebacterium* varies from strain to strain. In human infections it is therefore impossible to predict the severity of the delayed complications.

The major nerve damage due to the neurotoxin is usually delayed for 15–40 days after the onset of pharyngitis. Occasionally a precocious paralysis may develop 3–10 days after infection, being limited to the local area, particularly the palate, and is relatively benign. More severe paralysis often also begins in the palate but rapidly spreads into a generalised neuropathy, motor involvement predominating. The patient may require assisted ventilation, because of paralysis of bulbar and respiratory muscles.

The toxin is rapidly fixed in the body; 1 hour after injection into experimental animals its effect can no longer be neutralised by an injection of massive doses of antitoxin. The toxin is a potent inhibitor of elongation factor 2 and therefore of protein synthesis. It causes segmental demyelination by damaging the Schwann cells of the peripheral nerves in a patchy fashion. There is breakdown of the myelin sheaths, but the axons remain intact unless the neuropathy is very severe. This produces slowing of nerve conduction or a complete conduction block and paralysis. However, remyelination occurs quickly and the paralysis disappears in 15–30 days if death from complications does not supervene. In the experimental animal, clinical recovery occurs at a stage when nerve conduction remains slowed.

Exogenous toxins

A wide range of chemical agents may damage the peripheral nervous system (Table 25.2). Most cause a distal sensorimotor polyneuropathy affecting the longest and largest axons. However, others such as lead may produce pure muscle weakness. A diligent search for intoxication in a patient may allow withdrawal of the source of the neuropathy and hence recovery.

Care is required before accepting all reports of neuropathies due to toxic substances, particularly those recording uncommon reactions to drugs. The neuropathy may in fact be due to the underly-

Table 25.2 Some causes of toxic neuropathy

Metals	Lead, arsenic, mercury, thallium, gold
Industrial organic compounds	*Solvents*: *n*-hexane, methyl-*n*-butyl-ketone, trichlorethylene, carbon disulphide
	Others: TOCP, acrylamide, dimethylamino-dipropionitrile, ethylene oxide
Drugs	*Anticonvulsants*: phenytoin
	Chemotherapeutic: isoniazid, nitrofurantoin, dapsone, metronidazole ethambutol
	Antimitotic: Vinca alkaloids (vincristine, vinblastine), cisplatin
	Others: amiodarone disulfiram, hydrallazine, misonidazole, pyridoxine, thalidomide
Foods and intoxicants:	*Cyanogens* (cassaval) ethy alcohol. lathyrogens
Infective	Diphtheria

ing disease for which the drug was first given, or the association may be fortuitous. Moreover, allergic immunological reactions to almost any agent can occur. The agent acts as a hapten and binds to protein, which then becomes an antigen against which the body reacts. Such reactions are usually no more common with one agent than another, the 'allergic predisposition' being more a characteristic of the individual.

Other idiosyncratic reactions may indicate an underlying metabolic abnormality. Isoniazid intoxication occurs particularly in slow inactivators of the drug. In these individuals hepatic acetylation is slow and, consequently, blood levels are abnormally high, the major mechanism for drug elimination being urinary excretion (Evans et al 1960, Evans 1963). This tendency is inherited as an autosomal recessive trait, heterozygotes showing intermediate rates of inactivation.

Poisons may affect multiple sites and are rarely entirely specific, although many have a predilection for certain parts of the peripheral nervous system. Botulinum toxin blocks the release of trans-

mitter from vesicles at the neuromuscular junctions (Duchen 1970). Saxitoxin and tetrodotoxin block the depolarisation of axonal and neuronal membranes (Evans 1969). Diphtheria toxin has a particular effect on the Schwann cells (see above), causing demyelination with relative sparing of the axons. However, in most cases of toxic neuropathy the agent acts mainly on the perikaryon and axon, producing axonal degeneration. In triorthocresyl phosphate (TOCP) (Cavanagh 1964) and acrylamide neuropathies (Fullerton 1969) this has been particularly well studied. Frequently, the pattern of degeneration is the 'dying-back' type, affecting the distal parts of the largest fibres.

Vitamin deficiencies

Peripheral nerve damage occurs in several vitamin deficiencies, those with the greatest motor involvement being beriberi and alcoholism. Leaving aside vitamin B_{12} deficiency, lack of other vitamins usually occurs in the setting of malnutrition, when multiple deficiencies coexist. In experimental work it has been difficult to prove the need of an individual vitamin for peripheral nerve function, with the exception of thiamine (Victor 1965). For an extensive review of this problem the reader is referred to Windebank & Calloway (1993).

Thiamine — vitamin B_1. The active form of this vitamin is thiamine pyrophosphate which is the co-enzyme for at least three important enzymes of carbohydrate metabolism — pyruvate decarboxylase, alpha-ketoglutarate decarboxylase and transketolase. Deficiency causes an accumulation of pyruvate and lactate, with an impairment of energy metabolism in both the neurone and in Schwann cells. Although starvation alone in the presence of vitamin therapy may cause a peripheral neuropathy, a typical setting for thiamine deficiency was that occurring in the Japanese prisoner-of-war camps in the Second World War. The diet consisted predominantly of polished rice, which contains carbohydrate but not vitamins because of the removal of the rice husks. The result was damage to the peripheral nerves (dry beriberi) and to the heart with congestive cardiac failure (wet beriberi). The incidence of symptomatic neuropathy depended upon the severity of deprivation. Most of the patients showed signs of a distal, symmetrical polyneuropathy, which in 50% was mixed sensorimotor, in 30% mainly sensory, and in 20% mainly motor (Cruickshank 1952). Treatment with thiamine at a dose of more than 100 mg/day led to a slow recovery which often took more than 6 months. Those who had suffered prolonged and severe starvation made a lesser degree of recovery, residual dysaesthesiae being particularly common.

Vitamin B$_{12}$ is involved in the metabolism of methyl units, in nucleic acid metabolism, and probably in cell-membrane synthesis. Deficiency is most often due to loss of intrinsic factor produced by the gastric mucosa and required for intestinal absorption of vitamin B$_{12}$; this is usually due to autoimmune damage to gastric parietal cells by circulating autoantibodies. There is a familial tendency and the disease usually presents in middle age or later life. More rarely there is congenital absence of transcobalamin II, a serum protein that carries vitamin B$_{12}$, and the disease presents in the infant. Other causes of malabsorption of vitamin B$_{12}$ include the bowel blind loop syndrome, ileal resection, the fish tapeworm and the dietary habits of vegans. The mechanism of damage of the peripheral nerves in vitamin B$_{12}$ deficiency is uncertain. Clinically, central nervous system changes predominate, particularly those in the spinal cord, with progressive signs of damage to the pyramidal tracts and dorsal columns. In addition, many patients have paraesthesiae in the hands and feet and a mild glove and stocking impairment of the modalities of sensation conveyed by the larger fibres, together with loss of ankle jerks.

There is 10–20% slowing of maximum motor and sensory conduction velocities in the distal parts of the peripheral nerves, with no change in the proximal parts (Mayer 1965). The response to treatment with intramuscular vitamin B$_{12}$ at a dose of 1000 µg/day is relatively quick, the paraesthesiae sometimes disappearing within a few days and the distal reflexes returning within 1 or 2 months. Similarly, distal nerve conduction velocity returns to normal within 1 month (Mayer 1965). However, the spinal cord disease is much less responsive to therapy, and the prognosis is entirely dependent upon this. Physiological studies suggest that the neuropathy is a 'dying-back' type of axonal degeneration, and this suggestion is supported by pathological studies in man; there is loss of larger myelinated fibres in distal sensory nerves with changes of axonal degeneration in teased single fibres (McLeod et al 1969). However, in experimental vitamin B$_{12}$ deficiency in monkeys, segmental demyelination seems to predominate (Torres et al 1971).

Malabsorption and other causes of vitamin deficiencies. Several different nervous and muscular syndromes have been reported in association with diseases causing malabsorption, a progressive symmetrical distal mixed polyneuropathy being the commonest, with sensory ataxia, paraesthesiae and spontaneous pains (Cooke & Smith 1966, Erbsloh & Abel 1970). Malabsorption of all types may cause deficiencies, particularly of the fat-soluble vitamins and folic acid. Some are related to chronic vitamin E deficiency (Harding 1986) and, in these, there may be accompanying evidence of myopathy.

Alcoholism. These subjects frequently have a peripheral neuropathy similar in presentation to that of thiamine deficiency, and have been shown to have deficiencies of thiamine, folic acid, pyridoxine, pantothenic acid and riboflavine (Fennely et al 1964), with evidence of malabsorption of thiamine (Tomasulo et al 1968). The high calorie intake in the form of alcohol, with deficiency of thiamine, may be responsible for the nerve damage in many. Some, however, fail to improve with replacement of vitamins of the B group, and the direct toxic effect of alcohol and the possible effect of liver damage must also be considered.

Pyridoxine (vitamin B$_6$). Deficiency of pyridoxine, of which the active derivative pyridoxal-5-phosphate is a co-enzyme for many decarboxylases and transaminases, produces experimentally a peripheral neuropathy (Follis & Wintrobe 1945, Vilter et al 1953). This is predominantly a distal, symmetrical sensory polyneuropathy, although central nervous system changes also occur. In the pig it is probably mainly an axonal degeneration, although single-fibre studies have not been undertaken (Follis & Wintrobe 1945). Isoniazid produces an essentially identical neuropathy by interfering with pyridoxine metabolism, probably with the formation of the isonicotinyl hydrazone of pyridoxine (Aspinall 1964). The pathological changes of axonal degeneration in isoniazid neuropathy are well described (Cavanagh 1967, Ochoa 1970). Excessive (usually greater than 1 g/day) doses of pyridoxine produce a distal sensory polyneuropathy (Schaumburg et al 1983).

In pellagra, which is due to *nicotinic acid* deficiency, a painful, burning, distal symmetrical sensory polyneuropathy may occur, although the central nervous system changes predominate (Erbsloh & Abel 1970).

Ischaemic neuropathies and connective tissue disorders. Although the peripheral nerves have an extensive plexus of blood vessels, occlusion of several major feeding vessels or of many smaller vasa nervorum can cause a neuropathy. This is usually asymmetrical, acute and predominantly motor (Fujimura et al 1991). Large artery disease causes symptoms which are due to ischaemia of muscles (intermittent claudication) or gangrene of the whole limb, but 63% of patients with symptomatic arterial disease showed paraesthesiae, 87.5% had sensory abnormalities, 41% had depressed ankle jerks, 51% had weakness of one or both legs, and 31% had muscle wasting which was frequently asymmetrical (Eames & Lange 1967). Pathological examination often showed severe loss of myelinated fibres with both wallerian degeneration and segmental demyelination (Eames & Lange 1967, Chopra & Hurwitz 1968). An acute asymmetrical mononeuropathy may occur in subacute bacterial endocarditis because of embolisation of the major feeding vessels (Jones & Seikert 1968). The proximal ischaemic mononeuropathy of diabetes is described below.

Most of the connective tissue diseases can damage the nerves by ischaemia. The incidence of peripheral nerve involvement is highest in polyarteritis nodosa in which up to 20–30% of patients have a neuropathy (Lovshin & Kernohan 1948, Bleehen et al 1963). The picture is usually that of multifocal neuropathies with acute lesions of several individual nerves, although later it may blend into a progressive distal symmetrical sensorimotor polyneuropathy. Individual vascular lesions of the nerve are often painful. The treatment of polyarteritis nodosa with corticosteroids alone is not completely effective, and combination with cytotoxic immunosuppressive agents is usually required.

Estimates of the prevalence of involvement of the peripheral nervous system in systemic lupus erythematosus vary from 3 to 13% (Dubois 1966, Johnson & Richardson 1968), central nervous system involvement being considerably more frequent. Again the pattern is usually that of a multifocal neuropathy, although in some patients there is a distal symmetrical sensorimotor polyneuropathy. Occasionally a picture resembling an acute inflammatory polyneuropathy may develop. A peripheral neuropathy can occur in giant cell arteritis, scleroderma, dermatomyositis and Wegener's granulomatosis.

Several types of clinically symptomatic peripheral neuropathy have been described in rheumatoid arthritis. They were classified into four types by Pallis & Scott (1965):

Lesions of the major nerves of the upper and lower limbs (37%)
Distal symmetrical sensory polyneuropathy of the lower limbs (35%)
Digital neuropathy (22%)
Distal mixed sensorimotor polyneuropathy of upper and lower extremities.

This last category is the smallest group (6%) but is the most severe and has the poorest prognosis. It often presents initially with multiple mononeuropathies before progressing to a distal symmetrical sensorimotor polyneuropathy. The course is relatively rapid over a few months, and most patients die within 2 years from a widespread vasculitis.

Pathological studies have generally shown a diffuse vasculitis with occlusion of the vasa nervorum, more marked in the fourth type of neuropathy than in the second. Nerve fibre loss occurs, particularly at upper arm and mid-thigh levels, involving the centre of the fasciculi; these areas may constitute 'watershed territories' in the peripheral nerves (Dyck et al 1972a). The nerves may show segmental demyelination, although wallerian degeneration predominates, particularly in the more severe cases (Haslock et al 1970, Weller et al 1970, Dyck et al 1972b). Treatment is extremely difficult. In the fourth type of neuropathy, cytotoxic immunosuppressive agents such as cyclophosphamide are worthy of trial because of the poor prognosis.

Motor syndromes in diabetic neuropathy

The commonest type of peripheral neuropathy related to diabetes mellitus is a distal symmetrical sensory and autonomic polyneuropathy. There may be coexistent electromyographic evidence of denervation in peripheral muscles (Fagerberg et al 1963) or sometimes mild distal muscle wasting and weakness. Less commonly, syndromes occur in which motor deficits predominate.

Focal cranial and limb neuropathies. These are most frequently encountered in the older age groups. Among cranial mononeuropathies, the third and seventh are most common and usually have an abrupt onset. They are likely to have a vascular basis (Asbury et al 1970).

Focal neuropathies affecting the limbs and the thoraco-abdominal wall are commoner in patients with diabetes than in the general population. Those of acute onset probably have a vascular cause. Others occur at sites of entrapment or external compression, and it is likely that diabetics have an increased susceptibility to pressure palsies.

Diabetic amyotrophy. A proximal lower limb motor neuropathy may develop, usually in the older male diabetic, and can be the presenting feature in maturity-onset cases of non-insulin-dependent diabetes. Very occasionally the proximal muscles in the upper limbs are involved. Lower limb proximal motor neuropathy was originally recognised by Bruns (1890) but interest in the condition was reawakened by Garland (1955) who introduced the term 'diabetic amyotrophy'. Electromyography demonstrates denervation, and conduction time in the femoral nerve is prolonged (Chopra & Hurwitz 1968), clearly indicating a motor neuropathy. The site of damage is probably not only in nerve trunks, including the femoral (Skanse & Gydell 1956), but also in the lumbosacral plexus (Linden 1962).

Some cases are unilateral and of acute onset. They may recover, only to be followed by the same sequence on the opposite side. The onset is frequently associated with pain which may persist for several weeks and which is particularly troublesome at night. The territory of the femoral nerve is most often affected but muscles innervated by other lower limb nerves may also be involved simultaneously. The distribution often indicates lumbosacral plexus rather than nerve trunk involvement. The knee jerk is frequently lost but sensory impairment tends to be slight unless there is an accompanying distal sensory polyneuropathy. The prognosis for recovery is relatively good (Coppack & Watkins 1991). In other patients there is bilateral symmetrical or asymmetrical lower limb weakness of insidious onset, especially quadriceps muscle weakness. In this variant there is more likely to be an associated distal sensorimotor neuropathy (Subramony & Wilbourn 1982). The prognosis for recovery is probably less satisfactory in this form. As with other types of proximal motor neuropathy, confusion with myopathic disorders not infrequently occurs.

The cause in cases with an acute onset is probably vascular. It has been suggested that cases with an insidious onset and symmetrical distribution have a metabolic basis (Asbury 1977), but this clinical picture could be related to the cumulative effects of multiple small ischaemic lesions.

Porphyric neuropathy

Acute intermittent porphyria may produce severe episodes of abdominal pain, psychiatric disorders and peripheral neuropathy. An identical neuropathy may also develop in variegate porphyria and in the rare hereditary coproporphyria and ALA dehydratase deficiency. It is an acute, severe and chiefly motor neuropathy leading to flaccid paralysis and loss of reflexes. There is often a *proximal* predominance, the upper limbs being involved more than the lower. The cranial nerves, trunk and respiratory muscles and sphincters are also often involved. In about 50% of patients there is some sensory impairment, which may be either proximal or distal and which affects all modalities. The most classic picture is of a proximal muscle weakness with sensory loss in a bathing trunk distribution, and paradoxical preservation of the ankle jerks. Muscle wasting is rapid.

Pathological changes are predominantly of axonal degeneration, which in the motor nerves affects particularly the distal parts of the larger fibres in the intramuscular nerves and in the sensory fibres affects predominantly the centrally directed axons of the dorsal roots (Cavanagh & Ridley 1967). In both instances there is, therefore, a 'dying-back' distribution in individual axons, although the longest fibres are not involved as is usual in the 'dying-back' type of condition. It has been suggested that the effects fall particularly on those fibres with the largest motor units, although this appears unlikely in view of the similar distribution of damage in the sensory fibres.

In severe attacks, respiratory and bulbar paralysis may cause death, and assisted ventilation is often required. A few patients make a rapid recovery, although in most recovery is relatively slow, as might be expected after axonal degeneration. Sorensen & With (1971) reviewed 95 patients with acute intermittent porphyria, 41 of whom had suffered from paralytic episodes. Of these 41, 17 had died, and 12 of the 24 survivors had residual paralyses after 3 years which, in most cases, remained permanent thereafter. Recovery was less rapid and complete in males.

Attacks of acute intermittent porphyria occur either spontaneously or are precipitated by drugs, such as alcohol in excess, barbiturates and sulphonamides. The disease is of autosomal dominant inheritance with incomplete penetrance. It has been shown that the attacks are associated with the induction of high levels of delta-aminolaevulinic acid synthetase in the liver causing increased excretion of delta-aminolaevulinic acid and porphobilinogen in the urine (Sweeney et al 1970). The mechanism of production of the neuropathy remains obscure. Early diagnosis is vital in order to prevent the administration of drugs that aggravate the condition. Often, the diagnosis of a conversion syndrome may be made because of associated psychiatric features, or the predominant motor symptomatology and the proximal distribution of the weakness may lead to an erroneous diagnosis of acute polymyositis. Confirmation of acute intermittent porphyria is obtained by estimating urinary porphobilinogen and confirmed by measuring erythrocyte hydroxymethylbilane synthase, formerly known as porphobilinogen deaminase or uroporphyrinogen I synthase.

Treatment with glucose and haematin appears to be helpful in aborting an attack of porphyric neuropathy; the haematin probably produces feedback inhibition of the abnormally increased enzymes of the early parts of the pathway for haem synthesis (Bosch et al 1977).

Hereditary motor and sensory neuropathy (Charcot–Marie–Tooth disease)

The history of peroneal muscular atrophy goes back to the descriptions by Charcot & Marie (1886) and Tooth (1886) with progressive distal wasting and weakness producing a 'stork-leg' appearance, with motor involvement later spreading to the hands and relatively little involvement of the sensory nerves. It is clear that the clinical syndrome of peroneal muscular atrophy is genetically complex. The elucidation of this group of disorders was initiated by the seminal work of Dyck & Lambert (1968a, b) and has been elaborated in numerous later studies. In some cases there is a pure motor syndrome, constituting a hereditary distal spinal muscular atrophy (Harding & Thomas 1980a). In the remainder there is associated sensory involvement, although motor phenomena predominate. They have been categorised as hereditary motor and sensory neuropathy (HMSN) and are again subdivisible on clinical and genetic grounds (Harding & Thomas 1980b).

1. Hereditary motor and sensory neuropathy, type I (Charcot–Marie–Tooth disease type I). This group includes kinships similar to those described by Charcot & Marie (1886), and Roussy & Lévy (1926). Symptoms most often begin during the first decade. The earliest sign is usually pes cavus, and some gait disturbance often appears by the second decade due to progressive atrophy of the anterior tibial group of muscles. A progressive foot-drop develops, and later there is difficulty in manipulating the fingers. Significant sensory impairment appears late, affects especially the large fibre modalities, and is less severe than the motor involvement. The condition is very slowly progressive and most patients can still walk with aids 30 years after the onset. The maximum motor and sensory nerve conduction velocities are 10–40 m/s, and the nerve shows extensive segmental demyelination and hypertrophy with 'onion-bulb' formation. Signs of spinal cord dysfunction are sometimes present, probably resulting from compression by hypertrophic nerve roots (Symonds & Blackwood 1962).

The inheritance is usually autosomal dominant, but pedigrees with autosomal recessive inheritance are also recognised. In most autosomal dominant families the disease is now known to map to chromosome 17 (Vance et al 1989) and has been shown to be due to a segmental duplication at 17p11.2 (Lupski et al 1991, Raeymaekers et al 1991). This variant has been referred to as HMSN Ia (CMT Ia). In a small number of families linkage to the Duffy locus on chromosome 1 has been established (Bird et al 1982, Guiloff et al 1982) (HMSN Ib). These are related to mutations in the gene for PO myelin protein (Hayasaka et al 1993). In yet other families linkage to both chromosomes 17 and 1 appears to have been excluded.

2. Hereditary motor and sensory neuropathy, type II (neuronal form of Charcot–Marie–Tooth disease). The clinical pattern in this condition is similar to that in type I, but the onset is commonest in the second decade and is sometimes delayed to middle or late life; in addition, there is less upper limb involvement and the calf muscles are often affected as well as the anterolateral lower leg muscles. There is no enlargement of the peripheral nerves. Sensory loss is mild compared with motor impairment. Nerve conduction velocity is normal or modestly reduced. Sensory nerve biopsies show loss of the larger myelinated nerve fibres, little segmental demyelination and virtually no onion bulbs. The disorder probably represents a primary degeneration of anterior horn and primary sensory neurones. Inheritance is usually autosomal dominant. Families with autosomal recessive inheritance are also encountered. The cases described by Ouvrier et al (1981) and Gabreëls-Festen et al (1991) with an onset in early childhood and an aggresssive course are probably also recessively inherited.

3. X-linked hereditary motor and sensory neuropathy. X-linked dominant HMSN is uncommon but is now well documented (de Weerdt 1978, Rozear et al 1987, Hahn et al 1990). The manifestations in affected males resemble those of HMSN I. Carrier females are either asymptomatic or have less severe manifestations. The disorder has been mapped to the Xq13 region (Beckett et al 1986) and recently shown to be due to mutations in the gene for the gap junction protein connexin 32 (Fairweather et al 1994).

4. Hereditary motor and sensory neuropathy, type III (Dejerine–Sottas disease). The onset is usually in the first few years of life with delayed walking. The condition progresses slowly so that the patient becomes wheelchair-bound by 20–30 years of age. These is a progressive symmetrical glove-and-stocking loss of sensation. The peripheral nerves are thickened and nerve conduction velocity is severely reduced, usually to less than 10 m/s. Nerve biopsies show hypertrophic changes and hypomyelination (Dyck et al 1971). Inheritance is usually autosomal recessive. The condition is probably genetically heterogeneous.

The limits of HMSN are not yet fully defined and current classifications will have to be modified as individual genes are identified. The status of families with additional clinical features such as pyramidal signs (Harding & Thomas 1984) or optic atrophy and deafness (Rosenberg & Chutorian 1969) is still uncertain.

Refsum's disease. The disease was originally described by Refsum (1946), under the title of *heredopathia atactica polyneuritiformis*. Symptoms usually appear in the first and second decades of life, with the development of a chronic progressive symmetrical distal sensorimotor polyneuropathy which may show relapses and remissions. There is cerebellar dysfunction with ataxia and nystagmus, and a pigmentary retinopathy which lacks the classic 'bone corpuscle' pigment cells of typical retinitis pigmentosa. The CSF protein concentration is raised, and there are often anosmia, nerve deafness, ichthyosis, and cardiac and pupillary abnormalities. Inheritance is autosomal recessive. The condition is rare, but is important because of a knowledge in part of its underlying biochemistry and its treatment. There is an increased amount of the long-chain fatty acid, phytanic acid (3,7,11, 15-tetramethyl-hexadecanoic acid) in the blood and many tissues of the body (Klenk & Kahlke 1963); this accumulation is due to impaired metabolism of dietary phytol. The exclusion of phytol from the diet (Steinberg et al 1970), and plasma exchange to remove phytanic acid may produce considerable improvement.

Radiation-induced neuropathy

A virtually pure motor neuropathy that particularly affects the gluteal and peroneal muscles may be seen as a late sequel after irradiation of the para-aortic and inguinal lymph glands. The average latency is 12–14 months. Prominent muscle fasciculation may be a feature. Some cases with a shorter latency and in which sensation is also affected may be reversible. These syndromes have been reviewed by Thomas & Holdorff (1992).

Chronic cryptogenic polyneuropathy

In a significant proportion of patients with a chronic progressive peripheral neuropathy referred to a neurologist, no aetiology is found. In such cases the condition is usually termed chronic cryptogenic (idiopathic) polyneuropathy, and about half of these are predominantly motor in type. Dyck and coworkers (1981) found that very detailed investigation of the patients themselves and of their family members demonstrated that

about one-half of these patients have a familial neuropathy. With sufficient length of follow-up to identify cases of paraneoplastic neuropathy, the proportion of undiagnosed cases can be reduced to 12% (McLeod et al 1984).

CONCLUSIONS

Disorders of the peripheral nerves frequently enter into the differential diagnosis of conditions affecting skeletal muscle, the neuromuscular junction and the anterior horn cells. Careful clinical examination, full laboratory investigation and knowledge of the anatomy of the musculoskeletal system and the diseases which affect it allow the separation and identification of these conditions in most patients.

REFERENCES

Ad Hoc NINCDS Committee 1978 Criteria for diagnosis of Guillain–Barré syndrome. Annals of Neurology 3: 565

Arnason B G, Asbury A K 1968 Idiopathic polyneuritis after surgery. Archives of Neurology 18: 500

Asbury A K 1977 Proximal diabetic neuropathy. Annals of Neurology 2: 179

Asbury A K, Aldredge H, Herschberg R, Fisher C M 1970 Oculomotor palsy in diabetes mellitus: a clinicopathological study. Brain 93: 555

Aspinall D L 1964 Multiple deficiency state associated with isoniazid therapy. British Medical Journal 2: 1177

Austin J H 1958 Recurrent polyneuropathies and their corticosteroid treatment. Brain 81: 157

Beckett J, Holden J J A, Simpson N E, White B N, MacLeod P M 1986 Localization of X-linked dominant Charcot–Marie–Tooth disease (CMT 2) to Xq13. Journal of Neurogenetics 3: 225

Bird T D, Ott J, Giblett E R 1982 Evidence for linkage of Charcot–Marie–Tooth neuropathy to the Duffy locus on chromosome 1. American Journal of Human Genetics 34: 288

Bleehen S S, Lovelace R E, Cotton R E 1963 Mononeuritis multiplex in polyarteritis nodosa. Quarterly Journal of Medicine 32: 193

Bosch E P, Pierach C A, Bossenmaier I, Cardinal R, Thorson M 1977 Effect of hematin in porphyric neuropathy. Neurology (Minneapolis) 27: 1053

Bruns L 1890 Über neuritische Lahmungen beim Diabetes mellitus. Berlinen klinische Wochenschrift 27: 509

Cavanagh J B 1964 Peripheral nerve changes in orthocresyl phosphate poisoning in the cat. Journal of Pathology and Bacteriology 87: 365

Cavanagh J B 1967 Pattern of change in peripheral nerves produced by isoniazid intoxication in rats. Journal of Neurology, Neurosurgery and Psychiatry 30: 26

Cavanagh J B, Ridley A R 1967 The nature of the neuropathy complicating acute intermittent porphyria. Lancet ii: 1023

Charcot J M, Marie P 1886 Sur une forme particulière d'atrophie musculaire progressive souvent familial débutant par les pieds et les jambes et atteignant plus tard les mains. Revue de Médecine (Paris) 6: 97

Chopra J S, Hurwitz L J 1968 Femoral nerve conduction in diabetes and chronic occlusive vascular disease. Journal of Neurology, Neurosurgery and Psychiatry 31: 28

Cooke W T, Smith W T 1966 Neurological disorders associated with adult coeliac disease. Brain 89: 683

Coppack S W, Watkins P J 1991 The natural history of diabetic femoral neuropathy. Quarterly Journal of Medicine 79: 307

Cornblath D R, Sumner A J, Daube J et al 1991a Issues and opinions: conduction block in clinical practice. Muscle and Nerve 14: 869

Cornblath D R, Asbury A K, Albers J W et al 1991b Research criteria for diagnosis of chronic inflammatory demyelinating polyneuropathy (CIDP). Neurology 71: 617

Cruikshank E K 1952 Dietary neuropathies. Vitamins and Hormones 10: 1

Cusimano M D, Bilbao J M, Cohen S M 1988 Hypertrophic brachial plexus neuritis: a pathological study of two cases. Annals of Neurology 24: 615

de Weerdt C J 1978 Charcot–Marie–Tooth disease with sex-linked inheritance: linkage studies and abnormal serum alkaline phosphatase levels. European Neurology 17: 336

Dubois E L (ed) 1966 Lupus erythematosus. McGraw Hill, New York

Duchen L W 1970 Changes in motor innervation and cholinesterase localization induced by botulinum toxin and skeletal muscle of the mouse: difference between fast and slow muscles. Journal of Neurology, Neurosurgery and Psychiatry 33: 40

Dyck P J, Lambert E H 1968a Lower motor and primary sensory neuron diseases with peroneal muscular atrophy. I: Neurologic, genetic and electrophysiologic findings in hereditary polyneuropathies. Archives of Neurology 18: 603

Dyck P J, Lambert E H 1968b II: Neurologic, genetic and electrophysiologic findings in various neuronal degenerations. Archives of Neurology 18: 619

Dyck P J, Lambert E H, Sanders K, O'Brien P C 1971 Severe hypomyelination and marked abnormality of conduction in Dejerine–Sottas hypertrophic neuropathy: myelin thickness and compound action potential of sural nerve in vitro. Mayo Clinic Proceedings 46: 433

Dyck P J, Conn D L, Okazaki H 1972a Necrotizing angiopathic neuropathy. Mayo Clinic Proceedings 47: 461

Dyck P J, Schultz P W, O'Brien P C 1972b Quantitation of touch-pressure sensation. Archives of Neurology 26: 465

Dyck P J, Lais A C, Ohta M, Bastron J A, Okazaki H, Groover R V 1975 Chronic inflammatory polyneuropathy. Mayo Clinic Proceedings 50: 621

Dyck P J, Oviatt K F, Lambert E H 1981 Intensive evaluation of referred unclassified neuropathies yields improved diagnosis. Annals of Neurology 10: 222

Dyck P J, O'Brien P C, Oviatt K F et al 1982 Prednisone improves chronic inflammatory demyelinating polyradiculoneuropathy more than no treatment. Annals of Neurology 11: 136

Dyck P J, O'Brien P, Swanson C, Low P, Daube J 1985 Combined azathioprine and prednisone in chronic inflammatory demyelinating polyneuropathy. Neurology 35: 1173

Dyck P J, Daube J, O'Brien et al 1986 Plasma exchange in chronic inflammatory demyelinating polyradiculoneuropathy. New England Journal of Medicine 314: 461

Eames R A, Lange L S 1967 Clinical and pathological study of ischaemic neuropathy. Journal of Neurology, Neurosurgery and Psychiatry 30: 215

Elizan T S, Spire J P, Andiman R M, Baughman F A, Lloyd-Smith D L 1971 Syndrome of acute idiopathic ophthalmoplegia with ataxia and areflexia. Neurology (Minneapolis) 21: 281

Erbsloh F, Abel M 1970 Deficiency neuropathies. In: Vinken P J, Bruyn G W (eds) Handbook of clinical neurology, vol 7. North Holland, Amsterdam, pp 558–663

Evans D A P 1963 Pharmacogenetics. American Journal of Medicine 34: 639

Evans D A P, Manley K A, McKusick V A 1960 Genetic control of isoniazid metabolism in man. British Medical Journal 2: 485

Evans M H 1969 Mechanism of saxitoxin and tetrodotoxin poisoning. British Medical Bulletin 25: 263

Fagerberg S E, Petersen I, Steg G, Wilhelmsen L 1963 Motor disturbances in diabetes mellitus. A clinical study using electromyography and nerve conduction determination. Acta Medica Scandinavica 174: 711

Fairweather N, Bell C, Cochrane S et al 1994 Mutations in the connexin 32 gene in X-linked dominant Charcot-Marie-Tooth disease (CMTX1). Human Molecular Genetics 3: 29

Feasby T E, Gilbert J J, Brown W F et al 1986 An acute axonal form of Guillain–Barré polyneuropathy. Brain 109: 1115

Fennely J, Frank O, Baker H, Leevy C M 1964 Peripheral neuropathy of the alcoholic. Aetiologic role of aneurin and other B-complex vitamins. British Medical Journal 2: 1290

Fisher C M 1956 An unusual variant of acute idiopathic polyneuritis (syndrome of ophthalmoplegia, ataxia and areflexia). Journal of Medicine 255: 57

Follis R H Jr, Wintrobe M M 1945 A comparison of the effects of pyridoxine and pantothenic acid deficiency on nervous tissue of swine. Journal of Experimental Medicine 81: 539

Fujimura H, Lacroix C, Said G 1991 Vulnerability of nerve fibres to ischaemia: a quantitative light and electron microscope study. Brain 114: 1929

Fullerton P M 1969 Electrophysiological and histological observations on peripheral nerves in acrylamide poisoning in man. Journal of Neurology, Neurosurgery and Psychiatry 32: 186

Gabreëls-Festen A A W M, Joosten E M G, Gabreëls F J M, Jennekens F G I, Gooskens R H J M, Stegeman D 1991 Infantile motor and sensory neuropathy of neuronal type. Brain 114: 1855

Garland H 1955 Diabetic amyotrophy. British Medical Journal 2: 1287

Guillain G, Barré J, Strohl H 1916 Sur un syndrome de radiculonévrite avec hyperalbuminose du liquide cephalorachidien sans réaction cellulaire. Bulletin et memoires de la Société médicale des hôpitaux de Paris 1462

Guiloff R J, Thomas P K, Contreras M, Schwarz G, Sedgwick E M 1982 Linkage of autosomal dominant type I hereditary motor and sensory neuropathy to the Duffy locus on chromosome 1. Journal of Neurology, Neurosurgery and Psychiatry 45: 669

Hahn A F, Brown W F, Koopman W J, Feasby T E 1990 X-linked dominant hereditary motor and sensory neuropathy. Brain 113: 1511

Harding A E 1986 Vitamin E and the nervous system. CRC Critical Reviews in Neurobiology 3: 89

Harding A E, Thomas P K 1980a Hereditary distal spinal muscular atrophy. A report on 34 cases and a review of the literature. Journal of the Neurological Sciences 45: 337

Harding A E, Thomas P K 1980b The clinical features of hereditary motor and sensory neuropathy, types I and II. Brain 103: 259

Harding A E, Thomas P K 1984 Peroneal muscular atrophy with pyramidal features. Journal of Neurology, Neurosurgery and Psychiatry 47: 169

Haslock D I, Wright V, Harriman D G F 1970 Neuromuscular disorders in rheumatoid arthritis. A motor-point biopsy study. Quarterly Journal of Medicine 39: 335

Hayasaku K, Tabaka G, Ionasecu V V 1993 Mutation of the PO gene In Charcot-Marie-Tooth neuropathy type 1B. Human Molecular Genetics 2: 1369

Hewer R L, Hilton P J, Crampton-Smith A, Spalding J M K 1968 Acute polyneuritis requiring artificial respiration. Quarterly Journal of Medicine 37: 479

Hughes R A C 1990 Guillain–Barré syndrome. Springer, London

Hughes R A C, Newsom-Davis J M, Perkin J D, Pearce J M 1978 Controlled trial of prednisolone in acute polyneuropathy. Lancet ii: 750

Hughes R A C and the Guillain–Barré Syndrome Trial Group 1992a Multicentre trial of high dose intravenous methylprednisolone in Guillain–Barré syndrome. Journal of Neurology 239: S52

Hughes R A C, Sanders E, Hall S, Atkinson P, Colchester A 1992b Subacute idiopathic demyelinating polyneuropathy. Journal of Neurology 239: S53

Johnson R T, Richardson E P 1968 The neurological manifestations of systemic lupus erythematosus. Medicine (Baltimore) 47: 333

Jones H R, Siekert R G 1968 Embolic mononeuropathy and bacterial endocarditis. Archives of Neurology 19: 535

Kadlubowski M, Hughes R C, Gregson N A 1980 Experimental allergic neuritis in the Lewis rat:

characterization of the activity of peripheral myelin and its major basic protein, P_2. Brain Research 184: 439

Kaldor J, Speed B R 1984 GBS and *Campylobacter jejuni*: a serological study. British Medical Journal 288: 1867

Klenk E, Kahlke W 1963 Über das Vorkommen, der 3, 7, 11, 15-tetramethyl-Hexadecansäure in den Cholisterinestern und anderen Lipoidfraktionen der Organe bein einem Krankheitsfall unbebannter Genese (Verdacht auf Heredopathia atactica polyneuritiformis [Refsum-Syndrom]). Hoppe-Seyler's Zeitschrift für physiologische Chemie 333: 133

Lewis R A, Sumner A J, Brown M J, Asbury A K 1982 Multifocal demyelinating neuropathy with persistent conduction block. Neurology 72: 458

Linden L 1962 Amyotrophia diabetica. Svenska Läkertidningen 59: 3368

Linington C, Izumo S, Suzuki M, Uyemura K, Meyermann R, Wekerle H 1984 A permanent rat T-cell line that mediates experimental allergic neuritis in the Lewis rat in vivo. Journal of Immunology 133: 1946

Lovshin L L, Kernohan J W 1948 Peripheral neuritis in periarteritis nodosa. Archives of Internal Medicine 82: 321

Lupski J R, De Oca-Luna R M, Slaugenhaupt S et al 1991 DNA duplication associated with Charcot–Marie–Tooth disease type Ia. Cell 66: 219

McCombe P A, Pollard J D, McLeod J G 1987 Chronic inflammatory demyelinating polyradiculoneuropathy. Brain 110: 1617

McKhann G (The Guillain–Barré Study Group) 1985 Plasmapheresis and acute Guillain-Barré syndrome. Neurology (Cleveland) 35: 1096

McKhann G M, Cornblath D R, Ho T et al 1991 Clinical and electrophysiological aspects of acute paralytic disease of children and young adults in northern China. Lancet 338: 593

McLeod J G, Walsh J C, Little J M 1969 Sural nerve biopsy. Medical Journal of Australia ii: 1092

McLeod J G, Tuck R R, Pollard J D, Cameron J, Walsh J C 1984 Chronic polyneuropathy of undetermined cause. Journal of Neurology, Neurosurgery and Psychiatry 47: 530

Mayer R F 1965 Peripheral nerve function in vitamin B_{12} deficiency. Archives of Neurology 13: 355

Mitsumoto H, Levin K H, Wilbourn A J, Chou S M 1990 Hypertrophic mononeuritis clinically presenting with painful legs and moving toes. Muscle and Nerve 13: 215

Ochoa J 1970 Isoniazid neuropathy in man. Quantitative electron microscopic study. Brain 93: 831

Ouvrier R A, McLeod J G, Morgan G J, Wise G A, Conchin T E 1981 Hereditary motor and sensory neuropathy of neuronal type with onset in early childhood. Journal of the Neurological Sciences 51: 181

Pallis C A, Scott J T 1965 Peripheral neuropathy in rheumatoid arthritis. British Medical Journal 1: 1141

Parry G, Clark S 1985 Pure motor neuropathy with multifocal conduction block masquerading as motor neuron disease. Muscle and Nerve 8: 617

Pestronk A, Cornblath D R, Ilyas A A et al 1988 A treatable multifocal motor neuropathy with antibodies to GM1 ganglioside. Annals of Neurology 24: 73

Raeymaekers P, Timmerman V, Nelis E et al 1991 Duplication in chromosome 17p11.2 in Charcot–Marie–Tooth neuropathy type Ia (CMT Ia). Neuromuscular Disorders 1: 93

Refsum S 1946 Heredopathia atactica polyneuritiformis:

familial syndrome not hitherto described. Acta Psychiatrica et Neurologica Scandinavica 38

Ropper A H, Shahani B T 1984 Diagnosis and management of acute areflexic paralysis with emphasis on the Guillain–Barré syndrome. In: Asbury A K, Gilliatt R W (eds) Peripheral nerve disorders. A practical approach. Butterworths, London

Ropper A H, Wijdicks E F M, Traux B T 1991 Guillain–Barré syndrome. FA Davis, Philadelphia

Rosenberg R N, Chutorian A 1967 Familial opticoacoustic nerve degeneration and polyneuropathy. Neurology 17: 827

Roussy G, Lévy G 1926 Sept cas d'une maladie familiale particulière: Trouble de la marche, pied bots et aréfléxie tendineuse généralisée, avec accessoirement, légère maladresse des mains. Revue Neurologique 1: 427

Rozear M P, Pericak-Vance M A, Fischbeck K et al 1987 Hereditary motor and sensory neuropathy, X-linked: a half-century follow-up. Neurology 37: 1460

Saida T, Saida K, Dorfman S H et al 1979 Experimental allergic neuritis induced by sensitisation with galactocerebroside. Science 204: 1103

Schaumburg H, Kaplan J, Windebank A, Vick N, Rasmus S, Pleasure D, Brown M J 1983 Sensory neuropathy from pyridoxine abuse. New England Journal of Medicine 309: 445

Schonberger L B, Hurwitz E S, Katona P, Holman R C, Bergman D J 1981 Guillain–Barré syndrome: its epidemiology and associations with influenza vaccination. Annals of Neurology 9 (Suppl): 31

Skanse B, Gydell K 1956 A rare type of femoral sciatic neuropathy in diabetes mellitus. Acta Medica Scandinavica 155: 463

Sorensen A W S, With T K 1971 Persistent paresis after porphyric attacks. Acta Medica Scandinavica 190: 219

Steinberg D, Mize C E, Herndon J H Jr, Fales H M, Engel W K, Vroom F Q 1970 Phytanic acid in patients with Refsum's syndrome and response to dietary treatment. Archives of Internal Medicine 125: 75

Subramony S H, Wilbourn A J 1982 Diabetic proximal neuropathy. Clinical and electromyographic studies. Journal of the Neurological Sciences 53: 293

Sweeney V P, Pathak M A, Asbury A K 1970 Acute intermittent porphyria: increased ALA-synthetase activity during an acute attack. Brain 93: 369

Symonds C P, Blackwood W 1962 Spinal cord compression in hypertrophic neuritis. Brain 85: 251

Thomas P K, Lascelles R G, Hallpike J F, Hewer R L 1969 Recurrent and chronic relapsing Guillain–Barré polyneuritis. Brain 92: 589

Thomas P K, Holdoff B 1993 Neuropathy due to physical agents. In: Dyck P J, Thomas P K, Griffin J, Low P, Poduslo J (eds) Peripheral neuropathy, 3rd edn. WB Saunders, Philadelphia

Tomasulo P A, Kater R M H, Iber F L 1968 Impairment of thiamine resorption in alcoholism. American Journal of Clinical Nutrition 21: 1340

Tooth H H 1886 The peroneal type of progressive muscular atrophy (Thesis, University of London). H K Lewis, London

Torres I, Smith W T, Oxnard C E 1971 Peripheral neuropathy associated with vitamin B_{12} deficiency in captive monkeys. Journal of Pathology 105: 125

Trousseau A, Lassegue G 1851 Du nassonnement de la paralysie du voile de palais. L'Union Médicale 5: 471

Vance J M, Nicholson G A, Yamaoka L H et al 1989 Linkage of Charcot–Marie–Tooth neuropathy type Ia to chromosome 17. Experimental Neurology 104: 186

Van den Bergh P, Logigan E L, Kelly J 1989 Motor neuropathy with multifocal conduction blocks. Muscle and Nerve 11: 26

Van der Meché F G A, Schmitz P I M and the Dutch Guillain–Barré Study Group 1992 A randomized trial comparing intravenous immune globulin and plasma exchange in the Guillain–Barré syndrome. New England Journal of Medicine 326: 1123

Victor M 1965 The effects of nutritional deficiency on the nervous system. A comparison of the effects of carcinoma. In: Lord Brain, Norris F H Jr (eds) The remote effects of cancer on the nervous system. Grune and Stratton, New York, pp 134–161

Vilter R W, Muller J F, Glazer H S et al 1953 The effect of vitamin B_6 deficiency produced by desoxypyridoxine in human beings. Journal of Laboratory and Clinical Medicine 42: 335

Waksman B H, Adams R D 1955 Allergic neuritis: an experimental disease of rabbits induced by injection of peripheral nervous tissue and adjuvants. Journal of Experimental Medicine 102: 213

Weller R O, Bruckner F E, Chamberlain M A 1970 Rheumatoid neuropathy: a histological and electrophysiological study. Journal of Neurology, Neurosurgery and Psychiatry 33: 592

Windebank A, Callaway W 1993 Polyneuropathy due to nutritional deficiency and alcoholism. In: Dyck P J, Thomas P K, Griffin J, Low P, Poduslo J (eds) Peripheral neuropathy, 3rd edn. WB Saunders, Philadelphia

Winer J B, Hughes R A C, Osmond C 1988a A prospective study of acute idiopathic neuropathy. I. Clinical features and their prognostic value. Journal of Neurology, Neurosurgery and Psychiatry 51: 605

Winer J B, Hughes R A C, Anderson M J, Jones D M, Kangro H, Watkins R F P 1988b A prospective study of acute idiopathic neuropathy. II. Antecedent events. Journal of Neurology, Neurosurgery and Psychiatry 51: 613

26. Genetic aspects of neuromuscular disease

Katharine M. D. Bushby   *Alan E. H. Emery*

INTRODUCTION

Many of the diseases described in this book have a genetic basis. This chapter addresses aspects of some of these disorders which are relevant to genetic counselling. The diagnosis of an inherited disorder inevitably has an impact on the patient and his family beyond the immediate issues raised by the illness itself. They are anxious to understand why the disease came about, what its likely progression will be, whether there is any treatment, whether there is any risk to their offspring or the offspring of other family members, and whether any tests can help to clarify carrier risk or allow presymptomatic or prenatal diagnosis. The aim of genetic counselling is to present the answers to these questions in a way which will allow the family to make their own informed decisions about their future, and in particular their reproductive options. The sophisticated advances which have come about in molecular biology are an important component of what can be offered to patients, but no less important is the compassion which needs to be extended to these families, in many of whom the occurrence of an inherited neuromuscular disorder will have devastated their lives.

It is the process of 'positional cloning', previously described as 'reverse genetics' (Collins 1992) which has opened the way to a new understanding of the mechanisms involved in the pathogenesis of many of the inherited neuromuscular diseases. In many of these diseases, it had not been possible to discover the primary abnormality by standard biochemical techniques. The process of 'positional cloning' however, makes it possible to demonstrate the chromosomal position of a gene responsible for a particular disorder by linkage analysis. Linkage analysis relies on the existence of large families (or a large number of small families) with a clearly definable and homogeneous disease entity. These families are studied with polymorphic markers until evidence for linkage to a marker whose chromosomal location is already known establishes the chromosomal position of the gene. Mapping of the genes responsible for several of the muscular dystrophies, for example facioscapulohumeral muscular dystrophy (Wijmenga et al 1992) and myotonic dystrophy (Moraes et al 1992b), has been achieved by this approach. Where chromosomal rearrangements exist in association with the disease phenotype this provides additional evidence for the gene localisation, and speeds the search considerably, as for example with the X-autosome translocations in girls with Duchenne muscular dystrophy (Boyd & Buckle 1986). The exact position of the gene is then defined by finer genetic and physical mapping of the chromosomal region identified, and expressed transcripts from the area assessed as possible candidates for the gene itself by demonstrating expression in the expected tissues, conservation between species, and ultimately by finding mutations in the gene in affected individuals. The protein defective in the disease can then be deduced from the nucleotide sequence of the gene and its prediction of the amino-acid sequence of the protein. The numbers of disease genes mapped by this method have been increasing in an exponential fashion since the description of restriction fragment length polymorphisms and more recently through the use of 'microsatellite' polymorphisms (Weissenbach et al 1992). These random DNA sequence variations are generally much more polymorphic and therefore more informative than the systems previously available and allow greater coverage of the genome, increasing the likelihood of the success of the search.

A complementary approach to positional cloning and one which is likely to become more widely applicable as the Human Genome Project comes closer to a complete map of human chromosomes, is the 'candidate gene' approach. Here, a knowledge of the pathophysiology or biochemistry of a condition may provide a clue to the protein involved, or the genetic defect may have been identified in an appropriate animal model.

For a structural protein, abnormalities may be identifiable directly by immunostaining techniques. Alternatively, if the chromosomal position of the gene for the candidate protein is known, then this area of the genome can be targetted by linkage analysis, and relatively easily excluded or confirmed as a candidate area. The gene itself can then be analysed for disease-associated mutations segregating in affected families. Such an approach has been successful in a growing number of neuromuscular disorders, including malignant hyperthermia (Gillard et al 1991) and some of the myotonias (Koch et al 1991a).

The mapping and characterisation of the genes involved in many of the neuromuscular diseases should ultimately lead to a new understanding of the way muscle functions in health and disease. Work is under way to use this new understanding to develop potential therapies. In the meantime, each stage of the reverse genetics process leads to a significant advance in the strategies for carrier testing and prenatal diagnosis which can be offered to patients and their families (Fig. 26.1).

MODES OF INHERITANCE

An understanding of the modes of transmission of genetic disorders is obviously fundamental to offering correct counselling to the family. For any particular genetic characteristic which is not encoded by genes on the X or Y chromosomes, an individual will have inherited one gene from his mother and one from his father. In a classical autosomal dominant disorder, an individual need inherit only one faulty copy of the gene to manifest the disease. Dominant disorders may affect males and females, and there is a 50% risk that any offspring of an affected individual may also be affected. Dominant disorders often show considerable variation in severity, sometimes referred to as variable expressivity. Occasionally a gene carrier may show no manifestations of the disease at all, in which case the gene is said to be non-penetrant. For any dominant disorder the proportion of gene carriers (heterozygotes) who are affected to whatever extent, is referred to as the 'penetrance' of the gene.

In autosomal recessive disorders, an individual must inherit two faulty copies of the gene, one

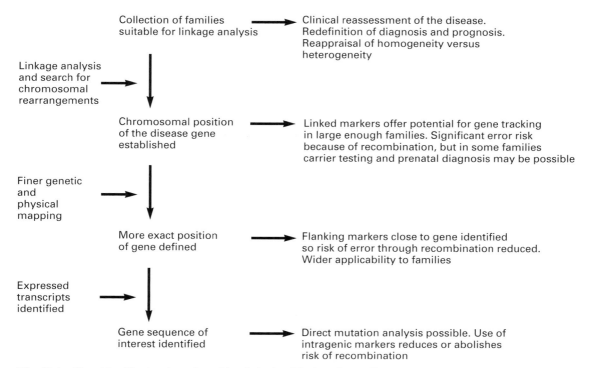

Linkage analysis
and search for
chromosomal
rearrangements

Finer genetic
and
physical
mapping

Expressed
transcripts
identified

Collection of families
suitable for linkage analysis → Clinical reassessment of the disease.
Redefinition of diagnosis and prognosis.
Reappraisal of homogeneity versus
heterogeneity

Chromosomal position
of the disease gene
established → Linked markers offer potential for gene tracking
in large enough families. Significant error risk
because of recombination, but in some families
carrier testing and prenatal diagnosis may be possible

More exact position
of gene defined → Flanking markers close to gene identified
so risk of error through recombination reduced.
Wider applicability to families

Gene sequence of
interest identified → Direct mutation analysis possible. Use of
intragenic markers reduces or abolishes
risk of recombination

Fig. 26.1 Gene identification through positional cloning. The benefits to affected individuals and their families of each stage of this process are shown on the right of the figure.

from each parent, in order to express the disease. Except in inbred populations, recessive disorders are rarely seen in more than one generation of a pedigree. After the birth of a child with a recessive disorder, the risk of recurrence in any subsequent pregnancy is 1 in 4. The children of affected individuals will all be carriers of the faulty gene, but will not have affected children themselves unless by chance they marry another carrier which, as long as their partner is unrelated, is very unlikely with a rare disorder. Similarly, although the siblings of an affected individual will be at 2/3 risk of carrying the faulty gene, their risk of affected offspring is also very low.

X-linked disorders are caused by mutant genes on the X-chromosome. Almost all X-linked diseases are recessive, so that female carriers do not usually manifest the disease, and only males are affected. As female carriers have one normal and one faulty copy of the gene, it follows that a carrier has a 1 in 4 chance of having an affected son in any pregnancy (i.e. half her sons will be affected and

half her daughters will be carriers). The phenomenon of X-inactivation explains why some female carriers of X-linked diseases show some degree of involvement which may help in determining carrier status (Lyon 1962). According to the Lyon hypothesis, one copy of the X-chromosome is inactivated in every female cell early in development. This process is usually random, and the pattern of X-inactivation in that particular cell is then stably inherited by its progeny. If by chance a greater proportion of cells express the mutant X (the normal X being inactivated), then a female carrier of an X-linked disease may show signs of that disease which may approach the severity of the full-blown disease in males. It is possible to study X-inactivation status through the identification of methylation differences between the active and inactive X-chromosomes.

The conditions discussed in this chapter are essentially those where there is a clear genetic aetiology. Other neuromuscular disorders may have a genetic predisposition, and may occasionally be seen in some families to be following a definable mode of inheritance. For example, myasthenia gravis in its adult form is most usually sporadic, but the much rarer congenital myasthenia syndromes probably represent autosomal recessive inheritance (see Chapter 20). Motor neurone disease is also usually sporadic, though 5–10% of cases are familial and are more likely to be early-onset (Emery & Holloway 1982). In most families presenting for genetic counselling, the mode of inheritance will be clear from an examination of the pedigree, and a knowledge of the most usual form of inheritance of the disease in question. With clinical and genetic heterogeneity, a feature of so many of the neuromuscular diseases, diagnostic precision is essential before any counselling can be offered.

As the genetic mechanisms underlying an increasing number of disorders are elucidated, it is becoming apparent that there are cases which do not follow the rules of mendelian inheritance. This applies most importantly in the field of neuromuscular disease to the mitochondrial myopathies: some are caused by defects in nuclear genes which encode mitochondrial enzymes and are inherited in a mendelian fashion, but others result from mutations of the mitochondrial genome itself. As mitochondria are almost exclusively maternally inherited, this accounts for the pattern of inheritance where both sexes can be affected but the disease is transmitted only by females.

A further mechanism which has been confirmed by direct mutation analysis and which has implications for genetic counselling is *germline mosaicism*. Here, a mutation is present in a proportion of the germ cells, often also in association with a degree of somatic mosaicism. The transmission of this mutation may lead to a new dominant or X-linked disorder in the offspring of apparently normal parents, and may explain some cases of what was previously believed to be non-penetrance. The chance of recurrence is difficult to assess, as it is dependent upon the proportion of ova or sperm bearing the mutation. However, the possibility of germline mosaicism must always be taken into account when counselling the family of an apparently isolated case of X-linked or dominant disease.

As the molecular background to so many dis-

eases becomes clearer, explanations are beginning to emerge for phenomena which could not previously be explained. It appears that *anticipation*, or worsening of the disease phenotype with successive generations can be at least partially explained in myotonic dystrophy by the presence of a mutation which expands as it is transmitted through each generation (Richards & Sutherland 1992). The relationship between Duchenne and Becker muscular dystrophy — very similar in their distribution of muscle weakness and wasting, but very different in the rate of progression of the disease — can now be understood in terms of the effect of different types of mutations on the function of the same gene and protein (Davies et al 1988). Different mutations in the same gene encoding the sodium-channel alpha-subunit in adult skeletal muscle (SCN4A) result in at least two phenotypically distinct disorders, paramyotonia congenita and hyperkalaemic periodic paralysis (McClatchey et al 1992), whereas the congenital myotonias are due to chloride-channel defects. In other diseases, it has been demonstrated that there are different genes ('locus heterogeneity') for clinically relatively similar disorders, such as the various types of hereditary motor and sensory neuropathy (Malcolm 1992).

THE MUSCULAR DYSTROPHIES

Until Walton & Nattrass (1954) attempted a classification of the muscular dystrophies based on genetic considerations, studies were handicapped by the use of categories which lumped together a number of disparate genetic entities. This classification based on genetic criteria has served well as the basis for both counselling and further research into these conditions, many of which can now be defined at the molecular level.

Duchenne and Becker muscular dystrophy

Duchenne and Becker muscular dystrophy (DMD and BMD) are X-linked recessive conditions. The clinical features of DMD have been well-established since the original descriptions of the disease in the nineteenth century by Meryon in England (Meryon 1852) and Duchenne in France (Duchenne 1868, Emery & Emery 1993).

Several reports had included patients with a milder clinical course but an identical pattern of muscle involvement, and this clinical entity was further delineated by Becker (Becker & Kiener 1955). Reports of several other families with a distinctly milder form of the disease confirmed its existence, but although in the original description of the milder form Becker had suggested that the two might be allelic, this could not be confirmed until the identification of the gene defects in these conditions. It is now known that various mutations at the gene locus result in a spectrum of disease severity. At the severe end is the DMD group with devastating early onset of proximal muscle weakness with confinement to a wheelchair usually by the age of 12, a high incidence of intellectual impairment and death often by the early 20s (Emery 1993). Approximately 10% of DMD patients in most series have disease of 'intermediate' severity with slightly less severe muscle involvement and usually longer survival (Brooke et al 1983). At the mild end of the spectrum is the BMD group, by definition wheelchair-bound after the age of 16. The severity of BMD is variable, though the majority of patients are ambulant into their forties or beyond (Emery & Skinner 1976, Bushby & Gardner-Medwin 1993). Creatine kinase levels are grossly elevated from birth in all forms of the disease allowing presymptomatic diagnosis, though levels fall with age (Zatz et al 1991).

Various estimates have been made of the population frequency of DMD and BMD. A world survey of population frequencies of the neuromuscular disorders showed considerable variability in the calculated prevalence and incidence in various parts of the world but with the incidence of DMD approaching $300/10^{-6}$ or roughly 1 in 3500 male births in recent and exhaustive studies (Emery 1991). Recent British estimates suggest that the current prevalence of DMD is $23.1/10^{-6}$ (Gardner-Medwin & Sharples 1989). It is likely that BMD has been under-diagnosed in the past because of difficulties in distinguishing clinically between it and some cases of spinal muscular atrophy and limb-girdle muscular dystrophy. However, with full ascertainment and diagnosis through direct gene and protein analysis, it has been shown in the North East of England that the

prevalence of DMD and BMD are almost the same, and the cumulative birth incidence of BMD is about one-third that of DMD (Bushby et al 1991). As the reproductive fitness in DMD is essentially zero (affected males almost never reproduce), it follows that as the disease gene is maintained at a constant level in the population, approximately one-third of cases are the result of new mutations. Using the figures for incidence of BMD and DMD in the North East of England, with biological fitness in BMD approximately 70% (Bushby & Gardner-Medwin 1993), the mutation rate for the gene as a whole is aproximately 6.55×10^{-5}. It is now known that the gene responsible for DMD and BMD is very large, which may explain the high mutation rate, which is apparently equal in males and females.

The molecular basis and investigation of DMD and BMD. The gene for DMD was initially localised to the short arm of the X-chromosome by the observation of several girls with symptoms similar to boys with DMD who were found to have chromosomal rearrangements involving a breakpoint at Xp21 (Boyd & Buckle 1986). Linkage analysis using probes from the same area established that BMD was localised to the same region of the X-chromosome and that the two were therefore likely to be allelic (Kingston et al 1983). Intensive study of a patient with a large deletion, and simultaneously a translocation patient led to the identification of genomic sequences which were deleted in other patients with DMD, and ultimately to the characterisation of the entire coding sequence (Koenig et al 1987). From this coding sequence the structure of the protein was predicted, and named dystrophin (Hoffman et al 1987). The gene encompasses over 2.5 megabases of genomic DNA, distributed over 79 exons (Roberts et al 1992b), from which a 14 kilobase mRNA is transcribed. Dystrophin, a previously unrecognised protein which comprises about 0.002% of total muscle protein, consists of some 3685 amino acids and has a molecular weight of approximately 427 kDa. The regulation and interactions of dystrophin are discussed in more detail in Chapter 3.

Information available from direct analysis of the dystrophin gene and protein has significantly altered the approach to diagnosis and carrier testing in the Xp21 muscular dystrophies. The diagnosis can be confirmed in a patient by direct gene or protein analysis. Each method has its advantages and, where possible, a combination of the two methods provides the maximum possible information.

Molecular diagnosis at the DNA level relies essentially on demonstrating a deletion of the dystrophin gene (present in 65–85% of cases). While point mutations of the dystrophin gene have been described (Bulman et al 1991, Roberts et al 1992a), their identification is not yet routine. The most widely used screening test for deletions is by the use of the polymerase chain reaction (PCR) by which multiple exons of the dystrophin gene are amplified simultaneously and can be directly visualised on a gel (Chamberlain et al 1988, Beggs et al 1990, Abbs et al 1991). This test is rapid and requires the use of only nanogram quantities of DNA, therefore having the potential to be used on DNA from blood spots or muscle biopsy samples stored from patients who had died before such tests were available. Alternatively, Southern blotting using probes from the dystrophin cDNA may be used to detect deletions or duplications. This method screens the entire dystrophin cDNA for rearrangements, and therefore has the advantage of detecting deletions of exons which are not amplified in the selected sets used for multiplex PCR (Multicentre study group 1992), and also of being able to define the full extent of a particular deletion or duplication.

At the protein level, the diagnosis may be confirmed by demonstrating an abnormal pattern of dystrophin labelling on immunostaining of muscle biopsy sections or immunoblotting. Immunocytochemistry allows the visualisation of dystrophin around the muscle fibre membrane, and the assessment of the pattern of staining (Nicholson et al 1989b), but is an essentially subjective analysis and cannot be used to determine the abundance of dystrophin produced. Western blotting allows the size of the dystrophin molecule detected to be determined compared to normal control samples run simultaneously and also an assessment of the abundance of dystrophin, provided allowance is made of the total amount of muscle protein present in the sample (Nicholson et al 1989a). A range of polyclonal or monoclonal antibodies to different domains extending over the entire dystrophin molecule is now available. Use of a range of antibodies can help to reduce the likelihood of a false-negative result where the epitope for a particular antibody has been removed in a patient's deletion. Abnormalities of dystrophin seem to be relatively specific to Xp21 muscular dystrophy, and to be present in all patients with this form of muscular dystrophy whether or not a dystrophin gene deletion can be identified.

The ability to detect abnormalities directly in the dystrophin gene and protein has led to the realisation that unusual features, such as cramps, may be the only manifestation of the gene mutation for many years (Gospe et al 1989). A few patients have also been identified who carry dystrophin gene mutations but who appear to have no signs of myopathy (Nordenskjöld et al 1990). The ability to make a precise diagnosis in BMD and sporadic manifesting carriers of dystrophin mutations especially, has had a major impact on counselling of these patients, as these conditions were often readily confused with limb-girdle muscular dystrophy and spinal muscular atrophy before the advent of a direct test for dystrophinopathy (Clarke et al 1989, Norman et al 1989, Vainzof et al 1991). Although it was known that up to 8% of known carriers of DMD had some muscle symptoms (Moser & Emery 1974, Norman & Harper 1989), it was impossible to estimate the numbers of sporadic cases of women with muscle disease who would in fact be manifesting carriers of dystrophin mutations. Dystrophin analysis is now apparently able to confirm the diagnosis of Xp21, or dystrophin-related, muscular dystrophy in such patients. At least 10% of isolated female cases of proximal myopathy with elevated serum creatine kinase (CK) activity probably fall into this category, and this may well be a considerable underestimate (Hoffman et al 1992). A spectrum of disease severity similar to that seen in male patients exists amongst the carriers of DMD and BMD who manifest the disease and present with symptoms (Bushby et al 1993b), and abnormalities of X-inactivation are present in some but not all of these cases.

The results of gene and protein analysis, in conjunction with the clinical status of the patient, may also help to give some guide as to the likely prognosis. The spectrum of clinical abnormalities seen in this group of patients is reflected by a spectrum of genetic and protein abnormalities. The deletions responsible for the disease in 60–85% of patients may occur anywhere in the gene, but tend to be clustered in two areas (Koenig et al 1987). The position and size of the deletion appears to have relatively little effect on the severity of the resultant phenotype, but a crucial factor appears to be the effect of a deletion on the translational reading frame of the gene (Monaco et al 1988). Deletions which remove exons so that the reading frame beyond the deletion is disrupted, leading to a premature stop codon and the production of an unstable and severely shortened protein, tend to be associated with a DMD phenotype and low or undetectable levels of dystrophin. However, where dystrophin is detected in DMD cases with frameshift deletions, it seems to be produced at a larger size than would be predicted from this model, as if some mechanism for alternative splicing or exon skipping existed to restore the reading frame to some extent in some fibres (Nicholson et al 1992). Even the low levels of dystrophin detected in some DMD patients appear to have some functional significance, with those having detectable dystrophin tending to remain ambulant on average longer than those without detectable dystrophin (Nicholson et al 1993). Patients of 'intermediate' clinical severity have deletions which may be in or out of frame, but generally produce more dystrophin than classical DMD patients (Bushby 1992b). Patients with BMD almost invariably have deletions which maintain the reading frame, allowing the production of an internally deleted protein, produced at relatively high abundance. Amongst those patients with the most typical mild BMD phenotype, there is a strong association with deletions of exons 45–47 and exons 45–48 particularly (Norman et al 1990, Bushby et al 1993a). While it holds true as a general rule across the Xp21 muscular dystrophy spectrum that increasing dystrophin abundance is correlated with a milder phenotype (Bushby 1992b), there is no one value for dystrophin abundance which will reliably predict a particular phenotype. Assessment of dystrophin abundance is necessarily based on a small muscle sample and may not be representative of the musculature as a whole.

Efforts are underway to enable the understanding of the genetic and protein defects in DMD to be translated into a potential cure, either through the use of myoblast transfer (Partridge 1991) or gene therapy (Acsadi et al 1991). While a significant breakthrough in therapy is awaited, at present genetic counselling is still concentrated on the identification of potential carriers of DMD and the provision of prenatal diagnosis if required. The high rate of new mutations in the dystrophin gene means that in one-third of cases, the mutation will have arisen in the affected boy himself, so that in a case with no previous family history, even the mother of an affected boy need not necessarily be a carrier of the dystrophin gene mutation. Most female carriers of DMD and BMD are asymptomatic, so many techniques have been used in the past to try to detect abnormalities in them, including electrocardiography, electromyography and muscle histology (Dubowitz 1963, Emery 1965, Gardner-Medwin 1968, Gardner-Medwin et al 1971, Roses et al 1977), but none of these techniques was reliable enough to be in regular use. Serum creatine kinase (CK) measurement has proved to be relatively useful in carrier testing providing the figures are not taken as absolute and the distribution of CK levels in a large number of carriers and normal women is available for the laboratory in which the test is performed. From this the relative probability of normal to carrier state can be determined and this can be incorporated into a likelihood calculation for the woman's overall risk of being a carrier which also takes into account all possible information from the pedigree (Emery 1993). Many different methods have been proposed to improve carrier testing using DNA or dystrophin analysis, but none is universally applicable (Fig. 26.2). The search for a deletion in an affected boy is of prime importance because of the ability to use this information to offer precise prenatal diagnosis and potentially direct carrier testing to females in the family. Theoretically, the identification of a deletion, either by PCR or Southern blotting, enables female relatives at risk to be analysed in a similar way to determine whether they carry the same mutation. In practise, the identification of deletions in females is less reliable than in males because of the need to use techniques which can detect a deletion in the

1. INFORMATION FROM PEDIGREE GIVES PRIOR RISK OF CARRIER STATUS

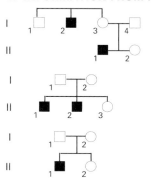

I_3 is an obligate carrier
II_2 is at 50% risk of being carrier

I_2 is a probable carrier, though the occurrence of the disease in both of her sons may be the result of germline mosaicism

I_2 is at $^2/_3$ risk of being a carrier
II_2 is at $^1/_3$ risk of being a carrier

2. (a) DIRECT CARRIER TESTING

If deletion known in affected individual, direct mutation analysis may be available using:
Southern blotting or PCR + dosage
Hemizygosity for polymorphisms within deletion
Identification of junction fragments
Chromosomal in situ hybridisation using cosmid clones lost in deletion
Lymphocyte mRNA PCR
Immunological assessment of dystrophin (value not proven in women without symptoms)

(b) INDIRECT TESTING

Information may be incorporated into Bayes theorem to reach an estimate of carrier risk for example:
Creatine kinase levels (in conjunction with graphs for laboratory where analysis performed)
Conditional information from pedigree (eg. presence of normal males)
Information from linked or intragenic polymorphisms if family structure suitable (but potential recombination risk even with intragenic probes)

Fig. 26.2   Carrier testing in DMD.

presence of a normal, non-deleted, X-chromosome; for example, dosage analysis in conjunction with PCR or Southern blotting (Mao & Cremer 1989, Bejjani et al 1991, Abbs & Bobrow 1992). In a proportion of affected boys, a deletion is associated with a 'junction fragment' which can also be identified in carrier females, allowing relatively straightforward carrier testing if the fragment can be identified on Southern blotting. Alternative techniques, such as pulsed field gel electrophoresis, chromosomal in situ hybridisation using cosmid clones and lymphocyte mRNA PCR (Ried et al 1990, Roberts et al 1990, Cockburn & Miciak 1992) also offer a specific test for deletions in carriers, though the methods are more specialised and expensive. It is not yet completely clear whether dystrophin analysis (which would of course necessitate a muscle biopsy) is reliable in identifying abnormalities in non-manifesting female carriers (Clerk et al 1991).

The situation is further complicated by the relatively high level of germline mosaicisms in DMD (Bakker et al 1987, Claustres et al 1990, Grimm et al 1990, Van Essen et al 1992). Both male and female germline mosaicism have been described. It has been calculated that there is a mean recurrence risk of 20% to a mother of an affected boy when the at-risk X-chromosome is transmitted, even when a deletion cannot be detected in the mother (Van Essen et al 1992). The level of germline mosaicism and therefore of subsequent transmission of the mutation is difficult to establish in an individual family, though there is some evidence that the position of the mutation in the gene may have some bearing on this risk, possibly related to the timing of mutations during embryonic development (Passos-Bueno et al 1993).

There remains, therefore, a relatively large number of potential carriers in whom no definitive answer can be given about their carrier status.

They include those where no deletion has been identified in their affected relative, or in whom the available techniques have been inconclusive. Others have no living affected relative. In these women a variety of indirect methods needs to be employed to arrive at a figure of their risk of being a carrier and therefore their risk of having an affected son, including serum CK analysis and linkage analysis using probes within and flanking the dystrophin gene to establish the X-chromosome at risk in a particular family. Because of the relatively high recombination rate (usually taken to be of the region of 5–10% even with intragenic probes) in and around the dystrophin gene, these indirect tests for carrier status and prenatal diagnosis carry a risk of error. This is incorporated into a bayesian calculation (Young 1991) whereby the best estimate of a woman's carrier status is calculated taking into account her prior probability of being a carrier (based on analysis of the pedigree) as well as conditional information such as the presence of normal or affected sons and derived from the use of serum CK analysis and linked or intragenic DNA markers. This methodology is considered in detail in Emery (Emery 1993).

The choice of how to proceed once a risk of being a carrier of DMD has been calculated remains of course in the hands of the individual women. The devastating nature of the disease, and the personal experience of the relatives of a DMD patient very often colour their perception of any given risk. Fortunately, direct carrier testing, and the incorporation of the maximum possible information from indirect carrier testing reduces the number of females to whom an 'intermediate' carrier risk still needs to be given (Emery 1993).

The methods available to determine carrier risk in any given situation may be extrapolated to offer prenatal diagnosis if requested. In most centres, chorionic villus biopsy can be performed in the first trimester. The sex of the fetus is determined by karyotyping, and further testing performed on male fetuses. If a direct test for a known mutation is available, then the situation is straightforward. When linked markers need to be used to establish the at-risk haplotype, then potential error due to recombination must always be considered. If a woman of uncertain carrier status decides to ter-minate a pregnancy on the basis of a prediction that a fetus has inherited the haplotype which is more likely to be at risk, then very valuable information may be obtained by dystrophin analysis of muscle from the terminated fetus, allowing a definitive assignment of carrier status, and potentially a precise prenatal test for the future (Ginjaar et al 1991).

Emery–Dreifuss muscular dystrophy

A clinically distinct form of X-linked recessive muscular dystrophy, Emery–Dreifuss muscular dystrophy (EDMD), is characterised by onset in childhood of a triad of features comprising early contractures, humeroperoneal muscle weakness and cardiac conduction defects (Emery 1989). The contractures are often present before significant weakness and involve primarily the Achilles tendons, elbows and spine. Muscle involvement begins in a predominantly humeroperoneal distribution, with or without weakness of the facial muscles and sternomastoids. Cardiac involvement is frequent from the twenties onwards and usually manifests as conduction defects with a significant risk of sudden death unless a pacemaker is inserted. Creatine kinase is usually elevated in the serum and may also be raised in some female carriers, who may also show some evidence of cardiac conduction defects. Linkage data suggests that the gene for EDMD maps to Xq 28 (Yates 1991). In families with definite evidence of X-linkage, probes are available which may be useful in carrier testing and prenatal diagnosis if required.

Several families have been described where the triad of features distinctive of EDMD were inherited in an autosomal dominant fashion, though with some slight variation in muscle involvement (Chakrabarti & Pearce 1981, Fenichel et al 1982). One family with autosomal dominant disease had evidence of neurogenic involvement on EMG and muscle biopsy (Witt et al 1988).

Facioscapulohumeral muscular dystrophy

Facioscapulohumeral muscular dystrophy (FSHD) is inherited as an autosomal dominant trait characterised by the onset of weakness (often asymmetrical) in the facial or shoulder-girdle muscles with progression in time to the abdominal and foot extensor muscles and pelvic girdle. The age at onset is highly variable, with even greater variability in the age at presentation, as expression of the disease may be very mild indeed and in fact be completely unrecognised by the patient or his relatives. For example, Walton (1955) emphasised the unreliability of family histories in his description of this family:

The affected girls in generation II were examined on two occasions and each time II4 was interviewed. It was only at a late stage of the second interview that the author's suspicions of facial involvement in II4 were aroused and examination subsequently revealed that she was undoubtedly an abortive case. She had insisted previously that all her sibs were well; however when they, too, agreed to be examined it was discovered that II9 was another abortive case, and that II7 was quite severely affected.

Facial weakness may sometimes not be a prominent feature, or in other cases may be the only finding (Hanson & Rowland 1971). Therefore in order to assess the numbers of individuals affected in a family prior to offering genetic counselling, it is advisable not to accept that an individual is unaffected without examination by someone familiar with the subtle signs of the disease. As serum CK activity is elevated in only 73% of affected men and 43% of affected women (Lunt & Harper 1991), its use as a presymptomatic test is limited. Retinal vascular abnormalities and hearing difficulties have been reported in association with FSHD, but their usefulness in screening for preclinical status has not been established.

Given these provisos, in a study of 41 families (Lunt & Harper 1991) six cases were identified in which there was no evidence of disease in either parent, representing presumably new mutations, complete non-penetrance in one of the parents or incorrect paternity. In the same study, penetrance of the disease was <5% under 4 years of age, 21% between 5 and 9, 58% between 10 and 14, 86% between 15 and 19 and 95% over 20 years. Given the difficulties of full ascertainment in a disease where expression may be minimal, it is not surprising that estimates of prevalence have varied widely, from 2.2 to 66.9 × 10^{-6} (Emery 1991). Lunt & Harper (1991) also addressed the question

of the severity of the disease. Their figures suggested that 19% of those affected with FSHD would require a wheelchair by the age of 40 or over, while 30% remained mildly affected throughout their life. Involvement of the pelvic-girdle musculature before the age of 20 years was an indication that the eventual disability might be severe enough to necessitate use of a wheelchair. There was no significant relationship between the severity of the disease in parents and offspring, nor any apparent difference in the severity of the disease with maternal or paternal transmission.

Close linkage of FSHD to markers on distal 4q is now established, with initially no evidence for heterogeneity (Wijmenga et al 1990, Upadhyaya et al 1991). However, there is now some evidence to suggest that some families with phenotypically indistinguishable disease may not be chromosome 4-linked (Gilbert et al 1993). A DNA rearrangement has been identified in a proportion of both sporadic and familial cases of FSHD using a cosmid clone mapping to chromosome 4q (Wijmenga et al 1992). While this initially showed promise as a direct diagnostic test for FSH dystrophy, it has now been established the rearrangement does not always segregate with the disease and that the association is therefore not absolute. The clinical applications of this test are limited until its nature is more clearly understood (Weiffenbach et al 1993).

The 'limb-girdle' muscular dystrophies

'Limb-girdle' muscular dystrophy (LGMD) comprises a group of diseases where genetic analysis is beginning to clarify areas which have been the subject of debate for many years. Suggested initially as a name for the group of muscular dystrophies that were not classifiable as X-linked or FSH (Walton & Nattrass 1954), the term has been applied to a variety of conditions where the only unifying characteristic has been the predominance of weakness in the limb-girdle musculature with sparing of the facial muscles. With the advent of direct testing for dystrophin abnormalities some patients with a previous diagnosis of LGMD have been shown to have BMD or be manifesting carriers of dystrophin mutations, and the identification of the gene product involved in the spinal muscular atrophies and possibly also FSHD will probably also reveal some misdiagnoses (Yates & Emery 1985, Arikawa et al 1991a). Therefore all previous figures for the prevalence and incidence of LGMD are likely to be overestimates (Emery 1991).

Essentially, muscular dystrophy which predominantly affects the limb-girdle musculature can have onset at any age and be inherited in a recessive or dominant manner. A preliminary subdivision of published and presented families tentatively suggested the following categories (Bushby 1992a), partly based on the results of linkage analysis in genetically homogeneous family groups and partly on clinical similarities between different families and groups of families.

1. Autosomal recessive LGMD linked to chromosome 15q. Families from the Reunion Island and Amish populations have both been shown to be linked to markers on chromosome 15q (Beckmann et al 1991, Young et al 1992), and preliminary analysis suggests that some families from elsewhere may also show linkage to the same markers. In both groups in whom linkage has been described the onset of the disease was in late childhood, though preclinical cases could be identified through significant elevation of serum CK, and the disease was of moderate progression (Jackson & Carey 1961, Jackson & Strehler 1968, Beckmann et al 1991).

2. Autosomal recessive muscular dystrophy of childhood. The Duchenne-like pattern of severe disease is most commonly seen in the North African population (Ben Hamida et al 1983) but is occasionally seen in other populations too, where it may be confused clinically with DMD (Passos-Bueno et al 1991). Dystrophin analysis allows the diagnosis to be excluded with certainty, as dystrophin is normal in the autosomal recessive muscular dystrophies. However, recent studies using antibodies to the components of the glycoprotein complex to which dystrophin binds via its C-terminus have shown a specific reduction of the 50 kDa dystrophin-associated glycoprotein in the muscle of patients with severe autosomal recessive muscular dystrophy of childhood (Matsumura et al 1992). The genetic defect in Tunisian families with Duchenne-like autosomal recessive muscular dystrophy has been mapped to the centromeric region of chromosome 13 (Ben Othmane et al 1992).

3. Other more slowly progressive autosomal recessive muscular dystrophies. Patients with recessive disease and a relatively benign clinical course have been described (Passos-Bueno et al 1991, Mahjneh et al 1993). At present, there are insufficient data on which to base a clinical distinction between families in this category which may turn out to be linked to chromosome 15 and those which are not. Whether there will be forms of relatively mild LGMD which turn out to be allelic to the more rapidly progressive forms is not yet known.

4. Autosomal dominant LGMD with late onset. Several families with an essentially similar pattern have been described (de Coster et al 1974, Gilchrist et al 1988, Marconi et al 1991). Progression of the disease in these families was very slow, and serum CK showed only marginal elevation, if at all, precluding its use as a presymptomatic test. The disease in one large American family (in which some affected individuals had dysarthria) has been shown to be linked to chromosome 5q (Speer et al 1992).

5. Autosomal dominant muscular dystrophy with early onset and contractures. This relatively specific disease entity (also known as Bethlem myopathy (Bethlem & Van Wijngaarden 1976, Tachi et al 1989), and which may or may not represent a true muscular dystrophy) is characterised by early onset, slow progression and prominent early contractures of the elbows, ankles and fingers.

Thus limb-girdle muscular dystrophy is the name given to a heterogeneous group of disorders, and genetic counselling is only straightforward in the presence of an established family history, or in an area with a high prevalence of any one of the recognised forms. The proportion of families with recessive disease linked to chromosome 15 has not yet been established, but is unlikely to be more than 35% (J. Beckmann, personal communication). In any case, most individual families are too small for linkage to be informative. The demonstration of linkage in other large families to other loci should help to clarify the situation and help establish the relative contributions of allelic and locus heterogeneity to the variability seen in these conditions. In the meantime, counselling of an isolated case remains difficult. Exclusion of all alternative diagnoses must be made as specifically as possible. On the basis of current knowledge, though it is likely that recessive disease is more common than the dominant form, it cannot be assumed that all sporadic cases are recessive with a correspondingly low recurrence risk to their offspring. There are few features which distinguish the two modes of inheritance, though the presence of early contractures does not seem to be a feature of recessive disease, and gross elevation of serum CK, even in presymptomatic cases, seems to be more a feature of recessive disease than dominant. However, in practice these distinctions are of limited value in individual cases.

Congenital muscular dystrophies

The provision of correct genetic counselling to families with a child diagnosed as having congenital muscular dystrophy relies heavily on the exclusion by histopathological techniques of the congenital myopathies in which inheritance patterns are variable (see later), the exclusion by dystrophin analysis of unusually early onset of DMD, and the examination of the mother to exclude congenital myotonic dystrophy. Congenital muscular dystrophy is characterised by hypotonia from birth associated with a severe weakness which is essentially non-progressive (Donner et al 1975). Patients often need calipers to aid walking, and many require aggressive management of contractures, which may be present from birth or become prominent later (Jones et al 1979). IQ is usually normal (except in Fukuyama muscular dystrophy, see below). Muscle biopsy shows severe histopathological changes suggestive of muscular dystrophy. CK activity in the serum is usually elevated in the first few years, and subsequently falls. Mortality is high in childhood. Individual cases or families have been described where a congenital muscular dystrophy has been associated with other features, for example congenital heart disease or abnormalities of cerebral white matter on a CT scan (Nogen 1980).

Cases of congenital muscular dystrophy are most often isolated or sib-pairs, with autosomal recessive inheritance likely. No specific prenatal or carrier testing is possible.

There are several forms of congenital muscular dystrophy where the geographical distribution and characteristic associated features suggest that they represent truly separate genetic entities. Ullrich's hypotonic-sclerotic form of congenital muscular dystrophy is most likely to be a distinct autosomal recessive condition, characterised by a non-progressive myopathy present from birth with thin muscles, proximal contractures but hyperextensible distal muscles, usually facial sparing and associated features such as a prominent calcaneus, hyperhidrosis and a high-arched palate. CK activity is not usually markedly elevated (Nihei et al 1979).

Other congenital muscular dystrophies are associated with relatively specific cerebral abnormalities. Fukuyama muscular dystrophy is most commonly seen in Japan, where its incidence is approximately half that of DMD in the same population (Fukuyama et al 1981). Cerebral gyral abnormalities are a feature of the condition, and the CT scan is usually abnormal, showing ventricular dilatation, cortical atrophy or diffuse low-density areas in the brain (Fukuyama et al 1981). The clinical course of Fukuyama muscular dystrophy is more severe than DMD with most patients never able to walk, and suffering a profound degree of mental handicap. Most die before the age of 10. While dystrophyn immunostaining is usually normal in the congenital muscular dystrophies, abnormalities of dystrophyn have been described in some Fukuyama patients investigated by immunocytochemistry. These dystrophin abnormalities are associated with a high incidence of spectrin abnormalites, suggesting that the plasma membrane is severely disrupted in Fukuyama patients, causing secondary disruption of dystrophin immunocytochemistry (Arikawa et al 1991b). In addition, some Fukuyama patients have been described where dystrophin is unexpectedly completely absent. This has led to the suggestion that there may be an interaction between the (still unknown) Fukuyama gene product and dystrophin, such that patients with X-linked DMD who are also by chance heterozygous for the autosomal recessive Fukuyama gene have a phenotype which is more severe than classical DMD, and also sometimes not entirely typical of Fukuyama MD (Beggs et al 1992). An abnormality of the

43 kDa dystrophin associated protein has now been identified in Fukuyama muscular dystrophy, which may explain the secondary disruption of dystrophin (Matsumura et al 1993).

A further group of disorders where congenital muscular dystrophy is associated with cerebral abnormalities is known variously as muscle–eye–brain disease, congenital cerebro-ocular muscle dysgenesis and Walker–Warburg syndrome (Leyton et al 1991). These abnormalities are felt to represent a yet more severe neuropathological disruption than Fukuyama muscular dystrophy (Leyton et al 1991, Miller et al 1991). Generalised hypotonia and very profound mental retardation are most commonly described, often with death in infancy, though families have been described where minor abnormalities in some family members may represent variable expression. Inheritance is most likely to be autosomal recessive. Fetal ultrasound allows a possible means for prenatal diagnosis, with hydrocephalus described in one fetus at 18 weeks' gestation (Miller et al 1991).

Other clinical patterns of muscular dystrophy

Various other apparently distinct clinical subtypes of muscular dystrophy are recognised, in some of which the mode of inheritance is clear, but in many of which it is not. The situation is further complicated by the occasional description in the literature of families where two types of muscular dystrophy co-exist (Udd et al 1991, Mahjneh et al 1993). A brief description of some of the remaining clinical subtypes of muscular dystrophy and their modes of inheritance is given in Table 26.1. A more complete description of these conditions may be found in Chapter 14.

ABNORMALITIES OF MUSCLE FIBRE EXCITABILITY — THE MYOTONIAS AND PERIODIC PARALYSES

Some form of electrical instability of the muscle fibre membrane is thought to be responsible for the diseases in this genetically heterogeneous group, in which there is sometimes some overlap of symptoms between the clinically recognisable phenotypes. Recent work in physiology and molecular biology is clarifying these relationships.

Conditions associated with myotonia

Myotonia is a failure of voluntary muscle to relax immediately following contraction. Several genetically heterogeneous disorders are associated with myotonia, including myotonic dystrophy, myotonia congenita, the Schwartz–Jampel syndrome and paramyotonia. Myotonia may also be found in hyperkalaemic periodic paralysis, which is dis-

Table 26.1   Clinical characteristics and modes of inheritance of some other forms of muscular dystrophy

Disease	Clinical characteristics	Mode(s) of inheritance	References
Distal muscular dystrophy	Involvement of small muscles of hands and feet. Benign progression to involve proximal muscles.	AD (seen mainly in Sweden) Homozygotes occasionally seen: more severely affected.	Welander 1951, Welander 1957
		Juvenile onset form also AD possibly some neuropathic features	Van der Does de Willebois et al 1968
	Onset of distal weakness in 2nd or 3rd decade with more rapid progression	Sporadic or autosomal recessive	Nonaka et al 1985
Scapulohumeral muscular dystrophy	Onset in early adulthood affecting shoulder girdle with later spread to proximal lower limbs	Usually sporadic. Some possibly dominant.	Dubowitz 1978
Scapuloperoneal muscular dystrophy	Onset in 2nd to 5th decade. Present often with foot-drop. Progression very slow	AD	Thomas et al 1975

AD, autosomal dominant.

cussed in the next section. Myotonic dystrophy is the only one of these conditions which is usually progressive and associated in the majority of cases with significant muscle weakness. In the non-dystrophic myotonias, there is no evidence to suggest multisystem involvement, and the prognosis is generally good. The molecular basis of these disorders, and their sometimes complex interrelationships, is becoming clearer through a combination of physiological studies and genetic linkage analysis. Candidate genes for some of these conditions have been identified. This has allowed a reclassification of the non-dystrophic myotonias according to their molecular basis as follows (Lehmǎnn-Horn et al 1993):

Muscle sodium channel diseases:

    Hyperkalaemic periodic paralysis
    Normokalaemic periodic paralysis
    Paramyotonia congenita
    Myotonia fluctuans

Muscle chloride channel diseases:

    Myotonia congenita (Thomsen's disease)
    Recessive generalised myotonia (Becker).

Myotonic dystrophy. Myotonic dystrophy is the most common disease in which myotonia is a prominent feature, with a prevalence ranging from 9.1 to 96.2×10^{-6} with an overall figure of around 50×10^{-6} (Emery 1991, Koch et al 1991a). The typical adult features of myotonic dystrophy include myotonia predominantly found in the small hand muscles, forearms and tongue. Facial and sternomastoid weakness are common, with weakness in the limbs involving essentially distal muscles. Frontal baldness and cataract are commonly seen and may be the only manifestations in mildly affected individuals. Inheritance is autosomal dominant, with almost complete penetrance, but frequently with only subtle signs in the older generations of a family, in whom electromyography, slit lamp examinaton or molecular biological studies may be required to make the diagnosis. The phenomenon of anticipation, with earlier age at onset and progressively more severe disease seen in successive generations of affected families has frequently been reported in myotonic dystrophy, though it was argued for many years that these observations were the result of bias of

ascertainment (Harper et al 1992). An additional complication in counselling in myotonic dystrophy is the risk of congenital myotonic dystrophy (Vanier 1960) in the children of heterozygous mothers (Harper & Dycken 1972). Children of affected males only very rarely seem to have this most severe form of the disease. Congenital myotonic dystrophy presents at or before birth with generalised hypotonia which may manifest as reduced fetal movements or feeding and breathing difficulties, and which may require the use of mechanical ventilation. Facial weakness is severe and is present from birth but myotonia is not a feature in the first 2 years of life. These children are usually globally retarded. Symptoms in the mother may be so slight as to have been unnoticed until the birth of a congenitally affected child but more severely affected mothers have an increased risk of a congenitally affected child, and there is some evidence for a birth order effect (Koch et al 1991a). Thus while the risk of passing on the faulty gene in any one pregnancy remains 50%, it has been recommended that women who are symptomatic at the time of contemplating pregnancy or who have already had a congenitally affected child should be counselled as having an approximately 40% risk of the severe form in their offspring, compared with approximately 10% for women who are known to be gene carriers, but who are asymptomatic (Koch et al 1991a).

The mutation responsible for myotonic dystrophy has recently been identified through the finding of an unstable repeat sequence on chromosome 19q13.3 (Aslandis et al 1992, Buxton et al 1992). Unaffected individuals have approximately 5–30 copies of the CTG repeat. Amplification of this repeat (50 to thousands of copies of the repeat may be found in affected individuals) segregates with the disease, with a tendency for expansion of the repeat from generation to generation, broadly correlating within families with increasing severity of the disease phenotype (Harley et al 1992, Tsilfidis et al 1992), thus providing a biological mechanism for the phenomenon of anticipation (Harper et al 1992). However, the specific maternal transmission of the mutation responsible for congenital myotonic dystrophy has yet to be explained. The repeat appears to be situated in the 3′ untranslated region of a gene which has homology to cyclic-AMP-dependent serine-threonine protein kinases (Brook et al 1992) and which is predominantly expressed in heart, skeletal muscle and brain (Jansen et al 1992). The mechanism whereby a repeat in an untranslated region of a gene produces a dominant phenotype is not yet understood, but may be through an effect on chromatin structure, gene dosage, splicing, or through an effect on transcription or RNA transport. Extensive alternative splicing in the gene has been demonstrated (Jansen et al 1992), which may have implications for the production of the phenotype. In addition, a second gene ending less than 1 kb upstream from the protein kinase gene has been described and may also be relevant (Jansen et al 1992).

The immediate effect of the discovery of the repeat sequence has been to be able to offer specific diagnosis and prenatal testing. Preliminary data suggest that an increase in expansion from parent to child will result in worsening of the phenotype (Tsilfidis et al 1992), but as yet a congenitally affected case cannot be predicted or excluded with certainty.

Myotonia congenita. Myotonia congenita is itself genetically heterogeneous, with dominant and recessive forms described. In addition, variable symptoms have been reported in association with both forms of inheritance.

Autosomal dominant myotonia congenita (Thomsen's disease). Motor problems are present from early childhood, and myotonia itself is the most prominent feature, usually affecting the arms and legs and eye muscles, with lid-lag a common feature. Speech may also be affected. Muscle mass is usually normal, or there may be some hypertrophy (Lipicky 1979). Different clinical subgroups of dominantly inherited myotonia may have myotonia demonstrable only electrically, with lid-lag the only symptom, or may have a highly variable course with some worsening on exposure to cold or in response to a potassium load. In the form described by Thomsen, there was no aggravation of myotonia with cold or potassium loading (Iaizzo et al 1991). Symptoms in all forms are non-progressive, and the lifespan is normal.

Electrophysiological and pathophysiological studies in myotonia congenita have implicated abnormalities of both skeletal muscle sodium channels (Iaizzo et al 1991) and chloride channels (Rudel 1986). These potential clues to the pathophysiology led to a search for the defective gene based on a candidate gene approach, targetting the adult skeletal muscle sodium channel on chromosome 17, and the cystic fibrosis transmembrane regulator (involved in chloride channel function) on chromosome 7q. Both areas were excluded (Abdalla et al 1992b), but further work based on a mouse model (the ADR mouse) where the genetic defect had been shown to be transposon inactivation of a muscle chloride channel gene mapped to mouse chromosome 6, showed linkage in four pedigrees to the syntenic region in humans on chromosome 7q35 (Abdalla et al 1992a), and mutations in the human skeletal muscle chloride channel gene have now been demonstrated in individuals with Thomsen's disease (George et al 1993).

Autosomal recessive myotonia congenita (Becker type). The recessive form of myotonia congenita is more common then the dominantly inherited disease, the myotonia is more severe, and progressive weakness may occur. The onset may be delayed beyond infancy and early childhood, but the symptoms tend to progress at least until puberty. The syndrome is also known as recessive generalised myotonia, as it usually affects all muscles, while the pattern of muscle involvement in the dominant form is often restricted. Transient stiffening of the muscles when used after a period of rest is a common feature of this condition, and this may be replaced by weakness, which may last long enough to be significantly disabling. In the upper limbs particularly, weakness tends to be the more disabling symptom, while myotonia is more prominent in the lower limbs (Rudel et al 1988). Muscle hypertrophy is more common than in the dominant forms. Low chloride conductance also appears to be the predominant conduction abnormality in this condition (Rudel et al 1988, Iaizzo et al 1991). Recessive generalised myotonia has also been localised to chromosome 7, and a mutation in the skeletal muscle chloride channel gene identified in an affected family (Koch et al 1992). The same gene is therefore implicated in both the recessive and dominant forms of the condition, with presumable total loss of function in the recessive form, and a more subtle disruption of function in the dominant form. This may explain some of the clinical and electrophysiological differences between the two forms.

Schwartz–Jampel syndrome (chondrodystrophic myotonia). Schwartz–Jampel syndrome is a rare recessive disorder in which myotonia is the prominent feature, along with generalised contractures, muscle stiffness, skeletal anomalies, short stature and facial dysmorphism (Vijoen & Peighton 1992). Malignant hyperthermia may be a fatal complication. Several different membrane defects have been demonstrated in muscle from a Schwartz–Jampel patient, including abnormal sodium channel gating, reduced chloride conductance and altered regulation of myoplasmic free calcium (Lehmann-Horn et al 1990). Prenatal diagnosis by ultrasound in the mid-trimester has been reported in a family with a previously affected child by demonstrating constant finger flexion, decreased fetal activity and mild shortening and bowing of the femora (Hunziker et al 1989).

Paramyotonia. Paramyotonia is another autosomal dominant condition of high penetrance in which myotonia is a characteristic feature. The major distinguishing feature of this form of myotonia is the extreme sensitivity to cold experienced by patients. Some patients with other myotonic conditions report some degree of cold sensitivity, but never to the same extent as in paramyotonia. In a warm environment, myotonia may be indistinguishable from that seen in myotonia congenita, but after a few minutes exposure to cold, myotonia, especially of the facial muscles and hands, worsens dramatically and is followed by weakness or flaccid paralysis. The contractions persist as long as exposure to cold continues and gradually disappear on rewarming. Weakness or paralysis follows the myotonia, and may persist for hours. Onset of the symptoms is in childhood, with no evidence of progression of the disease or reduction of life-span.

Defects in sodium channel behaviour, with abnormally high sodium conductance have been demonstrated in paramyotonia muscle, with more pronounced abnormalities shown under cold conditions (Lehmann-Horn et al 1987a). Therefore the genes involved in sodium regulation were likely to be candidate genes for abnormalities in this disorder. The gene for the alpha-subunit of the human adult skeletal muscle sodium channel (SCN4A) has been mapped to chromosome 17q (Fontaine et al 1990). Genetic linkage studies concentrating on this area of chromosome 17 have demonstrated linkage to this gene for both paramyotonia congenita and hyperkalaemic periodic paralysis (see next section) (McClatchey et al 1992). Haplotype analysis using polymorphisms within the SCN4 gene suggests that the two disorders are caused by different mutations in the gene, with allelic heterogeneity for both.

The periodic paralyses

This group of dominant disorders is characterised by episodic periods of weakness or paralysis and can be subdivided clinically according to whether attacks are associated with high potassium levels (hyperkalaemic periodic paralysis — HYPP), low potassium (hypokalaemic periodic paralysis — HOPP) or occur when the patient is normokalaemic, though the last group is the least well-defined. There is some overlap of symptomatology. Abnormal sodium conductance has been demonstrated in both HYPP and HOPP (Rudel et al 1984, Lehmann-Horn et al 1987b).

Hyperkalaemic periodic paralysis. Attacks tend to be preceded by prodromal feelings of heaviness or stiffness in the muscles and occur when patients rest after exercise or in the first few hours in bed at night. Paresis starts in the thighs and calves or back muscles and progresses to the arms and neck, though some residual mobility usually persists in affected muscles. Recovery may take minutes or up to 2 hours. The frequency of attacks is very variable and occasionally mild weakness may persist between attacks. Onset is usually in childhood and life expectancy is not reduced. Inheritance is autosomal dominant, probably with complete penetrance, and three clinical variants appear to breed true: HYPP with myotonia (the majority of cases — lid-lag and other eye signs tend to be especially prominent, and in some individuals from these families myotonia may be the only sign of disease), HYPP without myotonia, and HYPP with paramyotonia.

Electrophysiological evidence of abnormal inactivation of sodium channels in HYPP muscle

(Lehmann-Horn et al 1987b) suggested a defect in this channel, so that as in paramyotonia the SCN4 gene was an obvious candidate for this disease. Linkage analysis using a polymorphism within the gene confirmed tight linkage in several HYPP pedigrees (Fontaine et al 1990, Ptacek et al 1991, Koch et al 1991b, McClatchey et al 1992). All of the families investigated apparently had HYPP with myotonia. A single nucleotide mutation in SCN4 leading to a methionine-to-valine substitution in an evolutionarily conserved area has been decribed in a family and in a sporadic case with HYPP, suggesting that this same disease-causing mutation had arisen twice independently (Rojas et al 1991). The same mutation was not found in other HYPP families, despite linkage to SCN4, suggesting that several different mutations are responsible for the disease at this locus.

Hypokalaemic periodic paralysis. This form of periodic paralysis is more common than HYPP. Most attacks occur in the early morning, often with symmetrical and almost complete paralysis though speech, respiration and eye movements are usually spared. Less severe attacks are also described and may be more frequent. Reports of cardiac involvement may reflect the hypokalaemia rather than heart pathology per se. The age at onset and frequency of the attacks are variable, and there is usually some decrease in frequency with increasing age. Some patients have persistent muscle weakness between attacks, and some may develop permanent weakness and muscular atrophy which may be severely disabling and associated with vacuolar changes in the muscle biopsy. The disease is inherited in an autosomal dominant fashion, though there is extreme variation in the severity of the disorder, especially in females. This probably explains the preponderance of males to females reported by some authors as 3 : 1 or 4 : 1.

Although abnormal sodium conductance has been reported in HOPP as well as HYPP, families with HOPP do not show linkage to SCN4 on chromosome 17 (Fontaine et al 1991), suggesting that the two disorders are not allelic.

MALIGNANT HYPERTHERMIA

Volatile anaesthetic agents such as halothane and the muscle relaxant drug succinylcholine may each provoke muscle rigidity, hypermetabolism and ion imbalance in individuals susceptible to malignant hyperthermia (MH), a situation which may be fatal (Maclennan & Phillips 1992). Susceptibility to MH can be inherited as an autosomal dominant condition, where individuals are completely healthy unless challenged by an anaesthetic. Some patients with MH have elevated serum creatine kinase activity, but this alone is not a reliable test. Other tests for MH rely on studying muscle in vitro for sensitivity to caffeine or halothane, but require muscle biopsy, are expensive, and tend to err on the side of false-positive diagnoses (Ording 1988). A mutation in the gene for the calcium-release channel of skeletal muscle sarcoplasmic reticulum (the ryanodine receptor) has been identified in swine with porcine stress syndrome, a porcine homologue of MH (Maclennan et al 1990). Linkage to the human ryanodine receptor (on human chromosome 19, close to the myotonic dystrophy gene) has been demonstrated in some MH families (McCarthy et al 1990), with one having the same cysteine for arginine substitution found in affected pigs (Gillard et al 1991). Other families are apparently unlinked to the ryanodine receptor (Levitt et al 1991, Deufel et al 1992) suggesting genetic heterogeneity, though the possibility of incorrect assignment of affected status on the basis of in vitro tests remains a serious problem in linkage analysis of these families (Maclennan & Phillips 1992). Still, it would appear that up to 50% of British families do not show linkage to chromosome 19 (Ball and Johnson 1993). As there is no risk to individuals with MH except when challenged with an anaesthetic, the major impetus to determining the gene mutations responsible is to identify which family members need special care during anaesthesia and which can be treated normally. This will undoubtedly supplant the less reliable indirect tests in the future once the full spectrum of disease-associated genes and mutations is known. In the meantime such tests are applicable to a small number of families only where definitive linkage to chromosome 19q has been established.

Several separate conditions have been reported in which there is an apparent susceptibility to or association with MH (Brownell 1988). Central core disease (CCD) has particularly often been associated with MH, and in fact linkage of CCD to the ryanodine receptor has now been established (Kausch et al 1991a) suggesting a common genetic basis for the two conditions. Several neuromuscular conditions which are apparently genetically distinct have also been reported as conferring susceptibility to MH in some individuals, including the King-Denborough syndrome (Chitayat et al 1992), myodenylate deaminase deficiency, Schwartz–Jampel syndrome, Fukuyama muscular dystrophy, periodic paralysis, myotonia congenita and occasionally others (Brownell 1988), suggesting that the clinical phenotype recognised as MH susceptibilty may arise through a number of different mechanisms.

THE CONGENITAL MYOPATHIES

Congenital myopathies most often present with hypotonicity in infancy, though they may also be responsible for the later onset of relatively non-progressive muscle weakness, even in adult life. Genetic counselling in these disorders is complex as inheritance patterns for many of the recognised histological diagnoses are variable. In some of these cases dysmorphic features or other associated abnormalities may be helpful in assigning a clinical diagnosis (Heckmatt & Dubowitz 1990) and detailed examination and possibly muscle biopsy of relatives may shed light on the mode of inheritance. Many different classifications of the congenital myopathies have been proposed, based essentially on histological and histochemical characteristics. Progress has been made towards identifying the genes responsible for some of these conditions, and these and some features relevant to genetic counselling of the best characterised entities are presented in Table 26.2.

MITOCHONDRIAL MUSCLE DISEASE

Complex clinical syndromes with the common features of morphologically and biochemically abnormal mitochondria have been recognised since 1962 (Luft et al 1962). The presentation and underlying biochemical defects of the mitochondrial encephalomyopathies are heterogeneous, but most are associated with the presence of so-called 'ragged-red' fibres in muscle biopsy sections as demonstrated by the modified Gomori trichrome stain (Engel & Cunningham 1963). Muscle symptoms which have been particularly associated with mitochondrial disease include external ophthalmoplegia, exercise intolerance, and muscle weakness and wasting of variable distribution. Onset can be at any age and progression is variable. It is likely that at least some cases of so-called ocular or oculopharyngeal muscular dystrophy are in fact the result of mitochondrial abnormalities. Associated features found in varying combinations in the different delineated mitochondrial encephalomyopathies include cerebral abnormalities leading to ataxia, seizures or stroke-like episodes, ocular abnormalities including optic atrophy and retinal degeneration, and various other multisystem manifestations including short stature, cardiomyopathy, renal tubular pathology, endocrine abnormalities and liver failure (Petty et al 1986, Lombes et al 1989). These features are seen in variable combinations in the clinically recognised syndromes of the mitochondrial encephalomyopathies, which include the Kearns–Sayre syndrome, chronic progressive external ophthalmoplegia, MERFF (a syndrome of myoclonus, epilepsy and ragged-red fibres) and MELAS (mitochondrial myopathy, encephalopathy, lactic acidosis and stroke-like episodes).

The genetic basis for the mitochondrial encephalomyopathies is complex, and counselling in these disorders similarly so. Mitochondrial DNA encodes 13 of the approximately 67 subunits of the mitochondrial respiratory chain and oxidative phosphorylation system as well as two ribosomal RNAs and 22 transfer RNAs (Harding 1991). Mitochondrial DNA is almost exclusively maternally transmitted, which accounts for the observed 9:1 ratio of maternal to paternal transmission in familial cases of mitochondrial myopathy (Harding et al 1988). Under such a model of inheritance, theoretically all offspring of affected females might be expected to be affected. However, the observed situation is that this is not so, and furthermore, there is considerable variability in severity, even within sibships. This is explained by the presence of the variable proportions of mutant and normal populations of mitochondrial

Table 26.2 The congenital myopathies

Disease	Histopathological characteristics	Clinical pattern	Associated features	Mode of inheritance	Gene defect	References
Central core disease	Type I fibres show well-demarcated central cores on staining for oxidative enzymes. Type I fibre predominance	Variable. Usually mild myopathy from infancy causing mild disability. Legs usually weaker than arms	Malignant hyperpyrexia, kyphoscoliosis, congenital dislocation of hip, foot + joint contractures	AD. Some gene carriers may be identifiable only on muscle biopsy	Linked to chromosome 19q13.1 (see section on malignant hypothermia)	Kausch et al 1991a
Nemaline myopathy	Abundant thread or rod-like particles in myofibres seen in Gomori trichrome staining, often with type I fibre predominance. α-actinin is a major component of nemaline bodies	1. Congenital onset, may be rapidly fatal or more benign. Weakness most marked in face, neck, trunk and distal limbs	Dysmorphic features — long thin face, high-arched palate, chest deformity, pes cavus, scoliosis	AR. Some carriers have non-specific muscle biopsy abnormalities which may be difficult to interpret	Unknown	Wallgren-Petterson et al 1990
		2. Later onset but variability within families. May be progressive	Less frequently associated with dysmorphic features	AD	Linked in a large family to chromosome 1q21-23	Laing et al 1992
Centronuclear (myotubular) myopathy	Prominent central nuclei in many muscle fibres with aggregation of oxidative enzymes and glycogen. Often type I fibre predominance	1. Antenatal or neonatal onset often with death in first year. Feeding and respiratory problems in neonatal period	Facial weakness and ptosis. May be some dysmorphism and skeletal malformations	X-linked recessive. Carriers may show minor weakness or biopsy abnormalities. Clinically important to exclude myotonic dystrophy in mother	Some families show linkage to Xq28 markers	Heckmatt et al 1985, Starr et al 1990, De Angelis et al 1991
		2. Later childhood onset often with ptosis and ophthalmoplegia and affecting proximal muscle groups		AD cases well-documented. Recessive inheritance proposed for cases of intermediate severity but not proven. Sporadic cases may in fact be isolated X-linked or dominant mutations	No loci known for AD or AR forms	
Minicore/ multicore disease	Focal defects of oxidative and myofibrillar ATPase with disorganisation of myofilaments on electron microscopy. Type I fibre predominance, but minicores present in both fibre types	Early-onset weakness of neck muscles and proximal limbs. Strength may improve with time	Facial muscles may be involved. Scoliosis has been described	Most cases assumed to be sporadic or autosomal recessive. Some apparently dominant families described	Unknown	Penegyres & Kakulas 1991, Paljarvi et al 1987

Table 26.2 *Contd*

Disease	Histopathological characteristics	Clinical pattern	Associated features	Mode of inheritance	Gene defect	References
Congenital fibre-type disproportion	Normal or hypertrophied type II fibres and small type I fibres	Floppiness from birth. Generally good prognosis unless respiratory problems	Contractures, congenital dislocation of the hip, foot deformities, scoliosis, high-arched palate	Most cases sporadic. Families with apparently dominant and recessive inheritance have been described. Other diagnoses should be carefully excluded	Unknown; a translocation case has been described	Cavanagh et al 1979, Gerdes et al 1993

DNA in affected individuals (heteroplasmy). These different populations of mitochondrial DNA coexist in different proportions in different tissues including the ova.

The nuclear genome interacts with the mitochondrial genome at several levels. Most of the subunits of the respiratory chain and oxidative phosphorylation system are in fact encoded by nuclear genes (Zeviani 1992). Mutations in these genes, or abnormalities in the transfer and assembly of their products into the mitochondria, may therefore also be responsible for histological or biochemical mitochondrial abnormalities. Nuclear factors also play a role in the regulation of mitochondrial DNA itself. A defect at any of these levels may be responsible for autosomally inherited mitochondrial disease (Lombes et al 1989).

A review of 71 cases with a variety of histologically confirmed mitochondrial myopathies identified 18% with a similarly affected relative, and calculated an overall recurrence risk of 3% for sibs and 5.5% for the offspring of individual cases (Harding et al 1988). These overall risk estimates mask the situation for individual disorders manifesting with abnormalities of the respiratory chain and oxidative phosphorylation systems. It is now possible in some cases to define the defect at the DNA level, providing a more rational basis for counselling. For example, in Kearns–Sayre syndrome (KSS) about 90% of cases can be shown to have deletions of mitochondrial DNA in the tRNA genes detectable using Southern blotting from muscle or brain DNA, but only by more sensitive techniques (such as the polymerase chain reaction) in rapidly dividing tissue such as leucocytes or fibroblasts. Duplications of the mitochondrial genome have also been described in KSS, and large deletions of mitochondrial DNA have also been seen in progressive external ophthalmoplegia alone (Harding 1991). As KSS is almost never familial, these rearrangements of the mitochondrial DNA presumably arise in the mitochondria during oogenesis as a chance event. By contrast, the syndrome encompassing myoclonus, epilepsy and ragged-red fibres (MERRF) appears to follow the expected pattern for maternal inheritance (Wallace et al 1988). A point mutation in the lysine tRNA gene of the mitochondrial genome has been described in several large kindreds with MERRF with heteroplasmy for the mutated mitochondrial DNA species (Harding 1991). Maternal transmission has also been demonstrated in families with mitochondrial myopathy, encephalopathy, lactic acidosis and stroke-like episodes (MELAS) (Lombes et al 1989) and a heteroplasmic point mutation in the leucine tRNA gene has been identified in diverse populations (Moraes et al 1992a). Detectable abnormalities of mitochondrial DNA have also been described in families with autosomal inheritance which may be the result of a nuclear defect in the regulation of mitochondrial DNA replication (Zeviani & DiDonato 1991).

The ability to study the mitochondrial genome has caused a rapid expansion in knowledge about the diverse diseases associated with mitochondrial abnormalities. In any individual case, detailed biochemical and mitochondrial DNA studies of as many family members as possible may be necessary in order to provide reliable genetic counselling.

SPINAL MUSCULAR ATROPHY

The spinal muscular atrophies (SMAs) may be defined as a group of inherited disorders in which the primary defect is degeneration of the anterior horn cells of the spinal cord and often of bulbar motor nuclei, but with no evidence of peripheral nerve or long tract involvement. The classification of these disorders has been the subject of much debate owing to their heterogeneity, and several different classifications have been proposed (Emery 1971, Zerres 1989). Thus SMA has been described presenting at any age with fast or slow progression, with predominantly proximal or distal involvement, inherited as autosomal recessive, dominant or X-linked traits. The difficulties of differentiating between SMA and the muscular dystrophies on the basis of muscle histology and electrophysiology were highlighted by Bradley (Bradley et al 1978), and misdiagnoses have undoubtedly been made. For example, now that specific dystrophin gene and protein abnormalities can be identified, some apparently X-linked and sporadic adult-onset cases of SMA have been shown to be BMD (Clarke et al 1989). Families with diagnosed facioscapulohumeral SMA have been shown to be linked to chromosome 4q, suggesting that in fact they represent cases of FSH muscular dystrophy (Upadhyaya et al 1991). It is likely that even more progress in differentiating SMA and the muscular dystrophies at the molecular level will allow a further revision of the previously proposed classifications.

The best defined group of SMAs is that presenting with proximal weakness and inherited in an autosomal recessive fashion. The incidence of autosomal recessive SMA is approximately 1 in 25 000 live births, with a carrier rate of 1 in 80, making it the second most common recessive disease after cystic fibrosis (Pearn 1973). Even within this group, the great heterogeneity of age of onset and rate of progression has caused much controversy over the relationship of the various disorders (Dubowitz 1991). In order to provide a diagnostic framework for the molecular studies being carried out in SMA, an international SMA collaboration recently published guidelines for diagnosis and classification (Munsat 1991). Thus, diagnosis should be based on symmetrical predominantly proximal weakness of legs more than arms, with trunk involvement and evidence of denervation either on EMG, muscle biopsy or the presence of clinical fasciculations. Within this framework, cases are classified as severe (Type I) if the onset of symptoms is before 6 months of age, the child never sits unaided and death is before the age of 2 years (the pattern of disease frequently referred to as Werdnig–Hoffmann disease). Intermediate cases (Type II) present before the age of 18 months and the child is able to sit unaided, but not stand. Life expectancy depends on the degree of respiratory muscle weakness. In mild SMA (Type III, Kugelberg–Welander disease), the onset of symptoms is later than 18 months and the patient is able to walk unaided. The progression in this group is very variable, but may be very mild, compatible with a normal lifespan. While the clinical course in affected siblings is usually similar, some cases of intrafamilial variability have been decribed (Dubowitz 1991). Linkage analysis in pedigrees with all three forms of recessive SMA has demonstrated linkage to chromosome 5q11.2–13.3 (Gilliam et al 1990, Davies et al 1991), with no evidence to suggest a second locus once cases with features incompatible with a strict diagnosis of SMA were excluded (Dubowitz 1991). When families with different forms of SMA in the same sibship were analysed using probes from this area, there was evidence to suggest that the variation in severity may not be due to the inheritance of different alleles at the SMA locus (Muller et al 1992), suggesting that either the influence of a different gene or non-genetic factors were responsible for the variation in severity in these families.

The identification of closely linked and flanking markers has made it possible to offer prenatal diagnosis to a couple with a previously affected child, providing a sample is available from that child (Daniels et al 1992a,b). However, until the identification of the gene involved and the disease-associated mutations, care must be taken to incorporate the risk of potential misdiagnoses (particularly in the milder forms of SMA) or the possibility of other modes of inheritance before offering prenatal diagnosis in a small family (Muller & Clerget-Darpoux 1991, Daniels et al 1992a).

Though rare, dominantly inherited SMA shows a similar spectrum of disease severity to the recessive form, also with some evidence for intrafamilial variability (Rietschel et al 1992), and cannot be distinguished in an isolated case. The dominant form of the disease is not linked to chromosome 5q (Kausch et al 1991b).

While some cases of previously designated X-linked SMA are now known to be cases of BMD, the gene for a distinct form of X-linked SMA has been identified. In this form of SMA (Kennedy's disease), there is an adult onset of proximal weakness and wasting, together with bulbar weakness. The additional features of gynaecomastia and occasionally testicular atrophy and reduced fertility suggested decreased end-organ responsiveness to androgen, and through a combination of linkage analysis (Fischbeck et al 1986) and candidate gene studies (Fischbeck et al 1991) the defect in this condition has been localised to the androgen receptor gene (La Spada et al 1991). As with myotonic dystrophy, the nature of the mutation appears to be expansion of a trinucleotide repeat, but unlike myotonic dystrophy, there is no expansion of the repeat with its transmission, and the repeat is within the coding sequence of the gene (Richards & Sutherland 1992).

CONCLUSIONS

The continuing explosion of knowledge about the molecular basis of many of the inherited neuromuscular diseases is leading to an ever-expanding range of tests available for diagnosis, carrier detection and prenatal diagnosis. A major lesson of these rapid advances is that investigations are becoming more sophisticated all the time and even where no information about the molecular background of a disease is available at the time of seeing a patient, DNA should be stored if there is any likelihood of the patient or his family requiring counselling in the future. The availability of such specific analyses is not without some problems, in particular in relation to the ethical issues involved in the testing of children for adult-onset diseases, and these issues remain the subject of debate.

REFERENCES

Abbs S , Yau S C, Clark S, Mathew C G, Bobrow M 1991 A convenient multiplex PCR system for the detection of dystrophin gene deletions. A comparative analysis with cDNA hybridisation shows mistyping by both methods. Journal of Medical Genetics 28: 304

Abbs S, Bobrow M 1992 Analysis of quantitative PCR for the diagnosis of deletion and duplication carriers in the dystrophin gene. Journal of Medical Genetics 29: 191

Abdalla J A, Casley W L, Cousin H K et al 1992a Linkage of autosomal dominant myotonia congenita (Thomsen's disease) to the TCRB gene locus on chromosome 7q35. Neurology 42: 1426 (abstract)

Abdalla J A, Casley W L, Hudson A J et al 1992b Linkage analysis of candidate loci in autosomal dominant myotonia congenita. Neurology 42: 1561

Acsadi G, Dickson G, Love D et al 1991 Human dystrophin expression in mdx mice after intramuscular injection of DNA constructs. Nature 352: 815

Arikawa E, Hoffmann E P, Kaido M, Nonaka I, Sugita H, Arahata K 1991a The frequency of patients with dystrophin abnormalities in a limb-girdle patient population. Neurology 41: 1491

Arikawa E, Ishihara T, Nonaka I, Sugita H, Arahata K 1991b Immunocytochemical analysis of dystrophin in congenital muscular dystrophy. Journal of the Neurological Sciences 105: 79

Aslandis C, Jansen G, Amemiya C et al 1992 Cloning of the essential myotonic dystrophy region and mapping of the putative defect. Nature 355: 548

Bakker E, Van Broeckhoven C, Bontane J, Van de Vooren M J, Veanema H 1987 Germline mosaicism and Duchenne muscular dystrophy mutations. Nature 329: 55

Ball S P, Johnson K J 1993 The genetics of malignant hyperthermia. Journal of Medical Genetics 30: 89

Becker P E, Kiener F 1955 Eine neue X-chromosome muskeldystrophie. Archive fur Psychiatrie und Nervenkrankheiten 193: 427

Beckmann J S, Richard I, Hillaire D et al 1991 A gene for limb-girdle muscular dystrophy maps to chromosome 15 by linkage. Comptes Rendus de l'Academie de Science Paris 312: 141

Beggs A M, Koenig M, Boyce F M, Kunkel L M 1990 Detection of 98% of DMD/BMD gene deletions by polymerase chain reaction. Human Genetics 86: 45

Beggs A H, Neumann P E, Arahata K et al 1992 Possible influences on the expression of X chromosome-linked dystrophin abnormalities by heterozygosity for autosomal recessive Fukuyama congenital muscular dystrophy. Proceedings of the National Academy of Science USA 89: 623

Bejjani B, Finn P, Milunsky A, Amos J 1991 The value of deletion analysis for carrier detection in Duchenne muscular dystrophy (DMD). Clinical Genetics 39: 245

Ben Hamida M, Fardeau M, Attia N 1983 Severe childhood muscular dystrophy affecting both sexes and frequent in Tunisia. Muscle and Nerve 6: 469

Ben Othmane K, Ben Hamida M, Pericak-Vance M A et al

1992 Linkage of Tunisian autosomal recessive Duchenne-like muscular dystrophy to the pericentromeric region of chromosome 13q. Nature Genetics 2: 315

Bethlem J, Van Wijngaarden G K 1976 Benign myopathy with autosomal dominant inheritance: a report of three pedigrees. Brain 99: 91

Boyd Y, Buckle V J 1986 Cytogenetic heterogeneity of translocations associated with Duchenne muscular dystrophy. Clinical Genetics 29: 108

Bradley W G, Jones M Z, Mussini J M, Fawcett P R W 1978 Becker-type muscular dystrophy. Muscle and Nerve 1: 111

Brook J D, McCurrach M E, Harley H G et al 1992 Molecular basis of myotonic dystrophy: expansion of a trinucleotide (CTG) repeat at the 3' end of a transcript encoding a protein kinase family member. Cell 68: 799

Brooke M, Fenichel G, Griggs R et al 1983 Clinical investigation in Duchenne dystrophy: 2. Determination of the 'power' of therapeutic trials based on the natural history. Muscle and Nerve 6: 91

Brownell A K W 1988 Malignant hyperthermia: relationship to other diseases. British Journal of Anaesthetics 60: 303

Bulman D E, Gangopadhyay S B, Bebchuck K G, Worton R G, Ray P N 1991 Point mutation in the human dystrophin gene: identification through Western blot analysis. Genomics 10: 457

Bushby K 1992a Report on the 12th ENMC sponsored international workshop — the 'limb-girdle' muscular dystrophies. Neuromuscular Disorders 2: 3

Bushby K M D 1992b Genetic and clinical correlations of Xp21 muscular dystrophy. Journal of Inherited Metabolic Disease 15: 551

Bushby K M D, Thambyayah M, Gardner-Medwin D 1991 Prevalence and incidence of Becker muscular dystrophy. Lancet 337: 1022

Bushby K, Gardner-Medwin D, Nicholson L et al 1993a The clinical, genetic and dystrophin characteristics of Becker muscular dystrophy. 2: Correlation of phenotype with genetic and protein abnormalities. Journal of Neurology 240: 98

Bushby K, Goodship J A, Nicholson L V B, Johnson M A, Haggerty I D, Gardner-Medwin D 1993b Variability in clinical, genetic and protein abnormalities in manifesting carriers of Duchenne and Becker muscular dystrophy. Neuromuscular Disorders 3:57

Bushby K, Gardner-Medwin D 1993 The clinical, genetic and dystrophin characteristics of Becker muscular dystrophy. 1. Natural History. Journal of Neurology 240: 105

Buxton J, Shelbourne P, Davies J et al 1992 Detection of an unstable fragment of DNA specific to individuals with myotonic dytrophy. Nature 355: 547

Cavanagh N P C, Lake B D, McMeniman P 1979 Congenital fibre type disproportion myopathy. Archives of Disease in Childhood 54: 735

Chakrabarti A, Pearce J M S 1981 Scapuloperoneal syndrome with cardiomyopathy: report of a family with autosomal dominant inheritance and unusual features. Journal of Neurology, Neurosurgery and Psychiatry 44: 1146

Chamberlain J S, Gibbs R A, Ranvier J E, Nguyen P N, Caskey C T 1988 Deletion screening of the Duchenne muscular dystrophy locus via multiplex DNA amplification. Nucleic Acids Research 16: 11141

Chitayat D, Hodgkinson K A, Ginsburg O, Dimmick J, Watters G V 1992 King syndrome: a genetically

heterogeneous phenotype due to congenital myopathies. American Journal of Medical Genetics 43: 954

Clarke A, Davies K, Gardner-Medwin D, Burn J, Hudgson P 1989 Xp21 DNA probe in diagnosis of muscular dystrophy and spinal muscular atrophy. Lancet i: 443

Claustres M, Kjellberg P, Desgeorges M, Bellet H, Demaille J 1990 Germinal mosaicism from grand-paternal origin in a family with Duchenne muscular dystrophy. Human Genetics 86: 241

Clerk A, Rodillo E, Heckmatt J, Dubowitz V, Strong P N, Sewry C A 1991 Characterisation of dystrophin in carriers of Duchenne muscular dystrophy. Journal of the Neurological Sciences 102: 917

Cockburn D J, Miciak A 1992 Accurate carrier detection for Duchenne muscular dystrophy (DMD) by pulsed field gel electrophoresis. Clinical Cytogenetics Bulletin 2(6): 16 (abstract)

Collins F S 1992 Positional cloning: let's not call it reverse anymore. Nature Genetics 1: 3

Connor J M, Evans D A P 1982 Genetic aspects of fibrodysplasia ossificans progressiva. Journal of Medical Genetics 19: 35

Daniels R J, Suthers G K, Morrison K E et al 1992a Prenatal prediction of spinal muscular atrophy. Journal of Medical Genetics 29: 165

Daniels R J, Thomas N H, MacKinnon R N et al 1992b Linkage analysis of spinal muscular atrophy. Genomics 12: 335

Davies K E, Smith T J, Bundey S et al 1988 Mild and severe muscular dystrophy associated with deletions in Xp21 of the human X chromosome. Journal of Medical Genetics 25: 9

Davies K E, Thomas N H, Daniels R J, Dubowitz V 1991 Molecular studies of spinal muscular atrophy. Neuromuscular Disorders 1: 83

de Coster W, de Reuck J, Thiery E 1974 A late onset autosomal dominant form of limb-girdle muscular dystrophy. European Neurology 12: 159

De Angelis M S, Palmucci L, Leone M, Doriguzzi C 1991 Centronuclear myopathy: clinical, morphological and genetic characters. A review of 288 cases. Journal of the Neurological Sciences 103: 2

Deufel T, Golla A, Iles D et al 1992 Evidence for genetic heterogeneity of malignant hyperthermia susceptibility. Amerian Journal of Human Genetics 50: 1151

Donner M, Rapola J, Somer H 1975 Congenital muscular dystrophy: a clinicopathological and follow-up study of 15 patients. Neuropadiatrie 6: 239

Dubowitz V 1963 Myopathic changes in muscular dystrophy carriers. Proceedings of the Royal Society of Medicine 56: 810

Dubowitz V 1978 Muscle disorders in childhood. Saunders, London

Dubowitz V 1991 Chaos in classification of the spinal muscular atrophies of childhood. Neuromuscular Disorders 1: 77

Duchenne G B 1868 Recherches sur la paralysie musculaire pseudohypertrophique ou paralysie myo-sclérosique. Archives Générales de Médecine 11: 5

Emery A E H 1965 Carrier detection in sex-linked muscular dystrophy. Journal de Genetique Humaine 14: 318

Emery A E H 1971 The nosology of the spinal muscular atrophies. Journal of Medical Genetics 8: 481

Emery A E H 1989 Emery–Dreifuss muscular dystrophy. Journal of Medical Genetics 26: 367

Emery A E H 1991 Population frequencies of inherited

neuromuscular diseases — A World Survey. Neuromuscular Disorders 1: 19

Emery A E H 1993 Duchenne Muscular Dystrophy, 2nd edn. Oxford Medical Publications

Emery A E H, Skinner R 1976 Clinical studies in benign (Becker-type) X-linked muscular dystrophy. Clinical Genetics 10: 189

Emery A E H, Holloway S 1982 Familial motor neuron diseases. In: Rowland L P (ed) Human motor neuron diseases. Raven, New York, p 139

Emery A E H, Emery M 1993 Edward Meryon (1809–1880) and muscular dystrophy. Journal of Medical Genetics 30: 506

Engel W K, Cunningham G G 1963 Rapid examination of muscle tissue: an improved trichrome stain method for fresh-frozen biopsy sections. Neurology 13: 919

Fenichel G M, Sul Y C, Kilroy A W, Blouin R 1982 An autosomal dominant dystrophy with humeropelvic distribution and cardiomyopathy. Neurology 32: 1399

Fischbeck K H, Ionasescu V, Ritter A W et al 1986 Localisation of the gene for X-linked spinal muscular atrophy. Neurology 36: 1595

Fischbeck K H, Souders D, LaSpada A 1991 A candidate gene for X-linked spinal muscular atrophy. Advances in Neurology 56: 209

Fontaine B, Khurana T S, Hoffman E P et al 1990 Hyperkalemic periodic paralysis and the adult muscle sodium channel α-subunit gene. Science 250: 1000

Fontaine B, Trofatter J, Rouleau G A et al 1991 Different gene loci for hyperkalemic and hypokalemic periodic paralysis. Neuromuscular Disorders 1: 235

Fukuyama Y, Osawa M, Suzuki H 1981 Congenital progressive muscular dystrophy of the Fukuyama type: clinical, genetic and pathological considerations. Brain and Development 6: 373

Gardner-Medwin D 1968 Studies of the carrier state in the Duchenne type of muscular dystrophy 2. Quantitative electromyography as a method of carrier detection. Journal of Neurology, Neurosurgery and Psychiatry 31: 124

Gardner-Medwin D, Pennington R J, Walton J N 1971 The detection of carriers of X-linked muscular dystrophy. A review of some methods studied in Newcastle upon Tyne. Journal of the Neurological Sciences 13: 459

Gardner-Medwin D, Sharples P 1989 Some studies of the Duchenne and autosomal recessive types of muscular dystrophy. Brain and Development 11: 91

George A L, Crackower M A, Abdalla J A, Hudson A J, Ebers G C 1993 Molecular basis of Thomsen's disease (autosomal dominant myotonia congenita). Nature Genetics 3: 305

Gerdes A, Peterson M, Schroder H, Wulf K, Brondum-Nielson K 1992 Congenital myopathy with fibre-type disproportion: a family with a chromosomal translocation t(10;17) may indicate candidate gene regions. Journal of Medical Genetics 30: 348

Gilbert J R, Stajich J M, Wall S et al 1993 Evidence for heterogeneity in facioscapulohumeral muscular dystrophy. American Journal of Human Genetics 53: 401

Gilchrist J M, Pericak-Vance M A, Silverman L, Roses A D 1988 Clinical and genetic investigation in autosomal dominant limb-girdle muscular dystrophy. Neurology 38: 5

Gillard E F, Otsu K, Fuji J et al 1991 A substitution of cysteine for arginine 614 in the ryanodine receptor is potentially causative of human malignant hyperthermia. Genomics 11: 751

Gilliam T C, Brzustowicz L M, Castilla L H et al 1990 Genetic homogeneity between acute and chronic forms of spinal muscular atrophy. Nature 345: 823

Ginjaar I B, Soffers S, Moorman A F M et al 1991 Fetal dystrophin to diagnose carrier status. Lancet 338: 257

Gospe S M, Lazaro R P, Lava N S, Grootscholten P M, Scott A B, Fischbeck K H 1989 Familial X-linked myalgia and cramps: a non-progressive myopathy associated with a deletion in the dystrophin gene. Neurology 39: 1277

Grimm T, Muller B, Muller C R, Janka M 1990 Theoretical considerations on germline mosaicism in Duchenne muscular dystrophy. Journal of Medical Genetics 27: 683

Hanson P A, Rowland L P 1971 Mobius syndrome and facioscapulohumeral muscular dystrophy. Archives of Neurology 24: 31

Harding A E 1991 Neurological disease and mitochondrial genes. Trends in Neurosciences 14: 132

Harding A E, Petty R K H, Morgan-Hughes J A 1988 Mitochondrial myopathy: a genetic study of 71 cases. Journal of Medical Genetics 25: 528

Harley H G, Brook J D, Rundle S A et al 1992 Expansion of an unstable DNA region and phenotypic variation in myotonic dystrophy. Nature 355: 545

Harper P S, Dyken P R 1972 Early-onset dystrophia myotonica: evidence supporting a maternal environmental factor. Lancet ii: 53

Harper P S, Harley H G, Reardon W, Shaw D J 1992 Review article: anticipation in myotonic dystrophy: new light on an old problem. American Journal of Human Genetics 51: 10

Heckmatt J Z, Sewry C A, Hodes D, Dubowitz V 1985 Congenital centronuclear (myotubular) myopathy. Brain 108: 941

Heckmatt J Z, Dubowitz V 1990 Congenital myopathies (including glycogenoses). In: Emery A E H, Rimion D L (eds) Principles and practice of medical genetics. Churchill Livingstone, Edinburgh, p 513

Hoffman E P, Brown R H, Kunkel L M 1987 Dystrophin: the protein product of the Duchenne muscular dystrophy locus. Cell 51: 919

Hoffman E P, Arahata K, Minetti C, Bonilla E, Rowland L P, and 47 co-authors 1992 Dystrophinopathy in isolated cases of myopathy in females. Neurology 42: 967

Hunziker U A, Savoldelli G, Bolthauser E, Giedion A, Schinzel A 1989 Prenatal diagnosis of Shwartz–Jampel syndrome with early manifestations. Prenatal Diagnosis 9: 127

Iaizzo P A, Franke C, Hatt H et al 1991 Altered sodium channel behaviour causes myotonia in dominantly inherited myotonia congenita. Neuromuscular Disorders 1: 47

Jackson C E, Carey J H 1961 Progressive muscular dystrophy: autosomal recessive type. Pediatrics 28: 77

Jackson C E, Strehler D A 1968 Limb-girdle muscular dystrophy: clinical manifestations and detection of preclinical disease. Pediatrics 41: 495

Jansen G, Mahadevan M, Amemiya C et al 1992 Characterisation of the myotonic dystrophy region predicts multiple protein isoform-encoding mRNAs. Nature Genetics 1: 261

Jones R, Khan R, Hughes S, Dubowitz V 1979 Congenital muscular dystrophy: the importance of early diagnosis and orthopaedic management in the long term prognosis. Journal of Bone and Joint Surgery 61B: 13

Kausch K, Lehmann-Horn F, Janka M, Wieringa B, Grimm T, Muller C R 1991a Evidence for linkage of the central core disease locus to the proximal long arm of human chromosome 19. Genomics 10: 765

Kausch K, Muller C R, Grimm T et al 1991b No evidence for linkage of autosomal dominant proximal spinal muscular atrophies to chromosome 5q markers. Human Genetics 86: 317

Kingston H M, Thomas N S T, Pearson P L, SarFarabi M, Hoper P S 1983 Genetic linkage between Becker muscular dystrophy and a polymorphic DNA sequence on the short arm of the X chromosome. Journal of Medical Genetics 20: 255

Koch M C, Grimm T, Harley H G, Harper P S 1991a Genetic risks for children of women with myotonic dystrophy. American Journal of Human Genetics 48: 1084

Koch M C, Ricker K, Otto M et al 1991b Confirmation of linkage of hyperkalaemic periodic paralysis to chromosome 17. Journal of Medical Genetics 28: 583

Koch M C, Steinmeyer K, Lorenz C et al 1992 The skeletal muscle chloride channel in dominant and recessive human myotonia. Science 257: 797

Koenig M, Hoffman E P, Bertelson C J, Monaco A P, Feener C, Kunkel L M 1987 Complete cloning of the Duchenne muscular dystrophy (DMD) cDNA and preliminary genomic organization of the DMD gene in normal and affected individuals. Cell 50: 509

Laing N G, Majda B T, Akkari P A et al 1992 Assignment of a gene (NEM1) for autosomal dominant nemaline myopathy to chromosome 1. American Journal of Human Genetics 50: 576

La Spada A R, Wilson E M, Lubahn D B, Harding A E, Fischbeck K H 1991 Androgen receptor gene mutations in X-linked spinal and bulbar muscular atrophy. Nature 352: 77

Lehmann-Horn F, Rudel R, Ricker K 1987a Membrane defects in parmyotonia congenita (Eulenburg). Muscle and Nerve 10: 633

Lehmann-Horn F, Kuther G, Ricker K 1987b Adynamia episodica hereditaria with myotonia: a non-inactivating sodium current and the effect of extra-cellular pH. Muscle and Nerve 10: 363

Lehmann-Horn F, Iaizzo P A, Franke C, Hatt H, Spaans F 1990 Schwartz–Jampel syndrome: 11. Na^+ channel defect causes myotonia. Muscle and Nerve 13: 528

Lehmann-Horn F, Rudel R, Ricker K 1993 Workshop Report: non-dystrophic myotonias and periodic paralyses. Neuromusular Disorders 3: 161

Levitt R C, Nouri N, Jedlicka A E et al 1991 Evidence for genetic heterogeneity in malignant hyperthermia susceptibility. Genomics 11: 543

Leyton Q H, Renkawek K, Renier W O et al 1991 Neuropathological findings in muscle-eye-brain disease (MEB-D). Neuropathological delineation of MEB-D from congenital muscular dystrophy of the Fukuyama type. Acta Neuropathologica 83: 55

Lipicky R J 1979 Myotonic syndromes other than myotonic dystrophy. In: Vinken P J, Bruyn G W (eds) Handbook of clinical neurology, vol 40. Elsevier, Amsterdam, p 533

Lombes A, Bonilla E, Dimauro S 1989 Mitochondrial Encephalomyopathies. Revue Neurologique 145: 671

Luft R, Ikkos D, Palmieri G 1962 A case of severe hypermetabolism of nonthyroid origin with a defect in the maintenance of mitochondrial respiratory control: a correlated clinical, biochemical and morphological study. Journal of Clinical Investigation 41: 1776

Lunt P W, Harper P S 1991 Genetic counselling in facioscapulohumeral muscular dystrophy. Journal of Medical Genetics 28: 655

Lyon M F 1962 Sex chromatin and gene action in the mammalian X-chromosome. American Journal of Human Genetics 14: 135

Maclennan D H, Duff C, Zorzato F et al 1990 Ryanodine receptor gene is a candidate for predisposition to malignant hyperthermia. Nature 343: 559

Maclennan D H, Phillips M S 1992 Malignant hyperthermia. Science 256: 789

Mahjneh I, Vanelli G, Bushby K, Marconi GP 1993 A large inbred Palestinian family with two forms of muscular dystrophy. Neuromuscular Disorders 2: 277

Malcolm S 1992 Charcot–Marie–Tooth disease type 1. Journal of Medical Genetics 29: 3

Mao Y, Cremer M 1989 Detection of Duchenne muscular dystrophy carriers by dosage analysis using the DMD cDNA clone 8. Human Genetics 81: 193

McCarthy V T, Healy S J M, Heffron J J A et al 1990 Localisation of the malignant hyperthermia susceptibility locus to human chromosome 19q12–13.2. Nature 343: 562

McClatchey A I, Trofatter J, McKenna-Yasek D et al 1992 Dinucleotide repeat polymorphisms at the SCN4A locus suggest allelic heterogeneity of hyperkalemic periodic paralysis and paramyotonia congenita. American Journal of Human Genetics 50: 896

Marconi G, Pizzi A, Arimondi C G, Vanelli B 1991 Limb-girdle muscular dystrophy with autosomal dominant inheritance. Acta Neurologica Scandinavica 83: 234

Matsumura K, Tomé F, Collin H et al 1992 Deficiency of the 50 K dystrophin-associated glycoprotein in severe childhood autosomal recessive muscular dystrophy. Nature 359: 320

Matsumura K, Nonaka I, Campbell K 1993 Abnormal expression of dystrophin-associated proteins in Fukuyama-type congenital muscular dystrophy. Lancet 341: 521

Meryon E 1852 On granular and fatty degeneration of the voluntary muscles. Transaction of the Medical and Chirugical Society of London 35: 73

Miller G, Ladda R L, Towfighi J 1991 Cerebro-ocular dysplasia — muscular dystrophy (Walker-Warburg) syndrome. Findings in 20-week fetus. Acta Neuropathologica 82: 234

Monaco A P, Bertelson C J, Liechti-Gallati S, Moser H, Kunkel L M 1988 An explanation for the phenotypic differences between patients bearing partial deletions of the DMD locus. Genomics 2: 90

Moraes C T, Ricci E, Bonilla E, Dimauro S, Schon E A 1992a The mitochondrial tRNA mutation in mitochondrial encephalomyopathy, lactic acidosis and stroke like episodes (MELAS): genetic, biochemical, and morphological correlations in skeletal muscle. American Journal of Human Genetics 50: 934

Moraes C T, Ricci E, Petruzzella V et al 1992b Molecular analysis of the muscle pathology associated with mitochondrial DNA deletions. Nature Genetics 1: 359

Moser H, Emery A E H 1974 The manifesting carrier in Duchenne muscular dystrophy. Clinical Genetics 5: 271

Muller B, Melki J, Burlet P, Clerget-Darpoux F 1992 Proximal spinal muscular atrophy (SMA) types II and III in the same sibship are not caused by different alleles at the SMA locus on 5q. American Journal of Human Genetics 50: 892

Muller B, Clerget-Darpoux F 1991 Becker's model and prenatal diagnosis in proximal spinal muscular atrophy: a note of caution. American Journal of Human Genetics 49: 238

Multicentre study group. 1992 Diagnosis of Duchenne and Becker muscular dystrophies by polymerase chain reaction. Journal of the American Medical Association 267: 2609

Munsat T L 1991 Workshop report — international SMA collaboration. Neuromuscular Disorders 1: 81

Nicholson L V B, Davison K, Falkous G et al 1989a Dystrophin in skeletal muscle: I. Western blot analysis using a monoclonal antibody. Journal of the Neurological Sciences 94: 125

Nicholson L V B, Davison K, Johnson M A et al 1989b Dystrophin in skeletal muscle: II. Immunoreactivity in patients with Xp21 muscular dystrophy. Journal of the Neurological Sciences 94: 137

Nicholson L V B, Bushby K M D, Johnson M A, Den Dunnen J T, Ginjaar I B, Van Ommen G J B 1992 Predicted and observed sizes of dystrophin in some patients with deletions that disrupt the open reading frame. Journal of Medical Genetics 29: 892

Nicholson L V B, Johnson M A, Bushby K, Gardner-Medwin D 1993 The functional significance of dystrophin-positive fibres in Duchenne muscular dystrophy. Archives of Disease in Childhood 68: 632

Nihei K, Kamoshita S, Atsumi T 1979 A case of Ullrich's disease. Brain and Development 1: 61

Nogen A G 1980 Congenital muscle disease and abnormal findings on computerised tomography. Developmental Medicine and Child Neurology 22: 658

Nonaka I, Sunohara N, Satayoshi E, Terasawa K, Yonemoto K 1985 Autosomal recessive distal muscular dystrophy: a comparative study with distal myopathy with rimmed vacuole formation. Annals of Neurology 17: 52

Nordenskjöld M, Nicholson L V B, Edström L et al 1990 A normal male with an inherited deletion of one exon within the DMD gene. Human Genetics 84: 207

Norman A M, Harper P S 1989 A survey of manifesting carriers of Duchenne and Becker muscular dystrophy in Wales. Clinical Genetics 36: 31

Norman A M, Hughes H E, Gardner-Medwin D, Nicholson L V B 1989 Dystrophin analysis in the diagnosis of muscular dystrophy. Archives of Disease in Childhood 64: 1501

Norman A M, Thomas N S T, Kingston H M, Harper P S 1990 Becker muscular dystrophy: correlation of deletion type with clinical severity. Journal of Medical Genetics 27: 236

Ording H 1988 Diagnosis of susceptibility to malignant hyperthermia in man. British Journal of Anaesthesia 60: 287

Paljarvi L, Kalimo H, Lang H, Savontaus M-L, Sonninen V 1987 Minicore myopathy with dominant inheritance. Journal of the Neurological Sciences 77: 11

Partridge T A 1991 Invited review: myoblast transfer: a possible therapy for inherited myopathies? Muscle and Nerve 14: 197

Passos-Bueno M R, Vainzof M, de Cassia R et al 1991 Limb-girdle syndrome: a genetic study of 22 large Brazilian families. Comparison with X-linked Duchenne and Becker muscular dystrophies. Journal of the Neurological Sciences 103: 65

Passos-Bueno M R, Bakker E, Kneppers A L J et al 1993 Different mosaicism frequencies for proximal and distal Duchenne muscular dystrophy mutations indicate diference in etiology and recurrence risk. American Journal of Human Genetics 51: 1150

Pearn J H 1973 The gene frequency of acute Werdnig–Hoffman disease (SMA type I): a total population survey in north-east England. Journal of Medical Genetics 10: 260

Penegyres P K, Kakulas B A 1991 The natural history of minicore-multicore myopathy. Muscle and Nerve 14: 411

Petty R K H, Harding A E, Morgan-Hughes J A 1986 The clinical features of mitochondrial myopathy. Brain 109: 915

Ptacek L J, Tyler F, Trimmer J S, Agnew W S, Leppert M 1991 Analysis in a large hyperkalemic periodic paralysis pedigree supports tight linkage to a sodium channel locus. American Journal of Human Genetics 49: 378

Richards R I, Sutherland G R 1992 Heritable unstable DNA sequences. Nature Genetics 1: 7

Ried T, Mahler V, Vogt P et al 1990 Direct carrier detection by in situ hybridization with cosmid clones of the Duchenne/Becker muscular dystrophy locus. Human Genetics 85: 581

Rietschel M, Rudnik-Schoneborn S, Zerres K 1992 Clinical variability of autosomal dominant spinal muscular atrophy. Journal of the Neurological Sciences 107: 65

Roberts R G, Bentley D R, Barby T F M, Manners E, Bobrow M 1990 Direct diagnosis of carriers of Duchenne and Becker muscular dystrophy by amplification of lymphocyte RNA. Lancet 336: 1523

Roberts R G, Bobrow M, Bentley D R 1992a Point mutations in the dystrophin gene. Proceedings of the National Academy of Science USA 89: 2331

Roberts R G, Coffey A J, Bobrow M, Bentley D R 1992b Determination of the exon structure of the distal portion of the dystrophin gene by vectorette PCR. Genomics 13: 942

Rojas C V, Wang J, Schwartz L S, Hoffman E P, Powell B R, Brown R H 1991 A Met-to-Val mutation in the skeletal muscle Na^+ channel α-subunit in hyperkalaemic periodic paralysis. Nature 354: 387

Roses M S, Nicholson M T, Kircher C S, Roses A D 1977 Evaluation and detection of Duchenne's and Becker's muscular dystrophy carriers by manual muscle testing. Neurology 27: 20

Rudel R 1986 The pathophysiologic basis of the myotonias and the periodic paralyses. In: Engel A G, Banker Q (eds) Myology. McGraw-Hill, New York, p 1297

Rudel R, Lehmann-Horn F, Ricker K 1984 Hypokalaemic periodic paralysis: in vitro investigation of muscle fibre membrane parameters. Muscle and Nerve 7: 110

Rudel R, Ricker K, Lehmann-Horn F 1988 Transient weakness and altered membrane characteristic in recessive generalized myotonia (Becker). Muscle and Nerve 11: 202

Speer M C, Yamaoka L H, Gilchrist J H et al 1992 Confirmation of genetic heterogeneity in limb-girdle muscular dystrophy: linkage of an autosomal dominant form to chromosome 5q. American Journal of Humen Genetics 50: 1211

Starr J, Lamont M, Iselius L, Harvey J, Heckmatt J 1990 A linkage study of a large pedigree with X-linked centronuclear myopathy. Journal of Medical Genetics 27: 281

Tachi N, Tachi M, Sasaki K, Imamura S 1989 Early-onset benign autosomal dominant limb-girdle myopathy with contractures (Bethlem myopathy). Pediatric Neurology 5: 232

Thomas P K, Schott G D, Morgan-Hughes J A 1975 Adult onset scapuloperoneal myopathy. Journal of Neurology, Neurosurgery and Psychiatry 38: 1008

Tsilfidis C, MacKenzie A E, Mettler G, Barcelo J,

Korneluk R G 1992 Correlation between CTG trinucleotide repeat length and frequency of severe congenital myotonic dystrophy. Nature Genetics 1: 192

Udd B, Kaarianen H, Somer H 1991 Muscular dystrophy with separate clinical phenotypes in a large family. Muscle and Nerve 14: 1050

Upadhyaya M, Lunt P W, Sarfarazi M et al 1991 A closely linked DNA marker for facioscapulohumeral disease on chromosome 4q. Journal of Medical Genetics 28: 665

Vainzof M, Pavanello R C M, Pavanello-Filho I et al 1991 Screening of male patients with autosomal recessive Duchenne dystrophy through dystrophin and DNA testing. American Journal of Medical Genetics 39: 38

Van der Does de Willebois A/EM, Bethlem J, Meijer A E F H, Simons A J R 1968 Distal myopathy with onset in early infancy. Neurology 18: 383

Van Essen A J, Abbs S, Bauget M et al 1992 Parental origin and germline mosaicism of deletions and duplications of the dystrophin gene: a European study. Human Genetics 88: 249

Vanier T M 1960 Dystrophia myotonica in childhood. British Medical Journal 2: 1284

Vijoen D, Peighton P 1992 Schwartz–Jampel syndrome (chondrodystrophic myotonia). Journal of Medical Genetics 29: 58

Wallace D C, Zheng Z, Lott M T et al 1988 Familial mitochondrial encephalomyopathy (MERRF): genetic, pathophysiological and biochemical characterisation of a mitochondrial DNA disease. Cell 55: 601

Wallgren-Petterson C, Kaariainen H, Rapola J, Salmi T, Jaaskelainen J, Donner M 1990 Genetics of congenital nemaline myopathy: a study of 10 families. Journal of Medical Genetics 27: 480

Walton J N 1955 On the inheritance of muscular dystrophy. Annals of Human Genetics 20: 1

Walton J N, Nattrass F J 1954 On the classification, natural history, and treatment of the myopathies. Brain 77: 169

Weiffenbach B, Dubois J, Storvick D et al 1993. Mapping the facioscapulohumeral muscular dystrophy gene is complicated by chromosome 4q35 recombination events. Nature Genetics 4: 165

Weissenbach J, Gyapay G, Dib C et al 1992 A second-generation linkage map of the human genome. Nature 359: 794

Welander L 1951 Myopathia distalis tarda hereditaria. Acta Medica Scandinavica 264 (suppl. 1): 1

Welander L 1957 Homozygous appearance of distal myopathy. Acta Geneticae Medicae et Gemellologiae 7: 321

Wijmenga C, Frants R R, Brouwer O F, Moerer P, Padberg G W 1990 The facioscapulohumeral muscular dystrophy gene maps to chromosome 4. Lancet ii: 651

Wijmenga C, Hewitt J E, Sandkuijl L A et al 1992 Chromosome 4q DNA rearrangements associated with facioscapulohumeral muscular dystrophy. Nature Genetics 2: 26

Witt N, Garner C G, Pongratz D, Baur X 1988 Autosomal dominant Emery–Dreifuss syndrome: evidence of a neurogenic variant of the disease. European Archives of Psychiatry and the Neurological Sciences 237: 230

Yates J R W 1991 Workshop report — European workshop on Emery–Dreifuss muscular dystrophy. Neuromuscular Disorders 1: 393

Yates J R W, Emery A E H 1985 A population study of adult onset limb-girdle muscular dystrophy. Journal of Medical Genetics 22: 250

Young I 1991 Risk calculation in genetic counselling. Oxford Medical Publications, Oxford

Young K, Foroud T, Williams P et al 1992 Confirmation of linkage of limb-girdle muscular dystrophy, type 2, to chromosome 15. Genomics 13: 1370

Zatz M, Rapaport D, Vainzof M et al 1991 Serum creatine-kinase (CK) and pyruvate kinase (PK) activities in Duchenne (DMD) as compared with Becker (BMD) muscular dystrophy. Journal of the Neurological Sciences 102: 190

Zerres K 1989 Klassification und genetik spinaler muskelatrophien. Georg Thieme Verlag, Stuttgart

Zeviani M 1992 Nucleus-driven mutations of human mitochondrial DNA. Journal of Inherited Metabolic Diseases 15: 456

Zeviani M, DiDonato S 1991 Neurological disorders due to mutations of the mitochondrial genome. Neuromuscular Disorders 1: 165

27. The clinical features of some miscellaneous neuromuscular disorders

D. Hilton-Jones

INTRODUCTION

This chapter covers a diverse range of disorders with neuromuscular manifestations, many of which do not find a ready home elsewhere in the text. Included are conditions affecting the central nervous system, nerve roots, peripheral nerves, and the neuromuscular junction, with secondary effects on skeletal muscle, as well as disorders affecting voluntary muscle directly. Some are rare, others relatively common, but all are important in the differential diagnosis of neuromuscular disorders.

CENTRAL NERVOUS SYSTEM

Tetanus

As a result of active immunisation programmes, tetanus is rare in developed countries, but is still a cause of considerable morbidity and mortality in developing nations, and should be considered an entirely preventable disorder despite occasional reports of disease arising in immunised patients (Crone & Reder 1992).

The spores of *Clostridium tetani* gain access to the body through a wound, typically a dirty cutaneous injury, less commonly in neonates via the umbilical stump, puerperally through the genital tract, during elective surgery or, increasingly commonly, through self-innoculation in drug abusers. In up to one-quarter of cases no source of infection is identified.

At the site of infection a neurotoxin is produced that passes either directly or via the blood stream to skeletal muscle, from where it passes by retrograde transport up motor nerves to gain access to the CNS (Price et al 1975). It is taken up by inhibitory interneurones and blocks the release of inhibitory neurotransmitters, resulting in over-activity of spinal and bulbar motor neurones (Mellanby & Green 1981). Recent evidence suggests that the neurotoxin acts by cleaving synapto-brevin-2, which appears to be a key protein associated with neurotransmitter release (Schiavo et al 1992).

The incubation period is 4–21 days. Trismus, dysphagia, facial spasm and neck stiffness are common early symptoms, focal limb or trunk spasms and cranial nerve palsies less common. In most cases generalised and extremely painful muscle spasms, including respiratory muscle involvement, develop within a few days (Edmondson & Flowers 1979). Most patients need to be paralysed and ventilated, with an average duration of paralysis of 21 days, although a small number with milder disease may be managed with sedation and muscle relaxants (Edmondson & Flowers 1979). Even in experienced hands mortality is about 10%, and attributable to respiratory complications or autonomic disturbance, which may be profound (Kerr et al 1968).

The differential diagnosis includes drug-induced acute dystonic reactions, stiff-man syndrome, tetany and non-organic disease. *Cl. tetani* can be cultured from the wound in about one-quarter of cases. Cerebrospinal fluid examination is normal. Electromyography shows normal but continuous motor unit potential discharges in muscles in spasm.

In addition to supportive management, treatment includes intravenous, and possibly intra-thecal, globulin antitoxin, antibiotic therapy and wound toilet and initiation of a course of active immunisation, for the illness itself does not confer immunity.

The outlook in those who survive is usually good, with psychological sequelae being more common than significant physical disability (Flowers & Edmondson 1980).

Stiff-man syndrome

This extraordinary condition was first described by Moersch & Woltman (1956). Subsequently the literature became somewhat confused with a heterogeneous group of conditions being de-scribed under the same title. Important reviews delineating diagnostic criteria and reassessing earlier reported cases have tidied up some of this confusion, but a precise definition of the disorder will not be possible until its exact pathogenesis has been determined (Gordon et al 1967, Lorish et al 1989, Blum & Jankovic 1991). North American authors in particular have indicated a preference for the term stiff-person syndrome, purportedly to emphasise that females and children may also be affected but perhaps more in response to the current vogue for so-called 'political correctness'.

The disorder is currently defined on the basis of a number of clinical and electrophysiological criteria (Table 27.1). Most cases present in middle adult life and onset in childhood is exceptional. The first symptoms are usually intermittent stiffness and discomfort in axial muscles, but over a period of weeks or months the stiffness becomes more persistent and spreads to the limb-girdle and proximal-limb musculature. Distal limb muscle involvement is less frequent, and usually less severe, and in only a few cases are facial muscles affected. The axial muscle spasms produce spinal deformity, particularly a hyperlordotic posture, and limit neck movement, whilst the shoulder girdle involvement inhibits upper limb movement and the pelvic girdle involvement affects gait, producing a rather characteristic stiff or puppet-like walk. Most distressing to the patient are super-imposed and sometimes extremely painful muscle

Table 27.1   Criteria for diagnosing the stiff-man syndrome

1. *Prodromal* phase of aching and stiffness of axial muscles
2. Slow *progression*, usually symmetrical, of stiffness to involve limb girdle and then upper limb musculature, hindering volitional movements and mobility
3. Superimposed painful *muscle spasms* precipitated by movement, touch, noise and emotion
4. *Spinal* deformity
5. Partial or complete relief of spasms during *sleep*
6. *Physical examination* is normal except for the muscle spasms, spinal deformity, sometimes increased tendon reflexes and disuse atrophy in longstanding cases
7. Normal *cognitive function*
8. Typical *electromyographic* findings
9. Beneficial response, usually, to *diazepam*
10. Abolition of spasms in response to certain *neuromuscular blocking* procedures

After Gordon et al (1967) and Lorish et al (1989).

spasms, occurring either spontaneously or triggered by touch, sound, attempts at passive stretching of a muscle, movements such as chewing, talking or swallowing, and by emotional stimuli. Respiration may be affected by spasms of the respiratory muscles and dysphagia can occur. Paroxysmal autonomic dysfunction may occur in association with muscle spasms and is rarely a cause of sudden death (Mitsumoto et al 1991).

Physical examination is generally normal, excluding the hardness of affected muscles, the muscle spasms, spinal deformity, altered gait and, often, increased tendon reflexes.

Electromyography (EMG) shows continuous motor unit activity in affected muscles, despite all efforts by the patient to place the muscle at rest. The individual motor unit potentials are normal in appearance. The EMG appearance and the muscle stiffness are improved by sleep, general or spinal anaesthesia, peripheral nerve blockade, neuromuscular junction blockade, and intravenous diazepam, all of which point to the abnormal motor activity having a central rather than a peripheral cause.

On experimental and theoretical grounds it is suggested that the stiff-man syndrome is due to a disorder of GABAergic neurones in a descending spinal pathway, arising in the brain stem (Layzer 1988). Neurophysiological studies show gross enhancement of exteroceptive reflexes, quantitation of which may be valuable in monitoring progress and response to therapy (Meinck et al 1984). Further support for the GABAergic neurone hypothesis comes from recent evidence for an autoimmune basis for the syndrome.

The high incidence of serum autoantibodies and of autoimmune diseases, particularly diabetes, in patients with the stiff-man syndrome raises the possibility that it also has an autoimmune aetiology (Blum & Jankovic 1991). Further support for an autoimmune basis comes from the detection of an autoantibody directed against glutamic acid decarboxylase (GAD) in many patients, and the beneficial effects in some patients of plasmapheresis. GAD, responsible for synthesising GABA, is localised to GABAergic neurones. Recent studies have shown a high incidence of GAD autoantibodies in the serum, and sometimes in the CSF, of patients with the syndrome (Solimena et al 1988, Gorin et al 1990, Solimena et al 1990, Brashear & Phillips 1991). It remains uncertain whether the GAD autoantibodies have a direct pathogenetic role, or whether they are an epiphenomenon that arise in response to the release of GAD from its usual intracellular site in response to some other primary pathological process. The high frequency of these antibodies may strongly suggest a primary role, but if so an explanation has to be found for those cases in which autoantibodies are apparently absent.

That plasmapheresis benefits some patients (Vicari et al 1989, Brashear & Phillips 1991) adds further support to an autoimmune basis, and in one patient improvement was shown to be accompanied by a fall in GAD antibody titre (Brashear & Phillips 1991). However, not all patients have responded to plasmapheresis or immunosuppression (Harding et al 1989).

In summary, there is ever-growing, if not overwhelming, evidence for an autoimmune basis for the stiff-man syndrome, but the exact pathogenetic mechanisms remain to be determined. It may be that the clinical criteria currently used still result in our grouping together a heterogeneous population of disorders.

Diazepam is the mainstay of drug treatment and can be very effective, although symptoms are rarely abolished completely and sedation is often a problem at the high doses required. Other benzodiazepines, sodium valproate and baclofen are occasionally helpful. Currently, increasing attention is being given to plasmapheresis and immunosuppressive therapy.

Whilst a number of neurological disorders might superficially be confused with the stiff-man syndrome, careful clinical evaluation should exclude most of them. Conditions that have caused diagnostic confusion include cervical myelopathy with pronounced rigidity, parkinsonian syndromes, Wilson's disease, chronic tetanus, acquired neuromyotonia, myotonia congenita and Hoffman's syndrome.

NERVE ROOTS

Neuralgic amyotrophy

In its most typical form neuralgic amyotrophy is a

readily recognised clinical entity, although of obscure pathogenesis (Parsonage & Turner 1948). Men appear to be more frequently affected than women. The first symptom is pain, often severe, usually unilateral, and increasing in severity over several hours. It is in the shoulder girdle/scapular/upper arm region, infrequently below the elbows. Within a few days weakness develops, most often involving C5/6 innervated muscles, notably deltoid, spinati and serratus anterior, corresponding to involvement of the axillary and suprascapular nerves, and the nerve to serratus anterior. Sensory symptoms and signs are rarely conspicuous. Shortly after the onset of weakness the affected muscles start to atrophy. The pain starts to settle at this stage and has often resolved within a few weeks of the onset of symptoms, although rarely it may continue for much longer. Bilateral clinical involvement is infrequent, and curiously is rarely severe. However, EMG evidence of contralateral involvement and of muscles not clinically affected, is common.

In mild cases recovery occurs in a few weeks but in the majority is much more prolonged, typically over 1–2 years, with about 10% failing to make a complete recovery and with a small number of patients showing very poor recovery.

Even in severe cases cerebrospinal fluid examination is normal. Neurophysiological studies show features of denervation in affected muscles but lack of such changes in paraspinal muscle (Kimura 1983a). These several observations suggest that the main pathological process is in distal motor branches.

There has been much recent interest in what seem to be variants of the disorder described above. It is likely that many patients with mild forms of neuralgic amyotrophy do not reach specialist attention but are diagnosed as having 'a trapped nerve' secondary to degenerative cervical spine disease. In some patients nerves derived from the lower part of the brachial plexus are involved, producing forearm and hand weakness, or more localised lesions such as anterior interosseous or median nerve palsies, or damage to the nerve fibres to pronator teres (England & Sumner 1987). Weakness of an entire upper limb is rare.

Much mention has been made of phrenic nerve involvement and diaphragmatic paralysis. It is not that uncommon, usually unilateral but not always on the same side as the limb paralysis, and rarely causes respiratory embarrassment (Tsairis et al 1972). However, there are exceptions. Gregory et al (1990) described the case of a 40-year-old man with three episodes of shoulder pain, respiratory embarrassment and investigations suggesting isolated phrenic nerve palsy, presumed to be due to neuralgic amyotrophy. Looking at the problem in reverse, Lagueny et al (1992) identified four patients with unilateral diaphragmatic paralysis, three presenting with the sudden onset of breathlessness, in whom neurophysiological studies showed evidence of a neuropathic process in limb muscles consistent with the diagnosis of neuralgic amyotrophy but without the typical clinical accompaniments.

Otherwise typical limb involvement may be accompanied by laryngeal nerve palsy and involvement of the lower cranial nerves (Pierre et al 1990).

Finally, a similar disorder affecting the lumbosacral plexus has been described, but appears to be much rarer than the upper limb equivalent (Evans et al 1981, Sander & Sharp 1981).

Despite suspicions of an immune basis, the pathogenesis remains unknown and there are scant pathological data. In perhaps one-half of patients a potentially important antecedent event can be identified including infection, immunisation, surgery, trauma, pregnancy, exposure to a potential toxin, drug abuse, or an association with serum sickness. Four patients have been described recently who developed neuralgic amyotrophy whilst receiving radiotherapy for Hodgkin's disease (Malow & Dawson 1991). The acute painful onset during or shortly after radiotherapy made radiation plexopathy very unlikely. However, in the other one-half of all cases no antecedent event is apparent.

The differential diagnosis of neuralgic amyotrophy includes cervical radiculopathy, thoracic outlet syndrome, lung or breast carcinoma infiltrating the brachial plexus, and poliomyelitis. Acute rheumatological problems of the shoulder joint may cause confusion, but it must also be remembered that neuralgic amyotrophy can cause a frozen shoulder.

There is no good evidence that steroids are of

benefit, but anecdotal reports have suggested they may reduce pain. On present evidence there is no justification for their routine use. Physiotherapy is important, particularly in the prevention of frozen shoulder, and orthoses may be of value depending upon the distribution of weakness.

PERIPHERAL NERVE

Acquired neuromyotonia (Isaacs' syndrome, syndrome of continuous muscle-fibre activity)

This is yet another of those disorders which successive publications after the original description (Isaacs 1961) served to confuse rather than illuminate, because of the inclusion of patients with similar disorders of varying aetiology. Rowland (1985) has reviewed the salient clinical findings, and commented upon the difficulties of terminology with respect to the clinical and neurophysiological description of the abnormal muscle movements.

Onset can be at any age but is often in early adult life and males are more often affected. Symptoms have often been developing over several months prior to presentation. The most characteristic feature, and essential for the diagnosis, is continuous muscle twitching (myokymia), more marked in the limb than trunk muscles. Other symptoms, present in about one-half of patients (Rowland 1985), include abnormal posturing of the hands and feet, cramps, excessive sweating and impaired relaxation of muscles, most easily seen after forceful grasp (pseudomyotonia). There is rarely true percussion or EMG myotonia. Less common features include depression of tendon reflexes (Zisfein et al 1983), muscle hypertrophy, usually of the calves (Zisfein et al 1983, Sinha et al 1991), muscle atrophy (Isaacs 1961) and evidence of peripheral neuropathy (Rowland 1985).

There are several reports of acquired neuromyotonia in association with other conditions, or in response to drug therapy, but these may be describing a heterogeneous group of disorders. Associations include neoplasia (Partanen et al 1980), peripheral neuropathy (Vasilescu et al 1984, Hahn et al 1991), penicillamine (Reeback et al 1979) and gold salt treatment (Mitsumoto

et al 1982). Another condition that has to be considered in the differential diagnosis is the cramp-fasciculation syndrome described by Tahmoush et al (1991). This shows many similarities to acquired neuromyotonia, with cramps, myokymia and a response to carbamazepine, but without the *continuous* muscle contraction and EMG motor unit activity seen in acquired neuromyotonia. Whether these are truly separate disorders remains to be determined.

EMG studies show spontaneous activity at rest with single and multiplet discharges. Nerve stimulation produces numerous after-discharges following the M-response. Pseudomyotonia is not due to true myotonic discharges but to after-discharges of motor unit potentials. There is occasionally evidence of peripheral nerve dysfunction in the form of prolonged motor and sensory nerve conduction velocities (Rowland 1985).

There is considerable evidence that the site of origin of the abnormal discharges, and thus the site of the pathological process, is in the terminal network of motor neurones. Clinical evidence for this comes from the observations that the abnormal muscle activity persists in sleep, during general anaesthesia, spinal anaesthesia and proximal blockade with local anaesthesia, but is abolished by blockade of the neuromuscular junction with curare. Pathological, as opposed to physiological, data are lacking but intraterminal and ultraterminal nerve sprouting has been demonstrated, consistent with a disorder in the region of the neuromuscular junction (Oda et al 1989).

An autoimmune aetiology for acquired neuromyotonia had been suspected on the basis of the detection of immune complexes in one patient, the knowledge that penicillamine can induce other autoimmune disorders as well as neuromyotonia, and the existence of a possible paraneoplastic form of the disorder (Sinha et al 1991). Strong support for this hypothesis came from the demonstration of improvement in the clinical disorder following plasma exchange, and the ability of the patient's plasma or purified IgG to cause an increased resistance to tubocurarine at the neuromuscular junction of phrenic nerve-diaphragm preparations, following passive transfer to mice. It is postulated that the putative autoantibody might reduce the number of functional slowly activating potassium channels, that normally stabilise membrane excitability (Sinha et al 1991). A further example of improvement following plasma exchange has been reported (Bady et al 1991).

Carbamazepine or phenytoin help the majority of patients. Until recently the difficulty has been to know what to use in patients resistant to such therapy. On the basis of the information given above, it would seem reasonable to consider plasma exchange or immunosuppressive drugs.

Although usually a sporadic disorder, there are examples of dominantly inherited forms of continuous muscle fibre activity, some of which appear to be closely related if not identical to the sporadic form (Auger et al 1984, McGuire et al 1984), whereas others are less clearly related (Ashizawa et al 1983).

SITE UNCERTAIN

There are several disorders in which the site of involvement is uncertain or there appear to be several sites of disease activity.

Restless legs syndrome (Ekbom's syndrome)

'Restless legs' is a common symptom in clinical practice, is of uncertain pathogenesis, but is associated with a diverse range of pathologies suggesting multiple aetiologies. Since Ekbom's (1960) definitive review, useful synopses and suggestions for diagnostic criteria include those of Gibb & Lees (1986) and Clough (1987).

Patients describe a distressing deep creeping sensation in their lower legs, usually bilaterally, that develops at rest, particularly when first retiring to bed thus preventing sleep, and making it impossible for them to keep their legs still. Movement, either in bed or more typically by having to get up and walk around, eases the discomfort often within a few minutes but occasionally not until an hour or more has passed. Not infrequently a similar sensation is felt above the knees, but only very rarely are such symptoms also experienced in the upper limbs. Troublesome insomnia and secondary depression are common.

Clinical examination is normal and pathological studies have shown no abnormality in peripheral nerves, skeletal muscle or in the motor end-plate region (Harriman et al 1970).

Many possible clinical associations with Ekbom's syndrome have been reported (Clough 1987), but the only three that have a certain relationship are iron deficiency anaemia (Ekbom 1960), pregnancy (Ekbom 1960, Goodman et al 1988, McParland & Pearce 1988) and peripheral neuropathy, particularly that associated with renal failure (Callaghan 1966, Thomas et al 1971). Less certain associations include gastric surgery (Banerji & Hurwitz 1970), chronic pulmonary disease (Spillane 1970) and folate deficiency in pregnancy (Botez & Lambert 1977).

Patients with mild symptoms may require no specific treatment other than reassurance as to the benign nature of the condition. In all patients basic haematological and biochemical studies should be performed, including serum iron and folate studies, and any abnormality investigated and treated as appropriate.

If further treatment is required there is a wide range of drugs that have been reported to help, but most reports are anecdotal (Clough 1987). There is clear evidence of a response to placebo in many patients (Telstad et al 1984), further lessening the value of such anecdotal reports. Taking into account short-term and long-term side-effects, carbamazepine is probably the treatment of choice (Telstad et al 1984). Clonazepam (Montagna et al 1984) and levodopa (von Scheele 1986) have been demonstrated to be more effective than placebo and there is an anecdotal report of a favourable response to clonidine (Handwerker & Palmer 1985).

Painful legs and moving toes

There appear to be sufficient clinical features to identify this disorder as being distinct from Ekbom's restless-legs syndrome. Whilst these patients also complain of pain and some discomfort in their lower limbs, the most striking feature is of involuntary movement of the toes, which the patient may be able to suppress (Spillane et al 1971). It seems likely that this condition is often associated with physical disease affecting afferent fibres of the posterior nerve roots (Nathan 1978). A similar syndrome was seen in a patient with posterior tibial nerve mononeuropathy (Mitsumoto et al 1990).

Polymyalgia rheumatica

Not infrequently this disorder is misdiagnosed as polymyositis, but clinical features alone normally allow an easy distinction between them. Laboratory investigations and a different rate of response to treatment with steroids further distinguish between these two unrelated disorders.

Polymyalgia rheumatica (PMR) is very rare under the age of 55 years, is about twice as common in women as in men, and does not appear to be associated with any other clinical disorder except for giant cell arteritis (GCA). It is widely thought that the two disorders represent different manifestations of the same underlying primary disorder, but the aetiology remains obscure. Putative links with viral infection and HLA types have not been substantiated, and nor has the recent suggestion of an association with a mitochondrial myopathy (Harle et al 1992). The number of patients with PMR who go on to develop GCA, and vice versa, is uncertain but is perhaps in excess of 50% (Hunder & Allen 1978, Jones & Hazleman 1981).

The site of the primary pathological process in PMR is unclear, but the association with GCA and the demonstration of lymphocyte proliferation in response to exposure to arterial wall antigen suggests that vascular involvement is a key feature (Hazleman et al 1975). Pathological changes in muscle, described below, may be secondary, and the main features of PMR probably relate to joint involvement with chronic synovitis (O'Duffy et al 1980).

Clinical features. The major neuromuscular symptoms are of pain and stiffness, typically around the neck and shoulder girdle but sometimes involving the pelvifemoral region. The stiffness is exacerbated by inactivity and is often most pronounced first thing in the morning. The pain is exacerbated by movement, which is a much more striking feature than discomfort on palpation, and so patients try to restrict movement of the affected parts, resulting in a rather characteristic stiffness of movement. Systemic features are common and include low-grade fever and polyarthralgia, weight loss and night sweats. Some patients will have symptoms and signs of GCA. Symptoms usually develop over a period of weeks to months but occasionally a much more acute onset occurs over a few days.

On examination the characteristic stiffness of movement, and reluctance to move, will be apparent. These features can give rise to a false impression of weakness, which does not occur. However, it may not be until the pain has resolved that it can be shown beyond doubt that no weakness is present. Muscle tenderness is not a major feature and movement invariably produces more pain than can be induced by palpation.

Investigations. The erythrocyte sedimentation rate (ESR) is invariably elevated and the diagnosis of PMR should be made with considerable caution if it is not. Less specific abnormalities include an increase in the α_2-globulin fraction and the occasional presence of antinuclear antibodies. The serum creatine kinase (CK) activity is normal.

Electromyography is usually normal and the occasional abnormalities that have been reported are of uncertain significance (Bromberg et al 1990).

The most consistent finding on muscle biopsy is type II fibre atrophy (Brooke & Kaplan 1972) which may simply reflect disuse. Ragged-red fibres are seen occasionally but their significance is uncertain (Harle et al 1992).

Whilst joint studies may be abnormal (O'Duffy et al 1980) they do not form part of the routine assessment of patients with PMR.

Treatment. The mainstay of treatment is prednisolone and the response is usually impressive and often dramatic. Pain and stiffness resolve within a matter of days and it can then be demonstrated easily that weakness is not present. A typical starting dose of prednisolone is 40 mg daily, and the dose is reduced slowly at a rate depending upon clinical features and the level of the ESR. Maintenance therapy with a dose in the range of 5–15 mg daily may be required for 2–5 years (Kyle & Hazelman 1990). Alternate-day therapy is probably inadvisable in the early stages of treatment but may be used when the dose is low and withdrawal is being attempted.

Mildly affected patients may gain adequate symptomatic relief from non-steroidal anti-inflammatory drugs, and undoubtedly spontaneous remission without the use of steroids can occur although the time-course may be protracted. However, because of the risk of developing GCA most clinicians advocate the use of steroids to achieve clinical remission and reduction of the ESR, although even this approach will not always prevent the complications of GCA (Jones & Hazleman 1981).

Eosinophilia-myalgia syndrome

Since 1989 many thousands of cases in the USA, and much smaller numbers from other countries, have been reported of an acute syndrome characterised by severe myalgia and peripheral blood eosinophilia. The cause of this epidemic has been identified as the ingestion of L-tryptophan-containing compounds, taken either for insomnia or as self-medication as a 'health food'. Recent evidence has shown that the L-tryptophan preparations involved originated from a single manufacturer and it is likely that the cause is not the amino acid itself but a contaminant (Varga et al 1992). Whilst several impurities have been identified there is a strong association with a compound labelled peak E, identified by high pressure liquid chromatography, which is a dimeric form of L-tryptophan. Even taking into account a dose–effect relationship, not all patients who took the contaminated preparation developed symptoms, suggesting that additional factors are involved, perhaps individual variation or abnormalities in the metabolism of L-tryptophan. This disorder bears close similarities to the Spanish toxic oil syndrome epidemic of the early 1980s, presumed to be due to an as yet unidentified contaminant of rapeseed oil.

Clinical features. The clinical features can be divided into early and late manifestations (Kaufman et al 1991, Lamb et al 1992, Varga et al 1992). Early features of the syndrome include severe myalgia, skin rashes and oedema, dyspnoea, arthralgia, fatigue and weakness and systemic features including fever and weight loss. Late features, developing after several months, include scleroderma-like skin infiltration in about one-half of patients, persistent myalgia and weakness. The

weakness is in part attributable to myopathy and in part to a sensorimotor peripheral neuropathy, usually axonal in type (Heiman-Patterson et al 1990), but occasionally demyelinating (Freimar et al 1992). Neuropathy develops in about two-thirds and myopathy in about one-third of patients. A single case of an apparently associated acute encephalopathy has been described (Adair et al 1992).

Whilst the acute symptoms, and certainly the peripheral blood eosinophilia, respond to steroid treatment, there is no evidence of long-term benefit (Kaufman et al 1991). Chronic disability is common and in one series of 31 patients 93% still had symptoms after 1 year (Kaufman et al 1991). Although contaminated batches of L-tryptophan have been withdrawn, the disorder is likely to remain of some importance over the next few years, given that symptoms may progress even after cessation of therapy and that some patients may have hoarded supplies.

Investigations. The most striking finding in the blood is the eosinophilia, with most patients having eosinophil counts in excess of 1000/µl. Although the serum CK activity is normal the aldolase is elevated in 60% of patients (Kaufman et al 1991). Antinuclear antibodies are found in just over one-third of patients.

Neurophysiological studies commonly show features of an axonal peripheral neuropathy, often with additional myopathic features (Smith & Dyck 1990), but evidence of demyelination may also be found (Heiman-Patterson et al 1990, Freimar et al 1992).

Muscle biopsy shows fibre atrophy, small numbers of eosinophils and a T-cell-predominant lymphocytic infiltrate indicating a cell-mediated immune response against some connective tissue component (Emslie-Smith et al 1991, Hollander & Adelman 1991).

Sural nerve biopsy shows axonal degeneration and epineural and perivascular mononuclear cell inflammatory infiltrates, with occasional eosinophils (Heiman-Patterson et al 1990, Smith & Dyck 1990).

Full-thickness skin biopsy shows thickening of the fascia and dermis due to accumulation of collagen and mucopolysaccharides, together with an inflammatory infiltrate (Varga et al 1990).

Pathogenesis. It is tempting to think that eosinophils have a major role in the development of the multisystem manifestations of the eosinophilia-myalgia syndrome. Eosinophil activation leads to the release of several proteins, including major basic protein and eosinophil-derived neurotoxin, that could certainly explain some of the tissue damage seen in this syndrome. However, eosinophils may be scanty or absent, and their degranulation products absent, in damaged tissue, indicating that other mechanisms must be at work (Varga et al 1992). Furthermore, patients have been identified who have appropriate clinical and laboratory features to make a diagnosis of eosinophilia-myalgia syndrome, but who lack eosinophilia. Muscle biopsy studies certainly imply a role for cell-mediated immunity (Emslie-Smith et al 1991).

Identification of the contaminant and further laboratory studies should answer some of these uncertainties, and may also contribute to a better understanding of somewhat similar clinical disorders such as eosinophilic fasciitis and other disorders associated with eosinophilia and fibrosis.

NEUROMUSCULAR JUNCTION

Botulism

Clostridium botulinum, like its close relative *Cl. tetani*, produces a powerful exotoxin that acts on the nervous system. Whereas the clinical features of tetanus are related to central nervous system dysfunction, botulism causes skeletal muscle paralysis and parasympathetic blockade due to inhibition of the calcium-mediated release of acetylcholine from peripheral cholinergic neurones (Sellin 1981). The exact mechanism of inhibition of neurotransmitter release is uncertain but it has recently been shown that tetanus and botulinum B neurotoxins cleave synaptobrevin-2, which is a protein that appears to have a major role in the neurotransmitter release mechanism (Schiavo et al 1992).

Three clinical forms of botulism are recognised. In perhaps the best known form, food-borne, preformed toxin is ingested in tainted food. In infantile botulism, a probably underrecognised condition, and wound botulism, the rarest form, toxin is formed at the site of the infection, being the gastrointestinal tract and a dirty wound respectively.

Food-borne botulism is rare but tends to occur in outbreaks, making recognition somewhat easier. The spores of *Cl. botulinum* germinate at room or body temperature under anaerobic conditions and toxin production is greater the higher the pH. The foodstuffs most commonly associated with botulism are vegetables, fruits and fish and many cases relate to home-bottled or canned food that had been inadequately cooked, or not cooked, before consumption. Cooking for 30 minutes at 80°C inactivates the spores. Recent outbreaks affecting 36 and 27 people respectively were attributed to contaminated chopped garlic in soybean oil, and hazelnut yoghurt (St Louis et al 1988, Critchley et al 1989).

Symptoms of parasympathetic blockade may develop before or concurrently with paralytic symptoms, and the typical incubation period from ingestion to first symptoms is 6–36 hours. Autonomic symptoms include blurred vision from mydriasis, abdominal pain, vomiting, constipation, diarrhoea, fever and a dry mouth. Paralytic symptoms usually start in the cranial nerve territory with ptosis, diplopia, dysphagia, dysphonia and facial weakness. Fatigability in the limbs is followed by increasing weakness, depression of tendon reflexes, and breathing difficulties. In two recent series 8/27 and 7/36 patients required mechanical ventilation and curiously in the latter, Chinese patients had a more severe illness and 60% required ventilation compared with only 4% of other races (St Louis et al 1988, Critchley et al 1989). Weakness is usually symmetrical.

Symptoms may progress for up to 1 week, rarely longer, and start to improve over the next few weeks, sooner in milder cases. Depending upon severity, full recovery may take anything from a few months to over 1 year. Mortality relates to failure to make the diagnosis, which is perhaps more likely in sporadic than epidemic cases, failure to anticipate the development of respiratory failure and from infections, both systemic and pulmonary, secondary to mechanical ventilation.

The diagnosis is confirmed by the identification of *Cl. botulinum* in the contaminated food, by culturing the organism from the faeces, or by identifying the toxin in serum or faeces.

Infant botulism may be more common than food-borne botulism (Arnon 1980). It is commonest in the first 6 months of life and the infant presents with constipation, feeding difficulty, feeble cry, hypotonia, ptosis and generalized weakness. It may explain some cases of sudden infant death.

The disorder is due to intestinal colonization by *Cl. botulinum* and treatment includes sterilisation of the gut with antibiotics. Rarely, a similar disorder may develop in adults, particularly in the presence of achlorhydria or following gastric surgery (Chia et al 1986). The diagnosis is established by the demonstration of the *Cl. botulinum* and toxin in faeces.

Wound botulism is rare, which is perhaps surprising, given the behaviour of *Cl. tetani*. The clinical picture is similar to food-borne botulism but gastrointestinal symptoms are less frequent. Diagnosis depends upon recovery of spores from the wound or identification of the toxin in the serum.

Whilst specific tests are required to confirm the diagnosis, characteristic changes may be demonstrated neurophysiologically and, not surprisingly, given the pathophysiological basis of botulism, the findings are not dissimilar to those seen in the Lambert–Eaton myasthenic syndrome. In weak muscles the compound muscle action potential amplitude is low and post-tetanic potentiation can often be demonstrated. In severe cases, after several weeks, the EMG shows features of denervation consequent upon the severe block of neuromuscular transmission (Kimura 1983b).

Treatment of botulism is largely supportive, particularly of respiratory function. Antitoxins are available and may be valuable in the early stages in that they will prevent further binding of toxin, although they do nothing to remove toxin that is already bound. Although some patients may show a slight and/or brief response to anticholinesterase drugs, guanidine or 3,4-diaminopyridine, the results are generally disappointing. Autonomic instability may require treatment, as of course do secondary infections.

Botulinum toxin causes irreversible damage to the presynaptic calcium-mediated acetylcholine release mechanism. Recovery occurs due to axonal sprouting, the development of new end-plates, and the establishment of new synapses (Duchen 1970).

MUSCLE

Compartment syndromes

Ischaemic muscle swells. Causes of muscle ischaemia and swelling include arterial problems (compression due to a displaced fracture or limb haematoma, tourniquet pressure, penetrating injury and iatrogenic causes such as clamping during surgery), direct trauma to muscle (crush injury) including sustained pressure such as an unconscious patient's head resting on the forearm, and certain drugs which may cause rhabdomyolysis, such as heroin and alcohol.

In certain parts of the body, muscles are enclosed within a semi-rigid fibro-osseous compartment, the most important in clinical practice being the anterior tibial compartment and the volar compartment of the forearm. At these sites muscle swelling is constrained by the boundaries of the compartment and thus there is a rapid rise of pressure in the compartment in response to the swelling. The increased pressure further impedes capillary blood flow and so a vicious circle of ever-increasing ischaemia develops (Owen et al 1979). Furthermore, compression of nerves within the compartments (peroneal nerve, and anterior interosseous, median and ulnar nerves respectively) leads to weakness and sensory disturbance in the appropriate distribution, which may become permanent if the nerve infarcts.

The clinical picture is thus of increasing pain, weakness, and often sensory disturbance, with local swelling and tenderness evident, but often without typical distal signs of limb ischaemia such as reduced pulses or impaired cutaneous circulation. In such circumstances urgent decompression with subcutaneous fasciotomies is indicated to try and prevent irreversible damage. Compartment pressure measurements using a wick catheter may help assess the severity of the problem and whether the pressure is increasing or decreasing.

The contracture due to fibrosis of the damaged muscle, and sensorimotor disturbance due to damage to the nerve passing through the compartment, is referred to as Volkmann's ischaemic contracture, and is seen most frequently affecting the long flexors of the fingers following a supra-condylar fracture of the humerus.

A more benign form of anterior tibial compartment syndrome is also seen. Patients complain of anterior shin pain on exercise, especially unaccustomed exercise, eased by rest ('shin splints'). Increasing symptoms or the development of sensorimotor symptoms suggesting nerve embarrassment are an indication for decompression of the compartment. Such problems can occur apparently spontaneously, presumably relating to a particular anatomical configuration, or may develop following a tibial fracture.

Myositis ossificans

At least two forms of this condition exist, which differ clinically but show pathological similarities.

Localized myositis ossificans. This appears to be an acquired disorder, generally associated with trauma and restricted to a single site. The trauma to the affected muscle may have been obvious and direct, but can follow on from repeated activity of the muscle or minor repeated trauma, a situation most frequently met in sportsmen or women, or in an industrial setting. Rarely, a similar problem can develop in the pelvic-girdle musculature in patients with paraplegia.

The initial feature is a localised area of swelling and tenderness, which over a few weeks is replaced by a hard, sometimes painful, mass. Within 1 or 2 months radiological studies will demonstrate bone formation within the muscle.

The natural history of the condition is not entirely clear, but spontaneous resolution of small areas of damage may occur. Occasionally, the ossification is an incidental finding, for example seen in shoulder-girdle muscles on a chest radiograph, and the patient may have noted no more than slight discomfort attributed to a muscle strain. Larger areas of ossification may have a simple mechanical effect impeding muscle performance. In such cases, or if there is significant discomfort, surgical excision is indicated.

Myositis ossificans progressiva. This rare disorder, or group of disorders, generally appears as a sporadic condition but is probably inherited as an autosomal dominant trait with variable expressivity, with new mutations being common (McKusick 1960). Apart from muscle involvement, associated congenital abnormalities are frequent, including absence or smallness of digits, particularly the big toe and thumb, abnormalities of the teeth and ear lobules, deafness, exostoses and hypogonadism (Connor & Evans 1982).

Muscle involvement develops within the first decade of life, often in the first couple of years. Typically, the muscles around the neck and shoulder region are affected first, and the hips and legs later. An area of muscle becomes swollen, hot and tender, which then, as in the acquired form, settles over a few weeks to be replaced by a hard area of bone deposition. Also as in the acquired form, trauma may precipitate the development of an area of damage.

Progressive muscle involvement and contractures lead to restriction of movements. The spine may become rigid and joints may be locked in position, due in part to bony ankylosis. Most patients are wheelchair-bound by early adult life. Whilst involvement of the diaphragm appears to be rare, death in adult life may be due to respiratory failure or secondary infection because of progressive restriction of chest wall movement. Ulceration and secondary infection of ossified muscle may occur.

Pathologically, true myositis is not a prominent feature of either the generalised or localised form of myositis ossificans and although the pathological progression has not been fully delineated, muscle fibre involvement appears to be secondary. In the early lesion there may be inflammatory changes with haemorrhage and connective tissue proliferation. Subsequently, collagen proliferates and bone forms, typically around the periphery of the lesion. Muscle fibre atrophy is probably a secondary phenomenon, with fibres being surrounded by dense connective tissue (Satoyoshi & Nonaka 1982).

Treatment in the localised acquired form is by local excision, the indications being pain or if the mass is causing a mechanical impediment to movement. Surgery has a much smaller part to play in the generalised inherited form, in which a treatment to prevent recurrence is required, but lacking. Steroids are ineffective, but etidronate disodium may be of some value (Russel et al 1972).

Intramuscular calcification is also seen occasionally in the late stages of the idiopathic inflammatory myopathies, parathyroid disorders, vitamin D excess and in association with malignancy, but it is unlikely that these could be confused with the two disorders described above.

Tumours of muscle

Muscle tumours are rare and the classification of primary tumours has caused some confusion (Van Unnik 1982).

Rhabdomyomas in adults are rare and most frequently involve the head, neck and throat region. Cardiac rhabdomyomas in infancy may occur in isolation or in association with tuberous sclerosis, and carry a poor prognosis.

In early childhood *embryonal rhabdomyomas* may affect the head and neck region, and the genitourinary tract. The grape-like appearance at the latter site gives rise to the term sarcoma botryoides. The prognosis relates in part to the site of involvement, but overall the outcome has improved in response to aggressive treatment programmes (Liebner 1976).

In older children *alveolar rhabdomyomas* arise in the extremities or over the trunk and may show papillary-like alveolar structures histologically. They are aggressive tumours that may metastasise and have a poor prognosis.

In adults, *pleomorphic rhabdomyosarcomas* most frequently arise in the legs in middle-adult life, and are often highly aggressive, may metastasise early, and respond poorly to radiotherapy. About one-third of patients survive 5 years, although considerable variation in survival has been noted (Ariel & Briceno 1975).

With the exception of local invasion of pectoral muscles from breast carcinoma, skeletal muscle involvement by *secondary tumour* appears to be rare in clinical practice, perhaps surprisingly given that muscle is highly vascular and makes up as much as 40% of total body weight. Pathologically, Pearson (1959) has shown that skeletal muscle involvement is perhaps more frequent than one might think, with 16% of 38 cases of malignancy showing tumour emboli and growth

in skeletal muscle, but this is rarely identified clinically.

Doshi & Fowler (1983) reported two patients who presented with features of a proximal myopathy that proved to be due to metastatic spread to the muscle from a bronchogenic carcinoma in the one and breast carcinoma in the other. In both cases the weakness was initially presumed to be due to non-metastatic neuromyopathy. Given that many such patients in this situation are *in extremis* and are not likely to be subjected to muscle biopsy, it is possible that such cases are more frequent than is generally realised.

Tumours of skeletal muscle supporting tissues are also rare, but include *angiomata* and *dermoid tumours*. *Neurofibromata* may cause pain in response to palpation or contraction of adjacent muscles. Conditions that may mimic muscle tumour include pyogenic abscesses, for example in patients with diabetes mellitus, tropical myositis, muscle herniation through fascia, and tendon rupture (e.g. of biceps brachii).

Bornholm disease

Devil's grip, pleurodynia or epidemic myalgia (Sylvest 1934) is an acute viral illness usually due to Coxsackie B infection, less commonly to Coxsackie A or Echo virus. There may be a prodromal illness with upper respiratory tract symptoms, fever, malaise and headache, but the characteristic feature is pain, often severe, around the lower chest wall, roughly in the area of insertion of the diaphragm, and abdomen. The pain may be unilateral, is exacerbated by movement, and may have a pleuritic quality in that it is increased by coughing and respiratory movements. Pleuritic signs may occasionally be present. Back, shoulder-girdle and neck pain may be present, and many patients also complain of headache. Associated symptoms related to an aseptic meningitis, myocarditis, pericarditis, hepatitis and orchitis may be present. Symptoms typically resolve in a couple of weeks but relapses are common.

Physical signs may be absent but occasionally intercostal muscle swelling and tenderness may be evident.

There have been no adequate reports detailing serum enzyme, EMG or nerve conduction studies.

Apart from the clinical features, the evidence for primary muscle involvement is limited but is based upon knowledge of the myopathic potential of Coxsackie viruses in animals, and the occasional report of histological evidence of an acute inflammatory myopathy in patients (Lepine et al 1952). Viruses can often be cultured from faeces, and perhaps also from muscle (Lepine et al 1952).

It is a self-limiting disorder for which there is no specific treatment. Differentiation from other pleural and peritoneal inflammatory disorders is more likely to be a problem in sporadic cases than during an epidemic.

Chronic fatigue syndrome (CFS)

This is now the preferred term for a symptom-complex recognised throughout the developed world, but perhaps not in the Third World, that has previously carried many names including Royal Free disease, Icelandic disease and epidemic neuro-myasthenia to name but a few. The still popular term myalgic encephalomyelitis (ME) indicates the frequent presence of muscle symptoms, but is inappropriate because encephalomyelitis has never been demonstrated. Postviral fatigue syndrome presupposes the aetiology, which has not been proven, and similarly the label chronic infectious mononucleosis, once popular in America, has had to be dropped because of clear evidence that most patients do not have chronic Epstein–Barr virus infection.

Of the plethora of symptoms that have been described in CFS (and indeed it is difficult to think of many symptoms that have not been described in CFS), the most prominent are fatigue, often accompanied by myalgia, and disturbance of mental functions including poor memory, impaired concentration, sleep disturbance and emotional lability (Sharpe et al 1991).

In some patients, but by no means all, the precipitating event seems to be a viral infection, and some research groups have perhaps clouded the water by including only such patients, and excluding those with identical persistent symptoms but no evidence of an initiating infection. Particularly amongst sufferers, there is a very strong belief that most of the features of the condition are due to active physical disease, and the most popular theory is that of persistent viral infection.

In the USA the concept of chronic Epstein–Barr infection gained popularity, based largely on anecdotal reports, and is perhaps proving hard to dismiss despite publication of data that refute the concept (Gold et al 1990). In Britain several reports during the 1980s, mainly from the west of Scotland, suggested, on the basis of serum IgG antibody studies, that Coxsackie B virus infection might have an aetiological role, and these data are still much cited. However, more recent evidence published by many of the same authors, looking at serum IgM antibodies, have not provided support for a cause–effect relationship between Coxsackie infection and CFS, and show that the rates of infection are the same in patients and control subjects (Miller et al 1991). It is only to be hoped that this evidence will be as widely disseminated as the results of the earlier, inadequate, studies.

Despite the lack of evidence for persistent viral infection, chronic stimulation by a virus has been proposed as a possible explanation for the immune activation seen in some patients with CFS (Landay et al 1991). An equally attractive hypothesis is that CFS is primarily a psychological disorder, and there is good evidence that stress increases susceptibility to viral infection and may alter immune function (Cohen et al 1991).

The prominence of fatigue and myalgia has led many investigators to look for evidence of primary involvement of skeletal muscle in CFS, as opposed to more central mechanisms.

The report of abnormally early acidification of skeletal muscle during exercise (Arnold et al 1984), measured by phosphorus magnetic resonance spectroscopy, in a single patient has been referred to frequently, often erroneously implying that several patients have been shown to have this abnormality (Behan et al 1991). More recently, the laboratory responsible for this single case report has reported that in a study of 46 CFS patients it was not possible to demonstrate any specific metabolic abnormality (Barnes et al 1993).

Persistence of enteroviral RNA in skeletal muscle has been reported by two related groups (Archard et al 1988, Gow et al 1991). Inappropriate and inadequate selection of control subjects makes these studies difficult to interpret. Twenty of 96 CFS patients were positive using RNA hybridisation techniques, whereas all *four* controls were negative (Archard et al 1988). Using a more sensitive polymerase chain reaction technique, 53% of CFS patients were positive, against 15% of 41 controls (Gow et al 1991). Patients, but not controls, were included only if they gave a history of an acute, apparently viral, illness, so that even if not aetiologically important the patient group may not surprisingly have had a higher prevalence of evidence of viral infection.

Single fibre EMG abnormalities have been reported by the Glasgow group (Jamal & Hansen 1989), but not substantiated by others. No control subjects were studied.

With respect to muscle histology, the two largest series reported have come from the same Glasgow group (Behan et al 1985, Behan et al 1991). The major finding on light microscopy was type II fibre atrophy, present in 39 of 50 patients with CFS (Behan et al 1991). Whilst generally considered to be a non-specific finding, particularly associated with disuse and therefore not a surprising finding in patients with CFS, the authors took this to be a sign of muscle damage. Ultrastructural mitochondrial abnormalities were seen in 80% of patients whereas in control subjects 'even mild changes were rarely detected'. As is so often the case in studies of CFS, a major criticism can be levelled at the choice of control subjects. None showed type II atrophy, from whatever cause, and so it cannot be stated whether the mitochondrial abnormalities noted were primary or secondary. Given the known variability between different muscles, it was unfortunate that CFS patients had vastus lateralis biopsies whereas the control subjects had biopsies of pectoralis major, rectus abdominis and vastus medialis, but not of vastus lateralis. Finally, it appears that assessment of the biopsies was open rather than blind, which is a major criticism for this type of study.

Even if one accepts any or all of the information cited above as providing evidence for persistent disease of skeletal muscle, then there are still two major obstacles to be overcome. First, if these changes are important with respect to the pathophysiology of CFS, then why are they not present in all patients? Secondly, and much more importantly, if such changes are of significance, rather than simply being epiphenomena, it should be possible to show that they give rise to impaired muscle function. That is, that the symptomatic complaint of fatigue is related to impaired muscle contractile function. Such evidence does not exist, and those studies that have looked at muscle performance, voluntary activation, twitch properties, endurance and recovery have failed to show impaired physiological function (Lloyd et al 1988, Stokes et al 1988, Lloyd at al 1991). Furthermore, biochemical studies provide no evidence of a major defect in muscle intermediary energy pathways (Byrne & Trounce 1987).

In summary, the status of CFS remains in doubt. It is likely that several disparate factors may precipitate symptoms, including viral infection. Persistence of symptoms can readily be explained, invoking only psychological mechanisms, although this is a view strongly opposed by most of the self-help groups and many of their members. The evidence that has been widely cited as providing support for a physical basis for the symptoms of CFS is bedevilled by lack of appropriate control studies, lack of critical appraisal and biased selection of patients, and stands up poorly to close scrutiny.

There is no doubting the existence of the syndrome, nor the great misery that it causes. In Britain, the ME Association estimates that there are over 100 000 sufferers. Many patients are helped by tricyclic compounds, such as amitriptyline, which is not to say that CFS is a depressive disorder, although that is often the case. Unfortunately, patients may refuse such treatment, perhaps particularly if they have been advised by a self-help group, thus denying themselves effective treatment. This relates to the futile but continuing *organic vs non-organic* debate, with respect to the cause of CFS (Kendell 1991).

NEUROMUSCULAR DISORDERS ASSOCIATED WITH NEOPLASTIC DISEASES

Muscle wasting, weakness and fatigue are common features in patients with malignant disease and often represent a rather non-specific effect of a number of systemic factors including cachexia, malnutrition, infection, bone and joint disease and inactivity. However, direct involvement of nerve and muscle, and paraneoplastic involvement of nerve, muscle and the neuromuscular junction is well recognised and is described below. The incidence of paraneoplastic neuromuscular disorders is probably much underestimated, in part because investigations may be limited in a terminally ill patient. In one recent prospective study of 150 patients with small-cell lung cancer, neuromuscular or autonomic deficits occurred in up to 44% of cases (Elrington et al 1991).

Neuropathic disorders

Direct involvement. Neoplastic tissue may simply spread locally and involve adjacent nerves. Cranial nerves, spinal nerves and roots, the brachial and lumbosacral plexuses and peripheral nerves may all be involved in this fashion, and perhaps the commonest examples are Pancoast's syndrome and lumbosacral plexus involvement with pelvic tumours. Motor and sensory deficits appropriate to the distribution of the nerve develop often but not always accompanied by pain. The clinical features are the same, whether the spread is from a primary site or a secondary deposit. If the tumour is affecting nerves or roots within the leptomeningeal compartment then there may be a CSF reaction with pleocytosis and an increased protein content. Diffuse leptomeningeal spread produces carcinomatous meningitis with widespread cranial and spinal nerve involvement, headache and spinal pain. A rather characteristic syndrome is that of mental neuropathy, or the numb chin syndrome, most frequently associated with lymphoreticular malignancies. The patient presents with unilateral or, less commonly, bilateral chin and lower lip numbness. The syndrome may be due to diffuse infiltration of the mandibular nerve, direct compression of the mental nerve by a mandibular metastasis, or to leptomeningeal spread of tumour and involvement of the trigeminal nerve, when malignant cells may be found in the CSF (Massey et al 1981, Kuroda et al 1991).

Paraneoplastic disorders. The two main clinical types of paraneoplastic neuropathy are a sensory neuropathy and a sensorimotor neuropathy, the latter encompassing several different syndromes (McLeod 1993). Rarely, a disorder indistinguishable from classical motor neurone disease arises as a paraneoplastic disorder.

Sensory neuropathy (ganglioradiculitis). First described by Denny-Brown in 1948, this disorder is particularly associated with small-cell lung tumours, but occurs also with many other tumour types and lymphoreticular malignancies. Rather typically it precedes the discovery of the associated malignancy. The principal pathological findings are degeneration of dorsal root ganglion cells, posterior columns, and sensory fibres in the peripheral nerves.

Clinically, the onset is subacute with distal paraesthesiae and numbness which spread proximally over several weeks, limb incoordination and gait disturbance due to sensory ataxia. Limb pain may be prominent. Autonomic features are uncommon. Mild weakness may develop in later stages. On examination there is reduction of all sensory modalities, particularly vibration and joint position sense, and loss of the tendon reflexes. An associated encephalomyelitis may give rise to dementia, memory disturbance, pupillary and eye-movement disorders.

The CSF may show a slight lymphocytosis and the protein content is often elevated to 1–2 g/l. Treatment of the underlying malignancy has little effect on the neurological syndrome.

Sensorimotor neuropathy. Subacute, chronic, and relapsing and remitting sensorimotor polyneuropathies represent perhaps the commonest forms of paraneoplastic neurological disturbance (Croft & Wilkinson 1965), and bronchial carcinoma is the commonest underlying malignancy. Clinical evidence of polyneuropathy is evident in perhaps 5% of patients with carcinoma, but electrophysiological changes may be detected in nearly one-half of patients (Lipton et al 1991). In up to one-half of patients the onset of neurological symptoms may precede the detection of the malignancy, sometimes by several years.

The typical presentation is with a distal sensory and motor neuropathy, affecting the lower limbs more than the upper, sometimes with a trigeminal neuropathy, and with subacute or chronic progression. The commonest pathological finding is axonal degeneration.

A relapsing and remitting polyneuropathy with segmental demyelination may also occur, and is more common with lymphoma and other reticuloses than with carcinoma.

An inflammatory brachial plexopathy has been described in a patient with Hodgkin's disease and a diffuse sensorimotor peripheral neuropathy (Lachance et al 1991).

Typical Guillain–Barré syndrome may occur in association with lymphoma, and much more rarely in patients with carcinoma.

Motor neurone disease. Since the early descriptions of an association (Brain et al 1965, Norris & Engel 1965) there has been considerable controversy as to whether a paraneoplastic form of otherwise classical motor neurone disease/amyotrophic lateral sclerosis exists. It has been argued that the association is fortuitous, and although Norris & Engel (1965) showed that the prevalence of carcinoma in patients with amyotrophic lateral sclerosis was 10-fold greater than in a concurrent series of stroke patients, the design of the study was not ideal. Another argument is that a motor neurone disease-like disorder could arise through the development of a combined paraneoplastic encephalomyelitis and a pure motor, or predominantly motor, neuropathy.

Reports of patients whose motor neurone disease-like syndrome has improved following treatment of a neoplasm are difficult to interpret given the absence of pathological studies (Mitchell & Olczak 1979, Evans et al 1990).

Whatever the pathological features it is clear that neoplasia can produce a paraneoplastic disorder that looks like classical motor neurone disease to experienced observers.

Myopathic disorders

Direct involvement. Local spread of tumour into muscle is common but of little practical importance except with respect to planning surgery.

Marantic embolism causing muscle infarction has been described in three patients with adenocarcinoma of the gastrointestinal tract and nonbacterial thrombotic endocarditis (Heffner 1971).

Paraneoplastic disorders. Many paraneoplastic myopathic disorders have been identified, some better defined than others.

Carcinomatous neuromyopathy. This term was used by Brain & Henson (1958) to describe the whole group of central and peripheral nervous system disorders associated with carcinoma. It is now used in a more restricted sense to describe a syndrome of symmetrical proximal muscle weakness and wasting, affecting particularly the hip flexors, of subacute or chronic course, and with depressed tendon reflexes. Neurophysiological studies may show features of both neuropathic and myopathic dysfunction (Campbell & Paty 1974). Unfortunately, this and other studies have failed to correlate neurophysiological with pathological data and the exact nature of this condition has not been clarified. However, most evidence suggests that it is probably a neurogenic disorder.

Acute necrotising myopathy. Four patients have been described with rapid progression of generalised muscle weakness, with little or no pain, whose muscle showed a non-inflammatory necrotising myopathy (Smith 1969, Urich & Wilkinson 1970, Swash 1974). The pathogenesis of this disorder is unknown.

Dermatomyositis (DM) and polymyositis (PM). Until recently DM and PM have often been considered to be the same disorder, with respect to disease course and the muscle lesions, differing only in the presence or absence of a skin rash (Bohan & Peter 1975, Behan & Behan 1985). It is now appreciated that DM, PM and inclusion body myositis are each quite distinct disorders with characteristic clinical, immunopathological and morphological features (Dalakas 1991). Humoral immune factors predominate in DM, whereas in PM and inclusion body myositis T-cell-mediated cytotoxicity is more important. From a practical standpoint, the presence or absence of a rash is insufficient evidence alone to allow a distinction to be made between DM and PM.

It has long been appreciated that there is a link between carcinoma and inflammatory myopathy. Unfortunately, the most recent study to look at this association, examining a cohort of 788 patients, had a number of flaws, the most important of which was the use of outdated criteria to distinguish between DM and PM (Sigurgeirsson et al 1992). Using their criteria cancer was diagnosed in 15% of patients with DM and 9% of patients with PM. Given that misclassification will have lead to some patients with DM being considered as having PM, but not vice versa, the association with cancer is probably higher than stated for DM, and lower for PM, and it remains uncertain as to whether there is truly an increased relative risk of cancer in patients with PM (Hilton-Jones & Squier 1992).

Thus, patients with DM should be screened for the presence of malignant disease (general, rectal and vaginal examination, haematological studies, urinalysis, chest radiograph, CT scan of abdomen, and further appropriate investigations as directed by symptoms).

Metabolic and endocrine myopathies. Serum electrolyte changes induced by neoplastic disorders, including tumours of endocrine glands, may cause weakness (Table 27.2).

Tumours of endocrine glands may be functional causing hormone excess, or non-functional, but causing reduced hormone production. Hormone excess may also be due to ectopic production. Apart from the disorders associated with electrolyte disturbances noted above, weakness directly due to hormone excess or deficiency is common, and endocrine myopathies are discussed in more detail elsewhere (Ch 17), but are summarised in Table 27.3. The cause of weakness is often multifactorial. For example, parathormone excess may cause weakness because of the associated hypercalcaemia, but weakness can also occur with normal calcium levels. Similarly, ACTH excess causes glucocorticoid excess but evidence

Table 27.2 Electrolyte disorders, associated with neoplastic disease, causing muscle weakness

Hypokalaemia	Aldosterone-producing adrenal adenoma (Conn's syndrome)
	Renin-secreting tumours
	Cushing's syndrome
	Pituitary adenoma
	Ectopic ACTH production
	Acute leukaemia
	Villous adenoma of rectum
Hyperkalaemia	Addison's disease due to destruction of the adrenal glands by metastatic tumour
Hyponatraemia	Addison's disease due to destruction of the adrenal glands by metastatic tumour
	Any tumour causing the syndrome of inappropriate secretion of antidiuretic hormone
Hypercalcaemia	Parathormone-secreting parathyroid adenoma
	Parathormone-secreting tumours
	Bone metastases
	Myeloma

Table 27.3 Neoplastic endocrine disorders causing weakness

Hormone	Excess or deficiency	Cause
Anterior pituitary	↓	Panhypopituitarism due to: Pituitary adenoma Craniopharyngioma Secondary pituitary tumour
ACTH	↑	Cushing's syndrome due to: Pituitary adenoma Ectopic ACTH production
Growth hormone	↑	Pituitary adenoma
Glucocorticoids	↑	Cushing's syndrome due to: Pituitary adenoma Ectopic ACTH production Adrenal adenoma
Adrenocortical	↓	Addison's disease due to: Adrenal destruction by secondary tumour
Catecholamines	↑	Phaeochromocytoma
Thyroxine	↑	Functional thyroid tumour
Parathormone (PTH)	↑	Parathyroid adenoma Ectopic PTH production

suggests that both factors may contribute to the weakness.

Disorders of neuromuscular transmission

Lambert–Eaton myasthenic syndrome. This disorder is discussed in detail elsewhere (see Ch. 20). The major clinical features are proximal weakness, depressed tendon reflexes which show post-tetanic potentiation, diplopia, ptosis, dryness of the mouth and impotence. In about one-half of cases there is an underlying neoplasm, and about 80% of these are small-cell lung cancers (O'Neill et al 1988).

Myasthenia gravis. This disorder is also discussed in detail in Chapter 20. The only recognised association with tumour is with neoplasia of the thymus gland. Thymic hyperplasia is seen in about 75% of patients with myasthenia gravis, and thymoma, which may be locally invasive, in about 10%. Conversely, up to one-third of patients with thymoma may develop myasthenia. Malignant thymoma is rare. Thymectomy as treatment for myasthenia is less effective if a tumour is present.

REFERENCES

Adair J C, Rose J W, Digre K B, Balbierz J M 1992 Acute encephalopathy associated with the eosinophilia-myalgia syndrome. Neurology 42: 461

Archard L C, Bowles N E, Behan P O, Bell E J, Doyle D 1988 Postviral fatigue syndrome: persistence of enterovirus RNA in muscle and elevated creatine kinase. Journal of the Royal Society of Medicine 81: 326

Ariel M, Briceno M 1975 Rhabdomyosarcoma of the extremities and trunk: analysis of 150 patients treated by surgical resection. Journal of Surgical Oncology 7: 269

Arnold D L, Radda G K, Bore P J, Styles P, Taylor D J 1984 Excessive intracellular acidosis of skeletal muscle on exercise in a patient with post-viral exhaustion/fatigue syndrome. A ^{31}P nuclear magnetic resonance study. Lancet i: 1367

Arnon S S 1980 Infantile botulism. Annual Review of Medicine 31: 451

Ashizawa T, Butler I J, Harati Y, Roongta S M 1983 A dominantly inherited syndrome with continuous motor neuron discharges. Annals of Neurology 13: 285

Auger R G, Daube J R, Gomez M R, Lambert E H 1984 Hereditary form of sustained muscle activity of peripheral nerve origin causing generalized myokymia and muscle stiffness. Annals of Neurology 15: 13

Bady B, Chauplannaz G, Vial C, Savet J-F 1991 Autoimmune aetiology for acquired neuromyotonia. Lancet 338: 1330

Banerji N K, Hurwitz L J 1970 Restless legs syndrome, with particular reference to its occurrence after gastric surgery. British Medical Journal 4: 774

Barnes P R J, Taylor D J, Kemp G J, Radda G K 1993 Skeletal muscle bioenergetics in the chronic fatigue syndrome. Journal of Neurology, Neurosurgery and Psychiatry, 56: 579

Behan P O, Behan W M H, Bell E J 1985 The post-viral fatigue syndrome — an analysis of the findings in 50 cases. Journal of Infection 10: 211

Behan W M H, Behan P O 1985 Immunological features of polymyositis/dermatomyositis. Springer Seminars in Immunopathology 8: 267

Behan W H M, More A R, Behan P O 1991 Mitochondrial abnormalities in the postviral fatigue syndrome. Acta Neuropathologica 83: 61

Blum P, Jankovic J 1991 Stiff-person syndrome: an autoimmune disease. Movement Disorders 6: 12

Bohan A, Peter J B 1975 Polymyositis and dermatomyositis. New England Journal of Medicine 292: 344

Botez M I, Lambert B 1977 Folate deficiency and restless-legs syndrome in pregnancy. New England Journal of Medicine 297: 670

Brain R, Henson R A 1958 Neurological syndromes associated with carcinoma. Lancet ii: 971

Brain R, Croft P B, Wilkinson M 1965 Motor neurone disease as a manifestation of neoplasms. Brain 85: 479

Brashear H R, Phillips L H 1991 Autoantibodies to GABAergic neurons and response to plasmapheresis in stiff-man syndrome. Neurology 41: 1588

Bromberg M B, Donofrio P D, Segal B M 1990 Steroid-responsive electromyographic abnormalities in polymyalgia rheumatica. Muscle and Nerve 13: 138

Brooke M H, Kaplan H 1972 Muscle pathology in rheumatoid arthritis, polymyalgia rheumatica, and polymyositis: a histochemical study. Archives of Pathology 94: 101

Byrne E, Trounce I 1987 Chronic fatigue and myalgia syndrome: mitochondrial and glycolytic studies in skeletal muscle. Journal of Neurology, Neurosurgery and Psychiatry 50: 743

Callaghan N, 1966 Restless legs syndrome in uremic neuropathy. Neurology 16: 359

Campbell M J, Paty D W 1974 Carcinomatous neuromyopathy: 1. Electrophysiological studies. Journal of Neurology, Neurosurgery and Psychiatry 37: 131

Chia J K, Clarke J B, Ryan C A, Pollack M 1986 Botulism in an adult associated with food-borne intestinal infection with Clostridium botulinum. New England Journal of Medicine 315: 239

Clough C 1987 Restless legs syndrome. British Medical Journal 294: 262

Cohen S, Tyrrell D A J, Smith A P 1991 Psychological stress and susceptibility to the common cold. New England Journal of Medicine 325: 606

Connor J M, Evans D A P 1982 Genetic aspects of fibrodysplasia ossificans progressiva. Journal of Medical Genetics 19: 35

Critchley E M R, Hayes P J, Isaacs P E T 1989 Outbreak of botulism in north west England and Wales, June 1989. Lancet ii: 849

Croft P B, Wilkinson M 1965 The incidence of carcinomatous neuromyopathy with special reference to carcinoma of the lung and breast. In: Brain W R, Norris F H (eds) The remote effects of cancer on the nervous system. Grune & Stratton, New York, p 44

Crone N E, Reder A T 1992 Severe tetanus in immunized patients with high anti-tetanus titers. Neurology 42: 761

Dalakas M C 1991 Polymyositis, dermatomyositis, and inclusion-body myositis. New England Journal of Medicine 325: 1487

Denny-Brown D 1948 Primary sensory neuropathy with muscular changes associated with carcinoma. Journal of Neurology, Neurosurgery and Psychiatry 1: 73

Doshi R, Fowler T 1983 Proximal myopathy due to discrete carcinomatous metastases in muscle. Journal of Neurology, Neurosurgery and Psychiatry 46: 358

Duchen L W 1970 Changes in motor innervation and cholinesterase localization induced by botulinum toxin in skeletal muscle of the mouse: differences between fast and slow muscles. Journal of Neurology, Neurosurgery and Psychiatry 33: 40

Edmondson R S, Flowers M W 1979 Intensive care in tetanus: management, complications and mortality in 100 cases. British Medical Journal 1: 1401

Ekbom K A 1960 Restless legs syndrome. Neurology 10: 868

Elrington G M, Murray N M, Spiro S G, Newsom-Davis J 1991 Neurological paraneoplastic syndromes in patients with small cell lung cancer. A prospective survey of 150 patients. Journal of Neurology, Neurosurgery and Psychiatry 54: 764

Emslie-Smith A M, Engel A G, Duffy J, Bowles C A 1991 Eosinophilia myalgia syndrome: I. Immunocytochemical evidence for a T-cell-mediated immune effector response. Annals of Neurology 29: 524

England J D, Sumner A J 1987 Neuralgic amyotrophy: an increasingly diverse entity. Muscle and Nerve 10: 60

Evans B A, Stevens J C, Dyck P J 1981 Lumbosacral plexus neuropathy. Neurology 31: 1327

Evans B K, Fagan C, Arnold T, Dropcho E J, Oh S J 1990 Paraneoplastic motor neuron disease and renal cell carcinoma: improvement after nephrectomy. Neurology 40: 960

Flowers M W, Edmondson R S 1980 Long-term recovery from tetanus: a study of 50 survivors. British Medical Journal 1: 303

Freimar M L, Glass J D, Chaudhry V et al 1992 Chronic demyelinating polyneuropathy associated with eosinophilia-myalgia syndrome. Journal of Neurology, Neurosurgery and Psychiatry 55: 352

Gibb W R G, Lees A J 1986 The restless legs syndrome. Postgraduate Medical Journal: 62: 329

Gold D, Bowden R, Sixbey J et al 1990 Chronic fatigue: a prospective clinical and immunologic study. Journal of the American Medical Association 264: 48

Goodman J D S, Brodie C, Ayida G A 1988. Restless leg syndrome in pregnancy. British Medical Journal 297: 1101

Gordon E E, Januszko D M, Kaufman L 1967 A critical survey of stiff-man syndrome. American Journal of Medicine 42: 582

Gorin F, Baldwin B, Tait R, Pathak R, Seyal M, Mugnaini E 1990 Stiff-man syndrome: a GABAergic autoimmune disorder with autoantigenic heterogeneity. Annals of Neurology 28: 711

Gow J W, Behan W M H, Clements G B, Woodall C, Riding M, Behan P O 1991 Enteroviral RNA sequences detected by polymerase chain reaction in muscle of patients with postviral fatigue syndrome. British Medical Journal 302: 692

Gregory R P, Loh L, Newsom-Davis J 1990 Recurrent isolated alternating phrenic nerve palsies: a variant of brachial neuritis? Thorax 45: 420

Hahn A F, Parkes A W, Bolton C F, Stewart S A 1991 Neuromyotonia in hereditary motor neuropathy. Journal of Neurology, Neurosurgery and Psychiatry 54: 230

Handwerker J V, Palmer R F 1985 Clonidine in the treatment of 'restless legs' syndrome. New England Journal of Medicine 313: 1228

Harding A E, Thompson P D, Kocen R S, Batchelor J R, Davey N, Marsden C D 1989 Plasma exchange and immunosuppression in the stiff-man syndrome. Lancet ii: 915

Harle J R, Pellissier J-F, Desnuelle C, Disdier P, Figarella-Branger D, Weiller P-J 1992 Polymyalgia rheumatica and mitochondrial myopathy: clinicopathologic and biochemical studies in five cases. American Journal of Medicine 92: 167

Harriman D G F, Taverner D, Woolf A L 1970 Ekbom's syndrome and burning paraesthesiae. Brain 93: 393

Hazleman B L, MacLennan I C, Esiri M M 1975 Lymphocyte proliferation to artery antigen as a positive diagnostic test in polymyalgia rheumatica. Annals of the Rheumatic Diseases 34: 122

Heffner R R 1971 Myopathy of embolic origin in patients with carcinoma. Neurology 21: 840

Heiman-Patterson T D, Bird S J, Parry G J et al 1990 Peripheral neuropathy associated with eosinophilia-myalgia syndrome. Annals of Neurology 28: 522

Hilton-Jones D, Squier M V 1992 Risk of cancer in dermatomyositis or polymyositis. New England Journal of Medicine 327: 207

Hollander D, Adelman L S 1991 Eosinophilia-myalgia syndrome associated with ingestion of L-tryptophan: muscle biopsy findings in 4 patients. Neurology 41: 319

Hunder G G, Allen G L 1978 Giant cell arteritis: a review. Bulletin of Rheumatic Diseases 29: 980

Isaacs H 1961 A syndrome of continuous muscle-fibre activity. Journal of Neurology, Neurosurgery and Psychiatry 24: 319

Jamal G A, Hansen S 1989 Electrophysiological studies in the post-viral fatigue syndrome. Journal of Neurology, Neurosurgery and Psychiatry 48: 691

Jones J G, Hazleman B L 1981 Prognosis and management of polymyalgia rheumatica. Annals of Rheumatic Diseases 40: 1

Kaufman L D, Gruber B L, Gregersen P K 1991 Clinical follow-up and immunogenetic studies of 32 patients with eosinophilia-myalgia syndrome. Lancet 337: 1071

Kendell R E 1991 Chronic fatigue, viruses and depression. Lancet 337: 160

Kerr J H, Corbett J L, Prys-Roberts C, Crampton Smith A, Spalding J M K 1968 Involvement of the sympathetic nervous system in tetanus. Lancet ii: 236

Kimura J 1983a Electrodiagnosis in diseases of nerve and muscle. F A Davis, Philadelphia, p 452

Kimura J 1983b Electrodiagnosis in diseases of nerve and muscle. F A Davis, Philadelphia, p 179

Kuroda Y, Fujiyama F, Ohyama T et al 1991 Numb chin syndrome secondary to Burkitt's cell acute leukaemia. Neurology 41: 453

Kyle V, Hazelman B L 1990 Stopping steroids in polymyalgia rheumatica and giant cell arteritis. British Medical Journal 300: 344

Lachance D H, O'Neill B P, Harper C M, Banks P M, Cascino T L 1991 Paraneoplastic brachial plexopathy in a patient with Hodgkin's disease. Mayo Clinic Proceedings 66: 97

Lagueny A, Ellie E, Saintarailles J, Marathan R, Barat M, Julien J 1992 Unilateral diaphragmatic paralysis: an electrophysiological study. Journal of Neurology, Neurosurgery and Psychiatry 55: 316

Lamb M L, Murphy J J, Jones J L et al 1992 Eosinophilia-myalgia syndrome in L-tryptophan-exposed patients. Journal of the American Medical Association 267: 77

Landay A L, Jessop C, Lennette E T, Levy J A 1991 Chronic fatigue syndrome: clinical condition associated with immune activation. Lancet 338: 707

Layzer R B, 1988 Stiff-man syndrome — an autoimmune disease? New England Journal of Medicine 318: 1060

Lepine P, Desse G, Sautter V 1952 Biopsies musculaires examen histologique et isolement du virus coxsackie chez l'homme atteint de myalgie epidemique (Maladie de Bornholm). Bulletin De L'Académie Nationale De Médicine 136: 66

Liebner E J 1976 Embryonal rhabdomyosarcoma of head and neck in children: correlation of stage, radiation dose, local control and survival. Cancer 37: 2777

Lipton R B, Galer B S, Dutcher J P et al 1991 Large and small fibre type sensory dysfunction in patients with cancer. Journal of Neurology, Neurosurgery and Psychiatry 54: 706

Lloyd A R, Hales J P, Gandevia S C 1988 Muscle strength endurance and recovery in the post-infection fatigue syndrome. Journal of Neurology, Neurosurgery and Psychiatry 51: 1316

Lloyd A R, Gandevia S C, Hales J P 1991 Muscle performance, voluntary activation, twitch properties and perceived effort in normal subjects and patients with the chronic fatigue syndrome. Brain 114: 85

Lorish T R, Thorsteinsson G, Howard F M 1989 Stiff-man syndrome updated. Mayo Clinic Proceedings 64: 629

McGuire S A, Tomasovic J J, Ackerman N 1984 Hereditary continuous muscle fiber activity. Archives of Neurology 41: 395

McKusick V A 1960 Heritable disorders of connective tissue, 2nd edn. St Louis, Minneapolis

McLeod J G 1993 Paraneoplastic neuropathies. In: Dyck P J, Thomas P K (eds) Peripheral neuropathy, 3rd edn. Saunders, Philadelphia, p 1583

McParland P, Pearce J M S 1988 Restless legs syndrome in pregnancy. British Medical Journal 297: 1543

Malow B A, Dawson D M 1991 Neuralgic amyotrophy in association with radiation therapy for Hodgkin's disease. Neurology 41: 440

Massey E W, Moore J, Schold S C 1981 Mental neuropathy from systemic cancer. Neurology 31: 1277

Meinck H M, Ricker K, Conrad B 1984 The stiff-man syndrome: new pathophysiological aspects from abnormal exteroceptive reflexes and the response to clomipramine, clonidine and tizanidine. Journal of Neurology, Neurosurgery and Psychiatry 47: 280

Mellanby J, Green J 1981 How does tetanus toxin act? Neuroscience 6: 281

Miller N A, Carmichael H A, Calder B D et al 1991 Antibody to coxsackie B virus in diagnosing postviral fatigue syndrome. British Medical Journal 302: 140

Mitchell D M, Olczak S A 1979 Remission of a syndrome indistinguishable from motor neurone disease after resection of bronchial carcinoma. British Medical Journal 2: 176

Mitsumoto H, Wilbourn A J, Subramony S H 1982 Generalized myokymia and gold therapy. Archives of Neurology 39: 449

Mitsumoto H, Levin K H, Wilbourn A J, Chou S M 1990 Hypertrophic mononeuritis clinically presenting with painful legs and moving toes. Muscle and Nerve 13: 215

Mitsumoto H, Schwartzman M J, Estes M L et al 1991 Sudden death and paroxysmal autonomic dysfunction in stiff-man syndrome. Journal of Neurology 238: 91

Moersch F P, Woltman H W 1956 Progressive fluctuating muscular rigidity and spasm ('stiff-man' syndrome). Mayo Clinic Proceedings 31: 421

Montagna P, De Bianchi L S, Zucconi M, Cirignotta F, Lugaresi E 1984 Clonazepam and vibration in restless legs syndrome. Acta Neurologica Scandinavica 69: 428

Nathan P W 1978 Painful legs and moving toes: evidence on the site of the lesion. Journal of Neurology, Neurosurgery and Psychiatry 41: 934

Norris F H, Engel W K 1965 Carcinomatous amyotrophic lateral sclerosis. In: Brain W R, Norris F H (eds) The remote effects of cancer on the nervous system. Grune & Stratton, New York, p 24

O'Duffy J D, Hunder G G, Wahner H W 1980 A follow up study of polymyalgia rheumatica: evidence of chronic axial synovitis. Journal of Rheumatology 7: 685

O'Neill J H, Murray N M F, Newsom-Davis J 1988 The Lambert–Eaton myasthenic syndrome. Brain 111: 577

Oda K, Fukushima N, Shibasaki H, Ohnishi A 1989 Hypoxia-sensitive hyperexcitability of the intramuscular nerve axons in Isaacs' syndrome. Annals of Neurology 25: 140

Owen C A, Mubarak S J, Hargens A R, Rutherford L, Garetto L P, Akeson W H 1979 Intramuscular pressures with limb compression. New England Journal of Medicine 300: 1169

Parsonage M J, Turner J W A 1948 Neuralgic amyotrophy. The shoulder girdle syndrome. Lancet i: 973

Partanen V S J, Soininen H, Saksa M, Riekkinen P 1980 Electromyographic and nerve conduction findings in a patient with neuromyotonia, normocalcaemic tetany and small-cell lung cancer. Acta Neurologica Scandinavica 61: 216

Pearson C M, 1956 Incidence and type of pathologic alterations observed in muscle in a routine autopsy survey. Neurology 9: 757

Pierre P A, Laterre C E, Van Den Bergh P Y 1990 Neuralgic amyotrophy with involvement of cranial nerves IX, X, XI, and XII. Muscle and Nerve 13: 704

Price D L, Griffin J, Young A, Peck K, Stocks A 1975 Tetanus toxin: direct evidence for retrograde intraaxonal transport. Science 188: 945

Reeback J, Benton S, Swash M, Schwartz M S 1979 Penicillamine-induced neuromyotonia. British Medical Journal i: 1464

Rowland L P 1985 Cramps, spasms and muscle stiffness. Revue Neurologique 141: 261

Russel R G G, Smith R, Bishop M C, Price D A, Squire C M 1972 Treatment of myositis ossificans progressiva with a diphosphonate. Lancet i: 10

Sander J E, Sharp F R 1981 Lumbosacral plexus neuritis. Neurology 31: 470

Satoyoshi E, Nonaka I 1982 Myositis ossificans, myosclerosis and muscle contracture. In: Mastaglia F L, Walton J (eds) Skeletal muscle pathology. Churchill Livingstone, Edinburgh, p 621

Schiavo G, Benfenati F, Poulain J B et al 1992 Tetanus and botulinum-B neurotoxins block neurotransmitter release by proteolytic cleavage of synaptobrevin. Nature 359: 832

Sellin L C 1981 The action of botulinum toxin at the neuromuscular junction. Medical Biology 59: 11

Sharpe M, Archard L C, Banatvala J E et al 1991 A report on chronic fatigue syndrome: guidelines for research. Journal of the Royal Society of Medicine 84: 118

Sigurgeirsson B, Lindelof B, Edhag O, Allander E 1992 Risk of cancer in patients with dermatomyositis or polymyositis. New England Journal of Medicine 326: 363

Sinha S, Newsom-Davis J, Mills K, Byrne N, Lang B, Vincent A 1991 Autoimmune aetiology for acquired neuromyotonia (Isaacs' syndrome). Lancet 338: 75

Smith B 1969 Skeletal muscle necrosis associated with carcinoma. Journal of Pathology 97: 207

Smith B E, Dyck P J 1990 Peripheral neuropathy in the eosinophilia-myalgia syndrome associated with L-tryptophan ingestion. Neurology 40: 1035

Solimena M, Folli F, Dennis-Donini S, Comi G C, Pozza G, De Camilli P, Vicari A M 1988 Autoantibodies to glutamic acid decarboxylase in a patient with stiff-man syndrome, epilepsy and type I diabetes mellitus. New England Journal of Medicine 318: 1012

Solimena M, Folli F, Aparisi R, Pozza G, De Camilli P 1990 Autoantibodies to GABA-ergic neurons and pancreatic beta cells in stiff-man syndrome. New England Journal of Medicine 322: 1555

Spillane J D 1970 Restless legs syndrome in chronic pulmonary disease. British Medical Journal 4: 796

Spillane J D, Nathan P W, Kelly R E, Marsden C D 1971 Painful legs and moving toes. Brain 94: 541

St Louis M E, Peck S H S, Bowering D et al 1988 Botulism from chopped garlic: delayed recognition of a major outbreak. Annals of Internal Medicine 108: 363

Stokes M J, Cooper R G, Edwards R H T 1988 Normal muscle strength and fatiguability in patients with effort syndrome. British Medical Journal 297: 1014

Swash M 1974 Acute fatal carcinomatous neuromyopathy. Archives of Neurology 30: 324

Sylvest E 1934 Epidemic myalgia: Bornholm disease. Levin & Munksgaard, Copenhagen

Tahmoush A J, Alonso R J, Tahmoush G P, Heiman-Patterson T D 1991 Cramp-fasciculation syndrome: a treatable hyperexcitable peripheral nerve disorder. Neurology 41: 1021

Telstad W, Sørensen Ø, Larsen S, Lillevold P E, Stensrud P, Nyberg-Hansen R 1984 Treatment of the restless legs syndrome with carbamazepine: a double blind study. British Medical Journal 288: 444

Thomas P K, Hollinrake K, Lascelles R G et al 1971 The polyneuropathy of renal failure. Brain 94: 761

Tsairis P, Dyck P J, Mulder D W 1972 Natural history of brachial plexus neuropathy: report on 99 patients. Archives of Neurology 27: 109

Urich H, Wilkinson M 1970 Necrosis of muscle with carcinoma: myositis or myopathy? Journal of Neurology, Neurosurgery and Psychiatry 33: 398

Van Unnik A J M 1982 Muscle tumours: In: Mastaglia F L, Walton J (eds) Skeletal muscle pathology. Churchill Livingstone, Edinburgh, p 561

Varga J, Peltonen J, Uitto J, Jimenez S 1990 Development of diffuse fasciitis with eosinophilia during L-tryptophan treatment: Demonstration of elevated type I collagen gene expression in affected tissues. Annals of Internal Medicine 112: 344

Varga J, Uitto J, Jimenez S A 1992 The cause and pathogenesis of the eosinophilia-myalgia syndrome. Annals of Internal Medicine 116: 140

Vasilescu C, Alexianu M, Dan A 1984 Muscle hypertrophy and a syndrome of continuous motor unit activity in prednisone-responsive Guillain–Barré polyneuropathy. Journal of Neurology 231: 276

Vicari A M, Folli F, Pozza G et al 1989 Plasmapheresis in the treatment of stiff-man syndrome. New England Journal of Medicine 320: 1499

Von Scheele C 1986 Levodopa in restless legs. Lancet ii: 426

Zisfein J, Sivak M, Aron A M, Bender A N 1983 Isaacs syndrome with muscle hypertrophy reversed by phenytoin therapy. Archives of Neurology 40: 241

28. Drug-induced neuromuscular disorders in man

Z. Argov   F. L. Mastaglia

INTRODUCTION

An increasing number of drugs are known to have effects on the neuromuscular system when used therapeutically in man. Some have selective structural and functional effects on muscle (Lane & Mastaglia 1978), while others interfere with neuromuscular transmission or are neurotoxic. Certain drugs such as vincristine, colchicine and chloroquine are both myotoxic and neurotoxic.

The frequency of drug-induced neuromuscular disorders in clinical practice is difficult to establish because the association with drug therapy is not always recognised and subclinical forms are probably commoner than is generally appreciated. The recognition of such iatrogenic forms of neuromuscular disease is important, because early withdrawal of the offending agent often results in complete reversal of symptoms, while failure to do so may lead to serious disability. Awareness of the possibility of drug effects on the neuromuscular system is also of importance as the range of therapeutic agents introduced into clinical practice continues to expand. The increasing recognition of neuromuscular effects of drugs in widespread clinical use also has important implications with regard to the adequacy of laboratory testing of new therapeutic agents before they are released for general use.

MYOPATHIES

Muscle damage may result from the local effects of drugs administered by intramuscular injection, or from a more widespread effect on the skeletal muscles. The resulting clinical syndromes vary in severity, mode of onset and rate of progression.

Some are acute or subacute and are associated with muscle pain, while others are more protracted and painless (Table 28.1). Muscle involvement is usually widespread and symmetrical, the proximal muscles often being most severely affected, while those innervated by the cranial nerves are usually spared. The mechanisms involved may be either direct myotoxicity or indirect muscle damage through drug-induced electrolyte disturbances, immunological abnormalities, ischaemia, neural activation or muscle compression in drug-induced coma (Mastaglia 1982).

Focal myopathy

Intramuscular injections produce localised areas of muscle damage as a result of needle insertion ('needle myopathy') and local effects of the agent injected. Creatine kinase (CK) activity in the serum may be increased after injection of a variety of drugs including diazepam, lidocaine and digoxin; histological examination of the injection site in animals has shown extensive necrosis after injection of such drugs, but not after injection of saline (Steiness et al 1978). Other drugs which have a local toxic effect include chloroquine (Aguayo & Hudgson 1970), and the opiates and chlorpromazine which are thought to cause damage by inducing histamine release (Cohen 1972, Brumback et al 1982). Some drugs such as paraldehyde and cephalothin sodium, which are particularly irritant, may cause more severe tissue damage leading to abscess formation (Lane & Mastaglia 1978, Greenblatt & Allen 1978). These focal forms of muscle damage are usually of little clinical consequence apart from the fact that the finding of elevated serum enzyme activities may be misleading in patients with suspected myocardial infarction, unless isoenzyme studies are performed (Marmor et al 1978).

Marked muscle fibrosis leading to progressive induration and contractures may occur as a result of repeated intramuscular injections. This complication has occurred particularly in children following intramuscular injections of antibiotics (Saunders et al 1965, Battacharrya 1966, Hagen 1968), and in adults addicted to pethidine (Mastaglia et al 1971) or pentazocine (Steiner et al 1973, Levin & Engel 1975, Adams et al 1983,

Roberson & Dimon 1983). The quadriceps femoris and deltoid muscles are most often affected but more widespread involvement has been reported in some drug addicts (Aberfeld et al 1968, Mastaglia et al 1971, Steiner et al 1973, Choucair & Ziter 1984). Repeated needle trauma, toxic effects of the drug, haemorrhage and low-grade infection may all be contributory factors.

Acute or subacute painful myopathy

A number of drugs may cause a rapidly evolving syndrome characterised by muscle pain, tenderness and weakness involving proximal limb and axial muscles most severely. This may be due to a direct toxic effect of the drug or to the development of hypokalaemia or of an inflammatory myopathy. The tendon reflexes are usually preserved unless the myopathy is profound or is associated with peripheral neuropathy. Serum activities of CK and other enzymes are usually considerably raised and myoglobinuria may occur. Electromyography (EMG) shows the typical changes of primary muscle disease (see Ch. 29) and spontaneous potentials may be prominent (Lane et al 1979).

Toxic myopathy. The drugs which most frequently produce this syndrome as a result of a direct toxic effect are the cholesterol-lowering agents (clofibrate, gemfibrozil, lovastatin and nicotinic acid), epsilon-amino-caproic acid (EACA) and emetine, all of which cause a necrotising myopathy (Fig. 28.1a). An identical syndrome has also been reported in heroin addicts (Richter et al 1971) and alcoholics (Perkoff et al 1966).

Clofibrate. Many cases of clofibrate myopathy have been reported and were reviewed by Rimon et al (1984). The myopathy appears to be dose-dependent; it is uncommon when the drug is administered in conventional therapeutic doses but is more likely to develop in patients with renal failure (Pierides et al 1975), the nephrotic syndrome (Bridgeman et al 1972) or hypothyroidism, probably because plasma levels of the unbound drug are high in these conditions (Rumpf et al 1976). However 20 patients with normal renal function also developed this complication. Five patients with clofibrate-induced myopathy contin-

Table 28.1 Features of drug-induced myopathies

	Drugs implicated	Clinical features	Serum† CK	Myoglobinuria	Electromyography findings	Pathology
Focal myopathy	IM injections of various drugs	—	may be ↑	—	—	Focal necrosis
Muscle fibrosis and contractures	antibiotics pethidine pentazocine heroin	Induration and contracture of injected muscles	Normal may be ↑	—	BSAPPs; variable spontaneous activity	Marked fibrosis and myopathic changes in injected areas
Acute/subacute painful proximal myopathy Toxic effect	clofibrate lovastatin gemfibrozil EACA emetine heroin amiodarone ipamidol	Muscle pain, proximal or generalised weakness; reflexes usually preserved	↑↑	+/−	BSAPPs; spontaneous potentials may be prominent	Necrosis regeneration
	vincristine	Proximal pain, atrophy, weakness, absent reflexes	?	—	?	
	zidovudine	Myalgia, weakness loss of reflexes	↑↑	+/−	BSAPPs fibrillations	Mitochondrial abnormalities
	cyclosporin nicotinic acid clofibride isoetherine danazol cimetidine metolazone bumetadine lithium salbutamol labetalol mercaptopropionyl glycine suxamethonium nifedipine D-penicillamine gold	Myalgia/cramps/ myokymia/ weakness	Normal or ↑	—	Usually normal	
Hypokalaemia	diuretics purgatives liquorice fluoroprednisolone carbenoxolone amphotericin B	Weakness may be periodic; reflexes may be depressed or absent	↑↑	+/−	BSAPPS	Vacuolar myopathy ± necrosis/regeneration
Inflammatory myopathy	D-penicillamine L-tryptophan procainamide levodopa phenytoin penicillin cimetidine leuprolide propylthiouracil	Proximal muscle pain, weakness ± skin changes	↑↑	—	BSAPPs ± spontaneous activity	Necrosis/regeneration/ inflammation
Acute rhabdomyolysis	heroin cocaine caffeine overdose methadone amphetamine	Severe muscle pain, swelling flaccid quadriparesis, areflexia, renal	↑↑↑	+++	BSAPPs; prominent spontaneous discharges	Severe necrosis; ± regeneration

Table 28.1 *Contd*

	Drugs implicated	Clinical features	Serum† CK	Myoglobinuria	Electromyography findings	Pathology
	barbiturates diazepam meprobamate isoniazid amphotericin B phenformin fenfluramine carbenoxolone vasopressin phenylpropano- lamine loxapin lovastatin gemfibrozil clofibrate	failure				
Subacute or chronic painless proximal myopathy	corticosteroids	Predominantly proximal, atrophy and weakness	Normal	—	BSAPPs	Type II fibre atrophy
	steroids + muscle relaxants	Weakness, atrophy, areflexia	Normal or ↑	—	Myopathic neuropathic	thick filament loss
	chloroquine colchicine heroin perhexiline amiodarone alcohol	Reflexes may be lost due to associated neuropathy	↑↑↑	—	Myopathic/ neuropathic; spontaneous discharges may be prominent	Vacuolar myopathy Nonspecific myopathic changes
	squill oxymel (cardiac glycoside)	Proximal weakness ± myasthenic features	↑↑↑	—	Myopathic/ neuropathic	Necrosis
Myotonic syndrome	20, 25- diazacholesterol and analogues	Muscle cramps, weakness, myotonia	—	—	Myotonic and other spontaneous discharges	—
	suxamethonium propranolol pindolol fenoterol ritodrine furosemide acetazolamide	May aggravate myotonia	Normal	—		—
Malignant hyperpyrexia	suxamethonium halothane diethyl ether cyclopropane chloroform methoxyflurane ketamine enflurane	Rigidity, hyperpyrexia, acidosis, hyperkalaemia, disseminated intra-vascular coagulation, renal failure	↑↑↑ (↑ in some cases at risk)	+++	Variable myopathic changes in survivors and family members at risk	Necrosis (variable abnormalities in cases at risk)

† CK, Creatine Kinase. BSAPPs, brief duration, small amplitude, polyphasic motor unit action potentials.

ued to take the drug at lower doses and all recovered. Symptoms develop quite abruptly, usually within 3 weeks of the start of therapy, possibly when the concentration of the drug in the blood reaches a critical level (Teravainen et al 1977). In almost all patients muscle enzyme activity in the serum is increased. The mechanism whereby clofibrate causes muscle necrosis is uncertain, but the observation that the drug causes an increase in muscle lipoprotein-lipase activity may be relevant (Lithell et al 1978). Disturbances in muscle energy metabolism were found in rats treated with clofibrate (Paul & Abidi 1979).

Gemfibrozil. This is a derivative of fibric acid, like clofibrate, that has recently been used as a cholesterol-lowering drug. Painful muscle weakness with mild elevation of serum CK was found in one patient after 3 years of drug administration (Magarian et al 1991). This patient recovered when gemfibrozil was withdrawn, but a short rechallenge again led to myalgia and high CK activity. The mechanism of the myopathy is unknown. There are several other reports of painful myopathy with the combined use of lovastatin and gemfibrozil (see below); the relative contribution of each drug is uncertain.

Lovastatin. This is a competitive inhibitor of 3-hydroxy-3-methylglutaryl-Coenzyme A (HMG-CoA) reductase that has become a major drug in the treatment of hypercholesterolaemia, both familial and non-familial. Rhabdomyolysis was reported in several heart transplant patients who were receiving this drug in association with the usual immunosuppressive protocol (Corpier et al 1988, East et al 1988). The patients developed myalgia and muscle cramps after a few weeks to several months of therapy. Muscle weakness soon ensued. In all, serum CK was elevated more than 100-fold. Withdrawal of lovastatin was followed by slow recovery with return of CK levels to normal. All the first reported patients were also receiving cyclosporin, another potentially myotoxic agent, and the hypothesis was that the combined use of the two drugs led to the rhabdomyolysis. Exposure of rats to HMG-CoA reductase inhibitors produced a dose-related myopathy with myofibrillar necrosis, interstitial oedema and inflammatory infiltrates. These changes were augmented by combined administration of the HMG-

CoA reductase inhibitor and cyclosporin. Pharmacological studies in these rats suggest that the combined toxicity is due to altered clearance and increased tissue exposure induced by cyclosporin (Smith et al 1991).

A similar lovastatin-induced syndrome appeared in one patient who was not a heart transplant recipient and who subsequently responded to a rechallenge with a marked rise in serum CK (Ayanian et al 1988). Israeli et al (1989) found three out of 60 patients on lovastatin who had high CK activity without muscle symptoms. One showed a rise in CK activity after rechallenge. Pierce et al (1990), from the USA Food and Drug Administration, cited 63 reports of elevated CK with the use of lovastatin. Most patients had only a symptomless rise of CK, while three had rhabdomyolysis. It is thus clear that lovastatin by itself is myotoxic, although the mechanism of this side-effect is speculative.

Combined use of lovastatin and gemfibrozil has been associated with rhabdomyolysis in at least 14 patients (Goldman et al 1989, Pierce et al 1990, London et al 1991). Whenever combined use of these two cholesterol-lowering drugs is indicated, close follow-up of serum CK activity and muscle status is therefore essential.

Nicotinic acid. Three patients who were taking nicotinic acid for a few months developed muscle cramps associated with abdominal pain and nausea. CK activity was mildly elevated but no weakness was reported and neither EMG nor biopsy were performed. In one patient this was the only cholesterol-lowering drug given and in the others gemfibrozil was also used. Recovery occurred rapidly after withdrawal of nicotinic acid (Litin & Anderson 1989).

Epsilon-aminocaproic acid. The development of a myopathy is a well-recognised but uncommon complication of treatment with this antifibrinolytic agent. Brown et al (1982) reviewed 19 reported cases. This myopathy usually develops abruptly after weeks of treatment with daily doses of 10–30 g, suggesting that it is due to a cumulative dose-related effect of the drug (Lane et al 1979). It has been reported most frequently in patients with hereditary angioneurotic oedema (Korsan-Bengsten et al 1969) or subarachnoid haemorrhage (Lane et al 1979). The myopathy may be severe and acute rhabdomyolysis with renal failure has been recorded (Brodkin 1980). It has been suggested that complement abnormalities and lysine deficiency may possibly be predisposing factors. Active muscle regeneration occurs and complete recovery over a period of weeks is the rule (Lane et al 1979, Brown et al 1982). One patient with EACA-induced myopathy who was given a cyclic analogue of this drug, tranexamic acid, did not have this side-effect (Kane et al 1988). It is not clear how the structural differences between the two drugs relate to the mechanism of myotoxicity. Histological evidence of capillary occlusion was reported in some (Cullen & Mastaglia 1980, Kennard et al 1980) but not all cases (Britt et al 1980). Attempts to reproduce this myopathy in animals have been unsuccessful.

Cardiac glycosides. A myopathy characterised by muscle pain and tenderness with elevated serum CK levels and in some cases associated myasthenic features has been reported in the Australian literature in opiate addicts consuming large quantities of the cough suppressant Linctus Codeine (Kennedy 1981, Kilpatrick et al 1982, Seow 1984). Muscle biopsy shows evidence of a necrotising myopathy. One of the components of Linctus Codeine is squill (an extract of the bulb of *Urginea maritama*) which contains the cardiac glycosides scillarin A and B. The myopathy and associated cardiac abnormalities which occur in some cases have been attributed to the inhibitory effects of these glycosides on the muscle cell membrane Na^+–K^+ pump.

Emetine. Patients treated with this anti-amoebic agent frequently developed generalised muscle weakness during (Klatskin & Friedman 1948) or after a course of treatment (Young & Tudhope 1926). This is usually reversible, but the outcome may be fatal, particularly when there is an associated cardiomyopathy (Fewings et al 1973). Although emetine myopathy is usually painful and is associated with elevated serum CK activity, a painless case with no change in serum CK was described (Bennett et al 1982). Overdose of emetine may be responsible for a myopathy developing in some patients treated with ipecac syrup to induce emesis (Bennett et al 1982; Halbig et al 1988, Kuntzer et al 1989). The pathological features included sarcomeric changes such as Z-line streaming and sarcotubular breakdown (Halbig et al 1988, Kuntzer et al 1989). Early clinical reports suggested that there were both 'neuritic' and 'myositic' forms of emetine toxicity. However, experimental studies have shown a pure myotoxic effect with mitochondrial and myofibrillar changes followed by necrosis and regeneration (Duane & Engel 1970, Bradley et al 1976) and no evidence of damage to intramuscular nerves or motor endplates.

Vincristine. A painful proximal necrotising myopathy may occur in some patients treated with vincristine in addition to the severe polyneuropathy caused by the drug (Bradley et al 1970). Electron-microscopic studies in man (Bradley et al 1970) and in the experimental animal (Anderson et al 1967, Bradley 1970) have shown that the drug has a profound effect on membrane systems and causes severe autophagic degeneration of muscle fibres.

Zidovudine. This drug, formerly called azidothymidine (AZT), was introduced for the treatment of HIV infection in the mid-1980s. Zidovudine-induced myalgia occurred in 8% of patients (Richman et al 1987). During the succeeding years a distinctive myopathy associated with this drug was identified in dozens of patients and has been reviewed by several authors (Dalakas et al 1990, Chalmers et al 1991, Mhiri et al 1991). The myopathy develops after several months (usually more than 9 months) of full-dose therapy and is characterised by progressive muscle weakness and exercise-related myalgia. The limb girdle muscles are mainly affected but dysphagia is common. Facial and neck muscles are spared. In all patients serum CK is elevated, usually 2–5 times normal. The EMG is myopathic with the presence of fibrillations. There are two main features in the muscle biopsy of such patients: inflammatory infiltrates of $CD8^+$ cells and macrophages and abundant abnormal mitochondria with a tendency to produce ragged-red like fibres. Inflammatory myopathy is common in AIDS patients and usually responds only to immunomodulation (plasmapheresis and steroids). In the zidovudine myopathy, however, withdrawal of the drug leads to partial or almost full recovery. Mitochondrial abnormalities were not identified in AIDS-related myopathy without zidovudine (Dalakas et al 1990, Mhiri et al 1991) and are regarded as the distinctive feature of this myopathy. Zidovudine inhibits DNA polymerase and this is thought to be the mechanism of the mitochondrial changes, although the mitochondrial DNA showed no abnormality on Southern blots. It still remains to be shown that the toxic effect of zidovudine on muscle is solely due to the mitochondrial abnormality. T-cell-mediated cytotoxicity was implicated in one study (Dalakas et al 1990).

Cyclosporin. Normal therapeutic levels of this drug led to myalgia without weakness in five transplanted subjects (Noppen et al 1987, Fernandez-Sola et al 1990, Goy et al 1989). Serum CK activity remained normal or was slightly elevated and the EMG in painful muscles was normal. Muscle biopsy showed fibre atrophy, usually type II, which is non-specific. In all patients withdrawal of cyclosporin led to recovery and in one patient a rechallenge again caused myalgia (Noppen et al 1987). The mechanism of this side-effect is unknown.

Other drugs. A number of other drugs including lithium carbonate (Ghose 1977), cimetidine (Wade 1977, Treves et al 1985), propranolol and sotalol (Forfar et al 1979), tetracycline (Sinclair & Phillips 1982), mercaptoproprionyl glycine (Hales et al 1982), adenine arabinoside (Mak et al 1990), labetalol (Teicher et al 1981), nifedipine (Keidar et al 1982), gold (Mitsumoto et al 1982), D-penicillamine (Pinals 1983), clofibride, danazol, isoetherine, metolazone, bumetanide, cytotoxic agents (Dukes 1977) and salbutamol (Palmer 1978) have been reported to cause myalgia, muscle cramps, myokymia or weakness in some patients. Recovery has invariably followed withdrawal of the offending agent. Muscle pain following suxamethonium, usually after minor surgical procedures, is a relatively common complaint (Dottori et al 1965, Brodsky & Ehrenwerth 1980).

A patient developed severe myalgia and raised serum CK a few hours after administration of iopamidol 370, a non-ionic contrast agent, during urography (Stinchcombe & Davies 1989). Acute painful myopathy with muscle necrosis and phagocytosis was found in one man, 3 months after the onset of amiodarone treatment (Clouston & Donnelly 1989). The histological features were different from the more common amiodarone-induced lysosomal changes (see below). Recovery occurred upon withdrawal of the drug.

Myositis. A number of drugs have been associated with the development of an inflammatory myopathy (Mastaglia & Argov 1982) (Table 28.1).

D-penicillamine. A number of patients with rheumatoid arthritis or Wilson's disease treated with D-penicillamine in daily doses up to 1200 mg have developed acute or subacute polymyositis (Schraeder et al 1972, Halla et al 1984) or dermatomyositis (Fernandes et al 1977, Lund & Nielsen 1983, Carroll et al 1987). In some cases there has been associated myocardial involvement and a fatal outcome (Doyle et al 1983). Spontaneous recovery can occur after withdrawal of the drug but in several cases steroid therapy was required to induce a remission (Halla et al 1984). This complication is less frequent than the immunologically mediated myasthenia syndrome which develops in other patients treated with penicillamine. Interestingly, in three patients with D-penicillamine-induced myositis, antibodies against the acetylcholine receptor were detected in the serum without clinical signs of myasthenia (Carroll et al 1987). Other autoantibodies may also be found in such patients (Takahashi et al 1986). The immunogenetic profile of patients with penicillamine-associated myositis (HLA B18, B35 and DR4) is different from that of patients with idiopathic polymyositis and penicillamine-induced myasthenia gravis (Carroll et al 1987).

L-tryptophan. A form of interstitial eosinophilic myositis and fasciitis characterised by myalgia, muscle tenderness, weakness, cutaneous oedema and induration and a peripheral blood eosinophilia has recently been linked to the ingestion of certain preparations of L-tryptophan (*eosinophilia-myalgia syndrome*) (Kaufman 1990, Kaufman et al 1991). Over 1500 cases of this syndrome are known to have occurred in the USA alone. Some patients also had an ascending peripheral neuropathy or other systemic features (Smith & Dyck 1990). The syndrome is thought to be due to a contaminant in the preparations rather than to the L-trytophan itself (Belongia et al 1990).

Other drugs. An interstitial myositis may occur in some patients treated with procainamide (Fig. 28.1b) and is usually part of a lupus-like syndrome (Fontiveros et al 1980). A similar myopathy was described in a patient receiving levodopa therapy for Parkinson's disease (Wolf et al 1976). Other drugs which have been implicated as a possible cause of myositis, usually in single patients, include phenytoin (Harney & Glasberg 1983), penicillin (Hayman et al 1956), cimetidine (Feest & Read 1980, Watson et al 1983), leuprolide acetate used for the treatment of prostatic carcinoma (Crayton et al 1991) and propylthiouracil (Shergy & Caldwell 1988).

Hypokalaemic myopathy. Widespread muscle weakness, which may be painful, and which may be associated with depressed or absent tendon reflexes and a marked increase in serum CK activity and myoglobinuria, may result from hypokalaemia in patients taking diuretics (Jensen et al 1977), purgatives (Basser 1979), carbenoxolone (Mohamed et al 1966), or amphotericin B which causes renal tubular damage (Drutz et al 1970) and fluoroprednisolone-containing nasal sprays (Vita et al 1986). Hypokalaemic myopathy has also been reported in individuals consuming large quantities of liquorice, traditional Chinese medicines containing liquorice extracts, snuff or chewing tobacco (Gross et al 1966, Cumming et al 1980, Valeriano et al 1983). Histological studies in such cases usually show a vacuolar myopathy but, in severe cases, necrosis and regeneration may be present.

Acute rhabdomyolysis

Although several drugs already discussed may cause a severe necrotising myopathy and myoglobinuria, the features of the potentially fatal condition referred to as acute rhabdomyolysis are sufficiently distinctive to merit special consideration. It is characterised by the abrupt onset of severe generalised muscle pain, tenderness and flaccid areflexic paralysis, often with severe muscle swelling which may require fasciotomy. Gross myoglobinuria usually leads to acute oliguric renal failure which may be responsible for death. Serum levels of CK and of other enzymes are markedly raised and the EMG reveals myopathic changes, often with prominent spontaneous discharges. Muscle biopsy shows widespread necrosis with mild reactive inflammatory changes, and regener-

ative activity may be profuse in patients who survive. Recovery usually occurs over a period of weeks, but full muscle power may not be restored for several months.

Acute rhabdomyolysis has occurred in association with amphotericin B (Drutz et al 1970), carbenoxolone therapy (Mohamed et al 1966), intravenous vasopressin (Affarah et al 1984), several cholesterol lowering agents (see above), labetalol (Willis et al 1990), and high doses of the appetite suppressant phenylpropanolamine (Swenson et al 1982). Intoxication with barbiturates, meprobamate and diazepam (Nicolas et el 1970, Penn et al 1972, Wattel et al 1978), phencyclidine (Cogen et al 1978), loxapin (Tam et al 1980) and its analogue amoxapin (Abreo et al 1982), amphetamine poisoning (Grossman et al 1974), combined overdosage with phenformin and fenfluramine (Palmucci et al 1978), alcoholism (Perkoff et al 1966), heroin and methadone addiction (Richter et al 1971) and caffeine overdose (Wrenn & Oschner 1989) can all lead to rhabdomyolysis. Cocaine abuse has also been associated with rhabdomyolysis (Herzlich et al 1988, Reinhart & Stricker 1988, Anand et al 1989). Rubin & Neugarten (1989) reviewed 55 such patients. In one-half to two-thirds of patients there were other possible causative factors but in the rest only cocaine exposure could be associated with the rhabdomyolysis. The mechanisms of myotoxicity in these situations have not been investigated and it remains to be determined whether a direct toxic drug effect is involved, or whether individual idiosyncracy or other predisposing factors play a part.

A variety of other drugs have also been implicated in causing rhabdomyolysis (see Kakulas & Mastaglia 1992, Mastaglia 1993). However, few of these have been proven to be myotoxic and it is likely that in many of the reported cases other factors such as muscle compression and ischaemia, hypoxia and hypotension and intense muscular hyperactivity (e.g. in patients with drug-induced seizures, dyskinesias or acute dystonic reactions) have been responsible for causing the muscle damage.

Less severe forms of rhabdomyolysis have been recognised in apparently normal individuals (Gibbs 1978, Hool et al 1984) and in patients with Duchenne muscular dystrophy (Watters et al

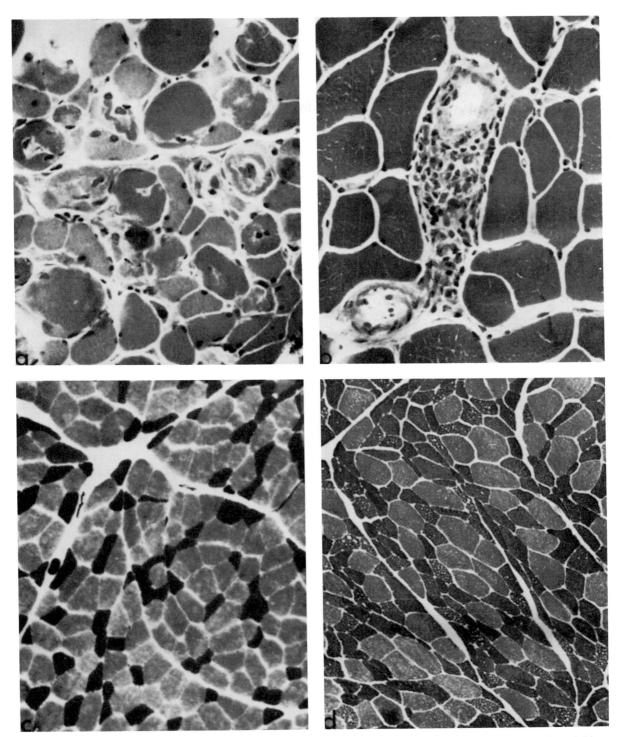

Fig. 28.1 **a**. Severe necrotising myopathy due to epsilon-aminocaproic acid in a 67-year-old female. Quadriceps femoris biopsy; H & E, × 320. **b**. Interstitial perivascular mononuclear cell infiltrate in a 54-year-old man with a procainamide-induced lupus-like syndrome. Quadriceps femoris biopsy; H & E, × 320. **c.** Type II fibre atrophy in a 26-year-old female treated with corticosteroids for systemic lupus erythematosus (SLE). Quadriceps femoris biopsy; myofibrillar ATPase (pH 9.4) ×125. **d.** Vacuolar myopathy with predominant involvement of intermediate and type II fibres in a 55-year-old female with suspected SLE who was treated with chloroquine. Quadriceps femoris biopsy; myofibrillar ATPase (pH 7.2) ×160.

1977) following administration of suxamethonium during anaesthesia.

Subacute or chronic painless proximal myopathy

This is probably the commonest form of drug-induced myopathy encountered in clinical practice and occurs most frequently in patients on long-term corticosteroid therapy.

Corticosteroids. Myopathy occurs particularly in patients treated with the fluorinated steroids triamcinolone (Williams 1959), betamethasone and dexamethasone (Golding & Begg 1960, Dropcho & Soong 1991) but has also been associated with cortisone, prednisone, prednisolone and methyl-prednisolone therapy (Askari et al 1976). Myopathy is more likely to develop in patients maintained on high doses of these drugs for prolonged periods (Askari et al 1976) and is unlikely to occur if the daily dose of steroid is kept below 10 mg of prednisone or its equivalent (Yates 1970, Bowyer et al 1985). Severe myopathy may occasionally follow parenteral treatment with high doses of hydrocortisone. A reversible form of myopathy of the laryngeal muscles resulting in dysphonia has been reported in patients treated with inhaled corticosteroids (Williams et al 1983). Severe corticosteroid myopathy is uncommon but the true frequency of the condition is difficult to determine because mild forms may be overlooked, particularly in patients with an underlying disorder such as rheumatoid arthritis, which may also cause muscle weakness and wasting. Quantitative studies of muscle function in such patients have shown significant reductions in muscle performance (Rothstein et al 1983, Khaleeli et al 1983). Electromyographic findings indicate that subclinical myopathy is common (Coomes 1965a, Yates 1970). In patients with brain tumours who were on daily dexamethasone therapy, the risk of steroid myopathy was found to be lower in those who were also taking phenytoin which increases the hepatic metabolism of dexamethasone (Dropcho & Soong 1991).

In the typical case there is symmetrical involvement of proximal limb muscles, particularly those of the pelvic girdle, and atrophy and weakness of the quadriceps femoris are prominent. Muscle pain is not usually a feature and the tendon reflexes are preserved. Serum enzyme levels are normal and, if found to be elevated, should suggest the possibility of some other myopathy. Creatinuria occurs and urinary creatine levels have been held to be useful in diagnosis and in monitoring progress (Askari et al 1976). The EMG shows the typical changes of primary muscle disease, particularly in proximal groups, spontaneous discharges usually being absent. In contrast to experimental corticosteroid myopathy (see Ch. 12), the histological changes in steroid myopathy in man are relatively inconspicuous. Muscle biopsy shows an atrophic process with particular involvement of the type II B fibres (Fig. 28.1c) as occurs in experimental corticosteroid myopathy (Livingstone et al 1981). Necrosis, regeneration and vacuolar change are not found. The myopathy is usually reversible on stopping the drug or, to some extent, on substituting prednisone for the offending steroid (Williams 1959, Walton 1977). Anabolic steroids and B group vitamins, which prevent the development of corticosteroid myopathy in the rat (Sakai et al 1978), are ineffective in the human condition (Coomes 1965b). However, a regular programme of physical activity can at least partially prevent or reverse the muscle atrophy and weakness (Hickson & Davis 1981, Horber et al 1985).

Although usually subacute or chronic, steroid myopathy can also be acute. There have been reports of patients with status asthmaticus who were treated with high doses of intravenous hydrocortisone, who developed a severe generalised myopathy with involvement of the respiratory muscles and elevation of serum CK activity (MacFarlane & Rosenthal 1977, Van Marle & Woods 1980, Mastaglia 1982). Biopsy showed vacuolar changes in both fibre types with evidence of regeneration. These features resembled experimental steroid myopathy in rabbits (Afifi & Bergman 1969). Recovery was slow in these cases.

Combined use of high-dose corticosteroids and prolonged administration of non-depolarizing muscle relaxants (pancuronium, vecuronium) can result in a unique myopathic condition and over 20 patients with this have been reported (Danon

& Carpenter 1991, Dalakas 1992). Typically, when the ventilation of such a patient is terminated severe diffuse muscle weakness, atrophy and areflexia are noted. Ophthalmoplegia can also be found (Sitwell et al 1991). Serum CK activity can be elevated or normal and the EMG shows a mixed pattern. Most patients recover within weeks to months. Selective thick filament loss was found in one patient (Danon & Carpenter 1991) and was thought to be the result of combined exposure of steroids and pharmacological denervation, similar to the effects of steroids on denervated rat muscle (Rouleau et al 1987). In other cases large areas of myofilament loss and resulting loss of staining are found in both major fibre types (Dalakas 1992).

The mechanism of steroid-induced myopathy has been clarified by experimental studies which have shown that specific steroid receptor proteins are present in muscle (Shoji & Pennington 1977a), and that steroids interfere with oxidative metabolism (Koski et al 1974), enhance glycogen synthesis (Shoji et al 1974) and protein synthesis and degradation (Shoji & Pennington 1977b). The basic cellular action of corticosteroids is to inhibit messenger RNA synthesis which in turn interferes with the translation and synthesis of muscle-specific proteins (Rannels et al 1978, Karpati 1984).

Chloroquine. A severe myopathy may result from the prolonged administration of chloroquine (Whisnant et al 1963). It may be indistinguishable clinically from steroid myopathy and there may be difficulty in deciding which drug is responsible, in patients receiving both chloroquine and corticosteroids (Mastaglia et al 1977). As the drug may also cause a mild peripheral neuropathy, sensory changes, reflex depression and abnormal nerve conduction may be found (Whisnant et al 1963). Cardiomyopathy can also occur in some cases (Estes et al 1987). In contrast to steroid myopathy, spontaneous potentials, including myotonic discharges, are commonly found in the EMG, in addition to the typical changes of primary muscle disease (Mastaglia et al 1977). Biopsy shows a vacuolar myopathy, type I fibres usually being more severely affected, although in some cases there is predominant involvement of intermediate or type II fibres (Fig. 28.1d) (Mastaglia

et al 1977). Electron-microscopic studies of human and experimental animal material have shown that the drug has a profound effect on intracellular membrane systems, leading to the formation of a variety of abnormal membranous structures and to autophagic degeneration of muscle fibres (MacDonald & Engel 1970, Mastaglia et al 1977). The myopathy is reversible after withdrawal of the drug, but recovery is slow (Mastaglia et al 1977).

A similar myopathy can be induced experimentally in animals by a number of drugs which are all amphiphilic cationic compounds (Drenckhahn & Lullman-Rauch 1979). These drugs have high affinity for polar lipids and form non-digestible drug-lipid complexes within lysosomal structures. The abnormal lysosomes form the lamellated membrane bodies which may also be present in other tissues, resulting in a drug-induced lipidosis (Lullman et al 1978).

Colchicine. Overdose of this anti-inflammatory drug was long known to be associated with myopathy (Kontos 1962, Riggs et al 1986). However, the observations of Kuncl and his associates (Kuncl et al 1987, Kuncl & Duncan 1988) in 14 patients indicate that colchicine myopathy can also occur with therapeutic doses of the drug. It usually occurs in patients with impaired renal function and is characterised by chronic or subacute painless weakness and markedly elevated serum CK activity. Usually a mild sensory neuropathy and areflexia are also present. The electrodiagnostic studies reveal an 'irritative' myopathy (spontaneous activity and myopathic potentials coexisting) and mild axonopathy. Drug withdrawal or even lowering the dose leads to recovery within weeks. The histological features are similar to those of chloroquine myopathy, namely lysosomal abnormalities and numerous autophagic vacuoles.

Amiodarone and perhexiline. These drugs also have amphiphilic cationic characteristics and are implicated as causing drug-induced neuropathy (see below). Two patients on amiodarone had in addition to the neuropathy a severe clinical myopathy with lysosomal changes (Meier et al 1979, Roth et al 1990). Perhexiline can also lead to a neuromyopathy of a similar type in man (Fardeau et al 1979).

Myotonia

Drug-induced myotonia is now no longer encountered in clinical practice. The classic example of a drug-induced myotonic syndrome was that produced by the hypocholesterolaemic agent 20,25-diazacholesterol (Somers & Winer 1966). Patients taking the drug in daily doses of 25–50 mg developed muscle spasms and weakness with clinical and EMG evidence of myotonia. Complete recovery occurred over a period of 2–3 months after withdrawal of the drug. A comparable syndrome occurs in rats and goats after administration of the drug or of its analogues. Accumulation of desmosterol has been demonstrated in the serum and sarcolemma (Winer et al 1966) and the altered sterol composition and enzyme activity of the sarcolemma are thought to be the basis for the myotonia (Peter & Fiehn 1973). Myotonia which resembles human myotonia congenita can also be induced in animals by other compounds, such as monocarboxylic aromatic acids, triparanol and clofibrate (Kwiecinski 1981). Clofibrate myotoxicity in humans is not associated with clinical or electrical myotonia.

A number of drugs may precipitate or exacerbate myotonia in patients with dystrophia myotonica or other myotonic disorders. These include the beta-blockers propranolol (Blessing & Walsh 1977) and pindolol (Ricker et al 1978), the beta-adrenergic agonists fenoterol (Ricker et al 1978) and ritodrine (Sholl et al 1985), and the depolarising muscle relaxant suxamethonium (Mitchell et al 1978). In contrast, non-depolarising muscle relaxants do not have this effect and are therefore preferable for use in myotonic patients (Mitchell et al 1978). A number of diuretics including frusemide and acetazolamide may be considered harmful in myotonic disorders because they have been shown to induce myotonic potentials in vitro (Bretag et al 1980).

Malignant hyperpyrexia

In this serious condition, various anaesthetic agents and other drugs may precipitate a potentially fatal state characterised by generalised muscular rigidity, severe hyperpyrexia, metabolic acidosis and myoglobinuria (King & Denborough 1973a, Britt 1979, Gronert 1983, Nelson & Fleweller 1983). The condition is usually familial, being inherited by an autosomal dominant mechanism, and susceptible individuals have either a clinically apparent or, more frequently, a subclinical myopathy (King et al 1972, Harriman et al 1973). Those who are clinically normal may be identified by the finding of elevated serum CK activities (King et al 1972, Ellis et al 1975), focal myopathic changes in the EMG or, most reliably, by the demonstration of abnormal in vitro sensitivity of muscle tissue to anaesthetic agents (Ellis et al 1972). Recent genetic investigations have localised the gene for malignant hyperpyrexia to chromosome 19q12–13.2 (McCarthy et al 1990) and it is likely that diagnostic DNA probes will soon be available for the identification of susceptible individuals. A second group of individuals with this susceptibility are young males of short stature with a progressive congenital myopathy, skeletal abnormalities and other dysmorphic features similar to those seen in the Noonan syndrome, and in whom an autosomal recessive mechanism of inheritance is probably involved (King & Denborough 1973b, Kaplan et al 1977). Malignant hyperpyrexia may rarely also occur in cases of myotonia congenita, myotonic dystrophy, Duchenne muscular dystrophy, central core disease and in osteogenesis imperfecta (Rowland 1980, Mastaglia 1982).

The drugs which may precipitate malignant hyperpyrexia in susceptible individuals include halothane, suxamethonium, diethyl ether, cyclopropane, chloroform, methoxyflurane (Newson 1972), ketamine (Page et al 1972) and enflurane (Knape 1977). Tricyclic antidepressants and monoamine oxidase inhibitors have also been reported to precipitate a similar syndrome (Newsom 1972). A safe anaesthetic regime for muscle biopsy in susceptible individuals comprises oral premedication with diazepam followed by thiopentone, fentanyl citrate and nitrous oxide (Ellis et al 1975). D-Tubocurarine and local, regional or spinal anaesthesia and neuroleptalgesia may also be used with safety (Denborough 1977).

The malignant hyperpyrexia crisis is thought to be initiated by the sudden excess release of calcium ions into the myoplasm leading to sustained myofibrillar contraction with excessive production of lactic acid and heat (Denborough 1977, Britt 1979). Recent evidence points to a basic defect in the calcium release channel (the ryanodine receptor) of the sarcoplasmic reticulum (Mickelson et al 1988), the gene for which has been located on chromosome 19q13:1 (Johnson 1990) and which is postulated to function abnormally in the presence of anaesthetic agents leading to an exaggerated release of calcium ions (MacLennan et al 1990).

Various drugs have been used in the treatment of the acute hyperpyrexia syndrome with the aim of reducing myoplasmic Ca^{2+} levels. These include procaine, procainamide, hydrocortisone, dexamethasone and dantrolene sodium which causes excitation-contraction uncoupling by reducing myoplasmic calcium levels by binding to the sarcoplasmic reticulum and reducing calcium release (Ward et al 1986, Harrison 1989). It is now the drug of choice (Nelson & Flewellen 1983, Gronert 1983).

Neuroleptic malignant syndrome. This is a severe form of drug-induced extrapyramidal disorder occurring in patients treated with drugs belonging to the phenothiazine, butyrophenone or thioxanthene groups (Knezevic et al 1984a, Gibb & Lees 1985). It is characterised by pyrexia, severe rigidity and akinesia and bulbar muscle dysfunction. The serum CK activity is often increased and overt myoglobinuria and renal failure have been reported in some cases (Hashimoto et al 1984).

DISORDERS OF NEUROMUSCULAR TRANSMISSION

A variety of drugs, in addition to the neuromuscular blocking agents used in anaesthesia, may interfere with neuromuscular transmission in man (Argov & Mastaglia 1979a, Kaeser 1984, Howard 1990). Drug-induced neuromuscular block may manifest clinically in the following ways.

Clinical presentations

Drug-induced myasthenic syndrome. As shown in Table 28.2, a number of drugs have been implicated in causing a myasthenic syndrome in patients with no evidence of pre-existing myasthenia gravis (MG). The disorder has usually developed within a short period of starting treatment and has been reversible after withdrawal of the drug. In spite of this, the possibility remains that, in at least some of these cases, a subclinical disorder of neuromuscular transmission was unmasked by the effects of the drug. This is a relatively uncommon complication of treatment with these drugs, probably because of the high safety factor for neuromuscular transmission which exists under normal circumstances (Desmedt 1973, Stalberg et al 1975). Clinically manifest neuromuscular block probably occurs only when this safety margin is reduced, as in hypocalcaemia or other electrolyte disturbances (Katz 1966), or when high blood levels of a drug develop, as in patients with renal failure (Lindesmith et al 1968).

With drugs such as the antibiotics, which have a direct effect at the neuromuscular junction, the onset is relatively acute and respiratory paralysis with variable involvement of other muscle groups is the rule. However with D-penicillamine, which induces neuromuscular block through an immunological mechanism, symptoms usually develop only after months or years, are generally less acute in onset and the resulting clinical syndrome resembles more closely classical MG.

Aggravation or unmasking of myasthenia gravis. It is well known that certain drugs may lead to clinical deterioration when administered to previously stable myasthenic patients (Table 28.2). This is probably caused by a further reduction in the already lowered safety margin for transmission in such cases (Desmedt 1973), because of the effects of the drug at the neuromuscular junction. In patients in whom an irreversible myasthenic syndrome develops, the drug has probably unmasked previously undeclared MG.

Postoperative respiratory depression. As shown in Table 28.2, several drugs may cause respiratory depression after anaesthesia through an effect on neuromuscular transmission. This may be due to a direct effect of the drug itself, to enhancement of the blockade induced by muscle relaxants, or to a combination of these effects. The commonest example is the respiratory depression which may occur in patients given certain antibiotics in the preoperative period or during operation. In addition, some patients are unduly

Table 28.2 Clinical symptoms of drug-induced neuromuscular blockade and drugs implicated

Clinical presentation	Antibiotics	Antirheumatic drugs	Cardiovascular drugs	Anticonvulsants	Psychotropic drugs	Anaesthetics	Other drugs
Drug-induced myasthenic syndrome	neomycin streptomycin kanamycin gentamycin polymyxin B colistins	D-penicillamine	oxprenolol practolol trimetaphan procainamide?	trimethadione phenytoin			DL-carnitine
Aggravation or unmasking of myasthenia gravis	streptomycin kanamycin gentamycin erythromycin colistin rolitetracycline oxytetracycline ampicillin	chloroquine	quinidine procainamide propranolol acebutolol propafenone verapamil	phenytoin	lithium chlorpromazine		methoxyflurane isoflurane halothane ACTH corticosteroids thyroid hormones ACh-esterase inhibitors timolol magnesium iodinated contrast media bretylium emetine pyrantel pamoate citrate anticoagulant
Postoperative respiratory depression	neomycin streptomycin kanamycin colistin lincomycin clindamycin tobramycin amikacin polymyxin B						
Potentiation of muscle relaxants		chloroquine D-penicillamine	quinidine trimetaphan		lithium promazine phenelzine	diazepam ketamine propanidid ether	oxytocin Trasylol ® cholinesterase inhibitors procaine lidocaine timolol magnesium

susceptible to the neuromuscular blocking action of certain drugs administered in the immediate postoperative period. For example, respiratory depression may occur following the administration of quinidine in patients who have recovered from the effects of muscle relaxants and have already been extubated, a phenomenon which has been called 'recurarisation' (Way et al 1967). Electrophysiological study has shown that partial curarisation in the postoperative period is common (Lennmarken & Lofstrom 1984) explaining why drug-induced neuromuscular block has been described as a common postanaesthetic complication.

Mechanisms of drug-induced neuromuscular block

Drugs may interfere directly with neuromuscular transmission through a presynaptic local anaesthetic-like action at the nerve terminal, a postsynaptic curariform action, a combined pre- and postsynaptic action, or by a separate effect on the muscle fibre membrane (Fig. 28.2). The mechanism of action of some of the drugs to be discussed has been determined by experimental studies, while that of others is still conjectural.

The side-effect of a drug may be indirectly mediated, as in the case of citrate anticoagulant used in plasmapheresis, which lowers serum free calcium and probably reduces the neuromuscular safety margin (Wirguin et al 1990). Another indirect mechanism is mediated by the immune system as in the case of D-penicillamine myasthenia.

Presynaptic action. A number of drugs with local anaesthetic properties are suspected to reduce transmitter release by interfering with the generation of the nerve terminal action potential (Table 28.3). Confirmation of such an action would require simultaneous extracellular recording of the nerve terminal potential and the end-plate current produced by nerve stimulation (Katz & Miledi 1965). Another possible presynaptic action is interference with calcium entry into the presynaptic terminal. This is probably the mechanism of aggravation of myasthenia gravis and the Lambert–Eaton myasthenic syndrome by the calcium channel blockers (Krendel & Hopkins 1986, Wirguin et al 1992).

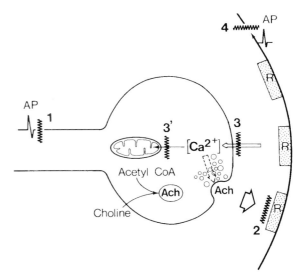

Fig. 28.2 Schematic representation of neuromuscular junction showing the possible sites of action of the drugs discussed. 1 — Presynaptic local anaesthetic-like effect on propagation of nerve action potential (AP); 2 — Postsynaptic receptor (R) blockade; 3, 3' — interference with acetylcholine (ACh) release through inhibiton of entry of Ca^{2+} ions into the nerve terminal (3) and into mitochondria (3'); 4 — Impairment of muscle action potential propagation.

Postsynaptic curariform block. A number of drugs exert their effect by competing for acetylcholine (ACh) receptor binding sites on the postsynaptic membrane (Table 28.3). Some of these drugs possess an ionised ammonium group which is thought to be the active binding site to the receptor (Koelle 1975). Such an effect has been demonstrated in vitro by the finding of a reduced end-plate electrical response to iontophoretically applied ACh (Werman & Wislicki 1971), or of a rapid reduction in miniature end-plate potential (mepp) amplitude after addition of the drug (Gissen et al 1966). The in vivo demonstration of potentiation of neuromuscular block by D-tubocurarine and reversal by neostigmine, although less conclusive, have been the basis for establishing a curare-like action of certain drugs such as the amphetamines (Skau & Gerald 1978), and procainamide (Galzigna et al 1972).

Combined pre- and postsynaptic block. A number of drugs have been shown to have both a presynaptic inhibitory effect on transmitter release and a postsynaptic curariform action. In the case

Table 28.3 Mechanisms of action of drugs which cause neuromuscular blockade

Mechanism	Antibiotics	Anti-inflammatory drugs	Cardiovascular drugs	Anticonvulsants	Psychotropic drugs	Anaesthetics	Other drugs
Presynaptic local anaesthetic-like action (1)*	clindamycin lincomycin kanamycin	chloroquine	propranolol quinidine		lithium imipramine		procaine
Postsynaptic curare-like action (2)*	Polymyxin B rolitetracycline lincomycin clindamycin	chloroquine	propranolol		amphetamines	ketamine ether halothane	emetine D,L-carnitine
Pre- and postsynaptic membrane stabilising action (2, 3)*	neomycin streptomycin gentamycin tobramycin polymyxins		procainamide	phenytoin	chlorpromazine amitriptyline droperidolol haloperidol barbiturates	methoxyflurane	ACTH (?) diphenydramine
Inhibition of muscle membrane conductance (4)*	polymyxin B (?) lincomycin (?)				imipramine		amantadine
Other mechanisms	colistin		verapamil ajmaline				citrate anticoagulant magnesium
Immunological		D-penicillamine		trimethadione			

* Refer to Figure 28.2

of drugs with so-called 'membrane-stabilising' properties, the presynaptic effect has been shown to be due to interference with the movement of Ca^{2+} ions into and within the nerve terminal (Fig. 28.2). Such drugs include phenytoin (Yaari et al 1977), chlorpromazine (Argov & Yaari 1979), and the aminoglycoside antibiotics (Elmqvist & Josefsson 1962, Dretchen et al 1973, Fiekers 1983a, b).

Interference with muscle membrane conductance. Certain drugs, such as amantadine, imipramine, and possibly polymyxin B and lincomycin, produce a postsynaptic block by interfering directly with ionic conductance across the muscle end-plate membrane rather than by binding to receptor sites. This has been demonstrated conclusively in the case of amantadine using the voltage clamp technique (Albuquerque et al 1978).

Immune-mediated block. This type of indirect block is typical of D-penicillamine-induced myasthenia but has also been hypothesised for other drugs (Table 28.3). The anti-ACh receptor antibodies induced by D-penicillamine (Masters et al 1977, Russell & Lindstrom 1978) reduce mepp amplitude (Vincent et al 1978) and are presumed to have a postsynaptic blocking effect similar to that in idiopathic myasthenia gravis.

Specific drugs

Antibiotics Aminoglycosides. Various antibiotics may interfere with neuromuscular transmission (Pittinger et al 1970). The most severe forms of neuromuscular block have occurred in patients treated with the aminoglycosides neomycin (Pridgeon 1956), kanamycin (Mullet & Keats 1961), streptomycin (Bodley & Brett 1962), gentamycin (Warner & Sanders 1971), tobramycin (Waterman & Smith 1977) and amikacin (Hashimoto et al 1978). This complication has developed either following introduction of one of these drugs into the peritoneal or pleural cavities during surgery, or after oral or parenteral administration of the drug, leading to postoperative respiratory depression. This has usually been seen as a delay in recovery of spontaneous respiration, both in patients in whom muscle relaxants had been administered and in some in whom inhalational anaesthetics alone were used (Pridgeon 1956, Bennetts 1964). In some cases, respiratory depression has occurred some time after apparently complete recovery from the effects of muscle relaxants (Pinkerton & Munro 1964). Involvement of the respiratory muscles has been the only, or predominant, manifestation of the neuromuscular block in some cases, while in others there was more generalised weakness. Some patients have had associated pupillary dilatation, blurring of vision, depression of corneal reflexes and paraesthesiae (McQuillen et al 1968).

Neomycin (Percy & Saef 1967), streptomycin (Loder & Walker 1959) and kanamycin (Ream 1963) may also produce a myasthenic syndrome unrelated to surgery, or may lead to transient deterioration in patients with MG (Hokkanen 1964). Gentamicin can severely aggravate MG (Agrov & Abramsky 1982) and of the currently used antibiotics is probably the most hazardous in this disorder. Streptomycin and neomycin have been shown to interfere with neuromuscular transmission by a combined pre- and postsynaptic effect (Elmqvist & Josefsson 1962, Tamaki 1978, Fiekers 1983a,b) and it is likely that the other closely related drugs act in a similar way.

Polypeptide antibiotics. Polymyxin B (Lindesmith et al 1968), colistin (Hokkanen 1964) and colistin methosulphonate (Perkins 1964, Zaunder et al 1966) may have similar effects to the aminoglycosides, but their mechanism of action has not been as well clarified. Colistin has been shown to reduce mepp amplitude and it has been suggested that this is due to a reduction in quantum size (McQuillen & Engbaek 1975). However, as these drugs have an ionised ammonium group at physiological pH, a postsynaptic effect seems more likely (Wright & Collier 1976a). Indeed a recent study has shown that these drugs have a predominantly postsynaptic action with an additional presynaptic effect (Viswanath & Jenkins 1978).

Other antibiotics. Oxytetracycline and rolitetracycline have been reported to aggravate MG in some patients (Gibbels 1967, Wullen et al 1967). The mechanism of action has been studied in the case of rolitetracycline, which has been shown to have a postsynaptic curare-like effect (Wright & Collier 1976a). Lincomycin (Duignan et al 1973, Samuelson et al 1975) and its derivative clindamycin (Fogdall & Miller 1974) have been shown to prolong the action of muscle relaxants in some patients. These drugs have been shown to have a postsynaptic effect and also a presynpatic local anaesthetic-like action in higher concentrations (Wright & Collier 1976b, Rubbo et al 1977). Argov et al (1986) reported two myasthenic patients who deteriorated after ampicillin administration. They also showed that high doses of this drug can aggravate experimental myasthenia. There has also been a single case report of aggravation of myasthenia gravis by erythromycin (May & Calvert 1990)

Anti-inflammatory drugs. *D-penicillamine.* A syndrome resembling classic MG may develop in patients with rheumatoid arthritis on long-term D-penicillamine therapy (Seitz et al 1976, Bucknall 1977). Although commonly reported in rheumatoid arthritis, D-penicillamine-induced myasthenia has also been reported in Wilson's disease (Czlonkowaska 1975), primary biliary cirrhosis (Marcus et al 1984) and progressive systemic sclerosis (Torres et al 1980); most reported cases were women. Involvement of the ocular muscles has usually been an early manifestation of such cases, and some have subsequently developed more widespread involvement. The duration of treatment before the appearance of myasthenic symptoms in the cases reported was between 4 months and 5 years. In about two-thirds of affected patients spontaneous recovery occurred after withdrawal of the drug, while the remainder required continuing anticholinesterase with or without steroid therapy or even thymectomy; one death has been recorded (Delrieu et al 1976, Delamere et al 1983).

It has been suggested that this complication may be more likely to develop in patients with rheumatoid arthritis, because most of the cases reported have been in patients with this condition (Bucknall 1977, Mastaglia & Argov 1982). That an immunological mechanism is involved has been shown by the finding of raised ACh receptor antibody levels in the serum in most cases (Masters et al 1977, Russell & Lindstrom 1978, Vincent et al 1978). In addition, antibody levels have been shown to fall with clinical improvement after withdrawal of the drug, suggesting that the antibody is directly involved in the pathogenesis of

the disorder (Vincent et al 1978, Fawcett et al 1982). The association of HLA A1, B8 and DR3 found in classic MG has been found in only some patients with the drug-induced disorder (Bucknall 1977, Russell & Lindstrom 1978). In fact, DR1 was increased in D-penicillamine-induced myasthenia in rheumatoid arthritis (Delamere et al 1983, Garlepp et al 1983), while DR 5 was associated with the complication in systemic sclerosis (Steen et al 1986). An association with thymoma has not been reported. It has been suggested that the development of myasthenia may be due to an independent effect of the drug on the immune system rather than to unmasking of subclinical MG.

The mechanism is not clear; D-penicillamine may stimulate B cells to secrete anti-acetylcholine receptor antibodies (Fawcett et al 1982), change the equilibrium between helper and suppressor T cells (Mastaglia & Argov 1982) or alter antigenic properties of the acetylcholine receptor (Bever et al 1982). A direct effect of D-penicillamine on neuromuscular transmission has also been found in animal studies (Burres et al 1979, Aldrich et al 1979), but is not relevant to the human condition.

Chloroquine has also been reported to aggravate or unmask MG (Robinson 1959, Robberecht et al 1989). In addition, respiratory depression has occurred in the immediate postoperative period in 14% of a series of 67 patients in whom the drug was introduced into the peritoneal cavity during abdominal surgery to prevent the formation of adhesions (Jui-Yen 1971). Experimental studies have shown that the drug may have both a presynaptic local anaesthetic-like effect (Vartanian & Chinyanga 1972) and a postsynaptic curariform action (Jui-Yen 1971).

Cardiovascular drugs. Quinidine, procainamide and a number of the beta-adrenergic blockers possess neuromuscular blocking properties. Quinidine has been reported to aggravate or to unmask MG in some patients (Weisman 1949, Kornfeld et al 1976). In addition this drug may interact with muscle relaxants and has been reported to cause delayed respiratory depression in the postoperative period (Grongono 1963, Schmidt et al 1963, Way et al 1967). The mechanism of action of the drug has not been fully investigated. Procainamide, which has been shown to have a postsynaptic blocking effect on neuromuscular transmission (Galzigna et al 1972), has also been reported to aggravate MG (Drachman & Skom 1965, Kornfeld et al 1976, Niakan et al 1981).

Propranolol, oxprenolol, acebutolol and practolol have been reported to induce a myasthenic syndrome or to unmask MG (Herishanu & Rosenberg 1975, Hughes & Zacharias 1976, Contavreux et al 1990). Interestingly, eye drops containing the potent beta-adrenergic blocker timolol have also been reported to unmask (Coppeto 1984) or aggravate MG (Shaivits 1979).

Experimental studies with propranolol (Werman & Wisicki 1971) have shown that, in concentrations comparable to those achieved during therapy, the drug has a postsynaptic curariform action, while at higher concentrations it has an additional presynaptic anaesthetic-like effect. Pindolol has both a pre- and a postsynaptic action (Larsen 1978).

The calcium channel blocker, verapamil, has been reported to induce respiratory failure in a postoperative setting (Swash & Ingram 1992, Zalman et al 1983), to impair neuromuscular transmission in myasthenic patients undergoing anaesthesia (Lee & Ho 1987) and to aggravate the Lambert–Eaton myasthenic syndrome (Krendel & Hopkins 1986). The potentiation of the action of conventional neuromuscular blockers by verapamil (Bikhazi et al 1988) and the aggravation of decrement in animal experimental myasthenia (Wirguin et al 1992) further support the notion that verapamil is hazardous in neuromuscular junction disorders. The mechanism of this drug-induced impairment is still under debate; some claim that verapamil causes a combined block (Baraka 1985) while others suggest that it facilitates spontaneous transmitter release (Policover & Duncan 1979).

Trimetaphan, which has postsynaptic curariform blocking properties (Gergis et al 1977), has been reported to induce a myasthenic syndrome (Dale & Schroeder 1976) or to increase the neuromuscular block produced by curare derivatives in man (Wilson et al 1976, Nakamura et al 1980).

Anticonvulsants. Phenytoin and trimethadione have been reported to induce myasthenia, probably through different mechanisms. In the case of trimethadione, this was associated with an SLE-like syndrome and high titres of antimuscle antibodies and antinuclear factor, suggesting that the myasthenia was part of a drug-induced autoimmune disorder (Peterson 1966, Booker et al 1970). A myasthenic syndrome has been associated with phenytoin therapy, usually with evidence of intoxication (Norris et al 1964, Regli & Guggenheim 1965, Brumlik & Jacobs 1974) but not always (Milonas et al 1983, Chi-Wan et al 1990). The effects of phenytoin on neuromuscular transmission have been studied in detail and the drug has been shown to have both a postsynaptic curariform and a presynaptic action, the latter being thought to predominate (Yaari et al 1977, 1979).

Psychotropic drugs. Lithium carbonate may unmask MG (Neil et al 1976, Granacher 1977) and has also been shown to prolong the neuromuscular blockade induced by pancuronium (Borden et al 1974) and suxamethonium (Hill et al 1976). The action of the drug is probably mainly a presynaptic one, resulting from substitution of Li^+ for Na^+ ions at the nerve terminal (Crawford 1975), but a postsynaptic effect has also been demonstrated (Onodera & Yamakawa 1966). Chlorpromazine, which has been shown in experimental studies to interfere with transmitter release and to have a lesser postsynaptic curare-like effect (Argov & Yaari 1979), may also aggravate MG (McQuillen et al 1963). Promazine (Regan & Aldrete 1967) and phenelzine (Bodley et al 1969) may potentiate the effect of suxamethonium. In the case of phenelzine this has been shown to be associated with reduced blood pseudocholinesterase levels.

Anaesthetic agents. The two major inhalational anaesthetics halothane (Nilsson et al 1989) and isoflurane (Nilsson & Muller 1990) have been shown to impair neuromuscular transmission in myasthenic patients. Methoxyflurane has been reported to unmask subclinical MG (Elder et al 1971) and has been shown experimentally to have a combined pre- and postsynaptic action, the latter predominating (Kennedy & Galindo 1975). Ketamine and propanidid have been shown to potentiate the neuromuscular blocking effect of suxamethonium (Clarke et al 1967, Bovill et al 1971) and diazepam that of gallamine (Feldman & Crawley 1970). Thus, one has to assume that any anaesthetic, even without neuromuscular blockers, may aggravate the condition of a myasthenic patient.

Carnitine. Four anuric patients on chronic haemodialysis who received D,L-carnitine developed a myasthenic syndrome with involvement of skeletal and bulbar but not of ocular muscles (De Grantis et al 1980). The condition resolved when D,L-carnitine was withdrawn and did not recur when L-carnitine alone was administered (Bazzato et al 1981). The mechanism of carnitine-induced myasthenia is not clear. Carnitine has been found to interfere competitively with neuromuscular transmission (Blum et al 1971) and to cause a presynaptic block (Bazzato et al 1981) in different preparations. The tendency for D-carnitine to accumulate selectively in renal insufficiency may explain the differential response to D,L and L-carnitine administration in the same patient.

Magnesium salts. Magnesium is known to block neuromuscular transmission through a presynaptic interference with calcium-mediated acetylcholine release. Thus, the use of magnesium-containing drugs in any situation where the synaptic safety factor is reduced, should be closely monitored. Reports that magnesium may potentiate neuromuscular blocking drugs (Ghoneim & Long 1970), interact with aminoglycosides to produce neuromuscular block (L'Hommedieu et al 1983), or aggravate the Lambert–Eaton syndrome (Gutmann & Takamori 1973, Streib 1977) have been published but there are no reports of adverse effects in MG. However, it is apparent that magnesium salts are potentially hazardous in this disorder.

Other drugs. A number of other drugs have been shown to have an effect on neuromuscular transmission when used therapeutically. These include oxytocin (Hodges et al 1959), Trasylol® (aprotinin) (kallikrein-trypsin inactivator) (Chasapakis & Dimas 1966), procaine and lidocaine (Usubiaga et al 1967) and eye drops containing potent anticholinesterases (Gesztes 1966), all of which have been reported to cause postoperative respiratory depression through potentiation of muscle relaxants. Pyrantel pamoate, which exerts its antihelminthic effects on the neuromuscular transmission of the worm by producing a depolarising type of block, was reported to

unmask myasthenia in a single patient (Bescansa et al 1991). Intravenous iodinated contrast agents may precipitate a myasthenic crisis (Canal & Franceschi 1983, Chagnac et al 1985. Frank et al (1987) questioned this side-effect because in their patients there were other possible causative factors. However, the aggravation of experimental myasthenia by iodinated contrast media (Eliashiv et al 1990) indicates that patients given large doses of these agents may be at risk. There have been single reports of the development of myasthenic syndromes in patients taking the oral contraceptive pill (Bickerstaff 1975) or busulphan (Djaldetti et al 1968) but these are difficult to evaluate. Thyroid hormones in doses affecting the basal metabolic rate may also aggravate MG (Engel 1961, Drachman 1962). Acetazolamide has been shown to prevent the increment induced by edrophonium in myasthenic patients and to have a similar action in vitro (Carmignani et al 1984). Two patients had transient worsening of their MG during plasmapheresis. This was probably due to reduction of serum free ionized calcium by the citrate anticoagulant. The detrimental effects of this agent were also shown in experimental MG (Wirguin et al 1990). It is well known that corticosteroids, ACTH and the anticholinesterases which are used in the treatment of MG may interfere with neuromuscular transmission in their own right and lead to exacerbation of the myasthenic state. This is discussed further in Chapter 20.

A number of other drugs which have not been implicated clinically, have been shown to interfere with neuromuscular transmission in experimental studies. The inhalational anaesthetic ether has been shown to have a postsynaptic curariform action (Watland et al 1957, Gissen et al 1966). The barbiturates (Proctor & Weakly 1976), amitriptyline (Lermer et al 1970), haloperidol and droperidol (Sokoll et al 1974, Boucher & Katz 1977) and certain of the antihistamines (Abdel-Aziz & Bakry 1973) have been shown to have combined pre- and postsynaptic blocking properties while the amphetamines (Skau & Gerald 1978) and emetine (Salako 1970) have a postsynaptic curariform action. Imipramine is thought to have a presynaptic anaesthetic-like effect (Chang & Chung 1972). Amantadine has been shown to interfere with muscle membrane conductance

(Albuquerque et al 1978) and ajmaline is thought to interfere with neuromuscular transmission by combining with ACh (Manani et al 1970).

Management. Recognition and withdrawal of the offending drug are the most important measures in the management of drug-induced neuromuscular block. When the clinical syndrome is typical and associated with a drug with known neuromuscular junction blocking properties recognition is relatively easy but is more difficult in the case of drugs which are not known to have such properties. Single case reports are at times hard to evaluate as there may be other factors that lead to deterioration in the myasthenic patient. Re-challenge carries practical and ethical problems but may sometimes be unavoidable (Argov et al 1986, Robberecht et al 1989). In vitro testing on isolated neuromuscular junction preparations has been used to evaluate the possible blocking activity of a drug, but the use of the experimental autoimmune myasthenia gravis model in animals may be more relevant to the human disease.

Avoidance of drug complications in myasthenia requires special attention in two situations: treating infection and anaesthesia for surgery. In the ambulatory patient, 'safe' antibiotics may be used orally (e.g. sulphamethoxazole-trimethoprim preparation). Since many antibiotics are hazardous in myasthenia, hospitalisation may be necessary if infection requires administration of another type of antibiotic (even if not previously reported to be deleterious in myasthenia gravis). Halothane is probably the preferred volatile anaesthetic (Nilsson & Muller 1990), although it also has neuromuscular blocking activity. Curariform muscle relaxants should not be used in patients with neuromuscular junction disorders. Treatment of acute severe blockade, as in patients with antibiotic-induced postoperative respiratory depression, involves assisted respiration and other supportive measures, as well as pharmacological attempts to reverse the block (Argov & Mastaglia 1979a, Sokoll & Gergis 1981). Calcium infusions may be effective in reversing presynaptic block and 4-aminopyridine may also be helpful in this situation. In the case of drugs with a primarily postsynaptic action, neostigmine should be administered parenterally. In many instances the block is of the combined form and both calcium and neostig-mine are required. If the respiratory muscles are not affected, discontinuation of the responsible drug and close monitoring of the patient will usually suffice. The form of myasthenia induced by D-penicillamine is usually slowly reversible after withdrawal of the drug but the treatment with oral anticholinesterases or corticosteroids may be required until remission occurs.

PERIPHERAL NEUROPATHIES

Many different drugs used in clinical practice may cause peripheral nerve damage in man (Le Quesne 1970, 1984, Argov & Mastaglia 1979b). Prompt recognition of this complication of drug therapy is important if severe neurological deficits are to be avoided. Mild forms of neuropathy are easily overlooked and subclinical involvement is not uncommon.

Clinical presentations

The common clinical forms of drug-induced neuropathy are shown in Table 28.4. While in most instances specific drugs produce fairly consistent and characteristic syndromes, this is not always the case and some drugs may cause either a sensorimotor neuropathy or a pure motor or sensory neuropathy.

Paraesthesiae and sensory neuropathy. A variety of drugs cause acroparaesthesiae, suggesting a disturbance of sensory nerve function, but clinical examination and electrophysiological studies fail to show objective evidence of peripheral nerve damage (Table 28.4). Some, such as acetazolamide and cytosine arabinoside, cause unpleasant and even painful paraesthesiae. Others, such as streptomycin and stilbamidine, cause facial paraesthesiae or other unpleasant sensations in the upper part of the body (Collard & Hargreaves 1947, Janssen 1960). A number of other drugs produce a sensory neuropathy with clinical and electrophysiological evidence of damage to sensory nerve fibres (Table 28.4) The resulting clinical syndrome is that of a symmetrical distal sensory disturbance, initially with paraesthesiae, and subsequently impairment, particularly of superficial sensory modalities, with relative sparing of vibration and proprioceptive sensation. The tendon reflexes are usually preserved but may be depressed or absent in some

Table 28.4 Drug induced peripheral neuropathies (clinical syndromes and drugs implicated)

Clinical presentation	Antimicrobial drugs	Antineoplastic drugs	Anti-inflammatory drugs	Hypnotics and psychotropics	Cardiovascular drugs	Other drugs
Sensory neuropathy	ethionamide chloramphenicol thiamphenicol diamines dideoxyinosine dideoxycytidine	procarbazine nitrofurazone misonidazole cisplatinum oxaliplatin taxol cytosine arabinoside	sulindac	thalidomide phenelzine		calcium carbimidine sulfoxone, ergotamine propylthiouracil, pyridoxine pyridoxine almitraine
Paraesthesiae only	colistin streptomycin nalidixic acid				propranolol	sulthiame, chlorpropamide methysergide, acetazolamide
Sensorimotor neuropathy	isoniazid ethambutol streptomycin nitrofurantoin clioquinol metronidazole	vincristine podophyllin chlorambucil laetrile cisplatin hexamethylmelamine	gold indomethacin colchicine chloroquine phenylbutazone mesalazine	thalidomide methaqualone gluthethimide amitriptyline lithium	perhexiline hydrallazine amiodarone disopyramide clofibrate	phenytoin, disulfiram carbutamide, tolbutamide chlorpropamide methimazole methylthiouracil, cimetidine D-penicillamine, tetanus toxoid, streptokinase
Predominantly motor	sulphonamides amphotericin B streptomycin dapsone	azathioprine suramin	sulindac	imipramine amitriptyline protriptyline lofepramine		almitrine

cases, presumably due to involvement of afferent fibres from the muscle spindles.

Sensorimotor neuropathy. Most cases of drug-induced neuropathy fall into this category (Table 28.4). Sensory manifestations usually appear first and are only followed by motor involvement at a later stage if the drug is not stopped. The onset and clinical progression of the disorder are usually gradual, but may be relatively acute and resemble the Guillain–Barré form of post-infective polyneuropathy in some cases. Sensory and motor involvement is usually distal and symmetrical and, with occasional exceptions in which there is predominant involvement of the upper limbs (Bruun & Hermann 1942), the lower limbs are usually involved first and most severely. Muscle pain and cramps may be prominent in some cases and may be the initial symptom (Steiner & Siegal 1989, Siegal & Haim 1990, Haim et al 1991). The tendon reflexes are usually depressed or absent even when motor involvement is absent or inconspicuous (Casey et al 1973). Exaggerated tendon reflexes in some cases suggest concomitant involvement of central motor pathways (Le Quesne 1984). Some drugs such as dapsone cause a motor neuropathy with absent or inconspicuous sensory abnormalities (Saquenton et al 1969, Epstein & Bohm 1976), while others such as nitrofurantoin, which usually produces a sensorimotor neuropathy, may rarely cause a pure motor neuropathy (Toole & Parrish 1973).

Localised neuropathies. Involvement of peripheral nerve trunks may occur as a complication of intramuscular injections of drugs, attributable either to direct needle trauma or to a local toxic effect of the drug itself. The best-known example is the sciatic nerve damage which may occur with injections into the buttock. Peripheral nerve involvement may also occur as a result of haemorrhage into confined spaces in patients on poorly controlled oral anticoagulant therapy. The femoral nerve trunk and the lumbosacral roots are most frequently affected in this way when the haemorrhage is retroperitoneal, but other peripheral nerves such as the median may also be involved (Dhaliwal et al 1976). Localised forms of neuropathy may also occur after intraarterial perfusion of cytotoxic agents such as nitrogen mustard or ethoglucid in the treatment of malignancy

(Scholes 1960, Westbury 1962, Bond et al 1964) or after streptokinase extravasation during intravenous administrarion (Blankenship 1991). In addition, local damage to nerves in the cubital fossa may occur as a result of intravenous infusions of certain drugs (Utz et al 1957).

Cranial neuropathies. Certain cranial nerves may be involved, either selectively or as part of a more generalised drug-induced neuropathy. The optic, trigeminal and eighth cranial nerve are the most commonly affected.

Pathogenesis

The mechanisms involved in the production of drug-induced neuropathies are poorly understood. Experimental animal studies have clarified the mechanism of action of certain drugs such as vincristine (Bradley 1970) and nitrofurantoin (Klinghardt 1967) while that of others remains to be determined. Few histological studies of peripheral nerve have been performed in patients with drug-induced neuropathy, but axonal degeneration appears to be the principal process in most cases. A predominantly demyelinating process has been described in some patients with neuropathy due to perhexiline (Said 1978) or amiodarone (Aronson 1978).

In general, the drugs which cause peripheral neuropathy do so either by interfering with axonal or Schwann cell metabolism or through a vascular effect. The neuropathy in which the nature of the metabolic disturbance is best understood is probably that caused by isoniazid in which peripheral nerve damage is secondary to an effect of the drug on pyridoxine metabolism (Biehl & Nimitz 1954, Biehl & Vilter 1954, McCormick & Snell 1959). Vitamin deficiency may also play a part in other drug-induced neuropathies, e.g. it has been shown that prolonged administration of chloramphenicol in the rat may lead to vitamin B_{12} deficiency, which in turn may play a part in causing the neuropathy which occasionally develops in patients treated with the drug (Satoyoshi & Wakata 1978). Thalidomide is thought to inhibit riboflavine (Leck & Millar 1962) and to interfere with pyruvate metabolism (Buckle 1963), while the nitrofurans interfere with pyruvate oxidation by competing with thiamine pyrophosphate (Paul et al 1954). Preliminary work has suggested that a disturbance of lipid metabolism may underlie the neuropathy caused by perhexiline (Pollet et al 1977). Vincristine and colchicine are neurotubular toxins (Schochet et al 1968, Rasmussen 1970). The neuropathy caused by laetrile is probably due to cyanide intoxication (Kalyanaraman et al 1983).

Some drugs cause peripheral nerve damage by an effect on neural blood vessels. This may result either from severe vasospasm, as in chronic ergotism (Merhoff & Porter 1974), or from a vasculitic process (Stafford et al 1975).

The possibility that certain drugs may produce a true allergic polyneuropathy has been considered (Cohen 1970), especially when a Guillain–Barré-like syndrome develops. Drugs reported to induce neuropathy via such mechanisms are cimetidine (Walls et al 1980), D-penicillamine (Knezevic et al 1984b), streptomycin (Janssen 1960), streptokinase (Eden 1983, Leaf et al 1984), sulindac (Lending et al 1984), tetanus and diphtheria toxoids (Halliday & Bauer 1983), the antidepressant zimeldine (Fagius et al 1985) and gangliosides (Lator et al 1991). A similar mechanism may be operative in patients developing a brachial plexopathy following administration of penicillin (Kolb & Gray 1946) or hepatitis B vaccine (Mastaglia unpublished).

Predisposing factors

Some drugs such as amitriptyline, clofibrate and disopyramide cause peripheral neuropathy only rarely and the possibility therefore arises that certain individuals are unduly susceptible to the effects of such drugs. By contrast, other drugs such as vincristine are highly neurotoxic and will consistently cause peripheral nerve damage if administered for long enough in high enough doses (Bradley et al 1970).

The best-known example of a genetic predisposition is the striking susceptibility of the Japanese to clioquinol neurotoxicity. The syndrome of subacute myelo-opticoneuropathy (SMON) developed in 17% of Japanese patients who took the drug (Sobue et al 1971, Tsubaki et al 1971) whereas very few cases were reported from other parts of the world where the drug was also freely used (Selby 1972, Le Quesne 1984). Variations

in the pharmacokinetics of certain drugs may also modify the susceptibility to neurotoxic effects. Impaired renal function may lead to toxic blood levels of drugs such as nitrofurantoin which are excreted through the kidneys, and thereby increase the likehood of neuropathy developing (Ellis 1962). Similarly, it is well known that slow acetylators of isoniazid are more likely to develop peripheral neuropathy if pyridoxine supplements are not given (Hughes et al 1954). Strenuous exercise was thought to predispose to the development of neuropathy in patients treated with the older sulphonamides (Bruun & Hermann 1942).

The underlying disease process may itself modify the susceptibility to drug-induced neuropathy, e.g. patients with lymphoma develop neuropathy more frequently when treated with vincristine than those with other forms of malignancy (Watkins & Griffin 1978). It is possible that the use of multiple drug regimens in oncology may augment the neurotoxicity, as in the case of intrathecal thiotepa (Martin-Algarra et al 1990). Hypomagnesaemia induced by cisplatinum is thought to increase the chances of developing cisplatinum neuropathy (Ashraf et al 1983). Whether or not drug-induced neuropathy is more likely to occur in patients with cancer, diabetes, vitamin deficiency or alcoholism, situations in which the peripheral nervous system may already be affected, is uncertain.

Specific drugs

It is beyond the scope of this chapter to discuss in detail each drug involved. Brief mention of the more important ones with relevant references will be given here.

Antimicrobial agents. Many drugs used in the treatment of bacterial, viral or protozoal infections may cause peripheral neuropathy (Snavely & Hodges 1984).

Isoniazid. The occurrence of peripheral neuropathy in patients treated with this antituberculous agent was first recognised soon after its introduction (Gammon et al 1953). The incidence of neuropathy was found to be dose-dependent, being as high as 17% in patients taking 400 mg of drug per day, and 35% during a second course of treatment (Mandel 1959). As indicated above, the neuropathy is due to pyridoxine deficiency (Biehl & Vilter 1954), being more likely to occur in individuals who inactivate the drug at slow rates in the liver, and being preventable when adequate supplements of vitamin B_6 are administered with the drug (10 mg per 100 mg of isoniazid) (Cohen 1970, Le Quesne 1984).

Other antituberculous agents. Ethambutol may also cause a sensorimotor neuropathy (Cohen 1970, Tugwell & James 1972) which responds favourably to withdrawal. Ethionamide, structurally similar to isoniazid, can also cause a mild sensory neuropathy (Poole & Schneeweiss 1961) and has other neurotoxic effects (Brouet et al 1959). Streptomycin has been reported to cause a peripheral neuropathy (Janssen 1960), but this is much less common than its ototoxic effects.

Nitrofurantoin. Peripheral neuropathy was a relatively frequent complication of treatment with this drug. A review of the literature by Toole & Parrish in 1973 disclosed 137 reported cases. With the exception of two patients who had a pure motor neuropathy (Morris 1966), most cases presented with distal sensory symptoms followed after a few days by pain and muscle weakness, the latter being profound in some cases and contributing to a fatal outcome (Rubenstein 1964, Yiannikas et al 1981).

Sulphonamides. Peripheral neuropathy was a well-recognised complication of treatment with sulphonamides in the 1940s. The clinical features were well documented in two Scandinavian reviews of over 100 patients, most of whom were treated with sulphanyldimethylsulfanilamide (Uliron®) (Bruun & Hermann 1942, Muller 1945). Although transient paraesthesiae occurred in some cases, the neuropathy was predominantly motor and usually developed 1–3 weeks after completing treatment. The mechanism of the neuropathy is uncertain, but it has been suggested that in some cases it is due to a toxic effect of the drug, while in others it may be allergic (Le Quesne 1970). None of the sulphonamides in current clinical use is known to have toxic effects on the peripheral nervous system (Weinstein et al 1974).

Clioquinol. The SMON syndrome, which was characterised by abdominal pain and the subsequent development of a neurological disorder involving the optic nerves, spinal cord and periph-

eral nerves, was prevalent in Japan during the 1950s and 1960s. Kono reviewed a total of 7856 probable cases of this syndrome in 1971. The association with clioquinol was recognised in 1971 (Tsubaki et al 1971), when it was found that 96% of a series of 969 affected patients had taken the drug before the onset of neurological symptoms.

Metronidazole. There have been a number of reports of a sensory neuropathy developing in patients with various conditions who were treated with this drug for prolonged periods (Ramsay 1968, Ingham et al 1975, Ursing & Kamme 1975, Coxon & Pallis 1976, Bradley et al 1977). Motor involvement has not been apparent clinically, but mild prolongation of distal motor latencies was found in one case (Bradley et al 1977). Misonidazole, etanidazole and related compounds, which are chemically similar to metronidazole, and are used as radio-sensitising agents in cancer therapy, can also induce a sensory neuropathy (Paulson et al 1984, Dische et al 1981, Coleman et al 1990).

Dideoxyinosine (ddI) and dideoxycytidine (ddC). These are two inhibitors of viral reverse transcriptase that were tried experimentally in AIDS. Peripheral neuropathy was found to be a major dose-limiting problem in all studies with ddI (Rozencweig et al 1990, Yarchoan et al 1990, Connolly et al 1991). Axonal type neuropathy developed in many AIDS patients treated with ddC (Dubinsky et al 1989). With both drugs the clinical picture was that of a painful sensory neuropathy, although a few patients also had motor involvement on electrophysiological testing (Dubinsky et al 1989). Slowly progressive sensory neuropathy can occur in AIDS patients with no drug treatment (Cornblath & McArthur 1988), but the acute onset of symptoms after starting one of these drugs and their disappearance after drug withdrawal point to a neurotoxic effect. A more commonly used nucleoside agent, zidovudine, was not found to be neurotoxic (Bozzette et al 1991) although it has myopathic side-effects (see above).

Griseofulvin. A case of reversible neuropathy induced by the antifungal agent griseofulvin was reported (Lecky 1990).

Antineoplastic agents *Vinca alkaloids.* These drugs, which have been used in the treatment of various malignancies, are extremely neurotoxic. Vincristine is particularly toxic and most patients who are on the drug for long enough will develop signs of peripheral nerve damage. The clinical features of vincristine neuropathy are well documented (Warot et al 1965, Bradley et al 1970, Casey et al 1973). Distal paraesthesiae, which are usually the earliest symptom, may involve the hands before the feet and may antedate sensory or motor deficits for long periods. Muscle cramps may be a prominent symptom which accompanies the onset of motor involvement. The latter often shows a predilection for the forearm extensor muscles (Casey et al 1973). The tendon reflexes are lost early, particularly in the lower limbs. Autonomic involvement may also occur and postural hypotension and constipation may be early symptoms (Warot et al 1965). Recovery may occur if the drug is stopped or even if the dose is reduced, but mild sensory impairment and reflex depression often persist.

Cisplatin. As with vincristine, the main dose-limiting side-effect of this heavy metal-based anti-neoplastic agent is peripheral neuropathy. It is primarily a large fibre sensory neuropathy with paraesthesiae and electric shock-like sensations (Lhermitte's sign), loss of vibration and proprioception sensation and 'spinal ataxia' (Ashraf et al 1983, Roelofs et al 1984, Thompson et al 1984, Mollman et al 1988a). The motor nerves are not involved, but muscle cramps were recently noted in about one-third of patients (Siegal & Haim 1990). Neural hearing loss is also frequent. As many as 50% of patients fail to recover after drug withdrawal (Mollman et al 1988a). Furthermore, off-therapy symptomatic deterioration has been described (Mollman et al 1988b, Siegal & Haim 1990). Oxaliplatin, another platinum-based drug, also causes a sensory neuropathy (Extra et al 1990).

Other cytotoxic drugs. A number of other drugs used in the treatment of malignancy may cause neuropathy. An extensive review of the neurotoxic effects of cancer therapy should be consulted for details (Kaplan & Wiernik 1982). Procarbazine, which is structurally similar to isoniazid, has occasionally been associated with a sensory neuropathy (Weiss et al 1974) as has nitrofurazone, a congener of nitrofurantoin which was used in the

treatment of testicular carcinoma (Le Quesne 1975). Cytosine arabinoside may cause a peripheral neuropathy of variable severity, especially after intravenous administration for haematological malignancies (Russell & Powles 1974, Baker et al 1991). A similar derivative, adenine arabinoside, used for advanced active liver disease, caused axonal neuropathy in one patient (Kanterewicz et al 1990). Podophyllin derivatives, which have been used in the treatment of disseminated malignancies, and which are also constituents of certain laxative preparations and topical agents, may cause a mild or severe peripheral neuropathy (Falkson et al 1975, Langman 1975, Filley et al 1982, Dobb & Edis 1984, O'Mahony et al 1990). Chlorambucil has also been reported to cause a sensorimotor neuropathy occasionally (Sandler & Gonsalkorale 1977). Carbetimer, a polymer derived from ethylene and maleic anhydride, was used experimentally in 26 patients with various solid tumours. Two of these patients developed a sensorimotor neuropathy (Dodion et al 1989). Taxol is a plant alkaloid which interferes with normal microtubule assembly. It was used mainly in breast cancer, but also in other solid tumours. Peripheral neuropathy is a very common, dose-related side-effect and is predominantly sensory, although sensorimotor neuropathy was also described (Lipton et al 1989, Holmes et al 1991). Suramin, a drug used in the treatment of trypanosomal infections, was tried in 38 patients with various malignancies. Four of these patients developed acute or subacute severe flaccid tetraparesis with a high CSF protein level and electrophysiological evidence of conduction block suggesting a drug-associated Guillain–Barré-like disorder (La-Rocca et al 1990).

Anti-inflammatory drugs. *Gold.* Peripheral neuropathy is a well-recognised complication of gold therapy in rheumatoid arthritis (Endtz 1958), occurring in 0.5–1% of patients treated in this way (Hartfall et al 1937, Doyle & Cannon 1950). Motor involvement is usually prominent and may be asymmetrical, and sensory signs may be inconspicuous. The onset may be abrupt and progression rapid, mimicking the Guillain–Barré form of postinfective polyneuropathy, particularly in some patients who also develop facial diplegia and have elevated cerebrospinal fluid protein levels (Le Quesne 1970, Katrak et al 1980). Fever and a skin rash may be associated with the neuropathy, indicating a more generalised reaction in some cases (Doyle & Cannon 1950).

Chloroquine. Evidence of peripheral nerve involvement has been found in some patients who developed a vacuolar myopathy while being treated with chloroquine (Loftus 1963, Whisnant et al 1963, Hicklin 1968). Nerve biopsy shows segmental demyelination and remyelination (Tegner et al 1988). The typical lysosomal cytoplasmic inclusions seen in muscle are also found in Schwann cells and other perineural cells but not in axons (Estes et al 1987, Tegner et al 1988).

Colchicine. There have been a few reports of neuropathy developing in patients with colchicine treatment (Prescott 1975, Riggs et al 1986, Kuncl et al 1987, Kuncl & Duncan 1988). This axonal sensory neuropathy is mild and usually resolves when the drug is withdrawn, The lysosomal changes are infrequent in nerve biopsies, unlike their abundance in muscle specimens of the same patients (Kuncl et al 1987).

Other anti-inflammatory drugs. Indomethacin has been implicated in causing a neuropathy (Eade et al 1975). There are occasional reports of peripheral neuropathy developing in patients treated with D-penicillamine (Meyboom 1977). Mesalazine treatment in ulcerative colitis may cause a mixed sensorimotor neuropathy (Woodward 1989).

Hypnotics and psychotropic drugs.
Thalidomide. This drug was first reported to cause neuropathy in 1960, 5 years after it was introduced into clinical use (Florence 1960). Although the drug was withdrawn from the market 2 years later, victims of its teratogenic and neurotoxic effects are still seen. The characteristics of thalidomide neuropathy were reviewed by Fullerton & Kremer (1961) and Fullerton & O'Sullivan (1968). The drug has also been used in dermatology and there have been reports of patients developing a neuropathy (Clemmensen et al 1984).

Methaqualone. A number of reports have suggested that methaqualone may be neurotoxic. At least 11 cases of a sensorimotor neuropathy have been reported in patients taking 200–600 mg of methaqualone nightly for periods of a few days to 2 years, either alone or with diphenhydramine, diazepam, meprobamate or promazine (McQuaker & Bruggen 1963, Finke & Spiegelberg 1973, Hoaken 1975, Markes & Sloggen 1976).

Glutethimide. Reports of two patients with sensory symptoms and areflexia after prolonged high-dose treatment with this drug (Bartholomew 1961), and of a suspected case of neuropathy in a glutethimide addict (Lingle 1966) raised suspicion that the drug, which has structural similarities to thalidomide, may be neurotoxic.

Tricyclic drugs. There have been occasional reports of a predominantly motor neuropathy developing in patients treated with imipramine (Collier & Martin 1960, Miller 1963, Cohen 1970), amytriptyline (Casarino 1977, Zampollo et al 1988), protriptyline (Stept & Subramony 1988) and lofepramine (Hewitt & Glinn 1989).

Lithium. Peripheral neuropathy with prominent motor involvement has rarely been described in patients with lithium intoxication (Brust et al 1979, Uchigata et al 1981, Chang et al 1988, Pamphlett & Mackenzie 1982, Vanhooren et al 1990). Some authors suggest that the more dramatic central nervous system signs prevent the recognition of the peripheral nerve involvement (Chang et al 1988, Pamphlett & Mackenzie 1982). Nerve conduction studies and sural nerve biopsy suggest an axonal neuropathy (Pamphlett & Mackenzie 1982, Vanhooren et al 1990).

Other drugs. Phenelzine has been associated with the development of primarily sensory neuropathy in two patients (Goodheart et al 1991).

Cardiovascular drugs. *Perhexiline.* The occurrence of neuropathy in patients treated with this coronary vasodilator is now well recognised (Bousser et al 1976, Lhermitte et al 1976, Fraser et al 1977, Geraud et al 1978, Sebille 1978). It was claimed that clinically manifest neuropathy occurred in about 0.1% of patients treated with the drug and that subclinical involvement was even commoner (Sebille 1978). Sensory symptoms, which are usually prominent, may appear as early as 3 weeks after commencement of treatment (Robinson 1978) and are followed by distal motor involvement in the limbs.

Amiodarone. There have been a number of reports of a demyelinating sensorimotor polyneuropathy developing in patients treated with this anti-arrhythmic agent (Robinson 1975, Aronson 1978, Meier et al 1979, Martinez-Arizala et al 1983, Lim et al 1984, Pellissier et al 1984, Anderson et al 1985, Fraser et al 1985, Jacobs & Costa-Jussa 1985, Rath et al 1990).

Hydrallazine. A number of cases of a mixed but predominantly sensory peripheral neuropathy have been reported in patients treated with this drug (Kirkendall & Page 1958, Le Quesne 1970, Perry 1973). The neuropathy appears to be unrelated to the lupus-like syndrome induced by the drug.

Clofibrate. Clinical and electrophysiological evidence of peripheral nerve involvement was found in two patients with clofibrate myopathy (Gabriel & Pearce 1976, Pokroy et al 1977). However, there is some doubt as to the cause of the neuropathy in these cases and further evidence is required before accepting that the drug is neurotoxic.

Other drugs *Phenytoin.* The occurrence of a mild peripheral neuropathy in patients on long-term phenytoin treatment is well recognised (Finkelman & Arieff 1942, Lovelace & Horwitz 1968). Sensory symptoms are present in some patients but most are asymptomatic, being found to have reflex depression or sensory impairment on clinical examination (Lovelace & Horwitz 1968). The frequency of polyneuropathy appears to increase with the duration of therapy (Lovelace & Horwitz 1968, Eisen et al 1974).

Disulfiram. The occurrence of a sensorimotor polyneuropathy in alcoholics treated with this drug is well established (Hayman & Wilkins 1956, Bradley & Hewer 1966, Gardner-Thorpe & Benjamin 1971, Nukada & Pollock 1981, Ansbacher et al 1982) although in some cases it has been difficult to be certain of the extent to which alcohol or nutritional deficiencies may have contributed to the neuropathy. Frisoni & Di Modena (1989) reviewed 37 patients with confirmed disulfiram neuropathy and suggested the following distinguishing features from alcoholic neuropathy: alcoholic patients on a balanced diet who develop a rapid onset neuropathy (weeks) after disulfiram (the onset and progression is dose-dependent) and have no muscle tenderness and no macrocytosis most probably have disulfiram-induced sensorimotor neuropathy. Nerve biopsy may distinguish between these disorders as axoplas-

mic neurofilamentous aggregates are at times seen in disulfiram neuropathy but not in alcoholic neuropathy. These authors hypothesize that there is a genetic predilection toward disulfiram neuropathy and provide evidence of the detrimental effect of chloral hydrate on this type of neuropathy.

Dapsone. This drug, which has been used in the treatment of leprosy and of a number of dermatological conditions, is known to cause an almost exclusively motor form of peripheral neuropathy (Saquenton et al 1969, Epstein & Bohm 1976, Gehlmann et al 1977). This has usually developed after prolonged high-dose therapy but has also occurred with lower doses of the drug (Rapoport & Guss 1972). Electrophysiological studies have shown mild impairment of motor conduction (Saquenton et al 1969, Fredericks et al 1976) with normal sensory conduction (Wyatt & Stevens 1972, Fredericks et al 1976).

Antithyroid agents. Several drugs which were used in the treatment of thyrotoxicosis have been associated with neurotoxic side-effects. Methimazole was reported to cause acute motor neuropathy (Accetta et al 1954) or sensory neuropathy (Roldan & Nigrin 1972) in single cases. Propyl-thiouracil caused sensory neuropathy (Crile 1947, Frawley & Koeppe 1950), while methyl-thiouracil was thought to be responsible for widespread sensorimotor neuropathy in one case (Barfred 1947).

Pyridoxine. Megadoses of pyridoxine, which in low doses is used to protect against isoniazid neuropathy, can cause a sensory neuropathy (Schaumburg et al 1983, Berensvein 1990).

Almitrine. Almitrine bismesylate, a drug which has been used in patients with cerebrovascular disease and chronic obstructive pulmonary disease, has recently been reported to cause a sensory polyneuropathy (Chedru et al 1985), or rarely combined sensorimotor neuropathy (Chedru et al 1985, Bouche et al 1989). The mechanism of this neuropathy is unclear but hypoxaemia and hypo-metabolism of the drug were excluded as contributing factors (Belec et al 1989).

CONCLUSIONS

It will be seen from the present review that drugs

used in various clinical situations may interfere with neuromuscular function. The possibility of such a complication should be considered in any patient who complains of muscle pain, weakness, fatiguability or sensory disturbances while on drug therapy; patients complaining of such symptoms should be subjected to a careful neurological examination and EMG study. In view of their potentially reversible nature, drug-induced disorders should enter into the differential diagnosis in any patient presenting with a myopathy, neuropathy or myasthenic syndrome and full details of drug therapy should be obtained in all such patients. The possibility of drug effects should be considered, particularly in patients with a pre-existing neuromuscular disorder, who may be more susceptible to, and less able to compensate for such effects.

In addition to their diagnostic role, electrophysiological and pathological studies of patients with drug-induced neuromuscular disorders help to provide a clearer indication of the true incidence of such complications. Such studies will also improve our understanding of the pathogenesis and pathophysiology of toxic forms of neuropathy and myopathy and of the basic pathological reactions of peripheral nerve and muscle.

Experimental studies in vivo and in vitro have elucidated the mechanisms whereby many drugs interfere with neuromuscular function. However, because of differences between the experimental and human situations, the results of such studies are not always directly applicable to man. Thus in the case of certain drugs such as amantadine, an effect on neuromuscular transmission has been identified in in vitro studies but has not been manifest clinically. Nevertheless, such studies are clearly important for the screening of newly introduced therapeutic agents and will serve to alert the clinician to possible effects on neuromuscular function.

ACKNOWLEDGEMENTS

The authors are grateful to Miss M. Jenkison who prepared the photomicrographs and provided technical assistance, and to Mrs S. Moncrieff for secretarial assistance.

REFERENCES

Abdel-Aziz A, Bakry N 1973 The action and interaction of diphenhydramine (Benadryl) hydrochloride at the neuromuscular junction. European Journal of Pharmacology 22: 169

Aberfeld D C, Bienenstock H, Shapiro M S, Namba T, Grob D 1968 Diffuse myopathy related to meperidine addiction in a mother and daughter. Archives of Neurology: 19: 384

Abreo K, Shelp W D, Kosseff A, Thomas S 1982 Amoxapin-associated rhabdomyolysis and acute renal failure: Case report. Journal of Clinical Psychiatry 43: 426

Accetta G S, Fitzmorris A O, Wettingfeld R F 1954 Toxicity of methimazole. Journal of the American Medical Association 155: 253

Adams E M, Horowitz H W, Sundstrom W R 1983 Fibrous myopathy in association with pentazocine. Archives of Internal Medicine 143: 2203

Affarah H B, Mars R L, Someren A, Smith H W B, Heymsfield S B 1984 Myoglobinuria and acute renal failure associated with intravenous vasopressin infusion. Southern Medical Journal 77: 918

Afifi A K, Bergman R A 1969 Steroid myopathy — a study of the evolution of the muscle lesion in rabbits. Johns Hopkins Medical Journal 124: 66

Aguayo A J, Hudgson P 1970 The short-term effects of chloroquine on skeletal muscle: An experimental study in the rabbit. Journal of the Neurological Sciences 11: 301

Albuquerque E X, Eldefrawi A T, Eldefrawi M E, Mansour N, Tsai M C 1978 Amantadine: neuromuscular blockade by suppression of ionic conductance of the acetylcholine receptor. Science 199: 788

Aldrich M S, Kim Y I, Sanders D B 1979 Effects of D-penicillamine on neuromuscular transmission in rats. Muscle and Nerve 2: 180

Anand V, Siami G, Stone W J 1989 Cocaine-associated rhabdomyolysis and acute renal failure. Southern Medical Journal 82: 67

Anderson N E, Lynch N M, O'Brien K P 1985 Disabling neurological complications of amiodarone. Australian and New Zealand Journal of Medicine 15: 300

Anderson P J, Song S K, Slotwiner P 1967 The fine structure of spheromembranous degeneration of skeletal muscle induced by vincristine. Journal of Neuropathology and Experimental Neurology 26: 15

Ansbacher L E, Bosch E P, Cancilla P A 1982 Disulfiram neuropathy: a neurofilamentous distal axonopathy. Neurology (NY) 32: 424

Argov Z, Mastaglia F L 1979a Disorders of neuromuscular transmission caused by drugs. New England Journal of Medicine 301: 409

Argov Z, Mastaglia F L 1979b Drug-induced peripheral neuropathies. British Medical Journal 1: 663

Argov Z, Yaari Y 1979 The action of chlorpromazine at an isolated cholinergic synapse. Brain Research 164: 227

Argov Z, Abramsky D 1982 Antibiotic treatment in myasthenia gravis. Harefuah 10: 225

Argov Z, Brenner T, Abramsky D 1986 Ampicillin may aggravate clinical and experimental myasthenia. Archives of Neurology 43: 255

Aronson J K 1978 Cardiac glycosides and drugs used in dysrhythmias. In: Dukes M N G (ed) Side effects of drugs. Excerpta Medica, Amsterdam, II, p 163

Ashraf M, Scotchel P L, Krall J M, Flink E B 1983 Cis-platinum-induced hypomagnesemia and peripheral neuropathy. Gynecologic Oncology 16: 309

Askari A, Vignos P J, Moskowitz R W 1976 Steroid myopathy in connective tissue disease. American Journal of Medicine 61: 485

Ayanian J Z, Fuchs C S, Stone R M 1988 Lovastatin and rhabdomyolysis. Annals of Internal Medicine 109: 682

Baker W J, Royer G L, Weiss R B 1991 Cytarabine and neurologic toxicity. Journal of Clinical Oncology 9: 679

Baraka A 1985 Action of verapamil at the neuromuscular junction: prejunctional or postjunctional? Anesthesiology 63: 234

Barfred A 1947 Methylthiouracil in the treatment of thyrotoxicosis. American Journal of Medical Sciences 214: 349

Bartholomew A A 1961 (In correspondence) British Medical Journal 2: 1570

Basser L S 1979 Purgatives and periodic paralysis. Medical Journal of Australia 1: 47

Battacharrya S 1966 Abduction contracture of the shoulder from contracture of the intermediate part of the deltoid. Report of three cases. Journal of Bone and Joint Surgery 46B: 127

Bazzato G, Coli U, Landini S, Mezzina C, Ciman M 1981 Myasthenia-like syndrome after D,L- but not L-carnitine Lancet i: 1209

Belec L, Larrey D, de Cremoux H et al 1989 Extensive oxidative metabolism of dextromethorphan in patients with almitrine neuropathy. British Journal of Clinical Pharmacology 27: 387

Belongia E A, Hedberg C W, Gleich G J et al 1990 An investigation of the cause of the eosinophilia-myalgia syndrome associated with tryptophan use. New England Journal of Medicine 323: 357

Bennett H S, Spiro A J, Pollack M A, Zucker P 1982 Ipecac-induced myopathy simulating dermatomyositis. Neurology 32: 91

Bennetts F E 1964 Muscular paralysis due to streptomycin following inhalation anaesthesia. Anaesthesia 19: 93

Berenstein A L 1990 Vitamin B6 in clinical neurology. Annals of the New York Academy of Sciences 585: 250

Bescansa E, Nicholas M, Aguado C, Toledano M, Vinals M 1991 Myasthenia gravis aggravated by pyrantel pamoate. Journal of Neurology, Neurosurgery and Psychiatry 54: 563

Bever C T, Chang H W, Penn A S, Jaffe I A, Bock E 1982 Penicillamine-induced myasthenia gravis: effects of penicillamine on acetylcholine receptor. Neurology 32: 1077

Bickerstaff E R 1975 Neurological complications of oral contraceptives. Clarendon Press, London, p 93

Biehl J P, Nimitz H J 1954 Studies on the use of a high dose of isoniazid. American Review of Tuberculosis 70: 430

Biehl J P, Vilter R W 1954 Effects of isoniazid on pyridoxine metabolism. Journal of the American Medical Association 156: 1549

Bikhazi G B, Leung I, Flores C, Mikati H M J, Foldes F F 1988 Potentiation of neuromuscular blocking agents by calcium channel blocker in rats. Anesthesia and Analgesia 67: 1

Blankenship J C 1991 Median and ulnar neuropathy after streptokinase infusion. Heart and Lung 20: 221

Blessing W, Walsh J C 1977 Myotonia precipitated by propranolol therapy. Lancet i: 73

Blum K, Seifter E, Seifter J 1971 The pharmacology of D- and L-carnitine. Comparison with choline and acetylcholine. Journal of Pharmacology and Experimental Therapeutics 178: 331

Bodley P O, Brett J E 1962 Post-operative respiratory inadequacy and the part played by antibiotics. Anaesthesia 17: 438

Bodley P O, Halwax K, Potts L 1969 Low pseudocholinesterase levels complicating treatment with phenelzine. British Medical Journal 3: 510

Bond M R, Clark S D, Neal F E 1964 Use of ethoglucid in treatment of advanced malignant disease. British Medical Journal 1: 951

Booker H E, Chun R W M, Sanguino M 1970 Myasthenia gravis syndrome associated with trimethadione. Journal of the American Medical Association 212: 2262

Borden H, Clarke M T, Katz N 1974 The use of pancuronium bromide in patients receiving lithium carbonate. Canadian Anaesthetic Society Journal 21: 79

Bouche P, Lacomblez L, Leger J M et al 1989 Peripheral neuropathy during treatment with almitrine: report of 46 cases. Journal of Neurology 236: 29

Boucher S D, Katz N I 1977 Effects of several 'membrane stabilizing' agents on frog neuromuscular junction. European Journal of Pharmacology 42: 139

Bousser M G, Bouche P, Brochard C, Herreman G 1976 Sept neuropathies périphériques après traitement par maleate de perhexiline. La Nouvelle Presse Médicale 5: 652

Bovill J G, Dundee J W, Coppel D L, Moore J 1971 Current status of ketamine anaesthesia. Lancet 1: 1285

Bowyer S L, LaMonthe M P and Hollister J R 1985 Steroid mopathy: incidence and detection in a population with asthma. Journal of Allergy and Clinical Immunology 76: 234

Bozzette S A, Santangelo J, Villasana D et al 1991 Peripheral nerve function in persons with asymptomatic or minimally symptomatic HIV disease: absence of zidovudine neurotoxicity. Journal of Acquired Immune Deficiency Syndrome 4: 851

Bradley W G 1970 The neuropathy of vincristine in the guinea pig. An electrophysiological and pathological study. Journal of the Neurological Sciences 10: 133

Bradley W G, Hewer R L 1966 Peripheral neuropathy due to disulfiram. British Medical Journal 1: 449

Bradley W G, Lassman L P, Pearce G W, Walton J N 1970 The neuromyopathy of vincristine in man. Clinical, electrophysiological and pathological findings. Journal of the Neurological Sciences 10: 107

Bradley W G, Fewings J D, Harris J B, Johnson M A 1976 Emetine myopathy in the rat. British Journal of Pharmacology 57: 29

Bradley W G, Karlsson I J, Rasool C G 1977 Metronidazole neuropathy. British Medical Journal 2: 610

Bretag A H, Dawe S R, Kerr D I B, Moskwa A G 1980 Myotonia as a side effect of diuretic action. British Journal of Pharmacology 71: 467

Bridgeman J F, Rosen A M, Thorp J M 1972 Complications during clofibrate treatment of nephrotic syndrome hyperlipoproteinaemia. Lancet 2: 502

Britt B A 1979 Etiology and pathophysiology of malignant hyperthermia. Federation Proceedings 38: 44

Britt C W, Light R R, Peters B H, Schochet S S 1980 Rhabdomyolysis during treatment with epsilon-aminocaproic acid. Archives of Neurology 37: 187

Brodkin H M 1980 Myoglobinuria following epsilon-aminocaproic acid (EACA) therapy. Journal of Neurosurgery 53: 690

Brodsky J B, Ehrenwerth J 1980 Postoperative muscle pains and suxamethonium. British Journal of Anaesthesia 52: 215

Brouet G, Marche J, Rist N, Chevallier J, Le Meur G 1959 Observation on the antituberculous effectiveness of alpha-ethyl-thiosonicotinamide in tuberculosis in humans. American Review of Tuberculosis 79: 6

Brown J A, Wollmann R L, Mullan S 1982 Myopathy induced by epsilon-aminocaproic acid. Journal of Neurosurgery 57: 130

Brumback R A, Empting L, Susag M E, Staton R D 1982 Muscle fibrosis associated with intramuscular chlorpromazine administration: A preliminary report. Journal of Pharmacy and Pharmacology 34: 526

Brumlik J, Jacobs R S 1974 Myasthenia gravis associated with diphenyl hydantoin therapy for epilepsy. Canadian Journal of Neurological Sciences 1: 127

Brust J C M, Hammer J S, Challenor Y, Healton E B, Lesser R P 1979 Acute generalized polyneuropathy accompanying lithium poisoning. Annals of Neurology 6: 360

Bruun E, Hermann K 1942 Polyneuritis after treatment with sulfonamide preparations. Acta Medica Scandinavica 111: 261

Buckle R M 1963 Blood pyruvic acid in thalidomide neuropathy. British Medical Journal 2: 973

Bucknall R C 1977 Myasthenia associated with D-penicillamine therapy in rheumatoid arthritis. Proceedings of the Royal Society of Medicine 70 (Suppl 3): 114

Burres S A, Richman D P, Crayton J W, Arnason B G W 1979 Penicillamine-induced myasthenia responses in the guinea pig. Muscle and Nerve 2: 186

Canal N, Franceschi M 1983 Myasthenic crisis precipitated by iothalmic acid. Lancet i: 1288

Carmignani M, Scoppetta C, Ranelletti F O, Tonali P 1984 Adverse interaction between acetazolamide and anticholinesterase drugs at the normal and myasthenic neuromuscular junction level. International Journal of Clinical Pharmacology, Therapeutics and Toxicology 22: 140

Carroll G J, Will R K, Peter J B, Garlepp M J, Dawkins R L 1987 Penicillamine induced polymyositis and dermatomyositis. Journal of Rheumatology 14: 995

Casarino J P 1977 Neuropathy associated with amitriptyline: bilateral footdrop. New York State Journal of Medicine 77: 2124

Casey E B, Jellife A M, Le Quesne P M, Millett Y L 1973 Vincristine neuropathy, clinical and electrophysiological observations. Brain 96: 69

Chagnac Y, Hadani M, Goldhammer Y 1985 Myasthenic crisis after intravenous administration of iodinated contrast agent. Neurology 35: 1219

Chalmers A C, Greco C M, Miller R G 1991 Prognosis in AZT myopathy. Neurology 41: 1181

Chang C C, Chuang S T 1972 Effects of desipramine and imipramine on the nerve, muscle and synaptic transmission of rat diaphragms. Neuropharmacology 11: 777

Chang Y C, Yip P K, Chiu Y N, Lin H N 1988 Severe generalized polyneuropathy in lithium intoxication. European Neurology 28: 39

Chasapakis G, Dimas C 1966 Possible interaction between muscle relaxants and the kallikrein-trypsin inactivator Trasylol. British Journal of Anaesthesia 38: 838

Chedru F, Nodzenski R, Dunand J F et al 1985 Peripheral neuropathy during treatment with almitrine. British Medical Journal 290: 896

Chi-Wan L A, Leppik I E, Jenkins D C, Sood P 1990 Epilepsy, myasthenia gravis and the effects of plasmapheresis on antiepileptic drug concentrations. Archives of Neurology 47: 66

Choucair A K, Ziter F 1984 Pentazocine abuse masquerading as familial myopathy. Neurology 34: 524

Clarke R S J, Dundee J W, Hamilton R C 1967 Interaction between induction agents and muscle relaxants. Anaesthesia 22: 235

Clemmensen O J, Olsen P Z, Andersen K E 1984 Thalidomide neurotoxicity. Archives of Dermatology 120: 338

Clouston P D, Donnelly P E 1989 Acute necrotising myopathy with amiodarone therapy. Australian and New Zealand Journal of Medicine 19: 483

Cogen F C, Rigg G, Simmons J L, Domino E F 1978 Phencyclidine-associated acute rhabdomyolysis. Annals of Internal Medicine 88: 210

Cohen L 1972 CPK test — effect of intramuscular injection in myocardial infarction. Journal of the American Medical Association 219: 625

Cohen M M 1970 Toxic neuropathies. In: Vinken P J, Bruyn G W (eds) Handbook of clinical neurology vol 7. North Holland, Amsterdam, p 527

Coleman C N, Wasserman T H, Urtason R C et al 1990 Final report of the phase 1 trial of the hypoxic cell radiosensitizer SR 2508 (etanidazole) radiation therapy oncology group 83–03. International Journal of Radiation, Oncology and Biological Physics 18: 389

Collard P J, Hargreaves W H 1947 Neuropathy after stilbamidine treatment of kala-azar. Lancet ii: 686

Collier G, Martin A 1960 Les effets sécondaires du tofranil. Revue générale à propos de trois cas de polynévrite des membres inferieurs. Annales Medicopsychologiques 118: 719

Confavreux C, Charles N, Aimard G 1990 Fulminant myasthenia gravis soon after initiation of acebutolo therapy. European Neurology 30: 279

Connolly K J, Allan J D, Fitch H et al 1991 Phase 1 study of 2'-3'-dideoxyinosine administered orally twice daily to patients with AIDs or AIDS-related complex and hematologic intolerance to zidovudine. American Journal of Medicine 91: 471

Coomes E N 1965a Corticosteroid myopathy. Annals of Rheumatic Diseases 24: 465

Coomes E N 1965b The rate of recovery of reversible myopathies and the effects of anabolic agents. Neurology (Minneapolis) 15: 523

Coppeto J 1984 Timolol-associated myasthenia gravis. American Journal of Ophthalmology 98: 244

Cornblath D R, McArthur J C 1988 Predominantly sensory neuropathy in patients with AIDS and AIDS-related complex. Neurology 38: 794

Corpier C L, Jones P H, Suki W N et al 1988 Rhabdomyolysis and renal injury with lovastatin use: Report of two cases in cardiac transplant recipient. Journal of the American Medical Association 260: 239

Coxon A, Pallis C A 1976 Metronidazole neuropathy. Journal of Neurology, Neurosurgery and Psychiatry 39: 403

Crawford A C 1975 Lithium ions and the release of transmitter at the frog neuromuscular junction. Journal of Physiology 246: 109

Crayton H, Bohlmann T, Sufit R, Graziano F M 1991 Drug induced polymyositis secondary to leuprolide acetate (Lupron) therapy for prostate cancer. Clinical and Experimental Rheumatology 9: 525

Crile G 1947 Treatment of hyperthyroidism. Canadian Medical Association Journal 57: 359

Cullen M J, Mastaglia F L 1980 Myopathy due to epsilon aminocaproic acid. Neuropathology and Applied Neurobiology 6: 78

Cumming A M M, Boddy K, Brown J J, Fraser R, Lever A F, Padfield P L, Robertson J I S 1980 Severe hypokalaemia with paralysis induced by small doses of liquorice. Postgraduate Medical Journal 56: 526

Czlonkowaska A 1975 Myasthenia syndrome during penicillamine treatment. British Medical Journal 2: 762

Dalakas M C 1992 Inflammatory and toxic myopathies. Current Opinion in Neurology and Neurosurgery 5: 645

Dalakas M C, Illa I, Pezeshkpour G H, Laukaitis J P, Cohen B, Griffin J L 1990 Mitochondrial myopathy caused by long-term zidovudine therapy. New England Journal of Medicine 322: 1098

Dale R C, Schroeder E T 1976 Respiratory paralysis during treatment of hypertension with trimetaphan camsylate. Archives of Internal Medicine 136: 816

Danon M J, Carpenter S 1991 Myopathy with thick filament (myosin) loss following prolonged paralysis with vecuronium during steroid treatment. Muscle and Nerve 14: 1131

De Grantis D, Mezzina C, Fiaschi A, Pinelli P, Bazzato G, Morachiello M 1980 Myasthenia due to carnitine treatment. Journal of the Neurological Sciences 46: 365

Delamere J P, Jobson S, Mackintosh L P, Wells, Walton K W 1983 Penicillamine-induced myasthenia in rheumatoid arthritis: its clinical and genetic features. Annals of the Rheumatic Diseases 42: 500

Delrieu F, Menkes C J, Sainte-Croix A, Baninet P, Chesneau A M, Delbarre F 1976 Myasthénie et thyroidite auto-immune au course du traitement de la polyarthrite rhümatoide par la D-penicillamine. Annales de Médecine Interne 127: 739

Denborough M A 1977 Malignant hyperpyrexia. Medical Journal of Australia 2: 757

Desmedt J E 1973 The neuromuscular disorder in myasthenia gravis. In: Desmedt J E (ed) New developments in electromyography and clinical neurophysiology, vol 1. Karger, Basel, p 305

Dhaliwal G S, Schlagenhauff R E, Megahed S M 1976 Acute femoral neuropathy induced by oral anticoagulation. Diseases of the Nervous System 37: 539

Dische S, Saunders M I, Stratfort M R 1981 Neurotoxicity with desmethylmisonidazole. British Journal of Radiology 54: 156

Djaldetti M, Pinkhas J, De Vries A, Kott E, Joshua H, Dollberg L 1968 Myasthenia gravis in a patient with chronic myeloid leukemia treated by busulfan. Blood 32: 336

Dobb G J, Edis R H 1984 Coma and neuropathy after ingestion of herbal laxative containing podophyllin. Medical Journal of Australia 140: 495

Dodian P, de Valeriola D, Body J J et al 1989 Phase 1 clinical trial with carbetimer. European Journal of Cancer and Clinical Oncology 25: 279

Dottori O, Lof B A, Yagge H 1965 Muscle pains after suxamethonium chloride. Acta Anaesthesiologia Scandinavica 9: 247

Doyle D R, McCurly T L, Sergent J S 1983 Fatal polymyositis in D-penicillamine-treated rheumatoid arthritis. Annals of Internal Medicine 98: 327

Doyle J B, Cannon E F 1950 Severe polyneuritis following gold therapy for rheumatoid arthritis. Annals of Internal Medicine 33: 1468

Drachman D A, Skom J H 1965 Procainamide — a hazard in myasthenia gravis. Archives of Neurology 13: 316

Drachman D B 1962 Myasthenia gravis and the thyroid gland. New England Journal of Medicine 266: 330

Drenckhahn D, Lullman-Rauch R 1979 Experimental myopathy induced by amphiphilic cationic compounds including several psychotropic drugs. Neuroscience 4: 549

Dretchen K L, Sokoll M D, Gergis S D, Long J P 1973 Relative effects of streptomycin on motor nerve terminal and endplate. European Journal of Pharmacology 22: 10

Dropcho E J and S Soong 1991 Steroid-induced weakness in patients with primary brain tumours. Neurology 41: 1235

Drutz D J, Fan J H, Tai T Y, Cheng J T, Hsieh W C 1970 Hypokalaemic rhabdomyolysis and myoglobinuria following amphotericin B therapy. Journal of the American Medical Association 211: 824

Duane D D, Engel A G 1970 Emetine myopathy. Neurology (Minneapolis) 20: 733

Dubinsky R M, Yarchoan R, Dalakas M, Broder S 1989 Reversile axonal neuropathy from the treatment of AIDS and related disorders with 2'-3'-dideoxycytidine (ddc). Muscle and Nerve 12: 856

Duignan N, Andrews J, Williams J D 1973 Pharmacological studies with lincomycin in late pregnancy. British Medical Journal 3: 75

Dukes M N G 1977 Side effects of drugs: Annual 1. Excerpta Medica, Amsterdam, p 118, 181, 292, 331, 339

Eade O E, Acheson E D, Cuthbert M F, Hawkes C H 1975 Peripheral neuropathy and indomethacin. British Medical Journal 3: 66

East C, Alivizatos P A, Grundy S M, Jones P H, Farmer J A 1988 Rhabdomyolysis in patients receiving lovastatin after cardiac transplantation. New England Journal of Medicine 318: 47

Eden K V 1983 Possible association of Guillain–Barré syndrome with thrombolytic therapy. Journal of the American Medical Association 249: 2020

Eisen A A, Woods J F, Sherwin A L 1974 Peripheral nerve function in long-term therapy with diphenylhydantoin. Neurology (Minneapolis) 24: 411

Elder B F, Beal H, De Wald W, Cobb S 1971 Exacerbation of subclinical myasthenia by occupational exposure to anaesthetic. Anaesthesia and Analgesia Current Researches 50: 383

Eliashiv S, Wirguin I, Brenner T, Argov Z 1990 Aggravation of human and experimental myasthenia gravis by contrast media. Neurology 40: 1620

Ellis F G 1962 Acute polyneuritis after nitrofurantoin therapy. Lancet 2: 1136

Ellis F R, Keaney N P, Harriman D G F et al 1972 Screening for malignant hyperpyrexia. British Medical Journal 3: 559

Ellis F R, Clarke, I M C, Modgill M, Currie S, Harriman D G F 1975 Evaluation of creatine phosphokinase in screening patients for malignant hyperpyrexia. British Medical Journal 3: 511

Elmqvist D, Josefsson J O 1962 The nature of the neuromuscular block produced by neomycin. Acta Physiologica Scandinavica 54: 105

Endtz L J 1958 Complications nerveuses du traitement aurique. Revue Neurologique 99: 395

Engel A G 1961 Thyroid function and myasthenia gravis. Archives of Neurology 4: 663

Epstein F W, Bohm M 1976 Dapsone-induced peripheral neuropathy. Archives of Dermatology 112: 1761

Estes M L, Ewing-Wilson D, Chou S M et al 1987 Chloroquine neuromyotoxicity: clinical and pathological perspective. American Journal of Medicine 82: 447

Extra J M, Espie M, Calvo F, Ferme C, Mignot L, Marty M 1990 Phase 1 study of oxaliplatin in patients with advanced cancer. Cancer Chemotherapy Pharmacology 25: 299

Fagius J, Osterman P O, Sidén A, Wiholm B-E 1985 Guillain–Barré syndrome following zimeldine. Journal of Neurology, Neurosurgery and Psychiatry 48: 65

Falkson G, van Dyk J J, van Eden E B, van der Merwe A M, van der Bergh J A, Falkson H C 1975 A clinical trial of the oral form of 4'-demethyl-epipodophyllotoxin-B-D ethylidene glucose (NSC 141540) VP 16–213. Cancer 35: 1141

Fardeau M, Tomé F M S, Simon P 1979 Muscle and nerve changes induced by perhexiline maleate in man and mice. Muscle and Nerve 2: 24

Fawcett P R W, McLachlan S M, Nicholson L V B, Argov Z, Mastaglia F L 1982 D-Penicillamine-associated myasthenia gravis: immunological and electrophysiological studies. Muscle and Nerve 5: 328

Feest T G, Read D J 1980 Myopathy associated with cimetidine? British Medical Journal 281: 1284

Feldman S A, Crawley B E 1970 Interaction of diazepam with the muscle-relaxant drugs. British Medical Journal 2: 336

Fernandes L, Swinson D R, Hamilton E B D 1977 Dermatomyositis complicating penicillamine treatment. Annals of Rheumatic Diseases 36: 94

Fernandez-Sola J, Campistol J, Casademont J, Grau J M, Urbano-Marquez A 1990 Reversible cyclosporin myopathy. Lancet 335: 362

Fewings J D, Burns R J, Kakulas B A 1973 A case of acute emetine myopathy. In: Kakulas B A (ed) Clinical studies in myology. Excerpta Medica, Amsterdam, p 594

Fiekers J F 1983a Effects of the aminoglycoside antibiotics, streptomycin and neomycin, on neuromuscular transmission. 1. Presynaptic considerations. Journal of Pharmacology and Experimental Therapeutics 225: 487

Fiekers J F 1983b Effects of the aminoglycoside antibiotics, streptomycin and neomycin, on neuromuscular transmission. II. Postsynaptic considerations. Journal of Pharmacology and Experimental Therapeutics 225: 496

Filley C M, Graff-Radford N R, Lacy J R, Heitner M A, Earnest M P 1982 Neurologic manifestations of podophyllin toxicity. Neurology (New York) 32: 308

Finke J, Spiegelberg U 1973 Polyneuropathy nach methaqualone. Nervenarzt 44: 104

Finkelman I, Arieff A J 1942 Untoward effects of phenytoin sodium in epilepsy. Journal of the American Medical Association 118: 1209

Florence A L 1960 Is thalidomide to blame? British Medical Journal 2: 1954

Fogdall R P, Miller R D 1974 Prolongation of pancuronium induced neuromuscular block by clindamycin. Anesthesiology 41: 407

Fontiveros E S, Cumming W J K, Hudgson P 1980 Procainamide-induced myositis. Journal of the Neurological Sciences 45: 143

Frank J H, Cooper G W, Black W C, Phillips L H 1987 Iodinated contrast agents in myasthenia gravis. Neurology 37: 1400

Forfar J C, Brown G J, Cull R E 1979 Proximal myopathy during beta blockade. British Medical Journal 279: 1331

Fraser A G, McQueen I N F, Watt A H, Stephens M R 1985 Peripheral neuropathy during longterm high-dose amiodarone therapy. Journal of Neurology, Neurosurgery and Psychiatry 48: 576

Fraser D M, Campbell I W, Miller H C 1977 Peripheral and autonomic neuropathy after treatment with perhexiline maleate. British Medical Journal 2: 75

Frawley T F, Koeppe G F 1950 Neurotoxicity due to thiouracil and thiourea derivatives. Journal of Clinical Endocrinology 10: 623

Fredericks E J, Kugelman T P, Kirsch N 1976 Dapsone-induced motor polyneuropathy. Archives of Dermatology 112: 1158

Frisoni G B, Di Modena V 1989 Disulfiram neuropathy: a review (1971–1988) and report of a case. Alcohol and Alcoholism 24: 429

Fullerton P M, Kremer M 1961 Neuropathy after intake of thalidomide (Distaval). British Medical Journal 2: 855

Fullerton P M, O'Sullivan D J 1968 Thalidomide neuropathy: a clinical, electrophysiological, and histological follow-up study. Journal of Neurology, Neurosurgery and Psychiatry 31: 543

Gabriel R, Pearce J M S 1976 Clofibrate-induced myopathy and neuropathy. Lancet 2: 906

Galzigna L, Manani G, Mammano S, Gasparetto A, Deana R 1972 Experimental study on the neuromuscular blocking action of procainamide. Agressologie 13: 107

Gammon G D, Burge F W, King G 1953 Neural toxicity in tuberculous patients treated with isoniazid (isonicotinic acid hydrazine). Archives of Neurology and Psychiatry 70: 64

Gardner-Thorpe C, Benjamin S 1971 Peripheral neuropathy after disulfiram administration. Journal of Neurology, Neurosurgery and Psychiatry 34: 253

Garlepp M J, Dawkins R L, Christiansen F T 1983 HLA antigens and acetylcholine receptor antibodies in penicillamine induced myasthenia gravis. British Medical Journal 286: 338

Gehlmann L K, Koller W C, Malkinson F D 1977 Dapsone-induced neuropathy. Archives of Dermatology 113: 845

Geraud G, Caussanel J P, Jauzac P H, Arbus L, Bes A 1978 Peripheral neuropathy after perhexiline maleate therapy. 4th International Congress on Neuromuscular Diseases, Montreal, Canada, Abstract 81

Gergis S D, Sokoll M D, Rubbo J T 1977 Effect of sodium nitro-prusside and trimetaphan on neuromuscular transmission in the frog. Canadian Anaesthetists Society Journal 24: 220

Gesztes T 1966 Prolonged apnoea after suxamethonium injection associated with eye drops containing an anticholinesterase agent. British Journal of Anesthesia 38: 408

Ghoneim M M, Long J P 1970 The interaction between magnesium and other neuromuscular blocking agents. Anesthesiology 32: 23

Ghose K 1977 Lithium salts: therapeutic and unwanted effects. British Journal of Hospital Medicine 18: 578

Gibb W R G, Lees A J 1985 The neuroleptic malignant syndrome — a review. Quarterly Journal of Medicine 220: 421

Gibbels E 1967 Weitere beobachtungen zur Nebenwirkung intravenoser reverin-gaben bei Myasthenia gravis pseudoparalytica. Deutsche Medizinische Wochenschrift 92: 1153

Gibbs J M 1978 A case of rhabdomyolysis associated with suxamethonium. Anaesthesia and Intensive Care 6: 141

Gissen A J, Karis J H, Nastuk W L 1966 Effect of halothane on neuromuscular transmission. Journal of the American Medical Association 197: 116

Golding D N, Begg T B 1960 Dexamethasone myopathy. British Medical Journal 2: 1129

Goldman J A, Fishman A B, Lee J E, Johnson R J 1989 The role of cholesterol-lowering agents in drug-induced rhabdomyolysis and polymyositis. Arthritis and Rheumatism 32: 358

Goodheart R S, Dunne J W, Edis R H 1991 Phenelzine associated peripheral neuropathy - clinical and electrophysiologic findings. Australian and New Zealand Journal of Medicine 21: 339

Goy J J, Stauffer J C, Deruaz J P et al 1989 Myopathy as a possible side-effect of cyclosporin. Lancet i: 1446

Granacher R P 1977 Neuromuscular problems associated with lithium. American Journal of Psychiatry 134: 702

Greenblatt D J, Allen D 1978 Intramuscular injection-site complications. Journal of the American Medical Association 240: 542

Gronert G A 1983 Malignant hyperthermia. Anesthesiology 53: 395

Grongono A W 1963 Anesthesia for atrial defibrillation. Effects of quinidine on muscular relaxation. Lancet 2: 1039

Gross E G, Dexter J D, Roth R G 1966 Hypokalemic myopathy with myoglobinuria associated with licorice ingestion. New England Journal of Medicine 74: 602

Grossman R A, Hamilton R W, Morse B M, Penn A S, Goldberg M 1974 Nontraumatic rhabdomyolysis and acute renal failure. New England Journal of Medicine 291: 807

Gutmann L, Takamori M 1973 Effects of Mg^{++} on neuromuscular transmission in the Eaton–Lambert syndrome. Neurology 23: 977

Hagen R 1968 Contracture of the quadriceps muscle. A report of 12 cases. Acta Orthopaedica Scandinavica 39: 565

Haim N, Barron S A, Robinson E 1991 Muscle cramps associated with vincristine therapy. Acta Oncologia 30: 707

Halbig L, Gutmann L, Goebel H H, Brick J F, Schochet S 1988 Ultrastructural pathology in emetine-induced myopathy. Acta Pathologica (Berlin) 75: 577

Hales D S M, Scott R, Lewi H J E 1982 Myopathy due to mercaptopropionyl glycine. British Medical Journal 285: 939

Halla J T, Fallahi S, Koopman W J 1984 Penicillamine-induced myositis. American Journal of Medicine 77: 719

Halliday P L, Bauer R B 1983 Polyradiculoneuritis secondary to immunization with tetanus and diphtheria toxoids. Archives of Neurology 40: 56

Harney J, Glasberg M R 1983 Myopathy and hypersensitivity to phenytoin. Neurology 33: 790

Harriman D G F, Sumner D W, Ellis F R 1973 Malignant hyperpyrexia myopathy. Quarterly Journal of Medicine 42: 639

Harrison G G 1989 Malignant hyperthermia. In Nunn J F, Utting J E, Brown B R (eds) General anaesthesia. Butterworths, ch 52, p 655

Hartfall S J, Garland H G, Goldie W 1937 Gold treatment of arthritis. A review of 900 cases. Lancet 2: 838

Hashimoto F, Sherman C B, Jeffrey W H 1984 Neuroleptic malignant syndrome and dopaminergic blockade. Archives of Internal Medicine 144: 629

Hashimoto Y, Shima T, Matsukawa S, Satou M 1978 A possible hazard of prolonged neuromuscular blockade by amikacin. Anesthesiology 49: 219

Hawkins R A, Eckhoff P J, MacCarter D K, Harmon C E 1983 Cimetidine and polymyositis. New England Journal of Medicine 309: 187

Hayman I, Abresman C E, Terplan K L 1956 Dermatomyositis following penicillin injections. Neurology 6: 63

Hayman M, Wilkins P A 1956 Polyneuropathy as a complication of disulfiram therapy of alcoholism. Quarterly Journal of Studies in Alcohol 17: 601

Herishanu Y, Rosenberg P 1975 β-Blockers and myasthenia gravis. Annals of Internal Medicine 83: 834

Herzlich B C, Arsura E L, Pagala M, Grob D 1988 Rhabdomyolysis related to cocaine abuse. Annals of Internal Medicine 109: 335

Hewitt J A, Glinn J 1989 Lofepramine and motor neuropathy. British Medical Journal 299: 1223

Hicklin J A 1968 Chloroquine neuromyopathy. Annals of Physical Medicine 9: 189

Hickson R C, Davis J R 1981 Partial prevention of glucocorticoid-induced muscle atrophy by endurance training. American Journal of Physiology 241: E226

Hill G, Wong K C, Hodges M R 1976 Potentiation of succinylcholine neuromuscular blockade by lithium carbonate. Anesthesiology 44: 439

Hoaken P C S 1975 Adverse effect of methaqualone. Canadian Medical Association Journal 112: 685

Hodges R J H, Bennett J R, Tunstall M E 1959 Effects of oxytocin on the response to suxamethonium. British Medical Journal 1: 413

Hokkanen E 1964 The aggravating effect of some antibiotics on the neuromuscular blockade in myasthenia gravis. Acta Neurologica Scandinavica 40: 346

Holmes F A, Walters R S, Theriault R L et al 1991 Phase 2 trial of taxol, an active drug in the treatment of metastatic breast cancer. Journal of the National Cancer Institute 83: 1797

Hool G J, Lawrence P J, Sivaneswaran N 1984 Acute rhabdomyolytic renal failure due to suxamethonium. Anaesthesia and Intensive Care 12: 360

Horber F F, Scheidegger J R, Grunig B E, Frey F J 1985 Thigh muscle mass and function in patients treated with glucocorticoids. European Journal of Clinical Investigation 15: 302

Howard J F 1990 Adverse drug effects on neuromuscular transmission. Seminars in Neurology 10: 89

Hughes H B, Biehl J P, Jones A P, Schmidt L H 1954 Metabolism of isoniazid in man as related to the occurrence of peripheral neuritis. American Review of Tuberculosis 70: 266

Hughes R O, Zacharias F J 1976 Myasthenic syndrome during treatment with practolol. British Medical Journal 1: 460

Ingham H R, Selkon J B, Hale J H 1975 The antibacterial activity of metronidazole. Journal of Antimicrobial Chemotherapy 1: 355

Israeli A, Raveh D, Arnon R, Eisenberg S, Stein Y 1989 Lovastatin and elevated creatine kinase: Results of rechallenge. Lancet i: 725

Jacobs J M, Costa-Jussa F R 1985 The pathology of amiodarone neurotoxicity. II. Peripheral neuropathy in man. Brain 108: 753

Janssen P J 1960 Peripheral neuritis due to streptomycin. American Review of Respiratory Diseases 81: 726

Jensen O B, Mosdal C, Reske-Nielsen E 1977 Hypokalaemic myopathy during treatment with diuretics. Acta Neurologica Scandinavica 55: 465

Johnson K 1990 Molecular genetics of malignant hyperthermia. Journal of the Neurological Sciences 98 (suppl) 134

Jui-Yen T 1971 Clinical and experimental studies on mechanism of neuromuscular blockade by chloroquine cliorotate. Japanese Journal of Anesthesia 20: 491

Kaeser H E 1984 Drug-induced myasthenic syndromes. Acta Neurologica Scandinavica 70: 39

Kakulas B A, Mastaglia F L 1992 Drug induced, toxic and nutritional myopathies. In: Mastaglia F L, Walton J N (eds) Skeletal muscle pathology, 2nd edn. Churchill Livingstone, Edinburgh, p 511

Kalayanaraman U P, Kalayanaraman K, Cullinan S A, McLean J M 1983 Neuromyopathy of cyanide intoxication due to 'laetrile' (amygdalin). Cancer 51: 2126

Kane M J, Silverman L R, Rand J H, Paciucci P A, Holland J F 1988 Myonecrois as a complication of the use of epsilon amino caproic acid: A case report and review of the literature. American Journal of Medicine 85: 861

Kanterewicz E, Bruguera M, Viola C, Lamarca J, Rodes J 1990 Toxic neuropathy after adenine arabinoside treatment in chronic HBsAg-positive liver disease. Journal of Clinical Gastroenterology 12: 90

Kaplan A M, Bergeson P S, Gregg S A, Curless R G 1977 Malignant hyperthermia associated with myopathy and normal muscle enzymes. Journal of Pediatrics 91: 431

Kaplan R S, Wiernik P H 1982 Neurotoxicity of antineoplastic drugs. Seminars in Oncology 9: 103

Karpati G 1984 Denervation and disuse atrophy of skeletal muscles — involvement of endogenous glucocorticoid hormones? Trends in Neurosciences: 61

Katrak S M, Pollock M, O'Brien C P et al 1980 Clinical and morphological features of gold neuropathy. Brain 103: 671

Katz B 1966 Nerve, muscle and synapse. McGraw-Hill, New York

Katz B, Miledi R 1965 Propagation of electric activity in motor nerve terminals. Proceedings of the Royal Society of London B161: 453

Kaufman L E 1990 Neuromuscular manifestations of the L-tryptophan-associated eosinophilia-myalgia syndrome. Current Opinion in Rhematology 2: 896

Kaufman L D, Grubeer B L, Gregersen P K 1991 Clinical follow-up and immunogenetic studies of 32 patients with eosinophilia-myalgia syndrome. Lancet 337: 1071

Keidar S , Binenboim C, Palant A 1982 Muscle cramps during treatment with nifedipine. British Medical Journal 285: 1241

Kennard C, Swash M, Henson R A 1980 Myopathy due to epsilon amino-caproic acid. Muscle and Nerve 3: 202

Kennedy, M 1981 Cardiac glycoside toxicity. An unusual manifestation of drug addiction. Medical Journal of Australia 1: 686

Kennedy R D, Galindo A D 1975 Comparative site of action of various anaesthetic agents at the mammalian myoneural junction. British Journal of Anesthesia 47: 533

Khaleeli A A, Edwards R H T, Gohil K et al 1983 Corticosteroid myopathy: A clinical and pathological study. Clinical Endocrinology 18: 115

Kilpatrick C, Braund W, Burns R 1982 Myopathy with myasthenic features, possibly induced by codeine linctus. Medical Journal of Australia 2: 410

King J O, Denborough M A, Zapf P W 1972 Inheritance of malignant hyperpyrexia. Lancet 1: 365

King J O, Denborough M A 1973a Malignant hyperpyrexia in Australia and New Zealand. Medical Journal of Australia 1: 525

King J O, Denborough M A 1973b Anesthetic-induced malignant hyperpyrexia in children. Journal of Pediatrics 83: 37

Kirkendall W M, Page E B 1958 Polyneuritis occurring during hydralazine therapy. Journal of the American Medical Association 167: 427

Klatskin G, Friedman H 1948 Emetine toxicity in man: studies on the nature of early toxic manifestations, their relation to the dose level, and their significance in determining safe dosage. Annals of Internal Medicine 28: 892

Klinghardt G W 1967 Schadigungen des nervensystems durch nitrofurane bei der ratte. Acta Neuropathologica (Berlin) 9: 18

Knape H 1977 In: Dukes M N G (ed) Side effects of drugs, vol 1. Excerpta Medica, Amsterdam, p 103

Knezevic W, Mastaglia F L, Lefroy R B, Fisher A 1984a Neuroleptic malignant syndrome. Medical Journal of Australia 140: 28

Knezevic W, Quintner J, Mastaglia F L, Zilko P J 1984b Guillain-Barré syndrome and pemphigus foliaceus associated with D-penicillamine therapy. Australian and New Zealand Journal of Medicine 14: 50

Koelle G B 1975 Neuromuscular blocking agents. In: Goodman L S, Gilman A (eds) The pharmacological basis of therapeutics, 5th edn. Macmillan, New York, p 577

Kolb L C, Gray S J 1946 Peripheral neuritis as a complication of penicillin therapy. Journal of the American Medical Association 132: 323

Kono R 1971 Subacute myelo-optico-neuropathy, a new neurological disease prevailing in Japan. Japanese Journal of Medical Science and Biology 24: 195

Kontos H A 1962 Myopathy associated with chronic colchicine toxicity. New England Journal of Medicine 266: 38

Kornfeld P, Horowitz S H, Genkins G, Papatestas A E 1976 Myasthenia gravis unmasked by antiarrhythmic agents. Mount Sinai Journal of Medicine 43: 10

Korsan-Bengsten K, Ysander L, Blohme G, Tibblin E 1969 Extensive muscle necrosis after long-term treatment with aminocaproic acid (EACA) in a case of hereditary periodic oedema. Acta Medica Scandinavica 185: 341

Koski C L, Rifenberick D H, Max S R 1974 Oxidative metabolism of skeletal muscle in steroid atrophy. Archives of Neurology 31: 407

Krendel D A, Hopkins L G 1986 Effect of verapamil in a patient with the Lambert Eaton syndrome. Muscle and Nerve 9: 519

Kuncl R W, Duncan G, Watson D, Alderson K, Rogawski M A, Peper M 1987 Colchicine myopathy and neuropathy. New England Journal of Medicine 316: 1562

Kuncl R W, Duncan G 1988 Chronic human colchicine myopathy and neuropathy. Archives of Neurology 45: 245

Kuntzer T, Bogousslavsky J, Deruaz J P, Janzer R, Regli F 1989 Reversible emetine-induced myopathy with ECG abnormalities: a toxic myopathy. Journal of Neurology 236: 246

Kwiecinski H 1981 Myotonia induced by chemical agents. CRC Critical Reviews in Toxicology 8: 279

Lane R J M, Mastaglia F L 1978 Drug-induced myopathies in man. Lancet 2: 562

Lane R J M, McLelland N J, Martin A M, Mastaglia F L 1979 Epsilon aminocaproic acid (EACA) myopathy. Postgraduate Medical Journal 55: 282

Langman M J S 1975 Gastrointestinal drugs. In: Dukes M N G (ed) Meyler's side-effects of drugs, vol 8. Excerpta Medica, Amsterdam, p 795

La-Rocca R V, Meer J, Gilliatt R W et al 1990 Suramin-induced polyneuropathy. 40: 954

Larsen A 1978 On the neuromuscular effects of pindolol and sotalol in the rat. Acta Physiologica Scandinavica 102: 35

Lator N, Koski C L, Walicke P A 1991 Guillain–Barré syndrome and parenteral gangliosides. Lancet ii: 757

Leaf D A, MacDonald I, Kliks B, Wilson R, Jones S R 1984 Streptokinase and the Guillain–Barré syndrome. Annals of Internal Medicine 100: 617

Leck I M, Millar E L M 1962 Incidence of malformation since the introduction of thalidomide. British Medical Journal 1: 16

Lecky B R F 1990 Griseofulvin-induced neuropathy. Lancet 335: 230

Lee S C, Ho S T 1987 Acute effects of verapamil on neuromuscular transmission in patients with myasthenia gravis. Proceedings of the National Science Council B (Republic of China) 11: 307

Le Quesne P M 1970 Iatrogenic neuropathies. In: Vinken P J, Bruyn G W (ed) Handbook of clinical neurology, North Holland, Amsterdam, p 527

Le Quesne P M 1975 Neuropathy due to drugs. In Dyck P J, Thomas P K, Lambert E H (eds) Peripheral neuropathy. Saunders, Philadelphia, p 1263

Le Quesne P M 1984 Neuropathy due to drugs. In: Dyck P J, Thomas P K, Lambert E H, Bunge R (eds) Peripheral neuropathy, 2nd edn. Saunders, Philadelphia, p 2162

Lending R E, Gall E P, Buchsbaum H W, Foote R A 1984 Hypersensitivity reaction to sulindac (Clinoril). Archives of Internal Medicine 144: 2259

Lennmarken C, Lofstrom J B 1984 Partial curarization in the postoperative period. Acta Anaesthesiologica Scandinavica 28: 260

Lermer H, Avni J, Bruderman I 1970 Neuromuscular blocking action of amitriptyline. European Journal of Pharmacology 13: 266

Levin B E, Engel W K 1975 Iatrogenic muscle fibrosis. Arm levitation as an initial sign. Journal of the American Medical Association 234: 621

Lhermitte F, Fardeau M, Chedru F, Mallecourt J 1976 Polyneuropathy after perhexiline maleate therapy. British Medical Journal 1: 1256

L'Hommedieu C S, Huber P A, Rasche D K 1983 Potentiation of magnesium-induced neuromuscular weakness by gentamicin. Critical Care Medicine 11: 55

Lim P K, Trewby P N, Storey G C A, Holt D W 1984 Neuropathy and fatal hepatitis in a patient receiving amiodarone. British Medical Journal 288: 1638

Lindesmith L A, Baines R D, Bigelow D B, Petty T L 1968 Reversible respiratory paralysis associated with polymyxin therapy. Annals of Internal Medicine 68: 318

Lingle F A 1966 Irreversible effects of glutethimide addiction. Journal of Psychiatry 123: 349

Lipton R B, Apfel S C, Dutcher J P et al 1989 Taxol produces a predominantly sensory neuropathy. Neurology 39: 368

Lithell H, Boberg J, Hellsing K, Lundqvist G, Vessby B 1978 Increase in the lipoprotein-lipase activity in human skeletal muscle during clofibrate administration. European Journal of Clinical Investigation 8: 67

Litin S C, Anderson C F 1989 Nicotinic acid-associated myopathy: A report of three cases. American Journal of Medicine 86: 481

Livingsone I, Johnson M A, Mastaglia F L 1981 Effects of dexamethasone on fibre subtypes in rat muscle. Neuropathology and Applied Neurobiology 7: 381

Loder R E, Walker G F 1959 Neuromuscular-blocking action of streptomycin. Lancet 1: 812

Loftus L R 1963 Peripheral neuropathy following chloroquine therapy. Canadian Medical Association Journal 89: 917

London S F, Gross K F, Ringel S P 1991 Cholesterol-lowering agent myopathy (CLAM). Neurology 41: 1159

Lovelace R E, Horwitz S J 1968 Peripheral neuropathy in long-term diphenylhydantoin therapy. Archives of Neurology 18: 69

Lullman H, Lullman-Rauch R, Wassermann O 1978 Lipidosis induced by amphiphilic cationic drugs. Biochemical Pharmacology 27: 1103

Lund H I, Nielsen M 1983 Penicillamine-induced dermatomyositis. Scandinavian Journal of Rheumatology 12: 350

McCarthy T V, Healy J M S, Heffron J J A et al 1990 Localization of the malignant hyperthermia susceptibility locus to human chromosome 19q12–13.2. Nature 343: 562

McCormick D B, Snell E E 1959 Pyridoxal kinase of human brain and its inhibition by hydrazine derivatives. Proceedings of the National Academy of Sciences USA 45: 1371

MacDonald R D, Engel A G 1970 Experimental chloroquine myopathy. Journal of Neuropathology and Experimental Neurology 29: 479

MacFarlane I A, Rosenthal F D 1977 Severe myopathy after status asthmaticus. Lancet ii: 615

MacLennan D H, Duff C, Zorsato F et al 1990 Ryanodine receptor gene is a candidate for predisposition to malignant hyperthermia. Nature 343: 559

McQuaker W, Bruggen P 1963 Side-effects of methaqualone. British Medical Journal 1: 749

McQuillen M P, Gross M, Johns R J 1963 Chlorpromazine-induced weakness in myasthenia gravis. Archives of Neurology 8: 286

McQuillen M P, Cantor H E, O'Rourke J R 1968 Myasthenic syndrome associated with antibiotics. Archives of Neurology 18: 402

McQuillen M P, Engbaek L 1975 Mechanism of colistin-induced neuromuscular depression. Archives of Neurology 32: 235

Magarian G J, Lucas L M, Colley C 1991 Gemfibrozil-induced myopathy. Archives of Internal Medicine 152: 1873

Mak K H, Wan S H, Boey M L, Lee Y S 1990 Myocardial and skeletal muscle injuries following adenine arabinoside therapy. Australia and New Zealand Journal of Medicine 20: 811

Manani G, Gasparetto A, Bettini V, Caldesi Valeri V, Galzigna G L 1970 Mechanism of action of ajmaline on neuromuscular junction. Agressologie 11: 275

Mandel W 1959 Pyridoxine and the isoniazid induced neuropathy. Diseases of the Chest 36: 293

Marcus S N, Chadwick D, Walker R 1984 D-Penicillamine-induced myasthenia gravis in primary biliary cirrhosis. Gastroenterology 86: 166

Markes P, Sloggen J 1976 Peripheral neuropathy caused by methaqualone. American Journal of the Medical Sciences 272: 323

Marmor A, Alpan G, Keider S, Grenadier E, Palant A 1978 The MB isoenzyme of creatine kinase as an indicator of severity of myocardial infarction. Lancet 2: 812

Martin-Algarra S, Henriquez I, Rebello J, Artieda J 1990 Severe polyneuropathy and motor loss after intrathecal thiotepa combination chemotherapy: description of two cases. Anticancer Drugs 1: 33

Martinez-Arizala A, Sobol S M, McCarty G E, Nichols B R, Rakita L 1983 Amiodarone neuropathy. Neurology 33: 643–645

Mastaglia F L 1982 Adverse effects of drugs on muscle. Drugs 24: 304–321

Mastaglia F L 1993 Toxic myopathies. In: Vinken P, Bruyn G, Klawans H L (eds) Handbook of Clinical Neurology, North Holland Publishing Company (in press).

Mastaglia F L, Argov Z 1982 Immunologically-mediated drug-induced neuromuscular disorders. In: Dukor P, Kallos P, Schlumberger H D, West G B (eds) Pseudo-allergic reactions — involvement of drugs and chemicals, vol 3, Cell mediated reactions. Karger, Basel, p 1–24

Mastaglia F L, Gardner-Medwin D, Hudgson P 1971 Muscle fibrosis and contractures in a pethidine addict. British Medical Journal 4: 532–533

Mastaglia F L, Papadimitriou J M, Dawkins R L, Beveridge B 1977 Vacuolar myopathy associated with chloroquine, lupus erythematosus and thymoma. Journal of the Neurological Sciences 34: 315

Masters C L, Dawkins R L, Zilko P J, Simpson J A, Leedman R J, Lindstrom J 1977 Penicillamine-associated myasthenia gravis, antiacetylcholine receptor and antistriatal antibodies. American Journal of Medicine 63: 689

May E F, Calvert P C 1990 Aggravation of myasthenia gravis by erythromycin. Annals of Neurology 128: 577

Meier C, Kauer B, Muller U, Ludin H P 1979 Neuromyopathy during chronic amiodarone treatment. A case report. Journal of Neurology 220: 231

Merhoff G C, Porter J M 1974 Ergot intoxication: Historical review and description of unusual clinical manifestation. Annals of Surgery 180: 773

Meyboom R H B 1977 Heavy metal antagonists. In: Dukes M N G (ed) Side effects of drugs, vol 1. Excerpta Medica, Amsterdam, p 192

Mhiri C, Baudrimont M, Bonne G et al 1991 Zidovudine myopathy: a distinctive disorder associated with mitochondrial dysfunction. Annals of Neurology 29: 606

Mickelson J R, Gallant E M, Litterer L A, Johnson K M, Rempel W E, Louis C F 1988 Abnormal sarcoplasmic reticulum ryanodine receptor in malignant hyperthermia. Journal of Biological Chemistry 263: 9310

Miller M 1963 Neuropathy, agranulocytosis and hepatotoxicity following imipramine therapy. American Journal of Psychiatry 120: 185

Milonas J, Kountouris D, Scheer E 1983 Myasthenic syndrome following long term diphenyhydantoin therapy for epilepsy. Nervenarzt 54: 437

Mitchell M M, Ali H H, Savarese J J 1978 Myotonia and neuromuscular blocking agents. Anesthesiology 49: 44

Mitsumoto H, Wilbourne A J, Subramony S H 1982 Generalized myokymia and gold therapy. Archives of Neurology 39: 449

Mohamed S D, Chapman R S, Crooks J 1966 Hypokalaemia, flaccid quadriparesis and myoglobinuria with carbenoxolone (Biogastrone). British Medical Journal 1: 1581

Mollman J E, Glover D J, Hogan M, Furman R E 1988a Cisplatin neuropathy: Risk factors, prognosis and protection by WR-2721. Cancer 612: 192

Mollman J E, Hogan W M, Glover D J, McClusky L F 1988b Unusual presentation of cis-platinum neuropathy. Neurology 38: 488

Morris J S 1966 Nitrofurantoin and peripheral neuropathy with megaloblastic anemia. Journal of Neurology, Neurosurgery and Psychiatry 29: 224

Muller R 1945 Polyneuritis following sulfanilamide therapy. Acta Medica Scandinavica 121: 95

Mullet R D, Keats A S 1961 Apnea and respiratory insufficiency after intraperitoneal administration of kanamycin. Surgery 49: 530

Nakamura K, Koide M, Imanaga T, Ogasawara H, Takahashi M, Yoshikawa M 1980 Prolonged neuromuscular blockade following trimetaphan infusion. Anaesthesia 35: 1202

Neil J F, Himmelhoch J M, Licata S 1976 Emergence of myasthenia gravis during treatment with lithium carbonate. Archives of General Psychiatry 33: 1090

Nelson T E, Flewellen E H 1983 The malignant hyperthermia syndrome. New England Journal of Medicine 309: 416

Newson A J 1972 Malignant hyperthermia: Three case reports. New England Journal of Medicine 75: 138

Niakan E, Bertorini T E, Acchiatdo S R, Werner M F 1981 Procainamide-induced myasthenia-like weakness in a patient with peripheral neuropathy. Archives of Neurology 38: 378

Nicolas F, Baron D, Dixneuf B, Visset J, Dubigeon P 1970 Les nécroses musculaires au cours des intoxications aigues. Presse Médicale 78: 751

Nilsson E, Paloheimo M, Muller K, Heinone J 1989 Halothane-induced variability in the neuromuscular transmission of patients with myasthenia gravis. Acta Anesthesiologica Scandinavica 33: 395

Nilsson E, Muller K 1990 Effects of isoflurane in patients with myathenia gravis. Acta Anaesthiologica Scandinavica 34: 126

Noppen M, Velkeniers B, Dierckx R, Bruyland M, Vanhaelst L 1987 Cyclosporin and myopathy. Annals of Internal Medicine 107: 945

Norris F H, Colella J, McFarlin D 1964 Effect of diphenylhydantoin on neuromuscular synapse. Neurology (Minneapolis) 14: 869

Nukada H, Pollock M 1981 Disulfiram neuropathy. A morphometric study of sural nerve. Journal of the Neurological Sciences 51: 51

O'Mahony S, Keohane C, Jacobs J, O'Riordain D, Whelton M 1990 Neuropathy due to podophyllin intoxication. Journal of Neurology 23: 110

Onodera K, Yamakawa K 1966 The effects of lithium on the neuromuscular junction of the frog. Japanese Journal of Physiology 16: 541

Page P, Morgan M, Loh L 1972 Ketamine anaesthesia in paediatric procedures. Acta Anaesthesiologica Scandinavica 16: 155

Palmer K N V 1978 Muscle cramp and oral salbutamol. British Medical Journal 3: 833

Palmucci L, Bertolotto A, Schiffer D 1978 Acute muscle

necrosis after chronic overdosage of phenformin and fenfluramine. Muscle and Nerve 1: 245

Pamphlett R S, Mackenzie R A 1982 Severe peripheral neuropathy due to lithium intoxication. Journal of Neurology, Neurosurgery and Psychiatry 45: 656

Paul H S, Abidi S A 1979 Paradoxical effects of clofibrate on liver and muscle metabolism in rats. Journal of Clinical Investigation 64: 405

Paul M F, Paul H E, Kopko F, Bryuson M J, Harrington C 1954 Inhibition by furacin of citrate formation in testis preparations. Journal of Biological Chemistry 206: 491

Paulson O B, Melgaard B, Hansen H S et al 1984 Misonidazole neuropathy. Acta Neurologica Scandinavica (Suppl) 100: 133

Pellissier J F, Pouget J, Cros D, De Victor B, Serratrice G, Toga M 1984 Peripheral neuropathy induced by amiodarone chlorhydrate. Journal of the Neurological Sciences 63: 251

Penn A S, Rowland L P, Fraser D W 1972 Drugs, coma and myoglobinuria. Archives of Neurology 26: 336

Percy A K, Saef E C 1976 An unusual complication of retrograde pyelography: neuromuscular blockade. Pediatrics 39: 603

Perkins R L 1964 Apnea with intramuscular colistin therapy. Journal of the American Medical Association 190: 421

Perkoff G T, Hardy P, Velez-Garcia E 1966 Reversible acute muscular syndrome in chronic alcoholism. New England Journal of Medicine 274: 1277

Perry H M 1973 Late toxicity to hydralazine resembling systemic lupus erythematosus or rheumatoid arthritis. American Journal of Medicine 54: 58

Peter J B, Fiehn W 1973 Diazacholesterol myotonia: Accumulation of desmosterol and increased adenosine triphosphatase activity of sarcolemma. Science 179: 910

Peterson H C 1966 Association of trimethadione therapy and myasthenia gravis. New England Journal of Medicine 274: 506

Pierce L R, Wysowski D K, Gross T P 1990 Myopathy and rhabdomyolysis associated with lovastatin-gemfibrozil combination therapy. Journal of the American Medical Association 264: 71

Pierides A M, Alvarez-Ude F, Kerr D N S, Skillen A W 1975 Clofibrate-induced muscle damage in patients with renal failure. Lancet ii: 1279

Pinals R S 1983 Diffuse fasciculations induced by D-penicillamine. Journal of Rheumatology 10: 809–810

Pinkerton H A, Munro J R 1964 Respiratory insufficiency associated with the use of streptomycin. Scottish Medical Journal 9: 256

Pittinger C B, Eryasa Y, Adamson R 1970 Antibiotic-induced paralysis. Anesthesia and Analgesia Current Researches 49: 487

Pokroy N, Ress S, Gregory M C 1977 Clofibrate-induced complications in renal disease. South African Medical Journal 52: 806

Policover S J, Duncan C J 1979 The action of verapamil on the rate of spontaneous release of transmitter at the frog neuromuscular junction. European Journal of Pharmacology 54: 119

Pollet S, Hauw J J, Escourolle R, Baumann N 1977 Peripheral nerve lipid abnormalities in patients on perhexiline maleate. Lancet i: 1258

Poole G W, Schneeweiss J 1961 Peripheral neuropathy due to ethionamide. American Review of Respiratory Diseases 84: 890

Prescott L F 1975 Anti-inflammatory analgesics and drugs

used in rheumatoid arthritis and gout. In: Dukes M N G (ed) Meyler's side effects of drugs, vol 8. Excerpta Medica, Amsterdam, p 228

Pridgeon J E 1956 Respiratory arrest thought to be due to intra-peritoneal neomycin. Surgery 40: 571

Proctor W R, Weakly J N 1976 A comparison of the presynaptic and post-synaptic actions of pentobarbitone and phenobarbitone in the neuromuscular junction of the frog. Journal of Physiology 258: 257

Ramsay I D 1968 Endocrine ophthalmopathy. British Medical Journal 4: 706

Rannels S R, Rannels D E, Pegg A E, Jefferson L S 1978 Glucocorticoid effects on peptide-chain initiation in skeletal muscle and heart. American Journal of Physiology 235: E134

Rapoport A M, Guss S B 1972 Dapsone-induced peripheral neuropathy. Archives of Neurology 27: 184

Rasmussen H 1970 Cell communication, calcium ion and cyclic adenosine monophosphate. Science 170: 404

Ream C R 1963 Respiratory and cardiac arrest after intravenous administration of kanamycin with reversal of toxic effects by neostigmine. Annals of Internal Medicine 59: 384

Regan A G, Aldrete J A 1967 Prolonged apnea after administration of promazine hydrochloride following succinylcholine infusion. Anesthesia and Analgesia Current Researches 46: 315

Regli F, Guggenheim P 1965 Myasthenisches syndrom als seltene komplikation unter hydantoinbehandlung. Nervenartz 36: 315

Reinhart W H, Stricker H 1988 Rhabdomyolysis after intravenous cocaine. American Journal of Medicine 85: 579

Richman D D, Fischl M A, Grieco M H et al 1987 The toxicity of azidothymidine (AZT) in the treatment of patients with AIDS and AIDS-related complex: a double-blind, placebo-controlled trial. New England Journal of Medicine 317: 192

Richter R W, Challenor Y B, Pearson J, Kagen L J, Hamilton L L, Ramsey W H 1971 Acute myoglobinuria associated with heroin addiction. Journal of the American Medical Association 216: 1172

Ricker K, Haass A, Glotzner F 1978 Fenoterol precipitating myotonia in a minimally affected case of recessive myotonia congenita. Journal of Neurology 219: 279

Riggs J E, Schochet Jr S S, Gutman L, Crosby T W, DiBartolomeo A G 1986 Chronic human neuropathy and myopathy. Archives of Neurology 43: 521

Rimon D, Ludatsher R, Cohen L 1984 Clofibrate-induced muscular syndrome. Israel Journal of Medical Sciences 20: 1082

Robberecht W, Bednarik J, Bourgeois P, van Hess J, Carton H 1989 Myasthenic syndrome caused by direct effect of chloroquine on neuromuscular junction. Archives of Neurology 46: 464

Roberson J R, Dimon J H 1983 Myofibrosis and joint contractures caused by injections of pentazocine. Journal of Bone and Joint Surgery 65: 1007

Robinson B F 1975 Drugs acting on the cardiovascular system. In: Dukes M N G (ed) Meyler's side effects of drugs, vol 8. Excerpta Medica, Amsterdam, p 447

Robinson B F 1978 Anti-anginal and beta adreno-receptor blocking drugs. In: Dukes M N G (ed) Meyler's side effects of drugs, vol 2. Excerpta Medica, Amsterdam, p 173

Robinson R G 1959 Leucotrichia totalis from chloroquine. Medical Journal of Australia 2: 460

Roelofs R I, Hrushesky W, Rogin J, Rosenberg L 1984
Peripheral sensory neuropathy and cisplatin chemotherapy.
Neurology 34: 934

Roldan E C, Nigrin G 1972 Peripheral neuritis after
methimazole therapy. New York State Journal of Medicine
72: 2898

Roth R F, Itabashi H, Louie J, Sanderson T, Narahara K A
1990 Amiodarone toxicity: myopathy and neuropathy.
American Heart Journal 119: 1223

Rothstein J M, Delitto A, Sinacore D R, Rose S J 1983
Muscle function in rheumatic disease patients treated with
corticosteroids. Muscle and Nerve 6: 128

Rouleau G, Karpati G, Carpenter S 1987 Glucocorticoid
excess induces preferential depletion of myosin in
denervated skeletal muscle fibres. Muscle and Nerve
10: 428

Rowland L P 1980 Malignant hyperpyrexia — A reply.
Muscle and Nerve 3: 443

Rozencweig M, McLaren C, Beltangady M et al 1990
Overview of phase 1 trails of 2′-3′-dideoxyinosine (ddI)
conducted on adult patients. Review of Infectious Disease
12 (suppl 5): S570

Rubbo J T, Gergis S D, Sokoll M D 1977 Comparative
neuromuscular effects of lincomycin and clindamycin.
Current Researches in Anesthesia and Analgesia 56: 329

Rubenstein C J 1964 Peripheral neuropathy caused by
nitrofurantoin. Journal of the American Medical
Association 187: 647

Rubin R B, Neugarten J 1989 Cocaine-induced
rhabdomyolysis masquerading as myocardial ischemia.
American Journal of Medicine 86: 551

Rumpf K W, Alberts R, Scheler F 1976 Clofibrate-induced
myopathy syndrome. Lancet 1: 249

Russell A S, Lindstrom J M 1978 Penicillamine-induced
myasthenia gravis associated with antibodies to
acetylcholine receptor. Neurology (Minneapolis) 28: 847

Russell J A, Powles R L 1974 Neuropathy due to cytosine
arabinosine. British Medical Journal 4: 652

Said G 1978 Perhexiline neuropathy: A clinicopathological
study. Annals of Neurology 3: 259

Sakai Y, Kobayashi K, Iwata N 1978 Effects of an anabolic
steroid and vitamin B complex upon myopathy induced
by corticosteroids. European Journal of Pharmacology
52: 353

Salako L A 1970 Inhibition of neuromuscular transmission in
the intact rat by emetine. Journal of Pharmaceutics and
Pharmacology 22: 69

Samuelson R J, Giesecke A H, Kallus F T, Stanley V F 1975
Lincomycin-curare interaction. Current Researches in
Anesthesia and Analgesia 54: 103

Sandler R M, Gonsalkorale M 1977 Chronic lymphatic
leukemia, chlorambucil and sensorimotor peripheral
neuropathy. British Medical Journal 2: 1265

Saquenton A C, Lorinz A L, Vick N A, Hamer R D 1969
Dapsone and peripheral motor neuropathy. Archives of
Dermatology 100: 214

Satoyoshi E, Wakata N 1978 Chloramphenicol neuropathy
and vitamin B_{12} deficiency. 4th International Congress on
Neuromuscular Diseases, Montreal, Canada, Abstract 89

Saunders F P, Hoefnagel D, Staples O S 1965 Progressive
fibrosis of the quadriceps muscle. Journal of Bone and Joint
Surgery 47A: 380

Schauburg H, Kaplan J, Windebank A et al 1983 Sensory
neuropathy from pyridoxine abuse. New England Journal of
Medicine 309: 445

Schmidt J L, Vick N A, Sadove M S 1963 The effect of
quinidine on the action of muscle relaxants. Journal of the
American Medical Association 183: 669

Schochet S S, Usar M C, Lampert P W 1968 Neuronal
changes induced by intrathecal vincristine sulfate. Journal
of Neuropathology and Experimental Neurology 27: 645

Scholes D M 1960 Pelvic perfusion with nitrogen mustard for
cancer: a neurological complication. American Journal of
Obstetrics and Gynecology 80: 481

Schraeder P L, Peters H A, Dahl D S 1972 Polymyositis and
penicillamine. Archives of Neurology 27: 456

Sebille A 1978 Prevalence of latent perhexiline neuropathy.
British Medical Journal 1: 1321

Seitz D, Hopf H C, Janzen R C W, Meyer W 1976 Penicillamin
induzierte Myasthenie bei chronischer Polyarthritis. Deutsche
Medizinische Wochenschrift 101: 1153

Selby G 1972 Subacute myelo-optic neuropathy in Australia.
Lancet 1: 123

Seow S S W 1984 Abuse of APF linctus codeine and cardiac
glycoside toxicity. Medical Journal of Australia 140: 54

Shaivits S A 1979 Timolol and myasthenia gravis. Journal of
the American Medical Association 242: 1611

Shergy W J, Caldwell D S 1988 Polymyositis after
propylthiouracil treatment for hyperthyroidism. Annals of
Rheumatic Diseases 47: 340

Shoji S, Takagi A, Sugita H, Toyokura Y 1974 Muscle
glycogen metabolism in steroid-induced myopathy of
rabbits. Experimental Neurology 45: 1

Shoji S, Pennington R J T 1977a Binding of dexamethasone
and cortisol to cytosol receptors in rat extensor digitorum
longus and soleus muscles. Experimental Neurology
57: 342

Shoji S, Pennington R J T 1977b The effect of cortisone on
protein breakdown and synthesis in rat skeletal muscle.
Molecular and Cellular Endocrinology 6: 159

Sholl J S, Hughey M J, Hirschmann R A 1985 Myotonic
muscular dystrophy associated with ritodrine tocolysis.
American Journal of Obstetrics and Gynecology 151: 83

Siegal T, Haim N 1990 Cisplatin-induced peripheral
neuropathy: Frequent off-therapy deterioration,
demyelinating syndromes and muscle cramps. Cancer
66: 1117

Sinclair D, Phillips C 1982 Transient myopathy apparently
due to tetracycline. New England Journal of Medicine
307: 821

Sitwell L D, Weinshenker B G, Monpetit V, Reid D 1991
Complete ophthalmoplegia as a complication of acute
corticosteroid- and pancuronium-associated myopathy.
Neurology 41: 921

Skau K A, Gerald M C 1978 Curare-like effects of the
amphetamine isomers on neuromuscular transmission.
Neuropharmacology 17: 271

Smith P F, Eydelloth R S, Grossman S J et al 1991 HMG-
CoA reductase inhibitor-induced myopathy in the rat:
cyclosporin A interaction and mechanism studies. Journal
of Pharmacology and Experimental Therapeutics 257: 1225

Smith B E, Dyck P J 1990 Peripheral neuropathy in the
eosinophilia-myalgia syndrome associated with
L-tryptophan ingestion. Neurology 40: 1035

Snavely S R, Hodges G R 1984 The neurotoxocity of
antibacterial agents. Annals of Internal Medicine 101: 92

Sobue I, Ando K, Iida M, Takayanagi T, Yamamura Y,
Matsuoka Y 1971 Myeloneuropathy with abdominal
disorders in Japan. Neurology (Minneapolis) 21: 168

Sokoll M D, Gergis S D, Post E L, Cronnelly R, Long J P

1974 Effects of droperidol on neuromuscular transmission and muscle membrane. European Journal of Pharmacology 28: 209

Sokoll M D, Gergis S D 1981 Antibiotics and neuromuscular function. Anesthesiology 55: 148

Somers J E, Winer N 1966 Reversible myopathy and myotonia following administration of a hypocholesterolaemic agent. Neurology (Minneapolis) 16: 761

Stafford C R, Bogdanoff B M, Green L, Spector H B 1975 Mononeuropathy multiplex as a complication of amphetamine angiitis. Neurology (Minneapolis) 25: 570

Stalberg E, Schiller H H, Schwartz M S 1975 Safety factor in single human motor end-plates studied in vivo with single fibre electromyography. Journal of Neurology, Neurosurgery and Psychiatry 38: 799

Steen V D, Blair S, Medsger Jr T A 1986 The toxicity of D-penicillamine in systemic sclerosis. Annals of Internal Medicine 104: 699

Steiner I, Siegal T 1989 Muscle cramps in cancer patients. Cancer 63: 574

Steiner J C, Winkelman A C, De Jesus P V 1973 Pentazocine-induced myopathy. Archives of Neurology 28: 408

Steiness E, Rasmussen F, Svendsen O, Nielsen P 1978 A comparative study of serum creatine phosphokinase (CPK) activity in rabbits, pigs and humans after intramuscular injection of local damaging drugs. Acta Pharmacologica et Toxicologica 42: 357

Stept M E, Subramony S H 1988 Peripheral neuropathy associated with protriptyline. Journal of the American Academy of Child and Adolescent Psychiatry 27: 377

Stinchcombe S J, Davies P 1989 Acute toxic myopathy: a delayed adverse effect of intravenous urography with iopamidol 370. British Journal of Radiology 62: 949

Streib E W 1977 Adverse effects of magnesium salt cathartics in a patient with the myasthenic syndrome (Lambert–Eaton syndrome). Annals of Neurology 2: 175

Swash M, Ingram D A 1992 Adverse effect of verapamil in myasthenia gravis. Muscle and Nerve 15: 396

Swenson R D, Golper T A, Bennett W M 1982 Acute renal failure and rhabdomyolysis after ingestion of phenylpropanolamine-containing diet pills. Journal of American Medical Association 248: 1216

Takahashi K, Ogita T, Okudaira H, Yoshinoya S, Yoshizawa H, Miyamoto T 1986 D-penicillamine-induced polymyositis in patients with rheumatoid arthritis. Arthritis and Rheumatism 29: 560

Tam C W, Olin B R, Ruiz A E 1980 Loxapin-associated rhabdomyolysis and acute renal failure. Archives of Internal Medicine 140: 975

Tamaki M 1978 The effect of streptomycin on the neuromuscular junction of the frog. 4th International Congress on Neuromuscular Diseases, Montreal, Canada, Abstract 48

Tegner R, Tomé F M S, Godeau P, Lhermitte F, Fardeau M 1988 Morphological study of peripheral nerve changes induced by chloroquine treatment. Acta Neuropathologica (Berlin) 75: 253

Teicher A, Rosenthal T, Kinnin E, Sarova I 1981 Labetalol-induced toxic myopathy. British Medical Journal 282: 1824

Teravainen H, Larsen A, Hillbom M 1977 Clofibrate-induced myopathy in the rat. Acta Neuropathologica (Berlin) 39: 135

Thompson S W, Davis L E, Korenfeld M, Hilgers R D, Standefer J C 1984 Cisplatin neuropathy. Cancer 54: 1269

Toole J F, Parrish M L 1973 Nitrofurantoin polyneuropathy. Neurology (Minneapolis) 23: 554

Torres C F, Griggs R C, Baum J, Penn A S 1980 Penicillamine-induced myasthenia gravis in progressive systemic sclerosis. Arthritis and Rheumatism 23: 505

Treves, R, Arnaud M, Tabaraud F, Burki F, Vallat J M 1985 Desproges–Gotterron: myopathie au cours d'un traitement a la cimetidine. Rev Rhum Mal Osteo-articulaires 52: 133

Tsubaki T, Honma Y, Hoshi M 1971 Neurological syndrome associated with clioquinol. Lancet 1: 696

Tugwell P, James S L 1972 Peripheral neuropathy with ethambutol. Postgraduate Medical Journal 48: 667

Uchigata M, Tanabe H, Hasue I, Kurihara M 1981 Peripheral neuropathy due to lithium intoxication. Annals of Neurology 9: 414

Urbano-Maquez A, Estruch R, Navarro-Lopez F, Grau J M, Mont L, Rubin E 1989 The effects of alcoholism on skeletal and cardiac muscle. New England Journal of Medicine 320: 409

Ursing B, Kamme C 1975 Metronidazole for Crohn's disease. Lancet 1: 775

Usubiaga J E, Wikinski J A, Morales R L, Usubiaga L E J 1967 Interaction of intravenously administered procaine, lidocaine and succinylcholine in anesthetized subjects. Current Researches in Anesthesia and Analgesia 46: 39

Utz J P, Louria D B, Feder N, Emmons C W, McCullough N B 1957 A report of clinical studies on the use of amphotericin in patients with systemic fungal diseases. Antibiotics Annals 65

Valeriano J, Tucker P, Kattah J 1983 An unusual cause of hypokalemic muscle weakness. Neurology (Cleveland) 33: 1242

Vanhooren G, Dehaene I, Van Zandycke M et al 1990 Polyneuropathy in lithium intoxication. Muscle and Nerve 13: 204

Van Marle W, Woods K L 1980 Acute hydrocortisone myopathy. British Medical Journal 281: 271

Vartanian G A, Chinyanga H M 1972 The mechanism of acute neuromuscular weakness induced by chloroquine. Canadian Journal of Physiology and Pharmacology 50: 1099

Vincent A, Newsom Davis J, Martin V 1978 Antiacetylcholine receptor antibodies in D-penicillamine-associated myasthenia gravis. Lancet i: 1254

Viswanath D V, Jenkins H J 1978 Neuromuscular block of the polymixin group of antibiotics. Journal of Pharmaceutical Sciences 67: 1275

Vita G, Bartolone S, Santoro M et al 1986 Hypokalemic myopathy induced by fluroprednisolone-containing nasal spray. Acta Neurologica (Napoli) 8: 108

Wade A 1977 Martindale — the extra pharmacopoeia, 27th edn. Pharmaceutical Press, London, p 1295

Walls T J, Pearce S J, Venables G S 1980 Motor neuropathy associated with cimetidine. British Medical Journal 281: 974

Walton J N 1977 Brain's diseases of the nervous system, 8th edn. Oxford University Press, Oxford, p 1032

Ward A, Chaffman M O, Sorkin E M 1986 Dantrolene: a review of its pharmacodynamic and pharmacokinetic properties and therapeutic use in malignant hyperthermia, the neuroleptic malignant syndrome and an update of its use in muscle spasticity. Drugs 32: 130

Warner W A, Sanders E 1971 Neuromuscular blockage associated with gentamycin therapy. Journal of the American Medical Association 215: 1153

Warot P, Goudemand M, Habay D 1965 Troubles

neurologiques provoqués par les alcaloïdes de Vinca rosea (la polynévrite de la pervenche). Revue Neurologique 113: 464

Waterman P M, Smith R B 1977 Tobramycin–curare interaction. Anesthesia and Analgesia 56: 587

Watkins S M, Griffin J P 1978 High incidence of vincristine-induced neuropathy in lymphomas. British Medical Journal 1: 610

Watland D C, Long J P, Pittinger C B, Cullen S C 1957 Neuromuscular effects of ether, cyclopropane, chloroform and fluothane. Anesthesiology 18: 883

Watson A J S, Dalbow M H, Stachura I et al 1983 Immunologic studies in cimetidine-induced nephropathy and polymyositis. New England Journal of Medicine 308: 142

Wattel F, Chopin C, Durocher A, Berzin B 1978 Rhabdomyolyses au cours des intoxications aigues. La Nouvelle Presse Médicale 7: 2253

Watters G, Karpati G, Kaplan B 1977 Post-anesthetic augmentation of muscle damage as a presenting sign in three patients with Duchenne muscular dystrophy. Canadian Journal of Neurological Sciences 4: 228

Way W L, Katzung B G, Larson C P 1967 Recurarization with quinidine. Journal of the American Medical Association 200: 163

Weinstein L, Madoff M A, Samet C M 1974 The sulfonamides. New England Journal of Medicine 291: 793

Weisman S L 1949 Masked myasthenia gravis. Journal of the American Medical Association 141: 917

Weiss H D, Walker M D, Wiernik P H 1974 Neurotoxicity of commonly used antineoplastic agents. New England Journal of Medicine 291: 127

Werman R, Wislicki L 1971 Propranolol, a curariform and cholinomimetic agent at the frog neuromuscular junction. Comparative General Pharmacology 2: 69

Westbury G 1962 Treatment of advanced cancer by extracorporeal perfusion and continuous intra-arterial infusion. Proceedings of the Royal Society of Medicine 55: 643

Whisnant J P, Espinosa R E, Kierland R R, Lambert E H 1963 Chloroquine neuromyopathy. Proceedings of the Mayo Clinic 38: 501

Williams R S 1959 Triamcinolone myopathy. Lancet i: 698

Williams A J, Baghat M S, Stableforth D E, Layton R M, Shenoi P M, Skinner C 1983 Dysphonia caused by inhaled steroids: recognition of a characteristic laryngeal abnormality. Thorax 38: 813

Willis J K, Tilton A H, Harkin J C, Boineau F G 1990 Reversible myopathy due to labetalol. Pediatric Neurology 6: 275

Wilson S L, Miller R N, Wright C, Haas D 1976 Prolonged neuromuscular blockade associated with trimetaphan: A case report. Current Researches in Anesthesia and Analgesia 55: 353

Winer N, Klachko D M, Baer R D, Langley P L, Burns T W 1966 Myotonic response induced by inhibitors of cholesterol biosynthesis. Science 153: 312

Wirguin I, Brenner T, Shinar E, Argov Z 1990 Citrate-induced impairment of neuromuscular transmission in

human and experimental autoimmune myasthenia gravis. Annals of Neurology 27: 328

Wirguin I, Brenner T, Sicsic C, Argov Z 1992 Effect of calcium channel antagonists (CCA) on neuromuscular transmission (NMT) in experimental autoimmune myasthenia gravis (EAMG). Neurology 42(suppl 3): 232

Wolf S, Goldberg L S, Verity A 1976 Neuromyopathy and periarteriolitis in a patient receiving levodopa. Archives of Internal Medicine 136: 1055

Woodward D K 1989 Peripheral neuropathy and Mesalazine. British Medical Journal 299: 1224

Wrenn K D, Oschner I 1989 Rhabdomyolysis induced by a caffeine overdose. Annals of Emergency Medicine 18: 94

Wright J M, Collier B 1976a The site of the neuromuscular block produced by polymyxin B and rolitetracycline. Canadian Journal of Physiology and Pharmacology 54: 926

Wright J M, Collier B 1976b Characterization of the neuromuscular block produced by clindamycin and lincomycin. Canadian Journal of Physiology and Pharmacology 54: 937

Wullen F, Kast G, Bruck A 1967 Uber nebenwirkungen bei tetracyclin-verabreichung an Myastheniker. Deutsche Medizinische Wochenschrift 92: 667

Wyatt E H, Stevens C 1972 Dapsone induced peripheral neuropathy. British Journal of Dermatology 86: 521

Yaari Y, Pincus J H, Argov Z 1977 Depression of synaptic transmission by diphenylhydantoin. Annals of Neurology 1: 334

Yaari Y, Pincus J H, Argov Z 1979 Phenytoin and transmitter release at the neuromuscular junction of the frog. Brain Research 160: 479

Yarchoan R, Mitsuya H, Pluda J M et al 1990 The National Cancer Institute phase 1 study of 2′, 3′-dideoxyinosine administration in adults with AIDS or AIDS-related complex: analysis of activity and toxicity profiles. Review of Infectious Diseases 12 (suppl 5): S522

Yates D A H 1970 Steroid myopathy. In: Walton J N, Canal N, Scarlato G (eds) Muscle diseases. Excerpta Medica, Amsterdam, p 482

Yiannikas C, Pollard J D, McLeod J G 1981 Nitrofurantoin neuropathy. Australian and New Zealand Journal of Medicine 11: 400

Young W A, Tudhope G R 1926 The pathology of prolonged emetine administration. Transactions of the Royal Society of Tropical Medicine and Hygiene 30: 93

Yousef G E, Bell E H J, Mann G F et al 1988 Chronic enterovirus infection in patients with postviral fatigue syndrome. Lancet i: 146

Zalman F, Perloff J K, Durant N N, Campion D S 1983 Acute respiratory failure following intravenous verapamil in Duchenne's muscular dystrophy. American Heart Journal 105: 510

Zampollo A, Sozzi G, Basso F 1988 Amitriptyline-related peripheral neuropathy. Case Report. Italian Journal of Neurological Sciences. 9: 89

Zaunder H L, Barton N, Benetts E J, Lore J 1966 Colistimethate as a cause of post-operative apnoea. Canadian Anesthetic Society Journal 13: 607

Electrodiagnosis

29. The clinical physiology of neuromuscular disease

Peter R. W. Fawcett   David D. Barwick

INTRODUCTION

An important property of muscle fibres is their ability to generate small voltages or action potentials, forming an essential link in the chain of events leading to contraction of the muscle fibre. Clinical electromyography (EMG) which is concerned with the recording and analysis of these electrical events in human muscle, effectively dates back to the introduction by Adrian & Bronk (1929) of the coaxial or concentric needle electrode. Subsequent development of the EMG as a clinical tool was carried out principally by workers in Scandinavia who defined the characteristics of the electrical signals derived from normal and diseased muscle. Studies in the laboratories of Kugelberg and of Buchthal did much to establish the foundation of concentric needle electromyography (CNEMG) which remains the most widely used technique. Recently there have been considerable developments in clinical neurophysiology, due largely to technological advances in electronics and particularly the availability of low-cost microcomputers. These have facilitated data acquisition, analysis and presentation, leading to improved quantitation, particularly in CNEMG. The introduction of several new recording techniques (single fibre EMG (SFEMG), scanning EMG and Macro EMG) has revealed new information about the organisation and function of the lower motor neurone in health and disease (Stålberg 1991).

The anatomy and physiology of the motor unit are described in Chapter 1. Only a brief recapitulation is given here. The motor unit (Sherrington 1926) consists of a lower motor neurone and all the individual muscle fibres innervated by its branches.

It forms the smallest element of a muscle capable of separate volitional activation when all of the constituent muscle fibres are excited almost synchronously. The number of muscle fibres innervated by a single neurone (the innervation ratio) has been estimated to vary from about six in the extraocular muscles to between 400 and 17 000 in normal limb muscles (Feinstein et al 1955, Christensen 1959).

Motor unit territory is the cross-sectional area over which the muscle fibres of a single motor unit are dispersed. In a normal muscle the diameter of the motor unit territory is less than 10 mm (Buchthal et al 1954a, Stålberg et al 1976, Stålberg & Antoni 1980). Individual muscle fibres of the unit are widely distributed throughout the territory and only rarely are two or three fibres found in propinquity (Edström & Kugelberg 1968). Each motor unit territory is extensively overlapped by those of other motor units. The diameter of individual muscle fibres shows some variation within a muscle; mean diameters are largest in the lower limbs (50–60 μm) and only 20–30 μm in the facial muscles (Polgar et al 1973). Normally each muscle fibre has a single neuromuscular junction, located in the central portion of the fibre. In many muscles the end-plates are distributed in a distinct area known as the end-plate zone. The muscle fibres of an individual motor unit are responsible for the motor unit action potential (MUP), the dimensions of which depend on a number of variables. The first of these is the form of the action potentials arising in individual muscle fibres. Parallel studies of intracellular and extracellular recordings of the single fibre action potential have been carried out in animals (Håkansson 1957, Katz & Miledi 1965). The extracellular recording resembles the second derivative of the intracellular action potential (Clark & Plonsey 1966, 1968). The extracellular action potential amplitude increases in proportion to 1.7 times the fibre diameter (Håkansson 1957). Muscle is a physical space permeable to electric currents; the spread of current in such a medium is termed volume conduction. In a homogeneous volume conductor (e.g. Ringer's solution) the amplitude of the extracellularly recorded action potential falls off linearly with the logarithm of the distance of the electrode from the fibre. When electrode to fibre distances exceed 0.15 mm the amplitude decreases with increasing distance by the power of -1.3. While the intracellular action potential is monophasic, the extracellular single fibre action potential is biphasic (Håkansson 1957). Volume conduction in muscle is more complex, as muscle is neither isotropic nor homogeneous. Various elements in the muscle tissue have different electrical resistivity. Anisotropy is also present, with the radial resistivity being some two to 10 times that parallel to the longitudinal axis of the muscle fibre in mammalian muscle (Geddes & Baker 1967).

Volume conduction of the action potentials of single fibres in human muscle has been studied by Gath & Stålberg (1977, 1978). The amplitude attenuation with distance was greater than predicted by mathematical models and although the discrepancy between forecast and actual results was greater for slow components, it was the fast components which showed the greatest decline. In the biceps brachii the mean distance over which the action potential declined to 90% of its original amplitude was 191 μm, s.e. (mean) 20 μm, when recorded with a 25 μm diameter electrode (Gath & Stålberg 1978).

Single fibre action potentials summate to form the MUP and this summation depends upon the degree of synchronisation of muscle fibre action potentials as recorded at the electrode employed. According to Buchthal et al (1957), the anatomical dispersion of the end-plate zone in the muscle plays the major role in determining the total duration of the MUP. Muscle fibre propagation velocity, terminal axonal velocity and neuromuscular transmission times are relatively unimportant in normal muscle. The form of the electrical activity recorded when a motor unit is excited, depends to a considerable extent on the type of electrode which is used to study the potential changes. These various electrodes are mentioned below.

Technical considerations

The technical specifications of amplifiers suitable for CNEMG recording have been detailed in a report by the Special Committee on EMG Instrumentation (Guld et al 1970). A recent review of the topic and an outline of the safety precautions required in EMG systems can be found in Kimura's textbook (see Seaba & Walker 1989).

COMPARISON OF DIFFERENT RECORDING TECHNIQUES

Concentric needle electromyography (CNEMG)

The concentric needle is the most widely used electrode, consisting of a stainless steel cannula resembling a hypodermic needle, through the centre of the shaft of which an insulated platinum (or nichrome silver) core is inserted (Fig 29.1a). The usual central core diameter is 0.1 mm, while the outer diameter of the shaft is about 0.5 mm. Recordings are made between the core tip and the cannula. A separate earth (ground) electrode is required during the recording process. The oblique, oval recording surface has an exposed tip area of the order of 150 μm × 580 μm (0.007 mm²). The electrode is relatively selective and has an effective pick-up area about 1 mm in diameter, within which only a portion of the activity of the whole motor unit is registered. The leading-off surface is large in relation to the muscle fibres, resulting in pronounced shunting of the electrical field, producing an average value of the isopotential lines crossing the electrode surface (Stålberg & Trontelj 1979). The recording electrode itself has marked directional properties, registering activity mainly from fibres situated in front of the bevelled surface (Nakao et al 1965). Simulation studies (Nandedkar et al 1984) indicate that the amplitude of the MUP is determined by the number and size of muscle fibres within 0.5 mm of the recording surface, while the area and duration mainly depend upon the number of fibres within 2 mm and 2.5 mm respectively of the electrode.

Dorfman et al (1985) have examined the electrical characteristics of a variety of commercial CNEMG electrodes, and demonstrated the value of electrolytic treatment. Untreated electrodes show considerable variation both in impedance and broadband-noise characteristics even between electrodes from the same manufacturer. Electrolytic treatment reduces impedance by a factor of up to four and reduces the variability. Broadband-noise is also reduced, often down to the level of

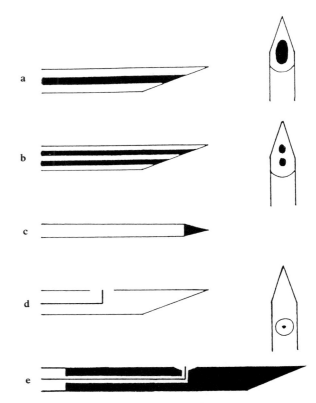

Fig. 29.1 Different types of intramuscular needle electrodes. **a** Concentric needle electrode (CNE); active recording surface 150 × 580 μm in bevel-cannula reference. **b** Bipolar needle electrode; recordings derived between the two surfaces in the bevel. **c** Monopolar electrode; recordings derived between the electrode tip and a remote reference electrode. **d** Single fibre electrode; active recording surface 25 μm in diameter placed in side-port behind tip of electrode–cannula reference. **e** Macro electrode; recordings derived between exposed terminal 15 mm portion of cannula and remote subcutaneous electrode. Separate SFEMG electrode 7.5 mm behind tip (modified from Stålberg & Trontelj 1979).

the instrumentation. Distortion is usually negligible but line interference from nearby power cables is suppressed only when the recording cables are fully shielded and the electromyographer earthed. The effect of electrolytic treatment is short-lived but repeatable.

The CNEMG electrode is inserted into a relaxed muscle and the presence or absence of insertional and spontaneous activity is determined. During gentle voluntary contraction, the MUPs of early recruiting motor units from a number of separate sites in the muscle can be examined and their firing rates and waveform recorded. A delay-line which allows display of the triggering MUP in the centre of the screen facilitates examination of MUP parameters. Various oscilloscope sweep-speeds are employed so that late components occurring many ms after the main MUP are detected. Fast sweep-speeds and a 500 Hz high-pass filter enable MUP stability to be assessed (Payan 1978). Increasing force of contraction results in the appearance of MUPs from more motor units firing asynchronously and rapidly building up to a pattern in which super-imposed activity completely obscures the oscilloscope base-line producing an 'interference pattern', the amplitude and density of which is noted.

Bipolar needle electrodes consist of two insulated wires with exposed tips inserted into a steel cannula which can act as the earth electrode (Fig. 29.1b). Potential changes are registered between the two wire tips and provide a relatively selective electrode. Activity from more distant sources arriving at the two recording surfaces simultaneously is not registered because of the common-mode rejection of the differential amplifier. As a consequence the initial and terminal elements of the MUP are cancelled and MUP duration is only 75% of the values obtained in CNEMG (Guld 1951, Buchthal et al 1954b). These electrodes are used for special purposes, where some selectivity of recording or stimulation is required.

The monopolar needle electrode is a solid steel needle insulated with varnish and bared at the tip (Fig. 29.1c). Recordings are made from the tip referred to a distant surface electrode or a subcutaneous needle electrode. They are more selective than the CNEMG electrodes and MUP duration and amplitude as measured with the monopolar electrodes tend to be somewhat greater and the shape more frequently complex than those determined in CNEMG (Guld 1951, Nandedkar & Sanders 1991). These electrodes are used in EMG in similar situations to the CNEMG electrode and are less expensive but also less easy to standardise.

Scanning electromyography

This recently introduced technique combines the technologies of CNEMG and SFEMG. Briefly, the SFEMG is used to lock on to a single muscle fibre action potential in a gently contracting muscle. At the same time a CNEMG electrode (the scanning electrode) is positioned between 10 and 20 mm from the SFEMG electrode. The position of the former is then adjusted so that it records a MUP synchronous with the single fibre action potential (i.e. from the unit to which the single fibre belongs). By appropriate delay-line settings the MUP is displayed in the centre of a 15 ms sweep of the oscilloscope. The scanning electrode is then advanced a further 10 mm into the muscle and scanning can begin. Gentle muscular contraction is required to give a constant, low firing rate. At the same time the electrode is pulled through the motor unit using a specially designed step-motor (linear actuator) to produce small, reproducible increments of movement of 50 μm. Between 150 and 400 sequential recordings of the MUP are obtained by the procedure and a computer or microprocessor is used to create a graphical display of the data on an XY plotter (utilising a special purpose program) as a contour map of the motor unit (Fig. 29.2a). The recording may consist of up to four separately identifiable action potentials which may demonstrate different temporal relationships. These have been called motor unit fractions and it is likely that each fraction is composed of a group of muscle fibres supplied by a large terminal branch of the motor axon (Stålberg & Fawcett 1984, Stålberg & Dioszeghy 1991).

Single fibre electromyography (SFEMG)

The electrode is a steel hypodermic needle with a 0.5 mm cannula diameter in which a 25 μm diameter leading-off surface of between 1 and 15 platinum wire recording electrodes are mounted in a side port opposite the bevel of the cannula (Fig. 29.1d) (Stålberg & Trontelj 1979). The small recording surface makes this a highly selective electrode. The SFEMG needle is inserted into the muscle at right angles to the long axis of the muscle fibres and its position is adjusted so as to record a single muscle fibre action potential (Fig. 29.3). Recordings use a fast oscilloscope

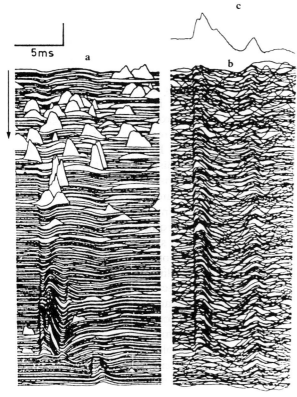

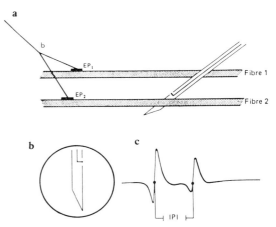

Fig. 29.2 **a** Scanning EMG recording from normal tibialis anterior muscle (deepest position at top of the plot). **b** Simultaneous recording between cannula and remote reference electrode. **c** Averaged recording from b with the needle at its deepest position; this corresponds to the Macro EMG. The plot shows that the cannula is also recording activity from the motor unit. This is seen as a 'trough' in the scan (a) which 'announces' the fibres before the action potentials are recorded at the tip of the electrode. Amplitude calibration: for a = 200 μV; for b = 100 μV; for c = 50 μV (from Stålberg & Antoni 1980).

Fig. 29.3 Single fibre EMG recording technique. **a** The SFEMG needle (insert **b**) recording from two muscle fibres. **c** The two fibre action potentials. The interpotential interval (IPI) is the time taken for the two nerve impulses from the branching point in the axon (b), transmission across the two motor end-plates (EP 1 & 2) and conduction of the two muscle fibre action potentials up to the electrode.

Macro electromyography

The recording electrode is relatively non-selective and consists of a modified SFEMG electrode in which the single fibre recording surface is exposed in a side port some 7.5 mm from the tip (Stålberg 1980a, Stålberg & Fawcett 1982). The steel cannula of 0.55 mm diameter is insulated to within 15 mm of the tip. The single fibre aperture is thus at the mid-point of the cannula recording surface (Fig. 29.1e). The electrode is placed in a muscle so that a single fibre from a motor unit can be recorded. If the fibre lies near the centre of the unit the Macro electrodes should span the whole motor unit territory in healthy as well as in diseased muscle. Macro MUPs are obtained by electronically averaging those potentials recorded by the Macro electrode time-locked to the single fibre trigger. It is possible to record from a variety of different motor units selecting different single fibres to act as triggers (Fig. 29.4). The Macro MUP represents the total activity of the individual motor unit. Considerable attenuation of high-frequency components arising from muscle fibres close to the cannula, as compared to more distant fibres, occurs so that recorded amplitudes are smaller than those seen in CNEMG and very much smaller than in SFEMG. Simulation studies

sweep, trigger and delay-line so that the delayed potentials can be centrally displayed on the oscilloscope. Recording selectivity may be further increased by using a 500 Hz high-pass filter which restricts activity from more distant fibres, attenuating their low-frequency components. An upper limit of 16 KHz is normally used. These settings are unsuitable for studies of the form of individual single fibre potentials. They distort the shape of the action potential even from the close fibres: settings for study of the shape of the potential should be from 2 Hz to 16 kHz.

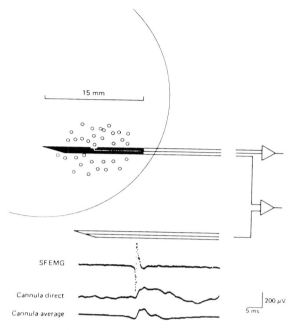

15 mm

SFEMG

Cannula direct

Cannula average

200 μV

5 ms

Fig. 29.4   Macro EMG recording technique. The electrode position is adjusted in order to record the action potential of a single muscle fibre with the small SFEMG recording surface. This triggers the oscilloscope and averager and the cannula signal is delayed and then averaged to extract the Macro motor unit potential (Macro MUP) (after Stålberg 1980a)

(Nandedkar & Stålberg 1983) indicated that the amplitude and area of the Macro MUP are principally determined by the number and mean diameter of the muscle fibres and are less sensitive to fibre distribution within the territory. The waveform corresponds with the findings in scanning EMG (Fig. 29.2b) and the major peaks and troughs seen in the latter technique can usually be identified in an attenuated form in the Macro EMG (Fig. 29.2c) (Stålberg & Fawcett 1982, Stålberg 1983). Macro MUP shape has also been shown by simulation studies (Nandedkar & Stålberg 1983) to be sensitive to end-plate scatter, differences in nerve branch conduction and the distribution of muscle fibre diameters.

Recently a modification of the technique has been reported using a concentric needle recording surface in the bevel of the electrode to trigger on the motor unit (Jabre 1988, 1991). However this technique has been shown to generate Macro MUPs with smaller amplitudes than those obtained

using the SFEMG recording in the side-port as trigger (Nix & Scherer 1992), probably because the majority of the bare cannula is outside the motor unit.

Surface electromyography

In the past, surface EMG has appeared to have little value for diagnostic electromyography and found its major application in long-term monitoring of muscle activity in kinesiology. High-frequency components tend to be lost and individual motor unit potentials are difficult to detect.

Special multiple surface electrodes were used by Hjorth et al (1973) to document the distribution and rate of occurrence of fasciculation potentials in motor neurone disease. Surface electrodes have been used in conjunction with SFEMG and averaging techniques to record single motor units (Milner-Brown & Stein 1975).

A series of special surface electrodes has been used to study the location of the neuromuscular junction and MUP propagation (Nishizono et al 1979, Masuda et al 1983, 1985). Nishizono et al used fine wire electrodes inserted in the middle of the belly of the biceps in healthy volunteers and a series of small, 8 mm diameter surface electrodes linearly disposed at 20 mm intervals on the longitudinal axis of the muscle. Computer averaging techniques were applied to the extraction of the contribution of the single motor unit, recorded by the wire electrode during gentle maintained voluntary contraction, to the surface recording. A conduction velocity of 4.6 m/s (s.e. (mean) 0.5 m/s) was found. Masuda et al (1983) used an elaborate array of surface electrodes consisting of 15 stainless steel wires parallel to each other with a 5 mm interelectrode gap and, in conjunction with computer analysis, studied the sites of neuromuscular junctional activity in the biceps in relation to muscular exertion. A still more elaborate surface electrode system was used by Hilfiker & Meyer (1984) to study normal and myopathic MUP propagation. During isometric contraction of the biceps brachii, using an array of 30 surface electrodes parallel to the long axis and centred on the end-plate zone, a computer program was used to display the action potentials and analyse their propagation pattern.

Motor Unit Count Technique

Surface electrodes are used in the technique of motor unit counting which was originally introduced by McComas et al (1971b) to estimate the number of functioning motor units in a muscle. Initially, extensor digitorum brevis (EDB) was employed (Fig. 29.5), but subsequently the method has been applied to other muscles (Brown 1972, Sica et al 1974). The recording electrodes consist of silver strips, an active or stigmatic electrode placed over the end-plate zone of the muscle under study and a remote reference electrode. Surface stimulating electrodes are placed over the nerve and by gradually increasing the stimulus strength, successive motor units are recruited and these can be identified by discrete increments in

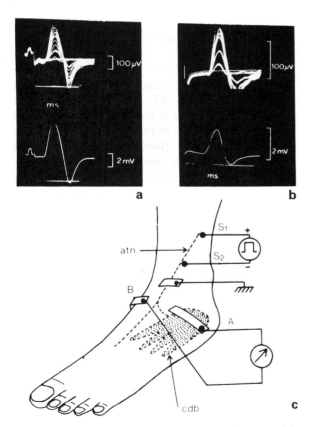

Fig. 29.5 Motor unit counting technique. Action potentials in extensor digitorum brevis evoked by stimulation of the deep peroneal nerve in control subject (**a**) and a 16-year-old boy with Duchenne dystrophy (**b**). The recording arrangements are illustrated in **c** (from McComas et al 1971b).

the evoked muscle action potential. Usually up to 10–15 such increments can be observed. The mean amplitude of these increments is calculated and divided into the amplitude of the muscle action potential evoked by a supramaximal nerve stimulus to give the number of motor units within the muscle.

The method depends upon a number of inherent assumptions: that each stepwise increase in the muscle action potential represents the additional response of a single motor unit; that the amplitudes summate in a simple manner; that the motor unit action potentials used to calculate the mean are representative of the whole population of motor units; and that the activity is derived solely from the muscle under study. A number of these assumptions have been questioned and various modifications of the technique have subsequently been developed. Ballantyne & Hansen (1974a,b,c) used a computerised system to measure not only the change in amplitude of each increment, but also the latency, duration and area of the potentials comprising the summated response. The motor unit potentials were each stored in digital form in a separate memory trace or template. Digital subtraction of succeeding templates from the preceding one yielded successive potentials in isolation, enabling the configuration of each motor unit potential to be determined. The area of each motor unit potential was calculated and this was divided into the area of the whole muscle action potential obtained after supramaximal nerve stimulation to give the number of motor units in the muscle. Other modifications of the method have been reported (Milner-Brown & Brown 1976, Stein & Yang 1990) and the present status of the technique and findings in normal muscles has been reviewed by McComas (1991).

Wire electrodes

Using a hypodermic needle it is possible to insert wire electrodes into a muscle where they may remain for long periods and are used in kinesiology (Basmajian & Stecko 1962). Wire electrodes have also been used for SFEMG studies. Very small recording surfaces can be obtained by using a spark to break through the insulation of a fine wire. Although selectivity is high, there are problems in the standardisation of recording surface size and impedance; in addition the form of the single fibre action potential is liable to distortion and fine adjustments to the electrode position are difficult (Stålberg & Trontelj 1979).

CLINICAL ELECTROMYOGRAPHY

CNEMG

Insertional activity. Injury to muscle fibres caused by movement of the exploring electrode evokes potentials referred to as insertion activity (Weddell et al 1944, Kugelberg & Petersén 1949). Brief bursts of short-duration, high-frequency spikes occur with each movement of the electrode, hardly outlasting the movement (Fig. 29.6a). The spike cluster is mainly positive and is due to the mechanical stimulation or injury of muscle fibres by the needle (Wiechers 1977). Where fibrous replacement of muscle has occurred in chronic atrophic disorders, insertional activity is reduced or absent. Increased insertional activity occurs when muscle fibres are abnormally excitable, as in denervation, myotonia, myositis, etc.

End-plate potentials. Spontaneous activity is recorded when the electrode is placed close to the end-plate zone (Fig. 29.6b). Often this appears as low-voltage irregularities of the base-line of 10–40 μV and is called end-plate noise. With fine adjustment of the electrode position it is possible to record monophasic negative potentials of 50–100 μV in amplitude and 0.5–5 ms duration occurring at high frequency and somewhat irregularly (Rosenfalck & Buchthal 1962). These spontaneous negative discharges are recorded when the CNEMG electrode tip is very close to the end-plate (Weiderholt 1970), and they correspond to miniature end-plate potentials as recorded intracellularly with a microelectrode (Buchthal & Rosenfalck 1966).

Also in the end-plate zone, biphasic spontaneous spike potentials (end-plate spikes) of 100–200 μV amplitude and 3–5 ms duration, firing irregularly at 5–50 Hz, may be seen (Jones et al 1955). Initially thought to originate from small intramuscular nerve bundles, it now appears that the activity is due to the firing of one or several muscle fibres activated by mechanical irritation

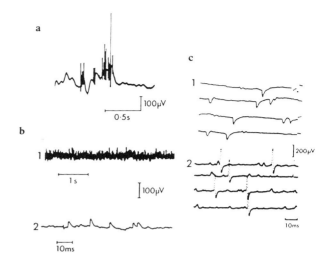

Fig. 29.6 CNEMG recordings. **a** Insertion activity recorded following needle movement. **b** Recordings from the region of the motor end-plate zone: (1) end-plate 'noise' recorded at a slow sweep speed; (2) miniature end-plate potentials recorded at faster sweep speed, showing characteristic initial sharp negative deflection and slow decay. **c** Positive sharp waves (1) and fibrillation potentials (2) recorded outside the end-plate zone.

of their intramuscular nerve terminals by the recording electrodes. These spikes have an initial negative deflection, unlike fibrillation potentials (Buchthal & Rosenfalck 1966). However, small positive potentials may be recorded in the end-plate zone and represent cannula pick-up of end-plate spikes with consequent reversed polarity and amplitude attenuation (Pickett & Schmidley 1980).

Spontaneous activity. *Positive sharp waves.* This activity is evoked by needle movement and consists of positive potentials, varying in voltage (50–400 μV) and duration (10–100 ms). They discharge at 2–50 Hz and have an abrupt positive intial deflection followed by a slow, almost exponential negative decay (Kugelberg & Petersén 1959, Jasper & Ballem 1949). A series of positive waves has a typical 'saw-tooth' appearance (Fig. 29.6c). The potential arises from the spontaneous or more often mechanical excitation of a non-propagated action potential at a damaged region of a single muscle fibre and is led-off from currents spreading from the inside of the fibre to the surrounding conducting tissue. Positive sharp waves are not seen when recording from normal muscle (Buchthal & Rosenfalck 1966), though they appear in the intrinsic foot muscles in apparently healthy subjects (Falk & Alaranta 1983) where they are probably related to the presence of a traumatic neuropathy. Positive waves are closely associated with fibrillation potentials and appear as frequently as fibrillations in the presence of complete denervation. With a partial lesion they occur only a third as often as fibrillation (Bachthal & Rosenfalck 1966). They precede by a day or two the appearance of fibrillation following nerve section (Wiechers 1977). Runs of positive sharp waves provoked by needle insertion have been reported in a number of patients in whom the remainder of the EMG examination and detailed clinical, metabolic and electrolyte assessment were normal (Wiechers & Johnson 1979, Nutter & Collins 1988). The positive sharp waves could be elicited in virtually all the muscles examined. The abnormality was found in other family members and appeared to show an autosomal dominant pattern of inheritance (Wiechers & Johnson 1979).

Fibrillation potentials. Spontaneous fibrillation potentials are bi- or tri-phasic waves of 20–300 µV amplitude, often less than 2 ms and not more than 5 ms in duration (Fig. 29.6c). They discharge either regularly or irregularly at rates varying from 2 to 20 Hz and are derived from the excitation of single muscle fibres (Denny-Brown & Pennybacker 1938, Jasper & Ballem 1949). While electrode insertion may produce profuse fibrillation, mechanical stimulation is not required for their production as they are recorded with subcutaneous electrodes (Rosenfalck & Buchthal 1967). Fibrillation potentials recorded in the end-plate region have an initial negative phase (Buchthal & Rosenfalck 1966). They may be detected in this region in normal individuals and the finding of an isolated fibrillation potential outside of the end-plate zone is not considered abnormal (Buchthal & Rosenfalck 1966). Falk & Alaranta (1983) have shown that fibrillation in the intrinsic foot muscles is seen in many apparently healthy individuals. In older subjects this may be due to an age-related neuropathy and in younger people the fibrillation is confined to the extensor digitorum brevis and may be due to local nerve trauma from footwear.

In denervation, the development of fibrillation potentials is closely associated with the time-course of wallerian degeneration and the fibrillations appear on average 10–21 days after nerve section. Denervated muscle shows an abnormal sensitivity to acetylcholine (ACh) (Denny-Brown 1949) and Denny-Brown & Pennybacker (1938) suggested that circulating ACh might excite the abnormally sensitive fibre. Axelson & Thesleff (1959) have demonstrated the appearance of extrajunctional cholinergic receptors following denervation. Fibrillation potentials continue to occur in the presence of curare and other neuromuscular blocking agents (Belmar & Eyzaguirre 1966). Recent evidence suggests that ACh is not directly involved in the generation of fibrillations which can be recorded from muscle in tissue culture where no ACh is present (Purves & Sakmann 1974, Thesleff 1982). In the denervated muscle fibre, a number of potentially reversible physical, biochemical and physiological changes occur, resulting from the synthesis of new protein and its insertion into the fibre membrane (Fambrough 1979). These changes appear as the nerve terminals degenerate and they can be prevented, in vitro, by protein synthesis inhibitors.

There are physiological differences in the genesis of regular, rhythmically discharging fibrillations and those which occur irregularly (Thesleff 1963, Thesleff & Ward 1975, Smith & Thesleff 1976). Rhythmical fibrillation tends to be maximal early in denervation, the irregular type appearing later. Fibrillation appears in a cyclical fashion in any one fibre and at any one time only a minority of denervated fibres are fibrillating (Smith & Thesleff 1976). Regular fibrillation is due to spontaneous biphasic oscillations of the membrane potential which increase in amplitude and on reaching a critical value, trigger an action potential in the muscle fibre which in turn initiates repetitive firing at a regular frequency of about 10 Hz (Li et al 1957). Although the precise cause of the oscillations is uncertain, it appears to be related to changes in sodium channels and resultant effects on sodium activation and inactivation. The reduction in resting membrane potential affects the threshold at which the oscillations generate an action potential (Thesleff 1982). Depolarisations responsible for the action potentials of irregularly discharging fibrillations occur randomly, arising in the region of the former end-plate. Their origin relates to alterations in sodium and potassium conductance in the transverse tubular system generating local discrete triggering depolarisations. These irregularly summate to reach threshold for the propagation of a fibrillation potential. This process appears less related to the level of the resting membrane potential than that generating rhythmical fibrillation (Thesleff 1982). Fibrillation will continue only as long as these mechanisms remain functional and in prolonged denervation; fibre atrophy results in the cessation of recurrent spontaneous action potentials.

Fibrillation and positive sharp wave activity are widespread and easy to detect in recently denervated muscle but also occur in other situations, such as botulism (Josefsson 1960) and in a variety of hereditary and acquired myopathies. Fibrillation seen in these conditions may be generated by mechanisms other than those responsible for the spontaneous activity in denervation. For example, the transient profuse fibrillation occurring in paramyotonia congenita on exposure to cold, the activity accompanying the onset of a paralytic attack in adynamia episodica hereditaria and the fibrillation sometimes seen in neuromyotonia show a clearly different electrogenesis (see below).

Fasciculation potentials. Fasciculation is the often visible muscle twitching accompanying the spontaneous contraction of some or all of the constituent fibres of motor units (Fig. 29.7). It occurs in healthy subjects, especially in the orbicularis oculi, and may be seen in conditions such as thyrotoxicosis, tetany and debilitating disorders. These fasciculation potentials are 'benign', i.e. they are not associated with a progressive lower motor neurone disorder. Fasciculation potentials are often a striking feature of anterior horn cell diseases, e.g. motor neurone disease, where they have a 'malignant' connotation. SFEMG evidence suggests that benign fasciculations are of primary myogenic origin while malignant fasciculations arise at various points in the nerve supply to the muscle (Stålberg & Trontelj 1982).

Fasciculation in motor neurone disease was first studied by Denny-Brown & Pennybacker (1938) who described it recurring at intervals of 2–10 s, apparently involving motor units still under voluntary control. Fasciculation is reduced but not abolished by peripheral nerve procaine block (Forster & Alpers 1944, Denny-Brown 1949) and

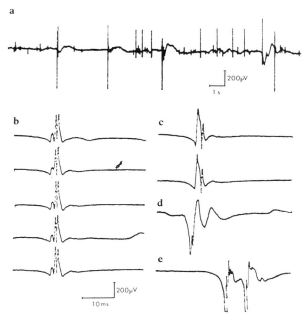

Fig. 29.7 CNEMG recordings of fasciculation potentials from a patient with motor neurone disease. **a** Displayed at slow sweep speed to show irregularity of discharge. **b – d** Examples of different fasciculation potentials which have a polyphasic shape. The potentials in b and c are relatively stable in successive discharges. **e** Fasciculation potential discharging as a doublet.

persists for 3–5 days following motor nerve division (Forster et al 1946). Fasciculations are reduced to about half by spinal anaesthesia (Swank & Price 1943). These observations suggest both a central and a peripheral neuronal origin for the fasciculation of motor neurone disease.

Conradi et al (1982) examined the fasciculations of motor neurone disease and showed that antidromic impulses occurred in the axons of fasciculating units as demonstrated by a collision technique. Lignocaine motor nerve blockade did not abolish fasciculation which was enhanced by neostigmine administration and abolished by a non-paralytic dose of a synthetic curare derivative. The fasciculation of motor neurone disease resembles that induced by cholinergic and anticholinesterase drugs (Meadows 1971). The mechanism of these drugs is to act on ACh receptors in the motor axon terminals, generating action potentials at these sites. Conradi et al (1982) postulate a similar site of origin in motor neurone disease.

The view that the majority of neurogenic fasciculations have an extremely peripheral origin in the axon terminal or preterminal has received much support (Stålberg & Trontelj 1970, Conradi et al 1982, Roth 1982). Distal ectopic excitation sites generate impulses which antidromically invade and thus excite the rest of the peripheral branches of the motor unit. The pattern of recruitment of the individual muscle fibres within the unit may differ, often considerably from that seen when the motor unit is activated centrally. If a fasciculation potential is generated at a single ectopic site, its waveform should be constant. Many fasciculations have unstable waveforms, due to the presence of multiple excitation sites or to variable axonal blocking in the preterminal neuronal network (Stålberg & Trontelj 1982). This may explain the different conclusions regarding the question of fasciculating motor units being or not being capable of voluntary recruitment; using CNEMG the shape of the action potential is a cardinal factor in its identification.

Fasciculations in the lower limb muscles have been reported in patients with cervical spondylotic myelopathy (King & Stoops 1973). These resolved following decompression in some patients and were attributed to impaired inhibitory influences.

The benign fasciculations of myogenic origin have been shown by SFEMG studies to be due to a hyperexcitable muscle fibre which fires spontaneously and ephaptically activates propinquitous muscle fibres which may belong to other motor units in the same fascicle. While there is a low jitter value between the fibres activated in the fasciculation when examined with SFEMG, suggesting ephaptic excitation, different muscle fibres may take part in the process on successive occasions so that these fasciculations may also appear unstable when recorded with CNEMG (Stålberg & Trontelj 1982). Fasciculation in normal muscle differs from that of motor neurone disease in having a shorter mean interval between successive potentials (Trojaborg & Buchthal 1965). The average interval between successive fasciculation potentials in motor neurone disease was 3.5 s ± s.e. (mean) 2.5 s, whereas in benign fasciculation the interval was 0.8 s ± s.e. (mean) 0.8 s. Distinction between benign fasciculation and that associated with progressive neurogenic lesions by study of

the form and discharge rate of the potentials using CNEMG remains difficult in an individual case. Using special surface electrodes, Hjorth et al (1973) studied the spatial and temporal distribution of fasciculations in motor neurone disease. They found that fasciculations occurred very irregularly at rates as slow as 1 per minute. The multilead surface recordings were highly sensitive means for demonstrating fasciculations (Howard & Murray 1992) and their widespread distribution, recorded at five or more of the eight electrodes, was a consistent finding in patients with motor neurone disease. Nevertheless the significance of fasciculation is best determined by the co-existence of fibrillation potentials or other signs of denervation.

Another form of spontaneous motor unit activity of uncertain nosology has been described by Buchthal & Olsen (1970) as the most consistent abnormality in the EMG in infantile spinal muscular atrophy. The units discharged regularly at rates from 5 to 15 Hz even during sleep, but the same units could be activated during voluntary contraction. The finding has been confirmed by Hausmanowa-Petrusewicz & Karwanska (1986).

High-frequency repetitive discharges (bizarre high-frequency discharges). Rapid discharges of constant frequency, amplitude and usually polyphasic wave form (Fig. 29.8b) may occur in muscle disease, particularly polymyositis (Walton & Adams 1958, Barwick & Walton 1963) and also in neuro-

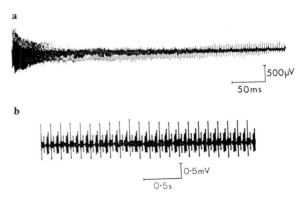

Fig. 29.8 **a** CNEMG recording of a myotonic discharge in a patient with dystrophia myotonica. **b** CNEMG recording of a repetitive high-frequency discharge in a patient with a chronic neurogenic disorder.

genic atrophy, especially anterior horn cell disease (Eisen & Karpati 1971). The discharge frequency, although constant for an individual train, may vary from 5 to 100 Hz. Repetitive discharges are evoked by needle movement and generally start and stop abruptly. They were previously called 'pseudomyotonic discharges', a term no longer approved. SFEMG studies have shed light on the genesis of this form of abnormal activity (see below).

Myotonic discharges. Myotonia is a sustained contraction of muscle fibres caused by repetitive depolarisation of their membranes (McComas & Johns 1981), recognised clinically by delayed muscular relaxation following a maintained contraction or twitch. The phenomenon may be elicited by movement of the exploring EMG electrode and by external percussion of the muscle. Myotonia is usually worsened by cooling and diminished by exercise. The hereditary myotonias include dystrophia myotonica, myotonia congenita and paramyotonia congenita. The condition may be acquired as a result of the administration of diazocholesterol and monocarboxylic acid groups of drugs and may rarely be a manifestation of hypothyroidism (Somers & Winer 1966, Venables et al 1978, Okuno et al 1981). Myotonia also occurs in hyperkalaemic periodic paralysis, malignant hyperpyrexia, acid maltase deficiency (Engel et al 1973) and chloroquine myopathy (Mastaglia et al 1977). The CNEMG shows prolonged trains of potentials occurring in profusion in response to electrode movement (Fig. 29.8a). Their frequency may reach 150 Hz, dropping subsequently to 20 or 30 Hz. They may resemble fibrillation potentials, positive sharp potentials or may be larger and more complex. An initial increase in frequency and amplitude is rapidly followed by a diminution in both, giving rise to a characteristic sound when the signal is relayed over a loudspeaker. The sound, increasing and decreasing in pitch, resembles the noise of a dive-bomber.

Myotonic activity is reduced by drugs such as phenytoin, quinine and procaine amide which interfere with voltage-dependent sodium channels. Extracellular electrolyte changes such as a rise in sodium or potassium concentration, or a fall in calcium or magnesium may increase the severity of the myotonia. Myotonic discharges arise from the repetitive activity of the single fibres or a number of muscle fibres, independent of neuronal activation as shown by the persistence of myotonia after curarisation (Landau 1952).

The underlying abnormalities in the myotonic muscle fibre membrane are discussed in detail elsewhere in this volume (see Chs 11, 15).

Neuromyotonia. Delayed muscular relaxation following a voluntary contraction deriving from abnormal impulse generation in nerve rather than muscle may be called neuromyotonia to differentiate it from true myotonia related to muscle fibre membrane abnormalities. The clinical disorders reported under this rubric are a heterogeneous group of conditions having in common a tendency to muscle stiffness and failure of muscle relaxation. Frequently muscle cramps and excessive sweating are seen and in severe generalised neuromyotonia postural abnormalities may develop (see Chs 20, 27). Although some reports indicate the presence of clinical myotonia as well as typical CNEMG myotonic trains, these are abolished by curare, indicating their origin proximal to the muscle fibre membrane. Other associated electrical change consists of continuous high-frequency asynchronous motor unit discharges often at 100–300 Hz. There is a marked decrement in the amplitude of these high-frequency trains, indicating a failure to keep abreast of the rapidly firing nerve impulses. Myokymia (see below) is often also present, as is fasciculation. Although fibrillation may be seen, unlike the fibrillation of denervation, it is abolished by curare and appears to be due to ectopic impulses arising in the terminal axon exciting single muscle fibres, and positive waves are not usually seen.

Extra discharges occasionally occur in normal motor units and are most common following initial recruitment of the unit or after an isolated electrical stimulus to the nerve. In neuromyotonia extra discharges are a striking feature and doublets, triplets and multiplets are seen (Fig. 29.9). Doublets or triplets may be recognised by the fact that the second or subsequent discharges have a similar form to that of the first, and that the amplitude depends on the time interval between the initial and extra discharge, decreasing as this falls below 10 ms due to refractoriness in the muscle fibres. The interval between the first and second

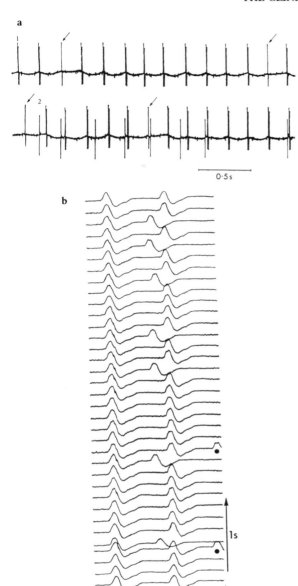

Fig. 29.9 CNEMG recording from tibialis anterior muscle in patient with peripheral neuropathy and neuromyotonia. **a** Spontaneously discharging units (1 and 2). Except for four occasions, indicated by arrows, unit 1 fires as a doublet or triplet (b, black circle). **b** This shows that the extra discharge in the doublet has two preferred intervals after the original discharge, suggesting that the extra discharges may originate at separate sites along the axon.

stimulation of the nerve, particularly by polarising currents, and may also be provoked by the mechanical stimulation of tapping over the motor point and are often seen in short spontaneous bursts. In addition to their occurrence in the neuromyotonias, multiple discharges are seen in tetany, motor neurone disease and some forms of polyneuropathy and compression neuropathies. They form grouped or repetitive motor unit discharges, formerly called 'iterative' discharges.

Neuromyotonic activity is at first accentuated, and later abolished, by ischaemia (Mertens & Zschocke 1965, Bergmans 1982). The effect is as pronounced when the cuff is applied distally as proximally, suggesting that the activity is generated at a distal site in the axon. This contrasts with the effects of ischaemia in normal individuals where the generators which will produce transient repetitive activity are predominantly proximal in situation (Kugelberg 1948). The neuromyotonic activity is abolished by curare (Harman & Richardson 1954), it persists during general anaesthesia and is uninfluenced by spinal anaesthesia or brachial anaesthetic nerve block but is progressively reduced as peripheral nerve block is induced more distally. These features exclude origin of the activity in the muscle fibre, the spinal cord or supraspinally and indicate that the proximal axon is not involved. Membrane stabilisers such as phenytoin and carbamazepine reduce or abolish the activity in some but not all cases. The site of origin of the high-frequency spontaneous activity probably lies in the distal portion of the motor axon. Isaacs (1961, 1967) believed that there was an excessive release of acetylcholine at the motor end-plate and coined the term 'quantal squander', but microelectrode studies of EPPs from a biopsy of intercostal muscles show no such excess (Lambert 1978). Evidence from recent studies suggests that some cases of acquired neuromyotonia may result from IgG autoantibodies to ion channels, most likely the potassium channel, involved with membrane excitability in peripheral nerves (Sinha et al 1991). Apart from the presence of neuromyotonia in overt peripheral neuropathy (Gamstorp & Wohlfart 1959, Welch et al 1972, Lancet et al 1979), patients with minor electrophysiological and histological abnormalities of distal motor nerve have been reported (Isaacs

potentials is from 4 to 10 ms and that between the second and third from 15 to 30 ms (Stålberg & Trontelj 1982). They may be evoked by electrical

1967, Hudson et al 1978, Lublin et al 1979, Bergmans 1982). Spontaneous activity in neuromyotonia may be generated in the distal motor axon which is in a hyperpolarised state, repetitive discharges being generated by a breakdown in nerve accommodation (Bergmans 1982). In a significant minority of patients sensory symptoms, typically peripheral paraesthesiae, have been present (Welch et al 1972). Microneurography (Lance et al 1979) in a single case demonstrated sensory as well as motor axonal hyperexcitability and sural nerve biopsy has indicated axonal degeneration in both myelinated and non-myelinated fibres (Wallis et al 1970, Welch et al 1972, Lance et al 1979).

Myokymia. The 'benign' fasciculations of myokymia are observable clinically as undulating contractions of narrow strips of a muscle along its long axis, likened to a subcutaneous bag of worms. Myokymia has been reported in thyrotoxicosis, peripheral neuropathy, multiple sclerosis, postirradiation damage to the spinal cord or nerve plexus, facial palsy, ischaemic neuropathy, diffuse vasculitis and the carpal tunnel syndrome (Daube et al 1979, Albers et al 1981, Auger et al 1984). The term has also been applied to the more transient fasciculations appearing around the eye or in the calf muscles in normal individuals (the benign myogenic fasciculations to which reference has already been made). Unfortunately, myokymia is also used by some workers to categorise patients who on electrophysiological grounds appear to have neuromyotonia or other disorders of muscular relaxation. The most widely studied form of myokymia affects the facial muscles, often in multiple sclerosis. The EMG shows groups of potentials with intervening periods of silence, the activity recurring in a quasi-rhythmical fashion producing a distinctive form of activity (Gamstorp & Wohlfart 1959). Considerable variation occurs in the number of individual discharges per burst, in the discharge frequency (usually 50 Hz or less) and in the duration and frequency of occurrence of each group. The activity in neuromyotonia shows a considerably higher discharge rate (200 Hz or more) and does not occur in the rhythmical or semirhythmical pattern of myokymia. The activity may resemble grouped motor unit discharge but is not susceptible to voluntary alter-

ation and persists in sleep. Unlike myotonia, the discharges are not influenced by needle movement or percussion and may be reduced or abolished by peripheral nerve block. Daube et al (1979) propose the term 'myokymic discharge' for activity of this type and suggest that classification should be on neurophysiological grounds. The myokymic discharge may be recorded in the absence of visible muscular abnormality, especially in radiation plexopathies but not in malignant infiltration of the plexus (Auger et al 1984). Although the exact origin of myokymia is not known, it often appears to be more proximal than the origin of neuromyotonia. In the carpal tunnel syndrome the origin appears to be at the wrist (Auger at al 1984) and ectopic impulse generation in a damaged nerve, plexus or root seems likely (Auger et al 1984). The status of the various myokymia and neuromyotonia syndromes is still subject to debate and there is no universal agreement on the neurophysiological or clinical nosology of these disorders (DeJong et al 1951, Harman & Richardson 1954, Greenhouse et al 1967, Gardner-Medwin & Walton 1969, Hughes & Matthews 1969, Daube et al 1979, Lublin et al 1979, Albers et al 1981, Bergmans 1982, Auger et al 1984).

Stiff-man syndrome. Spontaneous activity occurring in the stiff-man syndrome (Moersch & Woltman 1956) resembles physiological cramps but is widespread and continuous. CNEMG reveals a sustained interference pattern in affected muscles with normal individual MUPs. Sleep, general, spinal and local anaesthetic nerve block abolish the muscle fibre activity, suggesting a central origin (Price & Allott 1958, Werk et al 1961, Gordon et al 1967). Agents which suppress activity in spinal and supraspinal intraneurones, such as diazepam, baclofen and clonazepam, are effective therapies (Howard 1963, Martinelli et al 1978). Some similarities to tetanus have been remarked upon (Moersch & Woltman 1956, Gordon et al 1967). Excessive excitability of the motor neurone pool may develop because of a failure of recurrent inhibition, perhaps due to disturbed Renshaw interneurone function. The silent period is normal in the stiff-man syndrome, unlike tetanus where it is lost (Stohr & Heckl 1977). Clomipramine which inhibits the re-uptake of serotonin and noradrenaline, producing increased central serotoninergic and noradrenergic activity, severely aggravates the activity (Meink et al 1984). The presence of grossly exaggerated responses to exteroceptive stimuli and abnormally short transmission times with excessive reflex excitatory phases in face and limb muscles has been demonstrated (Meink et al 1984). The suggestion has been made that the disorder is the result of transmission of descending noradrenegic impulses from disordered medial brain-stem pathways impinging on the alpha motor neurone.

In tetanus, the toxin may impair Renshaw cell activity resulting in alpha motor neurone hyperexcitability (Brooks et al 1957). Renshaw cell failure would also explain the absence of the silent period. The spontaneous activity in the EMG is abolished by sleep, general and spinal anaesthesia and peripheral nerve block. The peripheral nerves have been shown to be affected by the disease (Shahani et al 1979) and the motor end-plate is also structurally abnormal (Duchen 1973), while SFEMG studies have shown abnormal neuromuscular jitter (Fernandez et al 1983). It is not yet clear how these peripheral defects contribute to the clinical picture.

When the serum ionised calcium is low, spontaneous muscular activity occurs (Kugelberg 1948). Ischaemia, hyperventilation or nerve percussion evoke or accentuate the muscular activity (Layzer & Rowland 1971). Increased sodium conductance is produced by low extracellular calcium, leading to repetitive nerve excitation and there is loss of nerve accommodation (Kugelberg 1948). The CNEMG shows MUPs often firing in groups, asynchronously at rates of 5–30 Hz, either in brief bursts or longer trains, with periods of relative silence between them. Many repetitive firing units show doublets, triplets and multiplets. The ectopic impulses appear to arise at a variety of levels in the motor axon and some may occur in muscle fibres (Stålberg & Trontelj 1982). Cramps and painful involuntary sustained contractions of muscles are associated with high-frequency motor unit discharge at 200–300 Hz. Synchronous involvement of large areas of muscle is usual (Layzer & Rowland 1971). Recurrent muscle cramps are often present in motor neurone disease and there are syndromes in which cramps are a major feature, including the familial and sporadic muscle

pain and fasciculation syndromes (Jusic et al 1972, Lazaro et al 1981). Mild abnormalities of nerve conduction are sometimes found but CNEMG is normal apart from the cramps. A syndrome has been described, mainly affecting females, where cramps are associated with diarrhoea and alopecia, later painful muscle spasms resembling tetany develop but the serum calcium is normal (Satoyoshi 1978).

Motor unit action potential (MUP)

Description, definition and methods of analysis. The MUP is the summation of the individual action potentials of its constituent muscle fibres. MUPs recorded with CNEMG electrodes can be described in terms of the duration, spike duration, amplitude, area, spike area, phases, turns, satellites and variability (Stålberg et al 1986)(Fig. 29.10) They have initial and terminal positive portions and a central negative spike and one or more phases, which are defined as one more than the number of base-line crossings. Smaller changes in polarity failing to cross the base-line are called turns. The spikes are derived from the action potentials of 2–12 muscle fibres of the motor unit lying within a 1 mm radius of the electrode's leading-off surface (Thiele & Boehle 1978). Simulation studies suggest that the MUP

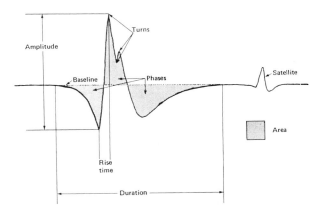

Fig. 29.10 Diagram of a motor unit potential (MUP) recorded with a CNEMG electrode. The duration, amplitude and number of phases are the most widely measured parameters. The satellite potential is excluded for measurement of the duration. Determination of the area requires the use of a computer.

amplitude depends on the number and size of muscle fibres within 0.5 mm of the recording surface and mainly the closest muscle fibre. Because of their distance from the recording electrode, action potentials from more remote muscle fibres in the unit may only appear in the smaller, lower frequency, initial or terminal portions of the MUP. Since the individual muscle fibres of the motor unit are dispersed and the concentric electrode has directional properties (Nakao et al 1965), MUP configuration varies with needle position. The degree of asynchrony between the arrival of individual muscle fibre action potentials at the electrode determines the number of phases or turns in the MUP recorded at a particular site. MUP duration varies less with changes in electrode position than the amplitude, the number of phases and the phase-relationships of the potential. Increasing dispersion of the action potentials of muscle fibres within 1 mm of the recording surface leads to a polyphasic waveform (Nandedkar et al 1988).

In up to 10% of MUPs in normal muscle, spikes separated from the main action potential are seen and are termed variously, linked, late, parasite or satellite components (Lang & Partanen 1976) (Fig. 29.9). They generally follow but may occasionally precede the main portion of the MUP. They are usually generated by single muscle fibres. Linked components are usually excluded from MUP duration measurements but their presence should be noted since they have important pathological implications, being frequently seen in neurogenic and certain myopathic conditions.

Most MUPs have amplitudes of from 250 µV to 2–4 mV and have diphasic or triphasic forms, with durations of 4–12 ms. In the majority of normal limb muscles up to 10% of units may be polyphasic (Caruso & Buchthal 1965), although in deltoid 25% may have a polyphasic shape. The time interval between the initial positive peak and the subsequent negative peak is the MUP rise-time and relates to the proximity of the electrode to the active muscle fibres.

The total duration of the MUP is measured from the departure of the initial positive deflection from the baseline to the return to the baseline of the terminal positive deflection. In manual analysis, these points, particularly the return to baseline

which is usually gradual, are strongly influenced by the gain setting. A standard gain and sweep speed (100 µV/cm, 10 ms/cm) should be employed (Stålberg et al 1986). The mean MUP duration of voluntary muscles varies with the muscle examined. Petersén & Kugelberg (1949) found a mean MUP duration in biceps brachii of 7.56 ms ± s.e. (mean) 0.14 ms compared with 2.28 ms ± s.e. (mean) 0.03 ms in facial muscles. Scattering of arrival times of individual action potentials making up the MUP depends on the distribution of motor end-plates. Normally these are arranged in one or sometimes two zones (Coërs & Woolf 1959), extending for about 1% of the total muscle length. For example in the biceps brachii there is a 20–30 mm longitudinal spread of the site of the end-plates and therefore of the origin of the muscle fibre action potentials. MUPs recorded deep within the muscle have comparable durations to those obtained with monopolar needle electrodes and are longer than those recorded close to the surface (Buchthal et al 1954b,c). The CNEMG cannula is not inert, it is a conductor which takes on a potential equal to the mean value of the tissue potential along its length. Thus the deeper the electrode is inserted, the lower is the cannula potential (Pollak 1971). When the electrode is superficial, the cannula potential is high and MUP durations no longer approximate to those found with a monopolar system.

In infants, mean MUP duration is shorter than in adults and in the elderly it is prolonged. The increase in duration occurring with maturation from infancy to adulthood is attributed to widening of the end-plate zones with growth, while that associated with advancing years appears to relate to an increased muscle fibre density within the motor units due to age-related denervation and reinnervation (Sacco et al 1962). MUP duration is also increased by cooling by about 5% for each degree Celsius fall; the amplitude of the potential drops between 2 and 5% and the number of polyphasic potentials rises by 1% (Buchthal et al 1954b,c). Differential cooling causes desynchronisation which more than offsets the facilitatory effect of cooling on the muscle fibre membrane. MUP amplitude has been shown to be greater in men than in women in the biceps brachii and tibialis anterior (Partanen & Lang 1982) but duration values appear to be the same in both sexes (Kaiser & Petersén 1965).

Quantification of MUP dimensions has a long history. Initial studies involved recording early-recruiting units on long lengths of film and MUPs identified as repeating free of artifact or interference from other units on at least three occasions were measured. The method ensures that polyphasic potentials are single MUPs and not superimpositions of more than one potential as can occur in tremor for example. This laborious procedure which involved collecting at least 20 different MUPs was made easier by the introduction of the delay-line. It is necessary to measure at least 20 separate, randomly recorded MUPs in order to derive the mean MUP duration (Buchthal & Rosenfalck 1955). When the same biceps brachii was examined on 20 separate occasions to validate the reproducibility of mean duration measurements based on a sample of about 20 different MUPs, a significant shortening occurred only on the final examination, attributed to the repeated needling (Buchthal et al 1954b,c). Because of variations in MUP amplitude with needle position, a much larger sample is needed if reproducible mean MUP amplitude measurements are to be made. The other feature studied is the percentage of polyphasic potentials (i.e. those with five or more phases) present. Manual determinations of MUP parameters may differ between individual electromyographers measuring the same material and biased selection of MUPs can occur during the recording process if random electrode repositioning is not strictly observed (Barwick & Gardner-Medwin 1967, Falk 1983).

Automatic and semiautomatic measurements of MUP characteristics have been introduced; in addition, methods of interference pattern analysis have also been developed. In many automated methods of MUP measurement the electromyographer still controls the selection of the units measured, first by siting the recording electrode, and in some methods, by choosing to accept or reject the particular action potential. Most systems require display of a delayed action potential after it has triggered the oscilloscope sweep. A window discriminator allows selection of a potential of a certain amplitude or slope in the presence of other activity, so that several different MUPs may be recorded at a single site. The electrode should be repositioned at a transverse distance of at least 10 mm in order to ensure that the same motor unit is not recorded twice from different parts of its territory. In smaller distal muscles this may not be possible and MUPs from different fractions of the same unit are registered. Electronic averaging makes it simpler to measure the dimensions of the motor unit potential free from noise or interference from other active units. Amplitude, phases, turns and rise-time are straightforward but problems in defining duration remain. MUP onset may be abrupt or more gradual when determination of its beginning may be difficult. The terminal portion of the MUP, due to volume conduction of action potentials travelling away from the recording site and towards the tendon, gradually disappears into the baseline. Its termination is particularly difficult to define and is a function of the gain in the recording system (Falk 1983). The automated methods so far reported (Bergmans 1971, Lee & White 1973, Kopec et al 1973, Kopec & Hausmanowa-Petrusewicz 1976) use arbitrary threshold levels of what constitutes a significant departure from the baseline. The lower this threshold is set, the longer will the MUP duration appear.

Four main methods for the identification of MUPs which are to be subject to automatic analysis have been described. First, the electromyographer selects the action potential and only then is the computer used to make the measurements. Second, there is the template technique in which the computer identifies one or more template MUPs and stores them. Each subsequent MUP is compared with the template until a predetermined number of identical MUPs have been collected; these are averaged and parameters defined by the particular program used are analysed and displayed (Bergmans 1971, 1973, Tanzi et al 1979, Hynninen et al 1979). Third, an individual MUP may be isolated using a suitable trigger, such as a peak-window or an adjustable level trigger (Lang et al 1971). The operator then decides after the potentials have been averaged and displayed whether to accept them for further analysis by the program. Fourth, a SFEMG port on the side of a CNEMG electrode is used to select a single fibre potential from the unit and locks on to this while the MUP is registered on the second channel

(Lang & Falk 1980). Comparison of the various manual and automated techniques for quantitative MUP analysis has shown a good correlation of the measurements of MUP duration among the different methods (Stålberg et al 1986).

The Polish minicomputer ANOPS 100 forms the basis of a MUP analysis system, the subject of several reports (Kopec & Hausmanowa-Petrusewicz 1969, 1976, 1983, Kopec et al 1973, Singh & Lovelace 1979, Wagner et al 1979). All potentials exceeding 100 μV are accepted for measurement and an amplitude criterion is used to measure duration (the onset and termination are 20 μV above the baseline). Peak-to-peak amplitude is also determined but the analysis of phases is unconventional. Phases are defined as polarity changes of over 50 μV rather than the number of baseline crossings plus one, so that some 'turns' are counted as phases. Recordings are made at 16 different sites and 64 signals from each site subjected to analysis. Although criticised because it may well analyse the same MUP several times and because it treats superimposed units as separate single MUPs (Ludin 1980), the values obtained for MUP amplitude and duration in normal subjects using this method correspond with those obtained manually (Wagner et al 1979). Moreover, there is a satisfactory differentiation between normal control values and those obtained in various neuromuscular diseases (Singh & Lovelace 1979).

The values obtained with automatic systems generally compare well with those obtained by manual measurements of the same material (Hirose et al 1974, Fuglsang-Frederiksen et al 1976, 1977). It has been pointed out (Sica et al 1978) that the durations established by Buchthal et al (1957) may differ from those produced by the automated methods. The analysis programs vary (Rathjen et al 1968, Bergmans 1971, 1973, Kunze 1971, 1973, Lee & White 1973, Kopec & Hausmanowa-Petrusewicz 1976, Hynninen et al 1979, Tanzi et al 1979, Stålberg & Antoni 1981, Falk 1983). There are now a number of commercial systems providing microprocessor-based automatic analysis of the standard motor unit potential parameters. Various workers have produced programs which will carry out the analysis on standard microcomputers to which many modern electromyographs can be linked (Rathjen et al 1968,

Stålberg & Antoni 1981). Using such devices it is possible to analyse many parameters not readily assessable manually, such as MUP area, duration and area of the spike component(s), spike slope, etc. The clinical utility of such extra measurements is yet to be demonstrated.

Interference pattern analysis

The motor units examined for quantitative motor unit potential analysis and in the SFEMG and Macro EMG techniques are generally recruited at low levels of contraction. Thus information concerning the larger, high-threshold motor units and of the interference pattern is lacking with these approaches. A number of different quantitative techniques have been developed for this purpose.

Frequency analysis. The frequency spectrum of the EMG as shown by Fourier analysis is dependent on both the mean duration of the motor units and the number of polyphasic units. Early studies (Richardson 1951, Walton 1952) involved the use of tuned circuits which enabled the frequency analysis to be displayed on an oscilloscope simultaneously with the interference pattern. Using this method the dominant frequency in limb muscles of normal subjects was found to be 100–200 Hz, tailing off to zero at 800 Hz. Larsson (1968, 1975) made use of an analyser developed by Kaiser & Petersén (1963), which employs four octave band filters with centre frequencies of 50, 200, 800 and 1600 Hz. It also includes a facility for statistical analysis and comparison of the values with control data. Recent interest has focused on the Fourier analysis applied to the EMG obtained through surface electrodes and its interpretation by means of mathematical models and computer simulation techniques (Lindström 1985). Surface electrode spectra appear to be highly reproducible and to be closely dependent on the propagation velocity of muscle fibres as well as the frequency and number of polyphasic motor units. The propagation velocity is slowed in fatigue (Stålberg 1966) and this is reflected in a shift towards the low-frequency end of the spectrum in fatigued muscle. These analyses are complex but non-invasive and with the increasing availability of microcomputers may become more widely used (Lindström & Petersén 1981, Lindström 1985).

Turns analysis. One of the most widely used approaches to quantification of the interference pattern depends upon counting the number of spikes or turn/s and amplitude/s in the signal (Willison 1964, Hayward 1983). A turn is defined as a point in the signal where a change in direction of either polarity occurs, with an amplitude difference between successive turns exceeding 100 μV. The number of turns was counted as one set of pulses (Fig. 29.11) and the number of 100 μV increments between the turns was determined as a second set of amplitude pulses, from which the total amplitude and mean amplitude in a given epoch could be derived (Fitch 1967). The turns count and mean amplitude are dependent on the level of activity in the muscle (Hayward & Willison 1973, Hayward 1983) and therefore analysis was performed at a standard load (2 kgf for biceps brachii, triceps brachii and tibialis anterior, 5 kgf for vastus lateralis). Fuglsang-Frederiksen & Månsson (1975) found that muscles of different strength may not give comparable results and that this could be corrected if a fixed percentage of maximum force (30%) was used for the examination. A further useful parameter which can be derived is the ratio between number of turns and mean amplitude which can be obtained without using any predetermined force. This is particularly valuable in the examination of children who may have difficulty in maintaining a sustained contraction at a given tension (Smyth & Willison 1982), and Fuglsang-Frederiksen et al (1984) have found this ratio to be the most sensitive index for differentiating between patients with myopathy and controls. Stålberg et al (1983) have further developed this approach, plotting turns against amplitude in order to obtain a relationship independent of force. Recordings are made at 20 different sites within the muscle over a range of force levels and epochs of 300 ms are analysed to give the number of turns and mean amplitude. A plot of the mean amplitude versus number of turns have been constructed for a number of muscles in control subjects and an area on this plot, called a cloud, has been defined to include more than 95% of all the data points. A study is considered to be abnormal if two or more data points lie outside the cloud for age-matched controls.

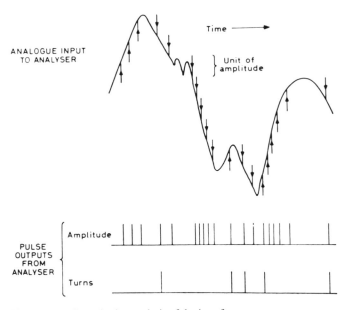

Fig. 29.11 Quantitative analysis of the interference pattern. Analysis of a typical waveform to show pulses derived from the analyser, each of which represents increments of voltage and changes of phase (from Fitch 1967).

In an attempt to analyse the interference pattern in a manner similar to that in which it is qualitatively assessed by an electromyographer, Nandedkar et al (1986a,b) have quantified the following parameters. The fullness of the interference pattern is represented by the parameter 'activity' which is the portion of the sweep that contains a signal. The 'upper centile amplitude' defines the upper limit of the maximum peak-to-peak amplitude of the motor unit action potentials contained in the interference pattern and the 'number of small segments' measures the complexity of the interference pattern, reflecting the polyphasicity of the component motor unit action potentials. The activity and logarithm of the upper centile amplitude are closely correlated with the force of muscle contraction, while the number of small segments initially increases with the force of contraction, levelling off at higher force levels.

INTERPRETATION OF THE EMG

CNEMG

In healthy muscle at rest, with the exploring electrode outside the end-plate zone, no electrical activity can be detected. In the end-plate zone electrical changes already described occur, including MEPPs and fibrillations. Electrical activity accompanying movement of the needle is brief. The initiation of volitional activity is associated with the recruitment of one or a small number of MUPs firing at low frequency with asynchrony between the units when more than one is present (Fig. 29.12a). The early recruiting units are generally smaller than those which appear at higher tensions and they recruit in an orderly fashion. The smallest anterior horn cells are responsible for the early units; this is the 'size principle' (Henneman 1957). Increasing force of contraction is associated with a rising firing rate of the early-recruited units and the appearance of additional MUPs (Fig. 29.12b). Initial firing rates are usually from 5–10 Hz and these rise considerably before it becomes impossible to follow individual MUPs and an interference pattern develops (Fig. 29.12c).

Upper motor neurone lesions. In upper motor neurone paralysis, in physiological hyper-

trophy of muscle and in the wasting of disuse atrophy, the EMG recorded with CNEMG electrode was thought to remain normal, apart from some increase in polyphasic potentials reported in the latter condition (Pinelli & Buchthal 1953).

Considerable controversy has developed over the changes occurring in pyramidal tract lesions. Goldkamp (1967) reported fibrillations in approximately two-thirds of the paretic muscles examined in a series of 116 hemiplegics. Spontaneous activity was more pronounced in distal muscles. This finding has been confirmed in a number of other studies (Johnson et al 1975, Segura & Sahgal 1981). Similar spontaneous activity has been reported in the lower limbs of paraplegics following spinal cord injuries (Van Alphen et al 1962, Spielholz et al 1972, Taylor et al 1974). There is argument as to the cause of these findings. It has been suggested that they are secondary to various compression or traction injuries to peripheral

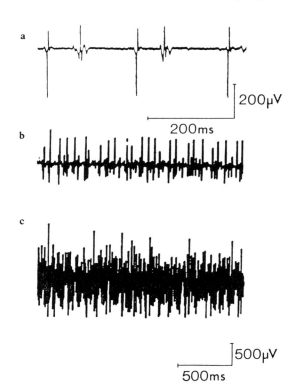

Fig. 29.12 CNEMG recordings of motor unit recruitment at different levels of activity in normal muscle. **a** Gentle contraction showing individual motor unit potentials. **b** Moderate contraction showing some overlap of potentials. **c** Maximal contraction showing an interference pattern.

nerves or plexuses consequent upon the paresis and immobility. While it is likely that such peripheral factors do play a part, the very widespread fibrillation recorded in some studies and its early onset between the second and fifth week following the development of the hemiplegia, suggest that unrecognised lower motor neurone pathology is not the only cause. Considerable change in the physiological properties of the motor unit occur in upper motor neurone lesions (Edström 1970, McComas et al 1973, Young & Rowley 1982). McComas et al (1973) reported a loss of 50% of motor units in hemiplegic muscle and histological evidence of denervation in hemiplegic muscle has been reported (Segura & Sahgal 1981). A greater decrement in the compound muscle action potential in response to repetitive stimulation in muscles on the hemiplegic side has been found (Brown & Wynn-Parry 1981). Trans-synaptic degeneration was proposed by McComas et al (1973) as the cause for the development of these features. For a fuller discussion of this controversial but important area see Brown (1984).

Lower motor neurone lesions. Following complete nerve section, total electrical silence of the denervated muscle ensues outside the end-plate-zone. Fibrillations appear following the time-course of wallerian degeneration and so take longer to appear in distal muscles when the nerve section is proximal (Luco & Eyzaguirre 1955). Positive sharp waves followed by fibrillation are seen, at first in relation to the mechanical stimulation of electrode movement and later spontaneously. By 3 weeks, fibrillation potentials and positive sharp waves are easily detected. Volitional potentials are absent from the time of onset of the nerve section. End-plate potentials eventually disappear from completely denervated muscle (Miledi & Slater 1963, Weiderholt 1970, Buchthal 1982).

The retention of some volitional MUPs in a lower motor neurone lesion indicates that the lesion is incomplete, an important finding in peripheral nerve injuries. Absence of MUPs indicates total dysfunction of the nerve, some of which may be axonal in type but conduction block due to demyelination may also contribute. The complete absence of excitability of the nerve distal to the site of injury may not indicate total section; the nerve

sheath may remain intact despite complete degeneration of its axonal content. Evidence of continuity may have to await the orderly return of motor unit activity consequent upon axonal regeneration at approximately 1–2 mm per day.

Fibrillations are profuse in acute and severe neurogenic lesions but may be less easy to identify in more chronic processes. Their absence can only be presumed after an exacting search. Buchthal (1982) reports being unable to detect fibrillation in a quarter to a third of partially denervated muscles. In longstanding partial denervation, absence of fibrillation may be due to reinnervation of many denervated fibres by collateral sprouting and severe atrophy of the remainder.

Incomplete lower motor neurone lesions cause a reduction of volitional MUPs which may preclude the development of an interference pattern on full volition. The interference pattern is deemed to be reduced when the baseline of the oscilloscope sweep is not continuously obscured by MUP activity but individual MUPs cannot be identified. More severe lesions result in the presence of so few units in the pick-up area of the CNEMG electrode that the beam returns to the isoelectric line between individual MUPs which can be identified; this is called discrete activity (Fig. 29.13a). The loss of motor units results in abnormally high firing-rates of the recruited surviving units. In severe partial denervation, the fall-out of motor units may be so extreme that a single MUP recurring at rates of 50–60 Hz may represent maximal effort. Quantification of the interference pattern shows a reduction in the turns count and increase in the mean amplitude (Hayward & Willison 1977), or reduction in the ratio of turns/mean amplitude (Fuglsang-Frederiksen et al 1977). With the cloud technique the data points show a shift to the upper border and an excess of points outside the limits (Stålberg et al 1983). The degree of change is related to the severity and chronicity of the underlying denervating process (Hayward & Willison 1977).

Changes occur in MUP morphology when partial denervation has been present for some time. Collateral sprouts from intramuscular nerve twigs of surviving motor units reinnervate adjacent muscle fibres. This first results in small late or satellite potentials of the MUP showing an unstable con-

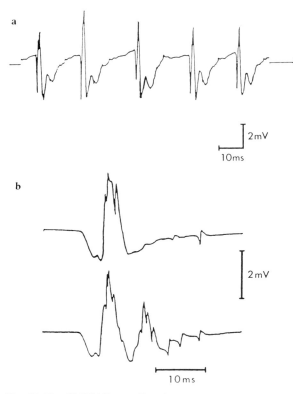

a

2mV
10ms

b

2mV

10ms

Fig. 29.13 CNEMG recordings in neurogenic atrophy.
a Discrete motor unit activity at maximal effort in patient with old poliomyelitis. The motor unit is firing at a frequency of about 60 Hz. **b** Motor unit potential of prolonged duration and with late components. In the lower trace there is an extra-discharge of the motor unit.

nection to the parent unit, evident with a delay-line and superimposition techniques (Borenstein & Desmedt 1973). The lateness of the component relates to slow conduction through an immature axon sprout, its frequent absence is due to trans-mission failure ('impulse blocking') at an imma-ture end-plate. These small spikes may follow the main MUP by 40–80 ms; later the connections become more mature and the components appear with less delay and more stability.

Collateral reinnervation results in increased fibre density (FD) as large numbers of muscle fibres are incorporated into the motor unit (Kugelberg 1973). When FD is increased in that part of the motor unit close to the leading-off surface of the recording electrode and there is close synchronisation between muscle fibre excitation, a large-amplitude MUP results (Fig. 29.13b). These

MUPs have been called 'giant' motor units as they commonly reach amplitudes of 10 or even 20 mV. This terminology is no longer approved; measure-ment of peak-to-peak amplitude and comparison with normal ranges for the particular muscle explored is preferred.

Prolonged MUP duration in reinnervation is mainly due to the increase in the number of fibres within the pick-up area of the electrode. Collateral sprouting widens the innervation zone leading to increased temporal dispersion of the muscle fibre action potentials, adding to MUP duration as well as increasing the number of polyphasic potentials (Buchthal & Clemmeson 1941). The collateral reinnervation capacity appears to be an important property of healthy anterior horn cells (McComas et al 1971a).

Nerve conduction studies and EMG comple-ment each other in the assessment of peripheral neuropathies. In acute axonal neuropathies, fibril-lation and positive sharp waves in distal muscles appear before reduction in CMAP amplitude or other conduction abnormalities can be confidently identified (Thage et al 1963, Trojaborg et al 1969). In severe postinfectious demyelinating neuropathy, there is profound slowing of conduc-tion but ultimately the prognosis depends upon the amount of axonal damage associated with the demyelination (Eisen & Humphries 1974). During recovery from axonal damage, the EMG may show the presence of long-duration (15–30 ms) poly-phasic MUPs consisting of many short spikes, due to axonal regeneration and reinnervation (Buchthal 1970).

The process of compensatory reinnervation may be complete in a year and remains stable thereafter if caused by a non-progressive lesion (Hakelius & Stålberg 1974). With ongoing disease, collateral reinnervation occurs but the disorder's progression ultimately causes its failure. A useful function of the EMG is to indicate the tempo and extent of the denervating process. Although SFEMG plays a major part in this, CNEMG may be useful. If profuse fibrillations and positive sharp waves accompany evidence of widespread remodelling of motor units with many unstable MUPs, a fairly rapidly evolving disease process is likely. If dener-vation is slowly progressive, florid spontaneous activity is less likely to be found, and the proportion of unstable MUPs may suggest the rate of progression. Complex, high-amplitude or long-duration but stable MUPs suggest that denervation and reinnervation have occurred but that the disorder is currently inactive. Using a CNEMG electrode and a 500 Hz high-pass filter, stability of individual motor units can be assessed. With a delay-line and a fast sweep speed, the time-relationships of individual spikes in the MUP can be observed. While it is not possible to measure jitter accurately, instability of the MUP and blocking of individual components can be identified. The technique provides an intermediate stage between CNEMG and SFEMG (Payan 1978).

Synchronisation of motor unit activity. The smoothness of muscular contraction is mainly due to asynchronous recruitment of motor units. However there is some apparent grouping of the MUPs which characteristically occurs at a frequency of about 9 Hz and is most striking during fatigue. The suggested cause for this is oscillation in the stretch reflex servo-loop which may account in part for physiological tremor (Lippold et al 1957). Apparent grouping of motor unit activity can occur in deafferented muscle so that not all grouping has a reflex basis. There is evidence (Taylor 1962) that under normal conditions a significant amount of grouping is a random occurrence.

In patients who have muscle weakness as a result of anterior horn cell disease such as poliomyelitis, action potentials can be recorded simultaneously from widely separated electrodes in the same muscle (Buchthal & Clemmeson 1941). The finding was regarded as evidence of a central (spinal cord) disorder. Denny-Brown (1949) suggested that there was a loss of the smaller, earlier recruiting motor units in anterior horn cell diseases and that the apparent synchronisation was due to the uncovering of larger units which in normal individuals were lost in the interference pattern.

Synchronous potentials are more frequent in muscle affected by anterior horn cell disease than peripheral nerve lesions (Buchthal & Madsen 1950). This may indicate an interaction between motor neurones leading to periods of synchronous firing (Simpson 1962, 1966, Norris 1965). Synchronisation may be due to the fact that each Renshaw interneurone receives fewer recurrent collateral fibres when there is a reduced anterior horn cell population promoting synchronous firing (Simpson 1966). There are alternative explanations; ephaptic excitation could occur proximally in the cord or motor root to explain the finding of synchronous motor unit activity in different muscles innervated by the same spinal segment, in advanced motor neurone disease as reported by Norris (1965).

Aberrant reinnervation and synkinesis. Regeneration and reinnervation following nerve damage is often misdirected, especially when the internal architecture of the nerve has been disrupted by the causative lesion. The axonal regrowth may result in the reinnervation of muscle fibres in quite separate muscles, such as the circumoral and circumocular muscles, following Bell's palsy, resulting in a permanent synchronisation (synkinesis) between different parts of what are pathologically dispersed single motor units. Aberrant reinnervation may also result in the presence of abnormal axon reflexes.

While studying axon reflex latencies in normal individuals to determine the sites of axonal branching, Stålberg & Trontelj (1979) found evidence suggesting that the branching began more proximally than previously suspected, some 10–15 cm proximal to the innervation zone. In chronic compressive nerve lesions, reinnervating axonal branches may occur distal to the site of the lesion allowing the possibility of widespread synkinesis (Fullerton & Gilliatt 1965). Esslen (1960) demonstrated synchronous 'volitional' motor unit activity in different muscles following aberrant reinnervation in facial and peripheral nerve lesions. Periodic recruitment of MUPs in the deltoid or biceps brachii, in phase with respiration, may develop after injuries to the brachial plexus, and is due to aberrant reinnervation by axons of the phrenic nerve (Swift et al 1980). Obstetric brachial plexus injury may cause extensive synkinesis and axon reflexes, sometimes involving antagonistic muscles (De Grandis et al 1979).

Primary myopathies. High-frequency discharges, positive sharp waves and fibrillations occur in some myopathies. McComas & Mrozek (1968) suggested that fibrillation in muscular dystrophy was due to functional denervation occurring when segmental necrosis separates a viable portion of a muscle fibre from its end-plate. Regenerating muscle fibres without an innervation may also discharge spontaneously. Because such fibres have a very small diameter their spontaneous discharges will be of low amplitude compared to fibrillations seen in recent denervation. The genesis of fibrillation potentials in myopathy is obscure but may be different from those mechanisms responsible for fibrillation in denervated muscle. Florid fibrillations may be recorded in polymyositis (particularly in the acute and subacute forms) which suggests that secondary involvement of the terminal nerve branches by the inflammatory process might be responsible (Richardson 1956). Functional denervation may also play a part, as may increased membrane irritability (Bohan et al 1977). In Duchenne dystrophy, fibrillation can be more easily recorded if the patient exercises prior to the examination (Buchthal & Rosenfalck 1966).

The alterations in CNEMG-recorded MUP parameters in myopathy are, first, a reduction in mean MUP duration (Kugelberg 1947). This is the most characteristic change and, to be considered significant, the reduction should be greater than 20% of that recorded from the same muscle of a normal subject of similar age. Secondly, there may be an increase in the number of polyphasic potentials present (Fig. 29.14a) and when this increase is combined with the finding of shortening of the mean MUP duration, the probability of myopathy is high. MUP amplitude may be reduced, but this is a less pronounced and more variable feature. The reduced MUP duration and amplitude seen in myopathy may have several causes. In myopathy the resting membrane potential may be reduced in amplitude (Lenman 1965) and consequently the action potential amplitude is also reduced. Extracellulary recorded action potentials from narrow diameter fibres are of low amplitude (Håkansson 1957). The initial and terminal portions of the MUP are of low amplitude and disappear into the baseline earlier.

Primary muscle disease may cause local increases in FD as a result of a number of processes including muscle fibre regeneration and reinnervation, fibre splitting, and perhaps closer packing of atrophied fibres. There is marked variation of fibre diameters resulting in increased scatter of action potential propagation velocities, causing desynchronisation of component spikes and temporal dispersion,

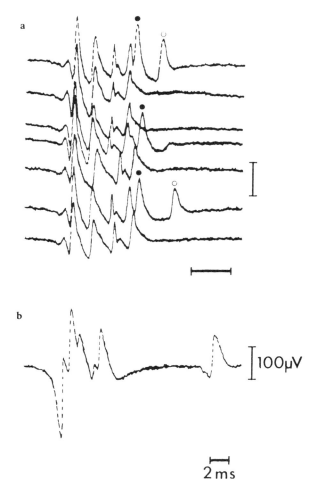

Fig. 29.14   CNEMG recordings in myopathy. **a** Polyphasic motor unit potential recorded from biceps in a patient with mitochondrial myopathy. Two potentials (closed and open circles) show increased jitter and blocking. **b** Recording from biceps in another patient with mitochondrial myopathy showing a polyphasic potential containing a late component 15 ms after the onset of the potential (from Fawcett et al 1982a).

leading to the presence of late components (Fig. 29.14b). Local increase in FD and the presence of hypertrophied fibres may account for the occasional high-amplitude potentials. Restriction of volume conduction due to fibrosis and fatty infiltration may result in an increase in the recorded amplitude of individual muscle fibre action potentials and hence an increased MUP amplitude (Stålberg & Trontelj 1979). Polyphasic potentials probably derive from the wider range of conduction velocities in immature nerve sprouts and smaller muscle fibres. In some recordings the effective MUP duration when all the satellite or late potentials are included, may be prolonged to values of 40–80 ms (Lang & Partanen 1976).

The fall in mean interference pattern amplitude may be explained by loss of individual muscle fibres within the units combined with fibrosis and fatty replacement which may alter the volume conduction characteristics of the muscle. The loss of muscle fibres, which would have contributed to the contractile process, accounts for the recruitment of more units to develop a given tension, resulting in an increased interference pattern density. As indicated above, in more severely affected dystrophic muscles, individual MUPs may have an excessively complex form and prolonged duration so that rapid discharge of a few such potentials will result in overlapping of the complexes. Thus a full interference pattern may be recorded during only moderate contractions but is of reduced amplitude. The finding of small, brief, often polyphasic MUPs, recruiting early in large numbers in myopathy, contrasts with MUPs of large amplitude and long duration showing reduced recruitment seen in chronic neurogenic disease.

Quantitative analysis of the interference pattern in patients with myopathy using a fixed load shows an increase in the number of turns (Rose & Willison 1967), while an elevation of the turns count and decrease in the mean amplitude is present when the technique employing a percentage of the maximum force is used (Fuglsang-Frederiksen et al 1976). A shift of data points towards the lower border of the cloud (high turns, small amplitudes) and an excess of points outside the limits has been found with the modified technique of Stålberg et al (1983). The degree of abnormality is related to the severity of the underlying myopathic process (Hayward 1983).

Differentiation of myopathy from neurogenic lesions may be less straightforward than suggested above (Gath et al 1969). Several neurogenic processes may result in an excess of low-amplitude, polyphasic, short-duration MUPs. In the early phase of reinnervation, neural connection may be established with a few muscle fibres within the motor unit. The resulting MUPs will resemble those found in myopathy, though conduction in the immature terminal innervation will be slow (Engel 1975). In distal neuropathy the sick axon may be unable to sustain innervation of all its muscle fibres and an apparently random dropout could produce a picture suggestive of myopathy.

Both histological and electrophysiological changes suggestive of a myopathy may be seen in longstanding partial denervation (Drachman et al 1967). Also in what appears to be a myopathic process, changes suggestive of denervation may occur and may be regarded as secondary neuropathic changes (Guy et al 1950). In muscles severely and chronically affected by myopathy or denervation, it may be impossible to decide, in the presence of findings suggestive of both a myopathic and neurogenic process, which of these is primary. The selection of mildly or moderately involved muscles for study is likely to be more profitable than examining those which are severely affected.

Scanning EMG

Normal muscle. The basis of this technique has already been mentioned (Stålberg & Antoni 1980). The biceps brachii and tibialis anterior have been most often studied. For any one position of the needle electrode, the MUP form remains relatively constant, the major spikes occurring at the same point along the sweep in successive recordings. Movement of the electrode through the motor unit territory gives information concerning the spatial and temporal distribution of the muscle fibres and their action potentials. MUPs which contain spike components are distributed over a distance of 5–10 mm for the biceps brachii and tibialis anterior muscles (Fig. 29.15a). In normal muscle there are usually no gaps or silent areas in the cross-section. A collection of adjacent spikes is called a 'peak'. In biceps brachii and tibialis anterior a single major negative peak is found in about 50% of recordings. Less often two, three or more rarely four peaks may be found, separated in the temporal domain by up to 9 ms. This appears to depend upon differing arrival-times of the muscle fibre action potentials at the electrode. Typically, the interpeak interval is about 3 ms.

These individual peaks derive from groups of muscle fibres called 'motor unit fractions'. They either have separate end-plate zones or may be innervated from different major axonal branches occurring relatively proximally. Each branch may have a different conduction time. The motor unit fraction concept should not be confused with the subunit theory (Buchthal 1961). There is no suggestion of anatomical subunits, the muscle fibres in each fraction being randomly scattered and intermingled with fibres of other motor units. The relationship of muscle fibres within the fraction is temporal rather than spatial.

Lower motor neurone lesions. Recordings with scanning EMG (Stålberg 1982, Stålberg & Dioszeghy 1991) show those features characteristic of the findings in CNEMG in neurogenic disease. These are increased mean duration, amplitude and number of phases of the MUP. As in normal muscle, the electrical front of MUPs within the whole motor unit is dispersed. No definite difference from the normal temporal dispersion of the

fractions occur. Some increase in the transverse distance over which spike components can be recorded is sometimes found. Because of volume conduction of action potentials of higher amplitude than normal, slow components of the motor unit can be recorded over a larger distance than found in normal muscle. Synchronous activity when found, occurs only within that area of muscle corresponding to the motor unit territory and there is no abnormally dispersed synchrony.

Primary myopathies. In primary myopathies, a normal or slightly reduced spatial dispersion together with increased temporal duration is found in scanning EMG. In addition, there may be silent areas in the territory (Fig. 29.15b). Individual action potentials recorded show either a reduced duration (due to fibre loss) or increased duration (due to the presence of late components) (Gootzen et al 1992). An increase in temporal duration is particularly striking in Duchenne dystrophy (Stålberg 1977, Hilton-Brown & Stålberg 1983a,b).

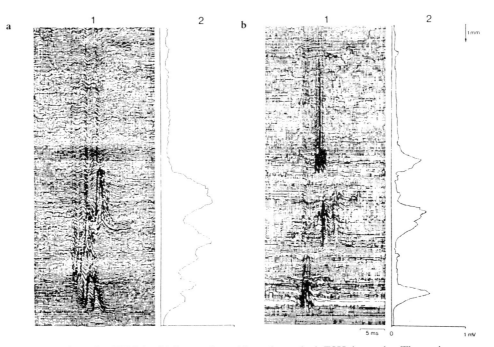

Fig. 29.15 Scanning EMG in tibialis anterior. **a** Normal muscle. **b** FSH dystrophy. The peak-to-peak amplitude in each sweep is measured and indicated to the right of the scans (a2, b2). Note in this example that the total length of the territory is slightly longer in the dystrophic muscle, but that the unit activity is interrupted by silent areas (reproduced with permission from Hilton-Brown & Stålberg 1983).

Single fibre EMG

The appearance of a single fibre action potential recorded by SFEMG electrodes has distinctive characteristics (Ekstedt 1964, Stålberg & Trontelj 1979). Single fibre potentials consist of smooth biphasic spikes, usually with an initial positive phase. The mean amplitude of single fibre potentials ranges from just under 1 mV to over 25 mV. A steep fall-off in the amplitude of the potentials occurs as the distance between the electrode and muscle fibre increases. The rise time of single muscle fibre action potentials is brief, ranging from 75 to 200 μs and total duration is about 1 ms.

Jitter. At about one in three sites where a single-fibre potential is recorded, a second potential clearly separate from the triggering spike is seen. The second wave form is not identical to the first, indicating that it is a separate muscle fibre action potential, not a repetitive discharge. The second spike fires with a fairly constant time relationship to the first, indicating that they both derive from a single motor unit. However, small variations in the time relationships occur between the two potentials which are termed 'jitter' (see Figs 29.24, 29.25a). The jitter value or interpotential interval variation relates to the safety-factor of neuromuscular transmission at the two neuromuscular junctions (see Part 2 below).

Jitter may be expressed as the mean of consecutive differences (MCD) of successive interpotential intervals (see Part 2 below). In normal muscle it varies between 5 and 55 μs MCD. Jitter of less than 5 μs between two action potentials and not increased by neuromuscular blocking agents, strongly suggests that the recordings come from a split portion of a single muscle fibre (Ekstedt & Stålberg 1969b). Similar low jitter values occur when one muscle fibre ephaptically excites another. Ephapsis is an insecure process and continued recording may demonstrate a sudden transmission failure, distinguishing the phenomenon from that due to fibre-splitting. Jitter in excess of 100 μs MCD is usually associated with transmission failure at one of the end-plates, manifesting as intermittent blocking of one of the spike components (see Fig. 29.26c). A recent collaborative study from many laboratories has reported reference values for jitter in many muscles obtained from control subjects of different ages (Ad Hoc Committee of the AAEM 1992).

Fibre density (FD). Single fibre electrodes are used to measure FD, the mean number of single muscle fibre spikes per recording site, at a minimum of 20 separate sites. Because two single fibre action potentials are recorded relatively infrequently at any one site, FD measured by this method is usually about 1.4–1.5 (Stålberg & Trontelj 1979, Gath & Stålberg 1982, Ad Hoc Committee of the AAEM 1992). There is some increase in FD with age, and a marked increase in the neurogenic disorders. In many myopathies muscle fibre degeneration, regeneration and reinnervation increase FD (Stålberg & Trontelj 1979, Hilton-Brown & Stålberg 1983a). The SFEMG electrode can also be used to deduce the presence of conduction block in motor axons. Thus SFEMG provides important insights into what has been termed the 'microphysiology' of the motor unit.

Muscle fibre propagation velocity. With a multilead SFEMG electrode the propagation velocity in single muscle fibres can be measured, since the action potential of one muscle fibre can be recorded at two sites along the electrode about 200 μm apart (Stålberg 1966). The conduction time between the two recording sites can be accurately assessed and the propagation velocity calculated. The major factor governing fibre velocity appears to be fibre size, the velocity being greater in larger fibres. Values range from 1.5 to 6.5 m/s, averaging about 3.5 m/s. In a majority of muscle fibres the velocity is also related to activity. The velocity falls during continuous activation and recovers after a brief rest. The relationship of velocity to prior activation is called the velocity recovery function (VRF). Two stimuli can be delivered to the fibre at different intervals and changes in response to the second or test stimulus observed. The muscle fibre is refractory for intervals of less than 3 ms. With interstimulus intervals of 3–10 ms the velocity in response to the test impulse is 80–100% of that of the conditioning stimulus. When interstimulus intervals from 10 to 500 ms are used, the test response velocity rises above that of the conditioning response reaching a maximum of 120% with interstimulus intervals of from 50 to 100 ms. The VRF reflects the process of repolarisation and provides information about the muscle fibre membrane characteristics while the velocity value gives an indirect measure of fibre diameter.

Lower motor neurone lesions. In denervated muscle, SFEMG shows that spontaneous fibrillations are the action potentials of single muscle fibres. At times, one denervated muscle fibre may trigger another by ephaptic excitation (Stålberg & Trontelj 1979, 1982). Using an intramuscular needle electrode to stimulate a denervated fibre electrically, ephaptic excitation of one or more muscle fibres adjacent to the stimulated fibre can be demonstrated. This explains the occasional more complex fibrillations sometimes recorded in CNEMG. SFEMG recordings have revealed the mechanisms underlying the generation of high-frequency repetitive discharges (Fig. 29.16a). The discharges originate in an abnormally excitable 'pacemaker' muscle fibre which drives ephaptically one or several adjacent fibres and is itself re-excited to continue the discharge until the onset of subnormal excitability in the pacemaker causes the cycle to halt abruptly (Stålberg & Trontelj 1982). The presence of ephaptic transmission is recognised by the finding of jitter of less than 5 μs MCD between individual spike components (Fig. 29.16b). This process may also cause the recruitment of a new muscle fibre or fibres during the discharge (Fig. 29.16c). Other fibres or groups of fibres may suddenly drop-out, the high discharge rate having resulted in the development of subnormal excitability.

Reinnervation. Increased FD occurs in partial denervation (Stålberg et al 1975). The FD reflects the balance between regenerative and degenerative processes and increases in FD of between two and five times normal are seen in chronic neurogenic disorders; smaller increases occur in more rapidly evolving states. Increased jitter and impulse blocking are characteristic of active neurogenic disorders, reflecting abnormal neuromuscular transmission at newly formed, functionally immature, motor end-plates (Fig. 29.17a). The jitter may be frequency-dependent, tending to be higher at faster discharge rates, and improves after intravenous edrophonium (Stålberg & Thiele 1972). Abnormal jitter and blocking are less striking in patients with slowly progressive diseases. In chronic spinal muscular atrophy there is usually a marked

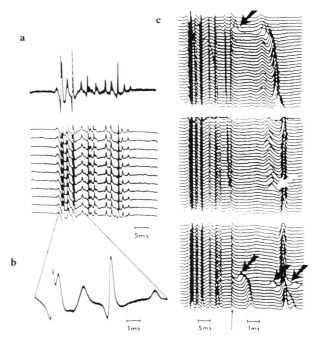

Fig. 29.16 Bizarre high-frequency repetitive discharges recorded by SFEMG. **a** Superimposed and rastered display of a complex containing 16 separate spikes. **b** Part of the recording presented at fast sweep speed to show abnormally low jitter (< 5 μs MCD) between components. **c** Complex showing recruitment of new components (black arrows) and blocking of one component (white arrow). Gaps in sequence correspond to interruptions in the recording.

increase in FD. Many complex potentials are present, often of prolonged duration (Fig. 29.17e–g). The final component of the complex may be 15–50 ms after the first. Extremely late potentials may result from slow conduction in new axonal sprouts, excessively long collaterals, end-plate formation at a distance from the main end-plate zone or to low propagation velocity in a reinnervated, atrophic muscle fibre. Marked increase in jitter and blocking are commonly seen in these complexes. The degree of jitter may vary in different complexes within the same muscle, being high with frequent blocking in some (Fig. 29.17a,b), consistent with recent reinnervation, and more moderate with less blocking in others (Fig. 29.17c) suggesting more advanced reinnervation. In yet other complexes (Fig. 29.17d) jitter is normal indicating that reinnervation has been completed (Stålberg & Fawcett 1984).

In the relatively rapidly progressive condition of

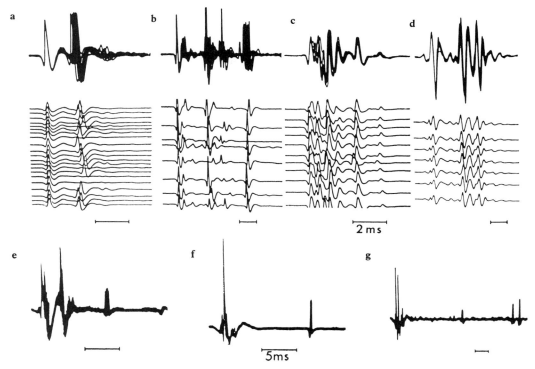

Fig. 29.17   SFEMG recordings in spinal muscular atrophy (SMA). **a–d** Fourteen-year-old girl with advanced disease. **a, b** Respectively show relatively simple and more complex potentials with increased jitter and blocking in all but the triggering spikes, indicating recent reinnervation of these muscle fibres. **c** Increased jitter in early components but no blocking, suggesting a more mature phase of reinnervation. **d** All the components are stable, indicating completed reinnervation. **e–g** Twenty-four-year-old man with chronic SMA. Complex potentials showing prolonged durations of between 14 and 44 ms.

motor neurone disease, FD is generally higher in muscles which are weak or showing wasting, but it is also increased in clinically normal muscles (Stålberg 1982). When symptoms present initially in the upper limb, they are associated with higher FD values, but individual values for different upper limb muscles do not differ significantly from one another (Swash 1980). An increase in FD is associated with reduced available muscle force suggesting that the reinnervation process is being outstripped by the rate of denervation.

In more slowly progressive neurogenic disorders, for example syringomyelia (Schwartz et al 1980), the action potential complexes show greater stability than those found in motor neurone disease. Depending on the muscle sampled, differing jitter values may be obtained. Higher values, often with blocking, occur in distal muscles of the arm where clinical weakness and wasting are more

likely. High jitter and frequent blocking is present in late components, being more marked the greater the delay in the late component.

Studies in patients with a previous history of poliomyelitis show increased jitter and blocking in affected muscles, indicating defective neuromuscular transmission (Wiechers & Hubbell 1981). Some of these patients are asymptomatic, but a significant proportion present with progressive muscle weakness, fatigue and muscle pain (the postpolio syndrome) following a period of clinical stability of 20–40 years after the acute poliomyelitis. It has been suggested that the neuromuscular transmission abnormality in these cases reflects metabolic failure of the anterior horn cells which have had to sustain a much enlarged motor unit. Fibres may then be lost from the motor unit which remains in a constant state of remodelling (Wiechers 1988). In severely affected muscles where only a few motor neurones survive, the overstretched motor neurone may never be able to supply the needs of normal transmission in all the fibres it has reinnervated. The extra fibres are thus maintained in a functional state at the expense of less than normal transmission (Wiechers 1988).

Various peripheral neuropathies have been studied by SFEMG (Thiele & Stålberg 1975). In the Guillain–Barré syndrome, for example, increased jitter may be found in a minority of patients as early as 14 days into the illness, before regeneration is established. The jitter is attributed to demyelination causing uncertain impulse transmission in the axon. If there is no associated axonal degeneration, there is no increase in FD, since collateral reinnervation will not take place without antecedent denervation. Axonal involvement is quite frequent and is signalled by the appearance of fibrillation. During recovery, FD increases with marked jitter at recently connected end-plates.

In chronic progressive peripheral neuropathies such as hereditary motor sensory neuropathy type I, both increased FD and jitter have been demonstrated (Thiele & Stålberg 1975). Surprisingly, in view of the mainly distal nature of the condition, increased FD occurs in the biceps brachii associated with increased jitter and impulse blocking. However, greater abnormality is present in the more distal tibialis anterior; here excess jitter can be seen in 25–50% of recordings and blocking in 5–20%. In other neuropathies, such as those related to alcohol and diabetes, similar changes in FD and jitter are found.

During reinnervation, when the SFEMG electrode is leading-off three or more spike components from one motor unit, two or more of them may disappear simultaneously (Fig. 29.18). This phenomenon is called concomitant blocking and appears to be due to transmission failure in a terminal nerve branch. Components showing concomitant blocking also share a common jitter value in relation to the other components recorded, called concomitant jitter. At low innervation rates, concomitant jitter is more likely; as the innervation rate increases concomitant blocking is manifest. The block may be improved by the injection of edrophonium chloride. Concomitant blocking can cause a fall in amplitude of the CMAP in response

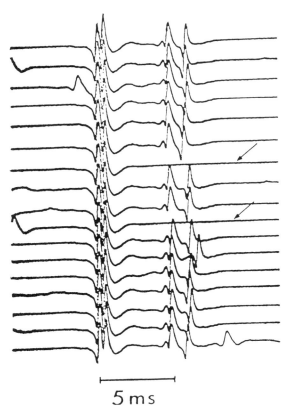

5 ms

Fig. 29.18 SFEMG recording from patient with motor neurone disease showing concomitant (paired) blocking of two components (arrows). Jitter between pairs of blocking spikes also increased, indicating that the concomitant blocking is occurring in the axon prior to the branching point to these fibres.

to repetitive nerve stimulation, simulating a defect in neuromuscular transmission when the actual defect is in the axon. At times, one or more late spike components occur with two latencies related to the remainder of the action potential complex. This phenomenon, which is called bimodal jitter, appears to relate to two differing transmission times along a single nerve branch, perhaps due to alternations between saltatory and continuous conduction along the fibre, occurring at a particular stage of axonal remyelination (Thiele & Staålberg 1974). The presence of an extra discharge of the motor unit within a brief interval has been noted in various lower motor neurone disorders (Fig. 29.19). These are usually followed by a compensatory pause at the next discharge. The

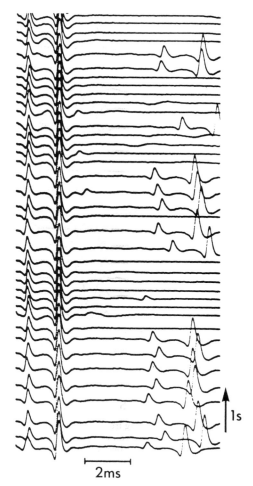

Fig. 29.19   SFEMG recording in tibialis anterior of a patient with HMSN type I showing extra discharges of a potential pair. The inter-discharge interval is prolonged following an extra discharge, helping to distinguish it from concomitant blocking. The interpotential interval is greater in the extra discharge than in the original discharge, due to the effects of refractoriness.

site of the generation of the extra discharge is thought to be at a point of hyperexcitability in the axon, possibly in an immature axonal sprout (Stålberg 1982).

Primary myopathies. SFEMG has contributed substantially to the understanding of the disturbances in the function in the motor unit brought about by primary muscle disease. The technique provides information concerning alterations in the anatomical arrangement of muscle fibres within the motor unit territory. Pathophy-

siological disturbances of neuromuscular transmission and muscle fibre function can be assessed.

The muscular dystrophies. SFEMG abnormalities have been described in all the commoner dystrophies including the Duchenne, Becker, facioscapulohumeral (FSH) and limb-girdle forms (Stålberg 1977, Hilton-Brown & Stålberg 1983a, Fawcett et al 1985a). FD is increased in Duchenne dystrophy from 2 to 2.5 times normal (Stålberg 1977). Multiple compound spikes are encountered in many recordings and may contain 3–6 or more rarely 10–15 separate action potentials derived from fibres in the same motor unit. In more advanced disease FD may decrease but remains above the normal range. The complex duration is prolonged and averages about 10 ms with a range of up to 40–50 ms between the first and last components. Unlike chronic neurogenic disorders, individual spikes tend to be well-dispersed throughout the complex, resulting in an increase in the mean interspike interval (MISI) of 1–3 ms (normal 0.6 ms). In Becker, FSH and limb-girdle dystrophies, FD is either normal or shows a mild to moderate increase and the mean duration of complex potentials and MISI are less prolonged (Figs 29.20, 29.21).

Increased jitter and blocking is commonly seen in Duchenne and Becker dystrophy with 20–40% of potentials showing increased jitter and 5–10% exhibiting blocking (Fig. 29.20e). In some recordings the magnitude of jitter may depend on the interdischarge interval (Fig. 29.21a). This effect tends to be especially marked in later components and results in slow trends, simultaneously affecting several elements of the multispike potential (Fig. 29.21b). This phenomenon probably relates to the propagation VRF and may be quite pronounced for the later spikes which tend to be generated by smaller muscle fibres. Rarely blocking may occur in the presence of normal jitter; more usually blocking of individual spikes is associated with very high jitter values. Concomitant jitter is seen occasionally and at times concomitant blocking of two or more spikes occurs. This may result from failure of axonal conduction (Fig. 29.20f) or from transmission failure at an end-plate supplying a split muscle fibre. (Fig. 29.20a) A rare occurrence is the recruitment of an additional fibre into the complex (Fig. 29.21c): this tends to

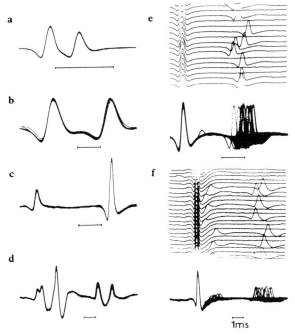

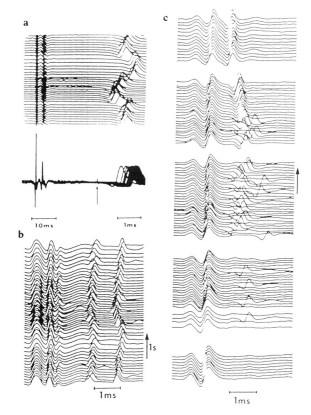

Fig. 29.20   SFEMG recordings in Becker muscular dystrophy. **a–d** Ten superimposed traces. **a** Abnormally low jitter, probably from a split muscle fibre. **b, c** Normal jitter. **d** Complex potential with five components and slightly increased duration (6.5 ms). **e** Increased jitter (235 μs MCD) and blocking (80%). **f** Concomitant jitter and blocking: relative jitter between pair is slightly increased (80 μs MCD), suggesting that the blocking is occurring in the nerve.

Fig. 29.21   SFEMG recordings in Becker muscular dystrophy. **a** Potential with a total duration of 22 ms. Influence of irregular discharge rate on IPI causing increased jitter in late component. **b** Multispike potential showing parallel changes in latencies to later components related to the discharge rate. **c** Recruitment of a third component, initially with high jitter and blocking and eventually normal jitter. Gaps in the sequence correspond to interruptions in the recording.

be seen at high discharge rates with disappearance of the spike as the rate decreases. Abnormally low jitter of less than 5 μs MCD, suggestive of split muscle fibres, may be seen in 2–16% of recordings from dystrophic muscle and is particularly common in Duchenne and Becker dystrophy (Hilton-Brown & Stålberg 1983a, Fawcett et al 1985a) (Fig. 29.20a).

Various factors may underlie the increase in FD in the muscular dystrophies. Closer packing of atrophic fibres may lead to an increase of their number within the pickup zone, although this effect will be countered by the fact that small fibres generate smaller action potentials which may not meet the required dimensions for inclusion in FD measurements. Most of the increase is probably accounted for by reinnervation of sequestered segments of fibres undergoing segmental necrosis and innervation of regenerated fibres originating from

satellite cells (Hilton-Brown & Stålberg 1983a). Reinnervation and the resultant immature endplates may also explain the presence of increased jitter in a proportion of the recordings. Split muscle fibres and fibres recruited by the process of ephaptic transmission also contribute to the increase in local FD within the motor unit.

Polymyositis. SFEMG findings vary between patients and even within the same patient in this condition, depending upon the stage and severity of the disease at the time of the investigation. In the early phases FD is usually only slightly increased and jitter is abnormal in many of the recordings, probably reflecting attempts at repair by the process of fibre regeneration and reinnervation. Neurogenic concomitant blocking and extra discharges occur suggesting neural involvement, most likely in newly formed and immature axonal sprouts. In later stages, more complex potentials may be recorded which tend to have increased durations. With successful treatment and recovery the FD increases and jitter improves, while the spike components of complex potentials become more synchronised and duration and MISI gradually shorten (Henriksson & Stålberg 1978).

Macro EMG

Normal muscle. An example of a Macro EMG recording from vastus lateralis in a normal subject is shown in Figure 29.22b. Normal values for Macro MUP amplitudes and areas have been obtained for the biceps brachii, vastus lateralis and tibialis anterior muscles in healthy subjects of various ages (Stålberg & Fawcett 1982). A strong positive correlation is found between amplitude and area measurements; therefore amplitude values are used since they can be manually determined if computer facilities are unavailable. In each individual a fairly wide scatter of values may be obtained, frequently with a positively skewed distribution. Consequently the median value is calculated in preference to the mean. The most important factor accounting for the wide range of amplitude values is that motor unit size is related to its recruitment threshold (size principle). This relationship is found in Macro EMG recordings (P. R. W. Fawcett, E. Stålberg & P. Hilton-Brown, unpublished results). Values in females appear to be slightly smaller than those for men. Macro MUP configuration is different in the three muscles, those in the biceps having a relatively simple shape with single or double peaks; in tibialis anterior two or more peaks are quite frequent. Most variation occurs in vastus lateralis where complex potentials are common. Despite this no significant difference is seen in the interval between the furthest peaks within each action potential. Mean interpeak interval is the same, being of the order of 3 ms. The median amplitude of the Macro MUPs varies from muscle to muscle and tends to increase with age over 60, particularly in vastus lateralis and tibialis anterior, probably reflecting age-related denervation and compensatory reinnervation.

Lower motor neurone lesions. In slowly progressive or longstanding partial denervation such as chronic spinal muscular atrophy, the Macro MUP is typically increased in amplitude (Stålberg & Fawcett 1984, Fawcett et al 1986)(Fig. 29.22c). In more rapidly progressive denervating processes, the Macro potential may remain of normal size despite SFEMG evidence of increased FD, indicating local collateral reinnervation. In adult motor neurone disease, increased amplitudes are found and there is an inverse correlation of amplitude with the degree of muscle weakness. Amplitudes of 10 times normal have been recorded from some motor units (Stålberg 1982). Longitudinal studies (Stålberg & Sanders 1984) have revealed an initial continuous increase in Macro MUP amplitude as compensatory reinnervation successfully keeps pace with the loss of motor units, followed by a decrease in amplitude and a parallel loss in muscle strength. The FD remains high, suggesting that there could be preferential loss of the largest motor units.

Primary myopathies. In muscular dystrophy the Macro MUP is usually either normal or slightly reduced in amplitude (Hilton-Brown & Stålberg 1983b) (Fig. 29.22a). Only occasionally is an increase in amplitude detected. The largest Macro MUPs are recorded in young patients with FSH dystrophy and may reflect compensatory hypertrophy. The relative preservation of the Macro MUP in dystrophy relates to the interaction of a variety of different pathophysiological processes as well as to inherent properties of the electrode. Loss of some muscle fibres and atrophy of others due to the dystrophy would be expected to reduce Macro MUP amplitude. The presence of fibres of widely differing diameters and different propagation velocities leading to desynchronisation of the motor unit would have a similar effect. Shrinkage of the muscle with closer packing of muscle fibres may increase the amplitude of the Macro MUP. The formation of new muscle fibres, fibre splitting and ephaptic transmission between muscle fibres will also increase Macro amplitude. Because there is a major contribution of relatively low-frequency components to the Macro MUP, the electrode is relatively insensitive

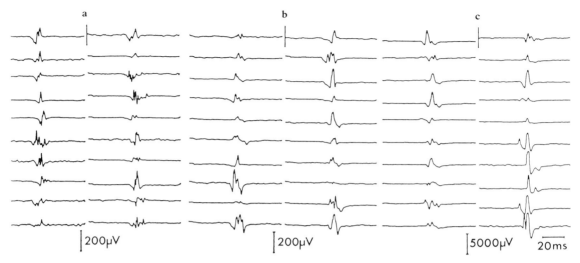

Fig. 29.22 Macro EMG recordings from vastus lateralis. **a** Becker muscular dystrophy. **b** Normal subject. **c** Spinal muscular atrophy (SMA). Note different amplitude calibration for SMA recording. Macro MUPs in dystrophic muscle are slightly smaller and tend to contain more peaks than normal. In SMA, Macro MUPs are frequently very large with amplitude in this case of between four and 50 times the normal median value for the decade. Median Macro MUP amplitude values: Becker 105 μV, normal 117 μV, SMA 2345 μV.

to alterations in volume conduction related to increased fibrosis or fatty infiltration.

Correlation between EMG and histology

Muscle and nerve biopsy may be employed in the investigation of neuromuscular disease and a number of reports have appeared in which the findings of muscle biopsy and EMG have been compared (Buchthal & Olsen 1970, Hausmanowa-Petrusewicz & Jedrzejowska 1971, Black et al 1974, Schwartz et al 1977, Schimrigk 1978, Buchthal & Kamieniecka 1982, Shields 1984). Hausmanowa-Petrusewicz & Jedrzejowska (1971) discuss the different roles of the EMG and biopsy; with the former it is possible to sample many muscles whereas biopsy is usually from a single site. A retrospective comparison of muscle biopsy, CNEMG and clinical data in 105 patients (Black et al 1974) showed in the 63 in whom both EMG and biopsy were needed to attempt a diagnosis, the overall agreement was greater than 90% with spinal muscular atrophy causing most difficulty. In a study of quantitative EMG and biopsy—with histology, histochemistry or both—EMG agreed with clinical diagnosis in 87% of patients with myopathy and 91% with neurogenic pathology

(Buchthal & Kamieniecka 1982). Muscle biopsy gave similar results but was more specific in identifying particular pathologies. When SFEMG is carried out with open muscle biopsy, correlations between FDs and histochemical evidence of fibre grouping is possible (Schwartz et al 1977). CNEMG has been used in a somewhat similar fashion (Petajan & Thurman 1981) with the use of an emulsion to localise the site of recording. Abnormal MUP duration, amplitude and recruitment intervals were seen to correlate with neurogenic atrophy in the biopsy.

Comparisons between SFEMG fibre density and quantitative estimates of histological fibre type grouping (Enclosed Fibre Count, EFC) in patients with various neuromuscular disorders showed a close correlation between FD and EFC in those with reinnervation (Fawcett et al 1985b). FD was found to be more sensitive to minor disturbances of motor unit architecture in myopathies and mild neurogenic states.

EMG findings in various myopathies

It is not suggested that these abnormalities necessarily allow differentiation between different disease entities.

Findings in Duchenne dystrophy depend on the stage of the disease at which the examination is made. Insertion activity may be increased early in the disease together with fibrillation and positive sharp waves (Buchthal & Rosenfalck 1966). In clinically weak muscle, short-duration, low-voltage, excessively polyphasic MUPs are seen (Kugelberg 1949, Pinelli & Buchthal 1953, Buchthal & Rosenfalck 1963). Complex, long-duration polyphasic potentials with variable or stable late components can be seen.

The use of a trigger and delay-line in CNEMG and information gained from SFEMG and other techniques allows a better understanding of the changes occurring in dystrophic muscle. Originally it was felt that the short-duration potentials indicated a marked loss of fibres from the motor unit. The increased FD and relatively normal Macro MUP amplitudes are at odds with this view, but scanning EMG has shown the probable explanation to be a redistribution of muscle fibres within the unit territory giving rise to local concentrations of fibres separated by silent areas (Hilton-Brown & Stålberg 1983a,b). The occasional high amplitude MUP may be due to a hypertrophied fibre close to the electrode, to restriction of volume conduction due to local fibrosis or most often to a locally increased FD. Increased recruitment at low tension is often a striking feature (Buchthal & Rosenfalck 1963). Macro MUP amplitudes are normal or reduced in contrast to the increased sizes seen in chronic neurogenic diseases. As the disease progresses, fatty replacement and fibrosis result in a reduction in insertional activity and spontaneous potentials become harder to find. Eventually in severely affected muscle the fall-out of fibres is such that there are many silent areas in the territory seen in the scanning EMG and the spatial dispersion of the unit is reduced. At this stage an isolated small amplitude potential may be the only activity seen at any one CNEMG recording site.

The suggestion in 1963 by Barwick and by Van den Bosch that some female carriers of the gene responsible for Duchenne muscular dystrophy showed minor CNEMG abnormalities, aroused considerable interest in detecting evidence of a mild myopathy in these subjects. The need to quantify small deviations from normal provided

an impetus to refining existing methods and to the development of new methods of EMG analysis (Willison 1968). There is a shortening of muscle refractory period in a proportion of carriers (Caruso & Buchthal 1965) and there are changes in the individual MUP parameters which allow identification of 50–70% of definite carriers (Davey & Woolf 1965, Emery et al 1966, Smith et al 1966, Gardner-Medwin 1968, Hausmanowa-Petrusewicz et al 1968, Willison 1968, Moosa et al 1972). However CNEMG has always played a subservient role to biochemical studies in carrier detection and recent developments in recombinant DNA technology should soon consign these observations to history.

In the Becker type muscular dystrophy (Bradley et al 1978) spontaneous fibrillation and positive waves are commonly recorded. Volitional activity consists of both low-amplitude short-duration and high-amplitude longer duration units. Interference pattern density and amplitude are often reduced and occasional high-frequency and myotonic discharges occur. Symmetrical involvement of proximal muscles is the rule and the paraspinal muscles often show complex repetitive discharges (Kimura 1989). SFEMG and Macro EMG studies (Fawcett et al 1985a) show a mild to moderate FD increase and abnormal jitter affecting around 10% of potential pairs. Blocking is seen in up to 5% and low jitter suggesting fibre splitting in about 6–13% of pairs. Concomitant jitter and blocking are infrequent. Both abnormally large and small Macro MUPs occur but the majority of amplitudes are normal. There is little evidence of a neurogenic component other than that related to muscle fibre regeneration and reinnervation. Carrier detection in Becker dystrophy is less satisfactory than in Duchenne and only a minority of carriers have CNEMG abnormalities (Gardner-Medwin 1968).

The 'limb-girdle syndrome' has been used to describe a heterogenous group of disorders having in common proximal muscle weakness and a sporadic or autosomal recessive pattern of occurrence. As well as a hereditary primary myopathy (dystrophy), diseases such as polymyositis, metabolic myopathies, some congenital myopathies and spinal muscular atrophy may present in this way. CNEMG may help in distinguishing neurogenic causes for the syndrome. Inflammatory myopathy tends to produce more florid EMG abnormalities than those seen in limb-girdle dystrophy which resemble those found in Duchenne dystrophy but are generally milder. SFEMG shows increased FD and jitter (Hilton-Brown & Stålberg 1983a). Scanning EMG shows silent areas in the motor unit territories but the corridors examined are of normal extent.

Facioscapulohumeral dystrophy may similarly be mimicked clinically by spinal muscular atrophy and by inflammatory and metabolic myopathies. CNEMG may aid in identifying neurogenic disorders but presently has a lesser role in distinguishing between the various myopathies. Facioscapulohumeral dystrophy shows CNEMG, SFEMG and scanning EMG abnormalities very similar to those of limb-girdle dystrophy (Hilton-Brown & Stålberg 1983a,b).

Oculopharyngeal dystrophy may resemble myasthenia clinically, with ptosis and dysphagia developing in late life but the CMAP, although sometimes of low amplitude, shows no significant alteration on repetitive stimulation. CNEMG shows brief, often polyphasic, low-amplitude MUPs and no spontaneous activity in proximal upper limb muscles (Murphy & Drachman 1968, Bosch et al 1979).

Hereditary distal myopathy (Welander 1951) is a dominantly inherited, or occasionally sporadic disorder, affecting mainly or exclusively distal limb muscles. CNEMG shows almost total loss of MUPs in the most severely affected muscles with abundant positive waves, fibrillation and scanty fasciculation. These findings suggest a neuropathy but distal motor and sensory nerve conduction is normal. Profuse recruitment of small, complex brief potentials in less affected muscles points to a myopathy, confirmed pathologically (Miller et al 1979). In the more severe sporadic form, similar, less florid CNEMG abnormalities also occur in proximal muscles (Markesbury et al 1974a).

Myotonic dystrophy is a dominantly inherited disorder which may be detected shortly after birth as congenital myotonic dystrophy or may present in later life. Infants present with neonatal hypotonia without clinical myotonia which is absent until later childhood (Zellweger & Ionasescu 1973,

Harper 1975, Swift et al 1975, Lazaro et al 1979). EMG myotonia is less distinct and easy to detect in the presence of prominent end-plate activity due to the multiple end-plates on single muscle fibres and the larger percentage of total muscle occupied by the end-plate zone in neonates. The infantile myotonic discharge is of lower voltage, briefer duration and shows less frequency variation than that seen in adults. Nerve conduction is in the normal range for the age of the infant. Only occasionally are low-voltage polyphasic MUPs found in infants and children; usually MUP parameters are normal (Zellweger & Ionasescu 1973). In childhood the electrophysiological expression of the disease is variable so that the absence of myotonic discharge in a child at risk does not exclude the diagnosis (Dodge et 1965).

Myotonic discharges occur in all affected adults and also appear in roughly half the relatives at risk, who have subclinical or mild disease (Bundey et al 1970, Polgar et al 1972), although an incomplete syndrome in which some individuals do not show myotonia has been reported in Labrador (Pryse-Philips et al 1982). In adults MUP abnormalities are found in distal muscles, polyphasic potentials being produced by regeneration and reinnervation. MUP amplitude may show progressive reduction when an isolated unit is followed with the delay-line, as sarcolemmal membrane changes cause progressive inactivation of individual muscle fibres of the unit. Recovery of MUP amplitude takes place with rest, though very gradual recovery may accompany continuing exertion. The effect of repetitive stimulation is discussed in Part 2. Abnormal nerve conduction has been reported in older patients, the changes being variable in severity (Messina et al 1976, Panayiotopoulos & Scarpalezos 1976, McComas et al 1978, Roohi et al 1981). Suggested causes for the neuropathy have included premature age-dependent neuropathy, the presence of associated disturbances such as alveolar hypoventilation and diabetes as well as the idea that the neuropathy is an integral part of the disease.

In myotonia congenita and paramyotonia no abnormalities in individual MUPs are seen and nerve conduction is normal. Myotonia is widespread both clinically and electrophysiologically. Other spontaneous activity such as fibrillation and positive discharges are also evident. In paramyotonia, exposure to cold has dramatic effects. It may produce increasing muscular stiffness and in some families this is paradoxical, being aggravated by muscular activity. The slow relaxation is not myotonic, there being no EMG after-discharge. Cooling to 30–25°C results in the disappearance of clinical and electrical myotonia and the falling temperature is associated with transient intense fibrillation. Flaccid muscle paralysis follows this phase, outlasting rewarming by several hours (Haass et al 1981). In vitro studies have shown a progressive depolarisation of paramyotonic muscle fibres from −80 to −40 mV: this is the probable explanation of the transient fibrillation, muscle weakness and paralysis as depolarisation first passes the electrical threshold and proceeds into inexcitability (Lehmann-Horn et al 1981). Cooling increases sodium conductance, possibly by a failure of proper closure of Na^+ channels after they open in the cold. Muscular activity accelerates the process by allowing Na^+ channel opening (Lehmann-Horn et al 1981). The lignocaine derivative, tocainide, a Na^+ channel blocker may prevent paramyotonic symptoms (Ricker et al 1980). The reason for the development of the muscle stiffness remains obscure. In myotonia congenita exposure to cold has no such effect, the severity of the myotonia is increased (Ricker et al 1977, Nielson et al 1982) but no paralysis or non-myotonic muscle stiffness occurs. Thomsen's disease is an autosomal dominant disorder but Becker (1977) has described a recessive form which he called recessive generalised myotonia. In this condition the EMG may be helpful in genetic counselling, as myotonic discharges may be present without clinical myotonia in heterozygotes (Harel et al 1979, Zellweger et al 1980). Decremental CMAP changes with repetitive stimulation and progressive reduction of individual MUP amplitudes with exercise are a feature of the recessive (Becker) variety of myotonia congenita (Aminoff et al 1977) (see Fig. 29.30). SFEMG shows that the MUP is reflecting similar changes in single fibre action potentials as the defective repolarisation capacity of the sarcolemmal membrane causes an extra negativity during the decaying phase of the potential (Stålberg 1977) (Fig. 29.23b). During high-frequency discharges there are continuous changes in the shape of the action potentials, often

with an initial increase in amplitude followed by a fall and prolongation of their rise-time and duration (Stålberg & Trontelj 1979) (Fig. 29.23a,b).

Although myotonic discharges are said to occur in the Schwartz–Jampel syndrome (Aberfeld et al 1956, Spaans et al 1990), other reports suggest that the activity is not truly myotonic (Taylor et al 1972, Fowler et al 1974, Cao et al 1978). Continuous, widespread, low-voltage activity is present, with no or only a slight tendency to wax and wane. The activity accounts for the persistent muscle contraction observed clinically and both continue during sleep, general and local anaesthesia. D-tubocurarine abolishes the discharge in most instances but persistence has been reported in a single case (Spaans et al 1990). In this patient, single fibre EMG studies showed a series of individual fibre discharges, firing at rates of 30–80 Hz. Some dis-

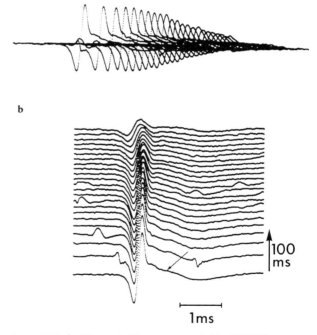

Fig. 29.23 **a** Myotonic discharge recorded by SFEMG showing progressive decline of the single muscle fibre action potential. **b** Raster display of same discharge. Note the extra negativity during the decaying phase (arrow) which probably corresponds to defective repolarisation of the muscle fibre membrane. The fall in amplitude is accompanied by prolongation of the rise time and total duration of the action potential.

charge series showed waxing and waning of the amplitude, while others were more constant. There were no signs of reinnervation on muscle histology and the authors concluded that the discharges were truly myogenic in origin. Further in vitro studies on a muscle sample from the same case (Lehmann-Horn et al 1990) showed evidence of abnormal sodium channel gating and reduced chloride conductance in the muscle fibre membrane which could account for the myotonic activity. Phenytoin reduces the discharges but procaine amide, quinidine and diazepam are ineffective. There is evidence of hyperirritability of the muscle fibre membrane but the bursts produced by needle movement are of constant frequency and cease abruptly, unlike those of myotonia (Taylor et al 1972). Nerve conduction velocities are normal and volitional MUPs have been described as small and brief or normal.

Congenital fibre-type disproportion is a genetically determined cause of infantile hypotonia often with associated contractures and skeletal deformities. CNEMG findings are variable, being normal in many patients, others show short-duration, low-amplitude and polyphasic MUPs with no spontaneous activity and in some the striking feature is fibrillation, positive waves and complex high-frequency discharges (Kimura 1989).

Myotubular or centronuclear myopathy is a rare disorder which may present as infantile hypotonia. Striking spontaneous activity occurs, fibrillations, positive waves, high-frequency repetitive activity and even myotonic discharges being present. MUPs are of low voltage, polyphasic and of brief duration (Munsat et al 1969, Hawkes & Absolon 1975, Radu et al 1977, Gil-Peralta et al 1978, Bill et al 1979). Clinical myotonia is a rare accompaniment (Gil-Peralta et al 1978). These abnormalities are much more florid than are those seen in other congenital myopathies.

Central core disease may also cause infantile hypotonia or be recognised in later life. There may be mild neurogenic features such as reduced CMAP amplitude, slight slowing of nerve conduction and the terminal innervation ratio is increased. No spontaneous activity is present and MUPs are often small, with excessive early recruitment but large polyphasic units also occur. An increased number of MUP late components is seen and

SFEMG reveals increased FD (Mrozek et al 1970, Isaacs et al 1975, Coërs et al 1976, Cruz Martinez et al 1979, Lopez-Terradas & Conde Lopez 1979).

Nemaline myopathy is another cause of a relatively non-progressive hypotonia evident early in life and often first suspected by associated dysmorphism. CNEMG reveals no spontaneous or abnormal insertion activity with short duration MUPs and increased polyphasia (Shy et al 1963, Kuitonnen et al 1972, Radu & Ionasescu 1972), which become more pronounced with increasing age (Wallgren-Pettersson et al 1989).

Acid maltase deficiency may present as a fatal infantile hypotonia and in childhood or in later life as a limb-girdle myopathy. Pathologically there is anterior horn cell involvement and a vacuolar myopathy. CNEMG shows the most florid changes in paraspinal and gluteal muscles with increased insertion activity, fibrillation, complex repetitive discharges and true myotonic discharges but no clinical myotonia. MUPs are of low voltage, recruit early and are generally brief with increased polyphasia. No disturbance of neuromuscular transmission has been found and nerve conduction is normal (Hogan et al 1969, Engel 1970, Engel et al 1973).

Debrancher enzyme deficiency causes hypotonia, failure to thrive, hepatomegaly and hypoglycaemia with a proximal myopathy. CNEMG reveals spontaneous activity, often profuse and small, brief MUPs (Brunberg et al 1971, DiMauro et al 1979).

Mitochondrial myopathies are an extremely heterogeneous group of disorders and may be familial, varying in mode of inheritance and clinical expression. A progressive external ophthalmoplegia with additional features may be seen and a facioscapulohumeral syndrome has been reported. CNEMG shows shortened MUP duration without spontaneous activity and SFEMG reveals increased FD and increased jitter in complex potentials and normal nerve conduction (Hudgson et al 1972, Olsen et al 1972, Fawcett et al 1982a, Krendel et al 1987). The presence of increased jitter in patients with fatiguability and ptosis should not therefore be automatically taken to indicate a diagnosis of myasthenia gravis and in equivocal cases a muscle biopsy may be indicated to exclude the possibility of a mitochondrial myopathy.

Lipid storage myopathies include those due to carnitine palmitoyl transferase deficiency and other defects of fatty acid oxidation. Recurrent myoglobinuria and painful muscle cramps are the clinical features of carnitine palmitoyl transferase deficiency. Nerve conduction and CNEMG are normal between attacks (Engel et al 1970). Other lipid storage disorders result in progressive weakness of limb-girdle muscles, with or without episodes of muscle pain and myoglobinuria. CNEMG shows spontaneous fibrillation in more than half of those affected. MUPs are brief, small with excessive early recruitment and nerve conduction is usually normal. The occasional presence of a neuropathy has been described (Markesbury et al 1974b).

Polymyositis and dermatomyositis are the commonest forms of inflammatory myopathy. In acute untreated patients, fibrillation and positive sharp waves are abundant and are most obvious in superficial layers of the paraspinal muscles. Fragility of the muscle fibre membrane as a result of inflammation is suggested as a reason for the very large numbers of positive sharp waves sometimes present (Streib et al 1979). Other spontaneous activity, high-frequency repetitive discharge in particular, together with myotonic discharge may be found. CNEMG examination reveals markedly polyphasic MUPs, initially of short duration. Regeneration and reinnervation result in long polyphasic units with variable late components. The excessive spontaneous activity tends to disappear with treatment but may recur with flare-ups of the disorder (Mechler 1974, Bohan et al 1977). In patients on corticosteroid drugs, increasing clinical weakness without EMG evidence of muscle fibre irritability should raise suspicion of a steroid myopathy (Sandstedt et al 1982). Response to corticosteroid treatment can be monitored by serial quantitative EMG study as increase in amplitude and duration of MUPs accompanies clinical improvement but polyphasia improves much more slowly (Mechler 1974, Sandstedt et al 1982). In acute myositis the EMG changes may be more localised within a single muscle than is the case in dystrophy; focal forms of myositis have also been recorded. SFEMG shows increased jitter and blocking where immature connections have been made with early regenerating muscle fibres and FD is increased. It is still not clear whether the denervation and reinnervation in this disease is simply due to muscle regeneration or whether damage to the terminal innervation by inflammation is a significant factor (Henriksson & Stålberg 1978).

CMAPs may show decrement or more rarely an incremental response on repetitive stimulation. Chronic polymyositis results in long-duration, often relatively stable MUPs (Mechler 1974). Fibrosis causes the development of silent areas with increased resistance to electrode movement and an apparent reduction in CNEMG recruitment may occur in late-stage disease. CNEMG abnormalities are more widespread and uniform in advanced disease. Occasional large amplitude potentials may be generated by local FD increase. Polymyositis may complicate connective tissue disorders and may be relatively mild with CNEMG changes limited to the paraspinal muscles. In these collagen diseases, peripheral neuropathy or mononeuritis may occur with reduced CMAP amplitude, altered nerve conduction and reduced or absent recruitment together with fibrillation.

Inclusion body myositis is slowly progressive and often mainly distal in distribution and EMG changes similar to those of polymyositis are seen. Parasitic and sarcoid myopathies show more scattered and more localised involvement than is usual in polymyositis. At the sites of involvement, CNEMG abnormalities, including evidence of local hyperirritability of muscle, can be seen. Patients infected with the human immunodeficiency virus (HIV) may occasionally present with a severe acute necrotising myopathy with evidence of florid spontaneous fibrillation and positive sharp wave activity on EMG (Lange et al 1988).

Various disorders of muscular function occur in endocrine disease. In hypothyroidism muscular manifestations are common (Rao et al 1980). Myoidema is a localised knot of contracting muscle occurring in response to percussion of the muscle or other direct mechanical stimulation. Brief contractions can be seen in normal subjects but gross and prolonged contractions occur in hypothyroidism (Salick & Pearson 1967). An initial short burst of action potentials accompanies the percussion and the whole fascicle tightens and remains in a state of electrically silent contraction for 30–60 s and then slowly disappears (Denny-

Brown & Pennybacker 1938). This form of electrically silent contraction, called a contracture, may be due to a prolongation of the active state due to excessive release or to slow re-accumulation of calcium by the sarcoplasmic reticulum (Mizusawa et al 1983). Enlargement of muscle may gradually develop in patients with myxoedema and pain and muscular stiffness are commonly present (Wilson & Walton 1959, Norris & Panner 1966). Evidence of muscular irritability with increased insertional activity, fibrillation, positive sharp activity and high frequency discharges may be recorded (Åström et al 1961) and true clinical and electromyographic myotonia has been observed (Venables et al 1978). Quantitative CNEMG of an unselected group of hypothyroid patients revealed shortened MUP duration in proximal muscles in 70% and excessive polyphasic potentials in 90% although only 20% of the patients had significant muscular weakness (Rao et al 1980).

Symptomatic thyrotoxic myopathy (Sanderson & Adey 1952) is a relatively infrequent presentation of thyrotoxicosis, but in hyperthyroidism quantitative CNEMG is almost always abnormal and the changes are most marked in patients with clinical weakness (Ramsay 1965, Buchthal 1970, Puvanendran et al 1979). Shortening of the mean MUP duration and an increased proportion of polyphasic MUPs are found. Spontaneous activity is infrequent.

Proximal myopathy is often a prominent feature of Cushing's syndrome and the CNEMG shows shortening of MUP duration without spontaneous activity (Muller & Kugelberg 1959). The iatrogenic disorder associated with the use of synthetic corticosteroids, especially triamcinolone, shows similar CNEMG changes (Williams 1959, Yates 1963, Coomes 1965).

Addison's disease is characterised by generalised muscular weakness which may be associated with shortened mean MUP duration (Buchthal 1970). Nelson's syndrome (increasing cutaneous pigmentation following adrenalectomy for Cushing's syndrome) may be associated with proximal muscle weakness. A pituitary tumour secreting high levels of ACTH is present and in the patients with weakness, Prineas et al (1968) demonstrated the presence of a lipid storage myopathy with quantitative CNEMG studies showing reduced mean MUP duration, an increased percentage of polyphasic MUPs and hyperirritability of the muscle with high frequency discharges, fibrillations and positive sharp waves.

Patients with acromegaly often complain of muscular weakness and of easy fatigability: these complaints are due to a myopathy (Lundberg et al 1970, Mastaglia et al 1970). Mastaglia et al (1970) showed a striking reduction in mean MUP duration in proximal muscles in more than half of a group of acromegalics including those without overt weakness. Spontaneous activity was not a feature of the CNEMG.

Vicale (1949) drew attention to the mild proximal weakness present in some patients with hyperparathyroidism. Other workers (Bischoff & Esslen 1965, Frame et al 1968) confirmed these observations and showed that there were changes in the CNEMG suggestive of a myopathy without spontaneous activity. Hudson et al (1970) described the familial variety of this disorder. Many diseases in which osteomalacia develops are associated with proximal muscle weakness and myopathic EMG abnormalities.

Although neuropathy is well recognised in chronic renal failure and in patients receiving regular haemodialysis, there are some in whom gross proximal weakness is due to a myopathy (Lindholm 1968, Floyd et al 1974, Hudgson & Barwick 1974) with shortening of the mean MUP duration and increased numbers of polyphasic potentials without spontaneous activity. Improvement in muscle function followed renal allografts and improvement was also produced by vitamin D therapy in undialysed patients.

Axonal neuropathy is the commonest toxic complication of alcoholism affecting the neuromuscular system but several types of myopathy may be seen. Acute muscular necrosis occurs in some chronic alcoholics during a drinking bout (Hed et al 1962). CNEMG shows copious spontaneous activity, reduced MUP duration and polyphasia. A syndrome of chronic proximal weakness and atrophy can also be seen in chronic alcoholism when signs of a neuropathy are absent or mild (Ekbom et al 1964, Perkoff et al 1967, Rossouw et al 1976). The CNEMG showed shortened MUP duration without spontaneous activity. Similar changes are seen in chronic alcoholics without overt clinical muscle involvement (Ekbom et al 1964, Faris & Reyes 1971). Another problem is the occasional development of acute hypokalaemic paralysis during an alcoholic debauch (Rubenstein & Wainapel 1977). This paralysis develops progressively over several days and spares the respiratory and bulbar muscles. The EMG abnormalities are florid with numerous spontaneous fibrillations resolving rapidly with potassium replacement.

The clinical features and the nature of the underlying defect in periodic paralysis are discussed elsewhere in this volume (see Ch. 17). The EMG changes seen in hyperkalaemic periodic paralysis are as follows. Between attacks there may be increased insertional activity with myotonic discharges and high-frequency complex repetitive activity. In attacks there is an increase in the myotonic activity and transient copious fibrillations occur in some patients (Morrison 1960) but neither mechanical nor electrical stimuli will excite the muscle. Jitter is usually normal between attacks but shows a significant increase as an attack begins and blocking rapidly develops. The abnormalities are increased by cooling and when the myotonia is pronounced, repetitive nerve stimulation may result in a decremental response (Lundberg et al 1974). A permanent myopathy sometimes develops. Recent in vitro studies (Lehmann-Horn et al 1983) suggest that the depolarisation of the fibre membrane, associated with the paralytic attacks, is connected to an increased sodium ion conductance.

In hypokalaemic periodic paralysis there is a reduction in the number of motor units available for voluntary recruitment and a reduced or absent muscle response to motor nerve stimulation (Gordon et al 1970). An incremental response to nerve stimulation at 10–25 Hz may be seen in muscles only mildly affected but does not occur in the weaker muscles (Grob et al 1957, Campa & Sanders 1974). Permanent progressive myopathy with associated EMG abnormalities occurs in some patients (Pearson 1964). Rüdel et al (1984) suggest on the basis of in vitro studies that the basic defect lies in a reduced membrane excitability and an increased sodium conductance and that both these defects are aggravated when the extracellular potassium concentration falls.

Chronic painless proximal myopathy is the commonest form of drug-induced myopathy and a particularly severe form occurs in some patients receiving chloroquine medication. In contrast to most other drug-induced myopathies, spontaneous activity abounds with fibrillations, positive waves, high-frequency repetitive activity and even true myotonic discharges are seen. In addition the typical volitional changes of a myopathy are seen and the presence of a neuropathy which may also complicate this therapy is revealed by abnormal nerve conduction (Mastaglia et al 1977 and see Ch. 28).

Neuromuscular transmission defects. Normal fatigue during voluntary contraction is accompanied by drop-out of motor unit potentials rather than change in their form. Lindsley (1935) found that the fatigue of myasthenia was accompanied by a marked fluctuation in amplitude of individual MUPs. Mean MUP duration is significantly shortened in myasthenia gravis (Oosterhuis et al 1972), especially in clinically weak muscles. Examination of MUPs isolated by use of a delay-line displays alterations in motor unit dimensions during sustained recruitment as more and more individual end-plates show conduction block. A high-pass filter (Payan 1978) assists in the demonstration of unstable motor units in the presence of abnormal neuromuscular transmission but CNEMG results are difficult to quantify and SFEMG and/or the response to repetitive nerve stimulation may be preferred. Studies of nerve conduction have shown an increase in terminal latency and prolongation of the CMAP at the end of a train of tetanic stimuli, greater than that which occurs in normal subjects. In some severely affected cases there is significant slowing of the motor conduction velocity during a tetanus (Preswick 1965). The distal latency of the CMAP may sometimes be prolonged in the resting state (Slomic et al 1968).

PART 2
TESTING OF NEUROMUSCULAR TRANSMISSION

INTRODUCTION

Primary disorders of neuromuscular transmission, such as myasthenia gravis and the myasthenic (Lambert–Eaton) syndrome are uncommon. However recent advances in understanding of their pathophysiology have led to improvements in management and prognosis. Early and accurate diagnosis is important if the patient is to benefit. Many treatments, e.g. long-term immunosuppression, using steroids or other drugs, thymectomy and plasmapheresis carry risks, so that diagnostic techniques must not only be sensitive but also objective and reliable.

The anatomy and physiology of the normal neuromuscular junction have been fully detailed elsewhere (see Chs 1 & 7). Normal and abnormal pharmacology of neuromuscular transmission has also been considered (see Ch. 5). Methods available for the study of neuromuscular transmission in man are described here and the results obtained both in the normal and in various disease states are discussed. Neuromuscular transmission defects may be divided into two broad groups according to whether the defect is presynaptic or postsynaptic. In the former, the problem may lie in the synthesis, storage, availability and release from the nerve terminal of ACh; postsynaptic disorders include abnormalities of ACh receptors, the phase of (end-plate) potential depolarisation, initiation of the muscle fibre action potential and ACh removal.

METHODS FOR STUDYING NEUROMUSCULAR TRANSMISSION IN MAN

In vitro microelectrode studies on muscle biopsy specimens

Much of our knowledge of the pathophysiology of various defects of neuromuscular transmission derives from intracellular recordings in the region of the motor end-plate. Microelectrodes inserted into resting muscle in this situation reveal intermittent small depolarisations across the postsynaptic membrane, so-called miniature end-plate potentials (mepps). These correspond to the random release of quanta of ACh, each of which is derived from one of the many vesicles situated in the presynaptic portion of the nerve terminal. In normal human muscle, mepp frequency is of the order of 0.2 Hz (Elmqvist 1973), while mepp amplitude is about 1 mV, much lower than the threshold for initiation of an action potential. Invasion of the terminal by a nerve impulse results in a marked increase in the number of quanta of ACh released, producing a much larger depolarisation called the end-plate potential (epp) which reaches threshold and gives rise to an action potential in the adjacent muscle fibre membrane.

The amplitude of the epp is variable and is influenced by preceding activity. During a high-frequency train of stimuli the first few epps show increasing amplitude (facilitation), soon followed by a progressive decline, or depressive phase (Katz 1966). At slower impulse rates, e.g. 1–3 Hz, there is no early increase; instead a steady reduction of epp amplitude occurs and eventually reaches a plateau. A few seconds after a tetanic train or period of intense activity, a longer-lasting increase in epp amplitude develops, corresponding to the phase of post-tetanic potentiation which may persist for 1–2 minutes. Subsequently during a period of depression (post-tetanic exhaustion), the epp amplitude gradually falls. The mechanisms underlying these events are not fully understood, but both facilitation and potentiation may relate to accumulation of calcium ions in the presynaptic region, leading to elevated ACh mobilisation by increasing vesicle fusion with the nerve terminal (Katz & Miledi 1968). Desensitisation of the ACh receptors has been suggested as the cause of the phase of exhaustion (Gage 1976), but the presence of normal-sized mepps would seem to be against this theory.

In normal muscle these fluctuations in epp size are of no consequence, because they remain well above the threshold for the generation of action potentials, reflecting the high safety-factor for neuromuscular transmission. However in pathological states in which the safety-factor is lowered either by reduced availability of ACh (presynaptic) or reduced effect of transmitter (postsynaptic), these normal phenomena become significant, resulting in defective neuromuscular transmission (Elmqvist et al 1964).

In man in vitro techniques for studying the neuromuscular junction have been developed, employing motor point biopsies, mainly from the intercostal muscles (Elmqvist et al 1964), but also more recently from anconeus (Maselli et al 1991) and vastus lateralis (Slater et al 1992).

Repetitive stimulation techniques

The observation by Harvey & Masland (1941) that repetitive nerve stimulation resulted in a decline in the amplitude of the compound muscle action potential (CMAP), in patients with myasthenia gravis, led to its development as a clinical neurophysiological test of disorders of neuromuscular transmission. Since its introduction, various modifications of the technique have been described, designed to increase its sensitivity when used in patients with localised or subclinical disease.

Supramaximal motor nerve stimulation is carried out as in determining motor conduction velocity (see Ch. 30). Conventional surface stimulating electrodes are satisfactory but must be very securely applied, as close as possible to the underlying nerve to ensure stimulation of the whole nerve trunk without using unduly high and unpleasant stimulus intensities. As it is essential that the stimulus remains supramaximal throughout the stimulus train an intensity of 1.5 times maximal is used. This allows for any slight electrode movement in relation to the nerve occurring during the course of the muscle contraction. Prior preparation of the overlying skin with spirit and mild abrasion will improve conductance and slightly lower the required stimulus intensity. Some authors (Slomic et al 1968) prefer subcutaneous needle electrodes inserted close to the nerve, reducing the stimulus strength needed and the degree of discomfort to the patient. A surface silver disc electrode may be placed over the motor point of the target muscle, where the muscle action potential has a sharp negative onset, together with a reference electrode over the tendon (often referred to as belly-tendon recording). The CMAP so recorded is an indication of the number of muscle fibres contributing to the response by summation relatively synchronously when stimulated. When the stimuli are repeated, changes in the CMAP may indicate a rise or fall in the number of muscle fibres responding.

Before coming to conclusions as to normal or abnormal behaviour of the muscle, it is vital to exclude artefacts. Electrode movement is a common problem with a surface electrode over an activated muscle; movement can also occur during the delivery of a long train of stimuli. Slomic et al (1968) prefer subcutaneous needle electrodes which are less prone to produce artefacts but most workers appear to prefer immobilisation of the stimulated muscle. At faster rates of stimulation of the nerve, an initial progressive increase in the size of the responses is due to shortening of the muscle fibres and improved synchronisation of the individual muscle fibre action potentials. The increase in amplitude is accompanied by a reduction in response duration, but little or no change in the CMAP area, indicating that this is a technical artefact or pseudofacilitation. Meticulous attention to technique is essential and results should be validated by the demonstration of their reproducibility in repeated trials.

Another factor requiring attention is temperature, as a lowering of the temperature at the end-plate improves the efficiency of impulse transmission (Borenstein & Desmedt 1974). Attempts should be made to maintain the temperature above 35°C, particularly when studying distal muscles. At higher temperatures the amplitude of the EPPs is reduced, despite an increase in MEPP frequency (Hubbard et al 1969). The timing and dosage of medications affecting neuromuscular transmission should be recorded and if possible these should be withheld prior to the testing session.

A variety of muscles are available for study: in myasthenia gravis, muscles showing clinical fatigability are most likely to give positive results on repetitive stimulation. Proximal muscles, such as trapezius, deltoid and biceps brachii or facial muscles, are more likely than the distal muscles of the hand to show a decrement (Özdemir & Young 1976). However, technical problems and patient discomfort are more prominent with the former and the hand muscles are more easily studied. A recent study has shown the vestigial muscle, anconeus, to be as diagnostically sensitive as deltoid, to be better tolerated and less troubled by artefact (Kennett & Fawcett 1990a). In botulism there may be a similar restriction of neurophysiological and clinical abnormalities to certain muscle groups in contrast to the myasthenic syndrome

where the changes are usually widespread. Kimura (1989) indicates those muscles commonly studied and suggests appropriate electrode placements.

After suitable amplification, the CMAP is displayed either on a storage oscilloscope, from which permanent photographic records may be obtained, or recorded directly on to light-sensitive paper. The amplitude of the negative phase of each response can then be measured. In some laboratories, the signals are fed directly into a computer which stores and displays the data in digital form and calculates the amplitude and area of the negative portion of the response.

A number of different stimulation paradigms may be used to test neuromuscular transmission; these will now be briefly considered in turn.

Paired stimuli may be delivered with short inter-stimulus intervals of 2.5 ms, 15 ms and 25 ms. When using the shortest of these intervals in a normal subject, the second response is reduced as it arrives during the relative refractory period for nerve and muscle. Similar responses are likely to be found in patients suffering from myasthenia gravis. In the myasthenic syndrome, however, the first response will be of subnormal amplitude, while the second response may be up to double the first. The defective ACh release in this condition results in small, subthreshold EPPs which fail to produce an action potential in most muscle fibres with the first shock. The arrival of the second stimulus allows the EPPs to summate, exciting muscle fibres not responsive to the initial shock. A similar response often occurs in botulism and may rarely be seen in myasthenia gravis (Cherington 1973).

Paired stimuli with longer interstimulus intervals such as 15–100 ms will result in no change in the second potential in normal individuals, in myasthenia and botulism. In the myasthenic syndrome true facilitation is to be expected when stimulating in this range. The decremental response to paired stimuli in myasthenia is best seen when applying inter-stimulus intervals of 100–700 ms.

Repetitive stimulation at slow rates. Stimuli delivered at slow rates are generally well tolerated by patients and technically satisfactory records are more easily obtained than with faster or tetanic rates. Stimulation at rates of 2–3 Hz should produce an identical series of responses in normal subjects. It is usual to compare the amplitude of the smallest of the first five responses with the first of a train. The largest percentage decrement usually occurs in the second response but as the process continues the largest absolute change in amplitude is evident when the fourth or fifth response is compared with the first, after which the amplitude increases to produce a 'U-shaped response' (Özdemir & Young 1971). When a reproducible percentage decrement between the first and fifth response of 10% or more can be obtained, the result is considered abnormal (Slomic et al 1968) (Fig. 29.24). If the abnormality can be reversed or reduced by drugs such as edrophonium or neostigmine which block the action of acetylcholinesterase, then the diagnosis of myasthenia is probable. A number of other diseases may produce abnormalities of neuromuscular transmission which give rise to decremental responses at slow stimulus rates. Motor neurone disease, botulism, multiple sclerosis, the myasthenic syndrome and reinnervating nerve have all been reported as showing decremental responses (Mulder et al 1959, Eisen et al 1978, Gilliatt 1966, Gilchrist & Sanders 1989). Both botulism and the Lambert–Eaton myasthenic syndrome (LEMS) are usually associated with small-amplitude responses to initial stimuli and a further fall in amplitude is usual.

Repetitive stimulation at faster rates. Here the effects of stimulation at rates of 20–30 Hz are considered. At these rates of stimulation the safety factor for neuromuscular transmission in the normal individual is sufficiently large that the amplitude of the response is maintained throughout the train. In LEMS the initial response is of low amplitude but there is a striking increase in the size of the response to the succeeding train (see Fig. 29.28); the amount of the increment at the end of the train is several times that of the first response, reflecting excitation of all or nearly all the muscle fibres in the muscle (Lambert et al 1961). In myasthenia gravis, particularly during steroid therapy or during spontaneous deterioration, a less striking incremental response may be detected and a similar slight increment may occur in botulism, both being more likely when the amplitude of the first response is normal (Mayer & Williams 1974, Pickett et al 1976). Prolonged stimulation is uncomfortable for the patient and is associated with increasing problems of artefact due to muscle contraction and electrode movement, particularly when proximal muscles are studied.

When the force of muscle contraction (twitch tension) is also measured in normal muscle sub-

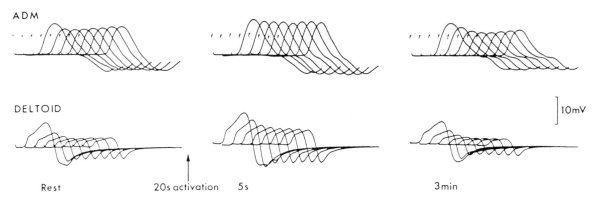

Fig. 29.24 Repetitive nerve stimulation studies in abductor digiti minimi (ADM) and deltoid in a patient with generalised myasthenia gravis. 3 Hz trains of stimuli at rest, 5 seconds and 3 minutes after 20 second maximal contraction. In both muscles a significant decrement (5th compared with 1st) occurred at rest (24% ADM, 53% deltoid). The decrement was abolished immediately after activation in ADM and was reduced in deltoid (33%) (postactivation potentiation); it was the same in ADM but more marked in deltoid 3 minutes later (59%) (postactivation exhaustion).

jected to a prolonged train of low frequency (1–2 Hz stimuli), there is a slow, progressive increase in the force of muscle twitch over the first minutes (positive staircase phenomenon); a less marked fall in twitch tension (negative staircase phenomenon) precedes the development of the positive staircase in about 50% of cases (Slomic et al 1968). This mechanical response is not accompanied by alteration in the size of the evoked action potential and its cause is uncertain but it appears to be independent of the number of active muscle fibres.

When patients with myasthenia are subject to an isolated supramaximal stimulus to the motor nerve, the twitch tension is often normal, though in those with moderate to severe disease there may be some reduction (Lambert et al 1961, Slomic et al 1968). When subject to a slow train of stimuli, however, the positive staircase response is said to be absent or reduced in myasthenics (Slomic et al 1968). Nevertheless, Grob & Namba (1976) found that the staircase phenomenon was present and usually normal in the myasthenic patients they studied. The position of the staircase phenomenon in myasthenia awaits further appraisal.

Tetanic stimulation. Shocks delivered at 50 Hz for 30 s will produce brief tetanic contractions of a muscle. Such stimulation is generally perceived as being most uncomfortable and few patients tolerate it for more than short periods. Because of this many laboratories no longer employ this rate and utilise the effect of exercise. However, the main features of interest are not the responses during the train but the changes in function over a period of up to 15 minutes after the tetany.

Post-tetanic potentiation is seen during the first 2 minutes. The response to an initial isolated supramaximal shock is compared to a similar response obtained shortly after a tetanic train has been delivered. Post-tetanic potentiation occurs when the second response is clearly greater than the first. Since all of the fibres in a normal muscle are excited by supramaximal stimulation, there is no change in the response size (i.e. there is no post-tetanic potentiation). Where there is a defect in ACh availability, the initial response would be smaller than normal and the tetany will increase the mobilisation of ACh; thus the amplitude of the post-tetanic response will exceed that of the first

response. This is the case in LEMS where the second response may show an increment of up to 200%.

In myasthenia gravis a smaller degree of potentiation may occur or the level of decrement may be less during the first 2 minutes due to the opposite effects of ACh depletion and post-tetanic potentiation. Instead of receiving an uncomfortable tetanic train, the patient can be asked to make a strong voluntary contraction over a time period of 20–30 s and this is the preferred routine in the authors' laboratory (Fig. 29.24). Activation of motor units at rates of up to 50 Hz can be achieved by the majority of patients. Post-tetanic exhaustion appears after potentiation, usually 2–4 minutes after the tetany or exercise.

After the stimulation it is usual to deliver single test shocks at 10 s and at 1 or 2 minute intervals over the succeeding 15 minutes. There is a large safety margin in normal muscle so that although there has been a marked reduction in the available store of ACh, the response to supramaximal shocks is maintained. The immature end-plates of the premature or newborn infant do not possess the same safety margin and post-tetanic exhaustion can be detected. Typically, patients with myasthenia gravis show progressively more impairment of neuromuscular transmission during the period, thought to be due to failure of mobilisation of ACh to cope with the demand during the tetanus/exercise leading to post-tetanic exhaustion. In LEMS, post-tetanic exhaustion produces responses of even lower amplitude than the first abnormally reduced action potential.

Additional stimulation techniques

Double step ischaemia. As patients with mild generalised myasthenia or ocular myasthenia may not show any definite abnormality when tested by the methods noted above, modifications of the test conditions have been introduced to increase diagnostic sensitivity. It has long been known that under ischaemic conditions there is a rapid increase in the amount of decrement to repetitive stimulation in patients with myasthenia gravis and that prolonged ischaemia causes failure of neuromuscular transmission in normal subjects (Harvey & Masland 1941).

A double-step ischaemic test has been described by Desmedt & Borenstein (1977a). The initial phase consists of recording the CMAP from the hypothenar muscles during a 4 minute period of continuous supramaximal stimulation of the ulnar nerve at a rate of 3 Hz. Thereafter further brief trains of 3 Hz stimuli are delivered at 30 second intervals and the presence or absence of decremental responses within each train is determined. If this first phase does not produce definite evidence of a defect, then the second ischaemic step is introduced. An occlusive cuff inflated to above arterial pressure is secured about the arm proximal to the site of nerve stimulation in order to induce ischaemia. The stimulation paradigm is then repeated.

In some normal subjects a progressive reduction of the CMAP amplitude may occur after 2–3 minutes of stimulation, whereas in others the action potential amplitude remains unchanged (Desmedt & Borenstein 1977a). However the subsequent short test periods of stimulation at 3 Hz produce no progressive decrement even in those individuals who had shown a diminution of the amplitude during the continuous conditioning period of ischaemic stimulation. Desmedt & Borenstein (1977a) suggest that the reduction in amplitude which occurs in some normal subjects is due to the production of a temporary conduction block in some of the nerve fibres by the ischaemia. If ischaemia is much more prolonged, to 7–15 minutes, a decremental response to the 3 Hz test stimuli is seen in normal individuals.

In patients with myasthenia gravis, evidence of a failure of neuromuscular transmission may be seen in the first step, that of 'exercise' induced by continuous 3 Hz stimulation. Where mild or mainly ocular disease is present this first phase may not reveal any abnormality. When stressed by both prolonged stimulation and ischaemia, many patients will show decremental responses during the initial ischaemic exercise period and more will show defects in transmission during the subsequent test periods.

Regional curare sensitivity. The use of neuromuscular blocking agents together with repetitive stimulation provide a further means of revealing mild disturbances of transmission by reducing the safety factor. The neuromuscular blocking drug D-tubocurarine is used for the procedure. In patients with ocular myasthenia the systemic injection of one-tenth of the normal curarising dose will often result in the development of weakness in previously clinically unaffected limb muscles (Rowland et al 1961). Such systemic injections are hazardous as they may induce respiratory failure and protracted generalised paralysis in myasthenic individuals. In order to overcome this danger, a small dose of curare may be injected into a forearm vein subsequent to the total occlusion of the circulation by inflating an occlusive cuff proximal to the injection site (Horowitz et al 1975). Alterations in CMAP amplitude produced by a stimulation programme are then assessed (Brown & Charlton 1975, Brown et al 1975). The concentration of curare at the neuromuscular junction varies from patient to patient, due to differing diffusion through the volume of tissue in the occluded region, and in consequence there may be difficulties in separating normal from pathological responses (Hertel et al 1977). Extra sensitivity to curare is not solely a feature of myasthenia. It is also seen in muscular weakness caused by certain antibiotics (Pittinger & Adamson 1972) and in motor neurone disease (Mulder et al 1959). There is also some risk of curare reaching the systemic circulation and affecting the respiratory muscles, after release of the tourniquet (Hertel et al 1977). For these reasons many investigators see no place for this test in the vast majority of myasthenic patients as the diagnosis can be reached using the safe methods now available (Özdemir & Young 1976).

Single-fibre electromyography (SFEMG)

Methods. The identification of disordered neuromuscular transmission depends upon demonstrating a failure of transmission during muscular activity. That failure appears in SFEMG as impulse blocking but abnormally high jitter values can indicate the presence of a disturbance before blocking develops. Thus, positive findings may be present in muscles which appear to be clinically unaffected (Ekstedt & Stålberg 1965, Stålberg & Ekstedt 1973, Stålberg et al 1974, Stålberg 1980b). Two different techniques are available, electrical stimulation and voluntary activation.

Electrical stimulation. A single fibre action potential evoked by repetitive supramaximal stimulation of its motor nerve shows, in successive appearances, small latency variations of the order of tens of microseconds. This phenomenon is due to variations in transmission times between the stimulus and recording sites. Normally neither the nerve action potential nor muscle fibre contribute to the variation by more than 3 μs, the major source being the neuromuscular junction (Stålberg & Trontelj 1979). The term 'jitter' has been coined for this phenomenon and is derived from technical electronic terminology, used to indicate the presence of instability in an oscilloscope display, as a result of varying trigger level or instability in the time-base generator. Two principal causes for jitter at the end-plate have been suggested: first, the steepness of the rising slope of the EPP may change, due to small-amplitude alterations in successive EPPs, causing variations in the time a muscle fibre action potential can be triggered; second, there may be temporal variations in the muscle fibre firing threshold leading to differing neuromuscular transmission times in the presence of constant amplitude EPPs.

Intramuscular nerve stimulation using a Teflon-coated monopolar needle is preferred to stimulation of the nerve trunk and the technique is useful in unconscious or very young patients. A number of methodological factors are important when testing neuromuscular function in this way (Trontelj et al 1986, Trontelj & Stålberg 1992). Supramaximal stimulus strength for the axon to the single fibre should be employed. This is ensured by the absence of further reduction in jitter with increments of stimulus intensity. The stimuli must not result in activation in adjacent motor units, of single fibre potentials with similar latency to the target single fibre potential, as false values for jitter would result from the 'rogue' fibre. At high rates of stimulation, nerve threshold may increase and a constant stimulus strength employed becomes subliminal, resulting in progressive increase in jitter and blocking. This phenomenon may be recognised and corrected by increasing the stimulus intensity which returns jitter to its former value and abolishes blocking (Stålberg & Trontelj 1979). Care is necessary to avoid direct muscle fibre stimulation, which may

be suspected in the presence of abnormally low jitter values of under 5 μs.

Voluntary activation. During gentle voluntary activation of a muscle (often the extensor digitorum communis (EDC)) the SFEMG electrode is sited so that it records the action potentials of a pair of fibres belonging to the same motor unit. One of the action potentials triggers the oscilloscope sweep and is used as a reference, the other potential appearing with a variable interval in relation to the triggering potential. In this situation the jitter represents the variability of neuromuscular transmission at both motor end-plates and may be expressed mathematically as:

$$\text{jitter} = \sqrt{\text{jitter } 1^2 + \text{jitter } 2^2}$$

For the assessment of jitter in an individual muscle at least 20 pairs are recorded and the jitter value in each pair is measured. In normal subjects, one of the potential pairs may show increased jitter or impulse blocking, but the remainder should have jitter values within the normal range of 5–55 μs; individual muscles have smaller ranges (Stålberg & Trontelj 1979). Considerable variation exists in the jitter found at normal end-plates both within single motor units and in muscles as a whole. The recording site does not influence the magnitude of jitter which is the same when recording near the insertion or end-plate region. Jitter in normal muscle is increased by a fall in intramuscular temperature below 35°C but an increase in temperature up to 38°C has no effect. Individuals over 70 show age-related increases in jitter in EDC but there is evidence of earlier increases in other muscles, usually accompanied by increase in FD and thought to have a neurogenic origin (Stålberg & Trontelj 1979). Continuous recording over several hours from a normal potential pair, utilising firing rates of 10–15 Hz, shows stable jitter. Fatigue prevents protracted recording at higher rates, such as over 30 Hz, but no change occurs with up to 10 minutes activation at these rates.

Jitter in a number of potential pairs within a single motor unit has been studied using a two-needle technique. The first needle is positioned in proximity to a single fibre potential which acts as the trigger throughout the study. The second electrode is moved to a series of positions where potentials time-locked to the trigger are detected. These potentials belong to the same motor unit and in this way the function of up to seven neuro-muscular junctions in a single motor unit has been studied (Stålberg et al 1976). The range of values for jitter determined for the muscle as a whole are the same as those within the single motor unit.

Quantifying neuromuscular jitter. Variation of the interpotential interval can be expressed in terms of the standard deviation (SD) of the mean interpotential interval (MIPI). However, during the recording of potential pairs, slow trends in the IPI quite frequently occur due to minor alterations in electrode position affecting action potential shape and short-term variability in neuromuscular trans-mission timing (Stålberg & Trontelj 1979), which renders the SD invalid as an accurate measure of jitter. Thus another method which measures the Mean value of Consecutive Differences (MCD) of the IPIs is recommended (Stålberg et al 1971) (Fig. 29.25a). In certain situations, especially those where the velocity recovery function of the muscle fibre comes into play, the IPI is affected by the preceding interdischarge interval (IDI). In such circumstances the MCD includes a spurious variability not due to end-plate jitter. To over-come this problem, the measured interpotential intervals are sorted in increasing order, according to the magnitude of the preceding interdischarge intervals, following which the mean value of con-secutive differences of this new sequence is esti-mated. This new value is called the mean sorted-data difference (MSD). In practice in order to determine in which way the data should be reported, an index is used; this is the ratio MCD/MSD. A ratio of more than 1.25 is an indi-cation that interdischarge intervals have so affected the variability that jitter should be expressed by the MSD. With ratios below 1.25 the results should be reported as the MCD.

Manual methods of jitter analysis. Manual methods of analysis consist of measurement of latency differences of baseline intersection points of the earliest and latest occurring second poten-tial when the first has been used to trigger the oscilloscope. A total of at least 50 successive dis-charges of the pair are recorded and superimposed on to photographic paper either in ten groups of five or five groups of ten. An oscilloscope sweep speed of at least 200 µs/cm should be used. The range of variations of the IPI in each group of recordings is measured between identical points on the rising positive-negative slope of the action potentials (Fig. 29.26b). The mean range from all of the groups of superimpositions is determined and converted into the MCD value using an appropriate conversion factor (0.49 for five and 0.37 for ten superimpositions). The manual me-thod is unable to assess the effects of irregular dis-charge rates on jitter, and in order to reduce this problem the patient should attempt to maintain a constant firing rate throughout the recording.

Automated methods of jitter analysis. As well as manual methods of SFEMG analysis, a number of automated methods have been des-cribed utilising mini or micro computers, and are incorporated into some of the recently developed commercial EMG systems. All systems use a trig-gering device to isolate the two potentials, and either a hardware interval counter or real-time clock within the computer to measure accurately the IPIs. The firing rate or IDI can also be mea-sured and the effect of IDI on jitter may be auto-matically assessed by determining the MSD value, after which the MCD/MSD index is obtained. The use of minicomputers and the storage capac-ity of hard-disc drives allows virtually continuous analysis and updating of both normal and patho-logical parameters for the SFEMG laboratory. Where such comprehensive facilities are lacking, the recording on to reel or cassette tape of the studies carried out provides a means of subse-quent off-line analysis and comparison of individ-ual results.

SFEMG findings in myasthenia gravis. In the presence of myasthenia gravis a 20-potential study may show some pairs with jitter values within the normal range, others with abnormal jitter and some where impulse blocking is present (Stålberg et al 1974, 1976) (Fig. 29.26). Blocking occurs in pairs showing higher jitter values and usually manifests itself when jitter has reached 100 µs. When a series of 50 consecutive dis-charges from a potential pair showing intermittent blocking is analysed, the range between minimal and maximal interpotential interval could be up to 4000 µs. Even when myasthenia is mild and restricted clinically, usually more than 30% of

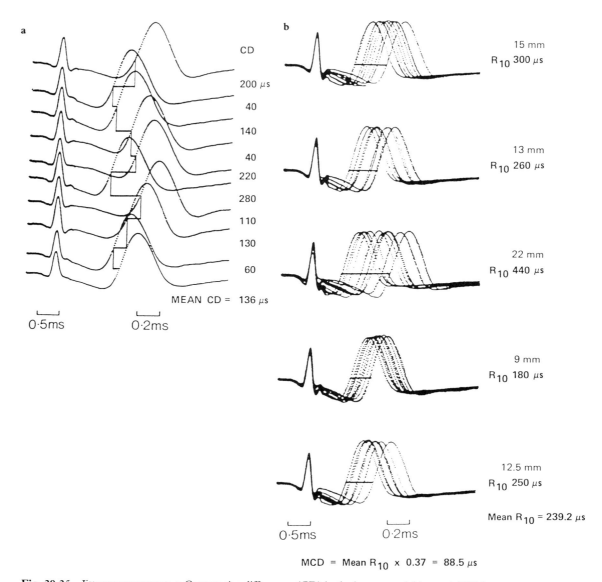

Fig. 29.25   Jitter measurement. **a** Consecutive differences (CD) in the interpotential interval (IPI) in μs (Horizontal lines). **b** Manual method for jitter measurement using five groups of 10 superimposed sweeps.

pairs show either increased jitter or blocking. Continuous activation, especially when accompanied by rising firing rates, will increase jitter and blocking at an affected neuromuscular junction. With a fall in firing rate, the proportion of blockings and magnitude of jitter declines. Occasionally the reverse will be true, with a fall in jitter and impulse blocking as the firing rate increases. This has also been found in stimulation jitter studies

which show that jitter and impulse blocking tend to be most abnormal at rates of 5–10 Hz stimulation and frequently improve at higher rates (20 Hz) (Kennett & Fawcett 1990b, Trontelj & Stålberg 1991). If an end-plate appears to have been spared, as indicated by an initial normal jitter, attempts to evoke an abnormality by continuous activity and increasing firing rate are usually fruitless. Although in myasthenia there is usually a

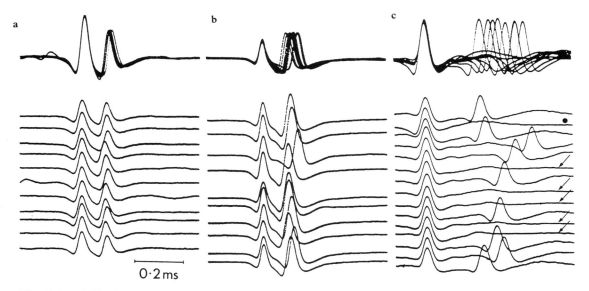

Fig. 29.26   SFEMG recordings from extensor digitorum communis muscle in a patient with myasthenia gravis. Upper trace, 10 superimposed sweeps; lower traces, raster display of successive sweeps. **a** Normal jitter (33 μs MCD). **b** Increased jitter (80 μs MCD). **c** Increased jitter associated with intermittent blocking of second potential (arrows) and first potential (closed circle).

variety of degrees of involvement of different end-plates in a muscle, from normal jitter at one to impulse blocking at another, this is not apparently due to selective involvement or sparing of individual motor units.

When a muscle shows clinical weakness at the time of the SFEMG study and jitter is normal, the diagnosis of myasthenia gravis is excluded (Stålberg & Trontelj 1979). In a minority of myasthenic patients (up to 30%), a recording from the EDC may be normal or show equivocal changes; these are usually patients with ocular myasthenia (Stålberg et al 1976, Sanders et al 1979). In this situation, SFEMG of the facial muscles will give an abnormal result in about 80–85% of patients (Stålberg 1980b, Sanders & Howard 1986). Conditions other than myasthenia may be associated with disturbed neuromuscular transmission and give rise to abnormal jitter values. In particular, the myopathy associated with mitochondrial abnormalities which may present with weakness of the external ocular muscles, frequently exhibit abnormal jitter (Fawcett et al 1982a, Krendel et al 1987) and a muscle biopsy will be needed to distinguish between mitochondrial myopathy and myasthenia.

Jitter in normal muscle is unaffected by the injection of edrophonium hydrochloride, whereas in myasthenia blocking may be abolished and jitter reduced. In patients receiving anticholinesterase therapy, some potential pairs may show the reverse effect with edrophonium, with increases in jitter and impulse blocking. These 'cholinergic crises' at isolated end-plates are an indication of the variations in severity of the disorder when looked at microphysiologically in an individual muscle (Stålberg & Trontelj 1979). Despite this, there is good overall correlation between severity of SFEMG changes and the clinical severity of the myasthenia (Sanders et al 1979). The number of potential pairs showing blocking matches the clinical fatigability both in untreated patients and in those receiving anticholinesterase or steroids. Serial studies in individual patients should show parallel changes in SFEMG abnormality and variations in clinical severity.

A minority of patients in remission, occurring spontaneously, after thymectomy or during corticosteroid therapy, show no SFEMG abnormality (Sanders et al 1979). In remission, impulse blocking is exceptional but abnormal numbers of pairs show elevated jitter levels. Where maintenance therapy with anticholinesterase preparations appears to have achieved complete control of the disorder clinically, the SFEMG remains unequivocally abnormal (Stålberg & Trontelj 1979). There is no need to discontinue therapy prior to SFEMG in a suspected case already on treatment.

Normal individuals receiving anticholinesterase drugs in the therapeutic range employed in the treatment of myasthenia, do not develop abnormal jitter. Chronic medication of this type fails to produce SFEMG abnormalities in normal subjects and people erroneously diagnosed and treated as myasthenics have been identified (Stålberg & Trontelj 1979).

The SFEMG in apparently normal first degree relatives of patients with myasthenia is of interest. Stålberg et al (1976) have examined a number of the relatives of patients with juvenile myasthenia and found abnormalities in a third of them. Increased jitter was found in 25% of the pairs examined and blocking in about 15%; overall, 25% of all the recordings were abnormal while in the clinically affected juveniles the abnormality rate was 75%.

SFEMG may be used to determine FD in patients with myasthenia and other disorders of neuromuscular transmission. Hilton-Brown et al (1982) reported the results of a study of 71 myasthenic patients and found a significant increase in FD compared to controls. Neither severity nor duration of the disease was correlated to the change in FD. Those individuals receiving anticholinesterase drugs had significantly higher FD values than untreated patients and controls. As many subjects in the study had a repeated examination, care was taken to avoid the possibility that needle injury to the muscle was a factor in the production of the FD increase. The problem of myasthenic drop-out of single fibres affecting FD was also addressed. The possibility of muscle fibre shrinkage leading to closer packing of the fibres appeared to be excluded by muscle biopsy. A direct effect of medication on the terminal innervation producing functional denervation and subsequent reinnervation appears possible. Morphological and physiological changes induced by anticholinesterase drugs administered experimentally to animal species, discussed elsewhere (see Ch. 5), support this hypothesis.

Stapedius reflex

In 1965 Blomberg & Persson described a new test for myasthenia gravis which depended on fatiguing the stapedius muscle. The stapedius muscle contracts reflexly in response to sound and prevents hyperacusis. Its contraction alters the acoustic impedance of the middle ear so that it is easy to monitor its contraction by impedance audiometry. In normal individuals sustained contractions in response to sound stimuli 70–100 dB above threshold at frequencies from 250 to 100 Hz can be maintained for up to 1 minute. In contrast, the myasthenic stapedius shows a rapid decrement and is unable to sustain reflex contraction, resulting in the rapid onset of hyperacusis. The response may be reversed or at least improved by intravenous edrophonium (Blom & Zakrisson 1974). The test appears well tolerated and in some myasthenics may be the only electrophysiological abnormality (Warrent et al 1977). It therefore may not only be of value as a diagnostic procedure but as an easy means of monitoring the response to treatment (Kramer et al 1981, Stålberg & Sanders 1981).

Saccadic eye movements

A number of methods for measuring the development of fatigue in the extraocular muscles by recording the fall-off in the velocity of angular movement during oculokinetic nystagmus or other eye movements (Baloh & Keesey 1976, Yee et al 1976) have been reported. In patients with myasthenia gravis there may be a fall-off in eye movement velocities improved by the administration of edrophonium. These tests require the cooperation of the patients and may be difficult to quantify.

NEUROPHYSIOLOGICAL FINDINGS IN VARIOUS DISORDERS OF NEUROMUSCULAR TRANSMISSION

Myasthenia gravis

Patients with myasthenia gravis may vary from those with mild restricted disease to those with severe widespread involvement, which by virtue of affecting bulbar and respiratory muscles may threaten life. The ease with which the diagnosis is made relates to the severity of the condition at presentation. Methods of repetitive stimulation are most widely available but will prove positive in only a quarter of patients with mild or restricted disease if distal muscles are tested. When the disease has resulted in moderate or severe weakness, the diagnostic yield reaches 90%. Utilising proximal muscles for repetitive stimulation studies produces positive results in 65–70% of all myasthenics. The double-step ischaemic test increases the detection rate dramatically even in mildly affected patients. Regional curare sensitivity testing now has no part to play in the routine diagnosis of myasthenia. Where SFEMG is available, examination of jitter and blocking in the EDC muscle will give abnormal results in 95% of myasthenics. If the patient has ocular myasthenia and shows no abnormality in EDC then SFEMG studies in the frontalis will demonstrate abnormal neuromuscular transmission in over 80% of these patients (Stålberg & Sanders 1981, Sanders & Howard 1986). Less widely available are the stapedius-reflex fatigue test which appears very sensitive, and tests of intraocular tension, ocular muscle fatigue and ocular EMG. Levels of antibody to ACh receptor are elevated in about 75–80% of myasthenics. The antibody level does not correlate with clinical severity which is better shown by the jitter in SFEMG studies (Konishi et al 1981). In occasional patients with characteristic clinical features of myasthenia gravis, electrophysiological testing shows a marked incremental response at high rates of repetitive nerve stimulation, typical of LEMS (Schwartz & Stålberg 1975).

Neonatal myasthenia. In about 15% of infants born to myasthenic mothers a transient disorder of neuromuscular transmission is seen. The condition appears to be due to the presence of ACh receptor antibodies which have been independently synthesised by the affected infants rather than, as previously thought, to the transplacental passive transfer of maternal antibodies (Lefvert & Osterman 1983). The main signs of the disorder are feeding difficulties, respiratory problems and hypotonia appearing within 3 days of birth, responding to anticholinesterase treatment. The neurophysiological findings (Desmedt & Borenstein 1977b) are identical with those of true myasthenia gravis and may still be present after apparent clinical recovery.

Congenital myasthenic syndromes

Several of these rare disorders of neuromuscular transmission have now been characterised and it is likely that other defects are still to be delineated. The first to be described is the myasthenic syndrome associated with end-plate acetylcholinesterase (AChE) deficiency, small nerve terminals and reduced ACh release (Engel et al 1977). After isolated nerve stimulation, the CMAP appears repetitively and there is a decremental response at all frequencies when trains of stimuli are delivered. Only a single case has been described and in vitro studies of muscle biopsy showed reduced mepp frequencies but preservation of mepp amplitude. The time-course of the mepp was prolonged. There was a reduced quantal content of the epp and a reduction in the stores of ACh immediately available for release. A total absence of AChE at the end-plate was demonstrated and normal numbers of acetylcholine receptors were present. The prolonged mepp duration and repetitive firing seemed to be due to the absence of AChE.

A familial infantile myasthenic syndrome possibly due to a presynaptic defect in transmitter resynthesis or mobilisation was first described by Hart et al in 1979. Further cases have been reported and the disorder is most often seen in the newborn but can affect older patients (Engel 1980, Lambert 1982, Matthes et al 1991). In the newborn, prolonged apnoeic attacks occur in relation to feeding and crying, sometimes leading to cerebral hypoxia and sudden infant death (Conomy et al 1975, Matthes et al 1991). When stimuli are applied to the nerve at 2 Hz there is a decrement in the CMAP only in muscles which are weak. Exercise or a tetanic train induces a significant decrement in the CMAP in other muscles (Fig. 29.27). Complex polyphasic motor unit potentials showing marked instability may be seen in proximal muscles, and satellite potentials, typical of a reinnervation state have been reported (Matthes et al 1991). The only in vitro abnormality is the presence of a marked fall in mepp and epp amplitudes when stimulated at 10 Hz; this is

A

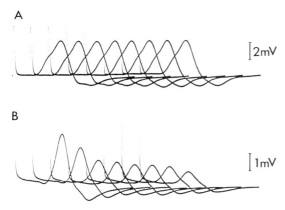

B

|2mV

|1mV

Fig. 29.27 Repetitive nerve stimulation study in a patient with familial myasthenic syndrome: recordings obtained from abductor digiti minimi using surface stimulating and recording electrodes. **a** 3 Hz stimulation at rest shows no decrement. **b** Four minutes after 2 minutes of continuous stimulation of the ulnar nerve at 10 Hz there was a decrement of 54% (5th/1st response) (from Matthes et al 1991).

similar to the effect when normal muscle is treated with hemicholinium suggesting defective re-uptake of choline by the nerve terminal. The condition usually responds well to treatment with pyrido-stigmine.

A congenital myasthenic syndrome attributable to a prolonged open time of the ACh-sensitive ion channels or 'slow channel syndrome' has been described (Engel et al 1982, Oosterhuis et al 1987). The disease may begin in infancy or appear later and is associated with the presence of repetitive discharges of the CMAP in response to single stimuli. In vitro studies have revealed the presence of very prolonged decay of the mepps and epps and prolonged mep currents together with a reduction in mepp amplitude. Other structural abnormalities which are thought to be secondary to the primary ion channel defect, include a reduction in the numbers of ACh receptors, decrease in the size of the nerve terminals and focal degeneration of the postjunctional folds. Small groups of atrophic muscle fibres and degenerative changes in the muscle fibres were also noted (Engel 1980, Engel et al 1982). The mepp currents are produced by opening of ACh-induced ion channels in response to a single quantum of transmitter; their prolonged decay in the presence of normal AChE activity suggests that the channels remain open too long.

The effect of this could be to allow an excessive calcium influx into the muscle cell which in turn could lead to the degenerative changes observed.

A familial myasthenic syndrome with possible abnormalities in the synthesis of ACh receptor (AChR) or its insertion into the postsynaptic membrane has been described (Vincent et al 1981, Lambert 1982, Lecky et al 1986). The results of neuromuscular testing in these patients were similar to those in myasthenia gravis, though no antibodies to ACh receptors were present. In another group of cases, a marked reduction in the number and size of the postsynaptic folds or clefts has been described (Smit et al 1988, Fawcett et al 1989, Wokke et al 1989). Small mepp amplitudes and a deficiency and abnormal distribution of the AChRs in the postsynaptic membrane were noted in one patient (Smit et al 1988), while a relatively normal mepp amplitude but a reduction in quantal content of the epp associated with a reduced density of AChRs was reported in another patient who showed a decrement of the CMAP response at low rates of stimulation and evidence of post-activation potentiation and exhaustion, similar to that seen in myasthenia gravis (Fawcett et al 1989).

Recently four other congenital myasthenic syndromes have been characterised (Engel et al 1990). In one patient a reduced number of synaptic vesicles in the nerve terminal, perhaps due to impaired axonal transport of preformed vesicles, was associated with a reduced quantal content of the epp. In a second case, evidence of a functionally abnormal AChR ion channel in the form of high channel conductance and reduced channel open time was found: a 'fast channel' syndrome. A reduced affinity of ACh for the AChR associated with small mepps and miniature endplate currents was demonstrated in a third patient while a deficiency of AChR and a short channel open time was observed in the fourth case. These and the other reported cases serve to highlight the highly heterogeneous nature of congenital myasthenia.

Lambert–Eaton myasthenic syndrome (LEMS)

In vitro studies (Elmqvist & Lambert 1968, Elmqvist 1973, Sanders et al 1980) demonstrate a defect in ACh release from nerve terminals. Spontaneously occurring mepps are normal in frequency and amplitude, demonstrating a normal postsynaptic response to a single ACh 'packet' and a normal ACh content of the packet. In the myasthenic syndrome epp amplitude is reduced, as instead of the usual 50 quanta of ACh being released in response to the nerve impulse, the epps are generated by only 2–10. The majority of the epps do not reach the level needed to generate muscle fibre action potentials and some nerve impulses fail to produce an epp. When stimulated repetitively, an increase in epp amplitude restores neuromuscular transmission. The resting mepp frequency, for reasons currently unclear, is about twice that seen in normal subjects. The findings on neuromuscular testing in LEMS may be summarised as follows. In distal limb muscles the response to an isolated supramaximal stimulus is a very low voltage CMAP. Repetitive stimulation at

low rates (2 or 3 Hz) is accompanied by a further decline in the amplitude of the response (Fig. 29.28a). A train of shocks at 10 Hz may result in an initial decline followed by recovery to the original amplitude (Fig. 29.28b). At 20 Hz and more strikingly at 50 Hz there is a rapid increase in CMAP amplitude to normal or nearly normal (Fig. 29.28c,d). Single shocks delivered immediately after such a train result in a much enhanced CMAP but the effect is short-lived. Similar results are produced by voluntary exercise for 30 seconds. CNEMG often reveals MUP instability similar to that seen in myasthenia gravis. There is no evidence of fibrillation, positive sharp waves or nerve conduction defects to suggest denervation. SFEMG shows that, in contrast to myasthenia gravis, jitter and impulse blocking are less at higher discharge rates and increase as the firing rate falls (Fig. 29.29). The maximum jitter (MCD) can be as high as 500 μs and the range of

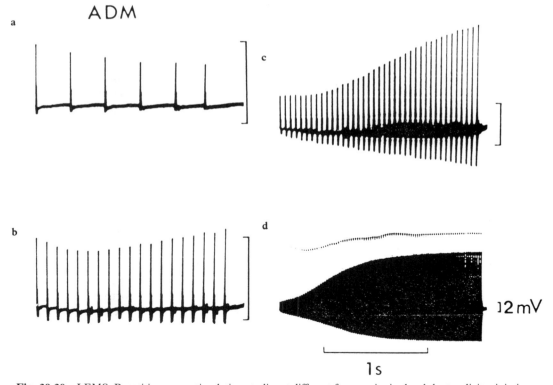

Fig. 29.28   LEMS. Repetitive nerve stimulation studies at different frequencies in the abductor digit minimi (ADM) muscle. Note low amplitude of the initial CMAP in each train. **a** 3 Hz, showing a decrement of 25% at the 5th response. **b** 10 Hz, showing an initial decrement followed by slight increment. **c, d** 20 Hz (c) 50 Hz (d) progressive increment of responses reaching 371% and 943% respectively.

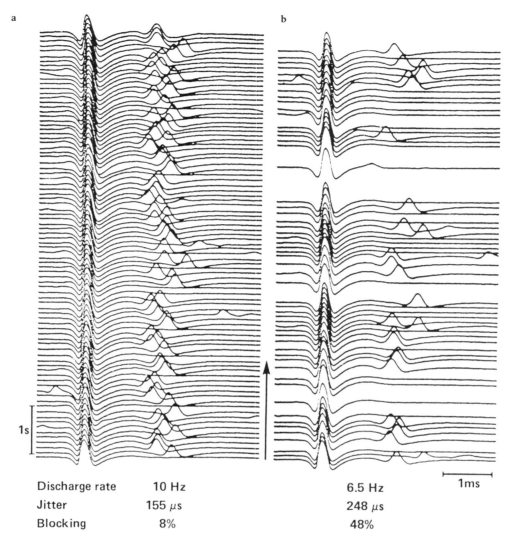

	a	b	
Discharge rate	10 Hz	6.5 Hz	
Jitter	155 μs	248 μs	
Blocking	8%	48%	

Fig. 29.29   LEMS. SFEMG recordings from extensor digitorum communis muscle showing increased jitter and blocking. Jitter and blocking are less marked at higher discharge (**a**) than lower discharge rates (**b**).

interpotential intervals for 50 discharges may reach 2000 μs (Stålberg & Trontelj 1979). The first impulse blocking tends to appear at somewhat higher jitter values than is the case with myasthenia gravis. Blocking is more probable if the preceding interpotential interval is long. Axonal stimulation jitter studies (Kennett & Fawcett 1990b, Trontelj & Stålberg 1991, Chaudhry et al 1991) demonstrate a dramatic reduction of the jitter and blocking at rates of 20 Hz compared with 2–5 Hz, at which rates it

may not be possible to obtain a response. Edrophonium chloride produces improvement as does guanidine hydrochloride and the less toxic 3,4-diaminopyridine, but anticholinesterase drugs are not very effective.

Botulism

The clinical features of the rapidly developing paralysis due to the blocking action on ACh release from motor nerve terminals caused by the exotoxin of *Clostridium botulinum* are described elsewhere (see Ch. 27). In vitro microelectrode studies in a case of botulism revealed (Maselli et al 1992) a marked variation in mepp amplitude although the mean value was normal. Quantal content of the epps was markedly reduced and the epp failed to reach the triggering threshold for an action potential. In affected individuals CNEMG examination of weak muscles shows short-duration, low-amplitude MUPs with reduced recruitment on effort. When examined 14 days or so after the onset of paralysis fibrillations are seen. These are believed to be due to the severity of the damage to the presynaptic region and they disappear as the patient recovers. Conduction velocity in motor nerves is normal and CMAP amplitude is normal or reduced in those muscles mildly involved. With rapid repetitive stimuli some facilitation may occur. In weak muscles CMAP amplitude to single shocks is low and falls further with 3 Hz stimulation; no facilitation is seen with rapid trains (Cherington 1973, 1974, 1982, Oh 1977). The duration of post-tetanic facilitation is prolonged, lasting 10–15 minutes after a conditioning stimulus train, much longer than in myasthenia or LEMS (Gutmann & Pratt 1976). Administration of guanidine or calcium gluconate may increase CMAP amplitudes (Oh 1977, Messina et al 1979). SFEMG studies in two patients revealed increased jitter and impulse blocking which were less pronounced at higher discharge frequencies (Schiller & Stålberg 1978). Over recent years, local muscular injection of botulinum toxin has become a popular treatment for focal dystonia. SFEMG studies performed in muscles distant from those which have been injected show an increase in jitter indicating spread of the effects of the botulinum toxin away from the treated muscles (Lange et al 1987, 1991, Sanders et al 1986, Olney et al 1988). Thus great care is required to avoid producing generalised weakness due to therapeutic overdose in these patients.

Drug-induced myasthenic syndromes

D-Penicillamine-induced myasthenia is a reversible disorder of neuromuscular transmission seen in patients receiving penicillamine treatment for rheumatoid arthritis, Wilson's disease or sclero-derma (Buchnall et al 1975). Anti-AChR antibodies can often be detected in these patients and the disorder is neurophysiologically identical to myasthenia gravis (Stålberg & Trontelj 1979, Fawcett et al 1982b).

Antibiotics have effects on neuromuscular transmission and especially in patients with renal failure, myasthenia gravis or other disorders of neuromuscular transmission may cause the development of weakness lasting for hours or days. The mechanism whereby the weakness is produced varies with the antibiotic used and is detailed elsewhere (see Ch. 28). Other drugs such as anticonvulsants, procainamide, quinidine, adrenergic blockers and lithium may also impair neuromuscular transmission.

Curare combines with the AChRs and reduces the number available for interaction with ACh. Clinically, curare in non-paralytic doses but in amounts sufficient to produce diplopia and ptosis is associated with increased jitter and impulse blocking, developing with jitter of the order of 70 µs. Muscle fibre conduction velocity is unaffected (Ekstedt & Stålberg 1969a).

Organophosphate poisoning results in irreversible inhibition of AChE and a depolarising block of the postsynaptic membrane. Repetitive discharges are seen following a single stimulus to the nerve, while repetitive nerve stimulation produces a decremental response (Besser et al 1989).

Transmission disorders in other neuromuscular diseases

Motor neurone disease is often associated with disordered neuromuscular transmission (Lambert & Mulder 1957, Mulder et al 1959, Simpson 1966, Lambert 1969, Brown & Jaatoul 1974, Bernstein & Antel 1981). A decrementing CMAP at low stimulus rates such as 1 Hz or less, improving only slightly with AChE administration, is found. Slight decremental responses may occur at higher stimulus rates. SFEMG shows increased jitter and blocking, especially in rapidly progressive disease (Stålberg et al 1975). Although transmission may be abnormal at the end-plates of anterior horn cells which are starting to degenerate, it is the presence of many immature junctions due to the abundant collateral reinnervation process which provides a situation where the uncertainty of neuromuscular transmission is increased. Neurogenic block due to intermittent axonal conduction is seen in 5–10% of potentials in motor neurone disease (Stålberg & Thiele 1972). In situations where nerve regeneration can be studied it can be shown that decremental responses to nerve stimulation occur frequently, especially in the early period of reinnervation. A typical U-shaped decremental response has also been reported in the deltoid muscle in a patient with a C5 radiculopathy (Gilchrist & Sanders 1989).

Peripheral neuropathies such as the Guillain–Barré syndrome, diabetic, chronic idiopathic neuropathy and postherpetic motor neuropathy have been shown to give a decremental response to stimulation (Simpson & Lenman 1959, Simpson 1966). No abnormalities in neuromuscular transmission were detected by SFEMG in uraemic or diabetic neuropathy but increased jitter and blocking were found in alcoholic neuropathy. With stimulus frequencies of up to 500 Hz, a decline in CMAP amplitude occurs earlier, and is more marked, in patients with diabetes mellitus than in normal subjects. This is the case even where there is no clinical evidence of a neuropathy (Miglietta 1971). In view of the high stimulus frequencies used, the presence of segmental demyelination of peripheral nerve in diabetes, and the absence of SFEMG abnormality, the finding may be due to defective axonal conduction. At present it is uncertain where the blocking occurs in these disorders and to what extent neurogenic rather than neuromuscular blocking is responsible (Thiele & Stålberg 1975).

Clinical fatigue, partially relieved by administration of AChE drugs and associated with a decremental response to repetitive stimulation, has been reported in some patients with multiple sclerosis (Patten et al 1972, Eisen et al 1978). There may be evidence of denervation and reinnervation and jitter may be increased. Involvement of motor axons within the spinal cord in the ventral horns may account for the denervation seen.

In Duchenne type muscular dystrophy SFEMG examination has shown increased jitter in about 30% of recordings and sometimes blocking in about 10% of those recordings where the largest jitter had been seen (Stålberg & Trontelj 1979). This is probably due to the presence on regenerated muscle fibres of immature neuromuscular junctions where the safety factor for neuromuscular transmission remains reduced for several months (Stålberg & Trontelj 1979). A high incidence of late, unstable, linked potentials lends support to this hypothesis (Borenstein & Desmedt 1973, Desmedt & Borenstein 1976, Stålberg 1977). Stålberg & Trontelj (1979) found a high incidence of concomitant blocking and a common value for jitter in two muscle fibres in relation to the rest of the complex. This suggests that the problem of transmission is situated in the terminal nerve twig. Another frequent finding was the presence of interdischarge interval-dependent jitter particularly affecting the later components, giving rise to the accordion phenomenon (see Fig. 29.19). The presence of abnormally small jitter values has been taken to indicate recording from a split muscle fibre.

In limb-girdle dystrophy (Stålberg & Trontelj 1979) jitter is increased in over 50% of sites in clinically affected muscle but blocking averaged only 4%. Similar findings were described in patients with facioscapulohumeral dystrophy.

In the myotonic disorders, particularly myotonia congenita, there is a decremental response to repetitive stimulation caused by increasing muscle fibre membrane refractoriness (Brown 1974, Özdemir & Young 1976, Aminoff et al 1977). This response differs from that of myasthenia in several respects (Fig. 29.30): first, it is steadily progressive with no evidence of a tendency to plateau or recover at the 5th or 6th stimulus; second, the decremental response develops later in the train than in myasthenia and is greater with higher stimulus frequencies; third, the response can be obtained when the muscle is stimulated directly, indicating that neuromuscular transmission is not involved. There is no decremental response when the stimulus frequency is 5 Hz. The response to single stimuli following exercise or a rapid train is reduced since most of the muscle fibres are refractory and it takes about 15–30 seconds for resting amplitudes to reappear.

In polymyositis, Henriksson & Stålberg (1978) showed that increased jitter and impulse blocking

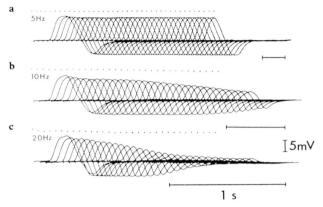

Fig. 29.30 Myotonia congenita (recessive Becker type). Repetitive nerve stimulation studies in abductor digiti minimi. **a** No change in amplitude at 5 Hz. **b** Progressive decline in amplitude at 10 Hz. **c** More rapid and marked decrement at 20 Hz to almost absence of response.

are frequent. When increased jitter was found on gentle contraction, a further rise in jitter and the development of blocking was produced by continuous activity and correlated with the presence of clinical fatigability. Low jitter values suggesting fibre splitting may be seen and concomitant blocking indicating impaired nerve conduction of the impulse is also present.

In McArdle's disease (myophosphorylase deficiency) a significant decremental response occurs at a stimulus frequency of 19 Hz accompanying the cramp after exercise (Dyken et al 1967). Even in the absence of cramp, a decrement develops, provided the stimulus train is continued for over 4 s (Delwaide et al 1968).

Increased jitter and impulse blocking have been reported in patients with mitochondrial myopathy (Fawcett et al 1982a, Krendel et al 1987) and this may make it difficult to distinguish between patients with chronic progressive external ophthalmoplegia and myasthenia gravis solely on the basis of the EMG.

Systemic disorders

In thyroid disease, weakness due to defective neuromuscular transmission is an occasional occurrence. A decremental response similar to that of myasthenia gravis is most common, the association between these disorders being well recognised. However, marked facilitation at rapid stimulus rates in a patient with thyrotoxicosis has been reported (Norris 1966). Changes characteristic of LEMS in a patient with myxoedema have been documented (Takamori et al 1972). A decremental response has been noted in patients with both thyrotoxicosis and myxoedema who were not clinically weak (Drechsler & Lastoukay 1969). The neurophysiological features of both the myasthenic syndrome and of myasthenia gravis have been detected in different muscles in a patient with hyperthyroidism (Mori & Takamori 1976). A significant decremental response to repetitive stimulation, particularly at rates of 20–30 Hz, has been found in a proportion of patients with intrinsic asthma (Basomba et al 1976). SFEMG studies have shown an increase in the 'jitter' phenomenon in patients in both the acute and convalescent phases of viral illnesses (Schiller et al 1977). The considerable functional reserve of the neuromuscular junction ensures that transmission is unaffected in most systemic illnesses. Disuse of muscle is associated with an abnormal decline in CMAP at rapid stimulus frequencies; it is therefore unsafe to infer that such changes are due to the effects of systemic illness on the neuromuscular junction.

REFERENCES

Aberfeld D C, Hinterbuchner L P, Schneider M 1956 Myotonia, dwarfism, diffuse bone disease and unusual ocular and facial abnormalities (a new syndrome). Brain 88: 313

Ad Hoc Committee of the AAEM Special Interest Group on Single Fibre EMG, Gilchrist J M, Coordinator 1992 Single fibre EMG reference values: a collaborative effort. Muscle and Nerve 15: 151

Adrian E D, Bronk D V 1929 Discharges of impulses in motor nerve fibres. Journal of Physiology 67: 119

Albers J W, Allen A A, Bastron J A, Daube J R 1981 Limb myokymia. Muscle and Nerve 4: 494

Aminoff M J, Layzer R B, Satya-Murti S, Faden A I 1977 The declining response of muscle to repetitive nerve stimulation in myotonia. Neurology 27: 812

Aström K E, Kugelberg E, Muller R 1961 Hypothyroid myopathy. Archives of Neurology 5: 472

Auger R G, Daube J R, Gomez M R, Lambert E H 1984 Hereditary form of sustained muscle activity of peripheral nerve origin causing generalised myokymia and muscle stiffness. Annals of Neurology 15: 13

Axelson J, Thesleff F A 1959 A study of supersensitivity in denervated mammalian muscle. Journal of Physiology 147: 178

Ballantyne J P, Hansen S 1974a A new method for estimation of motor units in a muscle. 1. Control subjects and patients with myasthenia gravis. Journal of Neurology, Neurosurgery and Psychiatry 37: 907

Ballantyne J P, Hansen S 1974b Computer method for the analysis of evoked motor unit potentials. 1. Control subjects and patients with myasthenia gravis. Journal of Neurology, Neurosurgery and Psychiatry 37: 1187

Ballantyne J P, Hansen S 1974c A new method for the estimation of motor units in a muscle. 2. Duchenne, limb-girdle and facioscapulohumeral, and myotonic muscular dystrophies. Journal of Neurology, Neurosurgery and Psychiatry 37: 1195

Baloh R W, Keesey J C 1976 Saccadic fatigue and response to edrophonium for the diagnosis of myasthenia gravis. Annals of the New York Academy of Sciences 274: 631

Barchi R L 1975 An evaluation of the chloride hypothesis. Archives of Neurology 32: 175

Barchi R L 1982 A mechanistic approach to the myotonic syndrome. Muscle and Nerve (Suppl) 5: 60

Barwick D D 1963 Investigations of the carrier state in the Duchenne type dystrophy. In: Proceedings of the 2nd Symposium on Research in Muscular Dystrophy. Pitman, London

Barwick D D, Walton J N 1963 Polymyositis. American Journal of Medicine 35: 645

Barwick D D, Gardner-Medwin D 1967 Observer bias in the measurement of motor unit action potentials. Electroencephalography and Clinical Neurophysiology 23: 490

Basmajian J V, Stecko G 1962 A new bipolar electrode for electromyography. Journal of Applied Physiology 17: 849

Basomba A, Permuy J, Pelaez A, Campos A, Villamanzo I G 1976 Myasthenia-like electrophysiological response in intrinsic bronchial asthma. Lancet ii: 968

Becker P E 1977 Myotonia congenita and syndromes associated with myotonia. Thieme, Stuttgart

Belmar J, Eyzaguirre C 1966 Pacemaker site of fibrillation potentials in denervated mammalian muscle. Journal of Neurophysiology 29: 425–441

Bergmans J 1971 Computer assisted on line measurement of motor unit parameters in human electromyography. Electromyography and Clinical Neurophysiology 11: 161

Bergmans J 1973 Computer assisted measurement of the parameters of single motor unit potentials in human electromyography. In: Desmedt J (ed) New developments in electromyography and clinical neurophysiology, vol 2. Karger, Basel

Bergmans J 1982 Repetitive activity induced in human motor axons: a model for pathological repetitive activity. In: Culp W J, Ochoa J (eds) Abnormal nerves and muscles as impulse generators. Oxford University Press, Oxford

Bernstein L P, Antel J P 1981 Motor neurone disease: decremental responses to repetitive nerve stimulation. Neurology 31: 202

Besser R, Gutmann L, Dillmann U 1989 End-plate dysfunction in acute organophosphate intoxication. Neurology 39: 561

Bill P L A, Cole G, Proctor N S F 1979 Centronuclear myopathy. Journal of Neurology, Neurosurgery and Psychiatry 42: 548

Bischoff A, Esslen E 1965 Myopathy with primary hyperparathyroidism. Neurology (Minneapolis) 15: 64–68

Black J T, Bhatt G P, DeJesus P V, Schotland D L, Rowland L P 1974 Diagnostic accuracy of clinical data, quantitative electromyography and histochemistry in neuromuscular disease. Journal of the Neurological Sciences 21: 59

Blom S, Zakrisson J E 1974 The stapedius reflex in the diagnosis of myasthenia gravis. Journal of the Neurological Sciences 21: 71

Blomberg L H, Persson T 1965 A new test for myasthenia gravis. Acta Neurologica Scandinavica 41 (suppl) 13: 363

Bohan A, Peter J B, Bowman R L, Pearson C M 1977 A computer-assisted analysis of 153 patients with polymyositis and dermatomyositis. Medicine 56: 255

Borenstein S, Desmedt J E 1973 Electromyographical signs of collateral reinnervation. In: Desmedt J E (ed) New developments in electromyography and clinical neurophysiology. Karger, Basel

Borenstein S, Desmedt J E 1974 Local cooling in myasthenia: Improvement of neuromuscular failure. Archives of Neurology 32: 152

Bosch E P, Gowans J D C, Munsat T 1979 Inflammatory myopathy in oculopharyngeal dystrophy. Muscle and Nerve 2: 73

Bradley W G, Jones M Z, Mussini J-M, Fawcett P R W 1978 Becker-type muscular dystrophy. Muscle and Nerve 1: 111

Brooks V B, Curtis D R, Eccles J C 1957 The action of tetanus toxoid on the inhibition of motoneurones. Journal of Physiology 135: 655

Brown J C 1974 Muscle weakness after rest in myotonic disorders: an electrophysiological study. Journal of Neurology, Neurosurgery and Psychiatry 37: 1336

Brown J C, Charlton J E 1975 Study of sensitivity to curare in certain neurological disorders using a regional technique. Journal of Neurology, Neurosurgery and Psychiatry 38: 34

Brown J C, Charlton J E, White D J K 1975 A regional technique for the study of sensitivity to curare in human muscle. Journal of Neurology, Neurosurgery and Psychiatry 38: 18

Brown J C, Wynn Parry C B 1981 Neuromuscular stimulation and transmission. In: Walton J N (ed)

Disorders of voluntary muscle, 4th edn. Churchill Livingstone, Edinburgh

Brown W F 1972 A method for estimating the number of motor units in thenar muscles and the changes in motor unit count with ageing. Journal of Neurology, Neurosurgery and Psychiatry 35: 845

Brown W F 1984 The physiological and technical basis of electromyography. Butterworth, London

Brown W F, Jaatoul N 1974 Amyotrophic lateral sclerosis. Electrophysiological study (number of motor units and rate of decay of motor units). Archives of Neurology 30: 242

Brunberg J A, McCormick W F, Schochet S S 1971 Type III glycogenosis. An adult with diffuse weakness and muscle wasting. Archives of Neurology 25: 71

Bryant R H 1982 Abnormal impulse production in myotonic muscle. In: Culp W J, Ochoa J (eds) Abnormal nerves and muscles as impulse generators. Oxford University Press, Oxford

Buchnall R C, Dixon A St J, Glick E N, Woodland J, Ztschi D W 1975 Myasthenia gravis associated with penicillamine treatment for rheumatoid arthritis. British Medical Journal 1: 600

Buchthal F 1961 The general concept of the motor unit. Research Publications of the Association of Nervous and Mental Diseases 38: 3

Buchthal F 1970 Electrophysiological abnormalities in metabolic myopathies and neuropathies. Acta Neurologica Scandinavica (suppl) 43: 129

Buchthal F 1982 Fibrillations: clinical electrophysiology. In: Culp W J, Ochoa J (eds) Abnormal nerves and muscles as impulse generators. Oxford University Press, New York

Buchthal F, Clemmesen S 1941 On the differentiation of muscle atrophy by electromyography. Acta Psychiatrica Neurologica Scandinavica 16: 143

Buchthal F, Kamieniecka Z 1982 The diagnostic yield of quantified electromyography and quantified muscle biopsy in neuromuscular disorders. Muscle and Nerve 5: 265

Buchthal F, Madsen A 1950 Synchronous activity in normal and atrophic muscle. Electroencephalography and Clinical Neurophysiology 2: 425

Buchthal F, Olsen P Z 1970 Electromyography and muscle biopsy in infantile spinal muscular atrophy. Brain 93: 15

Buchthal F, Rosenfalck P 1955 Action potential parameters in different human muscles. Acta Psychiatrica Scandinavica 30: 216

Buchthal F, Rosenfalck P 1963 Electrophysiological aspects of myopathy with particular reference to progressive muscular dystrophy. In: Bourne G H, Golarz M (eds) Muscular dystrophy in man and animals. Karger, New York

Buchthal F, Rosenfalck P 1966 Spontaneous electrical activity of human muscles. Electroencephalography and Clinical Neurophysiology 20: 321

Buchthal F, Erminio F, Rosenfalck P 1954a Motor unit territory in different human muscles. Acta Physiologica Scandinavica 54: 72

Buchthal F, Guld C, Rosenfalck P 1954b Action potential parameters in normal human muscle and their dependence on physical variables. Acta Physiologica Scandinavica 32: 200

Buchthal F, Pinelli P, Rosenfalck P 1954c Action potential parameters in normal human muscle and their physiological determinants. Acta Physiologica Scandinavica 32: 219

Buchthal F, Guld C, Rosenfalck P 1957 Multielectrode study of the territory of a motor unit. Acta Physiologica Scandinavica 32: 219

Bundey S, Carter C O, Solohill J F 1970 Early recognition of heterozygotes for the gene for dystrophia myotonica. Journal of Neurology, Neurosurgery and Psychiatry 33: 279

Campa J F, Sanders D B 1974 Familial hypokalemic periodic paralysis. Local recovery after nerve stimulation. Archives of Neurology 31: 110

Cao A, Cianchetti C, Calisti L, de Virgiliis S, Ferreli A, Tangheroni W 1978 Schwartz–Jampel syndrome: clinical, electrophysiological and histopathological study of a severe variant. Journal of the Neurological Sciences 35: 175

Caruso G, Buchthal F 1965 Refractory period of muscle and electromyographic findings in relatives of patients with muscular dystrophy. Brain 88: 29

Chaudhry V, Watson D F, Bird S J, Cornblath D R 1991 Stimulated single-fibre electromyography in Lambert–Eaton myasthenic syndrome. Muscle and Nerve 14: 1227

Cherington M 1973 Botulism: electrophysiological and therapeutic observations. In: Desmedt J (ed) New developments in electromyography and clinical neurophysiology. Karger, Basel

Cherington M 1974 Botulism. Ten year experience. Archives of Neurology 30: 432

Cherington M 1982 Electrophysiological methods as an aid in diagnosis of botulism: a review. Muscle and Nerve 5: s28

Christensen E 1959 Topography of terminal motor innervation in striated muscles from stillborn infants. American Journal of Physical Medicine 38: 17

Clark J, Plonsey R 1966 A mathematical evaluation of the core conductor model. Biophysical Journal 6: 95

Clark J, Plonsey R 1968 The extracellular potential field of the single active nerve fibre in a volume conductor. Biophysical Journal 8: 842

Coërs C, Woolf A L 1959 The innervation of muscle. Blackwell, Oxford

Coërs C, Telerman-Toppet N, Gerard J M, Szliwowski H, Bethlem J, Wijngaarlen G K V 1976 Changes in motor innervation and histochemical patterns in some congenital myopathies. Neurology (Minneapolis) 26: 1046

Conomy J P, Levingson M, Fanaroff A 1975 Familial infantile myasthenia gravis: a cause of sudden death in young children. Journal of Pediatrics 87: 428

Conradi S, Grimby L, Lundemo G 1982 Pathophysiology of fasciculation in ALS as studied by electromyography of single motor units. Muscle and Nerve 5: 202

Coomes E N 1965 Corticosteroid myopathy. Annals of the Rheumatic Diseases 24: 465

Cruz Martinez A, Ferrer M T, Lopez-Terradas J M, Pascual-Castroviejo I, Mingo P 1979 Single fibre electromyography in central core disease. Journal of Neurology, Neurosurgery and Psychiatry 42: 662

Cornblath D R, Sladky J T, Sumner A J 1983 Clinical electromyography of infantile botulism. Muscle and Nerve 6: 448

Cull-Candy S G, Lundh H, Thesleff S 1976 Effects of botulism toxin on neuromuscular transmission in the rat. Journal of Physiology 260: 177

Daube J R, Kelly J J, Martin R A 1979 Facial myokymia with polyradiculoneuropathy. Neurology 29: 662

Davey M R, Woolf A L 1965 An electromyographic study of carriers of muscular dystrophy. In: Proceedings of the 6th International Congress of Electroencephalography and Clinical Neurophysiology. Weiner Medizinische Akademie, Vienna

De Grandis D, Fiaschi A, Michieli G, Mezzina C 1979

Anomalous reinnervation as a sequel to obstetric brachial plexus palsy. Journal of the Neurological Sciences 43: 127

DeJesus P V, Slater R, Spitz L K, Penn A S 1973 Neuromuscular physiology of wound botulism. Archives of Neurology 29: 425

DeJong H H, Matzner I A, Unger A A 1951 Clinical and physiological studies in a case of myokymia. Archives of Neurology and Psychiatry 65: 181

Delwaide P J, Lemaire R, Reznik M 1968 EMG findings in a case of McArdle's myopathy. Electroencephalography and Clinical Neurophysiology 25: 414

Denny-Brown D 1949 Interpretation of the electromyogram. Archives of Neurology and Psychiatry 61: 99

Denny-Brown D, Pennybacker J B 1938 Fibrillation and fasciculation in voluntary muscle. Brain 61: 311

Desmedt J E 1978 Muscular dystrophy contrasted with denervation: different mechanisms underlying spontaneous fibrillation. Electroencephalography and Clinical Neurophysiology 34: 531

Desmedt J E, Borenstein S 1976 Regeneration in Duchenne muscular dystrophy. Archives of Neurology 33: 642

Desmedt J E, Borenstein S 1977a Double-step nerve stimulation test for myasthenic block: sensitisation of post-activation exhaustion by ischaemia. Annals of Neurology 1: 55

Desmedt J E, Borenstein S 1977b Time course of neonatal myasthenia gravis and unexpectedly long duration of neuromuscular block in distal muscles. New England Journal of Medicine 296: 633

DiMauro S, Hartwig G B, Hays A et al 1979 Debrancher deficiency: neuromuscular disorder in five adults. Annals of Neurology 5: 422

Dodge P R, Gamstorp I, Byers R K, Russell P 1965 Myotonic dystrophy in infancy and childhood. Pediatrics 35: 3

Dorfman L J, McGill K C, Cummins K L 1985 Electrical properties of commercial concentric EMG electrodes. Muscle and Nerve 8: 1

Drachman D B, Murphy S R, Nigam M, Hill J R 1967 'Myopathic' changes in chronically denervated muscles. Archives of Neurology 16: 14

Drechsler B, Lastoukay M 1969 An electrophysiological study of patients with thyreopathy. Electroencephalography and Clinical Neurophysiology 26: 234

Duchen L W 1973 The effects of tetanus toxin on the motor end-plates of the mouse. Journal of the Neurological Sciences 19: 160

Dyken M L, Smith D M, Peak R L 1967 An electromyographic screening test in McArdle's disease and a case report. Neurology (Minneapolis) 17: 45

Edström J, Kugelberg E 1968 Histochemical composition, distribution of fibres and fatiguability of single motor units. Journal of Neurology, Neurosurgery and Psychiatry 31: 424

Edström L 1970 Selective changes in the size of red and white muscle fibres in upper motor lesions and parkinsonism. Journal of the Neurological Sciences 11: 537

Eisen A, Karpati G 1971 Spontaneous electrical activity in muscle. Description of two patients with motor neurone disease. Journal of the Neurological Sciences 2: 137

Eisen A, Humphreys P 1974 The Guillain–Barré syndrome: a clinical and electrodiagnostic study of 25 cases. Archives of Neurology 30: 438

Eisen A, Yufe R, Trop D, Campbell I 1978 Reduced intramuscular transmission safety factor in multiple sclerosis. Neurology 28: 598

Ekbom K, Hed R, Kirstein L, Åström K E 1964 Muscular affections in chronic alcoholism. Archives of Neurology 10: 449

Ekstedt J 1964 Human single muscle fibre action potentials. Acta Physiologica Scandinavica 61 (Suppl) 226: 1

Ekstedt J, Stålberg E 1965 The diagnostic use of single muscle fibre recordings and the neuromuscular jitter in myasthenia gravis. In: the 6th International Congress of Electroencephalography and Clinical Neurophysiology Communications. Weiner Medizinische Akademie, Vienna

Ekstedt J, Stålberg E 1969a The effect of non-paralytic doses of D-tubocurarine on individual motor end-plates in man, studied with a new electrophysiological method. Electroencephalography and Clinical Neurophysiology 27: 557

Ekstedt J, Stålberg E 1969b Abnormal connections between skeletal muscle fibres. Electroencephalography and Clinical Neurophysiology 27: 607

Ekstedt J, Stålberg E 1973 Single fibre electromyography for the study of the microphysiology of the human muscle. In: Desmedt J E (ed) New developments in electromyography and clinical neurophysiology. Karger, Basel

Elmqvist D 1973 Neuromuscular transmission defects. In: Desmedt J E (ed) New developments in electromyography and clinical neurophysiology. Karger, Basel

Elmqvist D, Lambert E H 1968 Detailed analysis of neuromuscular transmission in a patient with the myasthenic syndrome sometimes associated with bronchogenic carcinoma. Mayo Clinic Proceedings 43: 689

Elmqvist D, Hofmann W W, Kugelberg E, Quastel D M J 1964 An electrophysiological investigation of neuromuscular transmission in myasthenia gravis. Journal of Physiology 174: 417

Emery A E H, Teasdall R D, Coombes E N 1966 Electromyographic studies in carriers of Duchenne muscular dystrophy. Bulletin of the Johns Hopkins Hospital 118: 439

Engel A G 1970 Acid maltase deficiency in adults: studies in four cases of syndromes which may mimic muscular dystrophy or other myopathies. Brain 93: 599

Engel A G 1980 Morphologic and immunopathologic findings in myasthenia gravis and in congenital myasthenic syndromes. Journal of Neurology, Neurosurgery and Psychiatry 43: 577

Engel A G, Gomez M R, Seybold M E, Lambert E H 1973 The spectrum and diagnosis of acid maltase deficiency. Neurology (Minneapolis) 27: 95

Engel A G, Lambert E H, Gomez M R 1977 A new myasthenic syndrome with end-plate acetylcholinesterase deficiency, small nerve terminals and reduced acetylcholine release. Annals of Neurology 1: 315

Engel A G, Lambert E H, Mulder D M et al 1982 A newly recognised congenital myasthenic syndrome attributed to a prolonged open time of the acetylcholine-induced ion channel. Annals of Neurology 11: 553

Engel A G, Walls T J, Nagel A, Uchitel O 1990 In: Aquilonius S M, Gillberg P G (eds) Progress in brain research, vol 84. Elsevier, Amsterdam

Engel W K 1975 Brief small, abundant motor unit action potentials. A further critique of electromyographic interpretation. Neurology 25: 173

Engel W K, Vick N A, Glueck C J, Levy R I 1970 A skeletal muscle disorder associated with intermittent symptoms and a possible defect of lipid metabolism. New England Journal of Medicine 282: 697

Esslen E 1960 Electromyographic findings in two types of misdirection of regenerating axons. Electroencephalography and Clinical Neurophysiology 12: 738

Falk B 1983 Automatic analysis of individual motor unit potentials recorded with a special two channel electrode. Academic Dissertation, University of Turku, Kirjapaino Pika Oy-Turku

Falk B, Alaranta H 1983 Fibrillation potentials, positive sharp waves and fasciculation in the intrinsic muscles of the feet of healthy subjects. Journal of Neurology, Neurosurgery and Psychiatry 46: 681

Fambrough D M 1979 Control of acetylcholine receptors in skeletal muscle. Physiological Reviews 59: 165

Faris A A, Reyes M G 1971 Reappraisal of alcoholic myopathy. Clinical and biopsy study on chronic alcoholics without muscle weakness or wasting. Journal of Neurology, Neurosurgery and Psychiatry 34: 86

Fawcett P R W, Mastaglia F L, Mechler F 1982a Electrophysiological findings including single fibre EMG in a family with mitochondrial myopathy. Journal of the Neurological Sciences 53: 397

Fawcett P R W, McLachlan S M, Nicholson L B V, Argov Z, Mastaglia F L 1982b D-penicillamine-associated myasthenia gravis: immunological and electrophysiological studies. Muscle and Nerve 5: 328

Fawcett P R W, Dick D J, Schofield I S 1985a SFEMG and macro EMG in Becker muscular dystrophy. Electroencephalography and Clinical Neurophysiology 61: 3 (S76)

Fawcett P R W, Dick D J, Schofield I S 1986 Single fibre EMG and macro EMG in spinal muscular atrophy. Electroencephalography and Clinical Neurophysiology 63: 33P

Fawcett P R W, Johnson M A, Schofield I S 1985b Comparison of electrophysiological and histochemical methods for assessing the spatial distribution of muscle fibres of a motor unit within muscle. Journal of the Neurological Sciences 69: 67

Fawcett P R W, Slater C R, Walls T J, Gardner-Medwin D 1989 Impaired transmitter release in a new congenital myasthenic syndrome with a paucity of post-synaptic folds. Journal of Neurology, Neurosurgery and Psychiatry 52: 1207

Feinstein B, Lindegard B, Nyman E, Wohlfart G 1955 Morphologic studies of motor units in normal human muscles. Acta Anatomica 23: 127

Fernandez J M, Fernandez M, Larrea L, Ramio R, Boada M 1983 Cephalic tetanus studied with single fibre EMG. Journal of Neurology, Neurosurgery and Psychiatry 46: 862

Fitch P 1967 An analyser for use in human electromyography. Electronic Engineering 39: 240

Floyd M, Ayyar D R, Barwick D D, Hudgson P, Weightman D 1974 Myopathy in chronic renal failure. Quarterly Journal of Medicine 53: 509

Forster F M, Alpers B J 1944 The site of origin of fasciculation in voluntary muscle. Archives of Neurology and Psychiatry 51: 254

Forster F M, Borkowski W J, Alpers B J 1946 Effects of denervation on fasciculation in human muscle. Archives of Neurology 56: 276

Fowler W M, Layzer R B, Taylor R G et al 1974 The Schwartz–Jampel syndrome: its clinical, physiological and histological expression. Journal of the Neurological Sciences 22: 127

Frame B, Heinze E G Jr, Block M A, Manson G A 1968 Myopathy in primary hyperparathyroidism. Observations in three patients. Annals of Internal Medicine 68: 1022

Fuglsang-Frederiksen A, Månsson A 1975 Analysis of electrical activity of normal muscle in man at different degrees of voluntary effort. Journal of Neurology, Neurosurgery and Psychiatry 38: 683

Fuglsang-Frederiksen A, Lo Monaco M, Dahl K 1984 Integrated electrical activity and number of zero crossings during a gradual increase in muscle force in patients with neuromuscular diseases. Electroencephalography and Clinical Neurophysiology 58(3): 211

Fuglsang-Frederiksen A, Scheel U, Buchthal F 1976 Diagnostic yield of analysis of the pattern of electrical activity and of individual motor unit potentials in myopathy. Journal of Neurology, Neurosurgery and Psychiatry 39: 742

Fuglsang-Frederiksen A, Scheel U, Buchthal F 1977 Diagnostic yield of the analysis of the pattern of electrical activity of muscle and of individual motor unit potentials in neurogenic involvement. Journal of Neurology, Neurosurgery and Psychiatry 40: 544

Fullerton P M, Gilliatt R W 1965 Axonal reflexes in human motor nerve fibres. Journal of Neurology, Neurosurgery and Psychiatry 28: 1

Gage P W 1976 Generation of end-plate potentials. Physiology Reviews 56: 177

Gamstorp I, Wohlfart G 1959 A syndrome characterised by myokymia, myotonia, muscular wasting and increased perspiration. Acta Psychiatrica Scandinavica 34: 181

Gardner-Medwin D 1968 Studies on the carrier state of the Duchenne type of muscular dystrophy. 2. Quantitative electromyography as a method of carrier detection. Journal of Neurology, Neurosurgery and Psychiatry 31: 124

Gardner-Medwin D, Walton J N 1969 Myokymia with impaired muscle relaxation Lancet ii: 127

Gath I, Sjaastad O, Løken A C 1969 Myopathic electromyographic changes correlated with histopathology in Wohlfart–Kugelberg–Welander disease. Neurology (Minneapolis) 19: 344

Gath I, Stålberg E 1977 On the volume conduction in human muscle: in situ measurements. Electroencephalography and Clinical Neurophysiology 43: 106

Gath I, Stålberg E 1978 The calculated radial decline of extracellular action potential compared with in situ measurements in the human brachial biceps. Electroencephalography and Clinical Neurophysiology 4: 547

Gath I, Stålberg E 1982 On the measurement of fibre density in human muscles. Electroencephalography and Clinical Neurophysiology 54: 699

Geddes L A, Baker L E 1967 The specific resistance of biologic material — a compendium for the biomedical engineer and physiologist. Medical Biological Engineering 5: 271

Gilchrist J M, Sanders D B 1989 Myasthenic U-shaped decrement in multifocal cervical radiculopathy. Muscle and Nerve 12: 64

Gilliatt R W 1966 Applied electrophysiology in nerve and muscle disease. Proceedings of the Royal Society of Medicine 59: 989

Gil-Peralta A, Rafel E, Bautista J, Alberrca R 1978 Myotonia in centronuclear myopathy. Journal of Neurology, Neurosurgery and Psychiatry 41: 1102

Goldkamp O 1967 Electromyography and nerve conduction studies in 116 patients with hemiplegia. Archives of Physical Medicine 48: 59

Gootzen T H J M, Vingerhoets D J M, Stegeman D F 1992 A study of motor unit structure by means of scanning EMG. Muscle and Nerve 15: 349

Gordon A M, Green J R, Lagunoff D 1970 Studies on a patient with hypokalemic familial periodic paralysis. American Journal of Medicine 48: 185

Gordon E E, Jauszko D M, Kaufman L 1967 A critical survey of the stiff-man syndrome. American Journal of Medicine 42: 582

Greenhouse A H, Bicknell J M, Pesch R N, Seelinger D F 1967 Myotonia, myokymia, hyperhidrosis and wasting of muscle. Neurology (Minneapolis) 17: 263

Greer M, Schotland M 1969 Myasthenia in the newborn. Paediatrics 26: 101

Grob D, Johns R J, Liljestrand A 1957 Potassium movement in patients with familial periodic paralysis. American Journal of Medicine 23: 356

Grob D, Namba T 1976 Characteristics and mechanism of neuromuscular block in myasthenia gravis. Annals of the New York Academy of Science 274: 143

Guld C 1951 On the influence of the measuring electrodes on the duration and amplitude of muscle action potentials. Acta Physiologica Scandinavica (Suppl) 89: 30

Guld C, Rosenfalck A, Willison R G 1970 Technical factors in recording electrical activity of muscle and nerve in man. Electroencephalography and Clinical Neurophysiology 28: 399

Gutman L, Pratt L 1976 Pathophysiologic aspects of human botulism. Archives of Neurology 33: 175

Guy E, Lefebre J, Lerique J, Scherrer J 1950 Le signes electromyographiques des dermatomyosites. Etude de 9 cas. Revue Neurologique 83: 278

Haass A, Ricker K, Rüdel R et al 1981 Clinical study of paramyotonia congenita with and without myotonia in a warm environment. Muscle and Nerve 4: 388

Håkansson C H 1957 Action potentials recorded intra and extracellularly from the isolated frog muscle fibre in Ringer's solution and in air. Acta Physiologica Scandinavica 39: 291

Hakelius L, Stålberg E 1974 Electromyographical studies of free autogenous muscle transplants in man. Scandinavian Journal of Plastic and Reconstructive Surgery 8: 211

Harel S, Chui L A, Shapira Y 1979 Myotonia congenita (Thomsen's disease): early diagnosis in infancy. Acta Pediatrica Scandinavica 68: 225

Harman J B, Richardson A T 1954 Generalised myokymia in thyrotoxicosis. Report of a case. Lancet ii: 473

Harper P S 1975 Congenital myotonic dystrophy in Britain. 1. Clinical aspects. Archives of Disease in Childhood 50: 505

Hart Z H, Sahashi K, Lambert E H, Engel A G, Lindstrom J M 1979 A congenital, familial myasthenic syndrome caused by a presynaptic defect of transmitter resynthesis or mobilisation. Neurology 29: 556

Harvey A M, Masland R L 1941 A method for the study of neuromuscular transmission in human subjects. Bulletin of the Johns Hopkins Hospital 69: 1

Hausmanowa-Petrusewicz I, Prot J, Niebrój-Dobosz I et al 1968 Studies of healthy relatives of patients with Duchenne muscular dystrophy. Journal of the Neurological Sciences 7: 465

Hausmanowa-Petrusewicz I, Jedrzejowska H 1971 Correlation between electromyographic findings and muscle biopsy in cases of neuromuscular disease. Journal of the Neurological Sciences 13: 85

Hausmanowa-Petrusewicz I, Karwanska A 1986 Electromyographic findings in different forms of infantile and juvenile proximal spinal muscular atrophy. Muscle and Nerve 9: 37

Hawkes C H, Absolon M J 1975 Myotubular myopathy associated with cataract and electrical myotonia. Journal of Neurology, Neurosurgery and Psychiatry 38: 761

Hayward M 1977 Automatic analysis of the electromyogram in healthy subjects of different ages. Journal of the Neurological Sciences 33: 397

Hayward M 1983 Quantification of interference patterns. In: Desmedt J E (ed) Progress in clinical neurophysiology, vol 10, Computer-Aided Electromyography. Karger, Basel, p 128

Hayward M, Willison R G 1973 The recognition of myogenic and neurogenic lesions by quantitative EMG. In: Desmedt J E (ed) New developments in electromyography and clinical neurophysiology, vol 2. Karger, Basel, p 448

Hayward M, Willison R G 1977 Automatic analysis of the electromyogram in patients with chronic partial denervation. Journal of the Neurological Sciences 33: 415

Hed R, Lundmark C, Fahlgren H, Orell S 1962 Acute muscular syndrome in chronic alcoholism. Acta Medica Scandinavica 171: 585

Henneman E 1957 Relation between size of neurons and their susceptibility to discharge. Science 126: 1345

Henriksson K G, Stålberg E 1978 The terminal innervation pattern in polymyositis: a histological and SFEMG study. Muscle and Nerve 1: 3

Hertel G, Ricker K, Hirsch A 1977 The regional curare test in myasthenia gravis. Journal of Neurology 24: 257

Hilfiker P, Meyer M 1984 Normal and myopathic propagation of surface motor unit action potentials. Electroencephalography and Clinical Neurophysiology 57: 21

Hilton-Brown P, Stålberg E, Osterman P O 1982 Signs of reinnervation in myasthenia gravis. Muscle and Nerve 5: 215

Hilton-Brown P, Stålberg E 1983a The motor unit in muscular dystrophy, a single fibre EMG and scanning EMG study. Journal of Neurology, Neurosurgery and Psychiatry 46: 981

Hilton-Brown P, Stålberg E 1983b Motor unit size in muscular dystrophy, a macro EMG and scanning EMG study. Journal of Neurology, Neurosurgery and Psychiatry 46: 996

Hilton-Brown P, Stålberg E, Trontelj J, Mihelin M 1985 Causes of the increased fibre density in muscular dystrophies studied with single fibre EMG during electrical stimulation. Muscle and Nerve 8: 383

Hirose K, Uono M, Sobue I 1974 Quantitative electromyography; comparison between manual values and computer ones on normal subjects. Electromyography and Clinical Neurophysiology 14: 315

Hjorth R J, Walsh J C, Willison R G 1973 The distribution and frequency of spontaneous fasciculations in motor neurone disease. Journal of the Neurological Sciences 18: 469

Hofmann W W, DeNardo G L 1968 Sodium flux in myotonic muscular dystrophy. American Journal of Physiology 214: 330

Hogan G R, Gutmann L, Schmidt R, Gilbert E 1969 Pompe's disease. Neurology (Minneapolis) 19: 894

Horowitz S H, Genkins G, Kornfeld P, Papatestas A E 1975 Regional curare test in evaluation of ocular myasthenia. Archives of Neurology 32: 84

Horowitz S H, Sivak M 1978 The regional curare test and electrophysiologic diagnosis of myasthenia gravis: further studies. Muscle and Nerve 1: 432

Howard F M 1963 A new and effective drug in the treatment of the stiff-man syndrome. Proceedings of the Staff of the Mayo Clinic 38: 203

Howard R S, Murray N M F 1992 Surface EMG in the recording of fasciculations. Muscle and Nerve 15: 1240

Hubbard J I, Llinas R, Quastel D M J 1969 Electrophysiological analysis of synaptic transmission. Edward Arnold, London

Hudgson P, Bradley W G, Jenkison M 1972 Familial 'mitochondrial' myopathy — a myopathy associated with disordered oxidative metabolism in muscle fibres. Journal of the Neurological Sciences 16: 343

Hudgson P, Barwick D D 1974 Myopathy in chronic renal failure. 3rd International Congress on Muscle Diseases. Excerpta Medica, Amsterdam 334: 172

Hudson A J, Cholod E J, Haust M D 1970 Familial hyperparathyroid myopathy. In: Walton J N, Canal C, Scarlato G (eds) Muscle disease: Exerpta Medica, Amsterdam, p 526

Hudson A J, Brown W F, Gilbert J J 1978 The muscular pain-fasciculation syndrome. Neurology 28: 1105

Hughes R C, Matthews W B 1969 Pseudomyotonia and myokymia. Journal of Neurology, Neurosurgery and Psychiatry 32: 11

Hynninen P, Philipson L, Manderson B, Elmqvist D 1979 A computer based method for automatic motor unit potential analysis. Acta Neurologica Scandinavica 60 (suppl) 73: 300

Isaacs H 1961 A syndrome of continuous muscle-fibre activity. Journal of Neurology, Neurosurgery and Psychiatry 24: 319

Isaacs H 1967 Continuous muscle fibre activity in an Indian male with additional evidence of terminal motor fibre abnormality. Journal of Neurology, Neurosurgery and Psychiatry 30: 126

Isaacs H, Heffron J J A, Badenhorst M 1975 Central core disease. Journal of Neurology, Neurosurgery and Psychiatry 38: 1177

Jabre J F 1988 Macro-electromyographic studies using a new electrode. Journal of Clinical Neurophysiology 5: 204

Jabre J F 1991 Concentric macro electromyography. Muscle and Nerve 14: 820

Jasper H, Ballem G 1949 Unipolar electromyograms of normal and denervated human muscle. Journal of Neurophysiology 12: 231

Johnson E W, Denny S T, Kelley J P 1975 Sequence of electromyographic abnormalities in stroke syndrome. Archives of Physical Medicine and Rehabilitation 56: 468

Jones R V, Lambert E H, Sayre G P 1955 Source of a type of 'insertion activity' in electromyography with evaluation of a histologic method of localisation. Archives of Physical Medicine 36: 301

Josefsson I O 1960 An electromyographic study of botulism intoxicated skeletal muscle. Acta Physiologica Scandinavica 49(suppl): 172

Jusic A, Dogan S, Stojanovic V 1972 Hereditary persistent distal cramps. Journal of Neurology, Neurosurgery and Psychiatry 35: 379

Kaiser E, Petersén I 1963 Frequency analysis of muscle action potentials during tetanic contraction. Electromyography 3: 5

Kaiser E, Petersén I 1965 Muscle action potentials studied by frequency analysis and duration measurement. Acta Neurologica Scandinavica 41 (suppl) 13: 213

Katz B 1966 Nerve, muscle and synapse. McGraw-Hill, New York

Katz B, Miledi R 1965 Propagation of electrical activity in motor nerve terminals. Proceedings of the Royal Scciety B 161: 453

Katz B, Miledi R 1968 The role of calcium in neuromuscular facilitation. Journal of Physiology 195: 481

Kelly J J, Daube J R, Lennon V A, Howard F M, Younge B R 1982 The laboratory diagnosis of mild myasthenia. Annals of Neurology 12: 238

Kennett R P, Fawcett P R W 1990a Repetitive nerve stimulation of the anconeus muscle. Muscle and Nerve 13: 975

Kennett R P, Fawcett P R W 1990b Effect of frequency on axonal stimulation jitter values in myasthenic disorders. Muscle and Nerve 13: 975

Kimura J 1989 Electrodiagnosis in diseases of nerve and muscle: principles and practice. Davis, Philadelphia

King R B, Stoops W L 1973 Cervical myelopathy with fasciculations in the lower extremity. Journal of Neurosurgery 20: 945

Konishi T, Nishitani H, Matsubara F, Ohta M 1981 Myasthenia gravis: relation between jitter in single fibre EMG and antibody to acetylcholine receptor. Neurology (New York) 31: 386

Kopec J, Hausmanowa-Petrusewicz I 1969 Histogram of muscle potentials recorded automatically with the aid of the averaging computer 'Anops'. Electromyography and Clinical Neurophysiology 9: 36

Kopec J, Hausmanowa-Petrusewicz I 1976 On-line computer application in clinical quantitative electromyography. Electromyography and Clinical Neurophysiology 16: 49

Kopec J, Hausmanowa-Petrusewicz I 1983 Computeranalyse des EMG und klinishe Ergebensse. EEG-EMG. 14: 28

Kopec J, Hausmanowa-Petrusewicz I, Rawaki M, Wolynski M 1973 Automatic analysis in electromyography. In: Desmedt J (ed) New developments in electromyography and clinical neurophysiology, vol 2. Karger, Basel

Kramer L D, Ruth R A, Johns M E, Sanders D B 1981 A comparison of stapedial reflex fatigue with repetitive stimulation and single fibre EMG in myasthenia gravis. Annals of Neurology 9: 531

Krendel D A, Sanders D B, Massey J M 1987 Single fibre electromyography in chronic progressive external ophthalmoplegia. Muscle and Nerve 10: 299

Kugelberg E 1947 Electromyogram in muscular disorders. Journal of Neurology, Neurosurgery and Psychiatry 10: 122

Kugelberg E 1948 Activation of human nerves by ischaemia. Archives of Neurology and Psychiatry 60: 140

Kugelberg E 1949 Electromyography in muscular dystrophy. Journal of Neurology, Neurosurgery and Psychiatry 10: 122

Kugelberg E 1973 Properties of the rat hind-limb motor units. In: Desmedt J E (ed) New developments in electromyography and clinical neurophysiology, vol 1. Karger, Basel

Kugelberg E, Petersén I 1949 'Insertion activity' in electromyography. Journal of Neurology, Neurosurgery and Psychiatry 12: 268

Kuitonnen P, Rapola J, Noponen A L, Donner M 1972 Nemaline myopathy. Report of 4 cases and review of the literature. Acta Pediatrica Scandinavica 61: 353

Kunze K 1971 Die automatische Analyse in der klinischen Electromyographie. Nervenarzt 42: 275

Kunze K 1973 Quantitative EMG analysis in myogenic and neurogenic muscle disease. In: Desmedt J E (ed) New developments in electromyography and clinical neurophysiology, vol 2. Karger, Basel

Lambert E H 1969 Electromyography in amyotrophic lateral sclerosis. In: Norris F H, Kurland L T (eds) Motor neurone disease. Grune and Stratton, New York

Lambert E H 1978 Muscle spasms, cramps and stiffness. American Academy of Neurology (Special Course) 17

Lambert E H 1982 Electrophysiological studies of the myasthenic syndrome and congenital neuromuscular syndromes. In: Didactic programme, 29th annual meeting. American Association of Electromyography and Electrodiagnosis, Minneapolis

Lambert E H, Mulder D W 1957 Electromyography studies in amyotrophic lateral sclerosis. Proceedings of the Staff Meetings of the Mayo Clinic 32: 441

Lambert E H, Rooke E D, Eaton L M, Hodgson C H 1961 Myasthenic syndrome occasionally associated with bronchial neoplasm–neurophysiologic studies. In: Viets H R (ed) Myasthenia gravis. Thomas, Springfield, Illinois

Lance J W, Burke D, Pollard J 1979 Hyperexcitability of motor neurones in neuromyotonia. Annals of Neurology 5: 523

Landau W M 1952 The essential mechanism in myotonia. Neurology (Minneapolis) 2: 369

Lang A H, Falk B 1980 A two-channel method for sampling, averaging and quantifying motor unit potentials. Journal of Neurology 223: 199

Lang A H, Nurkkanen P, Vaahtoranta K M 1971 Automatic sampling and averaging of electromyographic unit potentials. Electroencephalography and Clinical Neurophysiology 31: 404

Lang A H, Partanen V S J 1976 'Satellite' potentials and the duration of motor unit potentials in normal, neuropathic and myopathic muscles. Journal of the Neurological Sciences 27: 513

Lange D J, Brin M F, Warner C L, Lovelace R E, Fahn S 1987 Distant effects of local injection of botulinum toxin. Muscle and Nerve 10: 552

Lange D J, Britton C B, Younger D S, Hays A P 1988 The neuromuscular manifestations of human immunodeficiency virus infections. Archives of Neurology 45: 1084

Lange D J, Rubin M, Greene P E et al 1991 Distant effects of locally injected botulinum toxin: a double-blind study of single fibre EMG changes. Muscle and Nerve 14: 672

Larsson L E 1968 Frequency analysis of the EMG in neuromuscular disorders. Electroencephalography and Clinical Neurophysiology 24: 89

Larsson L E 1975 On the relation between the EMG frequency spectrum and the duration of symptoms in lesions of the peripheral motor neurone. Electroencephalography and Clinical Neurophysiology 38: 69

Layzer R B, Rowland L P 1971 Cramps. New England Journal of Medicine 285: 31

Lazaro R P, Fenichel G M, Kilroy A W 1979 Congenital muscular dystrophy: case reports and reappraisal. Muscle and Nerve 2: 349

Lazaro R P, Rollinson R D, Fenichel G M 1981 Familial cramps and muscle pain. Archives of Neurology 38: 22

Lecky B R F, Morgan-Hughes J A, Murray N M F, Landon D N, Wray D 1986 Congenital myasthenia: further evidence of disease heterogeneity. Muscle and Nerve 9: 233

Lee R G, White D G 1973 Computer analysis of motor unit action potentials in routine clinical electromyography. In: Desmedt J (ed) New developments in electromyography and clinical neurophysiology. Karger, Basel

Lefvert A K, Osterman P O 1983 New-born infants to myasthenic mothers: a clinical study and an investigation of acetylcholine receptor antibodies in 17 children. Neurology 33: 33

Lehmann-Horn F, Iaizzo P A, Franke C, Hatt H, Spaans F 1990 Schwartz–Jampel syndrome: II. Na^+ channel defect causes myotonia. Muscle and Nerve 13: 528

Lehmann-Horn F, Rudel R, Dengler R, Lorkovic H, Haass A, Ricker K 1981 Membrane defects in paramyotonia with and without myotonia in a warm environment. Muscle and Nerve 2: 109

Lehmann-Horn F, Rudel R, Ricker K, Lorkovic H, Dengler R, Hopf H C 1983 Two cases of adynamia episodica hereditaria: in vitro investigation of muscle cell membrane and contraction parameters. Muscle and Nerve 6: 113

Lenman J A R 1965 Effect of denervation on the resting membrane potential of healthy and dystrophic muscle. Journal of Neurology, Neurosurgery and Psychiatry 28: 525

Li C Y, Shy G M, Wells J 1957 Some properties of mammalian skeletal muscle fibres with particular reference to fibrillation potentials. Journal of Physiology 135: 522

Lindholm T 1968 The influence of uraemia and electrolyte disturbances on muscle action potentials and motor nerve conduction in man. Acta Medica Scandinavica Supplementum 491: 81

Lindsley D B 1935 Electrical activity of human motor units during voluntary contraction. American Journal of Physiology 114: 90

Lindström L 1985 Spectral analysis of EMG. In: Struppler A, Weindle A (eds) Electromyography and evoked potentials. Springer-Verlag, Berlin, p 103

Lindström L, Petersén I 1981 Power spectra of myoelectric signals: motor unit activity and muscle fatigue. In: Stålberg E, Young R R (eds) Neurology 1; clinical neurophysiology. Butterworth, London, p 66

Lippold O C J, Redfern J W T, Vuco J 1957 The rhythmical activity of groups of motor units in the voluntary contraction of muscle. Journal of Physiology 137: 473

Lopez-Terradas J M, Conde Lopez M 1979 Late components of motor units in central core disease. Journal of Neurology, Neurosurgery and Psychiatry 42: 461

Lublin F D, Tsairis P, Streletz L J, Chambers R A, Riker F, VanPosnak A, Duckett S W 1979 Myokymia and impaired muscular relaxation with continuous motor unit activity. Journal of Neurology, Neurosurgery and Psychiatry 42: 557

Luco J V, Eyzaguirre C 1955 Fibrillation and hypersensitivity to ACh in denervated muscle: effect of length of degenerating nerve fibre. Journal of Neurophysiology 18: 65

Ludin H P 1980 Electromyography in practice. Thieme Verlag, Stuttgart

Lundberg P O, Osterman P O, Stålberg E 1970 Neuromuscular signs and symptoms in acromegaly. In: Walton J N, Canal N, Scarlato G (eds) Muscle diseases. Exerpta Medica, Amsterdam

Lundberg P O, Stålberg E, Thiele B 1974 Paralysis periodica myotonica. A clinical and neurophysiological study. Journal of the Neurological Sciences 21: 309

McComas A J 1991 Invited review: motor unit estimation: methods, results, and present status. Muscle and Nerve 14: 585

McComas A J, Johns R F 1981 Potential changes in the normal and diseased muscle cell. In: Walton J N (ed) Disorders of voluntary muscle, 4th edn. Churchill Livingstone, Edinburgh

McComas A J, Mrozek K 1968 The electrical properties of

muscle fibre membranes in dystrophia myotonica and myotonia congenita. Journal of Neurology, Neurosurgery and Psychiatry 31: 441

McComas A J, Sica R E P, Campbell M J 1971a 'Sick motor neurones': a unifying concept of muscle disease. Lancet ii: 321

McComas A J, Fawcett P R W, Campbell M J, Sica R E P 1971b Electrophysiological estimates of the number of motor units within a human muscle. Journal of Neurology, Neurosurgery and Psychiatry 34: 121

McComas A J, Sica R E P, Upton A R M, Aguilera N 1973 Functional changes in motor neurones of hemiparetic patients. Journal of Neurology, Neurosurgery and Psychiatry 36: 183

McComas A J, Sica R E P, Toyonga K 1978 Incidence, severity and time-course of moto-neurone dysfunction in myotonic dystrophy. Journal of Neurology, Neurosurgery and Psychiatry 41: 882

Markesbury W R, Griggs R C, Leach R P, Lapham L W 1974a Late onset hereditary distal myopathy. Neurology (Minneapolis) 24: 127

Markesbury W R, McQuillen M P, Procois P G, Harrison A R, Engel A G 1974b Muscle carnitine deficiency. Association with lipid myopathy, vacuolar neuropathy and vacuolated leucocytes. Archives of Neurology 31: 320

Martinelli P, Pazzaglia P, Montagna P et al 1978 Stiff-man syndrome associated with nocturnal myoclonus and epilepsy. Journal of Neurology, Neurosurgery and Psychiatry 41: 58

Maselli R A, Mass D P, Distad B J, Richman D P 1991 Anconeus muscle: a human muscle preparation suitable for in-vitro microelectrode studies. Muscle and Nerve 14: 1189

Maselli R A, Burnett M E, Tonsgard J H 1992 In vitro microelectrode study on neuromuscular transmission in a case of botulism. Muscle and Nerve 15: 273

Mastaglia F L, Barwick D D, Hall R 1970 Myopathy in acromegalics. Lancet ii: 907

Mastaglia F L, Papadimitriou J M, Dawkins R L, Beveridge B 1977 Vacuolar myopathy associated with chloroquine, lupus erythematosus and thymoma. Journal of the Neurological Sciences 34: 315

Masuda T, Miyano H, Sadoyama T 1983 The propagation of motor unit action potentials and the location of neuromuscular junction by surface electrode array. Electroencephalography and Clinical Neurophysiology 55: 594

Masuda T, Miyano H, Sadoyama T 1985 A surface electrode array for detecting action potential trains of single motor units. Electroencephalography and Clinical Neurophysiology 60: 435

Matthes J W A, Kenna A P, Fawcett P R W 1991 Familial infantile myasthenia: a diagnostic problem. Developmental Medicine and Child Neurology 33: 924

Mayer R F, Williams I R 1974 Incrementing responses in myasthenia gravis. Archives of Neurology 31: 24

Meadows J C 1971 Fasciculation caused by suxamethonium and other cholinergic agents. Acta Neurologica Scandinavica 47: 381

Mechler F 1974 Changing electromyographic findings during the chronic course of polymyositis. Journal of the Neurological Sciences 23: 237

Mechler F, Fawcett P R W, Mastaglia F L, Hudgson P 1981 Mitochondrial myopathy. A study of clinically affected and asymptomatic members of a six-generation family. Journal of the Neurological Sciences 50: 191

Meink H M, Ricker K, Conrad B 1984 The stiff-man syndrome: new pathophysiological aspects from abnormal exteroceptive reflexes and the response to clomipramine, clonidine and tizanide. Journal of Neurology, Neurosurgery and Psychiatry 47: 280

Mertens H G, Zschocke S 1965 Neuromyotonia. Klinische Wochenschrift 43: 917

Messina C, Tonali P, Scopetta C 1976 The lack of deep reflexes in myotonic dystrophy: a neurophysiological study. Journal of the Neurological Sciences 30: 303

Messina C, Dattola R, Ginlanda P 1979 Effect of guanidine on the neuromuscular block of botulism. An electrophysiological study. Acta Neurologica Napoli 34: 459

Miglietta O E 1971 Myasthenic-like response in patients with neuropathy. American Journal of Physical Medicine 50: 1

Miledi R, Slater C R 1963 A study in rat nerve–muscle junctions after degeneration of the nerve. Journal of Physiology 151: 1

Miller R G, Blank N K, Layzer R B 1979 Sporadic distal myopathy with early adult onset. Annals of Neurology 5: 220

Milner-Brown H S, Brown W F 1976 New methods of estimating the number of motor units in a muscle. Journal of Neurology, Neurosurgery and Psychiatry 39: 258

Milner-Brown H S, Stein R B 1975 The relation between the surface electromyogram and muscular force. Journal of Physiology 246: 549

Mizusawa H, Takagi A, Sugita H, Toyokura Y 1983 Mounding phenomenon: an experimental study in vitro. Neurology 33: 90

Moersch F P, Woltman H W 1956 Progressive fluctuating muscular rigidity and spasm ('stiff-man' syndrome): report of a case and some observations on 13 other cases. Proceedings of the Staff of Mayo Clinic 31: 421

Moosa A, Brown B H, Dubowitz V 1972 Quantitative electromyography: carrier detection in Duchenne type muscular dystrophy using a new automatic technique. Journal of Neurology, Neurosurgery and Psychiatry 35: 841

Mori M, Takamori M 1976 Hyperthyroidism and myasthenia gravis with features of Eaton–Lambert syndrome. Neurology (Minneapolis) 26: 882

Morrison J B 1960 The electromyographic changes in hyperkalaemic familial periodic paralysis. Annals of Physical Medicine 5: 153

Mrozek K, Strugalska M, Fidzianska A A 1970 A sporadic case of central core disease. Journal of the Neurological Sciences 10: 339

Mulder D W, Lambert E H, Eaton L M 1959 Myasthenic syndrome in patients with amyotrophic lateral sclerosis. Neurology (Minneapolis) 9: 627

Muller R, Kugelberg E 1959 Myopathy in Cushing's syndrome. Journal of Neurology, Neurosurgery and Psychiatry 22: 314

Munsat T L, Thompson L R, Coleman R F 1969 Centrinuclear ('myotubular') myopathy. Archives of Neurology 20: 120

Murphy S F, Drachman D B 1968 The oculopharyngeal syndrome. Journal of the American Medical Association 203: 1003

Nakao K, Nakanishi T, Tsubaki T 1965 Action potentials recorded by co-axial needle electrodes in Ringer's solution. Electroencephalography and Clinical Neurophysiology 18: 412

Nandedkar S D, Sanders D B 1991 Recording characteristics of monopolar EMG electrodes. Muscle and Nerve 14: 108

Nandedkar S, Sanders D, Stålberg E 1984 Simulation of concentric needle EMG motor unit action potentials. Muscle and Nerve 7: 562

Nandedkar S, Sanders D, Stålberg E V 1986a Automatic analysis of the electromyographic interference pattern. Part I: Development of quantitative features. Muscle and Nerve 9: 431

Nandedkar S, Sanders D, Stålberg E V 1986b Automatic analysis of the electromyographic interference pattern. Part II: Findings in control subjects and in some neuromuscular disorders. Muscle and Nerve 9: 491

Nandedkar S, Sanders D, Stålberg E V, Andreassen S 1988 Simulation of concentric needle EMG motor unit action potentials. Muscle and Nerve 11: 151

Nandedkar S, Stålberg E 1983 Simulation of macro EMG motor unit potentials. Electroencephalography and Clinical Neurophysiology 56: 52

Nielson V K, Friis M L, Johnsen T 1982 Electromyographic distinction between paramyotonia congenita and myotonia congenita: effect of cold. Neurology 32: 827

Nishizono H, Saito Y, Miyshita M 1979 The estimation of conduction velocity in human skeletal muscle in situ with surface electrodes. Electroencephalography and Clinical Neurophysiology 46: 659

Nix W A, Scherer A 1992 Single fiber macro versus concentric trigger macro EMG: a comparison of methods. Muscle and Nerve 15: 193

Norris F H 1965 Central mechanisms of fasciculations. In: Proceedings of the 6th International Congress of Electroencephalography and Clinical Neurophysiology. Wiener Zinosche Akademie, Wien

Norris F H 1966 Neuromuscular transmission in thyroid disease. Annals of Internal Medicine 64: 81

Norris F H, Panner B J 1966 Hypothyroid myopathy, clinical electromyographic and ultrastructural observations. Archives of Neurology 14: 574

Nutter P, Collins K 1988 Diffuse positive waves: case report. Archives of Physical Medicine and Rehabilitation 69: 295

Oh S J 1977 Botulism: electrophysiological studies. Annals of Neurology 1: 481

Okuno T, Mori K, Furomi K, Takeoka T, Kondo K 1981 Myotonic dystrophy and hypothyroidism. Neurology 31: 91

Olney R K, Aminoff M J, Gell D J, Lowenstein D H 1988 Neuromuscular effects distant from the site of botulinum neurotoxin injection. Neurology 38: 1780

Olson W W K, Engel W K, Walsh G O, Einaugler R 1972 Oculocraniosomatic neuromuscular disease with 'ragged-red' fibres. Archives of Neurology 26: 193

Oosterhuis H J G H, Hoostmans W J M, Veenhuyzen H B, Van Zadelhoff 1972 The mean duration of motor unit potentials in patients with myasthenia gravis. Electroencephalography and Clinical Neurophysiology 12: 697

Oosterhuis H J G H, Newsom-Davis J, Wokke J H J et al 1987 The slow channel syndrome. Two new cases. Brain 110: 1061

Özdemir C, Young R R 1971 Electrical testing on myasthenia gravis. Annals of the New York Academy of Sciences 183: 287

Özdemir C, Young R R 1976 The results to be expected from electrical testing in the diagnosis of myasthenia gravis. Annals of the New York Academy of Sciences 274: 203

Panayiotopoulos C P, Scarpalezos S 1976 Dystrophia myotonica: peripheral nerve involvement and pathogenetic implications. Journal of the Neurological Sciences 27: 1

Partanen J, Lang H 1982 EMG dynamics in polymyositis. Journal of the Neurological Sciences 57: 221

Patten B M, Hert A, Lovelace R 1972 Multiple sclerosis associated with defects in neuromuscular transmission. Journal of Neurology, Neurosurgery and Psychiatry 32: 12

Payan J 1978 The blanket principle: a technical note. Muscle and Nerve 1: 423

Pearson C M 1964 The periodic paralyses. Brain 87: 341

Perkoff G T, Dioso M M, Blisch V, Klinkerfuss G 1967 A spectrum of myopathy associated with alcoholism. 1 Clinical and laboratory features. Annals of Internal Medicine 67: 481

Petajan J H, Thurman D J 1981 EMG and histochemical findings in neurogenic atrophy with electrode localisation. Journal of Neurology, Neurosurgery and Psychiatry 44: 1050

Petersén I, Kugelberg E 1949 Duration and form of action potentials in the normal human muscle. Journal of Neurology, Neurosurgery and Psychiatry 12: 124

Pickett J B, Schmidley J W 1980 Sputtering positive potentials in the EMG: an artefact resembling positive waves. Neurology (Minneapolis) 30: 215

Pickett J, Berg B, Chaplin E, Brunstetter-Shafer M A 1976 Syndrome of botulism in infancy: clinical and electrophysiologic study. New England Journal of Medicine 295: 770

Pinelli P, Buchthal F 1953 Muscle action potentials in myopathies with special regard to progressive muscular dystrophy. Neurology (Minneapolis) 3: 347

Pittinger G, Adamson R 1972 Antibiotic blockade of neuromuscular function. Annual Review of Pharmacology 12: 169

Polgar J, Bradley W G, Upton A R M et al 1972 The early detection of dystrophia myotonica. Brain 95: 761

Polgar J, Johnson M A, Weightman D, Appelton D 1973 Data on fibre size in thirty-six human muscles. An autopsy study. Journal of the Neurological Sciences 19: 307

Pollak V 1971 The waveshape of action potentials recorded with different types of electromyographic needles. Medical Biological Engineering 9: 657

Preswick G 1965 The myasthenic syndromes and their reactions. Proceedings of the Australian Association of Neurologists 3: 61

Price T M L, Allott E H 1958 The stiff-man syndrome. British Medical Journal 1: 682

Prineas J W, Hall R, Barwick D D, Watson A J 1968 Myopathy associated with pigmentation following adrenalectomy for Cushing's syndrome. Quarterly Journal of Medicine 37: 63

Pryse-Phillips W, Johnson G J, Larsen B 1982 Incomplete manifestations of myotonic dystrophy in a large kinship in Labrador. Annals of Neurology 11: 582

Purves D, Sakmann B 1974 Membrane properties underlying spontaneous activity of denervated muscle fibres. Journal of Physiology: 239 125

Puvanendran K, Cheah J S, Naganathan N, Wong P K 1979 Thyrotoxic myopathy. A clinical and quantitative analytic electromyographic study. Journal of the Neurological Sciences 42: 441

Radu H, Ionasescu V 1972 Nemaline (neuro-)myopathy: rodlike bodies and Type 1 fibre atrophy in a case of congenital hypotonia with denervation. Journal of the Neurological Sciences 17: 53

Radu H, Killyen I, Ionasescu V, Radu A 1977 Myotubular (centrinuclear) (neuro-)myopathy. European Neurology 15: 285

Ramsay I D 1965 Electromyography in thyrotoxicosis. Quarterly Journal of Medicine 34: 225

Rao S N, Katiyar B C, Nair K R P, Misra S 1980 Neuromuscular status in hypothyroidism. Acta Neurologica Scandinavica 61: 167

Rathjen R, Simons D G, Peterson C R 1968 Computer analysis of the duration of motor unit potentials. Archives of Physical Medicine and Rehabilitation 49: 524

Richardson A T 1951 Newer concepts of electrodiagnosis. St Thomas's Hospital Reports 7: 164

Richardson A T 1956 Clinical and electromyographical aspects of polymyositis. Proceedings of the Royal Society of Medicine 49: 111

Ricker K, Hertel G, Langsheid K, Stodieck G 1977 Myotonia not aggravated by cooling: force and relaxation of the adductor pollicis in normal subjects and in myotonia as compared to paramyotonia. Journal of Neurology 216: 9

Ricker K, Haass A, Rudel R, Bohlen R, Mertens H G 1980 Successful treatment of paramyotonia congenita (Eulenberg): muscle stiffness and weakness prevented by tocainide. Journal of Neurology, Neurosurgery and Psychiatry 43: 268

Roohi F, List T, Lovelace R E 1981 Slow motor nerve conduction in myotonic dystrophy. Electromyography and Clinical Neurophysiology 21: 97

Rose A L, Willison R G 1967 Quantitative electromyography using automatic analysis. Studies in healthy subjects and patients with primary muscle disease. Journal of Neurology, Neurosurgery and Psychiatry 30: 403–410

Rosenfalck P, Buchthal F 1962 Studies on the fibrillation potentials of denervated human muscle. Electroencephalography and Clinical Neurophysiology Supplement 22: 130

Rossouw J E, Keeton R G, Hewlett R H 1976 Chronic proximal muscular weakness in alcoholics. South African Medical Journal 50: 2095

Roth G 1982 The origin of fasciculations. Annals of Neurology 12: 542

Rowland L P, Aranow H, Hoefer P F A 1961 Observations on the curare test in the differential diagnosis of myasthenia gravis. In: Viets H R (ed) Myasthenia gravis. Thomas, Springfield

Rubenstein A E, Wainapel S F 1977 Acute hypokalemic myopathy in alcoholism. Archives of Neurology 34: 553

Rudel R, Lehmann-Horn F, Ricker K, Kuther G 1984 Hypokalemic periodic paralysis: in vitro investigation of muscle fibre membrane parameters. Muscle and Nerve 7: 110

Rudel R, Lehmann-Horn F 1985 Membrane changes in cells from myotonia patients. Physiology Review 65: 310

Sacco G, Buchthal F, Rosenfalck P 1962 Motor unit potentials at different ages. Archives of Neurology 6: 366

Salick A I, Pearson C M 1967 The electrical silence of myoedema. Neurology (Minneapolis) 17: 899

Sanders D B, Kim Y I, Howard J F 1980 Eaton–Lambert syndrome: a clinical and electrophysiological study of a patient treated with 4-aminopyridine. Journal of Neurology, Neurosurgery and Psychiatry 43: 978

Sanders D B, Howard J F Jr 1986 AAEE Minimonograph 25: single-fibre electromyography in myasthenia gravis. Muscle and Nerve 9: 809

Sanders D B, Howard J F, Johns T R 1979 Single fibre electromyography in myasthenia gravis. Neurology 29: 68

Sanders D B, Massey E W, Buckley E C 1986 Botulinum toxin for blepharospasm: single fibre EMG studies. Neurology 36: 545

Sanderson K V, Adey W R 1952 Electromyographic and endocrine studies in chronic thyrotoxic myopathy. Journal of Neurology, Neurosurgery and Psychiatry 15: 200

Sandstedt P E R, Henriksson K G, Larsson L E 1982 Quantitative electromyography in polymyositis and dermatomyositis. A long-term study. Acta Neurologica Scandinavica 65: 110

Satoyoshi E 1978 A syndrome of progressive muscle spasms, alopecia and diarrhoea. Neurology 28: 258

Schiller H H, Schwartz M S, Friman G 1977 Disturbed neuromuscular transmission in viral infection. New England Journal of Medicine 296: 258

Schiller H H, Stålberg E 1978 Human botulism studied with single fibre electromyography. Archives of Neurology 35: 346

Schimrigk K 1978 Combination of electromyographic and histological examination of skeletal muscle with an aspiration biopsy needle. European Neurology 17: 333

Schwartz M S, Moosa A, Dubowitz V 1977 Correlation of single fibre EMG and muscle histochemistry using an open biopsy recording technique. Journal of the Neurological Sciences 31: 369

Schwartz M S, Stålberg E 1975 Myasthenic syndrome studied with single fibre electromyography. Archives of Neurology 32: 815

Schwartz M S, Stålberg E, Schiller H H, Thiele B 1976 The reinnervated motor unit in man. A single fibre EMG multi-electrode investigation. Journal of the Neurological Sciences 27: 303

Schwartz M S, Stålberg E, Swash M 1980 Pattern of segmental motor fibre EMG study in syringomyelia: a single fibre EMG study. Journal of Neurology, Neurosurgery and Psychiatry 43: 150

Seaba P J, Walker D D 1989 Fundamentals of electronics and instrumentation. In: Kimura J (ed) Electrodiagnosis in disease of nerve and muscle. Davis, Philadelphia

Segura R P, Sahgal V 1981 Hemiplegic atrophy: electrophysiological and morphological studies. Muscle and Nerve 4: 246

Shahani M, Astur F D, Dastoor D H et al 1979 Neuropathies in tetanus. Journal of the Neurological Sciences 43: 173

Sherrington C S 1926 Remarks on some aspects of reflex inhibiton. Proceedings of the Royal Society B 97: 303

Shields R W 1984 Single fibre electromyography in the differential diagnosis of myopathic limb girdle syndromes and chronic spinal muscular atrophy. Muscle and Nerve 7: 265

Shields R W, Robbins N, Verrilli A A 1984 The effects of chronic muscular activity on age related changes in single fibre electromyography. Muscle and Nerve 7: 273

Shy G M, Engel W K, Somers J E, Wanko T 1963 Nemaline myopathy: a new congenital myopathy. Brain 86: 793

Sica R E P, McComas A J, Ferreira J C 1978 Evaluation of an automated method for analysing the electromyogram. Canadian Journal of Neurological Sciences 5: 275

Sica R E P, McComas A J, Upton A R M, Longmire D 1974 Motor unit estimations in the small muscles of the hand. Journal of Neurology, Neurosurgery and Psychiatry 37: 55

Simpson J A 1960 Myasthenia gravis: a new hypothesis. Scottish Medical Journal 5: 419

Simpson J A 1962 Recent studies on the physiology of the human spinal cord and its disturbance in poliomyelitis. Proceedings of the 8th Symposium of the European Association for Poliomyelitis. Masson, Paris, p 347

Simpson J A 1966 Control of muscle in health and disease.

In: Andrew B L (ed) Control and innervation of skeletal muscle. Livingstone, Edinburgh.

Simpson J A, Lenman J A R 1959 The effect of frequency of stimulation in neuromuscular disease. Electroencephalography and Clinical Neurophysiology 11: 604

Singh N, Lovelace R E 1979 Quantitative electromyography using on line computer. Acta Neurologica Scandinavica 60 (suppl 73): 309

Sinha S, Newsom-Davis J, Mills K, Byrne N, Lang B, Vincent A 1991 Autoimmune aetiology for acquired neuromyotonia (Isaacs' syndrome). Lancet 338: 75

Skaria J, Katiyar B C, Srivastava T P, Dube B 1975 Myopathy and neuropathy associated with osteomalacia. Acta Neurologica Scandinavica 51: 37

Slater C R, Lyons P R, Walls T J, Fawcett P R W, Young C 1992 Structure and function of neuromuscular junctions in the vastus lateralis of man. A motor point biopsy study of two groups of patients. Brain 115: 451

Slomic A, Rosenfalck A, Buchthal F 1968 Electrical and mechanical responses in normal and myasthenic muscle. Brain Research 10: 1

Smit L M E, Hageman G, Veldman H, Molenaar P C, Oen B S, Jennekens F G I 1988 A myasthenic syndrome with congenital paucity of secondary synaptic clefts: CPSC syndrome. Muscle and Nerve 11: 337

Smith H L, Amick L D, Johnson W W 1966 Detection of subclinical and carrier state in Duchenne muscular dystrophy. Journal of Paediatrics 69: 67

Smith J W, Thesleff S 1976 Spontaneous activity in denervated mouse diaphragm muscle. Journal of Physiology 257: 171

Smyth D P, Willison R G 1982 Quantitative electromyography in babies and young children with no evidence of neuromuscular disease. Journal of the Neurological Sciences 56 (2–3): 209

Somers J E, Winer N 1966 Reversible myopathy and myotonia following administration of a hypocholesterolemic agent. Neurology (Minneapolis) 16: 761

Spaans F, Theunissen P, Reekers A, Smit L, Veldman H 1990 Schwartz–Jampel syndrome: I. Clinical, electromyographic, and histologic studies. Muscle and Nerve 13: 516

Spielholz N I, Sell G H, Gold J, Rusk H A, Greens S K 1972 Electrophysiological studies in patients with spinal cord lesions. Archives of Physical Medicine and Rehabilitation 53: 558

Stålberg E 1966 Propagation velocity in human muscle fibres in situ. Acta Physiologica Scandinavica 70 (suppl) 287: 1

Stålberg E 1977 Electrogenesis in human dystrophic muscle. In: Rowland L (ed) Pathogenesis of human muscular dystrophies. Excerpa Medica, Amsterdam, 404: 570

Stålberg E 1980a Macro EMG, a new recording technique. Journal of Neurology, Neurosurgery and Psychiatry 43: 475

Stålberg E 1980b Clinical electrophysiology in myasthenia gravis. Journal of Neurology, Neurosurgery and Psychiatry 43: 622

Stålberg E 1982 Electrophysiological studies of reinnervation in ALS. In: Rowland L (ed) Human motor neurone diseases. Raven, New York, p 49

Stålberg E 1983 Macro EMG. Muscle and Nerve 6: 619

Stålberg E 1991 Invited review: electrodiagnostic assessment and monitoring of motor unit changes in disease. Muscle and Nerve 14: 293

Stålberg E, Andreassen S, Falk B, Lang H, Rosenfalck A,

Trojaborg W 1986 Quantitative analysis of individual motor unit potentials: a proposition for standardized terminology and criteria for measurement. Journal of Clinical Neurophysiology 3: 313

Stålberg E, Antoni L 1980 Electrophysiological cross section of the motor unit. Journal of Neurology, Neurosurgery and Psychiatry 43: 469

Stålberg E, Antoni L 1981 Microprocessors in the analysis of the motor unit and the neuromuscular transmission. In: Yamaguchi N, Fujisawa K (eds) Recent advances in EEG and EMG data processing. Elsevier/North-Holland Biomedical Press, Amsterdam, p 295

Stålberg E, Dioszeghy P 1991 Scanning EMG in normal muscle and in neuromuscular disorders. Electroencephalography and Clinical Neurophysiology 81: 403

Stålberg E, Ekstedt J 1973 Single fibre EMG and the microphysiology of the motor unit in normal and diseased muscle. In: Desmedt J E (ed) New developments in electromyography and clinical neurophysiology, vol 1. Karger, Basel

Stålberg E, Chu J, Bril V, Nandedkar S, Stålberg S, Ericsson M 1983 Automatic analysis of the EMG interference pattern. Electroencephalography and Clinical Neurophysiology 56: 672

Stålberg E, Fawcett P R W 1982 Macro EMG in healthy subjects of different ages. Journal of Neurology, Neurosurgery and Psychiatry 45: 870

Stålberg E, Fawcett P R W 1984 Electrophysiological methods for the study of the motor unit in spinal muscular atrophy. In: Gamstorp I, Sarnat H B (eds) Progressive spinal muscular atrophies. Raven, New York

Stålberg E, Hansson O 1973 Single fibre EMG in juvenile myasthenia gravis. Neuropadiatrie 4: 20

Stålberg E, Sanders D 1981 Electrophysiological tests of neuromuscular transmission. In Stålberg E, Young R R (eds) Clinical neurophysiology. Butterworths, London

Stålberg E, Sanders D B 1984 The motor unit in ALS studied with different neurophysiological techniques. In: Rose F C (ed) Research progress in motor neurone disease. Pitman, London

Stålberg E, Thiele B 1972 Transmission block in terminal nerve twigs: a single fibre electromyographic finding in man. Journal of Neurology, Neurosurgery and Psychiatry 35: 52

Stålberg E, Trontelj J V 1970 Demonstration of axon reflexes in human motor nerve fibres. Journal of Neurology, Neurosurgery and Psychiatry 33: 571

Stålberg E, Trontelj J V 1979 Single fibre electromyography Mirvalle Press, Old Woking, Surrey

Stålberg E, Trontelj J V 1982 Abnormal discharges generated within the motor unit as observed with single-fibre electromyography. In: Culp W J, Ochoa J (eds) Abnormal nerves and muscles as impulse generators. Oxford University Press, Oxford

Stålberg E, Ekstedt J, Broman A 1971 The electromyographic jitter in normal human muscles. Electroencephalography and Clinical Neurophysiology 31: 429

Stålberg E, Ekstedt J, Broman A 1974 Neuromuscular transmission in myasthenia gravis studied with single fibre electromyography. Journal of Neurology, Neurosurgery and Psychiatry 37: 540

Stålberg E, Schwartz M S, Trontelj J V 1975 Single fibre electromyography in various processes affecting the anterior horn cell. Journal of the Neurological Sciences 24: 403

Stålberg E, Trontelj J, Schwartz M S 1976 Single muscle fibre recording of the jitter phenomenon in patients with myasthenia gravis and in members of their families. Annals of the New York Academy of Sciences 274: 189

Stein R B, Yang J F 1990 Methods for estimating the number of motor units in human muscles. Annals of Neurology 28: 487

Stohr M, Heckl R 1977 Das stiff-man syndrome. Archiv für Psychiatrie und Nervenkrankheiten 223: 171

Streib E W, Wilbourn A J, Mitsumoto H 1979 Spontaneous electrical muscle activity in polymyositis and dermatomyositis. Muscle and Nerve 2: 14

Swank R L, Price J C 1943 Fascicular muscle twitchings in amyotrophic lateral sclerosis. Archives of Neurology and Psychiatry 49: 22

Swash M 1980 Vulnerability of lower brachial myotomes in motor neurone disease. Journal of the Neurological Sciences 47: 59

Swash M, Schwartz M S 1977 Implications of longitudinal muscle fibre splitting in neurogenic and myopathic disorders. Journal of Neurology, Neurosurgery and Psychiatry 40: 1152

Swift T R, Ignacio O J, Dyken P R 1975 Neonatal dystrophia myotonica: electrophysiological studies. American Journal of Diseases of Childhood 129: 374

Swift T R, Leshner R T, Gross J A 1980 Arm-diaphragm synkinesis. Neurology 30: 339

Takamori M, Gutmann L, Crosby T W, Martin J D 1972 Myasthenic syndromes in hypothyroidism. Electrophysiological study of neuromuscular transmission and muscle contraction in two patients. Archives of Neurology 26: 326

Tanzi F, Taglietti V, Zucca G et al 1979 Computerised EMG analysis. Electromyography and Clinical Neurophysiology 19: 495

Taylor A 1962 The significance of grouping of motor unit activity. Journal of Physiology 162: 259

Taylor R G, Kewalramani L S, Fowler W M 1974 Electromyographic findings in lower extremities of patients with high spinal cord injury. Archives of Physical Medicine and Rehabilitation 55: 16

Taylor R G, Layzer R B, Davis H S, Fowler W M 1972 Continuous muscle fibre activity in the Schwartz–Jampel syndrome. Electroencephalography and Clinical Neurophysiology 33: 497

Thage O, Trojaborg W, Buchthal F 1963 Electromyographic findings in polyneuropathy. Neurology (Minneapolis) 13: 273

Thesleff S 1963 Spontaneous electrical activity in denervated rat skeletal muscle. In: Gutmann E, Hnik P (eds) The effect of use and disuse on neuromuscular functions. Czechoslovak Academy of Sciences, Prague

Thesleff S 1982 Fibrillation in denervated mammalian skeletal muscle. In: Culp W J, Ochoa J (eds) Abnormal nerves and muscles as impulse generators. Oxford University Press, Oxford

Thesleff S, Ward M R 1975 Studies on the mechanism of fibrillation potentials in denervated muscle. Journal of Physiology 244: 313

Thiele B, Boehle A 1978 Anzahl der Spike-Komponenten im Motor-Unit Potential. EEG-EMG 9: 125

Thiele B, Stålberg E 1974 The bimodal jitter: a single fibre electromyographic finding. Journal of Neurology, Neurosurgery and Psychiatry 37: 403

Thiele B, Stålberg E 1975 Single fibre EMG findings in polyneuropathies of different aetiology. Journal of Neurology, Neurosurgery and Psychiatry 38: 881

Trojaborg W, Buchthal F 1965 Malignant and benign fasciculations. Acta Neurologica Scandinavica 41(Suppl) 13: 251

Trojaborg W, Franzen E, Andersen I 1969 Peripheral neuropathy associated with carcinoma of the lung. Brain 92: 71

Trontelj J V, Mihelin M, Fernandez J M, Stålberg E 1986 Axonal stimulation for end-plate jitter studies. Journal of Neurology, Neurosurgery and Psychiatry 49: 677

Trontelj J V, Stålberg E 1983a Responses to electrical stimulation of denervated human muscle fibres recorded with single fibre EMG. Journal of Neurology, Neurosurgery and Psychiatry 46: 305

Trontelj J V, Stålberg E 1983b Bizarre repetitive discharges recorded with single fibre EMG. Journal of Neurology, Neurosurgery and Psychiatry 46: 310

Trontelj J V, Stålberg E 1991 Single motor end-plates in myasthenia gravis and LEMS at different firing rates. Muscle and Nerve 14: 226

Trontelj J V, Stålberg E 1992 Jitter measurement by axonal micro-stimulation. Guidelines and technical notes. Electroencephalography and Clinical Neurophysiology 85: 30

Van Alphen H A, Lammers H J, Walder H A D 1962 On remarkable reaction of motor neurons of lumbosacral region after traumatic cervical transection in man. Neurochirugie 8: 328

Van Den Bosch J 1963 Investigation of the carrier state in the Duchenne type dystrophy. In: Proceedings of the 2nd Symposium on Research in Muscular Dystrophy. Pitman, London

Van Der Most, Van Spijk D 1964 Refractory and irresponsive period of muscle in myasthenia gravis. Electroencephalography and Clinical Neurophysiology 17: 103

Venables G S, Bates D, Shaw D A 1978 Hypothyroidism with true myotonia. Journal of Neurology, Neurosurgery and Psychiatry 41: 1013

Vicale C T 1949 The diagnostic features of a muscular syndrome resulting from hyperparathyroidism, osteomalacia owing to renal tubular acidosis, and perhaps to related disorders of calcium metabolism. Transactions of the American Neurological Association 74: 143

Vincent A, Cull-Candy S G, Newsom-Davis J, Trautman A, Molinar P C, Polak R L 1981 Congenital myasthenia: end-plate acetylcholine receptors and electrophysiology in five cases. Muscle and Nerve 4: 306

Wagner A, Kopec J, Szmidt Salkowska E 1979 Normal values obtained by automated system in analysis of electromyogram. Electromyography and Clinical Neurophysiology 19: 343

Wallgren-Pettersson C, Sainio K, Salmi T 1989 Electromyography in congenital nemaline myopathy. Muscle and Nerve 12: 587

Wallis W E, Van Poznak A, Plum F 1970 Generalised muscular stiffness fasciculations and myokymia of peripheral nerve origin. Archives of Neurology 22: 430

Walton J N 1952 The electromyogram in myopathy: analysis with the audio frequency spectrometer. Journal of Neurology, Neurosurgery and Psychiatry 15: 219

Walton J N, Adams R D 1958 Polymyositis. Livingstone, Edinburgh

Warmolts J R, Engel W K 1972 Open-biopsy electromyography. I. Correlation of motor unit behaviour with histochemical muscle fibre type in human limb muscles. Archives of Neurology 27: 512

Warmolts J R, Mendell J R 1980 Neurotonia: impulse-induced repetitive discharges in motor nerves in peripheral neuropathy. Annals of Neurology 7: 245

Warren W R, Gutmann L, Cody R C, Flowers P, Segal A T 1977 Stapedius reflex decay in myasthenia gravis. Archives of Neurology 34: 496

Weddell G, Feinstein B, Pattle R E 1944 The electrical activity of voluntary muscle in man under normal and pathological conditions. Brain 67: 178

Weiderholt W C 1970 'End-plate noise' in electromyography. Neurology (Minneapolis) 20: 214

Welander L 1951 Myopathia distalis tarda hereditaria. Acta Medica Scandinavica 141 (suppl) 265: 1

Welch L K, Appenzeller O, Bicknell J M 1972 Peripheral neuropathy with myokymia — sustained muscular contraction and continuous motor unit activity. Neurology 22: 161

Werk E E, Sholiton L J, Monell R J 1961 The stiff-man syndrome and hyperthyroidism. American Journal of Medicine 31: 647

Wiechers D O 1977 Mechanically provoked insertional activity before and after nerve section in rats. Archives of Physical Medicine and Rehabilitation 58: 402

Wiechers D O 1988 New concepts of the reinnervated motor unit revealed by vaccine-associated poliomyelitis. Muscle and Nerve 11: 356

Wiechers D O, Johnson E W 1979 Diffuse abnormal electromyographic insertional activity: a preliminary report. Archives of Physical Medicine and Rehabilitation 60: 419

Wiechers D O, Hubbell S L 1981 Late changes in the motor unit after acute poliomyelitis. Muscle and Nerve 4: 524

Williams R S 1959 Triamcinolone myopathy. Lancet i: 698

Williamson E, Brook M H 1972 Myokymia and the motor unit. Archives of Neurology 26: 11

Willison R G 1964 Analysis of electrical activity in healthy and dystrophic muscle in man. Journal of Neurology, Neurosurgery and Psychiatry 22: 320

Willison R G 1968 Quantitative electromyography: the detection of carriers of Duchenne dystrophy. Proceedings of the 2nd International Congress of Neurogenetics, Montreal

Wilson J, Walton J N 1959 Some muscular manifestations of hypothyroidism. Journal of Neurology, Neurosurgery and Psychiatry 22: 320

Wokke J H J, Jennekens F G I, Molenaar P C, Van den Oord C J M, Oen B S, Busch H F M 1989 Congenital paucity of secondary synaptic clefts (CPSC) syndrome in 2 adult sibs. Neurology 39: 648

Yates D A H 1963 The estimation of mean potential duration in endocrine myopathy. Journal of Neurology, Neurosurgery and Psychiatry 26: 458

Yee R D, Cogan D G, Zee D S, Baloh R W, Hornubia V 1976 Rapid eye movements in myasthenia gravis. Archives of Ophthalmology 94: 1465

Young J I, Rowley W F 1982 Physiological alterations of motor units in hemiplegia. Journal of the Neurological Sciences 54: 401

Zellweger H, Ionasescu V 1973 Early onset of myotonic dystrophy in infants. American Journal of Diseases of Childhood 125: 601

Zellweger H, Pavone L, Biondi A et al 1980 Autosomal recessive generalised myotonia. Muscle and Nerve 3: 176

30. Studies in nerve conduction

Peter R. W. Fawcett   Ian S. Schofield

INTRODUCTION

Primary disorders of the peripheral nerves constitute a large and important cause of neuromuscular dysfunction in patients of all ages. Following the introduction of motor and sensory nerve conduction measurement by Hodes et al (1948) and Dawson & Scott (1949) respectively, the techniques, combined with needle electromyography, have become well established in clinical practice for the investigation of peripheral nerve function in humans, enabling these disorders to be differentiated from primary diseases of the anterior horn cell, neuromuscular junction and muscle. While the basic concepts of the two techniques have changed little since their introduction, marked advances in instrumentation and quantitation of the techniques over the years has led to their widespread use for the provision of quantitative and objective data concerning the state of the peripheral nerves and muscles. Valuable information about the nature of the disease process can be obtained and the use of serial examinations enables its progress to be followed over time, documenting deterioration, or after the institution of a treatment regimen, any subsequent improvement in nerve function.

Since the first and subsequent editions of this book, many excellent texts dedicated to the description of nerve conduction techniques and their findings in different disorders have been published (Ludin 1980, Goodgold & Eberstein 1983, Notermans 1984, Kimura 1989). Accordingly the emphasis of this chapter reflects the place of nerve conduction and related techniques in the investigation of patients presenting with more generalised disorders of the neuromuscular systems.

Specific nerve lesions or nerve injuries have been omitted, and the reader should refer to the above-mentioned texts for expert guidance on these topics.

TECHNIQUE

Stimulation

There are two basic types of stimulator:

1. The constant voltage stimulator, which should be capable of delivering up to 250 V; this form of stimulation is satisfactory in most situations, but may be inadequate when electrode and/or skin impedances increase.

2. The constant current stimulator, which should provide a current output of up to 100 mA (Guld et al 1983).

The latter is preferable since the current remains relatively constant despite minor changes in impedance, which may be detected if current output is simultaneously monitored (Buchthal & Rosenfalck 1966). It is essential that the stimulator has a balanced output in order to reduce stimulus artefact and this is most conveniently achieved using a shielded transformer (Guld 1960).

The most common form of stimulus is a rectangular pulse, the duration of which may be varied between 0.05 and 1.0 ms. Stimulation is achieved by outflow of current at the cathode (–ve pole) which depolarises the underlying nerve, while at the anode (+ve pole) hyperpolarisation of the nerve occurs. The cathode must always be placed nearer to the recording electrodes to avoid the possibility of anodal conduction block. A wide range of stimulus frequencies (0.5–100 Hz) should be available, but for nerve conduction studies a frequency of 1 Hz is usually employed and is well tolerated by the patient.

The optimal site for stimulation of the nerve at each location may be found using a submaximal stimulus (usually 3.5 mA at 0.1 ms) and moving the stimulating electrode until a maximal response for that stimulus is obtained. Theoretically, larger diameter nerve fibres have lower stimulus thresholds than smaller fibres, but in practice the location of nerve fibres in the nerve trunk also in-fluences the order of excitation, with a tendency for those closer to the stimulating electrode to be excited before more distant fibres (McComas et al 1971).

For the purposes of conduction velocity measurement it is essential that the nerve is stimulated supramaximally in order that all the nerve fibres capable of contributing to the response are activated at each stimulus site. This is achieved by increasing the stimulus strength until the evoked muscle or sensory responses are maximal, following which the stimulus is further increased by about 25%. Too high a stimulus intensity, however, may result in spread of the effective stimulus point away from the stimulating cathode towards the recording electrode (Weiderholt 1970), giving erroneously short latencies.

Stimulating electrodes. Peripheral nerves may be stimulated using either surface or near-nerve needle electrodes, both of which have their advantages and disadvantages. Surface electrodes are more convenient, less time-consuming and non-invasive, but provide a less precise stimulus point and generally require higher stimulus intensities, which may be uncomfortable. With near-nerve needle electrodes the stimulus point may be more accurately localised and a much lower stimulus strength is needed. They may also be used when the nerve to be stimulated lies deeply (e.g. the sciatic) or when skin resistance is high due to hyperkeratosis. On the other hand, insertion of the needle may cause discomfort and there is a slight risk of injuring the nerve by direct puncture which may produce unpleasant persisting paraesthesiae. The use of needle electrodes also requires more time.

A convenient type of bipolar surface electrode which may be used to stimulate nerve trunks consists of saline-soaked felt pads of 3–5 mm diameter in contact with silver discs mounted 2.5 cm apart in a perspex holder, which may be either hand-held or strapped to the skin. Henriksen (1956) has shown that the effective stimulus point is the centre of the circular electrode. Various kinds of commercially available ring electrodes may be used to evoke sensory potentials by stimulation of digital nerves.

Conventional nerve conduction techniques employ brief electrical pulses to stimulate the peripheral nerves, but more recently high-voltage, low-output impedance electrical stimulation (Merton & Morton 1980) and magnetic stimulation (Barker et al 1985a,b, Chokroverty 1990) techniques have been developed. These have proved particularly valuable in the study of central motor pathways, which are beyond the scope of this chapter, and also for examining sites such as the spinal motor roots which are relatively inaccessible to conventional electrical stimulation (Mills & Murray 1986, de Noordhout et al 1988, Ugawa et al 1989, Schmid et al 1990). Attempts at stimulating peripheral nerves using magnetic coils have also been reported (Hallett et al 1990), but as yet they do not provide a sufficiently precise stimulus point to be of any clinical value.

Recording

Recording electrodes. Surface, subcutaneous needle, or intramuscular needle electrodes may be used to record motor responses and surface or near-nerve needle electrodes for recording sensory responses. In the case of motor conduction, surface electrodes are preferable since they avoid the need for needle puncture and pick up from a wider and more representative area of the muscle. It is also easier to reposition surface electrodes in order to obtain the optimum response. The intramuscular needle electrode records from a restricted region within the muscle and it is possible that the recorded activity may not arise from motor units supplied by the fastest-conducting motor fibres. There is also a tendency for the shape of the response to vary because of slight needle displacements caused by the accompanying mechanical twitch. Needle electrodes have the one advantage of being more selective, enabling the motor response to be isolated to a single muscle. Surface electrodes usually consist of 0.5–1 cm silver discs which are covered with electrode paste and attached to the skin with adhesive tape. For recording evoked nerve potentials, saline-soaked felt pads of 0.5–1 cm diameter set in silver cups mounted in a perspex holder with a fixed interelectrode distance of 2.5–3 cm are suitable, and may be conveniently applied in line with the underlying nerve trunk. In this situation Gilliatt et al (1965) have shown that the interelec-

trode distance significantly affects the amplitude and duration of the potential. It is therefore important that each laboratory should standardise on one type of recording electrode. Buchthal & Rosenfalck (1966) prefer needle electrodes which consist of stainless steel needles insulated with Teflon to within a short distance of the tip. The active recording electrode is inserted through the skin and positioned as closely as possible to the underlying nerve, while the reference electrode is inserted subcutaneously 2–4 cm perpendicularly to the nerve at the same level as the active electrode. With this arrangement a unipolar recording of the nerve action potential is obtained which gives rather shorter latency values than those obtained by bipolar recording.

Signal averaging

The size of sensory action potentials from normal and pathological nerves may be of the order of 5 μV or less and as a result may not be easily distinguished from noise. Considerable improvement in the signal-to-noise ratio may be obtained using the process of signal averaging, which allows the extraction of these small signals from the background noise. The method is based on the principle that stimulus-linked events will enhance as successive traces summate algebraically, while randomly occurring activity will cancel out. Improvement of the signal : noise ratio is a function of the square root of the number of sweeps averaged. Signals as low as 0.03 μV may be detected by averaging 1000 sweeps or more (Singh et al 1974), but such large numbers of stimuli may be unpleasant for the patient, and usually 16–128 sweeps are satisfactory.

METHODS

General

Ideally the patient and machine should be placed in a screened environment to reduce extraneous electrical interference to a minimum, but satisfactory recordings can often be obtained without these precautions. However, adequate earthing of the patient is essential, using a plate or strap-type electrode placed where possible between the stimulating and recording electrodes to minimise stimulus artefact.

Motor conduction

Motor conduction velocity may be most satisfactorily measured in the median, ulnar, radial, peroneal and posterior tibial nerves which are accessible for stimulation at two or more points along their course. When indicated, the velocity may also be determined in the musculocutaneous, femoral and sciatic nerves. Normally a small distal muscle supplied by the nerve under study is chosen to record the evoked compound muscle action potential (CMAP). The CMAP represents the summated electrical activity generated by all the motor units following a supramaximal stimulus of the motor nerve. Filter settings of 2–3 Hz to 10 kHz should be used.

Placement of the recording electrodes is crucial; it is essential that the active electrode is situated over the region of the end-plate zone in order to identify accurately the onset of the muscle action potential which will have an initial negative deflection. The reference electrode should be placed over the tendon of insertion. Failure to record from the end-plate zone will result in the inclusion of extra time taken for the much slower action potential conduction in the muscle fibres, and will give an erroneously prolonged terminal latency. This situation may be recognised by an initial positive deflection of the response. A relatively high gain (e.g. 0.2 or 0.5 mV/div.) should be used to identify the onset of the potential, while other characteristics of the response including amplitude, duration and shape may be assessed at a gain which allows the display of the whole signal (Fig. 30.1). With the above recording arrangement the CMAP is generally biphasic with initial negative and terminal positive phases. The motor terminal latency is measured between the stimulus delivered to the nerve at the most distal point and the onset of the muscle potential, and is accounted for by conduction in the tapering nerve trunk and progressively smaller nerve branches, invasion of the nerve terminals and finally transmission across the synapse at the neuromuscular junction. The amplitude, which is usually measured from baseline to negative peak (or peak-to-

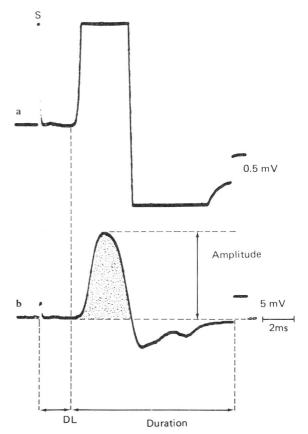

Fig. 30.1 Evoked muscle response (M-response) recorded from abductor pollicis brevis in **a** normal adult. **a** An amplifier gain of 0.5 mV/div. and sweep speed of 2 ms/div are used for latency measurement. **b** Measurement of the M-response, baseline to negative peak amplitude (or peak-to-peak amplitude) is performed with a gain of 5 mV/div. Estimation of the area of the negative peak requires the use of a computer.

peak), provides a measure of the volume of active muscle tissue. Duration of the response may be determined between the onset of the negative deflection and final return to baseline of the positive deflection, or be simply defined as the duration of the negative phase. Both the amplitude and duration are influenced by the synchronicity of impulse conduction in the population of motor axons. A more accurate measurement of the bulk of active muscle tissue may be obtained by estimating the CMAP area, usually the negative phase, which is now possible with some of the present computer-based systems. The area is measured in ms·mV.

Motor conduction velocity is determined by recording the CMAP following supramaximal stimulation of the motor nerve at two or more proximal sites. Differences in latency between the onset of these separate responses are determined and the velocities are calculated by dividing the distances between stimulus points by the appropriate latency differences (Fig. 30.2). The velocity is measured in metres per second. It should be stressed that this procedure gives the maximum motor conduction velocity since the onset of the CMAP probably represents activity derived from the largest and fastest conducting motor fibres. Comparison of the amplitudes, areas and shapes of the CMAPs elicited at each stimulus site is also important. As a consequence of the spectrum of motor nerve fibre diameters and hence conduction velocities, the volley of the action potentials from all the individual fibres becomes less syn-

chronised with increasing distance between the stimulus site and the muscle. The CMAP amplitude and area fall, due in part to phase cancellation, and the duration increases. The reduction is greater for amplitude than for area, and varies from nerve to nerve. A larger than normal reduction in amplitude (more than 20%) or area implies abnormal nerve conduction, involving the whole length of the nerve or of only a short segment as is seen in localised nerve compression.

Upper limb nerves. For median and ulnar nerves the active recording electrode is placed, over the belly of abductor pollicis brevis and abductor digiti minimi respectively, with the reference electrode over the tendon of insertion at the base of the appropriate digit. The nerves may be stimulated at the wrist, elbow, axilla and Erb's point, and the conduction velocity measured over each intervening segment. Spread of the stimulus from median to ulnar nerve and vice versa when stimulating at the wrist and axilla may give rise to misleading responses when recording from the small muscles of the hand. The shape of the muscle action potential, however, is helpful in avoiding any error of interpretation (Mavor & Libman, 1962). Other errors may arise from the anomalous innervation of the intrinsic muscles of the hand (Gassel 1964a, Kimura 1984). Motor conduction in the radial nerve may be determined by stimulating the nerve above the clavicle and in the mid-arm (Gassel & Diamantopoulos 1964), or in the axilla and 6 cm proximal to the lateral epicondyle of the humerus (Trojaborg & Sindrup 1969), recording the muscle response from brachioradialis or other forearm muscles innervated by the radial nerve. Motor and sensory conduction can be determined in the musculocutaneous nerve, the muscle response being recorded from biceps brachii (Trojaborg 1976). Measurement of the motor conduction velocity to other proximal shoulder girdle muscles is not possible and latency values from Erb's point to different muscles are therefore used (Gassel 1964a).

Lower limb nerves. Conduction velocities in fibres supplying the small muscles of the foot may be tested in the distribution of the common peroneal and posterior tibial nerves. The distal stimulus is applied to the deep peroneal or posterior tibial nerve at the ankle, and the proximal stimulus at the head of the fibula or in the lower

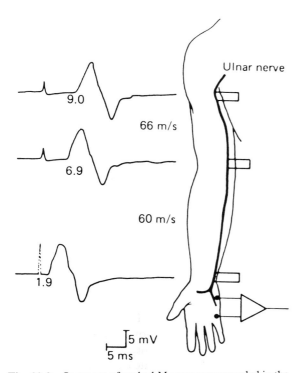

Fig. 30.2 Sequence of evoked M-responses recorded in the hypothenar muscles following stimulation of the ulnar nerve at the wrist, elbow and axilla for calculation of the motor conduction velocity in forearm and arm segments in a normal adult. Latencies to onset at each stimulus site are shown, together with the calculated conduction velocities in the intervening segments.

popliteal fossa respectively. The muscle action potential is usually recorded from the extensor digitorum brevis or abductor hallucis (Mavor & Atcheson 1966). Conduction rate in the sciatic nerve can also be estimated (Gassel & Trojaborg 1964) using needle electrodes placed deeply in the gluteal region to provide the proximal stimulus.

The F-response

Supramaximal stimulation of a peripheral motor nerve, as well as producing a direct M-response, often results in a small-amplitude late response of variable latency, amplitude and configuration, which Magladery & McDougal (1950) separated from the H-reflex and called the 'F-wave' (Fig. 30.3). It is best obtained from the distal muscles of the hand and foot and, in contrast to the latency of the M-response, that of the F-response decreases as the stimulus is applied more proximally, indicating a centripetal conduction of the impulse before distal transmission.

Despite early controversy surrounding its origins, there can now be little doubt that the F-response is produced by recurrent discharges of a few antidromically excited motor neurones (Dawson & Merton 1956). The F-response can be elicited in a deafferented limb (Mayer & Feldman 1967), and single motor unit studies (Thorne 1965, Trontelj & Trontelj 1973a, Schiller & Stålberg 1978) have shown it to occur only when preceded by an identical direct motor unit response. Moreover on single fibre EMG the variation in latency of the recurrent responses recorded from single muscle fibres is only slightly greater than that of the direct response from the same fibres (Trontelj 1973), and quite markedly less than that seen in a reflex response (Trontelj et al 1973). Although with surface recording techniques reflex components cannot be excluded completely, particularly in the presence of spasticity, it can be assumed that in the resting state and following supramaximal stimulation, most if not all of the late responses are recurrent discharges.

Not all motor neurones appear to respond to the antidromic stimulus, and in those that do, the production of an F-response is a relatively uncommon event (Schiller & Stålberg 1978, Yates &

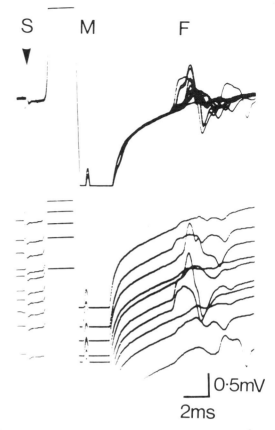

Fig. 30.3   Recordings from abductor pollicis brevis following supramaximal stimulation of the median nerve at the wrist in a normal adult. Note the initial large M-response followed by small F-responses which show variation of latency and configuration.

Brown 1979). On the basis of the amplitude ratio of the F-response and M-response it has been estimated that about 1% of the motor neurone pool participates in the production of each F-response (Kimura et al 1984). Using the collision technique Kimura et al (1984) have suggested that F-responses occur in both fast- and slow-conducting axons, and hence are generated by a relatively wide spectrum of motor neurone sizes. Fisher (1985) challenges this view and feels that there is selective activation of larger motor neurones with faster-conducting axons. Certainly the conduction velocities calculated using the earliest F-response latencies and the direct M-response latencies obtained at two sites of stimulation are almost identical, suggesting that they represent conduction in the same fastest-conducting axons.

Generation of the recurrent discharge depends upon a variety of factors, including the ability of the antidromic impulse to depolarise the initial segment of the axon hillock and the time required for repolarisation of the same segment before re-invasion by the soma-dendritic spike (Schiller & Stålberg 1978). This latter critical phase is influenced principally by the balance of excitatory and inhibitory postsynaptic potentials on individual anterior horn cells. Despite this the chances of an F-response occurring with each supramaximal stimulus to the nerve trunk are relatively high, with a frequency of between 50% and 95% in the ulnar nerve in different normal individuals (Peioglou-Harmoussi et al 1985a).

Over recent years the F-response has proved to be of considerable value in the investigation of peripheral nerve disorders, and in particular the examination of conduction in the proximal nerve segment which is inaccessible to conventional nerve conduction techniques. Kimura (1974) first described the method for calculating the conduction velocity in the proximal portion of the nerve using F-response latencies, but a number of assumptions upon which the method is based have been questioned by Young & Shahani (1978). The latter authors prefer to use the shortest F-response latency obtained following stimulation of the nerve at its most distal site to provide a measure of the F-response conduction time. This is the time taken for retrograde propagation of the impulse to the cord, turnabout at the cell body and finally orthodromic conduction to the muscle. This latency value is then compared with a nomogram relating F-response latency to arm length or height of the individual.

Opinions vary with regard to the number of F-responses required to obtain the 'correct' minimal latency value. Lachman et al (1980) suggest 10 responses are sufficient, while Panayiotopoulos et al (1977) state that at least 20 responses are necessary in order to establish the shortest latency. Even with this sample size the shortest latency may not be derived from the fastest conducting axon (Peioglou-Harmoussi et al 1985b). Fisher (1982) suggests that calculation of the mean latency of 10 responses is more reproducible than minimal latency. We feel that a sample of 20 is a satisfactory compromise and is generally well tolerated by most patients. The minimal and maximal latencies are determined for comparison with control data corrected for age and height (Peioglou-Harmoussi et al 1985b). Increases in F-response latency have been found in both axonal and demyelinating types of peripheral neuropathy and have proved more sensitive than maximal motor and sensory conduction velocity measurement in the demonstration of abnormal nerve function (Shahani & Sumner 1981, Fraser & Olney 1992). F-response abnormalities have also been reported in cervical and lumbar radiculopathies (Eisen et al 1977a, b).

Other F-response parameters. In addition to latency, a number of other characteristics of the F-response including frequency, presence and frequency of identical responses, amplitude, duration and shape, have been examined (Shahani & Sumner 1981, Peioglou-Harmoussi et al 1985a, b). F-response frequency varies quite considerably, even in healthy control subjects and also in different nerves (Peioglou-Harmoussi et al 1985b, Petajan 1985), factors which have to be taken into account when pathology is suspected. Identical or repeated responses normally account for up to 5% of the total number of responses, but their frequency increases in various neurogenic conditions such as motor neurone disease, cervical spondylosis and peripheral neuropathy (Petajan 1985, Peioglou-Harmoussi et al 1987).

Spectrum of motor axonal velocities

In conventional conduction studies, measurement of the latency to the onset of the evoked muscle action potential results in the conduction velocity being calculated for the fastest conducting motor fibres. It is possible in some conditions, that selective involvement of motor axons may occur according to their size, and therefore techniques have been devised to estimate the range of conduction velocities in different sizes of α-fibres within normal and diseased nerves (Thomas et al 1959, Hopf 1963).

These techniques employ the collision principle, and require two independently variable stimuli applied to the nerve at two points, one proximal, the other distal. In the method of Thomas et al (1959), a supramaximal stimulus applied at the proximal site is preceded at a set interval by a gradually increasing distal stimulus. Initially at low stimulus intensities low-threshold, fast-conducting axons will be excited distally, and the antidromically propagated action potentials will collide with the orthodromic impulses generated at the proximal site in the same axons. Further increases in stimulus intensity lead to occlusion in progressively smaller axons until the process is complete. In the Hopf technique supramaximal stimuli are applied at both sites and the time interval between the two stimuli is progressively decreased from a point at which there is no interaction to one at which complete blocking occurs. By these means conduction in the slowest fibres may be assessed as a percentage of the maximal conduction velocity. Thomas et al (1959) found that the majority of motor fibres have conduction velocities within 15–20% of the maximum, although the slowest fibres may conduct at rates of 35–40% below the maximum.

Gilliatt et al (1976) have slightly modified the technique of Thomas et al (1959), stimulating at two sites in the proximal part of the limb instead of one, the conduction velocity being calculated by subtraction in the usual way. The theoretical considerations upon which these methods are based are not entirely beyond dispute, but they do give a reflection of the spectrum of fibre velocities and by implication fibre size.

More recently a further modified version of the collision technique has been proposed which employs in sequence, a proximal stimulus, a distal stimulus and then a second proximal stimulus (Ingram et al 1987a,b). As the time interval between the first proximal and distal stimuli is increased, so an increasing proportion of the axon responses from the second proximal shock are blocked with a resulting progressive decline in the evoked muscle response. The spectrum of conduction velocities obtained with this technique is smaller than that seen with the other methods.

Sensory nerve conduction

Sensory conduction may be determined in various cutaneous nerves, and consequently the responses receive no contribution from muscle afferent fibres. The radial, median and ulnar nerves are usually studied in the upper limb, while in the lower limb the sural, medial plantar and superficial peroneal nerves are most suitable.

Characteristics of the sensory potential and measurement of the latency for calculation of the conduction velocity depend on the method of recording. With bipolar surface recording the volume conducted response has a triphasic appearance, with a small positive deflection preceding the larger negative depolarisation and a final positive deflection (Fig. 30.4). Filter settings of 8–10 Hz to 2–3.2 kHz are recommended. Gilliatt et al (1965) suggest that the latency should be measured to the onset of the negative deflection, as this represents the arrival of the action potentials in the fastest-conducting fibres at the first electrode.

In the case of monopolar needle recordings, the sensory potential may be biphasic or triphasic with an initial positive deflection (Buchthal & Rosenfalck 1966). Occasionally in normal subjects and more frequently in pathological nerves the main component may be followed by much smaller deflections which represent the activity from slower conducting fibres. Although theoretically the latency should be measured to the point where the negative deflection crosses the baseline (Buchthal & Rosenfalck 1966), the initial positive peak is

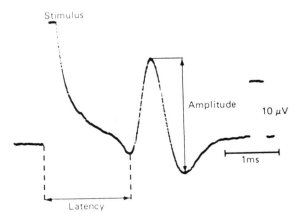

Fig. 30.4 Recording of the orthodromic sensory action potential from the median nerve at the wrist following stimulation of digit I. Latency is measured between stimulus artefact and initial positive peak; amplitude is measured between negative and positive peaks.

usually taken as it is more easily defined. Gilliatt et al (1965) observed that an accurate estimate of the conduction velocity can be obtained in the segment between the stimulating cathode and active recording electrode, provided that the stimulus is not more than 25% supramaximal. The velocity may also be calculated by the subtraction method, after recording the potential at two sites along the nerve. The size of the potential decreases with increasing distance away from the stimulating site due to dispersion of the action potentials of individual fibres with differing conduction velocities.

The amplitude of the sensory potential recorded with needle electrodes is much larger than the surface recorded potential (Dioszeghy 1986) but with both techniques the amplitude is rather variable and particularly in the case of needle electrodes, it is sensitive to electrode position. A close proximity between needle tip and nerve is usually obtained by using a weak stimulus to excite the nerve and adjusting the needle to produce the maximal perceived response.

In the upper limb, conduction in the median, ulnar and radial nerves may be performed with both orthodromic and antidromic techniques (Fig. 30.5). The digital nerve branches of the median and ulnar nerves are stimulated with ring electrodes placed over the first interphalangeal joint, while the recording is made over the mixed nerve trunk at the wrist or elbow (Dawson 1956). Reversal of this stimulation and recording arrangement produces a larger response (Sears 1959), probably because the nerve branches are more superficial. The response also has no initial positive component, and occasionally may be contaminated by volume conduction of simultaneously evoked muscle potentials. The radial nerve is accessible for stimulation and recording at several sites along its course, but usually the cutaneous superficial branch is examined either orthodromically or antidromically in the distal forearm segment (Downie & Scott 1967).

In the lower limb the medial plantar nerve may be stimulated with ring electrodes applied over the first toe, recording the response over the posterior tibial nerve trunk in the region of the medial malleolus (Mavor & Atcheson 1966, Guiloff & Sherratt 1977). Examination of the sural (Di Benedetto 1970, Burke et al 1974, Horowitz & Krarup 1992, Trojaborg et al 1992) and superficial peroneal nerves (Di Benedetto 1970) is best achieved antidromically, but because the potentials are often buried in noise, averaging techniques are usually necessary for their retrieval. The above authors have found the use of surface

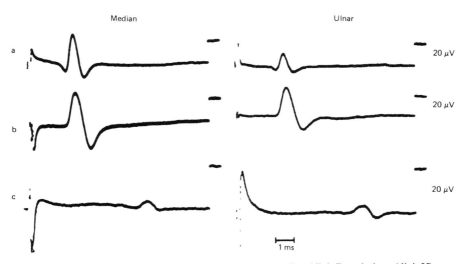

Fig. 30.5 Sensory action potentials recorded from the median (digit I) and ulnar (digit V) nerves in a normal adult. **a** Stimulus to digit, recording at wrist. **b** Stimulus to wrist, recording from digit. **c** Stimulus to digit, recording at elbow. S = stimulus. Calibration: 20 μV, 1 ms.

recording electrodes to be quite satisfactory, but Behse & Buchthal (1971) prefer needle recording electrodes and have reported their extensive findings on all of these nerves using this technique.

Di Benedetto (1970) and Burke et al (1974) suggested that measurement of the sensory action potential in the sural nerve may be a more sensitive index of peripheral neuropathy than the sensory potentials in the upper limbs. However, Guiloff & Sherratt (1977) found that changes in the medial plantar sensory action potential offered an even more sensitive test of peripheral nerve damage.

Compound nerve action potential

When the median or ulnar nerve is stimulated at the wrist, the compound action potential elicited above the elbow is formed by orthodromic conduction in sensory fibres and antidromic conduction in motor fibres. Dawson (1956) showed that the sensory fibres have a lower threshold and faster conduction rate than motor fibres. In some pathological situations, for example severe anterior horn cell disease, it is likely that the residual evoked potential seen at the elbow originates in sensory fibres only. Conduction within the brachial plexus may be assessed by recording potentials above the clavicle from the upper part of the plexus following stimulation of the median, ulnar or radial nerves at the wrist or elbow. This arrangement is particularly employed during cervical and cortical somatosensory potential recordings in order to ensure the integrity of the peripheral nerve pathway.

Refractory period

The refractory period of a nerve or muscle depends upon the recovery time of the fibre membrane after it has been depolarised. For a short interval after a stimulus the fibre will not respond to a second stimulus, however powerful; this is the absolute refractory period. The relative refractory period follows, in which a second stimulus of sufficient magnitude is effective. Finally, there may be a supernormal phase in which the fibre is hyperexcitable. The refractory period of sensory

or mixed nerves (0.6–0.7 ms (Gilliatt & Willison 1963)) is shorter than that of muscle (2.2–4.6 ms (Farmer et al 1960)). Determination of the refractory period in motor nerves is not readily carried out by direct measurement, but methods have been described using collision techniques (Kimura et al 1978, Ingram et al 1987a) which give the distribution of motor nerve refractory periods, while Borg (1984) has described a technique for determining the refractory period in single motor axons. Kopec et al (1978) have developed a subtraction technique for measuring the refractory period of the distal motor nerve branches and muscle fibres.

Increases in refractory period in the presence of normal nerve conduction velocities have been described in various peripheral neuropathies (Lowitzsch & Hopf 1975, Alderson & Petajan 1987), indicating that the technique is more sensitive than conventional nerve conduction measurement for identifying abnormal nerve function.

Conduction velocity distributions

Recently two methods have been reported for estimating the nerve fibre conduction velocity distributions by computer analysis of the compound action potential recorded from nerve trunks. Barker et al (1979) base their technique on analysis of the dispersion components present in two compound action potentials recorded from the same site following stimulation at two points along the nerve. Cummins and colleagues (Cummins et al 1979a,b) have developed a model of the compound action potential in terms of constituent single-fibre action potentials. They have applied this to the study of two compound action potentials separated by a known distance along the nerve, from which they are able to derive an estimate of the distribution of fibre conduction velocities. Both these techniques are extremely complex, requiring sophisticated analysis, and as yet their application in pathological situations is limited (Barker 1981, Cummins et al 1981).

Sources of errors

Problems of measurement and possible sources of errors in the estimation of nerve conduction velocities are discussed by Mavor & Libman (1962), Gassel (1964b), Simpson (1964) and Kimura (1984).

Errors in the measurement of conduction velocity may derive from both technical and biological causes. A number of the former have already been mentioned, including the use of differing stimulus strengths or amplifier gains at the different stimulus sites. It is important to ensure that the oscilloscope sweep is triggering correctly and to check for inaccuracies of the latency calibration.

Measurement of the distance between the two points of stimulation on the surface can only be an approximation of the true length of the underlying nerve, accounting for one of the most significant sources of error. Nevertheless, comparison of surface and true nerve measurement in cadavers has shown a close correlation between the two (Carpendale 1956). This relationship is less certain when the course of the nerve is non-linear, for example around the elbow and through the brachial plexus. In the latter situation measurement of the distance by obstetric calipers may be more accurate than with a surface tape (Jebsen 1967, London 1975). The error of measurement is more significant for shorter distances, and care should be taken to ensure as long a segment as possible, usually more than 10 cm, is examined. In some circumstances however, inclusion of a long section of normally conducting nerve may conceal the presence of a minor localised conduction defect, and estimation of conduction through the affected small segment may be necessary to reveal such a lesion.

Anatomical variations of nerves may also give rise to confusion if their presence is not appreciated. Communication between the median and ulnar nerves in the forearm occurs in 15–31% of the normal population (Buchthal et al 1974, Gutmann 1977), which may lead to simultaneous activation of ulnar-supplied muscles, the volume-conducted potentials of which may interfere with the response from median-innervated muscles. This is particularly apparent in the presence of a carpal tunnel syndrome (Iyer & Fenichel 1976). The same effect may be seen simply with distant spread of responses arising from more proximally situated muscles (Gassel 1964b).

REFLEX STUDIES

The H-reflex

Supramaximal stimulation of the posterior tibial nerve in the popliteal fossa evokes a muscle action potential in the triceps surae muscle with a relatively short latency, the M-response. If a weak stimulus is employed, a second muscle action potential may be recorded with a longer latency. As the stimulus strength is progressively increased, the second response becomes smaller and eventually disappears (Fig. 30.6). The latency of the second potential is long enough to suggest that it represents a spinal reflex, and this is supported by the fact that the latency increases as the stimulus site is moved distally. This late potential, first described by Hoffman (1918), is called the H-wave.

The reflex nature of the H-wave was established by Magladery and associates (1950) who stimulated the posterior tibial nerve in the popliteal fossa and recorded spinal root potentials from intrathecally

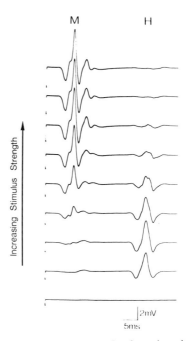

Fig. 30.6 Recording of the H-reflex from the soleus muscle in a normal adult following stimulation of the posterior tibial nerve in the popliteal fossa with stimuli of increasing intensity. When the stimulus is sufficient to evoke a direct M-response, the amplitude of the H-response is diminished.

placed electrodes. When these electrodes were placed close to the cord at L1, the time interval between anterior and posterior root potentials was only 1.5 ms. Allowing for the conduction time in the afferent and efferent arcs of the reflex, this is sufficient for passage through a single cord synapse (Magladery et al 1951). With increasing stimulus strength, an antidromic potential was recorded on the anterior roots which, with strong stimuli, occluded the anterior root potential. Conduction velocity studies showed that the afferent arc of the reflex is subserved by low-threshold, rapidly conducting group Ia fibres, and it seems that the H-reflex represents the electrical equivalent of the ankle jerk elicited by stimulation proximal to the muscle spindle.

Under normal circumstances the H-reflex is readily elicited only from the calf muscles (Magladery & McDougal 1950), but it may also be recorded in flexor carpi radialis (Schimscheimer et al 1985). The H-reflex has been most extensively used to examine motor neurone excitability (Magladery et al 1952), employing paired stimuli of progressively increasing intervals to establish a recovery curve. It has also proved valuable for assessing large sensory fibre function in peripheral neuropathies (Mayer & Mawdsley 1965, Adams et al 1973, Lefebvre-d'Amour et al 1979, Lachman et al 1980) and studying the integrity of the S1/S2 roots when recording from soleus (Braddom & Johnson 1974, Notermans & Vingerhoets 1974, Fisher et al 1978) and C6/C7 roots when flexor carpi radialis is used (Schimscheimer et al 1985).

The blink reflex

Electrical stimulation of the supraorbital nerve elicits a reflex response composed of two components, R1 and R2, in the orbicularis oculi muscle. The R1-response has a latency of about 10 ms, while the R2-component has a longer and more variable latency of 25–40 ms. The R1 appears only on the ipsilateral side whereas the R2 is recorded bilaterally. Side-to-side differences of the R1 latency should not exceed 1.2 ms. For the R2, the latency difference between the ipsilateral and contralateral responses elicited by stimulation

on one side should not be greater than 5 ms, while the difference in latency for the R2 evoked on the right and left sides should not exceed 7 ms (Kimura 1975).

There is clinical evidence that the R1 is conducted through the pons and relayed in the area of the principal sensory nucleus of the fifth nerve (Kimura 1970, Namerow & Etamadi 1970). Most of the evidence now indicates that it is exteroceptive, cutaneous and oligosynaptic in nature (Penders & Delwaide 1971, Shahani & Young 1973, Trontelj & Trontelj 1973b). The R2-component innervation descends along the spinal trigeminal tract to make connections via medullary polysynaptic pathways with both facial nuclei in the pons (Kimura & Lyon 1972).

Abnormalities of the blink reflex may occur in peripheral lesions affecting the trigeminal and facial nerves or their central connections, and in the presence of disturbances of suprasegmental function. In lesions of the trigeminal nerve, the first component may be small or absent, or have a prolonged latency (Ferguson 1978, Ongerboer de Visser & Kuypers 1978). In patients with Bell's palsy, conventional methods (distal conduction studies and facial EMG) are useful mainly in the detection of changes produced by wallerian degeneration and cannot localise proximal facial nerve segment lesions (Shahani & Young 1977). The blink reflex reflects conduction along the entire facial nerve. Kimura et al (1976) found serial testing a useful guide to determining a recovery pattern.

Significant prolongation of latency in both components of the blink reflex is observed in peripheral neuropathies of the segmental demyelinating type, including the Guillain–Barré syndrome (Shahani & Young 1977, Kimura 1982).

NORMAL FINDINGS

General

Because of variations in technique, it is highly desirable that each laboratory obtains its own control values for each nerve and segment of nerve. Tables 30.1 and 30.2 give a representative sample of results obtained by different authors, and show the considerable variation from segment to segment and the wide range of values even

Table 30.1 Normal values for motor conduction velocity in different nerves

Nerve and segment	Examinations (no.)	Conduction velocity (m/s) Mean	Range	Distal latency ms mean	Reference
Median					
Er-A	21	65.1	57.1–76.2	3.9	Ginzburg et al 1978
A-E	15	71.1	60.3–86.4	3.3	Mavor & Libman 1962
A-E (R)	58	69	(SD 6.5)		Peioglou-Harmoussi et al 1985a
E-W (R)	58	58	(SD 4.5)	3.5 (SD 0.35)	Peioglou-Harmoussi et al 1985a
E-W	145	58.8		3.5	Mulder et al 1961
Ulnar					
Er-A	22	63.0	55.0–73.2	3.5	Ginzburg et al 1978
Er-above E	30	58.9	50.0–67.7		London 1975
A-E	47	63.8			Trojaborg 1977
A-E (R)	64	68	(SD 6.8)		Peioglou-Harmoussi et al 1985a
E-W (R)	64	57	(SD 5.1)	2.7 (SD 0.32)	Peioglou-Harmoussi et al 1985a
E-W	225	59.9		2.7	Mulder et al 1961
Radial					
A-E	9	70.0	(SD 4.9)	2.5 (to brachioradialis)	Trojaborg & Sindrup (1969)
Sciatic	29	56.0	(SD 5.5)	5.4 (to soleus)	Gassel & Trojaborg 1964
Common peroneal	41	50.2	30.0–60.0	5.0	Mulder et al 1961
	172	50.1	(SD 7.2)		Johnson & Olsen 1960
Posterior tibial	12	48.7	(SD 3.5)	5.0	Mavor & Atcheson 1966
	30	43.2	(SD 4.9)		Thomas et al 1959

Er, Erb's point; A, axilla; E, elbow; W, wrist; (R), right; SD, standard deviation.

within one segment in normal nerves. Several studies have shown conduction to be slower in more distal than proximal segments for both motor and sensory nerves (Gilliatt & Thomas 1960, Trojaborg 1964, Kaeser 1975, Peioglou-Harmoussi et al 1985b). Conduction velocity is directly related to fibre diameter by a factor of about 6 m/s per μm (Hursch 1939), and therefore part of the distal slowing can be attributed to progressive tapering of axons (Magladery & McDougal 1950). A slight but significant decline in limb temperature distally may also be a contributory factor. Velocities are faster in the shorter upper limb than longer lower limb nerves, while a general inverse relationship between conduction velocity and height has been observed in an adult control population (Campbell et al 1981), although this has not been substantiated in a study on sural nerve conduction (Trojaborg et al 1992). Nerve action potential amplitudes are slightly higher on average in females than males (Casey & Le Quesne 1972a, Trojaborg et al 1992).

Variations due to age

Various studies (Thomas & Lambert 1960, Gamstorp 1963, Baer & Johnson 1965) have shown that conduction velocity in motor fibres at birth is only about half of that in adults. After an initial rapid increase in the first year, the velocity more gradually approaches that of adults by 3–5 years, with further more complex patterns of changes in velocity occurring in later childhood and adolescence (Lang et al 1985). The rate of increase in conduction velocity varies in different nerves, and appears to depend upon maturation of the axon, the process of myelination, and the actual length of the nerve (Lang et al 1985).

Slowing of conduction in motor fibres with increasing age in adult life has been demonstrated by several authors (Norris et al 1953, Mulder et al 1961). Buchthal & Rosenfalck (1966) observed a significant decrease in sensory conduction velocity in upper arm and forearm segments and also an increase in distal latency with advancing age; in addition, they, and more recently Andersen

Table 30.2   Normal values for sensory conduction velocity in different nerves

Nerve and segment	Examinations (no.)	Age (years)	Conduction velocity (m/s)	Amplitude (μV)	Reference
Median					
Digit II to wrist (S)	76	10–72	56.2 (SD 6.8)	18.6 (SD 8.8)	Fawcett et al 1982
Digit II to wrist (N)	13	18–25	50.2 (SD 5.2)	—	Buchthal & Rosenfalck 1966
Wrist to elbow (N)	10	70–88	44.1 (SD 3.6)	—	
	9	18–25	63.9 (SD 5.1)	—	
Ulnar					
Digit V to wrist (S)	59	19–76	55.1 (SD 5.7)	15.4 (SD 7.1)	Fawcett et al 1982
Digit V to wrist (N)	9	18–25	51.9 (SD 5.6)	—	Buchthal & Rosenfalck 1966
	10	70–89	50.2 (SD 3.7)	—	
Wrist to elbow (N)	9	18–25	63.9 (SD 5.1)	—	
Radial					
Digit I to wrist (S)	23	16–28	58 (SD 6.0)	13 (SD 7.5)	Trojaborg & Sindrup 1969
Wrist to elbow (S)	19	16–28	64 (SD 6.0)	31 (SD 11.7)	Sindrup 1969
Superficial peroneal					
Big toe to above (N)	19	15–25	46.1 (SD 4.1)	1.2	Behse & Buchthal 1971
Extensor retinaculum	17	40–65	42.2 (SD 6.3)	0.5	
Posterior tibial					
Big toe to (S)	11	20–29	34.9 (SD 2.6)	3.0 (SD 2.3)	Guiloff & Sherratt 1977
Medial malleolus	13	50–59	33.5 (SD 3.8)	1.7 (SD 0.6)	
Big toe to (N)	23	15–30	46.1 (SD 3.5)	—	Behse & Buchthal 1971
Medial malleolus	10	40–65	43.4 (SD 3.8)	—	
Sural calf to lateral	26	21–40	46.2 (SD 3.7)	16.4 (SD 5.5)	Burke et al 1974
malleolus (S)	23	41–60	46.4 (SD 3.7)	13.6 (SD 7.5)	Fawcett et al 1982
	34	17–52	49.5 (SD 4.3)	34.3 (SD 9.9)	
Dorsum of foot to	16	15–30	51.2 (SD 4.5)	—	Behse & Buchthal 1971
lateral malleolus (N)	15	40–65	48.3 (SD 5.3)	—	

S, Surface recording electrodes; N, needle recording electrodes.

(1985), have noted a reduction of the amplitude and increase in duration of the sensory evoked response.

tored by repeated measurements in the same patient at different times, when accurate temperature control is essential.

Effects of temperature

Studies by Henriksen (1956) and Johnson & Olsen (1960) in motor fibres, and by Buchthal & Rosenfalck (1966) in the larger sensory fibres, show that conduction rate slows with cooling by a factor of 2–2.4 ms/°C. Cooling also results in prolongation of the terminal motor latency (Fig. 30.7), and less well-appreciated changes in the muscle and nerve action potential, the amplitude and duration of which increase as the temperature falls (Denys 1977, Bolton et al 1981). In order to minimise the effect of temperature, the laboratory should be warm and the skin temperature should be maintained at about 34°C by either prior immersion in warm water or with a heating lamp. Particular care is required if the course of a progressive or recovering neuropathy is being moni-

ABNORMAL NERVE CONDUCTION

General considerations

The last two decades have seen considerable advances in our understanding of the major factors which determine impulse conduction in myelinated nerve fibres, and the ways in which pathological changes may influence this foremost of nerve functions (Rasminsky & Sears 1972, Bostock & Sears 1978, Waxman 1980, McDonald 1980, Sumner 1980). A number of studies have compared structural and electrophysiological changes in the nerve in various forms of neuropathy (Lambert & Dyck 1975, Behse & Buchthal 1977, Behse et al 1977, Buchthal & Behse 1977, Bolton et al 1979b), and while comparison of morphological aspects based on short segments of

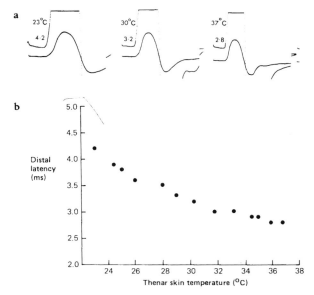

Fig. 30.7 Relationship between temperature and the distal latency, amplitude and duration of the M-response recorded from the thenar muscles following stimulation of the median nerve at the wrist in a normal adult. Note (in **b**) the progressive increase in latency as the overlying skin temperature falls from 37°C to 23°C. Associated with this (**a**) there is an increase in both the amplitude and duration of the M-response.

nerve with conduction characteristics obtained over a much longer segment may lead to inconsistencies, much valuable information has resulted from this type of study. Gilliatt (1966) has suggested that peripheral neuropathies can be separated into two groups according to the nerve conduction findings, which can be correlated pathologically with primary axonal degeneration and segmental demyelination. Although the majority of neuropathies can be categorised in this manner, it has become increasingly clear that a combination of both these features may be present in most neuropathies (Thomas 1971), reflecting a close functional relationship between the axons and Schwann cells. Nevertheless, one or other process may predominate, and in broad terms relatively distinctive patterns of change in clinical nerve conduction may be observed.

Axonal degeneration

Axonal disruption following direct nerve section

results in wallerian degeneration of the distal nerve portion. The earliest detectable change in motor nerves is failure of neuromuscular transmission (Miledi & Slater 1970), with little or no significant slowing of conduction in the motor fibres distal to the interruption for several days, after which conduction fails abruptly (Gilliatt & Taylor 1959, Gilliatt & Hjorth 1972). In many conditions axonal degeneration occurs in a centripetal fashion producing a 'dying-back' neuropathy (Cavanagh 1964), suggesting that the 'sick' parent cell body is unable to sustain the most distal portions of the long axon. In some hexacarbon neuropathies, abnormalities appear to occur simultaneously at numerous sites along the distal part of the axon, giving rise to the term distal axonopathy (Spencer & Schaumburg 1979).

Nerve conduction in axonal neuropathies is usually only minimally slowed, but is accompanied by a reduction in the size of either the evoked muscle response or nerve action potential, proportionate to the loss of functioning axons. In experimental acrylamide neuropathy, a 20% reduction in the maximum motor conduction velocity may occur, which has been attributed to selective loss of the largest and fastest conducting axons (Fullerton & Barnes 1966, Hopkins & Gilliatt 1971). More usually a wider spectrum of fibre sizes is involved by the degenerative process (Walsh & McLeod 1970, Behse & Buchthal 1977), and a sufficient number of large diameter axons remain so that the maximum velocity is little affected. With increasing severity of the neuropathy the velocity may decline further, but not to the degree seen with demyelination, and the evoked nerve or muscle potential may be lost.

One consequence of the dying-back process is that conduction slowing may be first detected in the most distal portions of the nerves, when velocity in more proximal segments is normal (Casey & Le Quesne 1972b). Because of the relatively minor changes in conduction and the wide range of evoked-response amplitudes in normal nerves and muscle, measurement of maximal conduction velocity is a rather insensitive method for identifying axonal neuropathies, particularly in the early stages. Determination of F-response latency may improve the diagnostic yield (Shahani & Sumner 1981), while electromyographic examination of the muscle for evidence of denervation is an essential part of the investigation. Serial studies may reveal a progressive decline in velocity and response amplitude even though the values remain within the normal range.

Demyelinating disorders

Disorders of the myelin sheath resulting in either paranodal or segmental demyelination produce much more dramatic changes in conduction than are seen in axonal neuropathies. This may take the form of either marked slowing of conduction, usually by more than 30% of their normal value to as low as 7 m/s, or conduction block (Feasby et al 1985). Terminal latencies are often strikingly prolonged, sometimes up to 35 ms, and the duration of the evoked response is often increased, particularly following proximal stimulation. Conduction block may be recognised by a reduction in the amplitude of the evoked response elicited from proximal sites. Lewis & Sumner (1982) recommend that the proximal response should be 50% or less of the amplitude following more distal stimulation in order to differentiate conduction block from the effects of impulse dispersion in variably affected nerve fibres, which may result in phase cancellation of responses from individual motor units.

The pathophysiological mechanisms relating conduction slowing or block and demyelination have been reviewed in detail by McDonald (1980). Loss or thinning of myelin in the region of nodes of Ranvier or internodal segments leads to a reduction in resistive and an increase in capacitive properties across the nerve fibre. This has the effect of reducing the longitudinal electrotonic flow of current preceding the active action potential, thereby delaying excitation at the next node or, if severe enough, resulting in failure of excitation and block of conduction. Experimental studies have revealed that segmental demyelination may in certain circumstances be associated with continuous rather than saltatory conduction through an affected segment, in which case conduction is markedly slowed (Bostock & Sears 1978). Whether this occurs in diseased human nerve is not known.

In addition to slowing of impulse propagation, demyelination renders the nerve fibre even more sensitive to changes in temperature. Rasminsky (1973) has shown that even slight increases of temperature within the physiological range can result in block of impulse conduction through demyelinated segments. The refractory period is also prolonged (Lehmann et al 1971), leading to a reduction in the capacity of the fibre to transmit repetitive trains of stimuli causing intermittent failure of conduction.

DISEASES OF THE ANTERIOR HORN CELL

Degeneration of the anterior horn cell occurs in a number of disorders including poliomyelitis, spinal muscular atrophy in its various forms, motor neurone disease (MND) and syringomyelia. Muscle atrophy in, for example, motor neurone disease and syringomyelia, may often begin in a focal manner and, while the clinical findings may point to a central lesion, patients are seen occasionally in whom it is not possible to exclude a disturbance of the peripheral nerves on clinical grounds. It is therefore important to know whether diseases involving the anterior horn cell have any effect on peripheral nerve function, other than the consequential loss of motor axons. Henriksen (1956) found only minor degrees of slowing amounting to no more than 10% in patients with poliomyelitis, provided that allowance was made for the lower temperature in the paretic limb. Similarly Lambert & Mulder (1957), Lambert (1962), Willison (1962) and Ertekin (1967) found maximal motor conduction velocity was within the normal range in most patients with motor neurone disease. Mild slowing of conduction was seen in those cases with severe muscular atrophy with correspondingly small M-response amplitudes, consistent with the loss of the fastest-conducting axons (Lambert & Mulder 1957, Hansen & Ballantyne 1978). In a recent study Cornblath et al (1992) stressed that the distal latency rarely exceeded 125% of the upper normal limit, while the motor conduction velocity was usually above 80% of the lower limit, helping to differentiate between motor neurone disease and chronic inflammatory demyelinating neuropathy which may present with a similar clinical picture (Parry & Clarke 1988, Kaji et al 1992).

Using the Hopf technique, Miglietta (1968) and Chaco (1970) found that the range of conduction velocities in MND was narrowed, suggesting perhaps an early loss of the slower conducting and therefore smaller axons. Hausmanowa-Petrusewicz & Kopec (1973) observed the same phenomenon in very severe cases, but in early cases the spectrum of velocities was normal, while it was increased due to slowing of the minimum conduction velocity value in an intermediate group. Ingram et al (1985) also found abnormal conduction velocity distributions in most cases, initially with slowing of conduction in some fibres, progressing eventually to involve all fibres in advanced patients. None of these studies has shown any evidence of preferential involvement of a particular class of anterior horn cell by the disease process in MND.

F-response studies in patients with MND (Peioglou-Harmoussi 1983, Petajan 1985) have shown increases in latency, suggesting either impaired conduction in surviving axons or, because the longest-latency response was more frequently abnormal (Peioglou-Harmoussi 1983), that changes in central excitability might cause F-responses to occur in a population of neurones with slower conduction velocities than is usually seen in control subjects. The presence of an excessive degree of segmental demyelination and remyelination of peripheral nerves in MND (Dayan et al 1969, Dyck et al 1975, Hanyu et al 1982) might account for the delayed F-responses. A decline in the frequency of F-responses was also found (Peioglou-Harmoussi et al 1987), particularly in the later stages when the muscles were markedly atrophic. Nevertheless the frequency with which individual F-responses occurred was increased (Petajan 1985, Peioglou-Harmoussi et al 1987), probably as a result of enhanced excitability in the remaining motor neurone pool due to upper motor neurone involvement. The amplitude of the F-response is generally slightly increased, reflecting an increase in the size of surviving motor units following collateral reinnervation (Argyropoulos et al 1978, Peioglou-Harmoussi 1983).

Several studies have shown normal sensory potentials and mixed nerve action potentials in motor neurone disease (Willison 1962, Fincham & Van Allen 1964, Ertekin 1967) and this finding will help to exclude a peripheral nerve lesion in patients presenting with muscle wasting. Others (Brown & Jaatoul 1974, Stålberg 1982, Peioglou-Harmoussi 1983) have demonstrated a reduction in sensory potential amplitudes and slowing of sensory conduction in some patients which suggests that the degenerative process may not be restricted to the motor system.

Motor conduction velocity is normal in the majority of patients with juvenile- and adult-onset spinal muscular atrophy (SMA) (Gardner-Medwin et al 1967, Meadows et al 1969, Buchthal & Olsen 1970, O'Sullivan & McLeod 1978, Harding & Thomas 1980a). Excluding cases with the distal form of SMA, the amplitude of the response evoked from intrinsic hand and foot muscles is usually within normal limits (personal observation), consistent with the predominant involvement of proximal muscle groups. Sensory conduction velocities and action potential amplitudes are also usually normal (O'Sullivan & McLeod 1978, Harding & Thomas 1980a), although Swift (1984) has observed abnormal sensory conduction in a proportion of juvenile-onset cases. Nevertheless the generally normal findings help to distinguish the distal form of SMA from the axonal variant of peroneal muscular atrophy (HMSN type II).

Motor conduction in infantile SMA (SMA types I, II) may be normal or slightly reduced according to the degree of muscle wasting (Hausmanowa-Petrusewicz et al 1975). Swift (1984) has also noted impaired sensory conduction in some of the infantile-onset group.

In syringomyelia, several studies have reported normal motor and sensory conduction velocities (Fincham & Cape 1968, Schwartz et al 1980, Peioglou-Harmoussi 1986), except when there is marked muscular atrophy and loss of larger neurones. Patients are at risk of developing ulnar nerve lesions at the elbow in relation to a Charcot arthropathy of the joint (Peioglou-Harmoussi et al 1986). Delayed F-responses have been observed in upper limb nerves in which conduction was normal in distal segments (Peioglou-Harmoussi et al 1986), suggesting either minor traumatic damage to the peripheral nerves, or abnormalities of the intraspinal portion of the motor nerve fibres and anterior horn cells. Normal sensory findings help to confirm that the characteristic sensory impairment seen in these individuals is due to a lesion in the sensory pathways which is proximal to the dorsal root ganglion.

PRIMARY MUSCLE DISEASES

Motor and sensory conduction is usually normal in patients with primary diseases of muscle, particularly in the Duchenne, Becker, limb-girdle and facioscapulohumeral forms of muscular dystrophy (Sica & McComas 1971, Hilton-Brown & Stålberg 1983, personal observations). Conduction is also normal in hereditary distal myopathy (Sumner et al 1971), helping to distinguish this rare disorder from the more common hereditary motor and sensory neuropathies.

Reduction in motor conduction velocity has been reported in some patients with myotonic dystrophy (Mongia & Lundervold 1975, Olson et al 1978, Panayiotopoulos 1978). Using the Hopf technique, Rossi et al (1983) were able to show slowing of both maximal and minimal velocities, implying that the whole spectrum of fibres was affected. There was no evidence of preferential involvement of smaller motor neurones supplying type I motor units which might have been expected from the histopathological findings of selective atrophy of type I muscle fibres (Brooke & Engel 1969). Abnormal peripheral sensory conduction has also been demonstrated by somatosensory evoked potential studies (Mongia & Lundervold 1975, Bartel et al 1984). These findings suggest that the peripheral nerve abnormality may be part of the more generalised disturbance of cellular function seen in this disorder.

While nerve conduction studies have been reported as normal in the vast majority of patients with mitochondrial myopathy, slight reductions in the motor and sensory velocities have occasionally been found, consistent with an axonal neuropathy (Spiro et al 1970, Berenberg et al 1977, Bertorini et al 1978, Markesbery 1979). More marked slowing of conduction has been described in other cases (Shy et al 1966, Drachman 1968, Peyronnard et al 1979), indicating a demyelinating neuropathy. The latter authors suggest that the mitochondrial abnormality may also impair Schwann cell function leading to a disturbance of myelin formation and axon maintenance. In a recent study Yiannikas & McLeod (1985) found neurophysio-logical evidence of a peripheral neuropathy in 45% of 20 cases of mitochondrial myopathy, suggesting more frequent involvement of the peripheral nerves than has been suspected. It should be noted however that in some cases of familial mitochondrial myopathy there is an increased incidence of diabetes mellitus (Mechler et al 1981) which may account for the peripheral neuropathy (Fawcett et al 1982).

A decrease in motor conduction velocity was reported in one patient with myopathic carnitine deficiency which was associated with an abnormal accumulation of lipid droplets in Schwann cells (Markesbery et al 1974).

NEUROMUSCULAR TRANSMISSION DISORDERS

Motor and sensory conduction velocities are normal in myasthenia gravis and congenital forms of myasthenia. The amplitudes of the resting CMAPs are also generally within the normal range, even in clinically weak muscles, although the average value may be less than normal. By contrast, in the Lambert–Eaton myasthenic syndrome and botulism, where low levels of acetylcholine are released, the CMAP amplitude following a single stimulus to the nerve is usually reduced. In this situation the finding of a further decrement at low rates of repetitive stimulation and marked postactivation facilitation identifies these patients as having a primary neuromuscular transmission defect.

In patients with the slow channel syndrome (Engel et al 1982) and acetylcholinesterase deficiency (Engel et al 1977), a repetitive CMAP is evoked by a single stimulus.

PERIPHERAL NEUROPATHIES

General considerations

The presentation of peripheral nerve disorders varies according to the nature and distribution of the abnormalities within the nerves. The principal clinical patterns seen include isolated lesions in individual nerves (mononeuropathy), isolated lesions in two or more separate nerves (mononeuropathy multiplex), or diffuse involvement of the peripheral nerves (polyneuropathy).

Compressive lesions of individual nerves, for example, the median nerve within the carpal tunnel and the ulnar nerve at the elbow are common, and may occur in isolation or complicating a more generalised disturbance of the peripheral nerves. Predominant involvement of the nerve roots is seen in some cases of acquired inflammatory neuropathy (see below), and in cervical and lumbar spondylosis. Isolated lesions in nerve trunks, as referred to above, may be associated with axonal degeneration, for example in the neuropathy of polyarteritis nodosa and in some cases of diabetes mellitus. Rarely focal demyelination sufficient to produce conduction block may present in this manner. Thus by appropriate assessment of nerve conduction velocity and nerve and muscle response characteristics in different peripheral nerves, the examiner may not only identify the presence of abnormal peripheral nerve function, but also provide information which is of primary diagnostic value.

Axonal neuropathies

Axonal degeneration represents the main pathological change in a large proportion of peripheral neuropathies. Included in this group are the neuropathies associated with diabetes mellitus, uraemia, chronic alcoholism, carcinoma, critically ill patients, primary amyloidosis, porphyria, malnutrition and vitamin deficiency, toxic chemicals and drugs, including some used in anticancer therapy. The axon is primarily affected in the type I variant of hereditary motor and sensory neuropathies, and in Friedreich's ataxia.

Demyelinating neuropathies

Segmental demyelination occurs as the principal pathological change in a number of neuropathies, including acute or subacute inflammatory polyradiculoneuropathy or the Guillain–Barré syndrome, chronic inflammatory polyneuropathy, the hypertrophic form of Charcot–Marie–Tooth disease (HMSN type I) and the neuropathies of Dejerine–Sottas, Refsum's disease, metachromatic leukodystrophy, Krabbe's leukodystrophy, hereditary neuropathies with liability to pressure palsy, some cases of diabetic and myeloma neuropathy, the

neuropathy associated with paraproteinaemia and leprosy.

The electrophysiological changes in some of these specific neuropathies are described in more detail below.

Diabetic polyneuropathy. This may present in various forms, with consequently different patterns of nerve conduction abnormalities. Several studies have revealed slowing of motor and sensory conduction in those with, and to a lesser extent those without, clinical evidence of neuropathy (Downie & Newell 1961, Lawrence & Locke 1961, Mulder et al 1961, Gilliatt & Willison 1962, Behse et al 1977), the changes being more marked in the lower limb nerves and in the distal segments (Kimura et al 1979). Some patients have a mononeuropathy of either the median, ulnar or common peroneal nerves at common sites of compression, with local slowing of conduction in the affected segment (Mulder et al 1961, Gilliatt & Willison 1962), conduction in the remaining nerves being normal or borderline. Others may present with a mononeuropathy of the femoral nerve or a polyradiculopathy (Bastron & Thomas 1981) and truncal mononeuropathy (Waxman & Sabin 1981) or radiculopathy (Streib et al 1986).

Slowing of motor conduction in the lower limbs and delayed F-response latencies (Dyck et al 1985) have been reported to be the earliest changes, while Lamontagne & Buchthal (1970) found abnormalities of the sensory potentials and the presence of fibrillation potentials in distal muscles to be sensitive indicators of a subclinical neuropathy. In studies of nerve-fibre conduction velocity distributions, asymptomatic patients with mild diabetes have been shown to demonstrate a shift towards the slower-conducting fibre populations, even when the maximal nerve conduction velocity was normal (Dorfman & Cummings 1980). The measurement of other parameters such as warming and vibration perception threshold have been found to be more sensitive than conventional nerve conduction studies for detecting early diabetic neuropathy (Le Quesne et al 1990, Kilma et al 1991).

The finding of fibrillation potentials in distal muscles reflects axonal degeneration (Thomas & Lascelles 1966, Behse et al 1977, Hansen & Ballantyne 1977), which may be particularly marked in chronic cases leading to loss of the evoked potentials. Nevertheless slowing of conduction is mainly accounted for by segmental demyelination and remyelination (Thomas & Lascelles 1966, Chopra et al 1969, Behse et al 1977). A small number of young adult patients with insulin-dependent diabetes have been reported to develop a severe polyneuropathy of relatively rapid onset (Said et al 1992). Electrophysiological studies revealed a marked reduction in the amplitude of the sural action potential, consistent with severe sensory axonal loss. Considerable slowing of motor conduction in the peroneal nerve with only a slight decrease in the evoked muscle action potential suggested demyelination of the motor axons, although in one case evidence of severe motor axonal loss was also found.

Uraemic polyneuropathy. Peripheral nerve abnormalities are well-recognised complications of chronic renal failure, usually taking the form of a mixed sensorimotor neuropathy. Moderate slowing of motor and sensory conduction occurs in both proximal and distal nerve segments of the upper and lower limbs (Neilsen 1973a). Conduction changes may precede clinical symptoms (Preswick & Jeremy 1964, Jennekens et al 1971, Neilsen 1973b), while the degree of slowing is correlated with a reducing creatinine clearance and the duration of renal failure (Jennekens et al 1971, Neilsen 1973b). H-reflex and F-response studies provide a sensitive means of identifying proximal conduction abnormalities in these patients (Panayiotopoulos & Lagos 1980).

Improved nerve conduction may lag behind clinical improvement following the institution of haemodialysis (Konatey-Ahulu et al 1965, Tenckhoff et al 1965, Neilsen 1974b), whereas renal transplantation usually results in considerable amelioration of both clinical and electrophysiological findings (Neilsen 1974a). Neilsen (1974a) found significant increases in conduction within weeks of transplantation, and suggests that this rapid change may reflect a restoration of the normal axon membrane potential, although early remyelination could not be excluded. A secondary, more protracted, phase of recovery was thought to be due to axonal regeneration, correlating with the main histological findings of axonal damage with secondary segmental demyelination (Dyck et al 1971a, Thomas et al 1971).

The creation of forearm and antebrachial arteriovenous fistulas have been reported to be associated with localised neuropathies of the median nerve at the wrist or forearm and ulnar nerve at the elbow (Warren & Otieno 1975, Harding & Le Fanu 1977, Bolton et al 1979a, Hamilton et al 1980, Knezevic & Mastaglia 1984). The mechanism(s) by which these lesions are produced is uncertain, but ischaemia due to shunting of the blood away from forearm tissues distal to the fistula and increased venous pressure leading to venous congestion and oedema have been proposed. It is also possible that aneurysmal dilatation of forearm veins may lead to localised nerve compression, particularly at the usual sites of entrapment beneath tendons or fascial bands (Knezevic & Mastaglia 1984).

Alcoholic polyneuropathy. Mild to moderate slowing of motor and sensory conduction (Mawdsley & Mayer 1965, Walsh & McLeod 1970, Behse & Buchthal 1977) and increased F-response latencies (Lefebvre-D'Amour et al 1979) have been demonstrated in alcoholic patients with and without clinical features of peripheral nerve disease. Changes are present in upper and lower limb nerves, but tend to be more pronounced in the lower extremities and in the most distal portions of the nerves (Casey & Le Quesne 1972b). Histological findings in sural nerve biopsies (Walsh & McLeod 1970, Behse & Buchthal 1977) indicate axonal degeneration of large and small fibres, which accounts for the main electrophysiological abnormality of a reduction in the sensory potential amplitude with only slight slowing of the maximal conduction velocity. An increase in the relative refractory period in the median sensory nerve has been reported to be the most sensitive indicator of axonal dysfunction in alcoholic neuropathy (Alderson & Petajan 1987). Increased F-response latencies and signs of minimal active denervation and compensatory reinnervation on electromyography in distal lower limb muscles have also been reported, indicating motor involvement (Shields 1985). Behse & Buchthal (1977) were unable to find any evidence of vitamin deficiency in their patients and concluded that the neuropathy was the result of a direct neurotoxic effect of alcohol.

Neuropathy in critically ill patients. A

peripheral polyneuropathy has been reported in up to 50% of patients who are critically ill through trauma, surgery or medical illness and this is usually associated with sepsis (Bolton et al 1984, Bolton 1987). The electrophysiological findings indicate that the neuropathy is due to distal axonal degeneration of both motor and sensory fibres.

HIV-related neuropathy. HIV infection is associated with a wide variety of neurological disorders of which peripheral neuropathy represents an important and increasingly recognised peripheral nervous system manifestation. Clinically evident neuropathy has been reported in 16–52% of patients with the acquired immunodeficiency syndrome (AIDS) (Snider et al 1983, Parry 1988, de la Monte et al 1988), although histopathological evidence suggests involvement of the peripheral nerves in up to 95% of patients (de la Monte et al 1988). The peripheral neuropathy may present as an acute or chronic inflammatory demyelinating polyneuropathy, mononeuropathy multiplex, autonomic neuropathy, polyradiculopathy, or a distal, mainly sensory, symmetrical polyneuropathy which manifests in the later stages of the disease in the setting of profound immunosuppression (Miller et al 1988, Simpson & Wolfe 1991).

In the distal symmetrical polyneuropathy, nerve conduction studies show slight slowing of maximal conduction velocity together with reduction of the sensory nerve action potentials and signs of minimal active denervation in distal muscles of the lower limb on needle electromyography, consistent with axonal degeneration (Cornblath & McArthur 1988, Parry 1988). Gross slowing of motor conduction and increased distal latencies indicative of demyelination have been reported in the acute and chronic demyelinating polyneuropathies (Miller et al 1988, Parry 1988).

Paraneoplastic neuropathy. Several studies have shown impairment of sensory and motor conduction in a small proportion of patients with various underlying neoplasms (Moody 1965, Trojaborg et al 1969, Campbell & Paty 1974, Walsh 1971). Generally only mild slowing of conduction was seen, a reduction in the amplitude of the sensory response (Walsh 1971, Campbell & Paty 1974) or the presence of fibrillation potentials (Trojaborg et al 1969) being the main changes.

These features suggested principally axonal degeneration, with secondary segmental demyelination occurring only at a late stage (Campbell & Paty 1974). In patients with primary sensory neuropathy, first described by Denny-Brown (1948), the sensory action potentials are absent and the motor velocities are generally normal (Horwich et al 1977), indicative of a primary dorsal root ganglionopathy. In three patients with small cell carcinoma of the lung and sensory neuropathy, the sera were found to contain neuronal antinuclear IgG antibodies, raising the possibility of a role for the antibodies in the pathogenesis of the sensory neuronopathy (Dick et al 1988).

While lymphoma is usually associated with axonal degeneration (Walsh 1971), some patients present with a subacute demyelinating neuropathy resembling the Guillain–Barré syndrome (Klingon 1965) and in another case with lymphomatous infiltration of the peripheral nerves associated with positive monoclonal IgM κ reactivity, a severe demyelinating polyneuropathy was found (Ince et al 1987). A causal relationship between the monoclonal IgM κ and demyelination was suggested (see also below).

A study on patients with bronchial carcinoma (Lenman et al 1981) showed only a slight but significant impairment of motor conduction velocity in the group as a whole, whereas rather more marked abnormalities of sensory conduction were found. EMG changes of fibrillations or positive sharp waves were recorded in just under half the patients, and tended to be more pronounced in distal muscles suggesting a 'dying-back' process. A slight but significant improvement in conduction was observed in a group of patients who had undergone successful treatment of their carcinoma.

Amyloid neuropathy. The neuropathy associated with primary systemic amyloidosis and inherited amyloidosis has been reported to be axonal in nature. Nerve conduction studies in the vast majority showed only minimal slowing of motor conduction and small or more usually absent sensory responses, while the EMG revealed fibrillation activity in distal lower limb muscles (Kelly et al 1979).

Myeloma neuropathy. Nerve conduction velocities in patients with myeloma neuropathy in the absence of amyloid showed moderate slowing of mainly motor conduction consistent with an axonal sensorimotor neuropathy (Kelly et al 1981). In patients with the sclerotic variety of myeloma, motor conduction was moderately to severely slowed, the evoked muscle reponses were markedly reduced and the EMG showed fibrillation activity. The sensory velocities were moderately slowed and the responses small or absent, indicating a mixture of axonal degeneration and demyelination (Kelly et al 1981).

Neuropathy associated with paraproteinaemia. Some patients with benign IgM and IgG paraproteinaemia develop a chronic slowly progressive sensorimotor neuropathy with moderate to marked slowing of motor conduction and absent sensory action potentials in the majority of cases, indicating demyelination (Swash et al 1979, Dalkas & Engel 1981, Smith et al 1983). In a recent study on polyneuropathies associated with monoclonal gammopathies, Kelly (1990) has reported a relationship between positive binding of the M-protein with a myelin-associated glycoprotein (MAG) and the presence of a demyelinating neuropathy, suggesting that the IgM-M protein is directed against an antigen in the myelin sheath.

Drug-induced and toxic neuropathies. Numerous drugs have been implicated as the cause of peripheral neuropathy, and the reader is referred to Chapter 28 which deals with this topic in detail. In most drug-induced neuropathies in which nerve conduction studies have been performed, mild to moderate slowing of motor and sensory conduction have been observed, consistent with axonal damage, e.g. nitrofurantoin (Toole et al 1968), metronidazole (Bradley et al 1977a), misonidazole (Mamoli et al 1979), disulfiram (Bradley & Hewer 1966), vincristine (Bradley et al 1970, Casey et al 1973), phenytoin (Lovelace & Horowitz 1968, Eisen et al 1974, Chokroverty & Sayeed 1975), lithium (Brust et al 1979, Vanhooren et al 1990). The neuropathy associated with dapsone appears to be purely motor, with normal or slightly reduced motor conduction together with EMG changes of denervation and normal sensory action potentials (Gutmann et al 1976). Thalidomide has recently been found to be an effective treatment in several dermatological conditions including aphthous ulcers and nodular prurigo. Apart from its now well-known mutagenic effects, it induces a peripheral axonal sensorimotor neuropathy which appears to be dose-related (Fullerton & O'Sullivan 1968). Serial nerve conduction studies are used to monitor the peripheral nerves (Wulff et al 1985, Lagueny et al 1986), a reduction in amplitude of the sural nerve action potential being the most sensitive indicator of the onset of the neuropathy. Progression of the electrophysiological abnormalities has been reported in some cases despite withdrawal of the drug, suggesting a prolonged action of the drug (Lagueny et al 1986).

In contrast to the above drug-induced neuropathies, that produced by perhexiline maleate is associated with moderate to severe slowing of motor conduction and reduction or loss of sensory evoked potentials (Bousser et al 1976, Said 1978), indicative of demyelination.

Nearly all neuropathies associated with exogenous chemical toxins such as heavy metals, solvents, organophosphates, etc. are axonal in nature (Cohen 1970) and are accompanied by minor changes in motor and sensory conduction. Lead, however, induces a mainly motor neuropathy (Buchthal & Behse 1979), affecting particularly the radial nerves, producing bilateral wrist-drop. An important exception to this general finding is seen in the neuropathy induced by n-hexane which is a constituent of many adhesive agents. 'Gluesniffing' has become an all-too-common habit in many countries and accounts for an increasing number of young people presenting with neuropathy. Nerve biopsy studies have revealed striking focal axonal swellings and accumulation of neurofilaments, together with thinning of the overlying myelin and widening of the nodes of Ranvier (Korobkin et al 1975). Motor conduction has been found to be moderately slowed and the distribution of sensory conduction velocities is increased (Yokoyama et al 1990), consistent with the abnormal myelination.

Inflammatory demyelinating polyneuropathies

Acute inflammatory demyelinating polyneuropathy (Guillain–Barré syndrome). The pattern of nerve conduction changes may show considerable variation in patients presenting with this disorder, and the findings in any one patient may differ according to the time interval between the onset of the neuropathy and the neurophysiological examination (Albers et al 1985). Usually there is slowing of motor conduction to about 60–70% of normal in one or more nerves. Proximal and distal segments may be affected to roughly the same extent (Kimura & Butzer 1975, King & Ashby 1976) although in some patients slowing may be patchy (Isch et al 1964) or most pronounced in common sites of nerve compression such as the carpal or cubital tunnel (Lambert & Mulder 1964, Eisen & Humphreys 1974). Prolonged distal motor latencies in the presence of normal or only slightly reduced conduction velocities may be the only abnormality in a proportion of patients. Figure 30.8 shows the motor and sensory conduction findings in a patient with Guillain–Barré syndrome (GBS) of recent onset.

Although slowing may be present early in the illness, it may not be apparent until after the condition has reached its peak. A number of studies (Lambert & Mulder 1964, McQuillen 1971, Eisen & Humphreys 1974, Albers et al 1985) have shown normal motor conduction in distal segments in about 10–20% of cases. However, using the F-response conduction technique to examine velocity over the proximal segments, including the roots, Kimura & Butzer (1975) and King & Ashby (1976) showed significant slowing restricted to this segment in some patients. Ambler et al (1985) also found delayed or absent F-responses to be the most sensitive parameter for detecting abnormal conduction in the early stages of the disease.

Evidence of conduction block is frequently seen in the acquired inflammatory demyelinating neuropathies, and together with multifocal conduction slowing, helps to distinguish this group from the familial demyelinating neuropathies (Lewis & Sumner 1982). In the acute form Ambler et al (1985) observed a reduction in M-response amplitude following proximal stimulation in a large proportion of cases, which they attributed to conduction block and/or temporal dispersion. Mills & Murray (1985) employing the recently introduced technique of direct percutaneous spinal cord stimulation, reported conduction block in the most proximal nerve segments in two

cases of GBS. Severe distal motor abnormalities with marked reduction in CMAP amplitudes and relative sensory sparing have also been described (Miller et al 1987). Although the electrophysiological finding of reduced conduction velocity correlates well with the predominantly demyelinating nature of the defect (Arnason 1984), a significant proportion of patients may demonstrate fibrillations and positive sharp waves in the EMG indicating axonal damage.

Sensory nerve conduction changes tend to be less marked and more variable than the motor findings, being normal or only slightly altered in distal nerve segments in milder cases. The distribution of affected nerves is often unusual for a polyneuropathy with abnormal median and ulnar nerve responses but normal or relatively spared radial and sural nerve responses (see Albers et al 1985 and Fig. 30.8). Abnormalities of the cervical and cortical evoked sensory responses have been reported in the early phase of the disease, suggesting defective conduction in proximal segments despite normal peripheral sensory function. In severe cases however, distal sensory conduction may be slowed and the responses lost (Bannister & Sears 1962, Eisen & Humphreys 1974, Raman & Taori 1976).

The electrophysiological features may have predictive value, for those patients with no conduction abnormalities tend to recover rapidly within about 4 weeks (Eisen & Humphreys 1974), whereas those with slowing of conduction generally take longer. In a large multicentre study the mean distal CMAP amplitude was found to be the single best prognostic indicator (Cornblath et al 1988). Recovery in the presence of axonal degeneration is more protracted and often incomplete, pronounced residual deficits being more common (Eisen & Humphreys 1974, Raman & Taori 1976).

An acute axonal form of Guillain–Barré syndrome has been reported (Feasby et al 1986) in which patients presenting with the clinical picture of an acute polyneuropathy were found to have primary axonal degeneration rather than demyelination on electrophysiological testing and, in one case which came to autopsy, on histological grounds. The prognosis is poorer in this group of patients, presumably because of the severity of the axonal involvement.

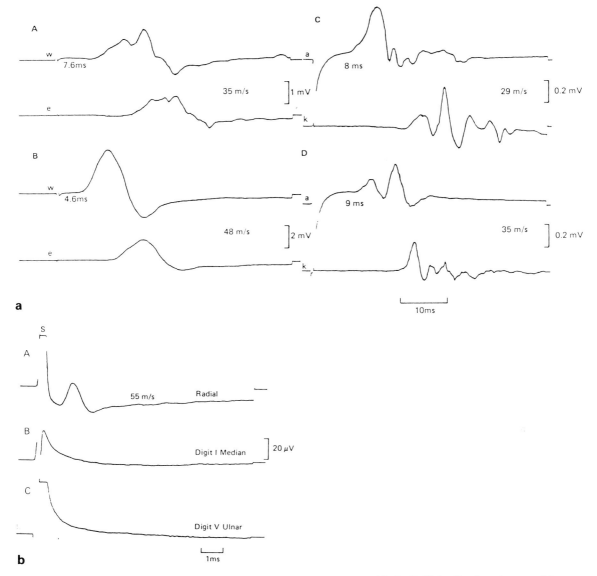

Fig. 30.8 Motor and sensory conduction findings in a 67-year-old woman with the Guillain–Barré syndrome. **a** Motor findings in median (A), ulnar (B), common peroneal (C) and posterior tibial (D) nerves (upper–distal stimulus, lower–proximal stimulus); note the small and dispersed M-responses, particularly following proximal stimulation. The large drop in amplitude of the proximal ulnar response suggests conduction block in addition to velocity dispersion. **b** Sensory recordings in radial (A), median (B) and ulnar nerves (C); the radial response is relatively well-preserved in contrast to absence of responses in the median and ulnar nerves.

Chronic inflammatory demyelinating polyneuropathy. In a smaller number of cases the inflammatory demyelinating polyneuropathy has a chronic and sometimes relapsing course. In some of these patients the clinical presentation may be with the pattern of a mononeuropathy multiplex due to the presence of multifocal persistent conduction block affecting different nerves (Lewis et al 1982) (Figs 30.9, 30.10). Cranial nerves as well as limb nerves may be affected (Kaji et al 1992) and the electrophysiological as well as clinical evidence demonstrates predominantly

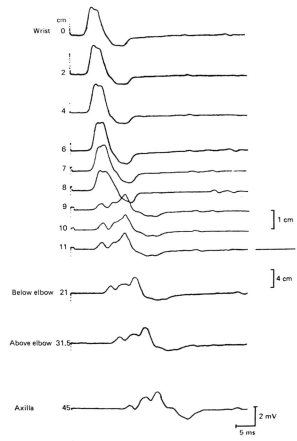

Fig. 30.9 Recordings of the M-response from the hypothenar muscles following stepwise stimulation of the ulnar nerve along its course in the forearm and arm in a patient with a multifocal demyelinating neuropathy. Note the abrupt change in shape and amplitude between 8 and 9 cm from the wrist, consistent with a focal demyelinating lesion and partial conduction block at this site. The patient had additional focal lesions in the ipsilateral radial and contralateral median and ulnar nerves.

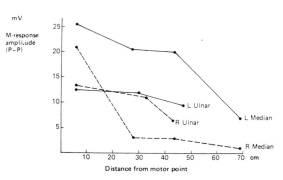

Fig. 30.10 Plots of M-response amplitude in the right and left median and ulnar nerves against distance from motor point in a patient with multifocal demyelinating neuropathy. Note the large drop in amplitude of the M-response in the forearm segment of the right median nerve and in the axilla to Erb's point segment of the left median nerve.

motor conduction abnormalities, with relative sparing of the sensory nerves. On clinical grounds, these cases may be mistaken for motor neurone disease (Parry & Clarke 1988, Kaji et al 1992) and thus it is essential to examine all such patients for evidence of motor conduction block.

Neuropathy associated with infectious agents

Leprosy. Peripheral nerve involvement is a characteristic feature of leprosy. Electrophysiological changes may be apparent in clinically normal nerves (McLeod et al 1975), or restricted to the enlarged segments (Swift et al 1973). Slowing of sensory conduction velocity has been found to occur in both tuberculoid and lepromatous leprosy, and velocity measurement in the superficial radial nerve has been proposed as a sensitive index of peripheral nerve involvement (Sebille 1978). Slowing of motor conduction velocities also occurs (Hackett et al 1968), and these conduction findings correlate with the principal pathological changes of segmental demyelination (Shetty et al 1977).

Lyme disease. The infectious agent is *Borrelia burgdorferi* and in common with a number of other diseases that may involve multiple systems, the clinical manifestations of Lyme disease are protean. Halperin et al (1990) have demonstrated that this agent can cause a variety of peripheral nerve disorders including radiculopathies, multifocal demyelinating and also axonal neuropathies. The condition is therefore of considerable clinical relevance as this is a treatable disorder (Halperin et al 1987).

Parasites. Parasitic infections usually cause peripheral nerve disorders by either direct involvement of peripheral nerve or as a secondary process. Primary involvement is, in general, not severe but *Trypanosoma* can cause a multifocal demyelinating neuropathy (Barreira et al 1981).

Diphtheria. The cause and effects of the neuropathy seen in diphtheria are well known and the toxin is very commonly used for experimental models of demyelinating neuropathies (McDonald 1973). Typically, the onset of the neuropathy is seen in the palate in the second or third week and then progressively involves more peripheral structures over the next 6–8 weeks. The neurophysiological findings are consistent with a demyelinating neuropathy with some degree of concomitant axonal loss if the degree of involvement is severe.

Hereditary motor and sensory neuropathies (HMSN)

Types I and II (Charcot–Marie–Tooth disease, peroneal muscular atrophy). Early studies of motor conduction velocity in this disorder revealed considerable slowing to about half the normal value or less (Gilliatt & Thomas 1957, Amick & Lemmi 1963, Dyck et al 1963). However, later reports on patients with a similar clinical picture showed some to have normal or only slightly reduced motor conduction velocities (Earl & Johnson 1963). This was confirmed by Dyck & Lambert (1968a,b), who separated two main groups on the basis of clinical, genetic, electrophysiological and histological findings — a hypertrophic group with slowed conduction, and a neuronal group with virtually normal conduction. Thomas & Calne (1974) also found that their patients displayed a bimodal distribution of the median motor conduction velocity with a cut-off point at about 40 m/s. By contrast others have observed a wide spectrum of motor conduction velocity (Salisachs 1974, Brust et al 1978) or have found evidence of an intermediate group (Bradley et al 1977b). However, Buchthal & Behse (1977) in a combined study of sensory conduction and biopsy findings in the sural nerve, supported the presence of two main groups, the hypertrophic and neuronal types, with no evidence of an intermediary type. More recently Harding & Thomas (1980b) in a large series of 228 patients, found clear evidence of two genetically distinct forms based on whether motor conduction in the median nerve was above or below 38 m/s. The hypertrophic and neuronal groups are now termed hereditary motor and sensory neuropathy (HMSN) types I and II respectively (Thomas et al

1974, Dyck 1975). In the majority of cases in both groups the pattern of inheritance is autosomal dominant, although sporadic cases occur and occasional families with an autosomal recessive pattern are seen (Harding & Thomas 1980b,c). Motor conduction in the recessive type I cases was shown to be significantly slower than in the dominantly inherited patients (Harding & Thomas 1980c). Sensory action potential amplitudes are abnormal in all cases, being absent or significantly reduced, even if the velocity in some of the type II patients is normal (Buchthal & Behse 1977, Harding & Thomas 1980b). This latter finding is of considerable importance for the differentiation of HMSN from distal spinal muscular atrophy, in which sensory conduction and the sensory action potentials are normal (Harding & Thomas 1980a). Figure 30.11 shows an example of a motor conduction study in a patient with type I HMSN.

Measurement of the conduction velocity may help to identify clinically normal carriers in a

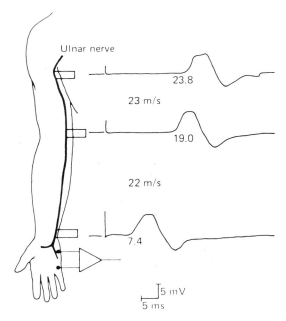

Fig. 30.11 Motor conduction study in the median nerve of a patient with HMSN type I. The distal latency is increased and there is marked slowing in distal and more proximal segments. Despite this, the M-response is relatively compact at each stimulus site, indicating that minimal temporal dispersion of individual nerve fibre conduction velocities has occurred, and that the surviving nerve fibres are affected to a similar degree by the demyelinating process.

family (Dyck et al 1963) and can also be of prognostic value as the neuropathy seems to progress more rapidly in the hypertrophic than the neuronal variety.

Type III (Dejerine–Sottas disease). Distal motor latencies are considerably prolonged and motor conduction is markedly slowed in this form of hypertrophic neuropathy with values ranging from 3 m/s to 22 m/s (Dyck & Lambert 1968a, Thomas & Lascelles 1967, Dyck et al 1971b), and usually below 10 m/s. The stimulus thresholds are greatly increased and there is evidence of temporal dispersion but no conduction block (Benstead et al 1990).

Type IV (Refsum's disease). Extreme slowing of motor conduction has also been reported in Refsum's disease, which after the patient had been on an appropriate diet to reduce the phytanic acid level, showed significant improvement, from a pretreatment value of 7 m/s to 19 m/s, one year later (Eldjarn et al 1966).

Type V (HMSN with spastic paraplegia). These patients generally have normal motor conduction velocities, but abnormal sensory conduction (Dyck & Lambert 1968a,b, Harding & Thomas 1984).

Friedreich's ataxia

Involvement of the peripheral nerves in this condition has been confirmed by the finding of slightly reduced motor conduction velocities and either very small or absent sensory action potentials (Preswick 1968, McLeod 1971, Oh & Halsey 1973, Dunn 1973, Salisachs et al 1975, Bouchard et al 1979, Caruso et al 1987). The conduction velocities show no significant change with age (Dunn 1973, Salisachs et al 1975, Peyronnard et al 1976), and large myelinated cutaneous fibres appear to be preferentially affected (Dyck 1984, Caruso et al 1987).

Hereditary pressure sensitive neuropathy

An increased sensitivity to compression and traction is associated with abnormally thickened myelin sheaths in the peripheral nerves of these patients. Slowing of motor and sensory conduction is found in the affected nerves (Behse et al 1973) and abnormal conduction may also be detected in clinically normal nerves and asymptomatic family members (Cruz Martinez et al 1977).

Hereditary sensory neuropathy

This condition presents clinically with loss of pain and temperature sensation, predominantly affecting the lower limbs, associated with perforating ulcers of the feet and deafness (Denny-Brown 1951). The dorsal root ganglia undergo degeneration (Denny-Brown 1951) and nerve conduction studies reveal absent sensory action potentials and slightly reduced motor conduction velocities (Dyck & Ohta 1975).

Acute intermittent porphyria

The neuropathy of this form of porphyria presents clinically as an acute or subacute and predominantly motor neuropathy, affecting proximal more than distal muscles. Motor conduction velocities are generally normal, but the evoked CMAP amplitudes are reduced and electromyography reveals spontaneous fibrillations and positive sharp waves in the weak proximal muscles (Albers et al 1978). The sensory action potentials and velocities are usually well preserved.

Metachromatic leukodystrophy (sulphatide lipidosis)

Peripheral nerve involvement is a well-described and generally early feature of the infantile and the less common adult forms of this disorder. The universal finding of quite markedly slowed conduction velocities reflects the presence of demyelination (Fullerton 1964, Yudell et al 1967, Pilz & Hopf 1972, Clark et al 1979), and the abnormal nerve conduction studies provide a useful screening test when the diagnosis is suspected (Cruz Martinez et al 1975), definite confirmation then being given by nerve biopsy and by assaying arylsulphatase A in leucocytes or fibroblasts.

Globoid leukodystrophy (Krabbe)

As in metachromatic leukodystrophy, slowing of conduction in peripheral nerves has also been demonstrated in this disorder (Hogan et al 1969).

REFERENCES

Adams R D, Shahani B T, Young R R 1973 A severe pansensory familial neuropathy. Transactions of the American Neurological Association 98: 67

Albers J W, Donofrio P D, McGonagle T K 1985 Sequential electrodiagnostic abnormalities in acute inflammatory demyelinating polyradiculopathy. Muscle and Nerve 8: 528

Albers J W, Robertson W C, Daube J R 1978 Electrodiagnostic findings in acute porphyric neuropathy. Muscle and Nerve 1: 292

Alderson M K, Petajan J H 1987 Relative refractory period: a measure to detect early neuropathy in alcoholics. Muscle and Nerve 10: 323

Ambler Z, Stålberg E, Fink R, Rydin E 1985 Electrodiagnosis in early stages of Guillain–Barré syndrome. Electroencephalography and Clinical Neurophysiology 61: S19

Amick L D, Lemmi H 1963 Electromyographic studies in peroneal muscular atrophy. Archives of Neurology 9: 273

Andersen K 1985 Surface recording of orthodromic sensory nerve action potentials in median and ulnar nerves in normal subjects. Muscle and Nerve 8: 402

Argyropoulos C J, Panayiotopoulos C P, Scarpalezos S 1978 F- and M-wave conduction velocity in amyotrophic lateral sclerosis. Muscle and Nerve 1: 479

Arnason B G W 1984 Acute inflammatory demyelinating polyradiculoneuropathies. In: Dyck P J, Thomas P K, Lambert E H, Bunge R (eds) Peripheral neuropathy, vol 2, 2nd edn. W B Saunders, Philadelphia, ch 90, p 2050

Baer R D, Johnson E W 1965 Motor nerve conduction velocities in normal children. Archives of Physical Medicine and Rehabilitation 46: 698

Bannister R G, Sears T A 1962 The changes in nerve conduction in acute idiopathic polyneuritis. Journal of Neurology, Neurosurgery and Psychiatry 25: 321

Barker A T 1981 Nerve conduction velocity distributions: an iterative method using two compound action potentials recorded from the same site. In: Dorfman L J, Cummins K L, Leifer L J (eds) Conduction velocity distributions: a population approach to electrophysiology of nerve. Alan R Liss, New York, ch 7, p 137

Barker A T, Brown B H, Freeston I L 1979 Determination of the distribution of conduction velocities in peripheral nerve trunks. IEEE Transactions of Biomedical Engineering 26: 76

Barker A T, Jalinous R, Freeston I L 1985a Non-invasive magnetic stimulation of the human motor cortex. Lancet i: 1106

Barker A T, Freeston I L, Jalinous R, Jarratt J A 1985b Noninvasive stimulation of motor pathways within the brain using time-varying magnetic fields. Electroencephalography and Clinical Neurophysiology 61: 245

Barreira A A, Said G, Krettli A V 1981 Multifocal demyelinative lesions of peripheral nerve in experimental Chagas' disease. Transactions of the Royal Society of Tropical Medicine and Hygiene 75: 751

Bartel P R, Lotz B P, van der Meyden C H 1984 Short-latency somatosensory evoked potentials in dystrophia myotonica. Journal of Neurology, Neurosurgery and Psychiatry 47: 524

Bastron J A, Thomas J E 1981 Diabetic polyradiculoneuropathy; clinical and electromyographic findings in 105 patients. Mayo Clinic Proceedings 56: 725

Behse F, Buchthal F 1971 Normal sensory conduction in the nerves of the leg in man. Journal of Neurology, Neurosurgery and Psychiatry 34: 404

Behse F, Buchthal F 1977 Alcoholic neuropathy: clinical, electrophysiological and biopsy findings. Annals of Neurology 2: 95

Behse F, Buchthal F, Carlsen F 1977 Nerve biopsy and conduction studies in diabetic neuropathy. Journal of Neurology, Neurosurgery and Psychiatry 40: 1072

Behse F, Buchthal F, Carlsen F, Knappers G G 1973 Conduction and histopathology of the sural nerve in hereditary neuropathy with a liability to pressure palsies. In: Desmedt J E (ed) New developments in electromyography and clinical neurophysiology. Karger, Basel, vol 2, p 286

Benstead T J, Kuntz N L, Miller R G, Daube J R 1990 The electrophysiologic profile of Dejerine–Sottas disease (HMSN III) Muscle and Nerve 13: 586

Berenberg R A, Pellock J M, DiMauro S et al 1977 Lumping or splitting? `Ophthalmoplegia-Plus' or Kearns–Sayre syndrome? Annals of Neurology 1: 37

Bertorini T, Engel W K, Di Chiro G, Dalakas M 1978 Leukoencephalopathy in oculocraniosomatic neuromuscular disease with ragged-red fibres. Archives of Neurology 35: 643

Bolton C F 1987 Electrophysiological studies of critically ill patients. Muscle and Nerve 10: 129

Bolton C F, Driedger A A, Lindsay R M 1979a Ischaemic neuropathy in uraemic patients caused by bovine arteriovenous shunt. Journal of Neurology, Neurosurgery and Psychiatry 42: 810

Bolton C F, Gilbert J J, Girvin J P, Hahn A F 1979b Nerve and muscle biopsy: electrophysiology and morphology in polyneuropathy. Neurology 29: 354

Bolton C F, Gilbert J J, Hahn A F, Sibbald W 1984 Polyneuropathy in critically ill patients. Journal of Neurology, Neurosurgery and Psychiatry 47: 1223

Bolton C F, Sawa G M, Carter K 1981 The effects of temperature on human compound action potentials. Journal of Neurology, Neurosurgery and Psychiatry 44: 407

Borg J 1984 Refractory period of single motor nerve fibres in man. Journal of Neurology, Neurosurgery and Psychiatry 47: 344

Bostock H, Sears T A 1978 The internodal axon membrane: electrical excitability and continuous conduction in segmental demyelination. Journal of Physiology 280: 273

Bouchard J P, Barbeau R, Bouchard R, Bouchard R W 1979 Electromyography and nerve conduction studies in Friedreich's ataxia and autosomal recessive spastic ataxia of Charlevoix–Saguenay (ARSACS). Canadian Journal of Neurological Sciences 6: 185

Bousser M G, Bouche P, Brochard C, Herreman G 1976 Neuropathies périphériques au maleate de perhexiline. A propos de 7 observations. Coeur Médicale Internal 15: 181

Braddom R I, Johnson E W 1974 Standardization of H-reflex and diagnostic use in S-1 radiculopathy. Archives of Physical Medicine and Rehabilitation 55: 161

Bradley W G, Hewer R L 1966 Peripheral neuropathy due to disulfiram. British Medical Journal 2: 449

Bradley W G, Karlsson I J, Rasool C G 1977a Metronidazole neuropathy. British Medical Journal 2: 610

Bradley W G, Lassman L P, Pearce G W, Walton J N 1970 The neuropathy of vincristine in man. Clinical, electrophysiological and pathological studies. Journal of the Neurological Sciences 10: 107

Bradley W G, Madrid R, Davis C J F 1977b The peroneal muscular atrophy syndrome. Clinical, genetic, electrophysiological and nerve biopsy studies. Part 3. Clinical, electrophysiological and pathological correlations. Journal of the Neurological Sciences 32: 123

Brooke M H, Engel W K 1969 The histographic analysis of human muscle biopsies with regard to fibre types. Neurology (Minneapolis) 19: 221

Brown W F, Jaatoul N 1974 Amyotrophic lateral sclerosis: electrophysiologic study (number of motor units and rate of decay of motor units). Archives of Neurology 30: 242

Brust J C M, Lovelace R E, Devi S 1978 Clinical and electrophysiological features of CMT syndrome. Acta Neurologica Scandinavica 58 (suppl) 68: 1

Brust J C M, Hammer J S, Challenor Y, Healton E B, Lesser R P 1979 Acute generalised polyneuropathy accompanying lithium poisoning. Annals of Neurology 6: 360

Buchthal F, Behse F 1977 Peroneal muscular atrophy (PMA) and related disorders. 1. Clinical manifestations as related to biopsy findings, nerve conduction and electromyography. Brain 100: 41

Buchthal F, Behse F 1979 Electrophysiology and nerve biopsy in men exposed to lead. British Journal of Industrial Medicine 36: 135

Buchthal F, Olsen P Z 1970 Electromyography and muscle biopsy in infantile spinal muscular atrophy. Brain 93: 15

Buchthal F, Rosenfalck A 1966 Evoked action potential and conduction velocity in human sensory nerves. Brain Research 3: 1

Buchthal F, Rosenfalck A, Trojaborg W 1974 Electrophysiological findings in entrapment of the median nerve at the wrist and elbow. Journal of Neurology, Neurosurgery and Psychiatry 37: 340

Burke D, Skuse N F, Lethlean A K 1974 Sensory conduction of the sural nerve in polyneuropathy. Journal of Neurology, Neurosurgery and Psychiatry 37: 647

Campbell M J, Paty D W 1974 Carcinomatous neuromyopathy: 1. Electrophysiological studies. An electrophysiological and immunological study of patients with carcinoma of the lung. Journal of Neurology, Neurosurgery and Psychiatry 37: 131

Campbell W W, Ward L C, Swift T R 1981 Nerve conduction velocity varies inversely with height. Muscle and Nerve 4: 520

Carpendale M T F 1956 Conduction time in the terminal portion of the motor fibres of the ulnar, median and peroneal nerves in healthy subjects and in patients with neuropathy. MS (Physical Medicine) Thesis, University of Minnesota

Caruso G, Santoro L, Perretti A et al 1987 Friedreich's ataxia: electrophysiologic and histologic findings in patients and relatives. Muscle and Nerve 10: 503

Casey E B, Jelliffe A M, Le Quesne P M, Millett Y L 1973 Vincristine neuropathy: clinical and electrophysiological observations. Brain 96: 69

Casey E B, Le Quesne P M 1972a Digital nerve action potentials in healthy subjects, and in carpal tunnel and diabetic patients. Journal of Neurology, Neurosurgery and Psychiatry 35: 612

Casey E B, Le Quesne P M 1972b Electrophysiological evidence for a distal lesion in alcoholic neuropathy. Journal of Neurology, Neurosurgery and Psychiatry 35: 624

Cavanagh J B 1964 The significance of the 'dying-back' process in experimental and human neurological disease. International Review of Experimental Pathology 3: 219

Chaco J 1970 Conduction velocity of motor nerve fibres in progressive spinal atrophy. Acta Neurologica Scandinavica 46: 119

Chokroverty S 1990 (ed) Magnetic stimulation in clinical neurophysiology. Butterworths, Boston

Chokroverty S, Sayeed Z A 1975 Motor conduction study in patients on diphenylhydantoin therapy. Journal of Neurology, Neurosurgery and Psychiatry 38: 1235

Chopra J S, Hurwitz L J, Montgomery D A D 1969 The pathogenesis of sural nerve changes in diabetes mellitus. Brain 92: 391

Clark J R, Miller R G, Vidgoff J M 1979 Juvenile-onset metachromatic leukodystrophy: biochemical and electrophysiological studies. Neurology 29: 346

Cohen M M 1970 Toxic neuropathy. In: Vinken P J, Bruyn G W (eds) Handbook of clinical neurology, vol 7. North Holland, Amsterdam, ch 20, p 510

Cornblath D R, McArthur J C 1988 Predominantly sensory neuropathy in patients with AIDS and AIDS-related complex. Neurology 38: 794

Cornblath D R, Kuncl R W, Mellits E D et al 1992 Nerve conduction studies in amyotrophic lateral sclerosis. Muscle and Nerve 15: 1111

Cornblath D R, Mellits E D, Griffin J W, McKhann G M, Albers J W, Miller R G, Feasby T E, Quaskey S A and The Guillain–Barré Syndrome Study Group 1988 Motor conduction studies in Guillain–Barré syndrome: description and prognostic value. Annals of Neurology 23: 354

Cruz Martinez A, Ferrer M T, Fueyo E, Galdos L 1975 Peripheral neuropathy detected on electrophysiological study as first manifestation of metachromatic leukodystrophy in infancy. Journal of Neurology, Neurosurgery and Psychiatry 38: 169

Cruz Martinez A, Perez Conde M C, Ramon y Cajal S, Martinez J 1977 Recurrent familial polyneuropathy with a liability to pressure palsies. Special regards to electrophysiological aspects of twenty-five members from seven families. Electromyography and Clinical Neurophysiology 17: 101

Cummins K L, Perkel D H, Dorfman L J 1979a Nerve fibre conduction-velocity distributions. I. Estimation based on the single-fibre and compound action potentials. Electroencephalography and Clinical Neurophysiology 46: 634

Cummins K L, Dorfman L J, Perkel D H 1979b Nerve fibre conduction-velocity distributions. II. Estimation based on two compound action potentials. Electroencephalography and Clinical Neurophysiology 46: 647

Cummins K L, Dorfman L J, Perkel D H 1981 Nerve conduction velocity distributions: a method for estimation based upon two compound action potentials. In: Dorfman L J, Cummins K L, Leifer L J (eds) Conduction velocity distributions: a population approach to electrophysiology of nerve. Alan R Liss, New York, ch 8, p 181

Dalkas M C, Engel W K 1981 Polyneuropathy with monoclonal gammapathy: studies of 11 patients. Annals of Neurology 10: 45

Dawson G D 1956 The relative excitability and conduction velocity of sensory and motor nerve fibres in man. Journal of Physiology 131: 436

Dawson G D, Merton P A 1956 'Recurrent' discharges from motor neurones. Abstract: 20th International Congress of Physiology, Bruxelles, p 221

Dawson G D, Scott J W 1949 The recording of nerve action potentials through the skin in man. Journal of Neurology, Neurosurgery and Psychiatry 12: 259

Dayan A D, Graveson G S, Illis L S, Robinson P K 1969 Schwann cell damage in motoneuron disease. Neurology (Minneapolis) 19: 639

de la Monte S M, Gabuzda D H, Ho D D et al 1988 Peripheral neuropathy in the acquired immunodeficiency syndrome. Annals of Neurology 23: 485

Denny-Brown D 1948 Primary sensory neuropathy with muscular changes associated with carcinoma. Journal of Neurology, Neurosurgery and Psychiatry 11: 73

Denny-Brown 1951 Hereditary sensory radicular neuropathy. Journal of Neurology, Neurosurgery and Psychiatry 14: 237

de Noordhout A M, Rothwell J C, Thompson P D, Day B L, Marsden C D 1988 Percutaneous electrical stimulation of lumbosacral roots in man. Journal of Neurology, Neurosurgery and Psychiatry 51: 174

Denys E H 1977 The effect of temperature on the compound action potential in neuromuscular disease and normal controls. Electroencephalography and Clinical Neurophysiology 43: 598

Di Benedetto M 1970 Sensory nerve conduction in the lower extremities. Archives of Physical Medicine 51: 253

Dick J D, Harris J B, Falkous G, Foster J B, Xuereb J H 1988 Neuronal anti-nuclear antibody in paraneoplastic sensory neuropathy. Journal of the Neurological Sciences 85: 1

Dioszeghy P 1986 Needle and surface recording electrodes in motor and sensory conduction studies. Electromyography and Clinical Neurophysiology 26: 117

Dorfman L J, Cummings K L 1980 Nerve-fibre conduction velocity distributions in normal and diabetic human nerves. Neurology 30: 415

Downie A W, Newell D J 1961 Sensory nerve conduction in patients with diabetes mellitus and controls. Neurology (Minneapolis) 14: 839

Downie A W, Scott T R 1967 An improved technique for radial nerve conduction studies. Journal of Neurology, Neurosurgery and Psychiatry 30: 332

Drachman D A 1968 Ophthalmoplegia plus. The neurodegenerative disorders associated with progressive external ophthalmoplegia. Archives of Neurology 18: 654

Dunn H G 1973 Nerve conduction studies in children with Friedreich's ataxia and ataxia-telangiectasia. Developmental Medicine and Child Neurology 15: 324

Dyck P J 1975 Inherited neuronal degeneration and atrophy affecting peripheral motor, sensory and autonomic neurones. In: Dyck P J, Thomas P K, Lambert E H (eds) Peripheral neuropathy, vol 2, W B Saunders, Philadelphia, ch 41, p 825

Dyck P J 1984 Neuronal atrophy and degeneration predominantly affecting peripheral sensory and autonomic neurons. In: Dyck P J, Thomas P K, Lambert E H, Bunge R (eds) Peripheral neuropathy, vol 2, 2nd edn. W B Saunders, ch 68, p 1557

Dyck P J, Karnes J L, Daube J, O'Brien P, Service F J 1985 Clinical and neuropathological criteria for the diagnosis and staging of diabetic polyneuropathy. Brain 108: 861

Dyck P J, Lambert E H 1968a Lower motor and primary sensory neuron diseases with peroneal muscular atrophy. 1. Neurologic, genetic, and electrophysiologic findings in hereditary polyneuropathies. Archives of Neurology 18: 603

Dyck P J, Lambert E H 1968b Lower motor and primary sensory neurone disease with peroneal muscular atrophy. 2. Neurologic, genetic, and electrophysiological findings in various neuronal degenerations. Archives of Neurology 18: 619

Dyck P J, Lambert E H, Mulder D W 1963 Charcot–Marie–Tooth disease: nerve conduction and clinical studies in a large kinship. Neurology (Minneapolis) 13: 1

Dyck P J, Johnson W J, Lambert E H, O'Brien P C 1971a Uraemic polyneuropathy–segmental demyelination secondary to axonal degeneration. Mayo Clinic Proceedings 46: 400

Dyck P J, Lambert E H, Sanders K, O'Brien P C 1971b Severe hypomyelination and marked abnormality of conduction in Dejerine–Sottas hypertrophic neuropathy: myelin thickness and compound action potential of sural nerve in vitro. Mayo Clinic Proceedings 46: 432

Dyck P J, Stevens J C, Mulder D W, Espinosa R E 1975 Frequency of nerve fibre degeneration of peripheral and motor sensory neurons in amyotrophic lateral sclerosis. Neurology (Minneapolis) 25: 781

Dyck P J, Ohta M 1975 Neuronal atrophy and degeneration predominantly affecting peripheral sensory neurons. In: Dyck P J, Thomas P K, Lambert E H (eds) Peripheral neuropathy, vol 2. W B Saunders, Philadelphia, p 791

Earl W C, Johnson E W 1963 Motor nerve conduction velocity in CMT disease. Archives of Physical Medicine 44: 247

Eisen A, Humphreys P 1974 The Guillain–Barré syndrome. A clinical and electrodiagnostic study. Archives of Neurology 30: 438

Eisen A, Schomer D, Melmed C 1977a The application of 'F' wave measurements in the differentiation of proximal and distal upper limb entrapments. Neurology (Minneapolis) 27: 662

Eisen A, Schomer D, Melmed C 1977b An electrophysiological method for examining lumbar root compression. Canadian Journal of Neurological Sciences 4: 117

Eisen A, Woods J F, Sherwin A L 1974 Peripheral nerve function in long term therapy with diphenyl hydantoin. Neurology (Minneapolis) 24: 411

Eldjarn L, Try K, Stokke O et al 1966 Dietary effects on serum-phytanic-acid levels and on clinical manifestations in hederopathia atactica polyneuritiformis. Lancet i: 691

Engel A G, Lambert E H, Gomez M R 1977 A new myasthenic syndrome with end-plate acetylcholinesterase deficiency, small nerve terminals and reduced acetylcholine release. Annals of Neurology 1: 315

Engel A G, Lambert E H, Mulder D M et al 1982 A newly recognised congenital myasthenic syndrome attributed to a prolonged open time of the acetylcholine-induced ion channel. Annals of Neurology 11: 553

Ertekin C 1967 Sensory and motor conduction in motor neurone disease. Acta Neurologica Scandinavica 43: 499

Farmer T W, Buchthal F, Rosenfalck P 1960 Refractory period of human muscle after the passage of a propagated action potential. Electroencephalography and Clinical Neurophysiology 12: 455

Fawcett P R W, Mastaglia F L, Mechler F 1982 Electrophysiological findings including single fibre EMG in a family with mitochondrial myopathy. Journal of the Neurological Sciences 53: 397

Feasby T E, Brown W F, Gilbert J J, Hahn A F 1985 The pathological basis of conduction block in human neuropathies. Journal of Neurology, Neurosurgery and Psychiatry 48: 239

Feasby T E, Gilbert J J, Brown W F et al 1986 An acute axonal form of Guillain–Barré polyneuropathy. Brain 109: 1115

Ferguson I T 1978 Electrical study of jaw and orbicularis oculi reflexes after trigeminal nerve surgery. Journal of Neurology, Neurosurgery and Psychiatry 41: 819

Fincham R W, Cape C A 1968 Sensory nerve conduction in syringomyelia. Neurology (Minneapolis) 18: 200

Fincham R W, Van Allen M W 1964 Sensory nerve conduction in amyotrophic lateral sclerosis. Neurology (Minneapolis) 14: 31

Fisher M A 1982 F response latency determination. Muscle and Nerve 5: 730

Fisher M A 1985 F waves. Muscle and Nerve 8: 71

Fisher M A, Shivde A J, Teixera C, Grainer L S 1978 Clinical and electrophysiological appraisal of the significance of radicular injury in back pain. Journal of Neurology, Neurosurgery and Psychiatry 41: 301

Fraser J L, Olney R K 1992 The relative diagnostic sensitivity of different F-wave parameters in various polyneuropathies. Muscle and Nerve 15: 912

Fullerton P M 1964 Peripheral nerve conduction in metachromatic leukodystrophy (sulphatide lipidosis). Journal of Neurology, Neurosurgery and Psychiatry 27: 100

Fullerton P M, Barnes J M 1966 Peripheral neuropathy in rats produced by acrylamide. British Journal of Industrial Medicine 23: 210

Fullerton P M, O'Sullivan D J 1968 Thalidomide neuropathy: a clinical, electrophysiological, and histological follow-up study. Journal of Neurology, Neurosurgery and Psychiatry 31: 543

Gamstorp I 1963 Normal conduction velocity of ulnar, median and peroneal nerves in infancy, childhood and adolescence. Acta Paediatrica Scandinavica Supplement 146: 68

Gamstorp I, Shelburne S A 1965 Peripheral sensory conduction in ulnar and median nerves of normal infants. Acta Paediatrica Scandinavica 54: 309

Gardner-Medwin D, Hudgson P, Walton J N 1967 Benign spinal muscular atrophy arising in childhood and adolescence. Journal of the Neurological Sciences 5: 121

Gassel M M 1964a A test of nerve conduction to muscles of the shoulder girdle as an aid in the diagnosis of proximal neurogenic and muscular disease. Journal of Neurology, Neurosurgery and Psychiatry 27: 300

Gassel M M 1964b Sources of error in motor nerve conduction studies. Neurology (Minneapolis) 14: 825

Gassel M M, Diamantopoulos E 1964 Pattern of conduction times in the distribution of the radial nerve. Neurology (Minneapolis) 14: 222

Gassel M M, Trojaborg W 1964 Clinical and electrophysiological study of the pattern of conduction times in the sciatic nerve. Journal of Neurology, Neurosurgery and Psychiatry 27: 351

Gilliatt R W 1966 Applied electrophysiology in nerve and muscle disease. Proceedings of the Royal Society of Medicine 59: 989

Gilliatt R W, Hjorth R J 1972 Nerve conduction during Wallerian degeneration in the baboon. Journal of Neurology, Neurosurgery and Psychiatry 35: 335

Gilliatt R W, Taylor J C 1959 Electrical changes following section of the facial nerve. Proceedings of the Royal Society of Medicine 52: 1080

Gilliatt R W, Thomas P K 1957 Extreme slowing of nerve conduction in peroneal muscular atrophy. Annals of Physical Medicine 4: 104

Gilliatt R W, Thomas P K 1960 Changes in nerve conduction with ulnar nerve lesions at the elbow. Journal of Neurology, Neurosurgery and Psychiatry 23: 312

Gilliatt R W, Willison R G 1962 Peripheral nerve conduction in diabetic neuropathy. Journal of Neurology, Neurosurgery and Psychiatry 25: 11

Gilliatt R W, Willison R G 1963 The refractory and supernormal periods of the human median nerve. Journal of Neurology, Neurosurgery and Psychiatry 26: 136

Gilliatt R W, Hopf H C, Rudge P, Baraitser M 1976 Axonal velocities of motor units in the hand and foot muscles of the baboon. Journal of the Neurological Sciences 29: 249

Gilliatt R W, Melville I D, Velate A S, Willison R G 1965 A study of normal nerve action potentials using an averaging technique (barrier grid storage tube). Journal of Neurology, Neurosurgery and Psychiatry 28: 191

Ginzburg M, Lee M, Ginzburg J, Alba A 1978 Median and ulnar nerve conduction determinations in the Erb's point-axilla segment in normal subjects. Journal of Neurology, Neurosurgery and Psychiatry 41: 444

Goodgold J, Eberstein A 1983 Electrodiagnosis of neuromuscular diseases, 3rd edn. Williams and Wilkins, Baltimore

Guiloff R J, Sherratt R M 1977 Sensory conduction in the medial plantar nerve. Journal of Neurology, Neurosurgery and Psychiatry 40: 1168

Guld C E 1960 Use of screened power transformers and output transformers to reduce stimulus artefacts. In: Medical electronics. Thomas, Springfield, IL

Guld C E, Rosenfalck A, Willison R G, 1983 Report of the committee on EMG instrumentation. In: Recommendations for the practice of clinical neurophysiology. Elsevier, Amsterdam, p 83

Gutmann L 1977 Median-ulnar nerve communications and carpal tunnel syndrome. Journal of Neurology, Neurosurgery and Psychiatry 40: 982

Gutmann L, Martin J D, Welton W 1976 Dapsone motor neuropathy — an axonal disease. Neurology 26: 514

Hackett E R, Shipley D, Livengood R 1968 Motor nerve conduction velocity studies of ulnar nerve in patients with leprosy. International Journal of Leprosy 36: 282

Hallett M, Cohen L G, Nilsson J, Panizza M 1990 In: Chokroverty (ed) Magnetic stimulation in clinical neurophysiology. Butterworths, Boston, p 275

Halperin J, Coyle P K, Little B W, Dattwyler R J 1987 Lyme disease. Cause of a treatable peripheral neuropathy. Neurology 37: 1700

Halperin J, Luft B J, Volkmann D J, Dattwyler R J 1990 Lyme neuroborreliosis. Peripheral nervous system manifestations. Brain 113: 1207

Hamilton D V, Evans D B, Henderson R G 1980 Ulnar nerve lesion as complication of Cimino–Brescia arteriovenous fistula. Lancet ii: 1137

Hansen S, Ballantyne J P 1977 Axonal dysfunction in the neuropathy of diabetes mellitus: quantitative electrophysiological study. Journal of Neurology, Neurosurgery and Psychiatry 40: 555

Hansen S, Ballantyne J P 1978 A quantitative electrophysiological study of MND. Journal of Neurology, Neurosurgery and Psychiatry 41: 773

Hanyu N, Oguchi K, Yanagisawa N, Tsukagoshi H 1982 Degeneration and regeneration of ventral root motor fibres in amyotrophic lateral sclerosis. Journal of the Neurological Sciences 55: 99

Harding A E, Le Fanu J 1977 Carpal tunnel syndrome related to antebrachial Cimino-Brescia fistula. Journal of Neurology, Neurosurgery and Psychiatry 40: 511

Harding A E, Thomas P K 1980a Distal spinal muscular atrophy: a report of 34 cases and review of the literature. Journal of the Neurological Sciences 45: 337

Harding A E, Thomas P K 1980b The clinical features of hereditary motor and sensory neuropathy types I and II. Brain 103: 259

Harding A E, Thomas P K 1980c Autosomal recessive forms of hereditary motor and sensory neuropathy. Journal of Neurology, Neurosurgery and Psychiatry 43: 669

Harding A E, Thomas P K 1984 Peroneal muscular atrophy with pyramidal features. Journal of Neurology, Neurosurgery and Psychiatry 47: 168

Hausmanowa-Petrusewicz I, Fidzianska A, Dobosz I, Drac H, Ryniewicz B 1975 The foetal character of the lesion in the acute form of Werdnig–Hoffmann disease. In: Bradley W G, Gardner-Medwin D, Walton J (eds) Recent advances in myology. Excerpta Medica, Amsterdam, p 546

Hausmanowa-Petrusewicz I, Kopec J 1973 Motor nerve conduction velocity in anterior horn lesions. In: Desmedt J E (ed) New developments in electromyography and clinical neurophysiology, vol 2. Karger, Basel p 298

Henriksen J D 1956 Conduction velocities of motor nerves in normal subjects and patients with neuromuscular disorders. MS (Physical Medicine) Thesis, University of Minnesota.

Hilton-Brown P, Stålberg E 1983 The motor unit in muscular dystrophy, single fibre EMG and scanning EMG study. Journal of Neurology, Neurosurgery and Psychiatry 46: 981

Hodes R, Larrabee M G, German W 1948 The human electromyogram in response to nerve stimulation and the conduction velocity of motor axons. Archives of Neurology and Psychiatry 60: 340

Hoffman P 1918 Über die Beziehungen der Sehnenreflex sur willkürlichen Bewegung und zum Tonus. Zeitschrift fur Biologie 68: 351

Hogan G R, Gutmann L, Chou S M 1969 The peripheral neuropathy of Krabbe's (globoid) leukodystrophy. Neurology (Minneapolis) 19: 1094

Hopf H C 1963 Electromyographic study on so-called mononeuritis. Archives of Neurology and Psychiatry 9: 307

Hopkins A P, Gilliatt R W 1971 Motor and sensory nerve conduction in the baboon: normal values and changes during acrylamide neuropathy. Journal of Neurology, Neurosurgery and Psychiatry 34: 415

Horowitz S H, Krarup C 1992 Conduction studies of the normal sural nerve. Muscle and Nerve 15: 374

Horwich M S, Cho L, Porro R S, Posner J B 1977 Subacute sensory neuropathy: a remote effect of carcinoma. Annals of Neurology 2: 7

Hursch J B 1939 Conduction velocity and diameter of nerve fibres. American Journal of Physiology 127: 131

Ince P G, Shaw P J, Fawcett P R W, Bates D 1987 Demyelinating neuropathy due to a primary IgM kappa B cell lymphoma of peripheral nerve. Neurology 37: 1231

Ingram D A, Davis G R, Swash M 1987a The double collision technique: a new method for measurement of the motor nerve refractory period distribution in man. Electroencephalography and Clinical Neurophysiology 66: 225

Ingram D A, Davis G R, Swash M 1987b Motor nerve conduction velocity distributions in man: results of a new computer-based collision technique. Electroencephalography and Clinical Neurophysiology 66: 235

Ingram D A, Davis G R, Schwartz M S, Swash M 1985 Motor nerve refractory period and conduction velocity distributions in motor neurone disease. Electroencephalography and Clinical Neurophysiology 61: S30

Isch F, Isch-Treussard C, Buchheit F, Delgado V, Kircher J P 1964 Measurement of conduction velocity of motor nerve fibres in polyneuritis and polyradiculitis. (Abstract) Electroencephalography and Clinical Neurophysiology, 16: 416

Iyer V, Fenichel G M 1976 Normal median nerve proximal latency in carpal tunnel syndrome: a. due to co-existing Martin–Gruber anastomosis. Journal of Neurology, Neurosurgery and Psychiatry 39: 449

Jebsen R H 1967 Motor conduction velocities in the median and ulnar nerves. Archives of Physical Medicine and Rehabilitation 48: 185

Jennekens F G I, Dorhout Mees E J, van der Most van Spiijk D 1971 Clinical aspects of uraemic polyneuropathy. Nephron 8: 414

Johnson E W, Olsen K J 1960 Clinical value of motor nerve conduction velocity determination. Journal of the American Medical Association 172: 2030

Kaeser H E 1975 Nerve conduction velocity measurements. In: Vinken P, Bruyn G W (eds) Handbook of Clinical Neurology, vol 7. North-Holland, Amsterdam, ch 5, p 116

Kaji R, Shibasaki H, Kimura J 1992 Multifocal demyelinating motor neuropathy: cranial nerve involvement and immunoglobulin therapy. Neurology 42: 506

Kelly J J 1990 The electrophysiological findings in polyneuropathies associated with IgM monoclonal gammopathies. Muscle and Nerve 13: 1113

Kelly J J, Kyle R A, Miles J M, O'Brien P C, Dyck P J 1981 The spectrum of peripheral neuropathy in myeloma. Neurology (New York) 31: 24

Kelly J J, Kyle R A, O'Brien P C, Dyck P J 1979 The natural history of peripheral neuropathy in primary systemic amyloidosis. Annals of Neurology 6: 1

Kilma R R, Weigand A H, DeLisa J A 1991 Nerve conduction studies and vibration perception thresholds in diabetic and uremic neuropathy. American Journal of Physical Medicine and Rehabilitation 70: 86

Kimura J 1970 Alteration of the orbicularis oculi reflex by pontine lesions: study in multiple sclerosis. Archives of Neurology (Chicago) 22: 156

Kimura J 1974 'F' wave velocity in the central segment of the median and ulnar nerve. A study in normal subjects and in patients with Charcot–Marie–Tooth disease. Neurology (Minneapolis) 24: 539

Kimura J 1975 Electrically elicited blink reflex in diagnosis of multiple sclerosis: review of 260 patients over a seven-year period. Brain 98: 413

Kimura J 1982 Conduction abnormalities of the facial and trigeminal nerves in polyneuropathy. Muscle and Nerve S139

Kimura J 1984 Principles and pitfalls of nerve conduction studies. Annals of Neurology 16: 415

Kimura J 1989 Electrodiagnosis in diseases of nerve and muscle: principles and practice. F A Davis, Philadelphia

Kimura J, Butzer J F 1975 'F' wave conduction velocity in Guillain–Barré syndrome. Assessment of nerve segment between axilla and spinal cord. Archives of Neurology 32: 524

Kimura J, Lyon L W 1972 Orbicularis oculi reflex in the Wallenberg syndrome: alteration of the late reflex by lesions of the spinal tract and nucleus of the trigeminal nerve. Journal of Neurology, Neurosurgery and Psychiatry 35: 228

Kimura J, Giron L T, Young S M 1976 An electrophysiological study of Bell's palsy. Archives of Otolaryngology 100: 140

Kimura J, Yamada T, Rodnitzky R L 1978 Refractory period of human motor nerve fibres. Journal of Neurology, Neurosurgery and Psychiatry 41: 784

Kimura J, Yamada T, Stevland N P 1979 Distal slowing of motor nerve conduction velocity in diabetic polyneuropathy. Journal of the Neurological Sciences 42: 291

Kimura J, Yanagisawa H, Yamada T, Mitsudome A, Sasaki H, Kimura A 1984 Is the F wave elicited in a select group of motoneurons? Muscle and Nerve 7: 392

King D, Ashby P 1976 Conduction velocity in the proximal segments of a motor nerve in the Guillain–Barré syndrome. Journal of Neurology, Neurosurgery and Psychiatry 39: 538

Klingon G H 1965 The Guillain–Barré syndrome associated with cancer. Cancer 18: 157

Knezevic W, Mastaglia F L 1984 Neuropathy associated with Brescia–Cimino arteriovenous fistulas. Archives of Neurology 41: 1184

Konatey-Ahulu F I D, Baillod R, Compty C M, Heron J R, Shaldon S, Thomas P K 1965 Effect of periodic dialysis on the peripheral neuropathy of end-stage renal failure. British Medical Journal 2: 1212

Kopec J, Delbeke J, McComas A J 1978 Refractory period studies in a human neuromuscular preparation. Journal of Neurology, Neurosurgery and Psychiatry 41: 54

Korobkin R, Asbury A K, Sumner A J, Neilsen S L 1975 Glue-sniffing neuropathy. Archives of Neurology 32: 158

Lachman T, Shahani B T, Young R R 1980 Late responses and aids to diagnosis in peripheral neuropathy. Journal of Neurology, Neurosurgery and Psychiatry 43: 156

Lagueny A, Rommel A, Vignolly B et al 1986 Thalidomide neuropathy: an electrophysiological study. Muscle and Nerve 9: 837

Lambert E H 1962 Diagnostic value of electrical stimulation of motor nerves. Electroencephalography and Clinical Neurophysiology (Supplement) 22: 9

Lambert E H, Dyck P J 1975 Compound action potentials of sural nerve in vitro in peripheral neuropathy. In: Dyck P J, Thomas P K, Lambert E H (eds) Peripheral neuropathy, vol 1. W B Saunders, Philadelphia, ch 20, p 241

Lambert E H, Mulder D W 1957 Electromyographic studies in amyotrophic lateral sclerosis. Proceedings of the Staff Meetings of the Mayo Clinic 32: 441

Lambert E H, Mulder D W 1964 Nerve conduction in the Guillain–Barré syndrome. Electroencephalography and Clinical Neurophysiology 17: 86

Lamontagne A, Buchthal F 1970 Electrophysiological studies in diabetic neuropathy. Journal of Neurology, Neurosurgery and Psychiatry 33: 442

Lang A H, Puusa A, Hynninen P, Kuusela V, Jantti V, Sillanpaa M 1985 Evolution of nerve conduction velocity in later childhood and adolescence. Muscle and Nerve 8: 38

Lawrence D G, Locke S 1961 Motor nerve conduction velocity in diabetes. Archives of Neurology 5: 483

Lefebvre-d'Amour M, Shahani B T, Young R R, Bird K T 1979 Importance of studying sural conduction and late responses in the evaluation of alcoholic subjects. Neurology (Minneapolis) 29: 1600

Lehmann H J, Lehmann G, Tackmann W 1971 Refraktarperiode und Ubermittlung von Serienimpulsen im N. tibialis des Meeerschweinchens bei experimenteller allergischer Neuritis. Z. Neurol. 199: 67

Lenman J A R, Fleming A M, Robertson M A H et al 1981 Peripheral nerve function in patients with bronchial carcinoma. Comparison with matched controls and effects of treatment. Journal of Neurology, Neurosurgery, and Psychiatry 44: 54

Le Quesne P M, Fowler C J, Parkhouse N 1990 Journal of Neurology, Neurosurgery and Psychiatry 53: 558

Lewis R A, Sumner A J 1982 The electrodiagnostic distinctions between chronic familial and acquired demyelinative neuropathies. Neurology (New York) 32: 592

Lewis R A, Sumner A J, Brown M J, Asbury A K 1982 Multifocal demyelinating neuropathy with persistent conduction block. Neurology (New York) 32: 958

London G W 1975 Normal ulnar nerve conduction velocity across the thoracic outlet: comparison of two measuring techniques. Journal of Neurology, Neurosurgery and Psychiatry 38: 756

Lovelace R E, Horowitz S J 1968 Peripheral neuropathy in long term diphenyl hydantoin therapy. Archives of Neurology 18: 69

Lowitzsch K, Hopf H C 1975 Propagation of compound action potentials of the mixed peripheral nerves in man at high stimulus frequencies. In: Kunze K, Desmedt J E (eds) Studies on neuromuscular diseases. Proceedings of an International Symposium, Giessen, 1973. Karger, Basel

Ludin H P 1980 Electromyography in practice. Georg Thieme Verlag, Stuttgart

McComas A J, Fawcett P R W, Campbell M J, Sica R E P 1971 Electrophysiological estimation of the number of motor units within a human muscle. Journal of Neurology, Neurosurgery and Psychiatry 34: 132

McDonald W I 1973 Experimental neuropathy: the use of

diphtheria toxin. In: Desmedt J E (ed) New developments in electromyography and clinical neurophysiology, vol 2. Karger, Basel, p 128

McDonald W I 1980 Physiological consequences of demyelination. In: Sumner A J (ed) The physiology of peripheral nerve disease. W B Saunders, Philadelphia, ch 8, p 265

MacLeod J G 1971 An electrophysiological and histological study in patients with Friedreich's ataxia. Journal of the Neurological Sciences 12: 333

McLeod J G, Hargrave J C, Walsh J C, Booth G C, Gye R S, Barron A 1975 Nerve conduction studies in leprosy. International Journal of Leprosy 43: 21

McQuillen M P 1971 Idiopathic polyneuritis: serial studies of nerve and immune functions. Journal of Neurology, Neurosurgery and Psychiatry 34: 607

Magladery J W, McDougal D D Jr 1950 Electrophysiological study of nerve and reflex activity in man. 1. Identification of certain reflexes in the electromyogram and the conduction velocity of peripheral nerve fibres. Bulletin of the Johns Hopkins Hospital 86: 265

Magladery J W, Porter W E, Park A M, Teasdall R D 1951 Electrophysiological studies of nerve and reflex activity in normal man. Bulletin of the Johns Hopkins Hospital 88: 499

Magladery J W, Teasdall R D, Park A M, Languth H W 1952 Electrophysiological studies of reflex activity in patients with lesions of the nervous system. Bulletin of the Johns Hopkins Hospital 91: 219

Mamoli B, Wessely P, Kogelnik H D, Muller M, Rathkolb O 1979 Electroneurographic investigation of misonidazole polyneuropathy. European Neurology 18: 405

Markesbery W R 1979 Lactic acidemia, mitochondrial myopathy, and basal ganglion calcification. Neurology 29: 1057

Markesbery W R, McQuillen M P, Procopis P G, Harrison A R, Engel A G 1974 Muscle carnitine deficiency. Association with lipid myopathy, vacuolar neuropathy and vacuolated leukocytes. Archives of Neurology 31: 320

Mavor H, Atcheson J B 1966 Posterior tibial nerve conduction. Archives of Neurology 14: 661

Mavor H, Libman I 1962 Motor nerve conduction velocity measurement as a diagnostic tool. Neurology (Minneapolis) 12: 733

Mawdsley C, Mayer R F 1965 Nerve conduction in alcoholic polyneuropathy. Brain 88: 335

Mayer R F, Mawdsley C 1965 Studies in man and cat of the significance of the H reflex. Journal of Neurology, Neurosurgery and Psychiatry 28: 201

Mayer R F, Feldman R G 1967 Observations on the nature of the 'F' wave in man. Neurology (Minneapolis) 17: 147

Meadows J C, Marsden C D, Harriman D G F 1969 Chronic spinal muscular atrophy in adults, part 1. The Kugelberg–Welander syndrome. Journal of the Neurological Sciences 9: 527

Mechler F, Fawcett P R W, Mastaglia F L, Hudgson P 1981 Mitochondrial myopathy. A study of clinically affected and asymptomatic members of a six-generation family. Journal of the Neurological Sciences 50: 191

Merton P A, Morton H B 1980 Stimulation of the cerebral cortex in the intact human subject. Nature (London) 285: 227

Miglietta O 1968 Motor nerve fibres in amyotrophic lateral sclerosis. American Journal of Physical Medicine 47: 118

Miledi R, Slater C R 1970 On the degeneration of rat neuromuscular junctions after nerve section. Journal of Physiology 207: 507

Miller R G, Peterson C, Rosenberg N L 1987 Electrophysiological evidence of severe distal nerve segment pathology in the Guillain–Barré syndrome. Muscle and Nerve 10: 524

Miller R G, Parry G J, Pfaeffl W, Lang W, Lippert R, Kiprov D 1988 The spectrum of peripheral neuropathy associated with ARC and AIDS. Muscle and Nerve 11: 857

Mills K R, Murray N M F 1985 Conduction in proximal nerve segments in demyelinating neuropathy. Electroencephalography and Clinical Neurophysiology 61: S70

Mills K R, Murray N M F 1986 Electrical stimulation over the human vertebral column: which neural elements are excited? Electroencephalography and Clinical Neurophysiology 63: 582

Mongia S K, Lundervold A 1975 Electrophysiological abnormalities in cases of dystrophia myotonica. European Neurology 13: 360

Moody J 1965 Electrophysiological investigations into the neurological complications of carcinoma. Brain 88: 1023

Mulder D W, Lambert E H, Bastron J A, Sprague R G 1961 The neuropathies associated with diabetes mellitus. Neurology (Minneapolis) 11: 275

Namerow N S, Etamadi A 1970 The orbicularis oculi reflex in multiple sclerosis. Neurology (Minneapolis) 20: 1200

Neilsen V K 1973a The peripheral nerve function in chronic renal failure. V. Sensory and motor conduction velocity. Acta Medica Scandinavica 194: 445

Neilsen V K 1973b The peripheral nerve function in chronic renal failure. VI. The relation between sensory and motor nerve conduction and kidney function, azotaemia, age, sex and clinical neuropathy. Acta Medica Scandinavica 194: 455

Neilsen V K 1974a The peripheral nerve function in chronic renal failure. IX. Recovery after renal transplantation. Electrophysiological aspects (sensory and motor conduction). Acta Medica Scandinavica 195: 171

Neilsen V K 1974b The peripheral nerve function in chronic renal failure — (a survey). Acta Medica Scandinavica (Supplement) 573

Norris A H, Shock N W, Wagman I H 1953 Age changes in the maximum conduction velocity of motor fibres in human ulnar nerves. Journal of Applied Physiology 5: 589

Notermans S L H (ed) 1984 Current practice of clinical electromyography. Elsevier, Amsterdam

Notermans S L H, Vingerhoets H M 1974 The importance of the Hoffman reflex in the diagnosis of lumbar root lesions. Clinical Neurology and Neurophysiology 97: 235

Oh S J, Halsey J H 1973 Abnormality in nerve potentials in Friedreich's ataxia. Neurology (Minneapolis) 23: 52

Olson N D, Jou M F, Quast J E, Nuttal Q 1978 Peripheral neuropathy in myotonic dystrophy. Archives of Neurology 35: 741

Ongerboer de Visser B W, Kuypers H G J M 1978 Late blink reflex changes in lateral medullary lesions. Brain 101: 285

O'Sullivan D J, McLeod J G 1978 Distal chronic spinal muscular atrophy involving the hands. Journal of Neurology, Neurosurgery and Psychiatry 41: 653

Panayiotopoulos C P 1978 F-wave conduction velocity in the deep peroneal nerve: Charcot–Marie–Tooth disease and dystrophia myotonica. Muscle and Nerve 1: 37

Panayiotopoulos C P, Lagos G 1980 Tibial nerve H-reflex and F-wave studies in patients with uremic neuropathy. Muscle and Nerve 3: 423

Panayiotopoulos C P, Scarpalezos S 1977 'F' wave studies on the deep peroneal nerve. Part 2 — 1. Chronic renal failure. 2. Limb-girdle muscular dystrophy. Journal of Neurological Sciences 31: 331

Panayiotopoulos C P, Scarpalezos S, Nastas P E 1977 F-wave studies on the deep peroneal nerve. Part 1. Control subjects. Journal of Neurological Sciences 31: 319

Parry G J 1988 Peripheral neuropathies associated with human immunodeficiency virus infection. Annals of Neurology 23(suppl): S49

Parry G J, Clarke S 1988 Multifocal acquired demyelinating neuropathy masquerading as motor neuron disease. Muscle and Nerve 11: 103

Peioglou-Harmoussi S 1983 Studies in F-response behaviour. PhD Thesis, University of Newcastle upon Tyne

Peioglou-Harmoussi S, Fawcett P R W, Howel D, Barwick D D 1985a F-responses: a study of frequency, shape and amplitude characteristics in healthy control subjects. Journal of Neurology, Neurosurgery and Psychiatry 48: 1159

Peioglou-Harmoussi S, Howel D, Fawcett P R W, Barwick D D 1985b F-response behaviour in a control population. Journal of Neurology, Neurosurgery and Psychiatry 48: 1152

Peioglou-Harmoussi S, Fawcett P R W, Howel D, Barwick D D 1986 F-responses in syringomyelia. Journal of the Neurological Sciences 75: 293

Peioglou-Harmoussi S, Fawcett P R W, Howel D, Barwick D D 1987 F-response frequency in motor neuron disease and cervical spondylosis. Journal of Neurology, Neurosurgery and Psychiatry 50: 593

Penders C A, Delwaide P L 1971 Blink reflex studies in patients with Parkinsonism before and during therapy. Journal of Neurology, Neurosurgery and Psychiatry 34: 674

Petajan J H 1985 F-waves in neurogenic atrophy. Muscle and Nerve 8: 690

Peyronnard J M, Bouchard J P, Lapointe L, Lamontagne A, Lemieux B, Barbeau A 1976 Nerve conduction studies and electromyography in Friedreich's ataxia. Canadian Journal of Neurological Sciences 3: 313

Peyronnard J-M, Charron L, Bellavance A, Marchand L 1979 Neuropathy and mitochondrial myopathy. Annals of Neurology 7: 262

Pilz H, Hopf H C, 1972 A preclinical case of late adult metachromatic leukodystrophy? Manifestation only with lipid abnormalities in urine, enzyme deficiency, and decrease of nerve conduction velocity. Journal of Neurology, Neurosurgery and Psychiatry 35: 360

Preswick G 1968 The peripheral neuropathy of Friedreich's ataxia. Electroencephalography and Clinical Neurophysiology 25: 399

Preswick G, Jeremy D 1964 Subclinical polyneuropathy in renal insufficiency. Lancet ii: 731

Raman P T, Taori G M 1976 Prognostic significance of electrodiagnostic studies in the Guillain–Barré syndrome. Journal of Neurology, Neurosurgery and Psychiatry 39: 163

Rasminsky M 1973 The effects of temperature on conduction in demyelinated single nerve fibres. Archives of Neurology 28: 287

Rasminsky M, Sears T A 1972 Internodal conduction in undissected demyelinated nerve fibres. Journal of Physiology 227: 323

Rossi B, Sartucci F, Stefanini A, Pucci G, Bianchi F 1983 Measurement of motor conduction velocity with Hopf's technique in myotonic dystrophy. Journal of Neurology, Neurosurgery and Psychiatry 46: 93

Said G 1978 Perhexiline neuropathy: a clinico-pathological study. Annals of Neurology 3: 259

Said G, Goulon-Goeau C, Salma G, Tchobroutsky G 1992 Severe early-onset polyneuropathy in insulin-dependent diabetes mellitus. New England Journal of Medicine 326: 1257

Salisachs P 1974 Wide spectrum of motor conduction velocity in Charcot–Marie–Tooth disease. An anatomic-physiological interpretation. Journal of the Neurological Sciences 23: 25

Salisachs P, Codina M, Pradas J 1975 Motor conduction velocity in patients with Friedreich's ataxia. Journal of the Neurological Sciences 24: 331

Schiller H H, Stålberg E 1978 'F' responses studied with single fibre EMG in normal subjects and spastic patients. Journal of Neurology, Neurosurgery and Psychiatry 41: 45

Schimscheimer R T, Ongerboer de Visser B W, Kemp B 1985 The flexor carpi radialis H reflex in lesions of the sixth and seventh cervical nerve roots. Journal of Neurology, Neurosurgery and Psychiatry 48: 445

Schmid U D, Walker G, Hess C W, Schmid J 1990 Magnetic and electrical stimulation of cervical motor roots: technique, site and mechanisms of excitation. Journal of Neurology, Neurosurgery and Psychiatry 53: 770

Schwartz M, Stålberg E, Swash M 1980 Pattern of segmental motor involvement in syringomyelia: a single fibre EMG study. Journal of Neurology, Neurosurgery and Psychiatry 43: 150

Sears T A 1959 Action potentials evoked in digital nerves by stimulation of the mechanoreceptors in the human finger. Journal of Physiology 148: 30

Sebille A 1978 Respective importance of different nerve conduction velocities in leprosy. Journal of the Neurological Sciences 38: 89

Shahani B T, Sumner A J 1981 Electrophysiological studies in peripheral neuropathy: early detection and monitoring. In: Stålberg E, Young R R (eds) Clinical neurophysiology. Butterworths, London, ch 6, p 117

Shahani B T, Young R R 1973 In: Desmedt J E (ed) New developments in electromyography and clinical neurophysiology, vol 3. Karger, Basel, p 641

Shahani B T, Young R R 1977 Blink, H and tendon vibration reflexes. In: Goodgold J, Aberstein A (eds) Electrodiagnosis of neuromuscular diseases, 2nd edn. Williams and Wilkins, Baltimore, p 11, 245

Shields R W 1985 Alcoholic polyneuropathy. Muscle and Nerve 8: 183

Shetty V P, Mehta L N, Antia A H, Irani P F 1977 Teased fibre study of early nerve lesions in leprosy and in contacts with electrophysiological correlates. Journal of Neurology, Neurosurgery and Psychiatry 40: 708

Shy G M, Gonatas N K, Perez M 1966 Two childhood myopathies with abnormal mitochondria. I. Megaconial myopathy. II. Pleoconial myopathy. Brain 89: 133

Sica R E P, McComas A J 1971 An electrophysiological investigation of limb-girdle and facioscapulohumeral dystrophy. Journal of Neurology, Neurosurgery and Psychiatry 34: 269

Simpson D M, Wolfe D E 1991 Neuromuscular complications of HIV infection and its treatment. Aids 5: 917

Simpson J A 1964 Fact and fallacy in measurement of conduction velocity in motor nerves. Journal of Neurology, Neurosurgery and Psychiatry 27: 381

Singh N, Behse F, Buchthal F 1974 Electrophysiological study of peroneal palsy. Journal of Neurology, Neurosurgery and Psychiatry 37: 1202

Smith I S, Kahn S N, Lacey B W et al 1983 Chronic demyelinating neuropathy associated with benign IgM paraproteinaemia. Brain 106: 169

Snider W D, Simpson D M, Nielsen S, Gold J W M, Metroka C E, Posner J B 1983 Neurological complications of acquired immune deficiency syndrome: analysis of 50 patients. Annals of Neurology 14: 403

Spencer P S, Schaumburg H H 1979 Neurotoxic chemicals as probes of cellular mechanisms of neuromuscular disease. In: Aguayo A J, Karpati G (eds) Current topics in nerve and muscle research. Excerpta Medica, Amsterdam, p 274

Spiro A J, Moore C L, Prineas J W, Strasberg P M, Rapin I 1970 A cytochrome-related inherited disorder of the nervous system and muscle. Archives of Neurology 23: 103

Stålberg E 1982 Electrophysiological studies of reinnervation in ALS. In: Rowland L P (ed) Advances in neurology, human motor neuron disease. Raven, New York, p 47

Streib E W, Sun S F, Paustian F F, Gallagher T F, Shipp J C, Eklund R E 1986 Diabetic thoracic radiculopathy: electrodiagnostic study. Muscle and Nerve 9: 548

Sumner A J 1980 Axonal polyneuropathies. In: Sumner A J (ed) The physiology of peripheral nerve disease. W B Saunders, Philadelphia, ch 11, p 340

Sumner D, Crawford M A, Harriman D G F 1971 Distal muscular dystrophy in an English family. Brain 94: 51

Swash M, Perrin J, Schwartz M S 1979 Significance of immunoglobulin deposition in peripheral nerve in neuropathies associated with paraproteinaemia. Journal of Neurology, Neurosurgery and Psychiatry 42: 179

Swift T R 1984 Commentary: electrophysiology of progressive spinal muscular atrophy. In: Gamstorp I, Sarnat H B (eds) Progressive spinal muscular atrophies. Raven, New York, p 135

Swift T R, Hackett D E, Shipley D E, Miner K M 1973 The peroneal and tibial nerves in lepromatous leprosy — clinical and electrophysiological observations. International Journal of Leprosy 41: 25

Tenckhoff H A, Boen F S T, Jebsen R H, Spiegler J H 1965 Polyneuropathy in chronic renal insufficiency. Journal of the American Medical Association 192: 1121

Thomas J E, Lambert E H 1960 Ulnar nerve conduction velocity and 'H' reflex in infants and children. Journal of Applied Physiology 15: 1

Thomas P K 1971 The morphological basis for alterations in nerve conduction in peripheral neuropathy. Proceedings of the Royal Society of Medicine 64: 295

Thomas P K, Calne D B 1974 Motor nerve conduction velocity in peroneal muscular atrophy: evidence for genetic heterogeneity. journal of Neurology, Neurosurgery and Psychiatry 37: 68

Thomas P K, Calne D B, Stewart G 1974 Hereditary motor and sensory polyneuropathy (peroneal muscular atrophy). Annals of Human Genetics (London) 38: 111

Thomas P K, Lascelles R G 1966 The pathology of diabetic neuropathy. Quarterly Journal of Medicine 35: 489

Thomas P K, Lascelles R G 1967 Hypertrophic neuropathy. Quarterly Journal of Medicine 35: 489

Thomas P K, Sears T A, Gilliatt R W 1959 The range of conduction velocity in normal motor nerve fibres to the small muscles of the hand and foot. Journal of Neurology, Neurosurgery and Psychiatry 22: 175

Thomas P K, Hollinrake K, Lascelles R G et al 1971 The polyneuropathy of chronic renal failure. Brain 94: 761

Thorne J 1965 Central responses to electrical activation of the peripheral nerves supplying the intrinsic hand muscles. Journal of Neurology, Neurosurgery and Psychiatry 28: 482

Toole J F, Gergen J A, Hayes D M, Felts J H 1968 Neural effects of nitrofurantoin. Archives of Neurology 18: 180

Trojaborg W 1964 Motor nerve conduction velocities in normal subjects with particular reference to the conduction in proximal and distal segments of median and ulnar nerves. Electroencephalography and Clinical Neurophysiology 17: 314

Trojaborg W 1976 Motor and sensory conduction in the musculocutaneous nerve. Journal of Neurology, Neurosurgery and Psychiatry 39: 890

Trojaborg W, Sindrup E H 1969 Motor and sensory conduction in different segments of the radial nerve in normal subjects. Journal of Neurology, Neurosurgery and Psychiatry 32: 354

Trojaborg W, Frantzen E, Andersen I 1969 Peripheral neuropathy and myopathy associated with carcinoma of the lung. Brain 92: 71

Trojaborg W, Moon A, Andersen B B, Trojaborg N S 1992 Sural nerve conduction parameters in normal subjects related to age, gender, temperature, and height: a reappraisal. Muscle and Nerve 15: 666

Trontelj J V 1973 A study of the F-responses by single fibre electromyography. In: Desmedt J E (ed) New developments in electromyography and clinical neurophysiology. Karger, Basel, p 318

Trontelj J V, Trontelj M 1973a 'F' responses of human facial muscles. A single motor neurone study. Journal of the Neurological Sciences 20: 211

Trontelj M A, Trontelj J V 1973b First component of human blink reflex studied on single facial motoneurones. Brain Research 53: 214

Trontelj J V, Trontelj M, Stålberg E 1973 The jitter of single human muscle fibre responses in certain reflexes. Electroencephalography and Clinical Neurophysiology 34: 825

Ugawa Y, Rothwell J C, Day B L, Thompson P D, Marsden C D 1989 Magnetic stimulation over the spinal enlargements. Journal of Neurology, Neurosurgery and Psychiatry 52: 1025

Vanhooren G, Dehaene I, Van Zandycke M et al 1990 Polyneuropathy in lithium intoxication. Muscle and Nerve 13: 204

Walsh J C 1971 Neuropathy associated with lymphoma. Journal of Neurology, Neurosurgery and Psychiatry 34: 42

Walsh J C, McLeod J G 1970 Alcoholic neuropathy. An electrophysiological and histological study. Journal of the Neurological Sciences 10: 457

Warren D J, Otieno L S 1975 Carpal tunnel syndrome in patients on intermittent haemodialysis. Postgraduate Medical Journal 51: 450

Waxman S G 1980 Determinants of conduction velocity in myelinated nerve fibres. Muscle and Nerve 3: 141

Waxman S G, Sabin T D 1981 Diabetic truncal polyneuropathy. Archives of Neurology 38: 46

Weiderholt W R 1970 Stimulus intensity and site of excitation in human median nerve sensory fibres. Journal of Neurology, Neurosurgery and Psychiatry 33: 438

Willison R G 1962 Electrodiagnosis in motor neurone disease. Proceedings of the Royal Society of Medicine 55: 1024

Wulff C H, Hoyer H, Asboe-Hansen G, Brodthagen H 1985 Development of polyneuropathy during thalidomide therapy. British Journal of Dermatology 112: 475

Yates S K, Brown W F 1979 Characteristics of the F response: a single motor unit study. Journal of Neurology, Neurosurgery and Psychiatry 42: 161

Yiannikas C, McLeod J G 1985 Peripheral neuropathy associated with mitochondrial myopathy. Electroencephalography and Clinical Neurophysiology 61: S20

Yokoyama K, Feldman R G, Sax D S, Salzsider B T, Kucera J 1990 Relation of distribution of conduction velocities to nerve biopsy findings in n-hexane poisoning. Muscle and Nerve 13: 314

Young R R, Shahani B T 1978 Clinical value and limitations of 'F' wave determination. Muscle and Nerve 1: 248

Yudell A, Gomez M R, Lambert E H, Dockerty M B 1967 The neuropathy of sulfatide lipidosis (metachromatic leukodystrophy). Neurology (Minneapolis) 17: 103

Index